The Complete Directory for People with Disabilities

2015

Twenty-Third Edition

The Complete Directory for People with Disabilities

A Comprehensive Source Book for Individuals and Professionals

A Sedgwick Press Book

Grey House Publishing

PUBLISHER: Leslie Mackenzie
EDITORIAL DIRECTOR: Laura Mars

PRODUCTION MANAGER & COMPOSITION: Kristen Thatcher
PRODUCTION ASSISTANT: Kate Hochswender
MARKETING DIRECTOR: Jessica Moody

A Sedgewick Press Book
Grey House Publishing, Inc.
4919 Route 22
Amenia, NY 12501
518.789.8700
FAX 845.373.6390
www.greyhouse.com
e-mail: books@greyhouse.com

First edition published 1991
Twenty-third edition published 2014

The complete directory for people with disabilities : products, resources, books, services.-1992-2013

1. People with disabilities-Services for-United States-Directories. 2. People with disabilities-Services for-United States-Periodicals. 3. Disabled Persons-United States-Bibliography. 4. Disabled Persons-United States-Directory. 5. Information Services-United States-Bibliography. 6. Information Services-United States-Directory. 7. Mental Retardation-Rehabilitation-United States-Bibliography. 8. Mental Retardation-Rehabilitation-United States-Directory. 9. Rehabilitation-United States-Bibliography. 10. Rehabilitation-United States-Directory. I. Title: Directory for people with disabilities.

HV1553.C58
362.4/048/02573

92-658843

Printed in Canada
ISBN 13: 1-61925-281-3 Softcover

Table of Contents

SECTION 1:
General Resources for People with Disabilities

SECTION 2:
Resources for People with Specific Disabilities

Introduction

This 23rd edition of the award-winning *Complete Directory for People with Disabilities* is an invaluable resource for all those living with a disability and all those committed to empowering these individuals. It offers thousands of ways for people with disabilities to succeed at work, in school, and in their community. Coverage includes Associations, Products, Camps, Living Facilities, Print and Electronic Resources and much more. The comprehensive Table of Contents guides you through the 27 chapters and more than 100 subchapters contained in this rich resource.

Praise for previous editions:

> *"...very helpful in fostering an increased understanding of the resources available to individuals with disabilities. The directory itself is very accessible...features...take...[it] from merely a sourcebook to something of added value."*
>
> —Doody's Book Reviews

> *"The strength of this source is in the information referral portion for each entry: the wide range of resources and organizations presented that can assist with additional information and support."*
>
> —ARBA

> *"...thousands of resources...covering a diverse range of services...separate section for specific disabilities...from aging to mobility and from the blind and deaf to speech and language disorders. Libraries...will want to consider..."*
>
> —Against the Grain

Careful research and compilation of the best data available maintains the reputation of *The Complete Directory for People with Disabilities* among educators, librarians and the disability community. This resource is a repeat recipient of the **National Mature Media Award** and the **National Health Information Award**.

Sure to save hours of Internet research time, *The Complete Directory for People with Disabilities* provides comprehensive, critical and immediate information in one source that can be accessed quickly and easily. This edition provides 8,993 descriptive listings, 23,782 key contacts, 8,026 fax numbers, 6,960 email addresses, and 8,516 web sites, thousands more pieces of valuable data than the last edition. Following this Introduction is a Glossary of Disability-Related Terms.

Three indexes provide quick, easy access to the data:

- **Entry Index**: Lists all directory listings alphabetically.
- **Geographic Index**: Organizes listings alphabetically by state.
- **Subject Index**: Organizes directory listings by relevant alphabetical topics, i.e. autism, language disorders.

In addition to the print directory, *The Complete Directory for People with Disabilities* is available for subscription on G.O.L.D., Grey House OnLine Databases. This gives you immediate access to the most valuable disability industry contacts in the United States, plus offers easy-to-use keyword searches, organization type and subject searches, hotlinks to web sites and emails, and so much more. Call 800-562-2139 for a free trial or visit http://gold.greyhouse.com for more information.

We welcome your comments, and look forward to another year of serving the disability community.

Glossary of Disability-Related Terms

Accessible: In the case of a facility, readily usable by a particular individual; in the case of a program or activity, presented or provided in such a way that a particular individual can participate, with or without auxiliary aids(s); in the case of electronic resources, accessible with or without the use of adaptive computer technology.

Access barrier: Any obstruction that prevents people with disabilities from using standard facilities, equipment and resources.

Accessible Web design: Creating World Wide Web pages according to universal design principles to eliminate or reduce barriers, including those that affect people with disabilities.

Accommodation: An adjustment to make a workstation, job, program, facility, or resource accessible to a person with a disability.

Adaptive technology: Hardware or software products that provide access to a computer that is otherwise inaccessible to an individual with a disability.

ALT attribute: HTML code that works in combination with graphical tags to provide alternative text for graphical elements.

Americans with Disabilities Act of 1990 (ADA): A comprehensive Federal law that prohibits discrimination on the basis of disability in employment, telecommunications, public services, public accommodations and services.

American Standard Code for Information Interchange (ASCII): Standard for unformatted text which enables transfer of data between platforms and computer systems.

Assistive technology: Technology used to assist a person with a disability (e.g., a handsplint or computer-related equipment).

Auxiliary aids and services: May include qualified interpreters or other effective methods of making aurally delivered materials available to individuals with hearing impairments; qualified readers, taped texts, or other effective methods of making visually delivered materials available to individuals with visual impairments; acquisition or modification of equipment or devices; and other similar services and actions.

Braille: A system of embossed characters formed by using a Braille cell, a combination of six dots consisting of two vertical columns of three dots each. Each simple Braille character is formed by one or more of these dots and occupies a full cell or space.

Browser: A program that runs on an Internet-connected computer and provides access to the World Wide Web. Web browsers may be text-only, such as Lynx, or graphical, such as Internet Explorer and Netscape Navigator.

Captioned film or videos: Transcription of the verbal portion of films or videos is displayed to make them accessible to people who have hearing impairments.

Closed Circuit TV Magnifier (CCTV): A camera used to magnify books or other materials on a monitor.

Cooperative education: Programs that work with students, faculty, staff, and employers to help students clarify career and academic goals, and expand classroom study by allowing students to participate in paid, practical work experiences.

Compensatory tools: Adaptive computing systems that allow people with disabilities to use computers to complete tasks that would be difficult without a computer (e.g., reading, writing, communicating, accessing information).

Disability: A physical or mental impairment that substantially limits one or more major life activities; a record of such an impairment; or being regarded as having such an impairment (Americans with Disabilities Act of 1990).

Discrimination: The act of treating a person differently in a negative manner based on factors other than individual merit.

Dymo Labeller: A device used to create raised print or Braille labels.

Electronic information: Any digital data for use with computers or computer networks, including disks, CD-ROMs, and World Wide Web resources.

Essential job functions: Those functions of a job or task which must be completed with or without an accommodation.

Facility: All or any portion of a physical complex, including buildings, structures, equipment, grounds, roads, and parking lots.

FM sound amplification system: An electronic amplification system consisting of three components: a microphone/transmitter, monaural FM receiver and a combination charger/carrying case. It provides wireless FM broadcasts from a speaker to a listener who has a hearing impairment.

Frame tags: A means of displaying Web pages. The browser reads the frame tags and produces an output that subdivides output within a browser into discrete windows.

Graphical user interface (GUI): Program interface that presents digital information and software programs in an image-based format as compared to a character-based format.

Hardware: Physical equipment related to computers.

Hearing impairment: Complete or partial loss of the ability to hear, caused by a variety of injuries or diseases, including congenital causes. Limitations, including difficulties in understanding language or other auditory messages and/or in production of understandable speech, are possible.

Independent study: A student works one-on-one with individual faculty members to develop projects for credit.

Informational interview: An activity where students meet with people working in careers to ask questions about their jobs and companies, allowing students to gain personal perspectives on career interests.

Input: Any method by which information is entered into a computer.

Internet: Computer network connecting governmental, educational, commercial, other organizations, and individual computer systems.

Internship: A time-limited, intensive learning experience outside of the typical classroom.

Interpreter: Professional person who assists a person who is deaf in communicating with hearing people.

Job shadowing: A short work-based learning experience where students visit businesses to observe one or more specific jobs to provide them with a realistic view of occupations in a variety of settings.

Keyboard emulation: Uses hardware and/or software in place of a standard keyboard.

Kinesthetic: Refers to touch-based feedback.

Large-print: Most ordinary print is six to ten points in height (about 1/16 to 1/8 of an inch). Large-print type is fourteen to eighteen points (about 1/8 to 1/4 of an inch) and sometimes larger.

Link: a connection between two electronic files or data items.

Lynx: A text-based World Wide Web browser.

Macro: A mini-program that, when run within an application, executes a series of predetermined keystrokes and commands to accomplish a specific task. Macros can automate tedious and often-repeated tasks or create special menus to speed data entry.

Mainstreaming: The inclusion of people with disabilities, with or without special accommodations, in programs, activities, and facilities with non-disabled people.

Major life activities: Functions such as caring for oneself, performing manual tasks, walking, seeing, hearing, speaking, breathing, learning, working, and participating in community activities (Americans with Disabilities Act of 1990).

Multimedia: A computer-based method of presenting information by using more than one medium of communication, such as text, graphics, and sound.

Optical Character Recognition (OCR): Machine recognition of printed or typed text. Using OCR software with a scanner, a printed page can be scanned and the characters converted into text in an electronic format.

Output: Any method of displaying or presenting electronic information to the user through a computer monitor or other device (e.g., speech synthesizer).

Portable Document Format (PDF): The file format for representing documents in a manner that is independent of the original application software, hardware and operating system used to create the documents.

Physical or mental impairment: Any physiological disorder or condition, cosmetic disfigurement, or anatomical loss affecting one or more, but not necessarily limited to, the following body systems: neurological; musculoskeletal; special sense organs; respiratory, including speech organs; cardiovascular; reproductive; digestive; genitourinary; hemic and lymphatic; skin and endocrine; or any mental or psychological disorder, such as mental retardation, organic brain syndrome, emotional or mental illness, and specific learning disabilities (Americans with Disabilities Act of 1990).

Plug-ins: Programs that work within a browser to alter, enhance, or extend the browser,s operation. They are often used for viewing video, animation or listening to audio files.

Proprietary software: Privately owned software based on trade secrets, privately developed technology, or specifications that the owner refuses to divulge, thus preventing others from duplicating a product or program unless an explicit license is purchased. The opposite of proprietary is open (publicly published and available for emulation by others).

Qualified individual with a disability: An individual with a disability who, with or without reasonable modification to rules, policies or practices, the removal of architectural, communication, or transportation barriers, or the provision of auxiliary aids and services, meets the essential eligibility requirements for the receipt of services or participation in programs or activities provided by a public entity (Americans with Disabilities Act of 1990).

Reader: Volunteer or employee of a blind or partially sighted individual who reads printed material in person or records to audiotape.

Relay service: A third-party service (usually free) that allows a hearing person without a TTY/TDD device to communicate over the telephone with a person who has a hearing impairment. The system also allows a person with a hearing impairment who has a TTY/TDD to communicate in voice through a third party, with a hearing person or business.

Screen reader: A text-to-speech system intended for use by computer users who are blind or have low vision that speaks the text content of a computer display using a speech synthesizer.

Service learning: A structured, volunteer work experience where students provide community service in non-paid, volunteer positions to give them opportunities to apply knowledge and skills learned in school while making a contribution to local communities.

Sign language: Manual communication commonly used by people who are deaf. Sign language is not universal; deaf people from different countries speak different sign languages. The gestures or symbols in sign language are organized in a linguistic way. Each individual gesture is called a sign. Each sign has three distinct parts: the hand shape, the position of the hands, and the movement of the hands. American Sign Language (ASL) is the most commonly used sign language in the United States.

Specific learning disability (SLD): A disorder of one or more of the basic psychological processes involved in understanding or in using language, spoken or written, which may manifest itself in difficulties listening, thinking, speaking, reading, writing, spelling, or doing mathematical calculations. Limitations may include hyperactivity, distractibility, emotional instability, visual and/or auditory perception difficulties and/or motor limitations, depending on the type(s) of learning disability.

Speech output system: A system that provides the user with a voice alternative to the text presented on the computer screen.

Speech impairment: A problem in communication and related areas, such as oral motor function, ranging from simple sound substitutions to the inability to understand or use language or use the oral-motor mechanism for functional speech and feeding. Some causes of speech and language disorders include hearing loss; neurological disorders; brain injury; mental retardation; drug abuse; physical impairments, such as cleft lip or palate; and vocal abuse or misuse.

Speech input system: A computer-based system that allows the operator to control the system using his/her voice.

Sticky keys: Enables a computer user to do multiple key combinations on a keyboard using only one finger at a time. The sticky keys function is usually used with the Ctrl, Alt, and Shift keys. Simultaneous keystrokes can be entered sequentially.

Telecommunications Device for the Deaf (TDD) or Teletypewriter (TTY): A device which enables someone who has a speech or hearing impairment to use a telephone when communicating with someone else who has a TDD/TTY. TDD/TTYs can be used with any telephone, and one needs only a basic typing ability to use them.

Trackball: A pointing device consisting of a ball housed in a socket containing sensors to detect the rotation of the ball " like an upside down mouse. The user rolls the ball with his thumb or the palm of his hand to move the pointer.

Traumatic Brain Injury (TBI): An open or closed head injury resulting in impairments in one or more areas, such as cognition; language; memory; attention; reasoning; abstract thinking; judgment; problem-solving; sensory, perceptual, and motor abilities; psychosocial behavior; physical functions; information processing; and speech. The term does not apply to brain injuries that are congenital or degenerative, or brain injuries induced by birth trauma.

Undue hardship: An action that requires significant difficulty or expense in relation to the size of the employer, the resources available, and the nature of the operation (Americans with Disabilities Act of 1990).

Universal design: Designing programs, services, tools, and facilities so that they are usable, without additional modification, by the widest range of users possible, taking into account a variety of abilities and disabilities.

Vocational Rehabilitation Act of 1973: An act prohibiting discrimination on the basis of disability which applies to any program that receives federal financial assistance. Section 504 of the act is aimed at making educational programs and facilities accessible to all people with disabilities. Section 508 of the act requires that electronic office equipment purchased through federal procurement meets disability access guidelines.

Voice input system: A computer-based system that allows the operator to control the system using his/her voice.

Vision impairments: A complete or partial loss of the ability to see, caused by a variety of injuries or diseases including congenital causes. Legal blindness is defined as visual acuity of 20/200 or less in the better eye with correcting lenses, on the widest diameter of the visual field subtending an angular distance no greater than 20 degrees.

World Wide Web (WWW, W3, or Web): Hypertext and multimedia gateway to the Internet.

DO-IT
University of Washington
Box 354842
Seattle, WA 98195-4842
doit@uw.edu
http://www.washington.edu/doit/
206-685-DOIT (3648) (voice/TTY)
888-972-DOIT (3648) (toll free voice/TTY)
206-221-4171 (FAX)
509-328-9331 (voice/TTY) Spokane

Director: Sheryl Burgstahler, Ph.D.

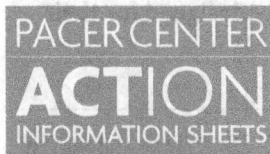

PACER CENTER
ACTION
INFORMATION SHEETS

Bullying and Harassment of Students with Disabilities

Top 10 facts parents, educators, and students need to know

1. The facts — Students with disabilities are much more likely to be bullied than their nondisabled peers.

Bullying of children with disabilities is significant but there is very little research to document it. Only 10 U.S. studies have been conducted on the connection between bullying and developmental disabilities but all of these studies found that children with disabilities were two to three times more likely to be bullied than their nondisabled peers. One study shows that 60 percent of students with disabilities report being bullied regularly compared with 25 percent of all students.

2. Bullying affects a student's ability to learn.

Many students with disabilities are already addressing challenges in the academic environment. When they are bullied, it can directly impact their education.

Bullying is not a harmless rite of childhood that everyone experiences. Research shows that bullying can negatively impact a child's access to education and lead to:

- School avoidance and higher rates of absenteeism
- Decrease in grades
- Inability to concentrate
- Loss of interest in academic achievement
- Increase in dropout rates

Learn more about other common misperceptions about bullying at PACER.org/bullying/resources/publications/

3. The definition — Bullying based on a student's disability may be considered harassment.

The Office for Civil Rights (OCR) and the Department of Justice (DOJ) have stated that bullying may also be considered harassment when it is based on a student's race, color, national origin, sex, or disability.

Harassing behaviors may include:

- Unwelcome conduct such as verbal abuse, name-calling, epithets, or slurs
- Graphic or written statements
- Threats
- Physical assault
- Other conduct that may be physically threatening, harmful, or humiliating

4. The Federal Laws — Disability harassment is a civil rights issue.

Parents have legal rights when their child with a disability is the target of bullying or disability harassment. Section 504 of the Rehabilitation Act of 1973 (often referred to as 'Section 504') and Title II of the Americans with Disabilities Act of 1990 (Title II) are the federal laws that apply if the harassment denies a student with a disability an equal opportunity to education. The Office for Civil Rights (OCR) enforces Section 504 and Title II of the ADA. Students with a 504 plan or an Individualized Education Program (IEP) would qualify for these protections.

According to a 2000 Dear Colleague letter from the Office for Civil Rights, "States and school districts also have a responsibility under Section 504, Title II, and the Individuals with Disabilities Education Act (IDEA), which is enforced by OSERS [the Office for Special Education and Rehabilitative Services], to ensure that a free appropriate public education (FAPE) is made available to eligible students with disabilities. Disability harassment may result in a denial of FAPE under these statutes."

The letter further outlines how bullying in the form of disability harassment may

PACER's National Bullying Prevention Center®

8161 Normandale Blvd
Minneapolis, MN 55437-1044
952.838.9000
952.838.0199 fax
PACER@PACER.org

PACER.org/Bullying
PACERKidsAgainstBullying.org
PACERTeensAgainstBullying.org

prevent a student with an IEP from receiving an appropriate education: "The IDEA was enacted to ensure that recipients of IDEA funds make available to students with disabilities the appropriate special education and related services that enable them to access and benefit from public education. The specific services to be provided a student with a disability are set forth in the student's individualized education program (IEP), which is developed by a team that includes the student's parents, teachers and, where appropriate, the student. Harassment of a student based on disability may decrease the student's ability to benefit from his or her education and amount to a denial of FAPE."

5. The State Laws — Students with disabilities have legal rights when they are a target of bullying.

Most states have laws that address bullying. Some have information specific to students with disabilities. For a complete overview of state laws, visit Olweus.org.

Many school districts also have individual policies that address how to respond to bullying situations. Contact your local district to request a written copy of the district policy on bullying.

6. The adult response is important

Parents, educators, and other adults are the most important advocates that a student with disabilities can have. It is important that adults know the best way to talk with someone in a bullying situation.

Some children are able to talk with an adult about personal matters and may be willing to discuss bullying. Others may be reluctant to speak about the situation. There could be a number of reasons for this. The student bullying them may have told them not to tell or they might fear that if they do tell someone, the bullying won't stop or may become worse.

When preparing to talk to children about bullying, adults (parents and educators) should consider how they will handle the child's questions and emotions and what their own responses will be. Adults should be prepared to listen without judgment, providing the child with a safe place to work out their feelings and determine their next steps.

It is never the responsibility of the child to fix a bullying situation. If children could do that, they wouldn't be seeking the help of an adult in the first place.

For more information, read PACER's "Talking With Your Child About Bullying."

7. The resources — Students with disabilities have resources that are specifically designed for their situation.

IEP

Students with disabilities, who are eligible for special education under the Individuals with Disabilities Education Act (IDEA), will have an Individualized Education Program (IEP).

The IEP can be a helpful tool in a bullying prevention plan. Remember, every child receiving special education is entitled to a free, appropriate public education (FAPE), and bullying can become an obstacle to that education.

For more information, read PACER's "Individualized Education Program (IEP) and Bullying."

Dear Colleague Letter

In 2000, a 'Dear Colleague' letter was sent to school districts nationwide from the U.S. Department of Education's Office for Civil Rights (OCR) and Office of Special Education and Rehabilitative Services (OSERS) that defined the term "disability harassment."

www2.ed.gov/about/offices/list/ocr/docs/disabharassltr.html

In 2010, another Dear Colleague letter from the Office for Civil Rights was issued that reminded school districts of their responsibilities under civil rights laws that prohibit discrimination and harassment on the basis of race, color, national origin, sex, disability, and religion.

www2.ed.gov/about/offices/list/ocr/letters/colleague-201010.html

Template Letters

PACER.org/bullying/resources/publications/

Parents should contact school staff each time their child informs them that he or she has been bullied. Parents may use one of these template letters as a guide for writing a letter to their child's school. These letters contain standard language and "fill-in-the-blank" spaces so that the letter can be customized for each child's situation.

PACER Center's sample letter(s) can serve two purposes:

- First, the letter will alert school administration of the bullying and your desire for interventions.
- Second, the letter can serve as your written record when referring to events. The record (letter) should be factual and absent of opinions or emotional statements.

The two letters — "Student with an IEP, Notifying School About Bullying" and "Student with a 504, Notifying School About Bullying" — are for parents who have a child with an Individualized Education Plan (IEP) or Section 504. The bullying law of the individual state applies to all students as noted in the law. When bullying is based on the child's disability, federal law can also apply under Section 504, Individuals with Disabilities Act (IDEA), and Title II of the Americans with Disabilities Act.

8. The Power of Bystanders – More than 50 percent of bullying situations stop when a peer intervenes.

Most students don't like to see bullying but they may not know what to do when it happens. Peer advocacy — students speaking out on behalf of others — is a unique approach that empowers students to protect those targeted by bullying.

Peer advocacy works for two reasons: First, students are more likely than adults to see what is happening with their peers and peer influence is powerful. Second, a student telling someone to stop bullying has much more impact than an adult giving the same advice.

Learn more about peer advocacy at PACER.org/bullying/resources/peer-advocacy.asp

9. The importance of self-advocacy

Self-advocacy means the student with a disability is responsible for telling people what they want and need in a straightforward way. Students need to be involved in the steps taken to address a bullying situation. Self-advocacy is knowing how to:

- Speak up for yourself
- Describe your strengths, disability, needs, and wishes
- Take responsibility for yourself
- Learn about your rights
- Obtain help, or know who to ask, if you have a question

The person who has been bullied should be involved in deciding how to respond to the bullying. This involvement can provide students with a sense of control over their situation, and help them realize that someone is willing to listen, take action, and reassure them that their opinions and ideas are important.

Learn more about self advocacy for students, PACER's "Tips for Teens: Use Your IEP Meetings to Learn How to Advocate for Yourself."

The Student Action Plan is a self-advocacy resource. It includes three simple steps to explore specific, tangible actions to address the situation:

1. Define the situation
2. Think about how the situation could be different
3. Write down the steps to take action

10. You are not alone

When students have been bullied, they often believe they are the only one this is happening to, and that no one else cares. In fact, they are not alone.

There are individuals, communities, and organizations that do care. **It is not up to one person to end the bullying** and it is never the responsibility of the child to change what is happening to them. **No one deserves to be bullied.** All people should be treated with dignity and respect, no matter what. Everyone has a responsibility — and a role to play — as schools, parents, students, and the community work together for positive change.

What is an Invisible Disability?

In general, the term *disability* is often used to describe an ongoing physical challenge. This could be a bump in life that can be well managed or a mountain that creates serious changes and loss. Either way, this term should not be used to describe a person as weaker or lesser than anyone else! Every person has a purpose, special uniqueness and value, no matter what hurdles they may face.

In addition, just because a person has a *disability*, does not mean they are *disabled*. Many living with these challenges are still fully active in their work, families, sports or hobbies. Some with disabilities are able to work full or part time, but struggle to get through their day, with little or no energy for other things. Others are unable to maintain gainful or substantial employment due to their disability, have trouble with daily living activities and/or need assistance with their care.

According to the Americans with Disabilities Act of 1990 (ADA) an individual with a disability is a person who: Has a physical or mental impairment that substantially limits one or more major life activities; has a record of such an impairment; or is regarded as having such an impairment (*Disability Discrimination*).

Furthermore, "A person is considered to have a disability if he or she has difficulty performing certain functions (seeing, hearing, talking, walking, climbing stairs and lifting and carrying), or has difficulty performing activities of daily living, or has difficulty with certain social roles (doing school work for children, working at a job and around the house for adults)" (*Disabilities Affect One-Fifth of All Americans*).

Often people think the term, disability, only refers to people using a wheelchair or walker. On the contrary, the 1994-1995 Survey of Income and Program Participation (SIPP) found that 26 million Americans (almost 1 in 10) were considered to have a severe disability, while only 1.8 million used a wheelchair and 5.2 million used a cane, crutches or walker (*Americans with Disabilities 94-95*). In other words, 74% of Americans who live with a severe disability do not use such devices. Therefore, a disability cannot be determined solely on whether or not a person uses assistive equipment.

The term *invisible disabilities* refers to symptoms such as debilitating pain, fatigue, dizziness, cognitive dysfunctions, brain injuries, learning differences and mental health disorders, as well as hearing and vision impairments. These are not always obvious to the onlooker, but can sometimes or always limit daily activities, range from mild challenges to severe limitations and vary from person to person.

Also, someone who has a *visible* impairment or uses an assistive device such as a wheelchair, walker or cane can also have *invisible disabilities*. For example, whether or not a person utilizes an assistive device, if they are debilitated by such symptoms as described above, they live with *invisible disabilities*.

Unfortunately, people often judge others by what they see and often conclude a person can or cannot do something by the way they *look*. This can be equally frustrating for those who may appear *unable*, but are perfectly capable, as well as those who appear *able*, but are not.

International Disability expert, Joni Eareckson Tada, explained it well when she told someone living with debilitating fatigue, “People have such high expectations of folks like you [with invisible disabilities], like, ‘come on, get your act together.’ but they have such low expectations of folks like me in wheelchairs, as though it’s expected that we can’t do much” (Joni).

The bottom line is that everyone with a disability is different, with varying challenges and needs, as well as abilities and attributes. Thus, we all should learn to listen with our ears, instead of judging with our eyes.

Sincerely,
The Invisible Disabilities Association

Reprinted from The Invisible Disabilities Association,
http://invisibledisabilities.org/what-is-an-invisible-disability/

American Association of People with Disabilities

Identifying Transition-Age Youth with Disabilities

The transition from youth to adult – and from home to independence - is difficult for many individuals, and youth with disabilities face even more challenges during this period due to issues with accessible environments, health care, and a change from youth to adult-based services. Programs that assist youth with disabilities during these transition years – defined here as ages 16 to 24 – are vital in ensuring their independence. Adequately identifying this population is important in order to assess needs and provide efficient and quality services.

According to a recent study issued by Mathematica Policy Research[1], a key problem in determining the issues that transition-age youth face is a lack of consistent data: surveys vary in the types of questions used to identify youth with disabilities. Due to this dearth of information, it is difficult not only to adequately identify the population, but also to determine how these youth are faring in transition.

Methods
The study reviewed twelve existing surveys related to disability and presented data from eight of those sources.[2] While several issues make it difficult to consistently count the population of youth with disabilities, the primary challenge is that there is no singular definition of disability used among the surveys. Rather, each survey uses different definitions and asks different questions. The numbers, obviously, then differ depending on which definition is used. Another factor is that most surveys do not specifically target youth with disabilities.

The study presents a framework—defining physical, activity, and participation difficulties, and special need indicators—that can assist in understanding how a survey defines youth with disabilities and why surveys differ.

Changing Disability Definitions from Childhood to Adult
The disability questions that are applied to youth, particularly those who are over age 16, are the ones used for adults. This is an issue because definitions of disability for youth are different than those used for adults in areas such as the kinds of daily activities considered (work is generally used in adult definitions, whereas questions regarding

---

[1] Todd Honeycutt and David Wittenburg, *Identifying Transition-Age Youth With Disabilities Using Existing Surveys*, Mathematica Policy Research, July 10, 2012.This study was supported by the National Institute on Disability and Rehabilitation Research, U.S. Department of Education, through its Rehabilitation Research and Training Center on Disability Statistics and Demographics grant to Hunter College.

[2] Data sources are shown from the Survey of Income and Program Participation (SIPP), National Longitudinal Survey of Youth 1997 (NLSY97), American Community Survey (ACS), Current Population Survey (CPS), National Health Interview Survey (NHIS), National Survey of Children's Health (NSCH), National Longitudinal Transition Survey 2 (NLTS2), and National Survey of SSI Children and Families (NSCF). Other data sources reviewed include the Medical Expenditure Panel Survey (MEPS), Panel Study of Income Dynamics (PSID), National Health and Nutrition Examination Survey (NHANES), and the National Survey of Children with Special Health Care Needs (NS-CSHCN).

school are generally more applicable to youth); certain conditions may be more common among youth than adults, such as learning disabilities and attention-deficit hyperactivity disorder; and youth may have specific needs or youth program indicators such as special education services and cash benefits from Social Security disability programs that differ from those for adults. Youth identified with these types of questions might therefore not be captured by adult definitions of disability

Among surveys that do specifically target youth, some include statistics on transition-age youth with disabilities as part of the larger population, which allows for comparison of youth with and without disabilities. Others focus just on youth with disabilities and thus provide more in-depth information regarding characteristics or outcomes of a specific group, such as youth in special education programs. Some surveys track individuals over a period of time; others just consider one point in time. Each type of survey has its advantages and disadvantages.

Prevalence Estimates Range

The typical categories included in most surveys – physical conditions (sensory, physical, or mental difficulties), activities (difficulties in identified daily activities) and participation (difficulties related to functions such as doing errands or preparing meals; work; school; and other activities such as housework and play) identify only a subset of those with disabilities. As part of its proposed disability framework for youth, the study added special needs indicators (whether an individual participates in special education services or has a special health need), which generally captures a broader population, including those with less severe disabilities. For instance, an individual may participate in a special education program due to a learning disability, but with the proper supports does not experience other difficulties in daily living that would necessitate a response to the survey by the youth as having a disability. It is therefore clear that who is counted as having a disability in a survey depends on what definition is used and whether the definition includes mild, moderate, or severe disabilities.

The range in disability prevalence across surveys— anywhere from 5 to 34 percent of youth have a disability—is largely driven by differences in survey content, structure, and questions used to identify disability. Of particular importance to prevalence is whether a survey includes more youth-based definitions, such as participation issues in school. Some surveys—such as the American Community Survey (ACS), which has a disability prevalence of 5 percent—use very broad definitions and ask very limited questions that may not capture all youth with disabilities and so have lower prevalence rates. Including special education and disability income indicators in the Survey of Income and Program Participation (SIPP) survey data increases the proportion with disabilities from 11 to 14 percent, and the disability prevalence is as high as 34 percent in the National Survey of Children's Health (NSCH) when including special education and special health need indicators.

Given these factors, and depending on the data need, it would be best to use multiple factors – physical, activity, and participation difficulties as well as special needs indicators – to identify youth with disabilities, and to consider functions that are applicable to transition- age youth – such as school, as opposed to work.

Institutional Group Facilities

The study found that most surveys do not include institutional group facilities, which is important because youth with disabilities make up a large proportion of those in institutional settings, mainly correctional facilities. Counting them is important and their overrepresentation in such facilities can have significant implications for programs and policies.

Variance Among States

The study also found a large difference in numbers across states. There is a threefold difference between the states with the highest rates of transition-age youth with disabilities and those with the lowest rates. This could be due to environmental factors, poverty, and the availability and quality of services provided.

Conclusions

These findings provide important guidance for future research. First, disability statistics for youth can vary across definitions, particularly whether a more youth or adult based set of concepts are available. Many of the adult definitions currently used in the literature, including the official disability estimates, do not capture people who might be considered having a disability as a youth because of differences between adult and youth measures (for example, a person with a learning disability). Because of differences between youth and adults, multiple and age-appropriate definitions should be used in identifying transition-age youth with disabilities. It would be useful to study the varied experiences of youth with different kinds of disabilities, and to examine their education and employment outcomes. This could provide valuable information to policymakers regarding programs for transition-age youth with disabilities and what works for different groups. It would also be useful to analyze data on at-risk behavior such as juvenile delinquency in order to determine whether and why youth with disabilities are overrepresented in institutional group settings such as correctional facilities, and how transition programs might reduce risky behavior. Studies should also compare the experiences of youth with disabilities to those of adults with disabilities in order to provide more insight and improve transitions to adulthood. Examining data and programs by state could provide insight into what services are available, which are effective, and which are needed. This research could, in turn, provide critical information for policymakers in determining how to best assist young people with disabilities in the transition from youth to adulthood.

User Guide

Descriptive listings in *The Complete Directory for People with Disabilities* are organized into 24 chapters, by either resource type or disability category type. You will find the following types of listings throughout the book:

- National Agencies & Associations
- State Agencies & Associations
- Camps & Exchanges Programs
- Manufacturers of Assistive Devices, Clothing, Computer Equipment & Supplies
- Print & Electronic Media
- Living Centers & Facilities
- Libraries & Research Centers
- Conferences & Trade Shows

Below is a sample listing illustrating the kind of information that is or might be included in an Association entry. Each numbered item of information is described in the paragraphs on the following page.

---

1 → 1234
2 → **Advocacy Center for Seniors with Disabilities**
3 → 1762 South Major Drive
New Orleans, LA 98087

4 → **800-000-0000**

5 → **058-884-0709**

6 → **Fax: 058-884-0568**

7 → **TDD: 800-000-0001**

8 → **email: info@sadvoc.com**

9 → **www.sadvoc.com**

10 → Barbara Pierce, Executive Director
Diane Watkins, Marketing Director
Robert Goldfarb, Administrative Assistant

11 → The mission of the Center is to advance the dignity, equality, self-determination and choices of senior citizens with disabilities. It provides referrals, publishes information, including a monthly newsletter, offers workshops and consultation on legal, social, travel, and medical issues. The Center works with various local organizations to help seniors with disabilities stay active in their community.

12 → Founded 1964

13 → 18 pages

14 → Monthly

User Key

1 → **Record Number**: Entries are listed alphabetically within each category and numbered sequentially. The entry numbers, rather than page numbers, are used in the indexes to refer to listings.

2 → **Organization Name**: Formal name of company or organization. Where organization names are completely capitalized, the listing will appear at the beginning of the alphabetized section. In the case of publications, the title of the publication will appear first, followed by the publisher.

3 → **Address**: Location or permanent address of the organization.

4 → **Toll Free Number**: This is listed when provided by the organization.

5 → **Phone Number**: The listed phone number is usually for the main office of the organization, but may also be for the sales, marketing, or public relations office as provided by the organization.

6 → **Fax Number**: This is listed when provided by the organization.

7 → **TDD Number**: This is listed when provided. It refers to Telephone Device for the Deaf.

8 → **E-Mail**: This is listed when provided by the organization and is generally the main office e-mail.

9 → **Web Site**: This is also referred to as an URL address. These web sites are accessed through the Internet by typing *http://* before the URL address.

10 → **Key Personnel**: Name and titles of department heads of the organization.

11 → **Organization Description**: This paragraph contains a brief description of the organization and their services.

12 → **Year Founded:** The year in which the organization was established or founded. If the organization has changed its name, the founding date is usually for the earliest name under which it was known.

13 → **Number of Pages**: Number of pages if the listing is a publication.

14 → **Frequency:** The frequency of the listing if it is a publication.

Arts & Entertainment

Resources for the Disabled

1 **AbleArts**
P.O. Box 831
Bear, DE 19701
302-368-7477
e-mail: ableartsinc@gmail.com
ablearts.org

2 **American Art Therapy Association (AATA)**
4875 Eisenhower Avenue
Suite 240
Alexandria, VA 22304
703-548-5860
888-290-0878
FAX: 703-783-8468
e-mail: info@arttherapy.org
www.americanarttherapyassociation.org

Sarah P. Deaver, PhD, ATR-BC, President
Michele Basham, Director, Membership Information & Programs
Barbara Florence, Director, Communication, Education & Conference
Dean Sagar, Director of Public Policy

Organization of professionals who believe the art process is a beneficial and healing process.

3 **American Council of the Blind**
2200 Wilson Boulevard
Ste 650
Arlington, VA 22201-3354
202-467-5081
800-424-8666
FAX: 703-465-5085
e-mail: info@acb.org
www.acb.org

Kim Charlson, President
Jeff Thom, First Vice President
Marlaina Lieberg, Second Vice President
Ray Campbell, Secretary

Aims to enlarge the art experience of blind people, encourages blind people to visit museums, galleries, concerts, the theater and other enjoyable public places, offers consultation to program planners in establishing accessible art and museum exhibits and presents Performing Arts Showcases at the American Council of the Blind's national convention.

4 **American Dance Therapy Association (ADTA)**
10632 Little Patuxent Pkwy
Ste 108
Columbia, MD 21044- 6258
410-997-4040
FAX: 410-997-4048
e-mail: info@adta.org
www.adta.org/

Sharon Goodill, President
Jody Wager, MS, BC-DMT, Vice President
Gail Wood, Secretary
Meghan Dempsey, Treasurer

Dance-movement therapy is a psychotherapeutic use of movement as a process which furthers the emotional, cognitive and physical integration of the individual.

5 **American Music Therapy Association (AMTA)**
8455 Colesville Road
Suite 1000
Silver Spring, MD 20910-3392
301-589-3300
FAX: 301-589-5175
e-mail: info@musictherapy.org
www.musictherapy.org

Andrea H. Farbman, Executive Director
Miss Angie K Elkins, Director of Membership Services & Information Systems
Al Bumanis, Director of Communications & Conferences
Jane P. Creagan, Director of Professional Programs

AMTA's purpose is the progressive development of the therapeutic use of music in rehabilitation, special education and community settings. Predecessors to the American Music Therapy Association included the National Association for Music Therapy founded in 1950 and the American Association for Music Therapy founded in 1971. AMTA is committed to the advancement of education, training, professional standards, credentials and research in support of the music therapy profession.

6 **Arena Stage**
1101 Sixth St. SW
Washington, DC 20024
202-554-9066
arenastage.org

Beth Newburger Schwartz, Chair
David E. Shiffrin, President
Molly Smith, Artistic Director
Edgard Dobie, Executive Producer

Arena Stage has played a pioneering role in providing access to all productions for people with disabilities. Access services and programs include wheelchair accessible seating; infrared assistive listening devices; Braille, large print, audio description and sign interpretation at designated performances.

7 **Art Therapy SourceBook**
McGraw-Hill Company
2 Penn Plaza
New York, NY 10121-101
212-904-2000
www.mhhe.com/hper/physed

Cathy Malchiodi, Author

An overview of the uses of art as a mentally therapeutic tool.
$18.00
272 pages
ISBN 1-565658-84-1

8 **Art and Disabilities**
Brookline Books
8 Trumbull Rd
Suite B-001
Northampton, MA 01060
413-584-0184
800-666-2665
FAX: 413-584-6184
e-mail: brbooks@yahoo.com
www.brooklinebooks.com

Florence Ludins-Katz, Author

A step-by-step guide to establishing creative arts centers for people with disabilities. Includes philosophy and making creative arts centers happen.

9 **Art and Healing: Using Expressive Art to Heal Your Body, Mind, and Soul**
Three Rivers Press/Crown Publishing-Random House
1745 Broadway
New York, NY 10019
212-782-9000
e-mail: crownpublicity@randomhouse.com
www.randomhouse.com/crown/trp.html

Barbara Ganim, Author
Markus Dohle, Chairman & CEO
Melanie Fallon-Houska, Dir., Corporate Contributions

The author believes creating a visual image through any medium can produce physical and emotional benefits for both the creator as well as those who view it. *$17.00*
256 pages
ISBN 0-609803-16-6

10 **Art for All the Children: Approaches to Art Therapy for Children with Disabilities**
Charles C. Thomas
2600 South First Street
Springfield, IL 62704-4730
217-789-8980
800-258-8980
FAX: 217-789-9130
e-mail: books@ccthomas.com
www.ccthomas.com

Frances E Anderson, Author
Sharon Moorman, Editorial Assistant

This second edition is for art therapists in training and for in-service professionals in art therapy, art education and special educa-

tion who have children with disabilities as a part of their case/class load. *$56.95*
398 pages Paperback
ISBN 0-398060-07-7

11 **Arts Unbound**
542/544 Freeman Street
Orange, NJ 07050
973-675-2787
FAX: 973-678-4408
e-mail: info@artsunbound.org
www.artsunbound.org
Margaret Mikkelsen, Executive Director
Catherine Lazen, Founder and Board Chair
Alan Hirsh, Executive Vice President
Tashea Patterson Carless, Director of Agency Operations
Arts Unbound is a nonprofit organization dedicated to the artistic achievement of youth, adults, and senior citizens with disabilities.

12 **Association of Mouth and Foot Painting Artists (AMPFA)**
2070 Peachtree Court
Suite 101
Atlanta, GA 30341
770-986-7764
877-637- 872
FAX: 770-986-8563
e-mail: mfpausa@bellsouth.net
www.mfpausa.com
Erich Stegmann, Founder
The AMPF is an international, for-profit association wholly owned and run by disabled artists to help them meet their financial needs. Members paint with brushes held in their mouths or feet as a result of a disability sustained at birth or through an accident or illness that prohibits them from using their hands.

13 **Brookline Books**
8 Trumbull Rd
Suite B-001
Northampton, MA 01060
413-584-0184
800-666-2665
FAX: 413-584-6184
e-mail: brbooks@yahoo.com
www.brooklinebooks.com

14 **Clinical Applications of Music Therapy in Developmental Disability, Pediatrics and Neurolog**
Taylor & Francis
400 Market Street
Suite 400
Philadelphia, PA 19106-4738
215-922-1161
866-416-1078
FAX: 215-922-1474
e-mail: hello.usa@jkp.com
www.jkp.com
Tony Wigram, Editor
Jessica Kingsley, Chairman, Managing Director
Jemima Kingsley, Director
Octavia Kingsley, Production Director
More and more, music therapy is being practiced as an intervention in medical and special educational settings. This book describes and explains the planning and evaluation of music therapy intervention and how it can be used for assessing complex organic and emotional disabilities. *$34.95*
312 pages
ISBN 1-853027-34-0

15 **Contemporary Art Therapy with Adolescents**
Taylor & Francis
400 Market Street
Suite 400
Philadelphia, PA 19106-4738
215-922-1161
866-416-1078
FAX: 215-922-1474
e-mail: hello.usa@jkp.com
www.jkp.com
Shirley Riley, Author
Jessica Kingsley, Chairman, Managing Director
Jemima Kingsley, Director
Octavia Kingsley, Production Director
Reviews contemporary theories on adolescent development and therapy and offers solutions to the treatment of young people. *$ 26.95*
285 pages
ISBN 1-853026-37-9

16 **Creative Arts Resources Catalog**
MMB Music
9051 Watson Road
Ste 161
St. Louis, MO 63126
314-531-9635
FAX: 314-531-8384
e-mail: info@mmbmusic.com
www.mmbmusic.com
Norm Goldberg, Founder & Chair
Publisher and distributor of creative arts therapy materials in the areas of music, dance, art, drama, and poetry. Free catalog contains hundreds of books, recordings, and videos.

17 **Creative Growth**
355 24th Street
Oakland, CA 94612
510-836-2340
FAX: 510-836-0769
e-mail: info@creativegrowth.org
www.creativegrowth.org
Jane Timberlake, President
Jessica Boncutter, Vice President
Jennifer Cooper, Secretary
Rob Forbes, Treasurer
Creative Growth Art Center serves adult artists with developmental, mental and physical disabilities, providing a professional studio environment for artistic development, gallery exhibition and representation and a social atmosphere among peers.

18 **Creativity Explored**
3245 16th Street
San Francisco, CA 94103
415-863-2108
FAX: 415-863-1655
e-mail: info@creativityexplored.org
www.creativityexplored.org
Jeff Spicer, President
Nina Sazevich, Vice President
Amy Taub, Executive Director
Ann Kappes, Marketing & Business Development Director
Creativity Explored is a nonprofit visual arts center for artists with developmental disabilities.

19 **Dancing from the Inside Out**
Fanlight Productions
c/o Icarus Films
32 Court Street, 21st Floor
Brooklyn, NY 11201
718-488-8900
800-876-1710
FAX: 718-488-8642
e-mail: info@fanlight.com
www.fanlight.com
Ben Achtenberg, Founder
This eloquent video looks at the lives and work of three talented dancers who dance professionally with the acclaimed AXIS Dance Troupe, which includes both disabled and non-disabled dancers. They discuss the process they went through in adapting to their disability and how they came to re-discover physical expression through dance.

20 **Deaf West Theatre**
5112 Lankershim Blvd.
North Hollywood, CA 91601
818-762-2998
FAX: 818-762-2981
e-mail: info@deafwest.org
deafwest.org
Ed Waterstreet, Founding Artistic Director
David Kurs, Artistic Director
Mark Freund, President
Deaf West Theatre, Inc., was founded in 1991 to directly improve and enrich the cultural lives of the 1.2 million deaf and hard-of-hearing individuals who live in the Los Angeles area. DWT provides exposure and access to professional theatre, filling a void for deaf artists and audiences.

21 **Dionysus Theatre, Inc.**
5300 North Braeswood #226
Houston, TX 77096 713-728-0041
FAX: 713-779-7483

Brandon Mark, President
Nicole Wycisio, Vice President
Diane Lee, Secretary
Michael Abbott, Treasurer

Dionysus Theatre is a non profit organization bringing the theatre experience to actors with disabilities and those that are non-disabled together using the theatre as our creative venue.

22 **Disability and Social Performance: Using Drama to Achieve Successful Acts**
Brookline Books
8 Trumbull Rd
Suite B-001
Northampton, MA 01060 413-584-0184
800-666-2665
FAX: 413-584-6184
e-mail: brbooks@yahoo.com
www.brooklinebooks.com

Bernie Warren, Author

This book makes a major contribution to the understanding of disability, people with disabilities and the creative power they possess which can be unleashed through performance. The books name is Disability and Social Performance: Using Drama to Achieve Successful Acts of Being. *$17.95*

23 **Expressive Arts for the Very Disabled and Handicapped of All Ages**
Charles C. Thomas
2600 S First Street
Springfield, IL 62704-4730 217-789-8980
800-258-8980
FAX: 217-789-9130
e-mail: books@ccthomas.com
www.ccthomas.com

Marilyn Wannamaker, Co-Author
Jane G. Cohen, Co-Author

The ideas presented are not only designed to hold the interest of the children and adults, but to meet the needs of professionals and volunteers working with the disabled artists. All crafts are rated on a sliding scale, are of a low difficulty rating, use inexpensive and safe materials, and include explicit instructions. *$ 49.95*

236 pages Spiral-Paper 1996
ISBN 0-398067-04-5

24 **Fanlight Productions**
c/o Icarus Films
32 Court Street, 21st Floor
Brooklyn, NY 11201 718-488-8900
800-876-1710
FAX: 718-488-8642
e-mail: info@fanlight.com
www.fanlight.com

Ben Achtenberg, Founder

Fanlight Productions is a leading distributor of innovative film and video works on the social issues of our time, with a special focus on healthcare, mental health, professional ethics, aging and gerontology, disabilities, the workplace, and gender and family issues. Select titles include Acting Blind, Autism: A World Apart, Dancing from the Inside Out, and Able to Laugh.

25 **Fountain Gallery**
702 Ninth Avenue at 48th Street
New York, NY 10019 212-262-2756
fountaingallerynyc.com

Jason Bowman, Director
Ariel Wilmott, Manager

Fountain Gallery provides an environment for artists living and working with mental illness to pursue their personal visions and to challenge the stigma that surrounds mental illness.

26 **Friends In Art (FIA)**
4317 Vermont Court
Columbia, MO 65203 573-445-5564
e-mail: paltschul@centurytel.net
www.friendsinart.com

Peter Altschul, President
Lynn Hedl, Vice President
Don Horn, Corresponding Secretary
Arlo Monthei, Treasurer

Friends in Art is a national organization for blind, visually impaired, and deaf-blind artists, musicians and writers, and art enthusiasts. The organization is dedicated to enhancing the skills and broadening the opportunities of the individuals involved with the organization.

27 **Future Horizons**
721 West Abram Street
Arlington, TX 76013-6995 817-277-0727
800-489-0727
FAX: 817-277-2270
www.fhautism.com

R. Wayne Gilpin, President
Jennifer Gilpin, VP, Foreign Translations
Kelly Gilpin, Editorial Dir.
Teresa Corey, Conference Administration

Founded in 1996, Future Horizons is devoted to supporting and fostering works and programs for those who live and work with autism and asperger's syndrome.

28 **Guide to the Selection of Musical Instruments**
MMB Music
9051 Watson Road
Ste 161
St. Louis, MO 63126 314-531-9635
800-543-3771
FAX: 314-531-8384
e-mail: info@mmbmusic.com
www.mmbmusic.com

Norm Goldberg, Founder & Chair

A marvelous resource book to aid therapists teaching those who are disabled to play musical instruments. *$7.75*

29 **In-Definite Arts Society**
8038 Fairmount Drive SE
Calgary, AB T2H0Y 403-253-3174
FAX: 403-255-2234
e-mail: ida@indefinitearts.com
www.indefinitearts.com

Darlene Murphy, Executive Director
Dijana Andric, Client Services Manager
Peter Kelsch, Accountant
Bernice Webb, Facility Coordinator

Promotes opportunities for people with developmental disabilities to express themselves and to grow and develop through their involvement in art.

30 **Infinity Dance Theater**
220 West 93rd Street
New York, NY 10025 212-877-3490
e-mail: info@infinitydance.com
infinitydance.com

Kitty Lunn, RDE, Founder/Artistic Director
Michael A. Fitch, Executive Director

Infinity has developed a curriculum for teaching this wheelchair dance technique which is deeply rooted in the principles of Classical Ballet and Modern Dance. The company includes dancers with and without disabilities, as well as dancers beyond the age traditionally associated with performing.

31 **Instrumental Music for Dyslexics: A Teaching Handbook**
Wiley & Sons
111 River Street
Hoboken, NJ 07030-5774
201-748-6000
FAX: 201-748-6088
e-mail: info@wiley.com
www.wiley.com

Sheila Oglethorpe, Author
Stephen M. Smith, President and CEO
Ellis E. Cousens, Executive Vice President, Chief Operations Officer
MJ O'Leary, Senior Vice President, Human Resources

Describes dyslexia in layman's terms and explains how the various problems that a dyslexic may have can affect all aspects of learning to play a musical instrument. It alerts the music teacher with a problem pupil to the possibilities of that pupil having some form of dyslexia. It offers suggestions as to how to teach dyslexics, with particular reference to piano teaching, and it suggests ways in which the music teacher may contribute to the welfare of a dyslexic pupil. *$ 34.95*
200 pages
ISBN 1-861562-91-8

32 **Interact Center**
Interact Center
212 Third Avenue N
Suite 140
Minneapolis, MN 55401
612-339-5145
e-mail: info@interactcenter.com
interactcenter.com

Jeanne Calvit, Artistic/Executive Director

Creates art in a spirit of radical inclusion; Inspires artists and audiences to explore the full spectrum of human potential; Transforms lives by expanding ideas of what is possible.

33 **Kaleidoscope: Exploring the Experience of Disability through Literature & the Fine Arts**
United Disability Services
701 South Main Street
Akron, OH 44311-1019
330-762-9755
FAX: 330-379-3342
e-mail: kaleidoscope@udsakron.org
www.udsakron.org/services/kaleidoscope

Gail Willmott, Editor in Chief
Gary Knuth, President/CEO
Howard Taylor, Vice President
Kay Shellenberger, Director of Adult Services

This magazine explores the experiences of disability through the lens of creative arts. Unlike rehabilitation, advocacy or independent living journals, this journal challenges and transcends stereotypical, patronizing and sentimental attitudes about disability. It offers a variety of articles, fiction, art and poetry relating to issues of disability, literature and the fine arts. *$10.00*
64 pages BiAnnually

34 **Keshet Dance Company**
4121 Cutler Avenue NE
Albuquerque, NM 87110
505-224-9808
keshetdance.org

Shira Greenberg, Artistic Director
Emily Thaler, President
Randy Trask, Vice President

Keshet's professional dancers conduct youth and adult classes and workshops for individuals with varying levels of physical disabilities and dance experience. Keshet pairs dancers with physical disabilities with able-bodied dancers, which often include siblings, parents, and peers, to create professional-quality dance works.

35 **Learning Disabilities Sourcebook, 3rd Ed.**
Omnigraphics
Order Department
PO Box 8002
Aston, PA 19014-8002
610-461-3548
800-234-1340
FAX: 800-875-1340
e-mail: contact@omnigraphics.com
www.omnigraphics.com

Joyce Brennfleck Shannon, Editor
Fred Ruffner, Founder
Peter Ruffner, Co-Founder

Learning Disabilities Sourcebook, Third Edition provides updated information about specific learning disabilities and other conditions that make learning difficult. These include dyscalculia, dysgraphia, dyslexia, auditory and visual processing, communication disorders, autism spectrum disorders, attention deficit/hyperactivity disorder, hearing and visual impairments, and brain injury. *$84.00*
600 pages Hard cover
ISBN 0-780810-39-6

36 **Manual of Sequential Art Activities for Classified Children and Adolescents**
Charles C. Thomas
2600 South First Street
Springfield, IL 62704-4730
217-789-8980
800-258-8980
FAX: 217-789-9130
e-mail: books@ccthomas.com
www.ccthomas.com

Rocco A L Fugaro, Author

Offers information to the special education professional on art therapy and management. *$41.95*
246 pages Softcover
ISBN 0-39805-85-6

37 **Mozart Effect: Tapping the Power of Music to Heal the Body, Strengthen the Mind**
Harper Collins Publishers
10 E 53rd St
New York, NY 10022-5244
212-207-7000
www.harpercollins.com

Don Campbell, Author
Brian Murray, President and CEO
Michael Morrison, President and Publisher, U.S. General Books and Canada
Susan Katz, President and Publisher, HarperCollins Children's Books

Offers dramatic accounts of how doctors, shamans, musicians, and others use music to deal with everything from anxiety, cancer, and chronic pain, to dyslexia and mental illness. *$14.95*
352 pages
ISBN 0-060937-20-3

38 **Music Therapy**
Future Horizons, Inc.
721 West Abram St
Arlington, TX 76013-6995
817-277-0727
800-489-0727
FAX: 817-277-2270
www.fhautism.com

Betsey King Brunk, Author
R. Wayne Gilpin, President
Jennifer Gilpin, VP, Foreign Translations
Kelly Gilpin, Editorial Dir.

Music therapy is the use of music to address non-musical goals. Parents and professionals are finding that music can break down barriers for children with autism in areas such as cognition, socialization, and communication. *$19.95*
123 pages
ISBN 1-885477-53-8

39 Music Therapy and Leisure for Persons with Disabilities
Sagamore Publishing
1807 N Federal Drive
Urbana, IL 61801
217-359-5940
800-327-5557
FAX: 217-359-5975
e-mail: books@sagamorepub.com
www.sagamorepub.com

Alicia L. Barksdale, Author
Joseph J. Bannon, Sr., Ph.D., Publisher & CEO
Peter L. Bannon, MBA, President
William Anderson, M.S., Director of Sales and Marketing

Explores the use of musical therapy in order to enhance the development of independent leisure skills with a variety of special populations. Suggestions are provided for alternative avenues through musical experiences enabling individuals to achieve their greatest potential for independence and a high quality of life. *$19.95*
ISBN 1-571675-11-6

40 Music Therapy for the Developmentally Disabled
Sage Publications
2455 Teller Road
Thousand Oaks, CA 91320
805-499-9774
800-818-7243
FAX: 800-583-2665
e-mail: info@sagepub.com
www.sagepub.com

S. Venkatesan, Author

Included are practical guidelines, case samples and step-by-step instructions that enable a music therapist to bring about dramatic improvements in developmentally disabled adults and children. *$40.00*
269 pages Hardcover
ISBN 0-890791-90-2

41 Music Therapy in Dementia Care
Jessica Kingsley Publishers
400 Market Street
Suite 400
Philadelphia, PA 19106-4738
215-922-1161
866-416-1078
FAX: 215-922-1474
e-mail: hello.usa@jkp.com
www.jkp.com

David Aldridge, Editor
Jessica Kingsley, Chairman, Managing Director
Jemima Kingsley, Director
Octavia Kingsley, Production Director

A comprehensive look at music therapy as a means of improving memory, health, and identity in those suffering from dementia, particularly Alzheimer's. For music therapists and those involved in psychogeriatry. *$29.95*
256 pages
ISBN 1-853027-76-6

42 Music Therapy, Sensory Integration and the Autistic Child
Jessica Kingsley Publishers
400 Market Street
Suite 400
Philadelphia, PA 19106-4738
215-922-1161
866-416-1078
FAX: 215-922-1474
e-mail: hello.usa@jkp.com
www.jkp.com

Dorita S. Berger, Author
Jessica Kingsley, Chairman, Managing Director
Jemima Kingsley, Director
Octavia Kingsley, Production Director

Examines the human physiologic function, the brain, information processing, functional adaption, and how that might be affected by music interventions in persons with sensory integration difficulties. *$23.95*
256 pages
ISBN 1-843107-00-7

43 Music and Dyslexia: A Positive Approach
Wiley & Sons
111 River Street
Hoboken, NJ 07030-5774
201-748-6000
FAX: 201-748-6088
e-mail: info@wiley.com
www.wiley.com

John Westcombe, Editor
Stephen M. Smith, President and CEO
Ellis E. Cousens, Executive Vice President, Chief Operations Officer
MJ O'Leary, Senior VP, Human Resources

This book shows how some people who have Dyslexia can be gifted musicians. The main point this books makes is that Dyslexic musicians can succeed provided only that they are given sufficient encouragement and understanding. *$34.95*
200 pages
ISBN 1-861562-05-5

44 Music for the Hearing Impaired
MMB Music
9051 Watson Road
Ste 161
St. Louis, MO 63126
314-531-9635
800-543-3771
FAX: 314-531-8384
e-mail: info@mmbmusic.com
www.mmbmusic.com

Norm Goldberg, Founder & Chair

A resource manual and curriculum guide. It is the product of a four-year developmental music program, placing emphasis on the needs of those with severe and profound losses. *$29.95*

45 Music: Physician for Times to Come
Quest Books
P.O.Box 270
Wheaton, IL 60187-270
630-665-0130
800-669-9425
FAX: 630-665-8791
e-mail: submissions@questbooks.net
www.questbooks.net

Don Campbell, Author

A resource guide for various types of music and their therapeutic outcome.
365 pages
ISBN 0-835607-88-7

46 National Arts and Disability Center (NADC)
Tarjan Center at UCLA
760 Westwood Plaza
Los Angeles, CA 90095-8346
310-825-2631
800-825-2631
FAX: 310-794-1143
e-mail: oraynor@mednet.ucla.edu
www.semel.ucla.edu/nadc

Peter Whybrow, Director
Fawzy Fawzy, Associate Director
Alan Han, Director of Development
Monica Rodriguez, Director of Human Resources

NADC has a database and website which deals with access to and participation in the arts by people with disabilities.

47 National Association for Drama Therapy
1450 Western Avenue
Suite 101
Albany, NY 12203
571-223-6440
888-416-7167
FAX: 518-463-8656
e-mail: office@nadta.org
www.nadt.org

Nadya Trytan, MA, RDT/BCT, President
Jeremy Segall, MA, RDT, LCAT, Vice President
Jason Butler, RDT/BCT, LCAT, President-Elect
Whitney Sullivan, RDT, LCSW, Secretary

The National Association for Drama Therapy (NADT) was incorporated in 1979 to establish and uphold rigorous standards of professional competence for drama therapists. The NADT promotes drama therapy through information and advocacy.

48 **National Endowment for the Arts: Office for AccessAbility**
1100 Pennsylvania Ave NW
Washington, DC 20506-0001
202-682-5034
FAX: 202-682-5666
TTY:202-682-5496
e-mail: webmgr@arts.gov
www.arts.gov/

Jane Chu, Chairman
Beth Bienvenu, Accessibility Director
Wendy Clark, Director of Museums, Visual Arts, and Indemnity
Ayanna N. Hudson, Arts Education Director

The National Endowment for the Arts Office for AccessAbility is the advocacy-technical assistance arm of the Arts Endowment to make the arts accessible for people with disabilities, older adults, veterans, and people living in institutions.

49 **National Institute of Art and Disabilities**
551 23rd St
Richmond, CA 94804-1626
510-620-0290
FAX: 510-620-0326
e-mail: admin@niadart.org
www.niadart.org

Deborah Dyer, Exec. Dir.
Tim Buckwalter, Director of Exhibitions and Marketing
Belinda Sifford, Director of Client Services
Judith Zoon, Administrative Coordinator

The National Institute of Art & Disabilities (NIAD) provides an art program that promotes creativity, independence, dignity, and community integration for people with developmental and other disabilities.

50 **National Library Service for the Blind And Physically Handicapped**
1291 Taylor St NW
Washington, DC 20011
202-707-5100
FAX: 202-707-0712
TTY:202-707-0744
e-mail: nls@loc.gov
www.loc.gov/nls

Karen Keninger, Dir.
Erica Vaughns, Exec. Assistant to the Dir.
Michael Martys, Automation Officer
Neil Bernstein, R & D Officer

Administers a national library service that provides Braille and recorded books and magazines on free loan to anyone who cannot read standard print because of visual or physical disabilities.
Annual

51 **National Theatre Workshop of the Handicapped (NTWH)**
535 Greenwich Street
New York, NY 10013-1004
212-206-7789
FAX: 212-206-0200
e-mail: admissions@ntwh.org
www.ntwh.org

Jason Matthews, Director of Admissions
Rick Curry, President & CEO
John Spalla, General Manager

A non-profit organization that provides individuals within the disabled community with the communication skills and the artistic discipline necessary to pursue a life in professional theatre.

52 **National Theatre of the Deaf**
139 N Main St
West Hartford, CT 06107-1264
860-236-4193
FAX: 860-574-9107
e-mail: Info@NTD.org
www.ntd.org

Betty Beekman, Executive Director
William C. Martin, Marketing/PR Director
George Ghista, Accountant
Kathy Strauss, Company Interpreter

The mission of the National Theatre of the Deaf is to produce theatrically challenging work of the highest quality, drawing from as wide a range of the world's literature as possible and to perform these original works in a style that links American Sign Language with the spoken word.

53 **New Music Therapist's Handbook, 2nd Ed. Berklee School of Music**
Berklee Press Publications
1140 Boylston Street
Boston, MA 02215
617-747-2146
866-237-5533
www.berkleepress.com

Suzanne B. Hanser, Author

Dr. Hanser's well-respected Music Therapist's Handbook has been revised and thoroughly updated to reflect the latest developments in the field of music therapy. *$29.95*
256 pages
ISBN 0-634006-45-2

54 **No Limits**
9801 Washington Boulevard
2nd Floor
Culver City, CA 90232
310-280-0878
FAX: 310-280-0872
e-mail: michelle@nolimitsfordeafchildren.org
nolimitsfordeafchildren.org

Michelle Christie, Founder/Executive Director
Liz Martinez, Program Manager

The mission of No Limits is to meet the auditory, speech and language needs of deaf children and enhance their confidence through the theatrical arts and individual therapy as well as provide family support and community awareness on the needs and talents of deaf children who are learning to speak.

55 **Non-Traditional Casting Project**
Ste 1600
1560 Broadway
New York, NY 10036-1518
212-730-4750
FAX: 212-730-4820
TTY:212-730-4913
e-mail: info@ntcp.org
www.ntcp.org/

Nancy Kim, Manager

The Non-Traditional Casting Project (NTCP) is a not-for-profit advocacy organization whose purpose is to address and seek solutions to the problems of racism and exclusion in theatre, film and television. NTCP's principal concerns are those of artists of color, female artists, Deaf and hard of hearing artists, and artists with disabilities.

56 **Nuvisions For Disabled Artists, Inc.**
C/O Rose Marcus
1319 Magee Street
Philadelphia, PA 19111
e-mail: hbedelstein@att.net
www.hbedelstein.home.att.net

Kaye E Schonbach, Executive Director

Nuvisions was established to enable physically challenged artists to pursue professional and semi-professional artistic opportunities. Nuvisions supports these artists by sponsoring accessible exhibitions, special projects and educational opportunities in Southeastern Pennsylvania and Southern New Jersey.

57 **Open Circle Theatre**
500 King Farm Blvd. #102
Rockville, MD 20850
240-683-8934
opencircletheatre.org

Suzanne Richard, Artistic Director
Ian Armstrong, Executive Producer

Open Circle Theatre is a professional theatre dedicated to producing productions that integrate the considerable talents of artists with disabilities. OCT was formed by a group of people with and without disabilities, who possess professional theater experience, love of the theater, and a commitment to full access for all persons in every opportunity our community has to offer.

58 **Pied Piper: Musical Activities to Develop Basic Skills**
Jessica Kingsley Publishers
400 Market Street
Suite 400
Philadelphia, PA 19106-4738
215-922-1161
866-416-1078
FAX: 215-922-1474
e-mail: hello.usa@jkp.com
www.jkp.com

John Bean, Author
Jessica Kingsley, Chairman, Managing Director
Jemima Kingsley, Director
Octavia Kingsley, Production Director

Describes 78 enjoyable music activities for groups of children or adults who may have learning difficulties. The emphasis is on using music, rather than learning songs or rhythms, so group members do not need any special skills to be able to participate. Full details are given about any equipment required for the games, as well as suggestions for variations or modifications. *$21.95*
96 pages
ISBN 1-853029-94-

59 **Project Onward**
Bridgeport Art Center
1200 W. 35th Street, 4th Floor
Chicago, IL 60609
773-940-2992
projectonward.org

60 **Pure Vision Arts**
114 West 17th Street
3rd Floor
New York, NY 10011
212-366-4263
FAX: 212-929-5754
e-mail: progers@shield.org
purevisionarts.org

Pamala Rogers, Director

Pure Vision Arts mission is to provide people with autism and developmental disabilities opportunities for artistic expression and to build public awareness of their important creative contributions.

61 **Reaching the Child with Autism Through Art**
Future Horizons, Inc.
721 W Abram St
Arlington, TX 76013-6995
817-277-0727
800-489-0727
FAX: 817-277-2270
www.fhautism.com

Toni Flowers, Author
R. Wayne Gilpin, President
Jennifer Gilpin Yacio, Vice President and Editorial Director
David Reasor, CPA and Administrative Director

This book uncovers how art encourages communication, positive self-image, concept development, spatial relationships, fine-motor skills, and many more facets of health child development.
$19.95
130 pages

62 **Survivors Art Foundation**
PO Box 383
Westhampton, NY 11977
e-mail: safe@survivorsartfoundation.com
www.survivorsartfoundation.org

Michael Herships, Ph.D, Project Leader & Board President
Candyce Brokaw, Art Director
Candyce M. Brokaw, Executive Director
Margaret Ashe Magistro, Secretary/Treasurer

Dedicated to encourage healing through the arts, committed to empowering Trauma-Survivors with Effective Expressive Outlets via Internet Art Gallery, Outreach Programs, National Exhibitions, Publications and Development of Employment Skills.

63 **Teaching Asperger's Students Social Skills Through Acting**
Future Horizons, Inc.
721 W Abram St
Arlington, TX 76013-6995
817-277-0727
800-489-0727
FAX: 817-277-2270
www.fhautism.com

Amelia Davies, Author
R. Wayne Gilpin, President
Jennifer Gilpin Yacio, Vice President and Editorial Director
David Reasor, CPA and Administrative Director

This book provides the theories and activities needed for setting up acting classes that double as social skills groups for individuals with Asperger's or high-functioning autism. Using these skills, students will be able to develop social understanding through repetition and generalization. *$19.95*
211 pages

64 **Teaching Basic Guitar Skills to Special Learners**
MMB Music
9051 Watson Road
Ste 161
St. Louis, MO 63126
314-531-9635
800-543-3771
FAX: 314-531-8384
e-mail: info@mmbmusic.com
www.mmbmusic.com

Norm Goldberg, Founder & Chair

The first-of-its-kind guitar book for use with persons who have difficulty learning to play via traditional methods. *$16.00*

65 **The Arts Of Life**
2010 W. Carroll Avenue
Chicago, IL 60612
312-829-2787
e-mail: info@artsoflife.org
artsoflife.org

Bronwyn Kelly, President
Chris McLaughlin, Treasurer
Rachel Edelshteyn, Secretary

We are people with and without disabilities creating an artistic culture to realize our full potential.

66 **The Awakenings Project**
PO Box 177
Wheaton, IL 60187
www.awakeningsproject.org

Robert Lundin, Co-Director
Irene O'Neill, President and Co-Director
Mary Lou Lowry, Secretary
John Rakow, Vice President

The Awakenings Project is an organization whose mission is to assist those artists with psychiatric illnesses in developing their talent and finding an outlet for their creative abilities through art in all forms.

67 **Theatre Without Limits**
P.O.Box 4002
Portland, ME 04101
207-607-4016
FAX: 207-761-4740
www.vsartsmaine.org

Kippy Rudy, Executive Director

VSA Maine is a 501(c)(3) non-profit organization providing educational, arts, and cultural opportunities to children and adults with disabilities in Maine.

68 **VSA - The International Organization on Arts and Disability**
2700 F Street, NW
Washington, DC 20566
202-467-4600
800-444-1324
FAX: 202-429-0868
TTY: 202-737-0645
e-mail: info@vsarts.org
www.kennedy-center.org/education/vsa/

Ambassador J Kennedy Smith, Founder
David M. Rubenstein, Chair
Michael M. Kaiser, President
Christoph Eschenbach, Music Director, NSO and Kennedy Center
VSA offers a large selection of guides, publications, and other resources dealing with a wide variety of subject matter in education, arts, and disabilities.

69 **VSA arts**
2700 F Street, NW
Washington, DC 20566
202-467-4600
800-444-1324
FAX: 202-429-0868
TTY: 202-737-0645
e-mail: info@vsarts.org
www.kennedy-center.org/education/vsa/

Ambassador J Kennedy Smith, Founder
David M. Rubenstein, Chair
Michael M. Kaiser, President
Christoph Eschenbach, Music Director, NSO and Kennedy Center
VSA arts is an international, nonprofit organization founded in 1974 by Ambassador Jean Kennedy Smith whose mission is to create a society where all people with disabilities learn through, participate in, and enjoy the arts. Most states offer local programs, such as Arts in Action, that showcases the accomplishments of artists with disabilities and promotes increased access to the arts for people with disabilities.

70 **We Are PHAMALY**
Fanlight Productions
c/o Icarus Films
32 Court Street, 21st Floor
Brooklyn, NY 11201
718-488-8900
800-876-1710
FAX: 718-488-8642
e-mail: info@fanlight.com
www.fanlight.com

Ben Achtenberg, Owner
Stands for Physically Handicapped Musical Actors League. This dynamic troupe doesn't cut any corners or make any compromises. The musicals they perform are chosen for their appeal to the audience, not because they are easy for the performers, who have a variety of sensory and mobility handicaps. *$199.00*
ISBN 1-572954-08-6

Assistive Devices

Automobile

71 **Ability Center**
Contact Technologies
11600 Western Ave
Stanton, CA 90680-3436
866-405-6806
FAX: 714-901-1492
e-mail: info@abilitycenter.com
www.abilitycenter.com
Darrell Heath, CEO
Dan Monahan, Manager
Offers rear or side entry designed with painstaking craftsmanship using steel.

72 **Acc-u-trol**
Ahnafield Corporation
9850 E. 30th Street
Indianapolis, IN 46229
877-223-5301
e-mail: info@acemobility.us
www.acemobility.us

73 **All View Mirror**
4335 S Santa Fe Dr
Englewood, CO 80110-5417
303-781-2062
800-782-4335
FAX: 303-761-6811
e-mail: info@handicapsinc.com
www.handicapsinc.com

74 **Arcola Mobility**
51 Kero Rd
Carlstadt, NJ 07072-2601
201-507-8500
800-272-6521
FAX: 201-507-5372
e-mail: info@arcolasales.com
www.arcolasales.com
Andrew Rolfe, Exec VP
Jeff Krane, Sales Mgr/Nat'l Accounts
John Akerlind, General Mgr
Teresa Smeriglio, Comml Bus Sales Coord
Arcola sells new and used accessible vehicles and adaptive driving equipment including hand controls, wheelchair lifts and securement systems. Daily, weekly and monthly vehicle rentals available. Stairway lift, porch elevators and ramps for the home sold and rented.

75 **Automobile Lifts for Scooters, Wheelchairs and Powerchairs**
Bruno Independent Living Aids
P.O.Box 84
Oconomowoc, WI 53066
262-567-4990
800-882-8183
FAX: 262-953-5501
www.bruno.com
Michael R. Bruno, II, President and CEO
Mike Krawczyk, Marketing Manager
Andrew Bayer, Product Manager
Over 18 different styles of automobile lifts for scooters, wheelchairs and power chairs for nearly any car, van, truck or sport utility vehicle that can raise most scooters or wheelchairs under 200 pounds and power chairs up to 300 pounds. All Bruno lifts are eligible for reimbursement of up to $1000.00 from GM, Saturn, Ford, and Chrysler under the terms of their Mobility Programs.

76 **Blinker Buddy II Electronic Turn Signal**
HARC Mercantile
5413 S. Westnedge Ave.
Suite A
Portage, MI 49002-5317
269-324-1615
800-445-9968
FAX: 269-324-2387
TTY: 800-445-9968
e-mail: info@harc.com
www.harc.com

77 **Braun Corporation**
631 West 11th Street
Winamac, IN 46996
574-946-6153
800-THE-LIFT
FAX: 574-946-4670
e-mail: mediaquestions@braunlift.com
www.braunability.com
Ralph Braun, Founder
Manufactures wheelchair lifts and lowered floor minivans as well as many other mobility products.

78 **Chevy Lowered Floor**
Ahnafield Corporation
9850 E. 30th Street
Indianapolis, IN 46229
877-223-5301
e-mail: info@acemobility.us
www.acemobility.us

79 **Classic**
Ricon
1135 Aviation Place
San Fernando, CA 91340
818-267-3000
800-322-2884
FAX: 818-962-1201
e-mail: sales@riconcorp.com
www.riconcorp.com

80 **DW Auto & Home Mobility**
1208 N Garth Ave
Columbia, MO 65203-4056
573-449-3859
800-568-2271
FAX: 573-449-4187
e-mail: contactus@dwauto.com
www.dwauto.com
Shawn Bright, Owner
Don Rothwell, General Manager
Brian Lutz, Service Manager
Paratransit conversions and personalized conversions for the physically challenged. Home elevators and lifts. Scooter, wheelchairs and DME.

81 **Dodge Lowered Floor**
Ahnafield Corporation
9850 E. 30th Street
Indianapolis, IN 46229
877-223-5301
e-mail: info@acemobility.us
www.acemobility.us

82 **Drive Master Company**
37 Daniel Rd West
Fairfield, NJ 07004-2521
973-808-9709
FAX: 973-808-9713
e-mail: sales@drivemaster.net
www.drive-master.com
Peter B. Ruprecht, President
Adrienne Ruprecht, Bookkeeping
Christina M. Knapik, General Office Manager
Vinnie Dalli-Cardillo, Dealer Relations
Full service mobility center, raised tops/doors, drop floors, custom driving equipment, distributor of name brand devices and systems for full sized and mini vans. Sister company Van Master rents mobility equipped vans.

83 **Dual Brake Control**
Kroepke Kontrols
104 Hawkins Street
Bronx, NY 10464
718-885-2100
FAX: 337-235-4181
e-mail: kroepke@mail.idt.net

84 **Entervan**
Braun Corporation
631 West 11th Street
Winamac, IN 46996
574-946-6153
800-THE-LIFT
FAX: 574-946-4670
e-mail: mediaquestions@braunlift.com
www.braunability.com

Ralph Braun, Founder
The Entervan accessible features are designed to blend seamlessly into the original design of the Chrysler minivan. In fact, you'll find the Entervan to be virtually indistinguishable from other minivans on the road, with the only differences being the easily accessible qualities of the van.

85 **Escort II XL**
Worldwide Mobility Products
Mesa, AZ
480-497-4692
800-848-3433
FAX: 480-497-3834
e-mail: service@worldwide-mobility.com
www.worldwide-mobility.com

86 **Foot Pedal Extensions**
4335 S Santa Fe Dr
Englewood, CO 80110-5417
303-781-2062
800-782-4335
FAX: 303-761-6811
e-mail: info@handicapsinc.com
www.handicapsinc.com

87 **Foot Steering**
Drive Master Company
37 Daniel Rd West
Fairfield, NJ 07004-2521
973-808-9709
FAX: 973-808-9713
e-mail: sales@drivemaster.net
www.drive-master.com

Peter B. Ruprecht, President
Adrienne Ruprecht, Bookkeeping
Christina M. Knapik, General Office Manager
Vinnie Dalli-Cardillo, Dealer Relations
Custom installed system to steer a vehicle with your foot.

88 **Foot Steering System**
Ahnafield Corporation
9850 E. 30th Street
Indianapolis, IN 46229
877-223-5301
e-mail: info@acemobility.us
www.acemobility.us

89 **Ford Lowered Floor**
Ahnafield Corporation
9850 E. 30th Street
Indianapolis, IN 46229
877-223-5301
e-mail: info@acemobility.us
www.acemobility.us

90 **Gear Shift Adaptor By Handicaps, Inc.**
4335 S Santa Fe Dr
Englewood, CO 80110-5417
303-781-2062
800-782-4335
FAX: 303-761-6811
e-mail: info@handicapsinc.com
www.handicapsinc.com

Jeanenne Phillips, Executive Director
Allows column mounted gear shift to be used with the left hand. *$90.00*

91 **Gresham Driving Aids**
30800 S Wixom Rd
Wixom, MI 48393-2418
248-624-1533
800-521-8930
FAX: 248-624-6358
e-mail: dave@greshamdrivingaids.com
www.greshamdrivingaids.com

David Ohrt, General Manager
Craig Wigginton, Sales Consultant
Dexter Jackson, Service Manager
Joyce Martell, Customer Service
Offers a full-service package to physically challenged individuals including lowered floors, raised roofs and doors and high-quad driver control systems. Dealer for Braun, Ricon, Crow River and Bruno wheelchair lifts.

92 **Hand Brake Control Only**
Kroepke Kontrols
104 Hawkins Street
Bronx, NY 10464
718-885-2100
FAX: 337-235-4181
e-mail: kroepke@mail.idt.net

93 **Hand Dimmer Switch**
Gresham Driving Aids
30800 S Wixom Rd
Wixom, MI 48393-2418
248-624-1533
800-521-8930
FAX: 248-624-6358
e-mail: dave@greshamdrivingaids.com
www.greshamdrivingaids.com

David Ohrt, General Manager
Craig Wigginton, Sales Consultant
Dexter Jackson, Service Manager
Joyce Martell, Customer Service
This switch is recommended for left leg handicaps or when a right leg handicap uses a left foot throttle. *$36.25*

94 **Hand Dimmer Switch with Horn Button**
Gresham Driving Aids
30800 S Wixom Rd
Wixom, MI 48393-2418
248-624-1533
800-521-8930
FAX: 248-624-6358
e-mail: dave@greshamdrivingaids.com
www.greshamdrivingaids.com

David Ohrt, General Manager
Craig Wigginton, Sales Consultant
Dexter Jackson, Service Manager
Joyce Martell, Customer Service
Attaches to the handle of control with a chrome plated steel insulated switch box, giving an instant warning without removing your hand from the steering wheel. *$28.75*

95 **Hand Gas & Brake Control**
Kroepke Kontrols
104 Hawkins Street
Bronx, NY 10464-288
718-885-2100
FAX: 337-235-4181
e-mail: kroepke@mail.idt.net
www.kroepkekontrols.com

96 **Hand Operated Parking Brake**
Gresham Driving Aids
30800 S Wixom Rd
Wixom, MI 48393-2418
248-624-1533
800-521-8930
FAX: 248-624-6358
e-mail: dave@greshamdrivingaids.com
www.greshamdrivingaids.com

David Ohrt, General Manager
Craig Wigginton, Sales Consultant
Dexter Jackson, Service Manager
Joyce Martell, Customer Service
Converts foot parking brake to a hand operation for easy access and maneuverability. *$30.20*

97 **Hand Parking Brake**
Kroepke Kontrols
104 Hawkins Street
Bronx, NY 10464-288
718-885-2100
FAX: 337-235-4181
e-mail: kroepke@mail.itd.net
www.kroepkekontrols.com

98 **Handicapped Driving Aids**
Handicapped Driving Aids of Michigan
3990 2nd Street
Wayne, MI 48184-1715
734-728-8808
FAX: 734-595-4520
Jim Bishop, President
Automobiles and vans customized, modified and equipped with industry approved handicapped equipment for ease of operation.

99 **Handicaps, Inc.**
4335 S Santa Fe Dr
Englewood, CO 80110-5417
303-781-2062
800-782-4335
FAX: 303-761-6811
e-mail: info@handicapsinc.com
www.handicapsinc.com
Jeanenne Phillips, Executive Director
Manufacturer of 'Superarm' wheelchair lifts, hand driving controls, and left foot gas pedals for vans & motor homes. *$120.00*

100 **Headlight Dimmer Switch**
Kroepke Kontrols
P.O.Box 288
Bronx, NY 10464-288
718-885-2100
FAX: 337-235-4181
e-mail: kroepke@mail.idt.net
www.kroepkekontrols.com

101 **Horizontal Steering**
Drive Master Company
37 Daniel Rd West
Fairfield, NJ 07004-2521
973-808-9709
FAX: 973-808-9713
e-mail: sales@drivemaster.net
www.drive-master.com
Peter B. Ruprecht, President
Adrienne Ruprecht, Bookkeeping
Christina M. Knapik, General Office Manager
Vinnie Dalli-Cardillo, Dealer Relations
Horizontal steering system is customized to meet the needs of the high-level, spinally injured and all others who experience limited arm strength and range of motion.

102 **Horn Control Switch**
Kroepke Kontrols
P.O.Box 288
Bronx, NY 10464-288
718-885-2100
FAX: 337-235-4181
e-mail: kroepke@mail.idt.net
www.kroepkekontrols.com

103 **Joystick Driving Control**
Ahnafield Corporation
9850 E. 30th Street
Indianapolis, IN 46229
877-223-5301
e-mail: info@acemobility.us
www.acemobility.us

104 **Kessler Institute for Rehabilitation**
1199 Pleasant Valley Way
West Orange, NJ 07052
973-731-3600
888-KES-SLER
FAX: 973-243-6819
www.kessler-rehab.com
Robert H. Brehm, President
Bruce M. Gans, MD, Executive Vice President and Chief Medical Officer
Karen Liszner, Chief Nurse Executive
Kim Ratner, AVP, Rehabilitation Services
Driver evaluation training for the physically/mentally challenged offering state certified driving instructors. Door-to-door pickup at home, work or rehab centers.

105 **Key Holders, Ignition & Door Keys**
Gresham Driving Aids
30800 S Wixom Rd
Wixom, MI 48393-2418
248-624-1533
800-521-8930
FAX: 248-624-6358
e-mail: dave@greshamdrivingaids.com
www.greshamdrivingaids.com
David Ohrt, General Manager
Craig Wigginton, Sales Consultant
Dexter Jackson, Service Manager
Joyce Martell, Customer Service
Easy for arthritic hands to handle. Easily installed. *$18.70*

106 **Kneelkar**
Mednet
923 E. Michigan Avenue
Battle Creek, MI 49014
269-660-1002
888-625-6335
FAX: 269-660-1296
e-mail: kneelvan@fminow.com
http://www.freedommotors.com
Mike Thompson, Vice President
Chet Baranski, Mobility Specialist-Midwest Vans
Danielle Baughman, Product Manager
Offers the ultimate van conversions with equipment that is easily installed and accessible for the physically challenged.

107 **Latchloc Automatic Wheelchair Tiedown**
Ahnafield Corporation
9850 E. 30th Street
Indianapolis, IN 46229
877-223-5301
e-mail: info@acemobility.us
www.acemobility.us

108 **Left Foot Accelerator**
Gresham Driving Aids
30800 S Wixom Rd
Wixom, MI 48393-2418
248-624-1533
800-521-8930
FAX: 248-624-6358
e-mail: dave@greshamdrivingaids.com
www.greshamdrivingaids.com
David Ohrt, General Manager
Craig Wigginton, Sales Consultant
Dexter Jackson, Service Manager
Joyce Martell, Customer Service
A custom pedal designed for left-foot usage. Stainless steel cross bar attaches above the throttle pedal and leaves right pedal free for right foot use. *$80.50*

109 **Left Foot Gas Pedal**
Kroepke Kontrols
P.O.Box 288
Bronx, NY 10464-288
718-885-2100
FAX: 337-235-4181
e-mail: kroepke@mail.itd.net
www.kroepkekontrols.com

110 **Left Foot Gas Pedal by Handicaps, Inc.**
4335 S Santa Fe Dr
Englewood, CO 80110-5417
303-781-2062
800-782-4335
FAX: 303-761-6811
e-mail: info@handicapsinc.com
www.handicapsinc.com

111 Left Hand Shift Lever
Gresham Driving Aids
30800 S Wixom Rd
Wixom, MI 48393-2418
248-624-1533
800-521-8930
FAX: 248-624-6358
e-mail: dave@greshamdrivingaids.com
www.greshamdrivingaids.com

David Ohrt, General Manager
Craig Wigginton, Sales Consultant
Dexter Jackson, Service Manager
Joyce Martell, Customer Service

Converts steering wheel lever or automatic transmission selector lever to left hand usage for right arm handicaps. *$34.50*

112 Low Effort and No Effort Steering
Drive Master Company
37 Daniel Rd West
Fairfield, NJ 07004-2521
973-808-9709
FAX: 973-808-9713
e-mail: sales@drivemaster.net
www.drive-master.com

Peter B. Ruprecht, President
Adrienne Ruprecht, Bookkeeping
Christina M. Knapik, General Office Manager
Vinnie Dalli-Cardillo, Dealer Relations

Reduced effort steering modifications available for nearly all vehicles. Additional products are pedal extensions which are 1 inch to 4 inch clamp-on aluminum blocks and 6 inch to 12 inch adjustable fold-down pedals.

113 Mini-Bus and Mini-Vans
Arcola Bus Sales
51 Kero Rd
Carlstadt, NJ 07072-2604
201-507-8500
800-272-6521
FAX: 201-507-5372
e-mail: JudyLongo@alliancebusgroup.com
www.arcolamobility.com

Andrew Rolfe, Exec VP
John Akerlind, General Mgr
Sam Garcia, Parts Manager
Cory Mahady, Vehicle Service & Repair

Offers a virtually unlimited choice of chassis size, body style, floor plan and optional features. We provide transporters for almost every use, including school buses, vans, mini-coaches, medium-duty buses and personalized vans for the disabled.

114 Mini-Rider
Ricon
1135 Aviation Place
San Fernando, CA 91340-6090
818-267-3000
800-322-2884
FAX: 818-962-1201
e-mail: sales@riconcorp.com
www.riconcorp.com

115 Mobility Vehicle Stairlifts and Ramps
Arcola Bus Sales
51 Kero Rd
Carlstadt, NJ 07072-2604
201-507-8500
800-272-6521
FAX: 201-507-5372
e-mail: JudyLongo@alliancebusgroup.com
www.arcolamobility.com

Andrew Rolfe, Exec VP
John Akerlind, General Mgr
Sam Garcia, Parts Manager
Cory Mahady, Vehicle Service & Repair

Arcola Mobility is a leading dealer of personal, accessible mini and full-size vans with custom conversions and modifications available. We offer a complete line of adaptive driving equipment, including wheelchair lifts, ramps, hand controls, steering devices, scooter lifters, car top wheelchair carriers and power transfer seats. In addition to new custom vehicles, we also have an extensive selection of used vehicles for the physically challenged.

116 Monarch Mark 1-A
Access Mobility Systems
7202 Evergreen Way
Everett, WA 98203
425-353-6563
800-854-4176
FAX: 425-355-6159
e-mail: info@accessams.com
www.accessams.com

117 Monmouth Vans, Access and Mobility
5105 New Jersey RT-33
Farmingdale, NJ 07727-4003
877-275-4907
e-mail: ask@mobilityworks
www.mobilityworks.com/

Gene Morton, President
Ray Morton, General Manager
Don Dufty, Certified Mobility Consultant
Nathan Ahrens, Care Center Director

Full vehicle modifications for driving and for transport of people with disabilities. Access equipment for buildings, e.g. ramps, stair lifts, pool lifts, automatic door openers and patient transfer lifts, pride jazzy portable and modular wheelchairs and scooters. Large selection of modified vans in stock.

118 New Quad Grip
Gresham Driving Aids
30800 S Wixom Rd
Wixom, MI 48393-2418
248-624-1533
800-521-8930
FAX: 248-624-6358
e-mail: dave@greshamdrivingaids.com
www.greshamdrivingaids.com

David Ohrt, General Manager
Craig Wigginton, Sales Consultant
Dexter Jackson, Service Manager
Joyce Martell, Customer Service

Automobile aids for the disabled. *$40.25*

119 PAC Unit
Ahnafield Corporation
9850 E. 30th Street
Indianapolis, IN 46229
877-223-5301
e-mail: info@acemobility.us
www.acemobility.us

120 Park Brake Extension By Handicaps, Inc.
4335 S Santa Fe Dr
Englewood, CO 80110-5417
303-781-2062
800-782-4335
FAX: 303-761-6811
e-mail: info@handicapsinc.com
www.handicapsinc.com

121 Pedal Ease
Ahnafield Corporation
9850 E. 30th Street
Indianapolis, IN 46229
877-223-5301
e-mail: info@acemobility.us
www.acemobility.us

122 Portable Hand Controls
Ahnafield Corporation
9850 E. 30th Street
Indianapolis, IN 46229
877-223-5301
e-mail: info@acemobility.us
www.acemobility.us

123 Portable Hand Controls By Handicaps, Inc.
4335 S Santa Fe Dr
Englewood, CO 80110-5417
303-781-2062
800-782-4335
FAX: 303-761-6811
e-mail: info@handicapsinc.com
www.handicapsinc.com

For those who have trouble getting in and out of a car. Sturdy bar slides into door striker and allows you better support to lift yourself out of the car. Stores easily under car seat. *$39.95*

138 **Tim's Trim**
25 Bermar Park
Rochester, NY 14624-1542
585-429-6270
888-468-6784
FAX: 585-429-6355
e-mail: Info@TimsTrim.com
www.timstrim.com/
Tim Miller, Owner
Offers vehicle modifications, drop floors, raised tops/doors, driving equipment, touch pads and lifts. Also is a member of NEMDA and QAP certified

139 **Transportation Equipment for People with Disabilities**
Drive Master Company
30800 S Wixom Rd
Wixom, MI 48393-2418
248-624-1533
800-521-8930
FAX: 248-624-6358
e-mail: dave@greshamdrivingaids.com
www.greshamdrivingaids.com
David Ohrt, General Manager
Craig Wigginton, Sales Consultant
Dexter Jackson, Service Manager
Joyce Martell, Customer Service
Wheelchair lifts and ramps, hand and foot controls, steering and braking modifications, complete van conversions, home modifications, wheelchairs and scooters and wheelchair accessible van rentals.

140 **Tri-Post Steering Wheel Spinner**
Gresham Driving Aids
37 Daniel Rd West
Fairfield, NJ 07004-2521
973-808-9709
FAX: 973-808-9713
e-mail: sales@drivemaster.net
www.drive-master.com
Peter B. Ruprecht, President
Adrienne Ruprecht, Bookkeeping
Christina M. Knapik, General Office Manager
Vinnie Dalli-Cardillo, Dealer Relations
Three nylon posts, adjustable for proper fit to drivers hand, to control the wheel, for use by persons with weak or limp wrists. *$40.25*

141 **Turn Signal Adapter By Handicaps, Inc.**
Handicaps
4335 S Santa Fe Dr
Englewood, CO 80110-5417
303-781-2062
800-782-4335
FAX: 303-761-6811
e-mail: info@handicapsinc.com
www.handicapsinc.com

142 **Ultra-Lite XL Hand Control**
Drive Master Company
30800 S Wixom Rd
Wixom, MI 48393-2418
248-624-1533
800-521-8930
FAX: 248-624-6358
e-mail: dave@greshamdrivingaids.com
www.greshamdrivingaids.com
David Ohrt, General Manager
Craig Wigginton, Sales Consultant
Dexter Jackson, Service Manager
Joyce Martell, Customer Service
Allows the driver to operate gas and brake by hand— push for brake— pull for gas. Can be installed in nearly every vehicle.

143 **United Access**
Wright-Way
175 E Interstate 30
Garland, TX 75043-4021
972-240-8839
877-503-9399
888-939-1010
FAX: 972-240-0412
e-mail: info@unitedaccess.com
www.unitedaccess.com

144 **Vantage Mini-Vans**
Vantage Mini-Vans
5202 S 28th Pl
Phoenix, AZ 85040-3799
602-243-2700
800-348-VANS
FAX: 602-304-3290
www.vantagemobility.com

145 **Velcro Peel-Off Shoes**
4335 S Santa Fe Dr
Englewood, CO 80110-5417
303-781-2062
800-782-4335
FAX: 303-761-6811
e-mail: info@handicapsinc.com
www.handicapsinc.com

146 **Voice Choice**
Ahnafield Corporation
9850 E. 30th Street
Indianapolis, IN 46229
877-223-5301
e-mail: info@acemobility.us
www.acemobility.us

147 **Voice Scan**
Ahnafield Corporation
9850 E. 30th Street
Indianapolis, IN 46229
877-223-5301
e-mail: info@acemobility.us
www.acemobility.us

148 **Warp Drive**
Ahnafield Corporation
9850 E. 30th Street
Indianapolis, IN 46229
877-223-5301
e-mail: info@acemobility.us
www.acemobility.us

149 **Wheelers Accessible Van Rentals**
Wheelers Accessible Van Rental
6614 West Sweetwater
Glendale, AZ 85304
623-776-8830
800-456-1371
FAX: 623-412-9920
e-mail: info@WheelersVanRentals.com
www.WheelersVanRentals.com

150 **XL Steering**
Ahnafield Corporation
9850 E. 30th Street
Indianapolis, IN 46229
877-223-5301
e-mail: info@acemobility.us
www.acemobility.us

Bath

151 **ARJO Inc.**
2349 West Lake Street
Suite 250
Addison, IL 60101
630-785-4490
800-323-1245
FAX: 888-389-2756
e-mail: usa.info@ArjoHuntleigh.com
www.arjohuntleigh.com

152 **Adjustable Bath Seat**
Arista Surgical Supply Company/AliMed
297 High St
Dedham, MA 02026-2852
781-329-2900
800-225-2610
FAX: 781-329-8392
e-mail: info@alimed.com
www.alimed.com

Julian Cherubini, President
Bath seat that fits easily in any size tub. Easily adjustable to any height for easier maneuverability. *$44.00*

153 **Adjustable Raised Toilet Seat & Guard**
Frohock-Stewart
1 Invacare Way
Elyria, OH 44035-4190
440-329-6000
800-333-6900
FAX: 877-619-7996
www.invacare.com

A Malachi Mixon III, Chairman
Gerald B. Blouch, President & CEO
Joseph B. Richey III, President - Invacare Technologies Division and SVP
Robert K. Gudbranson, Senior Vice President and Chief Financial Officer
The seat features an exclusive pivot locking system so it won't slip or tip and the adjustable guard rail fits all toilets.

154 **Bath Fixtures**
Crane Plumbing/Fiat Products
1000 Industrial Dr
Unit 2A
Bensenville, IL 60106-1260
630-350-7575
FAX: 630-350-7775
www.deery-pardue.com

Dave Pardue, Chairman Emeritus
Greg Pardue, Sales
Mark Nasuta, Sales
Matt Pardue, Sales
Manufacturers plumbing fixtures for the disabled. Products include toilets, lavatories, showers and tub/shower units.

155 **Bath Products**
Snug Seat
12801 E. Independence Blvd.
P.O. Box 1739
Matthews, NC 28106-1739
800-336-7684
FAX: 704-882-0751
e-mail: information@snugseat.com
www.snugseat.com

Kirk MacKenzie, President
Scott Crosswhite, Vice President
Greg Tilley, Controller
Angela Stegall, Purchasing
Offers a wide range of products to meet the transportation, mobility, seating and bath aid needs for people of all ages. From car seats and standers for children with special needs to versatile wheelchairs that offer adults customized options and the freedom to go anywhere with confidence.

156 **Bath Shower & Commode Chair**
7830 Steubenville Pike
Oakdale, PA 15071-9226
724-695-2122
888-347-4537
FAX: 724-695-2922
e-mail: info@clarkehealthcare.com
www.clarkehealthcare.com

157 **Bath and Shower Bench 3301B**
Mada Medical Products
625 Washington Ave
Carlstadt, NJ 07072-2901
201-460-0454
800-526-6370
FAX: 201-460-3509
e-mail: dianelind@mail.madamedical.com
www.madainternational.com

Jeffrey Adam, President
The bath and shower bench is corrosion resistant, has a cross brace design and angled legs to prevent tipping, and seat height adjustments.

158 **BathEase**
3815 Darston St
Palm Harbor, FL 34685-3119
727-786-2604
888-747-7845
FAX: 727-786-2604
e-mail: bathease@aol.com
www.bathease.com

Terry, Director of Design & Development
Gerry, Supervisor of Manufacturing
Bill, Supervisor of Operations
BathEase is the original, standard size, residential style, acrylic bathtub with a door. Ideal for use in private homes by all who are ambulatory, the award winning design was specially created as an aid to daily living for the elderly and physically challenged. *$ 1897.00*

159 **Bathroom Transfer Systems**
Columbia Medical Manufacturing
11724 Willake Street
Santa Fe Springs, CA 90670-5032
562-282-0244
800-454-6612
FAX: 310-305-1718
e-mail: info@columbiamedical.com
www.columbiamedical.com

Gary Werschmidt, CEO
Keith Wright, Dir. of Sales & Mktg
Sue Johnson, Dir. of Finance
Reese Regan, Dir. of Engineering
Offers a complete line of bathroom transfer systems, bath lifts, reclining bath chairs, bath/shower/commode chairs, wrap-around bath supports, toilet supports, positioning commodes, premium air, foam and gel seat cushions, giant trainers and positioning restraint car seats that accommodate individuals from 20-130 pounds.

160 **Bathtub Safety Rail**
Arista Surgical Supply Company/AliMed
297 High St
Dedham, MA 02026-2852
781-329-2900
800-225-2610
FAX: 781-329-8392
e-mail: info@alimed.com
www.alimed.com

Julian Cherubini, President
Made of stainless steel, this safety rail fits in any size bathtub and offers safety and independence at bathing time. *$55.00*

161 **Braun Corporation**
Braun Corporation
631 West 11th Street
Winamac, IN 46996
574-946-6153
800-843-5438
FAX: 574-946-4670
e-mail: mediaquestions@braunlift.com
www.braunability.com

Ralph Braun, Founder
Offers a variety of assistive devices for the bath and surrounding environment.

162 **Can-Do Products Catalog**
Independent Living Aids
137 Rano Rd
Buffalo, NY 14207
516-937-1848
800-537-2118
FAX: 516-937-3906
e-mail: can-do@independentliving.com
www.independentliving.com

Irwin Schneidmill, President
Fran Hennelly, Sales Director
Russell Pennington, Marketing Director
Provide essential aids and products for the blind and visually impaired.
84 pages Quarterly

163 Clarke Healthcare Products, Inc.
Clarke Health Care Products
7830 Steubenville Pike
Oakdale, PA 15071-9226
724-695-2122
888-347-4537
FAX: 724-695-2922
e-mail: info@clarkehealthcare.com
www.clarkehealthcare.com

164 Commode
Maxi Aids
42 Executive Blvd
Farmingdale, NY 11735-4710
631-752-0521
800-522-6294
FAX: 631-752-0689
TTY: 800-281-3555
e-mail: sales@maxiaids.com
www.maxiaids.com

Elliot Zaretsky, Founder & President
Adjustable seat height for patient comfort. *$65.95*

165 Deluxe Bath Bench with Adjustable Legs
Maxi Aids
42 Executive Blvd
Farmingdale, NY 11735-4710
631-752-0521
800-522-6294
FAX: 631-752-0689
TTY: 800-281-3555
e-mail: sales@maxiaids.com
www.maxiaids.com

Elliot Zaretsky, Founder & President
Bath bench with back support and adjustable legs. *$ 49.95*

166 Driving Systems
16141 Runnymede St
Van Nuys, CA 91406-2913
818-782-6793
FAX: 818-782-6485
e-mail: info@drivingsystems.com
www.drivingsystems.com

Rudolf Schinz, President
William C Butt, VP
DSI is the manufacturer of the Scott Driving Controls for the severely disabled driver. Also manufacturers of the 'Wave Grip' grab rails and bathroom accessories for the disabled and elderly. DSI is also the importers of the Carospeed Menox Hand Controls, Left Foot Pedals and other handicapped driving aids.

167 Electric Leg Bag Emptier and Tub Slide Shower Chair
RD Equipment
230 Percival Dr
West Barnstable, MA 02668-1244
508-362-7498
FAX: 508-362-7498
e-mail: info@rdequipment.com
www.rdequipment.com

Richard Dagostino, Owner and Founder
Designed for independence, this small, lightweight, battery-operated valve attaches to the bottom of the leg bag. A simple flip of the switch empties the leg bag, allowing the user to take in unlimited amounts of fluids. Tub Slide Shower Chair is a complete bathroom care system, with no need of costly renovations. Eliminates all transfers in the bathroom. *$200.00*

168 Freedom Bath
Arjo Inc
2349 West Lake Street
Suite 250
Addison, IL 60101
630-785-4490
800-323-1245
FAX: 888-389-2756
e-mail: usa.info@ArjoHuntleigh.com
www.arjohuntleigh.com

169 Great Big Safety Tub Mat
Maxi Aids
42 Executive Blvd
Farmingdale, NY 11735-4710
631-752-0521
800-522-6294
FAX: 631-752-0689
TTY: 800-281-3555
e-mail: sales@maxiaids.com
www.maxiaids.com

Elliot Zaretsky, Founder & President
Tub mat provides security against falls in the bath and shower. *$16.95*

170 Long Handled Bath Sponges
Therapro, Inc.
225 Arlington St
Framingham, MA 01702-8723
508-872-9494
800-257-5376
FAX: 508-875-2062
e-mail: info@therapro.com
www.therapro.com

Karen Conrad, Owner
Plastic-handled, 18-inch bath sponge. Handle may be heated and bent for easy reach. *$2.50*

171 Mariner Shower and Commode Chair
Maxi Aids
42 Executive Blvd
Farmingdale, NY 11735-4710
631-752-0521
800-522-6294
FAX: 631-752-0689
TTY: 800-281-3555
e-mail: sales@maxiaids.com
www.maxiaids.com

Elliot Zaretsky, Founder & President
The all aluminum frame and stainless steel hardware provides optimum rust resistance making it ideal for use in the shower. Lightweight; folds easily for transport or storage. Padded 4-position seat with easy access, swing-away front riggings with tool-less adjustable height footrests. *$699.95*

172 Modular Wall Grab Bars
Frohock-Stewart
1 Invacare Way
Elyria, OH 44035-4190
440-329-6000
800-333-6900
FAX: 877-619-7996
www.invacare.com

A Malachi Mixon III, Chairman
Gerald B. Blouch, President & CEO
Joseph B. Richey II, President, Invacare Technologies Division
Robert K. Gudbranson, Senior Vice President and Chief Financial Officer
Engineered for strength and beauty, these bars can be assembled in various combinations to fit any bath or shower.

173 Portable Shampoo Bowl
Ambulatory Cosmetology Technicians
JK Designs
4004 NE 4th Street suite #107-456
Renton, WA 98059
206-999-8226
e-mail: info@portableshampoobowl.com
www.portableshampoobowl.com

174 Prelude
Arjo Inc
2349 West Lake Street
Suite 250
Addison, IL 60101
630-785-4490
800-323-1245
FAX: 888-389-2756
e-mail: usa.info@ArjoHuntleigh.com
www.arjohuntleigh.com

175 **SLIDER Bathing System**
Assistive Technology
21279 Protecta Dr
Elkhart, IN 46516-9539
574-522-7201
800-478-2363
FAX: 574-293-0202
e-mail: info@pvcdme.com
www.pvcdme.com

176 **Suregrip Bathtub Rail**
Frohock-Stewart
1 Invacare Way
Elyria, OH 44035-4190
440-329-6000
800-333-6900
FAX: 877-619-7996
www.invacare.com

A Malachi Mixon III, Chairman
Gerald B. Blouch, President & CEO
Joseph B. Richey II, President, Invacare Technologies Division
Robert K. Gudbranson, Senior Vice President and Chief Financial Officer
Compact and versatile, the bars have a soft-touch, contoured, white vinyl gripping area for added safety.

177 **Talking Bathroom Scale**
Independent Living Aids
137 Rano Rd
Buffalo, NY 14207
516-937-1848
800-537-2118
855-746-7452
FAX: 516-937-3906
e-mail: can-do@independentliving.com
www.independentliving.com

Irwin Schneidmill, President
Michael Gutierrez, Director of Operations
Pamela Strauss, Director of Marketing
Ursula Izurieta, Director of Merchandising
Talking scale. *$59.95*

178 **Terry-Wash Mitt: Medium Size**
Therapro, Inc.
225 Arlington St
Framingham, MA 01702-8723
508-872-9494
800-257-5376
FAX: 508-875-2062
e-mail: info@therapro.com
www.therapro.com

Karen Conrad, Owner
Includes a thumb socket and a palm pocket to hold a bar of soap. *$8.00*

179 **Toilet Guard Rail**
Maxi Aids
42 Executive Blvd
Farmingdale, NY 11735-4710
631-752-0521
800-522-6294
FAX: 631-752-0689
TTY: 800-281-3555
e-mail: sales@maxiaids.com
www.maxiaids.com

Elliot Zaretsky, Founder & President
Made of chrome-plated, heavy gauge steel. Fits securely to the toilet for maximum sturdiness. *$43.95*

180 **Transfer Tub Bench**
Arista Surgical Supply Company/AliMed
297 High St
Dedham, MA 02026-2852
781-329-2900
800-225-2610
FAX: 781-329-8392
e-mail: info@alimed.com
www.alimed.com

Julian Cherubini, President
Curved padded backrest for comfortable support. Backrest also assists patient during lateral transfer. *$64.00*

181 **Tri-Grip Bathtub Rail**
Maxi Aids
42 Executive Blvd
Farmingdale, NY 11735-4710
631-752-0521
800-522-6294
FAX: 631-752-0689
TTY: 800-281-3555
e-mail: sales@maxiaids.com
www.maxiaids.com

Elliot Zaretsky, Founder & President
Two gripping heights for easy bathtub entrance or exit. *$36.95*

182 **Tub Slide Shower Chair**
RD Equipment
230 Percival Dr
West Barnstable, MA 02668-1244
508-362-7498
FAX: 508-362-7498
e-mail: info@rdequipment.com
www.rdequipment.com

Richard Dagostino, Owner and Founder
The tub slide shower chair was designed for the elderly and disabled to make any bathroom (at home or when travelling) accessible with little or no renovations. Go from the bed, to the commode and over to the bathtub for a shower using one product. No transfers in the bathroom whatsoever. *$2000.00*

Bed

183 **ASSISTECH Special Needs**
4801 W Calle Don Miguel
Tucson, AZ 85757-1400
520-883-8600
866-674-3549
FAX: 520-883-5926
TTY: 520-883-5926
www.assistech.com

Oliver Simoes, Owner
Sells hearing, visual and mobility aid devices. *$39.00*

184 **Adjustable Bed**
Golden Technologies
401 Bridge St
Old Forge, PA 18518-2323
570-451-7477
800-624-6374
FAX: 800-628-5165
www.goldentech.com

Richard Golden, CEO
Robert Golden, Co-Founder and Chairman
Fred Kiwak, Co-Founder and VP
Trouble-free gear motor, safety features, dual massage, variable speed timer and more, for the ultimate sleep experience.

185 **Bye-Bye Decubiti Air Mattress Overlay**
Ken McRight Supplies
401 Linden Center Drive
Fort Collins, CO 80524
970-484-7967
800-467-7967
FAX: 970-484-3800
e-mail: info@randscot.com
www.randscot.com

Joel Lerich, Co-Founder
Barbara, Co-Founder
Originally designed for hospital beds, converts any bed into an exceptionally therapeutic, flotation unit when used between the conventional mattress and pad. The complete overlay is comprised of five individually inflatable, 100 percent natural rubber, ventilated sections enclosed within separate pockets of a soft fleece cover. Conforms to any configuration of electric or manual beds. *$731.50*

186 **Cervical Support Pillow**
Wise Enterprises
5017 El Don Dr
Rocklin, CA 95677-4417
916-624-3848
888-947-3368
e-mail: sales@winsent.com
www.wisent.com

Tom Wise, Owner

These hypoallergenic, antimicrobial fiber pillows support the neck in a natural position. Standard, midsize and petite pillows support the neck while sleeping on the back or side. The compact travel pillow offers support while sitting or lying down. The cervical roll has a gentle center and firm ends to ensure maximum comfort and proper support. Position the roll under the neck, back or knees. Standard and midsize fits adults, petite fits children and small adults.

187 **Dual Security Bed Rail**
Maxi Aids
42 Executive Blvd
Farmingdale, NY 11735-4710
631-752-0521
800-522-6294
FAX: 631-752-0689
TTY: 800-281-3555
e-mail: sales@maxiaids.com
www.maxiaids.com

Elliot Zaretsky, Founder & President

Sleep without worry! Dual rails for double the safety. Steel with Powder Coat. Rails adjust up and down.

188 **Foam Decubitus Bed Pads**
Profex Medical Products
P.O.Box 140188
Memphis, TN 38114
800-325-0196
FAX: 901-454-9850
e-mail: customercare@ProfexMed.com
www.profexmed.com

Robert Gates Watel, Founder

Convoluted foam provides extra back support and comfort for wheelchair users.

189 **Global Assistive Devices, Inc.**
1121 East Commercial Blvd. #39
Oakland Park, FL 33334-3920
954-776-1373
888-778-4237
FAX: 954-776-8136
TTY:954-776-1373
e-mail: sales@GlobalAssistive.com
www.GlobalAssistive.com

Manufacturer of assistive devices designed to make life easier. Products include: vibrating watches/countdown timers, extra loud alarm clocks with adjustable tone and bed shaker option, door signalers, telephone ring signaler and caller identification for the television.

190 **Hard Manufacturing Company**
230 Grider St
Buffalo, NY 14215-3797
800-873-4273
www.hardmfg.com

191 **Jackson Cervipillo**
Wise Enterprises
5017 El Don Dr
Rocklin, CA 95677-4417
916-624-3848
888-947-3368
e-mail: sales@winsent.com
www.wisent.com

Tom Wise, Owner

The Jackson Cervipillo comfortably supports the neck vertebrae when sleeping on the side or on the back. Pillow measures 7 in diameter and is 17 long. A machine-washable cover is available separately.

192 **NeckEase**
Wise Enterprises
5017 El Don Dr
Rocklin, CA 95677-4417
916-624-3848
888-947-3368
e-mail: sales@winsent.com
www.wisent.com

Tom Wise, Owner

Microwave NeckEase for penetrating heat that sooths stiff necks and shoulders, easing tension. NeckEase features a unique filling of organic, long grain rice and aromatic herbs and spices. When heated, this filling provides soothing, moist aromatherapy. Heat lasts about 30-45 minutes. Available in two sizes: small fits snugly around the neck, applying gentle pressure at the base of the skull; Large may be worn for a snug fit, or loosely for application on the shoulder and upper back.

193 **Permaflex Home Care Mattress**
BG Industries
8550 Balboa Blvd
Ste 214
Northridge, CA 91325-3564
818-894-0744
FAX: 818-894-7972
e-mail: maxifloat@bgind.com
www.bgind.com

Larry Lankard, Director
Arnie Balonick, CEO/Director

Mattress with flame retardant upholstery material, water-repellant, anti-microbial and tear-resistant cover, for extra comfort.

194 **SleepSafe Beds**
3629 Reed Creek Drive
Bassett, VA 24055
276-627-0088
866-852-2337
FAX: 276-627-0234
e-mail: SleepSafeBed@SleepSafeBed.com
www.sleepsafebed.com

Gregg Weinschreider, President
Edward Hettig, Marketing
Casey Collins, Office Manager
Al Flora, Sales

Perfect for adult home or home care use. Offering twin or full size bed frames in classic style, these beds offer an attractive alternative to a hospital bed. Keeps the user safe during rest and electrically adjusts smoothly for user comfort and caregiver ease of use.

195 **Sonic Alert Bed Shaker**
ASSISTECH
4801 W Calle Don Miguel
Tucson, AZ 85757-1400
520-883-8600
866-674-3549
FAX: 520-883-5926
TTY: 520-883-5926
www.assistech.com

Oliver Simoes, Owner

Sells hearing, visual and mobility aid devices. *$49.00*

196 **Vibes Bed Shaker**
ASSISTECH
4801 W Calle Don Miguel
Tucson, AZ 85757-1400
520-883-8600
866-674-3549
FAX: 520-883-5926
TTY: 520-883-5926
www.assistech.com

Oliver Simoes, Owner

Sells hearing, visual and mobility aid devices.

197 **Waterproof Sheet-Topper Mattress and Chair Pad**
Pillow Talk
260 Madison Avenue
New York, NY 10016
732-780-9483
FAX: 732-780-0279
e-mail: info@PTIproductmarketing.com
www.pillowtalkusa.com

Dorothy Fajerman, President
Jack Fajerman, Marketing Director

This soft pad lies on the top sheet, absorbing accidents from incontinence, pregnancy or medical problems. Waterproof barrier locks out moisture, soiling and stains and eliminates midnight linen changes and the resulting laundry. Available in bed sizes W/4 Anchor, twin, full, queen, king, and crib.

Communication

198 **ADA Hotel Built-In Alerting System**
HARC Mercantile
5413 S. Westnedge Ave.
Suite A
Portage, MI 49002
269-324-1615
800-445-9968
FAX: 269-324-2387
TTY: 269-324-1615
e-mail: info@harc.com
www.harc.com

199 **Access Control Systems: NHX Nurse Call System**
Aiphone Corporation
1700 130th Ave NE
Bellevue, WA 98005-2203
425-455-0510
800-692-0200
FAX: 425-455-0071
e-mail: tech@aiphone.com.
www.aiphone.com

Futoshi Tanaka, President/CEO
AIPHONE manufactures audio and video intercom systems for home or business to help the physically disabled answer doors and communicate through physical barriers; also ADA-compliant emergency call intercom stations for use in public facilities and an Environmental Control System for persons with limited mobility.

200 **Adaptek Systems**
14224 Plank Street
Fort Wayne, IN 46818
260-637-8660
FAX: 260-637-8597
e-mail: info@adapteksystems.com
www.adapteksystems.com

201 **Akron Resources**
20 La Porte St
Arcadia, CA 91006-2827
626-254-9005
800-841-0884
FAX: 626-254-9266
www.arkon.com

Paul Brassard, Owner
Aaron Roth, VP, Marketing & Sales
Benjamin Arana, Sr. Account Manager
Cleber Gandra, Account Manager
Manufacturers of infrared amplification systems for televisions or stereos. $29-$69.00. The company name is Arkon Resources.

202 **Amplified Handsets**
HARC Mercantile
5413 S. Westnedge Ave.
Suite A
Portage, MI 49002
269-324-1615
800-445-9968
FAX: 269-324-2387
TTY: 269-324-1615
e-mail: info@harc.com
www.harc.com

203 **Amplified Phones**
HARC Mercantile
5413 S. Westnedge Ave.
Suite A
Portage, MI 49002
269-324-1615
800-445-9968
FAX: 269-324-2387
TTY: 269-324-1615
e-mail: info@harc.com
www.harc.com

204 **Amplified Portable Phone**
HARC Mercantile
5413 S. Westnedge Ave.
Suite A
Portage, MI 49002
269-324-1615
800-445-9968
FAX: 269-324-2387
TTY: 269-324-1615
e-mail: info@harc.com
www.harc.com

205 **Artificial Larynx**
HARC Mercantile
5413 S. Westnedge Ave.
Suite A
Portage, MI 49002
269-324-1615
800-445-9968
FAX: 269-324-2387
TTY: 269-324-1615
e-mail: info@harc.com
www.harc.com

206 **Assistive Technology**
333 Elm St
Dedham, MA 02026-4530
781-461-8200
800-793-9227
FAX: 781-461-8213
e-mail: sales@tobiiATI.com
www.tobii.com/

Henrik Eskilsson, CEO
John Elvesjo, CTO and deputy CEO
Mårten Skogo, Chief Science Officer
Torbjorn Moller, Chief Operating Officer
A premiere developer of innovative technology solutions for people with physical and learning disabilities. Breakthrough products enable people of all ages and abilities to live and learn independently. Supportive material for teachers, clinicians and those with disabilities.

207 **Big Red Switch**
AbleNet
2625 Patton Road
Roseville, MN 55113-1308
651-294-2200
800-322-0956
FAX: 651-294-2222
e-mail: customerservice@ablenetinc.com
www.ablenetinc.com

Bill Sproull, Chairman
Jennifer Thalhuber, CEO/President
William Mills, Board of Director
Five inches across the top and activates no matter where on its surface it is touched. It is made of shatterproof plastic and contains a cord storage compartment. Also available in green, yellow and blue. *$42.00*

208 **Cornell Communications**
7915 N 81st St
Milwaukee, WI 53223-3830
414-351-4660
800-558-8957
FAX: 414-351-4657
e-mail: sales@cornell.com
www.cornell.com

George, Management Staff
Gary, Management Staff
Jim, Management Staff
Cornell's Rescue Assistance Systems allow personnel to request emergency assistance. Applications include handicapped evacuations, parking garages and elevators. Voice, intercom and visual only signaling systems are available.

209 **Davis Center**
19 State Rte 10 E
Ste 25
Succasunna, NJ 07876
862-251-4637
FAX: 862-251-4642
e-mail: npdunn@thedaviscenter.com
www.thedaviscenter.com

Dorinne S. Davis, MA, CCC-A, FAAA, President
Elizabeth Meade, Head Sound Therapist
Nancy Puckett-Dunn, Office Manger
Offers sound-based therapies supporting positive change in learning, development and wellness. All ages/all disabilities. The Davis Model of Sound Intervention-an alternative approach. The company name is The Davis Center.

210 **Flashing Lamp Telephone Ring Alerter**
Independent Living Aids
137 Rano Rd
Buffalo, NY 14207
516-937-1848
800-537-2118
855-746-7452
FAX: 516-937-3906
e-mail: can-do@independentliving.com
www.independentliving.com

Irwin Schneidmill, President
Michael Gutierrez, Director of Operations
Pamela Strauss, Director of Marketing
Ursula Izurieta, Director of Merchandising
Once your phone is plugged into the Telephone Ring Alerter, the lamp light will flash with each ring, alerting you that there is a phone call. *$62.00*

211 **Harc Mercantile Ltd**
HARC Mercantile
5413 S. Westnedge Ave.
Suite A
Portage, MI 49002
269-324-1615
800-445-9968
FAX: 269-324-2387
TTY: 269-324-1615
e-mail: info@harc.com
www.harc.com

212 **Ideal-Phone**
IDEAMATICS
1364 Beverly Road
Suite 101
McLean, VA 22101-3617
703-903-4972
800-247-IDEA
FAX: 703-903-8949
e-mail: ideamatics@ideamatics.net
www.ideamatics.com

David L Danner, President
Michael A. Schwartz, Vice President
Mark A. Moore, Vice President of Operations
John R. Kaplar, Director of Applications Development
Integrates the personal computer and the telephone into a single, efficient workstation. It is ideal for mobility-impaired persons and others who need a hands-free operation of the phone. The Ideal-Phone includes one PC Board, a Plantronics headset, software for access and logging and complete documentation. It can be integrated into programs or pops-up over any application. MS-DOS based, version 3.0 or higher are available. *$195.00*

213 **IntelliKeys**
IntelliTools
24 Prime Parkway
Natick, MA 01760
303-651-2829
800-547-6747
FAX: 720-382-7438
e-mail: customerservice@cambiumlearning.com
www.intellitools.com

Arjan Khalsa, CEO
Card and cable to create keyboard port on Apple IIe computer to allow use of IntelliKeys alternative keyboard.

214 **LPB Communications**
960 Brook Rd
Norristown, PA 19401
856-365-8080
FAX: 856-365-8999
e-mail: info@LPBInc.com
www.lpbinc.com

John Devecka, VP Sales
Limited area AM and FM broadcast systems for hearing assistance and language translation manufacturing since 1960. Systems for small conference halls, churches and Olympic stadiums. Components or complete system. *$400.00*

215 **Language, Learning & Living**
Prentke Romich Company
1022 Heyl Rd
Wooster, OH 44691-9786
330-262-1984
800-262-1984
FAX: 330-263-4829
e-mail: info@prentrom.com
www.prentrom.com

David L Moffatt, President
Barry Romich, Co-Founder
Dave Moffatt, President & COO
A Minspeak application program designed for adolescent and adult individuals with developmental disabilities and associated learning difficulties. The software is used with Prentke Romich Company augmentative communication devices. *$355.00*

216 **Large Button Speaker Phone**
HARC Mercantile
5413 S. Westnedge Ave.
Suite A
Portage, MI 49002
269-324-1615
800-445-9968
FAX: 269-324-2387
TTY: 269-324-1615
e-mail: info@harc.com
www.harc.com

217 **Large Print Telephone Dial**
Maxi Aids
42 Executive Blvd
Farmingdale, NY 11735-4710
631-752-0521
800-522-6294
FAX: 631-752-0689
TTY: 800-281-3555
e-mail: sales@maxiaids.com
www.maxiaids.com

Elliot Zaretsky, Founder & President
Pressure sensitive dial with numbers that are easy to see for the disabled. *$69.00*

218 **Large Print Touch-Telephone Overlays**
Maxi Aids
42 Executive Blvd
Farmingdale, NY 11735-4710
631-752-0521
800-522-6294
FAX: 631-752-0689
TTY: 800-281-3555
e-mail: sales@maxiaids.com
www.maxiaids.com

Elliot Zaretsky, Founder & President
Pressure-sensitive and easy to apply overlays that make everyday phones accessible. *$49.00*

219 **Liberator**
Prentke Romich Company
1022 Heyl Rd
Wooster, OH 44691-9786
330-262-1984
800-262-1984
FAX: 330-263-4829
e-mail: info@prentrom.com
www.prentrom.com

David L Moffatt, President
Barry Romich, Co-Founder
Dave Moffatt, President & COO
A portable electronic communication device that uses Minspeak so that symbols are used to represent words, sentences or phrases.

Liberator can be accessed by pressing keys, optical headpointing and a wide variety of switch activated scans. It can be configured with 8, 32 or 128 locations. It offers a variety of unique features to permit the most effective communication possible. $7,345-$8,575.

220 Metropolitan Washington Ear
12061 Tech Road
Silver Spring, MD 20904-7826
301-681-6636
FAX: 301-625-1986
e-mail: information@washear.org
www.washear.org

Brother Hilary Mettes, Chairman
Freddie L Peaco, President Pro Tem
Dr. George Long, Vice President
Neely Oplinger, Executive Director

Multi-media reading service for blind and visually impaired. Offering 24 hour audio radio reading, dial-in newspapers and web casting, as well as audio description at theaters, museums and films.

221 Mini Teleloop
HARC Mercantile
5413 S. Westnedge Ave.
Suite A
Portage, MI 49002
269-324-1615
800-445-9968
FAX: 269-324-2387
TTY: 269-324-1615
e-mail: info@harc.com
www.harc.com

222 Multiple Phone/Device Switch
HARC Mercantile
5413 S. Westnedge Ave.
Suite A
Portage, MI 49002
269-324-1615
800-445-9968
FAX: 269-324-2387
TTY: 269-324-1615
e-mail: info@harc.com
www.harc.com

223 Personal FM Systems
HARC Mercantile
5413 S. Westnedge Ave.
Suite A
Portage, MI 49002
269-324-1615
800-445-9968
FAX: 269-324-2387
TTY: 269-324-1615
e-mail: info@harc.com
www.harc.com

224 Personal Infrared Listening System
HARC Mercantile
5413 S. Westnedge Ave.
Suite A
Portage, MI 49002
269-324-0301
800-445-9968
FAX: 269-324-2387
TTY: 269-324-1615
e-mail: info@harc.com
www.harc.com

225 Prentke Romich Company
1022 Heyl Rd
Wooster, OH 44691-9786
330-262-1984
800-262-1984
FAX: 330-263-4829
e-mail: info@prentrom.com
www.prentrom.com

David L Moffatt, President
Barry Romich, Co-Founder
Dave Moffatt, President / COO

The Prentke Romich Company is a full service company offering easy, yet powerful communication aids. The company believes in supporting customers before and after the sale by offering funding assistance, distance learning training, extended warranty, service assistance and much more. Visit our website to view our full line catalog, read about our success stories and to sign up for our online newsletter.

226 Push to Talk Amplified Handset
HARC Mercantile
5413 S. Westnedge Ave.
Suite A
Portage, MI 49002
269-324-0301
800-445-9968
FAX: 269-324-2387
TTY: 269-324-1615
e-mail: info@harc.com
www.harc.com

227 Room Valet Visual-Tactile Alerting System
HARC Mercantile
5413 S. Westnedge Ave.
Suite A
Portage, MI 49002
269-324-0301
800-445-9968
FAX: 269-324-2387
TTY: 269-324-1615
e-mail: info@harc.com
www.harc.com

228 Silent Call Communications
5095 Williams Lake Rd
Waterford, MI 48329-3553
248-673-7353
800-572-5227
FAX: 248-673-7360
TTY: 800-572-5227
e-mail: customerservice@silentcall.com
www.silentcall.com

George Elwell, President
Diana Elwell, President
Lisa DeLeuil, Director of Sales & Marketing

Alerting devices such as paging systems and smoke detectors for deaf and deaf-blind people.

229 Sonic Alert
Harris Communications
15155 Technology Dr
Eden Prairie, MN 55344-2273
952-906-1180
800-825-6758
FAX: 952-906-1099
TTY: 800-825-9187
e-mail: info@harriscomm.com
www.harriscomm.com

Dr.Robert Harris, Owner
Lori Foss, Marketing Director

Offers visual alerting devices that provide safety and convenience by turning vital sound into flashing light: telephone ring signalers, doorbell signalers, baby cry signalers and wake up alarms. Free catalog available.

230 Sound Induction Receiver
HARC Mercantile
5413 S. Westnedge Ave.
Suite A
Portage, MI 49002
269-324-0301
800-445-9968
FAX: 269-324-2387
TTY: 269-324-1615
e-mail: info@harc.com
www.harc.com

231 **SpeakEasy Communication Aid**
AbleNet
2625 Patton Road
Roseville, MN 55113-1308
651-294-2200
800-322-0956
FAX: 651-294-2259
e-mail: customerservice@ablenetinc.com
www.ablenetinc.com

Bill Sproull, Chairman of the Board
Jennifer Thalhuber, President/CEO
William Mills, Board of Director

SpeakEasy is a digitalized voice output communication Aid that is ideal for anyone who is beginning to develop communication skills such as making choices and identifying symbols. It holds 12 messages totaling four minutes and 20 seconds of recording time. It measures 7 1/2 inch by 1 3/4 inch and weighs only one pound. Activate messages using the built-in keyboard or via external switch. *$399.00*

232 **Speech Discrimination Unit**
HARC Mercantile
5413 S. Westnedge Ave.
Suite A
Portage, MI 49002
269-324-0301
800-445-9968
FAX: 269-324-2387
TTY: 269-324-1615
e-mail: info@harc.com
www.harc.com

233 **Speechmaker-Personal Speech Amplifier**
HARC Mercantile
5413 S. Westnedge Ave.
Suite A
Portage, MI 49002
269-324-0301
800-445-9968
FAX: 269-324-2387
TTY: 269-324-1615
e-mail: info@harc.com
www.harc.com

234 **Standard Touch Turner Sip & Puff Switch**
Access to Recreation
8 Sandra Ct
Newbury Park, CA 91320-4302
805-498-7535
800-634-4351
FAX: 805-498-8186
e-mail: customerservice@accesstr.com
www.accesstr.com

Don Krebs, President /Founder

A page turning device.

235 **Step-by-Step Communicator**
AbleNet
2625 Patton Road
Roseville, MN 55113-1308
651-294-2200
800-322-0956
FAX: 651-294-2259
e-mail: customerservice@ablenetinc.com
www.ablenetinc.com

Bill Sproull, Chairman of the Board
Jennifer Thalhuber, President/CEO
William Mills, Board of Director

Allows you to record a series of messages (as many as you want up to the 75 second limit). It has a 2 1/2 inches diameter switch surface and is 3 inches at its tallest point. Angled switch surface makes it easy to see and access. *$129.00*

236 **Strobe Light Signalers**
5413 S. Westnedge Ave.
Suite A
Portage, MI 49002
269-324-0301
800-445-9968
FAX: 269-324-2387
TTY: 269-324-1615
e-mail: info@harc.com
www.harc.com

237 **TTY's: Telephone Device for the Deaf**
HARC Mercantile
5413 S. Westnedge Ave.
Suite A
Portage, MI 49002
269-324-0301
800-445-9968
FAX: 269-324-2387
TTY: 269-324-1615
e-mail: info@harc.com
www.harc.com

238 **TalkTrac Wearable Communicator**
Ablenet
2625 Patton Road
Roseville, MN 55113-1308
651-294-2200
800-322-0956
FAX: 651-294-2259
e-mail: customerservice@ablenetinc.com
www.ablenetinc.com

Bill Sproull, Chairman of the Board
Jennifer Thalhuber, President/CEO
William Mills, Board of Director

The TalkTrac Wearable Communicator is a personal, portable communication aid that is wearable on the wrist. TalkTrac features: simple to use, 75 seconds of recording time, four 3/4 x 1/2 message locations, rechargeable, water resistant, adjustable 9 inch band, Boardmaker compatible.

239 **Talking Calculators**
ASSISTECH
4801 W Calle Don Miguel
Tucson, AZ 85757-1400
520-883-8600
866-674-3549
FAX: 520-883-5926
TTY: 520-883-5926
www.assistech.com

Oliver Simoes, Owner
Marsha Neilson, Sales Representative

Carries a complete line of assistive products for the deaf and hard of hearing, blind and visually impaired, speech impaired, and physically challenged . They also feature products for everyone such as medicine reminder watches and electronic language translators.

240 **Talking Clocks**
HARC Mercantile
5413 S. Westnedge Ave.
Suite A
Portage, MI 49002
269-324-0301
800-445-9968
FAX: 269-324-2387
TTY: 269-324-1615
e-mail: info@harc.com
www.harc.com

241 **Talking Watches**
HARC Mercantile
5413 S. Westnedge Ave.
Suite A
Portage, MI 49002
269-324-0301
800-445-9968
FAX: 269-324-2387
TTY: 269-324-1615
e-mail: info@harc.com
www.harc.com

242 **Telecaption Adapter**
HARC Mercantile
5413 S. Westnedge Ave.
Suite A
Portage, MI 49002
269-324-0301
800-445-9968
FAX: 269-324-2387
TTY: 269-324-1615
e-mail: info@harc.com
www.harc.com

243 **Touch Turner-Page Turning Devices**
Touch Turner Company
13621 103rd Ave NE
Arlington, WA 98223-8827
360-651-1962
888-811-1962
FAX: 360-658-9380
e-mail: touchturner@worldnet.att.net
www.touchturner.com

244 **Unity**
Prentke Romich Company
1022 Heyl Rd
Wooster, OH 44691-9786
330-262-1984
800-262-1984
FAX: 330-263-4829
e-mail: info@prentrom.com
www.prentrom.com

David L Moffatt, President
Barry Romich, Co-Founder
Dave Moffatt, President / COO
A Minspeak application program available for the Liberator and Delta Talker communication devices. Provides single word vocabulary to people of all ages at varying stages of language development, who may be either cognitively intact or challenged. *$355.00*

245 **Vantage**
Prentke Romich Company
1022 Heyl Rd
Wooster, OH 44691-9786
330-262-1984
800-262-1984
FAX: 330-263-4829
e-mail: info@prentrom.com
www.prentrom.com

David L Moffatt, President
Barry Romich, Co-Founder
Dave Moffatt, President / COO
Vantage is a portable communication aid that features the Unity Enhanced vocabulary software and a large high quality dynamic display. Vantage also employs the recently upgraded 4.0 operating system that makes system settings quick and easy. Vantage has synthesized speech powered by DECtalk Software, Spelling and Word Protection software, built-in visor (flip-up protective cover), digitized speech capability and built-in computer access and ECU controls. 15 and 45 location keyguards available. *$6295.00*

246 **Vibrotactile Personal Alerting System**
HARC Mercantile
5413 S. Westnedge Ave.
Suite A
Portage, MI 49002
269-324-0301
800-445-9968
FAX: 269-324-2387
TTY: 269-324-1615
e-mail: info@harc.com
www.harc.com

247 **Voice Amplified Handsets**
HARC Mercantile
5413 S. Westnedge Ave.
Suite A
Portage, MI 49002
269-324-0301
800-445-9968
FAX: 269-324-2387
TTY: 269-324-1615
e-mail: info@harc.com
www.harc.com

248 **WalkerTalker**
Prentke Romich Company
1022 Heyl Rd
Wooster, OH 44691-9786
330-262-1984
800-262-1984
FAX: 330-263-4829
e-mail: info@prentrom.com
www.prentrom.com

David L Moffatt, President
Barry Romich, Co-Founder
Dave Moffatt, President / COO
A portable direct selection communication device for active persons. The 16 location keyboard and speakers are carried in a belt that straps comfortably around the waist. The keyboard can be removed from its pouch to use by activating keys. Two versions are available, standard memory and expanded memory. *$1195.00*

Chairs

249 **Adjustable Chair**
Bailey Manufacturing Company
P.O.Box 130
Lodi, OH 44254-130
330-948-2655
800-321-8372
FAX: 800-224-5390
e-mail: baileymfg@baileymfg.com
www.baileymfg.com

Larry Strimple, President
Sandy Mooney, Customer Service
Judie Butler, Dealer Contact
The seat and footboard of this versatile chair can be adjusted to accommodate children of various sizes. A classroom-suitable variation of this model is also available.

250 **Adjustable Clear Acrylic Tray**
Bailey Manufacturing Company
P.O.Box 130
Lodi, OH 44254-130
330-948-2655
800-321-8372
FAX: 800-224-5390
e-mail: baileymfg@baileymfg.com
www.baileymfg.com

Larry Strimple, President
Sandy Mooney, Customer Service
Judie Butler, Dealer Contact
Adjusts for height and depth and is equipped with a spill rim for easy to clean edges.

251 **Adjustable Rigid Chair**
Kuschall North America
1811 Lefthand Cir
Ste B
Longmont, CO 80501-6785
303-682-2571
888-682-2571
FAX: 866-651-6973
www.kuschallna.com

Terry Mulkey, Owner
The Champion 3000 is a fully adjustable rigid frame chair weighing only 21 pounds with a new clamping system that adjusts seat height and angle without tools.

252 **Adjustable Tee Stool**
Bailey Manufacturing Company
P.O.Box 130
Lodi, OH 44254-130
330-948-2655
800-321-8372
FAX: 800-224-5390
e-mail: baileymfg@baileymfg.com
www.baileymfg.com

Larry Strimple, President
Sandy Mooney, Customer Service
Judie Butler, Dealer Contact
May be used to encourage balance as well as develop integrative and perceptual motor skills.

253 **BackSaver**
BackSaver Products Company
53 Jeffrey Ave
Holliston, MA 01746-2084
508-893-6990
800-251-2225
FAX: 508-429-8698
e-mail: stevek@backsaver.com
www.backsavercorp.com

Ed Foye, Owner
Eliminates slouching and extra pressure on your back and thighs which impairs circulation.

254 **Better Back**
Orthopedic Products Corporation
4100 1/2 Glencoe Ave
Marina Del Rey, CA 90292
323-584-6977
FAX: 310-306-0177

255 **Carendo**
Arjo Inc
2349 West Lake Street
Addison, IL 60101
630-785-4490
800-323-1245
FAX: 888-389-2756
e-mail: usa.info@ArjoHuntleigh.com
www.arjo.com

Philip M. Croxford, President/ CEO
The Carendo hygiene chair has been designed for caregivers.

256 **Century 50/60XR Sit**
Arjo Inc
2349 West Lake Street
Addison, IL 60101
630-785-4490
800-323-1245
FAX: 888-389-2756
e-mail: usa.info@ArjoHuntleigh.com
www.arjo.com

Philip M. Croxford, President/ CEO
This bathing system has a built-in cleaning/disinfectant injection system with adjustable flowmeter. The incorporation of an automatic hot water alarm/shut-off system, and digital temperature monitors, helps to assure resident safety and comfort.

257 **Convert-Able Table**
REAL Design
187 S Main St
Dolgeville, NY 13329-1455
315-429-3071
800-696-7041
FAX: 315-429-3071
e-mail: rdesign@twcny.rr.com
www.realdesigninc.com

Sam Camardello, Owner
This table has push button height adjustment and interchangeable tops so it can become a desk, art easel or a sensory stimulation bowl.

258 **Evac + Chair Emergency Evacuation Chair**
Evac + Chair North America LLC
3000 Marcus Ave
Ste 3E6
Lake Success, NY 11042-1012
516-502-4240
FAX: 516-327-8220
e-mail: sales@evac-chair.com
www.evac-chair.com

Richard Perl, VP Business Dev.
David Egen, Founder
Gravity driven evaluation chair allows one nondisabled person to smoothly glide a seated passenger down fire stairs and across landings to exit on a combination of wheels and track belts. Pivots in own width for tight landing turns. Aluminum; weight 19 pounds. Compactly stores on wall mount, 38 by 20 by 9 inches. Maximum capacity 330 pounds. Self braking features. No installation, works on all fire exit stairs. *$950.00*

259 **Golden Technologies**
401 Bridge St
Old Forge, PA 18518-2323
570-451-7477
800-624-6374
FAX: 800-628-5165
e-mail: johngcei@excite.com
www.goldentech.com

Richard Golden, CEO
Robert Golden, Chairman of the Board
Fred Kiwak, VP of R & D
The largest facility in the world dedicated solely to the manufacture of lift chairs.

260 **High-Low Chair**
Rehab and Educational Aids for Living
NY
800-696-7041
e-mail: rdesign@twcny.rr.com
www.realdesigninc.com/

Sam Camardello, President
Kris Wohnsen, Vice President
A high chair and mobile floor sitter in one. The high-low chair comes with colorful upholstered wipe clean seat and height adjustable tray. The chair has a single lever adjustment to change the seat height. Lateral and head supports are available as options. *$ 1199.00*

261 **Ladybug Corner Chair**
Rehab and Educational Aids for Living
NY
800-696-7041
e-mail: rdesign@twcny.rr.com
www.realdesigninc.com/

Sam Camardello, President
Kris Wohnsen, Vice President
For children 0-3 years. This chair is adjustable for long legs for conventional sitting.

262 **Lumex Recliner**
Graham-Field Health Products
2935 Northeast Pkwy
Atlanta, GA 30360-2808
678-291-3207
800-347-5678
FAX: 770-368-4702
e-mail: cs@grahamfield.com
www.grahamfield.com

Kenneth Spett, President & Chief Executive Officer
Cherie Antoniazzi, SVP Quality, Regulatory and Risk Management
Ivan Bielik, Senior Vice President, Business Analyst
Marc Bernstein, Senior Vice President, Consumer Sales
Combines therapeutic benefits of position change with attractive appearance.

263 **Modular QuadDesk**
Gpk
535 Floyd Smith Dr
El Cajon, CA 92020-1228
619-593-7381
800-468-8679
FAX: 888-755-5603
e-mail: sales@gpk.com
www.gpk.com

264 **Mulholland Positioning Systems**
P.O.Box 70
839 Albion Avenue
Burley, ID 83318
208-878-3840
800-543-4769
FAX: 208-878-3841
e-mail: info@mulhollandinc.com
www.mulhollandinc.com

Larry Mulholland, Owner
Dick Stepan, Sales Manager
Provides a full line of standing aids, seating systems, adaptive components and bath aids.

265 **Prime Engineering**
Prime Engineering
4202 W Sierra Madre Ave
Fresno, CA 93722-3932
559-276-0991
800-827-8263
FAX: 800-800-3355
e-mail: info@primeengineering.com
www.primeengineering.com

Bruce Boegel, CFO
Mary Wilson Boegel, President
Mark Allen, Vice President
Dawn Smith Cobb, Customer Service

Prime Engineering is a leading manufacturer of adult and pediatric standing devices and patient transfer equipment. Products include the all-new Support Standing System, Granstand III MSS Standing System Kidstand III MSS Standing System Superstand Multi-Position Pediatric Stander, the Lift, the CindyLift and the Original Lift Walker.

266 **Roll Chair**
Bailey Manufacturing Company
P.O. Box 130
Lodi, OH 44254-130
330-948-2655
800-321-8372
FAX: 800-224-5390
e-mail: baileymfg@baileymfg.com
www.baileymfg.com

Larry Strimple, President
Sandy Mooney, Customer Service
Judie Butler, Dealer Contact

The padded roll helps maintain proper hip abduction and prevents scissoring of the legs.

267 **Safari Tilt**
Convaid Products
2830 California Street
Torrance, CA 90503
310-618-0111
888-266-8243
FAX: 310-618-2166
www.convaid.com

Chris Braun, President

A semi-contour seat provides positioning with 5-45 degree tilt adjustment. One step design folds compactly into a lightweight chair.

268 **Spatial Tilt Custom Chair**
Redman Powerchair
Suite 107
1601 S Pantano Road
Tucson, AZ 85710-6791
520-546-6002
800-727-6684
FAX: 520-546-5530
e-mail: info@redmanpowerchair.com
www.redmanpowerchair.com

Don Redman, CEO
Paula Redman, CFO
Scott Evans, Regulatory affairs
Samuel Redman, General manager

Custom chair designed for comfort with a solid seat and back with modifications available for seat depth, height or width.

269 **Transfer Bench with Back**
Frohock-Stewart
1 Invacare Way
Elyria, OH 44035-4190
440-329-6000
800-333-6900
FAX: 877-619-7996
www.invacare.com

A. Malachi Mixon III, Chairman of the Board
Gerald B. Blouch, President and Chief Executive Officer
Joseph B. Richey, II, President - Invacare Technologies Division
Robert K. Gudbranson, Senior Vice President and Chief Financial Officer

This bench with air-cushioned seat sections has a full, reversible backrest for safety and comfort.

Cushions & Wedges

270 **Action Products**
954 Sweeney Drive
Hagerstown, MD 21740-4910
301-797-1414
800-228-7763
FAX: 301-733-2073
e-mail: service@actionproducts.com
www.actionproducts.com

Mistie Witt, President
Janet Kaplan, Marketing Director

Wheelchair pads, mattress pads, positioning cushions and insoles that aid in the prevention and cure of pressure sores by reducing pressure. All products are made of Akton viscoelastic polymer that does not leak, flow or bottom out. Manufacturer of the Xact line of positioning cushions for patients with high risk of skin breakdown.

271 **Adjustable Wedge**
Bailey Manufacturing Company
P.O. Box 130
Lodi, OH 44254-130
800-321-8372
FAX: 800-224-5390
e-mail: baileymfg@baileymfg.com
www.baileymfg.com

272 **Back-Huggar Pillow**
Bodyline Comfort Systems
3730 Kori Rd
Jacksonville, FL 32257-6036
904-262-4068
800-874-7715
FAX: 904-262-2225
e-mail: info@bodyline.com
www.bodyline.com

Dr.John W. Fiore, Owner

Exclusive design makes almost any seat more comfortable by exerting soothing pressure against back muscles and discs.

273 **Bye-Bye Decubiti (BBD)**
Ken McRight Supplies
7456 S Oswego Ave
Tulsa, OK 74136-5903
918-492-9657
FAX: 918-492-9694

Ken McRight, President

The BBD therapeutic wheelchair cushions have been market-proven since 1951 — in the prevention and cure of pressure sores (decubiti). These natural rubber inflatable products have recently been expanded to include pediatric, sports and double-valve models. Moderately priced, they offer a viable and cost-effective alternative in the market. $84.00-$112.00.

274 **Dynamic Systems**
104 Morrow Branch Rd
Leicester, NC 28748-9635
828-683-3523
855-786-6283
FAX: 844-270-6478
e-mail: dsi@sunmatecushions.com
www.sunmatecushions.com

Charles A Yost, CEO
Lewis McCrain, General Manager

SunMate orthopedic foam sheets and cushions, pudgee pads for pressure relief and skin breakdown prevention, laminar wheelchair cushions and Foam-in-Place Seating for custom molding seat inserts. Sample packs and literature available upon request.

275 **Econo-Float Water Flotation Cushion**
Jefferson Industries
1985 Rutgers Blvd
Lakewood, NJ 08701-4569
732-905-9001
800-257-5145
FAX: 732-905-9899

Charles Landa, General Manager

An inexpensive, yet effective approach to the problem of pressure ulcers for patients confined to wheelchairs, geriatric chairs, etc. *$15.00*

276 **Econo-Float Water Flotation Mattress**
Jefferson Industries
1985 Rutgers Blvd
Lakewood, NJ 08701-4569
732-905-9001
800-257-5145
FAX: 732-905-9899
Charles Landa, General Manager
Helps prevent and treat pressure ulcers by reducing and distributing pressure over the patient's bony prominences while supporting the body evenly over a greater surface area. *$39.00*

277 **Enhancer Cushion**
ROHO Group
100 North Florida Avenue
Belleville, IL 62221-5429
618-277-9173
800-851-3449
FAX: 618-277-9561
e-mail: tomb@therohogroup.com
www.therohogroup.com
Tom Borcherding, President
Bobby Graebe, CEO
Tim Richter, Vice President of Finance
Dave McCausland, Sr. VP of Planning & Gov Affairs
Uses AIR IN PLACE progressive positioning for enhanced midline channeling of the femurs, lateral stability and tissue protection.

278 **Functional Forms**
Consumer Care Products
1446 Pilgrim Rd
Plymouth, WI 53073-4969
920-893-4614
FAX: 800-977-2256
e-mail: ccpi@consumercareinc.com
www.consumercareinc.com
Terry Grall, Owner
These blocks, wedges, rolls, cervical pillows, head and leg supports and barrel rolls in resilient high density foam covered with durable antibacterial, antistatic, flame resistant, nonabsorbent vinyl are used to attain individualized support for the most difficult positioning needs for children and adults. Unique sizes allow fitting for almost any person. Use during exercise, feeding, therapy, recreation and rest at home, school and health care facilities. Packages available.

279 **Gaymar Industries**
Gaymar Industries
10 Centre Dr
Orchard Park, NY 14127-2295
716-662-2551
800-828-7341
FAX: 716-662-0748
e-mail: webmaster@gaymar.com
www.gaymar.com
Dan Kormowicz, International Sales & Mktg
Cindy Sylvia, Educational Svcs Administrator
Heather Lindstrom, Medical Res
Brian McLaughlin, International Order Coordinator
Gaymar offers a complete line of support surfaces, including low-air-loss mattresses, specialty foam mattresses, turning mattresses, air overlays and fluid therapy beds. These products economically prevent and treat bedsores. Clinical and reimbursement professionals are available to answer any question related to bedsores (decubitus ulcers). Also offers a complete line of temperature control devices. The T-Pump delivers warm therapy to effectively dilate vessels and increase blood flow.

280 **Geo-Matt for High Risk Patients**
Span-America Medical Systems
70 Commerce Ctr
Greenville, SC 29615-5814
864-288-8877
800-888-6752
FAX: 864-288-8692
www.spanamerica.com
James D Ferguson, CEO
Helps prevent pressure sores in high risk patients.

281 **High Profile Single Compartment Cushion**
ROHO Group
100 North Florida Avenue
Belleville, IL 62221-5429
618-277-9173
800-851-3449
FAX: 618-277-9561
e-mail: tomb@therohogroup.com
www.therohogroup.com
Tom Borcherding, President
Bobby Graebe, CEO
Tim Richter, Vice President of Finance
Dave McCausland, Sr. VP of Planning & Gov Affairs
With 4 inch cells, the HIGH PROFILE is the cushion of choice for individuals who suffer from ischemic ulcers (pressure sores) or who have a history of tissue breakdown.

282 **Inflatable Back Pillow**
Corflex
669 East Industrial Park Dr
Manchester, NH 03109-5625
603-623-3344
800-426-7353
FAX: 603-623-4111
e-mail: sales@corflex.com
www.corflex.com
Paul Lorenzetti, CEO
Folds flat to fit into its own carrying case, this inflatable back pillow ensures comfort while at home or traveling.

283 **Jobri**
520 N Division St
Konawa, OK 74849-2223
580-925-3500
800-432-2225
FAX: 580-925-3501
e-mail: support@jobri.com
www.jobri.com
Brian Gourley, CEO
Jobri manufactures ergonomic back supports, ergonomic chairs, orthopedic soft goods and sleep products.

284 **Lumex Cushions and Mattresses**
Graham-Field Health Products
2935 Northeast Pkwy
Atlanta, GA 30360-2808
678-291-3207
800-347-5678
FAX: 770-368-4702
e-mail: cs@grahamfield.com
www.grahamfield.com
Kenneth Spett, President & Chief Executive Officer
Cherie Antoniazzi, SVP Quality, Regulatory and Risk Management
Ivan Bielik, Senior Vice President, Business Analyst
Marc Bernstein, Senior Vice President, Consumer Sales
Line of cushions and pillows give comfort and independence to the physically challenged.

285 **Medpro Static Air Chair Cushion**
Medpro
1950 Rutgers Blvd
Lakewood, NJ 08701-4537
800-257-5145
FAX: 732-905-9899
Jody Gorran, President
Provides a protective layer of air beneath the patient helping prevent and treat pressure ulcers. *$94.95*

286 **Medpro Static Air Mattress Overlay**
Medpro
1950 Rutgers Blvd
Lakewood, NJ 08701-4537
800-257-5145
FAX: 732-905-9899
Jody Gorran, President
Supports the patient on a cushioned network of air designed to redistribute the patient's weight reducing tissue interface pressure. Medpro's design incorporates a series of 65 air-breather vents that maintain air circulation. Medpro effectively reduces pressure and helps prevent and treat pressure ulcers. *$164.95*

287 **Mini-Max Cushion**
ROHO
100 North Florida Avenue
Belleville, IL 62221-5429
618-277-9173
800-851-3449
FAX: 618-277-9561
e-mail: tomb@therohogroup.com
www.therohogroup.com

Tom Borcherding, President
Bobby Graebe, CEO
Tim Richter, Vice President of Finance
Dave McCausland, Sr. VP of Planning & Gov Affairs

Designed for the active individual with low risk of skin breakdown. The unique air cells of the MINI-MAX provide significant shock and impact absorption, skin protection and stability.

288 **NEXUS Wheelchair Cushioning System**
ROHO
100 North Florida Avenue
Belleville, IL 62221-5429
618-277-9173
800-850-7646
FAX: 618-277-9561
e-mail: tomb@therohogroup.com
www.therohogroup.com

Tom Borcherding, President
Bobby Graebe, CEO
Tim Richter, Vice President of Finance
Dave McCausland, Sr. VP of Planning & Gov Affairs

A unique modular cushion that mates a contoured polyurethane foam base with a dry flotation support pad. It is designed to give the user positioning and stability, while offering maximum protection to the ischia, sacrum and coccyx.

289 **Pediatric Seating System**
ROHO
100 N Florida Ave
Belleville, IL 62221-5429
618-277-9173
800-851-3449
FAX: 618-277-9561
e-mail: tomb@therohogroup.com
www.therohogroup.com

Tom Borcherding, President
Bobby Graebe, CEO
Tim Richter, Vice President of Finance
Dave McCausland, Sr. VP of Planning & Gov Affairs

ROHO Cushions for kids use individual air cells, creating the most versatile and dynamic cushioning products available. These cushions are designed to specifically fit pediatric wheelchairs.

290 **Quadtro Cushion**
ROHO
100 North Florida Avenue
Belleville, IL 62221-5429
618-277-9173
800-851-3499
FAX: 618-277-9561
e-mail: tomb@therohogroup.com
www.therohogroup.com

Tom Borcherding, President
Bobby Graebe, CEO
Tim Richter, Vice President of Finance
Dave McCausland, Sr. VP of Planning & Gov Affairs

For individuals who require special positioning of the pelvis or thighs and are at risk of skin breakdown, the Quadtro, with 4 inch cell height and air in place, progressive positioning is the cushion of choice.

291 **Silicone Padding**
Spenco Medical Group
P.O.Box 2501
Waco, TX 76702-2501
254-772-6000
800-877-3626
e-mail: spenco@spenco.com
www.spenco.com

Jeff Antonioli, VP Sales
Ryan Cruthirds, Vice President

For the management of pressure sores, this padding provides a special support system which allows even distribution of pressure and cool, comfortable, well-ventilated support.

292 **Soft-Touch Convertible Flotation Mattress**
Medpro
1950 Rutgers Blvd
Lakewood, NJ 08701-4537
800-257-5145
FAX: 732-905-9899

Jody Gorran, President

Gives the patient the option to choose between water and gel flotation depending on the needs of the patient. The mattress helps prevent and treat pressure ulcers by spreading the patient's weight over a greater surface area. $164.95-$239.95.

293 **Soft-Touch Gel Flotation Cushion**
Medpro
1940 Rutgers Blvd
Lakewood, NJ 08701-4537
732-905-9001
800-257-5145
FAX: 732-905-9899

Jody Gorran, President

Acts like an additional layer of fatty tissue beneath the patient to help prevent and treat pressure sores. *$99.95*

294 **Spenco Medical Group**
P.O.Box 2501
Waco, TX 76702-2501
254-772-6000
800-877-3626
e-mail: spenco@spenco.com
www.spenco.com

Jeff Antonioli, VP Sales
Ryan Cruthirds, Vice President

Wheel chair cushions, silicone mattress pads, wound dressings, second skin blister and burn pads, polysorb insoles, elbow, knee and wrist supports and walking shoes.

295 **Stop-Leak Gel Flotation Mattress**
Jefferson Industries
1989 Rutgers Blvd
Lakewood, NJ 08701-4538
732-905-9001
800-257-5145
FAX: 732-905-9899

Charles Landa, General Manager

Protects persons from messy leaks while it protects from pressure ulcers. *$54.00*

296 **Sun-Mate Seat Cushions**
Dynamic Systems
104 Morrow Branch Rd
Leicester, NC 28748-5710
828-683-3523
855-786-6283
FAX: 844-270-6478
e-mail: dsi@sunmatecushions.com
www.sunmatecushions.com

Charles A Yost, CEO
Lewis McCrain, General Manager

Line of cushions, pads and accessory items for personal comfort of the disabled. SunMate Orthopedic foam cushions and sheets that contours slowly to give uniform pressure distribution and soft spring back. Liquid SunMate for Foam-in-Place Seating (FIPS) to make custom molded seat inserts.

297 **Twin-Rest Seat Cushion & Glamour Pillow**
Better Sleep
57 Industrial Rd
Berkeley Heights, NJ 07922-1501
908-464-6568
FAX: 908-464-0058

William Emery Jr, President

Makes any seat more comfortable because it is ingeniously designed to soothe sensitive areas while at work, in the car or at home.

Dressing Aids

298 Button Aid
Maxi Aids
42 Executive Blvd
Farmingdale, NY 11735-4710
631-752-0521
800-522-6294
FAX: 631-752-0689
TTY: 800-281-3555
e-mail: sales@maxiaids.com
www.maxiaids.com

Elliot Zaretsky, Founder / President
Makes buttoning possible with the use of only one hand. *$9.95*

299 Deluxe Sock and Stocking Aid
Therapro, Inc.
225 Arlington St
Framingham, MA 01702-8723
508-872-9494
800-257-5376
FAX: 508-875-2062
e-mail: info@therapro.com
www.therapro.com

Karen Conrad, ScD, OTR/L, Owner
Flexible plastic, lined with blue nylon to reduce friction and outside with beige terry cloth to hold sock firmly until it is on the foot. *$12.95*

300 Dressing Stick
Maxi Aids
42 Executive Blvd
Farmingdale, NY 11735-4710
631-752-0521
800-522-6294
FAX: 631-752-0689
TTY: 800-281-3555
www.maxiaids.com

Elliot Zaretsky, Founder / President
Helps put on coats, sweaters and garments even when arm and shoulder movement is limited. *$7.95*

301 Elastic Shoelaces
Therapro, Inc.
225 Arlington St
Framingham, MA 01702-8723
508-872-9494
800-257-5376
FAX: 508-875-2062
e-mail: info@therapro.com
www.therapro.com

Karen Conrad, ScD, OTR/L, Owner
The elastic laces allow the wearer to slip tied shoes on and off. *$4.25*

302 Featherweight Reachers
Therapro, Inc.
225 Arlington St
Framingham, MA 01702-8723
508-872-9494
800-257-5376
FAX: 508-875-2062
e-mail: info@therapro.com
www.therapro.com

Karen Conrad, ScD, OTR/L, Owner
Useful in dressing or retrieving objects. *$17.95*

303 Mirror Go Lightly
AbleNet
2625 Patton Road
Roseville, MN 55113-1308
612-379-0956
800-322-0956
FAX: 612-379-9143
e-mail: customerservice@ablenetinc.com
www.ablenetinc.com

Bill Sproull, Chairman of the Board
Jennifer Thalhuber, President/CEO
William Mills, Board of Director
Framed in plastic, the mirror can be tilted to provide either a normal or magnified image or to direct its lights at, or away from, the user. *$22.00*

304 Molded Sock and Stocking Aid
Therapro, Inc.
225 Arlington St
Framingham, MA 01702-8723
508-872-9494
800-257-5376
FAX: 508-875-2062
e-mail: info@therapro.com
www.therapro.com

Karen Conrad, ScD, OTR/L, Owner
Sock or stocking is pulled over the molded plastic and then can be put on more easily. *$13.25*

305 Say What
Maxi Aids
42 Executive Blvd
Farmingdale, NY 11735-4710
631-752-0521
800-522-6294
FAX: 631-752-0689
TTY: 800-281-3555
www.maxiaids.com

Elliot Zaretsky, Founder / President
Braille the tag with information that the wearer wants on the tag and place the tag on a hanger. The custom-identification program makes it easier for the user to remember and identify just the right clothes. *$4.95*

306 Shoe and Boot Valet: Decreased Mobility Aid
Maxi Aids
42 Executive Blvd
Farmingdale, NY 11735-4710
631-752-0521
800-522-6294
FAX: 631-752-0689
TTY: 800-281-3555
www.maxiaids.com

Elliot Zaretsky, Founder / President
This is the perfect device to alleviate and in many cases eliminate the pain and embarrassment for millions of people who have a problem doing the simple everyday task of putting on and taking off their footwear. It works perfectly with shoes, boots, galoshes and slippers. *$49.95*

Health Aids

307 AMI
P.O.Box 808
Groton, CT 06340-808
860-536-3735
800-248-4031
FAX: 860-536-3735
e-mail: sales@aquamassage.com
www.aquamassage.com

David M. Cote, President
Dow Cote, Vice President Sales
Hilaire Cote, Senior Vice President
Scott Gilbert, Customer Service Manager
The Aqua PT provides the major benefits of Hydrotherapy, Massage Therapy and Dry Heat Therapy. 36 water jets provide continuous full body or localized massage while the client remains CLOTHED AND DRY! Adjustable water pressure, temperature and pulsation frequency can massage in either a two direction travel mode for musculoskeletal pain management or a one direction mode, flowing water from head to foot for a contrast massage-relax therapy. $25,000 to $30,000.

308 American Medical Industries
Ste 2
330 E 3rd St
Dell Rapids, SD 57022-1918
605-428-5501
801-618-0444
FAX: 605-428-5502
e-mail: info@ezhcare.com
www.ezhealthcare.com

Koby Jackson, Founder
Rick Martin, CEO
Kerina Blauer, VP Client Services
Jim Cannon, SVP Sales and Marketing

EZ-Swallow, EZ-Health, EZ-Home Care, Kleen-Handz, Kleen-Scent, EZ-Irrigator, EZ-VU, Pureshark, Gobot and AMI are all trademarks of American Medical Industries. Healthcare products made easy.

309 **BIPAP S/T Ventilatory Support System**
Respironics
1010 Murry Ridge Ln
Murrysville, PA 15668-8517 724-387-5200
FAX: 724-387-5010
e-mail: customerservice@respironics.com
www.respironics.com

John L Miclot, CEO
Gerald McGinnis, Chairman
Daniel Bevevino, VP/CFO
Craig Reynolds, Executive VP/COO
Respironics, a recognized resource in the medical device market, provides innovative products and unique designs to the health care provider while helping them to grow and manage their business efficiently.

310 **Bed Rails**
Mada Medical Products
625 Washington Ave
Carlstadt, NJ 07072-2901 201-460-0454
800-526-6370
FAX: 201-460-3509
e-mail: dianelind@mail.madamedical.com
www.madainternational.com

Jeffrey Adam, President
Chrome plated steel rails and crossbars, all welded construction, telescopic side rail length adjustable, and a standard rail height of 16 inches.

311 **Coast to Coast Home Medical**
Ste 4d
3381 Fairlane Farms Rd
Wellington, FL 33414-8711 561-792-4009
800-330-6316

Keri Suess, Owner
Home-delivered medical supplies for diabetes, respiratory, arthritis and impotence supplies.

312 **Drew Karol Industries**
P.O.Box 1066
Greenville, MS 38702-1066 662-378-2188
FAX: 601-378-3188
e-mail: dki@techinfo.com

Andrew K Hoszowski, Owner
Orally operated toothbrush and dental care system for persons with limited or complete loss of hand or arm use - wheelchair accessible. *$600.00*

313 **Duraline Medical Products Inc.**
P.O.Box 67
324 Werner Street
Leipsic, OH 45856-1039 419-943-2044
800-654-3376
FAX: 419-943-3637
e-mail: duraline@fairpoint.net
www.dmponline.com

Kathy Peck, General Manager
An assortment of quality incontinence products for adults and children.

314 **Duro-Med Industries**
1931 Norman Drive
Waukegan, IL 60085 800-526-4753
800-622-4714
FAX: 800-479-7968
www.mabisdmi.com

Mike Mazza, President
Tony D'Antonio, Senior VP of Sales
Alan Yefsky, Exec VP, Sales & Mktg
Manufacturers of a complete line of home health care products. Featured products are patient gowns, back and seat cushions, pillows and a complete line of aids for daily living.

315 **Easy Ply**
BioMedical Life Systems
P.O.Box 1360
Vista, CA 92085-1360 800-726-8367
FAX: 760-727-4220
e-mail: information@bmls.com
www.bmls.com

316 **Electronic Stethoscopes**
HARC Mercantile
5413 S. Westnedge Ave.
Suite A
Portage, MI 49002 269-324-0301
800-445-9968
FAX: 269-324-2387
TTY: 269-324-1615
e-mail: info@harc.com
www.harc.com

317 **Fold-Down 3-in-1 Commode**
Mada Medical Products
625 Washington Ave
Carlstadt, NJ 07072-2901 201-460-0454
800-526-6370
FAX: 201-460-3509
e-mail: dianelind@mail.madamedical.com
www.madainternational.com

Jeffrey Adam, President
The Fold-Down commode is constructed of heavy duty, 1 inch diameter, steel tubing with X frame, has folding features convenient for storage and transport, easily removable back rest, and full length armrests.

318 **Healing Dressing for Pressure Sores**
Baxter Healthcare Corporation
1 Baxter Pkwy
Deerfield, IL 60015-4625 800-422-9837
FAX: 800-568-5020
www.baxter.com

Robert L Parkinson Jr, Chairman of the Board/CEO
Jean-Luc Butel, Corporate Vice President - President, International
Ludwig N. Hantson, Corporate Vice President - President, BioScience
Robert J. Hombach, Corporate VP/CFO
A dressing specifically designed to promote healing of pressure sores and other dermal ulcers.

319 **Invacare Corporation**
1 Invacare Way
Elyria, OH 44035-4190 440-329-6000
800-333-6900
FAX: 877-619-7996
e-mail: info@invacare.com
www.invacare.com

A Malachi Mixon Iii, Chairman of the Board
Robert Gudbranson, Interim President & CEO; SVP & CFO
Joseph B. Richey, II, President - Invacare Technologies Division
Anthony C. LaPlaca, Senior Vice President /General Counsel
The world's leading manufacturer and distributor of innovative home and long-term care medical products which promote recovery and active lifestyles.

320 **MADAMIST 50/50 PSI Air Compressor**
Mada Medical Products
625 Washington Ave
Carlstadt, NJ 07072-2901 201-460-0454
800-526-6370
FAX: 201-460-3509
e-mail: dianelind@mail.madamedical.com
www.madainternational.com

Jeffrey Adam, President
The new compressor rated at 50 PSI is designed to drive humidifiers, nebulizers, mist tents and is ideal to administer pentamidine aerosol therapy.

321 **MedDev Corporation**
730 N Pastoria Ave
Sunnyvale, CA 94085-3522
408-730-9702
800-543-2789
FAX: 408-730-9732
e-mail: info@meddev-corp.com
www.meddev-corp.com

322 **Medi-Grip**
Therapro, Inc.
225 Arlington St
Framingham, MA 01702-8723
508-872-9494
800-257-5376
FAX: 508-875-2062
e-mail: info@therapro.com
www.therapro.com

Karen Conrad, ScD, OTR/L, Owner
Reasonably priced, nonskid material. This nonslip material is available in marine blue, desert sand and burgundy rolls 12 inches x 144 inches. *$11.95*

323 **Pocket Otoscope**
HARC Mercantile
5413 S. Westnedge Ave.
Suite A
Portage, MI 49002
269-324-0301
800-445-9968
FAX: 269-324-2387
TTY: 269-324-1615
e-mail: info@harc.com
www.harc.com

324 **Standard 3-in-1 Commode**
Mada Medical Products
625 Washington Ave
Carlstadt, NJ 07072-2901
201-460-0454
800-526-6370
FAX: 201-460-3509
e-mail: dianelind@mail.madamedical.com
www.madainternational.com

Jeffrey Adam, President
The standard commode is constructed of a heavy duty anodized aluminum frame, seat adjustment and an easily removable back rest.

325 **Strider**
Osborn Medical Corporation
7022 S. Revere Pkwy
Suite 240
Centennial, CO 80112
507-932-5028
800-535-5865
FAX: 507-932-5044
e-mail: info@osbornmedical.com
www.osbornmedical.com

Bill Davis, President and CEO
Keith Walli-Ware, Vice President of Sales and Marketing
Ian MacDonald, COO
Strider allows you to exercise in most chairs found in your home. No more small, uncomfortable bicycle seats to sit on while exercising. With Strider, your hands are free to read the paper or your favorite book while you exercise.

326 **Talking Clinical Thermometer**
Maxi Aids
42 Executive Blvd
Farmingdale, NY 11735-4710
631-752-0521
800-522-6294
FAX: 631-752-0689
TTY: 800-281-3555
www.maxiaids.com

Elliot Zaretsky, Founder / President
Audible clinical thermometer. *$199.95*

327 **Talking Thermometers**
Maxi Aids
42 Executive Blvd
Farmingdale, NY 11735-4710
631-752-0521
800-522-6294
FAX: 631-752-0689
TTY: 800-281-3555
www.maxiaids.com

Elliot Zaretsky, Founder / President
Clearly announces temperature in Fahrenheit or Celcius. *$17.95*

328 **Transfer Bench**
Mada Medical Products
625 Washington Ave
Carlstadt, NJ 07072-2901
201-460-0454
800-526-6370
FAX: 201-460-3509
e-mail: dianelind@mail.madamedical.com
www.madainternational.com

Jeffrey Adam, President
The transfer bench is a one piece bench with a wide base for stability, 1 inch diameter aluminum framework, corrosion resistant, and an adjustable seat.

Hearing Aids

329 **Auditech: Personal PA Value Pack System**
P.O.Box 821105
Vicksburg, MS 39182-1105
800-229-8293
FAX: 800-221-8639
e-mail: info@auditechusa.com
www.auditechusa.com

330 **Auditech: Pocketalker Pro**
P.O.Box 821105
Vicksburg, MS 39182-1105
800-229-8293
FAX: 800-221-8639
e-mail: info@auditechusa.com
www.auditechusa.com

331 **Battery Device Adapter**
AbleNet
2625 Patton Road
Roseville, MN 55113-1308
612-379-0956
800-322-0956
FAX: 651-294-2259
e-mail: customerservice@ablenetinc.com
www.ablenetinc.com

Bill Sproull, Chairman of the Board
Jennifer Thalhuber, President/CEO
William Mills, Board of Director
A cable which connects to and adapts battery-operated devices for external switch control. Two sizes are available to adapt devices with either AA or C and D size batteries. *$8.00*

332 **Custom Earmolds**
Lloyd Hearing Aid Corporation
P.O.Box 1645
4435 Manchester Dr
Rockford, IL 61109-1645
815-964-4191
800-323-4212
FAX: 815-964-8378
e-mail: info@lloydshearingaid.com
www.lloydhearingaid.com

Andy PalmQuist, President
Hearing aid molds, custom built to the exact fit of the customer. *$29.95*

333 **Digital Hearing Aids**
Lloyd Hearing Aid Corporation
P.O.Box 1645
4435 Manchester Dr
Rockford, IL 61109-1645
815-964-4191
800-323-4212
FAX: 815-964-8378
e-mail: info@lloydshearingaid.com
www.lloydhearingaid.com

Andy PalmQuist, President
Latest hearing technology. *$7.50*

334 **Doorbell Signalers**
HARC Mercantile
5413 S. Westnedge Ave.
Suite A
Portage, MI 49002
269-324-0301
800-445-9968
FAX: 269-324-2387
TTY: 269-324-1615
e-mail: info@harc.com
www.harc.com

335 **Double Gong Indoor/Outdoor Ringer**
HARC Mercantile
5413 S. Westnedge Ave.
Suite A
Portage, MI 49002
269-324-0301
800-445-9968
FAX: 269-324-2387
TTY: 269-324-1615
e-mail: info@harc.com
www.harc.com

336 **Duracell & Rayovac Hearing Aid Batteries**
Lloyd Hearing Aid Corporation
P.O.Box 1645
4435 Manchester Dr
Rockford, IL 61109-1645
815-964-4191
800-323-4212
FAX: 815-964-8378
e-mail: info@lloydhearingaid.com
www.lloydhearingaid.com

Andy PalmQuist, President
Batteries for hearing aids at discounted prices. As low as 45 cents each.

337 **Harris Communications**
Harris Communications
15155 Technology Dr
Eden Prairie, MN 55344-2273
800-825-6758
FAX: 952-906-1099
TTY:800-825-9187
e-mail: info@harriscomm.com
www.harriscomm.com

Dr.Robert Harris, Owner and President
A national distributor of assistive devices for the deaf and hard-of-hearing with many manufacturers represented. Catalog includes a wide range of assistive devices as well as a variety of books and video tapes related to deaf and hard-of-hearing issues. Products available for children, teachers, hearing professionals, interpreters and anyone interested in deaf culture, hearing loss and sign language.
180 pages Yearly

338 **Hearing Aid Batteries**
HARC Mercantile
5413 S. Westnedge Ave.
Suite A
Portage, MI 49002
269-324-0301
800-445-9968
FAX: 269-324-2387
TTY: 269-324-1615
e-mail: info@harc.com
www.harc.com

339 **Hearing Aid Battery Testers**
HARC Mercantile
5413 S. Westnedge Ave.
Suite A
Portage, MI 49002
269-324-0301
800-445-9968
FAX: 269-324-2387
TTY: 269-324-1615
e-mail: info@harc.com
www.harc.com

340 **Hearing Aid Dehumidifier**
HARC Mercantile
5413 S. Westnedge Ave.
Suite A
Portage, MI 49002
269-324-0301
800-445-9968
FAX: 269-324-2387
TTY: 269-324-1615
e-mail: info@harc.com
www.harc.com

341 **In the Ear Hearing Aid Battery Extractor**
HARC Mercantile
5413 S. Westnedge Ave.
Suite A
Portage, MI 49002
269-324-0301
800-445-9968
FAX: 269-324-2387
TTY: 269-324-1615
e-mail: info@harc.com
www.harc.com

342 **Micro Audiometrics Corporation**
655 Keller Rd
Murphy, NC 28906-5890
828-644-0771
800-729-9509
866-327-7226
FAX: 866-683-4447
e-mail: sales@microaud.com
www.microaud.com

Jason Keller, President
Manufacturer and distributor of hearing testing instruments, including the complete line of Earscan.

343 **Mushroom Inserts**
Lloyd Hearing Aid Corporation
P.O.Box 1645
4435 Manchester Drive
Rockford, IL 61109- 1645
815-964-4191
800-323-4212
FAX: 815-964-8378
e-mail: info@lloydhearingaid.com
www.lloydhearingaid.com

Andy PalmQuist, President
A universal earplug useful in wearing behind the ear type hearing instruments. *$2.50*

344 **Oval Window Audio**
33 Wildflower Ct
Nederland, CO 80466-9638
303-447-3607
FAX: 303-447-3607
TTY:303-447-3607
e-mail: info@ovalwindowaudio.com
www.ovalwindowaudio.com

Norman Lederman, Dir. of R & D
Paula Hendricks, Educational Dir.
Manufacturer of induction loop hearing assistance technologies compatible with hearing aids already used by many hard of hearing people. Also multisensory sound systems for use in speech and music therapy and science classes.

Kitchen & Eating Aids

345 **Bagel Holder**
Maxi Aids
42 Executive Blvd
Farmingdale, NY 11735-4710
631-752-0521
800-522-6294
FAX: 631-752-0689
TTY: 800-281-3555
www.maxiaids.com

Elliot Zaretsky, Founder / President
Holds bagels in place for easy slicing. *$3.95*

346 **Big Bold Timer Low Vision**
Maxi Aids
42 Executive Blvd
Farmingdale, NY 11735-4710
631-752-0521
800-522-6294
FAX: 631-752-0689
TTY: 800-281-3555
www.maxiaids.com

Elliot Zaretsky, Founder / President
Sixty-minute mechanical timer with large, easy-to-read numbers for the vision impaired. *$9.95*

347 **Box Top Opener**
Sammons Preston Rolyan
W68 N158 Evergreen Blvd.
Cedarburg, WI 53012
630-378-6000
800-228-3693
FAX: 262-387-8748
e-mail: sp@pattersonmedical.com
www.pattersonmedical.com

David P Sproat, President
Bruce Curtis, Sales Representative
This handy device exerts the pressure on those hard-to-open boxes of laundry/dishwasher soap, rice and prepared dinners. *$2.95*

348 **Capscrew**
Access with Ease
P.O.Box 1150
Chino Valley, AZ 86323-1150
928-636-9469
800-531-9479
FAX: 928-636-0292
e-mail: KMJC@northlink.com

349 **Cool Handle**
Maxi Aids
42 Executive Blvd
Farmingdale, NY 11735-4710
631-752-0521
800-522-6294
FAX: 631-752-0689
TTY: 800-281-3555
www.maxiaids.com

Elliot Zaretsky, Founder / President
A specially designed, heat-resistant handle, available in three sizes which can be affixed to the handles of most fry, sauce and saute pans. *$7.95*

350 **Cordless Receiver**
AbleNet
2625 Patton Road
Roseville, MN 55113-1308
612-379-0956
800-322-0956
FAX: 651-294-2259
e-mail: customerservice@ablenetinc.com
www.ablenetinc.com

Bill Sproull, Chairman of the Board
Jennifer Thalhuber, President/CEO
William Mills, Board of Director
The Cordless Receiver in conjunction with the Cordless Big Red Switch, can be used anywhere a switch is currently used to control battery or electrically-operated toys, games or appliances; augmentative communication systems; and computers (through a computer switch interface). *$79.00*

351 **Deluxe Long Ring Low Vision Timer**
Maxi Aids
42 Executive Blvd
Farmingdale, NY 11735-4710
631-752-0521
800-522-6294
FAX: 631-752-0689
TTY: 800-281-3555
www.maxiaids.com

Elliot Zaretsky, Founder / President
Bold black numerals on white background allows for easy reading at any distance. *$17.95*

352 **Deluxe Roller Knife**
Sammons Preston Rolyan
28100 Torch Parkway
Suite 700
Warrenville, IL 60555-3938
630-378-6000
800-323-5547
FAX: 630-393-7600
e-mail: sp@pattersonmedical.com
www.pattersonmedical.com

David P Sproat, President
Bruce Curtis, Sales Representative
Stainless steel blade rolls smoothly, cutting food cleanly. *$10.95*

353 **Dual Brush with Suction Base**
Sammons Preston Rolyan
28100 Torch Parkway
Suite 700
Warrenville, IL 60555-3938
630-378-6000
800-323-5547
FAX: 630-393-7600
e-mail: sp@pattersonmedical.com
www.pattersonmedical.com

David P Sproat, President
Bruce Curtis, Sales Representative
Two brushes clean the inside and outside of bottles and glasses at the same time using just one hand. *$14.50*

354 **Easy Pour Locking Lid Pot**
Maxi Aids
42 Executive Blvd
Farmingdale, NY 11735-4710
631-752-0521
800-522-6294
FAX: 631-752-0689
TTY: 800-281-3555
www.maxiaids.com

Elliot Zaretsky, Founder / President
Baked enamel and dishwasher safe, the pot comes with an easy lid that locks in place for extra safety. *$24.95*

355 **Electric Can Opener & Knife Sharpener**
Maxi Aids
42 Executive Blvd
Farmingdale, NY 11735-4710
631-752-0521
800-522-6294
FAX: 631-752-0689
TTY: 800-281-3555
www.maxiaids.com

Elliot Zaretsky, Founder / President
Features include a powerful magnetic lid holder, the ability to open odd-shaped cans, and easy operation for the physically challenged. *$19.95*

356 **Evio Plastics**
P.O.Box 2295
Sandusky, OH 44871-2295
419-621-1105
FAX: 419-626-2183

Doug Didion, Admininstrator Director
Danny Thomas, Owner
Handi Holder is a plastic holder for 1/2 gallon paper cartons of milk or juice. It is used to pour milk or juice without spills by using the handle.

357 Food Markers/Rubberbands
Maxi Aids
42 Executive Blvd
Farmingdale, NY 11735-4710
631-752-0521
800-522-6294
FAX: 631-752-0689
TTY: 800-281-3555
www.maxiaids.com

Elliot Zaretsky, Founder / President
These are durable plastic markers, easily identified by touch, texture, shape and form which help the visually impaired orient themselves to food location on the plate. *$11.95*

358 Good Grips Cutlery
Therapro, Inc.
225 Arlington St
Framingham, MA 01702-8723
508-872-9494
800-257-5376
FAX: 508-875-2062
e-mail: info@therapro.com
www.therapro.com

Karen Conrad, ScD, OTR/L, Owner
Stainless steel utensils have a special twist built into the metal to facilitate bending of a spoon or fork at any angle for right or left handed people. *$7.50*

359 H.E.L.P. Knife
Maxi Aids
42 Executive Blvd
Farmingdale, NY 11735-4710
631-752-0521
800-522-6294
FAX: 631-752-0689
TTY: 800-281-3555
www.maxiaids.com

Elliot Zaretsky, Founder / President
Adjustable food slicing system guides the knife for even, uniform slices while protecting the user. *$11.95*

360 Handy-Helper Cutting Board
Maxi Aids
42 Executive Blvd
Farmingdale, NY 11735-4710
631-752-0521
800-522-6294
FAX: 631-752-0689
TTY: 800-281-3555
www.maxiaids.com

Elliot Zaretsky, Founder / President
Laminated cutting board with unique features to hold food in place with corner ledge for cutting and spreading. *$19.95*

361 Innerlip Plates
Therapro, Inc.
225 Arlington St
Framingham, MA 01702-8723
508-872-9494
800-257-5376
FAX: 508-875-2062
e-mail: info@therapro.com
www.therapro.com

Karen Conrad, ScD, OTR/L, Owner
Food may be pushed to the side of the plate, then scooped up with a fork and spoon. Available in beige or blue. *$5.00*

362 Long Oven Mitts
Sammons Preston Rolyan
28100 Torch Parkway
Suite 700
Warrenville, IL 60555-3938
630-378-6000
800-323-5547
FAX: 630-393-7600
e-mail: sp@pattersonmedical.com
www.pattersonmedical.com

David P Sproat, President
Bruce Curtis, Sales Representative
Protect hands and forearms from heat, flames and oven grates with these practical mitts that allow a longer reach and less bending. *$8.95*

363 Magnetic Card Reader
Maxi Aids
42 Executive Blvd
Farmingdale, NY 11735-4710
631-752-0521
800-522-6294
FAX: 631-752-0689
TTY: 800-281-3555
www.maxiaids.com

Elliot Zaretsky, Founder / President
Produces audible labels so a recorded card can be taped on cans of food or a box of cake mix; even adding instructions for baking. *$159.95*

364 Maxi-Aids Braille Timer
Maxi Aids
42 Executive Blvd
Farmingdale, NY 11735-4710
631-752-0521
800-522-6294
FAX: 631-752-0689
TTY: 800-281-3555
www.maxiaids.com

Elliot Zaretsky, Founder / President
Three raised dots at 15, 30 and 45, two raised dots at remaining five minute intervals and one raised dot at remaining two and a half minute intervals, offers ease of operation to make this a helpful aid for the visually impaired. *$12.95*

365 Nosey Cup
Therapro, Inc.
225 Arlington St
Framingham, MA 01702-8723
508-872-9494
800-257-5376
FAX: 508-875-2062
e-mail: info@therapro.com
www.therapro.com

Karen Conrad, ScD, OTR/L, Owner
For those with a stiff neck or persons who can't tip their head back while drinking. *$6.00*

366 Paring Boards
Therapro, Inc.
225 Arlington St
Framingham, MA 01702-8723
508-872-9494
800-257-5376
FAX: 508-875-2062
e-mail: info@therapro.com
www.therapro.com

Karen Conrad, ScD, OTR/L, Owner
Suction feet stabilize board and stainless steel prongs hold food in place for easy, one-handed cutting. *$32.50*

367 PowerLink 2 Control Unit
AbleNet
2625 Patton Road
Roseville, MN 55113-1308
612-379-0956
800-322-0956
FAX: 651-294-2259
e-mail: customerservice@ablenetinc.com
www.ablenetinc.com

Bill Sproull, Chairman of the Board
Jennifer Thalhuber, President/CEO
William Mills, Board of Director
The PowerLink 2 Control Unit allows switch operation of electrical appliances. It can be used to activate 1 or 2 appliances (up to 1700 watts combined). If 2 appliances are used, they will activate simultaneously. There are four modes of control on the PowerLink 2; direct mode, timed (seconds) mode, timed (minutes) mode and latch mode. Meets safety standards from Underwriters Laboratory (UL) and Canadian Standards Association (CSA) for electrical appliances. *$159.00*

368 **Sammons Preston Rolyan**
28100 Torch Parkway
Suite 700
Warrenville, IL 60555-3938 630-378-6000
800-323-5547
FAX: 630-393-7600
e-mail: sp@pattersonmedical.com
www.pattersonmedical.com

David P Sproat, President
Bruce Curtis, Sales Representative
Sammons Preston Rolyan is a leading provider of rehabilitation and assistive devices to help those with disabilities meet daily physical challenges and achieve their greatest level of independence. With one of the industry's largest catalogs, Sammons Preston Rolyan offers a wide range of products available.
Annually

369 **Slicing Aid**
Snug Seat
12801 E. Independence Blvd.
P.O.Box 1739
Matthews, NC 28106-1739 704-882-0666
800-336-7684
FAX: 704-882-0751
e-mail: information@snugseat.com
www.snugseat.com

Scott Crosswhite, Vice President
Kirk Mackenzie, President
Greg Tilley, Controller
Angela Stegall, Purchasing
The design of these knives allows a better working posture and makes optimal use of strength in the arms and hands.

370 **Small Appliance Receiver**
AbleNet
2625 Patton Road
Roseville, MN 55113-1308 612-379-0956
800-322-0956
FAX: 651-294-2259
e-mail: customerservice@ablenetinc.com
www.ablenetinc.com

Bill Sproull, Chairman of the Board
Jennifer Thalhuber, President/CEO
William Mills, Board of Director
The Small Appliance Receiver, in conjunction with the Cordless Big Red Switch, allows you to control small electrical appliances in the environment without a cord. It should only be used with low-wattage appliances (under 500 watts) which have two prong plugs (i.e., radios, fans, lamps, blenders, etc.). It should not be used with heat generating appliances. *$32.00*

371 **Steel Food Guard**
Maxi Aids
42 Executive Blvd
Farmingdale, NY 11735-4710 631-752-0521
800-522-6294
FAX: 631-752-0689
TTY: 800-281-3555
www.maxiaids.com

Elliot Zaretsky, Founder / President
Provides stable area to push against while eating. *$ 10.95*

372 **Thick-n-Easy**
Therapro, Inc.
225 Arlington St
Framingham, MA 01702-8723 508-872-9494
800-257-5376
FAX: 508-875-2062
e-mail: info@therapro.com
www.therapro.com

Karen Conrad, ScD, OTR/L, Owner
Instant food thickener that sets in 30 seconds and will not become thicker even after refrigeration. *$6.50*

373 **Thumbs Up Cup**
Therapro, Inc.
225 Arlington St
Framingham, MA 01702-8723 508-872-9494
800-257-5376
FAX: 508-875-2062
e-mail: info@therapro.com
www.therapro.com

Karen Conrad, ScD, OTR/L, Owner
This cup is designed for those with limited strength or coordination or arthritis. The two backward-tilt handles and thumb rests allow finger joints to be used to their greatest mechanical advantage. *$9.50*

374 **Undercounter Lid Opener**
Sammons Preston Rolyan
28100 Torch Parkway
Suite 700
Warrenville, IL 60555-3938 630-378-6000
800-323-5547
FAX: 630-393-7600
e-mail: sp@pattersonmedical.com
www.pattersonmedical.com

David P Sproat, President
Bruce Curtis, Sales Representative
The gripper of this unit which installs under the counter can help unscrew any cap. *$5.75*

375 **Uni-Turner**
Sammons Preston Rolyan
28100 Torch Parkway
Suite 700
Warrenville, IL 60555-3938 630-378-6000
800-323-5547
FAX: 630-393-7600
e-mail: sp@pattersonmedical.com
www.pattersonmedical.com

David P Sproat, President
Bruce Curtis, Sales Representative
Odd shaped handles can be turned easily with one-handed, L-shaped Uni-Turner. *$16.50*

376 **Universal Hand Cuff**
Therapro, Inc.
225 Arlington St
Framingham, MA 01702-8723 508-872-9494
800-257-5376
FAX: 508-875-2062
e-mail: info@therapro.com
www.therapro.com

Karen Conrad, ScD, OTR/L, Owner
Comfortable cuff with Velcro strap holds utensils, toothbrushes, etc. *$9.95*

Lifts, Ramps & Elevators

377 **Accessibility Lift**
Inclinator Company of America
601 Gibson Blvd
Harrisburg, PA 17104-3215 717-939-8420
800-343-9007
FAX: 717-939-8075
e-mail: isales@inclinator.com
www.inclinator.com

Stephen Nock, President
An economical lift for restricted usage that provides barrier-free access that can be used by churches, schools, lodging halls and meeting halls to meet compliance requirements, with the dignified convenience and freedom they deserve.

378 Adjustable Incline Board
Bailey Manufacturing Company
P.O. Box 130
Lodi, OH 44254-130
800-321-8372
FAX: 800-224-5390
e-mail: baileymfg@baileymfg.com
www.baileymfg.com

379 AlumiRamp
855 E Chicago Rd
Quincy, MI 49082-9450
800-800-3864
FAX: 517-639-4314
e-mail: sales@alumiramp.com
www.alumiramp.com

Doug Cannon, General Manager

Complete line of modular, aluminum and portable ramps for both home and vehicle use. Welded construction and non-skid extruded surfaces are featured on all our ramps.

380 Area Access
7131 Gateway Court
Manassas, VA 20109-1015
703-396-4949
800-333-2732
FAX: 703-207-0446
www.areaaccess.com

381 Basement Motorhome Lift By Handicaps, Inc.
4335 S Santa Fe Dr
Englewood, CO 80110
303-781-2062
800-782-4335
FAX: 303-761-6811
e-mail: info@handicapsinc.com
www.handicapsinc.com

382 Bruno Independent Living Aids
P.O.Box 84
1780 Executive Drive
Oconomowoc, WI 53066
262-567-4990
800-882-8183
FAX: 262-953-5510
www.bruno.com

Michael R. Bruno, II, President/CEO
Andrew Bayer, Product Mgr, Automotive Div.
Mike Krawczyk, Mktg Svcs Mgr

An ISO 9001 Certified Manufacturer of automotive lifts for scooter, wheelchairs, and power chairs, three and four wheel scooters, and straight and custom curve stairlifts.

383 Butlers Wheelchair Lifts
Flinchbaugh Company
629 Lowther Road #C
Lewisberry, PA 17339
717-938-4253
888-847-0804
FAX: 717-938-4238
e-mail: hal@butlermobility.com
www.butlermobility.com

Hal Feinstein, VP Sales / Marketing

This wheelchair lift can be equipped with an end ramp and guard. Automatically retractable, it locks firmly into place when the lift is in operation.

384 Classique
Handi-Lift
730 Garden St
Carlstadt, NJ 07072-1625
201-933-0111
800-432-5438
FAX: 201-933-0050
e-mail: sales@handi-lift.com
www.handi-lift.com

Douglas Boydston, President

The Classique elevator answers access problems in churches, schools and small offices.

385 Columbus McKinnon Corporation
140 John James Audubon Pkwy
Amherst, NY 14228-1197
716-689-5400
800-888-0985
FAX: 716-689-5644
www.cmworks.com

Timothy T. Tevens, President/CEO
Gregory P. Rustowicz, VP/CFO
Charles R. Giesige, VP, Corporate Dev.
Richard A. Steinberg, VP, Human Resources

Supplies various lift and transfer systems for independent or attended applications including ceiling mounted or freestanding overhead track lifts and mobile floorbase units for homes, schools and healthcare facilities. Lift Systems for transferring between bed, chair, commode or bath are available with a variety of slings, scales and accessories.

386 Curb-Sider
Bruno Independent Living Aids
PO Box 84
1780 Executive Drive
Oconomowoc, WI 53066
262-567-4990
800-882-8183
FAX: 262-953-5501
www.bruno.com

Michael R. Bruno, II, President/CEO
Andrew Bayer, Product Mgr, Automotive Div.
Mike Krawczyk, Mktg Svcs Mgr

The lift of choice for storing your fully or partially assembled scooter or power chair weighing up to 400 pounds in the rear of your van or minivan, SUV, pickup truck or some station wagon applications.

387 Curb-Sider Super XL
P.O.Box 84
1780 Executive Drive
Oconomowoc, WI 53066
262-567-4990
800-882-8183
FAX: 262-953-5510
www.bruno.com

Michael R. Bruno, II, President/CEO
Andrew Bayer, Product Mgr, Automotive Div.
Mike Krawczyk, Mktg Svcs Mgr

388 Custom Lift Residential Elevators
Waupaca Elevator Company
1726 N Ballard Rd
Appleton, WI 54911-2444
920-991-9082
800-238-8739
FAX: 920-991-9087
e-mail: info@waupacaelevator.com
waupacaelevator.com

Bill Mc Michael, Owner

Waupaca Elevator residential elevators and dumbwaiters add value, convenience and reliability to today's homes.

389 Deluxe Convertible Exercise Staircase
Sammons Preston Rolyan
28100 Torch Parkway
Suite 700
Warrenville, IL 60555-3938
630-378-6000
800-323-5547
FAX: 630-393-7600
e-mail: sp@pattersonmedical.com
www.pattersonmedical.com

David P Sproat, President
Bruce Curtis, Sales Representative

Here's an exercise staircase to fit any department configuration. Just reposition a few nuts and bolts to change from a straight to a corner type staircase.

390 **E-Z Access Van Ramp**
Maxi Aids
42 Executive Blvd
Farmingdale, NY 11735-4710
631-752-0521
800-522-6294
FAX: 631-752-0689
TTY: 800-281-3555
www.maxiaids.com

Elliot Zaretsky, Founder / President
Telescopic ramps for manual and electric wheel chairs. Bridges gaps over steps and curbs and makes vans more accessible. Extends 7'ft. in length, locking securely in place with snap-button catches. Easy to store. Holds up to 600lbs. *$299.95*

391 **Easy Pivot Transfer Machine**
Rand-Scot
401 Linden Center Dr
Fort Collins, CO 80524-2429
970-484-7967
800-467-7967
FAX: 970-484-3800
e-mail: info@randscot.com
www.randscot.com

Joel Lerich, President
The Easy Pivot Patient Lifting System allows for strain-free, one-caregiver transfers of the disabled individual.

392 **Easy Stand**
Altimate Medical
262 W. 1st St.
Morton, MN 56270-180
507-697-6393
800-342-8968
FAX: 507-697-6900
e-mail: info@easystand.com
www.easystand.com

Andrew Gardeen, International Sales Manager
Designed to make standing fast and simple. The easy to operate, hydraulic lift system provides a controlled lifting and lowering. With the convenience of simply transferring to the chair and reaching a standing position in seconds with no straps to struggle with.

393 **Economical Liberty**
Handi-Lift
730 Garden St
Carlstadt, NJ 07072-1625
201-933-0111
800-432-5438
FAX: 201-933-0050
e-mail: sales@handi-lift.com
www.handi-lift.com

Douglas Boydston, President
Installs quickly and easily on most straight stairways. It uses regular household current and mounts over the carpet or directly to the stairs without marring.

394 **Electra-Ride**
Bruno Independent Living Aids
PO Box 84
1780 Executive Drive
Oconomowoc, WI 53066
262-567-4990
800-882-8183
FAX: 262-953-5501
www.bruno.com

Michael R. Bruno, II, President/CEO
Andrew Bayer, Product Mgr, Automotive Div.
Mike Krawczyk, Mktg Svcs Mgr
Bruno stairlifts can fit almost any custom curve or straight rail application and require no structural modification to the stairway. Plus, battery power allows for uninterrupted operation even during a power outage.

395 **Electra-Ride Elite**
Bruno Independent Living Aids
P.O.Box 84
1780 Executive Drive
Oconomowoc, WI 53066
262-567-4990
800-882-8183
FAX: 262-953-5510
www.bruno.com

Michael R. Bruno, II, President/CEO
Andrew Bayer, Product Mgr, Automotive Div.
Mike Krawczyk, Mktg Svcs Mgr
The new Electra-Ride Elite installs to within 5 inches of the wall and has a 350 pound weight capacity. Bruno stairlifts can fit almost any custom curve or straight rail application and require no structural modification to the stairway. Plus, battery power allows for uninterrupted operation even during a power outage.

396 **Electra-Ride III**
P.O.Box 84
1780 Executive Drive
Oconomowoc, WI 53066
262-567-4990
800-882-8183
FAX: 262-953-5510
www.bruno.com

Michael R. Bruno, II, President/CEO
Andrew Bayer, Product Mgr, Automotive Div.
Mike Krawczyk, Mktg Svcs Mgr

397 **Freedom Wheels**
580 Tc Jester Blvd
Houston, TX 77007
713-864-1460
888-422-5337
FAX: 713-864-1469
e-mail: info@freedomwheels.com
www.freedomwheels.com

Carlos Saez, Owner
An assistive technology and mobility equipment provider and is committed to people with disabilities and personal transportation options for an independent lifestyle.

398 **Handi Home Lift**
Handi-Lift
730 Garden St
Carlstadt, NJ 07072-1625
201-933-0111
800-432-5438
FAX: 201-933-0050
e-mail: sales@handi-lift.com
www.handi-lift.com

Douglas Boydston, President
An outdoor lift designed to provide access over porch stairs or other steps that impede movement.

399 **Handi Lift**
730 Garden St
Carlstadt, NJ 07072-1625
201-933-0111
800-432-5438
FAX: 201-933-0050
e-mail: sales@handi-lift.com
www.handi-lift.com

Douglas Boydston, President
Accessibility with Dignity. We create solutions that enable people with mobility impairments to live freely with products like wheelchair lifts and home elevators.

400 **Handi Prolift**
Handi-Lift
730 Garden St
Carlstadt, NJ 07072-1625
201-933-0111
800-432-5438
FAX: 201-933-0050
e-mail: sales@handi-lift.com
www.handi-lift.com

Douglas Boydston, President
Provides dependable vertical transportation for multi-level buildings.

401 Handi-Ramp
Handi-Ramp
510 North Ave
Libertyville, IL 60048-2025
847-680-7700
800-876-7267
FAX: 847-816-7689
e-mail: info@handiramp.com
www.handiramp.com

Thomas Disch, President/ CEO
Alicia C. Johns, Program Manager
Provides a complete line of economical, ADA Compliant access ramping products. Line includes van attachable and wheelchair tie downs; aluminum or expanded metal folding portables; aluminum channels; portable, sectional ramp systems; semi-permanent ramps, platforms and systems. All ramp series are available in varied lengths and widths in combination with platforms and optional hand railing, single or double bar construction with return ends. Special Order ramps and ramp systems.

402 Homewaiter
Inclinator Company of America
601 Gibson Blvd
Harrisburg, PA 17104-3215
717-939-8420
800-343-9007
FAX: 717-939-8075
e-mail: isales@inclinator.com
www.inclinator.com

Stephen Nock, President
With its roller truck riding in a specially formed monorail, it is easy to install and highly adaptable to existing conditions. It can travel up to 35 feet, opening on any or all three sides at different stations, whether at counter level or floor level.

403 Horcher Lifting Systems
324 Cypress Rd
Ocala, FL 34472-3102
352-687-8020
800-582-8732
FAX: 866-378-3318
e-mail: us-office@horcher.com
www.horcher.com

David Schultz, General Manager
Sharon Harbert, Administrative Assistant
Barrier Free Lifts by Horcher leads the industry for excellence in patient transfers and technology for over 18 years. They offer state of the art ceiling track systems, floor base lifts and bathing systems such as the Unilift, PC-2, Diana, Lexa, and Raisa to achieve greater mobility.

404 Inclinette
Inclinator Company of America
601 Gibson Blvd
Harrisburg, PA 17104-3215
717-939-8420
800-343-9007
FAX: 717-939-8075
e-mail: isales@inclinator.com
www.inclinator.com

Stephen Nock, President
Inclinette provides comfort and convenience in providing multi-floor access to persons who have difficulty climbing stairs.

405 Independent Driving Systems
580 T.C. Jester
Houston, TX 77007
713-864-1460
888-422-5337
FAX: 713-864-1469
e-mail: info@independentdrivingssytems.com
www.independentdrivingsystems.com

Chad Donnelly, Owner
Provides adaptive driving systems for individuals with disabilities with more severe higher levels of injury that require more sophisticated types of assistive technology to enable them to drive safely.

406 Joey Interior Platform Lift
Bruno Independent Living Aids
PO Box 84
1780 Executive Drive
Oconomowoc, WI 53066
262-567-4990
800-882-8183
FAX: 262-953-5501
www.bruno.com

Michael R. Bruno, II, President/CEO
Andrew Bayer, Product Mgr, Automotive Div.
Mike Krawczyk, Mktg Svcs Mgr
Lifts and stores your unoccupied scooter or powerchair in the back of your minivan at the touch of a button.

407 Lectra-Lift
La-Z-Boy
1284 N Telegraph Rd
Monroe, MI 48162-5138
734-242-1444
800-375-6890
FAX: 734-457-2005
www.lazboy.com

Kurt L Darrow, CEO
David M Risley, SVP/CFO
Patrick H Norton, Chairman
Kurt Darrow, CEO
This power recliner has a single motor drive that operates three distinct cycles: lifting, leg elevation and full power recline.

408 Liberty LT
Handi-Lift
730 Garden St
Carlstadt, NJ 07072-1625
201-933-0111
800-432-5438
FAX: 201-933-0050
e-mail: sales@handi-lift.com
www.handi-lift.com

Douglas Boydston, President
Stair lift with dual armrests that lock into position. The comfortable, contoured seat is designed to swivel and move forward at the bottom or top landings to facilitate transfer.

409 Lift-All
Amigo Mobility International
6693 Dixie Highway
Bridgeport, MI 48722-9725
989-777-0910
800-692-6446
800-248-9131
FAX: 800-334-7274
e-mail: info@myamigo.com
www.myamigo.com

Al Thieme, Chairman and Founder
Beth Thieme, CEO
Tim Drumhiller, President
Sandy Humpert, Sales Rep
Leading manufacturer of electric mobility; Amigo's Lift-All transports your wheelchair easily into the trunk of an automobile and neatly stores it for easy access. Also available is the Lift-It. *$965.00*

410 Lifts for Swimming Pools and Spas
Aquatic Access
1921 Production Dr
Louisville, KY 40299-2110
502-425-5817
800-325-5438
FAX: 502-425-9607
e-mail: info@AquaticAccess.com
www.aquaticaccess.com

Linda Nolan, President
David Nolan, Vice President
Aquatic Access manufacturers and sells water-powered lifts providing access to in-ground and above-ground swimming pools, spas, boats and docks. *$2310.00*

411 **Mac's Lift Gate**
2801 South Street
Long Beach, CA 90805-3751
562-634-5962
800-795-6227
FAX: 562-529-3466
e-mail: sales@macsliftgate.com
www.macsliftgate.com

Randy Maner, Training Mgr

Sales and service of van and truck lifts. Sales and service of wheel chair lifts for vans and automobiles. Sales, installation and service of vertical home lifts, scooter lifts and pool lifts. Sales of scooters.

412 **Mecalift Sling Lifter**
Arjo Inc
2349 West Lake Street
Addison, IL 60101
630-785-4490
800-323-1245
FAX: 888-389-2756
e-mail: usa.info@ArjoHuntleigh.com
www.arjo.com

Philip M. Croxford, President/ CEO

413 **Motorhome Lift By Handicaps, Inc.**
4335 S Santa Fe Dr
Englewood, CO 80110
303-781-2062
800-782-4335
FAX: 303-761-6811
e-mail: info@handicapsinc.com
www.handicapsinc.com

414 **One for All Lift All**
6693 Dixie Highway
Bridgeport, MI 48722-9725
989-777-0910
800-692-6446
800-248-9131
FAX: 800-334-7274
e-mail: info@myamigo.com
www.myamigo.com

Al Thieme, Chairman and Founder
Beth Thieme, CEO
Tim Drumhiller, President

Amigo Mobility designs and manufactures a complete line of power operated vehicles/mobility scooters and accessories in Bridgeport, Mich.

415 **Out-Sider III**
P.O.Box 84
1780 Executive Drive
Oconomowoc, WI 53066
262-567-4990
800-882-8183
FAX: 262-953-5510
www.bruno.com

Michael R. Bruno, II, President/CEO
Andrew Bayer, Product Mgr, Automotive Div.
Mike Krawczyk, Mktg Svcs Mgr

416 **Out-Sider Meridian**
Bruno Independent Living Aids
P.O. Box 84
1780 Executive Drive
Oconomowoc, WI 53066
262-567-4990
800-882-8183
FAX: 262-953-5501
www.bruno.com

Michael R. Bruno, II, President/CEO
Andrew Bayer, Product Mgr, Automotive Div.
Mike Krawczyk, Mktg Svcs Mgr

Lets you carry your scooter fully assembled and keeps your trunk space available for other things.

417 **Parker Bath**
Arjo Inc
2349 West Lake Street
Addison, IL 60101
630-785-4490
800-323-1245
FAX: 888-389-2756
e-mail: usa.info@ArjoHuntleigh.com
www.arjo.com

Philip M. Croxford, President/ CEO
Ross Scavuzzo, President

This involves no manual lifting, strain or stress for the caregiver.

418 **Patient Lifting & Injury Prevention**
Arjo Inc
2349 West Lake Street
Addison, IL 60101
630-785-4490
800-323-1245
FAX: 888-389-2756
e-mail: usa.info@ArjoHuntleigh.com
www.arjo.com

Philip M. Croxford, President/ CEO

Aids in patient lifting while protecting the caregiver from the risk of backstrain.

419 **Ramplette Telescoping Ramp**
Graham-Field Health Products
2935 Northeast Pkwy
Atlanta, GA 30360-2808
678-291-3207
800-347-5678
FAX: 770-368-4702
e-mail: cs@grahamfield.com
www.grahamfield.com

Kenneth Spett, President & Chief Executive Officer
Cherie Antoniazzi, SVP Quality, Regulatory and Risk Management
Ivan Bielik, Senior Vice President, Business Analyst
Marc Bernstein, Senior Vice President, Consumer Sales

A multi-functional, easily moved, economical ramp weighing 25 pounds.

420 **Rickshaw Exerciser**
Access to Recreation
8 Sandra Ct
Newbury Park, CA 91320-4302
805-498-7535
800-634-4351
FAX: 805-498-8186
e-mail: customerservice@accesstr.com
www.accesstr.com

Don Krebs, President/ Founder

This Exerciser develops the muscle used most by those in wheelchairs. It develops the strength you need to lift yourself for pressure relief, doing transfers and pushing your wheelchair.

421 **Ricon Corporation**
1135 Aviation Place
San Fernando, CA 91340-6090
818-267-3000
800-322-2884
FAX: 818-962-1201
e-mail: sales@riconcorp.com
www.riconcorp.com

John Condon, National Sales Manager
Mike O'Neill, Eastern Saler Manager
Peter Buckley, Central Area Sales Manager

Ricon corporation is a world leader in the manufacture of lifts and other mobility products for people with disabilities. The Ricon product line features the Activan (R) a lowered floor minivan conversion, wheelchair lifts power seat base and automatic door openers.

422 **Smart Leg**
Invacare Corporation
1 Invacare Way
Elyria, OH 44035-4190 440-329-6000
800-333-6900
FAX: 877-619-7996
e-mail: info@invacare.com
www.invacare.com

A Malachi Mixon Iii, Chairman of the Board
Gerald B. Blouch, President and Chief Executive Officer
Joseph B. Richey, II, President - Invacare Technologies Division
Robert K. Gudbranson, Senior Vice President and Chief Financial Officer
An ingenious elevating leg rest that automatically extends to correctly fit every outstretched leg.

423 **Smooth Mover**
Dixie EMS
10101 Foster Ave
Brooklyn, NY 11236-3425 718-257-6400
800-347-3494
FAX: 718-257-6401
e-mail: customerservice@dixieems.com
www.dixieems.com

Eva Silverstein, President
Patient mover is a board designed to transfer patients from bed to stretcher or table with one or two people. *$199.95*

424 **SpectraLift**
Inclinator Company of America
601 Gibson Blvd
Harrisburg, PA 17104-3215 717-939-8420
800-343-9007
FAX: 717-939-8075
e-mail: isales@inclinator.com
www.inclinator.com

Stephen Nock, President
A newly designed hydraulic wheelchair lift made of fiberglass construction suitable for commercial and residential use.

425 **Spectrum Aquatics**
7100 Spectrum Ln
Missoula, MT 59808-8416 406-543-6823
800-791-8056
FAX: 800-791-8057
e-mail: nkhaled@spectrumproducts.com
www.spectrumproducts.com

Nabil Khaled, Director of Sales
Rob Nelson, Manager of Logistics and Customer Service
Philip Frandsen, Customer Service Representative
Josh Hartley, Business Development Specialist (Southeast Region)

426 **Spectrum Products Catalog**
Spectrum Products
982 County Route 1
Pine Island, NY 10969-1205 406-542-9781
800-724-5305
FAX: 800-791-8057
e-mail: info@spectrumproducts.com
www.spectrumproducts.com

Nabil Khaled, Dir. of Sales
Chris Rhyne, Business Dev. Specialist
Rob Nelson, Mgr of Logistics
Manufacturers of swimming pool disabled access products such as lifts, ramps, railings, ladders, and stainless steel hydrotherapy tanks for the swimming pool and medical therapy markets.

427 **StairLIFT SC & SL**
Inclinator Company of America
601 Gibson Blvd
Harrisburg, PA 17104-3215 717-939-8420
800-343-9007
FAX: 717-939-8075
e-mail: isales@inclinator.com
www.inclinator.com

Stephen Nock, President
Simple, self-contained and efficient stair units.

428 **Stairway Elevators**
Bruno Independent Living Aids
P.O. Box 84
1780 Executive Drive
Oconomowoc, WI 53066 262-567-4990
800-882-8183
FAX: 262-953-5510
www.bruno.com

Michael R. Bruno, II, President/CEO
Andrew Bayer, Product Mgr, Automotive Div.
Mike Krawczyk, Mktg Svcs Mgr
Bruno offers a full line of stairway elevators, including the Electra-Ride II featuring access during power interruptions, convenient installation, comfort and a powerful drive system. The Electra-Ride which features battery-powered technology, a rail width of 25 inches and seat rotation for easy transfers. The Comfort-Ride AC stair lift which is battery operated, has a rail width of 7.25 inches and folded width of less than 14.5 inches.

429 **Straight and Custom Curved Stairlifts**
Bruno Independent Living Aids
P.O.Box 84
1780 Executive Drive
Oconomowoc, WI 53066 262-567-4990
800-882-8183
FAX: 262-953-5501
www.bruno.com

Michael R. Bruno, II, President/CEO
Andrew Bayer, Product Mgr, Automotive Div.
Mike Krawczyk, Mktg Svcs Mgr
Bruno stairlifts can fit almost any curve or straight rail application and requires little or no structural modification to the stairway. Normal rail position for a Bruno inside turn is 7 to 8 inches from the wall or obstruction which is the tightest radius of any stairlift manufacturing company in the world. The Bruno inside turn is ideal for bi-level homes or staircases with mid-level doors. Bruno's unique battery power allows for uninterrupted operation even during a power outage.

430 **Superarm Lift for Vans By Handicaps, Inc.**
4335 S Santa Fe Dr
Englewood, CO 80110 303-781-2062
800-782-4335
FAX: 303-761-6811
e-mail: info@handicapsinc.com
www.handicapsinc.com

431 **SureHands Lift & Care Systems**
982 County Route 1
Pine Island, NY 10969-1205 845-258-6500
800-724-5305
FAX: 845-258-6634
e-mail: info@surehands.com
www.surehands.com

Thomas F Herceg, President
Joyce Moraczewski, Marketing Coordinator
SureHands specializes in lift & care systems for both homecare and professional settings where the user's safety is most important. Offering a variety of lift and transfer options, SureHands provides the necessary tools to overcome physical and architectural barriers to deliver a system designed to meet the specific needs of the user.

432 **The Braun Corporation**
631 West 11th Street
Winamac, IN 46996-310 574-946-6153
800-843-5438
FAX: 574-946-4670
e-mail: mediaquestions@braunlift.com
www.braunability.com

Nick Gutwein, President
Greg Cook, Vice President Sales & Marketing
Joe Garnett, Director Of Marketing
Ralph Braun, Founder/ CEO
The Braun Corporation is the world's largest manufacturer of wheelchair-accessible vans, ramps and wheelchair lifts. Our

products enable people with physical disabilities to regain their mobility and to lead active and independent lives. Our companies broad product line includes the Chrysler/Dodge Entervan, the Honda Odyssey Entervan, and the Toyota Sienna Rampvan.

433 **Thyssen Krupp Access**
4001 E 138th St
Grandview, MO 64030-2837
816-200-1954
800-829-9760
FAX: 816-763-4467
e-mail: dealerinfo@tkaccess.com
www.tkaccess.com

Jurrien van Akker, CEO
Scott Zoetewey, Vice President of Operations
Thomas Hance, President

Whether you want to open your facility or stay in the home you love, Thyssen Krupp Access has the perfect wheelchair lift, stair lift or elevator to suit your budget and needs. Our lifts have the best warranties. Our nationwide network of dealers are close by and ready to help.

434 **Turning Automotive Seating (TAS)**
Bruno Independent Living Aids
P.O.Box 84
Oconomowoc, WI 53066-84
262-567-4990
800-882-8183
FAX: 262- 95- 550
e-mail: info@bruno.com
www.bruno.com

Michael R. Bruno, II, President/CEO
Cindy Schmidt, Customer Relations
Steve Nelson, Service Manager
Thomas Jacobson, Senior Vice President

Transfer in and out of a car, minivan, pickup truck and full size van without any lifting!

435 **Vangater, Vangater II, Mini-Vangater**
631 West 11th Street
Winamac, IN 46996-310
800-THE-LIFT
FAX: 574-946-4670
e-mail: mediaquestions@braunlift.com
www.braunability.com

Ralph Braun, Founder

Tri-fold and fold-in-half lifts represent a major innovation in the field of adapted van transportation.

436 **Versatrainer**
Pro- Max/ Division Of Bow- Flex Of America
2200 NE 65th Ave
Vancouver, WA 98661-6978
800-618-8853
800-952-7205
FAX: 360-993-3610
e-mail: customerservice@bowflex.com
www.bowflex.com

437 **Vestibular Board**
Bailey Manufacturing Company
P.O. Box 130
Lodi, OH 44254-130
800-321-8372
FAX: 800-224-5390
e-mail: baileymfg@baileymfg.com
www.baileymfg.com

438 **Wheelchair Carrier**
7325 Douglas Road
Lambertville, MI 48144-2624
734-568-6084
800-541-3213
FAX: 734-568-6705
e-mail: admin@WheelChairCarrier.com
wheelchaircarrier.com

David Makulinsky, President
Mike Siler, Engineer
Christina Makulinski, Office Manager

Wheelchair, scooter and powerchair carriers for hitch mount on vehicles, priced from $199 to $999.

Major Catalogs

439 **Access Store Products for Barrier Free Environments**
Access Store.Com
820 W 7th St
Chico, CA 95928-5011
530-893-1596
800-497-2003
FAX: 530-893-1560
e-mail: sales@accessstore.com
www.accessstore.com

Tim Vander Heiden, Owner
Lisa Bantum, Sales Administrator

One of the largest online ADA Compliance Catalogs available. Offers everything from innovative barrier removal products to survey equipment, to unique specialty products.

440 **Access to Recreation**
8 Sandra Ct
Newbury Park, CA 91320-4302
805-498-7535
800-634-4351
FAX: 805-498-8186
e-mail: customerservice@accesstr.com
www.accesstr.com

Don Krebs, President

The Access to Recreation catalog is full of recreation and exercise equipment. One can find items such as electric fishing reels and other fishing and hunting equipment for the disabled sportsman. There are also adapted golf clubs, swimming pool lifts, wheelchair gloves and cuffs and bowling equipment. There are devices to help with embroidery, knitting and card playing, videos, books and practical aides such as wheelchair ramps and book.

64 pages Bi-Annually

441 **Achievement Products**
P.O. Box 6013
Carol Stream, IL 60197-6013
800-373-4699
FAX: 800-766-4303
e-mail: Bids@achievement-products.com
www.specialkidszone.com

Teresa Cardon, VP

Offer a wide range of pediatric rehabilitation equipment and special education products including handwriting aids, weighted vests, positioning equipment, sensory integration products and adaptive furniture. Call for your free catalog.

442 **Adaptive Clothing: Adults**
Special Clothes
P.O.Box 333
E Harwich, MA 02645-333
508-430-2410
FAX: 508-430-2410
TTY:508-430-2410
e-mail: SPECIALCLO@aol.com
www.special-clothes.com

Judith Sweeney, President

Special Clothes produces a catalogue of garments for adults with disabilities and/or incontinence. Offerings include: undergarments, snap-crotch tee shirts, sleepwear, jumpsuits, bibs and some footwear. The catalogue is available without charge. Comparable to department store prices. Special Clothes produces a catalog of adaptive clothing for children in sizes from toddler through young adults. A full line of clothing is included from undergarments through wheelchair jackets and ponchos.

443 **Adaptive Technology Catalog**
Synapse Adaptive
14 Lynn Ct
San Rafael, CA 94901-5114
415-455-9700
800-317-9611
FAX: 415-455-9801
e-mail: info@synapse-ada.com
www.synapseadaptive.com

Martin Tibor, President

Adaptive technology for individuals with disabilities, ADA compliant workstations, and ergonomic furniture. Products accommodate blindness, low vision, mobility impairments or learning differences.

444 **Adult Long Jumpsuit with Feet**
Special Clothes
P.O.Box 333
E Harwich, MA 02645-333
508-896-7939
FAX: 508-896-7939
e-mail: specialclo@aol.com
www.special-clothes.com
Judith Sweeney, President
Line of clothing for people with disabilities. Child and adult catalog available.

445 **Adult Short Jumpsuit**
Special Clothes
P.O.Box 333
E Harwich, MA 02645-333
508-896-7939
FAX: 508-896-7939
e-mail: specialclo@aol.com
www.special-clothes.com
Judith Sweeney, President
This pull-on jumpsuit provides comfort and full coverage without bulk. Wide leg ribbing ends at mid-thigh, with snaps at the crotch. We use fine quality, comfortable cotton knit. 100% cotton knit. Made in USA. Option: long sleeves - add $3.00. Colors: white, navy, teal, light blue, light pink, red, burgundy, royal blue and black. Sm & Med: $36.50/3 for $104.00; L & XL: $39.00/3 for $111.25; and XXL: $42.00/3 for $119.25.

446 **AliMed**
297 High Street
Dedham, MA 02026
800-225-2610
FAX: 800-437-2966
e-mail: cust_serv@alimed.com
alimed.com

447 **American Discount Medical**
459 Main St
Ste 101-417
Trussville, AL 35173
205-467-6995
800-877-9100
FAX: 205-467-7095
e-mail: Sales@AmericanDiscountMed.com
www.americandiscountmed.com
Tom Ruf, President
Deeply discounts every major brand medical product available.

448 **Apria Healthcare**
26220 Enterprise Ct
Lake Forest, CA 92630-8405
949-639-2000
800-277-4288
e-mail: contact_us@apria.com
www.apria.com
Dan Starck, Chief Executive Officer
Nichola Denney, Executive Vice President, Revenue Management
Lisa M. Getson, EVP, Government Relations, Investor Relations and Compliance
Bill Guidetti, Executive Vice President, East Zone
Lifts, chairs, bathroom aids, bedroom aids, eating utensils and independent living aids for the physically challenged.

449 **Armstrong Medical**
575 Knightsbridge Parkway
P.O. Box 700
Lincolnshire, IL 60069-700
847-913-0101
800-323-4220
FAX: 847-913-0138
e-mail: csr@armstrongmedical.com
www.armstrongmedical.com
Armstrong, CEO
Diane Joseph, customer representative
Training aids, anatomical models, medical equipment, pediatrics equipment and rehabilitation equipment.

450 **Assistive Technology Journal**
1700 N Moore St
Suite 1905
Rosslyn, VA 22209-1905
703-243-1975
FAX: 703-524-6630
e-mail: info@technologistsinc.com
www.technologistsinc.com
Bi-Annually

451 **Assistive Technology Sourcebook**
Special Needs Project
Ste H
324 State St
Santa Barbara, CA 93101-2364
805-962-8087
818-718-9900
FAX: 818-349-2027
e-mail: editor@specialneeds.com
www.specialneeds.com
Hod Gray, Owner
Marian Hall, Editor
Provides you with 18 chapters of practical information on all aspects of assistive technology for individuals with functional limitations. *$60.00*
576 pages

452 **Bailey**
Bailey Manufacturing
P.O.Box 130
Lodi, OH 44254-130
800-321-8372
FAX: 800-224-5390
e-mail: baileymfg@baileymfg.com
www.baileymfg.com
70 pages

453 **Best 25 Catalog Resources for Making Life Easier**
Meeting Life's Challenges
9042 Aspen Grove Ln
Madison, WI 53717-2700
608-824-0402
FAX: 608-824-0403
e-mail: help@meetinglifeschallenges.com
www.meetinglifeschallenges.com
Shelley Peterman Schwarz, President
Deborah, Dir. of Mktg & Dev.
Unique reference guide to locate thousands of useful and hard-to-find adaptive devices to make dressing, eating, cooking, grooming, communicating, playing, exercising, etc. easier, safer and less frustrating for people of all ages and disabilities. A comprehensive, up-do-date reference for people with disabilities, caregivers and healthcare professionals. *$8.95*
36 pages
ISBN 1-891854-03-8

454 **Body Suits**
Special Clothes
P.O.Box 333
E Harwich, MA 02645-333
508-430-2410
FAX: 508-430-2410
e-mail: specialclo@aol.com
www.special-clothes.com
Judith Bari, President
Bodysuits, Jumpsuits, back opening garments, incontinence wear, bibs. Features include snap crotches and g-tube pockets.

455 **Cambridge Career Products Catalog**
Cambridge Educational
132 West 31st Street
17th Floor
New York, NY 10001
800-322-8755
800-468-4227
FAX: 609-679-0266
e-mail: custserv@films.com
www.cambridge.films.com/
Lisa Schmuclei, Marketing Director
A full color catalog featuring hundreds of products designed to aid people in career exploration, selecting specific occupations

and obtaining these jobs through resume and interview preparation.
64 pages BiAnnual

456 **Carex Health Brands**
P.O. Box 2526
Sioux Falls, SD 57101-2526
800-328-2935
FAX: 888-616-4297
e-mail: customerservice@carex.com
carex.com

457 **Carolyn's Low Vision Products**
3938 S Tamiami Trl
Sarasota, FL 34231-3622
941-373-9100
800-648-2266
FAX: 941-739-5503
e-mail: info@carolynscatalog.com
www.carolynscatalog.com
John Colton, Owner
Free mail-order catalog of items for visually impaired people. We also have a retail store.

458 **Communication Aids for Children and Adults**
Crestwood Communication Aids
6589 N
Crestwood Drive
Milwaukee, WI 53209
414-351-0311
FAX: 414-351-0311
e-mail: crestcomm@aol.com
www.communicationaids.com
Ruth B Leff, President
A free catalog of communication aids for children and adults with disabilities. Over 300 light and high tech switches and aids, and a large selection of adapted and voice-activated toys. Talking Pictures and Passports communication boards, easy to use and moderately priced talking aids.
32 pages Yearly

459 **Danmar Products**
221 Jackson Industrial Drive
Ann Arbor, MI 48103-9104
734-761-1990
800-783-1998
FAX: 734-761-8977
e-mail: sales@danmarproducts.com
www.danmarproducts.com
Dan Russo, President
Karen Green, Sales
Hidie Bowman, Sales
Manufactures adaptive equipment for persons with physical and mental disabilities, from seating and positioning equipment, flotation devices, toileting aids to hard and soft shell helmets.

460 **Dayspring Associates**
2111 Foley Rd
Havre De Grace, MD 21078-1703
410-939-5900
FAX: 410-939-6252
Benedict Schwartz, Manager
This publisher provides a directory of 1,000 rehabilitation aids.

461 **Disabilities Sourcebook**
Omnigraphics
155 West Congress
Suite 200
Detroit, MI 48226
313-961-1340
800-234-1340
FAX: 313-961-1383
e-mail: contact@omnigraphics.com
www.omnigraphics.com
Paul Rogers, Publicity Associate
Georgiann Fratoni, Customer Service Manager
Peter Ruffner
$78.00
616 pages
ISBN 0-780803-89-2

462 **Disability Bookshop Catalog**
P.O.Box 129
Vancouver, WA 98666-129
360-694-2462
800-637-2256
FAX: 360-696-3210
e-mail: twinpeak@pacifier.com
www.disabilitybookshop.virtualave.net/
40 pages

463 **Dressing Tips and Clothing Resources for Making Life Easier**
Attainment Company
504 Commerce Parkway
P.O.Box 930160
Verona, WI 53593-160
608-845-7880
800-327-4269
FAX: 608-845-8040
e-mail: info@attainmentcompany.com
www.attainmentcompany.com
Don Bastian, Founder and CEO
Scott Meister, Director of Software Development
Sue Lockard, Director of Operations/Dealer Sales
Karen Riley, Shipping/Receiving Manager
Learn hundreds of simple tips and techniques to make dressing easier. Learn how to adapt/modify ready-to-wear garments to accommodate your special dressing needs. Find out how to locate more than 100 resources offering specially designed or easy-on/easy-off clothing for men, women, children and/or wheelchair users. You'll find everything you need to look your best. An invaluable resource for people with special dressing needs, people with disabilities, caregivers and healthcare professionals. *$19.00*
144 pages 2000
ISBN 1-578611-19-9

464 **Enrichments Catalog**
Sammons Preston Rolyan
28100 Torch Parkway
Suite 700
Warrenville, IL 60555-3938
630-378-6000
800-323-5547
FAX: 630-393-7600
e-mail: sp@pattersonmedical.com
www.pattersonmedical.com
David P Sproat, President
Bruce Curtis, Sales Representative
Provides people with physical challenges with the products they need to help live their lives to the fullest. Includes items for everyday tasks and personal care; assistive products for home use; toileting and bathing aids; grooming and dressing devices; kitchen and dining aids. Also items for range of motion, mobility and exercise such as weights, therapy putty and exercise equipment; ergonomic gloves and supports; canes, crutches, walkers and wheelchair accessories. 36-page catalog.

465 **Equipment Shop**
34 Hartford Street
Bedford, MA 01730-33
781-275-7681
800-525-7681
FAX: 781-275-4094
e-mail: info@equipmentshop.com
www.equipmentshop.com
Ken Larson, Owner
Barbara Johnston, General Manager
Specializing in oral motor therapy equipment including flexi cut cups, maroon spoons, chewy tubes, ARK grabbers and z-vibes. Also tricycle foot peal attachments and trike back supports as well as fat wheels.

466 **Essential Medical Supply, Inc.**
6420 Hazeltine National Drive
Orlando, FL 32822
800-826-8423
FAX: 407-770-0624
essentialmedicalsupply.com

467 **Everest & Jennings**
Division of Graham-Field
2935 Northeast Parkway
Atlanta, GA 30360
678-291-3207
800-347-5678
FAX: 770-368-2386
e-mail: cs@grahamfield.com
www.grahamfield.com
Kenneth Spett, President & Chief Executive Officer
Cherie Antoniazzi, SVP Quality, Regulatory and Risk Management
Ivan Bielik, Senior Vice President, Business Analyst
Marc Bernstein, Senior Vice President, Consumer Sales
Manufactures more than 200 items for persons with physical disabilities, including wheelchairs, seat cushions, shower chairs, grab bars and more.

468 **Express Medical Supply**
218 Seebold Spur
Fenton, MO 63026
636-349-8448
800-633-2139
FAX: 800-633-9188
e-mail: sales@exmed.net
www.exmed.net
Bill Nahm, President
Offers a full line of medical and ostomy supplies at discounted prices. Order by phone or online.

469 **FlagHouse Rehab Resources**
601 FLAGHOUSE DRIVE
Hasbrouck Heights, NJ 07604-3116
201-288-7600
800-793-7900
FAX: 800-793-7922
www.flaghouse.com
George Carmel, President

470 **FlagHouse Special Populations**
601 FLAGHOUSE DRIVE
Hasbrouck Heights, NJ 07604-3116
201-288-7600
800-793-7900
FAX: 800-793-7922
e-mail: sales@flaghouse.com
www.flaghouse.com
Brigid de Lime, Sr Brand Manager
Diana Hohman, Brand Manager
Contains over 2,000 products of interest to therapy professionals.
Bi-Annually

471 **Freedom Rider**
Freedom Rider
5225 Tudor Ct
Naples, FL 34112
603-540-0933
888-253-8811
FAX: 866-522-4708
e-mail: info@freedomrider.com
www.freedomrider.com
Victoria Surr, President
A catalog of equipment for people with disabilities who ride and drive horses which includes instructional aids, vaulting equipment, and lots of hard to find items.

472 **HAC Hearing Aid Centers of America: HARC Mercantile**
Hearing Center
1111 W Centre Ave
Portage, MI 49024
269-324-0301
800-445-9968
888-426-6632
FAX: 269-324-2387
e-mail: info@harc.com
www.hacofamerica.com

473 **Health and Rehabilitation Products**
Luminaud
8688 Tyler Blvd
Mentor, OH 44060
440-255-9082
800-255-3408
FAX: 440-255-2250
e-mail: info@luminaud.com
www.luminaud.com
Thomas M Lennox, President
Dorothy Lennox, VP
Switches for limited capability, stoma and trach covers, shower protectors and thermo-stim oral motor stimulator. Personal voice amplifiers for people with weak voices. Artificial larynges for people with no voices. Small electronic communication boards. Books for laryngectomies and speech pathologists.

474 **HealthCare Solutions**
Blue Chip II
3478 Hauck Rd
Cincinnati, OH 45241
513-271-5115
800-417-5115
FAX: 513-527-3686
Michael Leabhart, Manager
Quality rehabilitation equipment sales and rental. Available equipment includes manual and powered mobility, positioning/seating equipment, vehicle modification, environmental controls, augmentative and alternative communication devices, adaptive computer access, ambulance aids and aids for daily living. Equipment provision is carried out through a total team approach. .

475 **Hear You Are**
98 Us Highway 46
Budd Lake, NJ 07828-1818
973-347-7662
FAX: 973-691-0611
Dorinne S Davis, President
A large catalog of various assistive and communication devices for people who are hearing impaired. *$3.00*
42 pages

476 **Hig's Manufacturing**
8375 Sunset Rd Ne
Minneapolis, MN 55418-3238
763-795-9478
FAX: 612-788-1926
Jim Murphy, Owner
Factory direct, lightweight aluminum, portable, 2 & 4-way folding, telescoping tracks, threshold, van, scooter and approach ramps.

477 **Huntleigh Healthcare**
2349, W Lake Street
Suite 250
Addison, IL 60101
630-785-4490
800-323-1245
FAX: 888-389-2756
e-mail: us.info@ArjoHuntleigh.com
www.huntleigh-healthcare.com

478 **Invacare Corporation**
1 Invacare Way
Elyria, OH 44035-4190
800-333-6900
FAX: 877-619-7996
e-mail: info@invacare.com
invacare.com
A. Malachi Mixon, III, Chair
Gerald B. Blouch, President/CEO
Joseph B. Richley, II, President
Robert K. Gudbranson, Senior Vice President/Chief Financial Officer
The global leader in the manufacture and distribution of innovative home and long-term care medical products that promote recovery and active lifestyles.

479 **Kleinert's**
433 Newton Street
Elba, AL 36323
800-498-7051
FAX: 305-937-0825
e-mail: customercare@kleinerts.com
www.hygienics.com
Michael Brier, President
Offers a complete line of incontinence products and skin care products consisting of disposable and reusable panties for women and pants for men. Also disposable liners, diapers and underpads.
16 pages Bi-Annual

480 **LS&S**
145 River Rock Drive
Buffalo, NY 14207
716-348-3500
800-468-4789
FAX: 877-498-1482
TTY: 800-317-8533
www.LSSproducts.com
Melissa Balbach, President
John K Bace, Executive Vice President.
Specializes in products for the blind, visually impaired, hearing impaired, and deaf. Free catalog upon request.

481 **Lighthouse Low Vision Products**
Lighthouse International
111 E 59th St
New York, NY 10022-1202
212-821-9200
800-829-0500
FAX: 212-821-9707
e-mail: info@lighthouse.org
www.lighthouse.org
Mark Ackermann, Chief Executive Officer
Joseph A Ripp, Chairman
Sarah Smith, Treasurer
This organization provides health care services related to vision loss; Career and academic services for people with vision loss; Music instruction and pre K curriculum for visually impaired students.

482 **Luminaud**
8688 Tyler Blvd
Mentor, OH 44060-4348
440-255-9082
800-255-3408
FAX: 440-255-2250
e-mail: info@luminaud.com
www.luminaud.com
Thomas M Lennox, President
Dorothy Lennox, VP
Offers a line of artificial larynx, personal voice amplifiers, special switches, stoma covers and other communication, health and safety items.

483 **MOMS Catalog**
9385 Dielman Ind Dr
Saint Louis, MO 63132-2214
800-269-4663
FAX: 314-997-0047
e-mail: custcare@hdis.com
www.hdis.com
Bruce Grench, President
MOMS catalog features high quality, incontinence supplies, mobility products, bath safety products urological products, aids for daily living products, ostomy supplies and many other adaptive items. MOMS offers low prices, excellent customer service and convenient home delivery to your doorstep.
52 pages

484 **Maddak Inc.**
661 Route 23 S
Wayne, NJ 07470
800-443-4926
FAX: 973-305-0841
e-mail: custservice@maddak.com
maddak.com

485 **Maxi Aids**
42 Executive Blvd
Farmingdale, NY 11735-4710
631-752-0521
800-522-6294
FAX: 631-752-0689
TTY: 800-281-3555
e-mail: sales@maxiaids.com
www.maxiaids.com
Elliot Zaretsky, Founder/ President
Products specially designed for the blind, low vision, visually impaired, deaf, deaf-blind, hard of hearing, arthritic, diabetic and individuals with special needs.

486 **New Vision Store**
919 Walnut Street
Philadelphia, PA 19107
215-627-0600
FAX: 215-922-0692
e-mail: asbinfo@asb.org
www.asb.org
Patricia C. Johnson, President & Chief Executive Officer
Derby Ewing, Director, Human Services
Brian Rusk, Public Relations Officer
Richard Forsythe, Director, Braille Division and Custom Audio
Catalog for individuals with visual impairments, listing visual aids, magnifiers, large print books and more.
30 pages

487 **Patterson Medical Holdings, Inc.**
1000 Remington Blvd. Suite 210
Bolingbrook, IL 60440-5117
800-323-5547
FAX: 800-547-4333
e-mail: customersupport@pattersonmedical.com
pattersonmedical.com

488 **Pearson Performance Solutions**
1 North Dearborn
Suite 1150
Chicago, IL 60602
800-922-7343
FAX: 312-242-4403
e-mail: HCM.info@vangent.com
hcrm.gdit.com
David Fabianski, Senior VP and General Mgr
Cindy Hotsky, finance Dir.
Julia McClung, VP, Talent Management Solutions
Publishes human resource assessment instruments for employment settings. The instruments include job analysis procedures to identify important characteristics for job success and objective assessment procedures to evaluate applicants and employees on these characteristics.

489 **Pearson Reid London House**
1 North Dearborn Street
Chicago, IL 60602-4335
FAX: 312-242-4403
e-mail: HCM.info@vangent.com
www.pearsonreidlondonhouse.com/index.htm
David Fabianski, Senior VP and General Mgr
Cindy Hotsky, finance Dir.
Julia McClung, VP, Talent Management Solutions

490 **Potomac Technology**
1500 Olympic Boulevard
Santa Monica, CA 90404
310-656-4924
800-233-9130
FAX: 310-450-9918
TTY: 800-233-9130
www.weitbrecht.com/
24 pages

491 Prentke Romich Company Product Catalog
1022 Heyl Rd
Wooster, OH 44691-9786
330-262-1984
800-262-1984
FAX: 330-263-4829
e-mail: info@prentrom.com
www.prentrom.com

David L Moffatt, President
Dave Moffatt, President/ COO
Barry Romich, Co-Founder

A full line, product catalog containing information on speech-output communication devices, environmental controls and computer access products.

492 Products for People with Disabilities
LS&S
145 River Rock Drive
Buffalo, NY 14207
716-348-3500
800-468-4789
FAX: 877-498-1482
TTY: 866-317-8533
e-mail: info@LSSproducts.com
www.LSSproducts.com

John K Bace, Executive Vice President

LS&S, LLC has a free catalog of products for the blind, deaf, visually and hearing impaired including: TTYs, computer adaptive devices, CCTVs, talking blood pressure, blood glucose and talking scales.

493 Rehabilitation Engineering and Assistive Technology Society of North America (RESNA)
1700 North Moore Street
Suite 1540
Arlington, VA 22209- 1903
703-524-6686
FAX: 703-524-6630
TTY:703-524-6639
e-mail: membership@resna.org
www.resna.org

Alex Mihailidis, PhD, P.Eng, President
Ray Grott, ATP, RET, President-Elect
Paul J. Schwartz, Treasurer
Jamie Arasz Prioli, ATP, Secretary

RESNA improves the potential of people with disabilities to achieve their goals through the use of technology. RESNA promotes research, development, education, advocacy and provision of technology; and by supporting the people engaged in these activities.

494 Sammons Preston Enrichments Catalog
Sammons Preston Rolyan
28100 Torch Parkway
Suite 700
Warrenville, IL 60555-3938
630-378-6000
800-323-5547
FAX: 630-393-7600
e-mail: sp@pattersonmedical.com
www.pattersonmedical.com

David P Sproat, President
Bruce Curtis, Sales Representative

Our Enrichments Catalog offers products that make the tasks and challenges of living at home— bathing, getting dressed, getting around— a little easier. Choose from personal care items to kitchen and dining aids, household helpers to mobility devices, plus a complete selection of pain-reducing products, exercise items, health monitoring equipment and more.
40 pages Yearly

495 Sportaid
78 Bay Creek Rd
Loganville, GA 30052
770-554-5033
800-743-7203
FAX: 770-554-5944
e-mail: stuff@sportaid.com
www.sportaid.com

Stacy Green, Owner
jimmy green, Owner

Offers an assortment of wheelchairs (everyday and racing), wheelchair sports equipment, replacement tires, hubs, spokes, pushrims, cushions and more. Call for free catalog.
68 pages Yearly

496 Store @ HDSC Product Catalog
Hearing, Speech & Deafness Center (HDSC)
1625 19th Ave
Seattle, WA 98122-2848
206-323-5770
888-222-5036
800-761-2821
FAX: 206-328-6871
TTY:206-452-7953
e-mail: seattle@hsdc.org
www.hsdc.org

Pamela Anderson, President
Ken Block, Vice President
Dan Bridge, Interim Executive Director
Deanna Aberle, Director of Speech

32 pages Yearly

497 Ultratec
450 Science Dr
Madison, WI 53711-1166
608-238-5400
800-482-2424
FAX: 608-238-3008
TTY: 800-482-2424
e-mail: service@ultratec.com
www.ultratec.com

Jackie Morgan, Marketing Director
Robert M Engelke, CEO

Works to make telephone access more convenient and reliable for people with hearing loss.
Yearly

498 WCI/Weitbrecht Communications
1500 Olympic Boulevard
Santa Monica, CA 90405
310-656-4924
800-233-9130
FAX: 310-450-9918
TTY: 800-233-9130
www.weitbrecht.com

24 pages

499 Walgreens Home Medical Center
7173 Cermak Rd
Berwyn, IL 60402-2103
708-795-1295
800-323-2828
FAX: 708-795-1308

Stan Kozlowski, Manager

Hospital supplies and home medical equipment with nationwide direct mail delivery. .

500 Walton Way Medical
1225 Walton Way
Augusta, GA 30901-2141
706-722-0276
FAX: 706-722-0279

Michael Bower, President

Offers medical, therapeutic, urological, hygiene and skin care products for disabled persons.

Miscellaneous

501 Access-USA
242 James St
PO Box 160
Clayton, NY 13624-160
800-263-2750
FAX: 800-563-1687
e-mail: info@access-usa.com
www.access-usa.com

Deborah Haight, PICOE

Access-USA provides one-stop alternate format transcription services for almost any type of document-reports, schedules, menus, monthly statements, brochures, reports, etc. Items may be submitted on computer disk, hard copy or email. Alternate formats include Braille, large print, Braille and print, audio recordings, adapted disks as well as video services-open/closed captioning and video descriptions. Accessible products also include Braille Business Cards and ADA signage.

502 **Access-USA: Transcription Services**
242 James St
PO Box 160
Clayton, NY 13624-160
800-263-2750
FAX: 800-563-1687
e-mail: info@access-usa.com
www.access-usa.com

Deborah Haight, PICOE

Access-USA produces Braille business cards as well as offering alternate format services and products to enhance accessibility. Braille, large print, captioning, audio-descriptive forms are available. We help business, government, education, corporations by providing brochures, menus, manuals, books, collateral materials, videos, specialties and promotion items that can be more accessible to more people.

503 **BeOK Key Lever**
Sammons Preston Rolyan
28100 Torch Parkway
Suite 700
Warrenville, IL 60555-3938
630-378-6000
800-323-5547
FAX: 630-393-7600
e-mail: sp@pattersonmedical.com
www.pattersonmedical.com

David P Sproat, President
Bruce Curtis, Sales Representative

Handy accessory helps position key to provide maximum leverage enabling the user to work the most stubborn lock. *$11.50*

504 **Big Lamp Switch**
Maxi Aids
42 Executive Blvd
Farmingdale, NY 11735-4710
631-752-0521
800-522-6294
FAX: 631-752-0689
TTY: 800-281-3555
e-mail: sales@maxiaids.com
www.maxiaids.com

Elliot Zaretsky, President

This big, three-spoke knob replaces small rotating knobs which are a problem for those with arthritis or other limitations of the fingers. *$6.75*

505 **Bookholder: Roberts**
Therapro, Inc.
225 Arlington St
Framingham, MA 01702-8723
508-872-9494
800-257-5376
FAX: 508-875-2062
e-mail: info@therapro.com
www.therapro.com

Karen Conrad, ScD, OTR/L, Owner

Gray plastic, ideal for hand free reading, adjusts to all sizes of books and prevents pages from flipping for the physically challenged. *$27.50*

506 **Brandt Industries**
4461 Bronx Blvd
Bronx, NY 10470-1496
718-994-0800
800-221-8031
FAX: 718-325-7995
e-mail: brandtequip@yahoo.com
www.brandtind.com

507 **Bus and Taxi Sign**
Maxi Aids
42 Executive Blvd
Farmingdale, NY 11735-4710
631-752-0521
800-522-6294
FAX: 631-752-0689
TTY: 800-281-3555
e-mail: sales@maxiaids.com
www.maxiaids.com

508 **Care Electronics**
3301 W 151 Court
Broomfield, CO 8002
303-444-2273
888-444-8284
FAX: 303-447-3502
e-mail: tmoody@careelectronics.com
www.medicalshoponline.com

Tom Moody, President

Care Electronics manufactures safety monitoring systems for caregivers, home-health care, and nursing homes. WanderCARE monitors loved ones who tend to wander away from home. Care Deluxe Occupancy systems monitor patients in bed and in wheelchairs to help prevent falls. WetSENSE provides incontinence monitors.

509 **Child Convertible Balance Beam Set**
Bailey Manufacturing Company
P.O. Box 130
Lodi, OH 44254-130
800-321-8372
FAX: 800-224-5390
e-mail: baileymfg@baileymfg.com
www.baileymfg.com

510 **Child Variable Balance Beam**
Bailey Manufacturing Company
P.O. Box 130
Lodi, OH 44254-130
330-948-1080
800-321-8372
FAX: 330-948-4439
e-mail: baileymfg@baileymfg.com
www.baileymfg.com

511 **Child's Mobility Crawler**
Bailey Manufacturing Company
P.O. Box 130
Lodi, OH 44254-130
800-321-8372
FAX: 800-224-5390
e-mail: baileymfg@baileymfg.com
www.baileymfg.com

512 **Choice Switch Latch and Timer**
AbleNet
2625 Patton Road
Roseville, MN 55113-1308
651-294-2200
800-322-0956
FAX: 651-294-2259
e-mail: customerservice@ablenetinc.com
www.ablenetinc.com

Bill Sproull, Chairman of the Board
Jennifer Thalhuber, President/CEO
William Mills, Board of Director

A Choice Switch Latch and Timer allows one user to learn to make choices. It has two switch inputs and can control two devices. Once one device has been activated, the other will not function until the first one is turned off or completes its timed cycle. *$83.00*

513 **Cordless Big Red Switch**
AbleNet
2625 Patton Road
Roseville, MN 55113-1308
651-294-2200
800-322-0956
FAX: 651-294-2259
e-mail: customerservice@ablenetinc.com
www.ablenetinc.com

Bill Sproull, Chairman of the Board
Jennifer Thalhuber, President/CEO
William Mills, Board of Director

The Cordless Big Red Switch, when used in conjunction with either the Cordless Receiver or the Small Appliance Receiver, gives you cordless control of toys, games, and appliances in your environment. *$89.00*

514 DEUCE Environmental Control Unit
APT Technology
236a N Main St
Shreve, OH 44676
330-567-2001
888-549-2001
FAX: 330-567-3073
e-mail: sales@apt-technology.com
www.apt-technology.com

Grace Miller, Office Manager

Allows a severely disabled person to control a variety of useful devices via a dual switch. DEUCE controls phone, 4 AC powered devices such as a radio, 4 switch controlled devices such as a page turner and up to 16 lights and or appliances distributed around the environment. Starts at $1,500. .

515 Dazor Manufacturing Corporation
2079 Congressiona
Saint Louis, MO 63146
314-652-2400
800-345-9103
FAX: 314-652-2069
e-mail: info@dazor.com
www.dazor.com

Kirk Cressey, Marketing Director
Bob Smith, National Sales Manager
Mark Hogrebe, President

Dazor is a US manufacturer of quality task lighting. Products include fluorescent, incandescent and halogen lighting fixtures. Illuminated magnifiers combine light and magnification to greatly enhance activities such as reading and make hobbies more enjoyable. All lamps come in a variety of mounting options to include desk bases, clamp on, floor stands and wall tracks. $95 - $450.

516 Digi-Flex
Therapro, Inc.
225 Arlington St
Framingham, MA 01702-8723
508-872-9494
800-257-5376
FAX: 508-875-2062
e-mail: info@therapro.com
www.therapro.com

Karen Conrad, ScD, OTR/L, Owner

This is a unique hand and finger exercise unit. Recommended for use of individuation of fingers, web space and general strengthening of work hands. Available in a variety of resistances. *$ 17.50*

517 Dorma Architectural Hardware
DORMA Drive, Drawer AC
Reamstown, PA 17567-411
717-336-3881
866-401-6063
FAX: 717-336-2106
e-mail: archdw@dorma-usa.com
www.dorma-usa.com

Larry O'Toole, CEO
Gary Phillips AHC, VP Regional Sales, East
Ken Theaker, VP Regional Sales West

DORMA provides a complete line of door controls, including barrier-free units that comply with the Americans with Disabilities Act. A wide variety of surface applied and concealed closers, low energy operators, exit devices and electronic access control systems are available to address these equipments.

518 Dual Switch Latch and Timer
AbleNet
2625 Patton Road
Roseville, MN 55113-1308
651-294-2200
800-322-0956
FAX: 651-294-2259
e-mail: customerservice@ablenetinc.com
www.ablenetinc.com

Bill Sproull, Chairman of the Board
Jennifer Thalhuber, President/CEO
William Mills, Board of Director

A Dual Switch Latch and Timer allows two users to activate two devices at a time in the latch. Timed seconds or timed minutes mode of control. *$88.00*

519 Enabling Devices
50 Broadway
Hawthorne, CA 10532
914-747-3070
800-832-8697
FAX: 914-747-3480
e-mail: customer_support@enablingdevices.com
www.enablingdevices.com

Elizabeth Bell, Marketing Manager
Karen O'Connor, VP Operations
Steven Kanor, Owner

For more than 25 years, Enabling Devices has been dedicated to providing affordable learning and assistive devices for the physically challenged. Products include augmentative communicators, adapted toys, capability switches, training and sensory devices and activity centers. Call for a free catalog.

520 Foot Inversion Tread
Bailey Manufacturing Company
P.O. Box 130
Lodi, OH 44254-130
800-321-8372
FAX: 800-224-5390
e-mail: baileymfg@baileymfg.com
www.baileymfg.com

521 Foot Placement Ladder
Bailey Manufacturing Company
P.O. Box 130
Lodi, OH 44254-130
800-321-8372
FAX: 800-224-5390
e-mail: baileymfg@baileymfg.com
www.baileymfg.com

522 HealthCraft SuperPole Traveller
Maxi Aids
42 Executive Blvd
Farmingdale, NY 11735-4710
631-752-0521
800-522-6294
FAX: 631-752-0689
TTY: 800-281-3555
e-mail: sales@maxiaids.com
www.maxiaids.com

Elliot Zaretsky, President

Central to the system is a stylish floor-to-ceiling grab bar, which provides a secure structure that can be installed in minutes between a floor and ceiling. Use it beside a bed, bath, toilet or chair. *$193.00*

523 Home Bed Side Helper
Maxi Aids
42 Executive Blvd
Farmingdale, NY 11735-4710
631-752-0521
800-522-6294
FAX: 631-752-0689
TTY: 800-281-3555
e-mail: sales@maxiaids.com
www.maxiaids.com

Elliot Zaretsky, President

The extra support you need getting in and out of bed is within your grasp with this easy to install Home Bed Side Helper. The rail itself features four easily accessible grasping points for the secure support you need when getting in or out of bed. *$126.75*

524 Hospital Environmental Control System
Prentke Romich Company
1022 Heyl Rd
Wooster, OH 44691-9786
330-262-1984
800-848-8008
800-262-1933
FAX: 330-263-4829
e-mail: sales@prentrom.com
www.prentrom.com

David L Moffatt, President

Permits the non-ambulatory patient to operate a variety of electrical items in a single room. A large liquid crystal display is mounted in front of the user and they scan through the menu of operations and make a selection using a sip-puff switch. Options include nurse call, standard telephone functions, electric bed control, hospital television operation and electrical appliance on and off. *$3860.00*

525 Knock Light
HARC Mercantile
5413 S. Westnedge Ave.
Suite A
Portage, MI 49002
269-324-0301
800-445-9968
FAX: 269-324-2387
TTY: 269-324-1615
e-mail: info@harc.com
www.harc.com

526 Leg Elevation Board
Bailey Manufacturing Company
P.O. Box 130
Lodi, OH 44254-130
800-321-8372
FAX: 800-224-5390
e-mail: baileymfg@baileymfg.com
www.baileymfg.com

527 Leveron
Lindustries
21 Shady Hill Rd
Weston, MA 02193-1407
781-237-8177
877-794-9511
FAX: 651-989-2131
www.trademarkia.com/leveron-73486756.html

Willard H Lind, Owner
Louise T Lind, VP

Leveron is a doorknob lever handle for ease of operation. Leveron converts standard doorknobs to lever action without removing existing hardware. No gripping, twisting or pinching when hands are wet, arthritic or arms are full. Leveron provides convenience. Available in five colors: almond, satin brass, silver metallic, dark bronze and Hi-Glow (glows in the dark) at low cost to comply with ADA access requirements in public and private places. *$16.95*

528 Longreach Reacher
Therapro, Inc.
225 Arlington St
Framingham, MA 01702-8723
508-872-9494
800-257-5376
FAX: 508-875-2062
e-mail: info@therapro.com
www.therapro.com

Karen Conrad, ScD, OTR/L, Owner

Reacher is useful when reaching, sitting or when standing. *$18.95*

529 Loop Scissors
Therapro, Inc.
225 Arlington St
Framingham, MA 01702-8723
508-872-9494
800-257-5376
FAX: 508-875-2062
e-mail: info@therapro.com
www.therapro.com

Karen Conrad, ScD, OTR/L, Owner

Pliable, plastic handles that allow for easy and controlled cutting. *$14.25*

530 Pedal-in-Place Exerciser
Thoele Manufacturing
475 County Road 100 N
Montrose, IL 62445-3019
217-924-4553
FAX: 217-924-4553
www.axistive.com/thoele-manufacturing.html

531 Plastic Card Holder
Therapro, Inc.
225 Arlington St
Framingham, MA 01702-8723
508-872-9494
800-257-5376
FAX: 508-875-2062
e-mail: info@therapro.com
www.therapro.com

Karen Conrad, ScD, OTR/L, Owner

For those with reduced finger control. *$4.00*

532 Power Door
11240 Gemini Ln
Dallas, TX 75229-4710
800-688-1758
FAX: 972-620-9875
e-mail: info@powerdoor.com
www.powerdoor.com

Jim Goldthwaite, National Sales Manager

Power door, low energy door operators.

533 ProtectaCap, ProtectaCap+PLUS, ProtectaChin Guard and ProtectaHip
Plum Enterprises
P.O.Box 85
Valley Forge, PA 19481-85
610-783-7377
800-321-PLUM
FAX: 610-783-7577
e-mail: info@PlumEnt.com
www.plument.com

Janice Carrington, CEO

Plum Enterprises award winning, exquisite, ergonomic protective wear keeps you safe from the dangers of falls. ProtectCap+Plus and ProtectHips are engineered for superior shock-absorption and designed for exquisite simplicity and amazing lightweight comfort. The perfect blend of style and function.

534 Quad Commander
Gpk
535 Floyd Smith Dr
El Cajon, CA 92020-1228
619-593-7381
800-468-8679
FAX: 888-755-5603
e-mail: info@gpk.com
www.gpk.com

535 Rocker Balance Square
Bailey Manufacturing Company
P.O. Box 130
Lodi, OH 44254-130
800-321-8372
FAX: 800-224-5390
e-mail: baileymfg@baileymfg.com
www.baileymfg.com

536 Scott Sign Systems
7525 Pennsylvania Ave
Suite 101
Sarasota, FL 34243
941-355-5171
800-237-9447
FAX: 941-351-1787
e-mail: info@scottsigns.com
www.scottsigns.com

Kathy Hannon, VP
Evelyn Brown, Sales

Call for a brochure.

537 Series Adapter
AbleNet
2625 Patton Road
Roseville, MN 55113-1308
651-294-2200
800-322-0956
FAX: 651-294-2259
e-mail: customerservice@ablenetinc.com
www.ablenetinc.com

Bill Sproull, Chairman of the Board
Jennifer Thalhuber, President/CEO
William Mills, Board of Director

Allows two-switch operation of any battery-operated device or electrical devices. *$13.00*

538 Signaling Wake-Up Devices
HARC Mercantile
5413 S. Westnedge Ave.
Suite A
Portage, MI 49002
269-324-1615
800-445-9968
FAX: 269-324-2387
TTY: 269-324-1615
e-mail: info@harc.com
www.harc.com

Ron Slager, Owner
Wake up devices. Vibrating alarm clocks, available with flashing lights, louder alarm noises and more. *$29.50*

539 Smoke Detector with Strobe
HARC Mercantile
5413 S. Westnedge Ave.
Suite A
Portage, MI 49002
269-324-1615
800-445-9968
FAX: 269-324-2387
TTY: 269-324-1615
e-mail: info@harc.com
www.harc.com

Ron Slager, Owner
Most of the smoke alarms are twice as loud, and have a 120+ candela strobe that will wake a person from a sound sleep. Mounting hardware for ceiling or wall. *$165.95*

540 Spinal Network: The Total Wheelchair Resource Book
No Limits Communications & New Mobility
75-20 Astoria Blvd.
East Elmhurst, NY 11370
800-404-2898
888-850-0344
www.newmobility.com

Josie Byzek, Managing Editor
Jean Dobbs, Editorial Director
Tim Gilmer, Editor
Ian Ruder, Senior Editor
Nearly 600 pages of profiles, articles and resources on every topic of interest to wheelchair users. Subjects include health, coping, relationships, sexuality, parenthood, computers, sports, recreation, travel, personal assistance services, legal rights, financial strategies, employment, and media images. *$34.95*
400 pages

541 SteeleVest
Steele
P.O.Box 7304
Kingston, WA 98346-7304
360-297-4555
888-783-3538
FAX: 360-297-2816
www.steelevest.com

Sandra Steele, President
Vest developed by NASA provides an external cooling system.

542 TV & VCR Remote
AbleNet
2625 Patton Road
Roseville, MN 55113-1308
651-294-2200
800-322-0956
FAX: 651-294-2259
e-mail: customerservice@ablenetinc.com
www.ablenetinc.com

Bill Sproull, Chairman of the Board
Jennifer Thalhuber, President/CEO
William Mills, Board of Director
Controls a TV, a VCR or a TV that is connected through a VCR tuner. It may be programmed to control functions such as on and off, channel up, preprogrammed TV channels and, if desired, other TV functions such as mute and pause. *$82.00*

543 Tactile Thermostat
Sense-Sations
919 Walnut Street
Philadelphia, PA 19107-5237
215-627-0600
FAX: 215-922-0692
e-mail: asbinfo@asb.org
www.asb.org

Patricia C. Johnson, President & Chief Executive Officer
Derby Ewing, Director, Human Services
Brian Rusk, Public Relations Officer
Richard Forsythe, Director, Braille Division and Custom Audio
Large embossed numbers on cover ring and raised temperature setting knob. *$31.50*

544 Therapy Putty
Therapro, Inc.
225 Arlington St
Framingham, MA 01702-8723
508-872-9494
800-257-5376
FAX: 508-875-2062
e-mail: info@therapro.com
www.therapro.com

Karen Conrad, ScD, OTR/L, Owner
Designed to exercise and strengthen hands, ranging from soft to firm for developing a stronger grasp. Available in two, four and six ounce sizes. Three ounce putty in unique clear fist shaped container.

545 Uppertone
535 Floyd Smith Dr
El Cajon, CA 92020-1228
619-593-7381
800-468-8679
FAX: 888-755-5603
e-mail: info@gpk.com
www.gpk.com

546 Visual Alerting Guest Room Kit
HARC Mercantile
5413 S. Westnedge Ave.
Suite A
Portage, MI 49002
269-324-1615
800-445-9968
FAX: 269-324-2387
TTY: 269-324-1615
e-mail: info@harc.com
www.harc.com

Ron Slager, Owner
ADA compliant visual alerting guest room kit for the hard of hearing and deaf. Includes visual smoke detector, phone alert, door knock sensor, tactile alarm clock and telephone amplifier. Variations include TTY.

547 Window-Ease
A-Solution
5505 Barranca Oso Ct NE
Albuquerque, NM 87111
505-856-6632
FAX: 505-856-6652
e-mail: info@windowease.com
www.windowease.com

Robert Gorrell, President
Jeff Dodd, Sales
Device adapts horizontally and vertically sliding windows to ANSI A117.1 standards. 10:1 mechanical advantage at the crank arm opens a 50lb window with 5lbs force. Price ranges from $350.00-$450.00.

Office Devices & Workstations

548 **Combination File/Reference Carousel**
Center for Rehabilitation Technology
Ste 118
490 10th St NW
Atlanta, GA 30318-5754
404-712-5667
800-457-9555
FAX: 404-875-9409
e-mail: rerc-br@scsn.net

TW Gannaway, Executive VP
Anthony Stringer PhD

Offers two reading platforms and file holders joined on one easily rotated carousel. The carousel is easily rotated by head, mouth or handstick. Page retainer adjusts to hold open a variety of books and magazines. *$299.00*

549 **Don Johnston**
26799 W Commerce Dr
Volo, IL 60073-9675
847-740-0749
800-999-4660
800-889-5242
FAX: 847-740-7326
e-mail: info@donjohnston.com
www.donjohnston.com

Don Johnston, President

A provider of quality products and services that enable people with special needs to discover their potential and experience success. Products are developed for the areas of Physical Access, Augmentative Communication and for those who struggle with reading and writing.

550 **Extensions for Independence**
6100 Center Drive
Suite 1190
Los Angeles, CA 90045
757-416-6575
888-321-4678
FAX: 866-632-7149
e-mail: support@inmotionhosting.com
www.mouthstick.net

Ted Sakis, Director of Operations

Develops, manufactures and markets special vocational equipment for the physically handicapped. Products: mouthsticks, computer mechanical aids: key locks and diskette loaders. Also, turntable desks, wheelchair portable desks, filing trays with slanted sides, telephone adapters, and motorized artist easel. All these products have been designed to solve the functional limitations of people with little or no use of hands and/or arms.

551 **Fairway Spirit Adaptive Golf Car: Model4852**
Fairway Golf Cars
Ste 300
3225 Gateway Rd
Brookfield, WI 53045-5139
262-790-9363
888-320-4850
888-320-4850
FAX: 262-790-9396
e-mail: bob_hansen@fairwaygolfcars.com
www.fairwaygolfcars.com

552 **Freedom Ryder Handcycles**
Brike International
20589 SW Elk Horn Ct
Tualatin, OR 97062-9518
503-692-1029
800-800-5828
FAX: 970-221-4308
e-mail: Mike@Freedomryder.com
www.freedomryder.com

Mike Lofgren, Owner
Brian Stewart, VP

The finest handcycle in the world. The cycles incorporate body, lean steering and the finest bicycle components to make this a three-wheeled vehicle without equal. Suitable for both recreation and competition. *$1995.00*

553 **Golf Xpress**
Emotorsports
4400 West M-61
Standish, MI 48658
989-846-6255
FAX: 989-846-6255
e-mail: mitch@golfxpress.com
www.golfxpress.com

554 **Infogrip: AdjustaCart**
1899 E. Main Street
Ventura, CA 93001-3411
805-652-0770
800-397-0921
FAX: 805-652-0880
e-mail: tech@infogrip.com
www.infogrip.com

555 **Infogrip: BAT Personal Keyboard**
1899 E. Main Street
Ventura, CA 93001-3411
805-652-0770
800-397-0921
FAX: 805-652-0880
e-mail: tech@infogrip.com
www.infogrip.com

556 **Maxi Marks**
Maxi Aids
42 Executive Blvd
Farmingdale, NY 11735-4710
631-752-0521
800-522-6294
FAX: 631-752-0689
TTY: 800-281-3555
e-mail: sales@maxiaids.com
www.maxiaids.com

Elliot Zaretsky, President

Braille writing and identification products. *$2.50*

557 **Pencil/Pen Weighted Holders**
Therapro, Inc.
225 Arlington St
Framingham, MA 01702-8723
508-872-9494
800-257-5376
FAX: 508-875-2062
e-mail: info@therapro.com
www.therapro.com

Karen Conrad, ScD, OTR/L, Owner

Securely hold any pencil or pen. These weighted holders allow for more control along with proprioceptive feedback to encourage better writing skills.

558 **Perkins Brailler**
Maxi Aids
42 Executive Blvd
Farmingdale, NY 11735-4710
631-752-0521
800-522-6294
FAX: 631-752-0689
TTY: 800-281-3555
e-mail: sales@maxiaids.com
www.maxiaids.com

Elliot Zaretsky, President

Can emboss 25 lines with 42 cells on an 11 x 11 1/2 sheet. *$495.00*

559 **PhoneMax Amplified Telephone**
Assistech
2738 N Campbell Ave
Tucson, AZ 85719-3141
520-883-8600
866-674-3549
FAX: 520-883-3172
www.assistivedevices.net

Oliver Simoes, Owner

560 Raised Line Drawing Kit
Maxi Aids
42 Executive Blvd
Farmingdale, NY 11735-4710
631-752-0521
800-522-6294
FAX: 631-752-0689
TTY: 800-281-3555
e-mail: sales@maxiaids.com
www.maxiaids.com

Elliot Zaretsky, President
For writing script or drawing graphs by the use of special plastic paper. *$24.45*

561 Reizen Braille Labeler
Maxi Aids
42 Executive Blvd
Farmingdale, NY 11735-4710
631-752-0521
800-522-6294
FAX: 631-752-0689
TTY: 800-281-3555
e-mail: sales@maxiaids.com
www.maxiaids.com

Elliot Zaretsky, President
Label everything in Braille with 3/8 or 1/2 wide labeling tape. *$47.95*

562 Sharp Calculator with Illuminated Numbers
Independent Living Aids
137 Rano Rd
Buffalo, NY 14207
516-937-1848
800-537-2118
855-746-7452
FAX: 516-937-3906
e-mail: can-do@independentliving.com
www.independentliving.com

Irwin Schneidmill, President
Michael Gutierrez, Director of Operations
Pamela Strauss, Director of Marketing
Ursula Izurieta, Director of Merchandising
A trim desktop calculator with large illuminated numbers that can be carried anywhere. *$34.95*

563 Signature and Address Self-Inking Stamps
Independent Living Aids
137 Rano Rd
Buffalo, NY 14207
516-937-1848
800-537-2118
855-746-7452
FAX: 516-937-3906
e-mail: can-do@independentliving.com
www.independentliving.com

Irwin Schneidmill, President
Michael Gutierrez, Director of Operations
Pamela Strauss, Director of Marketing
Ursula Izurieta, Director of Merchandising
Gives thousands of impressions before requiring re-inking. *$11.95*

564 Steady Write
Maxi Aids
42 Executive Blvd
Farmingdale, NY 11735-4710
631-752-0521
800-522-6294
FAX: 631-752-0689
TTY: 800-281-3555
e-mail: sales@maxiaids.com
www.maxiaids.com

Elliot Zaretsky, President
Furnishes the writer with increased holding capacity and stabilizes the hand. *$6.95*

565 Talking Desktop Calculators
Maxi Aids
42 Executive Blvd
Farmingdale, NY 11735-4710
631-752-0521
800-522-6294
FAX: 631-752-0689
TTY: 800-281-3555
e-mail: sales@maxiaids.com
www.maxiaids.com

Elliot Zaretsky, President
Unique voice synthesizers call out numerals and functions as they are keyed in or read out data stored in memory. *$467.95*

566 Talking Electronic Organizers
Independent Living Aids
137 Rano Rd
Buffalo, NY 14207
516-937-1848
800-537-2118
855-746-7452
FAX: 516-937-3906
e-mail: can-do@independentliving.com
www.independentliving.com

Irwin Schneidmill, President
Michael Gutierrez, Director of Operations
Pamela Strauss, Director of Marketing
Ursula Izurieta, Director of Merchandising
Electronic, portable, personal organizers that talk the user through all the functions and are totally voice interactive. $199.95 and up.

567 Television Remote Controls with Large Numbers
Independent Living Aids
137 Rano Rd
Buffalo, NY 14207
516-937-1848
800-537-2118
855-746-7452
FAX: 516-937-3906
e-mail: can-do@independentliving.com
www.independentliving.com

Irwin Schneidmill, President
Michael Gutierrez, Director of Operations
Pamela Strauss, Director of Marketing
Ursula Izurieta, Director of Merchandising
Large 5 1/2 inch x 8 1/2 inch unit that has easy to see and use buttons. Can be used on nearly every TV, VCR and cable boxes. *$39.95*

568 Wheelchair Activity/Computer Table
Maxi Aids
42 Executive Blvd
Farmingdale, NY 11735-4710
631-752-0521
800-522-6294
FAX: 631-752-0689
TTY: 800-281-3555
e-mail: sales@maxiaids.com
www.maxiaids.com

Elliot Zaretsky, President
This powered height-adjustable table is a wheelchair accessible activity table or computer workstation that's as stylish as it is functional. Adjusts with the push of a button from 27-39 inches, powered by an extremely quiet motor. ADA compliant computer workstation for assistive technology and school computer labs.

Scooters

569 Aerospace Compadre
Aerospace America
900 Harry Truman Pkwy.
Bay City, MI 48706-4171
989-684-2121
800-237-6414
FAX: 989-684-4486
www.aerospaceamerica.com

Mike Alley, President
Fully customized golf cart type vehicle for the physically impaired person. Fully equipped with hand controls, wheelchair

rack, storage racks, head and tail lights and full safety belts. *$2500.00*

570 Alante
Golden Technologies
401 Bridge St
Old Forge, PA 18518-2323
800-624-6374
FAX: 800-628-5165
www.goldentech.com

Robert Golden, Chairman
Richard Golden, CEO
Fred Kiwak, President
Rear-wheel-drive vehicle that represents the best in powered mobility.

571 Amigo Mobility International
Amigo Mobility International
6693 Dixie Highway
Bridgeport, MI 48722
989-777-0910
800-248-9131
800-692-6446
FAX: 800-334-7274
e-mail: info@myamigo.com
www.myamigo.com

Al Thieme, Chairman and Founder
Beth Thieme, CEO
Tim Drumhiller, President
An industry leader in power operated vehicles/scooters, Amigo provides innovative, durable, and customized mobility solutions for the disabled, injured, and seniors worldwide. Other services include healthcare, travel and transportation services. *$1295.00*

572 Amphibious ATV Distributors
Amphibious ATV Distributors
2760 Greendale Dr
Sarasota, FL 34232-3702
941-379-6186
800-843-2811
FAX: 941-377-8979
e-mail: CBeach1419@aol.com
www.maxsixwheel.com

Clay Beach, Owner
A two and four passenger, all-terrain vehicle that can provide you with year round activities the whole family can enjoy. Accessible and drivable for the physically disabled. Used in hunting, fishing and outdoor activities on land and in the water. Many options and accessories available. Delivery anwyhere in the US and worldwide. $5,000-$9,000.

573 Bravo! + Three-Wheel Scooter
EZ-International
W194 N11301 McCormick Drive
Germantown, WI 53022
262-250-7740
800-824-1068
FAX: 262-250-7741
e-mail: sales@ek-tech.com
www.ek-tech.com

574 Cruiser Bus Buggy 4MB
Convaid Products
2830 California Street
Torrance, CA 90503
310-618-0111
888-266-8243
FAX: 310-618-2166
www.convaid.com

rocio, Inside Sales Manager
In sizes from infant through young adult, this positioning buggy is crash-tested.

575 Cub, SuperCub and Special Edition Scooters
1780 Executive Dr
Oconomowoc, WI 53066
262-567-4990
FAX: 262-953-5502
www.bruno.com

Michael R. Bruno, II, President/CEO
Michael R Bruno II, President/CEO
Steve Nelson, Service Manager

576 Electric Mobility Corporation
P.O.Box 156
Sewell, NJ 08080-156
856-468-0083
800-257-7955
FAX: 856-468-3426
www.rascalscooters.com

Linda Autore, CEO
Manufactures Rascal Scooters.

577 Explorer+ 4-Wheel Scooter
EZ-International
W194 N11301 McCormick Drive
Germantown, WI 53022
262-250-7740
800-824-1068
FAX: 262-250-7741
e-mail: sales@ek-tech.com
www.ek-tech.com/

578 Featherlite
No Boundaries
1 Monster Way
Corona, CA 92879
714-891-5899
800-426-7367
FAX: 714-891-0658
e-mail: info@hansens.com
www.hansens.com

Hubert Hansen, Founder
Lightweight scooter folds in seconds without tools or bending down for hassle free travel on airplanes, cruise ships, trains, RVs, buses and more! Heaviest component weighs 27 pounds. Fits easily in almost any vehicle trunk.

579 Invacare Fulfillment Center
Invacare Corporation
1 Invacare Way
Elyria, OH 44035-4190
440-329-6000
800-333-6900
FAX: 877-619-7996
www.invacare.com

A Malachi Mixon Iii, Chairman of the Board
Gerald B. Blouch, President and Chief Executive Officer
Joseph B. Richey, II, President - Invacare Technologies Division
Robert K. Gudbranson, Senior Vice President and Chief Financial Officer
Invacare Corporation is the world's leading manufacturer and distributor of non-acute medical products which promote recovery and active lifestyles for people requiring home and other non-acute health care.

580 Invacare Lynx L-3 Scooter
Maxi Aids
42 Executive Blvd
Farmingdale, NY 11735-4710
631-752-0521
800-522-6294
FAX: 631-752-0689
TTY: 800-281-3555
e-mail: sales@maxiaids.com
www.maxiaids.com

Elliot Zaretsky, President
The L-3 model conveniently disassembles into four compact pieces for easy transport. With an estimated seven miles of range, a plug-in battery charger and flat-free tires, consumers can plan their schedule around what they want to do, not around the limitations of their scooter. *$795.00*

581 Leisure Lift
Leisure Lift
1800 Merriam Ln
Kansas City, KS 66106-4714
913-722-5658
800-255-0285
FAX: 913-722-2614
e-mail: Leisure-Lift@Leisure-Lift.com
www.pacesaver.com

Bill Burke, Founder
Leisure Lift offers light three wheel scooter models and seven power wheelchair models. *$2695.00*

582 MVP+ 3-Wheel Scooter
EZ-International
W194 N11301 McCormick Drive
Germantown, WI 53022
262-250-7740
800-824-1068
FAX: 262-250-7741
e-mail: sales@ek-tech.com
www.ek-tech.com/contact.php

583 Moxie
No Boundaries
1 Monster Way
Corona, CA 92879
714-891-5899
800-426-7367
FAX: 714-891-0658
e-mail: info@hansens.com
www.hansens.com

Hubert Hansen, Founder
Disassembles into three parts in less than a minute. Heaviest component weighs 41 pounds. Portable, affordable and downright snazzy!

584 Outdoor Independence
Palmer Industries
P.O.Box 5707
Endicott, NY 13763-5707
607-754-2957
800-847-1304
FAX: 607-754-1954
e-mail: palmer@palmerind.com
www.palmerind.com

Jack Palmer, President
The futuristic, one, two and three seater, electric three-wheeler designed to take you almost anywhere.

585 Pace Saver Plus II
Leisure-Lift
1800 Merriam Ln
Kansas City, KS 66106-4714
913-722-5658
800-255-0285
FAX: 913-722-2614
e-mail: Leisure-Lift@Leisure-Lift.com
www.pacesaver.com

Bill Burke, Founder
The scooter combines outdoor ruggedness with indoor maneuverability at a low price.

586 Palmer Independence
Palmer Industries
P.O.Box 5707
Endicott, NY 13763-5707
607-754-2957
800-847-1304
FAX: 607-754-1954
e-mail: palmer@palmerind.com
www.palmerind.com

Jack Palmer, President
Futuristic electric outdoor three wheeler designed to take the rider almost anywhere.

587 Palmer Twosome
Palmer Industries
P.O.Box 5707
Endicott, NY 13763-5707
607-754-2957
800-847-1304
FAX: 607-754-1954
e-mail: palmer@palmerind.com
www.palmerind.com

Jack Palmer, President
All electric two seat vehicle for those who can't pedal.

588 Phantom Compact Size Scooter
Maxi Aids
42 Executive Blvd
Farmingdale, NY 11735-4710
631-752-0521
800-522-6294
FAX: 631-752-0689
TTY: 800-281-3555
e-mail: sales@maxiaids.com
www.maxiaids.com

Elliot Zaretsky, President
Travel in style-ideal/affordable compact scooter. Great for both indoor and outdoor use. Three wheel design allows for small 32.3 turning radius. Top speed 4 miles per hour and a cruising range of 15 miles. Large carry basket.

589 Polaris Trail Blazer
Polaris Industries
2100 Highway 55
Medina, MN 55340-9770
763-542-0500
888-704-5290
FAX: 763-542-0599
www.polarisindustries.com

Scott Wine, Chairman and Chief Executive Officer
Bennett J. Morgan, President and Chief Operating Officer
Michael W. Malone, Vice President - Finance and Chief Financial Officer
Todd-Michael Balan, Vice President - Corporate Development
A four-wheeler that has many engineered innovations, features such as: full floorboards for full comfort, single lever breaking with auxiliary foot brake, electronic throttle control, parking brake and adjustable handlebars.

590 Quickie 2
Sunrise Medical/Quickie Designs
2842 Business Park Avenue
Fresno, CA 93727
800-333-4000
800-300-7502
www.sunrisemedical.com

Pete Coburn, President
Randi Binstock, VP- Business Dev.
Peter Riley, Senior VP - Corporate CFO
Kevin Marshman, North American Controller
This custom, ultralight, folding, everyday scooter offers portability and performance plus modular flexibility.

591 Rascal 3-Wheeler
Electric Mobility Corporation
P.O.Box 156
Sewell, NJ 08080-156
856-468-1000
800-257-7955
FAX: 856-468-3426
www.emobility.com

Scott Patrick, Manager
For primarily outdoor use, this three wheeler provides extra strength, durability and reliability.

592 Rascal ConvertAble
Electric Mobility Corporation
P.O.Box 156
Sewell, NJ 08080-156
856-468-1000
800-257-7955
FAX: 856-468-3426
www.emobility.com

Scott Patrick, Manager
An electric vehicle that's a compact mobile chair one minute and a rugged outdoor scooter the next. Use both indoors and outdoors. Also available with joystick controls.

593 Regal Scooters
Bruno Independent Living Aids
Ste 84
1780 Executive Dr
Oconomowoc, WI 53066-4830
262-567-4990
800-882-8183
FAX: 262-953-5510
e-mail: webmaster@bruno.com
www.bruno.com

Michael R. Bruno, II, President/CEO

This line includes the Regal Standard, the Regal Large Adult, the Regal Small Adult, the Regal Pediatric, The Regal Ten models 65 and 75, and The Regal Four. These scooters offer adjustable flip-up armrests, pneumatic tires front and rear, and more.

594 **Regent**
Golden Technologies
401 Bridge St
Old Forge, PA 18518-2323
570-451-7477
800-624-6374
FAX: 800-628-5165
e-mail: info@goldentech.com
www.goldentech.com
Richard Golden, CEO
Lisa Miller, Senior Customer Service
Top-rated performance scooter, with extra features and economically priced.

595 **Roadster 20**
ATV Solutions
Unit 4
4700 W 60th Ave
Arvada, CO 80003-6928
303-450-2881
866-777-9727
888-867-1159
FAX: 303-450-2880
e-mail: sales@atvsolutions.com
www.atvsolutions.com
Andrew Miro, Owner
Great for indoor or outdoor use. The powerful, quiet drive system, independent front suspension and fully reclining high-back seat make for a smooth, quiet ride. The Roadster is loaded with great features at a bargain price.

596 **Safari Scooter**
Ranger All Seasons Corporation
P.O.Box 132
George, IA 51237-132
712-475-2811
800-225-3811
FAX: 712-475-2810
www.rangerallseason.com

597 **Scoota Bug**
Golden Technologies
401 Bridge St
Old Forge, PA 18518-2323
570-451-7477
800-624-6324
FAX: 800-628-5165
e-mail: info@goldentech.com
www.goldentech.com
Richard Golden, CEO
A lightweight, completely modular scooter, that disassembles and fits into most auto trunks.

598 **Sierra 3000/4000**
EZ-International
W194 N11301 McCormick Drive
Germantown, WI 53022
262-250-7740
800-824-1068
FAX: 262-250-7741
e-mail: Sales@EK-Tech.com
www.ek-tech.com/

599 **Solo Scooter**
Ranger All Seasons Corporation
P.O.Box 132
George, IA 51237-132
712-475-2811
800-225-3811
FAX: 712-475-2810
e-mail: sales@rangerallseason.com
www.rangerallseason.com

600 **SoloRider Industries**
Regal Research & Manufacturing Company
1200 East Plano Parkway
Plano, TX 75074
972-422-5324
800-898-3353
FAX: 972-422-8010
e-mail: info@solorider.com
www.solorider.com
Roger Pretekin, Founder
Manufacturer and distributor of the Solorider Golf Cart. This revolutionary single rider adaptive cart is specifically designed to meet the needs of individuals with mobility impairments.

601 **Sportster 10**
ATV Solutions
Unit 4
4700 W 60th Ave
Arvada, CO 80003-6928
303-450-2881
866-777-9727
888-867-1159
FAX: 303-450-2880
e-mail: sales@atvsolutions.com
www.atvsolutions.com
Andrew Miro, Owner
Sportster 10 is our most maneuverable scooter, ideal for riders who must operate in tight spaces. Equipped with all of the great features of the Roadster 20, this three-wheeler is an exceptional buy.

602 **Systems 2000**
BioMedical Life Systems
P.O.Box 1360
Vista, CA 92085-1360
760-727-5600
800-726-8367
FAX: 760-727-4220
e-mail: information@bmls.com
www.bmls.com

603 **Terra-Jet: Utility Vehicle**
TERRA-JET USA
P.O.Box 918
Junction Hwy. 417 & 419
Innis, LA 70747-918
225-492-2249
800-864-5000
FAX: 225-492-2226
e-mail: Terra-Jet@Terra-Jet.Com
www.terra-jet.com
Larry Rabalais, President, General Manager and CEO
Shawn Oubre, Sales
TERRA-JET utility vehicles are unique in their ability to traverse many different types of terrain in remote areas otherwise inaccessible. It has a multitude of uses for industry, sportsmen or the whole family. Uniquely designed, industrial duty construction of low maintenance and low fuel consumption. $8,675-$21,995.

604 **Terrier Tricycle**
TRIAID
P.O.Box 1364
Cumberland, MD 21501-1364
301-759-3525
800-306-6777
FAX: 301-759-3525
e-mail: sales@triaid.com
www.triaid.com

605 **Trekker 40**
ATV Solutions
Unit 4
4700 W 60th Ave
Arvada, CO 80003-6928
303-450-2881
866-777-9727
888-867-1159
FAX: 303-450-2880
e-mail: sales@atvsolutions.com
www.atvsolutions.com
Andrew Miro, Owner
Our biggest, toughest scooter. With a huge 450 pound capacity and five inches of ground clearance, this machine is ideal for the daily outdoor user. The high top speed means you get there fast

and the four-wheel suspension makes the ride smooth and comfortable.

606 **Tri-Lo's**
TRIAID
P.O.Box 1364
Cumberland, MD 21501-1364
301-759-3525
800-306-6777
FAX: 301-759-3525
e-mail: sales@triaid.com
www.triaid.com

607 **Triumph 3000/4000**
EZ-International
W194 N11301 McCormick Drive
Germantown, WI 53022
262-250-7740
800-824-1068
FAX: 262-250-7741
e-mail: Sales@EK-Tech.com
www.ek-tech.com/

608 **Triumph Scooter**
EZ-International
W194 N11301 McCormick Drive
Germantown, WI 53022
262-250-7740
800-824-1068
FAX: 262-250-7741
e-mail: Sales@EK-Tech.com
www.ek-tech.com/

Stationery

609 **Access-USA**
242 James St
PO Box 160
Clayton, NY 13624-160
800-263-2750
FAX: 800-563-1687
e-mail: info@access-usa.com
www.access-usa.com

Deborah Webster, PICOE
Access-USA provides one-stop alternate format transcription services for almost any type of document-reports, schedules, menus, monthly statements, brochures, reports, etc. Items may be submitted on computer disk, hard copy or email. Alternate formats include Braille, large print, Braille and print, audio recordings, adapted disks as well as video services-open/closed captioning and video descriptions. Accessible products also include Braille Business Cards and ADA signage.

610 **Address Book**
Sense-Sations
919 Walnut Street
Philadelphia, PA 19107-5237
215-627-0600
FAX: 215-922-0692
e-mail: asbinfo@asb.org
www.asb.org

Patricia C. Johnson, President & Chief Executive Officer
Derby Ewing, Director, Human Services
Brian Rusk, Public Relations Officer
Richard Forsythe, Director, Braille Division and Custom Audio
The big print address book is the first personal book to provide enlarged writing spaces, making it easier to write down and retrieve information. *$12.50*

611 **Big Print Address Book**
Access with Ease
42 Executive Blvd
Farmingdale, NY 11735-4710
631-752-0521
800-522-6294
FAX: 631-752-0689
TTY: 800-281-3555
e-mail: sales@maxiaids.com
www.maxiaids.com

Elliott Zaretsky, Founder and President
Rods supported by two rubber blocks facilitate writing. *$16.95*

612 **Bold Line Paper**
Sense-Sations
919 Walnut Street
Philadelphia, PA 19107-5237
215-627-0600
FAX: 215-922-0692
e-mail: asbinfo@asb.org
www.asb.org

Patricia C. Johnson, President & Chief Executive Officer
Derby Ewing, Director, Human Services
Brian Rusk, Public Relations Officer
Richard Forsythe, Director, Braille Division and Custom Audio
This pad consists of 100 sheets of paper with bold lines to help guide the writing of an individual with limited vision. *$2.50*

613 **Braille Notebook**
Maxi Aids
42 Executive Blvd
Farmingdale, NY 11735-4710
631-752-0521
800-522-6294
FAX: 631-752-0689
TTY: 800-281-3555
e-mail: sales@maxiaids.com
www.maxiaids.com

Elliott Zaretsky, Founder and President
Made of heavy-duty board, covered with waterproof imitation leather and three rings for binding, including Braille paper and titles. *$12.95*

614 **Braille: Desk Calendar**
Maxi Aids
42 Executive Blvd
Farmingdale, NY 11735-4710
631-752-0521
800-522-6294
FAX: 631-752-0689
TTY: 800-281-3555
e-mail: sales@maxiaids.com
www.maxiaids.com

Elliott Zaretsky, Founder and President
Schedule appointments, remember birthdays or write messages for a particular day. *$39.95*

615 **Braille: Greeting Cards**
Sense-Sations
919 Walnut Street
Philadelphia, PA 19107-5237
215-829-9997
FAX: 215-922-0692
e-mail: asbinfo@asb.org
www.asb.org

Patricia C. Johnson, President & Chief Executive Officer
Derby Ewing, Director, Human Services
Brian Rusk, Public Relations Officer
Richard Forsythe, Director, Braille Division and Custom Audio
Birthday, anniversary, get well, sympathy and Christmas cards offering Braille print for the blind. *$.95*

616 **Clip Board Notebook**
Sense-Sations
919 Walnut Street
Philadelphia, PA 19107-5237
215-627-0600
FAX: 215-922-0692
e-mail: asbinfo@asb.org
www.asb.org

Patricia C. Johnson, President & Chief Executive Officer
Derby Ewing, Director, Human Services
Brian Rusk, Public Relations Officer
Richard Forsythe, Director, Braille Division and Custom Audio
Kit includes a pack of Bold Line paper and black ink pen. *$5.95*

617 **Deluxe Signature Guide**
Maxi Aids
42 Executive Blvd
Farmingdale, NY 11735-4710
631-752-0521
800-522-6294
FAX: 631-752-0689
TTY: 800-281-3555
e-mail: sales@maxiaids.com
www.maxiaids.com

Elliott Zaretsky, Founder and President

Rods supported by two rubber blocks facilitate writing. *$1.25*

618 **Highlighter and Note Tape**
Therapro, Inc.
225 Arlington St
Framingham, MA 01702-8723 508-872-9494
800-257-5376
FAX: 508-875-2062
e-mail: info@therapro.com
www.therapro.com

Karen Conrad, Owner
A great way to highlight and draw attention to words without damaging original. Price ranges from $4.00-$7.00.

619 **Letter Writing Guide**
Independent Living Aids
137 Rano Rd
Buffalo, NY 14207 800-537-2118
855-746-7452
FAX: 516-937-3906
www.independentliving.com

Irwin Schneidmill, President
Michael Gutierrez, Director of Operations
Pamela Strauss, Director of Marketing
Ursula Izurieta, Director of Merchandising
Sturdy plastic sheet with 13 apertures corresponding to standard line spacing. *$3.49*

620 **Lettering Guide Value Pack**
Independent Living Aids
137 Rano Rd
Buffalo, NY 14207 800-537-2118
855-746-7452
FAX: 516-937-3906
www.independentliving.com

Irwin Schneidmill, President
Michael Gutierrez, Director of Operations
Pamela Strauss, Director of Marketing
Ursula Izurieta, Director of Merchandising
Included in this useful pack are four durable plastic lettering and number guides for tracing letters when the individual is unable to write letters unassisted. *$6.29*

Visual Aids

621 **Aluminum Adjustable Support Canes for the Blind**
Maxi Aids
42 Executive Blvd
Farmingdale, NY 11735-4710 631-752-0521
800-522-6294
FAX: 631-752-0689
TTY: 800-281-3555
e-mail: sales@maxiaids.com
www.maxiaids.com

Elliott Zaretsky, Founder and President
Adjustable canes for the visually impaired. *$17.95*

622 **Audio Book Contractors**
P.O. Box 96
Riverdale, MD 20738-96 301-439-5830
FAX: 301-439-5830
e-mail: info@audiobookcontractors.com
www.audiobookcontractors.com

Flo Gibson, President
Over 950 titles of unabridged classic books on audio cassettes in sturdy vinyl covers with picture and spine windows. Discounted prices for disabled patrons.

623 **Beyond Sight**
5650 S Windermere St
Littleton, CO 80120-1240 303-795-6455
FAX: 303-795-6425
e-mail: jim@beyondsight.com
www.beyondsight.com

Scott Chaplick, Owner & President
Gina Whetzel, Sales & Merchandise Specialist
Products for the blind and visually impaired including talking clocks, watches and calculators, also carry a large selection of Braille products, magnifiers, reading machines and computer equipment.

624 **Big Number Pocket Sized Calculator**
Independent Living Aids
137 Rano Rd
Buffalo, NY 14207 516-937-1848
800-537-2118
855-746-7452
FAX: 516-937-3906
e-mail: can-do@independentliving.com
www.independentliving.com

Marvin Sandler, President
A handy pocket size calculator with big numbers that fits easily into purse or pocket. *$14.95*

625 **Braille Compass**
Maxi Aids
42 Executive Blvd
Farmingdale, NY 11735-4710 631-752-0521
800-522-6294
FAX: 631-752-0689
TTY: 631-752-0738
e-mail: sales@maxiaids.com
www.maxiaids.com

Elliott Zaretsky, Founder and President
The visually impaired can tell the direction by using this compass. *$42.95*

626 **Braille Plates for Elevator**
Maxi Aids
42 Executive Blvd
Farmingdale, NY 11735-4710 631-752-0521
800-522-6294
FAX: 631-752-0689
TTY: 800-281-3555
e-mail: sales@maxiaids.com
www.maxiaids.com

Elliott Zaretsky, Founder and President
The plates have curing type pressure sensitive material applied for metal to metal bonding. *$79.95*

627 **Braille Touch-Time Watches**
Independent Living Aids
137 Rano Rd
Buffalo, NY 14207 516-937-1848
800-537-2118
855-746-7452
FAX: 516-937-3906
e-mail: can-do@independentliving.com
www.independentliving.com

Marvin Sandler, President
White dial with black numerals and hands makes telling time possible quickly and easily for the visually impaired. *$44.95*

628 **Circline Illuminated Magnifer**
Dazor Manufacturing Corporation
2079 Congressional Dr.
St. Louis, MO 63146 314-652-2400
800-345-9103
FAX: 314-652-2069
e-mail: info@dazor.com
www.dazor.com

Mark Hogrebe,Ph.D, Past President
Provides even, shadow free light under the magnifying lens with a 22-watt circline fluorescent. The magnifier is mounted on a floating arm that allows you to position the light source and lens with the touch of a finger.

629 **Extra Loud Alarm with Lighter Plug**
HARC Mercantile
5413 S. Westnedge Ave.
Suite A
Portage, MI 49002
269-324-1615
800-445-9968
FAX: 269-324-2387
TTY: 269-324-1615
e-mail: info@harc.com
www.harc.com

Ron Slager, Owner
Battery operated, easy to read, digital clock with extra loud alarm. *$45.00*

630 **Low Vision Telephones**
2738 N Campbell Ave
Tucson, AZ 85719-3141
520-883-8600
866-674-3549
FAX: 520-883-3172
e-mail: info@assistivedevices.net
www.assistivedevices.net

Oliver Simoes, Owner

631 **Magni-Cam & Primer**
Innoventions
9593 Corsair Dr
Conifer, CO 80433-9317
303-797-6554
800-854-6554
FAX: 303-727-4940
e-mail: magnicam@magnicam.com
www.magnicam.com

Mark Freeman, President
Magni-Cam and Primer are hand-held, light weight, inexpensive auto-focus electronic magnification systems designed to meet the reading and writing needs of those with low vision. The systems present the image in black and white or in color with three different view modes. Connects to any TV monitor in minutes. Systems read any surface with no distortion. A battery powered system is available, providing total portability and flexibility.

632 **Magnifier Bookweight**
Levenger
420 S Congress Ave
Delray Beach, FL 33445-4693
901-566-5771
800-544-0880
FAX: 561-274-0263
e-mail: cservice@levenger.com
www.levenger.com

Steve Leveen, CEO
The Magnifier Bookweight features an optical quality magnifier and is long enough to enlarge the full width of most book pages while holing the pages open. This magnifier is encased in embossed leather and enlarges approximately four lines of text at a time to twice the original size.

633 **Man's Low-Vision Quartz Watches**
Independent Living Aids
137 Rano Rd
Buffalo, NY 14207
516-937-1848
800-537-2118
855-746-7452
FAX: 516-937-3906
e-mail: can-do@independentliving.com
www.independentliving.com

Marvin Sandler, President
An inexpensive, easy-to-read watch with chrome case. *$27.95*

634 **Men's/Women's Low Vision Watches & Clocks**
Maxi Aids
42 Executive Blvd
Farmingdale, NY 11735-4710
631-752-0521
800-522-6294
FAX: 631-752-0689
TTY: 800-281-3555
e-mail: sales@maxiaids.com
www.maxiaids.com

Elliott Zaretsky, Founder and President
Choose from a wide range of watches from Braille automatic to quartz pocket watches.

635 **MonoMouse Electronic Magnifiers**
Maxi Aids
42 Executive Blvd
Farmingdale, NY 11735-4710
631-752-0521
800-522-6294
FAX: 631-752-0689
TTY: 800-281-3555
e-mail: sales@maxiaids.com
www.maxiaids.com

Elliott Zaretsky, Founder and President
Simple and affordable magnifier for people with Low Vision. Just about the size of a standard computer mouse. Allows you to read books, newspapers, product labels, etc. on either a computer or TV screen.

636 **Rigid Aluminum Cane with Golf Grip**
Maxi Aids
42 Executive Blvd
Farmingdale, NY 11735-4710
631-752-0521
800-522-6294
FAX: 631-752-0689
TTY: 800-281-3555
e-mail: sales@maxiaids.com
www.maxiaids.com

Elliott Zaretsky, Founder and President
A straight, tubular, heavy gauge aluminum rigid cane for blind and visually impaired persons. *$12.95*

637 **Stretch-View Wide-View Rectangular Illuminated Magnifier**
Dazor Manufacturing Corporation
2079 Congressional Dr.
St. Louis, MO 63146
314-652-2400
800-345-9103
FAX: 314-652-2069
e-mail: info@dazor.com
www.dazor.com

Mark Hogrebe,Ph.D, Past President
Provides even, shadow free light under the magnifying lens with a 22-watt circline fluorescent. The magnifier is mounted on a floating arm that allows you to position the light source and lens with the touch of a finger.

638 **Timex Easy Reader**
Independent Living Aids
137 Rano Rd
Buffalo, NY 14207
516-937-1848
800-537-2118
855-746-7452
FAX: 516-937-3906
e-mail: can-do@independentliving.com
www.independentliving.com

Marvin Sandler, President
An easy-to-read large face watch that's water resistant. *$29.95*

639 **Unisex Low Vision Watch**
Independent Living Aids
137 Rano Rd
Buffalo, NY 14207
516-937-1848
800-537-2118
855-746-7452
FAX: 516-937-3906
e-mail: can-do@independentliving.com
www.independentliving.com

Marvin Sandler, President
Unisex watch with large numbers and wide hands. Gold-toned case with either expansion or leather band. *$31.95*

Walking Aids: Canes, Crutches & Walkers

640 **Air Lift Oxygen Carriers**
Air Lift Unlimited
1212 Kerr Gulch Rd
Evergreen, CO 80439-6397
800-776-6771
888-343-3352
FAX: 303-526-4700
e-mail: info@airlift.com
www.meridianmedicalusa.com

641 **Aluminum Crutches**
Arista Surgical Supply Company
297 High Street
Dedham, MA 02026-2852
781-329-2900
800-225-2610
FAX: 781-329-8392
e-mail: info@alimed.com
www.alimed.com

Julian Cherubini, President

Lightweight aluminum crutches with wood underarms and handgrips. *$25.00*

642 **Aluminum Walking Canes**
Maxi Aids
42 Executive Blvd
Farmingdale, NY 11735-4710
631-752-0521
800-522-6294
FAX: 631-752-0689
TTY: 800-281-3555
e-mail: sales@maxiaids.com
www.maxiaids.com

Elliott Zaretsky, Founder and President

Lightweight but strong, these walking canes are made of a heavy gauge aluminum tube with safety locknuts and heavy-duty rubber tips. *$10.75*

643 **Compact Folding Travel Rollator**
Maxi Aids
42 Executive Blvd
Farmingdale, NY 11735-4710
631-752-0521
800-522-6294
FAX: 631-752-0689
TTY: 631-752-0738
e-mail: sales@maxiaids.com
www.maxiaids.com

Elliott Zaretsky, Founder and President

Is perfect for someone on the go. Pull strap for quick folding and disassembly. Folds down to half its assembled size in seconds, to a manageable 26 inch L x 22 inch W x 8 inch D for easy storage. *$ 149.95*

644 **Crutches**
Mada Medical Products
625 Washington Ave
Carlstadt, NJ 07072-2901
201-460-0454
800-526-6370
FAX: 201-460-3509
e-mail: dianelind@mail.madamedical.com
www.madainternational.com

Jeffrey Adam, President

All aluminum construction, underarm crutch with double pushbutton height adjustment.

645 **Dapper Folding Adustable Cane**
Maxi Aids
42 Executive Blvd
Farmingdale, NY 11735-4710
631-752-0521
800-522-6294
FAX: 631-752-0689
TTY: 631-752-0738
e-mail: sales@maxiaids.com
www.maxiaids.com

Elliott Zaretsky, Founder and President

The Dapper walking stick can be folded and unfolded with only one hand and with minimum effort. The durable lanyard attached prevents loss and allows trailing of staff. Features a non-slip handle, non-skid rubber tip and is made of high quality sturdy aluminum. *$ 34.95*

646 **Dapper Walking Stick**
Maxi Aids
42 Executive Blvd
Farmingdale, NY 11735-4710
631-752-0521
800-522-6294
FAX: 631-752-0689
TTY: 631-752-0738
e-mail: sales@maxiaids.com
www.maxiaids.com

Elliott Zaretsky, Founder and President

The Dapper walking stick is safe durable and sturdy allowing the user to conveniently store it when not in use. It can be folded and unfolded with only one hand and with minimum effort. The durable lanyard attached prevents loss and allows trailing of staff. Features a non-slip handle, non-skid rubber tip and is made of high quality sturdy aluminum construction. *$34.95*

647 **Deluxe Nova Wheeled Walker & Avant Wheeled Walker**
Sammons Preston Rolyan
W68n158 Evergreen Blvd
Cedarburg, WI 53012-2637
262-387-8720
800-323-5547
FAX: 800-547-4333
e-mail: CustomerSupport@PattersonMedical.com
www.pattersonmedical.com/

Bruce Curtis, Sales Representative
David.P Sproat, President

Lightweight and simple to handle with an easy-to-operate braking system. *$425.40*

648 **Deluxe Standard Wood Cane**
Arista Surgical Supply Company/AliMed
297 High Street
Dedham, MA 02026-2852
781-329-2900
800-225-2610
FAX: 781-329-8392
e-mail: info@alimed.com
www.alimed.com

Julian Cherubini, President

A standard old-fashioned wooden cane for the physically challenged. *$10.00*

649 **EasyStand 6000 Glider**
Access To Recreation
8 Sandra Ct
Newbury Park, CA 91320-4302
800-634-4351
FAX: 805-498-8186
e-mail: customerservice@accesstr.com
www.accesstr.com

Don Krebs, President

Provides dynamic leg motion for individuals who are unable to stand upright or walk on their own.

650 **Freedom Three Wheel Walker**
Mada Medical Products
625 Washington Ave
Carlstadt, NJ 07072-2901
201-460-0454
800-526-6370
FAX: 201-460-3509
e-mail: dianelind@mail.madamedical.com
www.madainternational.com

Jeffrey Adam, President

The freedom walker has ultra light touch, locking loop brakes and sure grip hand grips.

651 **Liberty Lightweight Aluminum Stroll Walker**
Mada Medical Products
625 Washington Ave
Carlstadt, NJ 07072-2901
201-460-0454
800-526-6370
FAX: 201-460-3509
e-mail: dianelind@mail.madamedical.com
www.madainternational.com

Jeffrey Adam, President

The Liberty walker has a spring loaded push down braking system, adjustable handle height with locking system, a 12in wide fully padded seat, and a removable shopping basket.

652 **Maxi Superior Cane**
Maxi Aids
42 Executive Blvd
Farmingdale, NY 11735-4710
631-752-0521
800-522-6294
FAX: 631-752-0689
TTY: 800-281-3555
e-mail: sales@maxiaids.com
www.maxiaids.com

Elliott Zaretsky, Founder and President
Convenient folding cane designed for optimum balance. Tapered joints provide rigidity when open, and are made of heavy gauge aluminum. *$17.50*

653 **Out-N-About American Walker**
742 Market St
Oregon, WI 53575-1059
608-835-9255
FAX: 608-835-5234
Luann Smith, President
The lightweight Out-N-About is easy to handle. The four wheel design provides greater support and stability than any other walking aids. Its large rubber tires move effortlessly over most surfaces, indoors and out. The small turning radius makes it ideal for getting through confined spaces and narrow doorways. The attractive, burgundy colored, tubular steel frame is extremely durable. The Out-N-About folds flat and stands alone for easy storage. Made in USA.

654 **Patriot Extra Wide Folding Walkers**
Mada Medical Products
625 Washington Ave
Carlstadt, NJ 07072-2901
201-460-0454
800-526-6370
FAX: 201-460-3509
e-mail: dianelind@mail.madamedical.com
www.madainternational.com

Jeffrey Adam, President
The extra wide walkers have padded foam hand grips, two-stage push button folding mechanism, dual width adjustment, height adjustment, and nonskid tips.

655 **Patriot Folding Walker Series**
Mada Medical Products
625 Washington Ave
Carlstadt, NJ 07072-2901
201-460-0454
800-526-6370
FAX: 201-460-3509
e-mail: dianelind@mail.madamedical.com
www.madainternational.com
Jeffrey Adam, President
The patriot walker has high density, padded foam hand grips, high strength 1in lightweight, anodized, dull silver aluminum tube construction, adjustable height with push-button lock security, nonskid tips, and a single button folding mechanism.

656 **Patriot Reciprocal Folding Walkers**
Mada Medical Products
625 Washington Ave
Carlstadt, NJ 07072-2901
201-460-0454
800-526-6370
FAX: 201-460-3509
e-mail: dianelind@mail.madamedical.com
www.madainternational.com

Jeffrey Adam, President
The reciprocal folding walkers have padded foam hand grips, adjustable height with snap-in security, double front cross brace, and nonskid tips.

657 **Prone Support Walker**
Consumer Care Products
W282 N7109 Main Street
Merton, WI 53056
262-820-2300

e-mail: info@consumercarellc.com
www.consumercarellc.com

658 **Push-Button Quad Cane**
Arista Surgical Supply Company/AliMed
297 High Street
Dedham, MA 02026-2852
781-329-2900
800-225-2610
FAX: 781-329-8392
e-mail: info@alimed.com
www.alimed.com

Julian Cherubini, President
A reliable walking cane offering independence to the physically challenged user. *$25.00*

659 **Quad Canes**
Mada Medical Products
625 Washington Ave
Carlstadt, NJ 07072-2901
201-460-0454
800-526-6370
FAX: 201-460-3509
e-mail: dianelind@mail.madamedical.com
www.madainternational.com

Jeffrey Adam, President
There are large and small base quad canes with high density foam grips.

660 **Rand-Scot**
401 Linden Center Dr
Fort Collins, CO 80524-2429
970-484-7967
800-467-7967
FAX: 970-484-3800
TTY: 800-467-7967
e-mail: info@randscot.com
www.randscot.com
Joel Lerich, President
Barbara Hoehn, President
Manufactures the Easy Pivot patient lift, the BBD wheelchair cushion line and Saratoga Exercise products for the disabled. Offers a line of patient lifts and standers for the disabled. Rand-scot products are designed to help the disabled achieve independence, comfort, and stamina. A video or dvd is available at no charge for potential users, $800-$3,000.

661 **Secret Agent Walking Stick**
Gold Violin
PO BOX 147
Jessup, PA 18434
877-648-8466
FAX: 800-821-1282
goldviolin.blair.com
Connie Hallquist, CEO
The Secret Agent Walking Stick features a built-in flashlight, a red reflector and a built-in secret pill compartment. this folding aluminum cane is height adjustable and has a derby-style handle and a non-skid rubber tip. A nylon carrying case is included. The walking stick comes in a choice of gold, bronze, or black shaft with a faux burled walnut handle. . It has been taken over by Orchard Brands.

662 **StairClimber**
Martin Technology
29 N Main St
Gloversville, NY 12078-3006
518-725-1837
800-800-1410
FAX: 518-725-9522
Michael Lewy, Owner
A walker-capable person can climb and descend stairs with this walker-designed StairClimber.

663 **Standing Aid Frame with Rear Entry**
Consumer Care Products
W282 N7109 Main Street
Merton, WI 53056
262-820-2300
FAX: 920-459-9070
www.consumercarellc.com

664 **Stick Canes**
Mada Medical Products
625 Washington Ave
Carlstadt, NJ 07072-2901
201-460-0454
800-526-6370
FAX: 201-460-3509
e-mail: dianelind@mail.madamedical.com
www.madainternational.com

Jeffrey Adam, President
Mada's stick canes are adjustable with a locking security system.

665 **Torso Support**
Grandmar
5635 Peck Rd.
Arcadia, CA 91006-20
626-443-3143
800-447-6739
FAX: 800-767-3933
e-mail: info@posey.com
www.posey.com

Ernest Posey, CEO
Bob Kelleher, Senior Vice President of Supply Chain and Administration
Tracey Bertolina, CFO
Dale Clendon, President
An aid for people who are unable to maintain an upright position in an automobile or a wheelchair.

666 **U-Step Walking Stabilizer: Walker**
Maxi Aids
42 Executive Blvd
Farmingdale, NY 11735-4710
631-752-0521
800-522-6294
FAX: 631-752-0689
TTY: 631-752-0738
e-mail: sales@maxiaids.com
www.maxiaids.com

Elliott Zaretsky, Founder and President
If you want to feel as stable as you would while holding onto another person's arm, the U-Step Walking Stabilizer is for you. The innovative braking system is easy to use and puts you in complete control; roll only when you want to. Plus, it easily folds for transport. *$ 539.95*

667 **Ventura Enterprises**
4431 S. Eastern Avenue
Las Vegas, NV 89119
702-457-7676
FAX: 317-745-3179
e-mail: info@venturaenterprises.com
www.venturaenterprises.com

Sam Ventura, President, CEO
Ron Ventura, Vice President of Development
Galit Rozen, Vice President of Acquisitions
Ofir Ventura, ESQ., In House General Council
Manufacturer of everyday living mobility aids. Products include carrying aids for walkers and wheelchairs and also wheelchair cushions.

668 **WCIB Heavy-Duty Folding Cane**
Maxi Aids
42 Executive Blvd
Farmingdale, NY 11735-4710
631-752-0521
800-522-6294
FAX: 631-752-0689
TTY: 800-281-3555
e-mail: sales@maxiaids.com
www.maxiaids.com

Elliott Zaretsky, Founder and President
A four section aluminum folding cane with a golf-type grip handle and flexible wrist loop. Available in 34-60 lengths. *$17.95*

669 **Walker Leg Support**
Sammons Preston Rolyan
W68 N158 Evergreen Blvd
Cedarburg, WI 53012-2637
262-387-8720
800-228-3693
FAX: 262-387-8748
e-mail: CustomerSupport@PattersonMedical.com
www.pattersonmedical.com/

Bruce Curtis, Sales Representative
David.P Sproat, President
For lower extremity trauma. An alternative to crutches that allows safe, stable ambulation and frees hands and arms for daily tasks. *$11.50*

Wheelchairs: Accessories

670 **Advantage Wheelchair & Walker Bags**
Laurel Designs
TORRANCE, CA 90505
800-556-6307
FAX: 310-316-2561
e-mail: advantagebag@verizon.net
www.advantagebag.com/

671 **Automatic Wheelchair Anti-Rollback Device**
Alzheimer's Store
3197 Trout Place Rd
Cumming, GA 30041-8260
678-947-4001
800-752-3238
FAX: 678-947-8411
e-mail: cs@alzstore.com
www.alzstore.com

Ellen Warner, President
As a wheelchair user transfers to and from the chair, a pair of brake arms grabs the tires to prevent the chair from rolling backwards. Once the individual is seated, the device switches to stand-by mode and the wheelchair returns to standard function.

672 **Battery Operated Cushion**
DA Schulman
3827 Creekside Lane
Holmen, WI 54636
608-782-0031
866-782-9658
FAX: 608-782-0488
e-mail: aquila@aquilacorp.com
www.aquilacorp.com

673 **Dual-Mode Charger**
Lester Electrical
625 West A Street
Lincoln, NE 68522-1794
402-477-8988
FAX: 402-474-1769
e-mail: sales@lesterelectrical.com
www.lesterelectrical.com

674 **Equalizer 1000 Series**
Helm Distributing
P.O Box 25105 Deer Park P.O, Rd Dee
Alberta, T4R 2
403-309-5551
FAX: 403-342-5509
e-mail: james@equalizerexercise.com
www.equalizerexercise.com

675 **Equalizer 5000 Home Gym**
Helm Distributing
P.O Box 25105 Deer Park P.O, Rd Dee
Alberta, CA 45418-2713
403-309-5551
FAX: 403-342-5509
e-mail: info@equalizerexercise.com
www.equalizerexercise.com

676 **Featherspring**
105 W Lincoln Hwy
DeKalb, IL 60115
800-628-4693
FAX: 800-261-1164
e-mail: customerservice@luxis.com
www.luxis.com

677 **Gem Wheelchair & Scooter Service: Mobility & Homecare**
176-39 Union Turnpike
Flushing, NY 11366-1515 718-969-8600
800-943-3578
e-mail: help@gemwheelchairservice.com
www.gemwheelchairservice.com/

678 **Lifestand**
Frank Mobility Systems
300 Duke Drive
Lebanon, TN 37090 800-736-0925
FAX: 800-231-3256
e-mail: techsupport@permobil.com
www.lifestandusa.com
Larry Jackson, President and CEO
Tom Rolick, VP Sales North America
Darin Lowery, VP of Operations
Rick Haynes, Senior HR Manager
Lifestand offers a full line of standing wheelchairs for manual operation. Power assisted are fully motorized. *$7000.00*

679 **Mat Factory**
6726 North Figueroa Street
Los Angeles, CA 90042 800-628-7626
FAX: 323-254-4545
www.matfactoryinc.com

680 **One Thousand FS**
Fortress
P.O.Box 489
Clovis, CA 93613-489 559-322-5437
FAX: 559-323-0299

681 **Pac-All Wheelchair Carrier**
Pac-All Carriers
2321 Carolton Rd
Maitland, FL 32751-3624 407-830-6604
800-628-6672
FAX: 407-339-2847
LE Angel
No more lifting and no more pain wheelchair carrier. VA approved. Made in USA.
$158 - $226.40

682 **Safety Deck II**
Mat Factory
6726 North Figueroa Street
Los Angeles, CA 90042 800-628-7626
FAX: 323-254-4545
www.matfactoryinc.com

683 **Scooter & Wheelchair Battery Fuel Gauges and Motor Speed Controllers**
Curtis Instruments, Inc.
200 Kisco Ave
Mount Kisco, NY 10549-1407 914-666-2971
FAX: 914-666-2188
e-mail: gomezj@curtisinst.com
www.curtisinst.com
Stuart E Marwell, President and CEO
David Matthews, VP Sales Americas
Cheryl Leonaggeo, Customer Service Manager
Richard McFarlane, Customer Support Engineer
Provides a readable, accurate indication of battery in easy to read type of display. Innovative, efficient motor speed controllers for single or dual PM motor vehicles.

684 **Softfoot Ergomatta**
Mat Factory
6726 North Figueroa Street
Los Angelesa, CA 90042 949-645-3122
800-628-7626
FAX: 323-254-4545
www.matfactoryinc.com

685 **Tilt-N-Table**
Osterguard Enterprises c/o Jim's Shop
3228 W Olive Ave
Fresno, CA 93722-5733 559-275-4695
Jim Ostergaard Ii, Owner
These are lightweight tables for wheelchairs that are angle and height adjustable to your changing needs.

686 **Wheel Life News**
University of Virginia, Rehab Engineering Centers
3363 University Sta
Charlottesville, VA 22903 434-924-5118
www.medicine.virginia.edu
Kristine M. Garza, Ph.D., Executive Director of SACNAS
Steven T. DeKosky, Dean
Features tie downs and other adaptive technology for persons with disabilities.

687 **Wheelchair Accessories**
Diestco Manufacturing Company
P.O.Box 6504
Chico, CA 95927-6504 800-795-2392
e-mail: info@diestco.com
www.diestco.com

688 **Wheelchair Aide**
Graham-Field
400 Rabro Dr
Hauppauge, NY 11788-4258 631-348-1364

689 **Wheelchair Back Pack and Tote Bag**
Med Covers
320 Roebling Street
Suite 515
Brooklyn, NY 11211 718-302-1923
800-320-7140
FAX: 866-522-6967
e-mail: info@1800wheelchair.com
www.1800wheelchair.com

690 **Wheelchair Roller**
Access To Recreation
8 Sandra Ct
Newbury Park, CA 91320-4302 800-634-4351
FAX: 805-498-8186
e-mail: customerservice@accesstr.com
www.accesstr.com
Don Krebs, President
The McClain Wheelchair Roller allows you to build strength and stamina in the comfort of your own home.

691 **Wheelchair Work Table**
Bailey Manufacturing Company
P.O. Box 130
Lodi, OH 44254-130 800-321-8372
FAX: 800-224-5390
e-mail: baileymfg@baileymfg.com
www.baileymfg.com

Wheelchairs: General

692 **21st Century Scientific, Inc.Bounder Power Wheelchair**
4931 N Manufacturing Way
Coeur D Alene, ID 83815-8931 208-667-8800
800-448-3680
FAX: 208-667-6600
e-mail: 21st@wheelchairs.com
wheelchairs.com
Ronald E. Prior, Ph.D., President and Founder
RD Davidson, Sales/Marketing Director
Susan Harris, CFO and Webmaster

High performance power chairs for active individuals. Very fast (11+ MPH), OFF-ROAD and Bariatric options available. Power seating options include tilt, recline, 13-inch seat elevator, reverse tilt, leg rests, standing and front load (latitude). 6-drive programmable electronics standard; lights, horn, electric leg bag emptier and many other options available. Customization is our specialty.

693 **Arcoa Travel Chair**
Maxi Aids
42 Executive Blvd
Farmingdale, NY 11735-4710
631-752-0521
800-522-6294
FAX: 631-752-0689
TTY: 631-752-0738
e-mail: sales@maxiaids.com
www.maxiaids.com

Elliott Zaretsky, Founder and President
The unique Comfort Travel Chair collapses into an easy to manage 25in x 26in x 11in and includes a strap for easy carrying. It weighs just 16 lbs. but can hold up to 200 lbs., making it the perfect travel companion. You can rest assured that it will 'stay put' with a dual wheel lock, while you enjoy the comfort and support of the padded swing-back armrests and 16in seat. *$197.00*

694 **Bariatric Wheelchairs Regency FL**
Gendron
520 W. Mulberry St.
Suite 100
Bryan, OH 43506
800-537-2521
FAX: 419-636-9261
e-mail: sales@gendroninc.com
www.gendroninc.com

Roberta Jacobs, National Sales Manager
Bariatric wheelchairs, for users weighing up to seven hundred pounds. Manual and power styles built to order for specific needs.

695 **Breezy**
Sunrise Medical/Quickie Designs
2842 Business Park Avenue
Fresno, CA 93727
800-333-4000
800-300-7502
e-mail: webmaster@sunmed.com
www.sunrisemedical.com

Pete Coburn, President
Randi Binstock, VP, Business Dev.
Peter Riley, Senior VP/Corporate CFO
Roxane Cromwell, SVP, Operations North America
This lightweight chair is durable, comfortable and flexible enough to meet the needs of a wide range of wheelchair users.

696 **Champion 1000**
Kuschall of America
3601 Rider Trl S
Earth City, MO 63045-1116
314-512-7000
800-654-4768
FAX: 800-542-3567

697 **Champion 2000**
Kuschall of America
3601 Rider Trl S
Earth City, MO 63045-1116
314-512-7000
800-654-4768
FAX: 800-542-3567

698 **Champion 3000**
Kuschall of America
3601 Rider Trl S
Earth City, MO 63045-1116
314-512-7000
800-654-4768
FAX: 800-542-3567

699 **Choosing a Wheelchair: A Guide for Optimal Independence**
Patient-Centered Guides
1005 Gravenstein Hwy N
Sebastopol, CA 95472-3836
707-827-7019
800-889-8969
FAX: 707-824-8268
e-mail: order@oreilly.com
www.patientcenters.com

Linda Lamb, Series Editor
Shawnde Paull, Marketing
Tim O'Reilly, Publisher
Gary Karp, Author
With the right wheelchair, quality of life increases dramatically and even people with severe disabilities can have a considerable degree of independence and activity. Choosing the wrong chair can indeed the tantamount to confinement. This book describes technology, options, and the selection process to help you identify the chair than can provide you with optimal independence.
$9.95
186 pages Paperback
ISBN 1-565924-11-8

700 **Convaid**
2830 California Street
Torrance, CA 90503
310-618-0111
888-266-8243
FAX: 310-618-2166
e-mail: convaid@convaid.com
www.convaid.com

Rocio, Sales Manager
Monica, National Account Representative
Veronica, Export Department
Five different styles of wheelchairs.

701 **Custom**
Fortress
P.O.Box 489
Clovis, CA 93613-489
559-322-5437
FAX: 559-323-0299

702 **Custom Durable**
21279 Protecta Dr
Elkhart, IN 46516-9539
574-522-7201
800-478-2363
FAX: 574-293-0202
e-mail: info@pvcdme.com
www.pvcdme.com

703 **Edge**
Fortress
P.O.Box 489
Clovis, CA 93613-489
559-322-5437
FAX: 559-323-0299

704 **Etac USA: F3 Wheelchair**
Ste J
2325 Parklawn Dr
Waukesha, WI 53186-2938
262-717-9910
800-678-3822
FAX: 262-796-4605
e-mail: etac1usa@execpc.com
www.execpc.com/~etac1usa

Mark Samolyk, Manager
A Swedish wheelchair designed to provide function, comfort and flexibility. Seat frame and upholstery are adjustable to fit each individual. Swing away, detachable footrests are standard. Available in frame widths from 14, 18 and 20 inch. Numerous accessories are available in order to individualize each chair. Lifetime warranty on frame for original user.

705 **Evacu-Trac**
Garaventa Canada
7505 - 134 A Street, Surrey, BC V3W
Blaine, WA 98231-1769
866-824-8314
e-mail: productinfo@evacutrac.com

706 **Folding Chair with a Rigid Feel**
Kuschall of America
3601 Rider Trl S
Earth City, MO 63045-1116
314-512-7000
800-654-4768
FAX: 800-542-3567

707 **Formula Series Active Mobility Wheelchairs**
Everest & Jennings
3233 Mission Oaks Blvd
Camarillo, CA 93012-5047
805-389-7450

708 **Freestyle II**
Fortress
P.O.Box 489
Clovis, CA 93613-489
559-322-5437
FAX: 559-323-0299

709 **Gadabout Wheelchairs**
Gadabout Wheelchairs
1165 Portland Ave
Rochester, NY 14621-3945
585-338-2110
800-828-4242
FAX: 585-338-2696

Michael Fonte, Owner
Enjoy independence with the wheelchair that is lightweight, portable, convenient, comfortable and sturdy.

710 **Gem Wheelchair & Scooter Service: Mobility & Homecare**
176-39 Union Tpke
Flushing, NY 11366-1515
718-969-8600
800-943-3578
FAX: 718-969-8300
e-mail: help@gemwheelchairservice.com
www.gemwheelchairservice.com/

711 **Gendron**
520 W. Mulberry St. Suite 100
Bryan, OH 43506
419-445-6060
800-537-2521
FAX: 419-636-9261
e-mail: rbell@gendroninc.com
www.gendroninc.com

Roberta Jacobs, National Sales Manager
Manufacturer of wheelchairs for a variety of other applications, specializing in bariatric mobility products.

712 **HiRider**
Gaymar Industries
10 Centre Dr
Orchard Park, NY 14127-2280
716-662-2551
800-828-7341
FAX: 800-993-7890
www.gaymar.com

Frank L Lumbar, CEO
John.K Whitney, Founder
Cindy Sylvia, Educational Svcs Administrator
Dan Kormowicz, International Sales Coordinator
A wheelchair that provides mobility in both sitting and standing positions.

713 **Innovative Products**
4351 W College Ave
Appleton, WI 54914-3928
920-738-9090
800-424-3369
FAX: 920-738-9050
www.att.com

Fritz H Heerdt, President
Wheelchairs; accessories.

714 **Liberty**
Fortress
P.O.Box 489
Clovis, CA 93613-489
559-322-5437
FAX: 559-323-0299

715 **Lightweight Breezy**
Motion Design
2842 Business Park Avenue
Fresno, CA 93727
800-333-4000
FAX: 800-300-7502
e-mail: webmaster@sunmed.com
www.sunrisemedical.com

Pete Coburn, President
Randi Binstock, VP, Business Dev.
Peter Riley, Senior VP/Corporate CFO
Roxane Cromwell, SVP, Operations North America
A lightweight wheelchair. *$750.00*

716 **Majors Medical Equipment**
415 W Wilshire Blvd., Suite A
Oklahoma City, OK 73116
405-840-5272
1 8-8 4-4 01
FAX: 405-840-5274
e-mail: help@mmedsupply.com
www.majorsmedicalequipment.com

Pat Metz, Owner
America's largest selection of wheelchairs and homecare equipment.

717 **Natural Access**
PO Box 5729
Santa Monica, CA 90409
310-392-9864
800-411-7789
FAX: 310-392-3874
e-mail: john_egan_2000@yahoo.com
www.landeez.com

John Egan, Owner
Provides the Landeez all-terrain wheelchair, that can roll easily on sand, gravel and snow for outdoor fun. The entire chair can fit inside a travel bag!

718 **Patient Transport Chair**
Mada Medical Products
625 Washington Ave
Carlstadt, NJ 07072-2901
201-460-0454
800-526-6370
FAX: 201-460-3509
e-mail: dianelind@mail.madamedical.com
www.madainternational.com

Jeffrey Adam, President
Mada's lightweight design transport chair is constructed of heavy gauge chrome-plated, steel tubing with reinforced cross braces.

719 **Posture-Glide Lounger**
Graham-Field Health Products
2935 Northeast Pkwy
Atlanta, GA 30360-2808
678-291-3207
FAX: 770-368-2386
e-mail: cs@grahamfield.com
www.grahamfield.com

Kenneth Spett, President & CEO
Marc Bernstein, Senior Vice President, Consumer Sales
Cherie Antoniazzi, Senior Vice President, Quality, Regulatory & Risk Management
Ivan Bielik, Senior Vice President, Business Analyst
Provides all day comfort and safe, independent mobilization with feet or hands. The ergonomically engineered seat back provides correct support.

720 **Prairie Cruiser**
Wheelchairs of Kansas
204 West 2nd Street P.O.Box 32
Ellis, KS 67637-32
785-726-4885
800-537-6454
FAX: 800-337-2447
e-mail: workinfo@go2wok.com
www.wheelchairsofkansas.com

721 **Redman Apache**
Redman Powerchair
1601 S Pantano Road Suite 107
Tucson, AZ 85710
520-546-6002
800-727-6684
FAX: 520-546-5530
e-mail: info@redmanpowerchair.com
www.redmanpowerchair.com

Don Redman, CEO
Paula Redman, CFO
Scott Evans, Regulatory affairs
Samuel Redman, General Manager
These ultralight, active use wheelchairs offer quick release rear wheels, adjustable arm height and detachable arm swing-away.

722 **Redman Crow Line**
Redman Powerchair
1601 S Pantano Road Suite 107
Tucson, AZ 85710
520-546-6002
800-727-6684
FAX: 520-546-5530
e-mail: info@redmanpowerchair.com
www.redmanpowerchair.com

Don Redman, CEO
Paula Redman, CFO
Scott Evans, Regulatory affairs
Samuel Redman, General Manager
Reclining wheelchair that reclines a full 90 degrees to flat and can be stopped anywhere on the axis.

723 **Rolls 2000 Series**
Invacare Corporation
1 Invacare Way
Elyria, OH 44035-4107
440-329-6000
800-333-6900
FAX: 877-619-7996
e-mail: info@invacare.com
www.invacare.com

A. Malachi Mixon, III, Chairman of the Board
Gerald B. Blouch, President and Chief Executive Officer
Joseph B. Richey, II, President - Invacare Technologies Division & SVP
Robert K. Gudbranson, Senior Vice President and Chief Financial Officer
These wheelchairs are the first light-weight wheelchairs designed for rental use.

724 **Skyway**
Skyway Machine
4451 Caterpillar Rd
Redding, CA 96003-1496
530-243-5151
800-332-3357
FAX: 530-243-5104
e-mail: sales@skywaywheels.com
www.skywaytuffwheels.com

Ken Coster, Sales Department
Parrey Cremeans, Sales Department
Rein Stolz, Engineering Department
Patrick McEachen, Customer Service
For over 20 years Skyway has been the world leader in composite wheels. Supplying over 650 different wheel combinations for wheelchairs, lawn and garden products, bicycles and a large assortment of wheeled devices. Wheel sizes range from 4 inch to 24 inch diameter.

725 **Stand-Up Wheelchairs**
Lifestand
P.O.Box 232171
Encinitas, CA 92023-2171
800-782-6324
FAX: 610-586-0847
e-mail: dallery@msn.com

Jacques A Dallery, President
Offers a complete line of manual, electric and stand-up wheelchairs for the disabled.

726 **Standard Wheelchair**
Mada Medical Products
625 Washington Ave
Carlstadt, NJ 07072-2901
201-460-0454
800-526-6370
FAX: 201-460-3509
e-mail: dianelind@mail.madamedical.com
www.madainternational.com

Jeffrey Adam, President
Mada's standard wheelchairs are designed and built for long-lasting, reliable operation. Each wheelchair is constructed of heavy gauge, chrome plated, steel framework and tube in tube construction at stress points. Mada's state-of-the art engineering uses the most modern components to provide the strength needed while keeping the chair's weight down.

727 **Super Light Folding Transport Chair with Carry Bag**
Maxi Aids
42 Executive Blvd
Farmingdale, NY 11735-4710
631-752-0521
800-522-6294
FAX: 631-752-0689
TTY: 631-752-0738
e-mail: sales@maxiaids.com
www.maxiaids.com

Elliott Zaretsky, Founder and President
Folds like a conventional folding chair for added convenience and includes carry bag, fold-down footrests, padded flip back armrests, standard rear wheel locks and an attractive frame with durable lightweight nylon upholstery and limited lifetime warranty. Weighs only 18 pounds. Easy to push or transport. *$319.95*

728 **Surf Chair**
2052 S Peninsula Dr
Daytona Beach, FL 32118-5237
386-253-0986
800-841-6610
FAX: 386-253-7600

729 **Vista Wheelchair**
Arista Surgical Supply Company/AliMed
297 High Street
Dedham, MA 02026-2852
781-329-2900
800-225-2610
FAX: 781-329-8392
e-mail: info@alimed.com
www.alimed.com

730 **Wheelchair with Shock Absorbers**
Iron Horse Productions
3114 Strawberry Ln
Port Huron, MI 48060-1727
810-987-6700
800-426-0354

Wheelchairs: Pediatric

731 **Commuter & Kid's Commuter**
Fortress
P.O.Box 489
Clovis, CA 93613-489
559-322-5437
FAX: 559-323-0299

732 **Convaid**
2830 California St
Torrance, CA 90503-3908
310-618-0111
888-266-8243
FAX: 310-618-2166
e-mail: convaid@earthlink.net
www.convaid.com

Rocio, Sales Manager
Monica, National Account Representative
Veronica
Convaid manufactures Mobile Positioning Systems for children. The Expedition, Safari Tilt, Cruiser, EZ Rider and Metro offer a non-institutional styling and are lightweight and compact-folding. The steel/aluminum structure is engineered for maximum comfort and durability. The mobile positioning lines come with

more than 20 positioning features and a full range of positioning adaptations. All chairs have been successfully crash-tested and offer a limited lifetime warranty (except the Metro).

733 Imp Tricycle
TRIAID
P.O.Box 1364
Cumberland, MD 21501-1364
301-759-3525
800-306-6777
FAX: 301-759-3525
e-mail: sales@triaid.com
www.triaid.com

734 Kid's Custom
Fortress
P.O.Box 489
Clovis, CA 93613-489
559-322-5437
FAX: 559-323-0299

735 Kid's Edge
Fortress
P.O.Box 489
Clovis, CA 93613-489
559-322-5437
FAX: 559-323-0299

736 Kid's Liberty
Fortress
P.O.Box 489
Clovis, CA 93613-489
559-322-5437
FAX: 559-323-0299

737 Kid-Friendly Chairs
Vector Mobility
5030 E Jensen Ave
Fresno, CA 93725-4010
559-431-3334
800-441-0358
FAX: 559-431-5535

Dave Deatherage, Owner
Manual base offers the lowest available floor to seat height, growth capability, one-third the parts of a conventional chair and no welds to break. The power unit features standard shapes and personality designs from elephants to inch worms and autos to rainbows, lowest seat height, and smallest turning radius on the market.

738 Koala Miniflex
Permobil USA
300 Duke Drive
Lebanon, TN 37090
800-736-0925
FAX: 800-231-3256
e-mail: info@permobilus.com
permobilusa.com

739 Seven Fifty-Five FS
Fortress
P.O.Box 489
Clovis, CA 93613-489
559-322-5437
FAX: 559-323-0299

740 TMX Tricycle
TRIAID
P.O.Box 1364
Cumberland, MD 21501-1364
301-759-3525
800-306-6777
FAX: 301-759-3525
e-mail: sales@triaid.com
www.triaid.com

Wheelchairs: Powered

741 Amigo Mobility International Inc.
6693 Dixie Highway
Bridgeport, MI 48722-9725
989-777-0910
800-692-6446
FAX: 800-334-7274
e-mail: info@myamigo.com
myamigo.com

Al Thieme, Chairman/Founder
Beth Thieme, CEO
Tim Drumhiller, President
Amigo Mobility designs and manufactures a complete line of power operated vehicles/mobility scooters and accessories in Bridgeport, Michigan.

742 Bounder Plus Power Wheelchair
21st Century Scientific
4931 N Manufacturing Way
Coeur D Alene, ID 83815-8931
208-667-8800
800-448-3680
FAX: 208-667-6600
e-mail: 21st@wheelchairs.com
wheelchairs.com

Ronald E. Prior, Ph.D., President and Founder
RD Davidson, Sales/Marketing Director
Susan Harris, CFO and Webmaster
Available in widths of 16 to 20 inches for users up to 500 pounds with a 2 year warranty on the entire chair. It offers all the standard features of a BOUNDER, plus reinforced rear wheel mounts, reinforced caster barrels, and super duty upholstery (with double liner and web straps under every screw). The BOUNDER Plus also features tandem cross struts, middle vertical support strut, seat rails supported at five points and back upholstery attached with machine screws.

743 Bounder Power Wheelchair
21st Century Scientific
4931 N Manufacturing Way
Coeur D Alene, ID 83815-8931
208-667-8800
800-448-3680
FAX: 208-667-6600
e-mail: 21st@wheelchairs.com
wheelchairs.com

Ronald E. Prior, Ph.D., President and Founder
RD Davidson, Sales/Marketing Director
Susan Harris, CFO and Webmaster
Available in a variety of widths from 16 to 18 inches for users up to 250 pounds. The rugged frame is constructed with steel tubing. The standard 12 position Adjustable Front Forks, made of 1/4 inch thick steel, provides impact dampening and seat tilt adjustment. A Dual Group 27 Sliding Battery Box provides extended range and easy battery maintenance. *$8695.00*

744 Breez 1025
Electro Kinetic Technologies
W194 N11301 McCormick Drive
Germantown, WI 53022
262-250-7740
800-824-1068
FAX: 262-250-7741
e-mail: sales@ek-tech.com
ek-tech.com

745 Damaco D90
Damaco
28918 Hancock Parkway
Valencia, CA 91355
661-775-2020
877-528-2288
FAX: 661-775-2025
www.atbatt.com

746 **Gem Wheelchair & Scooter Service: Mobility & Homecare**
176-39 Union Turnpike
Flushing, NY 11366-1515 718-969-8600
800-943-3578
FAX: 718-969-8300
e-mail: help@gemwheelchairservice.com
www.gemwheelchairservice.com/

747 **Geronimo**
Redman Powerchair
Ste 202
3840 S Palo Verde Rd
Tucson, AZ 85714-2076 520-294-1466
800-727-6684
FAX: 520-294-1460
Arnie Johnson, Owner
Wheelchair offering direct drive, two year electronic guarantee and micro controls.

748 **Invacare IVC Tracer EX2 Wheelchair with Legrest**
Maxi Aids
42 Executive Blvd
Farmingdale, NY 11735-4710 631-752-0521
800-522-6294
FAX: 631-752-0689
TTY: 631-752-0738
e-mail: sales@maxiaids.com
www.maxiaids.com
Elliott Zaretsky, Founder and President
Bob Messenger, Clinical Respiratory Specialist
The Tracer EX2 combines the design and technology of the Invacare 9000 A true dual axle position allows for repositioning the 24 inch rear wheels and 8 inch casters for adult and hemi seat-to-floor heights. The new design also makes it possible to interchange components with the 9000 series chairs. *$189.95*

749 **Jet 3 Ultra Power Wheelchair**
Maxi Aids
42 Executive Blvd
Farmingdale, NY 11735-4710 631-752-0521
800-522-6294
FAX: 631-752-0689
TTY: 800-281-3555
e-mail: sales@maxiaids.com
www.maxiaids.com
Elliott Zaretsky, Founder and President
Delivers a broad range of standard performance features like Active-Trac Suspension and a powerful 50 amp PG VSI controller on a very compact and maneuverable frame.

750 **One Thousand FS**
Fortress
P.O.Box 489
Clovis, CA 93613-489 559-322-5437
FAX: 559-323-0299

751 **Permobil Max 90**
Permobil
4020 Christopher Way
Plano, TX 75024 877-394-3941
e-mail: mumu.moorthi@sigmabatteries.com
www.sigmabatteries.com

752 **Permobil Super 90**
Permobil
4020 Christopher Way
Plano, TX 75024 877-394-3941
e-mail: mumu.moorthi@sigmabatteries.com
www.sigmabatteries.com

753 **Power Wheelchairs**
LaBac Systems
3845 Forest St
Denver, CO 80207-2516 800-370-6808
www.falconrehab.net
Power tilt and recline seating systems for wheelchairs, offering more comfort and dependability for the physically challenged.

754 **Power for Off-Pavement**
Redman Powerchair
1601 S Pantano Road
Suite 107
Tucson, AZ 85710-2076 520-546-6002
800-727-6684
FAX: 520-546-5530
e-mail: info@redmanpowerchair.com
www.redmanpowerchair.com
Don Redman, CEO
Paula Redman, CFO
Scott Evans, Regulatory Affairs
Samuel Redman, General manager
Power-drive wheelchair has a solid seat and can handle safely and securely knolls and off-pavement terrain.

Wheelchairs: Racing

755 **Eagle Sportschairs, LLC**
2351 Parkwood Rd
Snellville, GA 30039-4003 770-972-0763
800-932-9380
FAX: 770-985-4885
e-mail: eaglesportschairs@gmail.com
www.eaglesportschairs.com
Barry Ewing, Owner
The Eagle line of custom lightweight performance chairs includes a range of options to fit all racing and sport needs including; track, baseball, quad-rugby, tennis, field events and waterskiing. Also popular for daily use. We are able to customize any chair to accommodate size and disability and all frames have a full five year warranty.

756 **East Penn Manufacturing Company**
East Penn Manufacturing Company
Deka Road P.O.Box 147
Lyon Station, PA 19536-147 610-682-6361
FAX: 610-682-4781
e-mail: contactus@eastpenn-deka.com
www.eastpenn-deka.com
Harold DeLight, Breidegam
Chairman
Specially engineered for demanding deep-cycle applications Gelled electrolyte Deka Dominator Batteries provides maintenance-free operation, longer battery life and hours of reliable performance. Their excellent recharge characteristics provide quick turn around time.

757 **Invacare Top End**
1 Invacare Way
Elyria, OH 44035-4107 440-329-6000
800-333-6900
FAX: 877-619-7996
e-mail: info@invacare.com
www.invacare.com
A. Malachi Mixon, III, Chairman of the Board
Gerald B. Blouch, President and Chief Executive Officer
Joseph B. Richey, II, President - Invacare Technologies Division & SVP
Robert K. Gudbranson, Senior Vice President and Chief Financial Officer
Manufacturers of light weight, rigid, sport-specific wheelchairs such as the Eliminator line of racing chairs, T-3 tennis and softball chairs, and the Terminator for quad rugby and basketball. The Excelerator, XLT three-wheel hand cycle for adults and juniors. Check out our full line of wheelchairs to fit every need. $1,895-$2,495

758 **Invacare Top End Excelerator XLT Gold Handcyle**
Maxi Aids
42 Executive Blvd
Farmingdale, NY 11735-4710 631-752-0521
800-522-6294
FAX: 631-752-0689
TTY: 631-752-0738
e-mail: sales@maxiaids.com
www.maxiaids.com

Elliott Zaretsky, Founder and President
It's been completely re-designed to be light and faster with more control than ever before. The 27 speeds operated by Shimano Rapid fire hands-on-shifter/brake delivers smooth, responsive shifting and braking right at your fingertips. No foot pedaling!
$3036.00

Associations

General Disabilities

759 **ACS Federal Healthcare**
5270 Shawnee Rd
Alexandria, VA 22312-2310
703-941-4387
FAX: 703-310-0126

Helene Fisher, VP

Project RSVP supports the SSA's initiative to expand operations vocational rehabilitation services through a national network of private providers. Rehabilitation companies interested in gaining access to a new client base, acquiring a new funding stream, and developing creative service delivery and entrepreneurial partnerships, may benefit from such a program.

760 **AHEAD Association**
107 Commerce Centre Drive
Suite 204
Huntersville, NC 28078-5870
704-947-7779
FAX: 704-948-7779
e-mail: information@ahead.org
www.ahead.org

Stephan J. Smith, Exec. Dir.
Richard Allegra, Professional Dev. Dir.
Bea Awoniyi, President-Elect
Scott Lissner, President

The premiere professional association committed to full participation of persons with disabilities in postsecondary education. AHEAD values diversity, personal growth and development and creativity. Promotes leadership and exemplary practices. Provides professional development and disseminates information. Orchestrates resources through partnership and collaboration. AHEAD dynamically addresses current and emerging issues with respect to disability, and education to achieve universal access.

761 **APSE**
416 Hungerford Dr., Suite 418
Rockville, MD 20850
301-279-0060
FAX: 301-279-0075
e-mail: membership@apse.org
apse.org

Susie Rinne, President
Derek Nord, Vice President
Heidi Maghan, Delegates Chair

Through advocacy and education, the Association of People Supporting EmploymentFirst advances employment and self-sufficiency for all people with disabilities.

762 **Abilities!**
201 I U Willets Rd
Albertson, NY 11507-1516
516-465-1400
FAX: 516-465-3358
e-mail: info@viscardicenter.org
www.abilitiesonline.org

John.D. Kemp, President/CEO
Sheryl P Buchel, Executive Vice President & Chief Financial Officer
Lauren M. Marzo, Chief Development Officer
Patrice McCarthy Kuntzler, Exec. Dir.

Dedicated to creating a world in which people with disabilities will live simply as people.

763 **Acupressure Institute**
1533 Shattuck Ave
Berkeley, CA 94709-1516
510-845-1059
800-442-2232
e-mail: info@acupressure.com
www.acupressure.com

Michael Gach, Ph. D., Exec. Dir.
Joseph Carter, B.S., L.Ac., Dir. of Acupressure Institute
Kathleen Davis, B.A., C.M.T. Di, Teacher
Katie Carrin, Instructor

Since 1976 the Acupressure institute has offered comprehensive acupressure trainings in the traditional Asian Bodywork Therapy (ABT)such as Thai massage and Shiatsu massage to students from around the world. In comparing other Acupressure schools, our trainings provide high quality education to support each student'sprofessional and personal goals, in a setting that encourages communication, respect, and confidentiality and safety for everyone.

764 **Advocacy Center**
590 South Ave
Rochester, NY 14620-1371
585-546-1700
800-650-4967
FAX: 585-546-7069
TTY: 585-546-1700
e-mail: info@advocacycenter.com
www.advocacycenter.com

Paul Shew, Executive Director
Joyce Steel, Director
Stepen G. Schwarz, President
Adam Anolik, Vice President

Is a non profit organization located in New York State that educates, supports, and advocates with people who have disabilities, their families and circles of support. A diverse consumer-driven organization leading New York State in shaping the future through the development of innovative, outcome-oriented, and quality initiatives for people with disabilities, their families, and circle of support.

765 **Advocacy Center for Persons with Disabilitites**
2728 Centerview Dr
Ste 102
Tallahassee, FL 32301-6298
800-342-0823
FAX: 850-488-8640
TTY:800-346-4127
e-mail: info@advocacycenter.org
www.advocacycenter.org

Bob Whitney, Executive Director
Paige Morgan, Executive Assistant

A non-profit organization providing protection and advocacy services in the State of Florida. The Center's mission is to advance the dignity, equality, self-determination and expressed choices of individuals with disabilities.

766 **Advocates for Children of New York**
151 W 30th St
5th Fl
New York, NY 10001
212-947-9779
FAX: 212-947-9790
e-mail: info@advocatesforchildren.org
www.advocatesforchildren.org

Kim Sweet, Executive Director
Jamie A Levitt, President
Barry Ford, Treasurer
Harriet Chan King, Secretary

AFC works on behalf of children from infancy to age 21 who are at greatest risk for school-based discrimination and/or academic failure. These include children with disabilities, ethnic minorities, immigrants, homeless children, foster care children, limited English proficient children and those living in poverty.

767 **Alliance for Technology Access**
1119 Old Humboldt Rd
Jackson, TN 38305
731-554-5282
800-914-3017
FAX: 731-554-5283
TTY: 731-554-5284
e-mail: atainfo@ataccess.org
www.ataccess.org

Margaret Doumitt, Executive Director
James Allison, President
Bob Van Der Linde, Vice President
Mike Hewitt, Secretary/Treasurer

The ATA is a growing national network of technology resource centers, organizations, individuals and companies. ATA encourages and facilitates the empowerment of people with disabilities to participate fully in their communities. Through public education, information and referral, capacity building in community organizations, and advocacy/policy efforts, the ATA enables millions of people to live, learn, work, define their futures, and achieve their dreams.

768 **American Academy of Environmental Medicine**
6505 E Central Ave #296
Wichita, KS 67206-1924
316-684-5500
FAX: 316-684-5709
e-mail: administrator@aaemonline.org
www.aaemonline.org

De Rogers Fox, Executive Director
Amy L. Dean D.O., President
Janette Hope, President-Elect
Jennifer Armstrong, Secretary
Environmental Medicine is the comprehensive, proactive and preventive strategic approach to medical care dedicated to the evaluation, management, and prevention of the adverse consequences resulting from Environmentally Triggered Illnesses.

769 **American Academy of Pediatrics**
141 NW Point Blvd
Elk Grove Village, IL 60007-1098
847-434-4000
800-433-9016
FAX: 847-434-8000
e-mail: kidsdocs@aap.org
www.aap.org

Rober.W. Block,MD,FAAP, President
Thomas K. McInerny, MD, FAAP, President-Elect
Errol Alden, MD, Executive Director/CEO
O. Marion Burton, MD, FAAP, Immediate Past President
Organization of 60,000 pediatricians committed to the attainment of optimal physical, mental, and social health and well-being for all infants, children, adolescents and young adults.

770 **American Association of Children's Residential Centers**
11700 W Lake Park Dr
Milwaukee, WI 53224-3021
877-332-2272
FAX: 877-362-2272
e-mail: info@aarc-dc.org
www.aacrc-dc.org

Kari Sisson, National Dir.
Margaret Vimont LCSW, President
Okpara Rice, Secretary
William P. Martone, MS, President
The American Association of Children's Residential Centers believes that children and adolescents, and their families, are entitled to treatment which offers the maximum opportunity for growth and change. AACRC believes that clinically crafted residential treatment options, ranging from community based homes through institutional environments, are essential components in a comprehensive system of behavioral health care.

771 **American Association of Oriental Medicine**
9650 Rockville Pike
Bethesda, MD 20814
866-455-7999
FAX: 301-634-7099
www.aaaomonline.org

Michael Jabbour, MS, LAc, President
Kimberley Benjamin, LAc, VP
Jane Yu, LAc, Secretary
John B. Barrett, CPA, LAc, Treasurer
Dedicated to the promotion and advancement of high ethical, educational, and professional standards in the practice of acupuncture and Oriental medicine (AOM) in the U.S.

772 **American Association of People with Disabilities**
2013 H Street, NW, 5th Floor
Washington, DC 20006-1675
202-457-0046
800-840-8844
FAX: 202-457-0473
TTY: 800-840-8844
e-mail: referrals@aapd.com
www.aapd.com

Mark Perriello, President/CEO
Helena Berger, Exec VP & COO
Jason Mida, VP of Dev.
Lara Schwartz, VP of External Affairs
The largest national nonprofit cross-disability member organization in the United States, dedicated to ensuring economic self-sufficiency and political empowerment for the more than 56 million Americans with disabilities. AAPD works in coalition with other disability organizations for the full implimentation and enforcement of disability nondiscrimination laws, particularly the Americans With Disabilities Act (ADA) of 1990 and the Rehabilitation Act of 1973.

773 **American Board of Clinical Metal Toxicology**
4889 Smith Rd
West Chester, OH 45069
513-863-6277
80- 35- 222
FAX: 513-942-3934
e-mail: treasurer@abcmt.org
www.abcmt.org

Rashid A Buttar, Chairman
James M. Holbert, MD, PhD, Vice Chairman
James Smith, DO, Treasurer
J Joseph Holliday, MD, Director
Dedicated to establishing and maintaining guidelines and standards for the practice of Clinical Metal Toxicology and to the assurance of a superior level of competence on the part of physicians treating patients with this psectrum of expanding global afflictions.

774 **American Board of Professional Disability Consultants**
Belle Meade Office Park. 4525 Hardi
3rd Fl
Nashville, TN 37205
615-327-2984
FAX: 615-327-9235
e-mail: americanbd@aol.com
www.americandisability.org

775 **American Botanical Council**
6200 Manor Rd
Austin, TX 78723-3754
512-926-4900
FAX: 512-926-2345
e-mail: abc@herbalgram.org
www.herbalgram.org

Mark Blumenthal, Executive Director/Founder
Lucy Bruno, Executive Assistant
Gayle Engels, Special Projects Director
The American Botanical Council (ABC) is the leading independent, nonprofit, international member-based organization providing education using science-based ad traditional information to promote the responsible use of herbal medicine.

776 **American Camping Association**
5000 State Road 67 N
Martinsville, IN 46151-7902
765-342-8456
800-428-2267
FAX: 765-342-2065
www.acacamps.org

Tisha Bolger, President
Peg Smith, CEO
Scott Brody, VP
Dayna Hardine, VP
The American Camp Association is a community of camp professionals who, for nearly 100 years, have joined together to share our knowledge and experience and to ensure the quality of camp programs. Because of our diverse 7,000 plus emmbership and exceptional programs, children and adults have the opportunity to learn powerful lessons in cmmunity, character-building, skill development, and healthy-living—-lessons that can be learned nowhere else.

777 **American Chiropractic Association**
1701 Clarendon Blvd
Arlington, VA 22209-2721
703-276-8800
FAX: 703-243-2593
e-mail: memberinfo@acatoday.org
www.acatoday.org

Keith S. Overland, DC, President
Bill O'Connelll, VP
Janet Ridgely, Deputy Exec VP
Dean Millard, Information Systems Senior Dir.
The ACA is a professional organization representing Doctors of Chiropratic. Its mission is to preserve, protect, improve, and promote the chiropractic profession and the services of Doctors of

Chiropratic for the benefit of the patients they serve. The purpose of the ACA is to provide leadership in health care and a positive vision for the chiropractic profession and its natural approach to health and wellness.

778 **American College of Advancement in Medicine**
8001 Irvine Center Dr
Ste 825
Irvine, CA 92618-2967
949-309-3520
800-532-3688
FAX: 949-272-3729
e-mail: guestservices@acam.org
www.acam.org

Mark O'Neal Speight, MD, President/CEO
Jeffrey Morrison, MD, Executive VP
Allen Green, MD, Treasurer and CFO
Dana Cohen, MD, Director

The American College for Advancement in Medicine (ACAM)is a not-for-profit society dedicated to educating physicians and other health care professionals on the latest findings and emerging procedures in preventive/nutritional medicine. ACAM's goals are to improve skills, knowledge and diagnostic procedures as they relate to complimentary and alternative medicine; to support research; and to develop awareness of alternative methods of medical treatment.

779 **American College of Nurse Midwives**
8403 Colesville Rd
Ste 1550
Silver Spring, MD 20910-6374
240-485-1800
FAX: 240-485-1818
e-mail: info@acnm.org
www.midwife.org

Holly Kennedy, President
Ginger Breedlove, President-Elect
Catherine A Collins-Fulea, Vice-President
Tanya Tanner, Treasurer

The American College of Nurse-Midwives (ACNM) is the oldest women's health care organization in the U.S. ACNM provides research, accredits midwifery education programs, administers and promotes continuing education programs, establishes clinical practice standards, creates liasons with state and federal agencies and members of Congress.

780 **American Counseling Association**
5999 Stevenson Ave
Alexandria, VA 22304-3304
703-823-0252
800-347-6647
FAX: 800-473-2329
TTY: 703-823-6862
e-mail: webmaster@counseling.org
www.counseling.org

Richard Yep, Executive Director
Marcheta Evans, Immediate Past President
Stacy Shaver, Executive Office
Brad Erford, President

The American Counseling Association is a not-for-profit, professional and educational organization that is dedicated to the growth and enhancement of the counseling profession.

781 **American Herbalists Guild**
PO Box 230741
Boston, M 02123
857-350-3128
e-mail: ahgoffice@earthlink.net
www.americanherbalistsguild.com

Bevin Clare, M.S., R.H., CN, VP
Roy Upton RH(AHG), Board of Advisors
KP Khalsa, RH(AHG), President
David N. Harder, RH (AHG), Treasurer

Founded in 1989 as a non-profit, educational organization to represent the goals and voices of herbalists specializing in the medicinal use of plants. Our primary goal is to promote a high level of professionalism and education in the study and practice of theraputic herbalism.

782 **American Holistic Medical Association**
27629 Chagrin Blvd. Suite 213
Woodmere, OH 44122
216-292-6644
FAX: 216-292-6688
e-mail: info@holisticmedicine.org
www.holisticmedicine.org

Molly Roberts, M.D., M.S, President
David Riley MD, Member at Large
Natalie Talis, BA, Marketing Manager
Steve.L Caldwell, Executive Director/CEO

The mission of the AMHA is to support practitioners in their evolving personal and professional development as healers and to educate physicians about holistic medicine.

783 **American Massage Therapy Association**
500 Davis St
Ste 900
Evanston, IL 60201-4695
847-864-0123
877-905-0577
FAX: 847-864-5196
e-mail: info@amtamassage.org
www.amtamassage.org

Winona Bontrager, President
Rachel Mann, VP
Nathan Nordstrom, VP
Jeff Smoot, VP

AMTA works to establish massage therapy as integral to the maintenance of good health and complementary to other therapeudic processes; to advance the profession through ethics and standards, certification, school accreditation, continuing education, professional publications, legislative efforts, public education, and fostering the development of members.

784 **American Occupational Therapy Association**
4720 Montgomery Lane
Suite 600
Bethesda, MD 20814-3449
301-652-2682
800-789-2682
FAX: 301-652-7711
TTY: 800-377-8555
e-mail: praota@aota.org
www.aota.org

Florence Clark, President
Ginny Stoffel, President-Elect
Amy Lamb, VP
Paul A Fontana, Secretary

Advances the quality, availability, use and support of occupational therapy through standard setting, advocacy, education, and research on behalf of its members.

785 **American Organization for Bodywork Therapies of Asia**
1010 Haddonfield Berlin Rd
Ste 408
Voorhees, NJ 08043- 3514
856-782-1616
FAX: 856-782-1653
e-mail: office@aobta.org
www.aobta.org

Wayne Mylin, President
Beverly Sonen, VP
Stuart Watts, Treasure/Secretary
Angela.H. McConnell, Director of Membership

The American Organization for Bodywork Therapies of Asia (AOBTA) is a professional membership organizaton which promotes Asian Bodywork Therapy and its practitioners while honoring a diversity of disciplines. AOBTA serves its community of members by supporting appropriate credentialing; defining scope of practice and educational standards; and providing resources for training, professional development and networking. AOBTA advocates public policy to protect its members.

786 **American Public Health Association**
800 I St NW
Washington, DC 20001-3710 202-777-2742
FAX: 202-777-2534
TTY:202-777-2500
e-mail: comments@apha.org
www.apha.org

George Benjamin, Executive Director
Adewale Troutman, President
Joyce R. Gaufin, President-Elect
Richard J. Cohen, PhD, FACHE, Treasurer

Founded in 1872, APHA is the oldest, largest and most diverse organization of public health professionals in the world. The association works to protect all Americans and their communities from preventable, seruious health threats. APHA represents a broad array of health officials, educators, environmentalists, policy-makers and health providers at all levels working both within and outside governmental organizations and educational institutions.

787 **American Red Cross**
2025 E Street
Washington, DC 20006-6434 202-303-5214
800-733-2767
FAX: 518-459-8268
e-mail: news@redcrossneny.org
www.redcrossneny.org

Gary Striar, CEO
Susan Rounds, COO
Gary Ferris, Executive Director
Lynn Gilbert, Executive Director

Today, in addition to domestic disaster relief, the American Red Cross offers compassionate services in five other areas: community services that help the needy; support and comfort for military members and their families; the collection, processing and distribution of lifesaving blood and blood products; educational programs that promote health and safety; and international relief and development programs.

788 **American Self-Help Clearinghouse**
50 Morris Avenue
St Clares Health Services
Denville, NJ 07834 973-625-7107
800-367-6274
FAX: 973-326-9467
e-mail: info@selfhelpgroups.org
www.selfhelpgroups.org

Edward J Madara MS, Director

Provides information on national self-help groups and offers training and technical assistance to exisiting and new self-help groups and clearinghouses. It has compiled a national database of over 800 of these model groups. Provides information on resource groups such as Violence Anonymous, Batterers Anonymous, and Stalkers' Victims Support Groups.

789 **American Society for the Alexander Technique**
PO Box 2307
Dayton, OH 45401-2307 937-586-3732
800-473-0620
FAX: 937-586-3699
e-mail: webteam@AmSATonline.org
www.amsat.ws

Kathryn Miranda, Chair
Ann Rodiger, Treasurer
Jennifer Sielicki, Secretary
Meg Jolley, Member at Large

The Alexander Technique is a proven, effective self help method for improving balance and coordination and increasing movement awareness by eliminating habitual reactions of misuse in every day activities. AmSats mission is to define, maintain and promote the Alexander Technique at its highest standard of professional practice and conduct.

790 **American Society of Bariatric Physicians**
2821 S Parker Rd
Ste 625
Aurora, CO 80014-2735 303-770-2526
FAX: 303-779-4834
e-mail: info@asbp.org
www.asbp.org

Laurie Traetow,CPA, Executive Director
Stacy Schmidt,PhD, Health Director
David Bryman, DO, President
Deborah Bade Horn DO, MPH, MS, Vice President

The American Society of Bariatric Physicians is an international association and allied health care professionals with special interest and experience in the comprehensive treatment of overweight, obesity and related disorders.

791 **American Society of Clinical Hypnosis**
140 N Bloomingdale Rd
Bloomingdale, IL 60108-1017 630-980-4740
FAX: 630-351-8490
e-mail: info@asch.net
www.asch.net

Michael White, Communication/Marketing Director
Erickson, MD Founder

To provide and encourage education programs to further, in every ethical way, the knowledge, understanding, and application of hypnosis in health care; to encourage research and scientific publication in the field of hypnosis; to promote the further recognition and acceptance of hypnosis as an important tool in clinical health care and focus for scientific research; to cooperate with other professional societies that share mutual goals, ethics, and interests

792 **Association for Applied Psychophysiology and Biofeedback**
10200 W 44th Ave
Ste 304
Wheat Ridge, CO 80033-2840 303-422-8436
800-477-8892
e-mail: info@aapb.org
www.aapb.org

Francine Butler, Executive Director
Richard Sherman, PhD, President
Richard Harvey, PhD, Treasurer
Stuart C. Donaldson, President-Elect

Provides names and phone numbers of local chapters. Mission is to advance the development, dissemination and utilization of knowledge about applied psychophysiology and biofeedback to improve health and the quality of life through research, education, and practice.

793 **Association for Persons in Supported Employment**
PO Box 1280
Rockville, MD 20849 301-279-0060
FAX: 301-251-3762
e-mail: jenny@apse.org
www.apse.org

David Hoff, President
Susan Rinne, VP
Laura.A. Owens,PhD, Executive Director
Vic Gable, Treasurer

Supported employment enables people with disabilities who have not been successfully employed to work and contribute to society. Focuses on a person's abiliities and provides the supports the individual needs to be successful on a long-term basis.

794 **Association for Persons with Severe Handicaps (TASH)**
1001 Connecticut Avenue, NW
Ste 235
Washington, DC 20036 202-540-9020
FAX: 202-540-9019
e-mail: info@tash.org
www.tash.org

David Westling, President
Barbara Trader, Executive Director
Jean Trainor, VP
Jonathan Riethmaier, Advocacy Communications Manager

International association of people with disabilities, their family members, other advocates and professionals, fighting for a society in which inclusion of all people in all aspects of society is the norm.

795 **Association of Educational Therapists**
7044 S. 13th St.
Oak Creek, WI 90064-5315 414-908-4949
FAX: 414-768-8001
e-mail: aet@aetonline.org
www.aetonline.org
Jeanette Rivera, MA, BCET, President
Susan Grama, MA, President
Jeanette Rivera, MA, BCET, Secretary
Vicki Bergoff, JD, ET/P, Director
Educational Therapy offers children and adults with learning disabilities and other learning challenges a wide range of intensive, individualized interventions designed to remediate learning problems.

796 **Association of University Centers on Disabilities**
AUCD
1100 Wayne Ave
Ste 1000
Silver Spring, MD 20910-5646 301-588-8252
FAX: 301-588-2842
e-mail: aucdinfo@aucd.org
www.aucd.org
George Jesien, Executive Director
Julie Fodor, PhD, President
Leslie Cohen, JD, Treasurer
Karen Edwards, MD, MPH, Secretary
The central office for the 61 University Centers for Excellence programs and 21 Mental Retardation and Developmental Disabilities Research Centers and is their representative to the federal government. UCEDD's are located at major universities and teaching hospitals in all 50 states, the District of Columbia and many US territories. UCCED's target their activities to support the independence, productivity and integration into the community of individuals with developmental disabilities.

797 **Association on Higher Education and Disability (AHEAD)**
107 Commerce Centre Dr
Ste 204
Huntersville, NC 28078- 5870 704-947-7779
FAX: 704-948-7779
e-mail: information@ahead.org
www.ahead.org
Richard Allegra, Director of Professional Dev.
Jean Ashmore, President
Michael Johnson, Treasurer
Scott Lissner, President-Elect
International, multicultural organization of proessionals committed to full participation in higher education for persons with disabilities. Plans and develops training programs, workshops, publications and conferences. Founded in 1977 to address the need and concern for upgrading the quality of services and support available to persons with disabilities in higher education.

798 **Bastyr University Natural Health Clinic**
3670 Stone Way N
Seattle, WA 98103-8004 206-834-4110
FAX: 206-834-4107
www.bastyrcenter.org

799 **Beach Center on Families and Disability**
University of Kansas
1200 Sunnyside Ave
Rm 3136
Lawrence, KS 66045-7534 785-864-7600
FAX: 785-864-7605
TTY:785-864-3434
e-mail: beachcenter@ku.edu
www.beachcenter.org
Ann Turnbull, Co-Founder, Co-Director
Rud Turnbull, Co-Founder, Co-Director
Victoria Cotsworth, Project Coordinator
Peter Griggs, Evaluation Coordinator
A federally funded center that conducts research and training in the factors that contribute to the successful functioning of families with members who have disabilities.

800 **Birth Defect Research for Children**
976 Lake Baldwin Lane, Suite 104
Orlando, FL 32814 407-895-0802
e-mail: staff@birthdefects.org
www.birthdefects.org
Betty Mekdeci, Manager/Founder
A nonprofit organization that provides information about birth defects of all kinds to parents and professionals. Offers a library of medical books and files of information on less common categories of birth defects and is involved in research to discover possible links between environmental exposures and birth defects.

801 **Bonnie Prudden Myotherapy**
4330 E. Havasu Road PO Box 65240
Tucson, AZ 85718 520-529-3979
800-221-4634
FAX: 520-529-6679
e-mail: info@bonnieprudden.com
www.bonnieprudden.com
Enid Whittaker, Associate Director
Myotherapy is a method for relaxing muscle spasm, improving circulation and alleviating pain. Pressure is applied using elbows, knuckled or fingers, and held for several seconds to defuse trigger points. The success of this method depends upon the use of specific corrective exercises of the freed muscles.

802 **Brain Injury Association of America**
1608 Spring Hill Rd
Ste 110
Vienna, VA 22812 703-761-0750
800-444-6443
FAX: 703-761-0755
e-mail: shconnors@biausa.org
www.biausa.org
Susan H Connors, President/CEO
Mary Ritter, Exec VP/COO
Marianna Abashian, Dir. of Professional Svcs
Amy C. Colberg, Dir. of Govt Affairs
Founded in 1980, the Brain Injury Association of America (BIAA) is the leading national organization serving and representing individuals, families and professionals who are touched by a life-altering, often devistating, traumatic brain injury (TBI) Together with its network of more then 40 charted state affiliates, as well as hundreds of local chapters and support groups across the country, the BIAA provides information, education and support to assist the 5.3 million living with brain injuries

803 **CAPP National Parent Resource Center Federation for Children with Special Needs**
45 Bromfield St
10th Fl
Boston, MA 02108 866-815-8122
FAX: 617-542-7832
e-mail: info@ppal.net
www.ppal.net
Lisa Lambert, Executive Director
Chip Wilder, Chair
Joanna Allison, Vice Chair
Anne Silver, Treasurer
A parent-run resource system designed to further the needs and goals of family-centered, community-based coordinated care for children with special health needs and their families. Offers written materials, training packages, workshops and presentations for parents and professionals on special education, health care financing and other topics.

804 **CARF Rehabilitation Accrediation Commission**
6951 E Southpoint Rd
Tucson, AZ 85756 520-325-1044
888-281-6531
FAX: 520-318-1129
TTY: 888-281-6531
e-mail: info@carf.org
www.carf.org

Brian J Boon, Ph.D., President/CEO
Amanda E Birch, Administrator of Operations
Cindy L. Johnson, CPA, Chief Resource
Darren M. Lehrfeld, Chief Accreditation Officer
CARF serves as the standards-setting and accrediting body for rehabilitation and life enhancement programs and services. The independent, not-for-profit commission provides accrediation of human service providers in the areas of aging services, behavioral health, child and youth services, DMEPOS, employment and community services, medical rehabilitation, and opioid treatment programs.

805 **Canine Companions for Independence**
National Offices
P.O.Box 446
Santa Rosa, CA 95402-0446 707-577-1700
800-572-2275
TTY:707-577-1756
e-mail: info@cci.org
www.cci.org

Alan Feinne, CFO
Corey Hudson, CEO
Paul Mundell, National Dir. of Canine Programs
Anne Gittinger, Chair of Board of Officers
A nonprofit organization that enhances the lives of people with disabilities by providing highly trained assistance dogs and ongoing support to ensure quality partnerships.

806 **Canine Helpers for the Handicapped**
5699 Ridge Rd
Lockport, NY 14094-9408 716-433-4035
FAX: 716-439-0822
e-mail: chhdogs@aol.com
www.caninehelpers.org

Beverly D. Underwood, Executive Director
A nonprofit organization devoted to custom training Assistance Dogs to assist people with disabilities to lead more independent, secure lives.

807 **Cape Organization for Rights of the Disabled (CORD)**
106 Bassett Ln
Hyannis, MA 02601-3800 508-775-8300
800-541-0282
FAX: 508-775-7022
TTY: 800-541-0282
e-mail: cordinfo@cilcapecod.org
www.cilcapecod.org

Cathy Taylor, ADA Specialist
The Cape Organization for the Rights of the Disabled (CORD) has been aggresively working since 1984 to advance the independence, productivity, and integration of people with disabilities into mainstream society. CORD is the Center for Independent Living (CIL) and is a member of the Aging and Disability Resources Consortium (ADRC) serving Cape Cod and the Islands.

808 **Case Management Society of America**
6301 Ranch Dr
Little Rock, AR 72223-4623 501-225-2229
800-216-2672
FAX: 501-221-9068
e-mail: cmsa@cmsa.org
www.cmsa.org

Nancy Skinner, RN-BC, CCM, President
Betty Overbey, RN-BC, CRRN,, Secretary
Jose Alejandro, RN-BC, MSN, Treasurer
Cheri A Lattimer, Executive Director
The Case Management Society of America is an international, non-profit organization founded in 1990 dedicated to the support and development of the profession of case management through educational forums, networking opportunities and legislative involvement.

809 **Center for Assistive Technology and Environmental Access**
490 Tenth St NW
Atlanta, GA 30332-0156 404-894-4960
800-726-9119
FAX: 404-894-9320
TTY: 404-894-4960
e-mail: catea@coa.gatech.edu
www.catea.org

Carrie Bruce, Research Scientist
Nagmesh Kumar, Research Engineer
Charlie Drummond, Administrative Assistant
Sarah Endicott, Research Scientist
CATEA supports individuals with disabilities of any age within the State of Georgia and beyond through expert services, research, design and technological development, information dissemination, and educational programs.

810 **Center for Disability Resources**
Pediatrics, School Of Medicine,Univ Of S. Carolina
8301 Farrow Rd
Columbia, SC 29208-1 803-216-3300
FAX: 803-935-5059
e-mail: steve.wilson@uscmed.sc.edu
www.uscm.med.sc.edu/cdrhome/

Jerome D. Odom Ph.D., Exec. Dir.
Susan Greer, Fiscal/Foundation Coordinator
Mechelle English, Senior Dev. Dir.
Kim E. Creek, PhD., Dir.
A University Affiliated Program which develops model programs designed to serve persons with disabilities and to train students in fields related to disabilities.

811 **Center for Mind/Body Studies**
5525 Connecticut Ave NW
Suite 415
Washington, DC 20015- 1813 202-966-7338
FAX: 202-966-2589
e-mail: center@cmbm.org
www.cmbm.org

Jim S. Gordon, MD, Founder & Dir.
Jo Cooper, Dir. of Nutrition Programs
Rosemary Murrain, Dir. of Administration & Finance
Amy Shinal, Clinical Dir.
The Center for Mind-Body Medicine is a non-profit educational organization dedicated to reviving the spirit and transforming the practice of medicine. The Center is working to create a more effective, comprehensive and compassionate model of healthcare and education. The Center's model combines the precision of modern science with the best of the world's healing traditions.

812 **Center for Universal Design**
NC State University
PO Box 8613
Raleigh, NC 27695-8613 919-515-3082
800-647-6777
FAX: 919-515-8951
e-mail: cud@ncsu.edu
www.design.ncsu.edu/cud

Sean Vance, Acting Director
Richard C Duncan, MRP:, Director of Training
Leslie Young, M.S.,, Director of Design
Angela Brockelsby, Director of Communications
A federally funded resource center that works toward improving housing for people with disabilities. Provides technical assistance, training and publications on accessible housing and universal design.

813 **Change**
1413 Park Rd NW
Washington, DC 20010-2801 202-387-3725
FAX: 202-387-3729
e-mail: changeinc@hotmail.com

Gracie Rolling, Executive Director
Therman Walker, President
Preston Hursey Jr., VP

Offers counseling/assessment, emergency food and clothing referrals, rental assistance and job assistance to disabled persons in the District of Columbia area.

814 Child and Parent Resource Institute
600 Sanatorium Road
London, ON, ON N6H-3W7
519-858-2774
877-494-2774
FAX: 519-858-3913
TTY: 519-858-0257
e-mail: Andrea.Wright@ontario.ca
www.cpri.ca

Dr. Shannon Stewart, Program Manager
Kim Arbeau, Research Coordinator
Liz Willits, Research Project Assistant
Melissa Currie, Manager (A)

Provides highly specialized services to children and youth from 0-18 years of age with complex mental health and/or developmental challenges on a short term inpatient and community basis.

815 Children's Alliance
420 Capitol Ave
Frankfort, KY 40601-2837
502-875-3399
FAX: 502-223-4200
e-mail: michelle@childrensallianceky.org
www.childrensallianceky.org

Michelle Sanborn, President
Mary Smither, Office Assistant
Melissa Muse, Member Services Director
Kathy Adams, Director of Public Policy

An association of individuals and human services organizations committed to being a voice for at-risk children and families. Interacts with the legislative and executive branches of government and assists members in developing services that most effectively meet the needs of at-risk children and families.

816 Children's National Medical Center
111 Michigan Ave NW
Washington, DC 20010-2916
202-476-2327
888-884-2327
FAX: 202-476-2270
e-mail: tbear@childrensnational.org
www.cnmc.org

Kurt Newman, MD, President/CEO
Raymond S. Sczudlo, Esq, Exec VP, Chief Legal Officer
Douglas Myers, Exec VP, CFO
Mark Batshaw, MD, Exec VP/CAO

Our mission is to be preeminent in providing health care services that enhance the health and well-being of children regionally, nationally and internationally. Through leadership and innovation, Children's will create solutions to pediatric health care problems. To meet the unique health care needs of children, adolescents and their families, Children's will excel in Care, Advocacy, Research and Education.

817 Clay Tree Society
838 Old Victoria Road
Nanaimo, BC V9R-6A1
250-753-5322
FAX: 250-753-2749
e-mail: claytree@shaw.ca
www.claytree.org

David Gaskill, President
Kim Chadwick, Vice President
Donna Browning, Treasurer
Veronica Harrison, Secretary

Non-profit society providing day programming for 75 adults with various developmental disabilities governed by an elected Board of Directors and funded by Community Living British Columbia and BC Gaming.

818 Community Enterprises
441 Pleasant Street
Northampton, MA 01060-598
413-584-1460
FAX: 413-586-1121
TTY:413-584-1460
e-mail: info@communityenterprises.com
www.communityenterprises.com

Dick Venne, President/CEO
William D. Donahue, Vice-Chair
Joanne Carlisle, Secretary/Clerk
Kate LaMay-Miller, Chair

Provide supported education services in a community college setting; supported employment including job training, placement and follow-up; transitional services from group homes and other settings to supported living within the community.

819 Council For Exceptional Children
2900 Crystal Drive, Suite 1000
Arlington, VA 22202
888-232-7733
e-mail: service@cec.sped.org
cec.sped.org

820 DB-Link
National Consortium on Deaf-Blindness
345 N. Monmouth Ave.
Monmouth, OR 97361-1329
503-838-8391
800-438-9376
FAX: 503-838-8150
TTY: 800-854-7013
e-mail: info@nationaldb.org
www.nationaldb.org

Kathy McNulty, Associate Director
D Jay Gense, Director
John W. Reiman, PhD., Associate Director
Joe McNulty, Co-Principal Investigator

Found at the National Consortium of Deaf-Blindness, DB-LINK is the largest collection of information related to deaf-blindness worldwide. A team of information specialists makes this extensive resource available in response to direct requests, via the NCDB website, through conferences, and via a variety of electronic medium.

821 Department of Physical Medicine & Rehabilitation at Sinai Hospital
2401 W Belvedere Ave
Baltimore, MD 21215-5271
410-601-9000
FAX: 410-601-9692
www.lifebridgehealth.org

Scott E. Brown, Department Chief
Neil Meltzer, President
Melanie C. Brown, M.D., Residency Program Dir.
Michael Anderson, Core Teaching Faculty

As one of largest, most comprehensive and most highly respected providers of health-related services to the people of the Northwest Baltimore region, LifeBridge heath advocates preventive services, wellness and fitness services and programs to educate and support the communities it serves. LifeBridge is dedicated to advancing the health of the community through a variety of health and wellness programs and services.

822 DisAbility LINK
755 Commerce Drive
Suite 105
Decatur, GA 30030-2613
404-687-8890
800-239-2507
FAX: 404-687-8298
TTY:711
e-mail: info@disabilitylink.org
www.disabilitylink.org

Larry Brown, Finance Director
Linda Pogue, Advocacy Director
Danny Housley, Social Media/I&R Coordinator
Michelle Lee, Youth Advocacy Coordinator

This center for rights and resources is committed to promoting the rights of all people with disabilities in allowing them to be independent, achieve goals, have access to their community and make decisions for themselves.

823 **Disability Funders Network**
14241 Midlothian Turnpike #151
Midlothian, VA 23113-6500 703-795-9646

e-mail: info@disabilityfunders.org
disabilityfunders.org

Kim Hutchinson, President/CEO
Kevin Webb, Chairman
Susan Olivo, Treasurer

Disability-inclusive grantmaking is the mission of DFN: inclusion of the disability in grantmaking programs and inclusion of people with disabilities in grantmaking organizations.

824 **Disabled Children's Relief Fund**
PO Box 89
Freeport, NY 11520-89 516-377-1605
FAX: 516-377-3978
www.dcrf.com

825 **Disabled and Alone/Life Services for the Handicapped**
61 Broadway
Suite 510
New York, NY 10006 212-532-6740
800-995-0066
FAX: 212-532-3588
e-mail: info@disabledandalone.org
www.disabledandalone.org

Lee Ackerman, Executive Director
Leslie D. Park, Chairman
Rex L. Davidson, Vice President
William G. Shannon, J.D., Treasurer

A national nonprofit humanitarian organization whose primary concern is the well-being of handicapped persons, particularly when their families can no longer care for them. Disabled and Alone 1) Helps families do sensible planning for and with their disabled children; 2) Provides advocacy and oversight when the parents cannot do so; 3) Advises families, attorneys and financial planners about life planning for a family member with a disability.

826 **Easter Seals**
233 South Wacker Drive, Suite 2400
Chicago, IL 60606 800-221-6827
easterseals.com

Richard W. Davidson, Chair
Sandra L. Bouwman, First Vice Chairman
Joseph G. Kern, Second Vice Chairman
Ralph F. Boyd Jr., Secretary

Easter Seals provides exceptional services, education, outreach and advocacy so that people living with autism spectrum disorders and other disabilities can live, learn, work, and play in our communities.

827 **Educational Accessibility Services**
Wayne State University
5155 Gullen Mall
1600 UGL
Detroit, MI 48202 313-577-1851
FAX: 313-577-4898
TTY:313-577-3365
e-mail: studentdisability@wayne.edu
www.eas.wayne.edu

Jane DePriester-Morandini,, Interim Dir.
Randie Kruman, M.A., University Counselor II
Kimberly Werth, M.A., LLPC, Professional Technician
Fran Marlowe, Program Specialist

To ensure a university experience in which individuals with disabilities have equitable access to programs and to empower students to self advocate i norder to fulfill their academic goals.

828 **Elwyn**
111 Elwyn Road
Elwyn, PA 19063 610-891-2000

elwyn.org

Joseph E. Pappano Jr.,M.D., Chair
Sandra S. Cornelius, Ph.D, President

our organization is recognized as a pioneer in developing groundbreaking programs for children and adults with disabilities and disadvantages.

829 **Enable America Inc.**
101 E. Kennedy Boulevard
Tampa, FL 33602 877-362-2533
FAX: 813-222-3298
e-mail: richard.salem@enableamerica.org
enableamerica.org

Richard J. Salem, Founder/CEO
Chris Jadick, Executive Director
Sandy Moonert, Program Director

Enable America's objective is to increase employment among people with disabilities in the United States.

830 **Esalen Institute**
55000 Highway 1
Big Sur, CA 93920-9546 831-667-3000
888-837-2536
FAX: 831-667-2724
e-mail: info@esalen.org
www.esalen.org

Gordon Wheeler, President/CEO
Michael Murphy, Founder
Dick Price, Founder
Tricia McEntee, CFO & CEO-elect

Founded in 1962 as an alternative education center devoted to the exploration of the world of unrealized human capacities that lies beyond the imagination. Blends East/West philosophies, experiential/didactic workshops, and a steady influx of philosophers, psychologists, artists, and religious thinkers.

831 **Family Resource Center on Disabilities**
20 E. Jackson Blvd.
Suite 300
Chicago, IL 60604-2265 312-939-3513
800-952-4199
FAX: 312-939-7297
TTY: 312-939-3519
e-mail: info@frcd.org
www.frcd.org

832 **Family Voices**
3701 SAN MATEO BLVD NE
Suite 103
Albuquerque, NM 87110 505-872-4774
888-835-5669
FAX: 505-872-4780
e-mail: lkeene@familyvoices.org
www.familyvoices.org

Molly Cole, President
Marcia O' Malley, Vice-President
Renee Turchi,MD, Secretary
Grace P Williams, Treasurer

Not-for-profit voluntary organization dedicated to ensuring that children's health issues are addressed as public and private healthcare systems undergo change in communities, states and the nation. National grassroots clearinghouse for information and education in ways to assure and improve health care for children with disabilities and chronic conditions. Provides materials including pamphlets, a newsletter and one-page papers on important topics.

833 **Favarh/Farmington Valley ARC**
225 Commerce Dr
PO Box 1099
Canton, CT 06019-1099 860-693-6662
FAX: 860-693-8662
e-mail: favarh@favarh.org
www.favarh.org

Rick Stanton, Creative Arts Coordinator
Stephen E. Morris MPA, Business Relations Manager
Annie George, Human Resources Director
Tim Hennessey, Recreation Director

Provides a variety of programs and services to adults with developmental, physical or mental disabilities and their families throughout the Farmington Valley communities of Avon,

Burlington and more. Favarh's programs are designed to enhance the personal, social, emotional, vocational and living capabilities of persons with disabilities.

834 **Fedcap Rehabilitation Services**
211 W 14th St
New York, NY 10011-7157 212-727-4225
FAX: 212-727-4303
TTY:212-727-4384
e-mail: homecare@fedcap.org
www.fedcap.org

Christine McMahon, President and CEO
Michael Kurtz, Chief Financial Officer
Joseph Giannetto, Chief Operating Officer
Lorrie Lutz, Chief Strategy Officer
Fedcap helps people with barriers achieve economic independence through employment. Through evaluation, vocational and soft-skills training, job placement, job creation and support programs, each year Fedcap helps thousands of Americans overcome obstacles, rebuild their lives, and find and keep meaningful employment.

835 **Federation for Children with Special Needs**
529 Main Street
Suite 1102
Boston, MA 02129 617-236-7210
800-331-0688
FAX: 617-241-0330
e-mail: fcsninfo@fcsn.org
www.fcsn.org

Rich Robison, Exec. Dir.
Mary Summers, Project Dir.
John Sullivan, Dir. of Information Technology
Mary Thompson, Dir. of Finance
The Federation for Children with Special Needs provides information, support, and assistance to parents of children with disabilities, their professional partners, and their communities. We are committed to listening to and learning from families, and encouraging full participation in community life by all people, especially those with disabilities.

836 **Federation of Families for Children's Mental Health**
Ste 280
9605 Medical Center Dr
Rockville, MD 20850-6390 240-403-1901
FAX: 240-403-1909
e-mail: ffcmh@ffcmh.org
www.ffcmh.org

Sandra Spencer, Executive Director
Teka Dempson, President
Sherri Luthe, Vice President
Josh Ross, Secretary
The FFCMH, a nationally family-run organization serves to provide advocacy at the national level for the rights of children and youth with emotional, behavioral and mental health challenges and their families. Provide leadership and technical assistance to a nation-wide network of family run organizations. Collaborate with family run and other child serving organizations to transform mental health care in America. The correct name is National Federation of Families for Children's Mental Health.

837 **Feingold Association of the US**
11849 Suncatcher Drive
Fishers, IN 46037 631-369-9340
800-321-3287
FAX: 631-369-2988
e-mail: help@feingold.org
www.feingold.org

Annette Miller, President
Kathleen Bratby MSN, RN, Secretary
Larisa Scarbrough, Vice President
Gail Wachsmuth, Treasurer
An organization of families and professionals, the Feingold Association of the United States is dedicated to helping children and adults apply proven dietary techniques for better behavior, learning and health.

838 **Feldenkrais Guild of North America (FGNA)**
5436 N Albina Ave
Portland, OR 97217 503-221-6612
800-775-2118
FAX: 503-221-6616
e-mail: executivedirector@feldenkrais.com
www.feldenkrais.com

Susan Marshall, Executive Director
Robert Black, BA, MSc, President
Jaclyn Boone, Vice President
Tom Bode, Treasurer
This is the organization which sets the standards for and certifies all FELDENKRAIS practitioners in North America. In order to practice, a practitioner must be a graduate of an FGNA accredited program (a minimum of 800 instruction hours over a three to four year period), and agree to follow both the Code of Professional Conduct and the Standards of Practice. FGNA may be contacted for further information about the FELDENKRAIS METHOD or for a list of FELDENKRAIS practitioners sorted by region.

839 **Focus Alternative Learning Center**
126 Dowd Avenue
PO Box 452
Canton, CT 06019 860-693-8809
FAX: 860-693-0141
e-mail: info@focuscenterforautism.org
www.focuscenterforautism.org

Marcia Bok, President
Claudia Godburn, Secretary
Rita Barredo, Treaurer
Carol Doiron, LCSW, Dir. of Education Svcs
A private non profit, licensed clinical and learning center specialized in the treatment of creatively wired and socially challenged kids. We treat kids on the autism spectrum who suffer from high anxiety, experience processing difficulties and learning problems. The name has been changed to FOCUS Center for Autism.

840 **George Washington University Health Resource Center**
2134 G St NW
Washington, DC 20052-0001
e-mail: askheath@gwu.edu
www.heath.gwu.edu

Stephen J Trachtenberg, CEO
Timothy W. Tong, Ph.D., Dean-School of Engineering
Rachelle Heller, Ph.D., Assoc. Dean, Academic Affairs
William Roper, Ph.D., Civil & Env Engineer
National clearinghouse for information about education after high school for people with disabilities. Also serves as an information exchange about educational support services, policies, procedures, adaptations and opportunities on American campuses, vocational-technical schools, adult education programs, independent living centers and other training entities after high school.

841 **Goodwill Industries International**
15810 Indianola Dr
Rockville, MD 20855-2674 301-530-6500
800-741-0186
FAX: 301-530-1516
TTY: 301-530-9759
e-mail: Contactus@goodwill.org
www.goodwill.org

Jim Gibbons, President/CEO
Lauren Lawson, Public Relations Director
Pat Boelter, Vice President of Marketing
Paul Spears, SCSEP Program Manager
Strives to achieve the full participation in society of disabled persons and other individuals with special needs by expanding their opportunities and occupational capabilities through a network of autonomous, nonproft, community-based organizations providing services throughout the world in response to local needs.

842 HRSA Information Center
PO Box 2910
Merrifield, VA 22116-2910
888-275-4772
FAX: 703-821-2098
TTY:877-489-4772
e-mail: ask@hrsa.gov
www.ask.hrsa.gov

843 Haldimand-Norfolk Resource Education and Counseling
101 Nanticoke Creek Parkway
Townsend, ON, ON N0A-1S0
519-587-2441
800-265-8087
FAX: 519-587-4798
e-mail: info@hnreach.on.ca
www.hnreach.on.ca

Mark Soppit, President
Ronelda Smith, VP
Lynda Nicholson, Secretary/Treasurer
Julianne West, Member at Large

Promote and support community well-being by providing co-ordinated access, planning, programs and services for individuals and families.

844 Health Action
5276 Hollister Ave
Ste 257
Santa Barbara, CA 93111
805-617-3390
FAX: 805-685-4710
e-mail: ha@healthaction.net.
www.healthaction.net

Dr. Roger Jahnke, Co Founder and CEO
Rebecca Mclean, Co Founder

Our mission is to foster innovation in health care that will increase health status, increase customer satisfaction, increase profitability, increase clinical efficacy and eliminate error, support provider efficiency and enhance clinical outcomes, and empower consumer self-managed care.

845 Health Resource Center for Women with Disabilities
Rehabilitation Institute of Chicago
345 E Superior St
Chicago, IL 60611-2654
312-238-1000
800-354-7342
FAX: 312-238-2208
e-mail: webmaster@ric.org
www.ric.org

Joanne C. Smith, MD, MBA, President/CEO
Edward B. Case, Exec VP/CFO
Nancy E. Paridy, JD, Senior VP, General Counsel
Peggy Kirk, Senior VP

RIC has earned a worldwide reputation as being a leader in patient health care, advocacy, research and educating health professionals in physical medicine and rehabilitation. People from around the globe choose RIC because of our expertise in treating a range of conditions, from the most complex conditions including cerebral palsy, spinal cord injury, stroke and traumatic brain injury, to the more common, such as arthritis, chronic pain, and sports injuries.

846 Homeopathic Educational Services
2124b Kittredge St
Berkeley, CA 94704
510-649-0294
800-359-9051
FAX: 510-649-1955
e-mail: email@homeopathic.com
www.homeopathic.com

Dana Ulman, MPH, Owner

Resource center for homeopathic products and services including books, tapes, research, medicines, medicine kits, software for the general public and the health professional and correspondence courses.

847 Human Ecology Action League (HEAL)
PO Box 509
Stockbridge, GA 30281-509
770-389-4519
FAX: 770-389-4520
e-mail: HEALNatnl @aol.com / HEAL3@aol.com
www.healnatl.org

848 Institute for Scientific Research
1000 Technology Dr
Ste 1000
Fairmont, WV 26554-8827
304-366-2577
877-363-5482
FAX: 304-366-2699
e-mail: info@wvhtf.org
www.wvhtf.org

James L. Estep, President/CEO
Dr Brian Lemoff, VP Advanced Technology
Brian Stolarik, VP, Mission Systems
Nancy E. Trudel, Esquire, General Counsel

Institute for Scientific Research, Inc. performs cutting-edge research across a variety of scientific and engineering disciplines. Our people participate in world-class projects from concept through development, in some of today's most fascinating scientific fields.

849 Institute of Transpersonal Psychology
1069 E Meadow Cir
Palo Alto, CA 94303-4231
650-493-4430
FAX: 650-493-6835
e-mail: itpinfo@itp.edu
www.itp.edu

Neal King, President
Brigitte Lindsey, Exec Assistant to President
Roger Ono, CFO
Paul Roy, Provost & VP

The Institute of Transpersonal Psychology is a private, non-sectarian graduate school accredited by the Western Association of Schools and Colleges. For over twenty-five years the Institute has remained a leader at the forefront of psychological research and education, probing the mind, body, spirit connection. The Institute's challenging and transformative educational paradigm has attracted students from all over the world.

850 International Association of Machinists
9000 Machinists Pl
Upper Marlboro, MD 20772-2687
301-967-4500
FAX: 301-967-4588
e-mail: websteward@iamaw.org
www.goiam.org

R Thomas Buffenbarger, President/CEO
Robert Roach, Jr., General Secretary-Treasurer
Dave Ritchie, General VP, Canada
Lynn D. Tucker, Jr., General VP, Eastern Territory

Placement programs for persons with disabilities.

851 International Association of Yoga Therapists
PO Box 12890
Prescott, AZ 86304
928-541-0004
FAX: 928-541-0182
e-mail: mail@iayt.org
www.iayt.org

John Kepner, MA, MBA, Executive Director
Eleanor Criswell Ed.D, President
Matra Raj,OTR, TYC,, Treasurer
Molly Lannon Kenny, Vice President

IAYT supports research and education in Yoga and serves Yoga practitioners, Yoga teachers, Yoga therapists, health care professionals, and researchers worldwide. Our mission is to establish Yoga as a recognised and respected therapy in the Western world. IAYT also serves members, the media, and the general public as a comprehensive source of information about contemporary Yoga education, research, and statistics.

852 International Chiropractors Association
6400 Arlington Blvd
Ste. 800
Falls Church, VA 22042
703-528-5000
800-423-4690
FAX: 703-528-5023
e-mail: chiro@chiropractic.org
www.chiropractic.org

Gary Walsemann, DC, President
W. Gene Cretsinger, DC, A LCP,, Vice President
Stephen P. Welsh, DC, Secretary-Treasurer
Corey B. Rodnick, DC, Central Regional Director

Established in 1926 to empower humanity in the expression of maximum health, wellness and human potential through the universal chiropractic expression and utilization. Strives to advance chiropractics throughout the world as a distinct health care profession predicated upon its unique philosophy, science and art.

853 International Clinic of Biological Regeneration
PO Box 509
Florissant, MO 63032-509
314-921-3997
800-826-5366
FAX: 314-921-8485
e-mail: icbr@aol.com
www.icbr.com

Dr. C. Tom Smith MD, HMD, D Hom (, Medical Director

The International Clinic of Biological Regeneration (ICBR) is a leading international cell therapy center that has been in continuous operation since 1981. During this time, Dr. Smith has constantly improved theraputic results of the treatment by selecting newer, safer and more effective formulations as delveloped by leading European research centers.

854 International Women's Health Coalition
333 7th Ave
6th Fl
New York, NY 10001-5004
212-979-8500
FAX: 212-979-9009
e-mail: info@iwhc.org
www.iwhc.org

Francoise Girard, President
Debora Diniz, Vice Chair
Ann Unterberg, Vice Chair
Brian A. Brink, MD, Chair

Information and pamphlets on sexually transmitted diseases and other health concerns. IWHC works to generate health and population policies, programs, and funding that promote and protect the rights and health of girls and women worldwide.

855 Invisible Disabilities Association
P.O. Box 4067
Parker, CO 80134
invisibledisabilities.org

Wayne Connell, President/Founder
Steve Tonkin, Vice President
Steve Durgin, Treasurer
Jim Calanni, Secretary

The Invisible Disabilities Association (IDA) encourages, educates and connects people and organizations touched by illness, pain and disability around the globe.

856 Job Accommodation Network
PO Box 6080
Morgantown, WV 26506-6080
304-293-7186
800-526-7234
FAX: 304-293-5407
TTY: 877-781-9403
e-mail: jan@askjan.org
www.jan.wvu.edu

Anne Hirsh, Co-Director
Louis Orslene, Co-Director
Linda Carter Batiste, Principal Consultants
Beth Loy, Principal Consultants

JAN's mission is to facilitate the employment and retention of workers with disabilities by providing employers, employment providers, people with disabilities, their family members and other interested parties with information on job accomodations, self-employment and small business opportunities and related subjects. JAN's efforts are in support of the employment, including self-employment and small business ownership, of people with disabilities.

857 Joni and Friends
PO Box 3333
Agoura Hills, CA 91376-3333
818-707-5664
800-736-4177
FAX: 818-707-2391
TTY: 818-707-9707
e-mail: jafmin@joniandfriends.org
www.joniandfriends.org

Joni Eareckson-Tada, Founder and CEO
Doug Mazza, President & COO
Billy C. Burnett, VP/CFO
Steve Bundy, VP

A nonprofit organization seeking to accelerate Christian ministry with people affected by disabilities. JAF educates churches and the community worldwide concerning the needs of the disabled and how those needs can be met. We sponsor family retreats for families with disabled members. Wheels for the World collects, restores and distributes used wheelchairs to disadvantaged populations around the world.

858 Juvenile Diabetes Research Foundation International
26 Broadway
14th Fl
New York, NY 10004
212-785-9500
800-533-2873
FAX: 212-785-9595
e-mail: info@jdrf.org
www.jdrf.org

Jeffrey Brewer, President/CEO
Gil King, VP, Internal Audit
Michael Malekoff, VP, Business Dev.
Cynthia Rice, VP, Govt Relations

The world's leading nonprofit, nongovernmental funder of diabetes research. It was founded in 1970 by parents of children with diabetes. JDF's mission is to find a cure for diabetes and its complications through the support of research. JDF also sponsors international workshops and conferences for biomedical researchers, individual chapters offer support groups and other activities for families affected by diabetes. JDF has more than 110 chapters and affiliates worldwide. Quarterly newsletter.

859 Lambton County Developmental Services
339 Centre St
PO Box 1210
Petrolia, ON N0N-1R0
519-882-0933
FAX: 519-882-3386
e-mail: administration@lcds.on.ca
www.lcds.on.ca

Frank Huybers, President
Tony Hogervorst, 1st Vice-President
Kari Lupton, 2nd Vice-President
Frank Back, Treasurer

A network of caring people, working together to provide services for people with developmental disabilities to facilitate the achievement of their life dreams.

860 LoSeCa Foundation
215-1 Carnegie Drive
St Albert, AB T8N-5B1
780-460-1400
FAX: 780-459-1380
e-mail: rbourret@telus.net
www.loseca.ca

Ron Bourret, Program Manager
Raymond Nkorimana, Program Manager
Francois Busque, Program Manager
Jules Lefebvre, Human Resources Manager

A non-profit organization that provides support services to adults with developmental disabilities

861 MCC Supportive Care Services
103-2776 Bourquin Circle W
Abbotsford, BC V2S-6A4
604-850-6608
800-622-5455
FAX: 604-850-2634
e-mail: office@communitascare.com
www.communitascare.com/

Steve Thiessen, CEO

A service provider, advocate and resource for persons living and dealing with mental, physical and/or emotional disabilities. The correct name is Communitas Supportive Care Society.

862 Mainstream
300 S Rodney Parham Rd
Ste 5
Little Rock, AR 72205-4774 501-280-0012
800-371-9026
FAX: 501-280-9267
TTY: 501-280-9262
www.mainstreamilrc.com

863 March of Dimes Birth Defects Foundation
1275 Mamaroneck Ave
White Plains, NY 10605-5201 914-997-4488
FAX: 914-428-8203
e-mail: nbrown@marchofdimes.com
www.marchofdimes.com/

Dr. Jennifer Howse, President
Richard Mulligan, Exec VP
Lisa Bellsey, Esq., SVP & General Counsel
The mission of the March of Dimes is to improve the health of babies by preventing birth defects and infant mortality.

864 Mental Health America
2000 N Beauregard St
6th Fl
Alexandria, VA 22311 703-684-7722
800-969-6642
FAX: 703-684-5968
e-mail: dshern@mentalhealthamerica.net
www.mentalhealthamerica.net

David Shern, Ph.D., President and CEO
Dianne Felton, Senior VP of Operations
Julie Nicholson Burke, VP of Finance
Mike Turner, VP of Dev
Nonprofit organization addressing all issues related to mental health and mental illness. With more than 340 affiliates nationwide, NMHA works to improve the mental health of all Americans, especially the 54 million individuals with mental disorders, through advocacy, education, research and service.

865 Metametrix Clinical Laboratory
3425 Corporate Way
Duluth, GA 30096-2552 770-446-5483
800-221-4640
FAX: 770-441-2237
e-mail: inquiries@metametrix.com
www.metametrix.com

Ted Hull, CEO
Robert M David PhD, Laboratory Director
Richard S Lord PhD, Chief Science Officer
Carolyn Bralley, President
Metametrix Clinical Laboratory has been a pioneer and leader in the development of nutritional, metabolic, and toxicant analyses since 1984. Metametrix is committed to helping health care professionals identify nutritional influences on health and disease, and is recognized internationally for its laboratory procedures in nutritional and biochemical testing.

866 Mind, Body, Health Sciences
393 Dixon Rd
Boulder, CO 80302-9769 303-440-8460
FAX: 303-440-7580
e-mail: luzie@joanborysenko.com
www.joanborysenko.com

Joan Borysenko, Founder
publish free annual newsletter/cataloge:Circle of Healing. Information about the works of Joan Borysenko.

867 Muscular Dystrophy Association - USA
3300 E Sunrise Dr
Tucson, AZ 85718-3299 520-529-2000
800-572-1717
FAX: 520-529-5454
e-mail: mda@mdausa.org
www.mdausa.org

Robert Ross, CEO
Valerie Cwik, M..D., Interim President
MDA provides comprehensive medical services to tens of thousands of people with neuromuscular diseases at some 230 hospital-affiliated clinics across the country. The Association's worldwide research program, which funds over 400 individual scientific investigations annually, represents the largest single effort to advance knowledge of neuromuscular diseases and to find cures and treatments for them. In addition, MDA conducts far-reaching educational programs for the public and professionals.

868 National Association for Holistic Aromatherapy
PO Box 27871
Raleigh, NC 27611-7871 919-917-7491
FAX: 919-594-1065
e-mail: info@naha.org
www.naha.org

Kelly Holland Azzaro, RA CCA, Vice President
Michele A. Miller, President
Shellie Enteen, BA, LMBT, Director Coordinator
Cheryl Hoard, Chairperson-Advisory Committee
The NAHA is an educational, nonprofit organization dedicated to enhancing public awareness of the benefits of true aromatherapy. It offers aromatherapy Tele-classes & membership benefits, and acts as a referral service.

869 National Association of Blind Merchants
1837 S Nevada Ave
PMB #243
Colorado Springs, CO 80905 719-527-0488
866-543-6808
e-mail: kevanwirkey@blindmerchants.org
www.blindmerchants.org

Nicky Gacos, President
Membership organization of blind persons employed in either self-employment work or the Randolph-Sheppard vending program. Provides information regarding rehabilitation, social security, tax and other issues which directly affect blind merchants. Serves as advocacy and support group.

870 National Association of Developmental Disabilities Councils
1825 K Street, NW
Suite 600
Washington, DC 20006 202-506-5813
FAX: 202-506-5846
e-mail: info@nacdd.org
www.nacdd.org

Claire Mantonya, President, Exec. Dir.
Michael Brogioli, CEO
John Morris, Treasurer, Exec. Dir.
Sheryl Matney, Senior Mgr, Council Svcs
The National Association of Councils on Developmental Disabilities (NACDD) is a national, member-driven organization consisting of 55 State and Territorial Councils. NACDD places high value on meaningful participation and contribution by Council members.

871 National Association of State Directors of Developmental Disabilities Services (NASDDDS)
113 Oronoco St
Alexandria, VA 22314-2015 703-683-4202
FAX: 703-684-1395
e-mail: cmosely@nasddds.org
www.nasddds.org

Nancy Thaler, Executive Director
Charles R Moseley, Ed.D., Associate Executive Director
Robin Cooper, Director of Technical Assistance
Barbara Brent, Director of State Policy
The association's goal is to promote and assist state agencies in developing effective, efficient service delivery systems that fur-

nish high-quality supports to people with developmental disabilities.

872 National Business & Disability Council
201 I U Willets Rd
Albertson, NY 11507-1516
516-465-1516
FAX: 516-465-3730
e-mail: jtowles@abilitiesonline.org
www.nbdc.com

John D. Kemp, President/CEO
Michael C. Pascucci, Exec. Leadership Team
Jennifer Towles, Membership Specialist
Sheryl P. Buchel, Senior VP

The NBDC is the leading resource for employers seeking to integrate people with disabilities into the workplace and companies seeking to reach them in the consumer marketplace.

873 National Center for Education in Maternal and Child Health
Georgetown University
PO Box 571272
Washington, DC 20057-1272
202-784-9770
877-624-1935
FAX: 202-784-9777
e-mail: mchlibrary@ncemch.org
www.ncemch.org

Rochelle Mayer, Research Professor and Director

Provides information on children with special health needs, child health and development, adolescent health, nutrition, violence and injury prevention and other issues of maternal and child health for health professionals and the public.

874 National College of Naturopathic Medicine
049 SW Porter St
Portland, OR 97201-4848
503-552-1555
FAX: 503-226-8133
e-mail: jstanard@ncnm.edu
www.ncnm.edu

David J. Schleich, President
Nancy W. Garbett, Board Chair
Richard Jones, Vice Chair of the Board
Don Drake, Chair Strategic Pathways Comm

NCNM offers two graduate professional degrees in accredited and recognized programs that prepare you for licensed practice in many states and provinces: Doctor of Naturopathic Medicine, a four-year program of clinical sciences and holistic methods of heal

875 National Council on Disability
1331 F Street Northwest
Suite 850
Washington, DC 20004- 1138
202-272-2004
FAX: 202-272-2022
TTY:202-272-2074
e-mail: ncd@ncd.gov
www.ncd.gov

Aaron Bishop, Exec. Dir.
Anne Sommers, Dir. of Legislative Affairs
Joan M. Durocher, General Counsel & Dir. of Policy
Sylvia Menifee, Dir. of Administration

NCD is a small, independent federal agency charged with advising the President, Congress, and other federal agencies regarding policies, programs, practices, and procedures that affect people with disabilities.

876 National Council on Independent Living
1710 Rhode Island Ave NW
5th Fl
Washington, DC 20036
202-207-0334
877-525-3400
FAX: 202-207-0341
TTY: 202-207-0340
e-mail: ncil@ncil.org
www.ncil.org

Kelly Buckland, Executive Director
Dan Kessler, President
Phil Pangrazio, Treasurer
Lou Ann Kibbee, Vice President

NCIL advances independent living and the rights of people with disabilities through consumer-driven advocacy.

877 National Deaf Education Network and Clearinghouse/Info To Go
Deaf Education Center/Gallaudet University
800 Florida Ave NE
Washington, DC 20002-3695
202-651-5051
FAX: 202-651-5704
TTY:202-651-5052
e-mail: clerc.center@gallaudet.edu.
www.gallaudet.edu/clerc_center

Dr T Alan Hurwitz, President
Edward Bosso, VP, National Deaf Education
Dr. Lynne Murray, VP for Dev. and Alumni Relations
Dr. Cynthia King, Chief Information Officer

Info to Go, from the Laurent Clerc National Deaf Education Center, provides information on topics dealing with deafness and hearing loss in children and young people under 21 years of age.

878 National Disability Rights Network
Ste 211
900 2nd St NE
Washington, DC 20002-3560
202-408-9514
FAX: 202-408-9520
TTY:202-408-9521
e-mail: info@ndrn.org
www.ndrn.org

Curtis L. Decker, JD, Exec. Dir.
Judith Stickle, Deputy Exec. Dir. for Finance
Janice K. Johnson Hunter, Deputy Exec. Dir.
Eric Buehlmann, Dir. of Public Policy

Voluntary national membership association of protection and advocacy systems and client assistance programs. Promoting and strengthening the role and performance of its members in providing quality legally based advocacy services.

879 National Dissemination Center for Children and Youth with Disabilities (NICHCY)
1825 Connecticut Ave NW
Ste 700
Washington, DC 20009
202-884-8200
800-695-0285
FAX: 202-884-8441
TTY: 800-695-0285
e-mail: nichcy@aed.org
www.nichcy.org

Suzanne Ripley, Director
Carol Valdivieso, Principal Investigator
Theresa Rebhorn, Writer / Designer
Lisa Kupper, Writer / Designer

NICHCY is the center that provides information to the nation on disabilities in children and youth; programs and services for infants, children, and youth with disabilities; IDEA, the nation's special education law; and research-based information on effective practices for children with disabilities.

880 National Early Childhood Technical Assistance Center
8040 Unc-Ch
Chapel Hill, NC 27599-8040
919-962-2001
FAX: 919-966-7463
e-mail: ectacenter@unc.edu
www.nectac.org

Lynne Kahn, Dir. & Principal Investigator
Joan Danaher, Associate Dir. Information
Christina Kasprzak, Associate Dir. Evaluation
Martha Diefendorfer, Associate Director

Assists states and other designated governing jurisdictions as they develop multidisciplinary, coordinated and comprehensive services for children with special needs.

881 **National Easter Seal Society**
233 S Wacker Drive
Ste 2400
Chicago, IL 60606-4851
312-726-6200
800-221-6827
FAX: 312-726-1494
TTY: 312-726-4258
www.easterseals.com

Alison A. Coady, Secretary
James E. Williams Jr, Assistant Secretary
Stephen F. Rossman, Chairman
Richard F. Vincent, Treasurer

Easter Seals provides exceptional services, education, outreach, and advocacy so that people living with autism and other disabilities can live, learn, work and play in our communities.

882 **National Guild of Hypnotists**
PO Box 308
Merrimack, NH 03054-0308
603-429-9438
FAX: 603-424-8066
e-mail: ngh@ngh.net
www.ngh.net

Dr. Dwight F Damon, DC, DNGH, OB, President
Don Mottin, NGH VP, CMI, D, Vice President
Melody Damon-Bachand, BCH, Executive Director
Dawn Huard, CH, Membership / Member Services

The National Guild of Hypnotists, Inc.is a not-for-profit, educational corporation in the State of New Hampshire. Officially founded in Boston, Massachusetts in 1950 the Guild is a professional organization comprised of dedicated individuals committed to advancing the field of hypnotism.

883 **National Information Center for Children**
1825 Connecticut Ave NW
Ste 700
Washington, DC 20009
202-884-8200
800-695-0285
FAX: 202-884-8441
TTY: 800-695-0285
e-mail: nichcy@fhi360.org
www.nichcy.org

Suzanne Ripley, Director
Carol Valdivieso, Principal Investigator
Theresa Rebhorn, Writer / Designer
Lisa Kupper, Writer / Designer

Information on disabilities and disibility-related issues for family, educators and professionals related to children and youth.

884 **National Institute on Disability and Rehabilitation Research**
Potomac Center Building
550 12 St., SW
Washington, DC 20202-7100
202-245-7640
800-872-5327
FAX: 202-245-7643
TTY: 800-437-0833
e-mail: nidrr-mailbox@ed.gov
www.ed.gov

Charlie Lakin, Dir.
Ruth Brannon, Acting Deputy Dir.
Tim Muzzio, Dir. Program Budget

Conducts comprehensive and coordinated programs of research and related activities to maximize the full inclusion, social integration, employment and independent living of individuals of all ages with disabilities. NIDRR's focus includes research in areas such as employment, health and function, technology for access and function, independent living and community integration, and other associated disability research areas.

885 **National Organization on Disability**
77 Water Street
Ste 204
New York, NY 10005
646-505-1191
FAX: 646-505-1184
e-mail: kbitting@wearenciman
www.nod.org

Carol Glazer, President
Kate Brady, Dir. of Res
Anne Fitzsimmons, Project & Business Associate
Howard Green, Deputy Director

The National Organization on Disability promotes the full and equal participation of men, women and children with disabilities in all aspects of American life. Founded in 1982, NOD is the leading national disability organization concerned with all disabil

886 **National Rehabilitation Association (NRA)**
P.O Box 150235
Alexandria, VA 22315-4109
703-836-0850
888-258-4295
FAX: 703-836-0848
TTY: 703-836-0849
e-mail: info@nationalrehab.org
www.nationalrehab.org

Beverlee Stafford, Executive Director
Sandra Mulliner, Administrative Assistant
Patricia Leahy, Governmental Affairs Director
Brian Coupe, Membership Director

NRA members work to eliminate barriers and increase employment opportunities for people with disabilities. We provide our members opportunities for advocacy and increased awareness of issues through professional development and access to current research topics.

887 **National Rehabilitation Information Center(NARIC)**
8400 Corporate Drive
Suite 500
Landover, MD 20785-2245
301-459-5900
800-346-2742
FAX: 301-459-4263
e-mail: naricinfo@heitechservices.com
www.naric.com

Mark Odum, Director

NARIC is a federally-funded library and information center that focuses on disability and rehabilitation information.

888 **National Vaccine Information Center**
407 Church St. NE
Ste H
Vienna, VA 22180-4737
703-938-3783
FAX: 703-938-5768
e-mail: contactnvic@gmail.com
www.nvic.org

Barbara Loe Fisher, Co-Founder/President
Kathi Williams, Co-Founder/VP
Theresa Wrangham, Executive Director
Paul Arthur, Director of Operations

A national nonprofit educational organization dedicated to preventing, through public education, vaccine injuries and deaths. NVIC represents vaccine consumers and health care providers, including parents whose children suffered illness or died following vaccination. NVIC supports the right of vaccine consumers to have access to the safest and most effective vaccine as well as the right to make informed, independent vaccination decisions.

889 **National Women's Health Network**
1413 K St NW
4th Fl
Washington, DC 20005-3459
202-682-2640
FAX: 202-682-2648
e-mail: nwhn@nwhn.org
www.nwhn.org

Cynthia Pearson, Executive Director
Heidi Gider, Director of Advancement
Amy Allina, Program & Policy Director
Latasha Jackson, Office Coordinator

The National Women's Health Network improves the health of all women by developing and promoting a critical analysis of health issues in order to affect policy and support consumer decision-making. The Network aspires to a health care system that is guided by social justice and reflects the needs of diverse women.

890 Native American Protection and Advocacy
PO Box 306
Window Rock, AZ 86515
928-871-4151
800-789-7287
FAX: 928-871-5036
www.nativelegalnet.org

Levon Henry, Executive Director
Sylvia Struss, Administrative Director
Kathy Gallagher, Development Director
Victoria Lee, Executive Assistant.

The Native American Protection & Advocacy which helps protect, promote, and expand the legal and human rights of Native Americans with disabilities. There are several goals for this organization, including quality legal representation for individuals with disabilities in various areas such as abuse and neglect, special education, civil rights and discrimination and employment.

891 New York Therapeutic Riding Center-Equestria
212-535-3917
FAX: 212-535-3917
e-mail: info@equestria.org
www.equestria.org

Richard Brodie, Board Of Director
Patricia Neal, Board Of Director
Karen Nielsen Esq., Board Of Director
Peter Rajsingh Esq., Board Of Director

The Therapeutic Riding Center has been conducting therapeutic horseback riding progams for children and adults with disabilites living in New York City for 11 years. Its riding facility is located at the well-equipped Chateau Stables, and staffed by volunteers with experience in physical therapy, osteopathy, art therapy and other areas designed to deal with various aspects of disabled individuals.

892 North America Riding for the Handicapped Association
PO Box 33150
Denver, CO 80233-150
303-452-1212
800-369-7433
FAX: 303-252-4610
e-mail: pathintl@pathintl.org
www.narha.org

Kay Green, CEO
Kaye Marks, Dir. of Mktg
Carolyn Malcheski, Finance/Human Resources Dir.
Megan Ream, Sponsorship/Dev. Mgr

National nonprofit equestrian organization dedicated to serving individuals with disability by giving disabled individuals the opportunity to ride horses. Establishes safety standards, provides continuing education and offers networking opportunities for both its individuals and center members. Produces educational materials including fact sheets, brochures, booklets, audio-visual tapes, a directory and NARHA's magazine Strides.

893 North Hastings Community Integration Association
2 Alice Street
Box 1508
Bancroft, ON K0L-1C0
613-332-2090
FAX: 613-332-4762
e-mail: communityliving@nhcia.ca
www.nhcia.ca

John Muro, President
Cathy Fulford, Vice President
Peter Stone, Treasurer
Barb Millar, Secretary

Supports people with an intellectual disability and their families.

894 Nurse Healers: Professional Associates International
TTIA Box 130
Delmar, NY 12054-419
518-325-1185
FAX: 509-693-3537
e-mail: info@therapeutic-touch.org
www.therapeutic-touch.org

Sue Conlin, QTTT, President
Lin Beilly, Communications
Cheri Brady, Education
David Shields, Membership

Cooperative among health professionals interested in healing. Sets the standards for the practice and teaching of Therapeutic Touch. Voluntary, not-for-profit organization.

895 PACER Center (Parent Advocacy Coalition for Educational Rights)
8161 Normandale Blvd
Bloomington, MN 55437-1044
952-838-9000
800-537-2237
FAX: 952-838-0199
TTY: 952-838-0190
e-mail: pacer@pacer.org
www.pacer.org

Paula F. Goldberg, Executive Director
Mary Schrock, Chief Operating/Development Off
Paul Luehr, Board President
Jessica Broyles, Board Treasurer

Mission is to expand opportunities and enhance the quality of life of children and young adults with disabilities and their families based on the concept of parents helping parents. Offers workshops, individual assistance and written information. Provides programs and materials that assist multicultural families, programs for students, schools and professionals with disability awareness puppet and child abuse prevention programs. Computer Resource Center/Software Lending Library available.

896 PEAK Parent Center
Ste 200
611 N Weber St
Colorado Springs, CO 80903-1072
719-531-9400
800-284-0251
FAX: 719-531-9452
e-mail: info@peakparent.org
www.peakparent.org

Barbara Buswell, Executive Director
Kent Willis, President Attorney
Sarah Billerbeck, Vice President
Delois Meyer, Secretary

PEAK Parent Center is Colorado's federally-designated Parent Training and Information Center (PTI). As a PTI, PEAK supports and empowers parents, providing them with information and strategies to use when advocating for their children with disabilities. PEAK works one-on-one with families and educators helping them realize new possibilities for children with disabilities by expanding knowledge of special education and offering new strategies for success.

897 Pacific Institute of Aromatherapy
PO Box 6723
San Rafael, CA 94903
415-479-9120
FAX: 415-479-0614
e-mail: contact@osapia.com
www.pacificinstituteofaromatherapy.com

898 Parent Professional Advocacy League
45 Bromfield St
10th Fl
Boston, MA 02108
617-542-7860
866-815-8122
FAX: 617-542-7832
e-mail: info@ppal.net
www.ppal.net

Lisa Lambert, Executive Director
Deborah A. Fauntleroy, MSW, Associate Director
Meri Viano, Senior Regional Manager
Chantell Albert, Outreach Coordinator

An organization that promotes a strong voice for families of children and adolescents with mental health needs. PAL advocates for supports, treatment and policies that enable families to live in their communities in an environment of stability and respect.

899 **Parents Helping Parents (PHP)**
1400 Parkmoor Ave
Ste 100
San Jose, CA 95126-3797 408-727-5775
855-727-5775
FAX: 408-286-1116
e-mail: info@php.com
www.php.com

Mary Ellen Peterson, M.A., CEO/Executive Director
Suzanne Cistulli, Board Chair
James Quaranta, Board Treasurer
Joyce Uggla, Board Secretary
Dedicated to assisting children with any type of special need: mental, physical, emotional, or learning disability. Mission is to help children with special needs receive love, hope, respect, and services needed to achieve their full potential by strengthening their families and the professionals who serve them. Developed and implemented numerous programs; produce a variety of educational and support materials, including information packets, brochures, database and a quarterly newletter.

900 **People First of Canada**
120 Maryland St
Suite 5
Winnipeg, MB R3G-1L1 204-784-7362
866-854-8915
FAX: 204-784-7364
e-mail: info@peoplefirstofcanada.ca
www.peoplefirstofcanada.ca

Shelley Rattai, Exec. Dir.
Catherine Rodgers, Community Inclusion
Shane Haddad, President
Patty Ward, Treasurer
People First of Canada is the national voice for people who have been labeled with an intellectual disability. People First is a movement of people who want all citizens to live equally in the country.

901 **People First of Oregon**
PO Box 12642
Salem, OR 97309-642 503-362-0336
FAX: 503-585-0287
e-mail: people1@people1.org
www.people1.org

Steven Kramer, President
Self-advocacy organization of developmentally disabled people who have joined together to learn how to speak for themselves. People first offers support, a united voice and advocacy to its members. Offers information and helps develop service projects in the communities they live in. Offers information and assistance to countries around the world in starting new chapters. Offers participation on DD boards, ARC boards, Transit Boards, and other boards in the community. .

902 **People-to-People Committee on Disability**
911 Main St
Ste 2110
Kansas City, MO 64105 816-531-4701
800-676-7874
FAX: 816-561-7502
e-mail: ptpi@ptpi.org
www.ptpi.org

Mary Eisenhower, President and CEO
Mark Stansberry, Chairman
Anita Manuel, Vice Chairman
Piya Radia, Secretary
Individuals concerned about the circumstances of handicapped people throughout the world. Disseminates information, acts as a consultant in promoting exchange activities, coordinates special assistance projects in developing countries and more.

903 **People-to-People International: Committee for the Handicapped**
911 Maint St
Ste 2110
Kansas City, MO 64105 816-531-4701
800-676-7874
FAX: 816-561-7502
e-mail: ptpi@ptpi.org
www.ptpi.org

Mary Eisenhower, President and CEO
Mark Stansberry, Chairman
Anita Manuel, Vice Chairman
Piya Radia, Secretary
Goals of this committee include: betterment of the handicapped through international unity; educating those with and without handicaps through technical assistance; opening access doors through sensory aids, prosthetic devices and travel tips; and coordination of major international cultural exchanges.

904 **Quan Yin Healing Arts Center**
965 Mission St
Ste 405
San Francisco, CA 94103-3416 415-861-4964
FAX: 415-644-0614
e-mail: info@qyhac.org
www.quanyinhealingarts.com

Carla Wilson, Exec. Dir.
Colin Howard, President
Hulda Brown, VP
Misha Cohen, Chair, Res & Education
The mission of Quan Yin Healing Arts Center is to provide accessable high quality, affordable acupuncture and Chinese medicine regardless of income. Collaborating with other healthcare providers, we support a holistic philosophy, empowering the individual to take responsibility for their health and well being.

905 **Rehabilitation International**
25 E. 21st Street
4th Floor
New York, NY 10010-6207 212-420-1500
FAX: 212-505-0871
e-mail: RI@riglobal.org
www.riglobal.org

Venus Ilagan, Secretary General
Iris Reiss, Rehabilitation Expert
Anne President
RI and its members develop and promote initiatives to protect the rights of people with disabilities and improve rehabilitation and other crucial services for disabled people and their families. RI also works toward increasing international collaboration and advocates for policies and legislation recognizing the rights of people with disabilities and their families, including the establishment of a UN Convention on the Rights and Dignity of Persons with Disabilities.

906 **Rehabilitation Services**
3075 Orchard Vista Drive SE
Grand Rapids, MI 49546 616-301-8000
800-695-7273
FAX: 616-301-8010
TTY: 800-649-3777
e-mail: mtanis@hopenetwork.org
www.hopenetwork.org

Dana DeVos, Chair
Joanne Voorhees, Vice Chair
Patrick A. Miles, jr., Secretary/Treasurer
Wilbur Lettinga, Ex Offico
An office of Hope Netowrk, one of the largest, private, nonprofit organization of its kind in Michigan. The purpose is to assist people with brain injuries and/or physical disabilities in achieving an optimal level of self determinations, dignity, and independence as they develop and attain goals to overcome environmental barriers and mobilize adaptive skills.

907 **Rolf Institute**
5055 Chaparral Ct
Ste 103
Boulder, CO 80301-3326
303-449-5903
800-530-8875
FAX: 303-449-5978
www.rolf.org

Ida P Rolf, Founder
Diana Yourell, Executive Director
Heidi Hauge, Membership Services Coordinator
Jim Jones, Director of Education

Established in 1971, The Rolf Institute is a nonprofit corporation, organized and existing under the laws of California and Colorado. It is recognized by the US Government as a tax-exempt educational and scientific research organization.

908 **Ronald McDonald House**
1500 17th St
Huntington, WV 25701-3956
304-529-1122
FAX: 304-529-2970
e-mail: margaret@mchouse.org
www.mchouse.org

Daniel Yon, Board Treasurer
Susan Barnes, Board President
Paul E. Smith, Board Vice President
Robert E. Yost, Board Secretary

A home-away-from-home, a temporary lodging facility for the families of seriously ill children being treated at nearby hospitals. Each house is run by a local nonprofit agency comprised of members of the medical community, McDonald's owners, businesses and civic organizations and parent volunteers.

909 **St. Paul Abilities Network**
4637-45 Avenue
St Paul, AB T0A-3A3
780-645-3441
866-645-3900
FAX: 780-645-1885
e-mail: mail@spanet.ab.ca
www.stpaulabilitiesnetwork.ca

Tim Bear, Exec. Dir.
Sam Chang, Finance Controller
Eugene McCafferty, Human Resources
Daina Foerster, Dir. of Residential Svcs

Provides support and opportunities to encourage the development of an individual's full potential through education, advocacy and community partnerships.

910 **Student Disability Services**
Wayne State University
5155 Gullen Mall
1600 UGL
Detroit, MI 48202-3919
313-577-1851
877-978-4636
FAX: 313-577-4898
TTY: 313-577-3365
e-mail: studentdisability@wayne.edu
www.studentdisability.wayne.edu

Jane DePriester-Morandini,, Interim Dir.
Randie Kruman, M.A., University Counselor II
Fran Marlowe, Program Specialist
Claressa Adams, M. A., Administrative Assistant II

Their mission is to ensure a university experience in which individuals with disabilities have equitable access to programs and to empower students to self-advocate in order to fulfill their academic goals.

911 **Teacher Preparation and Special Education**
2134 G St NW
Ste 416
Washington, DC 20052
202-994-8860
800-449-7343
FAX: 202-994-8613
e-mail: gsehdcom@gwu.edu
www.gsehd.gwu.edu

Michael J. Feuer, Dean
Carol Kochhar-Bryant, Senior Associate Dean
Maxine Freund, Associate Dean for Research
Phoebe Stevenson, Administrative Dean

Administers the Education of the Handicapped Act and related programs for the education of handicapped children, including grants to institutions of higher learning and fellowships to train educational personnel. Grants to states for the education of handicapped children, research and demonstration.

912 **Technology and Media Division**
Council For Exceptional Children
2900 Crystal Drive
Suite 1000
Arlington, VA 22202-3557
866-509-0218
888-232-7733
FAX: 703-264-9454
TTY: 866-915-5000
e-mail: service@cec.sped.org
www.cec.sped.org

Bruce Ramirez, Exec. Dir.
Margaret J. McLaughlin, President
James P. Heiden, Treasurer
Ken Dickson, Coordinator Gifted & Talented

To support educational participation and improved results for individuals with disabilities and diverse learning needs through the selection, acquisition, and use of technology. The secondary purpose is to provide services to members and other units of CEC, to federal, state and local education agencies, and to business and industry regarding the current and future uses if technology and media with individuals with exceptionalities

913 **The Davis Center**
19 State Route 10 E
Ste 25
Succasunna, NJ 07876
862-251-4637
FAX: 862-251-4642
e-mail: npdunn@thedaviscenter.com
www.thedaviscenter.com

Dorinne S Davis MA CCC-A FAAA, Director
Elizabeth Meade, Head Sound Therapist
Nancy Puckett-Dunn, Office Manger
Laura Darby, Part Time Sound Therapist

Offers sound-based therapies supporting positive change in learning, development, and wellness. All ages/all disabilities. The Davis Model of Sound Intervention-an alternative approach.

914 **Thresholds Psychiatric Rehabilitation Centers**
4101 N Ravenswood Ave
Chicago, IL 60613-2196
773-572-5500
888-997-3422
FAX: 773-880-6279
TTY: 773-880-6263
e-mail: thresholds@thresholds.org
www.thresholds.org

Gregory Hedges, Vice President
Michael Szkatulski, President
Jeffrey M. Josephs, Treasurer
Rand E. Arons, Secretary

A nationally-recognized psychosocial rehabilitation agency serving persons with severe and persistent mental illness. The agency offers its programming at 22 service locations and more than 40 residential facilities throughout Chicago and Northern Illinois. Also offers specialized programming for older adults, young adults, parents, the homeless and the hearing impaired and mentally ill.

Sliding scale

915 **United States Trager Association**
13801 W Center St
Ste C, P.O. Box 1009
Burton, OH 44021-9005
440-834-0308
FAX: 440-834-0365
e-mail: info@tragerus.org
www.tragerus.org

Anna Marie Bowers, Executive Director
Sharon Johnson, President
Sharon King Green, Vice President
Shelley Parker, Treasurer

The Trager approach is a pleasurable, gentle and effective approach to movement education and mind/body integration. The Trager approach helps release deep-seated physical and mental patterns and facilitates deep relaxation, increased physical mobility, and mental clarity. The benefits of a Trager session are long-lasting and cumulative, with subsequent sessions allowing for deeper and longer lasting changes.

916 **Universal Pediatric Services**
6750 Westown Parkway
Suite 115A
West Des Moines, IA 50266 800-383-0303
www.upsi.net

Tucker Anderson, President
Universal Pediatric Services, provides high tech care to medically fragile children and adults in the home setting. Emphasis is placed on the provision of services in the rural areas, the ability to service high tech needs and the promotion of primary nurse concept.

917 **Upledger Institute**
11211 Prosperity Farms Rd
Ste D-325
Palm Beach Gardens, FL 33410 561-622-4334
800-233-5880
FAX: 561-622-4771
e-mail: upledger@upledger.com
www.upledger.com

John M Upledger, CEO
Roy Desjarlais, VP
Alex Jozefyk, Director of Accounting
Steve Keller, Director of Distributions
A healthcare resource center recognized worldwide for its comprehensive education programs, advanced treatment options and unique outreach initiatives. The Institute has trained more than 100,000 healthcare professionals throughout the globe in the therapeutic approach.

918 **Women to Women**
PO Box 306
Portland, ME 04112-306 800-798-7902
FAX: 207-846-6167
e-mail: personalprogram@womentowomen.com
www.womentowomen.com

Marcelle Pick OB/GYN, NP, Co Founder/Director
Combination of alternative and conventional medicine in women's health, bring science and disipline to natural and preventative methods. Publishes the Creating Health Guide, a quarterly collection of articles written by the health care professionals at Women to Women.

919 **World Institute on Disability**
3075 Adeline Street
Suite 280
Berkeley, CA 94703 510-225-6400
FAX: 510-225-0477
TTY:510-225-0478
e-mail: wid@wid.org
www.wid.org

Cassandra Malry, Exec. Dir.
Thomas Foley, Deputy Dir/Access to Assets
Julia Day, Content Production Mgr
Bruce Curtis, Dir. of International Programs
The mission of the World Institute on Disability (WID) in communities and nations worldwide is to eliminate barriers to full social integration and increase employment, economic security and health care for persons with disabilities. WID creates innovative programs and tools; conducts research, public education, training and advocacy campaigns; and provides technical assistance.

920 **YAI: National Institute for People with Disabilities**
460 W 34th St
New York, NY 10001-2382 212-273-6100
FAX: 212-273-6200
www.yai.org

Stephen E. Freeman, L.C.S.W., CEO
Stephen Freeman, President/COO
Marco Damiani, M.A., Senior Dir.
Thomas A. Dern, L.C.S.W., Chief Operating Officer
Mission is to build brighter futures for people with developmental and learning disabilities and thier families. Every person, at every age and level of disability, has the potential for growth. Each individual is entitled to the same dignity, respect, and opportunities as all other members of society. Firmly committed to helping the people we serve to achieve their potential for independence, individuality, productivity, and inclusion in their communities.

Camps

Alabama

921 **Camp Merrimack**
Merrimack Hall Performing Arts Center
3320 Triana Blvd.
Huntsville, AL 35805
256-534-6455
FAX: 212-397-4684
www.merrimackhall.com

Debra Jenkins, Founder and President
Alan Jenkins, Vice President
Joe Ritch, Secretary / Treasurer
Kay Harrington, Financial Advisor
For children ages 3-12 with special needs including Down Syndrome, Cerebral Palsy, Autism and others. Camp includes theatre, visual arts and dance.

922 **Camp Rap-A-Hope**
2701 Airport Blvd
Mobile, AL 36606-2319
251-476-9880
FAX: 251-476-9495
e-mail: info@camprapahope.org
www.camprapahope.org

Laura Gibson, President
Sandy Blount, President Elect
Melissa McNichol, Executive Director
Roz Dorsett, Assistant Director
Camp Rap-A-Hope is a one-week summer camp for children and teenagers who are battling cancer or have ever been diagnosed with cancer and are 7 to 17 years of age. It is free of charge. Camp Rap-A-Hope strives to make sure every camper gets the opportunity to develop new skills and self-confidence. Camp activities are appropriate for our campers' ages and abilities and include, but are not limited to: swimming, music, arts and crafts, archery, fishing, canoeing and horseback riding.

923 **Camp Seale Harris**
Southeastern Diabetes Education Services
500 Chase Park South
Suite 104
Hoover, AL 35244-1869
205-402-0415
FAX: 205-402-0416
e-mail: info@southeasterndiabetes.org
www.southeasterndiabetes.org

Tip McAlpin, Chair
Cindy Freeman, Secretary
David Jamieson, JD, Vice Chair
Rhonda McDavid, Executive Director
A summer residential program that is located at Camp ASCCA (Alabama's Special Camp for Children and Adults), that encourages and motivates youth to reach their full potential despite diabetes, and teaches families how to serve as the primary educators and supporters for children and adolescents living with this illness. Four programs are offered: Senior Camp; Junior Camp; Family Camp; and Adventure Camps.

924 **Camp Shocco For The Deaf**
1314 Shocco Springs Road
Talledega, AL 35160
256-761-1100
800-280-1105
FAX: 256-761-1270
TTY: 256-474-0109
e-mail: campshocco@albcdeaf.org
www.campshocco.org

Chad Fleming, Director
Linnea Elliott, Assistant Dir. - Youth Camp
Mathew Dixon, Co-Director
Adam Schrimsher, Secretary / Director of Recreational Activities
One week camp of fun, games and spiritual growth for deaf children and teens.

925 **Camp Shocco for the Deaf**
AL Baptist State Board of Missions
1314 Shocco Springs Road
Talladega, AL 35160
256-761-1100
TTY:256-474-0109
e-mail: campshocco@albcdeaf.org
www.campshocco.org

Chad Fleming, Director
Linnea Elliott, Assistant Dir. - Youth Camp
Mathew Dixon, Co-Director
Adam Schrimsher, Secretary / Director of Recreational Activities
Camp Shocco gives each child and teenager attending camp the opportunity to have an unforgettable one week of fun, games, and spiritual growth. Campers also learn the essence of teamwork, while developing their own unique abilities and talents that can often be overlooked.

926 **Camp Smile-A-Mile**
P.O.Box 550155
Birmingham, AL 35255-155
205-323-8427
888-500-7920
FAX: 205-323-6220
e-mail: info@campsam.org
www.campsam.org

David L. Warren, Jr, President
Samuel H. Heide, Vice President
Ryan Weiss, Vice President
Fred Elliott, Secretary
Camp Smile-A-Mile is a non-profit organization for children who have or had cancer in Alabama. Camp Smile-A-Mile's mission is to provide challenging, unforgettable recreational and educational experiences for young cancer patients from across Alabama at no cost to their families. Our purpose is to provide these children with avenues for fellowship, to help them cope with their disease, and to prepare them for life.

927 **Camp WheezeAway**
American Lung Association Of Alabama
P. O. Box 2336
Bessemer, AL 36102
334-229-0035
e-mail: brendabasnight@yahoo.com
www.campchandler.org

Jeff Reynolds, Executive Director
Justin Castanza, Associate Camp Director
Art Mason, Operations Director
Daniel Blazer, Program Director
Camp WheezeAway is a 5 day overnight camp for children ages 8-12 with moderate to severe asthma, and is sponsored by the American Lung Association. Children are monitored while enjoying all the normal camp activities including ropes courses, canoeing, swimming, arts & crafts, horseback riding, fishing, tubing & more and above all learn to manage their asthma.

928 **Easter Seals Camp ASCCA**
Easter Seals
5278 Camp ASCCA Drive
Jackson's Gap, AL 36861
256-825-9226
FAX: 256-825-8332
e-mail: info@campascca.org
campascca.org

Matt Rickman, Camp Director
John Stephenson, Administrator
Camp ASCCA is Alabama's Special Camp for Children and Adults. ASCCA is a nationally recognized leader in therapeutic recreation for children and adults with both physical and intellectual disabilities. Providing weekend and week long sessions, Camp ASCCA is open year round.

Alaska

929 **ADA Camp Kushtaka**
American Diabetes Association
201 West Fireweed Lane
Suite 103
Anchorage, AK 99503- 1893
907-272-1424
800-342-2383
FAX: 907-272-1428
e-mail: askada@diabetes.org
www.childrenwithdiabetes.org

Michelle Cassano, Executive Director
Pam Bell, Organizer

ADA Camp Kushtaka is a five day camp for children & teens age 7-17 and their families (space permitting) and is held on the shores of Kenai Lake on the Kenai Peninsula in Cooper Landing. The camp combines ongoing and informal diabetes management and education along with the fun of outdoor activities such as hiking, canoeing, crafts and swimming.

930 **Camp Alpine**
Alpine Alternatives
2518 E. Tudor Road
Suite 105
Anchorage, AK 99507-1105
907-561-6655
800-361-4174
FAX: 907-563-9232
e-mail: alpinealternatives@arctic.net
www.alpinealternatives.org

Margaret Webber, Executive Director
Nancy Burnette, Bookkeeper/Program Administrator
Vanessa Hartley, Downhill Ski Program Director
LaVerne Lee, Day Outings Director & Camp Alpine Director

Our programs are designed to help people expand their horizons, master new skills, make new friends, and increase motor coordination. Most importantly, participants experience growth in self-confidence and independence that affects all aspects of an individual's life. Our services are open to all, regardless of type of disability or age. Activities include canoeing, hiking, swimming, outdoor games, sports, nature identification and much more.

931 **Camp Birchwood**
Muscular Dystrophy Association
17161 David Blackburn Drive
Chugiak, AK 99567
907-688-2734
FAX: 907-688-2734
e-mail: info@birchwoodcamp.org
www.birchwoodcamp.org

John Quinley, President
Rev. Doug Handlong, Vice President
Benee Braden, Treasurer
Nathan Woods, Secretary

A summer camp at Birchwood Camp in Chugiak, Alaska for individuals ages 6-21 who are affected by any of the 40-plus neuromuscular diseases in MDA's program. Common activities include: swimming, hockey, baseball, soccer, football, boating, horseback riding, fishing, music, cooking, arts and crafts, movies, dancing, talent shows, Harley-Davidson motorcycle sidecar or three-wheeled cycle rides, a visit from fire fighters and time for socializing and laughing.

932 **Champ Camp**
American Lung Association In Alaska
Glacier View Ranch
8748 Overland Rd
Ward, CO 80481
907-276-5864
800-586-4872
FAX: 907-565-5587
e-mail: champcamp@lungcolorado.org
www.lung.org/

Charles D. Connor, President and CEO
George Walker, Regional Director
Cindy Liverance, VP of Programs
Liz Toohey, Director of Development

Champ Camp is a week long summer recreation and asthma education program at Camp Kushtaka on the beautiful shores of Kenai Lake. Campers are able to explore their skills in outdoor activities including canoeing, hiking, swimming, archery, and arts and crafts. More importantly, Champ Camp boosts self-confidence and instills a sense of responsibility. It teaches preventive measures to improve asthma management, and avoid asthmatic episodes as well as increases a camper's sense of independence.

933 **Muscular Dystrophy Association Free Camp**
3300 E. Sunrise Dr.
Tucson, AZ 85718-3208
800-572-1717
e-mail: mda@mdausa.org
www.mda.org

Valerie A. Cwik, M..D., EVP, Chief Medical and Scientific Officer
Steven M. Derks, President and CEO
Julie Faber, Executive Vice President, Chief Financial Officer
Steven G. Ford, EVP, Chief Communications and Marketing Officer

MDA Camp provides a wide range of activities for those with limited mobility or are in wheelchairs. The camp offers many outdoor sporting events, arts & crafts and talent shows.

Arizona

934 **Arizona Camp Sunrise**
American Cancer Society
PO Box 27872
Tempe, AZ 85285
602-952-7550
FAX: 602-404-1118
e-mail: barb.nicholas@cancer.org
www.azcampsunrise.org

Barbara Nicholas, Dir.
Leigh Ansley, Mgr of Childhood Cancer Support
Melissa Lee, Camp Dir.
Jason Poulter, Technical Media Dir.

Provides one-week summer camping sessions to children aged 8-16 who have had, or currently have, cancer. The classes range from sports and outdoor games to dance and drama, arts, crafts, and cooking. Other activities planned for the campers include horseback riding, a trip to a lake, a dance, and learning to make friendship bracelets.

935 **Camp Abilities Tucson**
P.O. Box 86838
Tucson, AZ 85754-6838
520-235-2582
e-mail: campabilitiestucson@gmail.com
www.campabilitiestucson.org

Murry Everson, Camp Director

One week camp offering comprehensive developmental sports for children in middle and high school who are blind, deaf-blind or multiply disabled.

936 **Camp Candlelight**
Epilepsy Arizona
240 West Thomas Road
2nd Floor
Phoenix, AZ 85013-4407
602-406-3581
epilepsyaz.org/programs/camp-candlelight/

937 **Camp Civitan**
Civitan Foundation
3519 East Shea Blvd. #133
Phoenix, AZ 85028-3339
602-953-2944
FAX: 602-953-2946
e-mail: info@campcivitan.org
www.campcivitan.org

Mike Horne, Director, Partner & COO
John W Day, DMD, MS, Director Orthodontist
Kathy Spude, Director Credit Analyst
Gary Holliday, Director Pharmacy Director

We are the premier camp for developmentally disabled individuals of all ages. People from around Arizona and neighboring states come to Camp Civitan to enhance their quality of life, enjoy the multitude of outdoor experiences we offer and make lifelong friends.

938 **Camp Honor**
Hemophilia Association
826 North 5th Avenue
Phoenix, AZ 85003
602-955-3947
888-754-7017
e-mail: info@hemophiliaz.org
www.hemophiliaz.org

Steven Helm, President
Jim Durr, Vice President
Victor Alonzo, Treasurer
Sarah Fey, Secretary

Camp is located in Payson, Arizona at the Whispering Hope Ranch. One-week sessions for children with hemophilia or HIV and their siblings, as well as children of hemophiliacs. Coed, ages 7-17. Activities include swimming, canoeing, sports, archery and arts and crafts (to name a few fun things).

939 **Camp Not-A-Wheeze**
American Lung Association In Arizona
102 W McDowell Rd
Phoenix, AZ 85003-1213
602-258-7505
800-586-4872
FAX: 202-452-1805
e-mail: info@lungarizona.org
www.lung.org/

Larry Blumenthal, Chair
George Walker, Regional Dir.
Cindy Liverance, VP of Programs
Liz Toohey, Dir. of Dev

Camp Not-A-Wheeze is designed especially for kids ages 7-14 with moderate to severe asthma and was created to provide a traditional residential camp experience and teach children how to manage their asthma.

940 **Camp Rainbow**
Phoenix Childrens Hospital
1919 East Thomas Road
Phoenix, AZ 85016-7710
602-933-0157
888-908-5437
e-mail: msalloom@phoenixchildrens.com
www.phoenixchildrens.com/

Robert Meyer, President and CEO
David Cavazos, Chairman of the Board
Larry Clemmensen, Chairman of the Board
Steven S. Schnall, Senior VP

Camp is located in Prescott, Arizona. Offers one-week sessions for children who have had, or currently have, cancer. Boys and girls ages 7-17. Camp activities include swimming, horseback riding, arts and crafts, canoeing, performing arts, archery, rollerskating, fishing, an overnight camping trip and much more! It's a week filled with laughter, new experiences and new friends.

941 **Lions Camp Tatiyee**
Arizona Lions Clubs Multiple District 21
P.O.Box 6910
Mesa, AZ 85216-6910
480-380-4254
800-246-9771
FAX: 602-244-8667
e-mail: director@arizonalionscamp.org
www.arizonalionscamp.com

Pamela Swanson, Executive Director
Desirae Bender, RN BSN, Lead Nurse
Megan Anderson, Assistant Program Director

Camp is located in Lakeside, Arizona. Sessions are provided for campers of all ages, with a wide variety of disabilities/special needs and are divided by age and disability. Featured activities include arts and crafts, ceramics/pottery, climbing/rappelling, counselor training (CIT), drama, fishing, football, hiking, nature/environmental studies and team building.

942 **Summer Camp for Children with Muscular Dystrophy**
Muscular Dystrophy Association - USA
3300 E Sunrise Dr
Tucson, AZ 85718-3208
520-529-2000
800-572-1717
FAX: 520-529-5300
e-mail: mda@mdausa.org
www.mda.org

Valerie A. Cwik, M..D., EVP, Chief Medical and Scientific Officer
Steven M. Derks, President and CEO
Julie Faber, Executive Vice President, Chief Financial Officer
Steven G. Ford, EVP, Chief Communications and Marketing Officer

The MDA Summer Camp offers a wide range of activities specifically designed for young people with limited mobility or who use a wheelchair. Some of the activities include boating and canoeing, swimming, adaptive sports, fishing, archery, karaoke, scavenger hunts, arts & crafts, dances, talent shows and campfires.

943 **Triangle Y Ranch YMCA**
YMCA Of Southern Arizona
34434 S. Y Camp Road
P.O. Box 350
Oracle, AZ 85623
520-884-0987
e-mail: camp@tucsonymca.org
www.tucsonymca.org

Dane Woll, President and CEO
Kerry Dufour, V.P. Chief Dev. Officer
Cathy Scheirman, Chief Financial Officer
Deneiva Knight, Mktg and Communications Dir.

For children and young adults ages 6-17. The camp offers nature programs, swimming, horseback riding, sports, arts & crafts.

Arkansas

944 **Camp Aldersgate**
Camp Aldersgate, Inc.
2000 Aldersgate Road
Little Rock, AR 72205
501-225-1444
FAX: 501-225-2019
e-mail: info@campaldersgate.net
www.campaldersgate.net

Sarah C. Wacaster, CEO
Bill Faggard, Chief Operating Officer
Amy Frank, Dir. of Programs
Regina Riehl, Director of Finance and Human Resources

A non-profit camp for children and young adults with medical or physical conditions such as cerebral palsy, diabetes, arthritis, asthma, kidney disorders.

945 **Camp Funshine**
Camp Funshine Foundation, Inc.
P.O. Box 576
Pea Ridge, AR 72751
www.campfunshine.com

Jeff Brown, President
Aimee Albright, Vice President
Holly Floyd, Treasurer
Rain Sheppard, Secretary

A free camp for children ages 7 and up who have cystic fibrosis. The mission of the camp is to provide a fun, safe environment in which the kids can talk openly about themselves or their disease.

946 **Camp Kota**
Junior League Of Little Rock
401 South Scott Street
Little Rock, AR 72201
501-375-5557
FAX: 501-907-5296
www.jllr.org

Tisha Gribble, President
Maggie Young, President Elect
Brooke Hicks, Community Vice President
Jamie Jones, Membership Vice President

Camp Kota is for disabled and non-disabled children ages 6-16. Some of the activities include fishing, canoeing, swimming, archery, music and arts & crafts.

947 **Camp Quality Arkansas**
P.O. Box 9095
Jonesboro, AR 72403
870-931-2844
e-mail: chris.jennings@campqualityusa.org
www.campqualityusa.com

Chris Jennings, Camp Director
Betty Baureis, Treasurer
Shay Hankins, Secretary
Chris Jennings, Director

Camp Quality is for children with cancer and their siblings. The camp offers a stress-free environment that offers exciting activities and fosters new friendships, while helping to give the children courage, motivation and emotional strength.

California

948 **Bearskin Meadow Camp**
Diabetic Youth Foundation
5167 Clayton Road
Suite F
Concord, CA 94521-3163
925-680-4994
FAX: 925-680-4863
e-mail: info@dyf.org
www.dyf.org

Mats Wallin, Executive Director
Paula Gogin, Director of Development
Janet Kramschuster, Director of Programs
Dr. Mary Simon, Medical Director

Bear Skin Meadow Camp is for children, teens and families who are affected by diabetes. The Camp also teaches the children and teens diabetes management and education, skills for blood glucose checking and techniques for adjusting insulin, as well as food choices and how to have a fun, active life while living with diabetes.

949 **Camp Beyond The Scars**
Burn Institute
8825 Aero Drive
Suite 200
San Diego, CA 92123-2269
858-541-2277
FAX: 858-541-7179
e-mail: dkuhn@burninstitute.org
www.burninstitute.org

Chief David Ott, President
Chief Bob Pfohl, VP Chief Financial Officer
Dale Ganzow, VP Dev.
Michael D. Pierschbacher, Ph.D., VP Program

Summer camp for children who have suffered burns. The camp provides a relaxed social setting and helps to enhance the children's self esteem.

950 **Camp Bloomfield**
Junior Blind
35375 Mulholland Highway
Malibu, CA 90265
310-457-5330
FAX: 310-457-3952
e-mail: smanning@juniorblind.org
www.juniorblind.org

Shirley Manning, Director of Recreation
Joan Marason, Director of Wellness & Enrichment Programs
Laura M. Hardy, Senior VP of Dev. and Mktg
Kami Mann, Senior VP, Finance

Offers children and youth's who are blind, visually impaired or multi-disabled with a safe and natural environment where they can develop self esteem and build independence. The camp offers swimming, horseback riding, fishing, hiking, track and field, arts and crafts and more.

951 **Camp Christian Berets**
Christian Berets, Inc.
1317 Oakdale Road
Suite 340
Modesto, CA 95355
209-524-7993
FAX: 209-524-7979
www.christianberets.org

Tom Crooker, Chairman
Carletta Evans Steele, Treasurer
Kelly Luth, Secretary

Camp for children, students and adults with special needs.

952 **Camp Coelho**
The Epilepsy Foundation Of Northern California
155 Montgomery Street
Suite 309
San Francisco, CA 94104
416-677-4011
800-632-3532
FAX: 416-677-4190
www.epilepsynorcal.org

Michael A. Scott, Executive Director
Joseph McGrath, President
D. Andrew Neff, Vice President
Lane Auten, Treasurer

Camp for children and young adults ages 5-15 with epilepsy and seizure disorders.

953 **Camp Conrad-Chinnock**
Diabetic Youth Services
12045 E. Waterfront Drive
Playa Vista, CA 90094
310-751-3057
FAX: 888-800-4010
e-mail: rocky.wilson@dys.org
www.campconradchinnock.weebly.com/

Rocky Wilson, Ph.D., Executive And Camp Director
Dale Lissy, Camp Manager
Ryan Martz, Program Director
Tom Jenkins, Chief Operating Officer

Camp conrad-chinnock offers social, recreational and educational opportunities for youth and families with diabetes. Campers are taught diabetes self-management skills in an interactive, fun & safe environment.

954 **Camp Costanoan**
VIA Services West
2851 Park Avenue
Santa Clara, CA 95050
408-243-7861
e-mail: info@viaservices.org
www.viaservices.org

Leslie Davis, MA, Chief Executive Officer
Jacqueline Forsythe, MBA, Vice President of Advancement
Leslie Leger, Vice President of Administration
John Heagerty, Chair of the Board

Camp Costanoan is a residential, outdoor education, and recreational camp for children and adults, ages 5 and older, with physical and/or developmental disabilities and special needs. Camp Costanoan enhances camper self-esteem, improves socialization skills and provides hands-on learning and therapeutic recreation opportunities.

955 **Camp Del Corazon**
11615 Hesby St
North Hollywood, CA 91601-3620
818-754-0312
888-621-4800
FAX: 818-754-0377
e-mail: info@campdelcorazon.org
www.campdelcorazon.org

Lisa Knight, RN, Exec. Dir. and Co-Founder
Kevin Shannon, MD, Medical Dir. & Co-Founder
Tom Klitzner, MD, Exec. Board Member
Carl Schuster, Exec. Board Member

Active program for campers with heart disease, Camp del Corazon provides summer activities free of charge that include hiking and archery, arts and crafts, court and field games, waterfront activities and a beach barbecue.

956 **Camp Esperanza**
Southern California Chapter
800 West 6th Street
Suite 1250
Los Angeles, CA 90017
323-954-5760
800-954-2873
FAX: 323-954-5790
e-mail: jziegler@arthritis.org
www.arthritis.org

Manuel Loya, CEO
Victoria Fung, Chief Program Officer
Amy Daugherty, Chief Development Officer
Angele Price, VP, Development
A one-week camp in August that allows children with arthritis to participate in such activities as horseback riding, swimming, etc. in a fun-filled environment.

957 **Camp Firefly**
The Firefly Foundation
5737 Kanan Road
Suite 180
Agoura Hills, CA 91301
e-mail: mail@campfirefly.com
www.campfirefly.com

958 **Camp Forrest**
Angel View Crippled Children's Foundation
12379 Miracle Hill Rd
Desert Hot Springs, CA 92240-4010
760-329-6471
FAX: 760-329-9024
e-mail: angelview44@aol.com
www.angelview.org

David Thorton, Executive Director
Shelly Lee, Resale Shops
Catherine Rips, Director of Development
DeAnn Lubell Ames, Director of Public Relations
Camp is located in Joshua Tree, California. Offers to one-week sessions June-August to both able-bodied campers and those with a wide variety of disabilities. Coed, ages 10-25. Activities include archery, arts and crafts, cookouts, swimming, sports and games, hiking and star study.

959 **Camp Grizzly**
NorCal Services For Deaf & Hard Of Hearing, Inc.
4708 Roseville Road
Suite 111
North Highlands, CA 95660-5172
916-349-7500
FAX: 916-349-7580
TTY:916-349-7500
e-mail: info@nocalcenter.org
www.norcalcenter.org/

Sheri Farinah, CEO
Cheryl Bella, Chair
Michael D. Wilson, Vice Chair
Yim Orsi, Secretary
This camp is designed the deaf and hard of hearing youth or hearing youth with deaf or hard of hearing parent. The camp helps with social interaction, building self esteem, leadership skills while enriching the lives of the deaf and hard of hearing.

960 **Camp Kindle**
28245 Avenue Crocker
Suite 104
Santa Clarita, CA 91355
877-800-2267
FAX: 702-995-9186
e-mail: info@projectkindle.org
projectkindle.org

Eva Payne, Founder/Executive Director
Mandy Nickolite, Vice President/PsychoSocial Lead
Erin FitzGerald, Program Coordinator
The purpose of Camp Kindle is to enhance the overall well-being of children and young people living with a chronic or life threatening illness, disability, or other life challenge. Camp Kindle's primary mechanism for achieving its purpose is through camping events held in Nebraska and California.

961 **Camp Krem**
Camping Unlimited
4610 Whitesands Court
El Sobrante, CA 94803
510-222-6662
e-mail: campkrem@gmail.com
www.campingunlimited.com

Judy Simmons, President
Alex J. Krem, Treasurer
Mary Farfaglia, Executive Director
Year-round camp offering recreational activities and camping for children and adults with developmental disabilities.

962 **Camp Okizu**
Okizu Foundation
16 Digital Drive
Suite 130
Novato, CA 94949-5755
415-382-9083
FAX: 415-382-8384
e-mail: info@okizu.org
www.okizu.org

John H. Bell, Chairman
Michael D. Amylon, M.D., Vice-Chairman
Becca Horton, Administrative Assistant
Beth Dekker, Assistant Camp Director
Camp Okizu is located in Berry Creek, California, and offers children who are struggling with life threatening illnesses and their families a place to go and explore and enjoy a normal life experience. The camp also offers peer support, respite, mentoring as well as other programs designed to meet the needs of all members of families whom are affected by childhood cancer. The camp is open from April through October.

963 **Camp Pacifica, Inc.**
California Lions Camp
Mail Box 110
257 Belle Vue Rd
Atwater, CA 95301-209-
e-mail: ilybrookeb@yahoo.com
www.californialionscamp.org

Russ Custer, President
Jill Loving, Secretary
Ted Allan, Treasurer
Dee Heller, Vice President
Camp Pacifica has been developed to provide a unique environment where special needs children have opportunities to grow and understand themselves. The camp is open to special needs children ages 7-17 years old, and strives to promote greater independence and self confidence and provides opportunities for social interaction, further development of social skills and the opportunity to develop friendships.

964 **Camp Paivika**
AbilityFirst
600 Playground Drive
Cedarpines Park, CA 92322
909-338-1102
877-768-4600
FAX: 909-338-2502
e-mail: sramirez@abilityfirst.org
www.abilityfirst.org

Kelly Kunsek, Camp Director
Sonia Ramirez, Marketing Manager
Jane Garcia, Camper Services Coordinator
AbilityFirst has 24 locations throughout So. California, including a camp, serving children and adults with disabilities.

965 **Camp Quest**
The Epilepsy Foundation Of Northern California
155 Montgomery Street
Suite 309
San Francisco, CA 94104
416-677-4011
800-632-3532
FAX: 416-677-4190
www.epilepsynorcal.org

Michael A. Scott, Executive Director
Joseph McGrath, President
D. Andrew Neff, Vice President
Lane Auten, Treasurer

Summer camp for children and young adults ages 5-15 with epilepsy and seizure disorders.

966 Camp Ramah In California
17525 Ventura Blvd. #201
Encino, CA 91316
310-476-8571
888-226-7726
FAX: 310-472-3810
e-mail: info@ramah.org
www.ramah.org

Rabbi Joe Menashe, Executive Director
Randy Michaels, Director of Finance & Administration
Ariella Moss Peterseil, Associate Director
Ilana Ormond, Development Director
Camp for young adults ages 11-18 with learning, emotional and developmental disabilities.

967 Camp ReCreation
2110 Broadway
Sacramento, CA 95818
916-733-0136
FAX: 916-733-0195
e-mail: CampRec@scd.org
www.camprecreation.org

Kathy Barber, Administrator
A residential summer camp program for adults and children with developmental disabilities.

968 Camp Reach for the Sky
American Cancer Society c/o CR4TS
Ste 100
2655 Camino Del Rio N
San Diego, CA 92108-1633
619-682-7427
800-227-2345
FAX: 404-417-5974
TTY: 866-228-4327
www.cancer.org

Kimberly Wright, Dir., Mission Solutions & Tools
Kristina Thomson, LCSW, Division Director
Sheila G. Williamson, Regional VP
Tawana Thomas Johnson, Dir., Health Disparities
One-week sessions for children who have had, or currently have, cancer, and are residents of San Diego and Imperial counties. Coed, ages 4-18. Siblings are also invited to participate in activities.

969 Camp Ronald McDonald for Good Times
Ronald McDonald House Charities - Southern Calif.
1250 Lyman Place
Los Angeles, CA 90029
310-268-8488
800-625-7295
FAX: 310-473-3338
e-mail: bbaillie@campronaldmcdonald.org
www.campronaldmcdonald.org

Edward Lodgen, Esq., President
Jodie Lesh, Vice President
Sarah Orth, Executive Director
Chad Edwards, Program Director
Free year-round residential camping for children with cancer and their families.

970 Camp Ronald McDonald® at Eagle Lake
P.O. Box 172
Susanville, CA 96130
530-825-3158
FAX: 530-825-3158
e-mail: vflaig@rmhcnc.org
www.campronald.org

Vicky Flaig, MEd, RD, Camp Director
Supported by Ronald McDonald House Charities® Northern California-a fully accessible residential camp for kids with special needs. The goal of the camp is to provide confidence building experiences to children who are at risk, disadvantaged and/or living with physical, developmental or emotional disabilities.

971 Camp Rubber Soul
325A East Redwood Avenue
Fort Bragg, CA 95437
707-962-0906
e-mail: camp@camprubbersoul.org
www.camprubbersoul.org

Rachel Miller, Camp contact person
Sayre Statham, Camp contact person
The camp offers five one-week camping stays for children and young adults with special needs. Some of the activities include sports, wood working, painting, theatre, music and arts and crafts.

972 Camp Sunburst
Sunburst Projects
1025 19th Street
Suite 1A
Sacramento, CA 95814
916-440-0889
FAX: 916-440-1208
e-mail: admin@sunburstprojects.org
sunburstprojects.org/programs.shtml

973 Camp Sunshine Dreams
P.O. Box 28232
Fresno, CA 93729-8232
559-301-5419
e-mail: contact@campsunshinedreams.com
www.campsunshinedreams.com

Bryan Wood, Camp contact person
Anthony Aiello, Camp contact person
Camp Sunshine Dreams is open for children and young adults ages 8-15 years and their siblings. The camp focuses on providing an enjoyable, stimulating and supportive camping experience while also providing for each child's special emotional and physical needs.

974 Camp Taylor, Inc.
5424 Pirrone Road
Salida, CA 95368-9094
209-545-4715
FAX: 209-543-1861
e-mail: kimberlie@kidsheartcamp.org
www.kidsheartcamp.org

Kimberlie Gamino, Executive Director and Founder
Rollin A. Podwys, Camp Director
Steven Barbieri, Camp Counselor
Charlie Liamos, Venture Capitalist
Camp Taylor is open to children and young adults and their families who have heart disease and offers many recreational activities.

975 Camp Trinity
Star Route Box 150
Hayfork, CA 96041
530-628-5992
FAX: 530-628-9392
e-mail: camptrinity@bar717.com
www.bar717.com/

Emma Bundy, Staff Director
Casey Zarnes, Barn Director
Lucy A. Newell, Counseling Staff
Mitch Carter, Counseling Staff
Offers two, three and four-week camping sessions May-September. Accepts campers with diabetes and mobility limitation. Coed, ages 8-16. Also families, single adults and seniors.

976 Camp-A-Lot And Leisure Express (PALS Program)
Arc of San Diego
3030 Market Street
San Diego, CA 92102
619-685-1175
FAX: 619-234-3759
e-mail: info@arc-sd.com
www.arc-sd.com

Gerald W. Hansen, Chair
David W. Schneider, President and CEO
Anthony J. DeSalis, Esq, EVP & COO
Chad Lyle, VP of Finance/CFO
Recreational opportunities for children, teens and adults with developmental and intellectual disabilities. Programs include sum-

mer resident camp, San Diego local activities and trip/travel vacations.

977 **Camping Unlimited**
102 Brook Ln
Boulder Creek, CA 95006-9320
510-222-6662
FAX: 831-338-3210
e-mail: campkrem@gmail.com
www.campingunlimited.com
Judy Simmons, President
Mary Farfaglia, Executive Director
Alex J. Krem, Treasurer
Sharon Ardoin, Board Member
Camping Unlimited is a non-profit organization providing special needs children and adults a full program of recreation, education, fun and adventure. Our program encourages independence, nurtures responsibility, develops competence and builds lifelong friendships in a warm supportive atmosphere of planned permissiveness.
2 pages Monthly

978 **Camping Unlimited-Camp Krem**
Camping Unlimited for Children & Adults
102 Brook Ln
Boulder Creek, CA 95006
510-222-6662
e-mail: campkrem@gmail.com
www.campingunlimited.com
Judy Simmons, President
Mary Farfaglia, Executive Director
Alex J. Krem, Treasurer
Sharon Ardoin, Board Member
Camp is located in Boulder Creek, California in the Santa Cruz mountains. Offers one and two-week sessions June-August to campers with a variety of disabilities. Coed, ages 5-50. Camping unlimited also offers weekend programs and travel camps, year round programs and recreation. Boulder Creek is located 15 minutes from Santa Cruz, CA, and Pacific Ocean Beach.

979 **Camps for Children & Teens with Diabetes**
Diabetes Society
1701 N. Beauregard St.
Alexandria, VA 22311
408-287-3785
800-DIA-ETES
FAX: 408-287-2701
e-mail: camp@diabetessociety.org
www.diabetessociety.org
Dwight Holing, Chair
Larry Hausner, CEO
Debbie Johnson, CFO
Greg Elfers, Chief Field Development Officer
Since 1974, sponsors up to 20 day camps, family camps and resident camps for children 4 through 17. These camps provide an opportunity for children with diabetes to go to camp, meet other children and gain a better understanding of their diabetes. The total experience can help campers develop more confidence in their abilities to control their diabetes effectively while enjoying the traditional camp experience. Camps are located throughout CA and parts of Nevada.

980 **Deaf Kid's Kamp**
Sproul Ranch, Inc.
42263 50th Street West
Suite 610
Quartz Hill, CA 93536
661-675-3323
e-mail: deafkidskamp@earthlink.net
www.deafkidskamp.com
Buffy Sproul, Executive Director
Our purpose is to meet the needs of deaf children outside of the classroom setting. These needs, as we have defined them, would include but are not limited to: social contact with peers; contact with the culture of the Deaf Community; educational and recreational programs not available in most school settings.

981 **Dream Street Camp**
Dream Street Foundation
324 S. Beverly Drive
Suite 500
Beverly Hills, CA 90212
424-333-1371
FAX: 310-388-0302
e-mail: dreamstreetca@gmail.com
www.dreamstreetfoundation.org
Patty Grubman, Director
Louise Gonzales, Office Manager
Tiffany Alfaro, Director
For children and young adults with life threatening and chronic illnesses.

982 **Easter Seals Camp Harmon**
Easter Seals Central California
16403 Highway 9
Boulder Creek, CA 95006-9696
831-338-3383
800-400-0671
FAX: 831-338-0200
e-mail: campharmon@es-cc.org
www.centralcal.easterseals.com
Ruth Hutchison, Board Chair
Robert Guerin, Board Vice Chair
Tom Conway, CEO
Judy Anderson, Secretary / Treasurer
Camp is located in Boulder Creek, California. 6-10 day sessions for children and adults with physical and developmental disabilities. Coed, ages 8-65.

983 **Enchanted Hills Camp for the Blind**
Lighthouse for the Blind
214 Van Ness Ave
San Francisco, CA 94102
415-431-1481
888-400-8933
FAX: 415-863-7568
e-mail: info@lighthouse-sf.org
lighthouse-sf.org/
Joshua A. Miele, Ph.D., President
Chris Downey, 1st Vice President
Kathleen Knox, 2nd Vice President
Lisa Carvalho, 3rd Vice President
Camp is located in Napa, California. Half-week, one and two-week sessions for blind, deaf/blind children and adults, ages 5 and up. This program offers a basic camping experience. Activities include music, art, dance, hiking and riding. Camperships are available to California residents.

984 **Firefighters Kids Camp**
Firefighters Burn Institute
3101 Stockton Blvd.
Sacramento, CA 95820
916-739-8525
FAX: 916-455-4376
e-mail: website@ffburn.org
ffburn.org/
Brian Rice, President
Shannon Munoz, Executive Director
Pat Cook, Secretary-Treasurer
Svend Nance, Director of Membership Services
Provides children and young adults ages 6-17 who have had serious burn injuries the opportunity to continue their rehabilitation and recovery in an outdoor environment where they are safe and can have fun.

985 **Lions Wilderness Camp for Deaf Children, Inc.**
Lions Clubs of California and Nevada
P.O.Box 195
Knightsen, CA 94548
877-896-1598
888-613-1557
e-mail: campdirector@lionswildcamp.org
www.lionswildcamp.org
Richard A. Wilmot, President
Rachel Mix, Camp Program Director
Robin L. Nichol, Camp Manager
Dana Johnson, Secretary
A camp experience where a deaf child age 7 to 15 can learn outdoor skills and enjoy the wonder and beauty of nature to the fullest extent.

986 **New Horizons Summer Day Camp**
YMCA
13821 Newport Avenue
Suite 200
Tustin, CA 92780
714-549-9622
FAX: 714-838-5976
www.ymcaoc.org

Robert Traut, Board Chair
Jeff Black, Vice Chair
John Rochford, Vice Chair
Jeff McBride, President/CEO
One-week sessions for children with ADD and speech/communication impairment. Coed, ages 5-14.

987 **One Step At A Time Camp**
213 West Institute Place
Suite 511
Chicago, IL 60610
312-924-4220
FAX: 312-878-7374
onestepcamp.org

Jeff Infusino, President
Darryl Winston Perkins, Jr., Director Of Programs
Through our One Step programs, we offer camp experiences and other programs throughout the year that allow children with cancer to just be kids. Our programs offer fun, friendship and support in a safe and nurturing environment. Through the magic of childhood experiences, we help kids diagnosed with cancer reclaim their lives.

988 **Pilgrim Pines Camp & Conference Center**
United Church of Christ
39570 Glen Road
Yucaipa, CA 92399
909-797-1821
800-616-6612
800-678-5102
FAX: 909-797-2691
e-mail: info@pilgrimpinescamp.org
www.pilgrimpinescamp.org

June Boutwell, Executive Director
Christian camp offering one-week sessions for campers with developmental disabilities. Coed, ages 10-Adult. Also families.

989 **Quest Camp**
2355 San Ramon Valley Blvd.
Suite 208
San Ramon, CA 94583
925-743-2900
800-313-9733
FAX: 925-820-9761
e-mail: questcamps@mac.com
www.questcamps.com

Dr. Robert B Field, PhD., Founder/Executive Director
Debra Forrester-Field, M.A., Administrative Director
Adam Berman, Clinical Director
Jodie Knott, Ph.D., Director
Camp is located in Alamo, California. Day camp offering three to eight-week sessions including psychological treatment for children with ADD and other mild to moderate psychological disorders. Coed, ages 6-15.

990 **Special Camp For Special Kids**
31641 La Novia Avenue
San Juan Capistrano, CA 92675
949-661-0108
FAX: 949-661-8637
e-mail: lindsay.eres@smes.org
www.specialcamp.org

Lindsay Eres, Executive Director
Stefani Baker, Camp Operations Director
Patty Canright, RN, Nursing Director
Juliana Coleman, Program Assistant
Day camp for youths with disabilities offering arts & crafts, games, reading, and entertainment.

991 **The Painted Turtle**
1300 4th Street
Suite 300
Santa Monica, CA 90401
310-451-1353
866-451-5367
FAX: 310-451-1357
e-mail: info@thepaintedturtle.com
www.thepaintedturtle.org/

Page Adler, Founder/Chair
Lou Adler, Producer
Mary Brown, Board Member
Tom Amster, Board Member
This camp is the sixth edition to the 'Hole in the Wall' camps and is for seriously ill children in the California area. The Painted Turtle offers swimming, boating, fishing, horseback riding, art and crafts, and nature activities.

992 **Tuolumne Trails**
22988 Ferretti Road
Groveland, CA 95321
209-962-7534

e-mail: jerry@tuolumnetrails.org
tuolumnetrails.org

Colorado

993 **Adam's Camp**
6767 South Spruce Street
Suite 102
Centennial, CO 80112
303-563-8290
FAX: 303-563-8291
e-mail: laura@adamscamp.org
adamscamp.org/

Bill Harmon, President
Brian Simms, VP
Karel Horney, Executice Director
Laura Johnson, Billing & Finance Director
Adam's camp is designed for infants and children with special needs and their families, as well as young adults with mild to moderate developmental disabilities. The camp offers a variety of intensive, therapeutic programs and recreational programs.

994 **Aspen Camp of the Deaf & Hard of Hearing**
4862 Snowmass Creek Rd.
Snowmass, CO 81654
970-315-0513
FAX: 970-923-0643
TTY:970-315-0513
e-mail: info@aspencamp.org
www.aspencamp.org/

Kelly Krumrie, President
Ellen Roth, Board Member
Nick Stark, Board Member
Tim Whitsitt, Board Member
Provide enriching experiential educational and recreational experiences for Deaf and Hard of Hearing individuals.

995 **Breckenridge Outdoor Education Center**
P.O.Box 697
Breckenridge, CO 80424
970-453-6422
800-383-2632
800-383-BOEC
FAX: 970-453-4676
e-mail: boec@boec.org
www.boec.org

Tim Casey, Chair
John Ebright, Vice Chair
Bruce Fitch, Executive Director
Kristen Bennett, Finance Director
Provides year-round adventure based wilderness and adaptive ski programs for people with disabilities. The Center excels in offering challenging, rewarding outdoor experiences individually designed to the abilities and needs of participants.

996 CNI Cochlear Kids Camp
Colorado Neurological Institute
701 East Hampden Avenue
Suite 415
Englewood, CO 80113
303-783-4010
855-463-6264
FAX: 303-788-5469
e-mail: info@thecni.org
www.thecni.org

Tami Lack, MA, CFRE, Executive Director
Ellen Belle, MA-PT, Director of Patient Services
Luci Draayer, Director of Education and Support Services
Alicia Novak, Director of Research
Designed to bring together children ages 1-18 with cochlear implants and their families. Campers enjoy both indoor and outdoor recreational and educational programs.

997 Camp Paha Rise Above
City of Lakewood
480 S. Allison Pkwy
Lakewood, CO 80226
303-987-7000
FAX: 303-987-7832
TTY:303-987-7057
e-mail: marsno@lakewood.org
www.lakewood.org

Bob Murphy, Mayor
Kathy Hodgson, City Manager
Nanette Neelan, Deputy City Manager
Camp Paha is a City of Lakewood day camp for children ages 6-17 and young adults ages 18-25 with disabilities. We provide programs for campers with all disability types: developmental, physical, emotional, behavioral, and learning. Camp Paha offers safe, quality, fun and challenging activities. Camp provides campers an opportunity to participate in aquatics, sports, games, nature, music, drama, hiking, arts and crafts, and field trips into the community.

998 Camp Rocky Mountain Village
Easter Seals Colorado
P.O. Box 115
Empire, CO 80438
303-569-2333
FAX: 303-569-3857
e-mail: campinfo@eastersealscolorado.org
www.co.easterseals.com

Chris Whitley, Chair
Lynn Robinson, President/CEO
Nancy Hanson, VP, Human Resources
Bill Evert, Co-Treasurer
For children and adults with disabilities. Campers enjoy swimming, fishing, day trips, sports and recreation, arts and crafts.

999 Camp Wapiyapi
191 University Boulevard
Box 294
Denver, CO 80206
303-534-0883
FAX: 303-534-0874
e-mail: Wapiyapi@wapiyapi.org
www.wapiyapi.org

Jason Elbot, President
Darla Dakin, Executive Director
Kay Noser, Treasurer
Jeff Druck, M.D., Secretary
A no-cost respite for children with cancer and their families. The camp offers a wide variety of group and individual activities

1000 Challenge Aspen
P.O.Box 6639
Snowmass Village, CO 81615
970-923-0578
FAX: 970-923-7338
e-mail: possibilities@challengeaspen.com
www.challengeaspen.org

Jimmy Yeager, President
Jack Kennedy, VP
Kevin Berg, Board Member
Grayson Stover, Secretary
Challenge Aspen provides recreational and cultural experiences for individuals who have cognitive or physical challenges. Challenge Aspen offers a variety of recreational programs to fit a diversity of needs and interests. We offer both summer, winter and special events for both adults and children.

1001 Cheley/Children's Hospital Burn Camps Program
The Children's Hospital
Anschultz Medical Campus
13123 East 16th Avenue
Aurora, CO 80045
720-777-1234
800-624-6553
e-mail: boulter.trudy@tchden.org
www.thechildrenshospital.org

Jim Shmerling, DHA, FACHE, President and CEO
Camp is open for children ages 8 to 18 who have been hospitalized at The Children's Hospital or other burn units across the country. Campers gain life skills and confidence whether they are on a challenge course, catching a fish or climbing onto a horse.

1002 Colorado Lions Camp
P.O.Box 9043
Woodland Park, CO 80866
719-687-2087
FAX: 719-687-7435
e-mail: dsmith@coloradolionscamp.org
www.coloradolionscamp.org

Sharla F Westerman, President
Barbara Guest, VP
Dan Smith, Executive Director
Michelle Werner, Executive Administrative Assistant
Outdoor recreational camping for the visually and hearing impaired and developmentally delayed. All normal camp activities are offered at the year-round facility. Summer and winter programs. 1 to 4 staff supervision with a nurse or doctor in attendance.

1003 First Descents
3001 Brighton Boulevard
Suite 623
Denver, CO 80216
303-945-2490
FAX: 303-474-3005
e-mail: info@firstdescents.org
firstdescents.org

1004 Rocky Mountain Village
Easter Seals Colorado
PO Box 115
Empire, CO 80438
303-569-2333
FAX: 303-569-3857
e-mail: campinfo@eastersealscolorado.org
www.co.easterseals.com

Chris Whitley, Chair
Lynn Robinson, President/CEO
Nancy Hanson, VP, Human Resources
Bill Evert, Co-Treasurer
An 11 week summer camp for people with disabilities. After the summer season there is respite weekends for people with disabilities - once a month.

1005 Roundup River Ranch
8333 Colorado River Road
Gypsum, CO 81637
970-524-2267
FAX: 877-619-0323
roundupriverranch.org

Ruth B. Johnson, J.D., President/CEO
Tammy Argenbright, Chief Administrative Officer/Chief Financial Officer
Marita Bledsoe, M.D., Medical Director
Sterling Nell Leija, Camp Director
Roundup River Ranch is a medically supported camp for kids with chronic and life-threatening illnesses- the place where they can truly feel incredible, no matter what illness they're battling. We put the focus on their fun, not their conditions. And most importantly, we give kids an experience that encourages their lives, allowing them to simply enjoy the fun, games, and joys of childhood- for free.

1006 YMCA Camp Shady Brook
YMCA of the Pikes Peak Region (PPYMCA)
316 N. Tejon Street
Colorado Springs, CO 80903
719-329-7227
FAX: 719-272-7026
e-mail: campinfo@ppymca.org
www.campshadybrook.org

Sonny Adkins, Executive Director
Laura Petersen, Program Director
Patrick Casey, Facility Director
Michaela Eddleston, Conference & Retreat Director

Camp is located in Sedalia, Colorado. One-week sessions for campers with HIV. Boys and girls 7-16. Also families, seniors and single adults.

Connecticut

1007 Arthur C. Luf Children's Burn Camp
Connecticut Burns Care Foundation
601 Boston Post Road
Milford, CT 06460
203-878-6744
FAX: 203-878-4044
e-mail: ctburnscare@optonline.net
www.ctburnsfoundation.org

Frank Szivos, Executive Director
Susan M. Howard, Foundation Secretary
Frank Szivos, Executive Director

A safe outdoor environment for children ages 8-18 from around the world who have survived life altering burn injuries. Children learn to build self-confidence and self-esteem.

1008 Camp Harkness
Arc of New London County
P.O. Box 2545
Hartford, CT 06146-2545
www.sbacct.tripod.com/

1009 Camp Hemlocks
Easter Seals: Connecticut
733 Summer Street
Suite 104
Stamford, CT 6901
203-388-2192
800-832-4409
FAX: 203-388-2196
e-mail: campinfo@eastersealsct.org
www.eastersealscamphemlocks.org

Chris Whitley, Chair
Bill Evert, Co-Treasurer
Nancy Hanson, Corporate Secretary
Lynn Robinson, President/CEO

Camp is located in Hebron, Connecticut. One and two-week sessions June-August for campers with a variety of disabilities. Coed, ages 6 and up. Families, seniors, single adults. Campers can enjoy nature walks, swimming, boating arts & crafts and sing-a-longs around the campfire.

1010 Camp Horizons
127 Babcock Hill Rd
South Windham, CT 06266
860-456-1032
FAX: 860-456-4721
e-mail: scott.lambeck@camphorizons.org
www.camphorizons.org

Adam Milne, Board Chairperson
Chris McNaboe, President
Kathleen McNaboe, Board Vice President
L. Sanford (Sandy) Rice, Board Treasurer

Bordering Lake Probus, the facilities at the camp are equipped to accommodate a wide range of activities and programs for campers with developmental disabilities, or other challenging emotional and social needs. There is a 5:1 camper-counselor ratio with a schedule of three programs in the morning and four in the afternoon.

1011 Camp Isola Bella
American School for the Deaf
139 N Main St
West Hartford, CT 06107
860-570-2300
TTY:860-570-2222
e-mail: Steve.Borsotti@asd-1817.org
www.asd-1817.org

David W. Carter, President
Harold A. Smullen, 1st Vice President
Ed Peltier, Executive Director
Tom Wood, CFO

Hearing-impaired children, ages 6-19, blend educational instruction in communications with recreational activities. Qualified deaf and hearing staff members with experience in education, child care and counseling are employed at the camp.

1012 Hole in the Wall Gang Camp
565 Ashford Center Rd
Ashford, CT 06278
860-429-3444
FAX: 860-429-7295
e-mail: ashford@holeinthewallgang.org
www.holeinthewallgang.org

Raymond Lamontagne, Chairman
Ken Alberti, Chief Development Officer
James H. Canton, Chief Executive Officer
Kevin M. Magee, Chief Financial Officer

Low-cost eight-week sessions June-August for children with cancer and HIV. Coed, ages 7-15.

1013 Marvelwood Summer
Marvelwood School
476 Skiff Mountain Road
P.O. Box 3001
Kent, CT 06757- 3001
860-927-0047
FAX: 860-927-0021
e-mail: summerschool@marvelwood.org
www.marvelwood.org

Arthur F. Goodearl, Head of School
Bettyann Haskell, Business Office
Katherine Almquist, Director of Admission
Richard Becker, CFO

The emphasis in this summer program is on diagnosis and remediation of individual reading, spelling, writing, mathematics and study problems. Offered to ages 12-16.

1014 TSA CT Kid's Summer Event
Tourette Syndrome Association of Connecticut (TSA)
c/o Massachusetts Chapter
39 Godfrey Street
Taunton, MA 02780
617-277-7589
e-mail: info@tsa-ma.org
www.tsact.org

Peter Tavolacci, Vice Chairman
Paul Nazario, Treasurer
Jeanette Nazario, Board Member
Mike Tavolacci, Board Member

TSA of Connecticut sponsors summer events for children with TS/Tourette Syndrome activities of which include miniature golf in addition to an Annual Conference. The kids' program at this annual conference provides children who have TS a unique opportunity to meet other children like them who also struggle with TS. Entertainment includes puppeteers, magicians, learning karate from the experts, getting face paintings and more.
uniqu pages

1015 **YMCA Camp Jewell**
YMCA of Greater Hartford
6 Prock Hill Road
P.O. Box 8
Colebrook, CT 06021
860-379-2782
888-412-2267
FAX: 860-379-8715
TTY: 888-412-2267
e-mail: camp.jewell@ghymca.org
www.ghymca.org

Eric Tucker, Executive Director
Ray Zetye, Director
Marilyn Ducor, Camp Registrar
Kathie Reese, Office Manager

Camp is located in Colebrook, Connecticut. Two-week sessions for children with cancer. Coed, ages 8-16. Also families.

Delaware

1016 **Camp Fairlee Manor**
Easter Seals DE/MD Eastern Shore
61 Corporate Circle
New Castle, DE 19720
302-324-4444
800-677-3800
FAX: 302-324-4441
e-mail: contact@esdel.org
www.de.easterseals.com

Cynthia Morgan, Chair
Martha Rees, Vice Chair
Kenan Sklenar, President/CEO
Jeffery Gosnear, Treasurer

Residential camp at Fairlee Manor serves an average of 50 to 75 children and adults each week with physical disabilities and/or cognitive, behavioral impairments throughout the summer and on select weekends year-round.

1017 **Camp Manito/Camp Lenape**
United Cerebral Palsy Of Delaware
700 A River Road
Wilmington, DE 19809
302-764-2400
FAX: 302-764-8713
e-mail: ucpde@ucpde.org
www.ucpde.org

Donna M. Hopkins, President
D. Bruce McClenathan, Vice President
Michele M. Zonick, Recording Secretary
Daniel Edgar, Treasurer

For children & young adults aged 3-21 with orthopedic disabilities. Campers find a structured program of arts, crafts, sports, swimming, music and nature studies.

1018 **Childrens Beach House**
1800 Bay Ave
Lewes, DE 19958
302-645-9184
FAX: 302-655-4216
www.cbhinc.org

Martha P. Tschantz, President
Maryann Helms, Vice President
Linda M. Fischer, Secretary
Charles H. Sterner, Treasurer

Camp is located in Lewes, Delaware. Four-week sessions June-August for Delaware children with hearing impairment or speech/communication impairment, also fine or gross motor delays. Coed, ages 7-18. Also, serves children year round on weekends only.

1019 **Sandcastle Day Camp**
Children's Beach House
1800 Bay Ave
Lewes, DE 19958
302-645-9184
FAX: 302-655-4216
www.cbhinc.org

Martha P. Tschantz, President
Maryann Helms, Vice President
Linda M. Fischer, Secretary
Charles H. Sterner, Treasurer

Camp is located in Lewes, Delaware. Four-week sessions June-August for Delaware children with hearing impairment or speech/communication impairment. Coed, ages 6-12.

District of Columbia

1020 **Camp Quality George Washington University**
1444 Mockingbird Circle
Stow, OH 44224
330-671-0167
FAX: 866-285-5208
e-mail: patty@campqualityusa.org
www.campqualityusa.com

Lois Hartje, President
Vicki Irey, VP
Patricia Harris, Executive Director
Dennis Hart, Secretary

Camp Quality is for children with cancer and their siblings. The camp offers a stress-free environment that offers exciting activities and fosters new friendships, while helping to give the children courage, motivation and emotional strength.

1021 **Columbia Lighthouse for the Blind Summer Camp**
Columbia Lighthouse for the Blind
1825 K Street NorthWest
Suite 1103
Washington, DC 20006
202-454-6400
FAX: 877-595-9228
e-mail: info@clb.org
www.clb.org

Tony Cancelosi, K.M.,, President and CEO
Anthony Cancelosi, CEO
Jocelyn Hunter, Director of Communications
Cathy Miller, Director of Development

Helps enable the blind or visually impaired to obtain and maintain independence at home, school, work and in the community. Programs and services include early intervention services, training and consultation in assistive technology, career placement services, comprehensive low vision care and a wide range of rehabilitation services. Highly acclaimed summer camp, picnics and holiday activities encourage blind and visually impaired children to make new friends and experience the joys of childhood

1022 **Lab School of Washington**
4759 Reservoir Rd NW
Washington, DC 20007-1921
202-965-6600
e-mail: labschool@webmail.org
www.labschool.org

Sally Seawright, Interim Dir.
Robert Mathias, Chair
Mimi Dawson, Vice-Chair
Bill Tennis, Vice-Chair

The Lab School six week summer session includes individualized reading, spelling, writing, study skills and math programs. A multisensory approach addresses the needs of bright learning disabled children. Related services such as speech/language therapy and occupational therapy are integrated into the curriculum. Elementary/Intermediate; Junior High/High School.

Florida

1023 **Camp Amigo Burn Camp**
Children's Burn Camp Of North Florida, Inc.
P.O. Box 368
Tallahassee, FL 32302
850-509-6200
www.campamigo.com

Rusty Roberts, President
Stephanie Powell, Treasurer

Camp Amigo is open to burn survivors ages 6-18 living in North or Central Florida. The camp is free of charge and provides children who have physical and emotional scarring a place to be themselves and build a network of support.

1024 **Camp Boggy Creek**
30500 Brantley Branch Rd
Eustis, FL 32736
352-483-4200
866-462-6449
FAX: 352-483-0589
e-mail: info@campboggycreek.org
www.boggycreek.org

J. Patterson Cooper, Chair
Wendy Durden, Vice Chair
June Clark, President/CEO
Michelle Church, Treasurer

Year-round sessions for children with a variety of chronic or life-threatening illnesses including cancer, hemophilia, epilepsy, heart defects, HIV, spina bifida and asthma/respiratory ailments. Coed, ages 7-16.

1025 **Camp Challenge**
Easter Seals Of Florida
31600 Camp Challenge Road
Sorrento, FL 32776
352-383-4711
e-mail: camp@fl.easterseals.com
www.fleasterseals.com

1026 **Camp Thunderbird**
Quest, Inc.
P.O.Box 531125
Orlando, FL 32853
407-218-4300
888-80 -UEST
FAX: 407-218-4301
e-mail: webadmin@questinc.org
www.questinc.org/

David Canora, Chair
James Gallagher, Vice Chair
John Gill, President / CEO
Karenne Levy, COO

Residential summer camping program for children and adults with a developmental disability. Located on 19-acres of Wekiwa Springs State Park. Campers enjoy swimming, sports, nature hikes, an outdoor amphitheater, etc. One and two-week sessions June-August. Coed, ages 8-80.

1027 **Center Academy at Pinellas Park**
6710 86th Ave
Pinellas Park, FL 33782
727-541-5716
FAX: 727-544-8186
e-mail: infopp@centeracademy.com
www.centeracademy.com

Mack R Hicks PhD, Founder/Chairman of the Board
Eric V. Larson, Ph. D.,, President & COO
Andrew P Hicks PhD, CEO/Clinical Dir.
Lisa Hartmann, Dir. Education

Specifically designed for the learning disabled child and other children with difficulties in concentration, strategy, social skills, impulsivity, distractibility and study strategies. Programs offered include: attention training, visual-motor remediation, socialization skills training, relaxation training, horseback riding and more. The day camp meets weekdays from 9-3 for 3,4 or 5 week sessions.

1028 **Dream Oaks Camp**
Foundation For Dreams, Inc.
16110 Dream Oaks Place
Bradenton, FL 34212
941-746-5659
FAX: 941-745-1409
e-mail: jfranke@foundationfordreams.org
www.foundationfordreams.org

Jodi Franke, Executive Director
Elena Cassella, Director of Development
Gilda Poe, Administrative Assistant

Weekend camps and day residential programs open to children with physical and developmental disabilities and serious illnesses. Activities include horseback riding, nature programs, sports, game, swimming, talent shows, and arts and crafts.

1029 **Florida Diabetes Camp**
P.O.Box 14136
Gainesville, FL 32604
352-334-1321
FAX: 352-334-1326
e-mail: fccyd@floridadiabetescamp.org
www.floridadiabetescamp.org

Gary Cornwell, Executive Director
Chris Stakely, Assistant Director
Amy Soileau, Outrech Director
Robena Cornwell, Finance

Camp is located in Florida. One and two-week sessions June-August for children with diabetes. Coed, ages 6-18 and families. Camps throughout the year.

1030 **Florida Lions Camp**
Lions of Multiple District 35
2819 Tiger Lake Rd
Lake Wales, FL 33898
863-696-1948
FAX: 863-696-2398
e-mail: jrv113@gmail.com
www.lionscampfl.org

Barbara Cage, Executive Director
Liz Cage, Program Director/ Rentals
Carissa Moen, Bookkeeping/Registrar

One-week sessions June-August for youths and adults with visual impairments and other challenging disabilities. Coed, ages 5 and up. A variety of traditional summer camp activities which include: swimming, canoeing, fishing, hiking, camping out and cooking over a fire, games, arts & crafts, singing & dancing, hay-wagon rides, challenge course and much more. Activities are adapted to the age and ability of each camper to ensure maximum participation, safety and fun.

1031 **Florida Sheriffs Caruth Camp**
Florida Sheriffs Youth Ranches
2486 Cecil Webb Place
Live Oak, FL 32060
386-842-5501
800-765-3797
FAX: 386-842-2429
youthranches.org

Sheriff B. Stewart, Chair
Dan Hager, Vice Chairman
Roger Bouchard, President
Bill Frye, EVP

Camp is located in Inglis, Florida. One-week sessions for children with ADD. Coed, ages 10-15.

1032 **Hands To Love**
165 Montgomery Road
Altamonte, FL 32714
352-273-7382
FAX: 352-273-7388
e-mail: info@handstolove.org
www.handstolove.org

Jackie Hadala, President

Hands to Love (affectionately nicknamed H2L) is an organization for children with upper limb differences and their families.

1033 **Sertoma Camp Endeavor**
Sertoma Camp Endeavor
P.O.Box 910
Dundee, FL 33838-0910
863-439-1300
e-mail: info@sertomacampendeavor.com
www.sertomacampendeavor.org

1034 **VACC Camp**
Miami Childrens Hospital
3200 S.W. 60 Ct.
Suite 203
Miami, FL 33155-4076
305-662-8222
FAX: 305-663-8417
e-mail: bela.florentin@mch.com
www.vacccamp.com

Bela Florentin, Camp Coordinator

Free week-long overnight camp for ventilation assisted children and their families.

Georgia

1035 Aerie Experiences
Aerie Experiences
969 Golden Avenue
Dahlonega, GA 30533 404-285-0467
e-mail: mdweneta@aerieexperiences.com
aerieexperiences.com
Matthew D. Weneta, M.Ed.
We offer experiential, adventure-based, wilderness and therapeutic activities for children, individuals and families navigating Neurobiological Disorders, Aspergers, High Functioning Autism, Learning Disabilities and other special needs.

1036 Camp Breathe Easy
American Lung Association
2452 Spring Rd
Smyrna, GA 30080-3828 404-231-9887
e-mail: annie@camptwinlakes.org
www.campbreatheeasy.com/
Annie Garrett, Camp Director
Camp Breathe Easy is a seven-day, six-night overnight camp for children, ages 7-13, with asthma who need medication and are limited in summer camping opportunities. The children learn asthma self-management techniques and coping strategies to better handle their illness. Campers swim, repel off trees, fish, canoe, play soccer, basketball and miniature golf, and participate in ceramics and arts and crafts.

1037 Camp Caglewood
Caglewood, Inc.
P.O. Box 158
Flowery Branch, GA 30542 678-405-9000
FAX: 770-441-3406
e-mail: info@caglewood.org
www.caglewood.org

1038 Camp Dream
Camp Dream Foundation
4355 Cobb Parkway
Suite J117
Atlanta, GA 30339
www.campdreamga.org
JR Clark, President
Gary Marshall, Vice President
Beverly Taylor, Programs Director
Valarie Dunn, Secretary
Camp Dream is a free camp where special needs children can camp and have fun regardless of their physical and/or mental condition. The camp offers many recreational activities and programs.

1039 Camp Hawkins
GA Baptist Childrens Homes & Family Ministries,Inc
P.O. Box 329
Palmetto, GA 30268 770-463-3800
e-mail: ksewell@gbchfm.org
www.gbchfm.org
James Harper, D.Min, President/CEO
Kendra Sewell, Contact Person
Brian Hawkins, Administrator
Alan Mccumber, Vice President - Finance
Residential summer camp for youth's ages 8-12 coping with varying developmental disabilities such as down's syndrome, traumatic brain injuries, cerebral palsy, and learning disorders and/or developmental delays. Staff works one-on-one with each camper.

1040 Camp Independence
National Kidney Foundation
30 East 33rd Street
New York, NY 10016 770-452-1539
855-653-2273
855-NKF-CARE
FAX: 212-689-9261
e-mail: nkfcares@kidney.org
www.kidney.org
Gregory w. Scott, Chairman
Beth Piranio, President
Petros Gregoriou, VP, Finance
Ellie Schlam, VP, Communications
Camp Independence is Georgia's a overnight, week-long summer camp providing essential medical care, treatment & fun for kids with kidney disease and transplants. Camp Independence recognizes that campers are normal children but have special needs providing these children with opportunities for development & individual growth, peer support & normal life experiences. Activities include swimming, arts & crafts, fishing and horseback riding, in addition to archery, games and sports, and ceramics.

1041 Camp Juliena
Georgia Council for the Hearing Impaired
4151 Memorial Drive
Suite 103B
Decatur, GA 30032-1511 404-292-5312
866-873-2485
FAX: 404-299-3642
e-mail: info@fullcirclegrp.com
http://www.fullcirclegrp1.com
Thomas Galey, Executive Director
Bonna Lenyszyn, Camp Director
Ron Vickery, President
Deborah Douglin, Treasurer
A weeklong residential summer camp for youths and teens who are deaf or hard of hearing. Through challenging, team-oriented activities, campers form lasting friendships and acquire valuable leadership, social and communication skills.

1042 Camp Kudzu
Camp Kudzu, Inc.
5885 Glenridge Drive
Suite 160
Atlanta, GA 30328 404-250-1811
FAX: 404-250-1812
e-mail: info@campkudzu.org
www.campkudzu.org
Alex Allen, Executive Director
Ashley Conant, Camp Director
Maureen Warren, Medical Director
Cyndy McCoy Oastler, Camper Services Administrator
Camp for children, teens and families with type 1 diabetes. Besides teaching diabetes management, campers learn that they are not alone in their struggles and enjoy climbing, swimming and many other outdoor activities.

1043 Camp Sunshine
1850 Clairmont Road
Decatur, GA 30033-3405 404-325-7979
866-786-2267
FAX: 404-325-7929
www.mycampsunshine.com
Dorothy H. Jordan, Founder
Beth Abernathy, Chair
Sally Hale, Executive Director
J. Preston Byers, Treasurer
Camp sunshine gives children with cancer the opportunity to enjoy normal activities such as horseback riding, swimming, and arts & crafts.

1044 **Camp Twin Lakes**
1391 Keencheefoonee Rd
Rutledge, GA 30663
706-557-9070
FAX: 706-557-9147
e-mail: contact@camptwinlakes.org
www.camptwinlakes.org

Doug Hertz, Chairman and Founder
Lawrence Kenny, President
Elizabeth Richards, VP
Laura barnard, Treasurer

One-week sessions June-August for children with serious illnesses and life challenges. Works with over 40 different special needs organizations. Coed, ages 8-18. Two locations: Rutledge and Will-A-Way in Winder, GA.

1045 **Squirrel Hollow Summer Camp**
The Bedford School
5665 Milam Rd
Fairburn, GA 30213
770-774-8001
FAX: 770-774-8005
e-mail: bbox@thebedfordschool.org
www.thebedfordschool.org

Michael Vigil, Chair
Todd Weaver, Board Member
Aaron Turner, Board Member
Jimmy Collins, Board Member

A remedial summer program for children with academic needs held on the campus of The Bedford School in Fairburn, Georgia. It is a five week day camp held from June 19 to July 21 and serves ages 6-16. For more information contact Betsy Box at (770) 774-8001.

Hawaii

1046 **Camp Anuenue**
American Cancer Society
Waialua, HI 96791
818-788-9900
FAX: 808-595-7502
e-mail: editor@specialneeds.com
www.specialneeds.com/directory/camp/cancer/hi

Debra Glowik, Director

Camp Anuenue is for children ages 7-17 who have or have had cancer.

1047 **YMCA Camp Erdman**
YMCA Of Honolulu
1441 Pali Highway
Honolulu, HI 96813
808-531-9622
FAX: 808-533-1286
e-mail: camperdman@ymcahonolulu.org
www.ymcahonolulu.org

Lance Wilhelm, Chair
Keith Sakamoto, Vice Chair
Bruce Coppa, Vice Chair
Tim John, Vice Chair

Traditional Resident Camp program is five nights and six days of fun-filled activities that will create positive lifetime memories. Camp activities include: arts & crafts, swimming, kayaking, hiking, challenge course, snorkeling, athletics, nature, dance & drama, beach writing and archery. Traditional Resident Camp Experience (Ages 6-17) serving the needs of the disabled.

Idaho

1048 **Camp Hodia**
1701 N 12th St
Boise, ID 83702
208-891-1023
FAX: 208-891-1023
e-mail: lisa1@hodia.org
http://www.hodia.org

Natalie B. DelRio, Chair
Richard Christensen, Vice Chair
Lisa Gier, Executice Director
Vicki Cutshall, R.N., Director, Hodia Kids Camp

Camp is located in Alturas Lake, Idaho. One-week sessions for children with diabetes. Coed, ages 8-18. Ski Camp in Sun Valley in January, ages 12-18.

1049 **Camp Rainbow Gold**
216 West Jefferson Street
Boise, ID 83702
208-350-6435
e-mail: info@camprainbowgold.org
camprainbowgold.org

Tim Tyree, President
Elizabeth Lizberg, Executive Director
Doris F. Tunney, M.D., Treasurer
Meg Omel-Tyree, Secretary

Camp Rainbow Gold provides year round programs such as medically supervised camps, college scholarships and other emotionally empowering experiences to children diagnosed with cancer, their families and support network.

1050 **Camp Sawtooth**
Oregon-Idaho Conference Center
HC 64 BOX 8290
Ketchum
ID 83340
208-726-1155
e-mail: directorscampsawtooth@yahoo.com
www.campsawtooth.org/

Illinois

1051 **ADA Camp Grenada**
American Diabetes Association
1701 N. Beauregard St.
Alexandria, VA 22311
312-346-1805
888-342-2383
800-DIA-ETES
FAX: 317-594-0748
e-mail: wwallace@diabetes.org
www.diabetes.org

Dwight Holing, Chair
Larry Hausner, CEO
Debbie Johnson, CFO
Greg Elfers, Chief Field Development Officer

Camp Granada is an American Diabetes Association resident Camp located in Monticello, Illinois at the 4H Memorial Camp owned by the University of Illinois. For children with diabetes, ages 8-16. Activities include swimming, canoeing, wall climbing, tie-dying shirts, arts & crafts and fun filled evening programs.

1052 **ADA Teen Adventure Camp**
American Diabetes Association
4000 Ridgeway Drive
Birmingham, AL 35209
800-900-8086
FAX: 205-313-7475
e-mail: email@nchpad.org
http://www.ncpad.org

Sue Apsey, Program Director

Camping for teenagers with diabetes. Coed, ages 14 to 18. Camp dates are early in August. Located at the YMCA Camp Duncan in Ingleside, Illinois. Featured activities include archery and crafts, singing, outdoor movie night, and roller skating.

1053 **ADA Triangle D Camp**
American Diabetes Association
4000 Ridgeway Drive
Birmingham, AL 35209
800-900-8086
FAX: 205-313-7475
e-mail: email@nchpad.org
http://www.ncpad.org

Sue Apsey, Program Director

Triangle D Camp is a resident camp program located at the YMCA Camp Duncan in Ingleside, Illinois. Activities include swimming, row boating, canoeing, high ropes (11-13 yr. olds), climbing tower (9-10 yr. olds), Camp games, singing, archery, campfires, soccer, basketball, volleyball and diabetes education.

1054 ASCCA
Alabama Easter Seal Society
44 Montgomery St.
Suite 1605
San Francisco, CA 94104- 4602
415-296-6952
FAX: 415-296-6901
e-mail: socca@iars.org
www.socca.org/

Aryeh Shander, President
Laureen L. Hill, Director
Daniel R. Brown, Treasurer
Miguel A. Cobas, Secretary
The Society of Critical Care Anesthesiologists (SOCCA) formerly ASCCA, was founded in 1986 to address the unique concerns of intensivists before the American Society of anesthesiologists (ASA). The founding members of SOCCA believed and continue to believe that multidisciplinary critical care medicine is a desirable goal.

1055 Bright Horizons Summer Camp
Sickle Cell Disease Association of Illinois
200 Talcott Avenue South
Watertown, MA 02472
617-673-8000
e-mail: parents@brighthorizons.com
http://www.brighthorizons.com

David Lissy, CEO
Linda Mason, Chairman and Founder
Mary Ann Tocio, President and COO
Elizabeth Boland, CFO
Camping for children with blood disorders, ages 7-13. The joys of learning include instruction in first aid, swimming and water safety, boating, horseback riding and bowling plus arts and crafts. In addition, there is a traditional menu of camp pleasures, like hayrides, cookouts, nature hikes and sing-a-longs.

1056 Camp Callahan
Camp Callahan, Inc.
P.O. Box 5253
Quincy, IL 62305
217-833-2377
www.campcallahan.com

1057 Camp Discovery
American Academy Of Dermatology
930 E. Woodfield Road
Schaumburg, IL 60173
847-240-1280
866-503-SKIN
866-503-7546
FAX: 847-240-1859
e-mail: jmueller@aad.org
www.campdiscovery.org

Brett M. Coldiron, MD, President
Elise A. Olsen, VP
Suzanne M. Olbricht, Secretary-Treasurer
Neal D. Bhatia, Director
Free camp for ages 8-16 with chronic skin conditions such as psoriasis, eczema, scleroderma, epidermolysis bullosa, alopecia, Vitiligo, congenital nevus. Campers can enjoy boating, fishing, water skiing, swimming, arts and crafts.

1058 Camp Firefly
Jewish Child & Family Services
Attn: Melissa Newman
255 Revere Dr., Suite 200
Northbrook, IL 60062
FAX: 847-412-4360
www.campfireflyjcfs.com/index.html

Audra Kaplan, Psy.D., Camp Director
Andrew Rosenbloom, Psy.D., Assistant Camp Director
Dr Rachel Riley
Week-long camp for children with social disabilities. The camp offers all the experiences of an overnight camp that includes gaining a sense of autonomy and friendships. Staff members are there to help provide therapeutic and support assistance to help the children accomplish these goals.

1059 Camp Hug The Bear
Northern Suburban Special Recreation Association
3105 MacArthur Blvd.
Northbrook, IL 60062
847-509-9400
FAX: 847-509-1177
e-mail: info@nssra.org
www.nssra.org

Mary V. Arsdale, Chair
Steve Wilson, Vice Chair
Craig Culp, Executive Director
Caitlin Deptula, Registrar
For children who have sensory integration disorder or children who are on the autism spectrum. Children have the opportunity to take part in a unique camp experience which is vital in their growth and development. Recreation based programs include sports, arts and crafts, swimming, and games.

1060 Camp I Am Me
Illinois Fire Safety Alliance
P.O. Box 911
Mount Prospect, IL 60056
847-390-0911
800-634-0911
FAX: 847-390-0920
e-mail: ifsa@ifsa.org
www.ifsa.org

1061 Camp Little Giant
SIU:Carbondale Therapeutic Recreation Prgm
Southern Illinois University
Mail Code 6888
Carbondale, IL 62901
618-453-1121
FAX: 618-453-1188
e-mail: tonec@siu.edu
www.ton.siu.edu

Mary Anne Cunningham, Manager
Camp Little Giant is a summer program but the Therapeutic Program runs all year round. One and two week sessions for campers with a variety of disabilities. Coed, ages 8-80.

1062 Camp New Hope
P.O.Box 764
Mattoon, IL 61938-764
217-895-2341
FAX: 217-895-3658
e-mail: cnhinc@rr1.net
www.myfavoritecamp.org

Kim Carmack, Executive Director
Terri Taylor, Camp Director
Weekend Respite, advocacy services, social and recreational services and a summer camp for the disabled. The camp accommodates people of widely diverse needs and abilities including access for wheelchair users. Co-ed, for those 8 years and older, including adults. Facilities include a mini golf area; pontoon boat; fishing deck; playground; trails; swimmming pool; and sleeping cabins with air conditioning.

1063 Camp Quality Illinois
1444 Mockingbird Circle
Stow, OH 44224
330-671-0167
FAX: 866-285-5208
www.campqualityusa.com

Lois Hartje, President
Vicki Irey, VP
Dennis Hart, Secretary
Caleb Shannon, Treasurer
Camp Quality is for children with cancer and their siblings. The camp offers a stress-free environment that offers exciting activities and fosters new friendships, while helping to give the children courage, motivation and emotional strength.

1064 Camp Roehr
Epilepsy Foundation Greater Southern Illinois
8301 Professional Place
Landover, MD 20785-2353
301-459-3700
800-332-1000
FAX: 301-459-1569
e-mail: ContactUs@efa.org
www.epilepsyfoundation.org

Warren Lammert, Chair
Phil Gattone, President and CEO
May J. Liang, Secretary
Roger Heldman, Treasurer

A seven day residential camp for children diagnosed with epilepsy. The camp is held at the Pere Marquette State Park where children enjoy swimming, horseback riding, arts and crafts, nightly entertainment and the camaraderie of other children with epilepsy.

1065 JCYS Camp Red Leaf
Jewish Council for Youth Services
180 W Washington St.,
Suite 1100
Chicago, IL 60602
312-726-8891
FAX: 312-726-7920
www.jcys.org

Jeffery Friedman, President
Dan Brenner, VP of Programming
Liz Roberts, VP of Operations
Aaron Turner, VP of Development

Our special needs camp, serves adults and children with developmental disabilities in 8- one week sessions during the summer, several travel adventures for adults and ten respite weekends during the year for children and young adults.

1066 Rimland Services for Autistic Citizens
1265 Hartrey Ave
Evanston, IL 60202
847-328-4090
FAX: 847-328-8364
TTY:847-328-4090
rimland.org/

Lorraine Ganz, President
Bernice Gryczan, VP
Barbara Cooper, Secretary
Wiliam Egan, Board Member

An accessible camp facility that can be utilized by groups for day use or overnight camping experiences. Six winterized cabins, a meeting facility, indoor pool, full food service, and an excellent staff are available. Educational programs can be arranged or you can utilize the facility to manage your own programs.

1067 Shady Oaks Camp
16300 Parker Rd
Homer Glen, IL 60491
708-301-0816
FAX: 708-301-5091
e-mail: soc16300@sbcglobal.net
www.shadyoakscamp.org

Harry Burroughs, Chairman
Robert Szajkovics, President
Lori McAleavy, Vice President
Scott Steele, Executive Director

Shady Oaks Camp provides outdoor fun and recreation for children and adults with cerebral palsy and similar disabilities. Our camp is organized with the goal of providing stimulating life experiences that our campers may not have the opportunity to engage in elsewhere.

1068 Summer Wheelchair Sport Camps
University of Illinois
1207 S Oak St
Champaign, IL 61820-6901
217-333-4607
FAX: 212-333-0248
e-mail: sportscamp@illinois.edu
www.illinoiswheelchairathletics.com

Maureen Gilbert, Camp Director

Rigorous camps designed for individuals with lower extremity physical disabilities. Camp attendees will spend an average of 8-9 hours a day, focusing on development and refinement of fitness, techniques and strategies. Strength training, nutrition and mental training sessions will also be included in all camps. The camp staff is comprised of athletic staff and local wheelchair athletes with coaching experience from the University of Illinois Wheelchair Athletics Program.

1069 Timber Pointe Outdoor Center
Easter Seals UCP
507 East Armstrong Avenue
Peoria, IL 61603-3197
309-686-1177
FAX: 309-686-7722
www.ci.easterseals.com

Richard W. Davidson, Chair
Sandra L. Bouwman, 1st Vice President
Joseph G. Kern, 2nd Vice President
Ralph F. Boyd, Jr., Treasurer

One and two-week sessions for campers with a wide variety of disabilities. Coed, ages 6-99. Campers experience different activities each day such as arts and crafts, music, horses, field sports, outdoor nature, swimming, canoeing and fishing. Every night there is a different activity: skit night, casino night, boat night (campers go out on the lake on pontoon boats), night swim, camp fires, and of course, everyone's favorite - a dance on the last night.

1070 Triangle D Camp
American Diabetes Association
8216 Princeton-Glendale Rd.
PMB200
West Chester, OH 45069-1675
907-272-1424
800-342-2383
FAX: 907-272-1428
e-mail: JRoss@diabetes.org
www.childrenwithdiabetes.com

1071 YMCA Camp Duncan
32405 N Highway 12
Ingleside, IL 60041
847-546-8086
FAX: 847-546-3550
www.ymcacampduncan.org

Art Catrambone, Chair
Kim Kiser, Executive Director
Rona Roffey, Camp Director
Danielle Kiessel, Day Camp Director

The Tourette Syndrome/TS Camp USA, founded in 1994, is a residential camping program designed for girls and boys ages 8 - 16+ whose primary diagnosis is TS, and to a lesser degree, OCD and ADD/ADHD. The TS Camp is held at YMCA Camp Duncan which is located 30 miles north of Chicago. The goal of the camp is to allow children with TS an opportunity to meet other children, share similar experiences and coping mechanisms in a fun, safe and positive environment.

Indiana

1072 Autism Day Camp
Hillcroft Services: Isanogel
114 East Streeter Avenue
Muncie, IN 47304
765-284-4166
e-mail: bwilliamson@hillcroft.org
www.hillcroft.org

Ted Baker, Chair
Brenda Llyod, Vice Chair
Bruce Baldwin, Director
Julie Bering, Secretary/ Treasurer

The camp is designed to improve the academic, social skills, and behaviors of children with autism spectrum disorders. The day camp is an 8-week intensive experience for children classified with autism spectrum disorders.

1073 Bradford Woods: Camp Riley
Indiana University
5040 State Road 67 N
Martinsville, IN 46151 765-342-2915
FAX: 765-349-1086
e-mail: bradwood@indiana.edu
www.bradwoods.org

Shay Dawson, CTRS, Director
Melanie Wills, Director of Outdoor Education
Tim Street, Associate Director
Sheryl McGlory, Retreats Coordinator

One and two-week sessions for children with a variety of disabilities. Coed, ages 8-18.

1074 Brave Heart's Camp
The People's Burn Foundation
6337 Hollister Drive
Suite 2H
Indianapolis, IN 46224 317-803-2876
FAX: 317-692-0876
www.peoplesburnfoundation.org

Daryl Mickens, President
Matt Godbout, VP
Cindy Allison, Camp Director
Lora Hays, Adult, Child & Family Counselor

Specialized residential summer camp for burn survivor children. The camp gives the children an opportunity to heal from the physical and emotional scars by giving them the opportunity to just be kids.

1075 CHAMP Camp
1116 East Market St
Indianapolis, IN 46202 317-679-1860
FAX: 317-245-2291
e-mail: admin@champcamp.org
www.champcamp.org

Scott Beaty, President
Rick Adams, VP
Karen Mellen, Secretary
Scott Black, Treasurer

1076 Camp About Face
The Head's Up Foundation
P.O. Box 167
Medora, IN 47260 812-966-2761
FAX: 812-966-2927
e-mail: headsupfoundation2012@gmail.com
http://www.headsupfoundation.org

1077 Camp Alexander Mack
Indiana Deaf Camps Foundation
P.O.Box 158
Milford, IN 46542 574-658-4831
www.campmack.org

Galen Jay, Interim Executive Director
Lauren Carrick, Director of Development/Facility Manager
Amber Barrett, Food Service
Norma Miller, Ordained Minister

Our program is intentionally designed to provide campers with life changing experiences that lead to a formation of personal faith within a safe faith community.

1078 Camp Brave Eagle
Indiana Hemophilia And Thrombosis Center
8402 Harcourt Road
Suite 500
Indianapolis, IN 46260 219-834-2331
800-241-2873
www.campbraveeagle.org/

Briana Vieke, Program Director
Jennifer Maahs, Pediatric Nurse Practitioner

Summer camp for children with bleeding disorders and their siblings. Campers participate in a traditional summer camp experience with swimming, canoeing, fishing, and nature education. The goal is to encourage the children to have fun while learning to be self-sufficient, building their self confidence and self-esteem and promoting a positive outlook.

1079 Camp Challenge
8914 Us Highway 50 East
Bedford, IN 47421 812-834-5159
e-mail: info@gocampchallenge.com
www.gocampchallenge.com

Ralph Price, Executive Director
Camp Registr

One and two-week sessions for campers with developmental and or physical disabilities, hearing impairment and the blind/visually impaired. Ages 6-99 and families.

1080 Camp Crosley YMCA
165 Ems T2 Ln
North Webster, IN 46555-9378 574-834-2331
877-811-6189
FAX: 574-834-3313
e-mail: info@campcrosley.org
campcrosley.org/

Richard Armstrong, Executive Director
Mark Battig, Associate Executive Director
Naomi Thompson, Program Director
Pam Endicott, Office Manager/Registrar

Camp is located in North Webster, Indiana. Half-week, one, two and three-week sessions for campers with asthma/respiratory ailments and diabetes. Coed, ages 7-17. Also families and seniors.

1081 Camp John Warvel
American Diabetes Association
1701 N. Beauregard St.
Alexandria, VA 22311 312-346-1805
888-342-2383
800-DIA-ETES
FAX: 317-594-0748
www.diabetes.org

Dwight Holing, Chair
Larry Hausner, CEO
Debbie Johnson, CFO
Greg Elfers, Chief Field Development Officer

Camp is located in North Webster, Indiana. Provides an enjoyable, safe and educational out-of-doors experience for children with insulin-dependent diabetes. A unique learning atmosphere for children to acquire new skills in caring for their disease. The camp experience instills confidence for the child's self-management of diabetes. Offers one-week sessions and can accommodate 200 campers, boys and girls aged 7-16.

1082 Camp Little Red Door
Little Red Door Cancer Agency
1801 North Merideian Street
Indianapolis, IN 46202-1411 317-925-5595
FAX: 317-925-5597
www.littlereddoor.org

Jeff Henry, Chair
Erika Rager, Vice Chair
Tanya Shelburne, VP of Program
Zina Kumok, Media & Communications

Camp for pediatric cancer patients ages 8-19. The program is open to children diagnosed with or receiving treatment for cancer in the state of Indiana. Activities include swimming, fishing, canoeing, nature hikes, astronomy, arts and crafts.

1083 Camp Millhouse
25600 Kelly Rd
South Bend, IN 46614 574-233-2202
FAX: 574-233-2511
e-mail: campmillhouse@gmail.com
www.campmillhouse.org

Diana Breden, Executive Director
Scarlett Russell, Camp Director

Nestled in a rustic clearing surrounded by 45 acres of woods, Camp Millhouse is a retreat for children and young adults with mental and physical disabilities. Hiking trails, nature studies, crafts, swimming, and stories around the bonfire make up activities campers long remember. One-week session. Co-ed, ages 4 to 30.

1084 Camp Red Cedar
3900 Hursh Road
Fort Wayne, IN 46845 260-637-3608
FAX: 260-637-5483
e-mail: redcedar@awsusa.com
http://www.awsredcedar.com

Carrie Perry, Director
Shelly Detcher, HR Recruiter/Program Manager
Theresa Prentice, Barn Manager
Mallory Leatherman, Riding Instructor
Camp Red Cedar is open for children and adults with or without disabilities. Activities include, fishing, hiking, swimming and arts and crafts.

1085 Camp Riley
Camp Riley/Riley's Children Foundation
Attn: Camp Coordinator
30 S. Meridian Street, Suite 200
Indianapolis, IN 46204-3509 317-634-4474
877-867-4539
FAX: 317-634-4478
e-mail: campriley@rileykids.org
www.rileykids.org/camp

James T Morris, Chairman
Kristin G Fruehwald, Treasurer
Rebecca Kubacki, Secretary
Camp Riley is for youth's ages 8-18 with physical disabilities. The camp helps them to realize their potential as they become increasingly independent. Some of the activities that the camp offers is horseback riding and swimming.

1086 Englishton Park Academic Remediation
Englishton Park Presbyterian
P.O.Box 228
Lexington, IN 47138 812-889-2046
FAX: 812-934-4322
e-mail: ThomasLisaBarnett@etczone.com
www.englishtonpark.org

Lisa Barnett, Co-Directors
Thomas Barnett, Co-Director
Camp is located in Lexington, Indiana. Two-week sessions for children with ADD. Boys and girls, ages 7-12.

1087 Happiness Bag
3833 Union Rd
Terre Haute, IN 47802 812-234-8867
FAX: 812-238-0728
e-mail: jmexdir@aol.com
www.happinessbag.org/

Trudy Rupska, President
Cari Rohrmayer, VP
Jodi Moan, Executive Director
Caren Elrod, Program Director
Serves developmentally disabled age 5-adult; day and residential camp program; after school program; scouting; Special Olympic anticipation (basketball, athletics, bowling, softball and aquatics); and a bowling league.

1088 Hoosier Burn Camp
P.O. BOX 233
Battle Ground, IN 47920 765-567-0115
800-254-2878
FAX: 765-567-0195
e-mail: markkoopman@hoosierburncamp.org
www.hoosierburncamp.org

Mark Koopman, Director
Mark Koopman, Executive Director
Abby James, Program Manager
Kim Jones, Administrative Assistant
Held at Camp Tecumseh in Brookston, IN., the camp is for burn survivors ages 8-18. Campers learn how to have fun and just be kids, while building their self-esteem and self confidence, learning independence and the life skills they need to fully recover from burn injuries.

1089 Indiana Children's Deaf Camp
The Indiana Deaf Camps Foundation, Inc.
100 West 86th Street
Indianapolis, IN 46260 317-846-3404
FAX: 317-844-1034
e-mail: deafcamp@hotmail.com
www.deafcamps.org

1090 Residential Camp
Hillcroft Services: Isanogel
114 East Streeter Avenue
Muncie, IN 47303 765-284-4166
TTY:765-288-1073
e-mail: bwilliamson@hillcroft.org
www.hillcroft.org

Ted Baker, Board Chair
Brenda Lloyd, Vice Chair
Julie Bering, Secretary/Treasurer
Debbie Bennett, Chief Executive Officer
Programming at Isanogel includes creative arts, nature, recreation and aquatics. Individuals age 8 and older participate in one and two week programs.

1091 Twin Lakes Camp
1451 E Twin Lakes Rd
Hillsboro, IN 47949-8004 765-798-4000
FAX: 765-798-4010
e-mail: outdoors@twinlakescamp.com
www.twinlakescamp.com

Jon Beight, Executive Director
Dan Daily, Program Director
Natalie Eberhard, Outdoor Education Coordinator
Donna Beight, Secretary
Provides a summer camp program for special needs children and young adults. Campers suffer from a wide range of maladies including crippling accidents, Spina Bifida, epilepsy, Cerebral Palsy, Muscular Dystrophy, Quadriplegia, Paraplegia, and other disabling diseases. Campers range in age from 8 to 27.

Iowa

1092 Camp Albrecht Acres
14837 Sherrill Rd
Sherrill, IA 52073 563-552-1771
FAX: 563-552-2732
e-mail: info@albrechtacres.org
www.albrechtacres.org

Heidi Zwack Goin, President
Terry Mozena, Vice President
Paul Gorrell, Treasurer
Joe Vermeulen, Secretary
For children and adults with special needs. Campers enjoy swimming, fishing, nature studies, cookouts and dances.

1093 Camp Courageous of Iowa
P.O.Box 418
12007 190 th Street
Monticello, IA 52310- 0418 319-465-5916
FAX: 319-465-5919
e-mail: info@campcourageous.org
www.campcourageous.org

Jeanne Muellerleile, Camp Director
Charlie Becker, Executive Director
Shannon Poe, Respite Care/Volunteers Director
A year round residential and respite care facility for individuals with special needs and their families. Campers range in age from 1-99 years old. Activities include traditional activities like canoeing, hiking, swimming, nature and crafts plus adventure activities like caving, rock climbing, etc. Campers with disabilities have opportunities to succeed at challenging activities. This feeling of self-worth can transfer to home, work or school environments.

1094 **Camp Hertko Hollow**
101 Locust St
Des Moines, IA 50309-1720 515-897-9009
855-502-8500
FAX: 515-288-2531
e-mail: v.murray@camphertkohollow.com
www.camphertkohollow.com

Ann Wolf, Executive Director
Vivian Murray, Camp Director Emeritus
Deb Holwegner, Camp Director

Camp Hertko Hollow is a resident camp held at the Des Moines YMCA Camp site, located along the Des Moines River north of Boone, Iowa. Activities include horseback riding, swimming, canoeing, rappelling, crafts, ropes course, archery and riflery to name a few, plus special activities for different ages. Half-week and one-week sessions for children with diabetes. Coed, ages 6-16.

1095 **Camp L-Kee-Ta**
1308 Broadway Street
P.O. Box 190
West Burlington, IA 52655-190 319-752-3639
FAX: 319-753-1410
girlscoutstoday.org

Allison Johnson, Vice President of Performance Excellence/Regional Director
Angela Ventris, Assistant Director of Leadership Experiences
Brenda Lloyd, Vice President of Membership
Cheryl Noller, Vice President of Leadership Initiatives

Camp is located in Danville, Iowa. Half-week and one-week sessions June-August for children with asthma/respiratory ailments. Girls, ages 7-18 and families.

1096 **Camp Quality Heartland**
1444 Mockingbird Circle
Stow, OH 44224 330-671-0167
FAX: 866-285-5208
e-mail: patty@campqualityusa.org
www.campqualityusa.com

Lois Hartje, President
Vicki Irey, Vice-President
Dennis Hart, Secretary
Caleb Shannon, Treasurer

Camp Quality is for children with cancer and their siblings. The camp offers a stress-free environment that offers exciting activities and fosters new friendships, while helping to give the children courage, motivation and emotional strength.

1097 **Camp Sunnyside**
Easter Seals Of Iowa
401 N.E. 66th Avenue
Des Moines, IA 50313 515-289-1933
e-mail: krumpf@easterseals.org
www.easterseals.org

Claire LeCroy, Director, Camping & Respite Svcs
Kelsey Rumpf, Program Assistant

The camp is open year-round and is a place for children and adults with or without disabilities to gather and enjoy themselves while exploring their potentials. Activities include swimming, boating arts and crafts and games.

1098 **Camp Tanager**
Tanager Place
1614 W Mount Vernon Rd
Mount Vernon, IA 52314-9533 319-363-0681
FAX: 319-365-6411
e-mail: dpirrie@tanagerplace.org
www.camptanager.org

Donald Pirrie, Executive Director

Offers camp experiences for children 7 to 11 whose special social, economic or medical needs might not otherwise allow them to enjoy a summer camp experience. This private, non-profit camp serves over 600 children each summer with the staff-camper ratio being 1:6.

1099 **Camp Wyoming**
Presbyterian Church USA
9106 42nd Ave
Wyoming, IA 52362-7647 563-488-3893
FAX: 563-488-3895
e-mail: office@campwyoming.net
www.campwyoming.net

Kevin Cullum, Executive Director
Rev. Troy Winder, Board President
Matt LeClere, Board Vice President
Amy Saskowski, Board Secretary

Youth and adults, ages 16 and up, with mild to moderate mental and physical disabilities can take part in a one week experience of fun and fellowship in early July.

1100 **Diabetes Camp**
Tanager Place
1614 W Mount Vernon Rd
Mount Vernon, IA 52314-9533 319-363-0681
FAX: 319-365-6411
e-mail: dpirrie@tanagerplace.org
www.camptanager.org

Donald Pirrie, Executive Director

Provides children and adolescents with Diabetes a safe and healthy environment and healthy environment to enjoy a variety of recreational activities designed for fun and fitness. The camp held each July has an on-site 24-hour physician and nursing staff. Ages 6-13.

1101 **Easter Seals Camp Sunnyside**
Easter Seals Iowa
401 N.E. 66th Avenue
Des Moines, IA 50313 515-309-2375
FAX: 515-289-1281
TTY:515-289-4069
e-mail: krumpf@eastersealsia.org
www.easterseals.com

Richard W. Davidson, Chairman
Kelsey Rumpf, Program Assistant
Sandra L. Bouwman, 1st Vice Chairman
Joseph G. Kern, 2nd Vice Chairman

Each summer from June through August, campers with disabilities ages five and up, take part in one week camping sessions, gaining skills and independence by participating in activities like swimming, horseback riding, canoeing, fishing, camping and more. Coed, ages 4-95. Accepts seniors and single adults. Financial assistance available.

1102 **Wendell Johnson Speech And Hearing Clinic**
University Of Iowa
250 Hawkins Dr
Iowa City, IA 52242-1025 319-335-8736
FAX: 319-335-8851
e-mail: kathy-miller@uiowa.edu
www.uiowa.edu/~comsci/

Linda Souke, Clinic Director
Kathy Miller, Clinic Assistant

The clinic offers assessment and remediation for communication disorders in adults and children. The clinic also offers services during the Summer for school age children needing intervention services because of speech, language, hearing and/or reading problems.

1103 **Wesley Woods Camp and Retreat Center**
Iowa Conference United Methodist
10896 Nixon St
Indianola, IA 50125-7301 515-961-4523
866-684-7753
FAX: 515-961-4162
e-mail: wesleywoods.camp@iaumc.org
www.wesleywoodsiowa.org

Deke Rider, Executive Director
Suzanne Rider, Equestrian Coordinator

Camp is located in Indianola, Iowa. Half-week and one-week sessions June-August for campers with developmental disabilities. Coed, ages 18-99. Horses Helping People program is also available for developmentally and physically challenged persons age 4 and older.

1104 **Y Camp**
YMCA of Greater Des Moines
1192 166th Drive
Boone, IA 50036-1720
515-432-7558
FAX: 515-432-5414
e-mail: ycamp@dmymca.org
www.y-camp.org

Mike Havlik, Program Director- Environmental Education
David Sherry, Executive Director
Alex Kretzinger, Program Director- Summer Camp
Madi Short, Program Director- Retreats and Conferences
Camp is located in Boone, Iowa. Year-round one and two-week sessions for boys and girls with cancer, diabetes, asthma, cystic fibrosis, hearing impaired and other disabilities. Coed, ages 6-16 and families.

Kansas

1105 **Camp Discovery**
American Diabetes Association
837 S Hillside St
Wichita, KS 67211-3005
316-684-6091
800-362-1355
888-342-2838
FAX: 316-684-5675
e-mail: lthomas@diabetes.org
www.diabetescamps.org

Bill Dyar, Manager
Bridget Kroner, Associate Director
Camp is located in Junction City, Kansas. Offers young people with diabetes a week of fun at rock springs 4-H Center. Special attention to diabetes makes Camp Discovery a safe environment for active youth while providing valuable diabetes management education. Call the American Diabetes Association Kansas area office for more information. Coed, ages 8-17.

1106 **Camp Ka-Di-Da-Ca**
American Diabetes Association
608 West Douglas, Suite 100
Wichita, KS 67211
316-684-6091
FAX: 316-684-5675
http://www.diabetes.org

RaeAnn Moreno, Contact Person
Day camp for young adults ages 9-12 with diabetes.

1107 **Camp Quality Kansas**
2617 N. 75th Street
Kansas City, KS 66109
913-424-8355
FAX: 913-334-2802
e-mail: Susie.Mooney@CampQualityUSA.org
www.campqualityusa.com

Susie Mooney, Executive Director
Michelle Fields, Assistant Director
Jeff Coykendall, Personnel Chair
Sara Jolliff, Secretary
Camp Quality is for children with cancer and their siblings. The camp offers a stress-free environment that offers exciting activities and fosters new friendships, while helping to give the children courage, motivation and emotional strength.

1108 **Summer Camp for Physically & Mentally Challenged Children & Adults**
Kansas Jaycees' Cerebral Palsy Foundation
P.O.Box 267
Augusta, KS 67207-267
316-775-2421
e-mail: execdirector@cpranch.org
http://cpranch.cfsites.org

Cheryl Schmeidler, Executive Director
Sarah Walker, Camp Directo
Our mission is to provide a program which will allow individuals to enjoy their highest level of functioning and independence, consistent with their abilities, in a summer camp setting.

Kentucky

1109 **Anderson Woods**
4630 Adyeville Rd
Bristow, IN 47515
812-639-1079
e-mail: andersonwoodspsci.net
www.andersonwoods.org

Judy Colby, Administrative Office
Provides camping experience and residential services to persons with mental and/or physical disabilities. Campers learn self confidence, trust and responsibilities through working together, tending gardens, feeding animals all while enjoying natures beauty.

1110 **Bethel Mennonite Camp**
2773 Bethel Church Rd
Clayhole, KY 41317-9028
606-666-4911
FAX: 606-666-4216
e-mail: grow@bethelcamp.org
www.bethelcamp.org

Mark Driskill, Summer Camp Pastor
Roger Voth, Camp Director
Mary Driskill, Summer Camp Pastor
A Christ-centered ministry with an emphasis on Bible study and personal commitment to Christ. We offer a week long Special Needs Camp in June, with lodging for caregivers.

1111 **Camp Quality Kentuckiana**
P.O. Box 35474
Louisville, KY 40232
502-507-3235
e-mail: charlie.obranowicz@campqualityusa.org
www.campqualityusa.com

Charlie Obranowicz, Executive Director
Paul Eddie Bobbitt, Development Director
Amanda McClung, Secretary
Linda Wickliffe, Treasurer
Camp Quality is for children with cancer and their siblings. The camp offers a stress-free environment that offers exciting activities and fosters new friendships, while helping to give the children courage, motivation and emotional strength.

1112 **Cedar Ridge Camp**
4010 Old Routt Road
Louisville, KY 40299
502-267-5848
FAX: 502-297-0116
e-mail: info@cedarridgecamp.com
www.cedarridgecamp.com

Peter Ruys de Perez, Owner & Executive Director
Grayson Burke, Director
Jodie Campbell, Assistant Director
Alexandra Campbell, Director of Operations
Half-week, one and two-week sessions for children with diabetes, developmental disabilities and muscular dystrophy. Coed, ages 6-17.

1113 **Indian Summer Camp**
P.O. Box 24337
Louisville, KY 40224
502-365-1538
e-mail: Shelby.Dehner@gmail.com
www.iscamp.org

Shelby Dehner, Executive Director
Leah McComb, Program Director
Brandon Woehrle, Admin Assistant
Dr. Sherry Bayliff, Medical Director
Indian Summer Camp is open to boys and girls aged 6-18 years old who have had or are currently receiving treatment for cancer. Children can come to have fun, while having the opportunity to grow, learn and build self reliance.

1114 Lions Camp Crescendo, Inc.
1480 Pine Tavern Road
P.O. Box 607
Lebanon Junction, KY 40150-0607
502-833-3554
888-879-8884
FAX: 502-833-4249
e-mail: wibblesb@aol.com
www.lccky.org

Billie Flannery, Administrator
Kevin Patton, Resident Manager
Lion Paul Witten, Chairperson
Lion Cebert Gilbert, Vice-Chairperson

The enhancement of the quality of life for youth, especially those with disabilities, through the delivery of a traditional camp experience by caring individuals and to enable others to use our camping and retreat facilities to serve the larger communities humanitarian needs.

1115 Medical Camping
The Center For Courageouos Kids
1501 Burnley Road
Scottsville, KY 42164
270-618-2900
FAX: 270-618-2902
e-mail: info@courageouskids.org
www.courageouskids.org

Ed Collins, Camp Director
Roger Murtie, President and Executive Director
Joanie O'Bryan, Development Director
Stormi Murtie, Communications Director

A year-round, fun, safe camping experience for seriously ill and disabled children and their families.

1116 The Center For Courageous Kids
1501 Burnley Road
Scottsville, KY 42164
270-618-2900
FAX: 270-618-2902
e-mail: info@courageouskids.org
courageouskids.org

Roger Murtie, President/Executive Director
Emily Cosby, Program Director

The Center for Courageous Kids is a year round medical camp for children who have chronic or life threatening illnesses by creating experiences that are memorable, exciting, fun, build self-esteem, are physically safe and medically sound. Family retreats serve children 3-17 and summer camps serve children 7-15. No child or family will pay to attend camp.

Louisiana

1117 Camp Bon Coeur
Bon Coeur, Inc.
405 W. Main St.
Lafayette, LA 70501
337-233-8437
FAX: 337-233-4160
e-mail: info@heartcamp.com
www.heartcamp.com

Susannah Craig, Executive Director

Two-week sessions June-July for children with heart defects. Coed, ages 8-16.

1118 Camp Challenge
P.O.Box 10591
New Orleans, LA 70181
504-347-2267
e-mail: campdirector@campchallenge.org
www.campchallenge.org

Cathy Allain, Camp Director
Alaina Wertz, Public Relations

Camp Challenge is a grass roots non-profit organization dedicated to giving ill children and their siblings ages 6 through 18 a summer camp experience. Camp is open to all children who reside in Louisiana and have a form of cancer and chronic hematological disorders. These children do not have to pay for camp, it is free for all campers.

1119 Camp Pelican
Louisiana Lions Camp
P.O.Box 10235
New Orleans, LA 70181
504-466-7124
FAX: 866-295-3803
e-mail: tbone333@aol.com
www.lionscamp.org

Cathy Allain, Assistant Camp Director
Reverend R. Tony Ricard, Camp Director

Camp Pelican is an overnight residential camp for children with moderate to severe asthma or other pulmonary problems. Founded in 1977, Camp Pelican is jointly sponsored by the Louisiana Pulmonary Disease Camp Inc and the Louisiana Lions Camp. Over 100 children attend annually and participate in education, sports, arts and crafts, swimming and other camping activities. Medical staff including physicians, nurses, respiratory therapists and social workers participate in camp. Coed, ages 5-17.

1120 Camp Quality Louisiana
638 Ervin Cotton Rd
Eros, LA 71238
318-329-7993
e-mail: Michael.Brown@CampQualityUSA.org
www.campqualityusa.com

Carolyn Eads, Camp Director

Camp Quality is for children with cancer and their siblings. The camp offers a stress-free environment that offers exciting activities and fosters new friendships, while helping to give the children courage, motivation and emotional strength.

1121 Camp Victory
Lions Club And American Diabetes Association
2644 S. Sherwood Forest Blvd.
Suite 122
Baton Rouge, LA 70816
www.lionscamp.org

Lori Koonce, Manager
Treva Lincoln, Contact Person

Camp is for children with diabetes age 6-14 years old. The camp offers many outdoor activities as well as daily diabetes education classes.

1122 Louisiana Lions Camp
LA Lions League for Crippled Children
292 L. Beauford Drive
Anacoco, LA 71403
800-348-6567
FAX: 337-239-9975
e-mail: lalions@lionscamp.org
www.lionscamp.org

Raymond E Cecil III, Camp Director
Susan Todd, President

Free camp for boys and girls with mental and physical challenges, diabetes and pulmonary disorders.

1123 Louisiana Lions Camp - Camp Pelican
Lions Club Of Louisiana
292 L. Beauford Drive
Anacoco, LA 71403
800-348-6567
FAX: 337-239-9975
www.lionscamp.org

Jerry Adams, President

Free, residential summer camp for children with special needs, diabetes and pulmonary disorders.

1124 Med-Camps of Louisiana
102 Thomas Road
Suite 615
West Monroe, LA 71291
318-329-8405
e-mail: info@medcamps.com
www.medcamps.com

Caleb Seney, Executive Director
Erin Harper, Nursing Director
Bethany Gerfers, Administrative Assistant
Kacie Hobson, Events & Volunteer Coordinator

Serves children with severe asthma and allergies and many more.

Maine

1125 **Camp Waban**
Waban Projects, Inc.
5 Dunaway Drive
Sanford, ME 04073
207-324-7955
FAX: 207-324-6050
www.waban.org

Kathy Lane, President
Isabel Schmedemann, Vice President
Neal Meltzer, Executive Director
Cynthia Caron-Wilcox, Director of Day Services
Recreational opportunities in fully handicapped accessible waterfront facilities for children and adults with developmental disabilities. Activities include swimming, kayaking, pontoon boat rides, fishing and nightly camp fires.

1126 **Camp Bishopswood**
Diocese of Maine Episcopal
143 State St
Portland, ME 4101-3701
207-772-1953
800-244-6062
e-mail: mike@bishopswood.org
www.bishopswood.org

Georgia Koch, Director
Sara Foster, Assistant Director
Lisa Sholudko, Health Care Manager
Camp is located in Hope, Maine. One to seven-week sessions for hearing impaired children June-August. Coed, ages 7-16.

1127 **Camp Bloomfield**
Foundation For The Junior Blind
35375 Mulholland Highway
Malibu, CA 90265
310-457-5330
juniorblind.org

Shirley Manning, Director Of Recreation
Joan Marason, Director Of Wellness And Enrichment Programs
Junior Blind's Camp Bloomfield provides children and youth who are blind, visually impaired, or multi-disabled with a natural and safe environment to develop self-esteem, build independence and fully experience the joys of the great outdoors.

1128 **Camp Capella**
8 Pearl Point Road
Delham, ME 04429
207-843-5104
e-mail: dana@campcabella.org
www.campcapella.org

Dana Mosher, Religious Leader
Provides an opportunity for children with disabilities to engage in various recreational and social experiences.

1129 **Camp Lawroweld**
Northern New England Conference
228 West Side Road
Weld, ME 04285
207-585-2984
FAX: 207-585-2985
www.lawroweld.org

Harry Sabnani, Executive Director
Camp is located in Weld, Maine. Week sessions July for campers who are blind or visually impaired, all ages. Other camps coed, ages 9-16 and families, single adults, June - September.

1130 **Camp No Limits**
No Limits Limb Loss Foundation
265 Centre Road
Wales, ME 04280
207-240-5762
e-mail: campnolimits@yahoo.com
www.nolimitsfoundation.org

Mary Leighton, Founder/ Occupational Therapist
Kim Furlong, Physical Therapist
Loi Ho, Adult Amputee Volunteer/Prosthetist
Missy Moreau, Volunteer Coordinator/Office Administration
Camp No Limits is the leading camp for young people with limb loss and their families. The camp also has several other locations in California, Florida, Idaho, Maryland and Missouri.

1131 **Camp Pinecone**
Pine Tree Society
149 Front Street
P.O. Box 518
Bath, ME 04530-518
207-443-3341
FAX: 207-443-1070
TTY:207-443-3341
e-mail: info@pinetreesociety.org
www.pinetreesociety.org

Noel Sullivan, President & CEO
Teresa Berkowitz, Chief Operating Officer
RJ Gagnon, Finance Director
Denise Norko, Human Resources Director
A day camp for children with physical and/or developmental disabilities, ages 5 to 12. May through September.

1132 **Camp Sunshine**
35 Acadia Road
Casco, ME 04015
207-655-3800
FAX: 207-655-3825
e-mail: info@campsunshine.org
www.campsunshine.org

Gary Barron, Executive Director
Michael Katz, Campus Director
Michael Smith, Director of Special Events
Robert Butcher, Business Manager
This year round program provides respite, support, hope & joy to children with life threatening illnesses and their immediate families. The camp is open to families of children diagnosed with kidney disease, cancer, lupus, solid organ transplants and other life threatening illnesses. The camp is free of charge and includes onsite medical and psychosocial support, and bereavement groups.

1133 **Camp Waziyatah**
530 Mill Hill Rd
Waterford, ME 04088
207-583-2267
FAX: 509-357-2267
e-mail: info@wazi.com
www.wazi.com

Gregg Parker, Owner/Director
Mitch Parker, Owner/Director
Tim Ballard, Managing Director
Carl Acosta, New Family Liaison/Pines Division Director
Camp is located in Waterford, Massachusetts. Three, four and seven-week sessions June-August for campers with cancer and diabetes. Coed, ages 8-15 and families, single adults.

1134 **Camp Winnebago**
19708 Camp Winnebago Road
Caledonia, MN 55921
507-724-2351
FAX: 507-724-3786
e-mail: andy@campwinnebago.com
www.campwinnebago.org

Tommy Means, Co-Director, Program Director
Heather Johnson, RN, Co-Director, Health Center Director
Elise Hynek, Volunteer Coordinator
Michele Thompson, Office Assistant
A non profit organization specializing in the recreational needs of adults and children with developmental disabilities.

1135 **Indian Acres Camp for Boys**
1712 Main St
Fryeburg, ME 04037-4327
207-935-2300
e-mail: geoff@indianacres.com
www.indianacres.com

Michael Burness, Assistant Director
Lisa Newman, Director
Geoff Newman, Director
Mary Beth Wiig, Head Counselor, Camp Forest Acres
Camp is located in Fryeburg, Florida. Four and seven-week sessions June-August for boys with ADD ages 7-16.

1136 **Pine Tree Camp**
Pine Tree Society
149 Front Street
P.O. Box 518
Bath, ME 04530
207-443-3341
FAX: 207-397-5324
e-mail: ptcamp@pinetreesociety.org
www.pinetreesociety.org

Gerard Queally, Chair
Noel Sullivan, President & CEO
Teresa Berkowitz, Chief Operating Officer
Cheryl Timberlake, Secretary

Offers Maine children and adults with disabilities an extraordinary summer camp experience. The barrier-free setting and commitment of our staff allow campers to fully participate in activities that normally aren't available to them including swimming, fishing, boating, outdoor games, kayaking, arts and crafts and even camping in a tent under the stars. May through September.

1137 **YMCA Camp of Maine**
305 Winthrop Center Rd
P.O. Box 446
Winthrop, ME 04364
207-395-4200
FAX: 207-395-7230
e-mail: info@maineycamp.org
www.maineycamp.org

Barry W Costa, Executive Director

Activities include arts and crafts, nature study, hiking, and overnight camping, dancing, and singing. Summer session dates run from June through August; for ages 8-16.

Maryland

1138 **Camp Fairlee Manor**
Easter Seals Of Delaware
22242 Bay Shore Road
Chestertown, MD 21620
410-778-0566
FAX: 410-778-0567
e-mail: contact@esdel.org
www.de.easterseals.com

Amy Walls, Advisory Council Member

For children and adults with physical disabilities and/or cognitive impairments. Activities include arts and crafts, sports and games, nature walks, swimming, and fishing

1139 **Camp Glyndon**
American Diabetes Association
PO Box 56
Nanjemoy, MD 20662
301-870-5858
FAX: 301-246-9108
e-mail: info@LionsCampMerrick.org
www.lionscampmerrick.org

Wayne Magoon, President
Ray Shumaker, Vice President
Heidi A Fick, Executive Director
Donna Wadsworth, Camp Administrator

Camp is located in Nanjemoy, Maryland. One and two-week sessions July-August for children with diabetes and their families. Coed, ages 8-16.

1140 **Camp JCC**
Jewish Community Center of Greater Washington
6125 Montrose Rd
Rockville, MD 20852-4860
301-881-0100
FAX: 301-881-6549
e-mail: fgold@jccgw.org
www.jccgw.org

Bradley C. Stillman, President
Brian Pearlstein, Vice President for Administration/Treasurer
Heidi Hookman Brodsky, Vice President for Development
Mindy Berger, Vice President for Member & Guest Services

Camp JCC serves children with disabilities alongside their neighbors and friends. The American Camping Association has presented a National award to Camp JCC for its extraordinary model inclusion program. We also offer a program designed especially for 13-21 year olds with severe to profound disabilities. In order for us to afford to do these things, we count on contributions to our Inclusion Fund. Four and eight-week sessions general day camp program offering June-August for children.

1141 **Camp Milldale**
Jewish Community Center
3506 Gwynnbrook Avenue
Owings Mills, MD 21117
410-559-2390
FAX: 410- 58- 056
e-mail: info@campmilldale.org
www.campmilldale.org

Amy Bram, Camp Director
Stacy Deems, Camp Administrator
Amanda Max, Assistant Camp Director
Bill Kirkner, Aquatics Director

Camp is located in Reisterstown, MD. Four and eight week sessions, June - August. Inclusion program for children entering grades 5-13 with learning, developmental, social, emotional and physical disabilities. Self-contained program for teenagers with disabilities ages 14-21 focusing on recreational and vocational activities, including weekly field trips.

1142 **Camp Sunrise**
John Hopkins Hospital
750 East Pratt Street
Suite 1700
Baltimore, MD 21201
410-516-2385
e-mail: mscalf19@yahoo.com
www.hopkinsmedicine.org/kimmel_cancer_center/

Marilyn Scalf, Staffing Director
Jaclyn Young, Activities
Stephanie Davis, Donations
Jack Shipkoski, CEO

Camp Sunrise is open to children ages 6-18 who have or have had cancer. The camp also has a 'day camp' program for children ages 4-5 years old. Some of the camps activities include swimming, arts & crafts, nature walks, sports and games.

1143 **Camp Superkids**
John Hopkins Bayview Medical Center
P.O. Box 96
Maryland Line, MD 21105
410-550-0374
e-mail: campsuperkids@gmail.com
www.hopkinsbayview.org/campsuperkids

Ceal Curry, Camp Director
Heather Dougherty, Camp Administrator

Camp Superkids is an overnight camp for children between the ages of 8-14 with asthma.

1144 **Kamp A-Komp-Plish**
9035 Ironsides Rd
Nanjemoy, MD 20662-3432
301-870-3226
301-934-3590
FAX: 301-870-2620
e-mail: recreation@melwood.org
http://www.melwoodrecreation.org

Michael Glanz, Vice President, Community Services
Doria Fleisher, Associate Director, Recreation
Marisa Cucuzzella, Assistant Director, Operations & Enrollment
Hannah Rutt, Travel Coordinator

Camp is located in Nanjemoy, Maryland. Half-week, one-week and two-week sessions for blind/visually impaired children and those with developmental disabilities and mobility limitation. Coed, ages 8-16.

1145 **League at Camp Greentop**
The League for People with Disabilities
1111 E. Cold Spring Lane
Baltimore, MD 21239
410-323-0500
FAX: 410-323-3298
TTY:410-435-4298
e-mail: vfoster@leagueforpeople.org
www.leagueforpeople.org

Bill Morgan, VP, Camping & Therapeutic Recreat
David A. Greenberg, President & Chief Executive Officer
Margy Ryan, Vice President, Finance
Tom Schniedwind, Vice President, Marketing & Development

Camp is located in Thurmont, Maryland. Summer residential camp located in the Catoctin Mountain National Park. Since 1937, Greentop has been serving children and adults with physical and multiple disabilities in a completely accessible camp setting. Campers enjoy a traditional camping program. Medical facilities staffed 24 hours a day. Half-week/one/two-week sessions June-August. ACA/MD Youth Camp.

1146 **Lions Camp Merrick**
Lions Clubs of District 22-C
3650 Rick Hamilton Place
P.O. Box 56
Nanjemoy, MD 20662-56
301-870-5858
FAX: 301-246-9108
e-mail: info@LionsCampMerrick.org
www.lionscampmerrick.org

Wayne Magoon, President
Ray Shumaker, Vice President
Frank Culhan, Treasurer
Heidi A Fick, Executive Director

This recreational camp for special needs children offers a complete waterfront program including swimming, canoeing and fishing for ages 6-16. Designed for children who are deaf and hard of hearing, children of deaf parents, and children with diabetes. Also helps children to learn to deal with their special conditions.

1147 **Raven Rock Lutheran Camp**
17912 Harbaugh Valley Road
P.O.Box 136
Sabillasville, MD 21780-136
800-321-5824
e-mail: ravenrock@innernet.net

1148 **TLC's Summer Programs**
9975 Medical Center Drive
Rockville, MD 20850
301-738-9691
FAX: 301-738-8897
e-mail: enyang@ttlc.org
www.ttlc.org

Enda Elisabeth Nyang, Director, Camp Littlefoot Speech-Language Program
Brigid Baker, Director, Camp Littlefoot Occupational Therapy Programo
Sylvia Valdivia, Coordinator
Rhona Schwartz, Director

For children ages 3-13 and high school students in grades 9-12, who have special needs in the areas of speech, language, perceptual motor, sensory processing, academic development, and/or skill maintenance. Some programs also fulfill the requirements for Extended School Year Services (ESY). Extended Day is available for children 5 years or older in all programs (excluding the high school program). Extended day hours are 8:00 am to 9:00 am and 3:00 pm to 5:00 pm.

1149 **Youth Leadership Camp**
National Association of the Deaf
8630 Fenton Street
Suite 820
Silver Spring, MD 20910- 3819
301-587-1788
FAX: 301-587-1791
TTY:301-587-1789
e-mail: infor@nad.org
www.nad.org

Howard Rosenblum, Chief Executive Officer
Christopher Wagner, President
Melissa S. Draganac-Hawk, Vice-President
Joshua Beckman, Secretary

Sponsored by the National Association of the Deaf, this camp emphasizes leadership training for deaf teenagers and young adults. In addition to many recreational activities and sports, there are academic offerings and camp projects.

Massachusetts

1150 **Agassiz Village Camp**
Easter Seals: Massachusetts
484 Main St
Worcester, MA 01608
800-244-2756
FAX: 508-831-9768
TTY:800-564-9700
e-mail: info@eastersealsma.org
www.eastersealsma.org

Harry Salerno, Chairman
David Hoffman, Vice Chair
Anthony Tambone, Treasurer
Cheryl.E Mongell, Secretary

Operates a full inclusion residential summer camp that serves campers with disabilities (ages 8-13). Camp activities are facilitated with consideration to the needs of youth with disabilities.

1151 **Becket Chimney Corners YMCA Camps and Outdoor Center**
748 Hamilton Rd
Becket, MA 1223-9686
413-623-8991
FAX: 413-623-5890
e-mail: cburke@bccymca.org
www.bccymca.org

Phil Connor, CEO
Jim Brown, Chief Operations Officer
Christine Kalakay, Chief Financial Officer
Steve Turner, Director of Property & Maintenance

Half-week and one-week sessions for campers with asthma/respiratory ailments. Coed, ages 3 and up, families, seniors, single adults.

1152 **Camp Howe**
P.O.Box 326
Goshen, MA 01032
413-549-3969
e-mail: office@camphowe.com
www.camphowe.com

Heidi Gutekenst, Camp Director
Heather.B Baylis, President
Edlin Black, Vice President
Ramon Jon Black, Secretary/Treasurer

One and two-week sessions June-August for children with a variety of disabilities. Coed, ages 7-17.

1153 **Camp Jabberwocky**
200 Greenwood Avenue Ext.
P.O. Box 1357
Vineyard Haven, MA 02568
508-693-2339
e-mail: info@campjabberwocky.org
www.campjabberwocky.org

Kristin LB Oseychik, Chair
Jane Price, Vice Chair
Corby Reese, Treasurer
Melissa Mueller, Secretary

Residential vacation camp for people with disabilities.

1154 **Camp Joslin**
Barton Center for Diabetes Education
30 Ennis Road
PO Box 356
North Oxford, MA 01537-0356 508-987-2056
FAX: 508-987-2002
e-mail: info@bartoncenter.org
www.bartoncenter.org

Thomas.C Lynch, Chair
Mark W. Fuller, Treasurer
John Peri-Okonny, M.D., 1st Vice Chair
Fabrizio Aguirre, Camp Joslin Assistant Director

Camp is located in Charlton, Massachusetts. For boys, ages 7-16, with diabetes. This program offers active summer sports and activities, supplemented by medical treatment and diabetes education. Coed Winter Camp and Coed Weekend Retreats are offered during the school year.

1155 **Camp New Connections**
McLean Hospital
115 Mill Street
Belmont, MA 02478 617-855-2000
e-mail: kamadden@partners.org
www.mclean.harvard.edu/

Scott Rauch, MD, President and Psychiatrist in Ch

A four-week, summer day camp for children ages 7-17 who have Asperger's Syndrome, autism spectrum disorders, pervasive developmental disorders and non-verbal learning disabilities. Recreational activities include arts & crafts, swimming, field trips and communication games.

1156 **Camp Ramah in New England**
39 Bennett St
Palmer, MA 01069-9514 413-283-9771
FAX: 413-283-6661
e-mail: info@campramahne.org
www.campramahNE.org

Rabbi Ed Geld, Executive Director
Josh Edelglass, Assistant Director
Ed Pletman, Director of Finance and Operations
Talya Kalender, Director of Camper

8 week sleep-away camp for Jewish adolescents with developmental disabilities. Full camping program includes swimming, Hebrew singing and dancing, sports, arts and crafts, daily services, Kosher food and Jewish studies classes. Some mainstreaming and vocational opportunities.

1157 **Camp Starfish**
1121 Main Street
Lancaster, MA 01523 978-368-6580
FAX: 978-368-6578
e-mail: info@campstarfish.org
www.campstarfish.org

Emily Golinsky, Executive Director
Michele Cyr, MSW, Associate Director
Jill Connell, Administrative & Development Ass

Fosters the growth and success of children with emotional, behavioral and learning problems.

1158 **Camp Wee-Kan-Tu**
127 Worcester Street
Watertown, MA 02472
e-mail: info@campweekantu.org
www.campweekantu.org

Leslie G Brody, Ph.D, President and CEO
Charlene Sturgis, Director of Operations
Susan Welby, Director of Programs
Kristine Binette, Maine Field Service Coordinator

The camp offers children and teenagers aged 8-17 with epilepsy an overnight camping program full of fun and adventure. The camp strives to enhance the child's self esteem, confidence and independence.

1159 **Carroll School Summer Programs**
25 Baker Bridge Rd
Lincoln, MA 01773-3199 781-259-8342
FAX: 781-259-8842
e-mail: info@carrollscholl.org
www.carrollschool.org

Greely Summers, Director
Donna Brown, Manager
Linda Beneke, Adminstrator
Allison West, Academic Director

Academic and recreational programs designed to improve learning skills and build self-confidence. The school is a tutorial program for students not achieving their potential due to poor skills in reading, writing and math. The summer camp complements the summer school offering outdoor activities in a supportive, non-competitive environment.

1160 **Clara Barton Diabetes Camp**
Clara Barton for Girls with Diabetes
30 Ennis Road
PO Box 356
North Oxford, MA 01537-0356 508-987-2056
FAX: 508-987-2002
e-mail: info@bartoncenter.org
www.bartoncenter.org

Mark Bissell, Resident Camp Director
Lynn Butler, Executive Director
Sadie Vivenzio, Finance Director
Fabrizio Aguirre, Camp Joslin Assistant Director

Girls, ages 3-17, with diabetes participate in a well-rounded camp program with special education in diabetes, health and safety. Activities include swimming, boating, sports, dance, music and arts and crafts. Two week adventure camp for high school girls offering camping, hiking, canoeing, etc. Also a minicamp (one week) for girls 6-12. Day camps are offered in Worcester, Boston, and New York City.

1161 **Eagle Hill School: Summer Program**
242 Old Petersham Road
P.O. Box 116
Hardwick, MA 01037- 0116 413-477-6000
FAX: 413-477-6837
e-mail: admission@ehs1.org
www.ehs1.org

Robert M Breakell, B.A., M.A, ASSISTANT HEADMASTER
Marjorie E Castro, B.S., M.A., Ed, HEAD OF SCHOOL
Wendy G Salisbury, B.A., M.A, DIRECTOR OF EDUCATION
Tom Cone, B.A., M.A, DIRECTOR OF ADMISSIONS

For children ages 9-19 with specific learning (dis)abilities and/or Attention Deficit Disorder, this summer program is designed to remediate academic and social deficits while maintaining progress achieved during the school year. Electives and sports activities are combined with the academic courses to address the needs of the whole person in a camp-like atmosphere.

1162 **Edward J Madden Open Hearts Camp**
250 Monument Valley Road
Great Barrington, MA 01230 413-528-2229
888-611-1113
e-mail: hearts@openheartscamp.org
www.openheartscamp.org

David Zaleon, Executive Director
Jill Helme, Assistant Director
Jacqueline Reasor, Counselor
David Andrew, Counselor

Eight week program for children who have had and are fully recovered from open heart surgery or a heart transplant. Four two week sessions by age group. Small camp - 25 campers per session.

1163 **Handi Kids**
The Bridge Center
470 Pine St
Bridgewater, MA 02324-2112 508-697-7557
FAX: 508-697-1529
e-mail: info@TheBridgeCtr.org
www.bridgectr.com

Anita Howards, Director of Administration
Karen Ellis, Office Manager
Spencer Nichols, Program Director
Sarah Norris, Riding Programs Coordinator

A therapeutic recreational facility in Bridgewater, Massachusetts offering after-school programs, special events, school vacation full-week and summer day camp programs. Every individual is welcome. Two-week sessions July-August.

1164 **Kamp for Kids: Camp Togowauk**
Abilities Unlimited of Western New England
754 Russell Road
Westfield, MA 01085 413-562-5678
TTY:800-764-0200
e-mail: info@disabilityinfo.com
www.disabilityinfo.org

Anne Benoit, Director

Two-week sessions July-August for children and young adults with a variety of disabilities. Coed, ages 3-22.

1165 **PKU Camp**
YMCA Camp Burgess & Hayward
75 Stowe Road
Sandwich, MA 02563 508-428-2571
FAX: 508-420-3545
e-mail: pgorman@ssymca.org
www.ssymca.org

Paul Gorman, President
John Ireland, Executive Vice President
Jim Jarosz, Vice President of Finance and Systems
Jeanette Paul, Vice President of Human Resources & Leadership Development

Coed camp in August where children with PKU join other campers with or without PKU. This opportunity allows children to meet other children facing the same issues. Recreational activities include tennis, sailing, horseback riding and performing arts.

1166 **Tower Program at Regis College**
Regis College
235 Wellesley St
Weston, MA 2493-1545 781-768-7000
FAX: 781-899-7209
e-mail: admission@regiscollege.edu
www.regiscollege.edu

Antoinette M Hays, PhD, RN, President
Marla Botelho, MS, Chief Information Officer
Kara Kolomitz, MEd, Vice President, Student Affairs
Thomas Pistorino, MBA, Vice President, Finance and Business

Helps average and above average college-bound students, ages 16-17, having a diagnosed dyslexic learning disability, to adjust to a college setting. Emphasis is on instruction and academic reinforcement, affective support, awareness of support services available on most college campuses and strategy training.

Michigan

1167 **Camp Barakel**
P.O. Box 159
Fairview, MI 48621-0159 989-848-2279
FAX: 989-848-2280
e-mail: info@campbarakel.org
www.campbarakel.org

Paul Gardner, Resident Missionary Staff
Hannah Gardner, Resident Missionary Staff
Dan Haines, Resident Missionary Staff
Sarah Haines, Resident Missionary Staff

Five-day Christian camp experience in mid-August for campers ages 18-55 who are physically disabled, visually impaired, upper trainable mentally impaired or educable mentally impaired, bus transportation provided from locations in Lansing, Flint and Bay City, Michigan.

1168 **Camp Barefoot**
The Fowler Center For Outdoor Learning
2315 Harmon Lake Rd
Mayville, MI 48744-9737 989-673-2050
FAX: 989-673-6355
e-mail: info@thefowlercenter.org
www.thefowlercenter.org

Kyle L Middleton, CTRS, Executive Director
Lynn M Seeloff, CTRS, Assistant Director
Pat Jordan, Office Manager
Farrah Wojcik, Events Supervisor

Offered to adults with traumatic brain injuries/closed head injuries. A wide variety of activities are offered. The participants in Camp Barefoot request their week's activities, allowing each participant to design their own activity schedule.

1169 **Camp Catch-a-Rainbow**
American Cancer Society
1755 Abbey Road
East Lansing, MI 48823 248-302-8985
800-227-2345
FAX: 517-664-1349
e-mail: kwilson@ymcastorercamps.org
www.ymcastorercamps.org

Katie Wilson, Camp-Catch-A-Rainbow (CCAR) Coordinator
Becky Spencer, Vice President of Camping
Abimbola Fajobi, Program Executive
Nancy Burger, Senior Program Director

Camp Catch-a-Rainbow's programs are available completely free to any child in MI or IN who has or has had cancer, between the ages of 4 and 20, with their doctor's approval. Family Camp is reserved for those campers who have attended camp during that year's summer sessions and their families. Day, week, adult retreat, and family camp are available options.

1170 **Camp Chris Williams**
Lions 11 B-2 and MADHH
5236 Dumond Court
Suite C
Lansing, MI 48917-6001 586-778-4188
800-968-7327
e-mail: info@michdhh.org
www.michdhh.org

Nancy Asher, Executive Director
Office Manag

An exciting summer camp experience for deaf and hard of hearing youth and their siblings ages 8-14.

1171 **Camp Nissokone**
YMCA Camping Services
6836 F-41
Oscoda, MI 48750 248-887-4533
FAX: 248-887-5203
e-mail: camp@ymcadetroit.org
www.miymcacamps.org

Doug Grimm, Vice President Camping Services
David Marks, Director

A six week summer resident camp program for boys and girls whose learning and behavior styles have made successful participation in the traditional camp program difficult. All camp activities have a special emphasis on building self-esteem and peer relationships. Strong in waterfront, nature, campcrafts and a special arts program.

1172 **Camp Quality Michigan**
P.O. Box 345
Boyne City, MI 49712 231-582-2471
FAX: 866-564-7637
e-mail: mioffice@campqualityusa.org
www.campqualityusa.com

Kristyn Balog, Executive Director
Kim Ostrom, North Camp Director
Jeff Cram, South Camp Director

Camp Quality is for children with cancer and their siblings. The camp offers a stress-free environment that offers exciting activities and fosters new friendships, while helping to give the children courage, motivation and emotional strength.

1173 **Camp Roger**
8356 Belding Road
Rockford, MI 49341-9628
616-874-7286
FAX: 616-874-5734
e-mail: doug@camproger.org
www.camproger.org
Doug Vanderwell, Executive Director
Phil Warners, Director of Outdoor Education
Matt Zwiep, Director of Operations
Jack Heyboer, Director of Development
Camp Roger provides a fun top-notch summer program for disabled campers. Campers learn to love the woods, the water and the trails, getting to enjoy a wide variety of activities all designed to be fun, to build friendships, and develop self confidence.

1174 **Camp Tall Turf**
816 Madison Ave SE
Grand Rapids, MI 49507
616-452-7906
FAX: 616-452-7907
e-mail: info@turf.org
www.tallturf.org
Jack Kooyman, President
Camp is located in Walkerville, Michigan. Summer camping sessions for youth with asthma/respiratory ailments and ADD. Coed, ages 8-16.

1175 **Echo Grove Camp**
Salvation Army
1101 Camp Rd
Leonard, MI 48367-2812
248-628-3108
FAX: 248-628-7055
e-mail: vicky_purkey@usc.salvationarmy.org
www.echogrove.org
Mark Mc Clenaghan, Camp Director
Sharon McClenaghan, Associate Camp Director
Jeanie Engle, Program Director
Martin Soffran, Site & Facility Manager
Since 1921, the Army's Echo Grove Camp has offered a structured camping program for children, adults and seniors referred through Corps Community Centers. During the course of Echo Grove's 12 week season, the camp includes programs geared for every need and interest. In addition to outdoor recreation, camps may include religious, musical and skill-building instruction.

1176 **Indian Trails Camp**
0-1859 Lake Michigan Drive
Grand Rapids, MI 49534
616-677-5251
FAX: 616-677-2955
e-mail: info@indiantrailscamp.org
www.indiantrailscamp.org
Linda Barar, President
Cameron Young, Vice President
Nate Herrygers, Treasurer
Karol Belk, Secretary
Year round residential camping program for children and adults with physical disabilities. One and two-week sessions. Coed, ages 6-70.

1177 **Sherman Lake YMCA Outdoor Center**
6225 N 39th St
Augusta, MI 49012-9722
269-731-3000
FAX: 269-731-3020
e-mail: shermanlakeymca@ymcasl.org
www.shermanlakeymca.org
Luke Austenfeld, Executive Director
Lorrie Syverson, Director of Camping, Education & Retreat Services
Karen Stanley, Assist. Camp Director
Jean Henderson, Business Manager
Summer camping sessions for campers with ADD and spina bifida. Coed, ages 6-15 and families, seniors.

1178 **St. Francis Camp On The Lake**
10120 Murrey Road
Jerome, MI 49249
517-688-9212
FAX: 517-688-9298
e-mail: campadmin@saintfranciscamp.org
www.saintfranciscamp.org
Russell Kreinbring, President
Connie Quinn, Vice President
Michael Carpenter, Secretary
Bob Steinberger, Treasurer
The camp runs one-week sessions from June through August for cognitively impaired children and adults and is staffed with a 3-to-1 camper ratio. Campers are encouraged to plan their own activities and can partake in swimming, hiking, volleyball, and basketball. Camp staff also helps to emphasize the importance of daily living and socialization skills, and other activities such as helping in the kitchen, and making beds.

1179 **Trail's Edge Camp**
Mott Respiratory Care
200 E. Hospital Drive
Ann Arbor, MI 48109-0208
313-763-2420
e-mail: mdekeon@umich.edu
www.umich.edu/~tecamp
Mary Dekeon
Summer camp for children and young adults between the ages of 3-18 with special medical needs. Campers have tracheotomies or need ventilator assistance. Some of the camp activities include fishing, hiking, horseback riding, boating, swimming, nature & outdoor living skills.

1180 **YMCA Camp Copneconic**
10407 North Fenton Road
Fenton, MI 48430
810-629-9622
FAX: 810-629-2128
e-mail: request@campcopneconic.org
www.campcopneconic.org
John Carlson, Branch Executive Director
Brandon Dreffs, Associate Executive Director
Tom Correll, Director of School Programs/Overnight Camps
Katie O'Toole, Retreats and Partnership Manager
Camp is located in Fenton, Michigan. Summer sessions for campers with diabetes. Coed, ages 3-16 and seniors.

Minnesota

1181 **ADA Camp Needlepoint**
American Diabetes Association
532 County Road F
Hudson, WI 54016
763-593-5333
800-676-4065
FAX: 952-582-9000
e-mail: rbarnett@diabetes.org
www.diabetes.org
Becky Barnett, Camp Director
Carol Holten, Coordinator
Camping for children who have type 1 diabetes. Coed, ages 5-16.

1182 **Camp Benedict**
12459 Upper Sylvan Road SW
Pillager, MN 56473
612-424-2267
FAX: 763-592-8098
campbenedict.org
Connie Statz, President
Rob Andrews, Vice President
Camp Benedict is an educational/recreational family Camp. We strive to improve the quality of life for households who are infected or affected by HIV/AIDS.

1183 **Camp Buckskin**
PO Box 389
Ely, MN 55731 218-365-2121
FAX: 218-365-2880
e-mail: info@campbuckskin.com
www.campbuckskin.com

Thomas R Bauer CCD, Camp Director
Mary Bauer, Co-Director
Jared Griffin, Program Director

Camp is located in Ely, Minnesota. Buckskin assists LD, AD/HD, Asperger's, and adopted individuals to realize and develop the potentials and abilities which they possess. Teaches a combination of traditional camp, academic activities and social skills so the campers experience success in many areas. Ages 6-18.

1184 **Camp Confidence**
1620 Mary Fawcett Drive
Brainerd, MN 56401 218-828-2344
e-mail: info@campconfidence.com
www.campconfidence.com

Jeff Olson, Executive Director
Bob Slaybaugh, Program Director

Confidence Learning Center otherwise known as Camp Confidence is an outdoor center for persons with developmental disabilities. The program at Camp Confidence is aimed at promoting self-confidence and self-esteem, and the necessary skills to become full, contributing members of society.

1185 **Camp Courage North**
Courage Center
3915 Golden Valley Rd
Golden Valley, MN 55422-4249 763-588-0811
866-734-3273
TTY:763-520-0245
e-mail: couragekenny@allina.com
www.couragecenter.org

Jan Malcolm, CEO

Camp is located in Lake George, Minnesota. Summer sessions for campers who have blood disorders, hearing impairment, mobility limitation or are blind/visually impaired. Coed, ages 7-70.

1186 **Camp Friendship**
Friendship Ventures
10509 108th St NW
Annandale, MN 55302 952-852-0101
800-450-8376
FAX: 320-852-0123
e-mail: fv@friendshipventures.org
www.friendshipventures.org

Floyd Adelman, Chairman

Camp Friendship offers resident camp programs for children, teenagers and adults with developmental, physical or multiple disabilities, special medical conditions, Down Syndrome, Williams Syndrome, autism or other conditions. Summer camp offers archery, sailing, horseback riding, biking, fishing, creative arts, adventure challenge programs and other activities. Weekend camps and longer available. Other services available throughout the year. Coed, ages 5-90, families, seniors.

1187 **Camp Heartland**
One Heartland
2101 Hennepin Avenue
Suite 200
Minneapolis, MN 55405 888-216-2028
FAX: 612-824-6303
e-mail: helpkids@oneheartland.org
www.oneheartland.org

Colleen Brennan, President
John Adams, Vice President
W. Morgan Burns, Treasurer
Katherine Kellett, Secretary

Non-profit organization committed to improving the lives of children, youth and their families who have been impacted by HIV/AIDS.

1188 **Camp Knutson**
Camp Knutson And Knutson Point Retreat Center
1169 Whitefish Avenue
Crosslake, MN 56442 218-543-4232
www.lssmn.org/camp/

Rob Larson, Camp Director
Mary (Kate) Williams, Assistant Director
Susann Zeug-Hoese, Chairperson

Camp for children with autism, down syndrome, heart disease and skin disease. Activities include boating, swimming and other water activities.

1189 **Camp Sioux**
American Diabetes Association
106 Solid Rock Circle
Park River, ND 58270 763-593-5333
FAX: 952-582-9000
e-mail: rbarnett@diabetes.org
www.diabetes.org

Larry Hausner, MBA, CEO
Shereen Arent, Exec VP, Govt Affairs
Mary Vaneeda Bennett, Chief Revenue Officer
Becky Barnett, Camp Dir.

Camp Sioux, located in Park River, ND, is a week-long residential summer camp for children ages 8-14 who are living with diabetes. Programs encourage independence and self management with appropriate medical supervision to ensure the best possible experience for every camper. Nutrition activities, blood glucose monitoring, and injections/medications are integrated into the camp program.

1190 **Confidence Learning Center**
Confidence Learning Center
1620 Mary Fawcett Memorial Drive We
East Gull Lake, MN 56401 218-828-2344
FAX: 218-828-2618
e-mail: info@campconfidence.com
www.campconfidence.com/

Jeff Olson, Executive Director
Bob Slaybaugh, Program Director
Mary Harder, Volunteer Director
Jenni Bailey, Specialty Programs, Outdoor Education, Camp Sertoma Director

A year-round outdoor center for persons with developmental disabilities. Some of the summer activities include fishing, archery, beach activities, water volleyball and basketball. Also a specialty camps for deaf and hearing impaired campers.

1191 **Courage Center Camps**
Courage Center
3915 Golden Valley Road
Minneapolis, MN 55422 763-588-0811
866-734-3273
FAX: 320-963-3698
TTY: 763-520-0245
e-mail: couragekenny@allina.com
www.couragecenter.org/camps

Jan Malcolm, CEO
Pamela J. Lindemoen, Exec VP of Operations
Stephen Bariteau, Chief Dev. Officer
Alice Johnson, Chief Financial Officer

Camp is located in Maple Lake, Minnesota. Summer sessions for campers with a variety of disabilities. Coed, ages 6-99, families, seniors.

1192 **YMCA Camp Ihduhapi**
Minneapolis YMCA Camping Services
3425 Ihduhapi Rd
Loretto, MN 55357-9512 763-479-1146
FAX: 612-823-2482
e-mail: Kerry.pioske@ymcatwincities.org
www.ymcatwincities.org/camps/camp_ihduha pi/

Kerry Pioske, Camp Executive
Josh Cobb, Overnight Camp Director
Eric Wobschall, Building Superintendent

Camp is located in Loretto, Minnesota. Summer sessions for campers with asthma/respiratory ailments and epilepsy. Coed, ages 7-16.

Mississippi

1193 **Camp Dream Street**
Camp Dream Street, MS
3863 Morrison Road
Utica, MS 39175 601-885-6042
e-mail: info@dreamstreetms.org
www.dreamstreetms.org
Kimberly Evans, Program Director
Molly Fargotstein, Assistant Program Director
Scott Levy, Chairman
Cynthia Huff, Administrator
For children with physical disabilities. The camp is full of fun and excitement and offers activities such as swimming, art's and crafts, horseback riding and more.

Missouri

1194 **Camp Barnabas**
901 Teas Trail 2060
Purdy, MO 65734 417-476-2565
FAX: 417-486-2980
e-mail: info@campbarnabas.org
www.campbarnabas.org
Jason Brawner, CEO
Brittany Reed, Finance Officer
Mindy Frech, Director of Community Relations
Kylie Wright, Creative Director
Camp for people with developmental challenges, post traumatic burns, blood disorders, cancer, low vision/blindness, and physical challenges. The camp runs from June to August and provides activities such as canoeing, horseback riding and swimming.

1195 **Camp Encourage**
208 West Linwood Boulevard
Kansas City, MO 64111 816-830-7171
e-mail: info@campencourage.org
www.campencourage.org
Jenny Hines, President
Marita Burrow, Ph.D., Secretary
Kelly Lee, M.S.Ed., Executive Director
Alissa Jensen, MPA, Development Coordinator
Encourages social growth, independence and self esteem in children and young adults with autism spectrum disorders.

1196 **Camp Hickory Hill**
Central Missouri Diabetic Childrens Camp
P.O.Box 1942
Columbia, MO 65205-1942 573-445-9146
e-mail: camphickoryhill@yahoo.com
www.camphickoryhill.com
David Bernhardt, President
Pete Bakutes, Treasurer
Myia Custer, Vice President
Michael Gardner MD, Medical Director
Educates diabetic children concerning diabetes and its care. In addition to daily educational sessions on some aspects of diabetes, campers participate in swimming, sailing, arts and crafts and overnight camping. Coed, ages 7-17.

1197 **Camp MITIOG**
Share, Inc
7615 N. Platte Purchase Drive
Suite 116
Kansas City, MO 64118 913-522-9516
877-221-4450
FAX: 816-221-1420
e-mail: midlands@midlandsmc.org
www.campmitiog.org

1198 **Camp Quality Central Missouri**
P.O. Box 953
Jefferson City, MO 65012-953 636-795-7229
e-mail: cmo@campqualityusa.org
www.campqualityusa.com
Casey Bucher, Co-Director
Erin Carl, Co-Director
Camp Quality is for children with cancer and their siblings. The camp offers a stress-free environment that offers exciting activities and fosters new friendships, while helping to give the children courage, motivation and emotional strength.

1199 **Camp Quality Greater Kansas City**
434 NE Station Dr.
Lee's Summit, MO 64086 816-809-8600
FAX: 888-456-1611
e-mail: crystal.davison@campqualityusa.org
www.campqualityusa.com
Crystal Davison, Executive Director
Patricia Harris, CEO
Justin Bolton, Treasurer
Joe Manzo, Program Coordinator
Camp Quality is for children with cancer and their siblings. The camp offers a stress-free environment that offers exciting activities and fosters new friendships, while helping to give the children courage, motivation and emotional strength.

1200 **Camp Quality Missouri Ozarks**
P.O. Box 302
Joplin, MO 64802 417-437-6596
e-mail: zarks@campqualityusa.org
www.campqualityusa.com
Dave Adams, Assis. Director
Kevin Miller, Director
Megan Miller, Medical Director
James Lea, Camp Treasurer
Camp Quality is for children with cancer and their siblings. The camp offers a stress-free environment that offers exciting activities and fosters new friendships, while helping to give the children courage, motivation and emotional strength.

1201 **Camp Quality Northwest Missouri**
P.O. Box 9044
St. Joseph, MO 64508 816-232-2267
FAX: 816-232-2920
e-mail: nwmo@campqualityusa.org
www.campqualityusa.com
Gabe Bailey, Co-Director
Adam Nelson, Co-Director
Lynett Bingaman, Office Manager
Dennis Hart, Personnel Committee Chairman
Camp Quality is for children with cancer and their siblings. The camp offers a stress-free environment that offers exciting activities and fosters new friendships, while helping to give the children courage, motivation and emotional strength.

1202 **Concerned Care, Inc.**
320 Armour Rd
North Kansas City, MO 64116-3506 816-474-3026
FAX: 816-474-3029
www.concernedcarekc.org
Barbara Griggs, Executive Director
Gayle Bennett-Grant, Director of Residential Services
Jim Huffman, Director of Recreation
Carolyn Henry, Director of Development

Summer sessions for campers with developmental disabilities. Coed, ages 7-16. Residential facilities & programs; therapeutic recreation programs.

1203 **Kiwanis Camp Wyman**
Wyman Center
600 Kiwanis Dr
St. Louis, MO 63025-2212
636-938-5245
FAX: 636-938-5289
e-mail: info@wymancenter.org
www.wymancenter.org

Dave Hilliard, President/CEO
Kristine Ramsey, Sr. VP, Dev.
Claire Wyneken, Senior VP & Dir. of Partner Svcs
Tom Etzkorn, VP, Special Projects

Summer sessions for youth with diabetes. Coed, ages 8-16, run in conjunction with the American Diabetes Association. Call for program description.

1204 **Lions Den Outdoor Learning Center**
600 Kiwanis Dr
St. Louis, MO 63025-2212
636-938-5245
FAX: 636-938-5289
e-mail: info@wymancenter.org
wymancenter.org

Dave Hilliard, President/CEO
Kristine Ramsey, Sr. VP, Dev.
Claire Wyneken, Senior VP & Dir. of Partner Svcs
Tom Etzkorn, VP, Special Projects

Varied programs for mentally retarded children, ages 6 and up, includes daily living, socialization and language skills. Sports, tent camping, crafts, and nature study are also offered. Sliding scale tuition for 2 weeks.

1205 **Sunnyhill Adventure Center**
Council for Extended Care
6555 Sunlit Way
Dittmer, MO 63023-3306
636-274-9044
FAX: 636-285-1305
e-mail: dropin4fun@aol.com
www.sunnyhilladventures.org

Victoria James, President/CEO
Kathleen Branson, Director of Finance
Donald Mitchell, Director of ISLA
Rob Darroch, Director of Sunnyhill Adventures

Camp is located in Dittmer, Missouri. Summer sessions for campers with developmental disabilities and autism. Coed, ages 8-99. Sunnyhill Adventures is program that offers campers fun, exciting, educational experiences in a beautiful outdoor setting. Our residential summer camp combines traditional camping activities plus specially selected and adapted events to meet the needs of each camper group.

1206 **Wonderland Camp Foundation**
18591 Miller Circle
Rocky Mount, MO 65072-2400
573-392-1000
e-mail: info@wonderlandcamp.org
www.wonderlandcamp.org

Lori Miller, President
Dan Volmert, Vice President
Jill Wilke, Vice President
Jason Hynson, Executive Director

A residential camp for children and adults with mental and physical disabilities. 12 one week sessions. Coed. All Ages starting at age 6 through adult.

Montana

1207 **Big Sky Kids Cancer Camps**
Eagle Mount-Bozeman
6901 Goldenstein Lane
Bozeman, MT 59715
406-586-1781
FAX: 406-586-5794
e-mail: eaglemount@eaglemount.org
www.eaglemount.org

Mary Peterson, Executive Director
Maggee Harrison, Equestrian Program Director
Chad Biggerstaff, Big Sky Program Director
Heather Collins, Development Coordinator

Provides recreational opportunities for people of all ages with disabilities and children with cancer. Big Sky offers skiing, swimming, fishing, ice-skating, golf, cycling, and so much more.

1208 **Camp Mak-A-Dream**
P.O. Box 1450
Missoula, MT 59806
406-549-5987
FAX: 406-549-5933
e-mail: info@campdream.org
www.campdream.org

Dan Ortt, President
Margot O'Leary, Vice President
Laura Bianco Hanna, Executive Director
Beth Jones, Camp Director

A unique experience for young children in various stages of cancer therapy. The camp gives the children a chance to make new friends, try new things and experience how fun camp can be. Some of the activities include art projects, swimming, archery and campouts.

1209 **Charles Campbell Childrens Camp**
The Billings Lions Club
PO Box 23342
Billings, MT 59104
406-670-2496
e-mail: campbellcamp@msn.com
www.billingslions.org/ccc.htm

Doug Hanson, Director
Sue Hanson, Director

Camp is open to young adults with physical disabilities that include sight or hearing impairment, spina bifida, cerebral palsy, gross motor skill impairments and other disabilities. Campers enjoy hiking, swimming, fishing, dances, campfires and much more.

Nebraska

1210 **Camp Comeca & Retreat Center**
United Methodist Church
75670 Road 417
Cozad, NE 69130-4117
308-784-2808
e-mail: comeca@greatplainsumc.org
www.campcomeca.com

John Butler, Site Director

Camp is located in Cozad, Nebraska. Summer sessions for campers with diabetes and hearing impairment. Coed, ages 6-19, families, seniors, single adults.

1211 **Camp Floyd Rogers**
Floyd Rogers Foundation
P.O. Box 31536
Omaha, NE 68131-536
402-341-0866
e-mail: campers@campfloydrogers.com
www.campfloydrogers.com

1212 **Camp Kindle**
Project Kindle/Camp Kindle
PO BOX 81147
Lincoln, NE 68501
661-257-1901
877-800-2267
FAX: 702-995-9186
e-mail: info@projectkindle.org
www.campkindle.org

Eva Payne, Founder and Executive Director
Mandy Nickolite, Vice President and PsychoSocial Lead
Erin FitzGerald, Program Coordinator
Nikki Wiener, Medical Director

The camp offers children with HIV and AIDS a safe environment where they can go to strengthen their self esteem through interactive participation in educational and recreational programming.

1213 **Easter Seals Nebraska**
Easter Seals Nebraska
12565 West Center Road
Suite 100
Omaha, NE 68144-8144
402-345-2200
800-650-9880
FAX: 402-345-2500
www.ne.easterseals.com

James C. Summerfelt, President & CEO
Angela Howell, Vice President Easter Seals Nebraska
Lily Sughroue, Director of Camp, Respite & Recreation

Offers a variety of services to help people with disabilities address life's challenges and achieve personal goals. Terrific fun for campers and a much needed respite for families and caregivers from the daily challenges of caring for special needs individuals.

1214 **Kamp Kaleo**
46872 Willow Springs Rd
Burwell, NE 68823-8805
308-346-5083
FAX: 308-346-5083
e-mail: kampkaleo@gmail.com
www.kampkaleo.com

Gaylene O'Brien, Facilities Administrator
Sandy Denton, Minister of Faith Dev.
Jim Becker, Chairperson

Camp is located in Burwell, Nebraska. Summer sessions for campers who are blind/visually impaired or have developmental disabilities. Coed, ages 9-18 and families, seniors, single adults.

1215 **National Camps for Blind Children**
Christian Record Services
4444 S 52nd Street
Lincoln, NE 68516-1302
402-488-0981
FAX: 402-488-7582
e-mail: info@christianrecord.org
www.christianrecord.org

Larry Pitcher, President
Matthew Orian, VP for Finance
Dan Jackson, Chair
Tom Lemon, Vice Chair

Provides free Christian publications and programs, as well as new opportunities for people with visual impairments. Free services include subscription magazines available in Braille, large print and audio cassette, full-vision books combining Braille and print, lending library, gift bibles and study guides in Braille, large print and audio cassette, national camps for blind children and scholarship assistance for blind young people trying to obtain a college education.

1216 **YMCA Camp Kitaki**
Lincoln YMCA
570 Fallbrook Blvd.
Suite 210
Lincoln, NE 68521-3110
402-434-9200
FAX: 402-434-9226
e-mail: info@ymcalincoln.org
www.ymcalincoln.org

Barb Bettin, President/CEO
J.P. Lauterbach, Chief Operations Officer
Misty Muff, Chief Administrative Officer
Renee Yost, Chief Financial Officer

Camp is located in Louisville, Nebraska. Summer sessions for children with cystic fibrosis. Coed, ages 7-17 and families.

Nevada

1217 **Camp Buck**
Nevada Diabetes Association
1005 Terminal Way #170
Reno, NV 89502
775-856-3839
800-379-3839
FAX: 775-348-7591
e-mail: camp@diabetesnv.org
www.diabetesnv.org

Sarah Gleich, Associate State Exec. Dir.
Mylan Hawkins, State Exec. Dir.
Diana Kern, State Dir. of Dev.
Celeste Ochal, Southern Nevada Exec. Dir.

Co-ed summer camp for children with diabetes ages 8-17. While at the camp, the children develop a better understanding of their diabetes while enjoying a week filled with recreational and athletic activities such as swimming, kayaking, fishing and arts & crafts.

1218 **Camp Lotsafun**
3660 Baker Lane
Suite 103
Reno, NV 89509
775-827-3866
FAX: 775-827-0334
e-mail: camp@camplotsafun.com
www.camplotsafun.com

Gayla Ouellette, Director
Shannon Dressel, Chairman
Linda Barnes, Vice Chairman
Al Herak, Secretary/Treasurer

Provides therapeutic, educational, and recreational opportunities for individuals with developmental disabilities, while providing respite care for their families. Children, teens and adults with autism, down syndrome, traumatic brain injury, cerebral palsy and attention deficit hyperactive disorder are among some of the individuals who attend camp for fun and recreational activities such as swimming, kayaking, pet therapy, arts & crafts, drama and music.

1219 **Camp SignShine**
DHHARC
1150 Corporate Blvd.
Suite 1
Reno, NV 89502
775-434-0290
FAX: 775-355-8996
TTY:775-355-8994
www.dhharc.org

J. Farrell Cafferata Jenkins, President
Shannah Kanet, Secretary/Treasurer

Week long camp for children ages 7-19 who are deaf or hard of hearing and their siblings. Campers enjoy recreational and educational activities in a safe and comfortable environment.

1220 **CampCare**
P.O. Box 12155
Reno, NV 89510-2155
775-323-3737
FAX: 775-323-1019
e-mail: cmoore@campcarenevada.org
www.campcarenevada.org

New Hampshire

1221 **Camp Allen**
56 Camp Road
Bedford, NH 03110-6606
603-622-8471
FAX: 603-626-4295
e-mail: mary@campallennh.org
www.campallennh.org

Mary Constance, Executive Director
Michael Constance, Summer Camp Director
John Cronin, Director
Deb Schulte, Office Manager

A residential summer camp for individuals with disabilities. All of the activities are conducted by individual coordinators under the supervision of Program Director. Some of the activities include, aquatics, arts, crafts, games and nature programs. All camp events, special events, evening programs, and field trips are scheduled throughout the summer and are structured to meet the individual abilities and needs of each camper.

1222 **Camp Sno Mo**
Easter Seals: New Hampshire
555 Auburn St
Manchester, NH 03103-4803
603-623-8863
800-870-8728
FAX: 603-625-1148
e-mail: rkelly@eastersealsnh.org
www.easterseals.com/nh/

Jim Bee, Chairman
Christine Gordon, Vice Chairman
Andrew MacWilliam, Treasurer
Renee Walsh, Secretary

Mission is to create solutions that change the lives of children and adults with disabilities or special needs or their families. From campfire sing-a-longs and late night ghost stories, to boating, nature walks, swimming, and arts and crafts, Easter Seals camps provide the same excitement and activity available at other summer camp programs. Easter Seals campers experience the joys and challenges of camp in a fully-accessible setting.

1223 **Windsor Mountain American Sign Language Camp Program**
Windsor Mountain International
One World Way
Windsor, NH 03244
603-478-3166
800-862-7760
FAX: 603-478-5260
e-mail: Jake@WindsorMountain.org
www.windsormountain.org

Jake Labovitz, Director
Kerry Labovitz, Director
Pam Butler, Administrative Assistant
Richard Herman

Camp Windsor is for children from around the world who are deaf or hard of hearing.

New Jersey

1224 **Camp Carefree**
American Diabetes Association
275 Carefree Lane
Stokesdale, NC 27357
336-427-0966
e-mail: carefreedirectors@gmail.com
www.campcarefree.org/

Anne Jones, Founder & Executive Director
Tony McCallum, Program Director
Leah Sell-Goodhand, Program Director
Andrew Dippel, Program Director

Since 1986, Camp Carefree has provided a FREE, one week camping experience for kids with chronic illnesses. Our program also includes camps for well siblings of ill children, and a week for children with a sick parent.

1225 **Camp Chatterbox**
200 Portland Rd A-20
P.O. Box 8310
Highlands, NJ 07732- 2015
908-301-5451
e-mail: JBruno@childrens-specialized.org
www.campchatterbox.org

Joan Bruno, Ph.D., Director

Camp Chatterbox is an overnight camp for children who use augmentative communication devices. The camp offers recreational activities such as swimming, boating, sports and being with nature, and the camp activities programs are designed to facilitate device use throughout the day.

1226 **Camp Dream Street**
Kaplen JCC On The Palisades
411 East Clinton Avenue
Tenafly, NJ 07670
201-569-7900
FAX: 201-569-7448
e-mail: info@jccotp.org
www.jccotp.org

Danny Rocke, CFO
Avi A. Lewinson, Exec. Director
Deann Forman, COO
Lisa Robbins, Director

A one-week camp for children ages 4-14 who have cancer and other blood disorders. Campers and their siblings can enjoy a wide variety of activities such as arts and crafts, sports, nature, swimming, entertainment and music.

1227 **Camp Jotoni**
ARC of Somerset County
141 S Main St
Manville, NJ 08835-1803
908-725-8544
e-mail: lauraz@thearcofsomerset.org
www.thearcofsomerset.org

Ron Slahetka, President
Timothy McKeown, Vice President
Lauren Panarella, Executive Director
Christopher Corvino, Associate Executive Director

Sponsored by the Arc of Somerset County, Camp Jotoni is a day and residential camp for children and adults with developmental disabilities. Campers are ages five to adult. Set on 15 acres in Somerset County, the camp features a junior Olympic size pool, cabins, dining hall, playgrounds, open air pavilions, unspoiled woods, and wildlife. Coed, ages 5-99.

1228 **Camp Lou Henry Hoover**
Girl Scouts of Washington Rock Council
201 E Grove St
Westfield, NJ 07090-5614
908-518-4400
FAX: 908-232-2140
e-mail: girlscouts@gshnj.org
www.gshnj.org

Nancy Faulks, Chairman
Lydia Whitefield, Vice Chairman
Princess M. Palmer, Secretary
Michael Kzirian, Treasurer

Camp is located in Middleville, New Jersey. Sessions for girls who are blind/visually impaired, ages 7-18.

1229 **Camp Merry Heart**
Easter Seals: New Jersey
25 Kennedy Blvd
Suite 600
East Brunswick, NJ 08816
732-257-6662
FAX: 908-852-9263
e-mail: camp@nj.easterseals.com
www.easterseals.com/nj/

Michael Bisesti, Chairmna
Frank Lavadera, Vice Chairman/Operations
Ken Tsoi-A-Sue, Vice Chair/Treasurer
Eric Kunkel, Board Member

An organized program of swimming, arts and crafts, boating, nature study and travel offered to campers with a variety of disabilities. Coed, ages 5-80, families, seniors. Fall and spring travel programs for adults.

1230 **Camp Nejeda**
Camp Nejeda Foundation
910 Saddlebrook Road
P.O. Box 156
Stillwater, NJ 07875- 156
973-383-2611
FAX: 973-383-9891
e-mail: information@campnejeda.org
www.nejeda.convio.net

Henry Anhalt, DO, President
Scott Ross, Vice President
Bill Vierbuchen, Executive Director
Jim Daschbach, Camp Director
For children with diabetes, ages 7-15. Provides an active and safe camping experience which enables the children to learn about and understand diabetes. Activities include boating, swimming, fishing, archery, as well as camping skills.

1231 **Camp Oakhurst**
New York Service for the Handicapped
111 Monmouth Rd
Oakhurst, NJ 07755-1514
732-531-0215
FAX: 732-531-0292
e-mail: info@nysh.org
www.nysh.org/

Robert Pacenza, Executive Director
Charles Sutherland, Camp Director
Andy Arno, Board Member
Julian Bach, Board Member
Camp is located in Oakhurst, New Jersey. Summer sessions for campers with cerebral palsy, mobility limitation and spina bifida. Coed, age 8-18.

1232 **Camp Quality New Jersey**
1444 Mockingbird Circle
P.O. Box 264
Stow, OH 44224
330-671-0167
FAX: 866-285-5208
www.campqualityusa.com

Lois Hartje, President
Vicki Irey, Vice President
Dennis Hart, Secretary
Ptricia Harris, Executive Director
Camp Quality is for children with cancer and their siblings. The camp offers a stress-free environment that offers exciting activities and fosters new friendships, while helping to give the children courage, motivation and emotional strength.

1233 **Camp Sun'N Fun**
ARC of Gloucester
1555 Gateway Blvd.
West Deptford, NJ 08096-3486
856-848-8648
FAX: 856-875-1499
e-mail: camp@thearcgloucester.org
www.thearcgloucester.org

Robert H. Weir, Charter President
Dottie Weir, Charter President
Charles Funk, Vice President
Terri Wilson, Camp Director
Camp is located in Williamstown, New Jersey. Summer sessions for campers with developmental disabilities. Coed, ages 8-88. Activities include swimming, arts & crafts, nature, sports, games, music, dance and drama.

1234 **Camp Vacamas**
256 Macopin Rd
West Milford, NJ 07480-3718
973-838-0942
877-428-8222
e-mail: info@vacamas.org
www.vacamas.org

Felix A. Urrutia Jr, Executive Director
Kevin Ervin, Bronx Borough Supervisor
Seth Friedman, MPA., Director of Programs
Jennifer Thompson, MSW., Director of Strategic Development
Disadvantaged children with asthma or sickle cell anemia, ages 8-16, are offered special programs in canoeing, backpacking, camping, music and leadership training. Sliding scale tuition. Year round programs for youth at risk groups. Conference center facility open for group rentals.

1235 **New Jersey Camp Jaycee**
The Arc of New Jersey
985 Livingston Ave
North Brunswick, NJ 08902-1843
732-246-2525
FAX: 732-214-1834
e-mail: info@campjaycee.org
www.campjaycee.org

Frank Pirrello, President
John O'Brien, Vice President
Patricia Rhein, Secretary
Jason Brakeman, Camp Director
Camp Jaycee is located on 185 acres of forests, fields and streams located in the lovely Pocono Mountains, a short distance from the New Jersey border. Sessions for children and adults with autism and developmental disabilities. Goals of Camp Jaycee are centered around developing social skills, improving self esteem, increasing confidence, learning in a fun environment, developing physical fitness, and establishing meaningful relationships with new friends. Coed, ages 7-85.

1236 **New Jersey YMHA/YWHA Camps Milford**
21 Plymouth St
Fairfield, NJ 07004-1686
973-575-3333
800-776-5657
FAX: 973-575-4188
e-mail: info@njycamps.org
www.njycamps.org

Bruce L. Nussman, President
Silvio Berlfein, Assistant Director
Leonard Robinson, Executive Director
Hylton Wener, Director
Camp is located in Milford, Pennsylvania. Summer sessions for children with ADD. Coed, ages 6-17 and families.

1237 **Rolling Hills Country Day Camp**
P.O.Box 172
Marlboro, NJ 07746
732-308-0405
FAX: 732-780-4726
e-mail: info@rollinghillsdaycamp.com
www.rollinghillsdaycamp.com

Billy Breitner
Summer sessions for children with ADD. Coed, ages 3-12.

1238 **Round Lake Camp**
21 Plymouth Street
Fairfield, NJ 07004
973-575-3333

e-mail: rlc@njycamps.org
www.roundlakecamp.org

1239 **Summit Camp**
322 Route 46 West
Suite 210
Parisppany, NJ 07054
973-732-3230
800-323-9908
FAX: 973-732-3226
e-mail: info@summitcamp.com
www.summitcamp.com

Eugene Bell, Senior Director
Leah Love, Assistant Director
Kim Daum, Travel Director
Maryann Santora, Clinical Social Worker/Admissions Director
Camp is located in Honesdale, Pennsylvania. Summer sessions for children with ADD. Coed, ages 8-17.

New Mexico

1240 ADA Camp for Kids
American Diabetes Association
2625 Pennsylvania NE
Suite 225
Albuquerque, NM 87110- 3649 888-342-2383
e-mail: lbrown@diabetes.org
www.diabetes.org/living-with-diabetes/parents

Larry Hausner, MBA, CEO
Shereen Arent, Exec VP
Mary Vaneeda Bennett, Chief Revenue Officer
Greg Elfers, Chief Field Dev. Officer

One-week camping session for children with diabetes. Coed, ages 8-13. Camp will be held at Manzano Mountain Retreat, one hour from Albuquerque, New Mexico. Please call for exact dates.

New York

1241 ADA Camp Sunshine
American Diabetes Association
160 Allens Creek Rd
Rochester, NY 14618-3309 FAX: 585-458-3810
e-mail: dhumphreys@diabetes.org
www.diabetescamp.org

Terry Ackley, Exec. Dir.
Lorne Abramson, Consultant
Shelley Yeager, Dir. of Outreach & Dev.
Kathy Latimer, Administrative Assistant

The American Diabetes Association New York Area's Camp is a residential camp for children with diabetes. The program is held on the Rotary Sunshine Campus in Rush, only 15 miles from Rochester. The camp is located on 133 acres of land in a rural setting including modern year round cabins, an Olympic-sized swimming pool, nature trails, athletic fields and a fishing pond. Ages 8-16; held during July.

1242 Camp Abilities Brockport
The College At Brockport, State Univ Of New York
350 New Campus Drive
Brockport, NY 14420 585-395-5361
FAX: 585-395-2771
e-mail: llieberm@brockport.edu
www.campabilitiesbrockport.org

Dr. Lauren Lieberman, PhD, Camp Director
Tiffany Mitrakos, MEd, Assistant Director
Gina Pucci, Aquatic and Boating Director
Stacey Gibbins, Graduate Assistant

A one-week sports camp for children who are visually impaired, blind or deaf blind. Children learn to be more physically active, which in turn improves their health and well being.

1243 Camp Akeela
314 Bryn MawrAvenue
BalaCynwyd, PA 19004 866-680-4744
FAX: 866-462-2828
e-mail: info@campakeela.com
www.campakeela.com

Eric Sasson, Camp Director
Debbie Sasson, Camp Director
Kevin Trimble, Assistant Director and Program Director
Rob Glyn-Jones, Head Counselor

Co-ed, overnight camp for children and young adults ages 9-17 who have been diagnosed with Asperger's Syndrome or a non verbal learning disability.

1244 Camp Glengarra
Girl Scouts - Foothills Council
33 Jewett Pl
Utica, NY 13501-4715
e-mail: nbrown@girlscoutsfoothills.org

Karen Lubecki, Director

Camp Glengarra is located on 500+ acres of fields and forests, about eight miles west of Camden. This Girl Scout Camp hosts a myriad of programs throughout the year as well as summer day and resident camp. Summer sessions for girls 5-17 with ADD or asthma/respiratory ailments.

1245 Camp Good Days and Special Times
1332 Pitsford-Mendon Rd
PO Box 665
Mendon, NY 14506 585-624-5555
800-785-2135
FAX: 585-624-5799
www.campgooddays.org

Gary Mervis, Chairman and Founder
Wendy Bleier-Mervis, Exec. Dir.
Lisa Booz, Western New York Regional Dir.
Claire McKenney, Central New York Regional Dir.

The camp is dedicated to improving the quality of life for children, adults and their families whose lives have been touched by cancer and/or other life challenges.

1246 Camp Huntington
56 Bruceville Road
P.O. Box 37
High Falls, NY 12440 845-687-7840
866-514-5281
FAX: 845-213-4313
e-mail: mbednarz@camphuntington.com
www.camphuntington.com

Michael Bednarz, Executive Director
Alex Mellor, Program Director
Margaret Short, Health Director
Cathy Crowley, Program Supervisor

A co-ed residential summer camp specifically designed to focus on Adaptive and Therapeutic Recreation. Campers include those with learning and developmental disabilities, ADD/HD, Autism Spectrum Disorders, Asperger's, PDD, and other special needs. Three programs are offered that focus on: recreation and social skills; independence; and participation. Campers may attend for a week at a time with a full summer lasting nine weeks.

1247 Camp Jened
United Cerebral Palsy Association New York
P.O.Box 483
Rock Hill, NY 12775-483 845-434-2220
FAX: 845-434-2253
www.campjened.org

1248 Camp Mark Seven
Mark Seven Deaf Foundation
144 Mohawk Hotel Rd
Old Forge, NY 13420-4010 315-357-6089
e-mail: registrar@campmark7.org
www.campmark7.org

Andrew Brinks, Ph.D., Executive Director
Vicki Liggera, Registrar
Gregoire Youbara, Office Manager
Dave Staehle, Camp Director

Adirondack Mountain camp for hard-of-hearing, deaf and hearing people. Coed, ages 1-99, families, seniors and single adults.

1249 Camp Northwood
132 State Route 365
Remsen, NY 13438-5700 315-831-3621
FAX: 315-831-5867
e-mail: northwoodprograms@hotmail.com
www.nwood.com

Gordon W Felt, Director
Donna Felt, Director

Summer sessions for children with ADD. Coed, ages 8-18.

1250 **Camp Ramapo**
Route 52 Salisbury Turnpike
PO Box 266
Rt. 52 / Salisbury Turnpike
Rhinebeck, NY 12572 845-876-8403
FAX: 845-876-8414
e-mail: office@ramapoforchildren.org
www.ramapoforchildren.org

Richard Rosenthal, President
Teri Goldberg Horowitz, First Vice President
Claude Ann Mellins, Ph.D., Vice President
Deusdedi Merced, Esq., Vice President
Ramapo's specific focus is adventure-based, experiential learning programs that promote positive character values in children and teens with special needs.

1251 **Camp Sisol**
Jewish Community Center of Greater Rochester/JCC
1200 Edgewood Ave
Rochester, NY 14618-5408 585-461-2000
e-mail: jshellman@jccrochester.org
www.jccrochester.org

Jeremy Wolk, President
Burton Kleinman, Vice President
Dan Goldstein, Secretary
Justin Goldman, Treasurer
Camp is located in Honeoye Falls, New York. Summer sessions for children with autism. Coed, ages 5-16.

1252 **Camp Tova**
92nd Street Y
1395 Lexington Ave
New York, NY 10128-1612 212-415-5500
www.92y.org

Stuart J. Ellman, President
Sol Adler, Executive Director
Laurence D. Belfer, Vice President
Cheryl Minikes, Vice President
Children with learning and developmental disabilities thrive in Camp Tova's small group setting. Making friends and developing a wide variety of creative, social, and physical skills are the goals for Tova campers.

1253 **Camp Venture, Inc.**
25 Smith Street
Suite 510
Nanuet, NY 10954-2970 845-624-3860
www.campventure.org

John Murphy, President
Daniel Lukens, Exec. Dir.
Dorothy Cox, Deputy Exec. Dir.
Lisa Nolte, Associate Exec. Dir.
In more than a dozen Rockland neighborhoods, residential, employment, rehabilitation or recreation programs have arisen to help people with disabilities contribute to the life of the community. There are, for instance, more than a dozen Community Residential Facilities, Venture Industries, Venture Day Treatment, Day Habilitation, Venture Chorus, after school programs and more.

1254 **Camp Whitman on Seneca Lake**
Presbyterian Church USA
150 Whitman Road
Penn Yan, NY 14527-278 315-536-7753
FAX: 315-536-2128
e-mail: camp@campwhitman.org
www.campwhitman.org

Lindsey Jensen, Pine Camp Program Coordinator
Rhonda Everdyke, Communications and Interim Camp Director
Karen Jensen, Camp Registrar
Darwyn Jepsen, Property Manager
To give the developmentally disabled youth/adult, ages 10-60, the opportunity to enjoy him/herself in a camping program. Campers are encouraged to participate in a full range of activities including games, sports, swimming, singing, and dancing. Because the camps are fairly small, we have a low camper to counselor ratio, and all have a chance to know one another and form close friendships.

1255 **Casowasco Camp, Conference and Retreat Center**
158 Casowasco Dr
Moravia, NY 13118-3498 315-364-8756
855-414-6400
FAX: 315-364-7636
e-mail: info@campsandretreats.org
www.campsandretreats.org/index.php/casowasco/

David Little, Chair
Carmen Vianese, Vice Chair
Mike Huber, Executive Director, CRM
Demetrio Beach, Program Director, Casowasco
Camp is located in Moravia, New York. Summer sessions for children with ADD. Coed, ages 6-18 and families.

1256 **Clover Patch Camp**
Center for Disability Services
55 Helping Hand Ln
Glenville, NY 12302-5801 518-384-3080
FAX: 518-384-3001
e-mail: cloverpatchcamp@cfdsny.org
www.cloverpatchcamp.org

Laura Taylor, Camp Director
Christopher Schelin, Program Administrator
Camp is located in Scotia, NY. Summer sessions for campers with a variety of disabilities. Coed, ages 5-85.

1257 **Double H Ranch**
A Hole In The Wall Camp
97 Hidden Valley Road
Lake Luzerne, NY 12846 518-696-5676
FAX: 518-696-4528
e-mail: myurenda@doublehranch.org
www.doublehranch.org

Victor Hershaft, Chairman
Ed Lewi, Vice Chairman
Max Yurenda, CEO/Executive Director
Jacqui Royael, Director Of Operations
Summer residential camp and winter sports programs for children and young adults ages 6-16 who have cancer and other life threatening illnesses. The programs are free of charge and some of the recreational activities include bead making, arts & crafts, kickball, tennis, soccer, and volleyball.

1258 **Father Drumgoole Connelly Summer Camp**
MIV Mount Loretto
6581 Hylan Blvd
Staten Island, NY 10309-3830 718-317-2803
e-mail: srynn@mountloretto.org
www.mountloretto.org

Stephen Rynn, Exec. Dir.
Maryann Virga, Exec. Assistant
Ed Gani, Facilities Manager
Loretta Polanish, Exec. Secretary
Summer sessions for children with epilepsy, hearing impairment and developmental disabilities. Coed, ages 5-13.

1259 **Friends Academy Summer Camps**
Duck Pond Rd
Locust Valley, NY 11560 516-393-4207
FAX: 516-465-1720
e-mail: camp@fa.org
www.fasummercamp.org

Rich Mack, Camp Director
Summer sessions for children with diabetes. Coed, ages 3-14, families.

1260 **Friendship Circle Summer Camp**
121 West 19th Street
New York, NY 10011 646-820-1066
www.friendshipnyc.com

1261 **Gow School Summer Programs**
2491 Emery Road
P.O. Box 85
South Wales, NY 14139-0085 716-652-3450
FAX: 716-652-3457
e-mail: summer@gow.org
www.gow.org

Robert Garcia, Director of Admissions
Gayle Hutton, Director of Development
Eric Bray, Summer Program Director
Rosemary Shields, CPA, Director of Finance

Co-ed summer programs for students ages 8-16 with dyslexia or similar learning disabilities offer a balanced blend of morning academics, afternoon/evening traditional camp activities and weekend overnights. The primary purpose of these programs is to provide a positive experience while balancing these three elements. Committed to the creation of a positive and enjoyable experience for each participant by defining and merging the goals of the camp and the school with those of camper students.

1262 **Happiness Is Camping**
2169 Grand Concourse
Bronx, NY 10453-2201 718-295-3100
FAX: 718-295-0406
e-mail: hicoffice@happinessiscamping.org
www.happinessiscamping.org

Louis D'Agostino, President of the Board
James Kramer, Secretary/Treasurer
Kenneth Bertholf, Officer
Martin Elson, Esq., Counsel

Camp is located in Blairstown, New Jersey. Free camping sessions for children with cancer. Coed, ages 6-15. June 30 - July 31, 2008.

1263 **Hemophilia Camp**
Tanager Place
116 West 32nd Street, 11th Floor
New York, NY 10001-9533 212-328-3700
FAX: 212-328-3777
e-mail: dpirrie@tanagerplace.org
www.hemaware.org/story/hemophilia-summer-camp

Donald Pirrie, Executive Director
John Indence, Executive Editor
January Payne, Managing Editor

During the six-day camp children with Hemophilia and their siblings participate in individual and group activities designed for fun and fitness. The camp held each year in mid-June has a 24-hour physician and nursing staff. Ages 5-16.

1264 **Kamp Kiwanis**
New York District Kiwanis Foundation
9020 Kiwanis Rd
Taberg, NY 13471-2727 315-336-4568
FAX: 315-336-3845
e-mail: kamp@kampkiwanis.org
www.kamp-kiwanis.org

Rebecca O. Lopez, Executive Director

Kamp Kiwanis is a mainstream camp for underprivileged youth with and without special needs. 20 campers with disabilities are integrated into weekly sessions. Coed, ages 8-14, seniors and single adults.

1265 **Maplebrook School**
5142 Route 22
Amenia, NY 12501-5357 845-373-9511
FAX: 845-373-7029
e-mail: jscully@maplebrookschool.org
www.maplebrookschool.org

Mark J. Metzger, Chairman
Robert Audia, Vice Chairman
George T. Whalen, Jr, Treasurer
Charles F. Chiusano, Secreatry

A coeducational boarding school which offers a six week camp for children with learning differences and ADD.

1266 **Marist Brothers Mid-Hudson Valley Camp**
P.O.Box 197
Esopus, NY 12429-197 212-55- 123
e-mail: info@maristbrotherscenter.org
www.maristretreathouse.net

Michelle Flemen-Tung, Camp Director, Special Children
Brother Owen Ormsby, Executive Director
Matt Fallon, Director of Operations
Mike Trainor, Facilities Director

Serves special people: children who have cancer or who are HIV positive, deaf or mentally retarded.

1267 **Sunshine Campus**
Rochester Rotary Club
180 Linden Oaks
Suite 200
Rochester, NY 14625 585-546-7435
e-mail: tdreisbach@rochesterrotary.org
www.sunshinecampus.org

Tracey Dreisbach, Executive Director
Brandi Koch, Sunshine Campus Partner Director
Amy Nicolis

Camp is located in Rush, New York. Camping sessions for children and young adults with a variety of disabilities. Ages 7-21.

1268 **VISIONS Vacation Camp for the Blind**
VISIONS Center on Blindness
111 Summit Park Rd
Spring Valley, NY 10977-1221 212-625-1616
FAX: 888-245-8333
e-mail: info@visionsvcb.org
www.visionsvcb.org

Nancy T. Jones, President
Richard P. Simon, Vice President
Burton M. Strauss, Jr., Treasurer
Carol Spawn Desmond, Secretary

Is a non profit agency that promotes the independence of people of all ages who are blind or visually impaired. Camp offers Braille classes, computers with large print and voice output, support groups, discussions, mobility lesions, cooking classes, personal and home management training, large print and Braille books.

1269 **Wagon Road Camp**
Children's Aid Society
105 East 22ndStreet
New York, NY 10010-2000 212-949-4800
FAX: 914-238-0714
e-mail: webmaster@childrensaidsociety.org
www.childrensaidsociety.org

Richard R. Buery, Jr., President and CEO
William D. Weisberg, Ph.D., Exec VP
Dan Lehman, VP and Chief Financial Officer
Valerie Russo, VP of Strategy and Excellence

Wagon Road Day Camp is a co-ed program for children ages 6-13 with a variety of disabilities held within Chappaqua, New York. Uniquely qualified specialists in Project Adventure activities, athletics, horsemanship, theater arts, nature/ecology studies and arts/crafts complement the day camp staff. Special events including Carnival, Olympics, Crazy Hat Day, Western Day, and optional sleepovers add to the summer excitement providing children with an enriching multicultural experience.

1270 **YMCA Camp Chingachgook on Lake George**
Capital District YMCA
1872 Pilot Knob Rd
Kattskill Bay, NY 12844-1802 518-656-9462
FAX: 518-656-9362
e-mail: chingachgook@cdymca.org
www.cdymca.org

George Painter, Executive Director
Billy Rankin, Senior Program Director
Lesley Munshower, Summer Camp Program Director
Heather Siegel-Sawma, Groups Director

Sailing programs for people with disabilities. Sessions for campers who are blind/visually impaired. Coed, ages 7-16, families, seniors and single adults.

1271 **YMCA Camp Weona**
YMCA of Greater Buffalo
301 Cayuga Rd
Suite 100
Buffalo, NY 14225-1912 716-565-6000
FAX: 716-565-6007
e-mail: jczochara@ymcabuffaloniagara.org
www.ymcabuffaloniagara.org

Jeff Burghardt, Finance/Financial Dev. Chair
A.L. Ferreira, Camp Exec. Dir.
Tim Marble, Camp Ranger
Julie Czochara, Business and Sales Coordinator

Camp is located in Gainesville, New York. Camping sessions for children and adults with epilepsy. Coed, ages 7-16, families and single adults. Nestled in 1,000 acres of hardwood and pine forests, Weona has miles of picturesque hiking trails, brooks, a heated outdoor pool and a world class adventure ropes course. Our indoor facilities include arts and crafts studios, environmental classrooms and a challenging rock climbing wall. It is the ideal setting for hands-on fun, adventure and learning.

North Carolina

1272 **Camp Carefree**
275 Carefree Lane
Stokesdale, NC 27357 336-427-0966
e-mail: carefreedirectors@gmail.com
www.campcarefree.org

Anne Jones, Founder & Executive Director
Tony McCallum, Program Director
Leah Sell-Goodhand, Program Director
Andrew Dippel, Program Director

A free, one-week camp for youngsters with serious health problems. The camp gives the children a chance to have the freedom to play, learn and enjoy all the recreational and craft activities the camp has to offer.

1273 **Camp Carolina Trails**
American Diabetes Association
2418 Blue Ridge Rd
Suite 206
Raleigh, NC 27607 743-540-3217
888-342-2383
FAX: 704-373-9113
e-mail: jthomas@diabetes.org
www.diabetes.org

Dwight Holing, Chair
Marjorie Cypress, President
Elizabeth Seaquist, MD, President
Larry Hausner, MBA, CEO

The American Diabetes Association is the nation's leading non-profit health organization providing diabetes research, information, advocacy and year round programs for children with diabetes.

1274 **Camp New Hope**
FriendshipVentures
4805 N Carolina 86
Chapel Hill, NC 27514 919-942-4716
FAX: 919-942-3266
e-mail: info@newhopeccc.org
www.newhopeccc.org

Richard Stevens, Executive Director
Gerald Sigleton, Facilities Manager
Suzanne Blankfard, Office Staff
Minnilue Braverman, Office Administrator

A place for children, teens and adults to have the time of their lives. The program focuses on building self esteem, independence and provides opportunities to practice social skills specifically designed for persons with developmental, physical and multiple disabilities, special medical needs, Down Syndrome, autism, or other conditions.

1275 **Camp Royall**
Autism Society of North Carolina
505 Oberlin Road
Suite 230
Raleigh, NC 27605 919-743-0204
800-442-2762
e-mail: info@autismsociety-nc.org
www.autismsociety-nc.org

Sharon Jeffries-Jones, Chairman
Elizabeth Phillippi, Vice Chairman
Tracey Sheriff, Chief Executive Officer
Paul Wendler, Chief Financial Officer

The best source in North Carolina for connecting people who live with autism (and those who care about them) with resources, support, advocacy and information tailored to their unique needs.

1276 **Camp Sertoma**
1105 Camp Sertoma Dr
Westfield, NC 27053 336-593-8057
www.campsertoma.org

Keith Russell, Center Director
Mike Bowman, Property Director

Camp Sartoma is a place where deaf and hard of hearing children can come to meet people just like them, with out communication barriers. Activities include swimming, canoeing, fishing, hiking, hayrides, campfires, games, astronomy, and nature crafts.

1277 **Camp Sky Ranch**
634 Sky Ranch Rd
Blowing Rock, NC 28605-8231 828-264-8600
FAX: 828-265-2339
e-mail: jsharp1@triad.rr.com
www.campskyranchevents.com

Jack Sharp, Owner

A private, residential camp for the developmentally delayed. This season is the camp's 56th year of providing a real camping experience for the handicapped. Camp Sky Ranch was the first private camp for the handicapped in the Southeast. Activities include: swimming, boating, horseback riding, and more. Campers must be able to walk, dress and feed themselves, and toilet trained.

1278 **Camp Tekoa UMC**
Western NC Conference/United Methodist Church
UnitedMethodist Camp Tekoa
P.O. Box 160
Hendersonville, NC 28793-0160 828-692-6516
FAX: 828-697-3288
e-mail: ecampbell@camptekoa.org
www.camptekoa.org

James Johnson, Exec. Dir.
John Isley, Assistant Director
Karen Rohrer, Business Mgr
Melisa Coates, Administrative Assistant

Camping for children with asthma/respiratory ailments, hearing impairment and developmental disabilities. Coed, ages 6-17.

1279 **SOAR Summer Adventures**
NC Base Camp
226 SOAR Lane
P.O.Box 388
Balsam, NC 28707-388 828-456-3435
FAX: 828-456-3449
e-mail: admissions@soarnc.org
www.soarnc.org

Jonathan Jones, Dir. Emeritus
Wandajean Jones, Dir. Emeritus
John Willson, M.S., LRT/CTR, Exec. Dir.
Laura Pate, Dir. of North Carolina Programs

A nonprofit adventure program working with disadvantaged youth diagnosed with learning disabilities in an outdoor, challenge based environment. Focuses on esteem building and social skills development through rock climbing, backpacking, white-water rafting, mountaineering, sailing, snorkeling, and much more. Offers two week, one month, and semester programs available. SOAR programs utilize North Carolina, Florida, Colorado, American Southwest, Alaska, and Jamaica as program areas.

1280 **Talisman Summer Camp**
64 Gap Creek Rd
Zirconia, NC 28790-8791
828-697-6313
855-588-8254
FAX: 828-697-6249
e-mail: info@talismancamps.com
talismancamps.com

Doug Smathers, Camp Director & Owner
Linda Tatsapaugh, Operations Director & Owner
Robiyn Mims, Admissions Director
Cory Greene, Program Manager

Camp is located in Black Mountain, North Carolina. Offers a program of hiking, rafting, climbing, and caving for learning disabled ADD/ADHD and autistic young people. Coed, ages 9-18.

1281 **Victory Junction Gang Camp**
4500 Adam's Way
Randleman, NC 27317
336-498-9055
877-854-2268
e-mail: info@victoryjunction.org
www.victoryjunction.org

Pattie Petty, Founder, Chairman & CEO
Kyle Petty, Founder; Vice-Chairman
Brian Flynn, Treasurer & Chief Operating Officer
Carolyn Bechtel, Member

The camp serves children with Autism, cancer, Craniofacial Anomalies, Diabetes, Sickle Cell and Spina Bifida.

Ohio

1282 **CYO Day Camp: Wickliffe**
Catholic Charities Health and Human Services
7911 Detroit Avenue
Cleveland, OH 44102-2815
216-334-2963
e-mail: contactus@clevelandcatholiccharities.org
ccdocle.org

Andrew Schuler, Chairman
Gerald Elliot, Vice Chairman
Tom Novak, Treasurer
Kathleen Homyock, Manager

Welcomes children and young adults ages 6-21 with cognitive (mr/dd) and other developmental disabilities, regardless of race, religion, culture or economic background.

1283 **Camp Allyn**
Stepping Stones Center
5650 Given Rd
Cincinnati, OH 45243-3426
513-831-4660
FAX: 513-831-5918
e-mail: info@steppingstonescenter.org
www.steppingstonescenter.org

Chris Adams, Exec. Dir.
Sam Browne Allen, Programs/Operations Dir.
Tim Stitzer, Dev. Dir.
CAS Brockman, Facilities/Support Svcs Dir.

A residential camp in Batavia, Ohio for children and adults with disabilities. Coed, ages 7-60. Campers participate in crafts, swimming, hiking, nature, sports and motor activities. Camp sessions range from 3 to 10 days, are theme oriented, and geared to individual abilities and interests. Also offers day camps for children ages 5-22.

1284 **Camp Cheerful**
Achievement Centers For Children
15000 Cheerful Ln
Strongsville, OH 44136-5420
440-238-6200
FAX: 440-238-1858
e-mail: connie.boros@achievementctrs.org
www.achievementcenters.org

Mozelle Jackson, Chairwoman
Julie Boland, Vice Chairwoman
Marvin A. Thomas, Jr, Treasurer
Jennifer Vergilli, Secretary

Sessions for campers with developmental disabilities, mobility limitation and speech/communication impairment. Coed, ages 7-99.

1285 **Camp Courageous**
12701 Waterville-Swanton Rd
Whitehouse, OH 43571-9551
419-875-6828
FAX: 419-875-5598
e-mail: camping@campcourageous.com
www.campcourageous.com

Steve Kiessling, Executive Director
Chelsea Banas

Camp Courageous provides residential camping services for people with developmental disabilities from ages 7-75 years old. Our six day, 5 night programs give campers a chance to experience activities such as: aquatics, arts and crafts, animal programs, sports skills, hiking, recreational and leisure education programs, nature studies, drama, cookouts and campfires.

1286 **Camp Emanuel**
P.O. Box 752343
Dayton, OH 45475
937-477-5504
e-mail: nan33@sbcglobal.net
www.campemanuel.weebly.com

Stephanie Ackner, President
Brain Demarke, Vice President
Mary Foreman, Secretary
Nan Crawford, Executive Director

Camp for hearing impaired and normal hearing youth.

1287 **Camp Happiness**
Catholic Charities Health & Human Services
7911 Detroit Road
Cleveland, OH 44102-2815
216-334-2963
e-mail: contactus@clevelandcatholiccharities.org
ccdocle.org

Andrew Schuler, Chairman
Gerald Elliot, Vice Chairman
Tom Novak, Treasurer
Kathleen Homyock, Manager

Offers a summer camp program for persons with developmental disabilities. Camp Happiness is a six-week day camp at several sites throughout the Diocese for individuals six years of age to 21 years of age.

1288 **Camp Ho Mita Koda**
Diabetes Association Of Greater Cleveland
3601 South Green Road
Suite 100
Cleveland, OH 44122-5719
216-591-0800
FAX: 216-591-0320
e-mail: information@diabetespartnership.org
www.dagc.org

Roger Ruch, Chair
William Murman, Vice Chair
Christina R. Milano, President & CEO
Lori Weinstein, Secretary

Camp is located in Newbury, Ohio. Summer sessions for children with type 1 diabetes. Coed, ages 6-15. Type 2 diabetes, coed, ages 12-17. Bicycle adventure, coed, ages 13-19. Mini-day camp, ages 4-7, coed.

1289 **Camp Ko-Man-She**
American Diabetes Association
2555 S Dixie Drive
Suite 112
Dayton, OH 45409
937-220-6611
FAX: 937-224-0240
e-mail: dada@diabetesdayton.org
www.diabetesdayton.org

Terry Fague, President
Tyler Starline, Vice President
Becky Roberts, Secretary
Michael Martens, Treasurer

Camp is located in Bellefontaine, Ohio. Summer sessions for children with diabetes. Coed, ages 8-17. Held in July.

1290 **Camp Libbey**
Maumee Valley Girl Scout Center
2244 Collingwood Blvd
Toledo, OH 43620-1147
419-243-8216
800-860-4516
FAX: 419-245-5357
e-mail: roniluckenbill@girlscoutsofwesternohio.org
www.girlscoutsofwesternohio.o rg

Jody Wainscott, Chair
Ellen Lobst, 1st Vice Chair
Ann Hartmann, 2nd Vice Chair
Kimber Fender, Secretary

Camp for girls 7-18 with asthma/respiratory ailments, diabetes, epilepsy and muscular dystrophy is located in Defiance, Ohio.

1291 **Camp Nuhop**
404 Hillcrest Dr
Ashland, OH 44805-4152
419-289-2227
e-mail: info@campnuhop.org
www.nuhop.org

Trevor Dunlap, CEO
Ann Bell, Summer Camp Director
Chris Clyde, Associate Director
Kristin Feldman, Director of Outdoor Education

A summer residential program for any youngster from 6 to 18 with a learning disability, behavior disorder or Attention Deficit Disorder. 84 campers and 41 staff members live on site in groups of to seven campers to every three counselors. Activities focus on positive self-concept and behaviors and teaches children to learn how to find their strengths, abilities and talents from a positive, yet realistic viewpoint.

1292 **Camp Quality Ohio**
1444 Mockingbird Circle
P.O. Box 264
Stow, OH 44224
330-671-0167
FAX: 866-285-5208
www.campqualityusa.com

Lois Hartje, President
Vicki Irey, Vice President
Dennis Hart, Secretary
Ptricia Harris, Executive Director

Camp Quality is for children with cancer and their siblings. The camp offers a stress-free environment that offers exciting activities and fosters new friendships, while helping to give the children courage, motivation and emotional strength.

1293 **Camp Stepping Stone**
Stepping Stones Center
5650 Given Rd
Cincinnati, OH 45243-3499
513-831-4660
FAX: 513-831-5918
www.steppingstonescenter.org

Jeremy Vaughan, President
John Mongelluzzo, Vice President
Whitney Wckert, Treasurer
Mark Robertson, Secretary

Day camp for children ages 5-22, serving persons with autism, cognitive deficits, Down Syndrome, cerebral palsy, brain injury, and multiple disabilities.

1294 **Echoing Hills**
36272 County Road 79
Warsaw, OH 43844-9770
800-419-6513
FAX: 740-327-6371
e-mail: info@echoinghillsvillage.org
www.echoinghillsvillage.org/

Buddy Busch, President
Larry Armentrout, Board of Director
Charles Bethel, Board of Director
Todd Imhoff, Board of Director

Summer camp for children and adults with cerebral palsy. Coed, ages 7-70.

1295 **Highbrook Lodge**
Cleveland Sight Center
1909 East 101st Street
P.O.Box 1988
Cleveland, OH 44106-188
216-791-8118
877-776-9563
e-mail: camp@clevelandsightcenter.org
www.clevelandsightcenter.org

William L. Spring, Chairman
Thomas P. Furnas, Vice Chairman
Gary W. Latz Poth, Treasurer
Steven M. Friedman, Ph.D., Executive Director

Camp is located in Chardon, Ohio. Summer sessions for children, adults and families who are blind or have low vision. There are seven sessions held annually through June, July and August with an wide range of outdoor camp activities. Camp activities focus on gaining independent skills, mobility, orientation and self confidence in an accessible and traditional camp setting.
220-660/session

1296 **Leo Yassenoff JCC Specialty Day Camp**
Jewish Community Center of Greater Columbus
1125 College Ave
Columbus, OH 43209-7802
614-231-2731
FAX: 614-231-8222
e-mail: cfolkerth@columbusjcc.org
www.columbusjcc.org

Carol Folkerth, Executive Director
Mike Klapper, Assistant Executive Director
Louise Young, Finance Director
Melanie Butter, Program Director

Summer camping sessions for children and young adults with developmental, physical, emotional, mental and learning disabilities. Coed, ages 3-25.

1297 **Recreation Unlimited: Day Camp**
Recreation Unlimited Foundation
7700 Piper Rd
Ashley, OH 43003-9741
740-548-7006
FAX: 740-747-2640
e-mail: info@recreationunlimited.org
www.recreationunlimited.org

Paul L. Huttlin, Executive Director & CEO
Chris Link, Operations Manager
David D. Hudler, Business Development Manager
Michelle Higgins, Billing Coordinator

Camping sessions for children and adults with a variety of disabilities. Coed, ages 5-99, families, seniors and single adults.

1298 **Recreation Unlimited: Residential Camp**
Recreation Unlimited Foundation
7700 Piper Rd
Ashley, OH 43003-9741
740-548-7006
FAX: 740-747-2640
e-mail: info@recreationunlimited.org
www.recreationunlimited.org

Paul L. Huttlin, Executive Director & CEO
Chris Link, Operations Manager
David D. Hudler, Business Development Manager
Michelle Higgins, Billing Coordinator

Camping sessions for children and adults with a variety of disabilities. Coed, ages 5-99, families, seniors and single adults.

1299 **Recreation Unlimited: Respite Weekend Camp**
Recreation Unlimited Foundation
7700 Piper Rd
Ashley, OH 43003-9741
740-548-7006
FAX: 740-747-2640
e-mail: info@recreationunlimited.org
www.recreationunlimited.org

Paul L. Huttlin, Executive Director & CEO
Chris Link, Operations Manager
David D. Hudler, Business Development Manager
Michelle Higgins, Billing Coordinator

Camping sessions for children and adults with a variety of disabilities. Coed, ages 5-99, families, seniors and single adults.

1300 **Recreation Unlimited: Specialty Camp**
Recreation Unlimited Foundation
7700 Piper Rd
Ashley, OH 43003-9741
740-548-7006
FAX: 740-747-2640
e-mail: info@recreationunlimited.org
www.recreationunlimited.org

Paul L. Huttlin, Executive Director & CEO
Chris Link, Operations Manager
David D. Hudler, Business Development Manager
Michelle Higgins, Billing Coordinator
Camping sessions for children and adults with a variety of disabilities. Coed, ages 5-99, families, seniors and single adults.

1301 **Rotary Camp**
Akron Area YMCA
4460 Rex Lake Dr
Akron, OH 44319-3430
330-644-4512
FAX: 330-644-1013
e-mail: rotarycamp@akronymca.org
www.akronymca.com

Dan Reynolds, Dir. of Endless Possibilities
Dawn Housley, Dir. of First Impressions
Joshua Strelbicki, The Innovator
Kristen Dunbar, Dir. of S'more Programs
Offers camping experiences for children and adults with disabilities. Rotary Camp is American Camping Association (ACA) accredited and provides a nurturing and enriching atmosphere where campers develop friendships, skills and memories that will last a lifetime. Coed, ages 6-17.

1302 **St. Augustine Rainbow Camp**
Disability Ministries at St. Augustine Parish
2486 W 14th St
Cleveland, OH 44113-4407
216-781-5530
FAX: 216-781-1124
e-mail: staugch@earthlink.net
www.staugustine-west14.org

Sr. Corita Ambro, CSJ, Program Dir.
Terry Hogan, Dir. of Special Religious Ed
Mary Ellen Czelusniak, Education Specialist
Mary Smith, Disability Advocate
Day camp for all children, disabled and non-disabled working together.

1303 **YMCA Outdoor Center Campbell Gard**
105 North Second Street
P.O. Box 13029
Hamilton, OH 45011
513-887-0001
877-224-9622
FAX: 513-887-0960
e-mail: contact@gmvymca.org
www.gmvymca.org

Jim Sexstone, Exec. Dir.
Pete Fasano, Outdoor School Program Dir.
Darren Corns, Special Needs Coordinator
Tom Andrews, Properties & Facilities Mgr
Camp is located in Hamilton, Ohio. Camping sessions for children with ADD, autism, developmental disabilities and blindness/visual impairment. Coed, ages 6-17 and families.

Oklahoma

1304 **Camp Classen YMCA**
YMCA of Greater Oklahoma City
500 NorthBroadway
Suite 500
Okhlama City, OK 73102-9405
405-297-7777
FAX: 580-369-2284
e-mail: bdoherty@ymcaokc.org
www.ymcaokc.org

Rick Warren, Property Manager
Heather Doherty, Outdoor School Coordinator
Bradley Doherty, Director of Camping
Russel Gholson, Equine Director
Camp is located in Davis, Oklahoma. Sessions for children and adults with diabetes. Coed, ages 8-17, families, seniors and single adults.

1305 **Camp Perfect Wings**
3800 N. May Avenue
Oklahoma City, OK 73112
405-942-3800
e-mail: info@bgco.org
www.bgco.org/campperfectwings

Amanda Davis, Camp Director
Becka Johnson, Camp Director
Keith Burkhart, BGCO Family Ministry
Jeremy Davis, BGCO Family Ministry
Specifically for children ages 8-17 with special needs. Campers enjoy canoeing, pool games, low ropes challenges, and crafts.

1306 **Easter Seals Oklahoma**
701 NE 13th St
Oklahoma City, OK 73104-5003
405-239-2525
FAX: 405-239-2278
e-mail: vwasinger@eastersealsoklahoma.org
www.ok.easterseals.com/

Rodney Burgamy, Chairman
Matt Vance, Chairman-Elect
Paula K. Porter, President & CEO
Jeb Reid, Treasurer
A nationally accredited, full-day program welcoming all children, including those with disabilities and those at risk of disability. The center offers developmentally appropriate learning activities and services to meet the unique needs of each child. Our Adult Day Health Center provides solutions to meet the physical, social and emotional needs of adults from the ages of 21 to 100+.

Oregon

1307 **Adventures Without Limits**
1341 Pacific Avenue
Forest Grove, OR 97116
503-359-2568
FAX: 503-359-4671
awloutdoors.com

Brad Bafaro, Volunteer Executive Director
Todd Gilstrap, Program Director
Adventures Without Limits facilitates inclusive, outdoor adventure for people of all ages and ability levels.

1308 **Camp Christmas Seal**
American Lung Association of Oregon
7420 SW Bridgeport Road
Suite 200
Tigard, OR 97224-7790
503-924-4094
FAX: 503-924-4120
e-mail: info@lungoregon.org
www.lung.org/associations/states/oregon/

Kathryn A Forbes, Chairman
David Pogue, Vice Chair
Harold Wimmer, President and Chief Executive Officer
Penny J. Siewert, Secretary/Treasurer
Camp is located in Sisterhood, Oregon. Sessions for children with asthma/respiratory ailments. Coed, ages 8-15.

1309 **Camp Easter Seals**
Easter Seals: Oregon
5757 SW Macadam Ave
Portland, OR 97239-3765
503-228-5108
800-556-6020
FAX: 503-228-1352
www.easterseals.com

Donna Waller, Executive Vice President
Sue Wimmer, Medical Rehabilitation Manager
Camp is located in Corbett, Oregon. Summer sessions for children and adults with a variety of disabilities. Coed, ages 6-90.

1310 **Camp Latgawa Special Needs, Inc.**
Oregon-Idaho Conference Center
13250 S Fork Little Butte Cr Rd
Eagle Point, OR 97524-5593 541-826-9699
e-mail: camplatgawa@hotmail.com
www.latgawa.gocamping.org/
Eva LaBonty, Camp Director
Greg Clensy, Camp Director
We are located in a beautiful, wooded area of the Rogue National Forest. Two gentle flowing creeks and towering evergreens provide a peaceful setting just 35 miles east of Medford, Oregon.

1311 **Camp Magruder**
Oregon-Idaho Conference Center
17450 Old Pacific Hwy
Rockaway Beach, OR 97136-9609 503-355-2310
FAX: 503-355-8701
e-mail: director@campmagruder.org
www.campmagruder.org
Steve Rumage, Camp Director
Amy Wood, Program Services Director
Angela Nebeker, Food Service Manager
Mark Burley Manager, Burley Manager
Camp is located in Rockaway Beach, Oregon. Sessions for children and adults with cancer and developmental disabilities. Coed, ages 9-18, families, seniors and single adults.

1312 **Camp Starlight**
P.O. Box 80666
Portland, OR 97280 503-964-1516
e-mail: info@camp-starlight.org
camp-starlight.org
Randy Bodkin, Camp Director
Camp Starlight is a week-long sleep-away summer camp for children in Oregon and Washington whose lives are affected by HIV/AIDS. Some of our campers are HIV+ themselves while others have someone in their immediate family- a parent, a sibling, a care-taker- who is infected.

1313 **Camp Taloali**
Lions Club of Oregon and Washington
P.O. Box 32
Stayton, OR 97383-9619 971-239-8153
FAX: 503-769-6415
TTY:503-400-6547
e-mail: camptaloali@comcast.net
www.taloali.org
Jeffrey Howard, Chair
Dave Taylor, Vice Chair
Carleene Iverson, Secretary
Anna Meliza, Treasurer
Summer sessions for children with hearing impairment. Coed, ages 9-17.

1314 **Gales Creek Diabetes Camp**
Gales Creek Camp Foundation
7110 SW Fir Loop
Suite 170
Portland, OR 97223-8136 503-968-2267
FAX: 503-443-2313
e-mail: info@galescreekcamp.org
www.galescreekcamp.org
Cheryl Sheppard, Executive Director
Eric Hanson, Development Specialist
Joannie Kono, RN, CDE
Camp is located in Forest Grove, Oregon. Summer sessions for children with diabetes. Coed, ages 6-16, family and pre-school family camps also available.

1315 **Hull Park**
43233 SE Oral Hull Road
Sandy, OR 97055 503-668-6195
e-mail: oralhull@gmail.com
oralhull.org
Gilbert Rivero, President
The Oral Hull Foundation for the Blind is dedicated to providing a special place for persons with blindness or low vision and their friends to get away for a day, weekend, or week for an exceptional experience.

1316 **Meadowood Springs Speech and Hearing Camp**
Institute for Rehab., Research, & Recreation Inc
316-A SE Emigrant
P.O. Box 1025
Pendleton, OR 97801-30 541-276-2752
FAX: 541-276-7227
e-mail: info@meadowoodsprings.org
www.meadowoodsprings.org
Michael Ashton, Executive Director
Kathy Hosek, Administrative Assistant
Cliff Story, Property Manager
Missy Newcomb, MS, CCC-SLP, Clinical Director
On 143 acres in the Blue Mountains of Eastern Oregon, this camp is designed to help young people who have diagnosed clinical disorders of speech, hearing or language. A full range of activities in recreational and clinical areas is available.

1317 **Mt Hood Kiwanis Camp**
Kiwanis Club of Montavilla
10725 Sw Barbur Blvd.
Suite 50
Portland, OR 97219 971-230-2921
FAX: 503-452-0062
e-mail: Kenney@mhkc.org
www.mhkc.org
Andy Jones, President
Kaleen Deatherage, Exec. Dir.
Terri Hammond, Mktg/Communications Dir.
Skye Burns, Development Director
Camp is located in Government Camp, Oregon. Summer sessions for children and adults with a variety of disabilities. Coed, ages 9-35.

1318 **Strength for the Journey**
Oregon-Idaho Conference Center
1505 SW 18th Ave
Portland, OR 97201-2524 800-593-7539
FAX: 503-228-3196
e-mail: camping@gocamping.org
www.getmorestrength.org/
Rev. Lisa Jean Hoefner, Executive Director
Geneva Cook, Registrar
Susan Delaney, Camping Office Assistant
Camp is located near Sisters, Oregon. For adults living with HIV/AIDS.

1319 **Suttle Lake Camp**
Oregon/Idaho Conference Center
29551 Suttle Lake Rd
Sisters, OR 97759-9508 541-595-6663
FAX: 503-228-3196
e-mail: suttlelake@gocamping.org
www.gbgm-umc.org/suttlelake/
Jane Petke, Camp Director
Daniel Petke, Facilities Director
Wendy White, Food Service
Steven Willson, Camping Ministry Intern
Camp is located in Sisters, Oregon. Camping sessions for children and adults with HIV. Coed, ages 6-18, families, seniors and single adults.

1320 **Upward Bound Camp for Persons With**
P.O.Box C
Stayton, OR 97383-90 503-897-2447
FAX: 503-897-4116
e-mail: upward.bound.camp@gmail.com
www.upwardboundcamp.org

1321 **Wallowa Lake Camp**
Oregon-Idaho Conference Center
84522 Church Ln
Joseph, OR 97846
541-432-1271
e-mail: wallowa@gocamping.org
www.wallowalakecamp.org

David Cook, Manager
Ingrid Cook, Manager
Camp offers volleyball, baseball, badminton, horseshoes, crafts, nature viewing and more

1322 **YWCA Camp Westwind**
YWCA of Greater Portland
1111 SW 10th Ave
Portland, OR 97205-2496
503-294-7400
FAX: 503-794-7399
e-mail: connect@ywcapdx.org
www.ywcapdx.org

Robert Mccarthy, President
Susan Stoltenberg, Executive Director
Janette McMurran - Kunkel, Camp Director
Sarah Keplinger, Camp Westwind Office Manager
Promotes the understanding of racism and all forms of discrimination and fosters value, respect, and enjoyment of each person's unique contribution.

Pennsylvania

1323 **Achieva**
711 Bingham St
Pittsburgh, PA 15203-1007
412-995-5000
888-272-7229
FAX: 412-995-5001
e-mail: nmurray@achieva.info
www.achieva.info

Marsha S. Blanco, President and CEO
Gary K. Horner, Executive Vice President
Reid Wolfe, Senior Vice President
Nancy J. Murray, President
Life-long services for people with disabilities.

1324 **Camp AIM**
South Hills YMCA
51 McMurray Road
Pittsburgh, PA 15241
412-833-5600
FAX: 412-653-7115
e-mail: campaiminfo@gmail.com
www.campaim.org

Paulette Colonna, Camp Administrator
Tom DiPietro, Camp Director
Julie Blanc, Administrative Assistant
Sarah Kettell, Activities Director
It is the goal of our program to create an environment that offers a variety of activities centered on positive recreational and social interactions that enrich the lives of our campers. Our staff and volunteers are dedicated to this endeavor.

1325 **Camp Can Do**
Easter Seals: Southeastern Pennsylvania
233 South Wacker Drive
Suite 2400
Chicago, IL 60606-333
215-263-7000
800-221-6827
FAX: 215-368-1199
www.easterseals.com

Richard W. Davidson, Chairman
Sandra L. Bouwman, 1st Vice Chairman
Joseph G. Kern, 2nd Vice Chairman
Ralph F. Boyd, Jr., Treasurer
Camp is located in Kulpsville, Pennsylvania. Summer sessions for children and young adults with a variety of disabilities. Coed, ages 5-21

1326 **Camp Dunmoreia**
Easter Seals: Southeastern Pennsylvania
468 N Middletown Rd
Media, PA 19063-5506
610-565-2353
FAX: 610-565-5256
e-mail: recreation@easterseals-sepa.org
www.easterseals-sepa.org

Roy Yaffe, President
Linda A. McDevitt, Vice President
Cummins Catherwood, Secretary
Linda A. McDevitt, Vice President
Summer sessions for children and young adults with a variety of disabilities. Coed, ages 5-21.

1327 **Camp Joy**
9812 Falls Road
Ste. 114-331
Potomac, MD 20854-1518
610-754-6878
888-694-6735
FAX: 610-754-7880
e-mail: contact@DomainMarket.com
www.campjoy.com

1328 **Camp Kweebec**
P.O.Box 511
Narberth, PA 19072-511
610-667-2123
FAX: 610-667-6376
e-mail: info@kweebec.com
www.kweebec.com

Les Weiser, Director
Maddy Weiser, Director
Josh Weiser, Associate Director
Amy Weiser, Associate Director
Camp is located in Schwenksville, Pennsylvania. Sessions for children and adults with diabetes. Coed, ages 6-16, families, seniors and single adults.

1329 **Camp Lee Mar**
805 Redgate Rd
Dresher, PA 19025-1432
215-658-1708
FAX: 215-658-1710
e-mail: gtour400@aol.com
www.leemar.com

Ari Segal, Exec. Dir.
Lee Morrone, Dir. and Founder
Laura Leibowitz, Assistant Director
Lynsey Trohoske, Program Director
Seven week summer camp for children and young adults with mild to moderate developmental disabilities. 5-21 years of age

1330 **Camp Make-a-Friend**
Easter Seals: Southeastern Pennsylvania
233 South Wacker Drive
Suite 2400
Chicago, IL 60606-5426
215-263-7000
800-221-6827
FAX: 215-879-8424
e-mail: recreation@easterseals-sepa.org
www.easterseals.com

Richard W. Davidson, Chairman
Sandra L. Bouwman, 1st Vice Chairman
Joseph G. Kern, 2nd Vice Chairman
Ralph F. Boyd, Jr., Treasurer
Mission is to create solutions that change lives of children and adults with disabilities or other special needs and their families.

1331 **Camp Ramah in the Poconos Education, Inc.**
2100 Arch Street
Philadelphia, PA 19103
215-885-8556
FAX: 215-885-8905
e-mail: info@ramahpoconos.org
www.ramahpoconos.org

Rabbi Joel Seltzer, Director
Michelle Sugarman, Assistant Director
Bruce Lipton, Director of Finance & Operation
Susan Ansul, Director

The Camp Ramah Tikvah Family Camp is located in Lakewood, Pennsylvania. It has a week-long camp in mid-August for families who have children with special needs.

1332 Camp Setebaid
Setebaid Services
P.O.Box 196
Winfield, PA 17889-196
570-524-9090
e-mail: info@setebaidservices.org
www.setebaidservices.org

Mark Moyer, Executive Director
Suzanne Lee, Director
David E. Keefer, Vice President
Peggy Coleman, Director

Camping sessions for children with diabetes. Coed, ages 3-13 years. Family retreat for children with diabetes and their families.

1333 Camp Surefoot Center
Easter Seals: Southeastern Pennsylvania
233 South Wacker Drive
Suite 2400
Chicago, IL 60606-5426
215-263-7000
800-221-6827
FAX: 215-945-4073
e-mail: recreation@easterseals-sepa.org
www.easterseals.com

Richard W. Davidson, Chairman
Sandra L. Bouwman, 1st Vice Chairman
Joseph G. Kern, 2nd Vice Chairman
Ralph F. Boyd, Jr., Treasurer

Camp is located in Levittown, Pennsylvania. Sessions for children and young adults with a variety of disabilities. Coed, ages 5-21.

1334 Camp Victory
58 Camp Victory Road
Millville, PA 17846
570-458-6530
www.campvictory.org

Dennis Wolff, President
Paul Kettlewell, Vice President
Art Girio, Vice President
Kathy Fries, Secretary

At Camp Victory, partner groups with specialized knowledge and training provide camping opportunities for children with chronic health problems or physical or mental challenges. We believe that by sharing their challenges with each other in the relaxed atmosphere of a summer camp, the children become mutually supportive, teaching each other confidence, courage, and self-esteem.

1335 Camp Wesley Woods: Northeastern Pennsylvan
Western PA United Methodist Church
1001 Fiddlersgreen Rd
Grand Valley, PA 16420-4429
814-436-7802
FAX: 814-436-7669
e-mail: info@wesleywoods.com
www.wesleywoods.com

Rick Frederick, Exec. Dir.
Marie Goodwill, Mktg Asst.
Andy Blystone, Programs and Mktg Dir.

Exceptional children's camp for children with emotional and intellectual handicaps.

1336 Camp Woodlands
134 Shenot Road
Wexford, PA 15090
724-935-6533
FAX: 724-935-6511
www.woodlandsfoundation.org

1337 Dragonfly Forest Summer Camp
1485 Valley Forge Road
Phoenixville, PA 19460
610-298-1820
FAX: 267-434-0100
e-mail: info@dragonflyforest.org
www.dragonflyforest.org

Dennis Wolff, President
Paul Kettlewell, Vice President
Art Girio, Vice President
Kathy Fries, Secretary

Dragonfly Forest Summer Camp program, provides children with Autism and medical needs the opportunity to enjoy an overnight camp experience in an environment that is safe, equipped to meet a variety of physical, medical, and psychological needs, nurturing, and filled with activities that allow each child to reach their full fun.

1338 Elling Camps
1635 State Route 2036
Thompson, PA 18465-9100
570-756-2660
FAX: 570-756-3083
e-mail: info@camptioga.com
www.camptioga.com

Ron Kuznetz, President
Dale Kuznetz, Camp Director
Mike Wagenberg, Camp Director
Mike Kuznetz, Camp Director

For youth ages 6-21 with learning disabilities and accompanying difficulties. This camp allows them to learn to adjust socially in a community atmosphere. The structured camp program includes land and water sports, nature and forestry, industrial arts, construction and work programs, and arts and crafts.

1339 Handi Camp
Handi Vangelism Ministries International
P.O.Box 122
Akron, PA 17501-122
717-859-4777
FAX: 717-859-4505
e-mail: info@hvmi.org
www.hvmi.org

Tim Sheetz, Exec. Dir.
Steve Gentino, Chief Financial Officer
Kathy Sheetz, Exec. Secretary
Brian Robinson, Assistant Director

Christian, overnight camping program for people with disabilities, ages 7-50, in Eastern PA and Southern NJ. Sponsored by Handi Vangelism Ministries International.

1340 Innabah Camps
United Methodist Church: Eastern Pennsylvania
712 Pughtown Rd
Spring City, PA 19475-3311
610-469-6111
FAX: 610-469-0330
e-mail: camp@innabah.org
www.innabah.org

Dan Lebo, Director
Katie MacFarlan, Program Manager
Erin Slye, Registrar
Gina L. James, Business Manager

Sessions for children and young adults with developmental disabilities. Ages 4-18, families and seniors.

1341 Lions Camp Kirby
1735 Narrows Hill Rd
Upper Black Eddy, PA 18972-9712
610-982-5731
e-mail: info@lionscampkirby.org
www.lionscampkirby.org

Alice Breon, Camp Director

Offers 4-week camps for deaf and hearing impaired children and their siblings in eastern Pennsylvania.

1342 Mainstay Life Services Summer Program
200 Roessler Road
Pittsburgh, PA 15220
412-344-3640
FAX: 412-344-5486
mainstaylifeservices.org

James R. Kirk, CEO

Mainstay Life Services' Summer program is a unique, urban camping experience. The program runs for four weeks in July with extended, overnight stay on a college campus in Pittsburgh, Pennsylvania. One and two week sessions are offered.

1343 **Outside In School Of Experiential**
P.O.Box 639
Greensburg, PA 15601-639 724-837-1518
FAX: 724-837-0801
e-mail: administration@outsideinschool.com
www.myoutsidein.org
Michael C. Henkel, Executive Director
Camp is located in Bolivar, Pennsylvania. Sessions for children with ADD and substance abuse problems. Boys 11-18 and girls 13-18.

1344 **Phelps School Summer School**
583 Sugartown Rd
Malvern, PA 19355-2800 610-644-1754
FAX: 610-644-6679
e-mail: admis@thephelpsschool.org
www.thephelpsschool.org
Michael J. Reardon, Head of School
Stephany Phelps Fahey, President
Gerald D. Fahey, Treasurer
Andrew Wilmerding, Secretary
Open for grades 7-11 to make up academic deficiencies or complete studies in English, math and reading. Sports include riding, tennis and swimming. A program is also available to a limited number of international students in English as a Second Language.

1345 **Sequanota Lutheran Conference Center and Camp**
P.O. Box 245
Jennerstown, PA 15547 814-629-6627
FAX: 814-629-0128
e-mail: contact@sequanota.com
www.sequanota.com/
Rev. Carol Custead, President
David Shoemaker, Vice President
Bob Coleman, Treasurer
Megan Will, Secretary
Summer sessions for adults with developmental disabilities and speech/communication impairment.

1346 **Variety Club Camp & Developmental**
2950 Potshop Road
P.O.Box 609
Worcester, PA 19490-609 610-584-4366
FAX: 610-584-5586
www.varietyphila.org
Douglas I. Zeiders, Esq., President
John Bruke, Vice President
Donald F. Faul, Treasurer
Robert George, Secretary
Year-round camping and recreation facility for children with special needs and their families. Includes summer camping, aquatics, weekend retreats and other specialty programs. Coed, ages 5-21.

1347 **YMCA Camp Fitch**
The YMCA's Camp Fitch On Lake Erie
12600 Abels Rd
North Springfield, PA 16430-1014 814-922-3219
877-863-4824
FAX: 814-922-7000
e-mail: info@campfitchymca.org
www.varietyphila.org
Brian Rupe, Executive Director
Matt Poese, Associate Executive Director
Kelly Poese, Summer Program Director
Jim Campbell, Office Manager
Camp is located in North Springfield, Pennsylvania. Camping sessions for children and adults with diabetes, hearing impairment, developmental disabilities, mobility limitation and speech/communication impairment. Ages 8-16, families and seniors.

Rhode Island

1348 **Camp Mauchatea**
Rhode Island Lions Sight Foundation, Inc.
P.O. Box 284
Greenville, RI 02828 401-949-2442
e-mail: ralpheiannitelli@aol.com
www.lions4sight.org
Ralph E. Iannitelli, Development Director
Jay Ward Providence, President
Gary W. Latz Westerly, Secretary
William Scot Narragansett, Treasurer
Camp serving those who are blind/visually impaired. Campers enjoy developing and maintaining friendships with fellow campers. Some of the activities include boating and other water sports, as well as hiking and nature studies.

1349 **Camp Ruggles**
PO Box 353
Chepachet, RI 02814 401-567-8914
e-mail: info@ricamps.org
www.ricamps.org
Peter Swain, President
Camp Ruggles is located in Glocester, RI, and is a summer day camp for emotionally handicapped children. The Camp offers a 6 week co-ed summer session for 60 children ages 6-12.

1350 **Canonicus Camp**
American Baptist Churches Rhode Island
54 Exeter Road
Exeter, RI 02822-503 401-294-6318
800-294-6318
FAX: 401-294-7780
e-mail: camp@canonicus.org
www.canonicus.org
Linda Martin, Conference Coordinator
Shyral Wallis, Hospitality
Linda Martin, Conference Coordinator
Matt Black, Facilities Manager
Summer sessions for children with asthma/respiratory ailments. Coed, ages 4-18.

1351 **Hasbro Children's Hospital Asthma Camp**
593 Eddy Street
Providence, RI 02903 401-444-4000
e-mail: webteam@lifespan.org.
www.hasbrochildrenshospital.org/services/asth
Timothy J. Babineau,MD, President & CEO
Fred Macri, Executive Vice President
Mamie Wakefield, Executive Vice President
Myra Edens, RN, Administrative Director
Camp for children with asthma. Children learn about asthma and asthma management through interactive, educational and fun activities. The camp also offers activities such as swimming, canoeing and arts & crafts.

South Carolina

1352 **Burnt Gin Camp**
SC Department of Health and Environmental Control
P.O.Box 101106
Mills-Jarrett Complex
Columbia, SC 29011 803-898-0784
FAX: 803-898-0613
e-mail: aimonemi@dhec.sc.gov
www.scdhec.gov
Marie I Aimone, Camp Director
A residential camp for children who have physical disabilities and/or chronic illnesses. Camper/staff ratio is 2:1. Five seven-day sessions for 7-15 year olds and one six-day session for 16-19 year olds. Limited to residents of South Carolina.

1353 **Camp Adam Fisher**
P.O. Box 5226
Columbia, SC 29250
803-434-2442
e-mail: scottm14@earthlink.net
www.campadamfisher.com
Elizabeth Todd-Heckel, Program Director
Scott McFarland, Camp Director
For children with diabetes and their siblings. Campers enjoy swimming, horseback riding, tubing, basketball, volleyball and arts & crafts, while also learning how to manage their diabetes so they can live longer, healthier lives.

1354 **Camp Debbie Lou**
726 Lucky Run
Latta, SC 29565
843-752-5416
e-mail: info@campdebbielou.com
www.campdebbielou.com

1355 **Camp Gravatt**
1006 Camp Gravatt Rd
Aiken, SC 29805-8730
803-648-1817
FAX: 803-648-7453
e-mail: office@bishopgravatt.org
www.bishopgravatt.org
Lauri SoJourner Yeargin, Executive Director
Tammy Ayotte, Conference Center Director
Thomas K. Coleman, Program Director
Meredith Cook, Camp Director
Project adventure includes swimming, fishing, music and art and more in which disabled campers participate. Enjoy the fun and adventure of exploring a river in a canoe in the new canoe program. Title: Gravatt Camp and Conference Center

1356 **Camp Spearhead**
Greenville County Recreation District
4806 Old Spartanburg Road
Taylors, SC 29687
864-288-6470
FAX: 864-288-6499
e-mail: randy@gcrd.org
www.campspearhead.org
Gene Smith, Director
Gene Smith, Executive Director
Chanell Moore, Deputy Director
Don Shuman, Parks Director
Camp for children with disabilities age 8 years and up. The mission of Camp Spearhead is to provide an environment of unconditional acceptance for children and adults with disabilities. A caring staff, creative programming, and a state-of-the-art campsite all combine to offer a safe and nurturing camp experience for every camper.

South Dakota

1357 **Camp Friendship**
P.O. Box 1986
Rapid City, SD 57709
e-mail: campfriendshipdirector@hotmail.com
www.campfriendship.org
Kristi Berg, Camp Director
Nancy Clary, Camp Historian
Stacie Kellogg, Assistant Director in Training
Kathleen Haibeck
Held in the Black Hills of South Dakota, Camp Friendship is for individuals with physical and developmental disabilities. Campers go fishing, swimming, have cook outs and sing-a-longs, and just have fun!

1358 **Camp Gilbert**
Sanford Children's Specialty Clinic
1305 W. 18th Street
P.O. Box 89406
Sioux Falls, SD 57109-9406
605-328-0781
800-850-0064
e-mail: campgilbertinfo@gmail.com
www.campgilbert.com
Kay Schroeder, Pediatric Dietician
Nancy Hartung, Staffing/Treasurer
For children ages 8-18 with diabetes. Campers can enjoy a week of canoeing, swimming, sing-a-longs, crafts, and games, while also attending educational programs covering nutrition, exercise and lifestyle management.

1359 **NeSoDak**
Lutherans Outdoors in South Dakota
3285 Camp Dakota Dr.
Waubay, SD 57273
605-947-4440
800-888-1464
e-mail: nesodak@losd.org
www.losd.org/nesodak/index.html
Teri Gayer, Director
Rachel Nelson, Assistant Director
Nathan Skadsen, Program Director
Camp is located in Waubay, South Dakota. Sessions for children with diabetes. Coed, ages 8-18.

Tennessee

1360 **ACM Lifting Lives Music Camp**
Vanderbilt Kennedy Center
Vanderbilt University
110 Magnolia Circle
Nashville, TN 37203-5721
615-322-8240
www.kc.vanderbilt.edu/site/services/page.aspx
Tracy P. Beard, Assistant Director
Kylie Beck, Art Director
Tammy Day, Program Director
A camp for individuals with developmental disabilities where they can come to celebrate music by participating in songwriting workshops, recording sessions and live performances.

1361 **All Days Are Happy Days Summer Camp**
Boling Center
711 Jefferson Avenue
Memphis, TN 38105
901-448-6511
888-572-2249
FAX: 901-448-7097
TTY: 901-448-4677
www.uthsc.edu/bcdd/training/community/ADHDcam
Belinda Hardy, Director
Week long camp for children ages 6-11 years of age who have been diagnosed with ADHD. The primary goal is to educate campers and their parents about the diagnosis, treatment, and self-management of ADHD and related behaviors.

1362 **Bill Rice Ranch**
627 Bill Rice Ranch Road
Murfreesboro, TN 37128-4555
615-893-2767
800-253-7423
FAX: 615-898-0656
e-mail: info@billriceranch.org
www.billriceranch.org
Wil Rice IV, President
Troy Carlson, Director
Nathan McConnell, Deaf Ministries Director
Camping for hearing impaired children and youths ages 9-19.

1363 **Camp Discovery**
Tennessee Jaycees and Tennessee Jaycee Foundation
400 Camp Discovery Ln
Gainesboro, TN 38562-6161 931-268-0239
FAX: 931-268-6737
e-mail: director@jayceecamp.org
www.jayceecamp.org

Dawn Hickman, PhD., Vice President of Camp Operation
Paul Ottinger, Camp Director
Chester Lowe, Vice President of Camp Operations
Millie Dawkins, Camp Off Season Rentals
Serves children with skin conditions including: Epidermolysis Bullosa, Psoriasis, Alopecia, Vitiligo, Eczema, Scleroderma, Congenital Nevus, Ehlers-Danlos, Ichthyosis, Ectodermal Dysplasia and more. The Camp is located at 400 Camp Discovery Lane in Gainsboro, TN.

1364 **Camp Koinonia**
University Of Tennessee
1914 Andy Holt Avenue
HPER Building 361
Knoxville, TN 37996-2700 865-974-1288
FAX: 865-974-8981
e-mail: ghayes1@utk.edu
www.thecampkoinonia.com
Joseph L. Ortiz, President
J.D. King, Vice President
Dr. Gene A. Hayes, Executive Director
Angela Wozencroft, Secretary
Outdoor education program for children and young adults ages 7-22 who have multiple disabilities. The camp offers recreational activities such as canoeing, music and games.

1365 **Camp Okawehna**
1633 Church Street
Suite 500
Nashville, TN 37203 615-327-3061
FAX: 605-329-2513
e-mail: CampO@dciinc.org
www.dciinc.org/camp_info.php
Andy Parker, Camp Director
Week-long summer camp for critically ill children ages 6-18 years suffering from kidney disease. Children who have had kidney transplants as well as children on hemodialysis and peritoneal dialysis are welcome. The camp focuses on the critically ill child who needs to have fun and be in the company of other children who suffer from the same disease.

1366 **Camp Sugar Falls**
American Diabetes Association
4205 Hillsboro Road
Suite 200
Nashville, TN 37215 615-298-3066
888-342-2383
www.childrenwithdiabetes.com/camps/campsugarf
Devin Anna Bradford
Week long camp for children ages 6-12 who have diabetes and their siblings. Activities include education sessions, athletics and exercise.

1367 **Easter Seals Tennessee Camping Program**
Easter Seals Tennessee - State Headquarters
3011 Armory Drive
Suite 100
Nashville, TN 37204 615-292-6640
FAX: 615-251-0994
TTY:615-385-3485
www.easterseals.com

Mike Campbell, Chairman
John Pfeiffer, Vice Chairman
Jeff Bridges, Treasurer
Gay Bruner, Camp Director
Offers a variety of services to people with disabilities.

1368 **Indian Creek Camp**
Kentucky Tennessee Conference
150 Cabin Circle Dr.
Liberty, TN 37095 615-548-4411
FAX: 615-548-4029
e-mail: info@indiancreekcamp.com
www.indiancreekcamp.com

Ken Wetmore, Director
Marty Sutton, Assistant Director
Will Anderson, Business
Toni Stephens, Program Director
Camp is located in Liberty, Tennessee. Summer sessions for children and adults who are blind/visually impaired. Coed, ages 7-17, families and seniors.

1369 **LeBonheur Cardiac Kids Camp**
LeBonheur Children's Hospital
50 N. Dunlap
Memphis, TN 38103 901-287-6270
FAX: 901-287-4646
e-mail: cardiac@lebonheur.org
www.lebonheur.org/articles/registration-infor
Meri Armour, M.S.N., M.B.A., Camp Director
Bill May, M.D., M.B.A, Camp Administrator
Larry Spratlin, M.B.A
Dave Rosenbaum
Camp for children and young adults ages 8-16 with cardiac-related diagnoses. Children enjoy a fun-filled week at camp where they learn about their heart conditions and meet other children just like them.

1370 **Paddy Rossbach Youth Camp**
Amputee Coalition Of America
900 East Hill Avenue
Suite 290
Knoxville, TN 37915-2566 888-267-5669
TTY:865-525-4512
www.amputee-coalition.org
Dennis Strickland, Chairman
Jeffrey S. Lutz, Vice Chair
Kendra Calhoun, President & Chief Executive Offi
Mahesh Mansukhani, Secreatry
Georgia camp for youths ages 10-17 years of age who have limb loss or limb difference. Activities include sports, swimming, fishing, arts and crafts.

Texas

1371 **Camp CAMP**
P.O.Box 27086
San Antonio, TX 78227-86 210-671-5411
FAX: 210-671-5225
e-mail: campmail@campcamp.org
www.campcamp.org

Fred Swaney, Chairman
Mike Zerda, Vice Chairman
Jean Magargee, Treasurer
Toni Hill, Secretary
Camping for children and young adults with a variety of disabilities. Coed, ages 5-21. Respite services throughout calendar year. Adult camp ages 22-45.

1372 **Camp John Marc**
Special Camps for Special Kids
2824 Swiss Ave
Dallas, TX 75204-5956 214-360-0056
FAX: 214-368-2003
e-mail: mail@campjohnmarc.org
www.campjohnmarc.org

Vance C. Gilmore, Vice Chair
J. Marc Myers, Chairman
Bettye Slaven,, Executive Director
Dean A. Renkes
Camp is located in Meridian, Texas. Year-round camping for children with a variety of disabilities. Coed, ages 6-16 and families.

1373 **Camp Quality Texas**
1444 Mockingbird Circle
P.O. Box 264
Stow, OH 44224 330-671-0167
FAX: 866-285-5208
www.campqualityusa.com

Lois Hartje, President
Vicki Irey, Vice President
Dennis Hart, Secretary
Ptricia Harris, Executive Director

Camp Quality is for children with cancer and their siblings. The camp offers a stress-free environment that offers exciting activities and fosters new friendships, while helping to give the children courage, motivation and emotional strength.

1374 **Camp Summit**
17210 Campbell Road
Suite 180-W
Dallas, TX 75252-4202 972-484-8900
FAX: 972-620-1945
e-mail: camp@campsummittx.org
www.campsummittx.org

Carla R. Weiland, President/CEO
Lisa Braziel, Camp Director
Kristi Colunga, Executive Assistant
Dana Zimmerman, Assistant Camp Director

Camp is located in Argyle, Texas. Camping for children and adults with a variety of disabilities. Coed, ages 6-99.

1375 **Camp Sweeney**
Southwestern Diabetic Fund
P.O.Box 918
Gainesville, TX 76241-918 940-665-2011
FAX: 940-665-9467
e-mail: info@campsweeney.org
www.campsweeney.org

Ernie Fernandez

Teaches self-care and self-reliance to children ages 7-18 with diabetes. Campers participate in such activities such as swimming, fishing, horseback riding and arts and crafts while learning about how to self manage their diabetes.

1376 **Camp for All**
Camp for All Foundation
6301 Rehburg Rd
Burton, TX 77835-5675 979-289-3752
FAX: 979-289-5046
e-mail: campsite@campforall.org
www.campforall.org

Liz Rigney, Chairman
Pat Prior Sorrells, President and CEO
Belinda Munsell, Development Director
Kurt R. Podeszwa, Camp Director

Fully-accessible year round camp facility is located in Burton, Texas. Camping for children and adults with a variety of disabilities. Coed, ages 5-35 and up and families.

1377 **Dallas Academy**
950 Tiffany Way
Dallas, TX 75218-2743 214-324-1481
FAX: 214-327-8537
e-mail: mail@dallas-academy.com
www.dallas-academy.com

Troy Sturrock, Chair
Terrence S. Welch, Vice Chair
Dallas Cothrum, Secretary
Redonna Higgins, Treasurer

7-week summer session for students who are having difficulty in regular school classes.

1378 **Growing Together Diabetes Camp**
1000 S. Beckham
P.O. Box 6400
Tyler, TX 75711-6400 903-596-3645
800-232-8318
www.etmc.org/diabetes_day_camp.htm

Anjani Upponi, Camp Director
Vicki Jowell, Director
Dr. Stella Hecker, Medical Director

A summer camp for youths ages 6 to 15 with Type 1 or Type 2 diabetes.

1379 **Hill School of Fort Worth**
4817 Odessa Avenue
Fort Worth, TX 76133-1640 817-923-9482
FAX: 817-923-4894
e-mail: hillschool@hillschool.org
www.hillschool.org

Roxann Breyer, Principal
Audrey Boda-Davis, Executive Director
Janet Smith, Account & Record Manager
Meri Perryman, Business Manager

Provides an alternative learning environment for students having average or above-average intelligence with learning differences. Hill school is an established leader in North Texas with a 25 year history of effectively serving LD children. Beginning in 1961 as a tutorial service, Hill became a formal school in 1973. Our mission is to help those who learn differently develop skills and strategies to succeed. We do this by developing academic/study skills, and self-discipline.

1380 **Texas Lions Camp**
Lions Club Of Texas
P.O.Box 290247
Kerrville, TX 78029-247 830-896-8500
FAX: 830-896-3666
e-mail: tlc@ktc.com
www.lionscamp.com

Stephen Mabry, Executive Director

The primary purpose of the League shall be to provide, without charge, a camp for physically disabled, hearing/vision impaired and diabetic children from the State of Texas, regardless of race, religion, or national origin. Our goal is to create an atmosphere wherein campers will learn the can do philosophy and be allowed to achieve maximum personal growth and self-esteem. The camp welcomes boys and girls ages 7-16.

Utah

1381 **Camp Hobe**
P.O. Box 520755
Salt Lake City, UT 84152-755
e-mail: wapitimama@camphobekids.org
www.camphobekids.org

Chris Beckwith, Camp Director

A special summer camp for children with cancer and their siblings.

1382 **Camp Kostopulos**
Kostopulos Dream Foundation
4180 Emigration Canyon Road
Salt Lake City, UT 84108 801-582-0700
FAX: 801-583-5176
e-mail: information@campk.org
www.campk.org

Rex Wheeler, President
Brad Bruschke, Vice-President
David Traveller, Treasurer
Chris Agnello, Board Member

Summer camping for children and adults ages 7-65 with a variety of disabilities. Year round recreation on site and community based activities.

1383 **Camp Nah-Nah-Mah**
University Health Care Burn Camp Programs
50 N. Medical Drive
Salt Lake City, UT 84132 801-581-2121

www.uuhsc.utah.edu

Brad Wiggins, Burn Camp Director
For children ages 6-12 years of age that are burn survivors. Some of the activities include canoeing, rock climbing and archery.

1384 **FCYD Camp**
Foundation for Children and Youth with Diabetes
1995 West 9000 South
West Jordan, UT 84088 801-566-6913

www.fcydcamp.org

David Okubo, MD, Co-Founder, Trustee
Elizabeth Elmer, Co-Founder, Trustee
Sherrie Hardy, RD, MS, CDE, Co-Founder, Trustee
Nathan Gedge, Co-Founder, Trustee
Camping for children with diabetes. Coed, ages 1-18 and families.

1385 **Kris' Camp**
1132 Green Hill Trace
Tallahassee, FL 32317 850-445-4821
FAX: 877-267-9451
e-mail: info@kriscamp.org
www.kriscamp.org

Kathy Berger, PT, Executive Director
Michelle Hardy, MT-BC, NMT, Board of Director
Sue Yudovin, Board of Director
Chris McHorney, Board of Director
For children with autism.

Vermont

1386 **Camp Betsey Cox**
140 Betsey Cox Lane
Pittsford, VT 05763 802-483-6611

e-mail: info@campbetseycox.com
www.campbetseycox.com

Lorrie Byrom, Director and Co-Owner
Mike Byron, Co-owner and Associate Director
Devri Byrom, Winter Office Director
Camp is located in Pittsford, Vermont. Summer sessions for girls aged 9-15 with ADD.

1387 **Camp Thorpe**
680 Capen Hill Road
Goshen, VT 05733 802-247-6611

e-mail: cthorpe@sover.net
www.campthorpe.org

Lyle Jepson, Director
Elizabeth Giard, Board of Trustee
Richard Giard, Board of Trustee
Ralph O. Hathaway, Board of Trustee
Focuses on meeting the needs of each individual camper; showing each of them that they have the ability and potential. Also provides positive camping experience for children challenged with handicapping conditions.

1388 **Silver Towers Camp**
56 Silver Towers Rd
Ripton, VT 5766 802-388-6446
FAX: 877-417-7661
e-mail: info@vtelks.org
www.vtelks.org/programs/silver-towers/

Carolyn Ravenna, Camp Director
Carl Colburn, VEA State President, Camp Committee Chairman
Two-week residential camp for ages 6-75 who are physically or mentally challenged. Campers gain the social skills and personal enrichment they seek. Activities include swimming, horseback riding, music, sing-a-longs, dancing, nature studies and more.

Virginia

1389 **Adventure Camp**
Amputee Coalition Of America
P.O. Box 485
Lovingston, VA 22949 434-263-5432

e-mail: adventurecampinc@aol.com
www.adventurecampinc.org

Mary Grant, President
Karen Johnson, VP
Ed Hicks, Treasurer
Jennifer Puskaric, Secretary
Adventure Camp is held each summer for children and adolescents with limb loss. Activities include swimming, ropes course, canoeing, fishing, golf, scavenger hunts, karaoke and much more.

1390 **Adventure Day Camp**
3480 Commission Ct
Lake Ridge, VA 22192 703-491-1444

e-mail: office@princewilliamacademy.com
www.princewilliamacademy.com

Dr. Samia Harris, Founder, Executive Director
Joy Dwyer, Admissions Director
Rebecca Nykwest, PhD, Director of Communications
Lindsay Chickering, Office Manager
Camping for children with asthma/respiratory ailments and cancer. Coed, ages 2-13.

1391 **Camp Dickenson**
Holston Conference of United Methodist Church
801 Camp Dickson Ln
Fries, VA 24330-4348 276-744-7241

e-mail: campdickenson@centurylink.net
www.holston.org/

Michael Snow, Manager
Camp is located in Fries, Virginia. Camping for children and adults with developmental disabilities. Coed, ages 5-18, families, seniors and single adults.

1392 **Camp Easter Seals Virginia**
Easter Seals: Virginia
201 E Main Street
Salem, VA 24153 540-777-7325
800-365-1656
FAX: 540-777-2194
e-mail: info@va.eastersealsucp.com
www.nc.eastersealsucp.com/

Joseph E. Pizzi, Jr., Board Chair
C. L. Cochran, President & CEO
Tristan Robertson, Executive Director
Gayle M. Rose, Executive Director
Summer camp sessions for children and adults ages 5-99 with physical disabilities, cognitive disabilities and sensory impairments. Therapeutic recreation activities including swimming, fishing, sports, horseback riding, rock climbing, and more. Twenty-six-day speech therapy camp children with disabilities ages 8-16. Twelve-day Spina Bifida Self Help Skills Camp.

1393 **Camp Holiday Trails**
400 Holiday Trails Lane
Charlottesville, VA 22903 434-977-3781
FAX: 434-977-8814
e-mail: campisgood@campholidaytrails.org
www.campholidaytrails.org

Tina La Roche, Executive Director
Caitlin Farley, Program Director
Heather Mott, Development Director
Christine Shifflett, Camp Coordinator
Private, nonprofit camp for children with special health needs and various chronic illnesses. Residential, 2-week sessions are open June - August; camperships are available. Coed 7-17, nationwide and international. Canoeing, swimming, horseback rid-

ing, arts and crafts, drama, ropes course, etc. 24-hr. medical supervision by doctor and nursing staff. Air conditioned cabins.

1394 Camp Loud And Clear
Holiday Lake 4-H Educational Center
1267 4-H Camp Road
Appomattox, VA 24522
434-248-5444
FAX: 434-248-6749
e-mail: bgoin@vt.edu
holidaylake4h.com/camploud.php

1395 Camp Virginia Jaycee
2494 Camp Jaycee Road
P.O. Box 648
Blue Ridge, VA 24064
540-947-2972
800-865-0092
FAX: 540-947-2043
e-mail: info@campvajc.org
www.campvajc.org

Tom King, Chair
Kathleen King, Vice Chair
Lisa Parrish, Treasurer
Sabitha Venkatesh, Secretary
Summer camping for children and adults with developmental disabilities. Coed, ages 7-70. Weekend respite camps for children and adults with mental retardation.

1396 Civitan Acres for the Disabled
Eggleston Services
2210 Cedar Rd
Chesapeake, VA 23323-6303
757-487-6062
FAX: 757-487-4143
e-mail: info@egglestonservices.org
www.egglestonservices.org

Paul Atkinson, President and CEO
Dave Wilber, Senior VP
Josh Shockley, Senior VP
Tom Redmond, VP, Mktg and Dev.
Offers a summer camp for adult and children with disabilities. Participants can choose from day or overnight packages.

1397 Loudoun County Special Recreation Programs
Loudoun County Local Government
P.O. Box 7000
Leesburg, VA 20177
703-777-0100
FAX: 703-771-5354
TTY:703-711-0343
e-mail: prcs@loudoun.gov
www.loudoun.gov

Scott K. York, Chairman At-Large
Shawn M. Williams, Vice Chairman
Kenneth D. Reid, Board Member
Ralph M. Buona, Board Member
Offers and promotes integration opportunities for individuals with disabilities. Coordinates ADA issues and Very Special Arts and Special Olympics for Loudoun County. Summer camps, sports, socials and community trips.

1398 Makemie Woods Camp
Presbytery of Eastern Virginia
3700 Ropers Church Road
Lanexa, VA 23089
757-566-1496
800-566-1496
FAX: 757-566-8803
e-mail: makwoods@makwoods.org
www.makwoods.org

Mike Burcher, Director
Beth Martin, Office Assistant
Anthony Burcher, Storyteller in Residence
Fran Parkhurst, Food Services Manager
Residential Christian camp that tailors each group and individual goals. Counselors serve as teachers, friends and activity leaders. For children 8-18 with diabetes.

1399 Oakland School & Camp
Boyd Tavern
Keswick, VA 22947
434-293-9059
FAX: 434-296-8930
e-mail: information@oaklandschool.net
www.oaklandschool.net

Carol Williams, Head of School
Jamie Cato, Admissions Director
Amanda Baber, Education Director
Pete Cormons, Operations Director
A highly individualized program stresses improving reading ability. Subjects taught are reading, English composition, math and word analysis. Recreational activities include horseback riding, sports, swimming, tennis, crafts, archery and camping. For girls and boys, ages 8-14.

Washington

1400 Camp Fun in the Sun
Inland NorthWest Health Services
501 N. Riverpoint Blvd., Suite 245
P.O.Box 469
Spokane, WA 99202
509-232-8138
e-mail: randalll@cherspokane.org
wellness.inhs.org

Tom Fritz, CEO
Nicole Stewart, Dir. of Mktg & Communications
Jerrie Heyamoto, Communication Coordinator
Tamitha Anderson, Communication Coordinator
Summer camping for children with diabetes. Coed, ages 6-18.

1401 Camp Killoqua
Camp Fire USA
4312 Rucker Ave
Everett, WA 98203
425-258-KIDS
FAX: 425-252-CAMP
e-mail: killoqua@campfiresnoco.org
www.campfireusasnohomish.org

Dave Surface, Executive Director
Carol Johnson, Assistant Executive Director
Michael Deal, Operations Director
Barbara Georger, Development Director
Camp is located in Stanwood, Washington. Camping for children with developmental disabilities. Coed, ages 6-17.

1402 Camp Prime Time
6 S. 2nd Street
Suite 815
Yakima, WA 98901
509-248-2854
FAX: 509-248-5505
e-mail: families@campprimetime.org
www.campprimetime.org

Ralph Berthon, Founder
Dave Berthon, Founder
Dick Haapala, President
Mike Burnam, VP
Prime Time serves children and adults with disabilities or have terminal or serious illnesses.

1403 Camp Volasuca
Volunteers of America: Western Washington
2802 Broadway Ave
P.O. Box 839
Everett, WA 98206
425-259-3191
888-216-5459
FAX: 425-258-2838
e-mail: info@voaww.org
www.voaww.org

Phil Smith, President/CEO
Kim Conant, VicePresident - Human Resources
Mark Johnson, Vice President of Development & Communications
Bruce Keller, Chief Financial Officer
Camp is located in Sultan, Washington. Summer sessions for children and adults with a variety of disabilities. Coed, ages 6-13, families and single adults.

1404 **Easter Seals Camp Stand by Me**
Easter Seal Society of Washington
17809 S. Vaughn Road KPN
P.O.Box 289
Vaughn, WA 98394- 313
253-884-2722
800-678-5708
FAX: 253-590-0594
e-mail: mayer@wa.easterseals.com
www.wa.easterseals.com

Jennifer Ting, Board Chair
Matt Carson, Vice Chair
Steve Rummel, Treasurer
Cathy Bisaillon, Ex Officio, President/CEO

Camp is located in Vaughn, Washington. Summer camping for adults and children with developmental disabilities and mobility limitation. Coed, ages 7-65, seniors. Respite weekends October thru May.

1405 **Northwest Kiwanis Camp**
P.O.Box 1227
Port Hadlock, WA 98339-1227
360-732-7222
e-mail: nwkc@earthlink.net
www.kiwaniscamp.com

Sharron Sherfick, Camp Administrator
Katie Jackson, Program Director
Jean Edwards, Recreation Coordinator
Nadine Jonientz, Food Service Manager

Campers range from 6-60 in age, and includes those with developmental disabilities, cerebral palsy, autism, downs syndrome, and other physical and/or mental handicaps.

1406 **YMCA Camp Orkila**
YMCA of Greater Seattle
909 4th Ave
Seattle, WA 98104
206-382-5010
FAX: 203-382-4920
e-mail: websiteadmin@seattleymca.org
www.seattleymca.org

Robert G. Gilbertson, Jr., President/CEO
Julie L. Brown, SVP, Chief Financial Officer
Sue Camou Arrant, SVP, Chief Operating Officer
Keith Hall, SVP, Chief Human Resources Officer

Camping for children with blood disorders and diabetes, ages 8-18.

West Virginia

1407 **Mountaineer Spina Bifida Camp**
5100 Ohio Street
South Charleston, WV 25309
304-766-0383
800-642-9704
e-mail: info@drewsday.org
www.drewsday.org/

Susan Nelsen, 5K Coordinator
Stephanie Gregory, 5K run/walk/stroll coordinator
Suzie Humphreys, 5K run/walk/stroll coordinator

Is a non profit organization which pursues education and training and focuses on activities that promote independence and those that facilitate everyday life. The objectives are to build self esteem, promote independence and enhance the development of social skills.

1408 **YMCA Camp Horseshoe**
Ohio-West Virginia YMCA
Horseshoe Leadership Center
3309 Horseshoe Run Road
Parsons, WV 26287-9029
304-478-2481
FAX: 304-478-4446
e-mail: Horseshoe@YLA-youthleadership.org
www.yla-youthleadership.org

David King, Director
David Cooper, Horseshoe Director
Sharon Cassidy, Administrative Coordinator
Brad Long, Development Coordinator

Summer camping for children with cancer, ages 7-18.

Wisconsin

1409 **Easter Seal Camp Wawbeek**
Easter Seals: Wisconsin
1450 Highway 13
Wisconsin Dells, WI 53965
608-277-8288
800-422-2324
FAX: 608-277-8333
e-mail: wawbeek@wi.easterseals.com
camp.eastersealswisconsin.com/content/our-loc

Christine Fessler, CEO
Nanc Howard, Executive Assistant
Brian Schuetz, Director
Pam Ganser, Chief Financial Officer

Hundreds of people with mild to severe disabilities attend Easter Seals Wisconsin camps. The camp offers adventure programs, camp sessions for other health agencies, family camp opportunities and year round respite sessions. Coed, ages 8-99.

1410 **Lutherdale Bible Camp**
Lutherdale Ministries
N7891 Us Highway 12
Elkhorn, WI 53121
262-742-2352
FAX: 888-248-4551
e-mail: info@lutherdale.org
www.lutherdale.org

Jeff Bluhm, Exec. Dir.
David Box, Program Director
Jimmy Mcginness, Assistant Program Director
Ava Whitehead, Assistant Program Director

Summer camping for people with developmental disabilities. Coed, ages 9-18 and families, seniors.

1411 **Phantom Lake YMCA Camp**
S110W30240 YMCA Camp Road
Mukwonago, WI 53149
262-363-4386
FAX: 262-363-4351
e-mail: office@phantomlakeymca.org
www.phantomlakeymca.org

Ray Goodden, Chair of the Board
Walter Stewart, Vice Chair
James Scharine, Vice Chair
Mike Hase, Treasurer

Summer camping for children with epilepsy, ages 7-15.

1412 **Timbertop Nature Adventure Camp**
YMCA Camp Glacier Hollow
1000 Division Street
Stevens Point, WI 54481
715-342-2980
FAX: 715-342-2987
e-mail: pmatthai@spymca.org
www.glacierhollow.com

Pete Timber Matthai, Camp Director
Tiffany Gecko Praeger, Summer Camp Program Director

For children who can benefit from an individualized program of learning in a non-competitive outdoor setting under the skilled leadership of people who understand the environment and the unique potential of these children.

1413 **Wisconsin Badger Camp**
11815 Munz Lane
Prairie Du Chien, WI 53821
608-988-4558
FAX: 608-988-4586
e-mail: wiscbadgercamp@centurytel.net
www.badgercamp.org

Carol Beals, Chair
Gerry O'Rourke, Vice Chair
Michelle Eno, Treasurer
Kim Martens, Secretary

Wisconsin Badger Camp, established in 1966, is a summer camp that serves individuals with developmental disabilities. Badger camp offers eight one-week camps and one two-week camp for ages 3-93. One week is for ages 14-25, one week for ages 3-13 and all other weeks for ages 18 and older.

1414 **Wisconsin Lions Camp**
Wisconsin Lions Foundation
3834 County Road A
Rosholt, WI 54473
715-677-4969
FAX: 715-677-3297
TTY:715-677-6999
e-mail: info@wisconsinlionscamp.com
www.wisconsinlionscamp.com

Evett J. Hartvig, Executive Director
Andrea Yenter, Camp Director
Jamie Jannusch, Assistant Camp Director
Dale Schroeder, Facility Director

Serves children who have either a visual, hearing or mild cognitive disability, as well as diabetes types I and II. Program activities include sailing, ropes course, hiking and canoe trips, environmental education, swimming, camping, canoeing, outdoor living skills and handicrafts. ACA accredited, located in central Wisconsin, near Stevens Point.

1415 **Wisconson Badger Camp**
P.O. Box 723
Platteville, WI 53818
608-348-9689
FAX: 608-348-9737
e-mail: bbowers@badgercamp.org
www.badgercamp.org

Carol Beals, Chair
Gerry O'Rourke, Vice Chair
Michelle Eno, Treasurer
Kim Martens, Secretary

Badger Camp gives individuals with developmental disabilities a chance to experience camp and enjoy themselves in an outdoor setting.

Wyoming

1416 **Camp Hope**
3920 West 45th Street
Casper, WY 82604
307-265-5865
FAX: 307-472-5008
e-mail: camphopewy@yahoo.com
www.camphopewy.com

Steve Johnson, Director
Nancy Johnson, Director

Camp Hope is a camp for children and young adults with diabetes. Some of the activities include biking, swimming, sports and games.

1417 **Eagle View Ranch**
SOAR
184 Uphill Road
P.O. Box 584
Dubois, WY 82513
307-455-3084
FAX: 801-820-3050
e-mail: evr@soarnc.org
www.soarnc.org

Jonathan Jones, Founder, Director Emeritus
James Jones, Development Director
John Willson, M.S., LRT/CTR, Executive Director
Laura Pate, Director of Operations

Camp for youths with learning disabilities and attention deficit disorder. Campers enjoy a broad range of wilderness adventure experiences that help to empower them to overcome challenges, while helping them to learn how to develop problem solving skills, effective communication strategies and social skills.

Clothing

Dresses & Skirts

1418 **Budget Cotton/Poly Open Back Gown**
Buck & Buck
3111 27th Ave S
Seattle, WA 98144-6502
206-722-4196
800-458-0600
FAX: 800-317-2182
e-mail: info@buckandbuck.com
www.buckandbuck.com

Julie Buck, Owner
Short raglan sleeves, lace at neck and bodice over lapping snapback closure. *$14.00*

1419 **Budget Flannel Open Back Gown**
Buck & Buck
3111 27th Ave S
Seattle, WA 98144-6502
206-722-4196
800-458-0600
e-mail: info@buckandbuck.com
www.buckandbuck.com

Julie Buck, Owner
3/4 raglan sleeve, lace at neck and bodice. *$17.00*

1420 **Cotton/Poly House Dress**
Buck & Buck
3111 27th Ave S
Seattle, WA 98144-6502
206-722-4196
800-458-0600
e-mail: info@buckandbuck.com
www.buckandbuck.com

Julie Buck, Owner
Comes in short and long sleeves, assorted florals and plaids. *$36.00*

1421 **Dusters**
Buck & Buck
3111 27th Ave S
Seattle, WA 98144-6502
206-722-4196
800-458-0600
e-mail: info@buckandbuck.com
www.buckandbuck.com

Julie Buck, Owner
Three types: Floral, Budget Better. Snap front styles and gathered yokes, flannel $16.00-$24.00. *$36.00*

1422 **Flannel Gowns**
Buck & Buck
3111 27th Ave S
Seattle, WA 98144-6502
206-722-4196
800-458-0600
e-mail: info@buckandbuck.com
www.buckandbuck.com

Julie Buck, Owner
Comes in long or short with a deep button-front opening for ease of slipping on. Shorter long length. *$21.00*

1423 **Float Dress**
Buck & Buck
3111 27th Ave S
Seattle, WA 98144-6502
206-722-4196
800-458-0600
e-mail: info@buckandbuck.com
www.buckandbuck.com

Julie Buck, Owner
A safe bet for everyone from a size medium to a 3X. Gathered yoke front and back and literally yards of fabric for fullness. Comes in cotton or polyester. *$32.00*

1424 **Muu Muu**
Buck & Buck
3111 27th Ave S
Seattle, WA 98144-6502
206-722-4196
800-458-0600
e-mail: info@buckandbuck.com
www.buckandbuck.com

Julie Buck, Owner
Comes in long and short styles, assorted bright floral prints. $20.00-$22.00. *$31.00*

1425 **Polyester House Dress**
Buck & Buck
3111 27th Ave S
Seattle, WA 98144-6502
206-722-4196
800-458-0600
e-mail: info@buckandbuck.com
www.buckandbuck.com

Julie Buck, Owner
Comes in short and long sleeves, assorted florals. *$ 36.00*

Footwear

1426 **Booties with Non-Skid Soles**
Buck & Buck
3111 27th Ave S
Seattle, WA 98144-6502
206-722-4196
800-458-0600
FAX: 800-317-2182
e-mail: info@buckandbuck.com
www.buckandbuck.com

Julie Buck, Owner
Acrylic knit or quilted cotton/poly and shearling inner. *$17.00*

1427 **Foot Snugglers**
Buck & Buck
3111 27th Ave S
Seattle, WA 98144-6502
206-722-4196
800-458-0600
FAX: 800-317-2182
e-mail: info@buckandbuck.com
www.buckandbuck.com

Julie Buck, Owner
Quilted poly/cotton outers lined with plush shearling pile, provide a thick, comfortable cushion which helps minimize the pressure points on tender areas. *$.30*

1428 **Propet Leather Walking Shoes**
Buck & Buck
3111 27th Ave S
Seattle, WA 98144-6502
206-722-4196
800-458-0600
FAX: 800-317-2182
e-mail: info@buckandbuck.com
www.buckandbuck.com

Julie Buck, Owner
Two velcro straps, leather upper, shock-absorbing sole. *$58.00*

1429 **TRU-Mold Shoes**
42 Breckenridge St
Buffalo, NY 14213-1555
716-881-4484
800-843-6653
FAX: 716-881-0406
www.trumold.com

Husain Syed, Production Manager
Custom made, fully molded shoes, relieve pressure in sensitive areas by taking all of the weight off the painful areas.

1430 **Velcro Booties**
Buck & Buck
3111 27th Ave S
Seattle, WA 98144-6502
206-722-4196
800-458-0600
FAX: 800-317-2182
e-mail: info@buckandbuck.com
www.buckandbuck.com

Julie Buck, Owner
The high-domed toe, and extra-wide, non-skid sole design accommodates virtually every foot related problem. *$20.00*

1431 **Washable Shoes**
Buck & Buck
3111 27th Ave S
Seattle, WA 98144-6502
206-722-4196
800-458-0600
FAX: 800-317-2182
e-mail: info@buckandbuck.com
www.buckandbuck.com

Julie Buck, Owner
Vinyl upper with velcro closure, nonskid sole. *$20.00*

Miscellaneous & Catalogs

1432 **Adaptations by Adrian**
PO Box 7
San Marcos, CA 92079-0007
760-744-3565
888-214-8372
FAX: 760-471-7560
e-mail: adrians1@sbcglobal.net
www.adaptationsbyadrian.com

1433 **Adaptive Clothing: Adults**
Special Clothes
P.O.Box 333
E Harwich, MA 02645-333
508-430-2410
FAX: 508-430-2410
e-mail: specialclo@aol.com
www.special-clothes.com

Judith Sweeney, President
Special Clothes produces a catalogue of garments for adults with disabilities and/or incontinence. Offerings include: undergarments, snap-crotch tee shirts, jumpsuits, and denim travel cath. The catalogue is available without charge. Comparable to department store prices. Special Clothes produces a catalog of adaptive clothing for children in sizes from toddler through young adults. A full line of clothing is included from undergarments through wheelchair jackets and ponchos.

1434 **Adult Short Jumpsuit**
Special Clothes
P.O.Box 333
E Harwich, MA 02645-333
508-430-2410
FAX: 508-430-2410
e-mail: specialclo@aol.com
www.special-clothes.com

Judith Sweeney, President
This pull-on jumpsuit provides comfort and full coverage without bulk. Wide leg ribbing ends at mid-thigh, with snaps at the crotch. We use fine quality, comfortable cotton knit. 100% cotton knit. Made in USA. Option: long sleeves - add $3.00. Colors: white, navy, teal, light blue, light pink, red, royal blue, black, khaki and juvenile print. S,M & L $43.00; XL & XXL $45.00

1435 **Body Suits**
Special Clothes
P.O.Box 333
E Harwich, MA 02645-333
508-430-2410
FAX: 508-430-2410
e-mail: specialclo@aol.com
www.special-clothes.com

Judith Sweeney, President
These are one piece garments that can be used to protect skin under braces, to add warmth and to shield incisions. S,M & L $42.00; XL & XXL $44.00.

1436 **Buck and Buck Clothing**
3111 27th Ave S
Seattle, WA 98144-6502
206-722-4196
800-458-0600
FAX: 800-317-2182
e-mail: info@buckandbuck.com
www.buckandbuck.com

Julie Buck, Owner
Clothing for the disabled and elderly.
88 pages Yearly

1437 **Carolyn's Catalog**
3938 S Tamiami Trl
Sarasota, FL 34231-3622
941-373-9100
800-648-2266
FAX: 941-739-5503
e-mail: support@carolynscatalog.com
www.carolynscatalog.com

John Colton, Owner
Free, mail-order catalog of items for visually impaired people.

1438 **Exquisite Egronomic Protective Wear**
Plum Enterprises
P.O.Box 85
Valley Forge, PA 19481-85
610-783-7377
800-321-7586
FAX: 610-783-7577
e-mail: info@plument.com
www.plument.com

Janice Carrington, President/CEO
Egronomic Protective Wear; ProtectaCap custom-fitting headgear has earned an unparalleled reputation for quality, safety, and comfort. ProtectaCap+Plus technologically-advanced protective headgear closes the gap between hard and soft helmets. Comes with optional ProtectaChin Guard and new sporty design. Protectahip protective undergarment is the intelligent, innovative solution to the problem of hip injuries for both men and women. Ladies' styles are covered with attractive stretch lace.

1439 **Headliner Hats**
Designs for Comfort
PO Box 671044
Marietta, GA 30066-2429
770-565-8246
800-443-9226
FAX: 770-565-8425
e-mail: headliner@mindspring.com
www.headlinerhats.com

Curt Maurer, President
A patented cap and hairpiece combination, the Headliner is both a quick, stylish coverup and an upbeat wig alternative for women experiencing hair care problems or hair loss. Ideal for social gatherings and outdoor activities as well as for sleeping and hospital stays. *$ 25.00*

1440 **Knee Socks**
Buck & Buck
3111 27th Ave S
Seattle, WA 98144-6502
206-722-4196
800-458-0600
FAX: 800-317-2182
e-mail: info@buckandbuck.com
www.buckandbuck.com

Julie Buck, Owner
Comes in regular and large size. $3.00 - $8.00

1441 **M&M Health Care Apparel Company**
Fashion Collection
1541 60th St
Brooklyn, NY 11219-5023
718-871-8188
800-221-8929
FAX: 718-436-2067
e-mail: info@fashionease.com
www.fashionease.com

Abraham Klein, Owner
Specialized clothing for disabled people.

1442 **Professional Fit Clothing**
Ste 1
831 N Lake St
Burbank, CA 91502-1600
818-563-1975
800-422-2348
FAX: 818-563-1834
e-mail: sales@professionalfit.com
www.professionalfit.com

Kurt Rieback, Owner

Professional fit clothing caters to homes that care for people with developmental disabilities and individuals who are physically challenged. Our clothing is fashionable, affordable and can be adapted to each person's special needs.

1443 **Spec-L Clothing Solutions**
849 Performance Drive
Stockton, CA 95206
714-427-0781
800-445-1981
FAX: 800-683-6510
e-mail: rlfortun@clothingsolutions.com
www.clothingsolutions.com

Jim Lechner, Owner

The nation's leading designer and manufacturer of assistive clothing for men and women. Free 56 page catalog available.

1444 **Special Clothes Adult Catalogue**
Special Clothes
P.O.Box 333
E Harwich, MA 02645-333
508-430-2410
FAX: 508-430-2410
e-mail: specialclo@aol.com
www.special-clothes.com

Judith Sweeney, President

Produces a catalogue of adaptive clothing for adults with disabilities. Offers include undergarments, casual bottoms, jumpsuits, swimwear, footwear and bibs. Prices are comparable to deparment store prices. The catalogue is free.

1445 **Special Clothes for Special Children**
Special Clothes
P.O.Box 333
E Harwich, MA 02645-333
508-430-2410
FAX: 508-430-2410
e-mail: specialclo@aol.com
www.special-clothes.com

Judith Sweeney, President

All special adaptations, such as velcro closures, snap crotches, bib fronts and G-tube access openings. Every item is fully washable. Offering optional features to customize each item to meet the needs of your child.

1446 **Specialty Care Shoppe**
16126 E 161st St S
Bixby, OK 74008-7325
918-366-2901
FAX: 918-366-9445
e-mail: deb@specialtycareshoppe.com
www.specialtycareshoppe.com

K J Marshall, Owner

Catalog of attractive, affordable clothing and accessories for adults with special needs. Includes items for edema, incontinence, alzheimers, limited mobility, and hand impairment.

1447 **Super Stretch Socks**
Buck & Buck
3111 27th Ave S
Seattle, WA 98144-6502
206-722-4196
800-458-0600
FAX: 800-317-2182
e-mail: info@buckandbuck.com
www.buckandbuck.com

Julie Buck, Owner

This sock has been improved to stretch laterally throughout the foot area as well as at the top. *$3.75*

1448 **Thigh-Hi Nylon Stockings**
Buck & Buck
3111 27th Ave S
Seattle, WA 98144-6502
206-722-4196
800-458-0600
FAX: 800-317-2182
e-mail: info@buckandbuck.com
www.buckandbuck.com

Julie Buck, Owner

A sheer, full length stocking. *$4.50*

1449 **Waterproof Bib**
Buck & Buck
3111 27th Ave S
Seattle, WA 98144-6502
206-722-4196
800-458-0600
FAX: 800-317-2182
e-mail: info@buckandbuck.com
www.buckandbuck.com

Julie Buck, Owner

Made with 3 layers of fabric including waterproof backing, these attractive bibs will not soak through like most others, protecting clothing from stains. *$18.00*

1450 **Wishing Wells Collection**
Ste 965
11684 Ventura Blvd
Studio City, CA 91604-2699
818-840-6919
FAX: 818-760-3878
e-mail: wishingwells@dawn-wells.com
www.dawnwells.com

Dawn Wells, Owner
Lorraine Parker, General Manager

Features designs full of back overlap construction and all velcro closures clothing.

Robes & Sleepwear

1451 **Creative Designs**
3704 Carlisle Ct
Modesto, CA 95356-924
209-523-3166
800-335-4852
e-mail: robes4you@aol.com
www.robes4you.com

Barbara Arnold, Owner

Designer of the original Change-A-Robe and the new Handi-Robe, which allows the wearer to put it on without having to stand up. Robes are designed especially for physically challenged, disabled individuals, and wheelchair users. *$69.95*

1452 **Flannel Pajamas**
Buck & Buck
3111 27th Ave S
Seattle, WA 98144-6502
206-722-4196
800-458-0600
FAX: 800-317-2182
e-mail: info@buckandbuck.com
www.buckandbuck.com

Julie Buck, Owner
$25.00

1453 **His & Hers**
Wishing Wells Collection
Ste 965
11684 Ventura Blvd
Studio City, CA 91604-2699
818-840-6919
FAX: 818-760-3878
e-mail: wishingwells@dawn-wells.com
www.dawnwells.com

Dawn Wells, Owner

This sleep shirt is designed for him or her. *$21.99*

1454 Nightshirts
Buck & Buck
3111 27th Ave S
Seattle, WA 98144-6502
206-722-4196
800-458-0600
FAX: 800-317-2182
e-mail: info@buckandbuck.com
www.buckandbuck.com
Julie Buck, Owner
Come in flannel or cotton patterns and prints in sizes S/M, 4XL, 2XL/3XL *$29.00*

1455 Open Back Nightgowns
Buck & Buck
3111 27th Ave S
Seattle, WA 98144-6502
206-722-4196
800-458-0600
FAX: 800-317-2182
e-mail: info@buckandbuck.com
www.buckandbuck.com
Julie Buck, Owner
Come in cotton (sizes S-4X) or flannel (sizes S-3X). *$20.00*

1456 Seersucker Shower Robe
Buck & Buck
3111 27th Ave S
Seattle, WA 98144-6502
206-722-4196
800-458-0600
FAX: 800-317-2182
e-mail: info@buckandbuck.com
www.buckandbuck.com
Julie Buck, Owner
Totally covers a man or woman being wheeled to and from the shower or bath. A crisp, light weight shower robe. *$34.00*

Shirts & Tops

1457 Basic Rear Closure Sweat Top
Buck & Buck
3111 27th Ave S
Seattle, WA 98144-6502
206-722-4196
800-458-0600
FAX: 800-317-2182
e-mail: info@buckandbuck.com
www.buckandbuck.com
Julie Buck, Owner
Top opens completely down the back for ease of dressing with snaps. *$19.00*

1458 Cotton Full-Back Vest
Buck & Buck
3111 27th Ave S
Seattle, WA 98144-6502
206-722-4196
800-458-0600
FAX: 800-317-2182
e-mail: info@buckandbuck.com
www.buckandbuck.com
Julie Buck, Owner
Wide shoulder straps that don't slide off shoulders. *$5.00*

1459 Dutch Neck T-Shirt
Buck & Buck
3111 27th Ave S
Seattle, WA 98144-6502
206-722-4196
800-458-0600
FAX: 800-317-2182
e-mail: info@buckandbuck.com
www.buckandbuck.com
Julie Buck, Owner
Stretchy neck makes it easy to get over the head. *$ 5.50*

1460 Printed Rear Closure Sweat Top
Buck & Buck
3111 27th Ave S
Seattle, WA 98144-6502
206-722-4196
800-458-0600
FAX: 800-317-2182
e-mail: info@buckandbuck.com
www.buckandbuck.com
Julie Buck, Owner
Comes in assorted colors, plain or with animal motifs and snaps all the way down the back. *$28.00*

1461 Rear Closure Shirts
Buck & Buck
3111 27th Ave S
Seattle, WA 98144-6502
206-722-4196
800-458-0600
FAX: 206-722-1144
e-mail: info@buckandbuck.com
www.buckandbuck.com
Julie Buck, Owner
Snaps down the back on T-shirts and dress shirts. *$ 33.00*

1462 Rear Closure T-Shirt
Buck & Buck
3111 27th Ave S
Seattle, WA 98144-6502
206-722-4196
800-458-0600
FAX: 800-317-2182
e-mail: info@buckandbuck.com
www.buckandbuck.com
Julie Buck, Owner
Closes down the back with velcro snaps. *$10.00*

Slacks & Pants

1463 Jumpsuits
Special Clothes
PO Box 333
E Harwich, MA 02645-333
508-430-2410
FAX: 508-430-2410
e-mail: lou@lnrmusic.com
www.special-clothes.com
Judith Sweeney, President
Several styles of one-piece garments are available for dressing ease. Front opening styles are designed for easy access. Prices range from $32.20-$44.00. *$55.00*

1464 Side Velcro Slacks
Buck & Buck
3111 27th Ave S
Seattle, WA 98144-6502
206-722-4196
800-458-0600
FAX: 800-317-2182
e-mail: info@buckandbuck.com
www.buckandbuck.com
Julie Buck, Owner
Slacks open down both sides from waist to hip with snap closures at sides. *$36.00*

1465 Side-Zip Sweat Pants
Buck & Buck
3111 27th Ave S
Seattle, WA 98144-6502
206-722-4196
800-458-0600
FAX: 800-317-2182
e-mail: info@buckandbuck.com
www.buckandbuck.com
Julie Buck, Owner
Out-seam zippers un-zip 22-inch zippers down both sides to enable dressing a resident with severe leg contractures. *$25.00*

1466 **Trunks**
Buck & Buck
3111 27th Ave S
Seattle, WA 98144-6502
206-722-4196
800-458-0600
FAX: 800-317-2118
e-mail: info@buckandbuck.com
www.buckandbuck.com

Julie Buck, Owner

Come in cotton or nylon, flare leg, full cut. *$5.00*

Undergarments

1467 **Adult Absorbent Briefs**
Special Clothes
PO Box 333
E Harwich, MA 02645-333
508-430-2410
FAX: 508-430-2410
e-mail: lou@lnrmusic.com
www.special-clothes.com

Judith Sweeney, President

Soft, comfortable, 100% cotton knit brief is seven layers thick at the crotch. Sides of the brief are a non-bulky single layer. The waistband elastic is enclosed in a soft cotton knit casing and does not touch the skin. Comfortable cotton rib knit bands circle the leg. This brief will not replace a diaper, but provides absorbency for light incontinence. *$18.50*

1468 **Adult Lap Shoulder Bodysuit**
Special Clothes
PO Box 334
E Harwich, MA 02645-333
508-430-2410
FAX: 508-430-2410
TTY:508-430-2410
e-mail: lou@lnrmusic.com
www.special-clothes.com

1469 **Adult Sleeveless Bodysuit**
Special Clothes
PO Box 335
E Harwich, MA 02645-333
508-430-2410
FAX: 508-430-2410
e-mail: lou@lnrmusic.com
www.special-clothes.com

Judith Sweeney, President

Bodysuit styles fasten at the crotch with sturdy snaps to stay neatly tucked. All are made of soft, absorbent 100% cotton knit for maximum comfort. They are cut wide at the hip and seat for full coverage, and will accomodate a diaper if necessary. Soft knit rib circles the neck and leg. This cool tank style slips on easily. Deep armholes are banded with rib knit. All styles: S,M,L $42, XL,XXL $44. A choice of 12 colors.

1470 **Adult Swim Diaper**
Special Clothes
PO Box 336
E Harwich, MA 02645-333
508-430-2410
FAX: 508-430-2410
e-mail: lou@lnrmusic.com
www.special-clothes.com

Judith Sweeney, President

This pant is made of soft, silent, light-weight, impermeable fabric- waterproof and secure. It is a containment brief, designed to be used in the pool in place of cloth or disposable diapers, which can become waterlogged or disintegrate in the water. Waist and legbands should be snug for proper fit, so please consult sizing chart before ordering. Darlex with lining of 100% cotton knit. Lycra waist and legbands. Made in USA. *$40.00*

1471 **Adult Tee Shoulder Bodysuit**
Special Clothes
PO Box 337
E Harwich, MA 02645-333
508-430-2410
FAX: 508-430-2410
TTY:508-430-2410
e-mail: lou@lnrmusic.com
www.special-clothes.com

1472 **Adult Waterproof Overpant**
Special Clothes
PO Box 338
E Harwich, MA 02645-333
508-430-2410
FAX: 508-430-2410
e-mail: lou@lnrmusic.com
www.special-clothes.com

Judith Sweeney, President

Overpants are made of a soft, silent, lightweight fabric which is waterproof and very secure. It is designed to be used over our Adult Absorbent Brief, or cloth diapers. It is completely latex-free and is an excellent non-allergenic substitute for rubber or vinyl pants. Waist and legbands should be snug to minimize leakage, so please consult the sizing chart before ordering. Lycra waist and legbands. Made in USA. *$40.00*

1473 **Briefs**
Special Clothes
P.O.Box 333
E Harwich, MA 02645
508-430-2410
FAX: 508-430-2410
e-mail: specialclo@aol.com
www.special-clothes.com

Judith Sweeney, President

A variety of unique brief styles available for easy access and practicality.

1474 **Panties**
Buck & Buck
3111 27th Ave S
Seattle, WA 98144-6502
206-722-4196
800-458-0600
FAX: 800-317-2182
e-mail: info@buckandbuck.com
www.buckandbuck.com

Julie Buck, Owner

Come in nylon or cotton, band leg for comfort. *$5.00*

1475 **Safe and Dry-Feel and Sure-Toddler Dry**
Kleinerts
433 Newton Street
Elba, AL 36323
305-937-0824
800-498-7051
FAX: 305-937-0825
e-mail: customercare@kleinerts.com
www.hygienics.com

Michael Brier, President

A variety of stress incontinence disposable liners which absorb 8-10 oz. of fluid packaged in 20 and 40 counts. Also available are patented knit nylon panties in medium, large and extra large sizes. All products are priced for the mass market.

1476 **Support Plus**
5581 Hudson Industrial Parkway
PO Box 2599
Hudson, OH 44236-0099
508-359-2910
866-229-2910
FAX: 800-950-9569
www.supportplus.com

Ed Janos, President

Offers a selection of support undergarments, braces and shoes for the physically challenged and medical professionals.

Computers

Assistive Devices

1477 Ability Research
PO Box 1721
Minnetonka, MN 55345-721
952-939-0121
FAX: 952-227-5809
e-mail: info@abilityresearch.net
www.abilityresearch.net

Suzanne Severson, Administrator
Manufacturers and marketers of assistive technology equipment.

1478 Academic Software Inc
3504 Tates Creek Rd
Lexington, KY 40517-2601
859-552-1020
FAX: 253-799-4012
e-mail: asistaff@acsw.com
www.acsw.com

Warren E Lacefield PhD, President
Penelope Ellis, Marketing Director
Sylvia P Lacefield, Graphic Artist
Employs a unique, goal-oriented approach to aid individuals in identifying adaptive devices with potential to support various physical limitations. Devices are categorized in seven databases: Existence, Travel, In-situ Motion, Environmental Adaptation, Communication, and Sports & recreation. ADLS provides its users with device descriptions, pictures and lists of sources for locating products and product information.

1479 Adaptivation
Ste 100
2225 W 50th St
Sioux Falls, SD 57105-6536
605-335-4445
800-723-2783
FAX: 605-335-4446
e-mail: info@adaptivation.com
www.adaptivation.com

Jonathan Eckrich, President
Manufacturers of switches, voice output devices and enviromental controls.

1480 Analog Switch Pad
Academic Software
331 W 2nd St
Lexington, KY 40507-1113
859-233-2332
800-842-2357
FAX: 859-231-0725

Warren E Lacefield PhD, President
Penelope Ellis, Marketing Director
A touch-activated, force-adjustable, low-voltage DC, electronic switch designed to control battery-operated toys, environmental controls, and computer access interfaces. This device features a large activation area that is soft and compliant to the touch. Force sensitivity is adjusted by a small dial from approximately 1 ounce to 32 ounces activation pressure, applied over an area ranging from the size of a fingertip to the size of the entire switch surface.

1481 Arkenstone: The Benetech Initiative
480 S California Ave
Palo Alto, CA 94306-1609
650-644-3400
FAX: 650-475-1066
e-mail: hrdag@benetech.org
www.hrdag.org

Jim Fruthterman, CEO
Roberta G Brosnaha, General Manager/VP
Patrick Ball, Executive Director
Offers various models of ready-to-read personal computers for the disabled.

1482 Augmentative Communication Systems (AAC)
ZYGO-USA
48834 Kato Road
Suite 101A
Freemont, CA 94538
510-249-9660
800-234-6006
FAX: 510-770-4930
e-mail: zygo@zygo-usa.com
www.zygo-usa.com

Lawrence Weiss, President
Full range of AAC systems and assistive technology including computer-based systems and computer access programs and devices.

1483 Away We Ride IntelliKeys Overlay
Soft Touch Inc
12301 Central Ave NE
Ste 205
Blaine, NE 55434
763-755-1402
888-755-1402
FAX: 76- 86- 292
e-mail: sales@marblesoft.com
www.softtouch.com

Joyce Meyer, President
Four full color preprinted overlays to use with Away We Ride. Just put them on an IntelliKeys keyboard and you are ready to go.

1484 BIGmack Communication Aid
AbleNet
2625 Patton Road
Roseville, MN 55113
651-294-2200
800-322-0956
FAX: 651-294-2222
e-mail: customerservice@ablenetinc.com
www.ablenetinc.com

Jen Thalhuber, CEO
A single message communication aid, BIGmack has 2 minutes of memory and has a 5 inches in diameter switch surface. *$86.00*

1485 Close-Up 6.5
Norton- Lambert Corporation
PO Box 4085
Santa Barbara, CA 93140-4085
805-964-6767

e-mail: sales@norton-lambert.com
www.norton-lambert.com

Jeannie Vesely, Marketing Coordinator
Remotely controls PC's via modem. Telecommute from your home or laptop PC to your office PC. Run applications, update spreadsheets, print documents remotely and access networks on remote PCs. Features: fast screen and file transfers, synchronize files, unattended transfers, multi-level security, transaction logs, automated installation. *$99.95*

1486 Concepts on the Move Advanced Overlay CD
Soft Touch Inc
12301 Central Ave NE
Ste 205
Blaine, MN 55434
763-755-1402
888-755-1402
FAX: 763-862-2920
e-mail: sales@marblesoft.com
www.softtouch.com

Joyce Myer, President
Use this overlay CD with Concepts on the Move Advanced Preacademics. Overlays match the concepts and graphics in the program. Includes standard overlays with all the choices and SoftTouch's changeable format overlays. Print and laminate the blank templates. Then print and laminate the picture keys in all three sizes - small, medium and large. Includes Overlay Printer by IntelliTools for easy printing. *$115.00*

1487 Concepts on the Move Basic Overlay CD
Soft Touch Inc
12301 Central Ave NE
Ste 205
Blaine, MN 55434
763-755-1402
888-755-1403
FAX: 763-862-2920
e-mail: sales@marblesoft.com
www.softtouch.com

Joyce Meyer, President
Use this Overlay CD with Concepts on the Move Basic Preacademics. Overlays match the concepts and graphics in the program. Includes standard overlays with all the choices and SoftTouch's changeable format overlays. Print and laminate the blank templates. Then print and laminate the picture keys in all three sizes - small, medium and large. It is easy and fast to place the images on the blank templates. *$115.00*

1488 Darci Too
WesTest Engineering Corporation
810 Shepard Ln
Farmington, UT 84025-3846
801-451-9191
FAX: 801-451-9393
e-mail: larryk@westest.com
westest.com

Robert Lessmann, President
A universal device which allows people with physical disabilities to replace the keyboard and mouse on a personal computer with a device that matches their physical capabilities. DARCI TOO works with almost any personal computer and provides access to all computer functions. *$995.00*

1489 Eyegaze Computer System
LC Technologies Inc
10363A Democracy Lane
Fairfax, VA 22030
703-385-7133
800-393-4293
FAX: 703-385-7137
e-mail: info0309@eyegaze.com
www.eyegaze.com

Nancy Cleveland, Medical Coordinator
Enables people with physical disabilities to do many things with their eyes that they would otherwise do with their hands.

1490 Five Green & Speckled Frogs IntelliKeys Overlay
Soft Touch Inc
12301 Central Ave NE
Ste 205
Blaine, MN 55434
763-755-1402
888-755-1403
FAX: 763-862-2920
e-mail: sales@marblesoft.com
www.softtouch.com

Joyce Meyer, President
Seven full color preprinted overlays to use with Five Green and Speckled Frogs. Just put them on an IntelliKeys keyboard and you are ready to go. *$49.00*

1491 GW Micro
725 Airport North Office Park
Fort Wayne, IN 46825-6707
260-489-3671
FAX: 260-489-2608
e-mail: sales@gwmicro.com
www.gwmicro.com

Dan Weirich, Sales Executive
Marty Hord, Sales Manager
Computer hardware and software products for people with disabilities.

1492 InvoTek, Inc.
1026 Riverview Drive
Alma, AR 72921
479-632-4166
FAX: 479-632-6457
invotek.org

Thomas Jakobs, President
InvoTek, Inc. is a research and development company that improves the quality of life for people who find it difficult or impossible to use their hands by giving them new, efficient ways to access computers.

1493 Jelly Bean Switch
AbleNet
2625 Patton Road
Roseville, MN 55113-1308
651-294-2200
800-322-0956
FAX: 651-294-2259
e-mail: customerservice@ablenetinc.com
www.ablenetinc.com

Jen Thalhuber, CEO
A momentary touch switch made of shatterproof plastic, small and sensitive to 2-3 ounces of pressure, this switch is provided audible feedback when activated and is a compact version of the Big Red Switch. Choice of colors: red, blue, green and yellow.

1494 Large Print Keyboard Labels
Hooleon Corp
P.O.Box 589
Melrose, NM 88124-589
575-253-4503
800-937-1337
FAX: 928-634-4620
e-mail: sales@hooleon.com
www.hooleon.com

Shannen Aikman, Admin Manager/Sales
Joan Crozier, President/Sales
Pressure sensitive labels for computer keyboards.

1495 MessageMate
Words+ Inc
42505 10th Street W
Lancaster, CA 93534-7059
661-723-6523
800-869-8521
FAX: 661-723-2114
e-mail: www.prentrom.com
www.words-plus.com

Jeff Dahlan, President
Ginger Woltosz, General Manager
Lightweight, hand-held communicator providing high-quality analog recording capability using either direct select keyboards or 1 to 2 switch access. Price ranges from $549.00 to $999.00. *$1550.00*

1496 Mouthsticks
Sammons Preston Rolyan
1000 Remington Blvd
Suite 210
Bolingbrook, IL 60440-5117
630-378-6000
800-323-5547
FAX: 630-378-6010
e-mail: sp@patterson-medical.com
www.pattersonmedical.com

Sandra Brown, Customer Service Director
Wide offering of mouthsticks featuring various functions (BK 5380, 5381, 5383, 5385, 6002, or BK 5370 series).

1497 Old MacDonald's Farm IntelliKeys Overlay
Soft Touch Inc
12301 Central Ave NE
Ste 205
Blaine, MN 55434
763-755-1402
888-755-1403
FAX: 763-862-2920
e-mail: sales@marblesoft.com
www.softtouch.com

Joyce Meyer, President
Extend your students' learning with more than 45 pre-made overlays that support all of the skills learned at the farm. Use with the IntelliKeys keyboard. Simply print and use. Print an extra set to make off computer activities, too. Note: Requires Overlay Maker or Overlay Printer by IntelliTools.

1498 **Origin Instruments Corporation**
854 Greenview Drive
Grand Prairie, TX 75050
972-606-8740
FAX: 972-606-8741
e-mail: support@orin.com
www.orin.com

1499 **Perfect Solutions**
2685 Treanor Ter
Wellington, FL 33414-6460
561-790-1070
800-726-7086
FAX: 561-790-0108
e-mail: perfect@gate.net
www.perfectsolutions.com

Andrew Kramer, President

A computer for every student and it speaks! Wireless laptop computers starting at $299.00 are ideal for students to carry with them all day. Text-to-speech and web browsing are available. *$299.00*

1500 **Phillip Roy**
13064 Indian Rocks Road
PO Box 130
Indian Rocks Beach, FL 33785-130
727-593-2700
800-255-9085
FAX: 877-595-2685
e-mail: info@philliproy.com
www.philliproy.com

Ruth Bragman PhD, President
Phil Padol, VP

Offers multimedia materials appropriate for use with individuals with disabilities. Programs range from preschool through the adult level. Many of the programs are high interest topics/low vocabulary, ideal for transition and employability skills. Materials are also available which focus on social and personal development. Call for a free catalog.

1501 **SS-Access Single Switch Interface for PC'swith MS-DOS**
Academic Software
3504 Tates Creek Road
Lexington, KY 40517-2601
859-552-1020
800-842-2357
FAX: 253-799-4012
e-mail: asistaff@acsw.com
www.acsw.com

Warren E Lacefield PhD, President
Penelope Ellis, Marketing Director

A general purpose single switch hardware and software interface for DOS and the IBM and compatible PC family. It is designed to be easy to install, simple to use, and compatible with the widest possible range of computers and application software programs. SS-ACCESS! connects to one of the PC serial ports and provides a jack to connect an external switch. The DOS version of the software works by sending a user defined keystroke to the PC keyboard buffer whenever the switch is pressed. *$ 90.00*

1502 **Simplicity**
Words+
42505 10th Street W
Lancaster, CA 93534-7059
661-723-6523
800-869-8521
FAX: 661-723-2114
e-mail: info@words-plus.com
www.words-plus.com

Jeff Dahlan, President
Ginger Wolosz, General Manager

Swing-down mount for portable computers and other devices is made from high-quality aircraft aluminum. Simplicity contains very few moving parts and installs in minutes, providing a positive, secure support for computer/device in both the stored and overlap position. *$1199.00*

1503 **Slim Armstrong Mounting System**
AbleNet
2625 Patton Road
Roseville, MN 55113-1308
612-379-0956
800-322-0956
FAX: 651-294-2259
e-mail: customerservice@ablenetinc.com
www.ablenetinc.com

Jen Thalhuber, CEO

Slim Armstrong is a mounting system strong enough to hold up to five pounds in any position. Mix and match parts to create the system length you desire. *$188.00*

1504 **Songs I Sing at Preschool IntelliKeys Overlay**
Soft Touch
12301 Central Ave NE
Ste 205
Blaine, MN 55434
763-755-1402
888-755-1403
FAX: 763-862-2920
e-mail: sales@marblesoft.com
www.softtouch.com

Joyce Meyer, President

Pre-made overlays for use with Songs I Sing at Preschool. Simply print and use with an IntelliKeys keyboard. Print an extra set to make off computer activities, too.

1505 **Switch Basics IntelliKeys Overlay**
Soft Touch
12301 Central Ave NE
Ste 205
Blaine, MN 55434
763-755-1402
888-755-1403
FAX: 763-862-2920
e-mail: sales@marblesoft.com
www.softtouch.com

Joyce Meyer, President

Four preprinted overlays to use with Switch Basics. Just put them on an IntelliKeys keyboard and you're ready to go.

1506 **Teach Me Phonemics Blends Overlay CDSoftTouch Inc.**
12301 Central Ave NE
Ste 205
Blaine, MN 55434
763-755-1402
888-755-1403
FAX: 763-862-2920
e-mail: sales@marblesoft.com
www.softtouch.com

Roxanne Butterfield, Marketing
Joyce Meyer, President

Teach Me Phonemics Blends Overlay CD contains over 40 IntelliKeys overlays for use with Teach Me Phonemics - Blends program. Choose either 4-item or 9-item layout to match the presentation you use in the program. Print extra copies of the overlays for off computer activites, too.

1507 **Teach Me Phonemics Medial Overlay CD**
SoftTouch Incorporated
Ste C
17117 Oak Dr
Omaha, NE 68130-2193
402-330-1301
877-763-8868
FAX: 402-334-8478
e-mail: support@softtouch.com
www.softtouch.com

Kip Fisher, Manager
Roxanne Butterfield, Marketing

Teach Me Phonemics Medial Overlay CD contains over 40 IntelliKeys overlays for use with Teach Me Phonemics - Medial program. Choose either 4-item or 9-item layout to match the presentation you use in the program. Print extra copies of the overlays for off computer activites, too.

1508 Teach Me Phonemics Overlay Series Bundle
SoftTouch
Ste 401
4300 Stine Rd
Bakersfield, CA 93313-2352
661-396-8676
877-763-8868
FAX: 661-396-8760
e-mail: softtouch@funsoftware.com
www.softtouch.com

Roxanne Butterfield, Marketing
Joyce Meyer, President
Teach Me Phonemics Overlay Series Bundle includes one copy of each Teach Me Phonemics Overlay CD - Initial, Medial, Final and - four CD's in all.

1509 Teach Me to Talk Overlay CD
Soft Touch
12301 Central Ave NE
Ste 205
Blaine, MN 55434
763-755-1402
888-755-1403
FAX: 763-862-2920
e-mail: sales@marblesoft.com
www.softtouch.com

Joyce Meyer, President
For older version of Teach Me to Talk. Mac only version with red label and PC only version with yellow label. More than 48 pre-made overlays that match the activities on Teach Me to Talk. Simply print and use with an IntelliKeys keyboard. Print an extra set to make off computer activities, too.

1510 Teach Me to Talk: USB-Overlay CD
Soft Touch
12301 Central Ave NE
Ste 205
Blaine, MN 55434
763-755-1402
888-755-1403
FAX: 763-862-2920
e-mail: sales@marblesoft.com
www.softtouch.com

Joyce Meyer, President
Revised version of Teach Me to Talk Overlays for the newest version that is USB IntelliKeys compatible. This CD contains more than 48 overlays that match the activities and updated graphics of Teach Me to Talk. Includes Overlay Printer by IntelliTools for easy printing.

1511 Teen Tunes Plus IntelliKeys Overlay
Soft Touch
12301 Central Ave NE
Ste 205
Blaine, MN 55434
763-755-1402
888-755-1403
FAX: 763-862-2920
e-mail: sales@marblesoft.com
www.softtouch.com

Joyce Meyer, President
Seven full color, preprinted overlays to use with Teen Tunes Plus. Just put them on an IntelliKeys keyboard and you're ready to go. *$49.00*

1512 U-Control III
Words+
42505 10th St W
Lancaster, CA 93534-7059
575-253-4503
800-869-8521
FAX: 661-723-2114
e-mail: www.prentrom.com
www.words-plus.com

Jeff Dahlen, President
Ginger Wolosz, General Manager
Works with the Words+ system (EX Keys, Morse WSKE, Scanning WSKE, Talking Screen) to provide wireless, portable control of items which are already infrared-controlled such as a TV, VCR, CD player, etc. *$499.00*

1513 Universal Switch Mounting System
AbleNet
2625 Patton Road
Roseville, MN 55113-1308
612-379-0956
800-322-0956
FAX: 651-294-2259
e-mail: customerservice@ablenetinc.com
www.ablenetinc.com

Jen Thalhuber, CEO
Mounting system that allows switch placement in any position. A single lever locks all joints securely in place. Extends to 20 1/2 inches and holds up to five pounds. A mounting system for quick and easy positioning. *$210.00*

1514 WinSCAN: The Single Switch Interface for PC's with Windows
Academic Software
3504 Tates Creek Rd
Lexington, KY 40517-2601
859-522-1020
FAX: 253-799-4012
e-mail: asistaff@acsw.com
www.acsw.com

Warren E Lacefield, President
Penelope Ellis, Marketing Director/COO
A general purpose single-switch control interface for Windows. It provides single-switch users independent control access to educational and productivity software, multimedia programs, and recreational activities that run under Windows 3.1 and higher versions on IBM and compatible PC's. The user can navigate through Windows; choose program icons and run programs, games, and CD's; even surf the Internet with WinSCAN and his or her adaptive switch. *$349.00*

1515 Words+ IST (Infrared, Sound, Touch)
Words+
42505 10th St W
Lancaster, CA 93534-7059
575-253-4503
800-869-8521
FAX: 661-723-2114
e-mail: www.prentrom.com
www.words-plus.com

Jeff Dahlan, President
Ginger Wolosz, General Manager
A unique switch that is activated by slight movement or faint sound. The switch provides user control when connected to a device driven by a single switch. Individuals are currently accessing a wide variety of communication and computer systems with movement using the IST switch. *$395.00*

Braille Products

1516 Braille Keyboard Labels
Hooleon Corporation
PO Box 589
Melrose, NM 88124-589
928-634-7515
800-937-1337
FAX: 928-634-4620
e-mail: sales@hooleon.com
www.hooleon.com

Barry Green, Sales Manager
Joan Crozier, President/Sales
Also large print keyboard labels and large print with Braille.

1517 Brailon Thermoform Duplicator
American Thermoform Corporation
1758 Brackett St
La Verne, CA 91750-5855
909-593-6711
800-331-3676
FAX: 909-593-8001
e-mail: pnunnelly@americanthermoform.com
www.americanthermoform.com

Patrick Nunnelly, VP
Gary Nunnelly, Owner
This copy machine, for producing tactile images, copies any brailled or embossed original, by a vacuum forming process. This model is for the reproduction of teaching aids and mobility maps.

1518 **Computer Paper for Brailling**
Maxi Aids
42 Executive Blvd
Farmingdale, NY 11735-4710 631-752-0521
800-522-6294
FAX: 631-752-0689
TTY: 631-752-0738
e-mail: sales@maxiaids.com
www.maxiaids.com

Elliot Zaretsky, President
Specially made paper for braille printing. 1,500 sheets/case *$85.99*

1519 **Duxbury Braille Translator**
Duxbury Systems
Ste 6
270 Littleton Rd
Westford, MA 01886-3523 978-692-3000
FAX: 978-692-7912
e-mail: info@duxsys.com
www.duxburysystems.com

Joe Sullivan, President
A complete line of easy to use word processing and Braille translation software available for Windows (including 64 bit windows. Applications for anyone wanting to produce or communicate with Braille; signs, note cards, textbooks, business communications and forms, telephone bills, etc. Simple to use, FREE technical support. Free one year upgrades. DBT is for producing Braille in English, Spanish, French, Portuguese, Italian, Latin, Greek, German and 125 other languages. *$600.00*

1520 **Enabling Technologies Company**
1601 NE Braille Pl
Jensen Beach, FL 34957-5345 772-225-3687
800-777-3687
FAX: 772-225-3299
e-mail: info@brailler.com
www.brailler.com

Tony Schenk, President
Kate Schenk, Product Manager Western US
Greg Schenk, Sales & Marketing
Manufactures the most complete line of American made Braille embossers, including desktop or portable models capable of producing high quality single sided or interpoint Braille. Also carries a complete line of adaptive technology aids for the blind community at affordable prices.

1521 **Freedom Scientific Blind/Low Vision Group**
11800 31st Ct N
St Petersburg, FL 33716-1805 727-803-8000
800-444-4443
FAX: 727-803-8001
e-mail: info@freedomscientific.com
www.freedomscientific.com

Brad Davis, VP Hardware Product Management
Dr Lee Hamilton, President/CEO
Developer and manufacturer of assistive technology products for people who are blind or who have low vision. Innovative blindness products include: JAWS® screen reading software; the PAC Mate Omni™, an accessible Pocket PC; the SARA™ scanning and reading appliance; OpenBook™ scanning and reading software; FSReader™ DAISY player; FaceToFace™ deaf-blind communications solution; and PAC Mate and Focus Braille Displays. *$16.95*

1522 **Hooleon Corporation**
PO Box 589
Melrose, NM 88124-589 928-634-7515
800-937-1337
FAX: 928-634-4620
e-mail: sales@hooleon.com
www.hooleon.com

Kim Green, Manager
Joan Crozier, President/Sales
Large print and combination Braille adhesive keytop labels for computer keyboards. Helps visually impaired computer users access correct key strokes either by sight or by touch. Raised Braille meets ADA specifications and large print fills key top surface.

1523 **Infogrip: Large Print/Braille Keyboard Labels**
1899 E. Main Street
Ventura, CA 93001 805-652-0770
800-397-0921
FAX: 805-652-0880
e-mail: sales@infogrip.com
www.infogrip.com

Liza Jacobs, President
Aaron Gaston, VP
Makes a standard keyboard more accessible for visually impaired individuals with large print or Braille keyboard labels. Characters on the large print labels are .5 by .25 inches, about 3 times larger than standard keyboard characters. Braille labels are available as clear labels with Braille dots or large print with Braille. Each set includes all the keys used on a standard Windows keyboard. *$29.00*

1524 **Raised Dot Computing**
Duxbury Systems Incorporated
270 Littleton Rd.
Unit 6
Westford, MA 01886-3523 978-692-3000
FAX: 978-692-7912
e-mail: info@duxsys.com
www.duxburysystems.com

Joe Sullivan, President
Peter Sullivan, VP of Software Development
Genevieve Sullivan, Treasurer
Dana Winikates, Software Engineer
Software for the visually impaired.

1525 **Touchdown Keytop/Keyfront Kits**
Hooleon Corporation
P.O.Box 589
304 West Denby Ave
Melrose, NM 88124 575-253-4503
800-937-1337
FAX: 575-253-4299
e-mail: Sales@Hooleon.com
www.hooleon.com

Bob Crozier, Founder
Joan Crozier, President
Barry Green, Sales Manager
These kits enlarge the key legends of a computer and include Braille for easy recognition.

Information Centers & Databases

1526 **ABLEDATA**
103 West Broad St.
Suite 400
Falls Church, VA 22046 703-356-8035
800-227-0216
FAX: 703-356-8314
TTY: 703-992-8313
e-mail: abledata@neweditions.net
www.abledata.com

Katherine Belknap, Project Director
David Johnson, Publications Director
Juanita Hardy, Information Specialist
David Johnson, Publications Director
ABLEDATA is an electronic database of assistive technology and rehabilitation equipment products for children and adults with physical, cognitive and sensory disabilities. ABLEDATA staff can perform database searches or the database can be searched on the ABLEDATA website, database printouts, informed consumer guides and fact sheets are available at cost from the office or free from the website.

1527 **ATTAIN**
Division of Disability Aging & Rehab Services
Ste 1400
32 E Washington St
Indianapolis, IN 46204-3552 317-232-1147
800-528-8246
FAX: 317-486-8809
e-mail: attain@attaininc.org
www.attaininc.org

Gary R Hand, Executive Director
Peter Bisbecos, Manager
Nonprofit organization that creates system change by expanding the availability of community-based technology-related activities, outreach services, empowerment and advocacy activities through the development of a comprehensive, consumer-responsive, statewide program to serve individuals with disabilities, of all ages and all disabilities, their families, caregivers, educators and service providers. Provides training, information and referrals, system change and assessments for equipment needs.

1528 **Aloha Special Technology Access Center**
710 Green St
Honolulu, HI 96813-2119 808-523-5547
FAX: 808-536-3765
e-mail: astachi@yahoo.com
www.alohastac.org

Ali Silvert, President
Ms. Jacquely Brand, Founder
Computer technology center.

1529 **Audiogram/Clinical Records Manager**
19 State Route 10 E
Ste 25
Succasunna, NJ 7876 862-251-4637
FAX: 862-251-4642
e-mail: npdunn@thedaviscenter.com
www.thedaviscenter.com

Dorinne.S Davis,MA, CCC-A, FAAA, Director
Elizabeth Meade, Head Sound Therapist
Nancy Puckett-Dunn, Office Manager
Donna Warr, Office Assistant
Sound-based therapy—Uses sound vibration with special equipment, specific programs, modified music, and/or specific tones/beats, the need for which is identified with appropriate testing. Sound-based therapy fits under the term sound therapy so The Davis Center is considered a sound therapy center. *$414.75*

1530 **Birmingham Alliance for Technology Access Center**
Birmingham Independent Living Center
206 13th Street South
Birmingham, AL 35233-1317 205-251-2223
FAX: 205-251-0605
TTY:205-251-2223
e-mail: bilc@bellsouth.net
www.birminghamilc.org

Phil Klebine, President
Graham Sisson, VP
Daniel Kessler, Executive Director
Computer technology center.

1531 **Bluegrass Technology Center**
409 Southland Drive
Lexington, KY 40503 859-294-4343
800-209-7767
FAX: 866-576-9625
e-mail: office@bluegrass-tech.org
www.bluegrass-tech.org

Debbie Sharon, Acting Executive Director
Linnie Lee, Assistive Technology Specialist
Jean Isaacs, Assistive Technology Consultant
Linda Gassaway, PhD, Assistive Technology Consultant
Provides assistive technology information, consulting and training for education, health professionals, consumers and parents of consumers. Maintains extensive lending library of assistive devices and adapted toys. Statewide training such as; AAC, how to obtain funding for assistive technology, augmentative and alternate communication, equipment implementation strategies, specific to hardware and software, etc.

1532 **CITE: Lighthouse for Central Florida**
215 East New Hampshire Street
Orlando, FL 32804 407-898-2483
FAX: 407-898-0236
e-mail: csacca@lcf-fl.org
www.lighthousecentralflorida.org/Default.asp
Lee Nasehi, MSW, President/CEO
Donna Esbensen CPA,MBA, VP/CFO
Jeff Whitehead, MPA, MS, Director of Program Services
Casey Mathews, Access Technology Specialist
CITE promotes the independence of adults and children with blindness, low vision and other disabilities through technology, education, support and advocacy.

1533 **Carolina Computer Access Center**
P.O.Box 247
Cramerton, NC 28032 704-342-3004
FAX: 704-342-1513
e-mail: bellsluth.net
www.ccac.ataccess.org

Linda Schilling, Executive Director
Nonprofit, community-based technology resource center for people with disabilities, providing information about and demonstration of the technology tools that enable individuals with disabilities to control and direct their own lives. Services and programs include: assessments, demonstrations, resource information, lending library, workshops and outreach.

1534 **Center for Accessible Technology**
3075 Adeline
Suite 220
Berkeley, CA 94703 510-841-3224
FAX: 510-841-7956
e-mail: info@cforat.org
www.cforat.org

Dmitri Belser, Executive Director
Eric Smith, Associate Director
A consumer-based technology resource and demonstration center for adults and children with disabilities, families, teachers, and professionals. The primary focus is on assistive technology for computer access. Seen by appointment only.

1535 **Center for Applied Special Technology**
40 Harvard Mills Square
Suite 3
Wakefield, MA 01880-3233 781-245-2212
FAX: 781-245-5212
e-mail: cast@cast.org
www.cast.org/

Anne Meyer, Founder
David H. Rose, Founder
Lisa Poller, Co-President
Gabrielle Rappolt-Schlichtmann, Co-President
Expands opportunities for individuals with special needs through innovative use of computers and related technology. We pursue this mission through research and product development that further universal design for learning.

1536 **Center for Assistive Technology & Inclusive Education Studies**
2000 Pennington Rd.
P.O.Box 7718
Ewing, NJ 08628-0718 609-771-3016
FAX: 609-637-5179
e-mail: caties@tcnj.edu
caties.pages.tcnj.edu

Amanda Norvell, President
Matt Bender, VP
Regina Morin, Parliamentarian
Laurie Wanat, Secretary
Computer technology center offering resource time, workshops, technology, training and evaluations.

1537 Center on Evaluation of Assistive Technology
National Rehabilitation Hospital
102 Irving St NW
Washington, DC 20010 202-877-1000
TTY:202-726-3996
e-mail: justin.m.carter@medstar.net
www.medstarhealth.org

Kenneth A. Samet, FACHE, President, CEO
Michael J. Curran, EVP, Chief Administrative and Financial Officer
Christine Swearingen, EVP, Planning, Marketing and Community Relations
Stephen R.T. Evans, MD, EVP, Medical Affairs and Chief Medical Officer

The center develops ways of collecting, producing and distributing information to help users, prescribers and third-party payers make intelligent selections of devices.

1538 Compuserve: Handicapped Users' Database
5000 Arlington Centre Blvd
Columbus, OH 43220-2913 614-326-1002
800-848-8990
FAX: 614-538-4023
webcenters.netscape.compuserve.com

1539 Computer & Web Resources for People With Disabilities
Alliance for Technology Access
Ste 240
1304 Southpoint Blvd
Petaluma, CA 94954-7464 707-778-3011
FAX: 707-765-2080
TTY:707-778-3015
e-mail: atainfo@ataaccess.org
www.ataccess.org

Sharon Hall, Manager

A guide to maneuvering the growing world of computers, both the mainstream and the assistive technology.
ISBN 0-897933-00-1

1540 Computer Access Center
P.O. Box 12464
Albuquerque, NM 87195 505-242-9588
e-mail: info@cac.org
www.cac.org

Richard Barlow, Board of Director
Richard Rohr, Board of Director
Michael Poffenberger, Board of Director
Damien Faughnan, Board of Director

Computer technology center.

1541 Computer Center for Visually Impaired People: Division of Continuing Studies
Baruch College
1 Bernard Baruch Way
Box H-648
New York, NY 10010 646-312-1420
FAX: 646-312-5101
e-mail: judith.gerber@baruch.cuny.edu
www.baruch.cuny.edu/ccvip

Karen Gourgey, Director
Judith Gerber, Operations Manager
Lynette Tatum, Training Specialist
William Reed, Assistant Director

Offers courses, tutors, equipment and assistance.

1542 Computer Resources for People with Disabilities
Hunter House Publishers, Inc
424 Church Street
Suite 2240
Nashville, TN 37219 615-255-BOOK
e-mail: info@turnerpublishing.com
www.hunterhouse.com

Kiran Rana, Publisher
Chris Alexander, Author
Sheila Alson, Author
Peter Axt, Author

Part One describes conventional and assistive technologies and gives strategies for accessing the Internet. Part Two features easy-to-use charts organized by key access concerns, and provides detailed descriptions of software, hardware, and communication aids. Part Three is a gold mine of Web resources, publications, support organizations, government programs, and technology vendors.

1543 Computer-Enabling Drafting for People with Physical Disabilities
County College of Morris
214 Center Grove Road
Randolph, NJ 07869-2086 973-328-5000
888-226-8001
FAX: 973-328-5067
www.ccm.edu

Edward J Yaw, President
Dr. Dwight Smith, Vice President of Academic Affairs
Karen VanDerhoof, Vice President for Business and Finance
Dr. Bette M. Simmons, VP of Student Development & Enrollment Management

Since they opened in 1968, more than 40,000 graduates have passed through their halls. Many have become teachers, nurses, police officers, doctors and engineers. CCM has also been a community resource for those seeking to enhance their careers through additional education. They drafted a newsletter on Computer-Enabling Drafting for People with Physical Disabilities

1544 DIRLINE
National Library of Medicine
8600 Rockville Pike
Bethesda, MD 20894 301-594-5983
888-346-3656
FAX: 301-402-1384
TTY:800-735-2258
e-mail: custserv@nml.nih.gov
www.nlm.nih.gov/

Dr. Donald A B. Lindberg, Director
Milton Corn, Deputy Director
Betsy Humphreys, Deputy Director
Todd Danielson, Office of Administration

18,000 listings of organizations that serve as information resources, including libraries, professional associations and government agencies.

1545 Developmental Disabilities Council
626 Main Street, Suite A
P.O.Box 3455
Baton Rouge, LA 70821-3455 225-342-6804
800-450-8108
FAX: 225-342-1970
e-mail: shawn.fleming@la.gov
www.laddc.org

Sandee Winchell, Executive Director
Shawn Fleming, Deputy Director
Derek White, Program Manager
Robbie Gray, Program Monitor

The Louisiana Developmental Disabilities Council is made up of people from every region of the state who are appointed by the governor to develop and implement a five year plan to address the needs of persons with disabilities. Membership includes persons with developmental disabilities, parents, advocates, professionals, and representatives from public and private agencies.

1546 **Employment Resources Program**
330 South Grand Avenue West
Springfield, IL 62704
217-523-2587
800-447-4221
FAX: 217-523-0427
TTY: 217-523-2587
e-mail: scil@scil.org
www.scil.org

Pete Roberts, Executive Director
Susanne Cooper, Program Director
Robin Ashton- Hale, Reintegration Coordinator
Kathryn Cline, Business Manager

An information and referral service that encourages inquiries from professionals, individuals with disabilities, family members, organizations or anyone requesting information pertaining to disabilities. The staff at DRN uses both computer listings and in-house library files to provide the programs services. The DRN program is funded by a grant from the Illinois Department of Rehabilitation Services.

1547 **Functional Skills Screening Inventory**
Functional Resources
3905 Huntington Dr
Amarillo, TX 79109-4047
806-353-1114
FAX: 806-353-1114
e-mail: info@winfssi.com
www.winfssi.com

Ed Hammer, Owner
Heather Becker PhD, Owner

Assesses the individual's level of functional skills and identifies supports needed by educational, rehabilitation and residential programs serving moderately and severely disabled persons. Includes environmental assessments as well as profiles of jobs and training sites.

1548 **High Tech Center**
Sacremento State
6000 J Street
Sacramento, CA 95819
916-278-6011
e-mail: sswd@csus.edu
www.csus.edu

Alexander Gonzalez, President
Judy Dean, Co-Director
Melissa Repa, Co-Director
Terry Gomez, Office Manager

The Center offers assessment and training in adaptive hardware/software for eligible students with disabilities at Sacramento State upon referral from the Office of Services to Students with Disabilities.

1549 **Idaho Assistive Technology Project**
121 W 3rd St
Moscow, ID 83843-2268
208-885-3557
20- 88- 614
FAX: 208-885-3628
e-mail: rseiler@uidaho.edu
www.idahoat.org

Ron Seiler, Project Director
Sue House, Information Specialist

A federally funded program managed by the center on disabilities and human development at the university of Idaho. The goal of the IATP is to increase the availability of assistive technology devices and services for Idahoans with disabilities. The IATP offers free trainings and technical assistance, a low-interest loan program, assistive technology assessments for children and agriculture workers, and free informational materials.

1550 **Increasing Capabilities Access Network**
525 W.Capitol
Little Rock, AR 72201
501-666-8868
800-828-2799
FAX: 501-666-5319
TTY: 501-666-8868
e-mail: nfo@ar-ican.org
www.arkansas-ican.org

Bryen Ayres, Member of Advisory Council
Billy Altom, Member of Advisory Council
Adrienne Brown, Member of Advisory Council
Carolyn Boyles, Member of Advisory Council

A consumer responsive statewide systems change program promoting assistive technology for persons of all ages with disabilities. The program provides information on new and existing technology and maintains an equipment exchange free of charge. Training on assistive technology is also provided.

1551 **International Center for the Disabled**
340 E 24th St
New York, NY 10010-4019
212-585-6000
FAX: 212-585-6161
e-mail: info@icdnyc.org
www.icdnyc.org

Jill Bowman, Manager
Les Halpert, CEO

The ICD is a comprehensive outpatient rehabilitation facility, providing medical rehabilitation, behavioral health and vocational services to children and adults with a broad range of physical, communication, emotional and cognitive disabilities.

1552 **Kentucky Assistive Technology Service Network**
200 Juneau Dr.
Suite 200
Louisville, KY 40243
502-429-4484
800-327-5287
FAX: 502-429-7114
www.katsnet.org

Derrick Cox, Manager

Statewide network of four regional assistive technology centers with a central coordinating office in Louisville and two regional centers in eastern Kentucky. Network services include but are not limited to assistive technology of services, loan of assistive devices, funding information and referral, assessment and evaluations, consultations on appropriate technologies, training, and technical assistance.

1553 **Learning Independence Through Computers**
2301 Argonne Drive
Baltimore, MD 21218
410-554-9134
FAX: 410-261-2907
e-mail: info@linc.org
www.linc.org

Theo Pinette, Executive Director
Sandy Fishman, Office and ComputerCenter Coordinator
Angela Tyler, Volunteer Services Manager
Christy Wooden, AT Learning Specialist

V-LINC creates technological solutions to improve the independence and quality of life for individuals of all ages with disabilities in Maryland. We do this through a mix of off-the-shelf computer software and equipment, and one-of-a-kind, customized assistive technology.

1554 **MEDLINE**
Dialog Corporation
2250 Perimeter Park Drive
Suite 300
Morrisville, NC 27560
800-334-2564
919-804-6400
FAX: 919-804-6410
www.dialog.com

Tim Wahlberg, Genral Manager
Morten Nicholaisen, VP Global Sales and Account Mana
Libby Trudell, VP Strategic Initiatives
Tim Hall, Director Integration and Busines

Bibliographic citations to biomedical literature.

1555 **Maine CITE**
University of Maine at Augusta
46 University Avenue
Augusta, ME 04330
207-621-3195
FAX: 207-629-5429
TTY:877-475-4800
e-mail: iweb@mainecite.org
www.mainecite.org

Robert McPhee, Member of Advisory Council
Deborah Gardner, Member of Advisory Council
Anita Dunham, Member of Advisory Council
Sandra Jaeger, Member of Advisory Council

Computer technology center.

1556 **Maryland Technology Assistance Program**
Maryland Department of Disabilities
2301 Argonne Drive
Rm T-17
Baltimore, MD 21218
410-554-9361
800-832-4827
FAX: 410-554-9237
TTY: 866-881-7488
e-mail: MDOD@mdod.state.md.us
www.mdtap.org

James McCarthy, Executive Director
Denise Schuler, Assistive Technology Specialist
Tanya Goodman, Loan Program Assistant Director
Lori Markland, Director ofCommunications, Outreach &Program Development

Assistive technology center. Information and referral, equipment display loans and demonstration, funding sources, alternative media, training, workshops and seminars. Rural outreach for individuals with disability in Maryland.

1557 **Minnesota STAR Program**
358 Centennial Office Building 658
Saint Paul, MN 55155- 1402
651-201-2640
800-627-3529
888-234-1267
FAX: 651-282-6671
e-mail: star.program@state.mn.us
www.admin.state.mn.us/assistivetechnology

Chuck Rassbach, Program Director
Jennis Delisi, Program Staff
Jaoan Gillum, Program Staff
Kim Moccia, Program Staff

STAR's mission is to help all Minnesotans with disabilities gain access to and acquire the assistive technology they need to live, learn, work and lay. The Minnesota STAR program is federally funded by the Rehabilitation Services Administration.

1558 **Mississippi Project START**
2550 Peachtree Street
Jackson, MS 39216
601-987-4872
800-852-8328
FAX: 601-364-2349
e-mail: pgaltelli@mdrs.ms.gov
www.msprojectstart.org

Patsy Galtelli, Executive Director
Dorothy Young, Project Director
Nekeba Simmons, Administrative Assistant
Jason Mac McMaster, Repair Specialist

Project START is a Tech Act project established to bring about systems change in the field of assistive technology in the State of Mississippi. Activities include providing training opportunities for consumers and service providers on subjects such as state-of-the-art AT devices, their application and funding resources; referral information on AT evaluation centers; technical assistance to AT users; establishment of an AT equipment loan program and an Information and Referral Service.

1559 **National Technology Database**
American Foundation for the Blind/ AF B Press
2 Penn Plaza
Suite 1102
New York, NY 10121
212-502-7600
800-232-5463
FAX: 888-545-8331
e-mail: afbinfo@afb.net
www.afb.org

Carl.R Augusto, President and CEO
Robin Vogel, Vice President, Resource Development
Kelly Bleach, Chief Administrative Officer
Rick Bozeman, Chief Financial Officer

This database includes resources for visually impaired persons.
$99.00

1560 **New Jersey Department of Labor & Workforce Development**
Office of the Commissioner
1 John Fitch Plaza
P.O.Box 110
Trenton, NJ 08625-0110
609-292-7060
FAX: 609-633-1359
e-mail: cmycoff@dol.state.nj.us
www.state.nj.us/labor

Harold J. Wirths, Commissioner
Aaron R. Fichtner, Ph.D., Deputy Commissioner
Frederick J. Zavaglia, Chief of Staff
David Ramsay, Director

Oversees various federal and state vocational rehabilitation services including sheltered workshops and independent living centers; adjudication of permanent disability claims filed with the Social Security Administration; oversees New Jersey's temporary disability program covering non-work related illnesses and injuries

1561 **New Mexico Technology Assistance Program**
435 Saint Michaels Drive
Ste D
Santa Fe, NM 87505-7679
505-827-8535
800-866-2253
FAX: 505-954-8608
e-mail: julie.martinez1@state.nm.us
www.nmtap.com

Julie Martinez, Program Director

Examines and works to eliminate barriers to obtaining assistive technology in New Mexico. Has established a statewide program for coordinating assistive technology services; is designed to assist people with disabilities to locate, secure, and maintain assistive technology.

1562 **Northern Illinois Center for Adaptive Technology**
3615 Louisiana Rd
Rockford, IL 61108
815-229-2163
e-mail: davegrass@eartlink.net
www.nicat.ataccess.org

Dave Grass, President

Computer technology center.

1563 **OCCK**
1710 W. Schilling Road
Salina, KS 67402-1160
785-827-9383
800-526-9731
FAX: 785-823-2015
TTY: 785-827-9383
e-mail: occk@occk.com
www.occk.com

Shelia Nelson Stout, President, CEO
Carolee Miner, CEO

Computer technology center; training center for employment and independent living for people with disabilities; family support center. Kansas AgrAbility program coordinator, Kansas equipment exchange site.

1564 Parents, Let's Unite for Kids
516 N 32nd St
Billings, MT 59101-6003
406-255-0540
800-222-7585
FAX: 406-255-0523
TTY: 406-657-2055
e-mail: info@pluk.org
www.pluk.org

Roger Holt, Executive Director
Computer technology center. Parents, Let's Unite for Kids offers an assistive technology lab that is open to people of all ages. The lab is a computer and assistive technology demonstration site. There is no charge for services.

1565 Pennsylvania's Initiative on Assistive Technology
Temple University
1755 N. 13th St
Student Center, Room 4115
Philadelphia, PA 19122-6024
215-204-1356
800-204-7428
FAX: 215-204-6336
TTY: 866-268-0579
e-mail: ATinfo@temple.edu
www.disabilities.temple.edu

Amy S Goldman, Director
Pennsylvania's Initiative on Assistive Technology (PIAT) offers information and referral about assistive Technology (AT), device demonstrations, and awareness-level presentations. PIAT also operates Pennsylvania's AT Lending Library, a free, state-supported program that loans AT devices to Pennsylvanians of all ages. This program allows you to try a device for a limited time to be sure it meets your needs.

1566 Rehabilitation Engineering & Assistive Technology Society of North America (RESNA)
1700 North Moore Street
Suite 1540
Arlington, VA 22209
703-524-6686
FAX: 703-524-6630
TTY:703-524-6639
e-mail: membership@resna.org
www.resna.org

Alex Mihailidis, PhD, P.Eng, President
Ray Grott, ATP, RET, President-Elect
Paul J. Schwartz, Treasurer
Michael J. Brogioli, Executive Director
Improves the potential of people with disabilities to achieve their goals through the use of technology and disability. Promotes research, development, education, advocacy and provision of technology, and by supporting the people engaged in theses activities.

1567 Resource Center for Independent Living(RCIL)
409 Columbia St.
PO Box 210
Utica, NY 13503-210
315-797-4642
FAX: 315-797-4747
TTY:315-797-5837
e-mail: burt.danovitz@rcil.com
www.rcil.com

Burt Danovitz, Executive Director
The RCIL aggressively advocates for and defends the rights of persons with disabilities. RCIL believes in integration adn assisting people to reach their full potential, encouraging a culture of risk-taking, creativity and innovation through our programs and services. They monitor and assess the current legal climate around rights for persons with disabilities on an ongoing bases and are committed and deliberate in speaking about the problems and obstacles faced by persons with disabilities.

1568 SACC Assistive Technoloy Center
P.O.Box 1325
Simi Valley, CA 93062-1325
805-582-1881

www.semel.ucla.edu

Debi Schultze, CEO
SACC connects children, adults and seniors with special needs to computers, technologies and resources. We provide information and referral, assessments, tutoring, presentations and outreach awareness.

1569 South Dakota Department of Human Services: Computer Technology Services
Properties Plaza
500 East Capitol Avenue
Pierre, SD 57501
605-773-5990
800-265-9684
FAX: 605-773-5483
TTY: 605-773-6412
e-mail: infodhs@state.sd.us
dhs.sd.gov

Dan Lusk, Division Director
Ted Williams, Director
Eric Weiss, Director
Gaye Mattke, Director
Computer technology center.

1570 Star Center
1119 Old Humboldt Rd
Jackson, TN 38305-1752
731-668-3888
888-398-5619
FAX: 731-668-1666
TTY: 731-668-9664
e-mail: information@starcenter.tn.org
www.starcenter.tn.org

John Borden, CEO
Nation's largest assistive technology center dedicated to helping children and adults with disabilities achieve their goals for competitive employment, effective learning, returning to or starting school and independent living. Programs include: high-tech training, music therapy, art therapy, low vision evaluation, orientation and mobility evaluation and training, augmentative communication evaluation, vocational evaluations, assistive technology, job placement services and job skills training.

1571 Students with Disabilities Office
University of Texas at Austin
100 West Dean Keeton A5800
Austin, TX 78712-1100
512-471-5017
FAX: 512-471-7833
e-mail: deanofstudents@austin.utexas.edu
deanofstudents.utexas.edu

Soncia Reagins-Lilly, Ed.D., Senior Associate VP for Student Affairs & Dean of Students
Douglas Garrard, Ed.D., Senior Associate Dean of Students
Wanda Brune, Administrative Associate
Sara LeStrange, Manager of Communications

1572 TASK Team of Advocates for Special Kids
100 W Cerritos Ave
Anaheim, CA 92805
714-533-8275
866-828-8275
FAX: 714-533-2533
e-mail: task@taskca.org
www.taskca.org

Marta Anchondo, Executive Director
Tom Bratkovich, Treasurer
Leana Way, Director
Computer technology center.

1573 Tech Connection
35 Haddon Avenue
Shrewsbury, NJ 07702
732-747-5310
FAX: 732-747-1896
e-mail: info@frainc.org
www.frainc.org

Bill Sheeser, President
Nancy Phalanukom, Executive Director
Sue Levine, Program Administrator
Vicky Butler, EI Program Coordinator
Offers a noncommercial center to examine and try computers, adapted equipment, alternative input devices, and a variety of software. Program of Family Resource Associates and a member of the Alliance for Technology Access (ATA), a growing national coalition of computer resource centers, professionals, technol-

ogy developers and vendors, interacting with new technology to enrich the lives of people with disabilities. Tech Connection offers evaluations, for computer technology.

1574 Tech-Able
1451 Klondike Road, Suite D
Conyers, GA 30094 770-922-6768
FAX: 770-922-6769
e-mail: c.b.wright@techable.org
www.techable.org

Cassandra Baker, Executive Director
Pat Hanus, Program Assistant
Erika Ruffin-Mosley, Assistive Technology Trainer
Jason Chadwell, AT & Blind / Low Vision Trainer

Provide assistive technology to individuals with disabilities, toy-lending and software libraries, product demonstration, access to technology devices and fabrication of keyguards for keyboards. Low vision consultant on Thursdays; computer training for persons with disabilities.

1575 Technology Access Center of Tucson
P.O.Box 13178
Tucson, AZ 85732-3178 520-638-2733
FAX: 520-519-7954
e-mail: tact1@qwestoffice.net
http://www.uacoe.arizona.edu/tact/

1576 Technology Assistance for Special Consumers
1856 Keats Drive
Huntsville, AL 35810 256-859-8300
FAX: 256-859-4332
e-mail: tasc@ucphuntsville.org
http://www.ucptasc.org/

Linda Rags, Executive Director

T.A.S.C. is a computer resource center with 10 computers, which are equipped with special adaptations for those who are blind, visually impaired, or severely physically disabled. Our staff demonstrates and trains individuals on this equipment so that they can become more independent at home, school, and work. Over 2,500 pieces of educational software are available for individuals who are learning disabled, mentally retarded or who have developmental delays.

1577 Tidewater Center for Technology Access Special Education Annex
1415 Laskin Rd
Virginia Beach, VA 23451 757-424-2672
FAX: 757-263-2801
e-mail: tcta@aol.com
www.tcta.access.org

Pat Mc Gee, Manager
Myra Jessie Flint, Designee

Nonprofit organization providing persons with disabilities access, support, and knowledge—re: technology; organization contracts for consultations, workshops and training, or conventional and assistive technologies including computers, augmented communication devices and software; resources: extensive lending library of educational software; books and videotape library; yearly individual membership and corporate membership fees; working/presentation and evaluation fees available upon request.

1578 Vermont Assistive Technology Project: Department of Aging & Disabilities
Agency of Human Services
103 South Main Street
Weeks Building
Waterbury, VT 05671-2305 802-871-3353
800-750-6355
FAX: 802-871-3048
TTY: 802-241-1464
e-mail: amber.fulcher@state.vt.us
atp.vermont.gov

Amber Fulcher, Program Director
Sharon Alderman, Assistive Technology Reuse Coordinator
Emma Cobb, Assistive Technology Services Coordinator

Increase the awareness and change policies to insure assistive technology is available to all Vermonters with disabilities.

1579 Xerox Imaging Systems/Adaptive Products Department
Personal Reader Department
9 Centennial Dr
Peabody, MA 01960-7906 978-977-2000
800-248-6550
FAX: 978-977-2409

Keyboards, Mouses & Joysticks

1580 A4 Tech (USA) Corporation
5585 Brooks St
Montclair, CA 91763-4547 909-988-9633
e-mail: info@a4tech.com
www.a4tech.com

Robert C

Manufacturers of a cordless mouse, trackballs and joysticks that emulate mouse controls, flatbed scanners, modified keyboards, and other specialty mouses.

1581 Abacus
3150 Patterson Ave SE
Grand Rapids, MI 49512 616-698-0330
800-451-4319
FAX: 616-698-0325
e-mail: info@abacuspub.com
www.abacuspub.com

Arnie Lee, President

Designs a mouse software program that permits programs written for one computer to be run on another computer.

1582 Ability Center of Greater Toledo
5605 Monroe Street
Sylvania, OH 43560 419-885-5733
FAX: 419-882-4813
www.abilitycenter.org

Tim Harrington, Executive Director
Dale Abell, Director of Program Development
Debbie Andriette, Director of Human Resources
Kimberley Arnett, Director of Community Services

Manufactures keyboard wrist supports to help prevent repetitive motion disorders.

1583 Dreamer
TS Micro Tech
17109 Gale Ave
City of Industry, CA 91745-1810 626-939-8998
FAX: 626-839-8516
e-mail: sales@fancard.com
www.fancard.com

Steve Heung, Owner

An intelligent, add-on function keyboard providing single-keystroke access to multiple-keystroke functions.

1584 FlexShield Keyboard Protectors
Hooleon Corporation
P.O.Box 589
Melrose, NM 88124-589 928-634-7515
800-937-1337
FAX: 928-634-4620
e-mail: sales@hooleon.com
www.hooleon.com

Barry Green, Sales Manager
Joan Crozier, President

Transparent keyboard protectors allowing instant recognition of keytop legends. They have a matte finish to reduce glare. Also available are large print and braille keyboard labels and large print/braille combo labels.

1585 Infogrip: King Keyboard
1899 E. Main Street
Ventura, CA 93001
805-652-0770
800-397-0921
FAX: 805-652-0880
e-mail: support@infogrip.com
www.infogrip.com

Lisa Jacobs, President
Giant alternative keyboard that plugs directly into a computer—no special interface is required. The keys are 1.25 inches in diameter, slightly recessed, and provide both tactile and auditory feedback. The King has a built-in keyboard so that you can rest on its surface without activating keys. This keyboard allows you to control both keyboard and mouse functions, so it's great for people who have difficulty maneuvering a standard mouse. *$130.00*

1586 Infogrip: Large Print Keyboard
1899 E. Main Street
Ventura, CA 93001
805-652-0770
800-397-0921
FAX: 805-652-0880
e-mail: support@infogrip.com
www.infogrip.com

Lisa Jacobs, President
Standard Windows keyboard with large print keys. The keyboard and its keys are the same size as a standard keyboard; however, the print has been enhanced. The characters measure .5 by .25 inches, about 3 times larger than standard keyboard characters. *$130.00*

1587 Infogrip: OnScreen
1899 E. Main Street
Ventura, CA 93001
805-652-0770
800-397-0921
FAX: 805-652-0880
e-mail: support@infogrip.com
www.infogrip.com

Lisa Jacobs, President
OnScreen features word prediction/completion (with an editable dictionary), Key Dwell Timer (a timer that selects a key under the cursor), integrated Verbal Keys Feedback, Show and Hide Keys (turns on/off keys to prevent access and minimize confusion) a Smart Window (automatically re-positions the keyboard or panels off of the area in use). On Screen also offers edit, numeric, macro, calculator and Windows enhancement capabilities. *$200.00*

1588 IntelliKeys
Intelli Tools
1720 Corporate Circle
Petaluma, CA 94954
707-773-2000
800-899-6687
FAX: 707-773-2001
e-mail: info@intellitools.com
www.intellitools.com

Dayton Johnson, VP, Sales
Arjan Khalsa, CEO
Alternative, touch-sensitive keyboards; plugs into any Macintosh or Windows computer. *$395.00*

1589 IntelliKeys USB
Intelli Tools
1720 Corporate Circle
Petaluma, CA 94954
707-773-2000
800-899-6687
FAX: 707-773-2001
e-mail: info@intellitools.com
www.intellitools.com

Dayton Johnson, VP, Sales
Arjan Khalsa, CEO
IntelliKeys alternative keyboard for USB computers and Windows 2000, Mac OSX. *$69.95*

1590 Key Tronic KB 5153 Touch Pad Keyboard
KeyTronic
N. 4424 Sullivan Road
Spokane Valley, WA 99216
509-928-8000
FAX: 509-927-5555
e-mail: EMSsales@keytronicems.com
www.keytronic.com

Craig.D Gates, President/CEO
Ronald.F Klawitter, EVP of Administration and Chief Financial Officer
Douglas G. Burkhardt, Executive Vice President of Worldwide Operations
Philip S. Hochberg, Executive Vice President of Business Development
Integrates a regular full-function keyboard, a numeric keypad with a cursor key capability and a touch pad into one unit.

1591 Magic Wand Keyboard
In Touch Systems
11 Westview Road
Spring Valley, NY 10977
845-354-7431
800-332-6244
e-mail: sc@magicwandkeyboard.com
www.magicwandkeyboard.com

Jerry Crouch, President
Susan Crouch, VP
The magic wand keyboard allows your child to use a keyboard and mouse easily-no light beams, microphones, or sensors to wear of position. This miniature computer keyboard has zero-force keys that work with the slightest touch of a wand (hand-held of mouthstick). No strength required.

1592 McKey Mouse
In Touch Systems
11 Westview Road
Spring Valley, NY 10977
845-354-7431
800-332-6244
e-mail: sc@magicwandkeyboard.com
www.magicwandkeyboard.com

Jerry Crouch, President
Susan Crouch, VP
Microsoft compatible mouse for persons with little or no hand/arm movement; it's an option for the Magic Wand Keyboard and adds full mouse function without adding any extra devices.

1593 PortaPower Plus
Words+
42505 10th Street West
Lancaster, CA 93534-7059
661-723-7723
800-869-8521
FAX: 661-723-5524
e-mail: info@simulations-plus.com
www.simulations-plus.com

Walter S Woltosz, M.S., M.A.S., President, CEO
John A. DiBella, Vice President, Marketing & Sales
John R. Kneisel, Chief Financial Officer
Robert D. Clark, Ph.D., Director, Life Sciences
Rechargeable battery pack designed to give longer life and remote usage time to laptop computers and other portable battery-operated devices and accessories. Requires a 12 volt auto adapter. *$149.00*

1594 Step on It! Computer Control Pedals
Suite 118
1290 Carmead Pkwy
Sunnyvale, CA 94086
408-736-6086
FAX: 408-736-6083
e-mail: bilbo@bilbo.com
www.bilbo.com

Sergei Burkov, President
BILBO Innovations, Inc. manufactures and sells Step On It keyboard control pedals. Ergonomic foot switches to emulate keystrokes and mouse clicks. Designed for victims of Repetitive Strain Injury (RSI), Carpal Tunnel Syndrome (CTS), handicapped and disabled. *$99.00*

1595 **Unicorn Keyboards**
Intelli Tools
1720 Corporate Circle
Petaluma, CA 94954
707-773-2000
800-899-6687
FAX: 707-773-2001
e-mail: info@intellitools.com
www.intellitools.com

Dayton Johnson, VP, Sales
Arjan Khalsa, CEO
Alternative keyboards with membrane surface and large, user-defined keys. Large and small sizes are available. *$250.00*

Scanners

1596 **Scanning WSKE**
Words+
42505 10th Street West
Lancaster, CA 93534-7059
661-723-7723
888-266-9294
FAX: 661-723-5524
e-mail: info@simulations-plus.com
www.simulations-plus.com

Walter S Woltosz, M.S., M.A.S., President, CEO
John A. DiBella, Vice President, Marketing & Sales
John R. Kneisel, Chief Financial Officer
Robert D. Clark, Ph.D., Director, Life Sciences
A software and a hardware product designed to operate on an IBM compatible PC. The software provides dual word prediction, abbreviation expansion, five different methods of voice output, and access to commercial software applications.

1597 **System 2000/Versa**
Words+
42505 10th Street West
Lancaster, CA 93534-7059
661-723-7723
800-869-8521
FAX: 661-723-5524
e-mail: info@simulations-plus.com
www.simulations-plus.com

Walter S Woltosz, M.S., M.A.S., President, CEO
John A. DiBella, Vice President, Marketing & Sales
John R. Kneisel, Chief Financial Officer
Robert D. Clark, Ph.D., Director, Life Sciences
Provides all of the strategies currently being used in AAC, from dynamic display color pictographic language, to dual-word prediction text language, in a single system.

1598 **Zygo-UsaSvc Corporation**
48834 Kato Road Suite 101-A
Fremont, CA 94538
510-249-9660
800-234-6006
FAX: 510-770-4930
e-mail: zygo@zygo-usa.com
www.zygo-usa.com

Adam Weiss, Vp Sales & Marketing
ZYGO-USA has been involved in manufacturing and distributing assistive technologies since 1974. They specialize in augmentative and alternative computer access. They offer a wide range of technology products to our clients so they can achieve a greater independence and to enhance the quality of their lives. These soloutins improve and individual's ability to learn, work, and interact with family and friends.

Screen Enhancement

1599 **Boxlight**
Boxlight Corporation
151 State Highway 300, Suite A
P.O. Box 2609
Belfair, WA 98528
360-464-2119
866-972-1549
e-mail: sales@boxlight.com
www.boxlight.com

Herb Myers, CEO/Founder
Sloan Myers, Founder
Hank Nance, President
BOXLIGHT is a global presentation solutions partner for trainers, educators and professional speakers. Solutions include projector sales, national rental service, technical support, repair, and presentation peripherals. For more information visit us online.

1600 **FDR Series of Low Vision Reading Aids**
Optelec U S
Breslau 4
Barendrecht, LT 92081-8358
886-783-444
800-826-4200
FAX: 886-783-400
e-mail: info@optelec.com
in.optelec.com

Stephan Terwolbeck, President
Michiel van Schaik, VP
Janet Lennex, Director of Customer Excellence
Jade Arbelo, Director of Human Resources
The Low Vision Reading Aids features; high resolution, positive and negative display, a high-quality zoom lens, versatile swivel and a 12 inch or 19 inch high-resolution monitor, color or black and white, computer compatible, or portable.

1601 **InFocus**
AI Squared
130 Taconic Business Park Road
Manchester Center, VT 05255
802-362-3612
800-859-0270
FAX: 802-362-1670
e-mail: sales@aisquared.com
www.aisquared.com

David Wu, CEO
Jost Eckhardt, VP of Engineering
Scott Moore, VP of Marketing
Shawn Warren, VP of Product Support
A memory-resident program that magnifies text and graphics - the entire screen, a single line or a portion of the screen.

1602 **Portable Large Print Computer**
Human Ware
1800, Michaud street
Drummondville, CA 94520-1213
819-471-4818
888-723-7273
FAX: 925-681-4630
e-mail: ca.info@humanware.com
www.humanware.com/en-australia/home

Real Goulet, Chairman
Gilles Pepin, CEO
Michel Cote, Corporate Director
Georges Morin, Corporate Director
A portable large print computer which magnifies up to 64 times. It is linked to a PC and has a hand-held camera.

1603 **ZoomText**
A I Squared
130 Taconic Business Park Road
Manchester Center, VT 05255
802-362-3612
800-859-0270
FAX: 802-362-1670
e-mail: sales@aisquared.com
www.aisquared.com

David Wu, CEO
Jost Eckhardt, VP of Engineering
Scott Moore, VP of Marketing
Shawn Warren, VP of Product Support

A RAM-resident program that enlarges screen characters up to eight times. It runs on IBM PC, XT, AT and PS/2.

Speech Synthesizers

1604 Artic Business Vision (for DOS) and Artic WinVision (for Windows 95)
Artic Technologies
3456 Rodchester Road
Troy, MI 48083
248-689-9883
FAX: 248-588-2650
e-mail: info@ablezone.com
www.articannex.ws/artictec.htm

Dale McDaniel, Founder
Kathy Gargagliano, Founder

A speech processor for blind computer users featuring true interactive speech with spread sheets, word processors, database managers, etc. Now available with both Windows 3.1 and Windows 95 access. *$ 495.00*

1605 Computerized Speech Lab
Kay Elemetrics Corporation
3 Paragon Drive
Montvalle, NJ 07645
973-628-6200
800-289-5297
FAX: 201-391-2063
www.kaypentax.com

John Crump, President

Hardware/software for the acquisition, analysis/display, playback and storage of speech signals.

1606 DynaVox Technologies Speech Communication Devices
Dyna Vox Technologies
2100 Wharton St
Suite 400
Pittsburgh, PA 15203-1945
412-381-4883
866-396-2869
FAX: 412-381-5241
e-mail: Ray.Merk@dynavoxtech.com
www.dynavoxtech.com

Ed Donnelly, CEO
Michelle Heying, President and COO
Kenneth Misch, CFO
Ray Merk, VP Finance

Develops and manufactures speech communication devices that help individuals who are unable to speak due to speech, language and/or learning disabilities to communicate quickly and easily.

1607 Electronic Speech Assistance Devices
Luminaud
8688 Tyler Blvd
Mentor, OH 44060-4348
440-255-9082
800-255-3408
FAX: 440-255-2250
e-mail: info@luminaud.com
www.luminaud.com

Thomas M Lennox, President
Dorothy Lennox, VP

Offers a full line of speech aids, voice amplifiers, mini-vox amplifiers, laryngectomec products.

1608 Keywi
Hoffmann + Krippner Inc.
200 Westpark Drive
Suite 270
Peachtree City, GA 30269
770-487-1950
FAX: 770-487-1945
www.keywi-usa.com

1609 Little Mack Communicator
AbleNet
2625 Patton Road
Roseville, MN 55113-1308
651-294-2200
800-322-0956
FAX: 651-294-2259
e-mail: customerservice@ablenetinc.com
www.ablenetinc.com

Bill Sproull, Chairman
Jennifer Thalhuber, President/CEO
Paul Sugden, Former Vice President of Finance
William Mills, Board of Directors

The Little Mack Communicator has 2 minutes of memory and has an angled switch surface making it easy to see and access. The switch surface is 2 1/2 inches in diameter. Detachable mounting base makes it easy to position a single unit in a variety of locations. *$129.00*

1610 Mega Wolf Communication Device
Wayne County Regional Educational Service Agency
33500 Van Born Rd
Wayne, MI 48184-2474
734-334-1300
FAX: 734-334-1620
www.resa.net

Lynda S. Jackson, President
Kenneth E. Berlinn, Vice President
James Petrie, Secretary
Mary E. Blackmon, Treasurer

A low cost voice output communication device which is primarily intended to provide the power of speech to those individuals who are most severely challenged mentally and/or physically. The WOLF device is User programmable and uses the Texas Instruments' Touch and Tell case and touch panel; ADAMLAB electronics with synthesized (robotic) voice. For users able to point with approximately 6 ounces of pressure. *$400.00*

1611 Talking Screen
Words+
42505 10th St W
Lancaster, CA 93534-7059
661-723-7723
888-266-9294
FAX: 661-723-5524
e-mail: info@simulations-plus.com
www.simulations-plus.com

Walter S Woltosz, M.S., M.A.S., Chairman, President and Chief Ex
John R. Kneisel, Chief Financial Officer
John DiBella, Vice President, Marketing and Sales
Robert D. Clark, Ph.D, Director, Life Sciences

An augmentative communication program that allows the user to select graphic symbols on the display to produce speech output. Symbols can be used either singly or in sequence as picture abbreviations. *$ 1395.00*

1612 Turnkey Computer Systems for the Visually, Physically, and Hearing Impaired
E VA S
39 Canal St P.O. Box 371
Westerly, RI 02891-1511
401-596-3155
800-872-3827
FAX: 401-596-3979
TTY: 401-596-3500
e-mail: contact@evas.com
www.evas.com

Gerald Swerdlick, Owner
Jerry Swerdlick, CEO

Offers clear speech with pleasant inflection and tonal quality as well as variable pitch, intonation and voices.

1613 **Voice-It**
V XI Corporation Incorporated
271 Locust Street
Denver, NH 03820
603-742-2888
800-742-8588
FAX: 603-742-5065
e-mail: info@vxicorp.com
www.vxicorp.com

Michael Ferguson, President
Tom Manero, Chief Financial Officer
Phil Pane, Vice President Operations
Brian Cole, Vice President Engineering

Adds voice to popular spreadsheet and word processing applications on IBM PCs and compatibles, turning spreadsheets and word processing documents into talking documents.

1614 **Window-Eyes**
G W Micro
725 Airport North Office Park
Fort Wayne, IN 46825
260-489-3671
FAX: 260-489-2608
e-mail: sales@gwmicro.com
www.gwmicro.com

Dan Weirich, Owner/Vice President of Sales an
Doug Geoffray, Owner

Provides access to available software automatically reading information important to the user while ignoring the rest. A screen reader for the windows operative system.

Software: Math

1615 **AIMS Multimedia**
Discovery Education
8145 Holton Dr
Florence, KY 41042-3009
859-342-7200
FAX: 877-324-6830
e-mail: info@multimedia.com
www.aimsmultimedia.com

Mike Wright, Director
Lynn Fassett, Administrative Assistant
Cindy Vogt, Human Resources Executive

AIMS Multimedia is a leader in the production and distribution of training and educational programs for the business and K-12 communities via YHS, interactive CD-ROM, DVD and Internet streaming video.

1616 **Basic Math: Detecting Special Needs**
Allyn & Bacon
One Liberty Square
Suite 1200
Boston, MA 02109-3988
617-261-0040
800-852-8024
FAX: 617-944-7273
e-mail: samplingdept@pearson.com
www.greenellp.com

Thomas M Greene, Attorney at Law
Michael Tabb, Attorney at Law

Describes special mathematics needs of special learners.
180 pages
ISBN 0-205116-35-3

1617 **Campaign Math**
Mindplay
4400 E. Broadway Blvd
Suite 400
Tucson, AZ 85711-1726
520-888-1800
800-221-7911
FAX: 520-888-7904
e-mail: mail@mindplay.com
www.mindplay.com

Judith Bliss, CEO
Brian Williams, Development Manager
Lisa Garcia, Director of Educational Services
Chris Coleman, Vice President of Business Development

A complete program on the electoral process as well as a math package which teaches ratios, fractions and percentages.

1618 **Educational Activities Software**
5600 W 83rd Street
Suite 300, 8200 Tower
Bloomington, MN 55437
866-243-8464
FAX: 239-225-9299
e-mail: jwest@orchardlng.com
www.edmentum.com

Vin Riera, President & Chief Executive Officer
Rob Rueckl, Chief Financial Officer
Dave Adams, Chief Academic Officer
Paul Johansen, Chief Technology Officer

Comprehensive MATH SKILLS software tutorials teach concepts ranging from rounding and tables to measuring area. MAC/WIN compatible. *$369.00*
Per Unit

1619 **Fraction Factory**
Queue
80 Hathaway Drive
Stratford, CT 06615
800-232-2224
FAX: 800-775-2729
e-mail: jdk@queueinc.com
qworkbooks.com

Anna Christopoulos, General Manager
Peter Uhrynowski, Comptroller
Steve Pernett, Director of Printing and Graphic
Ann Pleszko, Shipping Manager

In 1980, Jonathan Kantrowitz started Queue, Inc. as an educational software company. After twenty thriving years publishing and distributing high-quality software to educators, Queue began transitioning from software to workbooks, focusing on state-specific test preparation.

1620 **Information & Referral Services**
Information + Referral Services
2590 N. Alvernon Way
Tucson, AZ 85712
520-323-1708
FAX: 520-325-8841
e-mail: inform@azinfo.org
www.azinfo.org

Patti Caldwell, Executive Director
Chuck Palm, Treasurer
Ben Rensvold, Vice President
Tom DeSollar, President

Provides information about health and human services for people in Arizona over the telephone. Information specialists help callers clarify their needs, and provide referrals to the appropriate service agency.

1621 **King's Rule**
WINGS for Learning
1600 Green Hills Rd
Scotts Valley, CA 95066-4981
831-426-2228
FAX: 831-464-3600

Ani Stocks, Owner

A software mathematical problem solving game. Students discover mathematical rules as they work their way through a castle and generate and test a working hypothesis by asking questions.

1622 **Learning About Numbers**
C&C Software
5713 Kentford Cir
Wichita, KS 67220-3131
316-683-6056
800-752-2086

Carol Clark, President

Three programs use the power of computer graphics to provide young children with a variety of experiences in working with numbers. *$50.00*

1623 Math Rabbit
Learning Company
Ste 1900
100 Pine St
San Francisco, CA 94111-5205
415-659-2000
800-825-4420
FAX: 415-659-2020
e-mail: thelearningco@hmhpub.com
www.hmhco.com

Linda K. Zecher, President, Chief Executive Officer and Director
Eric Shuman, Chief Financial Officer
William Bayers, Executive Vice President and General Counsel
Dr. Tim Cannon, Executive Vice President,

Teaches early math concepts by matching objects to numbers, then adding and subtracting up to 18.

1624 Math for Everyday Living
Educational Activities Software
5600 W 83rd Street
Suite 300, 8200 Tower
Bloomington, MN 55437
866-243-8464
FAX: 239-225-9299
e-mail: jwest@orchardlng.com
www.edmentum.com

Vin Riera, President & Chief Executive Officer
Rob Rueckl, Chief Financial Officer
Dave Adams, Chief Academic Officer
Paul Johansen, Chief Technology Officer

Real life math skills are taught with this tutorial and practice software program. Examples include Paying for a Meal (addition and subtraction), Working with Sales Slips (multiplication), Unit Pricing (division), Sales Tax (percent), Earning with Overtime (fractions) plus more. Software: CD-ROM, Windows, MAC, and DOS. *$159.00*

1625 Math for Successful Living
Siboney Learning Group
5600 W 83rd Street
Suite 300, 8200 Tower
Bloomington, MN 55437
866-243-8464
FAX: 239-225-9299
e-mail: jwest@orchardlng.com
www.edmentum.com

Vin Riera, President & Chief Executive Officer
Rob Rueckl, Chief Financial Officer
Dave Adams, Chief Academic Officer
Paul Johansen, Chief Technology Officer

These programs include managing a checking account, budgeting, shopping strategies and buying on credit.

1626 Piece of Cake Math
Queue Inc
80 Hathaway Drive
Stratford, CT 06615
800-232-2224
FAX: 800-775-2729
e-mail: jdk@queueinc.com
www.qworkbooks.com

Anna Christopoulos, General Manager
Peter Uhrynowski, Comptroller
Steve Pernett, Director of Printing and Graphic
Ann Pleszko, Shipping Manager

In 1980, Jonathan Kantrowitz started Queue, Inc. as an educational software company. After twenty thriving years publishing and distributing high-quality software to educators, Queue began transitioning from software to workbooks, focusing on state-specific test preparation.

1627 Puzzle Tanks
WINGS for Learning
1600 Green Hills Rd
Scotts Valley, CA 95066-4981
831-426-2228
FAX: 831-464-3600

Ani Stocks, Owner

A mathematical problem solving game that involves multi-step problems.

1628 Right Turn
WINGS for Learning
1600 Green Hills Rd
Scotts Valley, CA 95066-4981
831-426-2228
FAX: 831-464-3600

Ani Stocks, Owner

Requires students to predict, experiment and learn about the mathematical concepts of rotation and transformation.

1629 RoboMath
4400 E. Broadway Blvd
Suite 400
Tucson, AZ 85711-1726
520-888-1800
800-221-7911
FAX: 520-888-7904
e-mail: mail@mindplay.com
www.mindplay.com

Judith Bliss, CEO
Brian Williams, Development Manager
Lisa Garcia, Director of Educational Services
Chris Coleman, Vice President of Business Development

A complete program on the electoral process as well as a math package which teaches ratios, fractions and percentages.

1630 Stickybear Math I Deluxe
Optimum Resource
1 Mathews Drive
Suite 107
Hilton Head Island, SC 29926- 3689
843-689-8000
FAX: 843-689-8008
e-mail: info@stickybear.com
www.stickybear.com

Richard Hefter, President

Sharpen basic addition and subtraction skills with this captivating series of math exercises. Grades Pre-K to 2. Available in as single edition with sizing up to 30 users at a site. English/Spanish. *$59.95*

1631 Stickybear Math II Deluxe
Optimum Resource
1 Mathews Drive
Suite 107
Hilton Head Island, SC 29926- 3689
843-689-8000
FAX: 843-689-8008
e-mail: info@stickybear.com
www.stickybear.com

Richard Hefter, President

Multiplication and division, beginning with the elementary problems and developing into the more complex problems with regrouping. Grades 2-4. Available for single user through the 30 user site package. English/Spanish. *$59.95*

1632 Stickybear Math Splash
Optimum Resource
1 Mathews Drive
Suite 107
Hilton Head Island, SC 29926- 3689
843-689-8000
FAX: 843-689-8008
e-mail: info@stickybear.com
www.stickybear.com

Richard Hefter, President

Unique multiple activities keep the learning level high while children acquire skills in addition, subtraction, multiplication and division. K-5th grade. Available as single edition up to 30 user site package. English/Spanish. *$59.95*

1633 Stickybear Math Word Problems
Optimum Resource
1 Mathews Drive
Suite 107
Hilton Head Island, SC 29926- 3689
843-689-8000
FAX: 843-689-8008
e-mail: info@stickybear.com
www.stickybear.com

Richard Hefter, President

Hundreds of different word problems make it easy for students to practice basic math skills around analyzing and solving word problems. Grades 1-5. Available as single edition up to 30 user site package. English/Spanish. *$59.95*

1634 Stickybear Money
Optimum Resource
1 Mathews Drive
Suite 107
Hilton Head Island, SC 29926- 3667 843-689-8000
FAX: 843-689-8008
e-mail: info@stickybear.com
www.stickybear.com

Chris Gintz, President
Teaches children to recognize US coins and paper money and introduces simple counting. K to 3rd grade. Bilingual. *$59.95*

1635 Stickybear Numbers Deluxe
Optimum Resource
1 Mathews Drive
Suite 107
Hilton Head Island, SC 29926- 3689 843-689-8000
FAX: 843-689-8008
e-mail: info@stickybear.com
www.stickybear.com

Richard Hefter, President
Counting and number recognition are as easy as 1-2-3 with this award-winning program. Teaches number recognition of numbers 0-9 and 0-30. Pre-K to 2nd grade. Available as single edition up to 30 user site package. *$59.95*

1636 Tomorrow's Promise: Mathematics
Compass Learning
203 Colorado Street
Austin, TX 78701 512-478-9600
800-678-1412
866-586-7387
www.compasslearning.com

Eric Loeffel, President
Trey Chambers, Chief Financial Officer
ARTHUR VANDERVEEN, Vice President, Business Strategy and Development
CHIPP WALTERS, Chief Designer Officer
By integrating interdisciplinary content and real-world application of skills, this product emphasizes the practical value of fundamental math skills. It helps your students develop a problem-solving aptitude for ongoing mathematics achievement.

Software: Miscellaneous

1637 Adventures in Musicland
Electronic Courseware Systems
1713 S State St
Champaign, IL 61820-7258 217-359-7099
800-832-4965
FAX: 217-359-6578
e-mail: support@ecsmedia.com
http://ecsmedia.com.np/

G Peters, President
Jodie Varner, Marketing Manager
This unique set of music games features characters from Lewis Carroll's, Alice in Wonderland. Players learn through pictures, sounds, and animation which help develop understanding of musical tones, composers, and musical symbols. Games include MusicMatch, Melody Mixup, Picture Perfect and Sound Concentration. *$49.95*

1638 Ai Squared
130 Taconic Business Park Road
Manchester Center, VT 05255-669 802-362-3612
800-859-0270
FAX: 802-362-1670
e-mail: sales@aisquared.com
http://www.aisquared.com

David Wu, CEO
Jost Eckhardt, VP of Engineering
Scott Moore, VP of Marketing
Shawn Warren, VP of Product Support
Developers of software for the visually impaired.

1639 All About You: Appropriate Special Interactions and Self-Esteem
P CI Educational Publishing
P.O.Box 34270
San Antonio, TX 78265-4270 210-377-1999
800-594-4263
800-471-3000
FAX: 888-259-8284
e-mail: submissions@pcieducation.com
www.pcicatalog.com

Lee Wilson, President and CEO
Randy Pennington, Executive VP
Jeff McLane, Founder
David Keith, Vice President of IT
This game offers parents and game players a new line of communication when discussing various issues such as learning to be thoughtful, respecting the rights and feelings of others, how to make and keep friends and more. *$49.95*

1640 All Star Review
Tom Snyder Productions
100 Talcott Ave
Watertown, MA 02472-5703 800-342-0236
e-mail: dealer@tomsnyder.com.
www.tomsnyder.com

Rick Abrams, Manager
Tom Synder, Founder
Bridget Dalton, Ed.D., Author
Peggy Healy Stearns, Ph.D., Author
This package turns group review into a baseball game for small and large groups.

1641 Attainment Company
I ET Resources
P.O.Box 930160
Verona, WI 53593-160 608-845-7880
800-327-4269
FAX: 608-845-8040
e-mail: info@attainmentcompany.com
www.attainmentcompany.com

Don Bastian, President
Julie Denu, Technical Support
Theresa O'Connor, Office Manager
Augmentative/alternative communication, software, videos, print and hands-on functional life skills and basic acdemics materials for developmental and cognitive disabilities.

1642 Attention Getter
Soft Touch
12301 Central Ave NE Ste 205
4300 Stine Rd
Blaine, MN 55434 763-755-1402
888-755-1402
FAX: 763-862-2920
e-mail: support@marblesoft.com
www.softtouch.com

Joyce Meyer, President
The whimsical photos morph to another photo and then to a third photo in categories. Paired with interesting sounds and music, the photo animations are so engaging that the student is motivated to activate the computer to see and hear the next one. This is a perfect vehicle to achieve goals aimed at attention getting, activating a switch or intentionally. Compatible with USB IntelliKeys keyboards.

1643 Attention Teens
Soft Touch
12301 Central Ave NE Ste 205
Blaine, MN 55434 763-755-1403
888-755-1403
FAX: 763-862-2921
e-mail: support@marblesoft.com
www.softtouch.com

Joyce Meyer, President
Attention Teens (formerly known as Loony Teens) is a program for teens with disabilities who need powerful input to get their at-

tention. Attention Teens is a computer program to do just this. Paired with interesting sounds and music, the photo animations are so engaging that the student is motivated to activate the computer to see and hear the next one. Compatible with USB IntelliKeys keyboards.

1644 **Away We Ride**
Soft Touch
12301 Central Ave NE Ste 205
4300 Stine Rd
Blaine, MN 55434 763-755-1404
888-755-1404
FAX: 763-862-2922
e-mail: support@marblesoft.com
www.softtouch.com

Joyce Meyer, President
Software for children and teens. For Macintosh and PC.

1645 **Battenberg & Associates**
11135 Rolling Springs Dr
Carmel, IN 46033-3629 317-843-2208

Jan Battenberg, Owner
Offers various software programs that develop the user's visual memory, sequencing skills, word recognition, hand-eye coordination and more.

1646 **Behavior Skills: Learning How People Should Act**
PCI Education Publishing
P.O.Box 34270
San Antonio, TX 78265-4270 210-377-1999
800-471-3000
FAX: 888-828-
www.pcieducation.com

Jeff Clain, CEO
Erin Kinard, VP Product Development/Publisher
Helps players learn what behavior is acceptable and what behavior is not acceptable in the real world. *$49.95*

1647 **Blocks in Motion**
Don Johnston
26799 W Commerce Dr
Volo, IL 60073-9675 847-740-0749
800-999-4660
FAX: 847-740-7326
e-mail: info@donjohnston.com
www.donjohnston.com

Ruth Ziolkowski, President
Don Jhonson, Founder
This unique art and motion program makes drawing, creating and animating fun and educational for all users. Based on the Piagetian Theory for motor-sensory development, this program promotes the concept that the process is as educational and as much fun as the end result. *$79.00*

1648 **CINTEX: Speak to Your Appliances**
NanoPac
4823 S Sheridan Rd
Suite 302
Tulsa, OK 74145-5717 918-665-0329
800-580-6086
FAX: 918-665-0361
TTY: 918-665-2310
e-mail: info@nanopac.com
www.nanopac.com

Silvio Cianfrone, President
CINTEX, with a voice recognition program, will control up to 256 off/on appliances, dial and answer the phone, flash for call waiting, dial from a directory, control TV's, VCR's, stereos and more — all with your voice. CINTEX2 includes the necessary hardware and voice macros which you can use to immediately control your environment. You can tailor these macros to your personal needs and add new macros. Pops-up over current application allowing instant access. $695-$2,000.

1649 **Car Builder Deluxe**
Optimum Resource
1 Mathews Drive
Suite 107
Hilton Head Island, SC 29926- 3689 843-689-8000
FAX: 843-689-8008
e-mail: info@stickybear.com
www.stickybear.com

Richard Hefter, President
As design engineers, users build cars on screen, specifying chassis length, wheelbase, engine type, transmission, fuel tank size, suspension, steering, tires and brakes. All functional choices are interrelated and will affect the performance of the final design. Grades 3 & up. *$59.99*

1650 **Center for Best Practices in Early Childhood**
Horrabin Hall 32
Macomb, IL 61455 309-298-1634
FAX: 309-298-2305
e-mail: jk-johanson@wiu.edu
www.wiu.edu/thecenter/

Linda Robinson, Assistant Director
The Center, part of the College of Education and Human Services at Western Illinois University, provides products, training materials, and information related to best practices for educators and families of young children with disabilities.

1651 **Clock**
Compass Learning
203 Colorado Street
Austin, TX 78701-3922 512-478-9600
800-678-1412
866-586-7387
www.compasslearning.com

Eric Loeffel, President
Trey Chambers, Chief Financial Officer
ARTHUR VANDERVEEN, Vice President, Business Strategy and Development
CHIPP WALTERS, Chief Designer Officer
An extremely simple, easy-to-use program for children who are learning how to read the time of day from clocks and digital displays. Apple and MS-DOS and Mac available. *$39.95*

1652 **Community Skills: Learning to Function in Your Neighborhood**
Programming Concepts
8700 Shoal Creek Boulevard
Austin, TX 78757-6897 210-377-1999
800-594-4263
800-471-3000
FAX: 888-259-8284
e-mail: submissions@pcieducation.com
www.proedinc.com

Lee Wilson, President and CEO
Randy Pennington, Executive VP
Jeff McLane, Founder
David Keith, Vice President of IT
Offers parents and educators a functional way to teach community life skills. *$49.95*

1653 **Companion Activities**
Soft Touch
12301 Central Ave NE Ste 205
4300 Stine Rd
Blaine, MN 55434 763-755-1404
888-755-1404
FAX: 763-862-2922
e-mail: support@marblesoft.com
www.softouch.com

Joyce Meyer, President
Print your own books, worksheets, flash cards, board games, matching games, bingo games, card games and many more. This CD offers numerous companion activities to different SoftTouch software titles. Activities range from very easy to difficult. Companion activities are great tools to reinforce learning. Use the work sheets - black and white and color - in the inclusion class for students with special needs.

1654 **Concepts on the Move Advanced Preacademics**
Soft Touch
12301 Central Ave NE Ste 205
P.O.Box 490215
Blaine, MN 55449 763-862-2920
888-755-1402
FAX: 763-862-2922
e-mail: support@marblesoft.com
www.marblesoft.com

Joyce Meyer, President
Choose from five concepts groups: categories, occupations, functions, goes with and prepositions. Use our Steps to Learning Design to choose how many concepts to present at one time and where to place each one in the scan array, on screen keyboard or IntelliKeys keyboard. Watch and listen as the concept morphs or changes and music plays. The words are also shown to reinforce emerging literacy skills. Compatible with USB IntelliKeys.

1655 **Cooking Class: Learning About Food Preparation**
Programming Concepts
8700 Shoal Creek Boulevard
Austin, TX 78757-6897 512-451-3246
800-897-3202
800-471-3000
FAX: 800-397-7633
e-mail: general@proedinc.com
www.proedinc.com

Jeff McLane, Founder
Lee Wilson, President and CEO
Randy Pennington, Executive VP
David Keith, Vice President of IT
This game offers parents and educators a new way to teach basic preparation skills. Kitchen safety and sanitation are stressed throughout the game. *$49.95*

1656 **Dilemma**
Educational Activities Software
5600 West 83rd Street
Suite 300, 8200 Tower
Bloomington, MN 55437 800-447-5286
FAX: 239-225-9299
e-mail: info@edmentum.com
www.edmentum.com

Vin Riera, President/CEO
Dan Juckniess, SVP, Sales & Professional Services
Stacey Herteux, VP, Human Resources
Rob Rueckl, Chief Financial Officer
Realistic stories with a choice of different gripping endings, color graphics, a built-in dictionary and a user controlled reading rate make these computer programs compelling enough to interest all students. Comprehension and vocabulary questions follow each story. *$159.00*

1657 **Dino-Games**
Academic Software
3504 Tates Creek Road
Lexington, KY 40517-2601 859-552-1020
859-552-1040
FAX: 253-799-4012
e-mail: asistaff@acsw.com
www.acsw.com

Dr. Warren E Lacefield PhD, President
Penelope D. Ellis, COO, Sales & Marketing Director
Sylvia B. Lacefield, Graphic Artist
Cindy L George, Author
Dino-Games are single switch software programs for early switch practice. Dinosaur games provide practice in pattern recognition, cause and effect demonstration, directionality training, number concepts and problem solving. They are compatible with most popular switch interfaces and alternate keyboards. For Macintosh, IBM and compatibles. DINO-LINK is a matching game; DINO-MAZE is a series of maze games; DINO-FIND is a game of concentration; and DINO-DOT is a collection of dot-to-dot games.
$39.95 per game

1658 **Directions: Technology in Special Education**
DREAMMS for Kids
273 Ringwood Road
Freeville, NY 13068-5606 607-539-3027
FAX: 607-539-9930
e-mail: janet@dreamms.org
www.dreamms.org

Janet P. Hosmer, Editor/Publisher
Chester D. Hosmer, Jr., Technical Editor
Susan Lait, Regular Contributor
Lorianne Hoenninger, Regular Contributor
A CD containing all of 'Directions' past articles and information gathered from their newsletter which lists resources for assistive and adaptive computer ethnologies in the home, school and community. *$24.95*

1659 **ESI Master Resource Guide**
Educational Software Institute
4213 S 94th St
Omaha, NE 68127-1223 402-592-3300
800-955-5570
FAX: 402-592-2017
e-mail: info@edsoft.com
www.edsoft.com

Lee Myers, President
Kathy Cavanaugh, Catalog Manager
Educational Software Institute (ESI) provides a one-stop shop to purchase software titles by all of the best publishers. The ESI Master Gold Book catalog and CD-ROM represents more than 400 software publishers, with information on more than 8,000 software titles. Take the confusion out of software selection by calling ESI for all of your software needs - including competitive prices, software previews, knowledgeable assistance, and the largest selection available all in one place.
Yearly

1660 **EZ Keys**
Words+
42505 10th Street West
Suite 109
Lancaster, CA 93534- 7059 661-723-7723
888-266-9294
FAX: 661-723-5524
e-mail: info@simulations-plus.com
www.simulations-plus.com

Walter S Woltosz, M.S., M.A.S., Chairman, President and Chief Executive Officer
John A. Dibella, VP, Marketing & Sales
Virginia E. Woltosz. M.B.A., Secretary & Treasurer
John R. Kneisel, Chief Financial Officer
A software and hardware product designed to operate on an IBM compatible PC. The software provides dual word prediction, abbreviation expansion, five different methods of voice output and access to commercial software applications. *$1395.00*

1661 **Early Games for Young Children**
Queue Incorporated
80 Hathaway Drive
Stratford, CT 06615 800-232-2224
FAX: 800-775-2729
e-mail: jdk@queueinc.com
www.qworkbooks.com

Anna Christopoulos, General Manager
Peter Uhrynowski, Comptroller
Steve Perrett, Director of Printing and Graphics
Ann Pleszko, Shipping Manager
Software that includes nine activities that entertain preschoolers in honing basic math and language skills.

1662 **Early Music Skills**
Electronic Courseware Systems
1713 S State St
Champaign, IL 61820-7258
217-359-7099
800-832-4965
FAX: 217-359-6578
e-mail: support@ecsmedia.com
www.ecsmedia.com
G Peters, President
Jodie Varner, Marketing Manager
A tutorial and drill program designed for the beginning music student. It covers four basic music reading skills: recognition of line and space notes; comprehension of the numbering system for the musical staff; visual and aural identification of notes moving up and down; and recognition of notes stepping and skipping up and down. *$ 39.95*

1663 **Eating Skills: Learning Basic Table Manners**
PCI Education Publishing
P.O.Box 34270
San Antonio, TX 78265-4270
210-377-1999
800-594-4263
FAX: 210-377-1121
e-mail: pciinfo@pcieducation.com
www.pcieducation.com
Erin Kinard, VP Product Development/Publisher
Jeff Clain, CEO
Offers parents and educators a functional way to teach and reinforce basic table manners. *$49.95*

1664 **Electronic Courseware Systems**
1713 S State St
Champaign, IL 61820-7258
217-359-7099
800-832-4965
FAX: 217-359-6578
e-mail: support@ecsmedia.com
www.ecsmedia.com
Jodie Varner, Manager
G Peters, President
Offers a complete library of instructional software for music, math, science and social studies.

1665 **Fall Fun**
Soft Touch
12301 Central Ave NE Ste 205
P.O.Box 490215
Blaine, MN 55449
763-862-2920
888-755-1402
FAX: 763-862-2922
e-mail: support@marblesoft.com
www.marblesoft.com
Joyce Meyer, President
Your students can begin their day with the Pledge of Allegiance, Pumpkins, Owls, and Cats. Witches adorn Five Pumpkins Sitting on the Gate. Five Fat Turkeys out smart the pilgrims with song and antics. The owl and cat have songs of their own. A variety of activities reinforce concepts such as short, tall, first, second, third, same and different. Fall Fun includes cause and effect and easy to more difficult levels. Eight songs in all.

1666 **Five Green & Speckled Frogs**
Soft Touch
12301 Central Ave NE Ste 205
P.O.Box 490215
Blaine, MN 55449
763-862-2920
888-755-1402
FAX: 763-862-2922
e-mail: support@marblesoft.com
www.marblesoft.com
Joyce Meyer, President
Laugh, learn and sing with Five Humorous Frogs. Activities start with cause and effect and progress to teach directionality and simple subtraction. This classic song makes learning numbers and number worlds easy. Selections can be set to 2, 3, 4, 5, or 6 on-screen choices. Two games are included. One teaches direction on a number line. If the child moves the frog in the correct direction, the frog gets a point. The other game teaches beginning subtraction.

1667 **Free and User Supported Software for the IBM PC: A Resource Guide**
McFarland & Company
960 NC Highway 88 W
P.O.Box 611
Jefferson, NC 28640-8813
336-246-4460
800-253-2187
FAX: 336-246-5018
e-mail: info@mcfarlandpub.com
www.mcfarlandpub.com
Robert McFarland Franklin, Founder
Kenneth.J Ansley, Author
Victor.D Lopez, Author
A selection of word processing, database management, spreadsheets, and graphics programs are described and evaluated. Describes how the program works and its strengths and weaknesses. Rating charts cover such aspects as ease of use, ease of learning, documentation, and general utility. *$27.50*
224 pages Paperback
ISBN 0-89950 -99-0

1668 **GoalView: Special Education and RTI Student Management Information System**
Learning Tools International
2391 Circadian Way
Santa Rosa, CA 95407-5439
707-521-3530
800-333-9954
e-mail: info@goalview.com
www.ltools.com
Cathy Zier, President/CEO
Natalie Sipes, VP
Michael R. Paul, Director of IT/Senior Web Engine
A Web Based information system for students, educators and parents that enables accountability and achievement tracking; prepares IDEA compliant IEP's in minutes; provides over 250,000 education standards and special education goals and objectives in English and Spanish; generates Federal compliance reports; and creates IDEA GoalCard progress reports for students, schools and districts for every reporting period.

1669 **HELP**
V OR T Corporation
P.O.Box G (George)
Menlo Park, CA 94026
650-322-8282
888-757-8678
FAX: 650-327-0747
e-mail: custserv@vort.com
vort.com
Tom Holt, Owner
A software version of HELP, covers over 650 skills in 6 developmental areas; cognitive, motor skills, language, gross motor, social and self-help.

1670 **Handbook of Adaptive Switches and Augmentative Communication Devices**
Academic Software
3504 Tates Creek Road
Lexington, KY 40517-2601
859-552-1020
859-552-1040
FAX: 253-799-4012
e-mail: asistaff@acsw.com
www.acsw.com
Dr. Warren E Lacefield PhD, President
Penelope D. Ellis, COO, Sales & Marketing Director
Cindy L George, Author
Sylvia B. Lacefield, Graphic Artist
This second edition contains physical descriptions and laboratory test data for a variety of commercially available pressure switches and augmentative communication devices and chapters on physical interaction, seating and positioning, and control access. It is an essential tool for assistive technology professionals and therapists who make decisions concerning physical access.
$60.00
300 pages Hardcover

1671 **HandiWARE**
Microsystems Software
600 Worcester Rd
Framingham, MA 01702-5303
508-626-8511
800-828-2600
FAX: 508-879-1069
e-mail: infor@microsys.com
www.handiware.com

Terri McGrath, Sales/Marketing
Bill Kilroy, Product Manager
Adapted access software, assists persons with physical, hearing and visual impairments in accessing computers running DOS and Windows. HandiWARE is a suite of 8 software programs which provide users with screen magnification, alternate keyboard access, word prediction, augmentative communication, hands free telephone access, a visual beep. $20.00-$595.00.

1672 **How to Write for Everyday Living**
Educational Activities Software
5600 West 83rd Street
Suite 300, 8200 Tower
Bloomington, MN 55437-585
800-447-5286
FAX: 239-225-9299
e-mail: info@edmentum.com
www.edmentum.com

Vin Riera, President/CEO
Dan Juckniess, SVP, Sales & Professional Services
Stacey Herteux, VP, Human Resources
Rob Rueckl, Chief Financial Officer
An individualized Life Skills WRITING Software program emphasizing the reading, writing, communication and reference skills needed for real-life tasks: preparing a resume, an employment form, a business letter and envelope, a learner's permit, a social security application and banking forms. *$159.00*

1673 **I KNOW American History**
Soft Touch
12301 Central Ave NE Ste 205
P.O.Box 490215
Blaine, MN 55449-2352
763-862-2920
888-755-1402
FAX: 763-862-2922
e-mail: support@marblesoft.com
www.marblesoft.com

Joyce Meyer, President
The new I KNOW programs is the way students practice attending, choice making and turn-taking while uncovering learning puzzles. Each press reveals more of the image while the narrator reads the text on the screen. Offers three levels of language: short phrases, short sentences and longer sentences to match the student's learning level. Choose from the five topic areas: American Symbols, Westward Movement, Early Colonial Americans, Industrial Revolution and Biographies.

1674 **I KNOW American History Overlay CD**
Soft Touch
12301 Central Ave NE Ste 205
P.O.Box 490215
Blaine, MN 55449-2352
763-862-2920
888-755-1402
FAX: 763-862-2922
e-mail: support@marblesoft.com
www.marblesoft.com

Joyce Meyer, President
Use this Overlay CD with I KNOW American History program. Includes standard overlays and SoftTouch's changeable overlays. Includes Overlay Printer by IntelliTools. Use Overlay Maker by IntelliTools (not included) to modify the overlays or to make additional learning materials.

1675 **Incite Learning Series**
Don Johnston
26799 West Commerce Drive
Volo, IL 60073
847-740-0749
800-999-4660
FAX: 847-740-7326
e-mail: info@donjohnston.com
www.donjohnston.com

Don Johnston, Founder
Ruth Ziolkowski, President
A collection of original short films and a thought-provoking instruction model to engage every student in the critical thinking and feeling process. This research-based program was developed around the science of how students learn best using the theory of 'anchored instruction' and 'front-loading' standards-based curriculum. *$79.00*

1676 **Innovation Management Group**
179 Niblick Rd
Ste 454
Paso Robles, CA 93446
818-701-1579
800-889-0987
FAX: 818-936-0200
e-mail: cs@imgpresents.com
www.imgpresents.com

Jerry Hussong, VP of Marketing
Publisher of the Assistive Technology Suite. The ultimate set of general purpose, adaptive computer access available today. Site License includes ALL computers and ALL active students and teachers at a single or multi-site location.

1677 **IntelliPics Studio 3**
Intelli Tools
1720 Corporate Cir
Petaluma, CA 94954-6924
707-773-2000
800-547-6747
FAX: 707-773-2001
e-mail: info@intellitools.com
www.intellitools.com

Arjan Khalsa, CEO
Multimedia authoring tool for both students and teachers to create activities, games, quizzes, slide shows, reports and presentations. *$395.00*

1678 **KIDS (Keyboard Introductory Development Series)**
Electronic Courseware Systems
1713 S State St
Champaign, IL 61820-7258
217-359-7099
800-832-4965
FAX: 217-359-6578
e-mail: support@ecsmedia.com
www.ecsmedia.com

G Peters, President
Jodie Varner, Marketing Manager
A four disk series for the very young. Zoo Puppet Theater reinforces learning correct finger numbers for piano playing; Race Car Keys teaches keyboard geography by recognizing syllables or note names; Dinosaurs Lunch teaches placement of the notes on the treble staff; and Follow Me asks the student to play notes that have been presented aurally. *$49.95*

1679 **Keyboard Tutor, Music Software**
Electronic Courseware Systems
1713 S State St
Champaign, IL 61820-7258
217-359-7099
800-832-4965
FAX: 217-359-6578
e-mail: support@ecsmedia.com
www.ecsmedia.com

G Peters, President
Jodie Varner, Marketing Manager
Presents exercises for learning elementary keyboard skills including knowledge of names of the keys, piano keys matched to notes, notes matched to piano keys, whole steps and half steps. Each lesson allows unlimited practice of the skills. The program may be used with or without a midi keyboard attached to the computer. *$39.95*

1680 Keyboarding by Ability
Teachers Institute for Special Education
9933 NW 45th St
Sunrise, FL 33351-4744
954-235-7940
FAX: 866-843-0765
e-mail: Support@Special-Education-Soft.com
www.special-education-soft.com

Gary Byowitz, President
Allows the learning disabled or dyslexic student to acquire keyboarding skills through visually cued alphabetical approach designed and tested to meet the specific learning style needs of this unique population at every grade level. Package contains: IBM software, a set of lesson plans and instructional goals; supplemental graded data input exercises. *$148.95*

1681 Keyboarding for the Physically Handicapped
Teachers Institute for Special Education
9933 NW 45th Street
Sunrise, FL 33351
954-235-7940
FAX: 866-843-0765
e-mail: Support@Special-Education-Soft.com
www.special-education-soft.com

Jack Heller, Director/Owner
Gary Byowitz, President
Custom designed touch typing programs for any student. A person needs order by the number of usable fingers on each hand (not counting the thumb), and whether or not a one finger or a head-pointer edition is wanted. Package includes IBM software; a complete set of lesson plans and instructional goals. *$149.95*

1682 Keyboarding with One Hand
Teachers Institute for Special Education
P.O.Box 2300
Wantagh, NY 11793-140
FAX: 516-781-4070
e-mail: jackheller@aol.com
www.users.aol.com/jackheller

Jack Heller, Director
This 22 lesson tutorial developed through 25 years of research, testing and teaching allows a student with one hand to acquire employable keyboarding skills using a touch system designed for the standard IBM PC keyboard. *$79.95*

1683 LPDOS Deluxe
Optelec U S
3030 Enterprise Court
STE C
Vista, CA 92081-8358
800-826-4200
FAX: 800-368-4111
e-mail: info@optelec.com
us.optelec.com

Stephan Terwolbeck, President
Michiel van Schaik, VP
Janet Lennex, Director of Customer Excellence
Jade Arbelo, Director of Human Resources
Large print software programs. *$595.00*

1684 Large Print DOS
Optelec U S
3030 Enterprise Court
STE C
Vista, CA 92081-8358
800-826-4200
FAX: 800-368-4111
e-mail: info@optelec.com
us.optelec.com

Stephan Terwolbeck, President
Michiel van Schaik, VP
Janet Lennex, Director of Customer Excellence
Jade Arbelo, Director of Human Resources

1685 Laureate Learning Systems
110 E Spring St
Winooski, VT 05404-1898
802-655-4755
800-562-6801
FAX: 802-655-4757
e-mail: info@llsys.com
www.laureatelearning.com

Mary Wilson, Owner
Kathy Hollandsworth, Office Manager
Laureate publishes award-winning talking software for children and adults with disabilities. Programs cover cause and effect, language development, cognitive processing, and reading. High-quality speech, colorful graphics and amusing animation make learning fun. Accessible with touchscreen, single switch, keyboard and mouse. No reading required. Available on a hybrid CD-ROM for Windows and Macintosh. Visit our website for more information or call for a free catalog.

1686 Learning Company
Ste 400
222 3rd Ave SE
Cedar Rapids, IA 52401-1542
319-395-9626
888-242-6747
FAX: 319-395-0217
e-mail: info@riverdeep.net
http://web.riverdeep.net

Barry O'Callaghan, Executive Chairman & Chief Executive Officer
Tony Mulderry, Executive Vice President, Corporate Development
Ciara Smyth, Executive Vice President, Global Business Operations
Scott Campbell, Executive Vice President, Strategic Sales
Software for children. For Macintosh or Windows (3.1 DOS or Windows 95, Windows 98 required). The Learning Company has been added to Riverdeep.

1687 Little Red Hen
Compass Learning
203 Colorado Street
Austin, TX 78701
512-478-9600
800-678-1412
866-586-7387
FAX: 619-622-7873
e-mail: support@compasslearning.com
www.compasslearning.com

Eric Loeffel, President, CEO
Tammy Deal, VP, Human Resources
Eric Wasser, VP, Sales
Eileen Shihadeh, VP, Marketing
Children learn about the rewards of hard work when they discover who the Little Red Hen's friends miss out on freshly baked bread. Puzzles, rhymes, story writing and other interactive exercises enhance the creative learning process. *$34.95*

1688 Looking Good: Learning to Improve Your Appearance
Programming Concepts
8700 Shoal Creek Boulevard
Austin, TX 78757-6897
512-451-3246
800-897-3202
800-471-3000
FAX: 800-397-7633
e-mail: general@proedinc.com
www.proedinc.com

Jeff McLane, Founder
Lee Wilson, President and CEO
Randy Pennington, Executive VP
David Keith, Vice President of IT
This game offers a creative way to discuss all areas of grooming. *$49.95*

1689 Monkeys Jumping on the Bed
Soft Touch
12301 Central Ave NE Ste 205
P.O.Box 490215
Blaine, MN 55449-2352
763-862-2920
888-755-1402
FAX: 763-862-2922
e-mail: support@marblesoft.com
www.marblesoft.com

Joyce Meyer, President

This program combines a favorite preschool song with number and color activities. Children and adults will enjoy engaging music and delightful animation. Students with cognitive delays respond to upbeat music and interesting sounds. Large graphics help learners focus on the action. Several important concepts are presented in enjoyable activity formats. Students learn cause and effect in Let's Play and Just for Fun.

1690 Morse Code WSKE
Words+
42505 10th Street West
Suite 109
Lancaster, CA 93534- 7059 661-723-7723
888-266-9294
FAX: 661-723-5524
e-mail: info@simulations-plus.com
www.simulations-plus.com

Walter S Woltosz, M.S., M.A.S., Chairman, President and Chief Executive Officer
John A. Dibella, VP, Marketing & Sales
Virginia E. Woltosz. M.B.A., Secretary & Treasurer
John R. Kneisel, Chief Financial Officer

A software and hardware product designed to operate on an IBM compatible PC.

1691 Multi-Scan Single Switch Activity Center
Academic Software
3504 Tates Creek Road
Lexington, KY 40517-2601 859-552-1020
859-552-1040
FAX: 253-799-4012
e-mail: asistaff@acsw.com
www.acsw.com

Dr. Warren E Lacefield PhD, President
Penelope D. Ellis, COO, Sales & Marketing Director
Cindy L George, Author
Sylvia B. Lacefield, Graphic Artist

A single switch activity center containing four educational games: Match, Maze, Dot-to-Dot, and Concentration, along with six graphics libraries; Dinosaurs, Sports, Animals, Independent Living, Vocations, and Cosmetology. MULTI-SCAN allows you to select a graphic library, choose games for each user, and adjust the difficulty level and other settings for each game. Other features allow you to save the game setups under each user's name and print out individual performance reports after sessions.
$154.00

1692 Muppet Learning Keys
WINGS for Learning
1600 Green Hills Rd
Scotts Valley, CA 95066-4981 831-426-2228
FAX: 831-464-3600

Ani Stocks, Owner

Designed to introduce children to the world of the computer as they become familiar with letters, numbers and colors.

1693 My Own Pain
Soft Touch
12301 Central Ave NE Ste 205
P.O.Box 490215
Blaine, MN 55449-2352 763-862-2920
888-755-1402
FAX: 763-862-2922
e-mail: support@marblesoft.com
www.marblesoft.com

Joyce Meyer, President

Three activities - three levels. Press the switch and the paint brush chooses the color and paints the vehicle. Music reinforces the sounds when the picture is complete. A second activity allows the student to choose the color and paint the vehicle parts any color he or she wants. The third activity is a blueprint. Print the color that matches the one in the wire drawing. Color the drawing to complete the picture.

1694 Old MacDonald's Farm Deluxe
Soft Touch
12301 Central Ave NE Ste 205
P.O.Box 490215
Blaine, MN 55449-2352 763-862-2920
888-755-1402
FAX: 763-862-2922
e-mail: support@marblesoft.com
www.marblesoft.com

Joyce Meyer, President

Toddlers, preschoolers and early elementary students will be entertained and captivated by the six major activities and animations in the delightful program. Includes 18 real animation images or 9 cartoon like characters. The teacher or child can choose which animals they want to sing about. Some activities are designed for children within the normal population, others are designed for students with moderate and severe disabilities.

1695 Optimum Resource Educational Software
Optimum Resource
1 Mathews Drive
Suite 107
Hilton Head Island, SC 29926 843-689-8000
FAX: 843-689-8008
e-mail: info@stickybear.com
www.stickybear.com

Richard Hefter, President

A complete topical curriculum of reading, math, keyboard skills and science programs that are age and skill specific. Programs include: Early Learning for Pre-K to 1st grade with introductions to numbers, language, shapes, and time; Language Arts from Pre-K to 12; Math for Pre-K to 12; two distinct Science programs; Tools for Educators provides Spelling and Math generators; and Bilingual programs for Pre-K through 9th grade. All are available as single user up to 30 user site packages.

1696 Optimum Resources/Stickybear Software
1 Mathews Drive
Suite 107
Hilton Head Island, SC 29926 843-689-8000
FAX: 843-689-8008
e-mail: info@stickybear.com
www.stickybear.com

Richard Hefter, President

Publisher of award-winning educational software for thirty years. Programs in use by millions of students nationwide.
$59.95

1697 Please Understand Me: Software Program and Books
Cambridge Educational
132 West 31st Street
17th Floor
New York, NY 10001 800-322-8755
FAX: 800-678-3633
e-mail: custserv@films.com
www.films.com

209 pages BiAnnual
ISBN 0-927368-56-x

1698 Pond
WINGS for Learning
1600 Green Hills Rd
Scotts Valley, CA 95066-4981 831-426-2228
FAX: 831-464-3600

Ani Stocks, Owner

Software game that teaches pattern recognition and encourages observation, trial and error and the interpretation of data.

1699 **Print, Play & Learn #1 Old Mac's Farm**
Soft Touch Incorporated
12301 Central Ave NE Ste 205
P.O.Box 490215
Blaine, MN 55449-2352
763-862-2920
888-755-1402
FAX: 763-862-2922
e-mail: support@marblesoft.com
www.marblesoft.com

Joyce Meyer, President

Once your students have completed Old Mac's Farm, let them use the fun off-computer activities to continue learning. Over 25 activities with 250 sheets you print. Board games, dot-to-dot drawings, word puzzles, make a scene, flash cards. Concentration, sentence strips, worksheets and much more are available for teachers to expand their teaching goals. This CD is full of activities to print and use.

1700 **Print, Play & Learn #7: Sampler**
Soft Touch
12301 Central Ave NE Ste 205
P.O.Box 490215
Blaine, MN 55449-2352
763-862-2920
888-755-1402
FAX: 763-862-2922
e-mail: support@marblesoft.com
www.marblesoft.com

Joyce Meyer, President

Print, Play and Learn Sampler gives you over 200 activities organized by training, easy, medium and hard levels so you can ready to help your student advance. Activities cover a wide range of basic knowledge, including colors, shapes, numbers, letters and much, much more. Note: Requires Overlay Maker or Overlay Printer by IntelliTools and a color printer.

1701 **Puzzle Power: Sampler**
Soft Touch
12301 Central Ave NE Ste 205
P.O.Box 490215
Blaine, MN 55449-2352
763-862-2920
888-755-1402
FAX: 763-862-2922
e-mail: support@marblesoft.com
www.marblesoft.com

Joyce Meyer, President

Puzzle Power - Sampler offers a variety of puzzles in different themes. Each theme puzzle is followed by a puzzle of one item in this category. For example, first solve a puzzle for occupations. Then, solve a puzzle that is a baker. The pictures are large, clear and easily identifiable.

1702 **Puzzle Power: Zoo & School Days**
Soft Touch
12301 Central Ave NE Ste 205
P.O.Box 490215
Blaine, MN 55449-2352
763-862-2920
888-755-1402
FAX: 763-862-2922
e-mail: support@marblesoft.com
www.marblesoft.com

Joyce Meyer, President

Here is a program for all of our students who need puzzle skills, but cannot access commercial puzzles. Puzzle Power puzzles start with just two pieces and progress to 16 pieces. The pictures are large, clear and easily identifiable. Four different activities enable all students to be successful. Automatic Placement: the student just presses the switch or keyboard to place the pieces. Magnet Mouse: all the student needs to do is move the mouse and it drops into place.

1703 **Rodeo**
Soft Touch
12301 Central Ave NE Ste 205
P.O.Box 490215
Blaine, MN 55449-2352
763-862-2920
888-755-1402
FAX: 763-862-2922
e-mail: support@marblesoft.com
www.marblesoft.com

Joyce Meyer, President

Rodeo action and familiar tunes for teens and preteens. Four activities invite students to learn, laugh, and sing as they go to the rodeo with up to six age-peer friends. Age-appropriate graphics with surprising animations reinforce the learning. The graphics are large and colorful, the melodies familiar, and the words descriptive of the action on the screen.

1704 **Shop Til You Drop**
Soft Touch
12301 Central Ave NE Ste 205
P.O.Box 490215
Blaine, MN 55449-2352
763-862-2920
888-755-1402
FAX: 763-862-2922
e-mail: support@marblesoft.com
www.marblesoft.com

Joyce Meyer, President

Designed specifically for preteens and teens with moderate and severe disabilities, this program will become a staple for the classroom. The student goes shopping and can choose which outfits to put together. They may choose to purchase the outfit - of course, with mom's credit card. Another activity is a video arcade game about money. Shop 'Til You Drop can be adjusted from a single switch cause-and-effect program to row-and-column scanning to direct choice.

1705 **Songs I Sing at Preschool**
Soft Touch
12301 Central Ave NE Ste 205
P.O.Box 490215
Blaine, MN 55449-2352
763-862-2920
888-755-1402
FAX: 763-862-2922
e-mail: support@marblesoft.com
www.marblesoft.com

Joyce Meyer, President

Songs I Sing at Preschool offers many options for the teacher and the student. Over the years, our software has used music because our students really respond to the sounds and rhythms of songs. Teachers select which songs to present, how many to present at one time and where to place each song on the overlay, keyboard or scan array.

1706 **Stickybear Early Learning Activities**
Optimum Resource
1 Mathews Drive
Suite 107
Hilton Head Island, SC 29926
843-689-8000
FAX: 843-689-8008
e-mail: info@stickybear.com
www.stickybear.com

Richard Hefter, President

Two modes of play allow youngsters to learn through prompted direction or by the discovery method. Lively animation and sound keep attention levels high as children learn writing, counting, shapes, opposites and colors. Stickybear Early Learning Activities is bilingual, so youngsters can build skills in both English and Spanish. Pre-K to 1st grade. *$59.95*

1707 **Stickybear Kindergarden Activities**
Optimum Resource
1 Mathews Drive
Suite 107
Hilton Head Island, SC 29926
843-689-8000
FAX: 843-689-8008
e-mail: info@stickybear.com
www.stickybear.com

Richard Hefter, President

This dynamic new multifaceted program covers a wide range of preschool skills that go far beyond the strictly academic. At Stickybear's house, children discover the alphabet, numbers, shapes, colors, plus - social skills, important safety messages and delightful off-screen activities that foster creativity. Over three hours of original music can be composed by a child and saved for future use. *$59.95*

1708 Stickybear Science Fair Light
Optimum Resource
1 Mathews Drive
Suite 107
Hilton Head Island, SC 29926 843-689-8000
FAX: 843-689-8008
e-mail: info@stickybear.com
www.stickybear.com

Richard Hefter, President

The first in the new series of science-based programs Stickybear Science Fair Light presents a content rich environment which allows students in grades 7-12 to explore, experiment with and understand light and it's properties. The program presents experiments, both structured and free-form, which allow users to work with prisms, lenses, color mixing, optical illusions and more. *$59.95*

1709 Stickybear Town Builder
Optimum Resource
1 Mathews Drive
Suite 107
Hilton Head Island, SC 29926 843-689-8000
FAX: 843-689-8008
e-mail: info@stickybear.com
www.stickybear.com

Richard Hefter, President

Children learn to read maps, build towns, take trips and use a compass in this simulation program. *$59.95*

1710 Stickybear Typing
Optimum Resource
1 Mathews Drive
Suite 107
Hilton Head Island, SC 29926 843-689-8000
FAX: 843-689-8008
e-mail: info@stickybear.com
www.stickybear.com

Richard Hefter, President

Sharpen typing skills with three challenging activities: Stickybear Keypress, Stickybear Thump and Stickybear Stories. Pre-K to 5th. *$59.95*

1711 Storybook Maker Deluxe
Compass Learning
203 Colorado Street
Austin, TX 78701 512-478-9600
800-678-1412
866-586-7387
FAX: 619-622-7873
e-mail: support@compasslearning.com
www.compasslearning.com

Eric Loeffel, President, CEO
Tammy Deal, VP, Human Resources
Eric Wasser, VP, Sales
Eileen Shihadeh, VP, Marketing

Using Storybook Maker Deluxe and their imaginations, students can create and publish stories filled with exciting graphics. Students can write stories and watch as the text appears in the setting they've chosen. Engaging sounds and music, plus lively animations, provide positive learning reinforcement throughout the program. *$44.95*

1712 Super Challenger
Electronic Courseware Systems
1713 S State St
Champaign, IL 61820-7258 217-359-7099
800-832-4965
FAX: 217-359-6578
e-mail: support@ecsmedia.com
www.ecsmedia.com

Jodie Varner, Manager
G Peters, President

An aural-visual musical game that increases the player's ability to remember a series of pitches as they are played by the computer. The game is based on a 12-note chromatic scale, a major scale, and a minor scale. Each pitch is reinforced visually with a color representation of a keyboard on the display screen. Computer/software. *$39.95*

1713 Switch Basics
Soft Touch
12301 Central Ave NE Ste 205
P.O.Box 490215
Blaine, MN 55449-2352 763-862-2920
888-755-1402
FAX: 763-862-2922
e-mail: support@marblesoft.com
www.marblesoft.com

Joyce Meyer, President

Discover whimsical animations and real life pictures while learning switch operations. Intriguing and humorous, nine different programs offer a multitude of learning experiences for all ages. Program options include: cause and effect, scanning, step scanning, row and column activities for one or two players. Watch the clouds roll away revealing African animals; visit the beauty salon or barber shop; work two to sixteen piece puzzles; or add swimming fish to a huge aquarium.

1714 Switch Interface Pro 5.0
Don Johnston
26799 West Commerce Drive
Volo, IL 60073 847-740-0749
800-999-4660
FAX: 847-740-7326
e-mail: info@donjohnston.com
www.donjohnston.com

Don Johnston, Founder
Ruth Ziolkowski, President

Allows individuals with physical disabilities to access the computer. Five ports accommodate multiple switches and emulate everything from a single-click to a return. Consequently, individuals gain access to the widest variety of switch-accessible software available. It requires no software and can be used with both Windows and Macintosh computers. *$79.00*

1715 Teach Me Phonemics Series Bundle
SoftTouch
Ste 401
4300 Stine Rd
Bakersfield, CA 93313-2352 661-396-8676
877-763-8868
FAX: 661-396-8760
e-mail: support@softtouch.com
www.funsoftware.com

Joyce Meyer, President
Roxanne Butterfield, Marketing

The Teach Me Phonemics Series Bundle includes one copy of each Teach Me Phonemics program - Initial, Medial, Final and Blends - four CD's in all.

1716 **Teach Me Phonemics Super Bundle**
SoftTouch
Ste 401
4300 Stine Rd
Bakersfield, CA 93313-2352 661-396-8676
877-763-8868
FAX: 661-396-8760
e-mail: softtouch@funsoftware.com
www.funsoftware.com
Roxanne Butterfield, Marketing
Joyce Meyer, President
Teach Me Phonemics Super Bundle includes all 4 Teach Me Phonemics programs and all 4 Teach Me Phonemics overlay CD's - eight CD's in all.

1717 **Teach Me Phonemics: Blends**
SoftTouch
Ste 401
4300 Stine Rd
Bakersfield, CA 93313-2352 661-396-8676
877-763-8868
FAX: 661-396-8760
e-mail: softtouch@funsoftware.com
www.funsoftware.com
Roxanne Butterfield, Marketing
Joyce Meyer, President
Teach Me Phonemics - Blends helps students explore words and hear the initial blend sounds. It features musical interludes and movement to engage the student. Teachers select the best combination options to motivate and engage the student. Options turn off and on the fly so you can quickly make changes to keep the student engaged.

1718 **Teach Me Phonemics: Final**
SoftTouch
Ste 401
4300 Stine Rd
Bakersfield, CA 93313-2352 661-396-8676
877-763-8868
FAX: 661-396-8760
e-mail: softtouch@funsoftware.com
www.funsoftware.com
Roxanne Butterfield
Joyce Meyer, President
Teach me Phonemics - Final helps students explore words and hear the final sounds. It features musical interludes and movement to engage the student. Options turn off and on the fly so you can quickly make changes to keep the student engaged.

1719 **Teach Me Phonemics: Initial**
SoftTouch
12301 Central Ave NE
Ste 205
Blaine, MN 55434 763-755-1402
888-755-1403
FAX: 763-862-2920
e-mail: sales@marblesoft.com
www.softtouch.com
Roxanne Butterfield, Marketing
Joyce Meyer, President
Teach Me Phonemics - Initial helps students explore the words and hear the initial sounds. It features musical interludes and movement to engage the student. Teachers select the best combination options to motivate and engage the student. Options turn off and on the fly so you can quickly make changes to keep the student engaged.

1720 **Teach Me Phonemics: Medial**
SoftTouch
12301 Central Ave NE
Ste 205
Blaine, MN 55434 763-755-1402
888-755-1403
FAX: 763-862-2920
e-mail: sales@marblesoft.com
www.softtouch.com
Roxanne Butterfield, Marketing
Joyce Meyer, President
Teach Me Phonemics - Medial helps students explore the words and hear the medial sounds. It features musical interludes and movement to engage the student. Teachers select the best combination options to motivate and engage the student. Options turn off and on the fly so you can quickly make changes to keep the student engaged.

1721 **Teach Me to Talk**
Soft Touch
12301 Central Ave NE Ste 205
P.O.Box 490215
Blaine, MN 55449-2352 763-862-2920
888-755-1402
FAX: 763-862-2922
e-mail: support@marblesoft.com
www.marblesoft.com
Joyce Meyer, President
The first activity Teach Me to Talk is used as a springboard for the student to learn to speak the word. There are 150 real pictures. When a picture is chosen, it appears on a clear background with musical interludes, movement, written word and spoken word. It culminates by morphing to the corresponding black and white Mayer-Johnson symbol. The second activity Story Time, takes some of these nouns and puts them in four line poetry. This helps students hear the word in the midst of a sentence.

1722 **Teen Tunes Plus**
Soft Touch
12301 Central Ave NE Ste 205
P.O.Box 490215
Blaine, MN 55449-2352 763-862-2920
888-755-1402
FAX: 763-862-2922
e-mail: support@marblesoft.com
www.marblesoft.com
Joyce Meyer, President
Introduce switch use to older students with disabilities. Large interesting graphics, a variety of musical interludes, and surprising animations are combined with calm soothing music and beautiful pictures in the software specifically designed for preteens and teens with severe cognitive delays and/or physical disabilities, and older students learning to use a switch.

1723 **There are Tyrannosaurs Trying on Pants in My Bedroom**
Compass Learning
203 Colorado Street
Austin, TX 78701-3922 512-478-9600
800-678-1412
866-586-7387
FAX: 619-622-7873
e-mail: support@compasslearning.com
www.compasslearning.com
Eric Loeffel, President, CEO
Tammy Deal, VP, Human Resources
Eric Wasser, VP, Sales
Eileen Shihadeh, VP, Marketing
In this popular story, Saturday chores turn into fun-filled frolicking when dinosaurs come for a visit. Sounds, music and animation make learning about phonics and vocabulary dyno-mite. *$34.95*

1724 **Three Billy Goats Gruff**
Compass Learning
203 Colorado Street
Austin, TX 78701-3922 512-478-9600
800-678-1412
866-586-7387
FAX: 619-622-7873
e-mail: support@compasslearning.com
www.compasslearning.com
Eric Loeffel, President, CEO
Tammy Deal, VP, Human Resources
Eric Wasser, VP, Sales
Eileen Shihadeh, VP, Marketing
Motivating exercises and creative activities provide hours of learning fun while young students follow the adventure of The Three Billy Goats Gruff in this animated version of the timeless tale. *$ 34.95*

1725 Three Little Pigs
Compass Learning
203 Colorado Street
Austin, TX 78701-3922 512-478-9600
800-678-1412
866-586-7387
FAX: 619-622-7873
e-mail: support@compasslearning.com
www.compasslearning.com

Eric Loeffel, President, CEO
Tammy Deal, VP, Human Resources
Eric Wasser, VP, Sales
Eileen Shihadeh, VP, Marketing

Help young students build reading comprehension and writing skills with this interactive version of the children's classic, The Three Little Pigs. Animated storytelling and creative activities inspire children to read, write and rhyme. *$34.95*

1726 TouchCorders
Soft Touch
12301 Central Ave NE Ste 205
P.O.Box 490215
Blaine, MN 55449-2352 763-862-2920
888-755-1402
FAX: 763-862-2922
e-mail: support@marblesoft.com
www.marblesoft.com

Joyce Meyer, President

TouchCorders are the flexible and easy-to-use communicator designed by Jo Meyer and Linda Bidabe for reach classroom use. TouchCorders are sensitive to touch at every angle and give the student kinesthetic feedback. With the unique Add 'n Touch system, Jo connects the puzzles bases of 2 or more TouchCorders on the fly to present vocabulary, sequencing, story telling, social stories, concepts and other curriculum and communication opportunities.

1727 TouchWindow Touch Screen
Riverdeep Incorporated
100 Pine Street
Suite 1900
San Francisco, CA 94111 415-659-2000
800-542-4222
FAX: 415-659-2020
e-mail: info@riverdeep.net
www.riverdeep.net

Barry O'Callaghan, Executive Chairman & Chief Executive Officer
Tony Mulderry, Executive Vice President, Corporate Development
Ciara Smyth, Executive Vice President, Global Business Operations
Scott Campbell, Executive Vice President, Strategic Sales

Software for children. *$335.00*

1728 Turtle Teasers
Soft Touch
12301 Central Ave NE Ste 205
P.O.Box 490215
Blaine, MN 55449-2352 763-862-2920
888-755-1402
FAX: 763-862-2922
e-mail: support@marblesoft.com
www.marblesoft.com

Joyce Meyer, President

Three Games, Three Levels from Easy, Medium to Hard. The Shell Game - easy: Watch one of the three turtles get the tomato. Then watch carefully as they switch positions and pop shut. Choose incorrectly and the frog disappears until the correct one is displayed. The Pond - medium: Watch the tomato disappear somewhere in the pond scene. Tomato Dump - hard: Hit the shell and it turns into the tomato, giving a score. There are different difficulty levels to equalize all students.

1729 What Was That!
Compass Learning
203 Colorado Street
Austin, TX 78701-3922 512-478-9600
800-678-1412
866-586-7387
FAX: 619-622-7873
e-mail: support@compasslearning.com
www.compasslearning.com

Eric Loeffel, President, CEO
Tammy Deal, VP, Human Resources
Eric Wasser, VP, Sales
Eileen Shihadeh, VP, Marketing

In this bedtime story, noises in the night send three brother bears scurrying out of bed. Thoughtful questions test young readers' comprehension, while games, voice recording, writing practice and other playful activities stimulate their creativity.

1730 Wivik 3
Prentke Romich Company
1022 Heyl Road
Wooster, OH 44691 330-262-1984
800-262-1984
FAX: 330-263-4829
e-mail: info@prentrom.com
www.prentrom.com

David L Moffatt, President

On-screen keyboard provides access to any application in the latest Windows operating systems. Selections are made by clicking, dwelling or switch scanning. Enhancements include word prediction and abbreviation expansion.

1731 WordMaker
Don Johnston
26799 West Commerce Drive
Volo, IL 60073 847-740-0749
800-999-4660
FAX: 847-740-7326
e-mail: info@donjohnston.com
www.donjohnston.com

Don Johnston, Founder
Ruth Ziolkowski, President

The computer version of Dr Patricia Cunningham's book 'Systematic Sequential Phonics They Use.' The program systematically builds spelling and word decoding skills for struggling readers and writers. *$79.00*

1732 Write: Out Loud
Don Johnston
26799 West Commerce Drive
Volo, IL 60073 847-740-0749
800-999-4660
FAX: 847-740-7326
e-mail: info@donjohnston.com
www.donjohnston.com

Don Johnston, Founder
Ruth Ziolkowski, President

Write: Out Loud is an easy-to-use talking word processor that uses text-to-speech and revision and editing supports to help students write more effectively, more often and with more enthusiasm as they share creative thoughts on paper. *$79.00*

1733 You Tell Me: Learning Basic Information
Programming Concepts
8700 Shoal Creek Boulevard
Austin, TX 78757-6897 512-451-3246
800-897-3202
800-471-3000
FAX: 800-397-7633
e-mail: general@proedinc.com
www.proedinc.com

Jeff McLane, Founder
Lee Wilson, President and CEO
Randy Pennington, Executive VP
David Keith, Vice President of IT

This game teaches and reinforces basic information all individuals need to know. Questions asked in this game help prepare people to communicate personal identification information important to community survival. *$49.95*

Software: Professional

1734 Acrontech International
5500 Main St
Williamsville, NY 14221-6755 FAX: 716-854-4014

1735 DPS with BCP
V OR T Corporation
P.O.Box G (George)
Menlo Park, CA 94026 650-322-8282
888-757-8678
FAX: 650-327-0747
e-mail: custserv@vort.com
vort.com
Tom Holt, Owner
This program uses unique DPS branching techniques to access goals and objectives.

1736 Diagnostic Report Writer
Parrot Software
P.O. Box 250755
West Bloomfield, MI 48325 248-788-3223
800-727-7681
FAX: 248-788-3224
e-mail: support@parrotsoftware.com
www.parrotsoftware.com
Dr. Frederic Weiner, Ph. D., CCC-SP, President, Owner
Creates a three page single-spaced diagnostic report for a child with a communication disorder from a list of questions; sections of the report include developmental and background history, oral peripheral exam, speech and language analysis, summary and recommendations.

1737 Discriptive Language Arts Development
Educational Activities Software
5600 West 83rd Street
Suite 300, 8200 Tower
Bloomington, MN 55437 888-351-4199
800-447-5286
FAX: 239-225-9299
e-mail: info@edmentum.com
www.edmentum.com
Vin Riera, President/CEO
Dan Juckniess, SVP, Sales & Professional Services
Stacey Herteux, VP, Human Resources
Rob Rueckl, Chief Financial Officer
This multimedia language arts development program provides instruction and application of fundamental English skills and concepts. *$395.00*

1738 Draft: Builder
Don Johnston
26799 West Commerce Drive
Volo, IL 60073 847-740-0749
800-999-4660
FAX: 847-740-7326
e-mail: info@donjohnston.com
www.donjohnston.com
Don Johnston, Founder
Ruth Ziolkowski, President
A software-based graphic organizer that breaks down the writing process into manageable chunks to structure planning, organizing, and draft-writing. *$79.00*

1739 EZ Dot
CAPCO Capability Corporation
3910 S. Union Court
Spokane Valley, WA 99206-6345 509-927-8195
800-827-2182
FAX: 800-827-2182
e-mail: info@skilltran.com
www.skilltran.com
Jeff Truthan, President
A critical software tool used in vocational counseling, job restructuring, recruitment and placement, better utilization of workers, and safety issues. This software offers occupational data by title, code, industry, GEO, DPT, or OGA. *$295.00*

1740 EZ Keys for Windows
Words+
Ste 109
42505 10th St W
Lancaster, CA 93534-7059 661-723-6523
800-869-8521
FAX: 661-723-2114
e-mail: info@words-plus.com
www.words-plus.com
Jean Dobbs, Editorial Director
Tim Gilmer, Editor
Josie Byzek, Managing Editor
Doug Lathrop, Senior Correspondent
A software and hardware product designed to operate on an IBM compatible PC. The software provides dual word prediction, abbreviation expansion, five different methods of voice output and access to commercial software applications. *$1395.00*

1741 Goals and Objectives
JE Stewart Teaching Tools
P.O.Box 15308
Seattle, WA 98115-308 206-262-9538
FAX: 206-262-9538
Jeff Stewart, Owner
Goals and Objectives software helps teachers make student plans including IEP's, IPP's and IHP's. The system provides curricula for all students and programs to develop and evaluate plans, print reports and make data forms. Systems are available for Windows and Macintosh for $139.

1742 Goals and Objectives IEP Program Curriculum Associates LLC
153 Rangeway Road
P.O.Box 2001
North Billerica, MA 01862-0901 978-667-8000
800-225-0248
FAX: 800-366-1158
www.curriculumassociates.com
Frank E. Ferguson, Chairman
Renee Foster, President & Publisher
Woody Palk, Senior Vice President, Sales
Robert Waldron, CEO
BRIGANCE CIBS-R standardized scoring conversion software, is a teacher's tool that prints goal and objective pages of the IEP. In less than two minutes per student, a teacher types student data into the computer.

1743 Nasometer
Kay Elemetrics Corporation
3 Paragon Drive
Montvale, NJ 07645 973-628-6200
800-289-5297
FAX: 201-391-2063
e-mail: sales@kaypentax.com
www.kaypentax.com
John Crump, President
Steve Crump, Direct Sales
Measures the ratio of acoustic energy for the nasal and real-time visual cueing during therapy. Used clinically in the areas of cleft palate, motor speech disorders, hearing impairment and palatal prosthetic fittings.

1744 PSS CogRehab Software
Psychological Software Services
3304 W 75th St
Indianapolis, IN 46268-1664 317-257-9672
FAX: 317-257-9674
e-mail: nsc@neuroscience.cnter.com
www.neuroscience.cnter.com
Odie L Bracy, Executive Director
PSS CogRehab Software is a comprehensive and easy-to-use multimedia cognitive rehabilitation software available, for clinical and educational use with head injury, stroke LD/ADD and

other brain compromises. The packages include 64 computerized therapy tasks which contain modifiable parameters that will accommodate most requirements. Exercises include attention and executive skills, multiple modalities of visuosatial and memory skills, simple, complex, problem-solving skills.
$260 - $2500

1745 Parrot Easy Language Simple Anaylsis
Parrot Software
P.O.Box 250755
West Bloomfield, MI 48325
248-788-3223
800-727-7681
FAX: 248-788-3224
e-mail: support@parrotsoftware.com
www.parrotsoftware.com
Dr. Frederic Weiner, Ph. D., CCC-SP, President, Owner
Designed for grammatical analysis of language samples. The user types and translates language samples of up to 100 utterances.

1746 SOLO Literacy Suite
Don Johnston
26799 West Commerce Drive
Volo, IL 60073
847-740-0749
800-999-4660
FAX: 847-740-7326
e-mail: info@donjohnston.com
www.donjohnston.com
Don Johnston, Founder
Ruth Ziolkowski, President
Places all of the right tools, and a wide-range of embedded learning supports, at their fingertips. SOLO includes word prediction, a text reader, graphic organizer and talking word processor, putting students in charge of their own learning and accommodations. Students of varying ages and abilities have access to, and make progress in, the general education curriculum. *$79.00*

1747 TOVA
Universal Attention Disorders
3321 Cerritos Avenue
Los Alamitos, CA 90720
562-594-7700
800-729-2886
FAX: 800-452-6919
e-mail: info@tovatest.com
www.tovatest.com
Lawrence M. Greenberg, MD
A computerized assessment which, in conjunction with classroom behavior ratings, is a highly effective screening tool for ADD. TOVA includes software, complete instructions, and supporting data including norms.

1748 Visi-Pitch III
Kayelemetrics Corporation
3 Paragon Drive
Montvale, NJ 07645
973-628-6200
800-289-5297
FAX: 201-391-2063
e-mail: sales@kaypentax.com
www.kaypentax.com
John Crump, President
Steve Crump, Direct Sales
Assists the speech/voice clinician in assessment and treatment tasks across an expansive range of disorders.

Software: Reading & Language Arts

1749 Choices, Choices 5.0
Tom Snyder Productions
100 Talcott Avenue
Watertown, MA 02472-5703
800-342-0236
e-mail: Ask@tomsnyder.com
www.tomsnyder.com
Tom Snyder, Founder
Bridget Dalton, Ed.D, Author
Peggy Healy Stearns, Ph.D., Author
David Dockterman, Ed.D., Author
Teaches students to take responsibility for their behavior. Helps students develop the skills and awareness they need to make wise choices and to think through the consequences of their actions.

1750 Co: Writer
Don Johnston
26799 West Commerce Drive
Volo, IL 60073
847-740-0749
800-999-4660
FAX: 847-740-7326
e-mail: info@donjohnston.com
www.donjohnston.com
Don Johnston, Founder
Ruth Ziolkowski, President
A software-based writing assistant that uses word prediction to cut through writing barriers and improve written expression. It is intended for students who struggle to write because of difficulty with spelling, syntax, and translating thoughts into writing. As students type, Co: Writer learns the context of the sentence and accurately 'predicts' words even when spelled phonetically or inventively. *$79.00*

1751 Community Exploration
Compass Learning
203 Colorado Street
Austin, TX 78701-3922
512-478-9600
800-678-1412
866-586-7387
FAX: 619-622-7873
e-mail: support@compasslearning.com
www.compasslearning.com
Eric Loeffel, President, CEO
Tammy Deal, VP, Human Resources
Eric Wasser, VP, Sales
Eileen Shihadeh, VP, Marketing
An award-winning learning adventure takes students who are learning English as a second language on a field trip to the make-believe town of Cornerstone. More than 50 community locations come to life with sound and animation. While exploring places in this typical American community where people live, work and play, students also enhance important English language skills. Offers an exciting approach for any age student who needs to improve their English language proficiency. 4-12. *$19.95*

1752 Conversations
Educational Activities Software
5600 West 83rd Street
Suite 300, 8200 Tower
Bloomington, MN 55437
888-351-4199
800-447-5286
FAX: 239-225-9299
e-mail: info@edmentum.com
www.edmentum.com
Vin Riera, President/CEO
Dan Juckniess, SVP, Sales & Professional Services
Stacey Herteux, VP, Human Resources
Rob Rueckl, Chief Financial Officer
Using American digitized voices, CONVERSATIONS provides 14 different dialogues in which the student can participate. The topics offer learners important information about American culture and the workplace. Available for DOS. *$195.00*

1753 Core-Reading and Vocabulary Development
Educational Activities
P.O.Box 87
Baldwin, NY 11510
516-223-4666
800-797-3223
FAX: 516-623-9282
e-mail: learn@edact.com
www.edact.com
Alfred Harris, President
Carol Stern, VP
Students begin with 36 basic words and progress to more than 200. Reading and writing activities are coordinated and integrated throughout the program for more substantial permanent learning. Five units covering readability levels from pre-primer to grade three.
Full Program

1754 Friday Afternoon
203 Colorado Street
Austin, TX 78701-3922
512-478-9600
800-678-1412
866-586-7387
FAX: 619-622-7873
e-mail: support@compasslearning.com
www.compasslearning.com

Eric Loeffel, President, CEO
Tammy Deal, VP, Human Resources
Eric Wasser, VP, Sales
Eileen Shihadeh, VP, Marketing

Save hours of preparation time and dazzle your students with interesting new activities to supplement their classroom learning. With Friday afternoon, you'll produce flash cards, word puzzles, even customized bingo cards and more, all at the click of a mouse. MacIntosh diskette. *$99.95*

1755 How to Read for Everyday Living
Educational Activities Software
5600 West 83rd Street
Suite 300, 8200 Tower
Bloomington, MN 55437
888-351-4199
800-447-5286
FAX: 239-225-9299
e-mail: info@edmentum.com
www.edmentum.com

Vin Riera, President/CEO
Dan Juckniess, SVP, Sales & Professional Services
Stacey Herteux, VP, Human Resources
Rob Rueckl, Chief Financial Officer

Basic vocabulary and key words are taught and, when need, retaught using alternative teaching strategies. Passages that students read help put the vocabulary into context. Each lesson is followed by crossword and other puzzles check comprehension.

1756 Learning English: Primary
203 Colorado Street
Austin, TX 78701-3922
512-478-9600
800-678-1412
866-586-7387
FAX: 619-622-7873
e-mail: support@compasslearning.com
www.compasslearning.com

Eric Loeffel, President, CEO
Tammy Deal, VP, Human Resources
Eric Wasser, VP, Sales
Eileen Shihadeh, VP, Marketing

Four stories and rhymes help students familiarize themselves with essential English language concepts, recognize patterns in language and associate words with objects. *$49.95*

1757 Learning English: Rhyme Time
Compass Learning
203 Colorado Street
Austin, TX 78701-3922
512-478-9600
800-678-1412
866-586-7387
FAX: 619-622-7873
e-mail: support@compasslearning.com
www.compasslearning.com

Eric Loeffel, President, CEO
Tammy Deal, VP, Human Resources
Eric Wasser, VP, Sales
Eileen Shihadeh, VP, Marketing

Using classic children's rhymes in an animated multimedia program, students work on language skills, vocabulary and comprehension.

1758 Lexia I, II and III Reading Series
Lexia Learning Systems
200 Baker Ave Ext.
Concord, MA 01742
978-405-6200
800-435-3942
800-507-2772
FAX: 978-287-0062
e-mail: info@lexialearning.com
www.lexialearning.com

Nick Gaehde, President and CEO
Paul More, Vice President, Finance
Collin Earnst, Vice President of Marketing
Peter Koso, Vice President of Operations

Lexia's software helps children and adults with learning disabilities master their core reading skills. Based on the Orton Gillingham method, Lexia Early Reading, Phonics Based Reading and SOS (Strategies for Older Students) apply phonics principles to help students learn essential sound-symbol correspondence and decoding skills. The Quick Reading Tests generate detailed skill reports in only 5-8 minutes per student to provide data for further instruction. Price: $40-400 per workstation.

1759 Memory Castle
WINGS for Learning
1600 Green Hills Rd
Scotts Valley, CA 95066-4981
831-426-2228
FAX: 831-464-3600

Ani Stocks, Owner

Introduces a strategy to increase memory skills via an adventure Q198game. Set in a castle, the game requires memory, reading, spelling skills and more to win.

1760 On a Green Bus: A UKanDu Little Book
Don Johnston
26799 West Commerce Drive
Volo, IL 60073
847-740-0749
800-999-4660
FAX: 847-740-7326
e-mail: info@donjohnston.com
www.donjohnston.com

Don Johnston, Founder
Ruth Ziolkowski, President

This early literacy program that consists of several create-your-own 4-page animated stories that help build language experience on each page and then watch the page come alive with animation and sound. After completing the story, students can print it out to make a book which can be read over and over again. Because there are no wrong answers, all children can have a successful literacy experience. *$ 45.00*

1761 Open Book
Freedom Scientific
11800 31st Court North
St Petersburg, FL 33716
727-803-8000
800-444-4443
FAX: 727-803-8001
e-mail: info@freedomscientific.com
www.freedomscientific.com

Lee Hamilton, President, CEO, and Chairman of
Mike Self, Sales Representative (Alabama)
Joseph McDaniel, Sales Representative (Alaska and
Bobby Lakey, Sales Representative (Arkansas)

Software that reads scanned text allowed and includes other features that aid the vision-impaired. *$995.00*

1762 Optimum Resource Software
1 Mathews Drive
Suite 107
Hilton Head Island, SC 29926
843-689-8000
FAX: 843-689-8008
e-mail: info@stickybear.com
www.stickybear.com

Richard Hefter, President

Optimum Resource publishes over 100 K-12 education curriculum software titles under its varietal brands, StickyBear, MiddleWare, High School and Tools for Teachers. Most programs are available in Bilingual English/Spanish, and are offered with options for the single user through 30 users.

1763 **Parts of Speech**
Optimum Resource
1 Mathews Drive
Suite 107
Hilton Head Island, SC 29926
843-689-8000
FAX: 843-689-8008
e-mail: info@stickybear.com
www.stickybear.com

Richard Hefter, President
Designed to help students build grammar and vocabulary as they strengthen reading and writing ability. Grades 3 to 9. *$59.95*

1764 **Programs for Aphasia and Cognitive Disorders**
Parrot Software
P.O.Box 250755
West Bloomfield, MI 48325
248-788-3223
800-727-7681
FAX: 248-788-3224
e-mail: support@parrotsoftware.com
www.parrotsoftware.com

Dr. Frederic Weiner, Ph. D., CCC-SP, President, Owner
Over 50 different computer programs that facilitate language, memory and attention training. Programs are available for MS DOS, WINDOWS and Apple II.

1765 **Punctuation Rules**
Optimum Resource
1 Mathews Drive
Suite 107
Hilton Head Island, SC 29926
843-689-8000
FAX: 843-689-8008
e-mail: info@stickybear.com
www.stickybear.com

Richard Hefter, President
Punctuation Rules is designed to help students improve their punctuation skills. Students work with appropriate level sentences which follow common rules of punctuation. The program covers material ranging from categories of sentences to forming possessives and allows students to gain strength in their ability to correctly use periods, commas, apostrophes, question marks, colons, hyphens, quotation marks, exclamation points and more. Grades 3-9. Bilingual. *$59.95*

1766 **Quick Reading Test, Phonics Based Reading, Reading SOS (Strategies for Older Students)**
Lexia Learning Systems
200 Baker Ave Ext.
Concord, MA 01742
978-405-6200
800-435-3942
800-507-2772
FAX: 978-287-0062
e-mail: info@lexialearning.com
www.lexialearning.com

Nick Gaehde, President and CEO
Paul More, Vice President, Finance
Collin Earnst, Vice President of Marketing
Peter Koso, Vice President of Operations
Lexia's software helps children and adults with learning disabilities master their core reading skills. Based on the Orton Gillingham method, Phonics Based Reading and S.O.S. (Strategies for the Older Student) apply phonics principles to help students learn essential sound-symbol correspondence and decoding skills. The Quick Reading Tests generate detailed phonemic skills reports in only 5-8 minutes per student to provide teachers with accurate data to focus their instruction. Price: $67-$500.

1767 **Quick Talk**
Educational Activities Software
5600 West 83rd Street
Suite 300, 8200 Tower
Bloomington, MN 55437
888-351-4199
800-447-5286
FAX: 239-225-9299
e-mail: info@edmentum.com
www.edmentum.com

Vin Riera, President/CEO
Dan Juckniess, SVP, Sales & Professional Services
Stacey Herteux, VP, Human Resources
Rob Rueckl, Chief Financial Officer
Students will learn and use new vocabulary immediately: high-frequency, everyday vocabulary words are introduced and used contextually using human speech, graphics and text. Voice-interactive program (MS-DOS). *$65.00*

1768 **Race the Clock**
Mindplay
4400 E. Broadway Blvd
Suite 400
Tucson, AZ 85711
520-888-1800
800-221-7911
FAX: 520-888-7904
e-mail: mail@mindplay.com
www.mindplay.com

Dan Figurski, Senior Vice President of Business
Chris Coleman, VP, Business Development
Judith Bliss, CEO
Brian Williams, Development Manager
A matching game, uses the animation capabilities to teach verbs. The player chooses a matching game from a menu.

1769 **Read: Out Loud**
Don Johnston
26799 West Commerce Drive
Volo, IL 60073
847-740-0749
800-999-4660
FAX: 847-740-7326
e-mail: info@donjohnston.com
www.donjohnston.com

Don Johnston, Founder
Ruth Ziolkowski, President
An accessible text reader that provides access to the curriculum. It features high-quality text to speech and study tools that help students read with comprehension. *$79.00*

1770 **Reader Rabbit**
Learning Company
Ste 1900
100 Pine St
San Francisco, CA 94111-5205
415-659-2000
800-825-4420
FAX: 415-659-2020
e-mail: thelearningco@hmhpub.com
www.thelearningcompany.com

Linda K. Zecher, President and CEO
Eric Shuman, Chief Financial Officer
John K. Dragoon, Executive Vice President and Chi
William Bayers, Executive Vice President and Gen
Supports young students in building fundamental reading readiness skills in a playful, multi-sensory environment.

1771 **Reading Comprehension Series**
Optimum Resource
1 Mathews Drive
Suite 107
Hilton Head Island, SC 29926- 3765
843-689-8000
FAX: 843-689-8008
e-mail: info@stickybear.com
www.stickybear.com

Richard Hefter, President
The Reading Comprehension Series, includes seven volumes packed with intriguing multi-level stories. Each volume will capture the interest of children ages 8-14 while teaching them crucial reading comprehension skills. These open-ended programs are versatile and easy to use, and Bilingual. *$59.95*

1772 **Simon SIO**
Don Johnston
26799 West Commerce Drive
Volo, IL 60073
847-740-0749
800-999-4660
FAX: 847-740-7326
e-mail: info@donjohnston.com
www.donjohnston.com

Don Johnston, Founder
Ruth Ziolkowski, President
A researched and widely field-tested phonics program for beginning readers, developed in collaboration with Dr. Ted Hasselbring of Vanderbilt University. The program uses a personal tutor to deliver individualized instruction and corrective feedback. *$79.00*

1773 **Sound Sentences**
Educational Activities Software
5600 West 83rd Street
Suite 300, 8200 Tower
Bloomington, MN 55437
888-351-4199
800-447-5286
FAX: 239-225-9299
e-mail: info@edmentum.com
www.edmentum.com

Vin Riera, President/CEO
Dan Juckniess, SVP, Sales & Professional Services
Stacey Herteux, VP, Human Resources
Rob Rueckl, Chief Financial Officer
This sound-interactive program breaks away from traditional language instruction. Instead of formal concentration on verb and basic vocabulary, students meet everyday English with colloquialisms they will hear in real life situations. They reinforce their knowledge of sentence structure while acquiring the ability to communicate in daily settings. (For MAC, MS-DOS and Windows). *$65.00*

1774 **Spelling Rules**
Optimum Resource
1 Mathews Drive
Suite 107
Hilton Head Island, SC 29926- 3765
843-689-8000
FAX: 843-689-8008
e-mail: info@stickybear.com
www.stickybear.com

Richard Hefter, President
A curriculum based, easy-to-use program that provides students with the practice they need to build strong spelling skills. Concepts discussed include plurals, compounds, i-before-e, capitalization, and more. Grades 3 to 9. Bilingual. *$59.95*

1775 **Start-to-Finish Library**
Don Johnston
26799 West Commerce Drive
Volo, IL 60073
847-740-0749
800-999-4660
FAX: 847-740-7326
e-mail: info@donjohnston.com
www.donjohnston.com

Don Johnston, Founder
Ruth Ziolkowski, President
Offers struggling readers a wide selection of engaging narrative chapter books written at two readability levels (2-3rd and 4-5th grade) and delivered in three media formats. Professionally-narrated audio and computer supports help scaffold reading to ensure success. *$79.00*

1776 **Start-to-Finish Literacy Starters**
Don Johnston
26799 West Commerce Drive
Volo, IL 60073
847-740-0749
800-999-4660
FAX: 847-740-7326
e-mail: info@donjohnston.com
www.donjohnston.com

Don Johnston, Founder
Ruth Ziolkowski, President
A reading series intended for students with multiple disabilities who are in 3-12th grade, but reading at a beginning level. Dr. Karen Erickson developed this series, which combines switch-accessible software with three types of text. *$79.00*

1777 **Stickybear Reading Comprehension**
Optimum Resource
1 Mathews Drive
Suite 107
Hilton Head Island, SC 29926- 3765
843-689-8000
FAX: 843-689-8008
e-mail: info@stickybear.com
www.stickybear.com

Richard Hefter, President
This multi-level reading comprehension program helps children improve reading skills with 30 high-interest stories and question sets created by the Weekly Reader editors. Children learn to recognize main ideas, define sequence, using context to identify words, and more. Grades 2 to 4. Bilingual. *$59.95*

1778 **Stickybear Reading Fun Park**
Optimum Resource
1 Mathews Drive
Suite 107
Hilton Head Island, SC 29926- 3765
843-689-8000
FAX: 843-689-8008
e-mail: info@stickybear.com
www.stickybear.com

Richard Hefter, President
Children discover and practice critical reading skills as the Stickybear family guides users through unique, action-packed activities, each with multiple levels of difficulty and skills that address both the auditory and visual needs of budding readers. Pre-K through 3rd grade. *$59.95*

1779 **Stickybear Reading Room Deluxe**
Optimum Resource
1 Mathews Drive
Suite 107
Hilton Head Island, SC 29926- 3765
843-689-8000
FAX: 843-689-8008
e-mail: info@stickybear.com
www.stickybear.com

Richard Hefter, President
Children build vocabulary and reading comprehension skills using hundreds of word/picture sets and thousands of put-together sentence parts. K-3rd grade. Bilingual, English/Spanish. *$59.95*

1780 **Stickybear Spelling**
Optimum Resource
1 Mathews Drive
Suite 107
Hilton Head Island, SC 29926- 3765
843-689-8000
FAX: 843-689-8008
e-mail: info@stickybear.com
www.stickybear.com

Richard Hefter, President
Children discover and practice critical spelling skills as they work with three unique action-packed activities, each with four graded levels of difficulty. The program is open-ended and teachers may add, change and modify the word lists for each individual. Stickybear Spelling contains more than 2000 recorded words. Levels may be set to allow students of different ages or abilities to compete effectively. Grades 2 through 4. *$59.95*

1781 **Tomorrow's Promise: Language Arts**
Compass Learning
13500 Evening Creek Drive North
Suite 600
San Diego, CA 92128
858-668-2586
866-475-0317
FAX: 858-408-2903
e-mail: info@bridgepointeducation.com
www.bridgepointeducation.com

Andrew S. Clark, Founder, Chief Executive Officer
Diane Thompson, SVP, General Counsel
Charlene Dackerman, SVP, Human Resources
Daniel J. Devine, Executive Vice President & CFO

You'll strengthen students' grammar, usage and vocabulary skills and promote higher order thinking skills with this comprehensive Language Arts curriculum. It utilizes cross-curricular, thematic instruction engaging multimedia learning exercises that encourage writing, speaking and listening proficiency. Promotes higher order thinking skills. *$279.95*

1782 **Tomorrow's Promise: Reading**

Compass Learning
203 Colorado Street
Austin, TX 78701-3922
512-478-9600
800-678-1412
866-586-7387
FAX: 619-622-7873
e-mail: support@compasslearning.com
www.compasslearning.com

Eric Loeffel, President, CEO
Tammy Deal, VP, Human Resources
Eric Wasser, VP, Sales
Eileen Shihadeh, VP, Marketing

This multimedia curriculum balances thematic, interactive exploration with core skills development, increasing your students' early reading proficiency, building a solid literacy foundation and fostering a lifelong love for reading. *$279.95*

1783 **Tomorrow's Promise: Spelling**

Compass Learning
203 Colorado Street
Austin, TX 78701-3922
512-478-9600
800-678-1412
866-586-7387
FAX: 619-622-7873
e-mail: support@compasslearning.com
www.compasslearning.com

Eric Loeffel, President, CEO
Tammy Deal, VP, Human Resources
Eric Wasser, VP, Sales
Eileen Shihadeh, VP, Marketing

Lovable characters and engaging multimedia effects put young students on a fast-track to early spelling proficiency with fourteen activities and three games. A full year's instruction on each CD includes 30 world lists per grade, in story context, or create word lists to suit your needs. This program addresses students' multiple learning styles and rewards students as they progress through each stage of spelling skill acquisition. *$99.95*

1784 **Vocabulary Development**

Optimum Resource
1 Mathews Drive
Suite 107
Hilton Head Island, SC 29926- 3765
843-689-8000
FAX: 843-689-8008
e-mail: info@stickybear.com
www.stickybear.com

Richard Hefter, President

A featured program in the middle school series. Vocabulary Development is designed to help students increase vocabulary as they strengthen reading skills. Students relate their current knowledge of vocabulary to the context in which they discover an unfamiliar word. Utilizing a variety of contextual aids, this program illustrates synonyms, antonyms, prefixes, suffixes, homophones, multiple meanings and context clues, allowing students to apply experience and context. *$59.95*

1785 **Whoops**

Cornucopia Software
P.O.Box 6111
Albany, CA 94706
510-528-7000
e-mail: supportstaff@practicemagic.com
www.practicemagic.com

Christina Morua, Manager

Checks spelling three ways. It checks words as they are typed, it checks an entire screen and highlights the errors and it reads ASCII text files from a disk and lists errors.

Software: Vocational

1786 **Films Media Group**

Infobase Publishing
132 W 31st St, 17th Floor
New York, NY 10001
800-322-8755
FAX: 800-678-3633
e-mail: custserv@factsonfile.com
www.infobaselearning.com

Melinda Gallo, Senior Account Executive

Educational publisher of DVD programming for schools and libraries. *$64.86*

ISBN 0-927368-59-5

1787 **Functional Literacy System**

Conover Company
4 Brookwood Court
Appleton, WI 54914
920-231-4667
800-933-1933
FAX: 800-933-1943
e-mail: support@conovercompany.com
www.conovercompany.com

Terry Schmitz, Founder and Owner
Mike, Vice President of Operations
Art Janowiak, Vice President of Sales

Assessment and skill building for basic functional literacy. This multimedia software program is adult in format and uses live action video taken in actual community settings to help learners become more capable of functioning independently. Twenty different programs are currently available. *$99.00*

1788 **Learning Activity Packets**

4 Brookwood Court
Appleton, WI 54914
920-231-4667
800-933-1933
FAX: 800-933-1943
e-mail: support@conovercompany.com
www.conovercompany.com

Terry Schmitz, Founder and Owner
Mike, Vice President of Operations
Art Janowiak, Vice President of Sales

Demonstrates how basic academic skills relate to 30 major career areas. LAPs provide valuable diagnostics in applied academic applications and demonstrates to users the importance of academics as they relate to the workplace. Software. *$99.00*

1789 **Microcomputer Evaluation of Careers & Academics (MECA)**

Conover Company
4 Brookwood Court
Appleton, WI 54914
920-231-4667
800-933-1933
FAX: 800-933-1943
e-mail: support@conovercompany.com
www.conovercompany.com

Terry Schmitz, Founder and Owner
Mike, Vice President of Operations
Art Janowiak, Vice President of Sales

A cost-effective, technology-based, career development system which provides users with opportunities to get their hands dirty. The MECA system utilizes work simulations and is built around common occupational clusters. Each cluster, or career area, consists of hands-on WORK SAMPLES which provide a variety of career exploration and assessment experiences, linked to LEARNING ACTIVITY PACKETS, which integrate basic academic skills into the career planning and placement process. $580-$1,070.

1790 **OASYS**
Vertek
12835 Bellevue-Redmond Road
Suite 310
Bellevue, WA 98005
425-455-9921
800-220-4409
FAX: 425-454-7264
e-mail: sales@vertekinc.com
www.vertekinc.com

Debra Callahan, Sales Representative, Northern California
Tim Whitney, Sales Representative, Ohio, Michigan
Beverly Duncan, Sales Representative, Florida
Debbie Gordon, Sales Representative, Illinois

A software system that matches a person's skills and abilities to occupations and employers.

1791 **Reading in the Workplace**
Educational Activities Software
5600 West 83rd Street
Suite 300, 8200 Tower
Bloomington, MN 55437-585
888-351-4199
800-447-5286
FAX: 239-225-9299
e-mail: info@edmentum.com
www.edmentum.com

Vin Riera, President/CEO
Dan Juckniess, SVP, Sales & Professional Services
Stacey Herteux, VP, Human Resources
Rob Rueckl, Chief Financial Officer

A job-based, reading software program using real-life problems and solutions to capture students' attention and improve their vocabulary and comprehension skills. Units include: automotive, clerical, health care and construction. *$295.00*

1792 **Stickybear Typing**
Optimum Resource
1 Mathews Drive
Suite 107
Hilton Head Island, SC 29926- 3765
843-689-8000
FAX: 843-689-8008
e-mail: info@stickybear.com
www.stickybear.com

Richard Hefter, President

The award winning Stickybear Typing program allows users to sharpen typing skills and achieve keyboard mastery with three engaging and amusing multi-level activities. *$59.95*

1793 **Work-Related Vocational Assessment Systems: Computer Based**
Valpar International
P.O.Box 5767
Tucson, AZ 85703-767
262-797-0840
800-633-3321
FAX: 262-797-8488
e-mail: sales@valparint.com
www.valparint.com

Neal Gunderson, President

Criterion-referenced to Department of Labor standards. Evaluate academic levels for reading, spelling, math and language, interests, personalities, cognitive and physical aptitudes.

1794 **Workplace Skills: Learning How to Function on the Job**
Programming Concepts
8700 Shoal Creek Boulevard
Austin, TX 78757-6897
512-451-3246
800-897-3202
FAX: 800-397-7633
e-mail: general@proedinc.com
www.proedinc.com

Jeff McLane, Founder
Lee Wilson, President and CEO
Randy Pennington, Executive VP
David Keith, Vice President of IT

Offers parents and educators a functional means by which to discuss all aspects of finding and keeping a job. *$49.95*

Word Processors

1795 **DARCI**
Wes Test Engineering Corporation
810 Shepard Lane
Farmington, UT 84025
801-451-9191
FAX: 801-451-9393
e-mail: webmail@westest.com
westest.com

Robert Lessmann, President
James Lynds

Provides transparent access to all computer functions by replacing the computer's keyboard with a smart joystick. *$975.00*

1796 **Eye Relief Word Processing Software**
SkiSoft Publishing Corporation
P.O.Box 364
Lexington, MA 02420-4
781-863-1876
e-mail: info@skisoft.com
www.skisoft.com

Ken Skier, President
Cynthia Skier, CFO

Large-type word processing program for visually-impaired PC users. *$295.00*

1797 **IntelliTalk**
Intelli Tools
24 Prime Parkway
Natick, MA 01760
707-773-2000
800-547-6747
FAX: 707-773-2001
e-mail: customerservice@cambiumtech.com
www.intellitools.com

Beth Davis, Director Sales Operations
Lori Castle, Supervisor
Arjan Khalsa, CEO

Talking word-processing program available for MacIntosh, Apple IIe, IBM compatible and Windows computers. *$39.95*

1798 **Large Type**
P.O.Box T
Hewitt, NJ 07421-2088
973-853-6585
800-736-2216
FAX: 928-832-2894
e-mail: nire@theoffice.net
http://www.angelfire.com

Don Selwyn, Vice President
Rev. Tom Schwanda, President & Chairman
Robt. Fondiller, Ph.D., P.E, Vice President
Everett G. Ball, Treasurer

Display enlargement programs for visually impaired users. Consist of a variety of programs for different needs, ranging from basic to full-featured.

1799 **Pegasus LITE**
Words+
Ste 109
42505 10th St W
Lancaster, CA 93534-7059
661-723-6523
800-869-8521
FAX: 661-723-2114
e-mail: info@words-plus.com
www.words-plus.com

Phil Lawrence, VP

Provides all of the strategies currently being used in AAC, from dynamic display color pictographic language, to dual-word prediction text language, in a single system. *$6995.00*

1800 **Up and Running**
Intelli Tools
24 Prime Parkway
Natick, MA 01760
707-773-2000
800-547-6747
FAX: 707-773-2001
e-mail: customerservice@cambiumtech.com
www.intellitools.com
Beth Davis, Director Sales Operations
Lori Castle, Supervisor
Arjan Khalsa, CEO
Instantly use hundreds of popular commercial software programs with this custom collection of setups and overlays. *$69.95*

1801 **Write This Way**
Compass Learning Incorporated
203 Colorado St
Austin, TX 78701-3922
512-478-9600
800-678-1412
e-mail: support@compasslearning.com
www.compasslearning.com
Trey Chambers, Chief Financial Officer
Eric Loeffel, Chief Executive Officer
Anne Henson, Vice President, Curriculum & Instruction / Vice President, C
Quannah Hopper, Vice President, Compass Learning Impact Teacher Academy
An easy-to-use, versatile word processor designed with learning disabled or hearing-impaired individuals in mind. Apple or Mac available. *$99.95*

1802 **Write: OutLoud**
Don Johnston
26799 West Commerce Drive
Volo, IL 60073-9675
847-740-0749
800-999-4660
FAX: 847-740-7326
e-mail: info@donjohnston.com
www.donjohnston.com
Don Johnston, Founder
Ruth Ziolkowski, President
The award-winning feasible and user friendly talking word processor with talking spell checker. Text-to-speech technology provides multi-sensory learning and positive reinforcements for writers of all ages and ability levels. *$99.00*

Conferences & Shows

General

1803 AACRC Annual Meeting
American Assn. of Children's Residential Centers
11700 W Lake Park Drive
Milwaukee, WI 53224-3021
877-332-2272
FAX: 877-362-2272
e-mail: info@aacrc-dc.org
www.aacrc-dc.org

Christopher Bellonci, M.D., Past President
Laurah Currey, MA, LSW, LPC, President Elect
Gayle Wiler, Director
Joseph Whalen, Director
One-day program that addresses accreditation as it relates to current behavioral health care challenges held in Pasadena, CA.
October

1804 AADB National Conference
American Association of the Deaf-Blind
PO Box 8064
Silver Spring, MD 20907-8064
301-563-9064
FAX: 301-495-4404
TTY:301-495-4402
e-mail: aadb-info@aadb.org
www.aadb.org

Jill Gaus, President
Randall Pope, President, Maryland
Lynn Jansen, Vice President
Adam Drake, Treasurer
A week of general meetings, workshops, tours and evening recreational activities.

1805 AAIDD Annual Meeting
American Association on Mental Retardation
501 3rd Street
NW Suite 200
Washington, DC 20001
202-387-1968
800-424-3688
FAX: 202-387-2193
e-mail: maria@aaidd.org
www.aamr.org

James R. Thompson, PhD, President
Amy S. Hewitt, PhD, President Elect
Susan B. Palmer, PhD, Vice President
Patti N. Martin, Secretary, Treasurer
At The Crossroads: Ethics, Genetics, Leadership and self-determination, this annual meeting offers a full compliment of workshops, symposia, and multiperspective sessions that fill four days including social events.
May/June

1806 AAO Annual Meeting
American Academy Of Opthamology
655 Beach Street
San Francisco, CA 94109-1336
415-561-8500
FAX: 415-561-8567
e-mail: faao@aao.org
www.faao.org

Brad A. Wong, Executive Director
Shawn C. Fallon, Director, Administration
Todd Lyckberg, Director of Development
Jenny E. Benjamin, Director
Offers the most comprehensive program with more than 2000 scientific presentations and six subspecialty day programs
October

1807 ABD Winter Conference
American Board of Disability Analysts
Belle Meade Office Park, 4525 Hardi
Second Floor
Nashville, TN 37205
615-327-2984
FAX: 615-327-9235
e-mail: americanbd@aol.com
www.americandisability.org

Alexander Horowitz, MD, ABDA, Executive Officer Emeritus
Kenneth Anchor, Ph.D., ABPP, Administrative Offices
Dana Adair, MS, RN, C (ABDA, Professional Advisory Council
Francella W. Betancourt, MA, CRC (A, Professional Advisory Council
Joint Conference: American Board of Disability.
February

1808 ACA Annual Conference
American Counseling Association
5999 Stevenson Ave
Alexandria, VA 22304
703-823-9800
800-347-6647
FAX: 800-473-2329
e-mail: webmaster@counseling.org
www.counseling.org

Robert L. Smith, President
Thelma Duffey, President Elect
Brian Canfield, Treasurer
Richard Yep, CEO
Promotes the development of professional counselors, advancing the counseling profession, and using the profession and practice of counseling to promote respect for human dignity and diversity.
March/April

1809 ACB Annual Convention
American Council for the Blind
2200 Wilson Boulevard
Suite 650
Arlington, VA 22201-3354
202-467-5081
800-424-8666
FAX: 703-465-5085
e-mail: info@acb.org
www.acb.org

Kim Charlson, President
Mitch Pomerantz, Immediate Past President
Jeff Thom, First Vice President
Marlaina Lieberg, Second Vice President
Offers 50-75 booths of information for the blind.
June/July

1810 ADA Annual Scientific Sessions
American Diabetes Association
1701 North Beauregard St
Alexandria, VA 22311
703-549-1500
800-342-2383
FAX: 703-836-7439
e-mail: webmaster@diabetes.org
www.diabetes.org

Don Laing, Senior Vice President, Human Resources
Rodney Sampson, Senior Vice President, Chief Technology Officer
Lois A. Witkop, MBA, Senior Vice President, Marketing Communications
Shereen Arent, Executive Vice President, Government Affairs & Advocacy
Trade show featuring exhibits of equipment and supplies used by professionals involved in the treatment of diabetes.

1811 AER Annual International Conference
Assoc. for Educ. & Rehab of the Blind/Vis. Imp.
1703 N Beauregard Street
Suite 440
Alexandria, VA 22311
703-671-4500
877-492-2708
FAX: 703-671-6391
e-mail: aer@aerbvi.org
www.aerbvi.org

Jim Adams, President
Lou Tutt, Executive Director
Ginger Croce, Senior Director, Marketing & Office Operations
Barbara James, Director, Membership & Office Operations

Dedicated to rendering support and assistance to the professionals who work in all phases of education and rehabilitation of blind and visually impaired children and adults.

July

1812 AG Bell Convention
Alexander Graham Bell Association
3417 Volta Place, NW
Washington, DC 20007
202-337-5220
FAX: 202-337-8314
TTY:202-337-5221
e-mail: info@agbell.org
www.listeningandspokenlanguage.org

Meredith K. Sugar, Esq. (OH), President
Donald M. Goldberg, Immediate Past President
Ted A. Meyer, President-Elect, Secretary, Treasurer
Emilio Alonso Mendoza (DC), Chief Executive Officer

Over 60 booths offering information on resources and technology for the deaf and hard of hearing.

June

1813 AHEAD
Association on Higher Education And Disability
107 Commerce Centre Drive
Suite 204
Huntersville, NC 28078
704-947-7779
FAX: 704-948-7779
e-mail: information@ahead.org
www.ahead.org

Stephan J. Smith, Executive Director
Richard Allegra, Director, Professional Development
Jeremy Jarrell, Director, Innovation & Development
Oanh Huynh, Associate Executive Director

AHEAD is a professional membership organization for individuals involved in the development of policy and in the provision of quality services to meet the needs of persons with disabilities involved in all areas of higher education.

July

1814 APSE Conference: Revitalizing Supported Employment, Climbing to the Future
Association for Persons in Supported Employment
416 Hungerford Dr.
Suite 418
Rockville, MD 20850
301-279-0060
FAX: 301-279-0075
e-mail: jenny@apse.org
www.apse.org

David Hoff, President
Laura A. Owens, Ph.D., Executive Director
Jenny Levet, Communications/Membership Director
Boshia McRoy, Administrative Associate

A major conference on Supported Employment. The conference includes 130 sessions presented by nationally recognized leaders in the field. Conference attendees come from all 50 states, Canada and several foreign countries and include professionals in supported employment, occupational therapy, rehabilitation technology and other related fields.

July

1815 ASHA Convention
American Speech-Language-Hearing Association
2275 Research Blvd
Suite 500
Rockville, MD 20850
646-328-2552
800-638-8255
FAX: 301-296-8580
TTY: 301-897-5700
e-mail: convention@asha.org
www.synutra.com

Liang Zhang, Chairman of the Board and Chief Executive Officer
Weiguo Zhang, President
Ning Clare Cai, Chief Financial Officer
Lei Lin, Director

Exhibits by companies specializing in alternative and augmentative communication products, publishers, software and hardware companies, and hearing aid testing equipment manufacturers. Speech-Language Pathologists are professionals who identify, assess, and treat speech and language problems. Audiologists are hearing health care professionals who specialize in preventing, identifying and assessing hearing disorders as well as providing audiologic treatment including hearing aids and more.

November

1816 ASIA Annual Scientific Meeting
American Spinal Injury Association
2020 Peachtree Rd NW
Atlanta, GA 30309-1426
404-355-9772
FAX: 404-355-1826
e-mail: ASIA_Office@shepherd.org
www.asia-spinalinjury.org

Lesley M Hudson MA, Executive Director
Patricia Duncan, Administrative Coordinator

Professional association for physicans and other health professionals working in all aspects of spinal cord injury. Also holds an annual scientific that surveys the latest advancements in the field.

May

1817 ATIA Conference
Assistive Technology Industry Association
330 N Wabash Avenue
Suite 2000
Chicago, IL 60611-4267
312-321-5172
877-687-2842
FAX: 312-673-6659
e-mail: info@atia.org
atia.org

Daniel Hubbell, Board President
David Wu, Treasurer
Tara Rudnicki, Secretary

The ATIA Conference is the largest international conference showcasing excellence in assistive technology.

1818 Abilities Expo
2601 Ocean Park Boulevard
Suite 200
Santa Monica, CA 9040
310-450-8831
FAX: 424-238-6358
e-mail: dkorse@abilitiesexpo.com
abilitiesexpo.com

David Korse, President/CEO

Abilities Expo is the nation's leading event for people with disabilities, their families, caregivers, and healthcare professionals. Meets in Chicago, Houston, Boston, Bay Area, Los Angeles, and New York.

1819 American Academy for Cerebral Palsy and Developmental Medicine Annual Conference
555 East Wells
Suite 1100
Milwaukee, WI 53202
414-918-3014
FAX: 414-276-2146
e-mail: info@aacpdm.org
www.aacpdm.org

Richard Stevenson, MD, President
Darcy Fehlings, MD MSc FRCPC, First Vice President
Eileen Fowler, PhD PT, Second Vice President
Joshua Hyman, MD, Treasurer

The Annual Meeting is a 3-day event, held in the Fall, designed to provide targeted opportunities for dissemination of information in the basic sciences, prevention, diagnosis, treatment, and technical advances as applied to persons with cerebral palsy and development disorders.
September

1820 American Board of Disability Analysts Annual Conference
Disability Analyst
Belle Meade Office Park, 4525 Hardi
Second Floor
Nashville, TN 37205
615-327-2984
FAX: 615-327-9235
e-mail: americanbd@aol.com
www.americandisability.org

Alexander Horowitz, MD, ABDA, Executive Officer Emeritus
Kenneth Anchor, Ph.D., ABPP, Administrative Offices
Dana Adair, MS, RN, C (ABDA, Professional Advisory Council
Francella W. Betancourt, MA, CRC (A, Professional Advisory Council
Annual conference held for members to meet and discuss current events and attend seminars.

1821 Annual Conference on Dyslexia and Related Learning Disabilities
New York Branch International Dyslexia Association
71 West 23rd Street
Suite 1527
New York, NY 10010
212-691-1930
FAX: 212-633-1620
e-mail: info@everyonereading.org
www.everyonereading.org

Jo Anne Simon, P.C., President
Leonard Gubar, Esq., Treasurer
Lavinia Mancuso, Interim Administrative Director
Jo Anne Lense, Director, Professional Development
Provides educational support services to people concerned and affected by dyslexia and related learning disabilities.
March

1822 Attention Deficit Disorders Association, Southern Region: Annual Conference
12345 Jones Road
Suite 287-7
Houston, TX 77070
281-897-0982
FAX: 281-894-6883
e-mail: addaoffice@sbcglobal.net
www.adda-sr.org

Laura Peddicord, President
Pam Esser, Executive Director
Opal Harris, Secretary
Tina Peden, Office Manager
Mission is to: provide a resource network; to support individuals impacted by attention deficit disorders; and to advocate for the development of community resources and services that meet the educational, social, and health care needs of all individuals with ADD/ADHD.
February

1823 Believable Hope Conference
United Cerebral Palsy Association
Ste 700
1660 L St NW
Washington, DC 20036-5638
202-776-0414
800-872-5827
FAX: 202-776-0414
TTY: 202-973-7197
e-mail: info@ucp.org
www.ucpa.org

Stephen Bennett, CEO
National, not-for-profit self-help organization dedicated to providing information and support to individuals with cerebral palsy and other disabilities, and their families. Supports more than 160 local affiliates; these affiliates provide a variety of programs and services for affected families, including support groups. Offers several educational and support materials, including a quarterly magazine, regular newsletters, and research reports.

1824 Blazing Toward a Cure Annual Conference
National Parkinson Foundation
1150 NW 72 Ave.
Suite 760
Miami, FL 33126
305-592-9954
800-327-4545
FAX: 305-477-7379
e-mail: info@acfm-cpa.com
www.acfm-cpa.com

Daniel Arty, Partner
Joel L. Moskowits, Partner
Julia Alemany, Audit Manager
Lester Feuer
Purpose is to find the cause and cure for Parkinson's Disease and related neurodegenerative disorders through research, education and dissemination of current information to patients, caregivers and families.
July/August

1825 Blind Childrens Center Annual Meeting
Blind Childrens Center
4120 Marathon Street
Los Angeles, CA 90029-3584
323-664-2153
800-222-3567
FAX: 323-665-3828
e-mail: Info@blindchildrenscenter.org.
www.blindchildrenscenter.org

Midge Horton, Executive Director
Muriel Scharf, Director of Development
Jennifer Brown, President
Kristin Dark, Director
A family-centered agency which serves children with visual impairments from birth to school-age. The center-based and home-based services help the children to acquire skills and build their independence. The Center utilizes its expertise and experience to serve families and professionals worldwide through support services, education and research.
September

1826 Blinded Veterans Association National Convention
Blinded Veterans Association
477 H Street
Northwest Washington, DC 20001-2694
202-371-8880
800-669-7079
FAX: 202-371-8258
e-mail: bva@bva.org
www.bva.org

Mark Cornell, National President
Robert Dale Stamper, National Vice President
Paul Mimms, National Treasurer
Joe Parker, National Secretary
Conventions have a three-fold purpose, to conduct Association business, to educate blinded veterans about the resources available to them, and to provide a means whereby blinded veterans can better strengthen and help one another.
August

1827 CQL Accreditation
Council on Quality and Leadership
100 West Road
Suite 300
Towson, MD 21204
410-583-0060
FAX: 410-583-0063
e-mail: info@thecouncil.org
www.c-q-l.org

Cathy Ficker Terrill, President and CEO
Tammi Watkins, Vice President, Operations
Kerri Melda, Vice President, Research & Product Development
Becky Hansen, Vice President, Accreditation & Training
Prepares you for CQL Accreditation, addressing Shared Values, Basic Assurances®, Personal Outcomes, Service Responsiveness and Commitment to Community Life.

1828 Closing the Gap's Annual Conference
Assist. Tech. Resources for Children & Adults
526 Main Street
P.O.Box 68
Henderson, MN 56044 507-248-3294
FAX: 507-248-3810
e-mail: info@closingthegap.com
www.closingthegap.com
Dolores Hagen, Co-Founder
Budd Hagen, Co-Founder
Connie Kneip, Vice President/General Manager
Megan Turek, Managing Editor/Advertising and Exhibit Sales
Topics cover a broad spectrum of technology as it is being applied to all disabilities and age groups in education, rehabilitation, vocation and independent living. People with disabilities, special educators, rehabilitation professionals, administrators, service/care providers, personnel managers, government officials, and hardware/software developers share their experiences and insights at this significant networking experience.
October

1829 Council for Exceptional Children Annual Convention and Expo
2900 Crystal Drive
Suite 1000
Arlington, VA 22202-3557 703-620-3660
866-509-0218
888-232-7733
FAX: 703-264-9494
TTY:866-915-5000
e-mail: service@cec.sped.org
www.cec.sped.org
Robin D. Brewer, President
James P. Heiden, President Elect
Christy A. Chambers, Immediate Past President
Mikki Garcia, Executive Director
Works to improve the educational success of children with disabilities and/or gifts and talents.
April

1830 Disability Matters
EMC Corporation
14 Glenbrook Drive
Mendham, NJ 07945 973-813-7260
FAX: 973-813-7261
e-mail: jill@consultingspringboard.com

1831 Eye Bank Association of America Annual Meeting
Eye Bank Association of America
1015 18th Street, NW
Suite 1010
Washington, DC 20036 202-775-4999
FAX: 202-429-6036
e-mail: malene@restoresight.org
www.restoresight.org
Kevin Corcoran, CAE, President / CEO
Molly Georgakis, Vice-President of Member Services
Bernie Dellario, Director of Finance
Jennifer DeMatteo, Director of Regulations and Standards
A four day program, which includes a series of presentations in administrative, hospital development, scientific and technical fields that are relative to eye banking.
June

1832 IDF National Conference
Immune Deficiency Foundation
40 West Chesapeake Avenue
Suite 308
Towson, MD 21204 410-321-6647
800-296-4433
FAX: 410-321-9165
e-mail: idf@primaryimmune.org
www.primaryimmune.org
Marcia Boyle, President & Founder
Katherine Antilla, Vice President, Education & Volunteers
Christine Belser, Vice President, Programs & Communications
Lawrence A. LaMotte, Vice President, Public Policy
World-renowned immunologists will share their time and expertise with families. Attendees will learn about scientific advancements in the diagnosis and treatment of these diseases and gain skills needed to manage their healthcare.
June

1833 Joint Conference with ABMPP Annual Conference
American Board of Disability Analysts
Belle Meade Office Park, 4525 Hardi
Second Floor
Nashville, TN 37205 615-327-2984
FAX: 615-327-9235
e-mail: americanbd@aol.com
www.americandisability.org
Alexander Horowitz, MD, ABDA, Executive Officer Emeritus
Kenneth Anchor, Ph.D., ABPP, Administrative Offices
Dana Adair, MS, RN, C (ABDA, Professional Advisory Council
Francella W. Betancourt, MA, CRC (A, Professional Advisory Council
Joint Conference with ABMPP Annual Conference Charleston, South Carolina.
May

1834 Lowe's Syndrome Conference
Lowe's Syndrome Association
PO Box 864346
Plano, TX 75086-4346 972-733-1338
FAX: 612-866-3222
e-mail: info@lowesyndrome.org
www.lowesyndrome.org
Debbie Jacobs, President
Jane Gallery, Treasurer
Fiona Fisher, Secretary
Christine Knight, Board Member and Director
An international conference held approximately every two years where family, friends, medical and other professionals gather to exchange ideas and information.
June

1835 NADD
National Association for the Dually Diagnosed
132 Fair St
Kingston, NY 12401-4802 845-331-4336
800-331-5362
FAX: 845-331-4569
e-mail: info@thenadd.org
www.thenadd.org
Robert Fletcher, CEO
NADD is a non-for-profit membership organization designed to promote awareness of, and services for, individuals who have co-occuring intellectual disability and mental illness. NADD provides training, consultation services, and publishes journals and books.
November

1836 NASPAC Annual Conference Association Annual Convention/Expo
National Assoc. of Subacute and Post Acute Care
P.O.Box 65085
Washington, DC 20035-5085 202-429-2700
FAX: 202-429-2701
www.naspac.net
Lyle Williams, President
Totally dedicated to servicing the subacute arena and its major entities. Features 100+ booths and over 75 exhibitors.
March

1837 NASW-NYS Chapter
NASW
188 Washington Ave
Albany, NY 12210
518-463-4741
800-724-6279
FAX: 518-463-6446
e-mail: info@naswnys.org
www.naswnys.org

Peter Chernack, DSW, LCSW-R, President
Diane Bessel Matteson, Ph.D., Vice President
Brian Masciadrelli, Ph.D., Treasurer
Karen Rich, PhD, LCSW, Secretary
Workshops, keynote speakers, and presentations offered at this event will develop and enhance practice skills and knowledge in the provision of quality mental health and community services.
March

1838 National Council on the Aging Conference
Conference Department
1901 L Street, NW
4th Floor
Washington, DC 20036
202-479-1200
800-424-9046
800-677-1116
FAX: 202-479-0735
TTY:202-479-6674
e-mail: membership@ncoa.org
www.ncoa.org

James P Firman, EdD, President and CEO
Donna Whitt, Senior Vice President, Chief Financial Officer
Wendy Zenker, Vice President, Public and Private Partnerships
Ramsey Alwin, Vice President, Economic Security
Offers ideas and programs to increase program and administrative skills through NCOA's professional development tracks and offering of continuing education units.
May

1839 PVA Summit And Expo
Paralyzed Veterans Of America
801 Eighteenth Street NW
Washington, DC 20006-3517
800-424-8200
TTY:8007954327
e-mail: summit@pva.org
pva.org

1840 PWSA (USA) Conference
Prader-Willi Alliance Of New York
244 5th Avenue
Suite D-110
New York, NY 10001
718-846-6606
800-442-1655
FAX: 914-312-0142
e-mail: alliance@prader-willi.org
www.prader-willi.org

Amy McDougall, President, Fulton
Hon. Daniel Angiolillo, President Emeritus, Director, W. Harrison
Rachel Johnson, Vice President, Endicott
Nancy Finegold, Vice President, W. Hempstead
Through conferences, publications, electronic communication and networking (parent-to-parent, parent-to professional, and professional-to-professional), the Prader-Willi Alliance provides a valuable resource for individuals and families sharing the same concerns.
July

1841 Pacific Rim International Conference
1410 Lower Campus Road #171F
Honolulu, HI 96822
808-956-7539
www.pacrim.hawaii.edu

1842 RESNA Annual Conference
Rehab Engineering & Assistive Tech. North America
1700 North Moore Street
Suite 1540
Arlington, VA 22209
703-524-6686
FAX: 703-524-6630
TTY:703-524-6639
e-mail: conference@resna.org
www.resna.org

Alex Mihailidis, Ph.D, P.En, President
Jerry Weisman, Immediate Past-President
Ray Grott, ATP, RET, President Elect
Paul J. Schwartz, Treasurer
Sponsored by a multidisciplinary association for the advancement of rehabilitation and assistive technologies, this annual conference brings together a large number of rehabilitation professionals, products and services from around the world and has something to offer for both professionals and consumers. The conference provides an informative and thought provoking forum for anyone with interests in rehabilitation technology.
June

1843 Rehabilitation International
25 East 21st Street,
4th floor
New York, NY 10010-6207
212-420-1500
FAX: 212-505-0871
e-mail: ri@riglobal.org
riglobal.org

Venus Ilagan, Manager
RI is a global network of people with disabilities, service providers, researchers, government agencies, and advocates protecting and promoting the rights and inclusion of people with disabilities. RI has over 1,000 member organizations in all regions on the world.

1844 Rehabilitation Technology Association Conference
PO Box 1004
Institute, WV 25112-1004
304-766-4602
800-624-8284
FAX: 304-766-2689

Betty Jo Tyler, RTA Coordinator
Dave Whipp, Information Manager
RTA holds this annual conference for the rehab technology community. It also publishes a quarterly newsletter and houses the Project Enable computerized bulletin board system.
Spring

1845 Source-APTA Audio Conference
American Physical Therapy Association
1111 North Fairfax Street
Alexandria, VA 22314-1488
703-684-2782
800-999-2782
FAX: 703-706-8536
TTY: 703-683-6748
e-mail: consumer@apta.org
apta.org

Paul Rockar, Jr, PT, DPT, M, President
Sharon L. Dunn, PT, PhD, OCS, Vice President
Laurita M. Hack, Secretary
Elmer Platz, PT, Treasurer
The American Physical Therapy Association (APTA), a national professional organization representing more than 66,000 members, sponsors this annual conference. The goal is to foster advancements in physical therapy practice, research, and education.

1846 Southwest Conference On Disability
2300 Menaul Boulevard NE
Albuquerque, NM 87107
505-272-6231
FAX: 505-272-9594
e-mail: swdisabilityconference@salud.unm.edu
http://cdd.unm.edu/swconf/

1847 TSA National Conference
Tourette Syndrome Association
42-40 Bell Boulevard
Bayside, NY 11361
718-224-2999
800-237-0717
FAX: 718-279-9596
e-mail: ts@tsa-usa.org
www.tsa-usa.org

Judit Unger, President
Gary Frank, Executive VP

More than 400 attendees come together for this biennial conference that includes members of the TS community and their families, educators, TS advocates, physicians, researchers, allied professionals, and TSA staff members. Attendees interact, socialize, share ideas, discuss issues of concern, learn from experts, and in many instances meet face to face for the first time.
Spring

1848 The Annual TASH Conference
TASH
2013 H Street NW
Washington, DC 20006
202-540-9020
FAX: 202-540-9019
e-mail: info@tash.org
conference.tash.org

Barb Trader, Executive Director

The TASH Conference is the advocacy, networking, and educational event of the year, attracting speakers and attendees from all over the world. Each year, self-advocates, educators, service providers and others come together to learn, share and grow.

1849 The Arc National Convention
The Arc
1825 K Street Nw
Suite 1200
Washington, DC 20006
202-534-3700
800-433-5255
FAX: 202-534-3731
e-mail: info@thearc.org
thearc.org

1850 YAI Conference
YAI Network
460 West 34th Street
New York, NY 10001-2382
212-273-6100
TTY:2122902787
www.yai.org

Abbe Wittenberg, Conference Manager
Tina Sobel, Conference Director
Amanda Katz, Exhibit Coordinator

YAI's International Conference on Intellectual and Development Disabilities is a global gathering on the future of the field and serves as a major forum for the exchange of ideas and information pertaining to programs, policies, and strategies that enhance the lives of people with intellectual and developmental disabilities.

1851 Young Onset Parkinson Conference
National Parkinson Foundation & ADPF
200 SE 1st Street
Suite 800
Miami, FL 33131
305-243-6666
800-473-4636
FAX: 305-537-9901
e-mail: contact@parkinson.org
www.parkinson.org

Joyce Oberdorf, President and CEO
Amy Gray, Vice President, Chapter Relations & Community Partnerships
Jill Davidson, Vice President, Finance & Administration
Peter Schmidt, PhD, Vice President, Programs, Chief Information Officer

Purpose is to find the cause and cure for Parkinson's Disease and related neurodegenerative disorders through research, education and dissemination of current information to patients, care-givers and families.
Annual

Construction & Architecture

Associations

1852 **Adaptive Environments Center**
200 Portland Street
Suite 1
Boston, MA 02114 617-695-1225
FAX: 617-482-8099
e-mail: info@HumanCenteredDesign.org
www.humancentereddesign.org

Ralph Jackson, FAIA, President
Chris Pilkington, Vice President
Nancy Jenner, Treasurer
Valerie Fletcher, Executive Director
Develops educational programs and materials on universal design, Americans with Disabilities Act, home adaptation, and more. Central Adaptive Environments publication list also available.

1853 **Building Owners and Managers Association International**
1101 15th St., NW
Suite 800
Washington, DC 20005 202-408-2662
FAX: 202-326-6377
e-mail: info@boma.org
www.boma.org

John G. Oliver, Chair and Chief Elected Officer
Kent C. Gibson, CPM, Chair-Elect
Henry H. Chamberlain, President, COO
Brian Harnetiaux, Vice Chair
Conducts seminars nationwide and publishes resource guidebooks for building owners and managers on ADA requirements for commercial facilities and places of public accommodation.

1854 **Mark Elmore Associates Architects**
Ste 104
42 East St
Crystal Lake, IL 60014-4400 815-455-7260
800-801-7766
FAX: 815-455-2238
e-mail: mark@elmore-architects.com
www.elmore-architects.com

Mark A Elmore, Owner
Architectural designs for accessible residential and commercial buildings. ADA compliance reviews.

1855 **National Conference on Building Codes and Standards**
505 Huntmar Park Drive
Suite 210
Herndon, VA 20170 703-437-0100
FAX: 703-481-3596
e-mail: membership@ncsbcs.org
www.ncsbcs.org

Cynthia Wilk, President
Robert C. Wible, Executive Director
Debbie Becker, Administrative Assistant
Kevin Egilmez, Project Manager
Serves as a forum in the interchange of information and provides technical services, education and training to our members to enhance the public's social and economic well being through safe, durable, affordable, accessible and efficient buildings.

1856 **National Council of Architectural Registration Boards (NCARB)**
1801 K Street NW
Suite 700K
Washington, DC 20006 202-879-0520
FAX: 202-783-0290
e-mail: customerservice@ncarb.org
ncarb.org

Michael J. Armstrong, Chief Executive Officer
Mary S. de Sousa, CAE, Chief Operating Officer
Stephen Nutt, AIA, NCARB, CAE, Senior Architect and advisor to the CEO
Sandy Vasan, Director, Marketing & Communications
Research service in print and online information. Large collection of books and periodicals on the building/architectural environments.

1857 **Overcoming Mobility Barriers International**
1022 S 4st St
Omaha, NE 68105 402-342-5731
FAX: 402-342-5731

Kay Neil, Executive Director
Members are government officials, service consumers and providers, and other persons interested in removing mobility barriers for elderly, handicapped and disadvantaged persons. Advises and works in conjunction with other groups and government agencies to establish safety standards for special equipment used in retrofitting vehicles and works to retrain drivers in the use of nonconventional driving controls.

1858 **Paradigm Design Group**
Paralyzed Veterans of America
801 Eighteenth Street, NW
Washington, DC 20006-3517 202-872-1300
800-424-8200
FAX: 202-785-4432
e-mail: info@pva.org
www.pva.org

Bill Lawson, National President
Homer S. Townsend Jr., Executive Director
Al F. Kovach Jr., National Senior Vice Presedent
Craig F. Enenbach, National Treasurer
Specialized firm providing architectural consulting services related to accessible designs. Experience includes product design and building codes and standards.

1859 **United States Access Board**
Ste 1000
1331 F St NW
Washington, DC 20004-1111 202-272-0080
800-872-2253
FAX: 202-272-0081
TTY: 800-993-2822
e-mail: info@access-board.gov
www.access-board.gov

Dave Yanchulis, Public Affairs Specialist
Offers information and technical assistance to the public on accessible design under the Americans with Disabilities Act and other laws. Guidance and publications are available free that address access to facilities, transit vehicles and information technology.

Publications & Videos

1860 Access Currents
United States Access Board
1331 F Street, NW
Suite 1000
Washington, DC 20004-1111
202-272-0080
800-872-2253
FAX: 202-272-0081
TTY: 800-993-2822
e-mail: info@access-board.gov
www.access-board.gov

Michael K. Yudin, Chair, Department of Education
Sachin Dev Pavithran, Vice Chair, Logan, Utah
Regina Blye, Public Member
Patrick D. Cannon, Public Member

Offers information and referrals on architectural accessibility for architects, designers, government agencies, building owners and consumers. A list of free publications is available on request.
bi-monthly

1861 Access Equals Opportunity
Council of B BB s Foundation
3033 Wilson Blvd
Suite 600
Arlington, VA 22201
703-276-0100
e-mail: media@cbbb.bbb.org
www.bbb.org

Beverly Baskin, Senior VP, Chief Mission Officer
Genie Barton, Vice President and Director, Onl
Rodney L. Davis, Senior VP Enterprise Programs
Joseph E. Dillon, VP and CFO

These six Title III compliance guides for existing small businesses offer creative cheap and easy suggestions for complying with the public accommodations section of the ADA. Each guide is industry specific for: retail stores, car sales/service, restaurants/bars, medical offices and fun/fitness centers. They include suggestions for readily achievable removal of architectural barriers; effective communication; and guidance for nondiscriminatory policies or procedures. *$2.50*

1862 Access for All
Hospital Audiences
548 Broadway
3rd Floor
New York, NY 10012
212-575-7676
FAX: 212-575-7669
e-mail: info@hostau.org
www.hospitalaudiences.org

David Sweeny, Executive Director
Jane Kleinsinger, Director of Operations
Jill Bernard, Marketing & Outreach Manager
JoAnne Brockways, Chief Financial Officer

Provides physical and program accessibility information for people with disabilities to New York City cultural institutions including theaters, museums, galleries, etc.

1863 Accessible Home of Your Own
Accent Books & Products
P.O.Box 700
Bloomington, IL 61702-700
309-378-2961
800-787-8444
FAX: 309-378-4420
e-mail: acmtlvng@aol.com
www.accentonliving.com

Raymond C Cheever, Publisher
Betty Garee, Editor

This guide includes 14 articles that have appeared in the magazine on the popular subject of how to make a disabled persons home more accessible. *$5.95*
52 pages Paperback
ISBN 0-91570 -29-9

1864 Adaptable Housing: A Technical Manual for Implementing Adaptable Dwelling
H UD U SE R
P.O.Box 23268
Washington, DC 20026-3268
202-708-3178
800-245-2691
FAX: 202-708-9981
TTY: 800-927-7589
e-mail: helpdesk@huduser.org
www.huduser.org

Patrick J. Tewey, Director, Budget, Contracts, and Program Control Division
Jacqueline D Buford, Director, Management and Administrative Services Division
Jean Lin Pao, General Deputy Assistant Secretary
Katherine M. O'Regan, Assistant Secretary for Policy Development and Research

An illustrated manual describing methods for implementing adaptability in housing. *$3.00*

1865 Adaptive Environments Center Home Assessment Form
Ste 301
374 Congress St
Boston, MA 02210-1807
617-695-1225
FAX: 617-482-8099
e-mail: info@adaptiveenvironment.org
adaptiveenvironments.org

Valerie Fletcher, Executive Director

A handy checklist for evaluating a disabled person's abilities and his/her home limitations to determine what accessibility modifications will be most effective. *$5.00*

1866 Consumer's Guide to Home Adaptation
Adaptive Environments Center
200 Portland Street
Suite 1
Boston, MA 02114
617-695-1225
FAX: 617-482-8099
e-mail: info@HumanCenteredDesign.org
www.humancentereddesign.org

Ralph Jackson, FAIA, President
Chris Pilkington, Vice President
Nancy Jenner, Treasurer
Valerie Fletcher, Executive Director

A workbook that enables people with disabilities to plan the modifications necessary to adapt their homes. Describes how to widen doorways, lower countertops, etc. *$12.00*
52 pages Paperback

1867 Design for Acessibility
National Endowment for the Arts Office
400 7th Street, SW
Washington, DC 20506-0001
202-682-5400
FAX: 202-682-5715
e-mail: webmgr@arts.gov
arts.gov

Jane Chu, Chairman
Joan Shigekawa, Senior Deputy Chairman
Mike Burke, Chief Information Officer
Joseph Smith, Deputy Chief Information Officer

A handbook for compliance with Section 504 of the Rehabilitation Act of 1973 and the Americans with Disabilities Act of 1990 including technical assistance on making arts programs accessible to staff, performers and audience.
101 pages
ISBN 0-160042-83-6

1868 Directory of Accessible Building Products
N AH B Research Center
400 Prince George's Blvd
Upper Marlboro, MD 20774
301-249-4000
800-638-8556
FAX: 301-430-6180
www.homeinnovation.com

Michael Luzier, CEO & President
Michelle Desiderio, Vice President of Innovation Services
Tom Kenney, P.E, Vice President of Engineering & Research
Phil Davis, Senior Economist & Analyst

Contains descriptions of more than 200 commercially available products designed for use by people with disabilities and age-related limitations. Paperback. *$5.00*
104 pages Yearly

1869 **Do-Able Renewable Home**
A AR P Fulfillment
601 E Street NW
Washington, DC 20049 202-434-3525
888-687-2277
877-342-2277
FAX: 202-434-3443
e-mail: member@aarp.org
www.aarp.org
John Wider, President, CEO, AARP Services Inc.
Lisa M. Ryerson, President, AARP Foundation
Robert R. Hagans, Jr., Executive Vice President & Chief Financial Officer
Hollis Terry Bradwell III, Executive Vice President & Chief Information Officer
Describes how individuals with disabilities can modify their homes for independent living. Room-by-room modifications are accompanied by illustrations.

1870 **ECHO Housing: Recommended Construction and Installation Standards**
601 E Street NW
Washington, DC 20049 202-434-3525
888-687-2277
877-342-2277
FAX: 202-434-3443
e-mail: member@aarp.org
www.aarp.org
John Wider, President, CEO, AARP Services Inc.
Lisa M. Ryerson, President, AARP Foundation
Robert R. Hagans, Jr., Executive Vice President & Chief Financial Officer
Hollis Terry Bradwell III, Executive Vice President & Chief Information Officer
Illustrated design, construction, and installation standards for temporary dwelling units for elderly people on single family residential property.

1871 **Electronic House: Enhanced Lifestyles with Electronics**
Electronic House
111 Speen Street, Suite 200
P.O. Box 989
Framingham, MA 01701-2000 508-663-1500
800-375-8015
FAX: 508-663-1599
e-mail: eheditorial@ehpub.com
electronichouse.com
Kenneth D. Moyes, President
Karen Bligh, Marketing Director
John Brillon, Web Creative Director
Guy Caiola, Director of Internet Operations
Dedicated to home automation. Featuring both extravagant and affordable smart homes that can be controlled with one touch. EH covers electronic systems that give homeowners more security, entertainment, convenience, and fun. Articles cover whole house control and subsystems like residential lighting, security, home theater, energy management and telecommunications. *$23.95*
84 pages BiMonthly
ISSN 0886-66 3

1872 **Fair Housing Design Guide for Accessibility**
National Council on Multifamily Housing Industry
1201 15th Street NW
Washington, DC 20005 202-266-8200
800-368-5242
FAX: 202-266-8400
e-mail: ggsmith@nahb.org
www.nahb.com
Kevin Kelly, Chairman of the Board
Tom Woods, First Vice Chairman of the Board
Ed Brady, Second Vice Chairman of the Board
Gerald M. Howard, CEO
Specifically tailored to address the needs of architects and builders. The book includes a detailed technical analysis of the legislation's impact on multifamily design, highlights potential construction problems, and identifies possible solutions. *$29.95*

1873 **Ideas for Making Your Home Accessible**
Accent Books & Products
P.O.Box 700
Bloomington, IL 61702-0700 309-378-2961
800-787-8444
FAX: 309-378-4420
e-mail: acmtlvng@aol.com
www.accentonliving.com
Raymond C Cheever, Publisher
Betty Garee, Editor
Offers over 100 pages of tips and ideas to help build or remodel a home. Includes many special devices and where to get them. *$7.50*
94 pages Paperback
ISBN 0-91570 -08-6

1874 **North Carolina Accessibility Code**
North Carolina Department of Insurance
P.O.Box 26387
Raleigh, NC 27611-6387 919-833-2110
FAX: 919-833-1801
e-mail: lwright@ncdoi.net
Gregory Griggs, Executive VP
Making buildings and facilities accessible to and usable by the physically handicapped. *$20.00*
678 pages Triannually

1875 **Removing the Barriers: Accessibility Guidelines and Specifications**
A PP A
1643 Prince Street
Alexandria, VA 22314 703-684-1446
FAX: 703-549-2772
e-mail: webmaster@appa.org
www.appa.org
John F. Bernhards, Associate Vice President
E. Lander Medlin, Executive VP
Steve Glazner, Director of Knowledge Management
Suzanne M. Healy, Director of Professional Development
Offers site accessibility, building entrances, doors, interior circulation, restrooms and bathing facilities, drinking fountains and additional resources. *$45.00*
125 pages
ISBN 0-91335 -59-9

1876 **Smart Kitchen/How to Design a Comfortable, Safe & Friendly Workplace**
Ceres Press
P.O.Box 87
Woodstock, NY 12498-87 845-679-5573
FAX: 845-679-5573
e-mail: cem620@aol.com
healthyhighways.com
David Goldbeck, Owner
This book provides information about designing kitchens that may be helpful to people with disabilities as well as safe and energy efficient. *$16.95*
132 pages Paperback

1877 **United Spinal Association**
75-20 Astoria Blvd
Suite 120
East Elmhurst, NY 11370- 1177 718-803-3782
800-444-0120
FAX: 718-803-0414
e-mail: mkurtz@unitedspinal.org
www.unitedspinal.org
Paul Tobin, President
Maria Kurtz, Executive Assistant
Information on spinal cord injury and laws and regulations concerning people with disabilities, including veterans.
Monthly

Education

Aids for the Classroom

1878 **AEPS Child Progress Record: For Children Ages Three to Six**
Brookes Publishing
PO Box 10624
Baltimore, MD 21285-624 410-337-9580
800-638-3775
FAX: 800-638-3775
e-mail: custserv@brookespublishing.com
www.brookespublishing.com

Paul Brooks, President
Melissa Behm, Executive VP
George Stamathis, VP and Publisher

This chart helps monitor change by visually displaying current abilities, intervention targets, and child progress. In packages of 30. *$21.00*
8 pages Gate-fold
ISBN 1-557662-51-7

1879 **AEPS Curriculum for Three to Six Years**
Brookes Publishing
PO Box 10624
Baltimore, MD 21285-0624 410-337-9580
800-638-3775
FAX: 410-337-8539
e-mail: webmaster@brookespublishing.com
www.brookespublishing.com

Paul H. Brookes, Chairman of the Board
Jeffrey D. Brookes, President
George S. Stamathis, VP/Publisher
Melissa A. Behn, Executive Vice President

Used after the AEPS® Test is completed and scored, this developmentally sequenced curriculum allows professionals to match the child's IFSP/IEP goals and objectives with activity-based interventions — beginning with simple skills and moving on to more advanced skills. *$ 65.00*
304 pages Spiral-bound
ISBN 1-557665-65-6

1880 **AEPS Data Recording Forms: For Children Ages Three to Six**
Brookes Publishing
PO Box 10624
Baltimore, MD 21285-624 410-337-9580
800-638-3775
FAX: 800-638-3775
e-mail: custserv@brookespublishing.com
www.readplaylearn.com

Paul Brooks, President

These forms can be used by child development professionals on four separate occasions to pinpoint and then monitor a child's strengths and needs in the six key areas of skill development measured by the AEPS Test. Packages of 10. *$24.00*
36 pages Saddle-stiched
ISBN 1-557662-49-5

1881 **AEPS Family Interest Survey**
Brookes Publishing
PO Box 10624
Baltimore, MD 21285-624 410-337-9580
800-638-3775
FAX: 800-638-3775
e-mail: custserv@brookespublishing.com
www.brookespublishing.com

Paul Brooks, President
Tracy Gracy, Educational Sales Manager

This is a 30-item checklist that helps families to identify interests and concerns to address in a child's IEP/IFSP. Comes in packages of 30. *$15.00*
8 pages Saddle-stiched
ISBN 1-557660-98-0

1882 **Advanced Language Tool Kit**
School Specialty
625 Mt. Auburn Street, 3rd Floor
PO Box 9031
Cambridge, MA 02139-9031 617-547-6706
800-225-5750
FAX: 888-440-2665
e-mail: Feedback.EPS@schoolspecialty.com
eps.schoolspecialty.com

Rick Holden, President, EPS
Jean S Osman, Co-Author
Paula D Rome, Author

Provides an overview o the structure, organization, and sound units that are needed to develop skills for advanced reading and spelling. The kit contains a teacher's manual and 3 pack of cards, with features similar to the cards in the Language Tool Kit. *$60.00*
ISBN 0-838885-48-9

1883 **All Kinds of Minds**
School Specialty
625 Mt. Auburn Street, 3rd Floor
PO Box 9031
Cambridge, MA 02139-9031 617-547-6706
800-225-5750
FAX: 888-440-2665
e-mail: Feedback.EPS@schoolspecialty.com
eps.schoolspecialty.com

Rick Holden, President, EPS
Melvin D Levine, Author

A fictitious account of five different students who have learning disabilities. *$33.00*
296 pages
ISBN 0-838820-90-5

1884 **American Sign Language Handshape Cards**
T J Publishers, Distributor
Ste 206
817 Silver Spring Ave
Silver Spring, MD 20910- 4617 301-585-4440
800-999-1168
FAX: 301-585-5930
e-mail: tjpubinc@aol.com

Angela K Thames, President
Jerald A Murphy, VP

Durable flashcards illustrate basic handshapes, classifiers and the American manual alphabet. An instructional booklet describes games for differing skill levels to improve vocabulary, increase hand and eye coordination, sign recognition and usage. *$16.95*

1885 **Asthma Action Cards: Child Care Asthma/Allergy Action Card**
Asthma and Allergy Foundation of America
8201 Corporate Drive
Suite 1000
Landover, MD 20785 202-466-7643
800-727-8462
FAX: 202-466-8940
e-mail: info@aafa.org
www.aafa.org

Tom Flanigan, Chariman
William Mclin, President and CEO
Yolanda Miller, VP and CFO

Includes necessary information a provider needs to care for a young child who has asthma and allergies. The card includes a medication plan, a list of the child's specific signs and symptoms that indicate the child is having trouble breathing, and steps on how to handle an emergency situation.

1886 Asthma Action Cards: Student Asthma Action Card
Asthma and Allergy Foundation of America
1233 20th St NW
Suite 610
Washington, DC 20036-2330
202-833-1700
800-727-8462
FAX: 202-833-2351
e-mail: info@aafa.org
www.swmlaw.com

Bill Mc Lin, Executive Director
Ben C Hadden, VP Finance & Treasurer
Bill Lin, Executive Director
Tool for communicating school aged children's and teen's asthma managment plan to school personnel. Includes sections for asthma triggers, daily medications, and emergency directions.

1887 Auditech: Classroom Amplification System Focus CFM802
PO Box 821105
Vicksburg, MS 39182-1105
800-229-8293
FAX: 800-221-8639
e-mail: info@auditechusa.com
www.auditechusa.com

1888 Auditech: Personal FM Educational System
PO Box 821105
Vicksburg, MS 39182-1105
800-229-8293
FAX: 800-221-8639
e-mail: info@auditechusa.com
www.auditechusa.com

1889 Auditory-Verbal Therapy for Parents and Professionals
Alexander Graham Bell Association
3417 Volta Place, NW
Washington, DC 20007
202-337-5220
FAX: 202-337-8314
TTY:202-337-5221
e-mail: info@agbell.org
www.listeningandspokenlanguage.org

Meredith K. Sugar, Esq. (OH), President
Donald M. Goldberg, Immediate Past President
Ted A. Meyer, M.D., Ph.D. (SC, President-Elect, Secretary, Treasurer
Emilio Alonso Mendoza (DC), Chief Executive Officer
A must-have for hearing health professionals, students entering hearing health fields and parents who want to explore the theory and practices of auditory-verbal therapy. *$54.95*
313 pages Paperback

1890 Barrier Free Education
Center for Assistive Technology & Env Access
490 10th St NW
Atlanta, GA 30332-156
404-894-4960
800-726-9119
FAX: 404-894-9320
e-mail: catea@coa.gatech.edu
www.catea.org

Elizabeth Bryant, Project Director
Math and science activities pose unique accommodation challenges for students with disabilities. The Barrier Free Education resource on accessible science experiments was developed for high school chemistry and physics students with physical or visual disabilities under the National Science Foundation's Program for Persons with Disabilities.

1891 Beginning Reasoning and Reading
School Specialty
625 Mt. Auburn Street, 3rd Floor
PO Box 9031
Cambridge, MA 02139-9031
617-547-6706
800-225-5750
FAX: 888-440-2665
e-mail: Feedback.EPS@schoolspecialty.com
eps.schoolspecialty.com

Rick Holden, President, EPS
Joanne Carlisle, Author
This workbook develops basic language and thinking skills that build the foundation for reading comprehension. Workbook exercises reinforce reading as a critical reasoning activity. *$10.45*
ISBN 0-838830-01-3

1892 Buy!
JE Stewart Teaching Tools
PO Box 15308
Seattle, WA 98115-308
206-262-9538
FAX: 206-262-9538

Jeff Stewart, Owner
Teaches 50 words as they appear in commercial and community situations such as clinic, sale, receipt, price and cleaner. These words are functional at school, on the job and shopping. *$32.50*
116 pages
ISBN 1-877866-05-9

1893 Catalog for Teaching Life Skills to Persons with Development Disability
PCI Education Publishing
PO Box 34270
San Antonio, TX 78265-4270
210-377-1999
800-594-4263
FAX: 888-259-8284
www.pcieducation.com

Lee Wilson, President/CEO
Erin Kinard, VP Product Development/Publisher
Randy Pennington, VP, Sales & Marketing
Over 200 educational products that help individuals learn and maintain the life skills they need to succeed in an inclusive society.

1894 Classroom GOAL: Guide for Optimizing Auditory Learning Skills
Alexander Graham Bell Association
3417 Volta Pl NW
Washington, DC 20007-2737
202-337-5220
FAX: 202-337-8314
e-mail: info@agbell.org
www.agbell.org

Alexander Graham, Executive Director
Judy Harrison, Director of Programs
Susan Boswell, Communications and Marketing
This reader-friendly teacher's guide filled with tips, source materials and sample charts and plans is designed for educators who have yearned for a resource that explains how to incorporate auditory goals into academic learning for students with different degrees of hearing loss. *$34.95*
Paperback

1895 Classroom Notetaker: How to Organize a Program Serving Students with Hearing Impairments
Alexander Graham Bell Association
3417 Volta Pl NW
Washington, DC 20007-2737
202-337-5220
FAX: 202-337-8314
e-mail: info@agbell.org
www.agbell.org

Alexander Graham, Executive Director
Judy Harrison, Director of Programs
Susan Boswell, Communications and Marketing
This detailed manual for instructors, administrators and staff notetakers promotes classroom notetaking within long-term educational programs as absolutely vital for students who are deaf and hard of hearing from elementary school to college. *$24.95*
127 pages Paperback

1896 Community Services for the Blind and Partially Sighted Store: Sight Connection
9709 Third Ave NE
Ste 100
Seattle, WA 98115-2027
206-525-5556
800-458-4888
FAX: 206-525-0422
e-mail: info@sightconnection.org
www.sightconnection.org

Miles Otoupal, Chair
Jonathan Avedovech, Vice Chair
David McBride, Treasurer
Mary Lewis, Secretary
Over 400 products specifically designed to make life easier for people with vision loss.

1897 Community Signs
JE Stewart Teaching Tools
P.O.Box 15308
Seattle, WA 98115-308
206-262-9538
FAX: 206-262-9538

Jeff Stewart, Owner
Teaches 50 words like go, fire, rest room, men, women, danger and walk needed to successfully navigate our environment. *$ 32.50*

1898 Comprehensive Assessment of Spoken Language (CASL)
AGS
PO Box 99
Circle Pines, MN 55014-99
800-328-2560
FAX: 800-471-8457
e-mail: agsmail@agsnet.com
www.agsnet.com

Kevin Brueggeman, President
Robert Zaske, Market Manager
CASL is an individually and orally administered research-based, theory-drive oral language assessment battery for ages 3 through 21. Fifteen tests measure language processing skills - comprehension, expression, and retrieval - in four language structure categories: lexical/semantic, syntactic, supralinguistic and pragmatic. *$299.95*

1899 Creative Arts Therapy Catalogs
MMB Music
9051 Watson Road
Suite 161
Saint Louis, MO 63126-1019
314-531-9635
800-543-3771
FAX: 314-531-8384
e-mail: info@mmbmusic.com
www.mmbmusic.com

Marcia Goldberg, President
Catalogs of books, videos, recordings for the creative arts and wellness (music, art, dance, poetry, drama, theater, photography).

1900 Cursive Writing Skills
School Specialty
625 Mt. Auburn Street, 3rd Floor
PO Box 9031
Cambridge, MA 02139-9031
617-547-6706
800-225-5750
FAX: 888-440-2665
e-mail: Feedback.EPS@schoolspecialty.com
eps.schoolspecialty.com

Rick Holden, President, EPS
Diana Hanbury King, Author
Boosts writing achievement through handwriting skills. Handwriting instruction helps students become fluent writers, allowing them to focus on their thoughts and ideas rather than on letter and word formation. *$12.00*
ISBN 0-83881 -05-

1901 Don Johnston
26799 West Commerce Drive
Volo, IL 60073-9675
847-740-0749
800-999-4660
FAX: 847-740-7326
e-mail: info@donjohnston.com
www.donjohnston.com

Don Johnston, Founder
Ruth Ziolkowski, President
Kevin Johnston, Director of Product Design
Ben Johnston, Director of Marketing
A provider of quality products and services that enable people with special needs to discover their potential and experience success. Products are developed for the areas of Physical Access, Augmentative Communication and for those who struggle with reading and writing.

1902 Dyslexia Training Program
School Specialty
625 Mt. Auburn Street, 3rd Floor
PO Box 9031
Cambridge, MA 02139-9031
617-547-6706
800-225-5750
FAX: 888-440-2665
e-mail: Feedback.EPS@schoolspecialty.com
eps.schoolspecialty.com

Rick Holden, President, EPS
This 2-year, cumulative series of daily 1-hour video lessons and accompanying Student's Books and Teacher's Guides is a structured, multisensory sequence of alphabet, reading, spelling, cursive handwriting, listening, language history, and review activities. Written by the Texas Scottish Rite Hospital for Children.

1903 Exceptional Teaching Inc
Exceptional Teaching Inc
3994 Oleander Way
PO Box 2330
Castro Valley, CA 94546
510-889-7282
800-549-6999
FAX: 510-889-7382
e-mail: info@exceptionalteaching.com
www.exceptionalteaching.com

Helene Holman, Owner/manager
Providing educational products for those with special needs via catalog and online store.

1904 Explode the Code
School Specialty
625 Mt. Auburn Street, 3rd Floor
PO Box 9031
Cambridge, MA 02139-9031
617-547-6706
800-225-5750
FAX: 888-440-2665
e-mail: Feedback.EPS@schoolspecialty.com
eps.schoolspecialty.com

Rick Holden, President, EPS
Nancy M Hall, Author
Helps students build the essential literacy skills needed for reading success: phonological awareness, decoding, vocabulary, comprehension, fluency and spelling. *$6.20*
Grades K-4, 1-3
ISBN 0-83881 -60-

1905 Food!
JE Stewart Teaching Tools
PO Box 15308
Seattle, WA 98115-308
206-262-9538
FAX: 206-262-9538

Jeff Stewart, Owner
Teaches 50 words like salt, pepper, hamburger, fruit, milk and soup, seen commonly on menus, packages and in directions used at home and at play. *$32.50*

1906 Fun for Everyone
AbleNet
2625 Patton Road
Roseville, MN 55113-1308
651-294-2200
800-322-0956
FAX: 651-294-2259
e-mail: customerservice@ablenetinc.com
www.ablenetinc.com

Jen Thalhuber, CEO
Ann Meyer, Vice President
Paul Sugden, VP Finance
Jason Voiovich, VP Marketing

Today, simple technology allows children and adults with disabilities to participate in leisure activities they were limited or excluded from in the past. *$20.00*

1907 Fundamentals of Autism
Slosson Educational Publications Inc.
538 Buffalo Road
East Aurora, NY 14052-280
716-652-0930
800-655-3840
888-756-7760
FAX: 716-655-3840
e-mail: slossonprep@gmail.com
www.slosson.com

Steven Slosson, President
John Slosson, VP
David Slosson, VP

The Fundamentals of Autism handbook provides a quick, user friendly, effective and accurate approach to help in identifying and developing educationally related program objectives for children diagnosed as autistic. These materials have been designed to be easily and functionally used by teachers, therapists, special education/learning disability resource specialists, psychologists and others who work with children diagnosed as autistic. *$56.00*
72 pages

1908 GO-MO Articulation Cards- Second Edition
Sage Publications
2455 Teller Road
Thousand Oaks, CA 91320
805-499-9774
800-818-7243
FAX: 800-583-2665
e-mail: info@sagepub.com
www.sagepub.com

Blaise R Simqu, President & CEO
Tracey Ozmina, VP and COO
Chris Hickok, Senior VP and CFO
Stephen Barr, Managing Director

The most popular system used for remedying defective speech articulation in children and adults. This popular card set was the first and is still the best therapy tool of its kind, as it continues to produce results and maintains the interest of students of all ages.

1909 Gillingham Manaual
School Specialty
625 Mt. Auburn Street, 3rd Floor
PO Box 9031
Cambridge, MA 02139-9031
617-547-6706
800-225-5750
FAX: 888-440-2665
e-mail: Feedback.EPS@schoolspecialty.com
eps.schoolspecialty.com

Rick Holden, President, EPS
Anna Gillingham, Author
Bessie W Stillman, Co-Author

Remedial training for children with specific disability in reading, spelling, and penmanship.
352 pages 69.95
ISBN 0-83880 -00-

1910 Guide to Teaching Phonics
School Specialty
625 Mt. Auburn Street, 3rd Floor
PO Box 9031
Cambridge, MA 02139-9031
617-547-6706
800-225-5750
FAX: 888-440-2665
e-mail: Feedback.EPS@schoolspecialty.com
eps.schoolspecialty.com

Rick Holden, President, EPS
June Lyday Orton, Author

This flexible teacher's guide presents multisensory procedures developed in association with the late Dr. Samuel Orton. They consist of 100 phonograms for teaching phonetic elements and their sequences in words for reading, writing and spelling. Also contains coordinated Phonics Cards. *$19.25*
96 pages
ISBN 0-838802-41-9

1911 Homemade Battery-Powered Toys
Special Needs Project
Ste H
324 State St
Santa Barbara, CA 93101-2364
818-718-9900
800-333-6867
FAX: 818-349-2027
e-mail: editor@specialneeds.com.
www.specialneeds.com

Hod Gray, Owner
Laraine Gray, Coordinator

Describes how to make simple switches and educational devices for severely handicapped children. *$7.50*

1912 Idaho Assistive Technology Project
University of Idaho
PO Box 444061
Moscow, ID 83844-4061
208-885-6097
800-432-8324
FAX: 208-885-6145
e-mail: janicec@uidaho.edu
www.idahoat.org

Janice Carson, Project Director
Sue House, Information/Referral Specialist

A federally funded program managed by the Center on Disabilities and Human Development at the University of Idaho. The goal is to increase the availability of assistive technology devices and services for Idahoans with disabilities. *$15.00*

1913 If It Is To Be, It Is Up To Me To Do It!
AVKO Educational Research Foundation
3084 Willard Road
Birch Run, MI 48415-9404
810-686-9283
866-285-6612
FAX: 810-686-1101
e-mail: webmaster@avko.org
www.avko.org

Don McCabe, President, Research Director Emeritus, Birch Run, Michigan
Linda Heck, VP, Clio, Michigan
Michael Lane, Treasurer, Clio, Michigan
Amy Messer, Board Member, Flint, Michigan

A student and tutor's text, for use on dyslexics and non-dyslexics, by parents, spouses, or friends. *$29.95*
206 pages
ISBN 1-564007-42-1

1914 Inclusive Play People
Educational Equity Concepts
Fl 8
100 5th Ave
New York, NY 10011-6903
212-243-1110
FAX: 212-627-0407
TTY:212-725-1803
e-mail: information@edequity.org
www.iconcapital.com

Jacqueline Johnson, Manager

Six sturdy multiracial wooden figures that provide a unique variety of nonstereotyped work and family roles and are inclusive of disabled and nondisabled people of various ages. For block building and dramatic play. *$25.00*

1915 Individualized Keyboarding

AVKO Educational Research Foundation
3084 Willard Road
Birch Run, MI 48415-9404
810-686-9283
866-285-6612
FAX: 810-686-1101
e-mail: webmaster@avko.org
www.avko.org
Don McCabe, President, Research Director Emeritus, Birch Run, Michigan
Linda Heck, VP, Clio, Michigan
Michael Lane, Treasurer, Clio, Michigan
Amy Messer, Board Member, Flint, Michigan

Utilizes a multi-sensory approach to teach typing skills. It not only teaches typing skills, it also reinforces the reading patterns that are necessary for typing proficiency. *$14.95*

96 pages

ISBN 1-654004-01-5

1916 Instruction of Persons with Severe Handicaps

McGraw-Hill School Publishing
PO Box 182604
Columbus, OH 43272
877-833-5524
FAX: 614-759-3749
e-mail: customer.service@mcgraw-hill.com
www.mcgraw-hill.com
Harold McGraw, President and CEO
Jack Callahan, Executive VP
John Berisford, Executive VP of HR

A complete introduction to the status of education as it pertains to people with severe handicaps.

1917 Keeping Ahead in School

Educators Publishing Service
PO Box 9031
Cambridge, MA 2139-9031
617-547-6706
800-225-5750
FAX: 888-440-2665
e-mail: feedback@epsbooks.com
www.epsbooks.com
Charles H Heinle, VP
Alexandra S Bigelow, Author
Gunnar Voltz, President

This book helps students not only understand their own strengths and weaknesses but also more fully appreciate their individuality. He suggests specific ways to approach work, bypass or overcome learning disorders, and manage other struggles that may beset students in school. *$24.75*

320 pages Paperback

ISBN 0-838820-69-7

1918 KeyMath Teach and Practice

AGS
P.O.Box 99
Circle Pines, MN 55014-99
800-328-2560
FAX: 800-471-8457
e-mail: agsmail@agsnet.com
www.agsnet.com
Kevin Brueggeman, President
Robert Zaske, Market Manager

This set of materials provides all the tools needed to assess students' math skills...and the strategies to deal with problem areas. Three sets are available: Basic Concepts Package; Operations Package; and Applications Package. $219.95 each or $599.95 for whole set.

1919 Lakeshore Learning Materials

2695 E. Dominguez Street
Carson, CA 90895
310-537-8600
800-421-5354
FAX: 800-537-5403
e-mail: lakeshore@lakeshorelearning.com
www.lakeshorelearning.com
Bo Kaplan, President/CEO
Josh Kaplan, VP Merchandising
Mat, Vice President of Operations

Offers books, resources, testing materials, assessment information and special education materials for the professional in the field of special education.

190 pages

1920 Language Parts Catalog

School Specialty
625 Mt. Auburn Street, 3rd Floor
PO Box 9031
Cambridge, MA 02139-9031
617-547-6706
800-225-5750
FAX: 888-440-2665
e-mail: Feedback.EPS@schoolspecialty.com
eps.schoolspecialty.com
Rick Holden, President, EPS
Melvin D Levine, Author

Offers a humorous and informative explanation of the various aspects of language and how they operate. Laid out in the form of a catalog, the book presents various parts that can help students improve their language abilities. *$12.65*

ISBN 0-838819-80-X

1921 Language Tool Kit

School Specialty
625 Mt. Auburn Street, 3rd Floor
PO Box 9031
Cambridge, MA 02139-9031
617-547-6706
800-225-5750
FAX: 888-440-2665
e-mail: Feedback.EPS@schoolspecialty.com
eps.schoolspecialty.com
Rick Holden, President, EPS
Paula D Rome, Author
Jean S Osman, Co-Author

Designed for use by a teacher or parents, teaches reading and spelling to students with specific language disability. *$43.25*

32 pages English Edition

ISBN 0-838885-20-3

1922 Language, Speech and Hearing Services in School

American Speech-Language-Hearing Association
10801 Rockville Pike
Rockville, MD 20852-3226
301-296-5700
800-638-8255
FAX: 301-296-8580
e-mail: actioncenter@asha.org
www.asha.org
Paul Rao, President
Robert Augustine, VP of Finance
Arlene Pietranton, Executive Director

Professional journal for clinicians, audiologists and speech-language pathologists. *$30.00*

1923 Learning American Sign Language

Harris Communications
15155 Technology Dr
Eden Prairie, MN 55344-2273
952-906-1180
800-825-6758
FAX: 952-906-1099
e-mail: info@harriscomm.com
www.harriscomm.com
Robert Harris, President
Kevin Horsky, Business Director

Offers over 700 titles on ASL including books, videotapes, CDs & DVDs. Free catalog available. *$78.95*

350 pages Video & Book

1924 Learning to Sign in My Neighborhood
T J Publishers
2544 Tarpley Rd
Suite 108
Carrollton, TX 75006-2288
972-416-0800
800-999-1168
FAX: 301-585-5930
e-mail: tjpubinc@aol.com
Angela K Thames, President
Jerald A Murphy, VP
Beautifully illustrated coloring book lets children learn signs from kids just like themselves! Recommended for ages 4 and up, let children have fun while they learn signs for words typically used in day-to-day activities. *$3.50*
32 pages Softcover
ISBN 0-93266 -36-1

1925 Literacy Program
School Specialty
625 Mt. Auburn Street, 3rd Floor
PO Box 9031
Cambridge, MA 02139-9031
617-547-6706
800-225-5750
FAX: 888-440-2665
e-mail: Feedback.EPS@schoolspecialty.com
eps.schoolspecialty.com
Rick Holden, President, EPS
Paula D Rome, Author
Jean S Osman, Co-Author
Written by the Texas Scottish Rite Hospital for Children. A one-year course that consists of 160 one-hour videotaped lessons accompanied by student workbooks, designed for high school students and adults who read below sixth grade level.

1926 Literature Based Reading
Oryx Press
4041 N Central Ave
Phoenix, AZ 85012-3330
602-265-2651
800-279-6799
FAX: 800-279-4663

1927 Living an Idea: Empowerment and the Evolution of an Alternative School
Brookline Books
8 Trumbull Rd, Suite B-001
Northampton, MA 1060-4533
413-584-0184
800-666-2665
FAX: 413-584-6184
e-mail: brbooks@yahoo.com
www.brooklinebooks.com
William H Walters, Author
Esther Wilder, Co-Author
This book is about the creation and 14 year evolution of a public alternative inner-city high school. The school lived an idea - empowerment. Students were encouraged to participate in shaping many aspects of their education, teachers were responsible for running the school, and parents invited to help govern. *$27.95*
ISBN 0-91479 -68-9

1928 Low Tech Assistive Devices: A Handbook for the School Setting
Therapro, Inc.
225 Arlington Street
Framingham, MA 02139-8723
508-872-9494
800-257-5376
800-268-6624
FAX: 508-875-2062
e-mail: info@therapro.com
www.therapro.com
Karen Conrad, Owner
A how-to book with step by step directions and detailed illustrations for fabrication of frequently requested low-tech assistive devices. *$45.00*
320 pages Paperback

1929 MTA Readers
Educators Publishing Service
625 Mt. Auburn Street, 3rd Floor
PO Box 9031
Cambridge, MA 02139-9031
617-547-6706
800-225-5750
FAX: 888-440-2665
e-mail: Feedback.EPS@schoolspecialty.com
www.epsbooks.com
Rick Holden, President, EPS
Illustrated readers for grades 1-3 that accompany the MTA Reading and Spelling Program (Multisensory Teaching Approach). Phonetic elements in a structured, but entertaining context.
48+ pages $4.65 - $11.65
ISBN 0-83882 -33-3

1930 Making School Inclusion Work: A Guide to Everyday Practice
Brookline Books
8 Trumbull Rd, Suite B-001
Northampton, MA 2445-4533
413-584-0184
800-666-2665
FAX: 413-584-6184
e-mail: brbooks@yahoo.com
www.brooklinebooks.com
William H Walters, Author
Esther Wilder, Co-Author
This book tells the reader how to conduct a truly inclusive program, regardless of ethnic or racial background, economic level and physical or cognitive ability. *$24.95*
254 pages
ISBN 0-914791-96-4

1931 Making the Writing Process Work: Strategies for Composition and Self-Regulation
Brookline Books
8 Trumbull Rd, Suite B-001
Northampton, MA 2445-4533
413-584-0184
800-666-2665
FAX: 413-584-6184
e-mail: brbooks@yahoo.com
www.brooklinebooks.com
William H Walters, Author
Esther Wilder, Co-Author
This book is geared toward students who have difficulty organizing their thoughts and developing their writing. The specific stategies teach students how to approach, organize, and produce a final written product.. *$24.95*
240 pages Paperback
ISBN 1-571290-10-9

1932 Manual Alphabet Poster
TJ Publishers
Ste 108
2544 Tarpley Rd
Carrollton, TX 75006-2288
972-416-0800
800-999-1168
FAX: 972-416-0944
e-mail: TJPubinc@aol.com
www.TJpublishers.com
Pat O'Rourke, President
Poster presents the manual alphabet. *$4.50*

1933 Many Faces of Dyslexia
40 York Rd
4th Floor
Baltimore, MD 21204-5243
410-296-0232
FAX: 410-321-5069
www.interdys.org
Nancy Hennessy, President
Sandra Soper, Vice President
Thoman Viall, Executive Director
Gives information on the teaching and rehabilitation techniques for people with dyslexia. *$16.50*
Paperback

1934 **Match-Sort-Assemble Job Cards**
Exceptional Education
PO Box 15308
Seattle, WA 98115-308 206-262-9538

Jeff Stewart, Owner
Teaches workers to use a series of symbolic cues to control their own production cycles. *$565.00*
Class Set

1935 **Match-Sort-Assemble Pictures**
Exceptional Education
PO Box 15308
Seattle, WA 98115-308 206-262-9538

Jeff Stewart, Owner
People with profound, severe and moderate mental retardation have immediate access with MSA Pictures. Students work with pictures (and if necessary a template) to match, sort, assemble and disassemble parts that vary in shape, length and diameter. *$426.00*
Class Set

1936 **Match-Sort-Assemble SCHEMATICS**
Exceptional Education
PO Box 15308
Seattle, WA 98115-308 206-262-9538

Jeff Stewart, Owner
Students with moderate and mild mental retardation and those who have completed MSA Pictures are ready for MSA Schematics. It increases abstraction and displacement of instruction from the work clearly and simply. *$495.00*
Class Set

1937 **Match-Sort-Assemble TOOLS**
Exceptional Education
PO Box 15308
Seattle, WA 98115-308 206-262-9538
FAX: 475-486-4510

Jeff Stewart, Owner
Students and clients learn to use the tools required for many jobs in light industry. Mastery of the production cycle with independence, endurance and the ability to learn new tasks through pictures and schematics and basic hand functions will help clients acquire and maintain employment in a competitive field. *$595.00*
Class Set

1938 **Meeting-in-a-Box**
Asthma and Allergy Foundation of America
1233 20th St NW
Suite 610
Washington, DC 20036-7322 202-833-1700
800-7AS-THMA
FAX: 202-833-2351
e-mail: info@aafa.org
www.swmlaw.com

Bill Mc Lin, Executive Director
Bill Mclin, Executive Director
A series of self-contained, comprehensive kits that contain all the necessary components for a successful asthma presentation.

1939 **More Food!**
JE Stewart Teaching Tools
PO Box 15308
Seattle, WA 98115-308 206-262-9538
FAX: 206-262-9538

Jeff Stewart, Owner
Teaches 50 more words found in restaurants, grocery stores, cookbooks such as pizza, carrot, tacos, oysters and pineapple. These words are functional at home, going shopping and during leisure. *$32.50*

1940 **More Work!**
J E Stewart Teaching Tools
PO Box 15308
Seattle, WA 98115-308 206-262-9538
FAX: 206-262-9538

Jeff Stewart, Owner
Teaches 50 words as they appear on parts, tools, job instructions, signs and labels, such as fill, grasp, release, lock, search, position and select. These words are functional in school and on-the-job. *$32.50*

1941 **Multisensory Teaching Approach**
Educators Publishing Service
PO Box 9031
Cambridge, MA 2139-9031 617-367-2700
800-225-5750
FAX: 617-547-0412
www.epsbooks.com

$110 - $140
ISBN 0-83888 -10-9

1942 **Peabody Articulation Decks**
AGS
PO Box 99
Circle Pines, MN 55014-99 651-287-7220
800-328-2560
FAX: 763-786-9007
e-mail: agsmail@agsnet.com
www.agsnet.com

Keith Powel, Special Education Transition Coo
Robert Zaske, Marketing Manager
Complete kit of playing-card sized PAD decks let students focus on the 18 most commonly misarticulated English consonants and blends. *$115.95*
ISBN 0-88671 -75-4

1943 **Phonemic Awareness in Young Children: A Classroom Curriculum**
Brookes Publishing
PO Box 10624
Baltimore, MD 21285-624 410-337-9580
e-mail: custserv@brookespublishing.com
www.brookespublishing.com

Clary Creighton, Exhibits Coordinator
Tracy Gray, Educational Sales Manager
Paul Brooks, Owner
This is a supplemental, whole-class curriculum for improving pre-literacy listening skills. It contains activities that are fun, easy to use, and proven to work in any kindergarten classroom - general, bilingual, inclusive, or special education. This program takes only 15-20 minutes a day. *$24.95*
208 pages Spiral-bound
ISBN 1-557663-21-1

1944 **Phonics for Thought**
Educators Publishing Service
PO Box 9031
Cambridge, MA 2139-9031 617-367-2700
800-225-5750
FAX: 617-547-0412
www.epsbooks.com

Paperback

1945 **Phonological Awareness Training for Reading**
Sage Publications
2455 Teller Road
Thousand Oaks, CA 91320 805-499-9774
800-818-7243
FAX: 800-583-2665
e-mail: info@sagepub.com
www.sagepub.com

Blaise R Simqu, President & CEO
Tracey Ozmina, Executive VP
Chris Hickok, Executive VP and CFO
Stephen Barr, Managing Director

Designed to increase the level of phonological awareness in young children. Can be taught individually or in small groups and takes about 12 to 14 weeks to complete if children are taught in short sessions three or four times a week. *$129.00*

1946 **Play!**
JE Stewart Teaching Tools
PO Box 15308
Seattle, WA 98115-308 206-262-9538
FAX: 206-262-9538

Jeff Stewart, Owner
Teaches 50 more words as they appear at recreation sites, on signs and labels and in newspapers and magazines, such as movie, visitor, ticket, gallery and zoo. These words are functional in school and at leisure. *$32.50*

1947 **Power Breathing Program**
Asthma and Allergy Foundation of America
8201 Corporate Drive
Suite 1000
Landover, MD 20785 202-466-7643
800-727-8462
FAX: 202-466-8940
e-mail: info@aafa.org
www.aafa.org

Bill McLin, Executive Director
Devoloped the only asthma education program specifically designed for and pre-tested with teens. Teens with asthma have special challenges. This interactive program covers everything from the basics of asthma to dealing with their asthma in social situations, in college, and on the job. Includes everything you need to present this three-four session program. *$295.00*

1948 **Primary Phonics**
School Specialty
625 Mt. Auburn Street, 3rd Floor
PO Box 9031
Cambridge, MA 02139-9031 617-547-6706
800-225-5750
FAX: 888-440-2665
e-mail: Feedback.EPS@schoolspecialty.com
eps.schoolspecialty.com

Rick Holden, President, EPS
Barbara W Makar, Author
A program of storybooks and coordinated workbooks that teaches reading for grades K-2. A structured phonetic approach. Contains 8 student workbooks, with 8 sets of 10 coordinated storybooks; consonant workbooks; initial consonant blend workbooks; picture dictionary, and coloring book.
ISSN 0838-83 0

1949 **Reading for Content**
School Specialty
625 Mt. Auburn Street, 3rd Floor
PO Box 9031
Cambridge, MA 02139-9031 617-547-6706
800-225-5750
FAX: 888-440-2665
e-mail: Feedback.EPS@schoolspecialty.com
eps.schoolspecialty.com

Rick Holden, President, EPS
Carol Einstein, Author
A series of 4 books designed to help students improve their reading comprehension skills. Each book contains 43 reading passages followed by 4 questions. Two questions as for a recall of main ideas, and two ask the student to draw conclusions from what they have read. *$ 11.45*
96 pages

1950 **Reading from Scratch**
Educators Publishing Service
P.O.Box 9031
Cambridge, MA 2139-9031 617-367-2700
800-225-5750
FAX: 617-547-0412
www.epsbooks.com

$6.25 - $49.30
ISBN 0-83888 -75-5

1951 **Recipe for Reading**
School Specialty
625 Mt. Auburn Street, 3rd Floor
PO Box 9031
Cambridge, MA 02139-9031 617-367-2700
800-225-5750
FAX: 888-440-2665
e-mail: Feedback.EPS@schoolspecialty.com
eps.schoolspecialty.com

Rick Holden, President, EPS
Nina Traub, Author
Frances Bloom, Co-Author
Contains comprehensive, multisensory, phonics-based reading program presents a skill sequence and lesson structured designed for beginning, at-risk, or struggling readers.

1952 **Rewarding Speech**
Speech Bin
PO Box 1579
Appleton, WI 54912-1579 772-770-0007
888-388-3224
FAX: 888-388-6344
e-mail: customercare@schoolspecialty.com
www.speechbin.com

Jan J Binney, Senior Editor
Reproducible reward certificates for children. *$12.95*
32 pages

1953 **SAYdee Posters**
Speech Bin
PO Box 1579
Appleton, WI 54912-1579 772-770-0007
888-388-3224
FAX: 888-388-6344
e-mail: customercare@schoolspecialty.com
www.speechbin.com

Jan J Binney, Senior Editor
Colorful speech and language posters. *$20.00*
24 pages
ISBN 0-93785 -47-5

1954 **Sequential Spelling: 1-7 with 7 Student Response Books**
AVKO Educational Research Foundation
3084 Willard Rd
Birch Run, MI 48415-9404 810-686-9283
866-285-6612
FAX: 810-686-1101
e-mail: webmaster@avko.org
www.avko.org

Deborah Wolf, President
Aaron Miller, Vice President
Sequential Spelling uses immediate student self-correction. It builds from easier words of a word family such as all and then builds on them to teach; all, tall, stall, install, call, fall, ball, and their inflected forms such as: stalls, stalled, stalling, installing, installment. *$89.95*
72 pages $8.95 each
ISBN 1-56400 -11-6

1955 **Signing Naturally Curriculum**
Harris Communications
15155 Technology Dr
Eden Prairie, MN 55344-2273
952-906-1180
800-825-6758
FAX: 952-906-1099
e-mail: info@harriscomm.com
www.harriscomm.com

Robert Harris, President
Kevin Horsky, Business Director

A series based on the functional approach that is the most popular and widely used sign language curriculum designed for teaching American Sign Language. Book and videotape set for level 1 & 2. Teacher's curriculum is also available. *$59.95*

1956 **Small Wonder**
AGS
PO Box 99
Circle Pines, MN 55014-99
651-287-7220
800-328-2560
FAX: 763-786-9007
e-mail: agsmail@agsnet.com
www.agsnet.com

Kevin Brueggeman, President
Robert Zaske, Marketing Manager

This infant through toddler program offers a delightful array of activities to teach babies about themselves, others, their surroundings and the world outside. Level One - zero to 18 months; Level Two 18-36 months. Discount price of $389.95 when both levels ordered. *$229.95*
ISBN 0-91347 -62-5

1957 **Solving Language Difficulties**
School Specialty
625 Mt. Auburn Street, 3rd Floor
PO Box 9031
Cambridge, MA 02139-9031
617-547-6706
800-225-5750
FAX: 888-440-2665
e-mail: Feedback.EPS@schoolspecialty.com
eps.schoolspecialty.com

Rick Holden, President, EPS
Amey Steere, Author
Caroline Z Peck, Co-Author

This basic workbook can be used in any corrective reading program. It deals extensively with syllables, syllable division, prefixes, suffixes and accent. *$9.75*
176 pages
ISBN 0-838803-26-1

1958 **Speech Bin**
Abilitations
PO Box 1579
Appleton, WI 54912-1579
772-770-0007
800-513-2465
FAX: 80- 51- 246
e-mail: onlinehelp@schoolspecialty.com
www.speechbin.com

Jan J Binney, Senior Editor

Activities, worksheets and games to encourage practice of speech and language skills. *$25.00*
128 pages
ISBN 0-93785 -42-4

1959 **Speech-Language Delights**
1965 25th Ave
Vero Beach, FL 32960-3062
772-770-0007

1960 **Spell of Words**
School Specialty
625 Mt. Auburn Street, 3rd Floor
PO Box 9031
Cambridge, MA 02139-9031
617-547-6706
800-225-5750
FAX: 888-440-2665
e-mail: Feedback.EPS@schoolspecialty.com
eps.schoolspecialty.com

Rick Holden, President, EPS
Elsie T Rak, Author

Covers syllabication, word building along with prefixes, phonograms, word patterns, suffixes, plurals, and possessives. *$14.70*
128 pages Grades 7-Adult

1961 **Spellbound**
School Specialty
625 Mt. Auburn Street, 3rd Floor
PO Box 9031
Cambridge, MA 02139-9031
617-547-6706
800-225-5750
FAX: 888-440-2665
e-mail: Feedback.EPS@schoolspecialty.com
eps.schoolspecialty.com

Rick Holden, President, EPS
Elsie T Rak, Author

This workbook begins with teaching simple, consistent rules and then moves on to those that are more difficult. By an inductive process, students use their own observations to confirm the spelling rules they learn. Each portion of the text is followed by exercises for drill and kinesthetic reinforcement. *$12.85*
144 pages Grades 7-Adult
ISBN 0-838801-65-X

1962 **Spelling Dictionary**
School Specialty
625 Mt. Auburn Street, 3rd Floor
PO Box 9031
Cambridge, MA 02139-9031
617-547-6706
800-225-5750
FAX: 888-440-2665
e-mail: Feedback.EPS@schoolspecialty.com
eps.schoolspecialty.com

Rick Holden, President, EPS
Gregory Hurray, Author

Contains the most frequently used and misspelled words for students at these grade levels. Designed to be useable and reliable, to build research and writing skills, and to help teachers promote independent learning in a classroom setting *$6.35*
ISBN 0-838820-56-5

1963 **Starting Over**
School Specialty
625 Mt. Auburn Street, 3rd Floor
PO Box 9031
Cambridge, MA 02139-9031
617-547-6706
800-225-5750
FAX: 888-440-2665
e-mail: Feedback.EPS@schoolspecialty.com
eps.schoolspecialty.com

Rick Holden, President, EPS
Joan Knight, Author

For students who are ready to try to learn to read again, or for those who are learning English as a second language. *$38.40*
ISBN 0-838881-65-5

1964 **Studio 49 Catalog**
MMB Music
9051 Watson Road
Suite 161
Saint Louis, MO 63126-1019
314-531-9635
800-543-3771
FAX: 314-531-8384
e-mail: info@mmbmusic.com
www.mmbmusic.com

Marcia Goldberg, President
Michelle Greenlaw, VP

Percussion instruments for school, therapy, church and family.

1965 Syracuse Community-Referenced Curriculum Guide for Students with Disabilties
Brookes Publishing
PO Box 10624
Baltimore, MD 21285-624 410-337-9580
800-638-3775
FAX: 410-337-8539
e-mail: custserv@brookespublishing.com
www.readplaylearn.com

Paul Brooks, President
Serving learners from kindergarten through age 21, this field-tested curriculum is a for professionals and parents devoted to directly preparing a student to function in the world. it examines the role of community living domains, functional academics, and embedded skills and includes practical implementation strategies and information for preparing students whose learning needs go beyond the scope of traditional academic programs.
$54.95
416 pages Spiral-bound
ISBN 1-557660-27-1

1966 Teaching Individuals with Physical and Multiple Disabilities
McGraw-Hill, School Publishing
PO Box 182604
Columbus, OH 43272 877-833-5524
FAX: 614-759-3749
e-mail: customer.service@mcgraw-hill.com
www.mcgraw-hill.com

Harold McGraw, President and CEO
Jack Callahan, Executive VP
John Berisford, Executive VP of HR
Focuses on the functional needs of the handicapped and the teaching skills of background teachers that they need to help them reach the highest possible level of self-sufficiency.
410 pages

1967 Teaching Students Ways to Remember
Brookline Books
8 Trumbull Rd, Suite B-001
Northampton, MA 1060 60- 66- 703
800-666-2665
FAX: 413-584-6184
e-mail: brbooks@yahoo.com
www.brooklinebooks.com

ISBN 0-914797-67-0

1968 Teaching Test-Taking Skills: Helping Students Show What They Know
Brookline Books
8 Trumbull Rd, Suite B-001
Northampton, MA 1060 60- 66- 703
800-666-2665
FAX: 414-584-6184
e-mail: brbooks@yahoo.com
www.brooklinebooks.com

ISBN 0-914797-76-X

1969 To Teach a Dyslexic
AVKO Educational Research Foundation
3084 Willard Rd
Birch Run, MI 48415-9404 810-686-9283
866-686-9283
FAX: 810-686-1101
e-mail: webmaster@avko.org
www.avko.org

Deborah Wolf, President
Aaron Miller, Vice President
A video available in DVD or video CD that shows Don McCabe working with a dyslexic teenager. The video helps teachers learn more about dyslexia and how to go about teaching a dyslexic student using the AVKO methodology and philosophy. This is a free video.
288 pages Paperback

1970 Tools for Transition
AGS
PO Box 99
Circle Pines, MN 55014-99 651-287-7220
800-328-2560
FAX: 763-786-9007
e-mail: agsmail@agsnet.com
www.agsnet.com

Kevin Brueggeman, President
Robert Zaske, Marketing Manager
This program prepares students with learning disabilities for postsecondary education. *$129.95*

1971 VAK Tasks Workbook: Visual, Auditory and Kinesthetic
Educational Tutorial Consortium
4400 S 44th St
Lincoln, NE 68516-1109 402-489-8133
FAX: 402-489-8160
e-mail: etc@altel.net
www.etc-ne.com

T Elli Cross, Owner
A workbook emphasizing the multisensory approach to teaching vocabulary and spelling. It is intended for middle-grade and older students working with prefixes, roots, suffixes, homonyms, and the spelling of easily confused endings. Includes spelling posters. *$7.00*
96 pages Paperback

1972 Volunteer Transcribing Services
Ste 200
205 E 3rd Ave
San Mateo, CA 94401-4028 650-357-1571
FAX: 650-632-3510

Alanah Hoffman, Coordinator
VTS is a nonprofit California corporation that produces large print school books for visually impaired students in grades K-12.

1973 Wordly Wise 3000
School Specialty
625 Mt. Auburn Street, 3rd Floor
PO Box 9031
Cambridge, MA 02139-9031 617-547-6706
800-225-5750
FAX: 888-440-2665
e-mail: Feedback.EPS@schoolspecialty.com
eps.schoolspecialty.com

Rick Holden, President, EPS
Kenneth Hodkinson, Author
Sandra Adams, Co-Author
Cheryl Dressler, Co-Author
Begins with a word list of 8-12 words, followed by clear, brief definitions and sentences that illustrate the meaning of the word. Books B and C often present more than one meaning of a word. Throughout all three books, drawings illustrate the meanings.
ISSN 0838-84 8

1974 Work!
JE Stewart Teaching Tools
PO Box 15308
Seattle, WA 98115-308 206-328-7664
FAX: 206-262-9538

Jan Gleason, Executive Director
Teaches 50 words as they appear on parts, tools, job instructions, signs, labels such as: hard hat, assembly, clamp, cut, drill, package and schedule. These words are functional in school and on-the-job. *$32.50*

1975 Working Together & Taking Part
A GS
PO Box 99
Circle Pines, MN 55014-99 651-287-7220
800-328-2560
FAX: 763-786-9007
e-mail: agsmail@agsnet.com
www.agsnet.com

Kevin Brueggeman, President
Robert Zaske, Market Manager

Two programs to build children's social skills in grades 3-6 through folk literature. Has 31 activity-rich lessons, teaching skills like: following rules, accepting differences, speaking assertively and helping others. Discount price of $279.00 when ordering both. *$149.95*

Associations

1976 **AVKO Educational Research Foundation**
3084 Willard Rd
Birch Run, MI 48415-9404
810-686-9283
866-686-9283
FAX: 810-686-1101
e-mail: webmaster@avko.org
www.avko.org

Deborah Wolf, President
Aaron Miller, Vice President

Comprised of individuals interested in helping others learn to read and spell. Develops and sells materials for teaching dyslexics or others with learning disabilities using a method involving audio, visual, kinesthetic and oral (multi-sensory) techniques.

1977 **Alliance for Parental Involvement in Education**
PO Box 59
East Chatham, NY 12060-59
518-392-6900
FAX: 518-392-6900
e-mail: allpie@taconic.net
www.croton.com/allpie

1978 **Alternative Work Concepts**
PO Box 11452
Eugene, OR 97440-3652
541-345-3043
FAX: 541-345-9669
e-mail: awc@efn.com
www.alternativeworkconcepts.org

Liz Fox, Executive Director

To promote individualized, integrated, and meaningful employment opportunities in the community for adults with multiple disabilities; to improve the quality of life and provide continuous opportunities for personal growth for these individuals; and to assist businesses with workforce diversification.

1979 **American Council for Headache Education(ACHE)**
19 Mantua Rd
Mount Royal, NJ 8061-1006
856-423-0043
FAX: 856-423-0082
e-mail: achehq@talley.com
www.achenet.org

Fred Sheftell, Chairman

Nonprofit, patient-health, professional partnership dedicated to advancing the treatment and management of headaches and to raising the public awareness of headache as valid, biologically based illness.

1980 **American School Counselor Association**
American Counselling Association
1101 King St
Suite 625
Alexandria, VA 22314-2957
703-683-2722
800-306-4722
FAX: 703-683-1619
e-mail: asca@schoolcounselor.org
www.schoolcounselor.org

Richard Wong, Executive Director
Kathleen Rakestraw, Director of Communications
Carolyn Stone, Board President

ASCA focuses on providing professional devleopment, enhancing school counseling programs, and research effective school counseling practices. Mission is to promote excellence in professional school counseling and the development of all students.

1981 **Association on Higher Education and Disability**
107 Commerce Centre Dr
Suite 204
Huntersville, NC 28078-5870
704-947-7779
FAX: 704-948-7779
TTY:617-287-3882
e-mail: ahead@ahead.org
www.ahead.org

Jean Ashmore, President
Michael Johnson, Treasurer
Stephan Smith, Executive Director

Higher education for people with disabilities. A vital resource, promoting excellence through education, communication and training.

1982 **CARF International (Commission on Accreditation of Rehabilitation Facilities)**
CARF International
6951East Southpoint Road
Tucson, AZ 8575-9407
520-325-1044
888-281-6531
FAX: 520-318-1129
e-mail: info @carf.org
carf.org

Brian J Boon, CEO

An independent, nonprofit accreditor of human service providers in the areas of aging services, behavioral health, child and youth services, DMEPOS, employment and community services, medical rehabilitation, and opioid treatment programs.

1983 **CEC-Division for Early Childhood**
Council for Exceptional Children
27 Fort Missoula Road
Suite 2
Missoula, MT 59804
406-543-0872
888-232-7733
FAX: 406-543-0887
e-mail: dec@dec-sped.org
www.dec-sped.org

Sarah Mulligan, Executive Director
Cynthia Wood, Associate Executive Director
Natalie Forcier, Program/Accounting Assistant
Marina Zaleski, Program Assistant

Promotes policies and advances evidence-based practices that support families and enhance the optimal development of young children who have or are at risk for developmental delays and disabilities.

1984 **Council for Exceptional Children**
2900 Crystal Drive
Suite 1000
Arlington, VA 22202-3557
703-620-3660
866-509-0218
888-232-7733
FAX: 703-264-9494
TTY:866-915-5000
e-mail: service@cec.sped.org
www.cec.sped.org

Robin D. Brewer, President
James P. Heiden, President Elect
Christy A. Chambers, Immediate Past President
Mikki Garcia, Executive Director

The largest international professional organization dedicated to improving the educational success of individuals with disabilities and/or gifts and talents. Advocates for appropriate governmental policies, sets professional standards, provides professional development, advocates for individuals with exceptionalities, and helps professionals obtain conditions and resources necessary for effective professional practice

1985 **Division for Physical and Health Disabilities (DPHD)**
Council for Exceptional Children (CEC)
2900 Crystal Drive,
Suite 1000
Arlington, VA 22202
888-232-7733
FAX: 703-264-9494
TTY:866-915-5000
e-mail: service@cec.sped.org
www.cec.sped.org

Linda Thomas, President of DPHMD
Juliet Hart, Vice President
The DPHD is the official division of the CEC that advocates for quality education for all individuals with physical disabilities, multiple disabilities, and special health care needs served in schools, hospitals, or home settings. The goals of DPHD include: promoting the continued development adequate resources and programs; disseminating relevant and timely information on issues, instructional strategies, and research through meetings and publications; and many more services and activities.

1986 **Educational Referral Service**
Doctor Yvonne Jones and Associates
2222 Eastlake Ave E
Seattle, WA 98102-3419
206-325-2600
FAX: 206-328-9172

Yvonne Jones
Specializes in matching children with the learning environments that are best for them and works with families to help them identify concerns and establish priorities about their child's education.

1987 **International Association of Parents and Professionals for Safe Alternatives in Childbirth**
Box 646
Rr 4
Marble Hill, MO 63764-9418
573-238-4273
FAX: 573-238-2010
e-mail: napsac@clas.org
www.napsac.org

Lee Stewart, Publisher
David Stewart, Executive Director
Dedicated to exploring, implementing, and establishing safe, family-centered childbirth programs that meet the social and emotional needs of families as well as provide the safe, appropriate aspects of medical science.

1988 **International Childbirth Education Association**
1500 Sunday Drive
Suite 102
Raleigh, NC 27607-48
919-863-9487
800-624-4934
FAX: 919-787-4916
e-mail: info@icea.org
www.icea.org

Denise Wheatley, President
Nancy Lantz, President- Elect
Deborah Codde, Treasuer
Debra Tolson, Secretary
Offer teaching certificates, seminars, continuing education workshops, and a mail order center.

1989 **International Dyslexia Association**
40 York Road
4th Floor
Baltimore, MD 21204-5243
410-296-0232
800-222-3123
FAX: 410-321-5069
e-mail: info@interdys.org
www.interdys.org

Guinevere Eden, President
Stephen Peregoy, Executive Director
Sandra Soper, Vice President
IDA is a clearinghouse of scientific data and practice-based information related to dyslexia. We also provide community-based referrals and information fact sheets in response to thousands of emails, calls & letters. Our annual conference attracts thousands of researchers, clinicians, parents, teachers, psychologist, educational therapists and people with dyslexia.

1990 **International Organization for the Education of the Hearing Impaired**
Alexander Graham Bell Association
3417 Volta Pl NW
Washington, DC 20007-2737
202-337-5220
FAX: 202-337-8314
TTY:202-337-5221
e-mail: info@agbell.org
www.agbell.org

Kathleen Treni, President
Meredith Knueve, Secretary Treasurer
Alexander Graham, Executive Director/CEO
Professional educators of the hearing impaired make up the members of this organization which promotes the excellence in teaching the hearing impaired child.

1991 **Jewish Guild for the Blind**
15 W 65th St
New York, NY 10023-6601
212-769-6200
800-284-4422
FAX: 212-769-6266
e-mail: info@guildhealth.org
www.jgb.org

Pauline Raiff, Chairman
Aaron Kesselman, President
Eileen Hanley, Senior VP
Barbara Klein, Director of Development
Full service vision care agency for children, adults and elderly people who are blind or visually impaired.

1992 **Job Accommodation Network**
Office of Disability and Employment Policy
PO Box 6080
Morgantown, WV 26506-6080
800-232-9675
800-526-7234
FAX: 304-093-5407
TTY: 877-781-9403
e-mail: jan@jan.wvu.edu
www.jan.wvu.edu

DJ Hendricks, Director
International toll-free consulting service that provides information about job accommodations and the employability of people with disabilities. Also provides information regarding the Americans with Disabilities Act (ADA).

1993 **Michigan Psychological Association**
124 W Allegan St
Suite 1900
Lansing, MI 48933-1768
517-347-1885
FAX: 517-484-4442
e-mail: office@michiganpsychologicalassociation.org
www.michiganpsychologicalass ociation.org

William Nicholson, President
Judith Kovach, Executive Director
Nonprofit organization of over 1000 psychologists, working to advance psychology as a science and a profession and to promote the public welfare by encouraging the highest professional standards, offering public education and providing a public service, and by participating in the public policy process on behalf of the profession and health care consumers.

1994 **National Association of Colleges and Employers**
62 Highland Ave
Bethlehem, PA 18017-9481
610-868-1421
800-544-5272
FAX: 610-868-0208
naceweb.org

Vanessa Strauss, President
Donnie Brown, VP of Human Resources
A national association with services for career planning, placement and recruitment professionals.

1995 **National Association of Private Special Education Centers**
601 Pennsylvania Avenue
Suite 900, South Building
Washington, DC 20004-1202
202-434-8225
FAX: 202-434-8224
e-mail: napsec@aol.com
napsec.org
Sherry Kolbe, Executive Director
Membership directory offering information on NAPSEC member schools nationwide available.

1996 **National Center for Homeopathy**
101 S Whiting St
Alexandria, VA 22304-3418
703-548-7790
FAX: 703-548-7792
e-mail: info@homeopathic.org
nationalcenterforhomeopathy.org
Sharon Stevenson, Executive Director
Provides information, referral lists, online webinals to members, and an annual homeopathic conference.

1997 **National Clearinghouse for Professions**
2900 Crystal Drive
Suite 1000
Arlington, VA 22202
703-264-9454
888-232-7733
FAX: 703-264-1637
e-mail: service@cec.sped.org
www.cec.sped.org
Bruce Ramirez, Executive Director

1998 **National Council on Rehabilitation Education (NCRE)**
1099 E. Champlain Drive, Suite A
PMB # 137
Fresno, CA 93720
559-906-0787
FAX: 559-412-2550
e-mail: info@ncre.org
www.rehabeducators.org
Charles Degeneffe, President
Ken Hergenrather, First VP
Jared Schultz, Second VP
Members include academic institutions and organizations, professional educators, researchers, and students. Assists in the documentation of the effect of education in improving services to persons with disabilities; determines the skills and training necessary for effective rehabilitation services; develops role models, standards and uniform licensure and certification requirements for rehabilitation personnel.

1999 **National Education Association of the United States**
1201 16th St NW
Washington, DC 20036-3290
202-833-4000
FAX: 202-822-7974
www.nea.org
Dennis Van Roekel, President
Lily Eskelsen, Vice President
Rebecca Pringle, VP and Secretary
John Wilson, Executive Director
Offers information to educational professionals.

2000 **National Society for Experiential Education**
19 Mantua Rd
Mount Royal, NJ 8061-1006
856-423-3427
FAX: 856-423-3420
e-mail: nsee@talley.com
www.nsee.org
James Walters, President
Mary King, Vice President
Haley Brust, Executive Director
National nonprofit organization which advocates experiential learning and works with college administrators and high school and college internship programs.

2001 **President's Committee for People with Intellectual Disabilities**
Administration for Children & Families
370 L Enfant Promenade SW
Washington, DC 20447-1
202-619-0634
FAX: 202-205-9519
www.acf.hhs.gov/programs/pcpid
Sally Atwater, Executive Director
Dalls Rob Sweezy, Chairperson
MJ Karimi, Executive Director Assistant
Prepares an annual report to the president of the United States addressing issues concerning citizens with intellectual disabilities.

2002 **Rifin Family/Daughters of Israel**
JGB Audio Library for the Blind
15 W 65th St
New York, NY 10023-6601
212-769-6200
800-284-4422
FAX: 212-769-6266
e-mail: info@JGB.org
www.JGB.org
Pauline Raiff, Chairman
Aaron Kesselman, President
Eileen Hanley, Senior VP

2003 **SSD (Services for Students with Disabilities)**
College Board
45 Columbus Ave
New York, NY 10023-6917
212-713-8000
866-630-9305
FAX: 212-713-8255
e-mail: help@cssprofile.org
www.collegeboard.com
Gaston Caperton, President
National, nonprofit membership association dedicated to preparing, inspiring and connecting students to college and opportunity. Founded in 1900, the association is composed of more than 3,800 schools, colleges, universities and other educational organizations. Services for Students with Disabilities (SSD) provides special arrangements to minimize the possible effects of disabilities on test performance through it's Admissions Testing Program (ATP).

2004 **Target Teach**
Evans Newton
Ste 1
15941 N 77th St
Scottsdale, AZ 85260-1217
480-998-2777
800-443-0544
FAX: 480-951-2895
e-mail: info@evansnewton.com
www.target.com
Jamie Piotti, CEO
Gary Davis, Director of Curriculum and Instr
Aligns and monitors Special Education Instructional Materials to tests that are used to measure the effectiveness of Special Education Instructional Programs.

2005 **United Cerebral Palsy**
1825 K Street NW
Suite 600
Washington, DC 20006-5638
202-776-0406
800-872-5827
FAX: 202-776-0414
e-mail: info@ucp.org
www.ucp.org
Stephen Bennett, CEO
Bruce Fried, Chariman
Keith Green, Vice Chair
Grants are awarded to institutions or organizations on behalf of a principal investigator in support of biomedical and bioengineering research in areas which have a significant relationship to cerebral palsy. While most research on central nervous system structure, function and disorder may be useful, the Foundation requires that research proposals address issues of relevance to cerebral palsy.

Directories

2006 BOSC: Directory of Facilities for People with Learning Disabilities
Books on Special Children
PO Box 3378
Amherst, MA 1004-3378 413-256-8164
FAX: 413-256-8896
e-mail: irene@boscbooks.com
www.boscbooks.com
Michael Young, President
Directory of schools, independent living programs, clinics and centers, colleges and vocational programs, agencies and commercial products. Five sections in special post binder that can be updated annually. Hardcover. *$70.00*
300+ pages Yearly
ISSN 0961-3888

2007 Complete Directory for Pediatric Disorders
Sedgwick Press/Grey House Publishing
4919 Route 22
P.O. Box 56
Amenia, NY 12501 518-789-8700
800-562-2139
FAX: 518-789-0556
e-mail: books@greyhouse.com
www.greyhouse.com
Leslie Mackenzie, Publisher
Laura Mars, Editorial Director
Jessica Moody, Marketing Director
Diana Delgado, Editorial Assistant
An annual directory for professionals, parents and caregivers. Provides valuable information on more than 200 pediatric conditions, disorders, diseases and disabilities, including informative descriptions and a wide variety of resources, from associations to publications. *$165.00*
1000 pages Annual
ISBN 1-592374-30-1

2008 Complete Directory for People with Chronic Illness
Sedgwick Press/Grey House Publishing
4919 Route 22
P.O. Box 56
Amenia, NY 12501 518-789-8700
800-562-2139
FAX: 518-789-0556
e-mail: books@greyhouse.com
www.greyhouse.com
Leslie Mackenzie, Publisher
Laura Mars, Editorial Director
Jessica Moody, Marketing Director
Diana Delgado, Editorial Assistant
This directory is structured around the ninety most prevalent chronic illnesses. Each chronic illness chapter includes an informative description, plus a comprehensive listing of resources and support services available for people diagnosed with chronic illness and their network of supportive individuals. *$165.00*
1000 pages Annual
ISBN 1-592374-15-8

2009 Complete Learning Disabilities Directory
Sedgwick Press/Grey House Publishing
4919 Route 22
P.O. Box 56
Amenia, NY 12501 518-789-8700
800-562-2139
FAX: 518-789-0556
e-mail: books@greyhouse.com
www.greyhouse.com
Leslie Mackenzie, Publisher
Laura Mars, Editorial Director
Jessica Moody, Marketing Director
Diana Delgado, Editorial Assistant
A comprehensive educational guide offering over 6,500 listings on associations and organizations, schools, government agencies, testing materials, camps, products, books, newsletters, legal information, classroom materials and more. Includes separate chapters on ADD and Literacy, as well as informative articles. *$150.00*
800 pages Annual
ISBN 1-592375-86-3

2010 Complete Mental Health Directory
Sedgwick Press/Grey House Publishing
4919 Route 22
P.O. Box 56
Amenia, NY 12501 518-789-8700
800-562-2139
FAX: 518-789-0556
e-mail: books@greyhouse.com
www.greyhouse.com
Leslie Mackenzie, Publisher
Laura Mars, Editorial Director
Jessica Moody, Marketing Director
Diana Delgado, Editorial Assistant
This directory offers comprehensive information covering the field of behavioral health, with critical information for both the layman and the mental health professional. It covers, in depth, 25 specific mental disorders, and includes informative descriptions and a complete list of resources. *$165.00*
800 pages Annual
ISBN 1-592375-44-8

2011 Directory for Exceptional Children
Porter Sargent
2 LAN Drive
Suite 100
Westford, MA 01886 978-692-5092
800-342-7470
FAX: 978-692-4714
e-mail: info@carnegiecomm.com
www.carnegiecomm.com
Joe Moore, President, CEO
Mark Cunningham, SVP, Enrollment Marketing
Melissa Rekos, SVP, Digital Services
Gary Allen Williams, VP, Special Projects
Supports parents and professionals seeking the optimal educational, therapeutic or clinical environment for special-needs youth. *$75.00*
1120 pages Trienniel
ISBN 0-875581-50-1

2012 Educators Resource Directory
Sedgwick Press/Grey House Publishing
4919 Route 22
PO Box 55
Amenia, NY 12501 518-789-8700
800-562-2139
FAX: 845-373-6390
e-mail: books@greyhouse.com
www.greyhouse.com
Leslie Mackenzie, Publisher
Laura Mars, Editorial Director
Jessica Moody, Marketing Director
Kristen Thatcher, Production Manager
Gives education professionals immediate access to Associations and Organizations, Conferences and Trade Shows, Educational Research Centers, Employment Opportunities and Teaching Abroad, School Library Services, Scholarships, Financial Resources and much more. *$ 145.00*
650 pages Annual
ISBN 1-592377-43-5

2013 Increasing and Decreasing Behaviors of Persons with Severe Retardation and Autism
Research Press
P.O. Box 7886
Champaign, IL 61826 217-352-3273
800-519-2707
FAX: 217-352-1221
e-mail: orders@researchpress.com
www.researchpress.com
Robert W. Parkinson, Founder
Dr Richard M Foxx, Author

Shows how to increase desirable behaviors by using techniques such as shaping, prompting, fading, modeling, backward chaining and graduated guidance. Offers specific guidelines for arranging and managing the learning environment as well as standards for evaluating and maintaining success. *$21.95*
230 pages
ISBN 0-878222-65-0

2014 **Teaching Special Students in Mainstream**
Books on Special Children
P.O.Box 305
Congers, NY 10920-305
845-638-1236
FAX: 845-638-0847
e-mail: irene@boscbooks.com
515 pages Softcover

Educational Publishers

2015 **AFB Press**
American Foundation for the Blind / AFB Press
2 Penn Plaza
Suite 1102
New York, NY 10121
212-502-7600
FAX: 888-545-8331
e-mail: afbinfo@afb.net
www.afb.org
Carl R. Augusto, President and CEO
Paul Schroeder, Vice President, Programs and Policy
Rick Bozeman, Chief Financial Officer
Kelly Bleach, Chief Administrative Officer
Develops, publishes, and sells a wide variety of informative books, pamphlets, periodicals, and videos for students, professionals, and researchers in the blindness and visual impairment fields, for people professionally involved in making the mainstream community accessible, and for blind and visually impaired people and their families; publication and video orders.

2016 **American Counseling Association**
5999 Stevenson Ave
Alexandria, VA 22304
703-823-0252
800-347-6647
FAX: 800-473-2329
e-mail: webmaster@counseling.org
www.counseling.org
Robert L. Smith, President
Thelma Duffey, President Elect
Brian Canfield, Treasurer
Richard Yep, CEO
Offers tools and books for the professional.

2017 **Brookes Publishing Company**
PO Box 10624
Baltimore, MD 21285-0624
410-337-9580
800-638-3775
FAX: 410-337-8539
e-mail: webmaster@brookespublishing.com
www.brookespublishing.com
Paul H. Brookes, Chairman of the Board
Jeffrey D. Brookes, President
George S. Stamathis, VP/Publisher
Melissa A. Behn, Executive Vice President
Publishes highly respected resources in early childhood, early intervention, inclusive and special education, developmental disabilities, learning disabilities, communication and language, behavior and mental health.

2018 **Brookline Books**
34 University Rd
Brookline, MA 02445-4533
617-734-6772
800-666-2665
FAX: 617-734-3952
e-mail: brbooks@yahoo.com
www.brooklinebooks.com
William H Walters, Author
Esther Wilder, Co-Author
Offers books for teachers and parents on law and legislation, education, integration and mainstreaming for the disabled, their families, caregivers and teachers.

2019 **Brooks/Cole Publishing Company**
511 Forest Lodge Rd
Pacific Grove, CA 93950-5040
831-373-0728
800-354-9706
FAX: 831-375-6414

2020 **Charles C Thomas Publisher LTD**
2600 S 1st Street
Springfield, IL 62704-4730
217-789-8980
800-258-8980
FAX: 217-789-9130
e-mail: books@ccthomas.com
www.ccthomas.com
Michael P. Thomas, President
Publishes specialty titles and textbooks in medicine, dentistry, nursing, and veterinary medicine, as well as a complete line in the behavioral sciences, criminal justice, education, special education, and rehabilitation. Aims to accommodate the current needs for information.

2021 **ERIC Clearinghouse on Disabilities and Gifted Education**
2900 Crystal Drive
Suite 1000
Arlington, VA 22202-3557
703-264-9454
888-232-7733
FAX: 703-264-1637
e-mail: service@cec.sped.org
www.cec.sped.org
Bruce Ramirez, Executive Director

2022 **Eric Clearinghouse on Disabilities and Gifted Education**
Council for Exceptional Children
2900 Crystal Drive
Suite 1000
Arlington, VA 22202-3557
703-264-9454
888-232-7733
FAX: 703-264-1637
e-mail: service@cec.sped.org
www.cec.sped.org
Bruce Ramirez, Executive Director
Provides information on special and gifted education. Provides referrals, offers patient networking services and provides information on current research programs. Focuses its efforts on prevention, identification, assessment, intervention and enrichment both in special settings and within mainstream communities. Offers a variety of materials including brochures and Spanish language matereials.

2023 **Gallaudet University Press**
800 Florida Avenue, NE
Washington, DC 20002-3695
202-651-5488
FAX: 202-651-5489
e-mail: gupress@gallaudet.edu
gupress.gallaudet.edu
David F Armstrong, Executive Director
Publishes scholarly trade books and journals about deaf people and their language, history, and culture for deaf people, parents of deaf children, professionals, educators and the general public. Produces spring and fall catalogs.

2024 **Greenwood Publishing Group**
88 Post Rd W
Westport, CT 06880-4208
203-226-3571
FAX: 203-222-1502
e-mail: webmaster@greenwood.com
greenwood.com
Wayne Smith, President
Kirstin Olsen, Author
ABC-CLIO and Greenwood Press are recognized as industry-leading providers of the highest-quality reference materials. These imprints offer authoritative reference scholarship and in-

novative coverage of history and humanities topics across the secondary and higher education curriculum.

2025 **Grey House Publishing**
4919 Route 22
P.O. Box 56
Amenia, NY 12501
518-789-8700
800-562-2139
FAX: 518-789-0556
e-mail: books@greyhouse.com
www.greyhouse.com

Leslie Mackenzie, Publisher
Laura Mars, Editorial Director
Jessica Moody, Marketing Director
Diana Delgado, Editorial Assistant
Grey House Publishing publishes directories, handbooks and reference works for public, high school and academic libraries and the business and health communities. Most titles are available as online databases.

2026 **Information from HEATH Resource Center**
National Clearinghouse on Postsecondary Education
2134 G Street, N.W.
Washington, DC 20052
202-939-9320
800-544-3284
FAX: 202-833-5696
e-mail: heath@ace.nche.edu
www.HEATH-resource-center.org

2027 **McGraw-Hill Company**
PO Box 182605
Columbus, OH 43218
800-338-3987
FAX: 609-308-4480
e-mail: customer.service@mheducation.com
www.mcgraw-hill.com

David Levin, President, CEO
Ellen Haley, President, CTB
Peter Cohen, President, School Education
Mark Dorman, President, International
Offers a catalog of testing resources and materials for the special educator.

2028 **National Association of School Psychologists**
4340 East West Highway
Suite 402
Bethesda, MD 20814
301-657-0270
866-311-6277
FAX: 301-657-0275
TTY: 301-657-4155
e-mail: webmaster@naspweb.org
www.nasponline.org

Stephen E. Brock, President
Todd A. Savage, President-Elect
Laura Benson, Chief Operating Officer
Susan Gorin, Executive Director
Represents over 22,500 school psychologists and related professionals. It serves its members and society by advancing the profession of school psychology and advocating for the rights, welfare, education and mental health of children, youth and their families.

2029 **PEAK Parent Center**
611 N Weber
Suite 200
Colorado Springs, CO 80903-1072
719-531-9400
800-284-0251
FAX: 719-531-9452
e-mail: info@peakparent.org
www.peakparent.org

Barbara Buswell, Executive Director
PEAK Parent Center is a federally-designated Parent Training and Information Center (PTI). As a PTI, PEAK supports and empowers parents, providing them with information and strategies to use when advocating for their children with disabilities. PEAK works one-on-one with families and educators helping them realize new possibilities for children with disabilities by expanding knowledge of special education and offering new strategies for success.

2030 **Prufrock Press**
PO Box 8813
Waco, TX 76714-8813
254-756-3337
800-998-2208
FAX: 800-240-0333
e-mail: jmcintosh@prufrock.com
www.prufrock.com

Joel McIntosh, Publisher & Marketing Director
Lacy Compton, Senior Editor
Rachel Taliaferro, Editor
Raquel Trevino, Graphic Designer and Production Coordinator
Publishes books, textbooks, teaching aids, journals, and magazines supporting gifted education and gifted children.

2031 **Research Press**
P.O. Box 7886
Champaign, IL 61826
217-352-3273
800-519-2707
FAX: 217-352-1221
e-mail: orders@researchpress.com
www.researchpress.com

Robert W. Parkinson, Founder
Dr Richard M Foxx, Author
Jeffrey S. Allen, Author
Bryce Alvord, Author
Research Press is an independent, family-owned business founded in 1968 by Robert W. Parkinson (1920-2001). During the past 40 years, the company has earned a solid reputation for publishing practical and effective educational and mental health resources. Authors from the early years include well-known names in the field of psychology, such as B.F. Skinner, Albert Ellis, Gerald Patterson, Wesley Becker, John Guttmann, Richard Foxx, Arnold Lazarus, and Joseph Cautela.

2032 **Sage Publications**
2455 Teller Road
Thousand Oaks, CA 91320
805-499-0721
800-818-7243
FAX: 800-583-2665
e-mail: info@sagepub.com
www.sagepub.com

Sara Miller McCune, Founder, Publisher & Executive Chairman
Blaise R Simqu, President/CEO
Chris Hickok, Senior Vice President & Chief Financial Officer
Stephen Barr, Managing Director/SAGE London, President of SAGE Internation
Publishes books, text books, journals, reference books, and databases mainly related to psychology, special education and speech, language and hearing.

2033 **Special Needs Project**
324 State St
Ste H
Santa Barbara, CA 93101
818-718-9900
FAX: 818-349-2027
e-mail: hgray@specialneeds.com
www.specialneeds.com

Hod Gray, Owner
Publishes child development textbooks, books about aspergers syndrome, autism, and other disabilities.

State Agencies: Alabama

2034 **Alabama Department of Education: Division of Special Education Services**
50 North Ripley Street
PO Box 302101
Montgomery, AL 36104
334-242-9700
FAX: 334-262-2677
e-mail: speced@alsde.edu
www.alsde.edu

Governor Rob Bentley, President
Jeffery Newman, President Pro Term
Ella B. Bell, Vice President
Thomas R. Bice, Ed.D., Secretary & Executive Officer

Provides technical assistance to all education agencies serving Alabama's gifted children as well as children with disabilities.

2035 Getting Ready for the Outside World(G.R.O.W.)
Riverview School
551 Route 6A East Sandwich
Cape Cod, MA 2537-1448
508-888-0489
FAX: 508-833-7001
e-mail: admissions@riverviewschool.org
www.riverviewschool.org

Janice James, Vice Chairman
Deborah Cowan, Vice Chair
James Shallcross, Treasurer
Kathleen Yazbak, Secretary

Riverview School's G.R.O.W. Program is a unique ten month transitional prgoram (1-3 years) for young adults with complex language, learning and cognitive disabilities. This post secondary program is designed to further develop academic, vocational and independent living skills, to enable students to function as independently as possible.

State Agencies: Alaska

2036 Alaska Department of Education: Office of Special Education
State of Alaska
801 West 10th Street, Suite 200
PO Box 110500
Juneau, AK 99811-0500
907-465-2800
FAX: 907-465-4156
TTY:907-465-2815
e-mail: eed.webmaster@alaska.gov
www.eed.state.ak.us

Cynthia Curran, Division Director

Administers special educational programs to the disabled residents of Alaska, through the Division of Teaching & Learning Support.

State Agencies: Arkansas

2037 Arkansas Department of Special Education
1401 West Capitol Ave, Victory Bldg
Suite 450
Little Rock, AR 72201
501-682-4221
FAX: 501-682-3456
TTY:501-682-4222
e-mail: spedsupport@arkansas.gov
arksped.k12.ar.us

Tom Hicks, Interim Associate Director
Ella Albert, Management Project Analyst
Howie Knoff, Director
Tony Boaz, Director

Provides oversight of all educational programs for children and youth with disabilities, ages 3 to 21. Provides technical assistance to all public agencies providing educational services to this population.

State Agencies: California

2038 California Department of Education: Special Education Division
1430 N Street
Sacramento, CA 95814-5901
916-319-0800
FAX: 916-327-3516
e-mail: scheduler@cde.ca.gov
www.cde.ca.gov

Tom Torlakson, State Superintendent of Public Instruction and Director of E
Fred Balcom, Director
Gordon Jackson, Director
Phyllis Bramson, Director

Information and resources to serve the unique needs of persons with disabilities so that each person will meet or exceed high standards of achievement in academic and nonacademic skills.

State Agencies: Colorado

2039 Colorado Department of Education: Special Education Service Unit
Colorado Department of Education
201 E Colfax Ave
Denver, CO 80203-1704
303-866-6600
FAX: 303-830-0793
e-mail: steinberg_e@cde.state.co.us
www.cde.state.co.us

Ed Steinberg, Commissioner

Provides consultation on materials and educational services for visually handicapped children, supervises volunteer services, transcribes textbooks for visually handicapped students.

State Agencies: Connecticut

2040 Connecticut Department of Education: Bureau of Special Education
165 Capitol Avenue
Hartford, CT 06106
860-713-6543
FAX: 860-713-7014
e-mail: annelouise.thompson@ct.gov
www.sde.ct.gov

Anne Louise Thompson, Bureau Chief
Lisa Spooner, Administrative Assistant
Regina Gaunichaux, Secretary
Carol Leddy, Secretary, Due Process Unit

The State Board of Education believes each student is unique and needs an educational environment that provides for, and accommodates, his or her strengths and areas of needed improvement.

2041 Connecticut State Board of Education and Services for the Blind
State of Connecticut Agency
184 Windsor Ave
Windsor, CT 06095-4536
860-602-4000
800-842-4510
FAX: 860-602-4020
TTY: 860-602-4221
e-mail: brian.sigman@po.state.ct.us
www.besb.state.ct.us

Keith Maynard, Deputy Director
Brian Sigman, Executive Director
Alan Sylvestre, Chairman
Eileen Akers, Director

Provides consultation for the education of visually disabled children, provides Braille instruction, independent living skills training, vocational rehabilitation services and community outreach and advocacy.

State Agencies: Delaware

2042 Department of Public Instruction: Exceptional Children & Special Programs Division
Department of Education
Ste 2
401 Federal St
Dover, DE 19901-3639
302-739-5471
FAX: 302-739-2388
www.doe.k12.de.us

Martha Toomey, Executive Director

State Agencies: DC

2043 **District of Columbia Public Schools: Special Education Division**
1200 First Street, NE
Washington, DC 20002-4210
202-442-5885
202-442-5517
FAX: 202-442-5026
www.dcps.dc.gov

Paul L Vance MD, Superintendent

Committed to providing a continuum of services that offers students with disabilities the opportunity to actively participate in the learning environment of their neighborhood school.

2044 **National Clearinghouse on Family Support and Children's Mental Health**
Ste 800
1 Dupont Cir NW
Washington, DC 20036-1149
202-939-9320
800-544-3284
FAX: 202-833-4760
e-mail: heatah@ace.nche.edu
ncfy.acf.hhs.gov/

State Agencies: Florida

2045 **Florida Department of Education: Bureau of Exceptional Education And Student Services**
325 West Gaines Street
Turlington Building, Suite 1514
Tallahassee, FL 32399
850-245-0505
FAX: 850-245-9667
e-mail: Monica.Verra-Tirado@fldoe.org
www.fldoe.org/ese

Monica Verra-Tirado, Ed.D., Bureau Chief
Gerard Robinson, Commissioner
Randy Hanna, Chancellor
Pam Stewart, Chancellor

Administers programs for students with disabilities and for gifted students. Coordinates student services throughout the state and participates in multiple inter-agency efforts designed to strengthen the quality and variety of services to students with special needs.

State Agencies: Hawaii

2046 **Hawaii Department of Education: Special Needs**
Hawaii Department of Education
3430 Leahi Ave
Honolulu, HI 96815-4246
808-941-3894
FAX: 808-941-3894

Margaret Donovan MD, State Administrator

Provides consultation on educational services for local schools, offers psychological testing and evaluation, maintains resource rooms in district schools and more for the blind and handicapped throughout the state.

State Agencies: Illinois

2047 **Illinois State Board of Education: Department of Special Education**
100 N 1st St
Springfield, IL 62777
217-782-5589
FAX: 217-782-0372
www.isbe.net

Elizabeth Hanselman, Asst Superintendent Special Ed.

Mission is to advance the human and civil rights of people with disabilities in Illinois. Statewide advocacy organization providing self-advocacy assistance, legal services, education and public policy initiatives. Designated to implement the federal protection and advocacy system; has broad statutory power to enforce the rights of people with physical and mental disabilities, including developmental disabilities and mental illnesses.

State Agencies: Indiana

2048 **Indiana Department of Education: Special Education Division**
Indiana Department of Education
South Tower, Suite 600
115 W. Washington Street
Indianapolis, IN 46204-2731
317- 23- 661
877-851-4106
FAX: 317- 23- 800
e-mail: webmaster@doe.in.gov
www.doe.in.gov/

Robert A Marra, Manager
Tony Bennett, Chair

Provides consultation on educational services for local schools, offers psychological testing and evaluation, maintains resource rooms in district schools and more for the blind and handicapped throughout the state.

State Agencies: Iowa

2049 **Iowa Department of Public Instruction: Bureau of Special Education**
400 E 14th St
Des Moines, IA 50319-9000
515-457-2000
FAX: 515-242-6019
www.educateiowa.gov/

Tom Kuehl, CEO
Jason Glass, Director
Jeff Berger, Administrative Services

State Agencies: Kansas

2050 **Kansas State Board of Education: Special Education Services**
900 SW Jackson Street
Topeka, KS 66612-1212
785-296-3201
800-203-9462
FAX: 785-296-7933
TTY: 785-296-6338
e-mail: contact@ksde.org
www.ksde.org

Ethan Erickson, Director
Kathy Gosa, Director
Denise Kahler, Director
Scott Myers, Director

Provides leadership and support for exceptional learners receiving special education services throughout Kansas schools and communities.

State Agencies: Kentucky

2051 **Kentucky Department of Education: Divisionof Exceptional Children's Services**
500 Mero St
Capital Tower Plaza
Frankfort, KY 40601
502-564-4770
FAX: 502-564-7749
e-mail: darlene.jesse@kde.state.ky.us
www.education.ky.gov

Darlene Jesse, Director

Provides consultation on educational services for local schools, offers psychological testing and evaluation, maintains resource rooms in district schools and more for the blind and handicapped throughout the state.

State Agencies: Louisiana

2052 **Louisiana Department of Education: Office of Special Education Services**
Louisiana Department of Education
1201 North Third Street
Baton Rouge, LA 70802
225-342-0090
877-453-2721
FAX: 225-342-0193
www.doe.state.la.us
David Elder, Manager
Kim Fitch, Director Human Resources
George Nelson, President

State Agencies: Massachusetts

2053 **Massachusetts Department of Education: Program Quality Assurance**
Massachusetts Department of Education
75 Pleasant Street
Malden, MA 2148-4906
781-388-3300
FAX: 617-388-3476
e-mail: boe@doe.mass.edu
www.doe.mass.edu/pqa/
Pamela Kaufamann, Administrator

State Agencies: Maryland

2054 **Maryland State Department of Education: Division of Special Education**
200 West Baltimore Street
Baltimore, MD 21201-2595
410-767-0100
888-246-0016
FAX: 410-333-8165
e-mail: dmcmicha@msde.state.md.us
www.marylandpublicschools.org
Nancy S Grasmick, State Supertintendent
Dr. Lillian Lowery, Superintendent of Schools
James V. Foran, Assistant State Superintendent
Katharine Oliver, Assistant State Superintendent
Collaborates with families, local early intervention systems, and local school systems to ensure that all children and youth with disabilities have access to appropriate services and educational opportunities to which they are entitled under federal and state laws.

State Agencies: Michigan

2055 **Michigan Department of Education: Special Education Services**
608 W. Allegan Street
PO Box 30008
Lansing, MI 48909
517-373-3324
FAX: 517-373-7504
e-mail: DHS-OCS-PEP@michigan.gov
www.michigan.gov/mde
John C. Austin, President
Kathleen N. Straus, President of the State Board
Michelle Fecteau, Executive Director
Daniel Varner, Chief Executive Officer of Excellent Schools Detroit
Oversees the administrative funding of education and early intervention programs and services for young children and students with disabilities.

2056 **Services for Students with Disabilities**
University of Michigan
G-664 Haven Hall
505 South State St.
Ann Arbor, MI 48109-1045
734-763-3000
FAX: 734-936-3947
TTY:734-615-4461
e-mail: ssdoffice@umich.edu
www.ssd.umich.edu
Stuart Segal, Director
Offers information to students of the University of Michigan and their parents.

State Agencies: Minnesota

2057 **Community Supports for People with Disabilities (CSP)**
South Central Technical College (SCTC)
1920 Lee Blvd
North Mankato, MN 56003-2504
507-389-7200
800-722-9359
e-mail: online@southcentral.edu
www.southcentral.edu
Christensen Tami, Executive Director
Keith Stover, President
Human services program available as a physical or online program, designed for those wanting to earn a certificate, diploma or associate degree as a Direct Support Professional for use in the health and human services industries. The program comprises eight courses relating to professional services and support for people with disabilities.

2058 **Professional Development Programs**
6303 Osgood Ave. N.
Ste 104
Stillwater, MN 55082
651-439-8865
877-439-8865
FAX: 877-259-5906
e-mail: programs@pdppro.com
www.pdppro.com
Cindy Lacosse, VP
Lori Lacrosse, President
Sponsors cutting edge and popular continuing education workshops and symposia of interest to professionals who provide services to children and adults with special needs.

State Agencies: Missouri

2059 **Missouri Department of Elementary and Secondary Education: Special Education Programs**
205 Jefferson St
PO Box 480
Jefferson City, MO 65102
573-751-5739
FAX: 573-526-4404
TTY:800-735-2966
www.dese.mo.gov
Stephen Barr, Assistant Commissioner
The Office of Special Education administers state and federal funds to support services for students and adults with disabilities.

State Agencies: Mississippi

2060 **Mississippi Department of Education: Office of Special Services**
359 North West Street
P.O. Box 771
Jackson, MS 39201
601-359-3513
FAX: 601-987-3892
www.mde.k12.ms.us
Dr Tom Burnham, Superintendent
Key priorities are: reading, early literacy, student achievement, teachers/teaching, leadership/principals, safe and orderly

schools, parent relations/community involvement, and technology.

State Agencies: Montana

2061 **Department of Public Health Human Services**
PO Box 4210
Helena, MT 59604-4210
406-444-5622
FAX: 406-444-1970
e-mail: hhsea@mt.gov
www.dphhs.mt.gov

Anna Whitin Sorrell, Director
Bernie Jacobs, Chief Legal Counsel
Deb Sloat, Human Resources Office
Jon Ebelt, Public Information Office

Provides consultation on educational services for local schools, offers psychological testing and evaluation, maintains resource rooms in district schools and more for the blind and handicapped throughout the state.

State Agencies: North Carolina

2062 **North Carolina Department of Public Instruction: Exceptional Children Division**
301 N Wilmington St
Raleigh, NC 27601
919-807-3300
FAX: 919-715-1569
e-mail: lharris@dpi.state.nc.us
www.ncpublicschools.org

June St. Clair Atkinson, Ed.D, State Superintendent of Public Instruction
Mike McLaughlin, Senior Policy Advisor to the State Superintendent
Rachel Beaulieu, Legislative & Community Affairs Director
Jeani Allen, Director of Internal Auditing

The mission is to assure that students with disabilities develop mentally, physically, emotionally, and vocationally through the provision of an appropriate individualized education in the least restrictive environment.

State Agencies: North Dakota

2063 **North Dakota Department of Education: Special Education**
600 E. Boulevard Avenue, Dept. 201
Floors 9, 10, and 11
Bismarck, ND 58505-0440
701-328-2260
866-741-3519
FAX: 701-328-2461
TTY: 701-328-4920
e-mail: mdanderson@nd.gov
www.dpi.state.nd.us

Kirsten Baesler, State Superintendent
Jerry Coleman, Director, School Finance & Organization
Linda Schloer, Child Nutrition & Food Distribution, Director
Gerry Teevens, Director, Special Education

Provides consultation on educational services for local schools, offers psychological testing and evaluation, maintains resource rooms in district schools and more for the blind and handicapped throughout the state.

State Agencies: Nebraska

2064 **Nebraska Department of Education: Special Populations Office**
1200 N Street, Suite 400
PO Box 98922
Lincoln, NE 68509
402-471-2186
877-253-2603
FAX: 402-471-2909
e-mail: NDEQ.moreinfo@Nebraska.gov
deq.ne.gov

Rod Gangwish Shelton, Council Member
Douglas Anderson Aurora, Council Member
Mark Whitehead Lincoln, Council Member
Mark Czaplewski Grand Islan, Council Member

Assists school districts in establishing and maintaining effective special education programs for children with disabilities (date of diagnosis through the school year when a child reaches 21). Major function: provide technical assistance to school districts and to parents of children with disabilities, assist programs in meeting state and federal special education regulations. Also responsible for assuring that the rights of children with disabilities and their parents are protected.

State Agencies: New Hampshire

2065 **Institute on Disability**
University of New Hampshire
10 West Edge Drive
Suite 101
Durham, NH 03824
603-862-4320
FAX: 603-862-0555
e-mail: contact.iod@unh.edu
www.iod.unh.edu

Charles E. Drum, Director & Professor
Andrew Houtenville, Director of Research
Matthew Gianino, Director of Communications
Mary Schuh, Director of Development and Consumer Affairs

Provides coherent university-based focus for the improvement of knowledge, policies, and practices related to the lives of persons with disabilities and their families.

2066 **New Hampshire Department of Education: Bureau for Special Education Services**
101 Pleasant Street
Concord, NH 03301-3860
603-271-3494
FAX: 603-271-1953
e-mail: Lori.Temple@doe.nh.gov
www.education.nh.gov

Santina Thibedeau, Administrator
Virginia Barry, Commissioner
Linda Breden, Secretary
Traci Biron, Secretary

The mission of Special Education is to improve educational outcomes for children and youth with disabilities by providing and promoting leadership, technical assistance and collaboration statewide. Provides oversight and implementation of federal and state laws that ensure a free appropriate public education for all children and youth with disabilities in New Hampshire.

State Agencies: New Jersey

2067 **New Jersey Department of Education: Office of Special Education Program**
New Jersey Department of Education
PO Box 500
Trenton, NJ 8625-500
609-292-0147
FAX: 609-984-8422
www.nj.gov/education/specialed/info/

Barbara Gantwerk, Director
Alfred Murray, Executive Director

State Agencies: New Mexico

2068 **New Mexico State Department of Education**
300 Don Gaspar Ave
Santa Fe, NM 87501-2744 505-827-6508
FAX: 505-827-6696
www.sde.state.nm.us

Bill Trant, Assistant Director
Judy Parks, Assistant Director
Provides consultation on educational services for local schools, offers psychological testing and evaluation, maintains resource rooms in district schools and more for the blind and handicapped throughout the state.

State Agencies: Nevada

2069 **Nevada Department of Education: Special Eduction Branch**
700 E Fifth St
Carson City, NV 89701-5096 775-687-9800
FAX: 775-687-9101
www.doe.nv.gov

Nick Gakalatos, Manager
The Office of Special Ed and School Improvement Program of the Nevada State Department of Education is responsible for management of state and federal programs providing educational opportunities for students with diverse learning needs. Included are such programs as: special education/disabled (IDEA); disadvantaged/at-risk programs (Title I/IASA); early childhood programs (Title I/ESEA); early childhood programs; migrant education; English language learners; NRS 395 student placement program.

State Agencies: New York

2070 **New York State Education Department**
1606 One Commerce Plz
Albany, NY 12234-1 518-474-5930
FAX: 518-486-6880
e-mail: nysed@mail.gov
www.nysed.gov

Bernard Margolis, Manager
Provides vocational rehabilitation and educational services for eligible individuals with disabilities throughout New York State. Services include evaluation, counseling, job placement, and referral to other agencies.

State Agencies: Ohio

2071 **Ohio Department of Education: Division of Special Education**
Ohio Department of Education
25 S Front St
Columbus, OH 43215-4183 614-995-1545
877-644-6338
FAX: 614-728-1097
TTY: 888-886-0181
www.ode.state.oh.us

Mike Armstrong, Manager
Provides technical assistance to educational agencies for the development and implementation of educational services to meet the needs of students with disabilities and/or those who are gifted. Provides information to parents. Administers state and federal funds allocated to educational agencies for the provision of services to students with disabilities and/or those who are gifted.

State Agencies: Oklahoma

2072 **Oklahoma State Department of Education**
2500 N Lincoln Blvd
Oklahoma City, OK 73105-4599 405-521-3301
FAX: 405-521-6205
www.sde.state.ok.us

Misty Kimbrough, Manager
Sandy Garrett, Administrator
Janet Barresi, State Superintendent
Provides consultation on educational services for local schools, offers psychological testing and evaluation, maintains resource rooms in district schools and more for the blind and handicapped throughout the state.

State Agencies: Oregon

2073 **Oregon Department of Education: Office of Special Education**
Oregon Department of Education:
255 Capitol St NE
Salem, OR 97310-1300 503-945-5600
FAX: 503-378-2897
www.dpeducation.com

Bruce Goldberg, Manager
Heidi Cockrell, Executive Assistant
Katy Coba, Executive Director
State agency ensuring provision of special education services to children with disabilities from birth to age 21.

State Agencies: Pennsylvania

2074 **Pennsylvania Department of Education: Bureau of Special Education**
333 Market St
Harrisburg, PA 17126-333 717-783-6788
FAX: 717-783-6139
TTY:717-783-8445
e-mail: 00specialed@psupen.psu.edu
www.pde.state.pa.us

Linda Rhen, Administrator
John Tommasini, Assistant Director
Provides effective and efficient administration of the Commonwealth of Pennsylvania's resources dedicated to enabling school districts to maintain high standards in the delivery of special education services and programs for all exceptional students.

State Agencies: Rhode Island

2075 **Rhode Island Department of Education: Office of Special Needs**
255 Westminster St
Providence, RI 2903 401-222-4600
FAX: 401-784-9513
www.ride.ri.gov

Al Moscola, Manager
Alfred Moscola, Manager
Provides consultation on educational services for local schools, offers psychological testing and evaluation, maintains resource rooms in district schools and more for the blind and handicapped throughout the state.

State Agencies: South Carolina

2076 South Carolina Assistive Technology Program (SCATP)
Center for Disability Resources
8301 Farrow Rd
Columbia, SC 29208-3245 803-935-5263
800-915-4522
FAX: 800-935-5342
e-mail: evelyne@cdd.sc.edu
www.sc.edu/scatp

Carol Page, Program Director
Mary Bechter, Program Coordinator
SCATP is a federally funded project concerned with getting technology into th hands of people with disabilities so that they might live, work, learn and be a more independent part of the community.

2077 South Carolina Department of Education: Office of Exceptional Children
1429 Senate St
Suite 808
Columbia, SC 29201-3730 803-734-8224
FAX: 803-734-4824
e-mail: sdeservicedesk@sde.ok.gov
www.scschools.com

Susan Durant, State Director
Provides consultation on educational services for local schools, offers psychological testing and evaluation, maintains resource rooms in district schools and more for the blind and handicapped throughout the state.

State Agencies: South Dakota

2078 South Dakota Department of Education & Cultural Affairs: Office of Special Education
700 Governors Dr
Pierre, SD 57501-2291 605-773-3804
FAX: 605-773-6041

Chelle Somsen, Manager
Dorothy Liegl, Manager

State Agencies: Tennessee

2079 Tennessee Department of Education
710 James Robertson Pkwy
Nashville, TN 37243-1219 615-741-2731
888-212-3162
FAX: 615-741-1791
www.state.tn.us/education

Ruth S Letson, Manager
Kevin Huffman, Commissioner
Provides consultation on educational services for local schools, offers psychological testing and evaluation, maintains resource rooms in district schools and more for the blind and handicapped throughout the state.

State Agencies: Texas

2080 Texas Education Agency
1701 N Congress Ave
Austin, TX 78701-1494 512-463-8532
FAX: 512-463-8057
www.tealighthouse.org

Shirley J Neeley, Commissioner of Education
Provides consultation on educational services for local schools, offers psychological testing and evaluation, maintains resource rooms in district schools and more for the blind and handicapped throughout the state.

2081 Texas Education Agency: Special Education Unit
1701 Congress Ave
PO Box 420637
Austin, TX 77242-637 512-463-8532
FAX: 512-463-8057
e-mail: info@tdea.org
www.tdea.org

Gene Lenz, Deputy Associate Commissioner
Shirley Neeley, Administrator

2082 Texas School of the Deaf
1102 S Congress Ave
Austin, TX 78704-1791 512-462-5353
800-332-3873
FAX: 512-462-5424
e-mail: ercod@tsd.state.tx.us
tsd.state.tx.us

Claire Bugen, Superintendent
Russell West, Residential Services Director
Gary Bego, Business and Operations Director
Brenda Fraenkel, Special Education Director
Ensures that students excel in an environment where they learn, grow and belong. Supports deaf students, families and professionals in Texas by providing resources through outreach services.

State Agencies: Utah

2083 Utah State Office of Education: At-Risk and Special Education Service Unit
Utah State Office of Education
250 East 500 South
P.O.Box 144200
Salt Lake City, UT 84114-4200 801-538-7500
FAX: 801-538-7521
e-mail: webmaster@schools.utah.gov
schools.utah.gov

Sandra Cox, Financial Analyst
Mark Peterson, Director
Glenna Gallo, State Director of Special Educat
Rebecca Donovan, Administrative Secretary
Provides consultation on educational services for local schools, offers psychological testing and evaluation, maintains resource rooms in district schools and more for the blind and handicapped throughout the state.

State Agencies: Virginia

2084 Virginia Department of Education: Divisionof Pre & Early Adolescent Education
Virginia Department Of Education
James Monroe Building, 101, N. 14th
P.O.Box 2120
Richmond, VA 23219 804-236-3631
FAX: 804-236-3635
e-mail: webmaster@doe.virginia.gov
www.pen.k12.va.us

Dr. Steven R Staples, Superintendent of Public Instruction
Kent Dickey, Deputy Superintendent, Finance & Operations
Chris Sorensen, Director, Budget
Becky Marable, Director, Human Resources
Provides consultation on educational services for local schools, offers psychological testing and evaluation, maintains resource rooms in district schools and more for the blind and handicapped throughout the state.

State Agencies: Washington

2085 **Superintendent of Public Instruction: Special Education Section**
Old Capitol Building, 600 Washingto
P.O. Box 47200
Olympia, WA 98504-7200 360-725-6000
FAX: 360-586-0247
TTY:360-664-3631
e-mail: webmaster@k12.wa.us
www.k12.wa.us

Randy I. Dorn, State Superintendent of Public I
Alan Burke, Deputy Superintendent
Robert Butts, Assistant Superintendent
Bob Harmon, Assistant Superintendent
Provides leadership, service and support for the development and implementation of research-based curriculum to assure that all learners achieve at all levels.

State Agencies: West Virginia

2086 **West Virginia Department of Education: Office of Special Education**
Rm 6
1900 Kanawha Blvd E
Charleston, WV 25305-0001 304-558-3660
FAX: 304-558-3741
e-mail: http://wvde.state.wv.us/boe/
wvde.state.wv.us

Liza Cordeiro, Executive Director
Mary Nunn, Assistant Director
Marshall Patton, Executive Director
Brenda Williams, Executive Director
Provides consultation on educational services for local schools, offers psychological testing and evaluation, maintains resource rooms in district schools and more for the blind and handicapped throughout the state.

State Agencies: Wyoming

2087 **Wyoming Department of Education**
2300 Capitol Avenue
Hathaway Building, 2nd Floor
Cheyenne, WY 82002-2060 307-777-7690
FAX: 307-777-6234
edu.wyoming.gov

Cindy Hill, WDE Superintendent
Deb Lindsey, Division Administrator, Assessment
Teri Wigert, Division Administrator, Support Systems & Resources
Dianne Bailey, Division Administrator, Finance & Data
Mission is to lead, model, and support continuous improvement of education for everyone in Wyoming.

Magazines & Journals

2088 **Adapted Physical Activity Programs**
Human Kinetics
1607 N. Market Street
P.O.Box 5076
Champaign, IL 61820 800-747-4457
FAX: 217-351-1549
e-mail: info@hkusa.com
www.humankinetics.com

Patty Lehn, Publicity Manager
Lori Cooper, Marketing Manager
Bill Dobrik, Sales Associate
Dan Stebel, Sales Associate
Human Kinetics produces a variety of resources for adapted physical education practitioners, including books on activities, a research journal and higher education references. *$24.00*
Quarterly
ISSN 0736-58 9

2089 **Advance for Providers of Post-Acute Care**
Merion Publications
2900 Horizon Drive
King of Prussia, PA 19406 610-278-1400
800-355-5627
FAX: 610-278-1421
e-mail: webmaster@advanceweb.com
advanceweb.com

Timothy Baum, MS, CRNP, Author
A free magazine for providers of post-acute care.

2090 **CEC Catalog**
Council for Exceptional Children
2900 Crystal Drive
Suite 1000
Arlington, VA 22202-3557 703-620-3660
866-509-0218
888-232-7733
FAX: 703-264-9494
TTY:866-915-5000
e-mail: service@cec.sped.org
www.cec.sped.org

Robin D. Brewer, President
James P. Heiden, President Elect
Christy A. Chambers, Immediate Past President
Mikki Garcia, Executive Director
Semi-annual catalog from the Council for Exceptional Children offering books, guides, materials, products and services for the special educator.
18 pages

2091 **Case Manager Magazine**
Elsevier Health
3251 Riverport Lane
Maryland Heights, MO 63043 314-447-8070
800-222-9570
e-mail: textbook@elsevier.com
journals.elsevierhealth.com

Thomas Reller, Vice President Global Corporate
Harald Boersma, Senior Manager Corporate Relatio
Ylann Schemm, Corporate Relations Manager
Sacha Boucherie, Press Officer
This national magazine is for medical case managers, social workers, counselors and home health professionals who work with people with serious injury or illness. It is a membership benefit of CMSA, the national association for case managers. *$55.00*
84 pages BiMonthly

2092 **Catalyst**
The Catalyst
Ste 275
1259 El Camino Real
Menlo Park, CA 94025-4208 800-647-0314
e-mail: info@thecatalyst.us
www.thecatalyst.us

Sue Swezey, Editor
Digest of news and information on the use of computers in special education. *$15.00*
20 pages Quarterly

2093 **Clinical Connection**
American Advertising Dist of Northern Virginia
708 Pendleton St
Alexandria, VA 22314-1819 703-549-5126
FAX: 703-548-5563
www.onlineceus.com

Kathie Harrington, M.A., CCC, Author
Covers speech language pathology.

2094 **College and University**
AACRAO
One Dupont Circle NW
Suite 520
Washington, DC 20036
202-293-9161
FAX: 202-872-8857
e-mail: reillym@aacrao.org
aacrao.org

Brad Myers, President
Dan Garcia, President Elect
Adrienne McDay, Past President
Stan DeMerritt, VP, Finance

Scholarly research journal. American Association of Collegiate Registrars and Admissions Offers (AACRAO) is a nonprofit, voluntary, professional, educational association of degree-granting, postsecondary institutions, government agencies, private educational organizations and education-oriented businesses in the United States and abroad. $80 per year US; $90 per year international.

30 pages Quarterly
ISSN 0010-0889

2095 **Continuing Care**
Stevens Publishing Corporation
14901 Quorum Dr,
Suite 425
Dallas, TX 75254
972-687-6700
FAX: 972-687-6750
e-mail: info@1105media.com
1105media.com

Neal Vitale, President & Chief Executive Officer
Richard Vitale, Senior Vice President & Chief Financial Officer
Mike Valenti, Executive Vice President
Jeff Klein, Non-Executive Chairman of the Board

A national magazine for case management and discharge planning professionals published monthly except for December. *$119.00*

34 pages Monthly

2096 **Counseling Psychologist**
American Psychological Association
2455 Teller Road
Thousand Oaks, CA 91320
805-499-0721
800-818-7243
FAX: 800-583-2665
e-mail: info@sagepub.com
www.sagepub.com

Sara Miller McCune, Founder, Publisher & Executive Chairman
Blaise R Simqu, President/CEO
Chris Hickok, Senior Vice President & Chief Financial Officer
Stephen Barr, Managing Director/SAGE London

Thematic issues in the theory, research and practice of counseling psychology. *$78.00*

Bi-Monthly

2097 **Counseling and Values**
American Counseling Association
5999 Stevenson Ave
Alexandria, VA 22304
703-823-0252
800-347-6647
FAX: 800-473-2329
e-mail: webmaster@counseling.org
counseling.org

Robert L. Smith, President
Thelma Duffey, President Elect
Brian Canfield, Treasurer
Richard Yep, CEO

Counseling and Values is the official journal of the Association for Spiritual, Ethical, and Religious Values in Counseling (ASERVIC), a member association of the American Counseling Association. Counseling and Values s a professional journal of theory, research, and informed opinion concerned with the relationships among psychology, philosophy, religion, social values, and counseling. *$12.00*

TriAnnual

2098 **Directions: Technology in Special Education**
DREAMMS for Kids
273 Ringwood Road
Freeville, NY 13068-5606
607-539-3027
FAX: 607-539-9930
e-mail: Greetings@dreamms.org
www.dreamms.org

Janet P Hosmer, Publisher & Editor in Chief
Kathy S. Knight, Editor
Chester D. Hosmer, Jr, Technical Editor
Lorianne Hoenninger, Regular Contributor

Provides technology tips to ease home instruction and use; describes and reviews adaptive educational software and hardware; reviews pertinent literature and audio and videotapes; describes adaptive and assistive technology devices; provides on-line service information for the disabled; announces upcoming educational and technology conference; and reports on new Department of Education legislation. *$14.95*

Monthly

2099 **Early Intervention**
Early Childhood Intervention Clearinghouse
51 Gerty Drive
Room 20
Champaign, IL 61820-7469
217-333-1386
877-275-3227
FAX: 217-244-7732
e-mail: Illinois-eic@illinois.edu
www.eiclearinghouse.org

Susan Fowler, Director

Features articles, conference calendar, material reviews and news concerning early childhood intervention and disability.

4 pages Quarterly

2100 **Exceptional Children**
Council for Exceptional Children
2900 Crystal Drive
Suite 1000
Arlington, VA 22202-3557
703-620-3660
866-509-0218
888-232-7733
FAX: 703-264-9494
TTY:866-915-5000
e-mail: service@cec.sped.org
cec.sped.org

Robin D. Brewer, President
James P. Heiden, President Elect
Christy A. Chambers, Immediate Past President
Mikki Garcia, Executive Director

Articles include research, literature surveys and position papers concerning exceptional children, special education and mainstreaming. *$58.00*

96 pages BiMonthly

2101 **Focus on Autism and Other Developmental Disabilities**
Sage Publications
2455 Teller Road
Thousand Oaks, CA 91320
805-499-0721
800-818-7243
FAX: 800-583-2665
e-mail: info@sagepub.com
www.sagepub.com

Sara Miller McCune, Founder, Publisher & Executive Chairman
Blaise R. Simqu, President & CEO
Chris Hickok, Senior Vice President & Chief Financial Officer
Stephen Barr, Managing Director/SAGE London

Practical management, treatment and planning strategies; a must for persons working with individuals with autism and other developmental disabilities. *$43.00*

64 pages Quarterly

2102 **Focus on Exceptional Children**
Love Publishing Company
9101 East Kenyon Avenue
Suite 2200
Denver, CO 80237
303-221-7333
FAX: 303-221-7444
e-mail: lpc@lovepublishing.com
www.lovepublishing.com
Steve Graham, Consulting Editor
Ron Nelson, Consulting Editor
Eva Horn, Consulting Editor
Contains research and theory-based articles on special education topics, with an emphasis on application and intervention, of interest to teachers, professors and administrators. *$36.00*
Monthly

2103 **HomeCare Magazine**
Trimedia Publications
1900 28th Avenue South
Suite 200
Birmingham, AL 35209
205-212-9402
cahabamedia.com
Greg Meineke, VP, Sales
Michelle Sergrest, VP of Editorial
Wally Evans, Publisher
Terri Gray, Creative Director
The business magazine of the home medical equipment industry offering information on legislation and regulations affecting the homecare industry, monthly profiles of suppliers, operational tips, newest products in the industry, advice on sales, government regulations. *$ 65.00*
120 pages Monthly

2104 **I Wonder Who Else Can Help**
AARP
601 E Street NW
Washington, DC 20049
202-434-3525
888-687-2277
877-342-2277
FAX: 202-434-3443
e-mail: member@aarp.org
www.aarp.org
John Wider, President, CEO, AARP Services Inc.
Lisa M. Ryerson, President, AARP Foundation
Robert R. Hagans, Jr., Executive Vice President & Chief Financial Officer
Hollis Terry Bradwell III, Executive Vice President & Chief Information Officer
Contains information about crisis counseling, needs and resources, written in lay terms.

2105 **International Rehabilitation Review**
Rehabilitation International
41 Madison Avenue
Office 3141
New York, NY 10010
212-420-1500
FAX: 212-505-0871
e-mail: info@riglobal.org
riglobal.org
Anne Hawker, President
Patric Fougeyrollas, Deputy Vice President for the No
Marca Bristo, Vice President for the North Ame
Martin Grabois, Treasurer
International overview of activities and programs in vocational and medical rehabilitation, prosthesis and orthotics and special education. *$30.00*
TriAnnual

2106 **Intervention in School and Clinic**
Sage Publications
2455 Teller Road
Thousand Oaks, CA 91320
805-499-0721
800-818-7243
FAX: 800-583-2665
e-mail: info@sagepub.com
www.sagepub.com
Sara Miller McCune, Founder, Publisher & Executive Chairman
Blaise R. Simqu, President & CEO
Chris Hickok, Senior Vice President & Chief Financial Officer
Stephen Barr, Managing Director/SAGE London
A hands-on, how-to resource for teachers and clinicians working with students for whom minor curriculum and environmental modifications are ineffective. *$35.00*
64 pages

2107 **Journal for Vocational Special Needs Education**
University of Wisconsin
1025 W Johnson St
Madison, WI 53706-1706
608-263-9250
FAX: 608-262-3050
e-mail: jgugerty@education.wisc.edu
www.cew.wisc.edu/jvsne/
John Gugerty, Co-Editor
Articles on vocational education for special needs population, including persons with physical and mental disabilities. *$16.00*

2108 **Journal of Applied School Psychology**
Haworth Press
711 Third Avenue
New York, NY 10017
212-216-7800
800-354-1420
FAX: 212-244-1563
e-mail: subscriptions@tandf.co.uk.
www.haworthpress.com
BiAnnually

2109 **Journal of Counseling & Development**
American Counseling Association
5999 Stevenson Ave
Alexandria, VA 22304-3304
703-823-0252
800-347-6647
FAX: 800-473-2329
e-mail: webmaster@counseling.org
counseling.org
Robert L. Smith, President
Thelma Duffey, President Elect
Brian Canfield, Treasurer
Richard Yep, CEO
Publishes archival material, also publishes articles that have broad interest for a readership composed mostly of counselors and other mental health professionals who work in private practice, schools, colleges, community agencies, hospitals, and government. An appropriate outlet for articles that: critically integrate published research; examine current professional and scientific issues; report research, new techniques, innovative programs and practices; and examine ACA as an organization. *$140.00*
128 pages Quarterly

2110 **Journal of Emotional and Behavioral Disorders**
Sage Publications
2455 Teller Road
Thousand Oaks, CA 91320
805-499-0721
800-818-7243
FAX: 800-583-2665
e-mail: info@sagepub.com
www.sagepub.com
Sara Miller McCune, Founder, Publisher & Executive Chairman
Blaise R. Simqu, President & CEO
Chris Hickok, Senior Vice President & Chief Financial Officer
Stephen Barr, Managing Director/SAGE London
An international, multidisciplinary journal featuring articles on research, practice and theory related to individuals with emo-

tional and behavioral disorders and to the professionals who serve them. *$39.00*
64 pages Quarterly

2111 Journal of Learning Disabilities
Sage Publications
2455 Teller Road
Thousand Oaks, CA 91320
805-499-0721
800-818-7243
FAX: 800-583-2665
e-mail: info@sagepub.com
www.sagepub.com
Sara Miller McCune, Founder, Publisher & Executive Chairman
Blaise R. Simqu, President & CEO
Chris Hickok, Senior Vice President & Chief Financial Officer
Stephen Barr, Managing Director/SAGE London
An international, multidisciplinary publication containing articles on practice, research and theory related to learning disabilities. Published bi-monthly. *$49.00*
Magazine

2112 Journal of Motor Behavior
Heldref Publications
325 Chestnut Street
Suite 800
Philadelphia, PA 19106
215-625-8900
800-354-1420
FAX: 215-625-2940
e-mail: customer.service@taylorandfrancis.com
www.heldref.org
Emilli Pawlowsky, Marketing Manager
Laura Rosse, Assistant Marketing Manager
Douglas Kirkpatrick, Publisher
A professional journal aimed at psychologists, therapists and educators who work in the areas of motor behavior, psychology, neurophysiology, kinesiology, and biomechanics. Offers up-to-date information on the latest techniques, theories and developments concerning motor control. Titles previously published by Heldref Publications will be joining the T&F portfolio. *$77.00*
115 pages Quarterly

2113 Journal of Musculoskeletal Pain
Haworth Press
711 Third Avenue
New York, NY 10017
212-216-7800
800-354-1420
FAX: 212-244-1563
e-mail: subscriptions@tandf.co.uk.
www.haworthpress.com
110 pages Quarterly

2114 Journal of Postsecondary Education & Disability
AHEAD
107 Commerce Centre Drive
Suite 204
Huntersville, NC 28078
704-947-7779
FAX: 704-948-7779
e-mail: information@ahead.org
www.ahead.org/publications/jped
Stephan J. Smith, Executive Director
Richard Allegra, Director, Professional Development
Jeremy Jarrell, Director, Innovation & Development
Oanh Huynh, Associate Executive Director
Provides in-depth examination of research, issues, policies and programs in postsecondary education.

2115 Journal of Prosthetics and Orthotics
330 John Carlyle Street
Suite 210
Alexandria, VA 22314
703-836-7114
FAX: 703-836-0838
e-mail: info@abcop.org
www.abcop.org
Catherine Carter, Executive Director
Debbie Ayres, Director, Marketing & Public Relations
Stephen Fletcher, CPO, LPO, Director, Clinical Resources
Heather Harris, Director, Continuing Education Programs
Provides the latest research and clinical thinking in orthotics and prosthetics, including information on new devices, fitting techniques and patient management experiences. Each issue contains research-based information and articles reviewed and approved by a highly qualified editorial board. *$60.00*
64 pages Quarterly
ISSN 1040-88 0

2116 Journal of Reading, Writing and Learning Disabled International
Hemisphere Publishing Corporation
7625 Empire Drive
Florence, KY 41042-2919
800-634-7064
FAX: 800-248-4724
e-mail: orders@taylorandfrancis.com
www.taylorandfrancis.com

2117 Journal of School Health Association
Suite 403
4340 East West Highway
Bethesda, MD 20814
301-652-8072
FAX: 301-652-8077
e-mail: info@ashaweb.org
ashaweb.org
Jeffrey K. Clark, President
Stephen Conley, Executive Director
Julie Greenfield, Marketing and Conferences Direct
Beverly Samek, Chair of Advocacy
This is a monthly journal which offers information to professionals and parents on school health. Membership dues, $95.00.

2118 Journal of Special Education
Sage Publications
2455 Teller Road
Thousand Oaks, CA 91320
805-499-0721
800-818-7243
FAX: 800-583-2665
e-mail: info@sagepub.com
www.sagepub.com
Sara Miller McCune, Founder, Publisher & Executive Chairman
Blaise R. Simqu, President & CEO
Chris Hickok, Senior Vice President & Chief Financial Officer
Stephen Barr, Managing Director/SAGE London
Internationally known as the prime research journal in special education. JSE provides research articles of special education for individuals with disabilities, ranging from mild to severe. Published quarterly. *$39.00*
Magazine

2119 Journal of Vocational Behavior
Academic Press, Journals Division
www.academicpress.com/jvb

2120 MDA Newsmagazine
Muscular Dystrophy Association
3300 E. Sunrise Drive
Tucson, AZ 85718
520-529-2000
800-572-1717
FAX: 520-795-3989
e-mail: tusconservices@mdausa.org
alsn.mda.org
Danielle Trzyna, Manager
Presents news related to muscular dystrophy and other neuromuscular diseases including research, personal profiles, fundraising activities and patient services.

2121 Measurement and Evaluation in Counseling
5999 Stevenson Ave
Alexandria, VA 22304-3304 703-823-0252
800-347-6647
FAX: 800-473-2329
e-mail: webmaster@counseling.org
www.counseling.org

Robert L. Smith, President
Thelma Duffey, President Elect
Brian Canfield, Treasurer
Richard Yep, CEO

The American Counseling Association is a not-for-profit, professional and educational organization that is dedicated to the growth and enhancement of the counseling profession

2122 Our World
National Center for Learning Disabilities
381 Park Avenue South
Suite 1401
New York, NY 10016 212-545-7510
800-575-7373
888-575-7373
FAX: 212-545-9665
e-mail: help@ncld.org
ncld.org

Frederic M. Poses, Chairman, CEO
Mary Kalikow, Vice Chairman
John R. Langeler, Treasurer
William Haney, Secretary

Contains features, articles, human interest news and information and information, and other practical material to benefit the millions of children and adults with learning disabilities and their families, as well as educators and other helping professionals. Magazine.
Quarterly

2123 Psychiatric Staffing Crisis in Community Mental Health
Nat l Council for Community Behavioral Healthcare
76 Ninth Avenue
New York, NY 10011 201-559-3882
800-THE-BOOK
e-mail: amilevoj@bn.com
www.barnesandnoble.com

Andy Milevoj, Vice President, Investor Relations
Mary Ellen Keating, SVP, Corporate Communications & Public Affairs
Carolyn Brown, Director of Corporate Communications

Find out some of the simple, low-cost ways you can increase workplace satisfaction among staff psychiatrists and compete successfully for their talents. *$20.00*

2124 Readings: A Journal of Reviews and Commentary in Mental Health
American Orthopsychiatric Association
3524 Washington Avenue
P.O. Box 1048
Sheboygan, WI 53081-1048 920-457-5051
800-558-7687
FAX: 920-457-1485
e-mail: info@americanortho.com
www.americanortho.com

Michael Bogenschuetz, President
Randy Benz, Chief Executive Officer
Charles Achter, Assistant Controller
Deb Schmidt, Administrative Manager

Reviews of recent books in mental health and allied disciplines. Includes essay reviews and brief reviews. *$25.00*
32 pages Quarterly

2125 Rehab Pro
1926 Waukegan Rd
Suite 1
Glenview, IL 60025-1770 847-657-6964
FAX: 847-657-6963
e-mail: carlw@tcag.com
www.rehabpro.org

Carl Wangman, Executive Director

The magazine is to promote the profession and to inform the public about the activities of the national organization, its state chapter affiliates, and the work of its special interest sections.
38 pages BiMonthly

2126 Remedial and Special Education
Sage Publications
2455 Teller Road
Thousand Oaks, CA 91320 805-499-0721
800-818-7243
FAX: 800-583-2665
e-mail: info@sagepub.com
www.sagepub.com

Sara Miller McCune, Founder, Publisher & Executive Chairman
Blaise R. Simqu, President & CEO
Chris Hickok, Senior Vice President & Chief Financial Officer
Stephen Barr, Managing Director/SAGE London

A professional journal that bridges the gap between theory and practice. Emphasis is on topical reviews, syntheses of research, field evaluation studies and recommendations for the practice of remedial and special education. Published six times a year.
$39.00
64 pages

2127 Teaching Exceptional Children
Council for Exceptional Children
2900 Crystal Drive
Suite 1000
Arlington, VA 22202-3557 703-620-3660
866-509-0218
888-232-7733
FAX: 703-264-9494
TTY:866-915-5000
e-mail: service@cec.sped.org
www.cec.sped.org

Robin D. Brewer, President
James P. Heiden, President Elect
Christy A. Chambers, Immediate Past President
Mikki Garcia, Executive Director

Journal designed for teachers of gifted students and students with disabilities, featuring practical methods and materials for classroom use. *$58.00*
96 pages BiMonthly

Newsletters

2128 Alert
Association on Handicapped Student Service Program
P.O.Box 21192
Columbus, OH 43221 614-365-5216
FAX: 614-365-6718

2129 Camp Virginia Jaycee Newsletter
Dare Care Charity
2494 Camp Jaycee Rd
P.O. Box 648
Blue Ridge, VA 24064 540-947-2972
e-mail: info@campvajc.org
www.campvajc.org

Tom King, Chairman
Kathleen King, Vice Chair
Lisa Parrish, Treasurer
William Hartz, Past Chair

Summer camping for children and adults with developmental disabilities. Coed, ages 7-70. Weekend respite camps for children and adults with mental retardation.
8 pages quarterly

2130 Counseling Today
American Counseling Association
5999 Stevenson Ave
Alexandria, VA 22304-3304 703-823-0252
800-347-6647
FAX: 800-473-2329
e-mail: webmaster@counseling.org
counseling.org

Robert L. Smith, President
Thelma Duffey, President Elect
Brian Canfield, Treasurer
Richard Yep, CEO
Aims to serve individuals active in professional counseling, in the school and university, in the workplace and the marketplace, as well as other citizens, community leaders and policy makers who appreciate the importance of the role of professional counselors in today's society.
Monthly

2131 Counselor Education and Supervision
American Counseling Association
5999 Stevenson Ave
Alexandria, VA 22304-3304 703-823-0252
800-347-6647
FAX: 800-473-2329
e-mail: webmaster@counseling.org
www.counseling.org

Robert L. Smith, President
Thelma Duffey, President Elect
Brian Canfield, Treasurer
Richard Yep, CEO
Dedicated to the growth and development of the counseling profession and those who are served. *$18.00*
Quarterly

2132 Counterpoint
National Association of State Directors of Special
10860 Hampton Rd
Fairfax Station, VA 22039-2700 703-519-3800
FAX: 703-503-8627

Quarterly

2133 Disability Compliance for Higher Education
LRP Publications
P.O. Box 24668
West Palm Beach, FL 33416-4668 561-622-2423
800-341-7874
FAX: 561-622-1375
e-mail: custserve@lrp.com
lrp.com

Kenneth F. Kahn, Owner and President
Ed Chase, Vice President
The only newsletter that is dedicated to the exclusive coverage of disability issues that affect colleges and universities. *$195.00*
8 pages Monthly

2134 Disability Resources Monthly
Disability Resources
4 Glatter Ln
South Setauket, NY 11720-1032 631-585-0290
FAX: 631-585-0290
e-mail: pubs@disabilityresources.org
disabilityresources.org

Avery Klauber, Executive Director
A newsletter that monitors, reviews and reports on resources for independent living. A monthly newsletter that features short topical articles, news items and reviews of books, pamphlets, periodicals, videotapes, on-line services, organizations and other resources for and about people with disabilities. It is intended primarily for librarians, social workers, educators, rehabilitation specialists, disability advocates, ADA coordinators and other health and social service professionals. *$33.00*
4 pages Monthly
ISSN 1070-72 0

2135 Early Childhood Reporter
LRP Publications
P.O. Box 24668
West Palm Beach, FL 33416-4668 561-622-2423
800-341-7874
FAX: 561-622-1375
e-mail: custserve@lrp.com
www.lrp.com

Kenneth F. Kahn, Owner and President
Ed Chase, Vice President
Monthly reports with information on federal, state, and local legislation affecting the implementation of early intervention and preschool programs for children with disabilities. *$145.00*
12-16 pages $10 shipping

2136 Healthline
CV Mosby Company
1600 John F. Kennedy Boulevard
Suite 1800
Philadelphia, PA 19103-2822 215-239-3900
800-523-1649
FAX: 215-239-3990
www.us.elsevierhealth.com

Monthly

2137 Help Newsletter
Learning Disabilities Association of Arkansas
P.O. Box 23514
Little Rock, AR 72221 501-666-8777
FAX: 501-666-8777
e-mail: info@ldaarkansas.org
www.ldaarkansas.org

Nathan Green, President
Rebecca Walker, VP
Becca Green, Past President, Treasurer
Doris Pierce, Secretary
Information on how to overcome obstacles and to achieve in spite of learning disabilities. *$30.00*
8 pages Quarterly

2138 International Rolf Institute
5055 Chaparral Ct.
Suite 103
Boulder, CO 80301 303-449-5903
800-530-8875
FAX: 303-449-5978
e-mail: dyourell@rolf.org
rolf.org

Kevin McCoy, Chairperson
Diana Yourell, Executive Director
Jim Jones, Director of Education
Carah Wertheimer, Admissions Advisor
Information, practitioner training and certification.

2139 Learning Disabilities Consultants Newsletter
Learning Disabilities Consultants
P.O.Box 716
Bryn Mawr, PA 19010 610-446-6126
800-869-8336
FAX: 610-446-6129
e-mail: rcooper-ldr@comcast.net
www.thebrookhospitals.com/Resources/Childrens

Richard Cooper, Director
Newsletter providing information about learning disabilities and differences. It contains both local and national news items and includes in each issue articles about various aspects of learning problems encountered in both children and adults. *$10.00*
6 pages 5x Year

2140 MA Report
National Allergy and Asthma Network
Ste 200
3554 Chain Bridge Rd
Fairfax, VA 22030-2709 703-385-4403
FAX: 703-352-4354

Monthly

2141 NYALD News
New York Association for the Learning Disabled
90 S Swan St
Albany, NY 12210-2105 518-465-6115

Kelly Jarrard, Executive Director
Michael Vacek, Manager
Newsletter offering information on the learning disabled in the New York area.
Monthly

2142 O&P Almanac
American Orthotic & Prosthetic Association
330 John Carlyle Street
Suite 200
Alexandria, VA 22314 571-431-0876
FAX: 571-431-0899
e-mail: info@aopanet.org
www.aopanet.org

Anita Liberman-Lampear, MA, President
Charles H. Dankmeyer, Jr, CPO, President-Elect
James Campbell, CO, Ph.D., Vice President
Jim Weber, MBA, Treasurer
Offers in-depth coverage on orthotics and prosthetics to current professional, government, business and reimbursement activities affecting the orthotics and prosthetics industry. *$59.00*
80 pages Monthly

2143 Occupational Therapy in Health Care
Haworth Press
711 Third Avenue
New York, NY 10017 212-216-7800
800-354-1420
FAX: 212-244-1563
e-mail: subscriptions@tandf.co.uk
www.haworthpress.com

2144 Ohio Coalition for the Education of Children with Disabilities
165 W Center St, 3rd Floor, Chase B
Suite 302
Marion, OH 43302 740-382-5452
800-374-2806
FAX: 740-383-6421
e-mail: ocecd@ocecd.org
www.ocecd.org

Martha Lause, Manager
Lee Ann Derugen, Co-Director
Margaret Burley, Executive Director
Lee Ann Derugen, Co-Director
Forum is a newsletter reporting on educational, legislative and other developments affecting persons with disabilities.
8 pages

2145 SAMHSA News
U S Department of Health and Human Services
1 Choke Cherry Road
Rockville, MD 20857 202-690-7650
877-SAM-SA 7
TTY:800-487-4889
www.samhsa.gov

Pamela S. Hyde, J.D., Administrator
Kana Enomoto, M.A., Principal Deputy Administrator
Daryl W. Kade, M.A., Chief Financial Officer and Director,OFR
Marla Hendriksson, M.P.M., Director, Office of Communications
This quarterly agency newsletter reports on information on substance abuse, mental health treatment and prevention programs of the Substance Abuse and Mental Health Services Administration.
Quarterly

2146 Sibling Information Network Newsletter
AJ Pappanikou Center
270 Farmington Avenue
Suite 181
Farmington, CT 06030 860-679-1500
866-623-1315
FAX: 860-679-1571
TTY: 860-679-1502
e-mail: contact.us.ucedd@uchc.edu
www.uconnucedd.org

Mary Beth Bruder, PhD, UCEDD/LEND Director
Gerarda Hanna, J.D., M.Ed., Associate UCEDD Director
Gabriela Freyre-Calish, MSW, Coordinator, Director, Cultural Diversity
Linda Procko, Program Coordinator
Contains information aimed at the varying interested of our membership. Program descriptions, requests for assistance, conference announcements, literature summaries and research reports.
$8.50

2147 Sibpage
AJ Pappanikou Center
270 Farmington Avenue
Suite 181
Farmington, CT 06030 860-679-1500
866-623-1315
FAX: 860-679-1571
TTY: 860-679-1502
e-mail: contact.us.ucedd@uchc.edu
www.uconnucedd.org

Mary Beth Bruder, PhD, UCEDD/LEND Director
Gerarda Hanna, J.D., M.Ed., Associate UCEDD Director
Gabriela Freyre-Calish, MSW, Coordinator, Director, Cultural Diversity
Linda Procko, Program Coordinator
Developed specifically for children containing games, recipes, pen pals, and articles written by siblings relating to developmental disabilities.
4 pages

2148 Special Edge
Resources in Special Education
Fl 4
1107 9th St
Sacramento, CA 95814-3616 916-492-9999
877-493-7833
FAX: 916-492-4004
e-mail: rise@wested.org

Virigina Reynolds, President
Provides education news, collaborative programs, amendments to the laws, tools for accommodations, resource information, a calendar of events, and more.
BiMonthly

2149 Special Education Report
LRP Publications
P.O. Box 24668
West Palm Beach, FL 33416-4668 561-622-2423
800-341-7874
FAX: 561-622-1375
e-mail: custserve@lrp.com
lrp.com

Kenneth F. Kahn, Owner and President
Ed Chase, Vice President
Current, pertinent information about federal legislation, regulations, programs and funding for educating children with disabilities. Covers federal and state litigation on the Individuals with Disabilities Education Act and other relevant laws. Looks at innovations and research in the field. *$266.00*
8 pages BiWeekly
ISSN 0194-22 5

2150 Topics in Early Childhood Special Education
Sage Publications
2455 Teller Road
Thousand Oaks, CA 91320 805-499-0721
800-818-7243
FAX: 800-583-2665
e-mail: info@sagepub.com
www.sagepub.com
Sara Miller McCune, Founder, Publisher & Executive Chairman
Blaise R. Simqu, President & CEO
Chris Hickok, Senior Vice President & Chief Financial Officer
Stephen Barr, Managing Director/SAGE London
Designed for professionals helping young children with special needs in areas such as assessment, special programs, social policies and developmental aids. *$43.00*
Quarterly

2151 Treatment Review
AIDS Treatment Data Network
57 Willoughby St.
2nd Floor
Brooklyn, NY 11201 347-473-7400
800-734-7104
TTY:212-925-9560
e-mail: info@housingworks.org
www.housingworks.org
Charles King, Chair
Linney Smith, Vice Chair
Earl Ward, Vice Chair
Andrew Coarney, Secretary
Individual members receive treatment education, counseling, referrals and case management support. Services are available in both English and Spanish. The Treatment Review newsletter includes descriptions of approved, alternative and experimental treatments, as well as announcements of seminars and forums on treatments and clinical trials.
Quarterly

2152 VIP Newsletter
Blind Children's Fund
6761 West US 12
P.O. Box 363
Three Oaks, MI 49128 989-779-9966
FAX: 269-756-3133
e-mail: BCF@blindchildrensfund.org
www.blindchildrensfund.org
Karla B. Kwast, Executive Director
Jeremy Murphy, President
Robert R. Storrer Jr., Vice President
Carrie L. Owens, Director
Provides parents and professionals with information, materials and resources that help them successfully teach and nurture blind, visually and multi-impaired infants and preschoolers. *$10.00*

Professional Texts

2153 A Teacher's Guide to Isovaleric Acidemia
150 North 18th Avenue
Phoenix, AZ 85007 602-542-1025
FAX: 602-542-0883
www.azdhs.gov
Will Humble, Director
Thomas Salow, Manager
Resource book for preschool teachers and school staff on isovaleric academia basics and classroom activities. *$2.50*

2154 A Teacher's Guide to Methylmalonic Acidemia
Arizona State Department of Health Services
150 North 18th Avenue
Phoenix, AZ 85007 602-542-1025
FAX: 602-542-0883
www.azdhs.gov
Will Humble, Director
Thomas Salow, Manager
Resource book for preschool teachers and school staff on methylmalonic academia basics and classroom activities. *$2.50*

2155 A Teacher's Guide to PKU
Arizona Department of Health Services
150 North 18th Avenue
Phoenix, AZ 85007 602-542-1025
FAX: 602-542-0883
www.azdhs.gov
Will Humble, Director
Thomas Salow, Manager
Resource book for preschool teachers and school staff on PKU basics, NutraSweet warning, and classroom activities. *$2.50*
13 pages

2156 ADD Challenge: A Practical Guide for Teachers
2612 N. Mattis Ave.
P.O. Box 7886
Champaign, IL 61822 217-352-3273
800-519-2707
FAX: 217-352-1221
e-mail: orders@researchpress.com
www.researchpress.com
Robert W. Parkinson, Founder
Steven B. Gordon, Author
Dr Richard M Foxx, Author
Michael J. Asher, Author
Research Press is an independent, family-owned business founded in 1968 by Robert W. Parkinson (1920-2001).

2157 ADHD in the Classroom: Strategies for Teachers
Guilford Publication
72 Spring Street
New York, NY 10012 212-431-9800
800-365-7006
FAX: 212-966-6708
e-mail: info@guilford.com
www.guilford.com
Bob Matloff, President
Seymour Weingarten, Editor-in-Chief
Russell A. Barkley, Author
Gary Stoner, Author
Designed specifically to help teachers with their ADHD students, thereby providing a better learning environment for the entire class. *$95.00*
ISBN 0-898629-85-3

2158 ADHD in the Schools: Assessment and Intervention Strategies
72 Spring Street
New York, NY 10012 212-431-9800
800-365-7006
FAX: 212-966-6708
e-mail: info@guilford.com
www.guilford.com
Bob Matloff, President
Seymour Weingarten, Editor-in-Chief
George J. DuPaul, Author
Gary Stoner, Author
The landmark volume emphasizes the need for a team effort among parents, community-based professionals, and educators. Provides practical information for educators that is based on empirical findings. Chapters Focus on how to identify and assess students who might have ADHD, the relationship between ADHD and learning disabilities; how to develop and supplement classroom-based programs. Communication strategies to assist physicians and the need for community-based treatments *$36.00*
269 pages Paperback
ISBN 0-898622-45-X

2159 AEPS Curriculum for Birth to Three Years
Brookes Publishing
P.O.Box 10624
Baltimore, MD 21285-0624 410-337-9580
800-638-3775
FAX: 410-337-8539
e-mail: custserv@brookespublishing.com
readplaylearn.com
496 pages
ISBN 1-557660-96-4

2160 **Access to Health Care: Number 3&4**
World Institute on Disability
3075 Adeline Street
Suite 155
Berkeley, CA 94703 510-225-6400
FAX: 510-225-0477
TTY:510-225-0478
e-mail: wid@wid.org
www.wid.org

Paul W. Schroeder, Chairman
Linda M. Dardarian, Vice Chairman
Anita Shafer Aaron, Executive Director
Mary Brooner, Treasurer
These policy bulletins focus on the capacity of the private and public health insurance systems to respond to the health care needs of persons with disabilities or chronic illness. *$6.50*
91 pages Paperback

2161 **Activity-Based Approach to Early Intervention, 2nd Edition**
Brookes Publishing
P.O.Box 10624
Baltimore, MD 21285-0624 410-337-9580
800-638-3775
FAX: 410-337-8539
e-mail: webmaster@brookespublishing.com
www.brookespublishing.com

Paul H. Brookes, Chairman of the Board
Jeffrey D. Brookes, President
George S. Stamathis, VP/Publisher
Melissa A. Behn, Executive Vice President
Activity-based intervention shows how to use natural and relevant events to teach infants and young children, of all abilities, effectively and efficiently. *$24.00*
240 pages
ISBN 1-55766 -87-5

2162 **Adapted Physical Education for Students with Autism**
Charles C. Thomas
2600 S 1st St
Springfield, IL 62704-4730 217-789-8980
800-258-8980
FAX: 217-789-9130
e-mail: books@ccthomas.com
ccthomas.com

Kimberly Davis, Author
Focuses on the physical education needs and curriculum for autistic children. Available in cloth, paperback and hardcover. *$27.95*
142 pages Paper
ISBN 0-398060-85-1

2163 **Adapting Early Childhood Curricula for Children with Special Needs**
McGraw-Hill School Publishing
P.O. Box 182604
Columbus, OH 43272 877-833-5524
FAX: 614-759-3749
e-mail: customer.service@mcgraw-hill.com
mcgraw-hill.com

Harold McGraw III, Chairman, President and Chief Executive Officer
Jack F. Callahan, Jr., Executive Vice President, Chief Financial Officer
Douglas Peterson, President, Standard & Poor's
Lou Eccleston, President, McGraw-Hill Financial
Offers information on educating the disabled.

2164 **Adapting Instruction for the Mainstream: A Sequential Approach to Teaching**
McGraw-Hill School Publishing
P.O. Box 182605
Columbus, OH 43218 800-338-3987
FAX: 609-308-4480
e-mail: customer.service@mheducation.com
mcgraw-hill.com

David Levin, President, CEO
Ellen Haley, President, CTB
Peter Cohen, President, School Education
Mark Dorman, President, International
This text gives both regular and special education teachers everything they need to help mildly handicapped students succeed in the mainstream.
226 pages

2165 **Adaptive Education Strategies Building on Diversity**
Brookes Publishing Company
P.O.Box 10624
Baltimore, MD 21285-0624 410-337-9580
800-638-3775
FAX: 410-337-8539
e-mail: webmaster@brookespublishing.com
www.brookespublishing.com

Paul H. Brookes, Chairman of the Board
Jeffrey D. Brookes, President
George S. Stamathis, VP/Publisher
Melissa A. Behn, Executive Vice President
Based on more than two decades of systematic research, this comprehensive manual provides a road map to the effective implementation of adaptive education. *$35.00*
304 pages Paperback
ISBN 1-557880-84-0

2166 **Advanced Sign Language Vocabulary: A Resource Text for Educators**
Charles C. Thomas
2600 S 1st St
Springfield, IL 62704-4730 217-789-8980
800-258-8980
FAX: 217-789-9130
e-mail: books@ccthomas.com
www.ccthomas.com

Elizabeth E. Wolf, Author
Janet R. Coleman, Author
This book is a collection of advanced sign language vocabulary for use by educators, interpreters, parents or anyone wishing to enlarge their sign vocabulary. *$53.95*
202 pages Spiralbound
ISBN 0-398057-22-2

2167 **Advances in Cardiac and Pulmonary Rehabilitation**
Haworth Press
711 Third Avenue
New York, NY 10017 212-216-7800
800-354-1420
FAX: 212-244-1563
e-mail: subscriptions@tandf.co.uk.
www.haworthpress.com

74 pages Hardcover
ISBN 0-866869-86-3

2168 **Aging Brain**
Taylor & Francis Group
Ste 800
325 Chestnut St
Philadelphia, PA 19106-2608 215-625-8900
800-354-1420
FAX: 215-625-2940
www.taylorandfrancisgroup.com

225 pages Paperback
ISBN 0-85066 -78-0

2169 Aging and Disability: Crossing Network Lines
Springer Publishing
11 West 42nd Street
15th Floor
New York, NY 10036 212-431-4370
877-687-7476
FAX: 212-941-7842
e-mail: marketing@springerpub.com
springerpub.com

Theodore C. Nardin, CEO/Publisher
Jason Roth, VP/Marketing Director
Annette Imperati, Marketing/Sales Director
Stephanie Drew, Acquisitions Editor,Social Work

Michelle Putnam has set forth this volume to reflect the current research, facilitate collaboration across service networks, and encourage movement toward more effective service policies. Professional stakeholders evaluate the bridges and barriers to crossing network lines, and chapter on current websites, agencies, and coalitions provides the much needed tools to bring collaboration into practice.

2170 Aging and Rehabilitation II
Springer Publishing Company
15th Fl
11 W 42nd St
New York, NY 10036-8002 212-431-4370
877-687-7476
FAX: 212-941-7842
e-mail: marketing@springerpub.com
www.springerpub.com

Anette Imperati, Marketing/Sales Director
Ursula Springer, President
Theodore C. Nardin, CEO/Publisher
Jason Roth, VP/Marketing Director

Current, multidisciplinary investigations of various practice issues. Leading experts in the field use a practical perspective to provide specific comments on interventions. The scope of this work encompasses the autonomy of elderly disabled, mobility, mental health and value issues, as well as basic aspects in rehabilitation of the elderly. *$41.95*

367 pages Hardcover
ISBN 0-82617 -80-3

2171 Alphabetic Phonics Curriculum
Educators Publishing Service
625 Mount Auburn Street
3rd Floor
Cambridge, MA 02138- 3039 617-547-6706
800-225-5750
e-mail: Feedback.EPS@schoolspecialty.com
www.epsbooks.com

Rick Holden, President, EPS

Ungraded multisensory curriculum for teaching phonics and the structure of language. Uses Orton-Gillingham approach to teach handwriting, spelling, reading, reading comprehension, and oral and written expression. program includes basic manual, workbooks, tests, teachers' guides, drill cards and all cards. *$28.15*

ISSN 8388-42

2172 Alternative Educational Delivery Systems
National Association of School Psychologists
4340 East West Highway
Suite 402
Bethesda, MD 20814 301-657-0270
866-331-NASP
FAX: 301-657-0275
TTY: 301-657-4155
e-mail: webmaster@naspweb.org
nasponline.org

Stephen E. Brock, President
Todd A. Savage, President-Elect
Laura Benson, Chief Operating Officer
Susan Gorin, Executive Director

A book offering information to the professional on how to enhance educational options for all students.

2173 Alternative Teaching Strategies
Special Needs Project
324 State St
Ste H
Santa Barbara, CA 93101 818-718-9900
FAX: 818-349-2027
e-mail: hgray@specialneeds.com
www.specialneeds.com

Hod Gray, Owner

Offers help for teachers who teach behaviorally troubled students.

2174 Antecedent Control: Innovative Approaches to Behavioral Support
Brookes Publishing
P.O.Box 10624
Baltimore, MD 21285-0624 410-337-9580
800-638-3775
FAX: 410-337-8539
e-mail: webmaster@brookespublishing.com
www.brookespublishing.com

Paul H. Brookes, Chairman of the Board
Jeffrey D. Brookes, President
George S. Stamathis, VP/Publisher
Melissa A. Behn, Executive Vice President

This book explains the theory and methodology of antecedent control. The treatment techniques in this book are effective for both children and adults.

416 pages Paperback
ISBN 1-55766 -34-3

2175 Anxiety-Free Kids: An Interactive Guide for Parents and Children
Prufrock Press
PO Box 8813
Waco, TX 76714-8813 800-998-2208
FAX: 800-240-0333
e-mail: info@prufrock.com
www.prufrock.com

Joel McIntosh, Publisher & Marketing Director
Lacy Compton, Senior Editor
Rachel Taliaferro, Editor
Raquel Trevino, Graphic Designer and Production Coordinator

Offers parents strategies that help children happy and worry-free, methods that relieve a child's excessive anxieties and phobias, and tools for fostering interaction and family-oriented solutions. *$19.95*

280 pages Paperback
ISBN 1-593633-43-1

2176 Applied Rehabilitation Counseling
Springer Publishing Compn
15th Fl
11 W 42nd St
New York, NY 10036-8002 212-431-4370
877-687-7476
FAX: 212-941-7842
e-mail: contactus@springerpub.com
www.springerpub.com

Sheri W. Sussman, Vice President
Ursula Springer, President
Theodore C. Nardin, CEO/Publisher
Jason Roth, VP/Marketing Director

This comprehensive text describes current theories, techniques, and their applications to specific disabled populations. Perspectives on varying counseling approaches such as psychodynamic, existential, gestalt, behavioral and psychoeducational orientations are systematically outlined in an easy-to-follow format. Practical applications for counseling are emphasized with attention given to strategies, goal-setting and on-going evaluations. *$29.95*

400 pages Softcover
ISBN 0-82615 -70-4

2177 **Art-Centered Education and Therapy for Children with Disabilities**
Charles C. Thomas
2600 S 1st St
Springfield, IL 62704-4730 217-789-8980
800-258-8980
FAX: 217-789-9130
e-mail: books@ccthomas.com
ccthomas.com
Frances E. Anderson, Author
This book has been written to help both the regular education, and art and special education teachers, both pre- and in-service, better understand some of the issues and realities of providing education and remediation to children with disabilities. The book is also offered as model concept that has govern the author's personal and professional career of over thirty years. *$41.95*
284 pages Paperback
ISBN 0-398060-06-1

2178 **Assessing the Handicaps/Needs of Children**
Books on Special Children
P.O.Box 3378
Amherst, MA 01004-3378 413-256-8164
FAX: 413-256-8896
e-mail: irene@boscbooks.com
www.boscbooks.com
260 pages Hardcover
ISBN 0-12218 -02-0

2179 **Assessment & Management of Mainstreamed Hearing-Impaired Children**
Sage Publications
2455 Teller Road
Thousand Oaks, CA 91320 805-499-0721
800-818-7243
FAX: 800-583-2665
e-mail: info@sagepub.com
www.sagepub.com
Sara Miller McCune, Founder, Publisher & Executive Chairman
Blaise R. Simqu, President & CEO
Chris Hickok, Senior Vice President & Chief Financial Officer
Stephen Barr, Managing Director/SAGE London
The theoretical and practical considerations of developing appropriate programming for hearing-impaired children who are being educated in mainstream educational settings are presented in this book.

2180 **Assessment Log & Developmental Progress Charts for the Carolina Curriculum**
Brookes Publishing
P.O.Box 10624
Baltimore, MD 21285-0624 410-337-9580
800-638-3775
FAX: 410-337-8539
e-mail: webmaster@brookespublishing.com
www.brookespublishing.com
Paul H. Brookes, Chairman of the Board
Jeffrey D. Brookes, President
George S. Stamathis, VP/Publisher
Melissa A. Behn, Executive Vice President
This 28-page booklet allows the progress of children with skills in the 12-36 month development range to be easily recorded. Available in packages of 10. *$23.00*
28 pages Saddle-stiched
ISBN 1-557662-21-5

2181 **Assessment and Remediation of Articulatoryand Phonological Disorders**
McGraw-Hill School Publishing
PO Box 182604
Columbus, OH 43218 877-833-5524
800-338-3987
FAX: 609-308-4480
e-mail: customer.service@mheducation.com
www.mcgraw-hill.com
David Levin, President/Chief Executive Officer
David Stafford, Senior Vice President/General Counsel
Maryellen Valaitis, Senior Vice President Human Resources
Patrick Milano, Chief Financial Officer/Chief Administrative Officer
Offers comprehensive coverage of articulation disorders.

2182 **Assessment in Mental Handicap: A Guide to Assessment Practices & Tests**
Brookline Books
8 Trumbull Rd
Suite B-001
Northampton, MA 01060 413-584-0184
800-666-2665
FAX: 413-584-6184
e-mail: brbooks@yahoo.com
www.brooklinebooks.com
Esther Wilder, Co-Author
Helps professionals understand the rationale and uses for assessment practices, and provides details of appropriate instruments within each type: adaptive behavior scales, assessment of behavioral disturbances, early development and Plagetian tests. *$20.00*
Hardcover
ISBN 0-91479 -31-X

2183 **Assessment of Children and Youth**
Longman Education/Addison Wesley
1185 Avenue of the Americas
New York, NY 10036-2601 212-997-8500
866-203-6215
TTY:800-231-5469
www.hess.com
Dr. Mark R. Williams, Chairman of the Board
Gregory P. Hill, President/COO
John B. Hess, Chief Executive Officer
Gary Boubel, Senior Vice President-Developments
Introductory text for preservice and in-service special educators on assessment, based on the principle that every child is unique. Comprehensive coverage of both formal and informal assessment instruments. *$50.00*
640 pages Paperback
ISBN 0-80131 -02-5

2184 **Assessment of Individuals with Severe Disabilities**
Brookes Publishing Company
PO Box 10624
Baltimore, MD 21285-0624 410-337-9580
800-638-3775
FAX: 410-337-8539
e-mail: custserv@brookespublishing.com
www.brookespublishing.com
Paul H. Brookes, Chairman
Jeffrey D. Brookes, President
Melissa A. Behn, ExecutiveVice President
George S. Stamathis, Vice President & Publisher
This expanded text offers instructors guidelines to design a comprehensive educational assessment for individuals with severe disabilities. *$34.00*
432 pages Paperback
ISBN 1-557660-67-0

2185 **Assessment of the Technology Needs of Vending Facilitiy Managers In Tennessee**
Mississippi State University
108 Herbert - South
Room 150/PO Drawer 6189
Mississippi State Univers, MS 39762-6189 662-325-2001
800-675-7782
FAX: 662-325-8989
TTY: 662-325-2694
e-mail: nrtc@colled.msstate.edu
www.blind.msstate.edu

Jacqui Bybee, Research and Training Coordinato
Michele Capella McDonnall, Ph.D., Research Professor/Interim Director
Jessica Thornton, Business Manager
Marty Giesen, Ph.D., Senior Research Scientist
This report summarizes the results and recommendations of a survey conducted of vending facility managers throughout the state of Tennessee who participate in the Randolph-Sheppard program. *$15.00*
39 pages Paperback

2186 **Assessment: The Special Educator's Role**
Brookes Publishing Company
PO Box 10624
Baltimore, MD 21285-0624 410-337-9580
800-638-3775
FAX: 410-337-8539
e-mail: custserv@brookespublishing.com
www.brookespublishing.com

Paul H. Brooks, Chairman
Jeffrey D. Brookes, President
Melissa A. Behm, ExecutiveVice President
George S. Stamathis, Vice President & Publisher
Aimed at students with little or no classroom experience in assessment, the book focuses on the integration of dynamic, curriculum-based and norm-referenced data for diagnostic decisions and program planning.
580 pages Casebound
ISBN 0-53421 -32-1

2187 **Asthma Management and Education**
Asthma and Allergy Foundation of America
8201 Corporate Drive
Suite 1000
Landover, MD 20785 202-466-7643
800-727-8462
e-mail: info@aafa.org
www.aafa.org

Lynn Hanessian, Chair
Mitchell Grayson, MD, Chair, Research
Barbara Corn, Chair, Governance
Calvin Anderson, Chair/Finance/Treasurer
One session, two hour program developed to educate allied health professionals about up-to-date asthma care and patient education, information and materials. Includes hands on experience with peak flow meters and demonstrations of medical devices.

2188 **Aston-Patterning**
PO Box 3568
Incline Village, NV 89450-3568 775-831-8228
FAX: 775-831-8955
e-mail: office@astonkinetics.com
www.astonkinetics.com

J Aston, Owner
Angelina Calafiore, Office Manager
Integrated system of movement education, body assessment, environmental modification and fitness training.

2189 **Attention Deficit Disorder in Children**
Charles C. Thomas
2600 S 1st St
Springfield, IL 62704-4730 217-789-8980
800-258-8980
FAX: 217-789-9130
e-mail: books@ccthomas.com
www.ccthomas.com

2190 **Aural Habilitation**
Alexander Graham Bell Association
3417 Volta Pl NW
Washington, DC 20007-2737 202-337-5220
FAX: 202-337-8314
TTY:202-337-5221
e-mail: info@agbell.org
www.listeningandspokenlanguage.org

Meredith K. Sugar, Esq. (OH), President
Ted A. Meyer, M.D., Ph.D, President-Elect/Secretary-Treasurer
Emilio Alonso-Mendoza, Chief Executive Officer
Susan Boswell, Director of Communications and Marketing
This classic text for professionals, educators and parents discusses verbal learning and aural habilitation of young children with hearing losses to ensure that each child is educated in the best setting. It discusses communication, normal development of spoken language, speech audiologic assessment, hearing aids and use of residual hearing, and program designs for individualized needs, including the assessment and planning of IEPs. *$26.95*
324 pages

2191 **Behavior Analysis in Education: Focus on Measurably Superior Instruction**
Brookes Publishing Company
PO Box 10624
Baltimore, MD 21285-0624 410-337-9580
800-638-3775
FAX: 410-337-8539
e-mail: custserv@brookespublishing.com
www.brookespublishing.com

Paul H. Brookes, Chairman
Jeffrey D. Brookes, President
Melissa A. Behm, ExecutiveVice President
George S. Stamathis, Vice President & Publisher
Designed to disseminate measurably superior instructional strategies to those interested in advancing sound, pedagogically effective, field-tested educational practices, this book is intended for graduate-level courses and seminars in special education and/or psychology focusing on behavior analysis and instruction.
512 pages Casebound
ISBN 0-53422 -60-9

2192 **Behavior Modification**
Sage Publications
2455 Teller Rd
Thousand Oaks, CA 91320-2218 805-499-0721
800-818-7243
FAX: 800-583-2665
e-mail: info@sagepub.com
www.sagepub.com

Sara Miller McCune, Founder, Publisher and Executive Chairman
Blaise R. Simqu, President & CEO
Chris Hickok, Senior Vice President & Chief Financial Officer
Stephen Barr, Managing Director/SAGE London
Describes in detail for replication purposes assessment and modification techniques for problems in psychiatric, clinical, educational and rehabilitation settings. *$53.00*
640 pages Quarterly

2193 **Behavioral Disorders**
Council for Exceptional Children
2900 Crystal Drive
Suite 1000
Arlington, VA 22202-3557 703-620-3660
866-509-0218
888-232-7733
FAX: 703-264-9494
TTY:866-915-5000
e-mail: services@cec.sped.org
www.cec.sped.org

Robin D. Brewer, President
James P. Heiden, President Elect
Joni L. Baldwin, Director
Christy A. Chambers, Immediate Past President
Provides professionals with a means to exchange information and share ideas related to research, empirically tested educational in-

novations and issues and concerns relevant to students with behavioral disorders. Individual, $20; Institution, $50.
Quarterly

2194 Behind Special Education
Love Publishing Company
9101 E Kenyon Ave
Suite 2200
Denver, CO 80237-1854 303-221-7333
FAX: 303-221-7444
e-mail: lpc@lovepublishing.com
www.lovepublishing.com

ISBN 0-89108-17-4

2195 Biomedical Concerns in Persons with Down's Syndrome
Paul H Brookes Publishing Company
PO Box 10624
Baltimore, MD 21285-0624 410-337-9580
800-638-3775
FAX: 410-337-8539
e-mail: custserv@brookespublishing.com
www.brookespublishing.com

Paul H. Brookes, Chairman
Jeffrey D. Brookes, President
Melissa A. Behm, ExecutiveVice President
George S. Stamathis, Vice President & Publisher
Written by leading authorities and spanning many disciplines and specialties, this comprehensive resource provides vital information on biomedical issues concerning individuals with Down's Syndrome. *$45.00*
336 pages Hardcover
ISBN 1-557660-89-1

2196 Breaking Barriers
AbleNet
2625 Patton Road
Roseville, MN 55113-5423 651-294-2200
800-322-0956
FAX: 651-294-2259
e-mail: customerservice@ablenetinc.com
www.ablenetinc.com

Bill Sproull, Chairman of the Board
William Mills, Board of Directors, Chair
Jennifer Thalhuber, President/CEO
Paul Sugden, Vice President of Finance, IT & CFO, Trustee
A practical resource for parents, caregivers, teachers and therapists. *$15.00*

2197 Building the Healing Partnership: Parents, Professionals and Children
Brookline Books
Suite B-001
8 Trumbull Rd
Northampton, MA 01060 413-584-0184
800-666-2665
FAX: 413-584-6184
e-mail: brbooks@yahoo.com
www.brooklinebooks.com

Esther Wilder, Co-Author
Successful programs understand that the disabled child's needs must be considered in the context of a family. This book was specifically written for practitioner's who must work with families but who have insufficient training in family systems assessment and intervention. It is a valuable blend of theory and practice with pointers for applying the principles. *$24.95*
Paperback
ISBN 0-91479-63-8

2198 Career Assessment Inventories Learning Disabled
C FK R Career Materials
P.O.Box 99
Meadow Vista, CA 95722-99 530-889-2357
800-525-5626
FAX: 800-770-0433
e-mail: requestinfo@cfkr.com
www.cfkr.com

2199 Caring for Children with Chronic Illness
11 W 42nd St
15th Floor
New York, NY 10036-8002 212-431-4370
877-687-7476
FAX: 212-941-7842
e-mail: cs@springerpub.com
www.springerpub.com

Ursula Springer, President
Theodore C. Nardin, CEO/Publisher
Jason Roth, VP/Marketing Director
James C. Costello, Vice President, Journal Publishing
A critical look at the current medical, social, and psychological framework for providing care to children with chronic illnesses. Emphasizing the need to create integrated, interdisciplinary approaches, it discusses issues such as the roles of families, professionals, and institutions in providing health care, the impact of a child's illness on various family structures, financing care, the special problems of chronically ill children as they become adolescents and more. *$36.95*
320 pages Hardcover
ISBN 0-82615-00-1

2200 Carolina Curriculum for Infants and Toddlers with Special Needs, 2nd Edition
Brookes Publishing
PO Box 10624
Baltimore, MD 21285-0624 410-337-9580
800-638-3775
FAX: 410-337-8539
e-mail: custserv@brookespublishing.com
www.brookespublishing.com

Paul H. Brookes, Chairman
Jeffrey D. Brookes, President
Melissa A. Behm, ExecutiveVice President
George S. Stamathis, Vice President & Publisher
This book includes detailed assessment and intervention sequences, daily routine integration strategies, sensorimotor adaptations, and a sample 24-page assessment log that shows readers how to chart a child's individual progress. *$40.00*
384 pages Spiral-bound
ISBN 1-55766-74-3

2201 Carolina Curriculum for Preschoolers with Special Needs
Brookes Publishing
PO Box 10624
Baltimore, MD 21285-0624 410-337-9580
800-638-3775
FAX: 410-337-8539
e-mail: custserv@brookespublishing.com
www.brookespublishing.com

Paul H. Brookes, Chairman
Jeffrey D. Brookes, President
Melissa A. Behm, ExecutiveVice President
George S. Stamathis, Vice President & Publisher
This curriculum provides detailed teaching and assessment techniques, plus a sample 28-page assessment log that shows readers how to chart a child's individual progress. This guide is for children between 2 and 5 in their developmental stages who are considered at risk for developmental delay or who exhibit special needs. *$34.00*
352 pages Spiral-bound
ISBN 1-55766-32-8

2202 Challenge of Educating Together Deaf and Hearing Youth: Making Manistreaming Work
Charles C. Thomas
2600 S 1st St
Springfield, IL 62704-4730 217-789-8980
800-258-8980
FAX: 217-789-9130
e-mail: books@ccthomas.com
www.ccthomas.com

198 pages Hardcover
ISBN 0-398063-91-5

2203 **Challenged Scientists: Disabilities and the Triumph of Excellence**
Greenwood Publishing Group
130 Cremona Drive
Santa Barbara, CA 93117
805-968-1911
800-368-6868
FAX: 866-270-3856
e-mail: CustomerService@abc-clio.com
www.abc-clio.com

208 pages
ISBN 0-275938-73-5

2204 **Child Care and the ADA: A Handbook for Inclusive Programs**
Brookes Publishing
PO Box 10624
Baltimore, MD 21285-0624
410-337-9580
800-638-3775
FAX: 410-337-8539
e-mail: custserv@brookespublishing.com
www.brookespublishing.com

Paul H. Brookes, Chairman
Jeffrey D. Brookes, President
Melissa A. Behm, ExecutiveVice President
George S. Stamathis, Vice President & Publisher
This book is designed for educators and administrators in child care settings. It offers a straightforward discussion of the Americans with Disabilities Act including children with disabilities in community programs. *$25.95*
240 pages Paperback
ISBN 1-55766 -85-5

2205 **Child with Disabling Illness**
Lippincott, Williams & Wilkins
227 S 6th St
Suite 227
Philadelphia, PA 19106-3713
215-521-8300
800-777-2295
FAX: 301-824-7390
www.lpub.com

700 pages

2206 **Childhood Behavior Disorders: Applied Research & Educational Practice**
Sage Publications
2455 Teller Road
Thousand Oaks, CA 91320-2218
805-499-0721
800-818-7243
FAX: 800-583-2665
e-mail: info@sagepub.com
www.sagepub.com
Sara Miller McCune, Founder, Publisher, Chairperson
Blaise R. Simqu, President/CEO
Chris Hickok, Senior Vice President & Chief Fi
Stephen Barr, Managing Director/SAGE London, P
The only comprehensive overview of childhood behavior disorders. This book gives you the how and why for helping children with behavior disorders.

2207 **Childhood Disablity and Family Systems**
Haworth Press
711 Third Avenue
New York, NY 10017
212-216-7800
800-354-1420
FAX: 212-244-1563
e-mail: subscriptions@tandf.co.uk.
www.haworthpress.com

246 pages Hardcover
ISBN 0-866566-71-6

2208 **Children and Youth Assisted by Medical Technology in Educational Settings, 2nd Edition**
Brookes Publishing
PO Box 10624
Baltimore, MD 21285-0624
410-337-9580
800-638-3775
FAX: 410-337-8539
e-mail: custserv@brookespublishing.com
www.brookespublishing.com

Paul H. Brookes, Chairman
Jeffrey D. Brookes, President
Melissa A. Behm, ExecutiveVice President
George S. Stamathis, Vice President & Publisher
Contains detailed daily care guidelines and emergency-response techniques, including information on working with a range of students who have the HIV infection, that rely on ventilators, that utilize tube feeding, or require catheterization. Also covers every aspect of planning for inclusive classrooms, including information on personnel training, entrance planning and transition, legal requirements, and transportation issues. *$52.00*
432 pages Spiral-bound
ISBN 1-55766 -36-3

2209 **Children's Needs Psychological Perspective**
National Association of School Psychologists
8455 Colesville Rd
Suite 1000
Silver Spring, MD 20910- 3392
301-589-3300
FAX: 301-589-5175
www.musictherapy.org

637 pages

2210 **Choices: A Guide to Sex Counseling for the Physically Disabled Adult**
Krieger Publishing Company
1725 Krieger Drive
Malabar, FL 32950
321-724-9542
800-724-0025
FAX: 321-951-3671
e-mail: info@krieger-publishing.com
www.krieger-publishing.com

132 pages
ISBN 0-898749-03-4

2211 **Choosing Options and Accommodations for Children**
Brookes Publishing
PO Box 10624
Baltimore, MD 21285-0624
410-337-9580
800-638-3775
FAX: 410-337-8539
e-mail: custserv@brookespublishing.com
www.brookespublishing.com

192 pages
ISBN 1-55766 -06-5

2212 **Cirriculum Development for Students with Mild Disabilities**
Charles C. Thomas
2600 South 1st Street
Springfield, IL 62704-4730
217-789-8980
800-258-8980
FAX: 217-789-9130
e-mail: books@ccthomas.com
www.ccthomas.com

Carroll J. Jones, Author
This book was designed to provide the foundation from which to write cirrocumuli that will provide academic and social skills for Individual Education Programs (IEPs). *$38.95*
258 pages Spiral-Paper
ISBN 0-398070-18-2

2213 **Classroom Success for the LD and ADHD Child**
John F Blair Publishing
1406 Plaza Dr
Winston Salem, NC 27103-1470
336-768-1374
800-222-9796
FAX: 336-768-9194
blairpub.com

John F. Blair, Publisher
Suzanne H. Stevens, Author
This book offers suggestions on teaching techniques, adapting texts, recognition of children with disabilities and testing, grading and mainstreaming the learning disabled and ADHD child.
$12.95
314 pages Paperback
ISBN 0-895871-42-4

2214 **Clinical Alzheimer Rehabilitation**
Springer Publishing
11 W 42nd St
15th Floor
New York, NY 10036-8002
212-431-4370
877-687-7476
FAX: 212-941-7842
e-mail: cs@springerpub.com
www.springerpub.com

Theodore C. Nardin, CEO/Publisher
Jason Roth, VP/Marketing Director
Annette Imperati, Marketing/Sales Director
James C. Costello, Vice President, Journal Publishing
This comprehensive and easy-to-read guidebook contains the latest research on dementia and AD in the elderly population, including the causes and risk factors of AD, diagnosis information, and symptoms and progressions of the disease. Significant emphasis is given to the physical, mental, and verbal rehabilitation challenges of patients with AD. The authors outline specific rehabilitation goals for the physical therapist, speech-language pathologist, and general caregiver.

2215 **Clinical Management of Childhood Stuttering, 2nd Edition**
Sage Publications
2455 Teller Road
Thousand Oaks, CA 91320-2218
805-499-0721
800-818-7243
FAX: 800-583-2665
e-mail: info@sagepub.com
www.sagepub.com

Sara Miller McCune, Founder, Publisher, Chairperson
Blaise R. Simqu, President/CEO
Chris Hickok, Senior Vice President/CFO
Stephen Barr, Managing Director/SAGE London
Updates and integrates recent findings in childhood stuttering into a broad range of therapeutic strategies for assessing and treating the young dysfluent child. *$38.00*
336 pages

2216 **Cognitive Approaches to Learning Disabilities**
Sage Publications
2455 Teller Road
Thousand Oaks, CA 91320-2218
805-499-0721
800-818-7243
FAX: 800-583-2665
e-mail: info@sagepub.com
www.sagepub.com

Sara Miller McCune, Founder, Publisher, Chairperson
Blaise R. Simqu, President/CEO
Chris Hickok, Senior Vice President/CFO
Stephen Barr, Managing Director/SAGE London
The first to bridge the gap between cognitive psychology and information processing theory in understanding learning disabilities. *$39.00*
495 pages Hardcover

2217 **Cognitive Strategy Instruction That Really Improves Children's Academic Skills**
Brookline Books
8 Trumbull Rd
Suite B-001
Northampton, MA 01060
413-584-0184
800-666-2665
FAX: 413-584-6184
e-mail: brbooks@yahoo.com
www.brooklinebooks.com

Esther Isabe Wilder, Author
A concise and focused work that summarily presents the few procedures for teaching strategies that aid academic subject matter learning: decoding reading comprehension, vocabulary, math, spelling and writing. Learning unrelated facts and science. Completely revised in 1995. *$27.95*
Paperback
ISBN 1-571290-07-9

2218 **Collaborating for Comprehensive Services for Young Children and Families**
Brookes Publishing Company
PO Box 10624
Baltimore, MD 21285-0624
410-337-9580
800-638-3775
FAX: 410-337-8539
e-mail: custserv@brookespublishing.com
www.brookespublishing.com

Paul H. Brookes, Chairman
Jeffrey D. Brookes, President
Melissa A. Behm, ExecutiveVice President
George S. Stamathis, Vice President & Publisher
Taking collaboration a step beyond basic implementation, this useful book shows agency and school leaders how to coordinate their efforts to stretch human services dollars while still providing quality programs. Provides the building blocks needed to establish a local interagency coordinating council. *$37.00*
272 pages
ISBN 1-557661-03-0

2219 **Collaborative Teams for Students with Severe Disabilities**
Brookes Publishing
PO Box 10624
Baltimore, MD 21285-0624
410-337-9580
800-638-3775
FAX: 410-337-8539
e-mail: custserv@brookespublishing.com
www.brookespublishing.com

Paul H. Brookes, Chairman
Jeffrey D. Brookes, President
Melissa A. Behm, ExecutiveVice President
George S. Stamathis, Vice President & Publisher
How can educators, parents and therapists work together to ensure the best possible educational experience for students with severe disabilities? This resource describes how a collaborative team can successfully create exciting learning opportunities for students, while teaching them to participate fully at home, school, work and play. *$ 30.00*
304 pages
ISBN 1-55766 -88-3

2220 **Communicating with Parents of Exceptional Children**
Love Publishing Company
9101 E Kenyon Ave
Suite 2200
Denver, CO 80237-1854
303-221-7333
FAX: 303-221-7444
e-mail: lpc@lovepublishing.com
www.lovepublishing.com

Roger L. Kroth, Author
Denzil Denzil Edge, Author
This book shows how teachers can facilitate parent involvement with children's education. It presents the mirror model of parent involvement, family, dynamics, how to listen actively to parents, values and perceptions, problem-solving, parent conferences and training groups. *$19.95*
ISBN 0-89108 -67-4

2221 Communication & Language Acquisition: Discoveries from Atypical Development
Brookes Publishing
PO Box 10624
Baltimore, MD 21285-0624
410-337-9580
800-638-3775
FAX: 410-337-8539
e-mail: custserv@brookespublishing.com
www.brookespublishing.com

Paul H. Brookes, Chairman
Jeffrey D. Brookes, President
Melissa A. Behm, ExecutiveVice President
George S. Stamathis, Vice President & Publisher

This text demonstrates how the study of language acquisition in children with atypical development promotes advances in basic theory. *$44.00*

352 pages Hardcover
ISBN 1-557662-79-7

2222 Communication Skills for Working with Elders
Springer Publishing Company
11 W 42nd St
15th Floor
New York, NY 10036-8002
212-431-4370
877-687-7476
FAX: 212-941-7842
e-mail: cs@springerpub.com
www.springerpub.com

Ursula Springer, President
Theodore C. Nardin, CEO/Publisher
Jason Roth, VP/Marketing Director
James C. Costello, Vice President, Journal Publishing

How aging and illness affects communication. *$17.95*

160 pages Softcover
ISBN 0-82615 -20-7

2223 Communication Unbound
Teachers College Press
Ste 2115
14781 Memorial Dr
Houston, TX 77079-5210
415-738-4323
FAX: 415-738-4329
e-mail: tcc.orders@aidcvt.com
www.pearsonhighered.com

240 pages Paperback
ISBN 0-087737-21-4

2224 Complete Handbook of Children's Reading Disorders: You Can Prevent or Correct LDs
Gallery Bookshop
319 Kasten Street
PO Box 270
Mendocino, CA 95460-270
707-937-2215
FAX: 707-937-3737
e-mail: info@gallerybookshop.com
www.gallerybooks.com

Tony Miksak, Owner

The complete handbook of children's reading disorders. *$34.95*

732 pages Paperback
ISBN 0-80772 -83-3

2225 Computer Access/Computer Learning
Special Needs Project
324 State St
Suite H
Santa Barbara, CA 93101-2364
805-962-8087
800-333-6867
FAX: 805-962-5087
e-mail: editor@specialneeds.com
www.specialneeds.com

Mark Darrow, Founder,The Prolotherapy Institu

A resource manual in adaptive technology and computer training. *$22.50*

2226 Consulting Psychologists Press
1055 Joaquin Rd
Suite. 200
Mountain View, CA 94043-1243
650-969-8901
800-624-1765
FAX: 650-969-8608
e-mail: custserv@cpp.com
www.cpp-db.com

Carl E. Thoresen, Chairman
Jeffrey Hayes, President and Chief Executive Officer
Andrew Bell, Vice President of International
Catey DeBalko, Vice President of Marketing

Catalog offering job assessment software, career development reports, educational assessment information and books for the professional.

2227 Counseling Persons with Communication Disorders and Their Families
Sage Publications
2455 Teller Road
Thousand Oaks, CA 91320-2218
805-499-0721
800-818-7243
FAX: 800-583-2665
e-mail: info@sagepub.com
www.sagepub.com

Sara Miller McCune, Founder, Publisher, Chairperson
Blaise R. Simqu, President & CEO
Chris Hickok, Senior Vice President & Chief Fi
Stephen Barr, Managing Director/SAGE London, P

A learning manual for speech-language pathologists and audiologists on how to deal with the emotional issues facing them in their work with clients with communication disorders and their families. *$ 29.00*

187 pages

2228 Counseling in the Rehabilitation Process
Charles C. Thomas
2600 South 1st Street
Springfield, IL 62704-4730
217-789-8980
800-258-8980
FAX: 217-789-9130
e-mail: books@ccthomas.com
www.ccthomas.com

Gerald L. Gandy, Author
E. Davis Martin Jr, Author
Richard E. Hardy, Author

This text provides the reader with a comprehensive overview and introduction to the field of rehabilitation counseling and services, and also has applicability in the growing field of community counseling. *$51.95*

358 pages paper 1999
ISBN 0-398069-70-4

2229 Creating Positive Classroom Environments: Strategies for Behavior Management
Brooks / Cole Publishing Company
511 Forest Lodge Rd
Pacific Grove, CA 93950-5040
831-373-0728
800-354-9706
FAX: 831-375-6414
e-mail: bc-info@brookscole.com
www.cengage.com

448 pages Paperbound
ISBN 0-53422 -54-4

2230 **Critical Voices on Special Education: Problems & Progress Concerning the Mildly Handicapped**

State University of New York Press
22 Corporate Woods Boulevard
3rd Floor
Albany, NY 12211-2504
518-472-5000
866-430-7869
FAX: 518-472-5038
e-mail: info@sunypress.edu
www.sunypress.edu

James Peltz, Associate Director
Janice Vunk, Assistant to the Director
Scott B Sigmon, Editor

Problems and progress concerning the mildly handicapped. *$24.95*

265 pages Paperback 1990
ISBN 0-79140-20-3

2231 **Cultural Diversity, Families and the Special Education System**

Teachers College Press
1234 Amsterdam Ave
New York, NY 10027-6602
212-678-3929
800-575-6566
FAX: 212-678-4149
e-mail: tcpress@tc.columbia.edu
www.teacherscollegepress.com

Beth Harry, Author

This timely and thought-provoking book explores the quadruple disadvantage faced by the parents of poor, minority, handicapped children whose first language is not that of the school they attend. *$22.95*

296 pages Paperback
ISBN 0-807731-19-6

2232 **Curriculum Decision Making for Students with Severe Handicaps**

Teachers College Press
1234 Amsterdam Ave
New York, NY 10027-6602
212-678-3929
800-575-6566
FAX: 212-678-4149
e-mail: tspress@ts.columbia.edu.
www.teacherscollegepress.com

192 pages Paperback
ISBN 0-807728-61-6

2233 **Deciphering the System: A Guide for Families of Young Disabled Children**

Brookline Books
Suite B-001
8 Trumbull Rd
Northampton, MA 01060
413-584-0184
800-666-2665
FAX: 413-584-6184
e-mail: brbooks@yahoo.com
www.brooklinebooks.com

Esther Wilder, Co-Author

This book informs parents of disabled children (0-5) of their rights and the service system, e.g., ways to manage the cumulating information, tips on IEP and IFSP meetings and the educational assessment process, and how parents can work with multiple service providers. It includes contributions from both parents and professionals who have experience with the service system. *$21.95*

ISBN 0-914797-87-5

2234 **Defining Rehabilitation Agency Types**

Mississippi State University
108 Herbert - South
Room 150 Industrial Education Depar
Mississippi State, MS 39762-6189
662-325-2001
800-675-7782
FAX: 662-325-8989
TTY: 662-325-2694
e-mail: nrtc@colled.msstate.edu
www.blind.msstate.edu

Jacqui Bybee, Research Associate II
Michele Capella McDonnall, Ph.D., Research Professor/Interim Director
Jessica Thornton, Business Manager
Marty Giesen, Ph.D., Senior Research Scientist

Relationships of participant selection and cost factors of service delivery across rehabilitation agency types. A national survey of state agencies for the blind was conducted to examine factors that define the characteristics of different agencies; similar programs were grouped together. Classification criteria were developed to distinguish agencies into logical groups based on line of authority, funding and operating procedures. *$10.00*

15 pages Paperback

2235 **Designing and Using Assistive Technology: The Human Perspective**

Brookes Publishing
PO Box 10624
Baltimore, MD 21285-0624
410-337-9580
800-638-3775
FAX: 410-337-8539
e-mail: custserv@brookespublishing.com
www.brookespublishing.com

Paul H. Brookes, Chairman
Jeffrey D. Brookes, President
Melissa A. Behm, ExecutiveVice President
George S. Stamathis, Vice President & Publisher

Presented here is a holistic perspective on how and why people choose and use AT. Features personal insights and the latest research on design and development. *$31.00*

352 pages Paperback
ISBN 1-55766-14-9

2236 **Developing Cross-Cultural Competence:Guideto Working with Young Children & Their Families**

Brookes Publishing
PO Box 10624
Baltimore, MD 21285-0624
410-337-9580
800-638-3775
FAX: 410-337-8539
e-mail: custserv@brookespublishing.com
www.brookespublishing.com

Paul H. Brookes, Chairman
Jeffrey D. Brookes, President
Melissa A. Behm, ExecutiveVice President
George S. Stamathis, Vice President & Publisher

This enlightening book perceptively and sensitively explores cultural, ethnic, and language diversity in human services. For those who work with families whose infants and young children may have or be at risk for a disability or chronic illness. (Second Edition) *$ 32.00*

448 pages Paperback
ISBN 1-55766-31-9

2237 **Developing Individualized Family Support Plans: A Training Manual**

Brookline Books
Suite B-001
8 Trumbull Rd
Northampton, MA 01060
413-584-0184
800-666-2665
FAX: 413-584-6184
e-mail: brbooks@yahoo.com
www.brooklinebooks.com

Esther Wilder, Co-Author

This manual provides in-service training coordinators, administrators, supervisors and university personnel with a compact package of functional and practical methods to train profession-

als about implementing family-centered individualized family support plans (IFSP'S). Also, case studies provide concrete examples to aid in learning to write IFSP's. *$24.95*
ISBN 0-914797-69-7

2238 Developing Staff Competencies for Supporting People with Disabilities
Brookes Publishing
PO Box 10624
Baltimore, MD 21285-0624
410-337-9580
800-638-3775
FAX: 410-337-8539
e-mail: custserv@brookespublishing.com
www.brookespublishing.com

Paul H. Brookes, Chairman
Jeffrey D. Brookes, President
Melissa A. Behm, ExecutiveVice President
George S. Stamathis, Vice President & Publisher
This timely second edition, now in a new easier to read format, gives service providers helpful strategies for increasing effectiveness and maintaining well-being while working in the rewarding yet challenging field of human services. *$34.00*
480 pages Paperback
ISBN 1-55766 -07-3

2239 Development of Language
McGraw-Hill, School Publishing
220 E Danieldale Rd
Desoto, TX 75115-2490
800-648-2970
FAX: 800-593-4418
www.mhschool.com

464 pages

2240 Developmental Disabilities of Learning
Gallery Bookshop
319 Kasten Street
PO Box 270
Mendocino, CA 95460-270
707-937-2215
FAX: 707-937-3737
e-mail: info@gallerybookshop.com
www.gallerybooks.com

Tony Miksak, Owner
Manual for professionals on developmental and learning disabilities in the growing child. *$25.00*
224 pages Illustrated

2241 Developmental Disabilities: A Handbook for Occupational Therapists
Haworth Press
711 Third Avenue
New York, NY 10017
212-216-7800
800-354-1420
FAX: 212-244-1563
e-mail: subscriptions@tandf.co.uk.
www.haworthpress.com

268 pages Hardcover
ISBN 0-866569-59-6

2242 Developmental Disabilities: A Handbook for Interdisciplinary Practice
Brookline Books
8 Trumbull Rd
Suite B-001
Northampton, MA 01060
413-584-0184
800-666-2665
FAX: 413-584-6184
e-mail: brbooks@yahoo.com
www.brooklinebooks.com

Esther Wilder, Co-Author
Successful interdisciplinary team practice for persons with developmental disabilities that require each team member to understand and respect the contributions of the others. This handbook explains the professions most often represented on interdisciplinary teams: their natures, concerns and roles in the interdisciplinary context. *$29.95*
256 pages
ISBN 1-571290-03-6

2243 Developmental Variation and Learning Disorders
Educators Publishing Service
PO Box 9031
Cambridge, MA 02139-9031
617-367-2700
800-225-5750
FAX: 617-547-0412
e-mail: eps@schoolspecialty.com
www.epsbooks.com

Rick Holden, President
Discusses seven major areas of development and four major areas of academic proficiency and then ties this information together by examining factors that predispose a child to dysfunction and disability, offering guidelines to assessment and management, and analyzing long-range outcomes and factors that promote resiliency for parents, educators and clinicians. *$69.00*
640 pages Cloth
ISBN 0-838819-92-3

2244 Digest of Neurology and Psychiatry
Institute of Living: Hartford Hospital
80 Seymour Street
Hartford, CT 06106-3309
860-545-5000
800-673-2411
FAX: 860-545-5066
e-mail: Fishe@harthosp.org
www.harthosp.org

Douglas Elliot, Chair of the Board
Stuart K. Markowitz, MD, FACR, President/SVP
Gerald J. Boisvert, HHC Regional Vice President / Chief Financial Officer,
Peter Q. Fraser, Regional Vice President Human Resources
Abstracts and reviews of selected current literature in psychiatry, neurology and related fields.

2245 Disability Funding News
8204 Fenton St
Silver Spring, MD 20910-4502
301-588-6380
800-666-6380
FAX: 301-588-6385
e-mail: info@cdpublications.com,
www.cdpublications.com

Mike Gerecht, Publisher

2246 Disability and Rehabilitation
Taylor & Francis
7625 Empire Dr
Florence, KY 41042-2919
800-634-7064
FAX: 800-248-4724
e-mail: orders@taylorandfrancis.com
www.taylorandfrancis.com

Monthly
ISSN 0963-82 8

2247 Divided Legacy: A History of the Schism in Medical Thought, The Bacteriological Era
North Atlantic Books
2526 Martin Luther King Jr. Way
Berkeley, CA 94704
510-549-4270
800-337-2665
FAX: 510-549-4276
e-mail: orders@northatlanticbooks.com
www.northatlanticbooks.com

Alla Spector, Director of Finance & Office Operations
Doug Reil, Executive Director/Associate Publisher
Ed Angel, Director of Office Administration
Janet Levin, Senior Director of Sales & Distribution
Concluding volume of Coulter's history of medical philosophy, from ancient times to today. Covers the origins of bacteriology and immunology in world medicine; describes the clash between orthodox and alternative medicine.

2248 Dual Relationships in Counseling
5999 Stevenson Ave
Alexandria, VA 22304-3304
703-823-0252
800-347-6647
FAX: 800-473-2329
e-mail: webmaster@counseling.org
www.counseling.org

Robert L. Smith, President
Thelma Duffey, President-Elect
Brian Canfield, Treasurer
Catherine Roland, Representative

Publishes archival material, also publishes articles that have broad interest for a readership composed mostly of counselors and other mental health professionals who work in private practice, schools, colleges, community agencies, hospitals, and government. An appropriate outlet for articles that: critically integrate published research; examine current professional and scientific issues; report research, new techniques, innovative programs and practices; and examine ACA as an organization.

2249 Early Communication Skills for Children with Down Syndrome
Woodbine House
6510 Bells Mill Rd
Bethesda, MD 20817-1636
301-897-3570
800-843-7323
FAX: 301-897-5838
e-mail: info@woodbinehouse.com
www.woodbinehouse.com

Nancy Gray Paul, Acquisitions Editor
Libby Kumin, Author

An expert shares her knowledge of speech and language development in young children with Down syndrome. Intelligibility, hearing loss, apraxia and other factors that affect communications are discussed. It also covers speech-language assessments and alternative communication options and literacy. *$19.95*
368 pages
ISBN 1-890627-27-5

2250 Early Intervention, Implementing Child & Family Services for At-Risk Infants
Sage Publications
2455 Teller Road
Thousand Oaks, CA 91320-2218
805-499-0721
800-818-7243
FAX: 800-583-2665
e-mail: info@sagepub.com
www.sagepub.com

Sara Miller McCune, Founder, Publisher, Chairperson
Blaise R. Simqu, President & CEO
Chris Hickok, Senior Vice President & Chief Financial Officer
Stephen Barr, Managing Director/SAGE London, President of SAGE Internation

New directions and recent legislation have produced a need for this guide which is designed for professionals facing the challenge of program development for disabled and at-risk infants, toddlers and their families. *$36.00*
394 pages
ISBN 0-890796-21-1

2251 Ecology of Troubled Children
Brookline Books Publications
8 Trumbull Rd
Suite B-001
Northampton, MA 01060
413-584-0184
800-666-2665
FAX: 413-584-6184
e-mail: brbooks@yahoo.com
www.brooklinebooks.com

Esther Isabe Wilder, Author

Designed for frontline mental health clinicians working with children with serious emotional disturbances; shows how to make children's' worlds more supportive by changing the places, activities and people in their lives. *$15.95*
256 pages
ISBN 1-571290-57-5

2252 Educating Children with Disabilities: A Transdisciplinary Approach
Brookes Publishing
PO Box 10624
Baltimore, MD 21285-0624
410-337-9580
800-638-3775
FAX: 410-337-8539
e-mail: custserv@brookespublishing.com
www.brookespublishing.com

Paul H. Brookes, Chairman
Jeffrey D. Brookes, President
Melissa A. Behm, ExecutiveVice President
George S. Stamathis, Vice President & Publisher

Widely respected textbook presents you with the strategies you need for developing an inclusive curriculum, integrating health care and educational programs and addressing needs and concerns. *$38.00*
512 pages
ISBN 1-557662-46-0

2253 Educating Children with Multiple Disabilities: A Transdisciplinary Approach
Brookes Publishing
PO Box 10624
Baltimore, MD 21285-0624
410-337-9580
800-638-3775
FAX: 410-337-8539
e-mail: custserv@brookespublishing.com
www.brookespublishing.com

Paul H. Brookes, Chairman
Jeffrey D. Brookes, President
Melissa A. Behm, ExecutiveVice President
George S. Stamathis, Vice President & Publisher

Emphasizing transdisciplinary cooperation between teachers, therapists, nurses and parents, this book describes a general model and specific techniques for effectively educating children with multiple disabilities. *$29.00*
496 pages Paperback
ISBN 1-557662-46-0

2254 Educating Individuals with Disabilities
Springer Publishing
15th Fl
11 W 42nd St
New York, NY 10036-8002
212-431-4370
877-687-7476
FAX: 212-941-7842
e-mail: marketing@springerpub.com
springerpub.com

Theodore C. Nardin, CEO/Publisher
Jason Nardin, VP/Marketing Director
Annette Imperati, Marketing/Sales Director
Stephanie Drew, Acquisitions Editor,Social Work and Psychology

Grigorenko's new book discusses how learning-disabled students are identified and assessed today, in light of the 2004 Individuals with Disabilities Education Improvement Act. Grigorenko's interdisciplinary collection is the first to comprehensively review the IDEIA 2004 Act and distill the changes professionals working with learning-disabled students face. The text takes an overarching perspective, first discussing the IDEIA in its historical, political, and legal context.

2255 Educating Students Who Have Visual Impairments with Other Disabilities
Brookes Publishing
PO Box 10624
Baltimore, MD 21285-0624
410-337-9580
800-638-3775
FAX: 410-337-8539
e-mail: custserv@brookespublishing.com
www.brookespublishing.com

Paul H. Brookes, Chairman
Jeffrey D. Brookes, President
Melissa A. Behm, ExecutiveVice President
George S. Stamathis, Vice President & Publisher

This introductory text provides techniques for facilitating functional learning in students with a wide range of visual impairments and multiple disabilities. With a concentration on

educational needs and learning styles, the authors of this multidisciplinary volume demonstrate functional assessment and teaching adaptations that will improve students' inclusive learning experiences. *$49.95*
552 pages Paperback
ISBN 1-557662-80-0

2256 Educating all Students in the Mainstream
Brookes Publishing Company
PO Box 10624
Baltimore, MD 21285-0624 410-337-9580
800-638-3775
FAX: 410-337-8539
e-mail: custserv@brookespublishing.com
www.brookespublishng.com
Paul H. Brookes, Chairman
Jeff Brookes, President
Melissa A. Behm, ExecutiveVice President
Cary Gold, Educational Sales Representative
Incorporating the research and viewpoints of both regular and special educators, this textbook provides an effective approach for modifying, expanding, and adjusting regular education to meet the needs of all students. *$34.00*
304 pages
ISBN 1-557660-22-0

2257 Educational Audiology for the Limited Hearing Infant and Preschooler
Charles C. Thomas
2600 S 1st St
Springfield, IL 62704-4730 217-789-8980
800-258-8980
FAX: 217-789-9130
e-mail: books@ccthomas.com
ccthomas.com
Donald Goldberg, Author
Nancy Coleffe-Schenck, Author
Doreen Pollack, Author
Offers information on current concepts and practices in audio-logic screening and evaluation, development of the listening function, development of speech, development of language, the role of parents, parent education, mainstreaming of the limited-hearing child, and program modifications for the severely learning disabled child. Also includes information on auditory assessment, sensory aides, cochlear implants, acoupedics and auditory verbal programs. *$76.95*
430 pages Paperback
ISBN 0-39806 -28-1

2258 Educational Care
Educators Publishing Service
625 Mount Auburn St
3rd Floor
Cambridge, MA 02138-3039 617-547-6706
800-225-5750
e-mail: Feedback.EPS@schoolspecialty.com
www.eps.schoolspecialty.com
Paula Fabbro, Sales Consultant
Leo Micale, Sales Consultant
Kristen Colson, Sales Consultant
Flora Francis, Sales Consultant
This book, written for both parents and teachers, is based on the view that education should be a system of care that is able to look after the specific needs of individual students. Using case studies, it analyzes various types of learning disorders and then suggests ways to help students with these problems. *$31.50*
325 pages
ISBN 0-838819-87-7

2259 Educational Intervention for the Student
Charles C. Thomas
2600 S 1st St
Springfield, IL 62704-4730 217-789-8980
800-258-8980
FAX: 217-789-9130
e-mail: books@ccthomas.com
www.ccthomas.com

2260 Educational Prescriptions
Educators Publishing Service
625 Mount Auburn St
3RD Floor
Cambridge, MA 02138-3039 617-547-6706
800-225-5750
e-mail: Feedback.EPS@schoolspecialty.com
www.eps.schoolspecialty.com
Paula Fabbro, Sales Consultant
Leo Micale, Sales Consultant
Kristen Colson, Sales Consultant
Flora Francis, Sales Consultant
This book provides specific recommendations for the classroom management of students who are experiencing subtle developmental and/or learning difficulties. Intended for regular classroom teachers, specific examples of accommodations teachers can make are provided for grades 1-3 and 4-6. *$13.50*
64 pages
ISBN 0-838819-90-7

2261 Effective Instruction for Special Education
Sage Publications
2455 Teller Road
Thousand Oaks, CA 91320-2218 805-499-0721
800-818-7243
FAX: 800-583-2665
e-mail: info@sagepub.com
www.sagepub.com
Sara Miller McCune, Founder, Publisher, Chairperson
Blaise R. Simqu, President/CEO
Chris Hickok, Senior Vice President/CFO
Stephen Barr, Managing Director/SAGE London, P
This exciting and wide-ranging book provides special educators with effective methods for teaching students with mild and moderate learning and behavioral problems, as well as for teaching remedial students in general. *$37.00*
419 pages Paperback

2262 Effectively Educating Handicapped Students
Longman Publishing Group
9th Fl
Upper Saddle River, NJ 07458-1813 201-236-3281
800-922-0579
FAX: 201-236-3290
www.pearsoned.com
468 pages Paperback
ISBN 0-801303-17-6

2263 Emotional Problems of Childhood and Adolescence
McGraw-Hill School Publishing
PO Box 182604
Columbus, OH 43218 877-833-5524
800-338-3987
FAX: 609-308-4480
e-mail: customer.service@mhedducation.com
www.mcgraw-hill.com
David Levin, President/Chief Ex
David Stafford, Senior Vice President/General Counsel
Maryellen Valaitis, Senior Vice President Human Resources
Patrick Milano, Chief Financial Officer Chief Administrative Officer
For future special educators, psychologists and others who work with emotionally disturbed children and adolescents.

2264 Enabling & Empowering Families: Principles & Guidelines for Practice
Brookline Books
8 Trumbull Rd
Suite B-001
Northampton, MA 01060 413-584-0184
800-666-2665
FAX: 413-584-6184
e-mail: brbooks@yahoo.com
www.brooklinebooks.com
Esther Wilder, Co-Author
This book was written for practitioners who must work with families but who have insufficient training in family systems assess-

ment and intervention. The authors' system enables professionals to help the family identify its needs, locate the formal and informal resources to meet these needs and develop the abilities to effectively access these resources. *$24.95*

220 pages
ISBN 0-914797-59-X

2265 Evaluation and Educational Programming of Students with Deafblindness & Severe Disabilities

Charles C. Thomas
2600 S 1st St
Springfield, IL 62704-4730
217-789-8980
800-258-8980
FAX: 217-789-9130
e-mail: books@ccthomas.com
www.ccthomas.com

Carroll J. Jones, Author

Subtitle: Sensorimotor Stage. This second edition offers a very complete package of information on the special education of deaf-blind students; including detailed diagnostic information to assist the instructor in evaluating the physical, social, mental status of the student, as well as the educational progress. *$50.95*

265 pages Spiral-Paper 2001
ISBN 0-398072-16-2

2266 Evaluation and Treatment of the Psychogeriatric Patient

Haworth Press
711 Third Avenue
New York, NY 10017
212-216-7800
800-354-1420
FAX: 212-244-1563
e-mail: subscriptions@tandf.co.uk.
www.haworthpress.com

111 pages Hardcover
ISBN 1-560240-52-0

2267 Exceptional Children in Focus

McGraw-Hill School Publishing
PO Box 182604
Columbus, OH 43218
877-833-5524
800-338-3987
FAX: 609-308-4480
e-mail: customer.service@mheducation.com
www.mcgraw-hill.com

David Levin, President/Chief Ex
David Stafford, Senior Vice President/General Counsel
Maryellen Valaitis, Senior Vice President Human Resources
Patrick Milano, Chief Financial Officer Chief Administrative Officer

Combines a light, personal look at the problems of special educators experiences with the basic facts of exceptionality.

288 pages

2268 Exceptional Lives: Special Education in Today's Schools, 4th Edition

Pearson Education
1 Lake St
Upper Saddle River, NJ 07458-1813
201-236-3281
800-922-0579
FAX: 201-236-3290
www.pearsoned.com

592 pages
ISBN 0-131126-00-8

2269 Facilitating Self-Care Practices in the Elderly

Haworth Press
711 Third Avenue
New York, NY 10017
212-216-7800
800-354-1420
FAX: 212-244-1563
e-mail: subscriptions@tandf.co.uk.
www.haworthpress.com

185 pages Hardcover
ISBN 1-560240-13-X

2270 Family-Centered Early Intervention with Infants and Toddlers

Brookes Publishing
PO Box 10624
Baltimore, MD 21285-0624
410-337-9580
800-638-3775
FAX: 410-337-8539
e-mail: custserv@brookespublishing.com
www.brookespublishing.com

Paul H. Brookes, Chairman
Jeffrey D. Brookes, President
Melissa A. Behm, ExecutiveVice President
George S. Stamathis, Vice President & Publisher

This informative text provides professionals with insight and practical guidelines to help fulfill the federal requirements for provision of early intervention services. *$37.00*

368 pages Hardcover
ISBN 1-557661-24-3

2271 Feeding Children with Special Needs

Arizona Department of Health Services
150 North 18th Avenue
Phoenix, AZ 85007-2607
602-542-1025
FAX: 602-542-0883
www.azdhs.gov

Will Humble, Director
Jeff Bloomberg, J.D., Manager
Robert Lane, Esq., Administrative Counsel
Lynn Golder, Esq., Administrative Counsel & HIPAA Privacy Officer

Guide designed to help develop a greater awareness of the special challenges involved in the nutrition and feeding concerns for children with special health care needs, and ways to approach the issues. *$5.00*

2272 Focal Group Psychotherapy

New Harbinger Publications
5674 Shattuck Ave
Oakland, CA 94609-1662
510-652-0215
800-748-6273
FAX: 800-652-1613
e-mail: customerservice@newharbinger.com
www.newharbinger.com

Matthew McKay, Founder
Patrick Fanning, Co-Founder/Writer

Guide to leading brief, theme-based groups. This book offers an extensive week-by-week description of the basic concepts and interventions for 14 theme or focal groups for: codependency, rape victims, shyness, survivors of incest, agoraphobia, survivors of toxic parents, depression, child molesters, anger control, domestic violence offenders, assertiveness, alcohol and drug abuse, eating disorders, and parent training. *$59.95*

544 pages Cloth
ISBN 1-879237-18-0

2273 Free Hand: Enfranchising the Education of Deaf Children

TJ Publishers
www.amazon.com

Margaret Walworth, Author
Donald F. Moores, Author
Terrence J. O'Rourke, Author

A select group of nationally prominent educators, linguists and researchers met at Hofstra University to consider the most vital and controversial question in education of the deaf: what role should ASL play in the classroom? Become part of that discussion with A Free Hand. *$16.95*

204 pages Softcover
ISBN 0-93266 -40-X

2274 Functional Assessment Inventory Manual
Stout Vocational Rehab Institute
655 15th St. NW
Suite 800
Washington, DC 20005 715-232-1411
800-538-3742
FAX: 715-232-2356
e-mail: botterbuschd@uwstout.edu
www2.epa.gov

Gina McCarthy, Administrator
Gwen Keyes Fleming, Chief of Staff
Bob Perciasepe, Deputy Administrator
Craig E. Hooks, Office of Administration and Resource Management (OARM)

The Functional Assessment is a systematic enumeration of a client's vocationally relevant strengths and limitations. *$12.00*
96 pages Paperback
ISBN 0-916671-53-4

2275 Global Perspectives on Disability: A Curriculum
Mobility International U SA
132 E Broadway
Suite 343
Eugene, OR 97401-3155 541-343-1284
FAX: 541-343-6812
TTY:541-343-1284
e-mail: info@miusa.org
www.miusa.org

Susan Sygall, CEO/Founder
Cerise Roth-Vinson, Chief Operating Officer
Cindy Lewis, Director of Programs
Stephanie Gray, Program Managers

Designed for secondary and higher education instructors. Includes five lesson plans covering disability awareness, disability rights and international perspectives on disability. Available in alternative formats. *$40.00*

2276 Glossary of Terminology for Vocational Assessment/Evaluation/Work
Rehabilitation Resource University
University of Wisconsin-Stou
Menomonie, WI 54751 715-232-2236
FAX: 715-232-2356
e-mail: gundlachj@uwstout.edu

Ronald Fry, Manager
Jennifer Gundlach Klatt, Program Assistant

This glossary contains 254 terms and their definitions. Primary focus is on the terminology related to the practice and professionals of vocational assessment, vocational evaluation and work adjustment. *$9.50*
40 pages Softcover

2277 Graduate Technological Education and the Human Experience of Disability
Haworth Press
711 Third Avenue
New York, NY 10017 212-216-7800
800-354-1420
FAX: 212-244-1563
e-mail: subscriptions@tandf.co.uk.
www.haworthpress.com

115 pages Hardcover
ISBN 0-789060-08-6

2278 HIV Infection and Developmental Disabilities
Brookes Publishing
PO Box 10624
Baltimore, MD 21285-0624 410-337-9580
800-638-3775
FAX: 410-337-8539
e-mail: custserv@brookespublishing.com
www.brookespublishing.com

Paul H. Brookes, Chairman
Jeffrey D. Brookes, President
Melissa A. Behm, ExecutiveVice President
George S. Stamathis, Vice President & Publisher

A resource for service providers pinpointing the most crucial medical, legal and educational issues to control HIV infection.
$47.00
320 pages
ISBN 1-557660-83-2

2279 Handbook for Implementing Workshops for Siblings of Special Children
Special Needs Project
324 State St
Suite H
Santa Barbara, CA 93101-2364 805-962-8087
800-333-6867
FAX: 805-962-5087
e-mail: editor@specialneeds.com
www.specialneeds.com

Mark Darrow, Founder,The Prolotherapy Institu

Based on three years of professional experience, this handbook provides guidelines and techniques for those who wish to start and conduct workshops for siblings. *$40.00*

2280 Handbook for Speech Therapy
Psychological & Educational Publications
PO Box 520
Hydesville, CA 95547 800-523-5775
FAX: 800-447-0907
e-mail: psych-edpublications@suddenlink.net
www.psych-edpublications.com

143 pages paperback

2281 Handbook for the Special Education Administrator
Edwin Mellen Press
PO Box 450
Lewiston, NY 14092-1205 716-754-2266
FAX: 716-754-4056
e-mail: jrupnow@mellenpress.com
www.mellenpress.com

Arthur R. Crowell, Author
Bonnie Crogan, Marketing
Irene Miller, Accounting
Patricia Schultz, Production

Organization and procedures for special education. *$ 49.95*
96 pages Hardcover
ISBN 0-88946 -22-9

2282 Handbook of Developmental Education
Greenwood Publishing Group
130 Cremona Drive
Santa Barbara, CA 93117 805-968-1911
800-368-6868
FAX: 866-270-3856
e-mail: CustomerService@abc-clio.com
www.abc-clio.com

This comprehensive handbook has brought together the leading practitioners and researchers in the field of developmental education to focus on the developmental learning agenda. Hardcover.
400 pages $65 - $75
ISBN 0-275932-97-4

2283 Handbook on Supported Education for Peoplewith Mental Illness
Brookes Publishing
PO Box 10624
Baltimore, MD 21285-0624 410-337-9580
800-638-3775
FAX: 410-337-8539
e-mail: custserv@brookespublishing.com
www.brookespublishing.com

Paul H. Brookes, Chairman
Jeffrey D. Brookes, President
Melissa A. Behm, ExecutiveVice President
George S. Stamathis, Vice President & Publisher

Here you will find all necessary information that mental health professionals need in order to provide supported education services. There are specific suggestions on how to help people with mental illness return to or remain in college, trade school, or GED

programs. Also addressed are funding and legal issues, accommodations, and specific interventions.
208 pages Paperback
ISBN 1-55766-52-1

2284 Head Injury Rehabilitation: Children
Taylor & Francis
47 Runway Dr
Ste G
Levittown, PA 19057-4738
267-580-2622
FAX: 215-785-5515
460 pages Cloth
ISBN 0-85066-67-1

2285 Health Care Management in Physical Therapy
Charles C. Thomas
2600 S 1st St
Springfield, IL 62704-4730
217-789-8980
800-258-8980
FAX: 217-789-9130
e-mail: books@ccthomas.com
www.ccthomas.com

2286 Health Care for Students with Disabilities
Brookes Publishing Company
PO Box 10624
Baltimore, MD 21285-0624
410-337-9580
800-638-3775
FAX: 410-337-8539
e-mail: custserv@brookespublishing.com
www.brookespublishing.com
Paul H. Brookes, Chairman
Jeffrey D. Brookes, President
Melissa A. Behm, ExecutiveVice President
George S. Stamathis, Vice President & Publisher
This practical guidebook provides detailed descriptions of the 16 health-related procedures most likely to be needed in the classroom by students with disabilities. *$25.00*
304 pages Paperback
ISBN 1-557660-37-9

2287 Helping Learning Disabled Gifted Children
Charles C. Thomas
2600 S 1st St
Springfield, IL 62704-4730
217-789-8980
800-258-8980
FAX: 217-789-9130
e-mail: books@ccthomas.com
ccthomas.com
James Harry Humphrey, Author
CC Thomas has been producing a strong list of specialty titles and textbooks in the biomedical sciences since 1927.

2288 Helping Students Grow
American College Testing Program
500 ACT Drive
PO Box 168
Iowa City, IA 52243-0168
319-337-1000
e-mail: info@keytrain.com
www.act.org
Jon Whitmore, Chief Executive Officer
Tom J. Goedken, Chief Financial Officer/Senior Vice President
Patricia C. Steinbrech, Chief Information Officer
Janet E. Godwin, Chief of Staff/Accountability Officer
Designed to assist counselors in using the wealth of information generated by the ACT Assessment.

2289 Home Health Care Provider: A Guide to Essential Skills
Springer Publishing
11 W 42nd St
15th Floor
New York, NY 10036-8002
212-431-4370
877-687-7476
FAX: 212-941-7842
e-mail: cs@springerpub.com
www.springerpub.com
Theodore C. Nardin, CEO/Publisher
Jason Roth, VP/Marketing Director
Annette Imperati, Marketing/Sales Director
James C. Costello, Vice President, Journal Publishing
This book is designed to foster quality care to home care recipients. Prieto provides information, tips, and techniques on personal care routines as well as additional responsibilities, including home safety and maintenance, meal planning, errand running, caring for couples, and making use of recreational time. The book focuses on the psycho-social needs of home care recipients, stressing the need to maintainthe house as a home, and sustaining the recipient's way of life throughout caregiving.

2290 How to Teach Spelling/How to Spell
Educators Publishing Service
625 Mount Auburn St
3rd Floor
Cambridge, MA 02138-3039
617-547-6706
800-225-5750
e-mail: Feedback.EPS@schoolspecialty.com
www.eps.schoolspecialty.com
Paula Fabbro, Sales Consultant
Leo Micale, Sales Consultant
Kristen Colson, Sales Consultant
Flora Francis, Sales Consultant
This is a comprehensive resource manual based on the Orton-Gillingham approach to reading and spelling. It recommends what and how much to teach at each grade level at the beginning of each lesson or section. There are four student manuals that accompany this. *$22.50*
Teachers Manual
ISBN 0-838818-47-1

2291 Human Exceptionality: Society, School, and Family
Allyn & Bacon
75 Arlington St
Suite 300
Boston, MA 02116-3988
e-mail: ab_webmaster@abacon.com
www.home.pearsonhighered.com
615 pages
ISBN 0-20528-39-0

2292 I Can't Hear You in the Dark: How to Lean and Teach Lipreading
Charles C. Thomas
2600 South 1st Street
Springfield, IL 62704-4730
217-789-8980
800-258-8980
FAX: 217-789-9130
e-mail: books@ccthomas.com
www.ccthomas.com
Betty Woerner Carter, Author
The goal of this text is to improve communication and strengthen relationships with others. *$40.95*
226 pages Spiral-Paper 1997
ISBN 0-398067-89-2

2293 I Heard That!
3417 Volta Pl NW
Washington, DC 20007-2737
202-337-5220
FAX: 202-337-8314
TTY:202-337-5221
e-mail: info@agbell.org
www.listeningandspokenlanguage.org

Meredith K. Sugar, Esq. (OH), President
Ted A. Meyer, M.D., Ph.D, President-Elect/Secretary-Treasurer
Emilio Alonso-Mendoza, Chief Executive Officer
Susan Boswell, Director of Communications and Marketing

Provides a framework for teachers, clinicians and parents when writing objectives and designing activities to develop listening skills in children with hearing loss from newborn to 3 years. *$7.95*
36 pages

2294 I Heard That!2
Alexander Graham Bell Association
3417 Volta Pl NW
Washington, DC 20007-2737
202-337-5220
FAX: 202-337-8314
TTY:202-337-5221
e-mail: info@agbell.org
www.listeningandspokenlanguage.org

Meredith K. Sugar, Esq. (OH), President
Ted A. Meyer, M.D., Ph.D, President-Elect/Secretary-Treasurer
Emilio Alonso-Mendoza, Chief Executive Officer
Susan Boswell, Director of Communications and Marketing

Provides a framework for teachers, clinicians and parents when writing objectives and designing activities to develop listening skills in children who are deaf or hard of hearing. *$7.95*
36 pages

2295 If It Is To Be, It Is Up To Us To Help!
AVKO Educational Research Foundation
3084 Willard Rd
Ste W
Birch Run, MI 48415-9404
810-686-9283
866-285-6612
FAX: 810-686-1101
e-mail: webmaster@avko.org
www.avko.org

Don Mc Cabe, President
Ted A. Meyer, M.D., Ph.D, Vice-President
Michael Lane, Treasurer
Birch Run, Research Director Emeritus

A book of lesson plans for an Adult Community Education Course for Volunteer Tutors. Contains information on how to go about establishing such a course and how to secure cooperation from local and national organizations. Free as an e-book for Foundation members. *$ 14.95*
ISBN 1-56400 -42-1

2296 Images of the Disabled, Disabling Images
Greenwood Publishing Group
130 Cremona Drive
Santa Barbara, CA 93117
805-968-1911
800-368-6868
FAX: 866-270-3856
e-mail: CustomerService@abc-clio.com
www.greenwood.com

Combines an examination of the presentation of persons with disabilities in literature, film and the media with an analysis of the ways in which these images are expressed in public policy concerning the disabled. *$55.00*
227 pages Hardcover
ISBN 0-275921-78-6

2297 Implementing Family-Centered Services in Early Intervention
Brookline Books
8 Trumbull Rd
Suite B-001
Northampton, MA 01060
413-584-0184
800-666-2665
FAX: 413-584-6184
e-mail: brbooks@yahoo.com
www.brooklinebooks.com

180 pages Paperback
ISBN 0-91479 -62-

2298 Including All of Us: An Early Childhood Curriculum About Disability
Educational Equity Concepts
71 Fifth Avenue
6th Floor
New York, NY 10003
212-243-1110
FAX: 212-627-0407
e-mail: lcolon@fhi360.org
www.edequity.org

Frank Schneiger, President
Antonia Cottrell Martin, Founder and President
Merle Froschl, Co-director
Barbara Sprung, Co-director

The first nonsexist, multicultural, mainstreamed curriculum. Step-by-step activities incorporate disability into three curriculum areas: Same/Different (hearing impairment), Body Parts (visual impairment), and Transportation (mobility impairment). *$14.95*
144 pages
ISBN 0-93162 -00-4

2299 Including Students with Severe and Multiple Disabilites in Typical Classrooms
Brookes Publishing
PO Box 10624
Baltimore, MD 21285-0624
410-337-9580
800-638-3775
FAX: 410-337-8539
e-mail: custserv@brookespublishing.com
www.brookespublishing.com

Paul H. Brookes, Chairman
Jeffrey D. Brookes, President
Melissa A. Behm, ExecutiveVice President
George S. Stamathis, Vice President & Publisher

This straightforward and jargon free resource gives instructors the guidance needed to educate learners who have one or more sensory impairments in addition to cognitive and physical disabilities. *$32.95*
224 pages Paperback
ISBN 1-55766 -39-8

2300 Including Students with Special Needs: A Practical Guide for Classroom Teachers
Allyn & Bacon
75 Arlington St
Suite 300
Boston, MA 02116-3988
e-mail: ab_webmaster@abacon.com
www.home.pearsonhighered.com

544 pages
ISBN 0-20528 -85-4

2301 Inclusive & Heterogeneous Schooling: Assessment, Curriculum, and Instruction
Brookes Publishing
PO Box 10624
Baltimore, MD 21285-0624 410-337-9580
800-638-3775
FAX: 410-337-8539
e-mail: custserv@brookespublishing.com
www.brookespublishing.com
Paul H. Brookes, Chairman
Jeff Brookes, President
Melissa A. Behm, ExecutiveVice President
Cary Gold, Educational Sales Representative
Presents methods for successfully restructuring classrooms to enable all students, particularly those with disabilities, to flourish. Provides specific strategies for assessment, collaboration, classroom management, and age-specific instruction. *$34.95*
448 pages Paperback
ISBN 1-55766-02-9

2302 Independent Living Approach to Disability Policy Studies
World Institute on Disability
3075 Adeline Street
Suite 155
Berkeley, CA 94703 510-225-6400
FAX: 510-225-0477
TTY:510-225-0478
e-mail: wid@wid.org
www.wid.org
Paul W. Schroeder, Chairman
Linda M. Dardarian, Vice Chairman
Mary Brooner, Treasurer
Cassandra Malry, Secretary
This collection of essays and bibliographies attempts to build a framework for understanding how the relationship between public policy, disability studies and disability policy studies will impact us in the future. *$17.50*
240 pages Paperback

2303 Information & Referral Center
Mississippi State University
108 Herbert - South
Room 150/PO Drawer 6189
Mississippi State Univers, MS 39762-6189 662-325-2001
800-675-7782
FAX: 662-325-8989
TTY: 662-325-2694
e-mail: nrtc@colled.msstate.edu
www.blind.msstate.edu
Jacqui Bybee, Research and Training Coordinato
Michele Capella McDonnall, Ph.D., Research Professor/Interim Director
Jessica Thornton, Business Manager
Marty Giesen, Ph.D., Senior Research Scientist
A comprehensive website that includes information about client assistance programs, vocational rehabilitation agencies, low vision clinics and information about blindness and low vision. *$25.00*
150 pages

2304 Instructional Methods for Students
Allyn & Bacon
75 Arlington St
Suite 300
Boston, MA 02116-3988
e-mail: ab_webmaster@abacon.com
www.home.pearsonhighered.com
450 pages
ISBN 0-205087-35-3

2305 Interactions: Collaboration Skills for School Professionals
Longman Education/Addison Wesley
75 Arlington St
Suite 300
Boston, MA 02116-3988
e-mail: ab_webmaster@abacon.com
www.longman.awl.com
270 pages Paperback
ISBN 0-80131-21-2

2306 International Journal of Arts Medicine
MMB Music
9051 Watson Road
Suite 161
Saint Louis, MO 63126 314-531-9635
800-543-3771
FAX: 314-531-8384
e-mail: info@mmbmusic.com
www.mmbmusic.com
Norm Goldberg, Founder/chairman
Exploration of the creative arts and healing. Presents peer-reviewed articles clearly written by educators in the creative arts, as well as internationally prominent physicians, therapists and health care professionals.

2307 Interpreting Disability: A Qualitative Reader
Teachers College Press
1234 Amsterdam Avenue
New York, NY 10027 212-678-3929
800-575-6566
FAX: 212-678-4149
e-mail: tcpress@tc.columbia.edu
www.tcpress.com
Brian Ellerbeck, Executive Acquisitions Editor
Marie Ellen Larcada, Senior Acquisitions Editor
Emily Spangler, Acquisitions Editor
Meg Hartmann, Acquisitions Assistant
This book offers a collection of exemplary qualitative research affecting people with disabilities and their families. Instead of focusing upon methodological details, the chapters illustrate the variety of styles and formats that interpretive research can adopt in reporting its results. *$24.95*
328 pages Paperback
ISBN 0-807731-21-8

2308 Intervention Research in Learning Disabilities
Gallery Bookshop
319 Kasten Street
PO Box 270
Mendocino, CA 95460-270 707-937-2215
FAX: 707-937-3737
e-mail: info@gallerybookshop.com
www.gallerybooks.com
Tony Miksak, Owner
Based on the Symposium on Intervention Research, this volume presents 12 papers addressing issues in intervention research, academic interventions, social and behavioral interventions, and postsecondary interventions. *$30.00*
347 pages

2309 Introduction to Learning Disabilities
Allyn & Bacon
75 Arlington St
Suite 300
Boston, MA 02116-3988
e-mail: ab_webmaster@abacon.com
www.pearsonhighered.com
608 pages
ISBN 0-20529-43-4

2310 Introduction to Mental Retardation
Allyn & Bacon
75 Arlington St
Suite 300
Boston, MA 02116-3988
e-mail: ab_webmaster@abacon.com
www.pearsonhighered.com

350 pages Casebound
ISBN 0-134879-27-9

2311 Introduction to Special Education: Teaching in an Age of Challenge, 4th Edition
Allyn & Bacon
75 Arlington St
Suite 300
Boston, MA 02116-3988
e-mail: ab_webmaster@abacon.com
www.pearsonhighered.com

640 pages cloth
ISBN 0-20526 -94-4

2312 Introduction to the Profession of Counseling
McGraw-Hill School Publishing
PO Box 182604
Columbus, OH 43218
877-833-5524
800-338-3987
FAX: 609-308-4480
e-mail: customer.service@mheducation.com
www.mcgraw-hill.com

David Levin, President/Chief Executive Officer
David Stafford, Senior Vice President/General Counsel
Maryellen Valaitis, Senior Vice President Human Resources
Patrick Milano, Chief Financial Officer/Chief Administrative Officer
Offers information, theories and techniques for counseling numerous cases from drug addiction to special populations.
464 pages

2313 Issues and Research in Special Education
Teachers College Press
PO Box 20
Williston, VT 05495-0020
800-575-6566
FAX: 802-664-7626
e-mail: tcp.orders@aidcvt.com
www.teacherscollegepress.com

264 pages Hardcover
ISBN 0-807731-95-1

2314 Kendall Demonstration Elementary School Curriculum Guides
Gallaudet University Bookstore
800 Florida Ave NE
Washington, DC 20002-3695
202-651-5488
800-621-2736
FAX: 202-651-5489
TTY: 888-630-9347
e-mail: gupress@gallaudet.edu
www.gupress.gallaudet.edu

Dr. T Alan Hurwitz, President
Edward Bosso, Vice President for Administration
Dr. Lynne Murray, Vice President for Development
Donald Beil, Chief of Staff
KDES is a day school serving students from birth through age 15, beginning with the Parent-Infant Program and ending in grade 8. Students come from the Washington, D.C., metropolitan area.

2315 Language Arts: Detecting Special Needs
Allyn & Bacon
75 Arlington St
Suite 300
Boston, MA 02116-3988
617-848-7500
800-852-8024
FAX: 617-944-7273
www.home.pearsonhighered.com

Bill Barke, Chairman/CEO
Nancy Forfyth, President
Kevin Stone, Vice President, National Sales M
Thomas A. Rakes, Author
Describes special language arts needs of special learners.
180 pages paperback
ISBN 0-205116-36-1

2316 Language Learning Practices with Deaf Children
Sage Publications
2455 Teller Road
Thousand Oaks, CA 91320
805-499-9774
800-818-7243
FAX: 800-583-2665
e-mail: books.claim@sagepub.com
www.sagepub.com

Sara Miller McCune, Founder, Publisher, Chairperson
Stephen P. Quigley, Co-Author
Susan Rose, Co-Author
Patricia L. McAnally, Co-Author
This new edition describes the variety of language-development theories and practices used with deaf children without advocating anyone. *$38.00*
321 pages Hardcover

2317 Language and Communication Disorders in Children
McGraw-Hill School Publishn
PO Box 182604
Columbus, OH 43218
877-833-5524
800-338-3987
FAX: 609-308-4480
e-mail: customer.service@mheducation.com
www.mcgraw-hill.com

David Levin, President/Chief Executive Officer
David Stafford, Senior Vice President/General Counsel
Maryellen Valaitis, Senior Vice President Human Resources
Patrick Milano, Chief Financial Officer/Chief Administrative Officer
Comprehensive coverage encompassing all aspects of children's language disorders.
512 pages

2318 Learning Disabilities, Literacy, and Adult Education
Brookes Publishing
PO Box 10624
Baltimore, MD 21285-0624
410-337-9580
800-638-3775
FAX: 410-337-8539
e-mail: custserv@brookespublishing.com
www.brookespublishing.com

Paul H. Brookes, Chairman
Jeffrey D. Brookes, President
Melissa A. Behm, ExecutiveVice President
George S. Stamathis, Vice President & Publisher
This book focuses on adults with severe learning disabilities and the educators who work with them. Described are the characteristics, demographics, and educational and employment status of adults with LD and the laws that protect them in the workplace and in educational settings.
450 pages Paperback
ISBN 1-55766 -47-5

2319 Learning Disabilities: Concepts and Characteristics

McGraw-Hill School Publishing
220 E Danieldale Rd
Desoto, TX 75115-2490
972-224-4772
800-442-9685
FAX: 972-228-1982
www.mhschool.com

Harold McGraw III, Chairman/ President/ Chief Ex
Jack F. Callahan, Executive Vice President, Chief
James A. McLoughlin, Co-Author
Gerald Wallace, Co-Author

Covers the conceptual basis of learning disabilities, identification, etiology and diagnosis.
448 pages

2320 Learning Disability: Social Class and the Cons of Inequality In American Education

Greenwood Publishing Group
130 Cremona Drive
Santa Barbara, CA 93117
805-968-1911
800-368-6868
FAX: 866-270-3856
e-mail: CustomerService@abc-clio.com
www.abc-clio.com

James Carrier, Author

Presents a detailed historical description of the social and educational assumptions integral to the idea of learning disability.
167 pages $43.95 - $47.95
ISBN 0-313253-96-X

2321 Learning and Individual Differences

National Association of School Psychologists
8455 Colesville Rd
Suite 1000
Silver Spring, MD 20910- 3392
301-589-3300
FAX: 301-589-5175
e-mail: info@musictherapy.org
www.musictherapy.org

Andrea Farbman, EdD, Executive Director
Judy Simpson, MT-BC, Director of Government Relations
Jane Creagan, MME, MT-BC, Director of Professional Program
E.L. Grigorenko, Editor

A multidisciplinary journal in education.

2322 Learning to See: American Sign Language asa Second Language

Gallaudet University Press
800 Florida Ave NE
Washington, DC 20002-3695
202-651-5206
800-621-2736
FAX: 800-621-8476
TTY: 888-630-9347
e-mail: clerc.center@gallaudet.edu.
www.gupress.gallaudet.edu

Dr. T Alan Hurwitz, President
Edward Bosso, Vice President for Administration
Phyliss Wilcox, Co-Author
Sherman Wilcox, Co-Author

This important book has been updated to help teachers teach American Sign Language as a second language, including information on Deaf culture, the history and structure of ASL, teaching methods and issues facing educators. *$19.95*
160 pages Softcover

2323 Let's Write Right: Teacher's Edition

AVKO Educational Research Foundation
3084 Willard Rd
Ste W
Birch Run, MI 48415-9404
810-686-9283
866-285-6612
FAX: 810-686-1101
e-mail: webmaster@avko.org
www.avko.org

Barry Chute, President
Julie Guyette, Vice President
Don Mc Cabe, Research Director
Clifford Schroeder, Treasurer

A manuscript and cursive writing program designed not only to teach handwriting but help with reading and spelling patterns as well. Teaches students to learn to read cursive as manuscript is being taught and ease the transition to cursive by using a D'Nealian-like script. Exercises involve phoically consistent patterns to help reinforce fluency with spelling and handwriting.
$39.95
164 pages

2324 Library Manager's Guide to Hiring and Serving Disabled Persons

Mc Farland & Company
960 NC Hwy 88 W
Jefferson, NC 28640
336-246-4460
800-253-2187
FAX: 336-246-5018
e-mail: infoinso@mcfarlandpub.com
www.mcfarlandpub.com

Kieth C. Wright, Co-Author
Judith F. Davie, Co-Author

Information for library staff on hiring and serving disabled persons. *$35.00*
171 pages Illustrated
ISBN 0-89950 -16-3

2325 Life-Span Approach to Nursing Care for Individuals with Developmental Disabilities

Brookes Publishing
PO Box 10624
Baltimore, MD 21285-0624
410-337-9580
800-638-3775
FAX: 410-337-8539
e-mail: custserv@brookespublishing.com
www.brookespublishing.com

Paul H. Brookes, Chairman
Jeffrey D. Brookes, President
Melissa A. Behm, ExecutiveVice President
George S. Stamathis, Vice President & Publisher

This reference book was written by and for nurses. This guide addresses fundamental nursing issues such as health promotion, infection control, seizure management, adaptive and assistive technology, and sexuality. Also offered are in-depth case studies, helpful charts and tables, and problem-solving strategies. *$49.95*
464 pages Hardcover
ISBN 1-557661-51-0

2326 Mainstreaming Deaf and Hard of Hearing Students: Questions and Answers

Gallaudet University Bookstore
800 Florida Ave NE
Washington, DC 20002-3600
202-651-5000
800-451-1073
FAX: 202-651-5489
TTY: 888-630-9347
e-mail: clerc.center@gallaudet.edu.
www.gupress.gallaudet.edu

Dr. T Alan Hurwitz, President
Debra S. Lipkey, University Budget Director
Donald Beil, Chief of Staff
Edward Bosso, Vice President for Administratio

This booklet presents mainstreaming as one educational option and suggests some considerations for parents, teachers and administrators. *$6.00*
40 pages

2327 Mainstreaming Exceptional Students: A Guide for Classroom Teachers
Allyn & Bacon
75 Arlington St
Suite 300
Boston, MA 02116-3988 617-848-7500
800-852-8024
FAX: 617-944-7273
www.home.pearsonhighered.com

Nancy Forfyth, President
Bill Barke, CEO
Jane B. Schulz, Co-Author
C. Dale Carpenter, Co-Author
Covers the various categories of exceptional students and discusses educational strategies and classroom management.
464 pages paperback
ISBN 0-20515 -24-6

2328 Mainstreaming: A Practical Approach for Teachers
McGraw-Hill School Publishing
PO Box 182604
Columbus, OH 43218 877-833-5524
800-338-3987
FAX: 609-308-4480
e-mail: customer.service@mheducation.com
www.mcgraw-hill.com

David Levin, President/Chief Executive Officer
David Stafford, Senior Vice President/General Counsel
Maryellen Valaitis, Senior Vice President Human Resources
Patrick Milano, Chief Financial Officer/Chief Administrative Officer
Provides teachers, administrators and school psychologists with the background, techniques and strategies they need to offer appropriate services for mildly handicapped students in the mainstream classroom.

2329 Managing Diagnostic Tool of Visual Perception
Gallery Bookshop
319 Kasten Street
PO Box 270
Mendocino, CA 95460-270 707-937-2215
FAX: 707-937-3737
e-mail: info@gallerybookshop.com
www.gallerybooks.com

Constantine Mangina, Author
For diagnosing specific perceptual learning abilities and disabilities. *$14.00*
ISBN 0-80580 -83-4

2330 Medical Rehabilitation
Lippincott, Williams & Wilkins
227 S 6th St
Suite 227
Philadelphia, PA 19106-3713 215-545-5630
800-777-2295
FAX: 215-732-9988
www.lpub.com

Cheryl Murkey, Manager
Information for the professional on new techniques and treatments in the medical rehabilitation fields. *$80.50*
368 pages Illustrated
ISBN 0-88167 -85-5

2331 Meeting the ADD Challenge: A Practical Guide for Teachers
Research Press
PO Box 7886
Champaign, IL 61826-9177 217-352-3273
800-519-2707
FAX: 217-352-1221
e-mail: rp@researchpress.com
www.researchpress.com

Robert W. Parkinson, Founder
Dr. Michael Asher, Co-Author
Dr. Steven B Gordon, Co-Author
$24.95
ISBN 0-878223-45-9

2332 Mental & Physical Disability Law Digest
A BA Commission on Mental and Physical Disability
1050 Connecticut Ave. N.W.
Suite 400
Washington, DC 20036-1019 202-662-1000
800-285-2221
FAX: 202-442-3439
e-mail: cmpdl@abanet.org
www.americanbar.org

Robert M. Carlson, Chair, House of Delegates:
James R. Silkenat, President
William C. Hubbard, President-Elect
Cara Lee, Secretary
Provides comprehensive, summary and analysis of federal and state disability and state disability laws from mental disability law and disability discrimination law perspectives. *$60.00*
376 pages
ISBN 1-590310-05-5

2333 Mental Health Concepts and Techniques for the Occupational Therapy Assistant
Lippincott, Williams & Wilkins
227 S 6th St
Suite 227
Philadelphia, PA 19106-3713 215-521-8300
800-777-2295
FAX: 301-824-7390
www.lpub.com

J Lippincott, CEO
This text offers clear and easily understood explanations of the various theoretical and practiced health models. *$36.00*
344 pages
ISBN 0-88167 -53-X

2334 Mental Health and Mental Illness
Lippincott, Williams & Wilkins
227 S 6th St
Suite 227
Philadelphia, PA 19106-3713 215-592-5400
800-777-2295
FAX: 301-824-7390
www.lpub.com

Kathy Sykes, Manager
Concise, comprehensive and completely up to date, this book presents the most current theory in mental health nursing for the student and the new practitioner. *$28.95*
480 pages
ISBN 0-39755 -73-7

2335 Mentally Ill Individuals
Mainstream
Ste 830
3 Bethesda Metro Ctr
Bethesda, MD 20814-6301 301-961-9299
800-247-1380
FAX: 301-654-6714
e-mail: info@mainstreaminc.org

Charles Moster
Mainstreaming mentally ill individuals into the workplace. *$2.50*
12 pages

2336 Midland Treatment Furniture
Sammons Preston Rolyan
W68 N158 Evergreen Blvd
Cedarburg, WI 53012-2637 262-387-8720
800-228-3693
FAX: 262-387-8748
e-mail: CustomerSupport@PattersonMedical.com
www.pattersonmedical.com

Free

2337 Multidisciplinary Assessment of Children With Learning Disabilities and Mental Retardation
Gallery Bookshop
319 Kasten Street
PO Box 270
Mendocino, CA 95460-270
707-937-2215
FAX: 707-937-3737
e-mail: info@gallerybookshop.com
www.gallerybooks.com

David L. Wodrich, Author
James E. Joy, Editor
Assessment of children with learning disabilities and mental retardation. *$24.00*
346 pages Illustrated
ISBN 0-93371 -62-1

2338 Multisensory Teaching of Basic Language Skills: Theory and Practice
Brookes Publishing
PO Box 10624
Baltimore, MD 21285-0624
410-337-9580
800-638-3775
FAX: 410-337-8539
e-mail: custserv@brookespublishing.com
www.brookespublishing.com

Paul H. Brookes, Chairman
Jeffrey D. Brookes, President
Melissa A. Behm, ExecutiveVice President
George S. Stamathis, Vice President & Publisher
This book presents specific multisensory methods for helping students who are having trouble learning to read due to dyslexia or other learning disabilities. Recommended techniques are offered for teaching alphabet skills, composition, comprehension, handwriting, math, organization and study skills, phonological awareness, reading and spelling. *$59.00*
608 pages Hardcover
ISBN 1-557663-49-1

2339 No Longer Immune: A Counselor's Guide to AIDS
American Counceling Association
5999 Stevenson Ave
Alexandria, VA 22304-3304
703-823-9800
800-347-6647
FAX: 703-823-0252
e-mail: membership@counseling.org
www.counseling.org

Robert L. Smith, President
Thelma Duffey, President-Elect
Cirecie A. West-Olatunji, Past-President
Brian Canfield, Treasurer
Covers a broad range of issues such as working with specific populations, handling pre and post testing situations, coping with fear, grief and survivor guilt, struggling with spiritual issues and dealing with counter transference. *$26.95*
295 pages
ISBN 1-55620 -64-1

2340 Occupational Therapy Across Cultural Boundaries
Haworth Press
711 Third Avenue
New York, NY 10017
212-216-7800
800-354-1420
FAX: 212-244-1563
e-mail: subscriptions@tandf.co.uk.
www.taylorandfrancisgroup.com

Derek Mapp, Non-Executive Chairman
Roger Horton, CEO
Emma Blaney, Group HR Director - Head of Corporate Responsibility
Isobel Peck, Group Chief Marketing Officer
Examines the concept of culture from a unique perspective, that of individual occupational therapists who have worked in environments very different from those in which they were educated or had worked previously. Journal publications formerly published by Haworth Press are now listed on the Taylor & Francis Journals website. *$74.95*
107 pages Hardcover
ISBN 1-560242-23-X

2341 Occupational Therapy Approaches to Traumatic Brain Injury
Haworth Press
711 Third Avenue
New York, NY 10017
212-216-7800
800-354-1420
FAX: 212-244-1563
e-mail: subscriptions@tandf.co.uk.
http://www.taylorandfrancisgroup.com/

Laura H Krefting, Co-Author
Jerry A Johnson, Co-Author
Focuses on the disabled individual, the family, and the societal responses to the injured, this comprehensive book covers the spectrum of available services from intensive care to transitional and community living. Journal publications formerly published by Haworth Press are now listed on the Taylor & Francis Journals website. *$74.95*
137 pages Hardcover
ISBN 1-560240-64-4

2342 Overcoming Dyslexia in Children, Adolescents and Adults
Sage Publications
2455 Teller Road
Thousand Oaks, CA 91320
805-499-9774
800-818-7243
FAX: 800-583-2665
e-mail: books.claim@sagepub.com
www.sagepub.com

Sara Miller McCune, Founder, Publisher, Chairperson
Blaise R Simqu, President/CEO
Tracey A. Ozmina, Executive Vice President & Chief
Dale R. Jordan, Author
This book describes some forms of dyslexia in detail and then relates those problems to the social, emotional and personal development of dyslexic individuals. *$34.00*
350 pages Paperback

2343 Oxford Textbook of Geriatric Medicine
Oxford University Press
198 Madison Ave
New York, NY 10016-4308
212-726-6000
800-445-9714
FAX: 919-677-1303
e-mail: custserv.us@oup.com
www.global.oup.com

Rebecca Seger, Director, Institutional Sales, Americas
Lesa Moran Owen, Library Sales Operations Manager
Lenny Allen, Director, Institutional Accounts
Nancy Roy, Library Sales Manager
This comprehensive text brings together extensive experience in clinical geriatrics with a strong scientific base in research. *$125.00*
784 pages

2344 PKU for Children: Learning to Measure
University of Washington PKU Clinic
PO Box 357920
University of Washington
Seattle, WA 98195-7920
206-598-1800
877-685-3015
FAX: 206-598-1915
e-mail: pku@u.washington.edu
www.depts.washington.edu/pku
C. Ronald Scott, MD, Professor, Pediatrics, Division
Michael J. Bamshad, MD, Division Chief and Professor
Eileen Chin, BA (Acc), Division Administrator
Susanna Ngai, BS, Fiscal Specialist 2 - Administra
Lesson format for parents and teachers.

2345 Pain Centers: A Revolution in Health Care
Lippincott Williams And Wilkins
227
227 S 6th St
Philadelphia, PA 19106-3713
215-521-8300
800-777-2295
FAX: 301-824-7390
www.lpub.com
J Lippincott, CEO
$103.00
280 pages

2346 Parental Concerns in College Student Mental Health
Haworth Press
711 Third Avenue
New York, NY 10017
212-216-7800
800-354-1420
FAX: 212-244-1563
e-mail: subscriptions@tandf.co.uk.
www.taylorandfrancisgroup.com
Derek Mapp, Non-Executive Chairman
Roger Horton, CEO
Emma Blaney, Group HR Director - Head of Corporate Responsibility
Isobel Peck, Group Chief Marketing Officer
An instructive guide for parents and mental health professionals regarding the most important issues about psychological development in college students. Journal publications formerly published by Haworth Press are now listed on the Taylor & Francis Journals website. *$74.95*
204 pages Hardcover
ISBN 0-866567-20-8

2347 Parents and Teachers
Alexander Graham Bell Association
3417 Volta Pl NW
Washington, DC 20007-2737
202-337-5220
866-337-5220
FAX: 202-337-8314
TTY: 202-337-5221
e-mail: info@agbell.org
www.listeningandspokenlanguage.org
Kathleen S. Treni, M.Ed., M.A., President
Meredith K. Knueve, Esq., Secretary-Treasurer
Alexander T. Graham, Executive Director/CEO
Corrine Altman, Director
This excellent book offers in-depth guidance to parents and teachers whose partnership can foster language in school-aged children with hearing impairments. The first section examines roles of parents, teachers, professionals and children in language acquisition, residual hearing and audiological management, language development stages and readying children for preschool. The second portion of the book presents specific objectives and teaching strategies to use at school and at home. *$27.95*
386 pages

2348 Patient and Family Education
Springer Publishing Company
11 W 42nd St
15th Floor
New York, NY 10036-8002
212-431-4370
877-687-7476
FAX: 212-941-7842
e-mail: cs@springerpub.com
www.springerpub.com
Dr. Ursula Springer, President
Ted Nardin, CEO
James C. Costello, Vice President, Journal Publishi
James C. Costello, Vice President, Journal Publishing
This guide outlines the actual clinical content needed to develop, implement and maintain patient education programs. Conveniently arranged in one-hour long lesson plans, each disease or condition is organized in an easy-to-follow format. *$26.95*
272 pages Softcover
ISBN 0-82615 -41-7

2349 Person to Person: Guide for Professionals Working with the Disabled
Paul H Brookes Publishing Company
PO Box 10624
Baltimore, MD 21285-0624
410-337-9580
800-638-3775
FAX: 410-337-8539
e-mail: custserv@brookespublishing.com
www.brookespublishing.com
Paul H. Brookes, Chairman
Jeffrey D. Brookes, President
Melissa A. Behm, ExecutiveVice President
George S. Stamathis, Vice President & Publisher
This second edition of an already-popular book helps professionals approach interactions with a people-first, disability second attitude. *$29.00*
288 pages Paperback
ISBN 1-557661-00-6

2350 Personality and Emotional Disturbance
Taylor & Francis
Ste G
47 Runway Dr
Levittown, PA 19057-4738
267-580-2622
FAX: 215-785-5515
Richard Roberts, CEO
The brain injured person has unique needs. Recent findings have highlighted that it is the personality, behavioral and emotional problems which most prohibit a return to work, create the greatest burden for the long-term care and rehabilitation of physical and cognitive functions. *$72.00*
260 pages Cloth
ISBN 0-85066 -71-3

2351 Peterson's Guide to Colleges with Programsfor Learning Disabled Students
Special Needs Project
Ste H
324 State St
Santa Barbara, CA 93101-2364
805-962-8087
818-718-9900
FAX: 805-962-5087
e-mail: books@specialneeds.com
www.specialneeds.com
B. B. Moose Peter, Author
Charles T. Mangrum, Editor
Stephen S. Strichart, Editor
The most complete and accurate guide to the more than 900 colleges with programs for the learning disabled. *$19.95*
406 pages

2352 Phenomenology of Depressive Illness
Human Sciences Press
233 Spring St
New York, NY 10013-1522
212-229-2859
877-283-3229
FAX: 212-463-0742
e-mail: ainy@aveda.com
www.aveda.edu
263 pages Cloth
ISBN 0-89885 -69-9

2353 Physical Disabilities and Health Impairments: An Introduction
McGraw-Hill School Publishing
PO Box 182604
Columbus, OH 43218
877-833-5524
800-338-3987
FAX: 609-308-4480
e-mail: customer.service@mheducation.com
www.mcgraw-hill.com
David Levin, President/Chief Executive Officer
David Stafford, Senior Vice President/General Counsel
Maryellen Valaitis, Senior Vice President Human Resources
Patrick Milano, Chief Financial Officer/Chief Administrative Officer

A comprehensive text which presents a wealth of up-to-date medical information for teachers.

2354 Physical Education and Sports for Exceptional Students
McGraw-Hill Company
2460 Kerper Blvd
Dubuque, IA 52001-2224 800-338-3987
FAX: 614-755-5654
e-mail: customer.service@mcgraw-hill.com
www.mhhe.com/hper/physed

Michael Horvat, Author
Harold McGraw III, Chairman, President and Chief Ex
Jack F. Callahan, Executive Vice President, Chief
John Berisford, Executive Vice President, Human
Physical education for exceptional students and teaching students with learning and behavior exceptionalities.
Cloth

2355 Physical Management of Multiple Handicaps: A Professional's Guide
Brookes Publishing Company
PO Box 10624
Baltimore, MD 21285-0624 410-337-9580
800-638-3775
FAX: 410-337-8539
e-mail: custserv@brookespublishing.com
www.brookespublishing.com

Paul H. Brookes, Chairman
Jeffrey D. Brookes, President
Melissa A. Behm, ExecutiveVice President
George S. Stamathis, Vice President & Publisher
Comprehensive guide, takes a transdisciplinary approach to therapeutic/technological management of persons with multiple handicaps. *$36.00*
352 pages Hardcover
ISBN 1-557660-47-6

2356 Physically Handicapped in Society
Ayer Company Publishers
Ste 322
400 Bedford St
Manchester, NH 03101-1195 603-669-9307
888-267-7323
FAX: 603-669-7945
e-mail: stg@ncia.net
www.ayerpub.com

Kathy Train, Office Manager
Ellie Phipps, Customer Service
A group of 39 books. Biographies that offer studies on attitudes, sociological and psychological. Please write or call for catalog. *$965.00*
Hardcover
ISBN 0-40513 -00-3

2357 Practicing Rehabilitation with Geriatric Clients
Springer Publishing Company
11 W 42nd St
15th Floor
New York, NY 10036-8002 212-431-4370
877-687-7476
FAX: 212-941-7842
e-mail: cs@springerpub.com
www.springerpub.com

Dr. Ursula Springer, President
Ted Nardin, CEO
James C. Costello, Vice President, Journal Publishi
James C. Costello, Vice President, Journal Publishing
Physical therapy in the geriatric client, psychological and psychiatric considerations in the rehabilitation of the elderly. *$32.95*
256 pages Hardcover
ISBN 0-82616 -80-5

2358 Pragmatic Approach
Educators Publishing Service
625 Mount Auburn St
3RD Floor
Cambridge, MA 02138-3039 617-547-6706
800-225-5750
FAX: 617-547-0285
www.eps.schoolspecialty.com

Paula Fabbro, Sales Consultant
Leo Micale, Sales Consultant
Kristen Colson, Sales Consultant
Flora Francis, Sales Consultant
Monograph on evaluation of children's performances on Slingerland Pre-Reading Screening Procedures to Identify First Grade Academic Needs. *$6.00*
56 pages
ISBN 0-838816-85-1

2359 Preschoolers with Special Needs: Children At-Risk, Children with Disabilities
Allyn & Bacon
75 Arlington St
Suite 300
Boston, MA 02116-3988 617-848-7500
800-852-8024
FAX: 617-944-7273
www.home.pearsonhighered.com

Bill Barke, CEO
Janet W. Lerner, Co-Author
Barbara Lowenthal, Co-Author
Rosemary W. Egan, Co-Author
Explores ways of providing preschool children with special needs and their families with a learning environment that will help them develop and learn. Emphasizes the needs of preschoolers age three to six and provides information to teachers and others who work with young children in all settings. Current models of curricula, which incorporate new features from research and practical expreiences with children who have special needs, are described and discussed. *$59.00*
336 pages cloth
ISBN 0-205358-79-9

2360 Preventing Academic Failure
Educators Publishing Service
3rd Floor
625 Mount Auburn St
Cambridge, MA 02138-3039 617-547-6706
800-225-5750
FAX: 617-547-0285
www.epsbooks.com

284 pages Paperback
ISBN 0-838852-71-8

2361 Preventing School Dropouts
Sage Publications
2455 Teller Road
Thousand Oaks, CA 91320 805-499-9774
800-818-7243
FAX: 800-583-2665
e-mail: books.claim@sagepub.com
www.sagepub.com

Sara Miller McCune, Founder, Publisher, Chairperson
Blaise R Simqu, President/ CEO
Tracey A. Ozmina, Executive Vice President & Chief
Thomas C. Lovitt, Author
For secondary teachers, special education and regular, who have difficulty teaching youth in their classes. Presented are 120 tactics, specific instructional techniques, for helping adolescents to stay in school. Each tactic is written in a format that includes five sections. *$38.00*
509 pages

2362 Prevocational Assessment
Exceptional Education
P.O.Box 15308
Seattle, WA 98115-308 206-262-9538
FAX: 475-486-4510

Jeff Stewart, Owner
Use the PACG to assess your students in nine areas (attendance and endurance, learning and behavior, communication skills, social skills, grooming and eating and toileting) covering 46 specific workshop experiences. *$12.00*
16 pages Complete Set
ISBN 1-87786 -23-7

2363 Progress Without Punishment: Approaches for Learners with Behavior Problems
Teachers College Press
1234 Amsterdam Ave
New York, NY 10027-6602 212-678-3929
800-575-6566
FAX: 212-678-4149
e-mail: tcpress@tc.columbia.edu
www.teacherscollegepress.com

Anne M. Donnellan, Author
In this volume, the authors argue against the use of punishment, and instead advocate the use of alternative intervention procedures. *$17.95*
184 pages Paperback
ISBN 0-807729-11-6

2364 Promoting Postsecondary Education for Students with Learning Disabilities
Sage Publications
2455 Teller Road
Thousand Oaks, CA 91320 805-499-9774
800-818-7243
FAX: 800-583-2665
e-mail: books.claim@sagepub.com
www.sagepub.com

Sara Miller McCune, Founder, Publisher, Chairperson
Stan F. Shaw, Co-Author
Joan M. McGuire, Co-Author
Loring Cowles Brinckerhoff, Co-Author
Primarily designed for postsecondary service providers who are responsible for serving college students with learning disabilities. *$41.00*
440 pages

2365 Psychiatric Mental Health Nursing
Lippincott, Williams & Wilkins
227 S 6th St
Suite 227
Philadelphia, PA 19106-3713 215-521-8300
800-777-2295
FAX: 301-824-7390
www.lpub.com

J Lippincott, CEO
This text emphasizes and contrasts the roles of the generalist nurse and the psychiatric nurse specialist. *$52.00*
1120 pages Illustrated

2366 Psychoeducational Assessment of Visually Impaired and Blind Students
Sage Publications
2455 Teller Road
Thousand Oaks, CA 91320 805-499-9774
800-818-7243
FAX: 800-583-2665
e-mail: books.claim@sagepub.com
www.sagepub.com

Sara Miller McCune, Founder, Publisher, Chairperson
Blaise R Simqu, President/CEO
Tracey A. Ozmina, Executive Vice President & Chief
Sharon Bradley-Johnson, Author
Professional reference book that addresses the problems specific to assessment of visually impaired and blind children. Of particular value to the practitioner are the extensive reviews of available tests, including ways to adapt those not designed for use with the visually handicapped. *$29.00*
140 pages Paperback
ISBN 0-890791-08-2

2367 Psychological and Social Impact of Illness and Disability
Springer Publishing
11 W 42nd St
15th Floor
New York, NY 10036-8002 212-431-4370
877-687-7476
FAX: 212-941-7842
e-mail: cs@springerpub.com
www.springerpub.com

Dr. Ursula Springer, President
Ted Nardin, CEO
Ph.D. Orto Arthur E. Dell, Editor
James C. Costello, Vice President, Journal Publishing
The newest edition of Psychological and Social Impact of Illness and Disability continues the tradition of presenting a realistic perspective on life with disabilies and then improves upon its predecessors with the inclusion of illness as a major influence on client care needs. Further broadening the scope of this edition is the inclusion of personal perspectives and stories from those living with illness or disabilities. These stories offer a look into what it is like to cope with these issues.

2368 Reading and Deafness
Sage Publications
2455 Teller Road
Thousand Oaks, CA 91320 805-499-9774
800-818-7243
FAX: 800-583-2665
e-mail: books.claim@sagepub.com
www.sagepub.com

Sara Miller McCune, Founder, Publisher, Chairperson
Beverly J Trezek, Co-Author
Peter V. Paul, Co-Author
Ye Wang, Co-Author
Three areas are looked at in this book: deaf children's prereading development of real-world knowledge, cognitive abilities and linguistic skills. *$39.00*
422 pages

2369 Readings on Research in Stuttering
Longman Publishing Group
1 Penn Plaza
Suite 2222
New York, NY 10119 646-556-8401
FAX: 646-556-8415
e-mail: coffee@rothfos.com
www.rothfos.com

Dan Dwyer, CEO
Thomas Minogue, CFO
Maria Tanpinco-Queyquep, Traffic Manager
Joseph P. Thomas, Traffic Coordinator
Collection of the key journal articles published on stuttering over the past decade, addressing trends in recent research in the field.
231 pages Paperback
ISBN 0-801304-10-5

2370 Recreation Activities for the Elderly
Springer Publishing Company
11 W 42nd St
15th Floor
New York, NY 10036-8002 212-431-4370
877-687-7476
FAX: 212-941-7842
e-mail: cs@springerpub.com
www.springerpub.com

Dr. Ursula Springer, President
Ted Nardin, CEO
James C. Costello, Vice President, Journal Publishi
James C. Costello, Vice President, Journal Publishing
Included in this volume are simple crafts that utilize easily obtainable, inexpensive materials, hobbies focusing on collections,

nature, and the arts' and games emphasizing both mental and physical activity. *$23.95*
240 pages Softcover
ISBN 0-82616-30-1

2371 Reference Manual for Communicative Sciences and Disorders
Pro- Ed Publications
8700 Shoal Creek Blvd
Austin, TX 78757-6897 512-451-3246
800-897-3202
FAX: 512-451-8542
e-mail: info@proedinc.com
www.proedinc.com
Raymond D. Kent, Author
An indispensable guide to standards and values essential in the assessment of communication disorders. *$54.00*
393 pages

2372 Rehabilitation Interventions for the Institutionalized Elderly
Haworth Press
711 Third Avenue
Floor 8th
New York, NY 10017 212-216-7800
800-354-1420
FAX: 212-564-7854
e-mail: subscriptions@tandf.co.uk.
www.taylorandfrancisgroup.com
Derek Mapp, Non-Executive Chairman
Roger Horton, CEO
Emma Blaney, Group HR Director - Head of Corporate Responsibility
Isobel Peck, Group Chief Marketing Officer
Gerontology professionals offer suggestions to enrich the quality of rehabilitation services offered to the institutionalized elderly. This volume examines up to the minute ideas, some that would have been unlikely even a few years ago, that focus exclusively on rehabilitation services for the institutionalized elderly. Journal publications formerly published by Haworth Press are now listed on the Taylor & Franc *$44.95*
77 pages Hardcover
ISBN 0-866568-33-6

2373 Rehabilitation Nursing for the Neurological Patient
Springer Publishing Company
15th Fl
11 W 42nd St
New York, NY 10036-8002 212-431-4370
877-687-7476
FAX: 212-941-7842
e-mail: cs@springerpub.com
www.springerpub.com
Dr. Ursula Springer, President
Ted Nardin, CEO
James C. Costello, Vice President, Journal Publishing
Marcia Hanak, Author
A practical new reference written especially for practicing nurses who work with neurologically disabled persons. *$ 32.95*
240 pages

2374 Rehabilitation Resource Manual: VISION
Resources for Rehabilitation
22 Bonad Rd
Winchester, MA 01890-1302 781-368-9094
FAX: 781-368-9096
e-mail: info@rfr.org
www.rfr.org
Marshall E. Flax, MS, Author
A desk reference that enables service providers, librarians and others to make effective referrals. Includes guidelines on establishing self-help groups, information on research and service organizations, and chapters on assistive technology, for special population groups and by eye condition. *$44.95*
Biennial

2375 Rehabilitation Technology
Haworth Press
711 Third Avenue
New York, NY 10017 212-216-7800
800-354-1420
FAX: 212-244-1563
e-mail: subscriptions@tandf.co.uk.
http://www.taylorandfrancisgroup.com/
Glenn E Hedman, Author
Learn how the use of technological devices can enhance the lives of disabled children. Informs physical therapists, occupational therapists, and rehabilitation technologists about the devices that are available today and provides important background information on these devices. Journal publications formerly published by Haworth Press are now listed on the Taylor & Francis Journals website. *$74.95*
173 pages Hardcover
ISBN 1-560240-33-4

2376 Report Writing in Assessment and Evaluation
Stout Vocational Rehab Institute
University of Wisconsin-Stout
712 South Broadway
Menomonie, WI 54751 715-232-1478
FAX: 715-232-2356
e-mail: giffordj@uwstout.edu
www.uwstout.edu
Charles W. Sorensen, Chancellor
Judy Gifford, Director
Stephen W. Thomas, Author
Linda Vanderloop, CFSC Office
This examines questions of who are you writing for and what does the referral source want. Defines characteristics of good reports, common problems, writing in different settings, types of reports, getting ready to write, and writing prescriptive recommendations. *$ 17.75*
188 pages Softcover

2377 Resources for Rehabilitation
22 Bonad Rd
Winchester, MA 01890-1302 781-368-9094
FAX: 781-368-9096
e-mail: info@rfr.org
www.rfr.org

2378 Restructuring High Schools for All Students: Taking Inclusion to the Next Level
Brookes Publishing
PO Box 10624
Baltimore, MD 21285-0624 410-337-9580
800-638-3775
FAX: 410-337-8539
e-mail: custserv@brookespublishing.com
www.brookespublishing.com
Paul H. Brookes, Chairman
Jeffrey D. Brookes, President
Melissa A. Behm, ExecutiveVice President
George S. Stamathis, Vice President & Publisher
Details the process of creating an inclusive, collaborate community of learners and teachers at the secondary level. *$29.95*
304 pages Paperback
ISBN 1-557663-13-0

2379 Restructuring for Caring and Effective Education: Administrative Guide
Brookes Publishing
PO Box 10624
Baltimore, MD 21285-0624 410-337-9580
800-638-3775
FAX: 410-337-8539
e-mail: custserv@brookespublishing.com
www.brookespublishing.com
Paul H. Brookes, Chairman
Jeffrey D. Brookes, President
Melissa A. Behm, ExecutiveVice President
George S. Stamathis, Vice President & Publisher

In this empowering book, leading general and special education schools reform experts synthesize the major school restructuring initiatives and describe the processes and rationale for changing the organizational structure and instructional practices of schools. *$ 29.00*

384 pages Paperback

ISBN 1-55766-91-3

2380 **Scoffolding Student Learning**

Brookline Books
8 Trumbull Rd
Suite B-001
Northampton, MA 01060
413-584-0184
800-666-2665
FAX: 413-584-6184
e-mail: brbooks@yahoo.com
www.brooklinebooks.com

Paul H. Brookes, Chairman
Jeffrey D. Brookes, President
Melissa A. Behm, ExecutiveVice President
George S. Stamathis, Vice President & Publisher

Collection of papers on the theory and practice of scoffolding—an interactive style of instructions that helps students develop more powerful thinking tools. *$21.95*

180 pages Paperback

ISBN 1-571290-36-2

2381 **Selective Nontreatment of Handicapped**

Oxford University Press
2001 Evans Rd
Cary, NC 27513-2009
919-677-0977
800-445-9714
FAX: 919-677-1303
e-mail: custserv.us@oup.com
www.global.oup.com

Lesa Moran Owen, Library Sales Operations Manager
Rebecca Seger, Director, Institutional Sales, Americas
Lenny Allen, Director, Institutional Accounts
Nancy Roy, Library Sales Manager

Information on selective nontreatment of handicapped newborns, moral dilemmas in neonatal medicine. *$17.95*

304 pages Paperback

2382 **Semiotics and Dis/ability: Interogating Categories of Difference**

State University of New York Press
22 Corporate Woods Boulevard
3rd Floor
Albany, NY 12210-2314
518-472-5000
866-430-7869
FAX: 518-472-5038
e-mail: info@sunypress.edu
www.sunypress.edu

James Peltz, Associate Director
Linda Rogers, Editor
Beth Blue Swadener, Editor

Examines the ways the words disability and difference and socially and culturally constructed. *$25.95*

265 pages Paperback 1990

ISBN 0-791449-06-6

2383 **Service Coordination for Early Intervention: Parents and Friends**

Brookline Books
8 Trumbull Rd
Suite B-001
Northampton, MA 01060
413-584-0184
800-666-2665
FAX: 413-584-6184
e-mail: brbooks@yahoo.com
www.brooklinebooks.com

Deborah D. Hatton, Co-Author
R. A. McWilliam, Co-Author
P. J. Winton, Co-Author

This book helps administrators and professionals to structure early intervention and ongoing services so that professionals work collaboratively with parents to promote the health, well being and development of children with special needs. *$19.95*

110 pages Paperback

ISBN 0-91479-91-3

2384 **Services for the Seriously Mentally Ill: A Survey of Mental Health Centers**

Nat'l Council for Community Behavioral Healthcare
12300 Twinbrook Pkwy
Ste 320
Rockville, MD 20852-1606
301-984-6200
FAX: 301-881-7159
www.nccbh.org

Linda Rosenberg, CEO
Dale K Klatzker, Board Chair

This ground-breaking report documents what administrators and practitioners have maintained for many years: community mental health organizations devote a significant percentage of the human and financial resources to serving the seriously mentally ill. *$30.00*

2385 **Shop Talk**

PO Box 7886
Champaign, IL 61826-9177
217-352-3273
800-519-2707
FAX: 217-352-1221
e-mail: rp@researchpress.com
www.researchpress.com

Robert W. Parkinson, Founder
Philip Roth, Author

2386 **Signed English Schoolbook**

Gallaudet University Press
800 Florida Ave NE
Washington, DC 20002-3600
202-651-5488
800-451-1073
FAX: 202-651-5489
TTY: 888-630-9347
e-mail: clerc.center@gallaudet.edu.
www.gupress.gallaudet.edu

Harry Bornstein, Co-Author
Karen L. Saulnier, Co-Author
Dr. T Alan Hurwitz, President
Edward Bosso, Vice President for Administratio

The Signed English Schoolbook provides vocabulary for teachers and others who serve school-age children and adolescents and covers the full range of school activities. *$13.95*

184 pages Softcover

2387 **Social Studies: Detecting and Correcting Special Needs**

Allyn & Bacon
75 Arlington St
Suite 300
Boston, MA 02116-3988
617-848-7500
800-852-8024
FAX: 617-944-7273
www.home.pearsonhighered.com

Harry Bornst Barke, CEO
Nancy Forfyth, President
Lana J. Smith, Co-Author
Dennie L. Smith, Co-Author

Describes social studies and special needs for special learners.

180 pages

ISBN 0-205121-51-9

2388 **Social and Emotional Development of Exceptional Students: Handicapped**

Charles C. Thomas
2600 S 1st St
Springfield, IL 62704-4730
217-789-8980
800-258-8980
FAX: 217-789-9130
e-mail: books@ccthomas.com
www.ccthomas.com

Michael P. Thomas, President
Carroll J. Jones, Author

Sixteen years after the passage of P.L. 94-142, the dream of special educators to educate the handicapped and nonhandicapped children and youth together resulting in increased academic gains and age-appropriate school skills for handicapped children and youth has not yet materialized. This book helps eliminate an existing void by providing teachers with understandable information regarding the social and emotional development of exceptional students. Also in cloth at $41.95 (ISBN# 0-398-05781-8) *$29.95*
218 pages Softcover
ISBN 0-398061-94-7

2389 Special Education Today
LifeWay Christian Resources Southern Baptist Conv.
One LifeWay Plaza
Nashville, TN 37234 615-251-2000
800-458-2772
FAX: 615-532-9412
e-mail: specialed@lifeway.com
www.lifeway.com

Thom S. Rainer, President/CEO
Brad Waggoner, Executive Vice President
Eric Geiger, Vice President, Church Resources Division
Tim Hill, Vice President/Chief Information Officer
This unique quarterly publications ministers to people with special education needs and to their families, the church, and other caregivers. It offers a variety of helps and encouragement, including: What's working in churches, Suggestions for adapting teaching techniques, inspirational stories about people who have disabilities, Parenting and family issues, Ideas for reaching, witnessing, worship, and recreation. *$4.25*
36 pages Quarterly

2390 Special Education for Today
Allyn & Bacon
75 Arlington St
Suite 300
Boston, MA 02116-3988 617-848-7500
800-852-8024
FAX: 617-944-7273
www.home.pearsonhighered.com

See search r Barke, CEO
Michael S. Rosenberg, Co-Author
David L. Westling, Co-Author
James McLeskey, Co-Author
An undergraduate introduction to special education covering all major areas of exceptionality. Contains pedagogical features designed to make the book accessible to the undergraduate.
576 pages hardcover
ISBN 0-138264-53-8

2391 Speech and the Hearing-Impaired Child
Alexander Graham Bell Association
3417 Volta Pl NW
Washington, DC 20007-2737 202-337-5220
866-337-5220
FAX: 202-337-8314
TTY: 202-337-5221
e-mail: info@agbell.org
www.listeningandspokenlanguage.org

Meredith K. Sugar, Esq. (OH), President
Ted A. Meyer, M.D., Ph.D, President-Elect/Secretary-Treasurer
Emilio Alonso-Mendoza, Chief Executive Officer
Susan Boswell, Director of Communications and Marketing
This textbook for professionals deals with basic theoretical issues in the acquisition of speech and the form of language (phonetics and phonology) in children with hearing losses. It provides a systematic framework to develop and evaluate speech target behaviors and their underlying subskills. *$29.95*
402 pages Paperback

2392 Speech-Language Pathology and Audiology: An Introduction
McGraw-Hill School Publishing
PO Box 182604
Columbus, OH 43218 877-833-5524
800-338-3987
FAX: 609-308-4480
e-mail: customer.service@mheducation.com
www.mcgraw-hill.com

David Levin, President/Chief Executive Officer
David Stafford, Senior Vice President/General Counsel
Maryellen Valaitis, Senior Vice President Human Resources
Patrick Milano, Chief Financial Officer & Chief Administrative Officer
Offers classroom-tested coverage of clinical objectives and functioning.
301 pages

2393 Spinal Cord Dysfunction
Oxford University Press
2001 Evans Rd
Cary, NC 27513-2009 919-677-0977
800-451-7556
FAX: 919-677-1303
e-mail: humanres@oup-usa.org
www.global.oup.com

Lesa Moran Owen, Library Sales Operations Manager
Rebecca Seger, Director, Institutional Sales, Americas
Lenny Allen, Director, Institutional Accounts
Nancy Roy, Library Sales Manager
Offers information on restoration of function after spinal cord damage as seen from the point of view of identification of impaired or absent function in the nerve cells and processes which survive after the initial insult, intact but with impaired functions. *$95.00*
368 pages

2394 Strategies for Teaching Learners with Special Needs
McGraw-Hill School Publishing
PO Box 182604
Columbus, OH 43218 877-833-5524
800-338-3987
FAX: 609-308-4480
e-mail: customer.service@mheducation.com
www.mcgraw-hill.com

David Levin, President/Chief Executive Officer
David Stafford, Senior Vice President/General Counsel
Maryellen Valaitis, Senior Vice President Human Resources
Patrick Milano, Chief Financial Officer & Chief Administrative Officer
This is a text that helps special educators develop the full range of teaching competencies needed to be effective.
560 pages

2395 Strategies for Teaching Students with Learning and Behavior Problems
Allyn & Bacon
75 Arlington St
Suite 300
Boston, MA 02116-3988 617-848-7500
800-852-8024
FAX: 617-944-7273
www.home.pearsonhighered.com

Bill Barke, CEO
Nancy Forfyth, President
Sharon R. Vaughn, Co-Author
Candace S. Bos, Co-Author
Provides descriptions of methods and strategies for teaching students with learning and behavior problems, managing professional roles, and collaborating with families, professionals, and paraprofessionals.
544 pages
ISBN 0-205113-89-3

2396 Students with Acquired Brain Injury: The School's Response
Brookes Publishing
PO Box 10624
Baltimore, MD 21285-0624 410-337-9580
800-638-3775
FAX: 410-337-8539
e-mail: custserv@brookespublishing.com
www.brookespublishing.com
Ann Glang, Editor
Bonnie Todis, Editor
Paul H. Brooks, Chairman of the Board
Cary Gold, Educational Sales Representative
This book is designed for school professionals and describes a range of issues that this population faces and presents proven means of addressing them in ways that benefit all students. Included topics are hospital-to-school transitions, effective assessment strategies, model programs in public schools, interventions to assist classroom teachers, and ways to involve family members in the educational program. *$29.95*
424 pages Paperback
ISBN 1-55766-85-1

2397 Students with Mild Disabilities in the Secondary School
Longman Group
75 Arlington St
Suite 300
New York, NY 10036-2601 212-782-3300
800-852-8024
www.home.pearsonhighered.com
William Hitchings, Co-Author
Michael Horvath, Co-Author
Bonnie Schmalle, Co-Author
Paul Retish, Co-Author, Editor
Provides methods and strategies for curriculum delivery to students with mild disabilities at the secondary school level.
2313G pages Paperback
ISBN 0-801301-66-1

2398 Supporting and Strengthening Families
Brookline Books
8 Trumbull Rd
Suite B-001
Northampton, MA 01060 413-584-0184
800-666-2665
FAX: 413-584-6184
e-mail: brbooks@yahoo.com
www.brooklinebooks.com
Carl J Dunst, Author
A collection of papers addressing the theory, methods, strategies, and practices involved in adopting an empowerment and family-centered resources approach to supporting families and strengthening individual and family functioning. *$30.00*
252 pages Paperback
ISBN 0-91479-94-8

2399 TESTS
Slosson Educational Publications
538 Buffalo rd
PO Box 280
East Aurora, NY 14052 716-652-0930
888-756-7766
FAX: 800-665-3840
e-mail: slossonprep@gmail.com
www.slosson.com
Steven W. Slosson, President
Dr. Georgina Moynihan, Office Personnel
Slosson Educational Publications, Inc. offers educators an extensive selection of testing products, along with books on autism. ADED and other special needs materials. Our catalog includes 30 pages of speech-language testing and language rehabilitation products. The behavioral conduct. Special needs section includes checklist and scales on aberrant/disruptive behavior, tapes on ADD, as well as products for dyslexia and remediation of reversals.

2400 Teacher's Guide to Including Students with Disabilities in Regular Physical Education
Brookes Publishing
PO Box 10624
Baltimore, MD 21285-0624 410-337-9580
800-638-3775
FAX: 410-337-8539
e-mail: custserv@brookespublishing.com
www.brookespublishing.com
Martin E. Block, Author
Melissa A. Behm, Executive Vice President
Paul H. Brooks, Chairman of the Board
Cary Gold, Educational Sales Representative
Provides simple and creative strategies for meaningfully including children with disabilities in regular physical education programs. *$39.00*
288 pages Paperback
ISBN 1-557661-56-1

2401 Teachers Working Together
Brookline Books
8 Trumbull Rd
Suite B-001
Northampton, MA 01060 413-584-0184
800-666-2665
FAX: 413-584-6184
e-mail: brbooks@yahoo.com
www.brooklinebooks.com
Carol Davis, Co-Author
Alice Yang, Co-Author
This collection of papers describes collaboraborative efforts for such classroom settings as preschools, elementary, middle and high schools, for content area teaching and into the transition to work. Each chapter describes actual practice and analyzes what is required to accomplish this collaboration. *$19.95*
Paperback
ISBN 1-57139-66-4

2402 Teaching Adults with Learning Disabilities
Krieger Publishing Company
1725 Krieger Drive
Malabar, FL 32902 321-724-9542
800-724-0025
FAX: 321-951-3671
e-mail: info@krieger-publishing.com
www.krieger-publishing.com
Dale R. Jordan, Author
R Krieger, Owner
Designed to teach literacy providers and classroom instructors how to recognize specific learning disability (LD) patterns and block reading, spelling, writing and arithmetic skills in students of all ages. One of the major problems faced by literary providers is keeping low-skill adults involved in basic education programs long enough to increase their literacy skills to the level of success. Shows instructors in adult education how to modify teaching strategies. *$25.50*
160 pages
ISBN 0-894649-10-8

2403 Teaching Children With Autism in the General Classroom
Prufrock Press
PO Box 8813
Waco, TX 76714-8813 254-756-3337
800-998-2208
FAX: 254-756-3339
e-mail: gbates@prufrock.com
www.prufrock.com
Joel McIntosh, Publisher & Marketing Director
Ginny Bates, Customer Service and Office Manager
Lacy Compton, Senior Editor
Rachel Taliaferro, Editor
Provides an introduction to inclusionary practices that serve children with autism, giving teachers the practical advice they need to ensure each students receives the quality education he or she deserves. *$39.95*
350 pages Paperback
ISBN 1-593633-64-6

2404 Teaching Disturbed and Disturbing Students: An Integrative Approach

Sage Publications
2455 Teller Road
Thousand Oaks, CA 91320 805-499-9774
800-818-7243
FAX: 800-583-2665
e-mail: books.claim@sagepub.com
www.sagepub.com

Sara Miller McCune, Founder, Publisher, Chairperson
Blaise R Simqu, President & CEO
Tracey A. Ozmina, Executive Vice President & Chief
Paul Zionts, Author

Using an integrative approach, this text provides teachers with step-by-step details of how to implement and use the methods and theories discussed in each chapter. *$37.00*

465 pages

2405 Teaching Every Child Every Day: Integrated Learning in Diverse Classrooms

Brookline Books
8 Trumbull Rd
Suite B-001
Northampton, MA 01060 413-584-0184
800-666-2665
FAX: 413-584-6184
e-mail: brbooks@yahoo.com
www.brooklinebooks.com

Karen R. Harris, Editor
Steve Graham, Editor
Don Deshler, Editor

Collection of articles addressing various issues in teaching to diverse classrooms—varied in need for special educational services, English proficiency, and socioeconomic and racial backgrounds. *$19.95*

224 pages Paperback
ISBN 0-57129 -40-0

2406 Teaching Infants and Preschoolers with Handicaps

Mc Graw- Hill, School Publishing
PO Box 182604
Columbus, OH 43218 877-833-5524
800-338-3987
FAX: 609-308-4480
e-mail: customer.service@mheducation.com
www.mcgraw-hill.com

David Levin, President/Chief Executive Officer
David Stafford, Senior Vice President/General Counsel
Maryellen Valaitis, Senior Vice President Human Resources
Patrick Milano, Chief Financial Officer & Chief Administrative Officer

Builds a solid background in early childhood special education.

380 pages

2407 Teaching Language-Disabled Children: A Communication/Games Intervention

Brookline Books
8 Trumbull Rd
Suite B-001
Northampton, MA 01060 413-584-0184
800-666-2665
FAX: 413-584-6184
e-mail: brbooks@yahoo.com
www.brooklinebooks.com

Susan Conant, Co-Author
Milton Budoff, Co-Author
Barbara Hecht, Co-Author

Describes exactly how to play the communication games. It does not simply exhort practitioners to give topic-relevant responses and take advantage of opportunities. It provides specific teaching methods and not simply a new perspective on language remeditation. *$22.95*

Hardcover
ISBN 0-91479 -38-7

2408 Teaching Learners with Mild Disabilities: Integrating Research and Practice

Brooke Publishing
PO Box 10624
Baltimore, MD 21285-0624 410-337-9580
800-638-3775
FAX: 410-337-8539
e-mail: custserv@brookespublishing.com
www.brookespublishing.com

Ruth Lyn Meese, Author
Melissa A. Behm, Executive Vice President
Paul H. Brooks, Chairman of the Board
Cary Gold, Educational Sales Representative

The authors illustrate interactions among regular teachers, special education teachers and students with mild disabilities through the use of hypothetical case studies of students and teachers.

496 pages Paperbound
ISBN 0-53421 -02-0

2409 Teaching Mathematics to Students with Learning Disabilities

Sage Publications
2455 Teller Road
Thousand Oaks, CA 91320 805-499-9774
800-818-7243
FAX: 800-583-2665
e-mail: books.claim@sagepub.com
www.sagepub.com

Sara Miller McCune, Founder, Publisher, Chairperson
Blaise R Simqu, President & CEO
Nancy S. Bley, Co-Author
Carol A. Thornton, Co-Author

New trends in school mathematics have surfaced in the teaching world. Problem-solving, estimation and the use of computers are receiving considerably greater emphasis than in the past and these areas are included in the new text. *$38.00*

486 pages Paperback

2410 Teaching Mildly and Moderately Handicapped Students

Allyn & Bacon
75 Arlington St
Suite 300
Boston, MA 02116-3988 617-848-7500
800-852-8024
FAX: 617-944-7273
www.home.pearsonhighered.com

Bill Barke, CEO
Nancy Forfyth, President
B. R. Gearheart, Author
Kevin Stone, Vice President, National Sales M

A cross-categorical text providing teaching ideas and techniques. Focuses on the theme of learning as a constructive process in which the learner interacts with the environment, constructing new systems of knowledge, Behavioral techniques and research are also presented.

hardcover
ISBN 0-138939-00-4

2411 Teaching Reading to Children with Down Syndrome: A Guide for Parents and Teachers

Woodbine House
6510 Bells Mill Rd
Bethesda, MD 20817-1636 301-897-3570
800-843-7323
FAX: 301-897-5838
e-mail: info@woodbinehouse.com
www.woodbinehouse.com

Irvin Shapell, Publisher
Patricia Logan Oelwein, Author
Beth Binns, Special Marketing Manage
Fran Marinaccio, Marketing Manager

Guide includes lessons customized to meet the unique interests and learning style of each child. *$16.95*

371 pages Paperback
ISBN 0-933149-55-7

2412 Teaching Reading to Disabled and Handicapped Learners
Charles C. Thomas
2600 S 1st St
Springfield, IL 62704-4730
217-789-8980
800-258-8980
FAX: 217-789-9130
e-mail: books@ccthomas.com
ccthomas.com

Michael P. Thomas, President
Freddie W. Litton, Co-Author
Harold D. Love, Co-Author
Designed as a text for undergraduate and graduate students, it's aim is to help the many children, adolescents, and adults who encounter difficulty with reading. It guides prospective and present special education teachers in assisting and teaching handicapped learners to read. The text integrates traditional methods with newer perspectives to provide and effective reading program in special education. *$37.95*
260 pages Paperback
ISBN 0-398062-48-X

2413 Teaching Reading to Handicapped Children
Love Publishing Company
9101 E Kenyon Ave
Suite 2200
Denver, CO 80237-1854
303-221-7333
FAX: 303-221-7444
e-mail: lpc@lovepublishing.com
www.lovepublishing.com

Charles H. Hargis, Author
The author covers skills teaching through letter sound association, word identification, synthetic and analytic methods and others, plus testing and assessment. *$24.95*
ISBN 0-89108 -13-5

2414 Teaching Self-Determination to Students with Disabilities
Brookes Publishing
PO Box 10624
Baltimore, MD 21285-0624
410-337-9580
800-638-3775
FAX: 410-337-8539
e-mail: custserv@brookespublishing.com
www.brookespublishing.com

Michael L. Wehmeyer, Co-Author
Martin Agran, Co-Author
Paul H. Brooks, Chairman of the Board
Cary Gold, Educational Sales Representative
Basic skills for successful transition. This teacher-friendly source will help educators prepare students with disabilities with the specific skills they need for a satisfactory, self-directed life once they leave school. *$34.95*
384 pages Paperback
ISBN 1-55766 -02-5

2415 Teaching Students with Learning Problems
McGraw-Hill School Publishing
PO Box 182604
Columbus, OH 43218
877-833-5524
800-338-3987
FAX: 609-308-4480
e-mail: customer.service@mheducation.com
www.mcgraw-hill.com

David Levin, President/Chief Executive Officer
David Stafford, Senior Vice President/General Counsel
Maryellen Valaitis, Senior Vice President Human Resources
Patrick Milano, Chief Financial Officer & Chief Administrative Officer
Expanded coverage of learning strategies, generalization training, self-monitoring techniques, and techniques for increasing the time students spend on academic tasks.
608 pages

2416 Teaching Students with Learning and Behavior Problems
Sage Publications
2455 Teller Road
Thousand Oaks, CA 91320
805-499-9774
800-818-7243
FAX: 800-583-2665
e-mail: books.claim@sagepub.com
www.sagepub.com

Sara Miller McCune, Founder, Publisher, Chairperson
Blaise R Simqu, President & CEO
Sharon R. Vaughn, Co-Author
Candace S. Bos, Co-Author
$65.00
444 pages Paperback
ISBN 0-890799-28-4

2417 Teaching Students with Mild and Moderate Learning Problems
Allyn & Bacon Longman College Faculty
75 Arlington St
Suite 300
Boston, MA 02116-3988
617-367-0025
800-852-8024
FAX: 617-367-2155
www.home.pearsonhighered.com

Bill Barke, CEO
John Langone, Author
Kevin Stone, Vice President, National Sales M
Kevin Stone, Vice President, National Sales M
Provides teachers with skills for assisting students with mild to moderate handicaps in making successful transitions in school and community environments.
496 pages
ISBN 0-205123-62-7

2418 Teaching Students with Moderate/Severe Disabilities, Including Autism
Charles C. Thomas
2600 S 1st St
Springfield, IL 62704-4730
217-789-8980
800-258-8980
FAX: 217-789-9130
e-mail: books@ccthomas.com
www.ccthomas.com

Michael P. Thomas, President
Elva Duran, Author
This resource and guide was written to help teachers, parents, and other caregivers provide the best educational opportunities for their students with moderate and severe disabilities. The author addresses functional language and other language intervention strategies, vocational training, community based instruction, transition and postsecondary programming, the adolescent student with autism, students with multiple disabilities, parent and family issues, and legal concerns. *$58.95*
416 pages Paperback
ISBN 0-398067-01-5

2419 Teaching Students with Special Needs in Inclusive Settings
Allyn & Bacon
75 Arlington St
Suite 300
Boston, MA 02116-3988
617-848-7500
800-852-8024
FAX: 617-944-7273
www.home.pearsonhighered.com

Tom E.C. Smith, Co-Author
Edward A. Polloway, Co-Author
James Patton, Co-Author
Carol A. Dowdy, Co-Author
This text is intended to be a survey text providing practical guidance to general education teachers. It will help them to meet the diverse needs of students with disabilities.
544 pages
ISBN 0-20527 -16-6

2420 **Teaching Young Children to Read**
Brookline Books
8 Trumbull Rd
Suite B-001
Northampton, MA 01060
413-584-0184
800-666-2665
FAX: 413-584-6184
e-mail: brbooks@yahoo.com
www.brooklinebooks.com

Dolores Durkin, Author
John P.
Detailed instructions on teaching reading to preschoolers. Gradually develops full fluency. *$16.95*
192 pages Paperback
ISBN 0-57129 -48-6

2421 **Teaching the Bilingual Special Education Student**
Ablex Publishing Corporation
P.O.Box 811
Stamford, CT 06904-811
FAX: 201-767-6717
ISBN 0-89391 -23-4

2422 **Teaching the Learning Disabled Adolescent**
Love Publishing Company
9101 E Kenyon Ave
Ste 2200
Denver, CO 80237-1813
303-221-7333
FAX: 303-221-7444
e-mail: lovepublishing@compuserve.com
lovepublishing.com

Gordon R. Alley, Author
This book gives expert strategies and methods for teaching learning disabled adolescents how, rather than what, to learn. *$34.95*
ISBN 0-89108 -94-5

2423 **Teaching the Mentally Retarded Student: Curriculum, Methods, and Strategies**
Allyn & Bacon
75 Arlington St
Suite 300
Boston, MA 02116-3988
617-367-0025
800-852-8024
FAX: 617-367-2155
www.home.pearsonhighered.com

Bill Barke, CEO
Richard L. Luftig, Author
Nancy Forfyth, President
Kevin Stone, Vice President, National Sales M
Represents a comprehensive approach to curriculum, methods and strategies for teaching the mildly mentally retarded student.
640 pages hardcover
ISBN 0-205102-62-X

2424 **Technology and Handicapped People**
Springer Publishing Company
11 W 42nd St
15th Floor
New York, NY 10036-8002
212-431-4370
877-687-7476
FAX: 212-941-7842
e-mail: cs@springerpub.com
www.springerpub.com

Dr. Ursula Springer, President
Ted Nardin, CEO
James C. Costello, Vice President, Journal Publishi
James C. Costello, Vice President, Journal Publishing
Important information for concerned professionals about new rehabilitation techniques and treatments for handicapped people. *$29.95*
224 pages Hardcover
ISBN 0-82614 -10-8

2425 **Textbooks and the Student Who Can't Read Them: A Guide for Teaching Content**
Brookline Books
8 Trumbull Rd
Suite B-001
Northampton, MA 01060
413-584-0184
800-666-2665
FAX: 413-584-6184
e-mail: brbooks@yahoo.com
www.brooklinebooks.com

Paperback
ISBN 0-91479 -57-3

2426 **The Resource Room**
State University of New York Press
22 Corporate Woods Boulevard
3rd Floor
Albany, NY 12210-2314
518-472-5000
866-430-7869
FAX: 518-472-5038
e-mail: info@sunypress.edu
www.sunypress.edu

Barry Edwards McNamara, Author
Provides teachers and administrators with helpful, practical information and explores the role of the resource room teacher as it relates to three major functions: assessment, instruction and consultation. It will also assist supervisors and administrators in evaluating their resource programs. *$28.95*
148 pages Paperback
ISBN 0-887069-84-0

2427 **There's a Hearing Impaired Child in My Class**
Gallaudet University Bookstore
800 Florida Ave NE
Washington, DC 20002-3600
202-651-5000
800-451-1073
FAX: 202-651-5489
TTY: 888-630-9347
e-mail: clerc.center@gallaudet.edu.
www.bookstore.gallaudette.edu

Debra Nussbaum, Author
Dr. T Alan Hurwitz, President
Edward Bosso, Vice President for Administratio
Donald Beil, Chief of Staff
This complete package provides basic facts about deafness, practical strategies for teaching hearing impaired children, and the question-and-answer information for all students. *$16.95*
44 pages

2428 **Toward Effective Public School Program for Deaf Students**
Teachers College Press
525 W 120th St
New York, NY 10027-6605
212-678-3000
800-575-6566
FAX: 212-678-4149
e-mail: webcomments@tc.columbia.edu
www.tc.columbia.edu

Susan H. Fuhrman, Ph.D., President of the College
Harvey Spector, Vice President for Finance and Administration
Suzanne M. Murphy, Vice President for Development and External Affairs
Janice S. Robinson, Vice President for Diversity and Community Affairs
This book translates research and data into useable recommendations and possible courses of action for organizing effective public school programs for deaf students. *$22.95*
272 pages Paperback
ISBN 0-807731-59-5

2429 Treating Adults with Disabilities: Access and Communication
World Institute on Disability
3075 Adeline Street
Suite 155
Berkeley, CA 94703
510-225-6400
FAX: 510-225-0477
TTY:510-225-0478
e-mail: wid@wid.org
www.wid.org

Paul W. Schroeder, Chairman
Linda M. Dardarian, Vice Chairman
Mary Brooner, Treasurer
Cassandra Malry, Secretary

This training curriculum is for medical professionals who want to improve the quality of care for people with disabilities and chronic illnesses. Also covers architectural, communication, attitudinal and economic policy barriers to quality health care and specific skills to increase good communication and rapport. *$6.50*
63 pages Paperback

2430 Treating Cerebral Palsy for Clinicians by Clinicians
Sage Publications
2455 Teller Road
Thousand Oaks, CA 91320
805-499-9774
800-818-7243
FAX: 800-583-2665
e-mail: books.claim@sagepub.com
www.sagepub.com

Sara Miller McCune, Founder, Publisher, Chairperson
Blaise R Simqu, President & CEO
Tracey A. Ozmina, Executive Vice President & Chief
Eugene T. McDonald, Editor

A clinical manual for professionals beginning to work with persons who have cerebral palsy. *$31.00*
312 pages

2431 Treating Disordered Speech Motor Control
Sage Publications
2455 Teller Road
Thousand Oaks, CA 91320
805-499-9774
800-818-7243
FAX: 800-583-2665
e-mail: books.claim@sagepub.com
www.sagepub.com

Sara Miller McCune, Founder, Publisher, Chairperson
Blaise R Simqu, President & CEO
Deanie Vogel, Author
Michael Cannito, Editor

This book about neuromotor disturbances of speech production is aimed at practicing professionals and advanced graduate students interested in the neuropathologies of communication. *$36.00*
410 pages

2432 Treating Families of Brain Injury Survivors
Springer Publishing Company
11 W 42nd St
15th Floor
New York, NY 10036-8002
212-431-4370
877-687-7476
FAX: 212-941-7842
e-mail: cs@springerpub.com
www.springerpub.com

Dr. Ursula Springer, President
Ted Nardin, CEO
James C. Costello, Vice President, Journal Publishi
James C. Costello, Vice President, Journal Publishing

Provides the mental health practitioner with a comprehensive program for helping families of head injury survivors cope with the change in their lives. Includes background on medical aspects of head injury, family structure functioning and special needs of various family members.
220 pages
ISBN 0-82616-20-1

2433 Understanding and Teaching Emotionally Disturbed Children & Adolescents
Sage Publications
2455 Teller Road
Thousand Oaks, CA 91320
805-499-9774
800-818-7243
FAX: 800-583-2665
e-mail: books.claim@sagepub.com
www.sagepub.com

Sara Miller McCune, Founder, Publisher, Chairperson
Blaise R Simqu, President & CEO
Tracey A. Ozmina, Executive Vice President & Chief
Phyllis L. Newcomer, Author

The teacher's handbook provides information that will change misconceptions about children who are frequently labeled as emotionally disturbed. It also gives information about a wide variety of intervention methods and approaches for use in educational settings. *$41.00*
620 pages Hardover

2434 Using the Dictionary of Occupational Titles in Career Decision Making
Stout Vocational Rehab Institute
University of Wisconsin Stou
Menomonie, WI 54751
715-232-2470
FAX: 715-232-5008
e-mail: luij@uwstout.edu
www.svri.uwstout.edu

John Lui, Contact Person

This is a self-study manual for learning how to use the 1991 U.S. Department of Labor's Dictionary of Occupational Titles. It gives the DOT user a tool to understand the DOT and then put its information to work. Shows how to quickly obtain information about the work performed in 12,741 occupations listed and described in the DOT and the worker requirements for those occupations. *$24.00*
142 pages Softcover

2435 VBS Special Education Teaching Guide
Life Way Christian Resources Southern Baptist Conv
1 Lifeway Plz
Nashville, TN 37234-1001
615-251-2000
e-mail: specialed@lifeway.com
www.lifeway.com

Tom Hellam, VP of Executive Communications a
Thom Rainer, President & CEO

This book contains teaching plans for five bible study sessions with reproducible handouts for learners. The plans use multisensory, experiential-based learning activities designed for adults and older youth who have mental retardation. Suggestions for Bible learning, crafts, recreation, snacks and theme interpretation are included. Designed primarily for Vacation Bible School, but may be used in camp/retreat settings. *$9.95*
56 pages Yearly

2436 Vermont Interdependent Services Team Approach (VISTA)
Brookes Publishing
PO Box 10624
Baltimore, MD 21285-624
410-337-9580
800-638-3775
FAX: 410-337-8539
e-mail: custserv@brookespublishing.com
www.brookespublishing.com

Paul Kelly, National Textbook Sales Manager
Tracy Gray, Educational Sales Manager
Paul Brooks, President

A guide to coordinating educational support services. This manual enables IEP team members to fulfill the related services provisions of IDEA as they make effective support services decisions using a collaborative team approach. *$27.95*
176 pages Spiral bound
ISBN 1-55766-30-4

2437 When You Have a Visually Impaired Student in Your Classroom: A Guide for Teachers
American Foundation for the Blind
2 Penn Plaza
Suite1102
New York, NY 10121
212-502-7600
800-232-5463
FAX: 888-545-8331
e-mail: afbinfo@afb.net
afb.org
Carl Augusto, President
This guide provides information on students' abilities and needs, resources and educational team members, federal special education requirements, and technology materials used by students. *$9.95*
84 pages
ISBN 0-891283-93-5

2438 Working Bibliography on Behavioral and Emotional Disorders
Natl. Clearinghouse for Alcohol & Drug Information
1 Choke Cherry Road
Rockville, MD 20857
301-468-2600
877-SAM-SA 7
FAX: 301-468-6433
e-mail: info@health.org
www.health.org
Lizabeth J Foster, Librarian/Info. Resource Manager
Pamela S. Hyde, Administrator
NCADI is a service of the U.S. Substance Abuse and Mental Health Services Administration. As the national focal point for information on alcohol and other drugs, NCADI collects, prepares, classifies, and distributes information about alcohol, tobacco and other drugs, prevention strategies and materials, research, treatment, etc.
40 pages

2439 Working Together with Children and Families: Case Studies
Brookes Publishing Company
PO Box 10624
Baltimore, MD 21285-624
410-337-9580
800-638-3775
FAX: 410-337-8539
e-mail: custerv@brookespublishing.com
www.brookespublishing.com
Paul Kelly, National Textbook Sales Manager
Tracy Gray, Educational Sales Manager
Paul Brooks, Owner
Early interventionists will be able to bridge the gap between theory and practice with this edited collection of case studies. *$23.00*
336 pages
ISBN 1-557661-23-5

2440 Working with Visually Impaired Young Students: A Curriculum Guide for 3 to 5 Year Olds
Charles C. Thomas
2600 S 1st St
Springfield, IL 62704-4730
217-789-8980
800-258-8980
FAX: 217-789-9130
e-mail: books@ccthomas.com
www.ccthomas.com
Michael P. Thomas, President
Ellen Trief, Editor
The first step in the education process of a visually impaired child is the early identification and treatment by an eye care specialist. This book is geared to the age of birth through 3-years. Available in cloth, paperback and hardcover. *$42.95*
194 pages Paperback
ISBN 0-398068-75-2

Testing Resources

2441 AEPS Child Progress Report: For Children Ages Birth to Three
Brookes Publishing
PO Box 10624
Baltimore, MD 21285-624
410-337-9580
800-638-3775
FAX: 410-337-8539
e-mail: custserv@brookespublishing.com
www.brookespublishing.com
Paul Kelly, National Textbook Sales Manager
Tracy Gray, Educational Sales Manager
Paul Brooks, Owner
This chart helps monitor change by visually displaying current abilities, intervention targets, and child progress. In packages of 30. *$18.00*
6 pages Gate-fold
ISBN 1-55766-65-0

2442 AEPS Data Recording Forms: For Children Ages Birth to Three
Brookes Publishing
PO Box 10624
Baltimore, MD 21285-624
410-337-9580
800-638-3775
FAX: 410-337-8539
e-mail: custserv@brookespublishing.com
readplaylearn.com
Paul Brooks, Owner
Melissa Behm, Executive Vice President
These forms can be used by child development professionals on four separate occasions to pinpoint and then monitor a child's strengths and needs in the six key areas of skill development measured by the AEPS Test. Packages of 10. *$23.00*
36 pages Saddle-stiched
ISBN 1-55766-97-2

2443 AEPS Measurement for Birth to Three Years
Brookes Publishing
PO Box 10624
Baltimore, MD 21285-624
410-337-9580
800-638-3775
FAX: 410-337-8539
e-mail: custserv@brookespublishing.com
www.brookespublishing.com
Paul Kelly, National Textbook Sales Manager
Tracy Gray, Educational Sales Manager
Paul Brooks, Owner
This dynamic volume explains the Assessment, Evaluation and Programming System, provides the complete AEPS Test and parallel assessment/evaluation tools for families and includes the forms and plans needed for implementation. *$39.00*
352 pages

2444 AEPS Measurement for Three to Six Years
Brookes Publishing
PO Box 10624
Baltimore, MD 21285-624
410-337-9580
800-638-3775
FAX: 410-337-8539
e-mail: custserv@brookespublishing.com
www.brookespublishing.com
Paul Kelly, National Textbook Sales Manager
Tracy Gray, Educational Sales Manager
Paul Brooks, Owner
Resources in early childhood, early intervention, inclusive and special education, developmental disabilities, learning disabilities, communication and language, behavior, and mental health. *$57.00*
400 pages Spiral-bound
ISBN 1-55766-87-1

2445 **AIR: Assessment of Interpersonal Relations**
Sage Publications
2455 Teller Road
Thousand Oaks, CA 91320
805-499-0721
800-818-7243
FAX: 800-583-2665
e-mail: info@sagepub.com
www.sagepub.com
Sara Miller McCune, Founder, Publisher, Chairperson
Blaise R Simqu, President & CEO
A thoroughly researched and standardized clinical instrument assessing the quality of adolescents' interpersonal relationships in a hierarchical fashion, including global relationship quality and relationship quality with three domains: Family, Social and Academic. *$89.00*

2446 **ALST: Adolescent Language Screening Test**
Sage Publications
2455 Teller Road
Thousand Oaks, CA 91320
805-499-0721
800-818-7243
FAX: 800-583-2665
e-mail: info@sagepub.com
www.sagepub.com
Sara Miller McCune, Founder, Publisher, Chairperson
Blaise R Simqu, President & CEO
Provides speech/language pathologists and other interested professionals with a rapid thorough method for screening adolescents (ages 11-17). *$119.00*

2447 **Adaptive Mainstreaming: A Primer for Teachers and Principals, 3rd Edition**
Longman Publishing Group
1330 Avenue of the Americas
New York, NY 10019
212-641-2400
800-745-8489
e-mail: wendy.spiegel@pearsoned.com
www.pearson.com
Glen Moreno, Chairman
Marjorie Scardino, Chief Executive Officer
An introduction to education for handicapped and gifted students. Presents research-based rationales for teaching exceptional students in the least restrictive environment. Provides historical perspectives, offers realistic descriptions of prevailing practices in the field, and reviews trends and new directions.
366 pages Paperback
ISBN 0-582285-04-6

2448 **Ages & Stages Questionnaires**
Brookes Publishing
PO Box 10624
Baltimore, MD 21285-624
410-337-9580
800-638-3775
FAX: 410-337-8539
e-mail: custserv@brookespublishing.com
www.brookespublishing.com
Paul Kelly, National Textbook Sales Manager
Tracy Gray, Educational Sales Manager
Paul Brooks, Owner
ASQ is an economical and field-tested system for identifying whether infants and young children may require further developmental evaluation and offers a screening and tracking program that helps early intervention professionals, service coordinators, and administrators maximize financial resources while promoting the health and growth of the children they serve. Set includes 11 color-coded, reproducible questionnaires, 11 reproducible, age appropriate scoring sheets. *$135.00*

2449 **American College Testing Program**
500 Act Drive
PO Box 168
Iowa City, IA 52243-168
319-337-1000
FAX: 319-339-3021
act.org
John Whitmore, CEO
Mark D Musik, President Emeritus
An independent, nonprofit organization that provides a variety of educational services to students and their parents, to high schools and colleges, and to professional associations and government agencies.

2450 **Assessing Students with Special Needs**
Longman Publishing Group
10 Bank Street
9th Floor
White Plains, NY 10606-1933
914-993-5000
www.ablongman.com
Joanne Dresner, President
Step-by-step guide to informal, classroom assessment of students with special needs.
174 pages Paperback
ISBN 0-801301-77-7

2451 **Assessment Log & Developmental Progress Charts for the CCPSN**
Brookes Publishing
P.O.Box 10624
Baltimore, MD 21285-624
410-337-9580
800-638-3775
FAX: 410-337-8539
e-mail: custserv@brookespublishing.com
www.brookespublishing.com
Paul Kelly, National Textbook Sales Manager
Tracy Gray, Educational Sales Manager
Paul Brooks, Owner
This 28-page booklet allows readers to actually chart the ongoing progress of each preschool child. Available in packages of 10. *$22.00*
28 pages Saddle-stiched
ISBN 1-55766-39-5

2452 **Assessment of Learners with Special Needs**
Allyn & Bacon
75 Arlinton Street
Ste 300
Boston, MA 2116-3988
617-848-7500
800-852-8024
FAX: 617-944-7273
www.ablongman.com
Bill Barke, CEO
Thomas Longman, Founder
The central goal of this book is to help teachers become sophisticated, informed test consumers in terms of choosing, using and interpreting commercially prepared tests for their special needs students.
508 pages Casebound
ISBN 0-205227-33-3

2453 **Benchmark Measures**
Educators Publishing Service
PO Box 9031
Cambridge, MA 2139
617-547-6706
800-225-5750
FAX: 888-440-2665
e-mail: feedback@epsbooks.com
www.epsbooks.com
Charles H Heinle, VP
Alexandra S Bigelow, Author
Gunnar Voltz, President
Ungraded test containing three sequential levels that assess alphabet and dictionary skills, reading, handwriting and spelling, and correspond to the first three schedules of the Alphabetic Phonics curriculum. The tests can be used at any level to measure a student's general knowledge of phonics. *$64.40*
Kit

2454 CREVT: Comprehensive Receptive and Expressive Vocabulary Test
Sage Publications
2455 Teller Road
Thousand Oaks, CA 91320
805-499-0721
800-818-7243
FAX: 800-583-2665
e-mail: info@sagepub.com
www.sagepub.com
Sara Miller McCune, Founder, Publisher, Chairperson
Blaise R Simqu, President & CEO
A new, innovative, efficient measure of both receptive and expressive oral vocabulary. The CREVT has two subtests and is based on the most current theories of vocabulary development, suitable for ages 4 through 17. *$174.00*
Complete Kit

2455 Carolina Curriculum for Preschoolers with Special Needs
Brookes Publishing
P.O.Box 10624
Baltimore, MD 21285-624
410-337-9580
800-638-3775
FAX: 410-337-8539
e-mail: custserv@brookespublishing.com
www.brookespublishing.com
Paul Kelly, National Textbook Sales Manager
Tracy Gray, Educational Sales Manager
Paul Brooks, Owner
This curriculum provides detailed teaching and assessment techniques, plus a sample 28-page Assessment Log that shows readers how to chart a child's individual progress. This guide is for children between 2 and 5 in their developmental stages who are considered at risk for developmental delay or who exhibit special needs. *$35.95*
352 pages Spiral-bound
ISBN 1-557660-32-8

2456 DAYS: Depression and Anxiety in Youth Scale
Sage Publications
2455 Teller Road
Thousand Oaks, CA 91320
805-499-0721
800-818-7243
FAX: 805-376-9443
e-mail: info@sagepub.com
www.sagepub.com
Sara Miller McCune, Founder, Publisher, Chairperson
Blaise R Simqu, President & CEO
A unique battery of three norm-references scales useful in identifying major depressive disorder and overanxious disorders in children and adolescents. *$129.00*
Complete Kit

2457 DOCS: Developmental Observation Checklist System
Pro- Ed Publications
8700 Shoal Creek Blvd
Austin, TX 78757-6897
512-451-3246
800-897-3202
FAX: 800-397-7633
e-mail: general@proedinc.com
www.proedinc.com
Donald D Hammill, Owner
Courtney King, Marketing Coordinator
A three-part system for the assessment of very young children with respect to general development, adjustment behavior and parent stress and support. *$124.00*

2458 Developmental Services Center
Therapeutic Nursery Program
4525 Lee St NE
Washington, DC 20019
202-388-3216
FAX: 202-576-8799
Alice Anderson
Offers assessment information and evaluation for developmentally delayed students.

2459 Frames of Reference for the Assessment of Learning Disabilities
Brookes Publishing
P.O.Box 10624
Baltimore, MD 21285-624
410-337-9580
800-638-3775
FAX: 410-337-8539
e-mail: custserv@brookespublishing.com
www.brookespublishing.com
Paul Kelly, National Textbook Sales Manager
Tracy Gray, Educational Sales Manager
Paul Brooks, Owner
New views on measurement issues. Here you'll find an in=depth look at the fundamental concerns facing those who work with children with learning disabilities - assessment and identification. *$55.00*
672 pages Hardcover
ISBN 1-55766-38-3

2460 How to Conduct an Assessment
FSSI
3905 Huntington Dr
Amarillo, TX 79109-4047
806-353-1114
FAX: 806-353-1114
e-mail: webmaster@winfssi.com
www.winfssi.com
Ed Hammer, Owner
The Functional Skills Screening Inventory,this behavioral checklist allows for parents and professionals to observe critical behaviors in individuals with multiple disabilities (7 years to adult years).

2461 Inclusive & Heterogeneous Schooling: Assessment, Curriculum, and Instruction
Brookes Publishing
P.O.Box 10624
Baltimore, MD 21285-624
410-337-9580
800-638-3775
FAX: 410-337-8539
e-mail: custserv@brookespublishing.com
www.brookespublishing.com
Paul Kelly, National Textbook Sales Manager
Tracy Gray, Educational Sales Manager
Paul Brooks, Owner
Presents methods for successfully restructuring classrooms to enable all students, particularly those with disabilities, to flourish. Provides specific strategies for assessment, collaboration, classroom management, and age-specific instruction. *$34.95*
448 pages Paperback
ISBN 1-557662-02-9

2462 Infant & Toddler Convection of Fairfield: Falls Church
Joseph Willard Health Center
3750 Old Lee Hwy
Fairfax, VA 22030-1806
703-246-7180
FAX: 703-246-7307
Susan Sigler, Program Coordinator
Allan Phillips, Director Early Intervention
Offers assessments, evaluations and educational/therapeutic infant programs for parents infants and toddlers birth to age 3.
Sliding Scale

2463 K-BIT: Kaufman Brief Intelligence Test
AGS
Ste 1000
5910 Rice Creek Pkwy
Shoreview, MN 55126-5023
651-287-7220
800-328-2560
FAX: 800-471-8457
e-mail: agsmail@agsnet.com
www.agsnet.com
Kevin Brueggeman, President
Robert Zaske, Market Manager
Quick and easy-to-use, KBIT assesses verbal and non-verbal abilities through two reliable subtests - vocabulary and matricies. *$ 124.95*
Ages 4-90

2464 **K-FAST: Kaufman Functional Academic Skills Test**
AGS
Ste 1000
5910 Rice Creek Pkwy
Shoreview, MN 55126-5023
651-287-7220
800-328-2560
FAX: 800-471-8457
e-mail: agsmail@agsnet.com
www.agsnet.com

Robert Zaske, Market Manager
Helps assess a person's capacity to function effectively in society regarding functional reading and math skills. *$99.95*
Ages 15-85+

2465 **K-SEALS: Kaufman Survey of Early Academic and Language Skills**
AGS
5910 Rice Creek Pkwy
Shoreview, MN 55126-5025
651-287-7220
800-328-2560
FAX: 800-471-8457
e-mail: agsmail@agsnet.com
www.agsnet.com

Kevin Brueggeman, President
Robert Zaske, Market Manager
An individually administered test of children's of both expressive and receptive skills, pre-academic skills and articulation. K-SEALS offers reliable scores usually in less than 25 minutes. *$ 179.95*
Ages 3-0; 6-11

2466 **KLST-2: Kindergarten Language Screening Test Edition, 2nd Edition**
Sage Publications
2455 Teller Road
Thousand Oaks, CA 91320
805-499-9774
800-818-7243
FAX: 800-583-2665
e-mail: info@sagepub.com
www.sagepub.com

Paul Kelly, National Textbook Sales Manager
Blaise R Simqu, President & CEO
Identifies children who need further diagnostic testing to determine whether or not they have language deficits that will accelerate academic failure. *$94.00*

2467 **Kaufman Test of Educational Achievement(K-TEA)**
AGS
PO Box 99
Circle Pines, MN 55014-99
800-328-2560
FAX: 800-471-8457
e-mail: agsmail@agsnet.com
www.agsnet.com

Robert Zaske, Marketing Manager
Kevin Brueggeman, President
K-TEA is an individually administered diagnostic battery that measures reading, mathematics, and spelling skills. Setting the standards in achievement testing today, K-TEA Comprehensive provides the complete diagnostic information you need for educational assessment and program planning. The Brief Forum is indispensable for school and clinical psychologists, special education teachers when a quick a measure of achievement is needed. *$249.95*

2468 **Life Centered Career Education: A Contemporary Based Approach, 4th Edition**
Council for Exceptional Children
2900 Crystal Drive
Suite1000
Arlington, VA 22202-3557
703-264-9454
888-232-7733
FAX: 703-264-1637
e-mail: president@cec.sped.org
www.cec.sped.org

Marilyn Friend, President
Provides a framework for building 97 functional skill competencies appropriate for preparing for adult life and special education students. *$28.00*
175 pages

2469 **Measure of Cognitive-Linguistic Abilities(MCLA)**
Speech Bin
PO Box 1579
Appleton, VA 54912-1579
772-770-0007
888-388-3224
FAX: 888-388-6344
e-mail: onlinehelp@schoolspecialty.com
www.speechbin.com

Jan J Binney, Senior Editor
A diagnostic test of cognitive-linguistic abilities of adolescents and adults with traumatically induced brain injuries. High level. Normed. *$89.00*
100 pages
ISBN 0-93785 -72-

2470 **ONLINE**
West Virginia Research and Training Center
P.O.Box 1004
Institute, WV 25112-1004
304-766-9495
800-624-8284
FAX: 304-766-2689
e-mail: info@icdi.wvu.edu
www.icdi.wvu.edu

Clifford Lantz, President
A quarterly newsletter offering information about hardware technology, software (commercial and home grown); applications that work and bonuses such as an exchange program for copyright-free software. *$25.00*
Quarterly

2471 **OWLS: Oral and Written Language Scales LC/OE & WE**
AGS
P.O.Box 99
Circle Pines, MN 55014-99
800-328-2560
FAX: 800-471-8457
e-mail: agsmail@agsnet.com
www.agsnet.com

Kevin Brueggeman, President
Robert Zaske, Market Manager
One kit provides an assessment of listening comprehension while the other assesses oral expression tasks: semantic, syntactic, pragmatic, and supralinguistic aspects of language. Written Expression may be administered individually or in small groups. *$249.95*

2472 **PAT-3: Photo Articulation Test**
Sage Publications
2455 Teller Road
Thousand Oaks, CA 91320
805-499-9774
800-818-7243
FAX: 800-583-2665
e-mail: info@sagepub.com
www.sagepub.com

Paul Kelly, National Textbook Sales Manager
Blaise R Simqu, President & CEO
This test consists of 72 color photographs. The first 69 photos test consonants and all but one vowel and one diphthong. The remaining pictures test connected speech and the remaining vowel and diphthong. *$144.00*
Complete Kit

2473 **Peabody Early Experiences Kit (PEEK)**
AGS
P.O.Box 99
Circle Pines, MN 55014-99
800-328-2560
FAX: 800-471-8457
e-mail: agsmail@agsnet.com
www.agsnet.com

Kevin Brueggeman, President
Robert Zaske, Market Manager
1,000 activities and all the materials you need to build youngsters' cognitive, social and language skills. Manuals, puppets,

manipulatives, picture card deck, picture mini decks and more to teach early development concepts. *$789.95*

2474 Peabody Individual Achievement Test-Revised Normative Update (PIAT-R-NU)

AGS
P.O.Box 99
Circle Pines, MN 55014-99
800-328-2560
FAX: 800-471-8457
e-mail: agsmail@agsnet.com
www.agsnet.com

Kevin Brueggeman, President
Robert Zaske, Market Manager

PIAT-R-NU is an efficient individual measure of academic achievement. Reading, mathematics, and spelling are assessed in a simple, non-threatening format that requires only a pointing response for most items. This multiple choice format makes the PIAT-R ideal for assessing individuals who hesitate to give a spoken response, or have limited expressive abilities. *$289.98*

2475 Peabody Language Development Kits (PLDK)

AGS
P.O.Box 99
Circle Pines, MN 55014-99
800-328-2560
FAX: 800-471-8457
e-mail: agsmail@agsnet.com
www.agsnet.com

Kevin Brueggeman, President
Robert Zaske, Market Manager

The main goals of the Peabody Kit language program are to stimulate overall language skills in Standard English and, for each level of the program, advance children's cognitive skills about a year. *$ 649.95*

Level P
ISBN 0-88671 -25-1

2476 Pediatric Early Elementary (PEEX II) Examination

Educators Publishing Service
625 Mount Auburn Street
3rd Floor
Cambridge, MA 2138- 3039
617-547-6706
800-225-5750
FAX: 888-440-2665
e-mail: feedback@epsbooks.com
www.epsbooks.com

Charles H Heinle, VP
Alexandra S Bigelow, Author
Gunnar Voltz, President

Assesses the second-fourth grade child's performance on thirty-two tasks in six specific areas of development: fine-motor function, language, gross-motor function, memory, visual processing, and delayed recall. At three points during the exam, the child is rated on selective attention and behavior and effect.

$15.40 - $93
ISBN 0-83888 -80-6

2477 Pediatric Exam of Educational-PEERAMID Readiness at Middle Childhood

Educators Publishing Service
625 Mount Auburn Street
3rd Floor
Cambridge, MA 2138- 3039
617-547-6706
800-225-5750
FAX: 888-440-2665
e-mail: feedback@epsbooks.com
www.epsbooks.com

Charles H Heinle, VP
Alexandra S Bigelow, Author
Gunnar Voltz, President

Assesses the 4th-10th grade child's performance on thirty-one tasks in six specific areas: minor neurological indicators, fine-motor function, language, gross-motor function, temporal-sequential organization, and visual processing. Complete set.

$15.40 - $109
ISBN 0-83888 -99-3

2478 Pediatric Examination of Educational Readiness

Educators Publishing Service
625 Mount Auburn Street
3rd Floor
Cambridge, MA 2139- 3039
617-547-6706
800-225-5750
FAX: 888-440-2665
e-mail: feedback@epsbooks.com
www.epsbooks.com

Charles H Heinle, VP
Alexandra S Bigelow, Author
Gunnar Voltz, President

Assesses the Pre-1st grade child's performance on twenty-nine tasks in six specific areas of development: orientation, gross-motor, visual-fine motor, sequential, linguistic and preacademic learning. The child is rated on ten dimensions of selective attention/activity processing efficiency and adaptation. Complete set.

$12.85 - $86.40
ISBN 0-83888 -80-1

2479 Pediatric Extended Examination at-PEET Three

Educators Publishing Service
625 Mount Auburn Street
3rd Floor
Cambridge, MA 2138- 3039
617-547-6706
800-225-5750
FAX: 888-440-2665
e-mail: feedback@epsbooks.com
www.epsbooks.com

Charles H Heinle, VP
Alexandra S Bigelow, Author
Gunnar Volta, President

Assesses the preschool-age child's performance on twenty-eight tasks in five basic areas of development: gross-motor, language, visual-fine motor, memory, and intersensory integration. Complete set.

$13.75 - $126
ISBN 0-83888 -79-4

2480 Pre-Reading Screening Procedures

Educators Publishing Service
625 Mount Auburn Street
3rd Floor
Cambridge, MA 2138- 3039
617-547-6706
800-225-5750
FAX: 888-440-2665
e-mail: feedback@epsbooks.com
www.epsbooks.com

Charles H Heinle, VP
Alexandra S Bigelow, Author
Gunnar Voltz, President

This revised group test, for grades K-1, evaluates auditory, visual and kinesthetic strengths in order to identify children who may have some form of dyslexia or specific language disability. *$ 18.00*

Grades K-1
ISBN 0-83885 -23-4

2481 Preparing for ACT Assessment

American College Testing Program
500 Act Drive
PO Box 168
Iowa City, IA 52243-168
319-337-1000
FAX: 319-339-3021
act.org

Richard L Ferguson, CEO

Designed to help high school students ready themselves for the ACT Assessment's subject area tests, explains the purposes of the four tests, describes their content and format, provides tips and exercises to improve student's test-taking skills and includes a complete sample text with scoring key.

2482 Psycho-Educational Assessment of Preschool Children
National Association of School Psychologists
Ste 105
4340 East West Hwy
Bethesda, MD 20814-4468 301-657-0270
866-331-NASP
FAX: 301-657-0275
e-mail: ADMIN@SOELIN.COM
soelin.com

Susan Gorin, Executive Director
This is a contributed text on assessing specific skills of preschool children.
592 pages

2483 RULES: Revised
Speech Bin
PO Box 1579
Appleton, VA 54912-1579 772-770-0007
888-388-3224
FAX: 888-388-6344
e-mail: customercare@schoolspecialty.com
www.speechbin.com

Jan J Binney, Senior Editor
Treatment program for young children who have phonological disorders. *$43.95*
280 pages
ISBN 0-93785 -51-3

2484 Receptive-Expressive Emergent-REEL-2 Language Test, 2nd Edition
Sage Publications
2455 Teller Road
Thousand Oaks, CA 91320 805-499-9774
800-818-7243
FAX: 800-583-2665
e-mail: info@sagepub.com
www.sagepub.com

Paul Kelly, National Textbook Sales Manager
Blaise R Simqu, President & CEO
A revision of the popular scale used for the multidimensional analysis of emergent language. The REEL-2 is specifically designed for use with a broad range of at risk infants and toddlers in the new multidisciplinary programs developing under P.L. 99-457. *$79.00*

2485 Slingerland Screening Tests
Educators Publishing Service
625 Mount Auburn Street
3rd Floor
Cambridge, MA 2138- 3039 617-547-6706
800-435-7728
FAX: 888-440-2665
e-mail: feedback@epsbooks.com
www.epsbooks.com

Charles H Heinle, VP
Alexandra S Bigelow, Author
Gunnar Voltz, President
These tests, by Beth Slingerland, for individuals or groups of children, grades 1-6, identify children who show indications of having specific language disability in reading, handwriting, spelling or speaking. Form D evaluates personal orientation in time and space as well as the ability to express ideas in writing.
$14.80 - $27.45
ISBN 0-83882 -02-2

2486 Special Needs Advocacy Resource Book
Prufrock Press
PO Box 8813
Waco, TX 76714-8813 800-998-2208
FAX: 800-240-0333
e-mail: info@prufrock.com
www.prufrock.com

Joel McIntosh, Publisher & Marketing Director
Rich Weinfield, Author
Michelle Davis, Author
Subtitle: What You Can Do Now to Advocate for Your Exceptional Child's Education. This is a unique hadnbook that teaches parents how to work with schools to achieve optimal learning situations and accommodations for their child's needs. *$19.95*
328 pages
ISBN 1-593633-09-7

2487 Speech Bin
PO Box 1579
Appleton, VA 54912-1579 772-770-0007
888-388-3224
FAX: 888-388-6344
e-mail: customercare@schoolspecialty.com
www.speechbin.com

Jan J Binney, Senior Editor
Catalog offering test materials, assessment information, books and special education resources for speech-language pathologists, occupational and physical therapists, audiologists, and other rehabilitation professionals in schools, hospitals, clinics and private practices.
ISSN 4773-324

2488 Stuttering Severity Instrument for Children and Adults
Psychological & Educational Publications
P.O.Box 520
Hydesville, CA 95547-520 707-768-1807
800-523-5775
FAX: 800-447-0907
e-mail: psych-edpublications@cox.net
www.psych-edpublications.com

Morrison Gardner, President
With this tool teachers can determine whether to schedule a child for therapy or to evaluate the effects of treatment.

2489 Taking Part: Introducing Social Skills to Young Children
AGS
P.O.Box 99
Circle Pines, MN 55014-99 800-328-2560
FAX: 800-471-8457
e-mail: agsmail@agsnet.com
www.agsnet.com

Kevin Brueggeman, President
Robert Zaske, Market Manager
The first social skills curriculum to be linked directly to an assessment tool. More than 30 lessons correlate with the skills assessed by the Social Skills Rating System, a multirater approach to assessing prosocial and problem behaviors. *$149.95*

2490 Test Critiques: Volumes I-X
Sage Publications
2455 Teller Road
Thousand Oaks, CA 91320 805-499-9774
800-818-7243
FAX: 800-583-2665
e-mail: info@sagepub.com
www.sagepub.com

Paul Kelly, National Textbook Sales Manager
Blaise R Simqu, President & CEO
Provides the professional and nonprofessional with in-depth, evaluative studies of more than 800 of the most widely used of these assessment instruments. *$649.00*

2491 Test of Early Reading Ability Deaf or Hard of Hearing
Pro- Ed Publications
8700 Shoal Creek Blvd
Austin, TX 78757-6816 512-451-3246
800-897-3202
FAX: 800-397-7633
e-mail: general@proedinc.com
www.proedinc.com

Donald D Hammill, Owner
Courtney King, Marketing Coordinator
This adaptation of the TERA-2 for simultaneous communication of American Sign Language is the ONLY individually administered test of reading designed for children with moderate to profound sensory hearing loss. *$169.00*
Complete Kit

2492 Test of Language Development: Primary
Sage Publications
2455 Teller Road
Thousand Oaks, CA 91320
805-499-9774
800-818-7243
FAX: 800-583-2665
e-mail: info@sagepub.com
www.sagepub.com
Paul Kelly, National Textbook Sales Manager
Blaise R Simqu, President & CEO
TOLD P:2 and TOLD I:2 are the most popular tests of spoken language used by clinicians today. They are used to identify children who have language disorders and to isolate the particular types of disorders they have. Primary Edition for ages 1-4 to 8-11: Intermediate Edition for ages 8-6 to 12-11.

2493 Test of Mathematical Abilities, 2nd Edition
Sage Publications
2455 Teller Road
Thousand Oaks, CA 91320
805-499-9774
800-818-7243
FAX: 800-583-2665
e-mail: info@sagepub.com
www.sagepub.com
Paul Kelly, National Textbook Sales Manager
Blaise R Simqu, President & CEO
The latest version was developed for use in grades 3 through 12. It measures math performance on the two traditional major skill areas in math as well as attitude, vocabulary and general application of math concepts in real life. *$84.00*

2494 Test of Nonverbal Intelligence, 3rd Edition
Sage Publications
2455 Teller Road
Thousand Oaks, CA 91320
805-499-9774
800-818-7243
FAX: 800-583-2665
e-mail: info@sagepub.com
www.sagepub.com
Paul Kelly, National Textbook Sales Manager
Blaise R Simqu, President & CEO
A language-free measure of intelligence, aptitude and reasoning. The administration of the test requires no reading, writing, speaking or listening on the part of the test subject. The items included in this test are problem-solving tasks that increase in difficulty. Each item presents a set of figures in which one or more components is missing. The test items include one or more of the characteristics of shape, position, direction, rotation, contiguity, shading, size, movement or pattern. *$229.00*
Complete Kit

2495 Test of Phonological Awareness
Sage Publications
2455 Teller Road
Thousand Oaks, CA 91320
805-499-9774
800-818-7243
FAX: 800-583-2665
e-mail: info@sagepub.com
www.sagepub.com
Paul Kelly, National Textbook Sales Manager
Blaise R Simqu, President & CEO
Measures young children's awareness of the individual sounds in words. Children who are sensitive to the phonological structure of words in oral language have a much easier time learning to read than children who are not. *$143.00*

2496 Test of Written Spelling, 3rd Edition
Pro- Ed Publications
8700 Shoal Creek Blvd
Austin, TX 78757-6897
512-451-3246
800-897-3202
FAX: 800-397-7633
e-mail: general@proedinc.com
www.proedinc.com
Donald D Hammill, Owner
Courtney King, Marketing Coordinator
This revised edition assesses the student's ability to spell words whose spellings are readily predictable in sound-letter patterns, words whose spellings are less predictable and both types of words considered together. *$74.00*

2497 The Teaching of Reading: A Continuum from Kindergarten through College
AVKO Educational Research Foundation
3084 Willard Rd
Birch Run, MI 48415-9404
810-686-9283
866-285-6612
FAX: 810-686-1101
e-mail: webmaster@avko.org
avko.org
Don Mc Cabe, Executive Director
A textbook for teaching teachers how to teach language arts with lessons about dyslexia, phonics, learning to write, the connection between reading and spelling, and diagnostic and prescriptive tests. Free as an e-book for Foundation members. *$49.95*
364 pages

2498 Treatment and Learning Centers
2092 Gaither Road
Suite 100
Rockville, MD 20850
301-424-5200
FAX: 301-424-8063
TTY:301-424-5203
e-mail: info@ttlc.org
www.ttlc.org
Dr Lisa Lenhart, Tutoring/Testing Services Dir
Diagnostic evaluations are provided on an individual basis to identify the learning differences and needs of students who may have learning disabilities, or who are struggling with the academic environment.

2499 Woodcock Reading Mastery Tests
Pearson
5601 Green Valley Dr
Bloomington, MN 55437-1099
800-627-7271
FAX: 800-232-1223
e-mail: pearsonassessments@pearson.com
www.pearsonassessments.com
Christine Carlson, Product Manager
Doug Kubach, President & CEO
The Woodcock Reading Mastery Tests - Revised provides an interpretive system and age range to help you assess reading skills of children and adults. Two forms, G and II, make it easy to test and retest, or you can combine the results of both forms for a more comprehensive assessment. Revised with recent updates. *$329.95*

2500 Young Children with Special Needs: A Developmentally Appropriate Approach
Allyn & Bacon
75 Arlington Street
Ste 300
Boston, MA 2116-3988
617-848-7500
800-852-8024
FAX: 617-944-7273
www.ablongman.com
Bill Barke, CEO
Thomas Longman, Founder
This book is designed to prepare students in making curriculum decisions in order to care for and foster the development of young children with special needs in normal early childhood settings.
270 pages
ISBN 0-20518 -94-X

Treatment & Training

2501 ABLE Program MCC-Longview
3200 Broadway
Kansas City, MO 64111-2105
816-604-1000
FAX: 816-672-2719
e-mail: joan.bergstrom@mcckc.edu
mcckc.edu/ABLE
Joan Bergstrom, Director
Kay Owens, Administrative Assistant

Intensive support services program for post secondary students with neurological disabilities. The ABLE Program can be reached at http://mcckc.edu/ABLE

2502 Academy for Guided Imagery
30765 Pacific Coast Hwy
Ste 355
Malibu, CA 90265-3643
800-726-2070
FAX: 800-727-2070
e-mail: info@acadgi.com
www.acadgi.com

David E Bresler, President
The Academy aims to teach people to access and use the power of the mind/body connection for healing, and to further understanding of the imagery process in human life and development. They provide systematic training and guidance to health professionals who are interested in the use of Guided Imagery in their practice. The Academy's Imagery Store offers guided imagery CDs, DVDs and books for self-healing.

2503 Asthma & Allergy Education for Worksite Clinicians
Asthma and Allergy Foundation of America
8201 Corporate Drive
Suite 1000
Landover, VA 20785
202-466-7643
800-727-8462
FAX: 202-466-8940
e-mail: info@aafa.org
aafa.org

Bill Mc Lin, President & CEO
Helen Taylor, Information Specialist
Developed to teach health professionals in the worksite about asthma and allergies and ultimately improve the health of the employees who have theses de\iseases. The program gives worksite clinicians the knowledge and tools they need to give employees guidance on how to control environmental factors both in the home and in the workplace, self-manage thier asthma and/or allergies and to determaine if ti is necessary for employees to see an allergist if symptoms persist.

2504 Asthma & Allergy Essentials for Children's Care Provider
Asthma and Allergy Foundation of America
8201 Corporate Drive
Suite 1000
Landover, VA 20785
202-466-7643
800-727-8462
FAX: 202-466-8940
e-mail: info@aafa.org
aafa.org

Bill Mc Lin, President & CEO
Helen Taylor, Information Specialist
Course gives child care providers the tools and knowledge they need to care for children with asthma and allergies. During the interactive, three hour program, a trained health professional teaches providers how to recognize the signs and symptoms of an asthma or allergy episode, how to institute environmental control measures to prevent these episodes, and how to properly use medication and the tools for asthma management. In areas of the country serviced by AAFA's 14 chapters.

2505 Asthma Care Training for Kids (ACT)
Asthma and Allergy Foundation of America
8201 Corporate Drive
Suite 1000
Landover, VA 20785
202-466-7643
FAX: 202-466-8940
e-mail: info@aafa.org
www.aafa.org

Bill Mc Lin, President & CEO
Helen Taylor, Information Specialist
Interactive program for children ages seven to 12 and their families. Children and their families attend three group sessions seperately to learn their own unique styles and then come together at the end of each session to share their knowledge.

2506 Ayurvedic Institute
PO Box 23445
Albuquerque, NM 87292-1445
505-291-9698
800-863-7721
FAX: 505-294-7572
e-mail: registrar@ayurveds.com
ayurveda.com

Wynn Werner, Administrator
Directed by Dr. Vasant Lad, trains people in Ayurveda.

2507 Harriet & Robert Heilbrunn Guild School
JGB Audio Library for the Blind
15 W 65th St
New York, NY 10023-6601
212-769-6200
800-284-4422
FAX: 212-769-6266
e-mail: info@JGB.org
www.JGB.org

Allen R Morse, JD, PhD, President & CEO
Ken Stanley, Manager
A Jewish Guild for the blind.

2508 Lake Michigan Academy
West Michigan Learning Disabilities Foundation
2428 Burton St SE
Grand Rapids, MI 49546-4806
616-464-3330
FAX: 616-285-1935
e-mail: info@wmldf.org
www.wmldf.org

Amy Barto, Executive Director
Is a private day school for children with learning disabilities.

2509 Mad Hatters: Theatre That Makes a World of Difference
P.O.Box 50002
Kalamazoo, MI 49005-2
FAX: 269-385-5868
Bobbe A Luce, Executive Director
A nationally-known theater which has presented effective and innovative programs to more than 175,000 people in over 1,150 performances in the past 15 years. Our presentations and training programs are a proven method of changing attitudes and behaviors. The Mad Hatters is a leader in the field of sensitivity training to build community and foster the inclusion of all people in society. Fees: $500-$4000 per program, depending on topic and audience.

2510 Ramapo Training
Ramapo for Children
Route 52/Salisbury Turnpike
PO Box 266
Rhinebeck, NY 12572
845-876-8403
FAX: 845-876-8414
e-mail: office@ramapoforchildren.org
www.ramapoforchildren.org

Richard Rosenthal, President
Teri Goldberg Horowitz, First Vice President
Claude Ann Mellins, Ph.D., Vice President
Deusdedi Merced, Esq., Vice President
Ramapo Training was established to provide staff training and program support for educational and recreational programs, especially those that serve children-at-risk and those with special needs.

2511 Sandhills School
1500 Hallbrook Dr
Columbia, SC 29209-4021
803-695-1400
FAX: 803-695-1214
e-mail: info@sandhillsschool.org
www.sandhillsschool.org

Anne Vickers, Head of School
Erika Senneseth, Asst Head of School
Angela Daniel, Director of Development
Carmen Kennedy, Business Manager
Exists to provide educational programs and intellectual development for average to above average students, six to 15, who learn differently and to promote the development of self-awareness, joy in learning and a vision of themselves as life-long learners.

2512 Senior Program for Teens and Young Adults with Special Needs
Camp J CC
6125 Montrose Rd
Rockville, MD 20852-4860
301-881-0100
FAX: 301-881-6549
e-mail: jcccamp@jccgw.org
www.jccgw.org

Scott Cohen, President
Mindy Burger, Vice President for Development

The senior Program is a transitional program for teens and young adults with mental retardation, severe learning disabilities and multiple disabilities. Socialization, recreation and independent living skills are enhanced ina fun enviroment. Activities include art, music, recreational swim and more.

2513 The Howard School
1192 Foster St NW
Atlanta, GA 30318-4329
404-377-7436
FAX: 404-377-0884
e-mail: admissions@howardschool.org
howardschool.org

Marifred Cilella, Head Of School

The Howard School educates students 5 years old through 12th grade with language learning disabilities and learning differences. Small student/teacher ratios allow for instruction that is personalized to complement the individual learning styles and to help each student understand his/her learning process. Students gain the tools and strategies needed to become independent, life-long learners.

2514 The Vanguard School
Valley Forge Specialized Educational Services
1777 N Valley Rd
Paoli, PA 19301
610-296-6700
FAX: 610-640-0132
e-mail: info@vanguardschool_pa.org
www.vanguardschool-pa.org

Tim Lanshe, Director of Education
James Kirkpatrick, CFO
Peg Osborne, Admissions Director

An Approved Private School (APS) for students aged 4-21 years with exceptionalities including autism spectrum disorder, mild emotional disturbances and/or neurological impairments.

2515 Worthmore Academy
3535 Kessler Boulevard East Dr
Indianapolis, IN 46220-5154
317-902-9896
877-700-6516
FAX: 317-251-6516
e-mail: bjackson@worthmoreacademy.org
www.worthmoreacademy.org

Brenda Jackson, Director
Alyssa Blaire Cook, Assistant Director

A place where children with learning disabilities receive individualized instruction to help remediate his or her condition. The most common learning disabilities we work with are Dyslexiz, A.D.D, A.D.H.D, Autism Spectrum (including Asperger's Syndrome), and communication disorders.

Exchange Programs

General

2516 A Guide to International Educational Exchange
Mobility International USA
132 E. Broadway
Suite 343
Eugene, OR 97401-2767
541-343-1284
FAX: 541-343-6812
e-mail: info@miusa.org
www.miusa.org

Susan Sygall, CEO
A Guide to International Educational Exchange, Community Service and Travel for People with Disabilities includes information travel and international programs, as well as personal experience stories from people with disabilities who have had successful international experiences. *$45.00*
600 pages
ISBN 1-880034-24-7

2517 American Institute for Foreign Study
River Plaza 9 W Broad St
Stamford, CT 6902-3788
203-399-5000
866-906-2437
FAX: 203-399-5590
e-mail: info@aifs.com
www.aifs.com

William L Gertz, CEO
Organizes cultural exchange programs throughout the world for more than 50,000 students each year and arranges insurance coverage for our own participants as well as participants of other organizations. Also provides summer travel programs overseas and in the US ranging from one week to a full academic year.

2518 American Universities International Programs
307 S College Ave
Fort Collins, CO 80524-2801
970-495-0084
888-730-2847
FAX: 970-495-0114
e-mail: info@auip.com
www.auip.com

Laurie Klith, Executive Director
Study abroad organization sending students to universities in Australia and New Zealand.

2519 American-Scandinavian Foundation
58 Park Ave
38 Street
New York, NY 10016-3007
212-779-3587
FAX: 212-686-1157
e-mail: info@amscan.org
scandinaviahouse.org

Edward Gallagher, President
Promotes international understanding through educational and cultural exchange between the United States and Denmark, Finland, Iceland, Norway and Sweden.

2520 Antioch College
One Morgan Place
Yellow Springs, OH 45387-1635
937-319-6082
FAX: 937-319-6085
e-mail: aea@antioch-college.edu
www.antioch-college.edu

Mark Roosevelt, President
Thomas Brookley, CFO & COO
Gariot Louima, Chief Communications Officer
Education abroad offers numerous programs which can be included in undergraduate and graduate study programs.

2521 Army and Air Force Exchange Services
PO Box 660202
Dallas, TX 75266-202
214-312-2011
800-527-2345
FAX: 800-446-0163
TTY: 800-423-2011
www.aafes.com

James Moore, Senior VP
MG Bruce Casella, Commander/CEO
Brings a tradition of value, service, and support to its 11.5 million authorized customers at military installations in the United States, Europe and in the Pacific.

2522 Association for International Practical Training
10400 Little Patuxent Pkwy
Suite 250
Columbia, MD 21044-3519
410-997-2200
FAX: 410-992-3924
e-mail: aipt@aipt.org
aipt.org

Elizabeth Chazottes, CEO
Nonprofit organization dedicated to encouraging and facilitating the exchange of qualified individuals between the US and other countries so they may gain practical work experience and improve international understanding.

2523 Basic Facts on Study Abroad
International Education
809 United Nations Plz
New York, NY 10017-3503
212-883-8200
FAX: 212-984-5452
e-mail: publications@un.org
iie.org

Allen E Goodman, CEO
Peggy Blumenthal, Executive Vice President
Information book including foreign study planning, educational choices, finances and study abroad programs. *$35.00*
30 pages

2524 Beaver College
Arcadia University
450 S Easton Rd
Glenside, PA 19038-3215
215-572-2901
888-232-8379
FAX: 215-572-2174
e-mail: cea@beaver.edu
www.beaver.edu/cea

Lorna Stern, Deputy Director
One of the largest college-based study abroad programs in the country. Prices from $8000.00 semester to $22000.00 a year.

2525 Buffalo State (SUNY)
1300 Elmwood Ave
South Wing 410
Buffalo, NY 14222-1095
716-878-4620
FAX: 716-878-3054
e-mail: intleduc@buffalostate.edu
www.buffalostate.edu/studyabroad
Lee Ann Grace, Asst Dean Int'l/Exchange Program
Provides international educational exchange opportunities for students of university age and older through its Office of International Education.

2526 Building Bridges: Including People with Disabilities in International Programs
Mobility International USA
132 E Broadway
Suite 343
Eugene, OR 97401-3155
541-343-1284
FAX: 541-343-6812
e-mail: info@miusa.org
miusa.org

Susan Sygall, CEO
Michele Scheib, Project Specialist
Melissa Mitchell, Public Relations Coordinator
Empowers people with disabilities around the world through international exhange and international development to achieve

their human rights. The international exchange programs usually last two-four weeks and are held throughout the year in the US and abroad. Activities include living with homestay families, leadership seminars, disability rights workshops, cross cultural learning and teambuilding activities such as river rafting and challenging courses.

2527 **Davidson College, Office of Study Abroad**
Davidson College
PO Box 7171
Davidson, NC 28035-7171 704-894-2000
FAX: 704-894-2005
e-mail: kocampbell@davidson.edu
www3.davidson.edu

Carol Quillen, President
Recognizes the value of study abroad for both the devlopment of worl understanding and the development of the student as a broadminded, objective and mature individual.

2528 **High School Students Guide to Study, Travel, and Adventure Abroad**
300 Fore Street
Portland, ME 4101 207-553-4000
FAX: 207-553-4299
e-mail: contact@ciee.org
www.ciee.org

Robert E. Fallon, CEO & President
Kenton Keith, Senior Vice President for Progra
This guide provides high school students with all the information they need for a successful trip abroad. Included are sections to help students find out if they're ready for a trip abroad, make the necessary preparations and get the most from their experience. Over 200 programs are described including language study, summer camps, homestays, study tours and work camps. The program descriptions include information for people with disabilities.
ISSN 0312-11

2529 **International Christian Youth Exchange**
134 W 26th St
New York, NY 10001-6803 212-206-7307
FAX: 212-633-9085

Ed Gragert
Offers participants a unique experience to learn about another culture and make friends from different countries.

2530 **International Partnership for Service-Learning and Leadership**
1515 SW 5th Avenue
Suite 606
Portland, OR 97201 503-954-1812
FAX: 503-954-1881
e-mail: info@ipsl.org
ipsl.org

Nevin Brown, President
A not for profit educational organization incorporated in New York State serving students, colleges, universities, service agenices and related organizations around the world by fostering programs that link volunteer service to the community and academic study.

2531 **International Student Exchange Programs (I SEP)**
1655 N Fort Myer Drive
Suite 400
Arlington, VA 22209 703-504-9960
FAX: 703-243-8070
e-mail: info@isep.org
www.isep.org

Dr. Thomas Hochstettler, Chair
Dr. Tony Atwater, President
ISEP is a network of 275 post-secondary institutions in the United States and 38 other countries cooperating to provide affordable international educational experiences for a diverse student population.

2532 **International University Partnerships**
University of Pennsylvania
1011 South Dr
Indiana, PA 15705-1046 724-357-2100
FAX: 724-357-6213
iup.edu

David Werner, President
Offers a variety of international educational exchange programs to students who wish to study overseas.

2533 **Lake Erie College**
391 W. Washington St.
Painesville, OH 44077 440-296-1856
800-533-4996
FAX: 440-375-7005
e-mail: admissions@lec.edu
www.lec.edu

Michael Victor, President
Michael Keresman lll, Director
Sends students abroad for a term or longer to develop intellectual awareness and individual maturity.

2534 **Lane Community College**
4000 E 30th Ave
Eugene, OR 97405-640 541-463-3000
FAX: 541-463-5201
e-mail: asklane@lanecc.edu
www.lanecc.edu

Mary Spilde, President
Lane Community Colloege offers a wide variety of instructional programs including transfer credit programs, career and technical degree and certificate programs, continuing education noncredit courses, programs in English as a Second Language and International ESL, GED programs, and customized training for local businesses.

2535 **Lions Clubs International**
300 W 22nd St
Oak Brook, IL 60523-8842 630-571-5466
FAX: 630-571-8890
e-mail: lions@lionsclub.org
www.lionsclubs.org

Joe Preston, International President
Jitsuhiro Yamada, First Vice President
Robert E. Corlew, Second Vice President
Eric R. Carter, First Year Directors
Over 46,000 individual clubs in over 194 countries and geographical areas which provide community service and promote better international relations. Clubs work with local communities to provide needed and useful programs for sight, diabetes and hearing, and aid in study abroad.

2536 **Lisle**
900 County Road 269
Leander, TX 78641-1633 512-259-4404
e-mail: lisle2@io.com
www.lisle.utoledo.edu

Barbara E Bratton, Owner
Educational organization which works toward world peace and better quality of human life through increased understanding between persons of similar and different cultures.

2537 **National 4-H Council**
7100 Connecticut Ave
Chevy Chase, MD 20815-4934 301-961-2800
FAX: 301-961-2894
www.4-h.org

Donald Floyd, President
Jennifer Sirangelo, Executive Vice President
4-H opened the door for young people to learn leadership skills and explore ways to give back. 4-H revolutionized how youth connected to practical, hands-on learning experiences while outside of the classroom.

2538 New Directions for People with Disabilities
5276 Hollister Avenue
Suite 207
Santa Barbara, CA 93111-3068
805-967-2841
888-967-2841
FAX: 805-964-7344
e-mail: hello@newdirectionstravel.org
www.newdirectionstravel.org

Dee Duncan, Executive Director
Jeanne Mohle, Director of Operations
Danna Mead, Program Director
Colette Piacentini, Business Manager

Provides high quality local, national, and international travel vacations and holiday programs for people with mild to moderate developmental disabilities. Through these programs, people with disabilities are increasingly understood, appreciated and more accepted as important and contributing members of our world.

2539 People to People International
911 Main Street
Suite 2110
Kansas City, MO 64105-2246
816-531-4701
FAX: 816-561-7502
e-mail: ptpi@ptpi.org
www.ptpi.org

Mary Eisenhower, CEO
Roseanne Rosen, Senior Vice President of Operati
Brian Hueben, Senior Director, Administration
Stacey Chance, Director, Publications

Exchanges international understanding and friendship through educational, cultural and humantarian activities involving the exchange of ideas and experiences directly among people of different countries and diverse cultures. Is also dedicated to enhancing cross cultural communication within each communityand across communities and nations.

2540 Rotary Youth Exchange
Rotary International
1560 Sherman Ave
Evanston, IL 60201-4818
847-866-3000
866-976-8279
FAX: 847-328-4101
e-mail: youthexchange@rotary.org
www.rotary.org

Kalyan Banerjee, International President
Noel A Bajat, Vice President
Kenneth R Boyd, Director
Elizabeth Demaray, Director

This worldwide organization of business and professional leaders provides humanitarian service, encourages high ethical standards in all vocations, and helps build goodwill and peace in the world. Approximately 1.2 million Rotarians belong to more than 31,000 Rotary clubs located in 167 countries for exchange opportunities.

2541 Scandinavian Exchange
24 Dickinson Street
Amherst, MA 1002
413-253-9737
FAX: 413-253-5282
e-mail: howery@scandinavianseminar.org
www.scandinavianseminar.org

Jacqueline D Waldman, CEO
William Kaufmann, Chair

Student exchange program founded in 1949.

2542 Sister Cities International
915 15th Street, NW
4th Floor
Washington, DC 20005
202-347-8630
FAX: 202-393-6524
e-mail: info@sister-cities.org
sister-cities.org

Patrick Madden, President
Jim Doumas, Executive Vice President, & Inte

A non profit citizen diplomacy network creating and strengthening partnerships between US and international communities in an effort to increase global cooperation at the municipal level, to promote cultural understnading and to stimulate economic development. Encourages local community development and volunteer action by motivating and empowering private citizens, municipal officials and business leaders to conduct long term programs of mutual benefits including exchange situations.

2543 State University of New York
1400 Washington Ave
Albany, NY 12222-100
518-442-3300
FAX: 518-442-5383
e-mail: ugadmissions@albany.edu
www.albany.edu

George Philip, President
Alain Kaloyeros, Senior Vice President & CEO
Susan Phillips, Provost & VP for Academic Affai
James Dias, VP for Research

Offers over 150 international educational exchange programs in 37 different countries. Broad mission of excellence in undergraduate and graduate education, research and public service engages 17,000 diverse students in nine schools and colleges across three campuses.

2544 University of Minnesota at Crookston
2900 University Ave
Crookston, MN 56716-5000
218-281-6510
800-862-6466
FAX: 218-281-8050
e-mail: UMCinfo@umn.edu
www.crk.umn.edu

Charles Casey, CEO
Eric Kaler, President

The University of Minnesota, Crookston (UMC) is a public, baccalaureate, coeducational institution and a coordinate campus of the University of Minnesota

2545 University of Oregon
5000 N Willamette Blvd
Portland, OR 97203-5798
503-943-8000
FAX: 503-725-3067
e-mail: webmaster@up.edu
up.edu

Patricia Esley, Manager
Rev.E.Willia Beauchamp, President
James Lyons, VP University Relations
Jim Ravelli, VP for University Research

Study/cultural experience is available in Tokyo and other Japanese cities as part of the Japan Studies Program at the University.

2546 Western Washington University
516 High St
Bellingham, WA 98225-5996
360-650-3000
FAX: 360-650-3022
www.wwu.edu

Bruce Shepard, President
Paul Dunn, Senior Executive Asst. to the Pr
Barbara Stoneberg, Assistant to the President
Mary Lacher, Receptionist, President & Provis

2547 World Experience Teenage Exchange Program
2440 S Hacienda Blvd
Suite 116
Hacienda Heights, CA 91745-4763
626-330-5719
800-633-6653
FAX: 626-333-4914
e-mail: info@worldexperience.org
worldexperience.org

Kerry Gonzales, President
Marge Archaumbault, President

Offers a quality and affordable program for over two decades and continues to provide students and host families a youth exchange program based on individual attention, with the help of an international network of overseas directors and USA coordinators.

2548 World of Options
Mobility International USA
132 E Broadway
Suite 343
Eugene, OR 97401-3155
541-343-1284
FAX: 541-343-6812
e-mail: info@miusa.org
miusa.org

Susan Sygall, CEO
Cerise Roth-Vinson, COO
Susan Dunn, Executive Asst. to the CEO
Alison Eker, Project Assistant

Empowering people with disabilities around the world through international exchange and international development to achieve their human rights. *$16.00*
338 pages
ISBN 1-880034-01-8

2549 Youth for Understanding International Exchange
6400 Goldsboro Road
Suite 100
Bethesda, MD 20817-5841
240-235-2100
800-833-6243
FAX: 240-352-2104
e-mail: admissions@yfu.org
yfu.org

Rachel Andreson, Founder
Samantha Brizzolara, Chair

Youth for Understanding (YFU) International Exchange, an educational, nonprofit organization, prepares young people for the opportunities and responsabilities in a changing, independent world. With YFU, students can choose a year, semenster, or summer program in one or more than 35 countries worldwide. More than 200,000 young people from more than 50 nations in Asia, Europe, North and South America, Africa and the Pacific have participated in YFU exchanges.

Foundations & Funding Resources

Alabama

2550 Alabama Power Foundation
PO Box 2641
Birmingham, AL 35291-11
205-257-2508
800-245-2244
FAX: 205-257-1860
www.alabamapower.com/foundation

Charles D McCrary, President & CEO

Honoring its mission to strengthen the communities the company serves, the foundation focuses its efforts on organizations that support education, civic activities, health services, the environment and the arts. By supporting the state's educational system from pre-K to universities the foundation is investing in Alabama's future and the well-being of its residents.

2551 Andalusia Health Services
700 River Falls Street
PO Box 667
Andalusia, AL 36420- 1213
334-222-6591
FAX: 334-222-6567
e-mail: dreeves@andalusiachamber.com
www.andalusiachamber.com

Janna McGlamory, President
Debbie Marcum, Vice President
Ashley Eiland, Executive Vice President
Gail Hayes, Treasurer

Only offers grants to the residents of Covington County in Alabama who are pursuing a degree in a medical field.

2552 The Arc Of Alabama
557 S Lawrence St
Montgomery, AL 36104-4611
334-262-7688
866-243-9557
FAX: 334-834-9737
e-mail: info@thearcofalabama.com
www.thearcofalabama.com

Thomas B. Holmes

The Arc of Alabama, Inc. is a volunteer-based membership organization made up of individuals with intellectual (such as mental retardation, an old and outdated term seldom used anymore), developmental and other disabilities, their families, friends, interested citizens, and professionals in the disability field.

Alaska

2553 Arc of Alaska
The Arc of Anchorage
2211 Arca Dr
Anchorage, AK 99508-3462
907-277-6677
800-258-2232
FAX: 907-272-2161
TTY: 907-277-0735
e-mail: info@thearcofanchorage.org
www.thearchofanchorage.com

Rod Shipley, President
Dave Falsey, Vice President
Meredith Parham, Secretary
Sharon Purkis, Treasurer

The Arc helps Alaskans who experience developmental disabilities, behavioral health concerns or deafness achieve lives of dignity and independence as valued members of our community.

2554 Rasmuson Foundation
301 West Northern Lights Blvd.
Suite 400
Anchorage, AK 99503-2648
907-297-2700
877-366-2700
FAX: 907-297-2770
e-mail: rasmusonfdn@rasmuson.org
www.rasmuson.org

Diane Kaplan, President & CEO
Sammye Pokryfki, Senior Program Officer

The Rasmuson Foundation invests both in individuals and well managed organizations dedicated to improving the quality of life for Alaskans.

Arizona

2555 Arizona Community Foundation
2201 E Camelback Road
Suite 202
Phoenix, AZ 85016-3481
602-381-1400
800-222-8221
FAX: 602-381-1575
e-mail: sseleznow@azfoundation.org
www.azfoundation.org

Steven Seleznow, President & CEO
Jim Pitofsky, Chief Strategy Officer
Megan Brownell, Chief Communications Officer

The mission of the Arizona Community Foundation is to empower and align philanthropic interests with community needs and build a legacy of living.

2556 Arizona Autism ResourcesThe Arc of Arizona
The Arc of Arizona
PO Box 90714
Phoenix, AZ 85066
602-234-2721
800-252-9054
FAX: 602-234-5959
e-mail: thearcaz@gmail.com
www.arcarizona.org

Ginger Pottenger, President
Richard Travis, Vice President
Sandra Malloy, Secretary

The Arc, a national organization on mental retardaion, is committed to securing for all people with developmental disabilities the opportunity to choose and realize their goals in regard to where they live, learn, work and play.

2557 Margaret T Morris Foundation
PO Box 592
Prescott, AZ 86302-592
928-445-6633
FAX: 928-445-6633
www.archive.naccho.org

Susan Rheem, Executive Director

2558 The Arizona Instructional Resource Center for Students who are Blind or Visually Impaired
Foundation For Blind Children
1235 E. Harmont Drive
Phoenix, AZ 85020
602-678-5816
FAX: 602-678-5811
e-mail: idurre@seeitourway.org
www.seeitourway.org

Inge Durre, Director, AIRC

The Foundation for Blind Children contracts with the Arizona Department of Education to provide statewide media services for students between pre-kindergarten and 12th grade who have a visual impairment or are blind andEneed their instructional materials in a specialized medium such as braille, large print, or electronic files as well as adaptive equipment.

Arkansas

2559 Arc of Arkansas
2004 Main St
Little Rock, AR 72206-1526
501-375-2039
FAX: 501-372-4621
e-mail: shitt@arcark.org
www.arcark.org
Steve Hitt, Chief Executive Officer
Cynthia Stone, Chief Operating Officer
Roger Williams, Chief Financial Officer
Serving people with disabilites and their families for over fourty years.

2560 Winthrop Rockefeller Foundation
225 East Markham Street
Suite 200
Little Rock, AR 72201
501-376-6854
FAX: 501-374-4797
e-mail: webfeedback@wrfoundation.org
www.wrfoundation.org
Sherece Y. West, Ph.D, President & CEO
Cory Anderson, Vice President
Andrea M. Dobson, COO & CFO
Angela Kremers, Senior Associate, Education
Mission is to improve the quality of life in Arkansas. It focuses its grantmaking efforts in three areas: education, economic development and civic affairs. Education projects funded in the past have included grants to schools that are working to involve teachers and parents in making decisions about what happens at their schools, projects that work to remove prejudice from the educational process and more. Major grants are made to support the development of new programs.

California

2561 Ahmanson Foundation
9215 Wilshire Blvd
Beverly Hills, CA 90210-5538
310-278-0770
e-mail: info@theahmansonfoundation.org
www.theahmansonfoundation.org
William Ahmanson, President
Karen Ahmanson Hoffman, Managing Director
Kristen K. O'Connor, CFO & Treasurer
Jennie Chin, Senior Accountant
The Foundation primarily gives in Southern California with major emphasis in Los Angeles County. The Foundation focuses on the arts and humanities, education, mental health and support for a broad range of social welfare programs.

2562 Alice Tweed Touhy Foundation
205 E Carrillo Street
Suite 219
Santa Barbara, CA 93101-7186
805-962-6430
Jeanne Mc Kay, Manager
Rehabilitation, recreation and building funds are given to organizations only within the Santa Barbara area.

2563 Alternating Hemiplegia of Childhood Foundation
2000 Town Center
Suite 1900
Livonia, MI 48075
919-569-5200
e-mail: sharon@ahckids.org
www.ahckids.org
Jeff Wuchich, President
Lynn Egan, Vice President
Vicky Platt, Secretary
Voluntary not-for-profit organizations dedicated to promoting professional and public awareness of Alternating Hemiplegia of Childhood (AHC) and providing current information to affected individuals and their families. Supports ongoing medical research into the cause, treatment and potential cure of AHC. Disseminates information about this disorder to promote proper diagnosis and maintains a registry of families, affected chidren and physicians who are familiar with AHC.

2564 Arc of California
1225 9th Street
Suite 350
Sacramento, CA 95815
916-552-6619
800-698-6619
FAX: 916-441-3494
e-mail: arcca@arccalifornia.org
www.arccalifornia.org
Tony Anderson, Executive Director
Carlos Palacios, Membership Services
Jordan Lindsey, Director, Public Policy
Advocates for people with intellectual and all developmental disabilities since 1953. The ARC of California is committed to securing for all people with developmental disabilities, in partnership with thier families, legal guardians or conservators the opportunity to choose and realize their goals of where and how they learn, live, work and play.

2565 Atkinson Foundation
1720 S. Amphlett Blvd
Suite 100
San Mateo, CA 94402-2710
650-357-1101
FAX: 650-357-1101
e-mail: atkinfdn@aol.com
www.atkinsonfdn.org
Elizabeth Curtis, Administrator
The Foundation focuses and awards grants to community service and civic organizations serving the residents of San Mateo County, California through programs that benefit children, youth, seniors, the disadvantaged and those in need of rehabilitation. Grants are also made to local churches and schools, and overseas for sustainable development, health education and family planning. No grants to individuals or for research, travel, special events, annual campaigns, media and publications.

2566 Baker Commodities Corporate Giving Program
4020 Bandini Blvd
Vernon, CA 90023
323-268-2801
FAX: 323-268-5166
www.bakercommodities.com
Jim Andreoli, President
Baker Commodities has been one of the nation's leading providers of rendering, and grease removal services. Baker Commodities, Inc. is a completely sustainable company, recycling animal by-products and kitchen waste into valuable products that can be used to feed livestock, power vehicles, and act as a base for everyday items.

2567 Bank of America Foundation
315 Montgomery St
Fl 8
San Francisco, CA 94104-1803
415-622-8248
888-488-9802
FAX: 704-386-6444
www.bankamerica.com/foundation
Ilana Orin, Manager
The Foundation will consider grants in four categories including: Health & Human Services, which provides support to health & human service organizations primarily through grants to the United Way campaigns; Education, with the focus on preparing people to become productive employees and participating citizens; Conservation & Environment, the improvement of California communities for the benefit of their citizens; and Culture & The Arts, supporting the leading performing and visual arts groups.

2568 Blind Babies Foundation
1814 Franklin Street
Suite 300
Oakland, CA 94612 510-446-2229
FAX: 510-446-2262
e-mail: bbfinfo@blindbabies.org
www.blindbabies.org
Dottie Bridge, President
Sharon Sacks, PhD, 1st Vice President
Clare Friedman, PhD, 2nd Vice President
Deborah Orel-Bixler, PhD, OD,, Secretary
Founded in 1949, the foundation provides home-based early intervention services to families with young children with vision impairment in the Northern and Central regions of California.

2569 Bothin Foundation
1660 Bush Street
Suite 300
San Francisco, CA 94109-5308 415-561-6540
FAX: 415-561-6477
e-mail: info@pfs-llc.net
www.pfs-llc.net/bothin/index.html
Charles Casey, President
Mary Gregory, Vice President
Eric Sloan, Senior Program Staff
Annie Yates, Program Officer
The Bothin Foundation makes grants for capital, building, and equipment needs to organizations providing direct services to low-income, at risk children, youth and families, the elderly, and the disabled in San Francisco, Marin, Sonoma, and San Mateo counties.

2570 Briggs Foundation
1969 Lancewood Ln
Carlsbad, CA 92009-6826 760-704-6481
FAX: 760-704-6483
Blaine A Briggs, President
Private non-operating foundation.

2571 Burns-Dunphy Foundation
5 3rd Street
Suite 528
San Francisco, CA 94103-3213 415-421-6995
FAX: 415-882-7774
Walter Gleason
Cressey Nakagawa
Grants are given to promote wellness for the visually impaired, physically and mentally disabled and to promote research in these areas.

2572 California Community Foundation
221 S. Figueroa Street
Suite 400
Los Angeles, CA 90012 213-413-4130
FAX: 213-383-2046
e-mail: info@ccf-la.org
www.calfund.org
Antonia Hernandez, President
Nichole Baker, Vice President, BD
Maria Blanco, Vice President, Civic Engagement
Areas of funding priority include grants for the disabled, child welfare, rehabilitation, developmentally disabled, employment projects, research and computer projects. Giving is limited to the greater Los Angeles area.

2573 California Endowment
1000 N Alameda St
Los Angeles, CA 90012-1804 213-628-1001
800-449-4149
FAX: 213-703-4193
e-mail: questions@calendow.org
www.calendow.org
Robert Ross, President & CEO
B. Kathlyn Mead, Executive Vice President & COO
California Endowment's mission is to expand access to affordable, quality health care for underserved individuals and communities, and to promote fundamental improvements in the health status of all Californians.

2574 Carrie Estelle Doheny Foundation
707 Wilshire Boulevard
Suite 4960
Los Angeles, CA 90017-3608 213-488-1122
FAX: 213-488-1544
e-mail: doheny@dohenyfoundation.org
www.dohenyfoundation.org
Nina Shepherd, Chief Administrative Officer
Peggy Morrison, Grants Administrator
The Foundation primarily funds local, not-for-profit organizations endeavoring to advance education, medicine and religion, to improve the health and welfare of the sick, aged, incapacitated, and to aid the needy.

2575 Coeta and Donald Barker Foundation
3740 Cahuenga Blvd
Studio City, CA 91604 760-340-1162
818-980-3630
FAX: 760-340-1255
www.scga.org
Nancy Harris, President
It is an independent organization that gives its attention to organizations that are charitable or nonprofit under the laws of the state of Oregon or California.

2576 Crescent Porter Hale Foundation
655 Redwood Highway
Suite 301
Mill Valley, CA 94941-3028 415-388-2333
FAX: 415-381-4799
www.crescentporterhale.org
Ulla Davis, Executive Director
E. William Swanson, Vice President
Robert S. Kelling, Jr., Secretary/Treasurer
Serves organizations in the San Francisco Bay Area who are involved in the following areas of concern: education in the fields of art and music; private elementary, high school and university education; capital funding; and other worthwhile programs which can be demonstrated as serving broad community purposes, leading toward the improvement of the quality of life.

2577 David and Lucile Packard Foundation
343 Second Street
Los Altos, CA 94022-3632 650-948-7658
FAX: 650-948-5793
e-mail: communications@packard.org
www.packard.org
Carol S Larson, President & CEO
Susan Packard Orr, Chairman
Julie E. Packard, Vice Chairman
This foundation provides grants to nonprofit organizations in the following areas: conservation; population; science; children, familes, and communities; arts and organizational effectiveness; and philanthropy. It provides national and international grants and also has a special focus on the Northern California Counties.

2578 Deutsch Foundation
5454 Beethoven St
Los Angeles, CA 90066-7017 310-862-3000
877-340-7700
FAX: 310-862-3100
deutschinc.com
Mike Sheldon, Manager
Learning disabled, visually impaired, mental health, eye research, child welfare, speech and hearing impaired, physically disabled and independence projects are funded through this Foundation. Giving is limited to California.

2579 **East Bay Community Foundation**
De Domenico Building
200 Frank H Ogawa Plaza
Oakland, CA 94612-2005 510-836-3223
FAX: 510-836-7418
e-mail: operations@eastbaycf.org
www.ebcf.org
Nicole Taylor, President & CEO
A collection of funds created by many people, organizations and businesses, the Foundation helps those people and groups to support effective nonprofit organizations to the East Bay and beyond.

2580 **Evelyn and Walter Hans JrHaas Jr**
114 Sansome Street
Suite 600
San Francisco, CA 94104 415-856-1400
FAX: 415-856-1500
www.haasjr.org
Ira S. Hirschfield, President
Jennie Lehua Watson, VP Communications
Michael Smith, Manager Information Services
Randall Miller, Senior Program Officer
A private foundation interested in programs which assist people who are hungry, homeless, or at risk of homelessness; enable older adults to maintain independent lives in the community and support Hispanic community development in San Francisco's Mission District. The Foundation also encourages proposals for corporate social responsibility efforts within the business community.

2581 **Family Caregiver Alliance**
180 Montgomery Street
Suite 900
San Francisco, CA 94104-4240 415-434-3388
800-445-8106
FAX: 415-434-3508
e-mail: info@caregiver.org
www.caregiver.org
William N Hancock, Owner

2582 **Financial Aid for the Disabled and Their Families**
Reference Service Press
5000 Windplay Dr
Suite 4
El Dorado Hills, CA 95762 916-939-9620
FAX: 916-939-9626
e-mail: info@rspfunding.com
www.rspfunding.com
Gail Schlachter, Author/Owner
R David Weber, Author
This directory, which Children's Bookwatch calls invaluable describes more than 1,100 financial aid opportunities available to support persons with disabilities and members of their families. Updated ever 2 years. *$39.50*
300 pages
ISBN 1-588410-31-5

2583 **Firemans Fund Foundation**
Firemans Fund Insurance Companies
777 San Marin Dr
Novato, CA 94998 415-899-2000
800-227-1700
FAX: 415-899-3600
e-mail: customerrelations@ffic.com
www.firemansfund.com
Lori Dickerson Fouche, President & CEO
Jill Paterson, Chief Financial Officer
Eleanor Barnard, Chief Distribution & Sales
Sally Narey, Chief Counsel, Corp. Secretary
Provides discretionary grants to the disabled only in Marin and Sonoma counties in the San Francisco Bay area.

2584 **Fred Gellert Foundation**
1038 Redwood Highway
Building B, Suite 2
Mill Valley, CA 94941 415-381-7575
FAX: 415-381-8526
e-mail: patty@fgffoundation.com
www.foundationcenter.org/grantmaker/fredgelle
Fred Gellert, Founder
Patty Oday, Administrator
Focuses on organizations and programs serving residents of San Mateo and San Francisco and Marin counties in California, with the exception of environmentally concerned organizations.

2585 **Gallo Foundation**
P.O. Box 1130
Modesto, CA 95353-1130 209-579-3204
FAX: 209-341-3307
www.ejgallo.com
John Gallo, Senior VP Operations
Physically and mentally disabled, child welfare, Special Olympics, United Cerebral Palsy and Easter Seal Society are among the grants provided by this foundation.

2586 **Glaucoma Research Foundation**
251 Post Street
Suite 600
San Francisco, CA 94108-5017 415-986-3162
800-826-6693
FAX: 415-986-3763
e-mail: question@glaucoma.org
www.glaucoma.org
Andrew Iwach, MD, Board Chair
Robert L. Stamper, MD, Vice Chair
Thomas M. Brunner, President/CEO
Fred H. Brinkmann, Treasurer
A national organization dedicated to protecting the sight of people with glaucoma through research and education. The Foundation conducts and supports research that contributes to improved patient care and a better understanding of the disease process. Provides education, advocacy and emotional support to patients and their families.

2587 **Harden Foundation**
1636 Ercia Street
Salinas, CA 93906 831-442-3005
FAX: 831-443-1429
e-mail: joe@hardenfoundation.org
www.hardenfoundation.org
Patricia Tynan Chapman, President
C. Bill Elliott, Vice President/Treasurer
Linda Taylor, Secretary
Bruce C. Taylor, Advisory Director
Founded to assist charitable organizations in the Salinas Valley.

2588 **Henry J Kaiser Family Foundation**
2400 Sand Hill Rd
Menlo Park, CA 94025-6941 650-854-9400
FAX: 650-854-4800
www.kff.org
Drew E Altman, President/CEO
Gary Claxton, Vice President
Mollyann Brodie, Senior Vice President for Executive Operations
Samantha Artiga, Director, Disparities Policy Project
A non-profit, private operating foundation focusing on the major health care issues facing the US, with a growing role in global health. Kaiser develops and runs its own research and communications programs, sometimes in partnership with other non-profit research organizations or major media companies.

2589 **Henry W Bull Foundation**
Santa Barbara Bank & Trust
P.O. Box 2340
Santa Barbara, CA 93120-2340 805-884-8637
FAX: 805-884-1404
Janice Gibbons, VP/Senior Trust Officer
Grant given to a wide range of organizations that include those which provide services for the disabled; arts, education, services

for elderly and youth grants awarded two times a year. Grant size ranges from $500 to $5,000. Proposal deadlines April 1, Sept 1.

2590 Irvine Health Foundation
18301 Von Karman Avenue
Suite 440
Irvine, CA 92612-0120
949-253-2959
FAX: 949-253-2962
e-mail: info@ihf.org
www.ihf.org

Timothy L. Strader, Sr., Chairman
Carol Mentor McDermott, Vice Chairman
Jeffrey E. Flocken, Treasurer
Thomas C. Cesario, M.D., Secretary

Mission is to improve the physical, mental and emotional well-being of all Orange County residents.

2591 Joseph Drown Foundation
1999 Avenue of the Stars
Suite 2330
Los Angeles, CA 90067-6043
310-277-4488
FAX: 310-277-4573
e-mail: staff@jdrown.org
www.jdrown.org

Norman C Obrow, President

Giving is focused primarily in California. No support for religious purposes or to individuals. Goal is to assist individuals in becoming successful, self-sustaining, contributing citizens.

2592 Junior Blind of America
5300 Angeles Vista Blvd
Los Angeles, CA 90043-1648
323-295-4555
800-352-2290
FAX: 323-296-0424
e-mail: info@juniorblind.org
www.juniorblind.org

Miki Jordan, President/CEO
Laura M Hardy, SVP, Development & Marketing
Kami Mann, SVP, Finance/CFO
Jay Allen, EVP/Chief Operating Officer

Junior Blind provides programs and services for children and adults who are blind or visually impaired and their families to achieve independence and self-esteem. Programs include; Camp Bloomfield, Visions: Adventures in Learning, Infant-Family Program, Early Childhood Program, Special Education School, Children's Residential Program, Davidson Program for Independence, and Student Transition and Enrichment Program, Vision Screening and After School enrichment.

2593 Kenneth T and Eileen L Norris Foundation
11 Golden Shore
Suite 450
Long Beach, CA 90802-4274
562-435-8444
FAX: 562-436-0584
e-mail: grants@ktn.org
www.norrisfoundation.org

Lisa D Hanson, Chairman
Ronald R Barnes, Executive Director & Trustee
Walter J Zanino, Controller
William G Corey, Medical Advisor

The Foundation is primarily focused on medicine and education. To a lesser extent the foundation contributes to community programs including visually impaired, autism, mentally and physically disabled, deaf and mental health in the Southern California area. Average grant size in this area is $5,000-$10,000. Grants are also given in the area of culture and youth.

2594 Koret Foundation
33 New Montgomery Street
Suite 1090
San Francisco, CA 94105-4526
415-882-7740
FAX: 415-882-7775
e-mail: info@koretfoundation.org
www.koretfoundation.org

Susan Koret, Board Chair
Tad Taube, President
Jeffrey A. Farber, Chief Executive Officer
Claudia Hardin, Chief Financial Officer

Koret seeks to fund outstanding examples of innovative approaches to community challenges and opportunities.

2595 LA84 Foundation
2141 W Adams Blvd
Los Angeles, CA 90018-2040
323-730-4600
FAX: 323-730-9637
e-mail: info@la84.org
www.la84.org

Frank M. Sanchez, Chair
Anita L. DeFrantz, President
F. Patrick Escobar, Vice President, Grants & Programs
Robert Wagner, Vice President, Partnerships

The LA84 Foundation was established to manage Southern California's share of the surplus from the highly successful 1984 Olympic Games in Los Angeles and offers sports programs, a premier sports library and meeting facilities. The foundation currently serves two million youth in eight Southern California counties.

2596 LJ Skaggs and Mary C Skaggs Foundation
1221 Broadway
21st Floor
Oakland, CA 94612-1837
510-451-3300
FAX: 510-451-1527
e-mail: skaggs@fablaw.com
www.skaggs.org

Philip M Jelley, President
Jayne C Davis, Vice President
Robert N Janopaul, Director
Joseph W Martin, Jr., Secretary, Treasurer

The Foundation presently makes grants under four program categories: performing arts, social concerns, projects of historic interest and special projects.

2597 LK Whittier Foundation
Whittier Trust Company Foundations Office
1600 Huntington Dr
S Pasadena, CA 91030-4709
626-441-5111
FAX: 626-441-0420
e-mail: hrdept@whittiertrust.com
www.whittiertrust.com

Michael J Casey, President/CEO
David A. Dahl, Managing Director/Chief Operating Officer
James A. Jeffs, Executive Vice President, Chief
Harold J. Depoali, Vice President, Client Administr

Giving is primarily offered to preselected organizations. No grants are given to individuals.

2598 Legler Benbough Foundation
2550 Fifth Avenue
Suite 132
San Diego, CA 92103-6622
619-235-8099
FAX: 619-235-8077
e-mail: peter@benboughfoundation.org
www.benbough.org

Peter K. Elsworth, President
Thomas Cisco, Treasurer
Hugh C. Carter, Director
Thomas E. Cisco, Director

The mission of the foundation is to improve the quality of life of the people of San Diego. The foundation focuses on three target areas for funding, one in the area of providing economic opportunity, one in the area of enhancing cultural opportunity, and one that provides focus for health, education and welfare funding.

2599 Levi Strauss Foundation
1155 Battery St
San Francisco, CA 94111-1264
415-501-7208
800-872-5384
FAX: 415-544-3490
www.levistrauss.com/about/foundations

Chip Bergh, President & CEO
Roy Bagattini, EVP/President of Asia, Middle East and Africa
Lisa Collier, Executive Vice President/President
James Curleigh, Executive Vice President/President

Has a funding initiative to support organizations which provide services for people with AIDS, and/or educational programs which help prevent the further spread of the HIV virus. The Foundation will assist in the development and enhancement of such services only in those communities where Levi Strauss & Co. has plants and distribution centers.

2600 Louis R Lurie Foundation
555 California Street
Suite 5100
San Francisco, CA 94104-1707 415-392-2470
FAX: 415-421-8669
www.foundationcenter.org/grantmaker/lurie

Nancy Terry, Foundation Administrator
Visually impaired, hard-of-hearing and physically disabled in the San Francisco Bay Area and Metropolitan Chicago areas only.

2601 Luke B Hancock Foundation
360 Bryant St
Palo Alto, CA 94301-1409 650-321-5536
FAX: 650-321-0697

Ruth Ramel, Director
Has concentrated its resources over the past year on programs which provide job training and employment for at-risk youth. Consortium funding with other foundations in areas where there is unmet need; emergency and transitional funding; and selected funding for music education. .

2602 Marin Community Foundation
5 Hamilton Landing
Suite 200
Novato, CA 94949-8263 415-464-2500
FAX: 415-464-2555
e-mail: info@marincf.org
www.marincf.org

Thomas Peters, President & CEO
Sid Hartman, Chief Financial and Operating Officer
Alexandra Derby, VP, Philanthropic Services
Vikki Garrod, Vice President for Marketing and Communications
Mission is to encourage and apply philanthropic contributions to help improve the human condition, embrace diversity, promote a humane and democratic society, and enhance the communities quality of life, now and for future generations.

2603 Mary A Crocker Trust
364 Bush Street
5 Hamilton Landing
San Francisco, CA 94108-2805 650-576-3384
FAX: 415-982-0141
e-mail: staff@mactrust.org
www.mactrust.org

2604 National Center on Caregiving at Family Caregiver Alliance (FCA)
785 Market Street
Suite 750
San Francisco, CA 94103 415-434-3388
800-445-8106
FAX: 415-434-3508
e-mail: info@caregiver.org
www.caregiver.org

Ping Hao, President
Jacquelyn Kung, Vice President
Jeff Kumataka, Treasurer
Kathleen Kelly, Executive Director
FCA offers programs at national, state and local levels to support and sustain caregivers. The National Center on Caregiving (NCC) program works to advance the development of high-quality, cost-effective policies and programs for caregivers in every state of the country. Uniting research, public policy and services, the NCC serves as a central source of information on caregiving and long term care issues for policy makers, service providers, media, funders and family caregivers.

2605 National Foundation of Wheelchair Tennis
940 Calle Amanecer
Suite B
San Clemente, CA 92673-6218 714-361-3663
FAX: 714-361-6603
e-mail: nfwt@aol.com
www.nfwt.org

Bill Butler
Founded in January of 1980, the intention of this foundation is to assist the newly physically disabled individual to realize his full potential in society by enhancing his esteem, independence productivity and physical capabilities regardless of age, sex, creed or disability extent.

2606 Optometric Extension Program Foundation
1921 Cernegie Avenue
Suite 3-L
Santa Ana, CA 92705-5510 949-250-8070
FAX: 949-250-8157
e-mail: rwilliams@oep.org
www.oepf.org

Gregory Kitchener, President
Paul A. Harris, Vice President
Robin D. Lewis, Secretary - Treasurer
Robert A. Williams, Executive Director
Vision care for learning disabilities and head trauma patients.

2607 Parker Foundation
2604-B El Camino Real
Suite 244
Carlsbad, CA 92008 760-720-0630
FAX: 760-720-1239
www.theparkerfoundation.org

Judy McDonald, President
William E. Beamer, Vice President
Ann Davies, Secretary
Raymond Ellis, Treasurer
The assets are directed to projects which will contribute to the betterment of any aspect of the people of San Diego County, California and solely to entities which, among other things, are organized exclusively for charitable purposes and are operating in San Diego County, California.

2608 Pasadena Foundation
260 S. Los Robles Avenue
Suite 119
Pasadena, CA 91101- 2824 626-796-2097
FAX: 626-583-4738
e-mail: pcfstaff@pasadenacf.org
www.pasadenacf.org

David M. Davis, Chair
Judy Gain, Vice Chair
Jennifer Fleming DeVoll, Executive Director
Mariver Copeland, Director of Finance
The mission of the Pasadena Foundation is to improve the quality of life for citizens of the Pasadena area through support of non-profit organizations that provide services beneficial to the community.

2609 RC Baker Foundation
P.O. Box 6150
Orange, CA 92863-6150 714-750-8987

F L Scott, Manager
Established in 1952, for general philanthropic purposes. The bulk of assistance and support has been to religious, scientific, educational institutions and youth organizations.

2610 Ralph M Parsons Foundation
888 West Sixth Street
Suite 700
Los Angeles, CA 90017- 2733
213-362-7600
FAX: 213-482-8878
www.rmpf.org

Franklin E. Ulf, Chairman
Walter B. Rose, Vice Chairman
Elizabeth Lowe, Community Leader
James Thomas, CEO

The Foundation is concerned with the encouragement and support of projects and programs deemed beneficial to mankind in several major areas of interest such as: education; social impact; civic and cultural; health and special products. Only funds in Los Angeles County.

2611 Robert Ellis Simon Foundation
312 S Canyon View Drive
Los Angeles, CA 90049-3812
310-275-7335

Joan Willens

Mental health and visually impaired grants are the main concerns of this organization.

2612 San Francisco Foundation
225 Bush Street
Suite 500
San Francisco, CA 94104-4224
415-733-8500
FAX: 415-477-2783
e-mail: info@sff.org
www.sff.org

Sandra R Hernandez, CEO
Nick Hodges, VP for Philanthropic Services
Bobbie Chapman, Director of Business Development
Shona Carter, Donor Relations Officer

The Foundation's purpose is to improve life, promote greater equality of opportunity and assist those in need or at risk in the San Francisco Bay Area. The Foundation strives to protect and enhance the unique resources of the Bay Area, committed to equality of opportunity for all and the elimination of any injustice, seeks to enhance human dignity and seeks to establish mutual trust, respect and communication among the Foundation.

2613 Santa Barbara Foundation
1111 Chapala Street
Suite 200
Santa Barbara, CA 93101- 2780
805-963-1873
FAX: 805-966-2345
e-mail: info@sbfoundation.org
www.sbfoundation.org

Ron Gallo, CEO
Guille Gil-Reynoso, Executive Special Projects Asst.
Jan Campbell, VP of Philanthropic Services
Amanda Kastelic, Donor Relations Officer

The Foundations mission is to enrich the lives of the people of Santa Barbara County through philanthropy. The Foundation awards grants to nonprofits within the County in the areas of education, health, human services, personal development, cluture, recreation, community enhancement and environment. No support is given to individuals except through student aid.

2614 Sidney Stern Memorial Trust
860 Via de la Paz
PO Box 457
Pacific Palisades, CA 90272
310-459-2117

e-mail: info@sidneysternmemorialtrust.org
www.sidneysternmemorialtrust.org

Betty Hoffenberg, Director

A Southern California-based foundation providing grants to nonprofit organizations for various projects. The foundation gives priority to the following areas of interest: education, health and science, community service projects, youth, services to the mentally and emotionally disabled, the arts, organizations and activities serving California. The Board prefers to make contributions to organizations that use the funds directly in the furtherance of their charitable and public purposes.

2615 Sierra Health Foundation
1321 Garden Hwy
Sacramento, CA 95833-9754
916-922-4755
FAX: 916-922-4024
e-mail: info@sierrahealth.org
www.sierrahealth.org

Chet Hewitt, CEO
Joan Kassis, Controller
Gil Alvarado, VP Administration / CFO
Amy Birthwhistle, Program Associate

The Foundation strives to establish a collaborative relationship with its grantees, and with other funders and foundations, through an open dialogue. The Foundation approaches each grant as a partnership, with opportunities for the grantee and grantor to work cooperatively to enhance the effectiveness of the grant project.

2616 Silicon Valley Community Foundation
2400 West El Camino Real
Suite 300
Mountain View, CA 94040-1498
650-450-5400
FAX: 650-450-5401
e-mail: info@siliconvalleycf.org
www.siliconvalleycf.org

Emmitt Carson, CEO
Eleanor Clement Glass, Chief Donor Engagement & Giving
Erica Wood, VP Community Leadership
Vera Bennett, CFO & Administrative Officer

Serving all of San Mateo & Santa Clara counties, Silicon Valley Foundation has more than $1.5B in assets under management and 1500 philanthropic funds. The community provides grants through donor advised and corporate funds in addition to its own Community Endowment Fund. In addition, the community foundation serves as a regional center for philanthropy, providing donors simple and effective ways to give locally & globally.

2617 Sonora Area Foundation
362 S Stewart Street
Sonora, CA 95370-577
209-533-2596
FAX: 209-533-2412
e-mail: edwyllie@sonora-area.org
www.sonora-area.org

Greg Applegate, Executive Director
Jim Johnson, President SAF
Roger Francis, Vice President
Tricia Gardella, Secretary, Treasurer

The Sonora Area Foundation strengthens its community through assisting donors, making grants, and providing leadership.

2618 Stella B Gross Charitable Trust C/O Bank of The West Trust Department
PO Box 1121
San Jose, CA 95108-1121
408-947-5203

e-mail: gpadilla@bankofthewest.com

Gabe Padilla, Trust Admin

Organization must be federal and state tax-exempt and reside within the bounds of Santa Clara County, California to be eligible.

2619 Teichert Foundation
3500 American River Dr
Sacramento, CA 95864-5893
916-484-3011
FAX: 916-484-6506
www.teichert.com

Frederick Teichert, Executive Director

Awards grants to community organizations and provides employee matching grants. Teichert Foundation expresses the companie's commitment to build and preserve a healthy and prosperous region.

2620 WM Keck Foundation
550 South Hope Street
Suite 2500
Los Angeles, CA 90071- 2617 213-680-3833
FAX: 213-614-0934
e-mail: info@wmkeck.org
www.wmkeck.org

Allison Keller, Executive Director & CFO
Maria Pellegrini, Ph.D, Executive Director of Programs
Thomas Everhart, Ph.D, Senior Scientific Advisor
Matesh Varma, Ph.D, Senior Program Director
Created to support accredited colleges and universities with particular emphasis on the sciences, engineering and medical research. The Foundation also maintains a Southern California Grant Program that provides support for non-profit organizations in the field of civic and community services, health care, precollegiate education and the arts.

2621 Willam G Gilmore Foundation
1660 Bush Street
Suite 300
San Francisco, CA 94109 415-984-0650
FAX: 415-434-3508
www.pfs-llc.net/gilmore/index.html
William N Hancock, Owner

Colorado

2622 AV Hunter Trust
650 South Cherry Street
Suite 535
Glendale, CO 80246- 1897 303-399-5450
FAX: 303-399-5499
www.avhuntertrust.org

Bruce K. Alexander, President
Allan B. Adams, Vice President
Mary K. Anstine, Treasurer
Barbara L. Howie, Executive Director
Donated nearly $50 million to nonprofit organizations serving those who captured Mr. Hunter's attention and sparked his compassion. Trust gives aid, comfort, support, or assistance to children or aged people or indigent adults.

2623 Adolph Coors Foundation
4100 E. Mississippi Avenue
Suite 1850
Denver, CO 80246- 3074 303-388-1636
FAX: 303-388-1684
e-mail: generalinfo@acoorsfdn.org
www.coorsfoundation.org
John W. Jackson, Executive Director
Jeanne L. Bistranin, Senior Program Officer
Carrie C. Tynan, Program Officer
Carol S. Strathman, Financial/Special Projects Coord
Applicant organizations must be classified as 501 and must operate within the United States. The areas covered by the Foundation are health, education, youth, community services, civic and cultural and public affairs.

2624 Arc of Colorado
1580 Logan Street
Suite 730
Denver, CO 80203-1942 303-864-9334
800-333-7690
FAX: 303-864-9330
e-mail: mrymer@thearcofco.org
www.thearcofco.org

Marijo Rymer, Executive Director
A private not-for-profit, membership-based, grassroots association. The Arc of Colorado is the state office whith local units located in various areas throughout the state.

2625 Bonfils-Stanton Foundation
Daniels and Fisher Tower
1601 Arapahoe
Suite 500
Denver, CO 80202-2015 303-825-3774
FAX: 303-825-0802
e-mail: webinfo@bonfils-stanton.org
www.bonfils-stantonfoundation.org

Dorothy A Horrell, President
Susan H. France, Vice President of Programs
Ann M. Hovland, CFO/Treasurer
Grants limited to Colorado 501 (c) (3) organizations. Grants are for general, charitable philanthropic activities within the State. Major categories include education, scientific (including hospital and health services), civic and cultural, community and human services. Organizations should request foundation guidelines before submitting a proposal.

2626 Comprecare Foundation
PO Box 740610
Arvada, CO 80006-610 303-432-2808
FAX: 303-432-2808
www.comprecarefoundation.org

Frederick G. Ihrig, Chairman of the Board
Milford H. Schulhof II, Vice Chairman
Milton W. Bollman, Secretar/Treasurer
M. Eugene Sherman M.D., Director
The purpose of the Comprecare Foundation is to encourage, aid or assist specific health related programs and to make grants to support the activities of organizations which are designed to advance and promote health care education, the delivery of health care services, and the improvement of community health and welfare.

2627 Denver Foundation
55 Madison Street
8th Floor
Denver, CO 80206-5419 303-300-1790
FAX: 303-300-6547
e-mail: lbarrett@denverfoundation.org
www.denverfoundation.org
David M Miller, President & CEO
Pamela Kenney Basey, Community Leader
Neighbors helping neighbors, that's what the foundation is for. As Denver's only community foundation we've been accepting charitable donations since 1925. Those funds have been given back to the community in ongoing grants to nonprofit organizations - organizations that touch nearly every meaningful artistic, cultural, civic, health and human services interest of metro Denver's citizens.

2628 El Pomar Foundation
10 Lake Circle
Colorado Springs, CO 80906-4201 719-633-7733
800-554-7711
FAX: 719-577-5702
e-mail: grants@elpomar.org
www.elpomar.org
William Hybl, Chairman/CEO
R. Thayer Tutt, Jr., President/Chief Investment
Dave Palenchar, COO & Trustee
Kyle Hybl, SVP/General Counsel
Mission of El Pomar is to enhance, encourage and promote the current and future well being of the people of Colorado through grantmaking and community stewardship.

2629 Helen K and Arthur E Johnson Foundation
1700 Broadway
Suite 1100
Denver, CO 80290-1718 303-861-4127
800-232-9931
FAX: 303-861-0607
e-mail: info@www.johnsonfoundation.org
www.johnsonfoundation.org
John H Alexander Jr, President
Cindy Willard, Senior Program Officer
Suzanne Bruce, Program Officer

A nonprofit, grantmaking private foundation incorporated under the laws of the State of Colorado in 1948. The Foundation is a general purpose foundation whose grant program consists of a wide variety of creative efforts to solve problems and to enrich the quality of life. The areas of interest are: education, youth, health, community services, civic and culture and senior citizens. Grants limited to the state of Colorado.

Connecticut

2630 **Aetna Foundation**
151 Farmington Ave
Hartford, CT 6156 860-273-6382
www.aetnahealthinsurance.com

Marilda L Gandara, President
The Aetna Foundation is the independent charitable and philanthropic arm of Aetna Inc. The Foundation helps build healthy communities by promoting volunteerism, forming partnerships and funding initiatives that improve the quality of life where our employees and customers live and work.

2631 **Arc of Connecticut**
43 Woodland Street
Suite 260
Hartford, CT 6105-2300 860-246-6400
FAX: 860-246-6406
e-mail: arcct@aol.com
www.arcct.com

Leslie Simoes, Interim Executive Director
The Arc of Connecticut is an advocacy organization committed to protecting the rights of people with intellectual, cognitive, and developmental disabilities and to promoting opportunities for their full inclusion in the life of thier communities.

2632 **Community Foundation of Southeastern Connecticut**
147 State St
New London, CT 6320-6302 860-442-3572
877-442-3572
FAX: 860-442-0584
e-mail: alice@cfsect.org
www.cfect.org

Alice Fitzpatrick, President
Edward Wozniak, Chief Financial Officer
Allison Woods, Director of Gift Planning
Kip Parker, Division Director
Provides donors with an easy and convenient way to give back to our community with joy and impact. We make grants to nonprofit organizations and support their efforts to strengthen our community.

2633 **Connecticut Mutual Life Foundation**
140 Garden St
Hartford, CT 6154 860-727-3000

Astrida Olds, Executive Director
Distinguished throughout its long history by unusual commitment to high principles of corporate purpose and business ethics. That commitment has been reflected not only in the firm belief that normal business functions must be carried out with a sense of responsibility beyond that required by the marketplace. Maintains an ongoing program of corporate contributions, a nationwide matching gifts plan for all employees on behalf of private and public education, skills training programs, and more.

2634 **Cornelia de Lange Syndrome Foundation**
302 West Main Street
#100
Avon, CT 6001-4331 860-676-8166
800-753-2357
FAX: 860-676-8337
e-mail: info@cdlsusa.org
www.cdlsusa.org

Liana Fresher, Executive Director
Antonie Kline, MD, Medical Director
Marie Concklin-Malloy, Assistant Executive Director
Alexi Dahlstrom, Communications Coordinator
Provides information about birth defects caused by Cornelia de Lange Syndrome.

2635 **Fidelco Guide Dog Foundation**
103 Old Iron Ore Rd
Bloomfield, CT 6002-1424 860-243-5200
FAX: 860-243-7215
e-mail: info@fidelco.org
www.fidelco.org

Eliot D. Russman, CEO & Executive Director
Mary P. Craig, DVM, MBA, Director, Strategic Initiatives
Louise C. England, Ownership & Development
Stephen H. Matheson, Chairman
The Fidelco Guide Dog Foundation, located in Bloomfield, Conn., is dedicated to providing increased freedom and independence to men and women who are blind by providing them with the highest quality guide dogs. We rely solely on the gifts and the generosity of individuals, foundations, corporations and organizations that partner with Fidelco to 'Share the Vision.'

2636 **GE Foundation**
General Electric Company
3135 Easton Tpke
Fairfield, CT 6828 203-373-3216
FAX: 203-373-3029
e-mail: gefoundation@ge.com
www.ge.com

Jeffrey R. Immelt, CEO
Michael J. Cosgrove, Treasurer
Paul Bueker, Secretary & Controller
Nani Beccalli, President & CEO GE International
Believes that our greatest national resource is the work force. If we are to successfully compete in the global arena, then we become involved in improving the education of all of our citizens. The Foundation sets examples for others to emulate helping people with their international grant program to higher education and to health care for children in developing countries.

2637 **Hartford Foundation for Public Giving**
10 Columbus Blvd
8th Floor
Hartford, CT 6106-1985 860-548-1888
FAX: 860-524-8346
e-mail: hfpg@hfpg.org
www.hfpg.org

Linda Kelly, President
Deborah Battit, Research Associate
Donna E. Jolly, VP, Communications & Marketing
Maria I. Mojica, VP for Programs
Developmentally disabled, housing, deaf, recreation and education grants.

2638 **Hartford Insurance Group**
1 Hartford Plz
Hartford, CT 6155-1708 860-547-5000
www.thehartford.com

Liam McGee, Chairman, President & CEO
Greg McGreevey, EVP & Chief Investment Officer
Lizabeth H. Zlatkus, EVP & Chief Risk Officer
Alan J. Kreczko, EVP & General Counsel
Giving is primarily in the Hartford, CT area and in communities where the company has a regional office. No support is available for political or religious purposes. Grants are given in the areas of education, health and United Way organizations.

2639 **Henry Nias Foundation**
20 Carmen Rd
Milford, CT 6460-7508 203-874-2787

Charles D Fleischman, President

Giving limited to NY metropolitan area. Arts, cultural programs, medical school/education, and children and youth.

2640 **Jane Coffin Childs Memorial Fund for Medical Research**
333 Cedar St, SHM
L300
New Haven, CT 6510-3206 203-785-4612
FAX: 203-785-3301
e-mail: jccfund@yal.edu
www.jccfund.org

Dr Randy Schekman, Director

The Fund awards fellowships to suitably qualified individuals for full time postdoctoral studies in the medical and related sciences bearing on cancer.

2641 **John H and Ethel G Nobel Charitable Trust**
Bankers Trust Company
1 Fawcett Pl
PO Box 1297
New York, NY 1008-1297 203-629-7120
FAX: 203-629-7170
john-h-ethel-g-noble-charitable-trust.idilogi

Paul J Bisset, VP

2642 **Scheuer Associates Foundation**
960 Lake Ave
Greenwich, CT 6831-3032 203-622-5002
FAX: 203-622-5002
scheuer-associates-foundation-inc.idilogic.ai

Thomas Scheuer, President

2643 **Swindells Charitable Foundation Trust**
Shawmut Bank
1211 SW Fifth Avenue, Suite 2340
Portland, OR 97204-2303 503-222-0689
FAX: 503-222-0726
www.swindellstrust.org

Maggie Willard, President

Grants made to charitable organizations or societies incorporated for the relief of sick and suffering poor children and/or the relief of sick suffering and indigent aged men and women and/or the support of public charitable hospitals. Geographic area includes Hartford, CT area primarily. Application is required, deadlines are Feb. 1 and Aug. 1.

Delaware

2644 **Arc of Delaware**
2 S Augustine Street
Suite B
Wilmington, DE 19804-2504 302-996-9400
FAX: 302-996-0683
TTY:800-232-5460
e-mail: eraign@arcde.org
www.thearcofdelaware.org

Terry Reilly, President
Bill Seufert, Vice President
Ruth Lavelle, Secretary
Margo Johnson, Treasurer

The Arc of Delaware is a non-profit organization of volunteers and staff who work together to improve the quality of life for people with disabilitiesand their families. We strive to include all children and adults with cognitive, intellectual and developmental disabilities in every community.

2645 **Longwood Foundation**
100 W 10th St
Suite 1109
Wilmington, DE 19801-1694 302-654-2477
FAX: 302-654-2323
www.longwoodfoundation.com

Peter Morrow, Executive Director

Offers grants to the mentally and physically disabled - capital, program, education and housing grants in the state of Delaware.

District of Columbia

2646 **Alexander and Margaret Stewart Trust**
Brawner Building
888 17th Street NW
Suite 1250
Washington, DC 20006-3321 202-333-1277
FAX: 202-333-3128
e-mail: aplatt@projectsinternational.com
www.projectsinternational.com

Alexander H. Platt, Executive Vice President
Imtiaz T. Ladak, Managing Director & CFO

Grants are given only to the Washington, DC area organizations providing care or treatment to cancer patients or those with childhood afflictions.

2647 **Arc of the District of Columbia**
415 Michigan Avenue, NE
Suite 400
Washington, DC 20017- 2144 202-636-2950
FAX: 202-635-7086
e-mail: arcdc@arcdc.net
www.arcdc.net

Mary Lou Meccariello, Executive Director
Michael Gonzales, Chief Operating Officer
Ed Cabatic, Director of Finance
Matt Rosen, Dir. Advocacy & Public Policy

Advocating for and providing services to persons with mental retardation. Mission is to improve the quality of life of all persons with mental retardation and their families through supports and advocacy.

2648 **Eugene and Agnes E Meyer Foundation**
The Meyer Foundation
1250 Connecticut Ave NW
Suite 800
Washington, DC 20036- 2620 202-483-8294
FAX: 202-328-6850
e-mail: meyer@meyerfdn.org
www.meyerfoundation.org

Julie Rogers, President & CEO
Danielle M. Reyes, Senior Program Officer
Jane Robinson Ward, Grants Manager & Program Officer
Jennifer Burke, Business Operations Assistant

Awards grants to projects dealing with the learning disabled, blind, mental health and vocational training in the Washington metropolitan area.

2649 **Federal Student Aid Information Center**
US Department of Education
400 Maryland Ave SW
Washington, DC 20202 202-275-5446
800-433-3243
www.ed.gov

Arne Duncan, Secretary of Education
Tony Miller, Deputy Secretary
Martha Kanter, Under Secretary

Answers questions about Federal student aid from students, parents and Members of Congress, as well as financial aid administrators.

2650 GEICO Philanthropic Foundation
1 Geico Plz
Washington, DC 20076
301-986-3000
800-841-3000
FAX: 301-986-2851
www.geico.com

Tony M Nicely, CEO
Hospitals, physically disabled and Special Olympics.

2651 Giant Food Foundation
8301 Professional Pl
Ste 115
Landover, MD 20785-2351
301-341-4100
888-469-4426
e-mail: jmiller@giantfood.com
www.giantfood.com

Anthony Hucker, President
Brian Beatty, Md. Director of Marketing and Ex
Stefanie Cain, Md. District Director
Bob Haas, Md. District Director
Offers grants in the areas of mental health, recreation, community and cultural programs, art, and educational programs for the health and prosperity of the greater Washington area.

2652 Jacob and Charlotte Lehrman Foundation
1836 Columbia Rd NW
Washington, DC 20009-2002
202-328-8400
FAX: 202-338-8405
www.lehrmanfoundation.org

Elizabeth Berry, Director
Robert Lehrman, Trustee
Samuel Lehrman, Trustee
Barbara Ferguson, Administrative/Program assistant
The Jacob & Charlotte Lehrman Foundation supports and seeks to enrich Jewish life in Washington DC, Israel and around the world. It is committed to making Washington a better place for all people and supports the arts, education and undeserved children, the environment, and healthcare.

2653 John Edward Fowler Memorial Foundation
Ste 206
4340 East West Hwy
Bethesda, MD 20814-4467
301-654-2700
www.foundationcenter.org

Richard H Lee, President
Ann Matikan, Grant Consultant
Although not a program priority, the foundation does offer grants to the physically disabled in the Washington, DC area only.

2654 Joseph P Kennedy Jr Foundation
1133 19th Street NW
12th Floor
Washington, DC 20036-3604
202-393-1250
FAX: 202-824-0351
e-mail: jpkf@jpkf.org
www.jpkf.org

Rebecca Salon, President
Steven Eidelman, Executive Director
Has two firm objectives: to seek the prevention of mental retardation, and to improve the way society deals with its citizens who are already mentally retarded. The Foundation uses its funds in areas where a multiplier effect can be achieved through development of innovative models for the prevention and amelioration of mental retardation, through provision of seed money that encourages new researchers, and thorough use of the Foundation's influence to promote public awareness.

2655 Kiplinger Foundation
1729 H St NW
Washington, DC 20006-3938
202-887-6400
FAX: 202-778-8976
e-mail: foundation@kiplinger.com
www.kiplinger.com

Knight Kiplinger, VP
Limited to the greater Washington, DC area, the grants focus primarily on education, social welfare, cultural activities and community programs. Matching grants to eligible secondary or higher education institutions are provided on behalf of employees and retirees of Kiplinger Washington Editors, Inc. The Foundation does not fund scholarships.

2656 Morris and Gwendolyn Cafritz Foundation
1825 K St NW
Ste 1400
Washington, DC 20006-1271
202-223-3100
800-544-0155
FAX: 202-296-7567
e-mail: info@cafritzfoundation.org
www.cafritzfoundation.org

Calvin Cafritz, Chairman/President/ CEO
John E. Chapoton, Vice Chairman and Treasurer
Ed McGeogh, Vice President - Asset Managemen
Rohan Rodrigo, Vice President - Finance
Grants are awarded to only 501(c)(3) organizations that are in the DC area. Grants are not awarded for capitol purposes, special events, endowments, or to individuals.

2657 Paul and Annetta Himmelfarb Foundation
4545 42nd St NW
Ste 203
Washington, DC 20016-4623
202-966-3796

M Preston, Executive Director
Primary areas of interest include health, children, human need, and Israel.

2658 Public Welfare Foundation
1200 U St NW
Washington, DC 20009-4443
202-965-1800
e-mail: info@publicwelfare.org
www.publicwelfare.org

Lydia M. Marshall, Chair
Mary E. McClymont, President
Phillipa Taylor, Chief Financial and Administrative Officer
Alyssa Piccirilli, Manager of Administration
The foundation's funding is specifically targeted to economically disadvantaged populations. Proposals must fall within one of the following categories: criminal justice, disadvantaged elderly, disadvantaged youth, environment, health and population and reproductive health, human rights and global security, and community economic developmental and participation. Proposals should be addressed to the Review Committee.

Florida

2659 Able Trust
3320 Thomasville Road
Suite 200
Tallahassee, FL 32308
850-224-4493
FAX: 850-224-4493
TTY:850-224-4493
e-mail: info@abletrust.org
www.abletrust.org

Susanne Homant, President
Guenevere Crum, Senior Vice President
Kathryn McManus, MA, Chief Development Director
Allison Chase, MS, State Director, Florida High Sch
The Able Trust is a non-profit, public/private partnership that supports non-profit vocational rehabilitation programs throughout Florida with fundraising, grant making and public awareness of disability issues.

2660 Arc of Florida
2898 Mahan Dr
Ste 1
Tallahassee, FL 32308-5462
850-921-0460
800-226-1155
e-mail: info@arcflorida.org
www.arcflorida.org

Pat Young, President
Dick Bradley, Vice President Administration
Linda Bloom, Vice President Advocacy
Greg Roe, Treasurer
Promotes, for all people with mental retardation and other developmental disablilities, through education, awareness, research, advocacy and the support of families, friends and community.

2661 BCR Foundation
83 Mussey Rd.
Scarborough, ME 04074
207-883-8000
800-227-6111
FAX: 207-883-0100
e-mail: solutions@bcr.net
www.bcr.net

2662 Bank of America Client Foundation
50 Central Avenue
Suite 750
Sarasota, FL 34236-5900
941-951-4103
e-mail: maryann.l.smith@ustrust.com
www.fdnweb.org/boacf/
Maryann L. Smith, Vice President, Senior Trust Off
Committed to creating meaningful change in the communities we serve through our philanthropic efforts, associate volunteerism, community development activities and investing, support of arts and culture programming and environmental initiatives.

2663 Barron Collier Jr Foundation
2600 Golden Gate Pkwy
Naples, FL 34105-3227
239-262-2600
FAX: 239-262-1840
e-mail: ContactUs@BarronCollier.com
www.barroncollier.com
Karen V. Triplett, Director of Property Management
Jose Medina, Facilities Manager
Barron Collier Companies - dedicated to the responsible development, management and stewardship of its extensive land holdings and other assets in the businesses of agriculture, real estate, and mineral management.

2664 Camiccia-Arnautou Charitable Foundation
Ste 402
980 N Federal Hwy
Boca Raton, FL 33432-2712
561-368-5757
FAX: 561-368-8505
Ronda Gluck, President

2665 Chatlos Foundation
PO Box 915048
Longwood, FL 32791-5048
407-862-5077
e-mail: info@chatlos.org
www.chatlos.org
Bill Chatlos, Trustee
Funds nonprofit organizations in the USA and around the globe. Funding is provided in the following areas of giving: Bible Colleges/Seminaries, Religious Causes, Medical Concerns, Liberal Arts Colleges and Social Concerns. Category of placement is determined by the organizations overall mission rather than the project under consideration. The Foundation does not make scholarship grants directly to individuals but rather to educational institutions which in turn select recipients.

2666 Dade Community Foundation
200 S Biscayne Blvd
Ste 505
Miami, FL 33131-2343
305-371-2711
FAX: 305-371-5342
e-mail: ruth.shack@dadecommunityfoundation.org
www.dadecommunityfoundation.org
Ruth Shack, President
The Foundation approaches all of its program activities with a focus on building the community. We conduct acticvities and support efforts that build community assets and relationships among individuals, organizations, and communities that connect people with resources and opportunities to improve their quality of life.

2667 Edyth Bush Charitable Foundation
199 E Welbourne Ave
Ste 100
Winter Park, FL 32789-4365
407-647-4322
888-647-4322
FAX: 407-647-7716
e-mail: dodahowski@edythbush.org
www.edythbush.org
Gerald F. Hilbrich, Chairman
Herbert W. Holm, Vice Chairman
David A. Odahowski, President/CEO
Mary Ellen Hutcheson, Vice-President/Treasurer
Funding is resrticted to 501c3 nonprofit organizations located and operating in Orange, Osceola, Seminole and Lake Counties, Florida. Visit www.edythbush.org for a list of funding policies.

2668 FPL Group Foundation
700 Universe Blvd
Juno Beach, FL 33408-2657
561-694-4000
888-488-7703
FAX: 561-694-4620
e-mail: PoweringFlorida@FPL.com
www.fpl.com
Maria V. Fogarty, Senior Vice President, Internal
James L. Robo, President and Chief Operating Of
Joseph T. Kelliher, Executive Vice President, Federa
Antonio Rodriguez, Executive Vice President, Power
The company consistently outperforms national averages for service reliability while customer bills are below the national average. A clean energy leader, FPL has one of the lowest emissions profiles and one of the leading energy efficiency programs among utilities nationwide. FPL is a subsidiary of Juno Beach, Fla.-based NextEra Energy, Inc.

2669 Frank Stanley Beveridge Foundation
19 Homestead Park
Needham, MA 02494
800-229-9667
e-mail: administrator@beveridge.org
www.beveridge.org
Ward Slocum Caswell, President
Philip Caswell, Chairman and Vice President
Ruth S. DuPont, Treasurer
Leah Beveridge Richardson, Clerk
The mission of The Frank Stanley Beveridge Foundation, Inc. is to preserve and enhance the quality of life by embracing and perpetuating Frank Stanley Beveridge's philanthropic vision through grantmaking initiatives in support of The Stanley Park of Westfield, Inc. and programs in youth development, health, education, religion, art and environment primarily in Hampden and Hampshire Counties, Massachusetts.

2670 Jefferson Lee Ford III Memorial Foundation
9600 Collins Ave
Bal Harbour, FL 33154-2202
305-868-2609
FAX: 305-868-2640
Sanford L King, Director
Yvonne Quatrale, President
Disabled children, hearing and speech center. Grants are only given to tax exempt organizations, no individual grants are offered.

2671 Jessie Ball duPont Fund
1 Independent Dr
Ste 1400
Jacksonville, FL 32202-5011
904-353-0890
800-252-3452
FAX: 904-353-3870
e-mail: contactus@dupontfund.org
www.dupontfund.org

Sherry P. Magill, President
Mark D. Constantine, Vice President for Strategy, Pol
Barbara Roole, Senior Program Officer
Katie Ensign, Senior Program Officer

Established under the terms of the will of the late Jessie Ball duPont. The fund is a national foundation having a special though not exclusive interest in issues affecting the South. The Fund works with the approximately 325 individual institutions to which Mrs. duPont personally contributed during the five-year period, 1960 through 1964.

2672 Lost Tree Village Charitable Foundation
8 Church Lane
North Palm Beach, FL 33408-2908
561-622-3780
FAX: 561-841-6773
e-mail: info@losttreefoundation.org
www.losttreefoundation.org

Pam Rue, Executive Director
Teresa Elu, Executive Assistant
Bob Heon, Controller

The Lost Tree Village Charitable Foundation is dedicated to building a stronger community and improving the quality of life for all local residents. Grants are awarded annually to local non-profit health and human service organizations providing information, expertise and assistance to those in need. Applications are only accepted from organizations located in Palm Beach and Southern Martin Counties. Visit the website for guidelines and further information.

2673 National Parkinson Foundation
200 SE 1st Street
Suite 800
Miami, FL 33131-1494
305-243-6666
800-473-4636
FAX: 305-537-9901
e-mail: contact@parkinson.org
www.parkinson.org

John W. Kozyak, Chairman
Joyce Oberdorf, President/CEO
Jill Davidson, Vice President, Chapter and Comm
Peter Schmidt, PhD, Vice President, Programs, Chief

The mission of the NPF is to improve the quality of care for people with Parkinson's disease through research, education, and outreach.

2674 Publix Super Markets Charities
Publix Super Market Corporation Office
PO Box 407
Lakeland, FL 33802-0407
800-242-1227
www.publix.com

Gino DiGrazia, Vice President of Finance
Maria Brous, Director of Media & Community R
Kimberly Reynolds, Media & Community Relations

In addition to giving to thousands of local projects, Publix annually supports five organizations in companywide campaigns: Special Olympics, March of Dimes, Children's Miracle Network, United Way and Food for All

2675 Richard W Higgins Charitable Foundation
Marshall & Ilsley Trust of Florida
800 Laurel Oak Dr
Ste 100
Naples, FL 34108-2713
877-202-9234
www.applebees.com

Ken Krei, President

Gives primarily for medical research with geographical focus on New York and Florida.

Georgia

2676 Arc Of Georgia
100 Edgewood Ave NE
Ste 1675
Atlanta, GA 30303-3068
678-733-8969
888-401-1581
FAX: 678-733-8970
e-mail: info@thearcofgeorgia.org
www.thearcofgeorgia.org

Torin Togut, President
David Glass, Vice President
Julie Lee, Secretary
Will Hudson, Treasurer

The Arc of Georgia advocates for the rights and full participation of all children and adults with intellectual and developmental disabilities. Together with our network of members and other local Chapters, we improve systems of supports and services, connect families, inspire communities, and influence public policy.

2677 Community Foundation for Greater Atlanta
50 Hurt Plz SE
Ste 449
Atlanta, GA 30303-2915
404-688-5525
FAX: 404-688-3060
e-mail: info@cfgreateratlanta.org
www.cfgreateratlanta.org

Suzanne Boas, Board Chair
Alicia Philipp, President
Robert Smulian, Vice President of Philanthropic
Lesley Grady, Senior Vice President of Community Partnerships

The Community Foundation for Greater Atlanta is a creative, cost-effective and tax-efficient way for people to invest in our community. We help donors and their families meet their charitable goals by educating them or critical issues and by matching them with organizations that serve their interests. By working with donors and the community, we improve the quality of life for residents in our region.

2678 Florence C and Harry L English Memorial Fund
Sun Trust Bank Atlanta
PO Box 4418
Mail Code 041
Atlanta, GA 30302
404-588-8250
FAX: 404-724-3082
e-mail: raymond.king@suntrust.com
www.suntrustatlantafoundation.org

Anil T. Cheriyan, Chief Information Officer
Kenneth J. Carrig, Chief Human Resources Officer
Rilla S. Delorier, Chief Marketing and Client Exper
Thomas E. Freeman, Chief Risk Officer

Grants only made to Metro Atlanta non-profit organizations; no grants to churches or individuals.

2679 Georgia Power
605 Boulevard NE
Atlanta, GA 30308-3374
404-506-6526
888-655-5888
www.georgiapower.com

W. Paul Bowers, Chairman/ President/ CEO
John L. Pemberton, Senior VP/SPO,
Mike Anderson, Senior VP, Charitable Giving
Ron Hinson, Executive VP/Chief Financial Officer/ Treasurer/ Comptroller

Georgia Power is an investor-owned, tax-paying utility that serves 2.25 million customers in all but four of Georgia's 159 counties.

2680 **Grayson Foundation**
1701 Willa Place Drive
Kernersville, NC 2728
336-650-9914
e-mail: graysonfoundation@gmail.com
www.graysonfoundation.net

Donna Sherrell, Finance- Public Relations
Tricia Gladstone, Behavior Analyst-Finance Public
Roger Sherrell, Information Technology-Web Manag
Bob Sherrell, Finance

Grayson Foundation enhances the quality of public educationfor the students of the Grayson cluster of schools by providing funds which enrich and extend educational oppurtunities.

2681 **Harriet McDaniel Marshall Trust in Memory of Sanders McDaniel**
Sun Trust Bank Atlanta
PO Box 4418
Mail Code 041
Atlanta, GA 30302
404-588-8250
FAX: 404-724-3082
e-mail: raymond.king@suntrust.com
www.suntrustatlantafoundation.org

Anil T. Cheriyan, Chief Information Officer
Kenneth J. Carrig, Chief Human Resources Officer
Rilla S. Delorier, Chief Marketing and Client Exper
Thomas E. Freeman, Chief Risk Officer

Grants only made to Metro Atlanta non-profit organizations, no grants to churches or individuals.

2682 **IBM Corporation**
1 New Orchard Rd
Armonk, NY 10504-1772
914-499-1900
800-426-4968
TTY:800-426-3383
e-mail: ews@us.ibm.com
www.ibm.com

Samuel J Palmisano, Chairman
Virginia M. Rometty, President and Chief Executive Of
Rodney C. Adkins, Senior Vice President
Michael E. Daniels, Senior Vice President and Group

Manages disability programs (which leverage IBM resources through partnerships) designed to train persons with disabilities and assist them in gaining employment. Also, disseminates information regarding products and resources for persons with disabilities with those of other companies and organizations.

2683 **John H and Wilhelmina D Harland Charitable Foundation**
3565 Piedmont Road, NE
Two Piedmont Center, Suite 710
Atlanta, GA 30305-1502
404-264-9912
FAX: 404-266-8834
e-mail: info@harlandfoundation.org
www.harlandfoundation.org

Margaret C. Reiser, President
Winifred S. Davis, Vice President/Treasurer
Robert E. Reiser, Secretary
Jane G. Hardesty, Executive Director

The Harland Charitable Foundation was established in 1972 by John H. and Wilhelmina D. Harland to support worthy local causes in Atlanta, with a particular interest in improving the welfare of children and youth as well as support of community services and arts and culture.

2684 **Lettie Pate Whitehead Foundation**
191 Peachtree Street NE
Suite 3540
Atlanta, GA 30303- 2951
404-522-6755
FAX: 404-522-7026
e-mail: fdns@woodruff.org
www.woodruff.org

James B. Williams, Chairman
James M. Sibley, Vice Chairman
P. Russell Hardin, President
J. Lee Tribble, Treasurer

Non-profit organization dedicated to the support of needy women in nine southeastern states.

2685 **Rich Foundation**
222 Summer Street
Stamford, CT 06901
203-359-2900
FAX: 203-328-7980
e-mail: info@fdrich.com
www.fdrich.com

2686 **SunTrust Bank, Atlanta Foundation**
Sun Trust Bank Atlanta
PO Box 4418
Mail Code 041
Atlanta, GA 30302
404-588-8250
FAX: 404-724-3082
e-mail: raymond.king@suntrust.com
www.suntrust.com

Anil T. Cheriyan, Chief Information Officer
Kenneth J. Carrig, Chief Human Resources Officer
Rilla S. Delorier, Chief Marketing and Client Exper
Thomas E. Freeman, Chief Risk Officer

Hawaii

2687 **Arc of Hawaii**
3989 Diamond Head Rd
Honolulu, HI 96816-4413
808-737-7995
FAX: 808-732-9531
e-mail: info@thearcinhawaii.org
www.thearcinhawaii.org

Thomas Huber, President
Lee Moriwaki, Vice President
Leolinda Parlin, Secretary
Noelle Liew, Treasurer

The Arc is a national, grassroots organization of and for people with intellectual and related developmental disabilities. With more then 140,000 members in 1000 local and state chapters. The Arc is the largest volunteer organization devoted soley to working on behalf of people with intellectual disabilities.

2688 **Atherton Family Foundation**
827 Fort Street Mall
Honolulu, HI 96813-2817
808-566-5524
888-731-3863
FAX: 808-521-6286
e-mail: foundations@hcf-hawaii.org
www.atherton.hawaiicommunityfoundation.org

Patricia R. Giles, Vice President
Judith M. Dawson, President
Frank C. Atherton, Vice President and Treasurer
Paul F. Morgan, Vice President

Supports educational projects, programs and institutions as the highest priority, with the enterprises of a religious nature and those concerned with health and social services given careful attention. The Foundation is one of the largest private resources in the State devoted exclusively to the support of activities of a charitable nature.

2689 **GN Wilcox Trust**
Bank of Hawaii
PO Box 3170
Honolulu, HI 96802-3170
808-649-4945
800-272-7262
FAX: 808-538-4006
e-mail: paula.boyce@boh.com
www.boh.com

Paul Boyce, AVP and Grants Administrator
Elaine Moniz, Trust Specialist
William "Bill" L. Carpenter, Senior Vice President
Diane W. Murakami, Senior Vice President

Benefits the people of Hawaii by funding programs that support social services, education, culture, the arts, youth services, religion, health and rehabilitation.

2690 Hawaii Community Foundation
827 Fort Street Mall
Honolulu, HI 96813-2817
808-537-6333
888-731-3863
FAX: 808-521-6286
e-mail: info@hcf-hawaii.org
www.hawaiicommunityfoundation.org

Kelvin Taketa, President/CEO
Chris van Bergeijk, Vice President/Chief Operating Officer
Joseph Martyak, Vice President of Communications
Tom Kelly, Vice President for Knowledge, Evaluation and Learning

The Hawaii Community Foundation is a public, statewide, charitable services and grantmaking organization supported by donor contributions for the benefit of Hawaii's people.

2691 McInerny Foundation Bank Of Hawaii,Corporate Trustee
PO Box 3170
Honolulu, HI 96802-3170
808-538-4945
800-272-7262
FAX: 808-538-4006
e-mail: paula.boyce@boh.com
www.boh.com

Paula Boyce, Avp And Grants Administrator
Elaine Moniz, Trust Specialist
William "Bill" L. Carpenter, Senior Vice President
Diane W. Murakami, Senior Vice President

Although the Trust is broad-purposed, it does not make grants to churches or individuals, nor for endowments, reserve purposes, deficit financing, or for the purchase of real estate.

2692 Sophie Russell Testamentary Trust Bank Of Hawaii
PO Box 3170
Honolulu, HI 96802-3170
808-538-4944
800-272-7262
FAX: 808-538-4006
e-mail: paula.boyce@boh.com
www.boh.com

Paula Boyce, Asst. Vice President
Elaine Moniz, Trust Specialist
William "Bill" L. Carpenter, Senior Vice President
Diane W. Murakami, Senior Vice President

Supports qualified tax-exempt charitable organizations, in the State of Hawaii only. Offers grants to the Humane Society and institutions giving nursing care and serving the physically and mentally handicapped.

Illinois

2693 Alzheimer's Association
225 N Michigan Ave
Fl 17
Chicago, IL 60601-7633
312-335-8700
800-272-3900
FAX: 312-335-5886
TTY: 312-335-5886
e-mail: info@alz.org
www.alz.org

Gerald Sampson, Chair
Stewart Putnam, Chair Elect
Harry Johns, President /CEO
Deborah Jones, Secretary

Mission is to eliminate Alzheimer's disease through the advancement of research, to provide and enhance care and support for all affected, and to reduce the risk of dementia through the promotion of brain health.

2694 American National Bank and Trust Company
33 N La Salle St
Chicago, IL 60602-2650
312-661-6000
800-240-8190
FAX: 815-961-7745
www.amnb.com

Charles H. Majors, Chairman & Chief Executive Offic
Jeffrey V. Haley, President
Charles T. Canaday, Jr., Senior Vice President
R. Helm Dobbins, Senior Vice President

Supports the endeavors of organizations working to meet the critical needs of the city and its surrounding communities. Success is greatly affected by the well-being of the communities the company serves, thus the foundation seeks to fulfill the social obligations both through financial funding and human resources. The Foundation funding categories include organizations and programs involved in economic development, education, community and social services, healthcare and culture and the arts.

2695 Amerock Corporation
P.O.Box 7018
Rockford, IL 61125-7018
815-963-9631
800-618-9559
FAX: 815-969-6029
www.amerock.com

Robert Bailey, President

Grants are given to organizations promoting wellness, health and rehabilitation of the visually impaired and physically disabled.

2696 Arc of Illinois
The Illinois Life Span Project
20901 S La Grange Rd
Ste 209
Frankfort, IL 60423-3213
815-464-1832
800-588-7002
FAX: 815-464-5292
e-mail: mike@illinoislifespan.org
www.thearcofil.org

Tony Paulauski, Executive Director
Janet Donahue, Director of Development
Katherine Hamann, Family Transition Program Director
Faye Manaster, Project Director

The Arc of Illinois is committed to empowering persons with disabilities to achieve full participation in community life thru informed choices.

2697 Benjamin Benedict Green-Field Foundation
18313 Greenleaf Ct
Tinley Park, IL 60487-2176
708-444-4241
FAX: 708-614-0496
e-mail: kathy@greenfieldfoundation.org
www.greenfieldfoundation.org

Colin Fisher, Chairman of the Board
Kathryn Groenendal, President
Dan Jarke, Vice President
Sheldon K. Rachman, Secretary

A privately endowed grantmaking organization trying to improve the qaulity of life for children and the elderly in the city of chicago.

2698 Blowitz-Ridgeway Foundation
Ste 201
1701 E Woodfield Rd
Schaumburg, IL 60173-5127
847-330-1020
FAX: 847-330-1028
e-mail: laura@blowitzridgeway.org
www.blowitzridgeway.org

Daniel L Kline, President
Pierre R. LeBreton, Ph.D., Vice-President
Anthony M. Dean, Treasurer
Sandra Swantek, M.D., Secretary

Provides limited program, capital and research grants to organizations aiding the physically and mentally disabled, and agencies serving children and youth. Grants generally limited to Illinois.

2699 Chaddick Institute for Metropolitan Development
243 S Wabash Ave
Ste 9000
Chicago, IL 60604-2302
312-362-5731
FAX: 312-362-5506
e-mail: chaddick@depaul.edu
www.las.depaul.edu

Joseph P Scwieterman PhD, Director
Marisa Schulz, LEED AP, Assistant Director
Justin Kohls, Program Manager
Susan Aaron, Civic Program Design

Advances the principals of effective land use, transportation, and community planning. Offers planners, attorneys, developers, and entrepreneurs a forum to share expertise on difficult land-use issues through workshops, conferences, and policy studies.

2700 **Chicago Community Trust**
225 North Michigan Avenue
Suite 2200
Chicago, IL 60601- 4501 312-616-8000
FAX: 312-616-7955
e-mail: alla@cct.org
www.cct.org

Frank M. Clark, Chairman
Terry Mazany, President /CEO
Jamie Phillippe, Vice President-Development and Donor Services
Chae Dawning, Sr. Director of Human Resources & Administration
A community foundation established in 1915, which receives gifts and bequests from individuals, families or organizations interested in providing through the community foundation, financial support for the charitable agencies or institutions which serve the residents of metropolitan Chicago.

2701 **Chicago Community Trust and Affiliates**
225 North Michigan Avenue
Suite 2200
Chicago, IL 60601- 4501 312-616-8000
FAX: 312-616-7955
TTY:312-853-0394
e-mail: alla@cct.org
www.cct.org
Frank M. Clark, Chairman
Terry Mazany, President /CEO
Jamie Phillippe, Vice President-Development and Donor Services
Chae Dawning, Sr. Director of Human Resources & Administration
Provides critical charitable resources in the arts, community and economic development, education, health and wellness, hunger and homeless alleviation, legal services, programs for youth, the elderly, and people with disabilities, and services to assure that basic human needs are met for all members of our community.

2702 **Community Foundation of Champaign County**
307 W University Ave
Champaign, IL 61820-3411 217-359-0125
FAX: 217-352-6494
e-mail: cfcc@soltec.net
www.cfeci.org

Steve Whitsitt, Chair
Jeff Davis, Vice-Chair
Menah Pratt-Clarke, Secretary
David Parkhill, Treasurer
A network of cultural resource providers and educational organizations who collaborate in the creation, coordination, and promotion of cultural resource programs for Champaign County Schools.

2703 **Dr Scholl Foundation**
1033 Skokie Blvd
Ste 230
Northbrook, IL 60062-4109 847-559-7430

www.drschollfoundation.com
Pamela Scholl, President
The Foundation is dedicated to providing financial assistance to organizations committed to improving our world. Grants are made annually after an executive review by the staff and all the directors.

2704 **Duchossois Foundation**
Chamberlain Group
845 N Larch Ave
Elmhurst, IL 60126-1114 630-279-3600
FAX: 630-530-6091
e-mail: employment@duch.com
www.duch.com
Richard L. Duchossois, Chairman
Robert L. Fealy, President /COO
Craig J. Duchossois, Chief Executive Officer
Michael E. Flannery, Executive Vice President/Chief Financial Officer
Established in 1984, the foundation returns dollars to the communities supporting its facilities and employees. Within these following areas, organizations are carefully selected on the basis of community needs and the organization's value and performance. Areas aimed at include: medical research, children/youth programs and cultural institutions.

2705 **Evenston Community Foundation**
1560 Sherman Ave
Suite 535
Evanston, IL 60201-5910 847-492-0990
FAX: 847-492-0904
e-mail: info@evanstonforever.org
www.evanstonforever.org
Sara Schastok, Phd., President and CEO
Gwen Jessen, Vice President for Philanthropy
Marybeth Schroeder, Vice President for Programs
Jan Fischer, Chief Financial Officer
The Foundation is a publicly supported plilanthropic organization dedicated to enriching Evanston and the lives of its people, now and in the future. The Foundation builds and manages its own and other community endowments, addresses Evanston's changing needs through grant making, and provides leadership on important community needs.

2706 **Field Foundation of Illinois**
200 S Wacker Dr
Ste 3860
Chicago, IL 60606-5848 312-831-0910
FAX: 312-831-0961
e-mail: byoung@fieldfoundation.org
www.fieldfoundation.org

Lyle Logan, Board Chair
Aurie A. Pennick, Executive Director and Treasurer
Sarah M. Linsley, Secretary
Mark C. Murray, Program Director
The Field Foundation seeks to provide support for community, civic and cultural organizations in the Chicago area, enabling both new and established programs to test innovations, to expand proven strengths or to address specific, time-limited operational needs.

2707 **Francis Beidler Charitable Trust**
53 W Jackson Blvd
Ste 530
Chicago, IL 60604-3422 312-922-3792
FAX: 312-922-3799

Francis Beidler, Owner
Children/youth, services. Community development, business promotion, crime and violence prevention. Federated giving programs, higher education, human services and family planning.

2708 **Fred J Brunner Foundation**
9300 King St
Franklin Park, IL 60131-2114 847-678-3232
FAX: 847-678-0642
www.fjbfoundation.com

Fred J Brunner, CEO
General disability grants.

2709 **George M Eisenberg Foundation for Charities**
Ste 480
2340 S Arlington Heights Rd
Arlington Heights, IL 60005-4507 847-981-0545
FAX: 847-941-0548
James Marousis, Manager

2710 **Grover Hermann Foundation**
233 S Wacker Dr
Suite 6600
Chicago, IL 60606-6473 312-258-5500
FAX: 312-258-5600
e-mail: rsafer@schiffhardin.com
www.schiffhardin.com
Ronald S. Safer, Managing Partner, Executive Comm

Provides funds for educational, health, public policy, community and religious organizations throughout the United States. Its major interests are in higher education and health.

2711 John D and Catherine T MacArthur Foundation
Office of Grants Management
140 S Dearborn St
Chicago, IL 60603-5285 312-726-8000
FAX: 312-920-6258
TTY:312-920-6285
e-mail: 4answers@macfound.org
www.macfound.org

Marjorie M. Scardino, Chair
Julia Statch, Interim President
Cecilia A. Conrad, Vice President-MacArthur Fellows Program
Susan E. Manske, Vice President/Chief Investment Officer

The Foundation supports creative people and effective institutions committed to building a more just, verdant, and peaceful world. In addition, we work to defend human rights, advance global conservation, & security, make cities better places, and understand how technology is affecting children and society.

2712 Les Turne Amyotrophic Lateral Sclerosis Foundation
5550 Touhy Ave
Ste 302
Skokie, IL 60077-3254 847-679-3311
888-257-1107
FAX: 847-679-9109
e-mail: info@lesturnerals.org
www.lesturnerals.org

Ken Hoffman, President
Wendy Abrams, Executive Director
Shari Diamond, RN, BSN, Director of Patient ServicesSupport Group Facilitator
Kim McIver, Director of Athletic Events

Voluntary health organization dedicated to raising funds for ALS research, patient services and public awareness. Provides educational materials for affected individuals and family members, health care professionals, and the general public. Program services include referrals and counseling; audio-visual aids and periodic newsletters. Offers support groups and patient networking to affected individuals, family members, and caregivers.

2713 Little City Foundation
1760 W Algonquin Rd
Palatine, IL 60067-4799 847-358-5510
FAX: 847-358-3291
e-mail: info@littlecity.org
www.littlecity.org

Matthew B. Schubert, President
B. Timothy Desmond, Executive Vice President
David Rose, Vice President
Douglas A. Wilson, Vice President

We offer innovative and personalized programs to fully assist and empower children & adults with autism and other intellectual and developmental disabilities. With a commitment to attaining a greater quality of life for Illinois most vulnerable citizens, we actively promote choice, person-centered planning and a holistic approach to health and wellness. 'ChildBridge' services include in-home personal & family supports, clinical behavior intervention, 24/7 residential services and much more.

2714 MAGIC Foundation for Children's Growth
6645 North Ave
Oak Park, IL 60302-1057 708-383-0808
800-362-4423
FAX: 708-383-0899
e-mail: dianne@magicfoundation.org
www.magicfoundation.org

Rich Buckley, Chairman
Ken Dickard, Vice Chairman
Mary Andrews, CEO and Co-Founder
Dianne Kremidas, Executive Director

This is a national nonprofit organization providing support and education regarding growth disorders in children and related adult disorders, including adult GHD. Dedicated to helping children whose physical growth is affected by a medical problem by assisting families of afflicted children through local support groups, public education/awareness, newsletters, specialty divisions and programs for the children.

2715 McDonald's Corporation Contributions Program
2111 McDonalds Dr
Oak Brook, IL 60523-5500 630-623-3000
800-244-6227
FAX: 630-623-5700
www.mcdonalds.com

Don Thompson, President and Chief Executive Of
Tim Fenton, Chief Operating Officer
Peter J. Bensen, Executive Vice President and Chi
Jose Armario, Corporate Executive Vice Preside

2716 Michael Reese Health Trust
150 N Wacker Dr
Ste 2320
Chicago, IL 60606-1608 312-726-1008
e-mail: wpalmer@healthtrust.net
www.healthtrust.net

Herbert S. Wander, Chairman
The Hon. How Carroll, Vice Chairman
Walter R. Nathan, Secretary
Gregory S. Gross, EdD, President

The trust seeks to improve the health of people in Chicago's metropolitan communities through effective grantmaking in health care, health education, and health research.

2717 National Eye Research Foundation
910 Skokie Blvd
Ste 207a
Northbrook, IL 60062-4033 847-564-9400
800-621-2258
FAX: 847-564-0807
e-mail: info@nerf.org
www.subway.com

Joel Tenner, Manager

Dedicated to improving eye care for the public and meeting the professional needs of eye care practitioners; sponsors eye research projects on contact lens applications and eye care problems. Special study sections in such fields as orthokertology, primary eyecare, pediatrics, and through continuing education programs. Provides eye care information for the public and professionals. Educational materials including pamphlets. Program activities include education and referrals.

2718 National Foundation for Ectodermal Dysplasias
6 Executive Dr
Suite 2
Fairview Heights, IL 62208-1360 618-566-2020
FAX: 618-566-4718
e-mail: info@nfed.org
www.nfed.org

Judy Woodruff, C.F.R.E, Executive Director
Gale Hoedebeck, Director of Administration
Kelley Atchison, Director of Support
Jodi Edgar Reinhardt, Director of Marketing and Communication

To empower and connect people touched by ectodermal dysplasias through education, support, and research.

2719 National Headache Foundation
820 N Orleans St
Ste 411
Chicago, IL 60610-3498 312-274-2650
888-643-5552
FAX: 312-640-9049
e-mail: info@headaches.org
www.headaches.org

Seymour Diamond, M.D., Executive Chairman
Roger K. Cady, M.D., Associate Executive Chairman
Arthur H. Elkind, M.D., President
Vincent Martin, M.D., Vice President

Foundation exists to enhance the healthcare of headache sufferers. It is a source of help to sufferers' families, physicians who treat headache sufferers, allied healthcare professionals and to the public.

2720 OMRON Foundation OMRON Electronics
1 Commerce Dr
Schaumburg, IL 60173-5330
847-843-7900
800-556-6766
FAX: 847-884-1866
e-mail: aoisales@omron.com
www.omron247.com

Tastu Goto, CEO

Supports local community projects through direct donations and matching employee-directed contributions.

2721 Parkinson's Disease Foundation
1359 Broadway
Suite 1509
New York, NY 10018-2331
212-923-4700
800-457-667
FAX: 212-923-4778
e-mail: info@pdf.org
www.pdf.org

Howard D. Morgan, Chair
Constance Woodruff Atwell, Ph.D., Vice Chair
Robin Anthony Elliott, President
James Beck, Ph.D., Vice President

International voluntary not-for-profit organization dedicated to patient services; education of affected individuals, family members, and healthcare professionals; and promotion and support of research for Parkinson's Disease and related disorders. Offers an extensive referral service to guide affected individuals to proper diagnosis and clinical care. Provides referrals to genetic counseling and support groups; promotes patient advocacy; and offers a variety of educational and support materials
Quarterly

2722 Peoria Area Community Foundation
331 Fulton St
Ste 310
Peoria, IL 61602-1449
309-674-8730
FAX: 309-674-8754
e-mail: jim@communityfoundationci.org
www.communityfoundationci.org

Bashir Ali, Chair
Cathy Butler, Vice Chair
Donna Marcacci, Secretary
Mark Roberts, CEO

Established to meet a wide variety of social, cultural, educational and other charitable needs throughout Central Illinois.

2723 Polk Brothers Foundation
20 W Kinzie St
Ste 1110
Chicago, IL 60654-5815
312-527-4684
FAX: 312-527-4681
e-mail: questions@polkbrosfdn.org
www.polkbrosfdn.org

Sandra P. Guthman, Chair
Raymond F. Simon, Vice Chair
Gordon S. Prussian, Secretary
Sidney Epstein, Treasurer

The Polk Brothers Foundation seeks to improve the quality of life for the people of Chicago. We partner with local nonprofit organizations that work to reduce the impact of poverty and provide area residents with better access to quality education, preventive health care and basic human services.

2724 Retirement Research Foundation
8765 W Higgins Rd
Ste 430
Chicago, IL 60631-4170
773-714-8080
FAX: 773-714-8089
e-mail: info@rrf.org
www.rrf.org

Nathaniel P. McParland, M.D., Chairman
Ruth Ann Watkins, Secretary
Downey R. Varey, Treasurer
Irene Frye, Executive Director

A private philanthropy with primary interest in improving the quality of life of older persons in the United States.

2725 Sears-Roebuck Foundation
3333 Beverly Rd
Hoffman Estates, IL 60179
847-286-2500
800-932-3188
FAX: 800-326-0485
www.sears.com

W Bruce Johnson, CEO

Has a special interest in projects that address women, families, and diversity, but awards most of its funding to disease-specific charities and United Way in the Chicago area.

2726 Siragusa Foundation
1 E Wacker Dr
Ste 2910
Chicago, IL 60601-1912
312-755-0064
FAX: 312-755-0069
www.siragusa.org

Irene S Phelps, President
Sharmila Rao Thakkar, Senior Program Officer
Kyla M. Evans, Adminstrative Assistant/ Grants
John E. Hicks, Jr., Chair

The Siragusa Foundation, is a private family foundation that is committed to honoring its founder by sustaining and developing Chicago's extraordinary nonprofit resources.

2727 Square D Foundation
1415 S Roselle Rd
Palatine, IL 60067-7337
847-397-2600
FAX: 847-925-7500
www.schneider-electric.com/site/home/i

2728 WP and HB White Foundation
540 W Frontage Rd
Ste 3240
Northfield, IL 60093-1232
847-446-1441

Margaret Blandford, Executive Director

The Foundation's funds are allocated on a continuing basis within the metropolitan area of Chicago where our founder's business prospered. The Foundation helps organizations specializing in the visually impaired, mental health, youth and recreation.

2729 Washington Square Health Foundation
875 N Michigan Ave
Ste 3516
Chicago, IL 60611-1957
312-664-6488
FAX: 312-664-7787
e-mail: washington@wshf.org
www.wshf.org

William N. Werner, MD, MPH, Board Chair
Howard Nochumson, Executive Director/President
William B. Friedeman, Secretary
James M. Snyder, Treasurer

Grants funds in order to promote and maintain access to adequate healthcare for all people in the Chicagoland area regardless of race, sex, creed or financial need.

2730 Wheat Ridge Ministries
1 Pierce Pl
Ste 250 E
Itasca, IL 60143-2634
630-766-9066
800-762-6748
FAX: 630-766-9622
e-mail: wrmail@weatridge.org
www.wheatridge.org

Richard Herman, President
Brian Becker, Senior Vice President
Holly Harrison Fiala, Vice President of Advancement
Ann Brandt, Director of Annual Giving and Advancement Services

Weat Ridge supports more then 100 new health-related ministries each year through a variety of grant programs

Indiana

2731 **Arc of Indiana**
107 N Pennsylvania St
Suite 800
Indianapolis, IN 46204- 2423
317-977-2375
800-382-9100
FAX: 317-977-2385
e-mail: thearc@arcind.org
www.arcind.org

Mark Hisey, President
Kerry Fletcher, Vice President
Mike Foddrill, Treasurer
Marlene Lu, Secretary
Arc of Indiana is commited to people with cognitive and developmental disabilities realizing their goals of learning, living, working, and playing in the community.

2732 **Ball Brothers Foundation**
222 S Mulberry St
Muncie, IN 47305-2802
765-741-5500
FAX: 765-741-5518
e-mail: info@ballfdn.org
www.ballfdn.org

James A. Fisher, Acting Chairman/Chief Executive Officer
Jud Fisher, President/Chief Operating Officer
Terry L. Walker, Secretary
Tammy Phillips, Treasurer, ex-officio
The Ball Brothers Foundation is dedicated to the stewardship legacy of the Ball brothers and to the pursuit of improving the quality of the Muncie, Delaware County, east Central Indiana and Indiana, through philanthropy and leadership.

2733 **Community Foundation of Boone County**
60 E. Cedar Street
PO Box 92
Zionsville, IN 46077
317-873-0210
FAX: 317-873-0219
e-mail: info@communityfoundationbc.org
www.communityfoundationbc.org

Marc Applegate, Chairman of the Board
Ray Ingham, Vice Chair
Mike Harlos, Treasurer
Suzy Rich, Secretary
The Community Foundation of Boone County provides pathways for connecting people who care with causes that matter for now and in the future.

2734 **John W Anderson Foundation**
402 Wall St
Valparaiso, IN 46383-2562
219-462-4611
FAX: 219-531-8954
e-mail: andersonfnd@aol.com

Bruce Wargo, Manager
Physically and mentally disabled, recreation and youth agencies in Northwest Indiana area.

Iowa

2735 **Arc of Iowa**
130 S. Sheldon Ave
Ste 302
Ames, IA 50014-3259
515-232-9330
800-362-2927
FAX: 515-309-0860
e-mail: casey@thearcofiowa.org
www.thearcofiowa.org

Casey Westhoff, Executive Director
The Arc of Iowa exists to ensure that people with intellectual disabilities and developmental disabilities receive the services, supports and opportunities necessary to fully realize their right to live, work and enjoy life in the community without discrimination.

2736 **Hall-Perrine Foundation**
115 3rd St SE
Ste 803
Cedar Rapids, IA 52401-1222
319-362-9079
FAX: 319-362-7220
e-mail: kristin@hallperrine.org
www.hallperrine.org

William Whipple, Chairman
Jack Evans, President
Darrel Morf, Vice President
Iris Muchmore, Secretary
This foundation is dedicated tio improving the quality of life for peole in Linn County, IA by responding to the changing social, economic, and cultural needs of the community.

2737 **Mid-Iowa Health Foundation**
3900 Ingersoll Ave
Ste 104
Des Moines, IA 50312-3535
515-277-6411
FAX: 515-271-7579
e-mail: info@midiowahealth.org
www.midiowahealth.org

Becky Miles-Polka, Chairman
Rob Hayes, Vice Chair
Suzanne Mineck, President
Cheryl Harding, Secretary/Treasurer
Mission is to serve as a partner and catalyst for improving the health of vulnerable people in greater Des Moines.

2738 **Principal Financial Group Foundation**
711 High St
Des Moines, IA 50392
515-247-5111
800-986-3343
FAX: 515-235-5724
www.principalfinancialgroup.com

Larry Zimpleman, Chairman/ President/ CEO
Daniel J. Houston, President - Retirement, Insuranc
James P. McCaughan, President - Principal Global Inv
Luis Valdes, President - Principal Internatio
The Principal Financial Group is a leading global financial company offering businesses, individuals and industrial clients a wide range of financial products and services.

2739 **Siouxland Community Foundation**
505 5th St
Suite 412
Sioux City, IA 51101-1507
712-293-3303
FAX: 712-293-3303
e-mail: office@siouxlandcommunityfoundation.org
www.siouxlandcommunityfoundation .org

Matthew J. Basye, President
Richard J. Dehner, Vice President/Co-Chair Investment/Finance Committee Chair
Marilyn J. Hagberg, Secretary
Paul A. Bergmann, Treasurer
The Siouxland Community Foundation strives to enhance the quality of life in the greater Siouxland tri-state area by seeking charitable gifts to build permanent endowments as charitable capital for the community, providing a flexable vehicle to receive and distribute gifts of any size, making grants in response to community needs, and providing services that will help shape the well-being of Siouxland.

Kansas

2740 **Arc of Kansas**
2701 SW Randolph Ave
Topeka, KS 66611-1536
785-232-0597
FAX: 785-232-3770
e-mail: info@tarcinc.org
www.tarcinc.org

Angela Cool, President
Ann Shelton, Vice President
Travis Stryker, Secretary
Kim Savage, Treasurer

Organzation works to ensure that the estimated 7.2 million Americans with intellectual and developmental disabilities have the services and supports they need to grow, develop, and live in communities across the nation.

2741 Hutchinson Community Foundation
1 North Main, Suite 501
PO Box 298
Hutchinson, KS 67504-0298 620-663-5293
FAX: 620-663-9277
e-mail: info@hutchcf.org
www.hutchcf.org

Aubrey Abbot Patterson, President and Executive Director
Terri L. Eisiminger, Vice President of Administration
Janet Hamilton, Community Investment Officer
Maria G. Kicklighter, Finance Assistant

Connects donors to community needs and opportunities, increases philanthropy and provides community leadership.

Kentucky

2742 Arc of Kentucky
706 E. Main Street
Suite A
Frankfort, KY 40601-2408 502-875-5225
800-281-1272
FAX: 502-875-5226
e-mail: arcofky@aol.com
arcofky.org

Patty Dempsey, Executive Director

The Arc of Kentucky works to ensure a quality of life for children and adults with intellectual and developmental disabilities to help in securing a positive future. The Arc values services and supports that enhance the quality of life through independence, friendship, choice and respect for individuals with intellectual and developmental disabilities.

Louisiana

2743 Arc of Louisiana
606 Colonial Dr
Ste G
Baton Rouge, LA 70806-6535 225-383-1033
FAX: 225-383-1092
e-mail: info@thearcla.org
www.thearcla.org

Dr. Duane Superneau, President
Kelly Serrett, Executive Director
Ashley Courville, Program Director

The Arc of Louisiana advocates for and with individuals with intellectual and developmental disabilities and their families that they shall live to their fullest potential.

2744 Baton Rouge Area Foundation
402 N 4th St
Baton Rouge, LA 70802-5506 225-387-6126
877-387-6126
FAX: 225-387-6153
e-mail: mverma@braf.org
www.braf.org

C. Kris Kirkpatrick, Chair
S. Dennis Blunt, Vice Chair
John G. Davies, President/CEO
Suzanne L. Turner, Secretary

The Foundation provides grants to nonprofits to make lives better in the region. It also takes on projects, often with parters, to remake Baton Rouge.

2745 Community Foundation of Shreveport-Bossier
401 Edwards St
Ste 105
Shreveport, LA 71101-5551 318-221-0582
FAX: 318-221-7463
e-mail: info@cfnla.org
www.cfnla.org

Edward J. Crawford, III, Chairman
Janie D. Richardson, Vice Chairman
Terry C. Davis, Ph.D, Secretary
Thomas H. Murphy, Treasurer

Provides a variety of charitable funds and gift options to help our partners achieve their vision for a stronger, more vibrant community. By bringing together fund donors, their financial advisors and non profit agencies, the Foundation is a powerful catalyst for building charitable giving and effecting positive change in our area

Maine

2746 UNUM Charitable Foundation
Maine Association of Non Profits
565 Congress St
Ste 301
Portland, ME 04101-3308 207-871-1885
FAX: 207-780-0346
e-mail: Manp@NonprofitMaine.org
www.nonprofitmaine.org

Ellen Golden, Board President
Doug Woodbury, Board Vice President
Cathy Ramsdell, Board Treasurer
Lisa Miller, Board Secretary

The Foundation encourages projects that: stimulate others in the private or public sector to participate in problem solving; advance innovative and cost-effective approaches for addressing defined, recognized needs; and demonstrate ability to obtain future project funding, if needed. The foundation generally limits its consideration of capital campaign requests to the Greater Portland, Maine area.

Maryland

2747 American Health Assistance Foundation
22512 Gateway Center Dr
Clarksburg, MD 20871-2005 301-948-3244
800-437-2423
FAX: 301-258-9454
e-mail: info@ahaf.org
www.ahaf.org

Stacy Pagos Haller, President / CEO
Donna Callison, Vice President of Development
Michael Buckley, Vice President of Public Affairs
Guy Eakin, Ph.D., Vice President of Scientific Affairs

The American Health Assistance Foundation (AHAF) is a registered non-profit organization that funds research into cures for Alzheimer's disease, macular degeneration and glaucoma, and provides the public with informantion about risk factors, preventative lifestyles, availiable treatments and coping strategies.

2748 American Occupational Therapy Foundation
4720 Montgomery Lane
P.O.Box 31220
Bethesda, MD 20814- 1220 301-652-6611
FAX: 301-656-3620
e-mail: aotf@aotf.org
aotf.org

Charles Christiansen, Executive Director
Diana Ramsay, President

AOFT provides advanced research, education and public awareness for occupational therapy, so that all people may participate fully in life regardless of their physical, social, mental or developmental circumstances.

2749 **Arc of Maryland**
PO Box 1747
Annapolis, MD 21401-1747 410-571-9320
888-272-3449
FAX: 410-974-6021
e-mail: info@thearcmd.org
www.thearcmd.org

Richard Dean, President
Aileen O'Hare, Vice President
Annette Hinkle, Treasurer
Adam Vanderhook, Secretary

The Arc of Maryland works to create a world where children and adults with cognitive and developmental disabilities have and enjoy equal rights and opportunities.

2750 **Baltimore Community Foundation**
2 E Read Street
Floor 9
Baltimore, MD 21202-6903 410-332-4171
FAX: 410-837-4701
e-mail: questions@bcf.org
www.bcf.org

Raymond L. Bank, Chair
Tedd Alexander, Vice Chair
Laura L. Gamble, Vice Chair
Thomas E. Wilcox, President

Makes grants in Baltimore City and Baltimore County; see website for how to apply. BCF is governed by a 30-member board of trustees, made up of a cross section of Baltimore.

2751 **Candlelighters Childhood Cancer Foundation**
PO Box 498
Kensington, MD 20895-0498 301-962-3520
855-858-2226
FAX: 301-962-3521
e-mail: staff@acco.org
www.acco.org

Naomi Bartley, President
Janine Lynne, Vice President
Ken Phillips, Treasurer
Judy Mendoza, Secretary

An international organization providing information and support, and advocacy to parents of children with cancer and survivors of childhood cancer.Health and Education professionals also welcome as members.Network of local support groups. Information on disabilities related to treatment of childhood cancer. Publications.

2752 **Children's Fresh Air Society Fund**
Baltimore Community Foundation
2 E Read St
Baltimore, MD 21202-2470 410-332-4171
FAX: 410-837-4701
e-mail: grants@bcf.org
bcf.org

Tom E. Wilcox, President
Danista Hunte, Vice President, Community Investment
Ralph M. Serpe, CFRE, Vice President, Development
Amy T. Seto, CPA, Vice President, Finance and Administration

Makes grants to nonprofit camps to provide tuition for disadvantaged and disabled Maryland children to attend summer camp. See website for how to apply.

2753 **Clark-Winchcole Foundation**
3 Bethesda Metro Ctr
Suite 550
Bethesda, MD 20814-5358 301-654-3607

Laura Phillips, President

Supported tax-exempt charitable organizations operating in the metropolitan area of Washington, DC in the following areas: deaf, higher education and physically disabled.

2754 **Columbia Foundation**
10630 Little Patuxent Parkway
Century Plaza, Suite 315
Columbia, MD 21044 410-730-7840
FAX: 410-997-6021
e-mail: info@columbiafoundation.org
www.cfhoco.org

Beverley White Seal, President / CEO
Priscilla Reaver, Senior Program Officer
Debbie Daskaloff, Development Officer
Tracy Locke-Kitt, Program Officer

The Columbia Foundation serves as a catalyst for building a more caring, creative and effective community in Howard County by promoting and creating opportunities for personal and corporate philanthropy, managing endowments, anticipating and responding to community needs, and strategically granting funds.

2755 **Corporate Giving Program**
Ryland Group
11000 Broken Land Pkwy
Columbia, MD 21044 410-715-7022
800-267-0998
FAX: 410-715-7909

Bruce N Haas, President

Contributions of equipment, volunteers and financial support to organizations working to meet the challenges and needs of modern society.

2756 **Cystic Fibrosis Foundation**
6931 Arlington Rd
2nd floor
Bethesda, MD 20814-5200 301-951-4422
800-344-4823
FAX: 301-951-6378
e-mail: info@cff.org
www.cff.org

Catherine C. McLoud, Board Chair
Robert J. Beall, Ph.D., President/Chief Executive Officer
C. Richard Mattingly, Executive Vice President/Chief Operating Officer
Preston W. Campbell, III, M.D., Executive Vice President for Medical Affairs

The mission of the Cystic Fibrosis Foundation, a nonprofit donor-supported organization is to assure the development of the means to cure and control cystic fibrosis and to improve the quality of life for those with the disease.

2757 **Foundation Fighting Blindness**
7168 Columbia Gateway Drive
Suite 100
Columbia, MD 21046 410-423-0600
800-683-5555
FAX: 410-363-2393
TTY: 800-683-5551
e-mail: info@fightblindness.org
www.blindness.org

William T. Schmidt, CEO
Annette Hinkle, CPA, Chief Financial Officer
James W. Minow, Chief Development Officer
Stephen M. Rose, Ph.D., Chief Research Officer

The urgent mission is to drive the research that will provide preventions, treatments, and cures for people affected by retinitis pigmentosa, macular degeneration, Usher syndrome and the entire spectrum of retinal degenerative diseases.

2758 **George Wasserman Family Foundation**
Grossberg Company
6707 Democracy Blvd
Suite 300
Bethesda, MD 20817-1176 301-571-4977
FAX: 301-571-6250

Helen Salud, Manager
Anthony Cpa, Partner

2759 Harry and Jeanette Weinberg Foundation
7 Park Center Ct
Owings Mills, MD 21117-4200 410-654-8500
FAX: 410-654-4900
e-mail: cdemchak@hjweinberg.org
hjweinbergfoundation.org
Ellen M. Heller, Chair
Barry I. Schloss, Treasurer
Alvin Awaya, Vice-President
Rachel Garbow Monroe, President and Chief Executive Officer
The Harry & Jeanette Weinberg Foundation, Inc. is dedicated to assisting the poor, primarily through operating and capital grants to direct service organizations located in Baltimore, Hawaii, Northeastern Pennsylvania, New York, Israel and the Former Soviet Union. These grants are focused on meeting basic needs such as shelter, nutrition, health & socialization & on enhancing an individual's ability to meet those needs. Within that focus, emphasis is placed on the elderly & Jewish community.

2760 Miracle-Ear Children's Foundation
5000 Cheshire Ln N
Minneapolis, MN 55446-3706 763-268-4000
800-464-8002
FAX: 763-268-4365
miracle-ear.com

2761 National Federation of the Blind
200 East Wells Street
at Jernigan Place
Baltimore, MD 21230-4998 410-659-9314
FAX: 410-685-5653
e-mail: nfb@nfb.org
nfb.org
John Berggren, Executive Director for Operation
John G. Paré Jr., Executive Director for Strategic Initiatives
Mark Riccobono, Executive Director, NFB Jernigan Institute
Joanne Wilson, Executive Director for Affiliate Action
The National Federation of the Blind (NFB) is the largest organization of the blind in the world. The Federation's purpose is to help blind people achieve self-confidence, self-respect, and self-determination. Their goal is the complete integration of the blind into society on a basis of equality.

2762 Sjogren's Syndrome Foundation
6707 Democracy Blvd
Suite 325
Bethesda, MD 20817-1164 301-530-4420
800-475-6473
FAX: 301-530-4415
e-mail: tms@sjogrens.org
www.sjogrens.org
Kenneth Economou, Chairman of the Board
Stephen Cohen, OD, Chairman-Elect
Vidya Sankar, DMD, MHS, Treasurer
Janet Ee. Church, Secretary
Provides patients practical information and coping strategies that minimize the effects of Sjogren's syndrome. In addition, the Foundation is the clearinghouse for medical information and is the recognized national advocate for Sjogren's syndrome.
$25.00
Monthly

Massachusetts

2763 Abbot and Dorothy H Stevens Foundation
P.O. Box 111
North Andover, MA 01845 978-688-7211
FAX: 978-686-1620
Josh Miner, Executive Director
Established in 1953, Purpose is giving primarily to the arts, education, conservation, and health and human services.

2764 Arc of Northern Bristol County
141 Park St
Attleboro, MA 02703-3020 508-226-1445
888-343-3301
FAX: 508-226-1476
e-mail: info@arcnbc.org
arcnbc.org
Richard Harwood, Chairperson
Valerie Zagami, Vice Chairperson
Paul Oliveira, Treasurer
D. Randall Hays, III, Secretary/Clerk
Mission is to strive for the right of all people with developmental disabilities to be valued as individuals, to experience choice, and to be fully included in all aspects of community life

2765 Boston Foundation
75 Arlington St
10th Fl
Boston, MA 02116-3992 617-338-1700
FAX: 617-338-1604
e-mail: info@tbf.org
tbf.org
Michael Keating, Esq., Chair
Catherine D'Amato, Vice Chair
Paul S. Grogan, President & CEO
Alfred F. Van Ranst, Jr., CFO and Treasurer
The Foundation's grantmaking, special initiatives and civic leadership promote innovation across a broad range of compelling community issues, from educational excellence to affordable housing to workforce development and the arts.

2766 Boston Globe Foundation
P.O. Box 55819
Boston, MA 02205-5819 617-929-2000
e-mail: lbailey@globe.com
bostonglobe.com
Mary Jacobus, President
The mission of the Boston Globe Foundation is to empower community-based organizations to effect real change in the ares of greatest need, where the Globe is uniquely postioned to add the most value. Priority focus areas: strengthen the reading, writing and critical thinking of young people, while fostering their inherent love of learning. Strengthen the roads that link people to culture. Strengthen the civic fabric of the city. Be responsive to the needs of our immediate community.

2767 Bushrod H Campbell and Ada F Hall Charity Fund
Palmer & Dodge
111 Huntington Ave
Boston, MA 02199-7610 617-239-0540
FAX: 617-227-4420
Brenda Taylor, Foundation Administrator
The fund's areas of interest include organizations and/or their projects supporting aid to the elderly, healthcare and population control. Medical research grants are administered through the Medical Foundation. No grants are awarded to individuals and the geographical area of support is limited to organizations located in Massachusetts within the area of Boston and Route 128.

2768 Clipper Ship Foundation
77 Summer St
Boston, MA 02110-1006 617-391-3088
FAX: 617-426-7087
e-mail: hblaisdell@gmafoundations.com
clippershipfoundation.org
Ron Ancrum, President
Makes grants to federally tax-qualified non-profit organizations offering human services to individuals living in Greater Boston and the cities of Lawrence and Brockton.

2769 **Community Foundation of Western Massachusetts**
P.O. Box 15769
1500 Main Street, Suite 2300
Springfield, MA 01115-5769 413-732-2858
FAX: 413-733-8565
e-mail: wmass@communityfoundation.org
www.communityfoundation.org

Katie Allan Zobel, President and CEO
Nancy Reiche, M.S.W., Vice President for Programs
Donna Roseman David, Chief Financial Officer/Chief Administrative Officer
Kristin Leutz, Vice President of Philanthropic Services
Provides a simple way to achieve the charitable objectives of donors most effectively; supports nonprofit organizations that offer programs in the arts, education, human services, healthcare, housing, and the environment; and works to improve the quality of life in our region.

2770 **Frank R and Elizabeth Simoni Foundation**
1401 Boston Providence Tpke
Norwood, MA 02062-5053 781-762-3449
FAX: 781-769-6166

Matthew Mac Donald, President
Ann Mac Donald, Secretary
Robert Mac Donald, Clerk

2771 **Friendly Ice Cream Corp Contributions Program**
1855 Boston Rd
Wilbraham, MA 01095-1002 413-543-3544
800-966-9970
FAX: 413-731-4467
friendlys.com

John Maguire, Chief Financial Officer
Steve Weigel, EVP, Chief Operating Officer
Pat Hickey, EVP, Chief Financial Officer
Tim Hopkins, EVP, Retail and Manufacturing

2772 **Greater Worcester Community Foundation**
370 Main St
Ste 650
Worcester, MA 01608-1738 508-755-0980
FAX: 508-755-3406
e-mail: info@greaterworcester.org
greaterworcester.org

Gerald Gaudette III, Chair
Warner S. Fletcher, Vice Chair
Thomas J. Bartholomew, Treasurer
Carolyn Stempler, Clerk
By focusing on the entire community rather then on any specific issue, the community foundation is able to address matters of greater importance to the people of the region. The Foundation has built a permanent, flexable endowment and has distributed grants and awards to a broad range of organizations and people throughout the region.

2773 **Hyams Foundation**
50 Federal St
Fl 9
Boston, MA 02110-2241 617-426-5600
FAX: 617-426-5696
e-mail: info@hyamsfoundation.org
hyamsfoundation.org

Martella Wilson-Taylor, Chair
Adam D. Seitchik, Treasurer
Roslyn M. Watson, Assistant Treasurer
Iris Gomez, Clerk
Mission is to increase economic and social justice and power within low-income communities in Boston and Chelsea, Massachusetts.

2774 **Raytheon Company Contributions Program**
870 Winter St
Waltham, MA 02451-1449 781-522-3000
FAX: 781-860-2172
raytheon.com

Thomas A. Kennedy, Chief Financial Officer
David C. Wajsgras, Senior Vice President and Chief Financial Officer
Keith J. Peden, Senior Vice President - Human Resources and Security
Jay B. Stephens, Senior Vice President - General Counsel and Secretary
Industry leader in defense and government electronics, space, information technology, technical services, and business aviation and special mission aircraft.

2775 **TJX Foundation**
TJX Companies
770 Cochituate Rd
Framingham, MA 01701-4666 508-390-1000
FAX: 508-390-2091
www.tjx.com

Carol Meyrowitz, CEO
The purpose of the TJX Foundation's Giving Program is to support qualified, tax-exempt nonprofit organizations that provide services which promote and improve the quality of life for children, women and families in need.

2776 **The Arc of Massachusetts**
217 South St
Waltham, MA 02453-2710 781-891-6270
FAX: 781-891-6271
e-mail: arcmass@arcmass.org
www.arcmass.org

Leo Sarkissian, Executive Director
Joshua Komyerox, Government Affairs Director
Brenda Asis, Development Director
Quarterly newsletter for The Arc of Massachusetts is Advocate.

2777 **Vision Foundation**
8901 Strafford Cir
Knoxville, TN 37923-1500 865-357-4603
FAX: 865-690-9322
e-mail: gordon@visionfoundation.net
www.visionfoundation.net

Gordon Adams, President
Offers counseling, support groups, seminars and transportation for the blind providing 600 members.

Michigan

2778 **Ann Arbor Area Community Foundation**
301 N Main St
Ste 300
Ann Arbor, MI 48104-1296 734-663-0401
FAX: 734-663-3514
e-mail: info@aaacf.org
aaacf.org

Bhushan Kulkarni, Chair
Michelle Crumm, Vice Chair
Brian P. Campbell, Treasurer
Cheryl W. Elliott, President & CEO
Interested in funding projects which will improve the quality of life for citizens of the Ann Arbor area. Eligible projects generally fall within these categories: education, culture, social service, community development, environmental awareness and health and wellness. The Foundation aims to support creative approaches to community needs and problems by making grants which will benefit the widest possible range of people.

2779 **Arc of Michigan**
State of Michigan
1325 S Washington Ave
Lansing, MI 48910-1652
517-487-5426
800-292-7851
FAX: 517-487-0303
e-mail: dhoyle@arcmi.org
arcmi.org

Dohn Hoyle, Executive Director
Sherri Boyd, Coordinator of Grants
Lisa Hertzer, Executive Assistant
Sybil Spencer, Communications Analyst
The Arc Michigan empowers local chapters to assure that citizens with disabilities are valued and that they and their families participate fully in and contribute to the life of their community.

2780 **Berrien Community Foundation**
2900 S State St
Ste 2e
Saint Joseph, MI 49085-2467
269-983-3304
FAX: 269-983-4939
e-mail: bcf@BerrienCommunity.org
berriencommunity.org

Tim Passaro, Chair
Hillary Bubb, Vice Chair
Jeffrey Dorn, Treasurer
Hon. Mabel Mayfield, Secretary
The Foundation is a union of numerous gifts, bequests and other contributions that form permanent endowments and other funds.

2781 **Blind Children's Fund**
6761 West 45-12
P.O. Box 363
Three Oaks, MI 49128
989-779-9966
FAX: 269-756-3133
e-mail: bcf@blindchildrensfund.org
www.blindchildrensfund.org

Karla B. Kwast, Executive Director
Provides parents and profesionsals informaion materials and resources that help them scuccesfullly teach and nurture blind, visually and multi-impaired infants and preschoolers.

2782 **Community Foundation of Monroe County**
P.O. Box 627
28 S. Macomb St.
Monroe, MI 48161-627
734-242-1976
FAX: 734-242-1234
e-mail: info@cfmonroe.org
cfmonroe.org

Kathleen Russeau, MBA, Executive Director
Michele Sandiefer, Office Manager
Julie Rhinehart, YAC Coordinator
Doug Redding, Project Manager
The mission of the Community Foundation of Monroe County is to encourage and facilitate philanthropy in Monroe County.

2783 **Cowan Slavin Foundation**
7881 Dell Rd
Saline, MI 48176-9744
734-944-1439
FAX: 734-944-3529
David Bovee, Owner

2784 **Daimler Chrysler**
Automobility Program
P.O. Box 5080
Troy, MI 48007-5080
800-255-9877
FAX: 855-409-0475
e-mail: rebates@chrysler.com
www.chryslerautomobility.com

2785 **Frank & Mollie S VanDervoort Memorial Foundation**
4646 Okemos Rd
Okemos, MI 48864-1795
517-349-7232

Ann L Gessert, Secretary

2786 **Fremont Area Community Foundation**
4424 W. 48th Street
Fremont, MI 49412-176
231-924-5350
FAX: 231-924-5351
e-mail: info@tfacf.org
tfacf.org

Carla Roberts, President & CEO
Robert Jordan, Vice President of Philanthropic
Gina Van Bruggen, Vice President of Program
Kathy Pope, Vice President of Finance
A local nonprofit organization serving the residence of Newaygo County. We connect the needs of the community with those who have the conviction to make a lasting impact. Our mission is to improve the quality of life for the people of Newaygo County.

2787 **Grand Rapids Foundation**
185 Oakes St SW
Grand Rapids, MI 49503-4008
616-454-1751
FAX: 616-454-6455
e-mail: grfound@grfoundation.org
grfoundation.org

Diana R. Sieger, President
Roberta F. King, APR, Vice President PR & Marketing
Marcia Rapp, Vice President, Programs
Laurie Craft, Program Director
Grand Rapids Community Foundation leads the community in making positive, sustainable change. Through our grantmaking and leadership initiatives we help foster academic achievement, build economic prosperity, achieve healthy ecosystems, encourage healthy people, support social enrichment, and create vibrant neighborhoods.

2788 **Granger Foundation**
6267 Aurelius Rd
Lansing, MI 48909-2187
517-393-1670
FAX: 517-393-1382
e-mail: elee@grangerconstruction.com
grangerconstruction.com

Alton Granger, Chairman
Glenn D. Granger, President & CEO
The primary purpose of the Granger Foundation is to enhance the quality of life within the Greater Lansing, Michigan Area. Our mission is to support Christ-centered activities. We also support efforts that enhance the lives of youth in our community.

2789 **Harvey Randall Wickes Foundation**
4800 Fashion Square Blvd
Saginaw, MI 48604-2677
989-799-1850
FAX: 989-799-3327

James Finkbeiner
Grants for rehabilitation.

2790 **Havirmill Foundation**
3503 Greenleaf Blvd
Ste 203
Kalamazoo, MI 49008-2580
269-375-1193

millenniumrestaurants.com

Ken Miller, CEO, Principal Partner
Shelly Pastor, CFO, Partner
Bob Lewis, COO, Partner
Matthew Burian, CBDO, CPO, F&B, Partner

2791 **Kelly Services Foundation**
999 W Big Beaver Rd
Troy, MI 48084-4782
248-362-4444
FAX: 248-244-4588
e-mail: kfirst@kellyservices.com
kellyservices.com

George S. Corona, Chief Operating Officer
Carl T. Camden, Chief Executive Officer
Patricia Little, Chief Financial Officer
Michael S. Webster, Global Solutions and General Manager, Americas

2792 Kresge Foundation
3215 W Big Beaver Rd
Troy, MI 48084-2818
248-643-9630
FAX: 248-643-0588
e-mail: info@kresge.org
kresge.org

Rip Rapson, President and CEO
Amy B. Coleman, Vice President and Chief Financial Officer
Ariel H. Simon, Chief Strategy Officer and Deputy to the President
Marcus L. McGrew, Director of Grants Management

This foundation offers challenge grants for capital projects, most often for construction or renovation of buildings, but also for the purchase of major equipment and real estate. As challenge grants, they are intended to stimulate new, private gifts in the midst of an organized fund raising effort. Offers special opportunities to build capacity, both in providing enhanced facilities in which to present programs and in generating private support. Only charitable organizations may apply.

2793 Lanting Foundation
1575 S Shore Dr
Holland, MI 49423-4436
616-355-2740

Arlyn Lanting, Partner

2794 Rollin M Gerstacker Foundation
PO Box 1945
Midland, MI 48641-1945
989-631-6097
www.gerstackerfoundation.org

Gail E. Lanphear, Chairperson
Lisa J. Gerstacker, President
E. N. Brandt, Vice President /Secretary
Alan Ott, Vice President /Treasurer

The Rollin M. Gerstacker Foundation was founded by Mrs. Eda U. Gerstacker in 1957, in memory of her husband. Its primary purpose is to carry on, indefinitely, financial aid to charities of all types supported by Mr. and Mrs. R.M. Gerstacker during their lifetimes. These charities are concentrated in the states of Michigan and Ohio.

2795 Steelcase Foundation
PO Box 1967
GH-4E
Grand Rapids, MI 49501-1967
616-246-4695
FAX: 616-475-2200
e-mail: pgebben@steelcase.com
steelcase.com

Phyllis Gebben, Coordinator of Donations
James P. Hackett, President & CEO

Established in 1951, the Foundation focuses on the areas of human service, health, education, community development, the arts and the environment – giving particular concern to people who are disadvantaged, disabled, young and elderly as they attempt to improve the quality of their lives.

Minnesota

2796 Arc of Minnesota
800 Transfer Road
Suite 7A
St. Paul, MN 55114
651-523-0823
800-582-5256
e-mail: mail@arcmn.org
www.arcmn.org

Pat Mellenthin, Executive Director
Steve Larson, Director of Public Policy
Mike Gude, Communications Manager

Your membership in The Arc of Minnesotta benefits persons with developmental disabilities and their families as they live, learn, work and play. Please join today!

2797 Deluxe Corporation Foundation
Deluxe Corporation
3680 Victoria St N
Shoreview, MN 55126-2966
651-483-7111
FAX: 651-483-7270
e-mail: feedback@deluxe.com
ww.deluxe.com

Lee J Schram, CEO
Terry D. Peterson, CFO /Senior VP
Malcolm J. McRoberts, Senior Vice President, Small Business Services
John D. Filby, Senior Vice President, Financial Services

Funds programs such as schools, museums, programs for the disadvantaged. We believe programs and services like these represent the heart and soul of our communities.

2798 General Mills Foundation
P.O. Box 9452
Minneapolis, MN 55440-9452
800-248-7310
FAX: 763-764-8330
e-mail: corporate.response@genmills.com
generalmills.com

Kendall J. Powell, Chairman / CEO
Mark W. Addicks, Senior Vice President/ Chief Marketing Officer
Kofi Bruce, Vice President, Treasurer
John Church, Vice President, Treasurer

2799 Hugh J Andersen Foundation
342 5th Ave N
Bayport, MN 55003-4502
651-439-1557
888-439-9508
FAX: 651-439-9480
e-mail: contact@srinc.biz
www.srinc.biz

Brad Kruse, Program Director

Established in 1962, this fund is a nonprofit charitable corporation classified as a private foundation. The Foundation was established as a general charitable fund, but now identifies projects that build individual and community capacity to be a priority. Giving is focused primarily in the counties of Washington, Minnesota, & St, Croix, Polk and Pierce of Wl. Grants are given in the areas of human services, health, education, arts and culture, community services and the environment.

2800 James R Thorpe Foundation
318 W 48th St
Minneapolis, MN 55419-5418
612-822-3412
e-mail: kerrieblevins@jamesrthorpefoundation.org
www.jamesrthorpefoundation.org

Tim Thorpe, President
Robert C. Cote, Treasurer
Kerrie Blevins, Foundation Manager
S. Ruggles Cote, Board Member

Foundation based on values of respect and compassion, and is dedicated to making the greater Minneapolis area better for all its citizens.

2801 Jay and Rose Phillips Family Foundation
615 First Ave. NE
Ste. 330
Minneapolis, MN 55413
612-623-1654
FAX: 612-623-1653
e-mail: info@phillipsfamilyfoundationmn.org
www.phillipsfnd.org

Patrick Troska, Executive Director
Joel Luedtke, Senior Program Officer
Tracy Lamparty, Grants and Operations Manager
Salena Acox, Vista Program Manager

2802 **Minneapolis Foundation**
80 S 8th St
Minneapolis, MN 55402-2100
612-672-3878
FAX: 612-672-3846
e-mail: email@mplsfoundation.org
www.mplsfoundation.org

Sandra L. Vargus, President and CEO
Jean M. Adams, Chief Operating Officer/Chief Financial Officer
Teresa Morrow, Vice President, External Relations and Marketing
Luz Maria Frias, Vice President, Community Impact

Provides a variety of charitable fund and gift options to help Minnesotans make a difference.

2803 **Ordean Foundation**
424 W Superior St
Duluth, MN 55802-1591
218-726-4785

Steve Mangan, Executive Director

Grants are given for a variety of purposes including: treatment and rehabilitation for persons who are chronically or temporarily mentally ill, persons whose physical capacity is impaired by injury or illness, promotes mental and physical health of the elderly, provides for youth guidance programs designed to avoid delinquency, and provides relief, aid and charity to people with no or low incomes. Grants are only offered to certain cities and townships near and around St. Louis County/Duluth.

2804 **Otto Bremer Foundation**
445 Minnesota St
Ste 2250
Saint Paul, MN 55101-2161
651-227-8036
888-291-1123
FAX: 651-312-3665
e-mail: obf@ottobremer.org
www.ottobremer.org

Kari Suzuki, Director of Operations
Randi Ilyse Roth, Executive Director
Danielle Cheslog, Grants Manager
Lue Her, Program Officer

Mission is to assist people in achieving full economic, civic and social participation in and for the betterment of their communities.

2805 **Rochester Area Foundation**
400 South Broadway
Suite 300
Rochester, MN 55904
507-282-0203
FAX: 507-282-4938
e-mail: info@rochesterarea.org
rochesterarea.org

JoAnn Stormer, President
Max Evans, Administration/Communications
Ann Fahy-Gust, Grants and Donors Manager
Paul Harkess, Development Officer

The mission of the Rochester Area Foundation is to strengthen community philanthropy by promoting responsible and informed giving and to assist donors in meeting their charitable objectives.

Mississippi

2806 **Arc of Mississippi**
704 North President Street
Jackson, MS 39202
601-355-0220
800-717-1180
FAX: 601-355-0221
e-mail: info@arcms.org
www.arcms.org

Kim Duffy, President
Ronnie Raggio, Senior Vice-President
Cherri Hedglin, Secretary
Christy Dunnaway, Treasurer

The Arc is Committed to securing for all people with developmental disabilities the opportunity to choose and realize their goals of where and how they learn live work and play.

Missouri

2807 **Allen P & Josephine B Green Foundation**
1055 Broadway
Suite 130
Kansas City, MO 64105
816-627-3420
FAX: 816-268-3420
e-mail: greenfoundation@gkccf.org
www.greenfdn.org

Matthew Fuller, Manager of Community Investment

While the Foundation makes grants in a variety of fields, in the past its major support was in the field of medical research. During a 20-year period, 1951-71, it contributed over $900,000 to research in Parkinson's and related diseases of the nervous system; $600,000 for research in pediatric neurology and lesser amounts in other areas of medical research, but the board is now trending in other directions. Grants are limited to Missouri and none are offered to individuals.

2808 **Anheuser-Busch**
1 Busch Pl
Saint Louis, MO 63118-1852
314-577-2000
800-342-5283
FAX: 314-577-2900
www.abcorpaffairs.com

August A Busch Iv, President

Supports education, helped fund health and human services organizations, provided disaster relief, and worked to preserve the environment.

2809 **Arc of the US Missouri Chapter**
PO Box 7823
Columbia, MO 65205
573-552-7648
e-mail: angela@arcofmissouri.org
www.arcofmissouri.org

2810 **Greater Kansas City Community Foundation & Affiliated Trusts**
1055 Broadwat St
Suite 130
Kansas City, MO 64105-1595
816-842-0944
FAX: 816-842-8079
e-mail: info@gkccf.org
gkccf.org

Robert D. Regnier, Chair
Dr. Jim Hinson, Vice Chair
Debbie Wilkerson, President/ CEO
Jeannine Strandjord, Treasurer

Mission is to improve the quality of life in Greater Kansas City by increasing charitable giving, connecting donors to community needs they care about, and providing leadership on critical community issues.

2811 **Greater St Louis Community Foundation**
319 N 4th St
Ste 300
Saint Louis, MO 63102-1930
314-588-8200
FAX: 314-588-8088
e-mail: dluckes@gstlcf.org
gstlcf.org

Amelia A.J. Bond, President/ CEO
Dwight D. Canning, Vice President & CFO
Christine G. Burghoff, Director of Gift Planning
Amy Basore Murphy, Director of Scholarships & Donor Services

To improve the quality of life across the region by helping individuals, families and businesses make a difference through charitable giving.

2812 H&R Block Foundation
1 H and R Block Way
Kansas City, MO 64105-1905 816-854-4361
FAX: 816-854-8025
e-mail: foundation@hrblock.com
www.blockfoundation.org

Henry W. Bloch, Chairman, Treasurer, and Directo
David P. Miles, President
Carey Wilker Looney, Vice President and Secretary
Robert L. Bloch, Program Officer

A charitable organization under the not-for-profit corporation law of the state of Missouri. Grants are made only to organizations which are tax exempt from Federal Income taxation and which are not classified as private foundations. Major emphasis is placed in the metropolitan areas of Kansas City, Missouri: and Columbus, Ohio. The goal is to provide proportionately significant support of relatively few activities, as opposed to minor support for a great many.

2813 James S McDonnell Foundation
1034 S Brentwood Blvd
Suite 1850
Saint Louis, MO 63117- 1284 314-721-1532
FAX: 314-721-7421
e-mail: info@jsmf.org
jsmf.org

John T. Bruer, Ph.D., President
Susan M. Fitzpatrick, Ph.D., Vice President
Cheryl A. Washington, Grants Manager
M. Brent Dolezalek, Senior Program Associate

The Foundation supports scientific, educational, and charitable causes locally, nationally and internationally.

2814 Lutheran Charities Foundation of St Louis
8860 Ladue Road
Suite 200
Saint Louis, MO 63124 314-231-2244
FAX: 314-727-7688
e-mail: info@lutheranfoundation.org
www.lutheranfoundation.org

Karl A. Dunajcik, Chairperson of the Board
Ann L. Vazquez, President/ CEO
Melinda K. McAliney, Program Director
Donna Luker, Office/Grants Manager

Seeks the improved care of people in the greater St. Louis metropolitan region. Lutheran Foundation of St. Louis manages the endowment established upon the sale of the Lutheran Medical Center and provides grant awards for health, human care, Lutheran congregations' community service programs, and Lutheran education.

2815 RA Bloch Cancer Foundation
1 H and R Block Way
Kansas City, MO 64105-1905 816-854-5050
800-433-0464
FAX: 816-854-8024
e-mail: hotline@blochcancer.org
www.blochcancer.org

Vangie Rich, Executive Director
Rosanne Wickman, Hotline Director

Provides a hotline that matches newly diagnosed cancer patients with someone who has survived the same kind of cancer. Offers free infomration, resources and support groups, and distributes lists of multidisciplinary second opinion centers. Also supplies three books at no charge: Fighting Cancer; Cancer... There's Hope; and A Guide for Cancer Supporters. All services and books are free of charge.

2816 Victor E Speas Foundation
10434 Indiana Ave
Kansas City, MO 64137-1532 816-868-9300
e-mail: vccmetro@crn.org
www.vcckcmetro.org

Latricia Scott Adams, President

VCC is a membership-based organization that brings together area volunteer managers and others interested in volunteerism for mutual support, exchange of ideas and information, and educational programs of timely interest.

Nebraska

2817 Arc of Nebraska
215 Centennial Mall South
Suite 508
Lincoln, NE 68508 402-475-4407
FAX: 402-475-0214
e-mail: info@arc-nebraska.org
www.arc-nebraska.org

Debbie Salomon, President
David Rowe, 1st Vice President
Kadi Holmberg, 2nd Vice President
Melissa Mazzulla, Treasurer

Arc of Nebraska is commited to helping children and adults with disabilities secure the oppurtunity to choose and realize their goals of where and how they learn, live, work, and play.

2818 Cooper Foundation
1248 O St
870 Wells Fargo Center
Lincoln, NE 68508-1493 402-476-7571
FAX: 402-476-2356
e-mail: info@cooperfoundation.org
cooperfoundation.org

Jack Campbell, Chair
Brad Korell, Finance Director
Art Thompson, President
Norton E. Warner, President

Serves only Nebraska with the primary interest in education, arts and humanities and the human services area.

2819 Mosaic
4980 S 118th St
Omaha, NE 68137-2200 402-896-9988
877-366-7242
FAX: 402-896-1511
www.mosaicinfo.org

Linda Timmons, President / CEO
Cindy Schroeder, Chief Financial Officer
Keith Schmode, Sr VP of Mission Advancement & CEO of The Mosaic Foundation
Raul Saldivar, Chief Operating Officer and Chief Integrity Officer

Headquarters for the faith-based organization providing services to people with disabilities in communities nationwide, and in conjunction with international partners. Mosaic was born of a merger of these two Lutheran organizations: Bethpage and Martin Luther Homes Society.

2820 Slosburg Family Charitable Trust
10040 Regency Cir
Ste 200
Omaha, NE 68114-3734 402-391-7900
FAX: 402-391-2991
richdale.com

David Slosburg, Owner

2821 Union Pacific Foundation
1400 Douglas St
Omaha, NE 68179 402-544-5000
888-870-8777
FAX: 402-501-0021
www.up.com

John J. Koraleski, Chairman and Chief Executive Officer
Lance M. Fritz, President & COO of Union Pacific Railroad
Eric L. Butler, Executive Vice President - Marketing and Sales
Diane K. Duren, Executive Vice President and Corporate Secretary

The Union Pacific Foundation is the philanthropic arm of the Union Pacific Corporation and Union Pacific Railroad. Union Pacific believes that the quality of life in the commuinities in which its employees live and work is an integral part of its own success.

Nevada

2822 Conrad N Hilton Foundation
30440 Agoura Road
Agoura Hills, CA 91301
818-851-3700
FAX: 310-694-9051
e-mail: cnhf@hiltonfoundation.org
hiltonfoundation.org

Steven M. Hilton, Chairman, President & CEO
Patrick J. Modugno, Vice President, Administration & CFO
Taryn Lee, Human Resources Director
Katherine Miller, Facilities and Office Services Manager

Our grant-making style is to initiate and develop major long-term projects and then seek out the organizations to implement them. As a consequence of this proactive approach, the Foundation does not generally consider unsolicited proposals. Our major projects currently include: blindness prevention and treatment, support the work of the Catholic Sisters, drug abuse prevention among youth, support of the Conrad N. Hilton College of Hotel and Restaurant Management, and much more.

2823 EL Wiegand Foundation
165 W Liberty St
Suite 200
Reno, NV 89501-1955
775-333-0310
FAX: 775-333-0314

Kristen A Avansino, President/Executive Director

2824 Nell J Redfield Foundation
PO Box 61
Reno, NV 89504
775-323-1373
FAX: 775-323-4476

Jerry Smith, Manager

2825 William N Pennington Foundation
441 W Plumb Ln
Reno, NV 89509-3766
775-333-9100
FAX: 775-333-9111

William Pennington, Owner

New Hampshire

2826 Agnes M Lindsay Trust
660 Chestnut St
Manchester, NH 03104-3550
603-669-1366
866-669-1366
FAX: 603-665-8114
e-mail: admin@lindsaytrust.org
lindsaytrust.org

Susan E. Bouchard, Administrative Director
Ernest E. Dion, CPA, Trustee
Alan G. Lampert, Esq., Trustee
Michael S. Delucia, Esq., Trustee

Funding for health and wefare organizations, special needs, mental health, blind, deaf and cultural programs to organizations, specifically for capital needs, not operating funds, located in the New England states of Maine, Massachusetts, New Hampshire and Vermont. We highly recommend you visit our web site.

2827 Foundation for Seacoast Health
100 Campus Dr
Ste 1
Portsmouth, NH 03801-5892
603-422-8200
FAX: 603-422-8206
e-mail: ffsh@communitycampus.org
ffsh.org

Debra S. Grabowski, Executive Director
Kathleen Taylor, Finance Director
Eligio Santana, Facility Manager
Noreen Hodgdon, Executive Assistant

Giving limited to Portsmouth, Rye, New Castle, Greenland, Newington, North Hampton, NH; and Kittery, Eliot, and York, ME.

New Jersey

2828 Arc of New Jersey
985 Livingston Ave
N Brunswick, NJ 8902-1843
732-246-2525
FAX: 732-214-1834
e-mail: info@arcnj.org
arcnj.org

Thomas Baffuto, Executive Director
Celine Fortin, Associate Executive Director
Sharon Levine, Director, Governmental Affairs
Ashley Scott, Communications Coordinator

The Arc of New Jersey is committed to enhancing the quality of life of children and adults with intellectual and developmental disabilities and their families, through advocacy, empowerment, education and prevention.

2829 Arnold A Schwartz Foundation
15 Mountain Blvd
Warren, NJ 7059-5611
908-757-7800
FAX: 908-757-8039
e-mail: skunzmannewjerseylaw.net

Steven A Kunzman, President

2830 Campbell Soup Foundation
1 Campbell Pl
Camden, NJ 08103-1701
800-257-8443
e-mail: media@campbellsoup.com
campbellsoup.com

Denise M. Morrison, President /Chief Executive Officer
Anthony P. DiSilvestro, Senior Vice President and Chief Financial Officer
Mark Alexander, Senior Vice President and President - Campbell North America
Carlos J. Barraso, Senior Vice President - Global Research & Development

Goal of this foundation is to match the company's assets with community needs in order to help forge solutions to community challenges. The Foundation believes that involvement at the community level can play a catalytic role in improving the quality of life. Giving is located in the areas of education, nutrition and health, cultural and youth related programs. The major focus of the foundation is on nutrition and health related matters, and places a high priority on Camden, New Jersey areas.

2831 Children's Hopes & Dreams Wish Fulfillment Foundation
280 US Highway 46
Dover, NJ 07801-2084
706-482-2248
FAX: 706-482-2289
e-mail: info@chddover.org
www.helpingnow.org

2832 Community Foundation of New Jersey
PO Box 338
Morristown, NJ 07963-388
973-267-5533
800-659-5533
FAX: 973-267-2903
e-mail: hdekker@cfnj.org
www.cfnj.org

Hans Dekker, President
Nancy Hamilton, Program Officer
Karen Arias, Grants Administrator
Patty Heath, Financial Assistant

The Community Foundation of New Jersey is an alliance of families, businesses, and foundations that work together to create lasting differences in lives and communities today and tomorrow.

2833 FM Kirby Foundation
PO Box 151
Morristown, NJ 07963-0151
973-538-4800

www.fdncenter.org/grantmaker/kirby

S. Dillard Kirby, President and Director
Jefferson W Kirby, Vice President and Director
Alice Kirby Horton, Assistant Secretary and Director
Wilson M. Compton, M.D.M.P.E., Director

Family foundation, grants made to a wide range of nonprofit organizations in education, health and medicine, the arts and humanities, civic and public affairs, as well as religious, welfare and youth organizations.

2834 Fannie E Rippel Foundation
14 Maple Avenue
Suite 200
Morristown, NJ 07960 973-540-0101
FAX: 973-540-0404
e-mail: info@rippelfoundation.org
www.rippelfoundation.org

Laura K Landy, President/ CEO
Chana Fitton, CFO & Vice President, Administration
Kimberly Hines Hart, JD, Legal Associate
Patricia MacBain, Office Manager

Core purposes: research and treatment related to cancer and heart disease, the health of women and the elderly, and the quality of our nation's hospitals.

2835 Fund for New Jersey
One Palmer Square East
Suite 303
Princeton, NJ 08542 609-356-0421
e-mail: lmandell@fundfornj.org
fundfornj.org

Kiki Jamieson, President
Lucy Vandenberg, Senior Program Officer
Laura Mandell, Office Manager
Brandon McKoy, Program Associate

Our grants promote projects that share a high purpose of furthering effective democracy through a range of methods encompassing education, advocacy, public policy analysis, and community problem-solving.

2836 Merck Company Foundation
PO Box 100
Whitehouse Station, NJ 08889 908-423-1000
merck.com

Kenneth C. Frazier, Chairman of the Board, Chief Executive Officer
Robert M. Davis, Executive Vice President and Chief Financial Officer
Willie A. Deese, EVP and President, Merck Manufacturing Division
Clark Golestani, Executive Vice President and Chief Information Officer

Mission of the foundation is to support organizations and innovative programs in alignment with four strategic profiles: Improving access to quality health care and the appropriate use of medicines and vaccines,building capacity in the biomedical and health sciences, promoting environments that support innovation, economic growth and development in and ethical and fair context, and supporting communities where Merck employees work and live.

2837 Nabisco Foundation
7 Campus Dr
Parsippany, NJ 07054-4413 973-682-7096
FAX: 973-503-3018

Henry Sandbach, Director

2838 Ostberg Foundation
PO Box 1098
Alpine, NJ 07620-1098 201-569-6800
FAX: 201-767-8006

2839 Prudential Foundation
Prudential Financial
751 Broad St
15th Floor
Newark, NJ 07102-3714 973-802-6000
FAX: 973-802-7486
e-mail: community.resources@prudential.com
prudential.com

John R Strangfeld, Chairman and CEO
Mark B. Grier, Vice Chairman
Charles Lowrey, Executive Vice President, Chief Operating Officer, Internati
Sharon C. Taylor, Senior Vice President, Corporate Human Resources

Gives priority to national programs that further our objectives and programs serving areas where The Prudential has a substantial employee presence. Places special emphasis on the home state of New Jersey and the headquarters city, Newark.

2840 Robert Wood Johnson Foundation
PO Box 2361
Route 1 and College Road East
Princeton, NJ 08543-2361 609-452-8701
877-843-7953
FAX: 888-727-1966
e-mail: mail@rwjf.org
rwjf.org

Risa Lavizzo-Mourey, President and CEO
Robin E. Mockenhaupt, Chief of Staff
Joan F. McKay, Executive Assistant, Executive Office
Wilma L. Packard, Administrative Coordinator, Executive Office

Our mission is to assure that all Americans have access to basic health care at reasonable cost, improve care and support for people with chronic health conditions, promote healthy communities and lifestyles and also, reduce the personal, social and economic harm caused by substance abuse.

2841 Victoria Foundation
31 Mulberry Street
5th Floor
Newark, NJ 07102-1397 973-792-9200
FAX: 973-792-1300
e-mail: info@victoriafoundation.org
www.victoriafoundation.org

Irene Cooper-Basch, Executive Officer
Dale Anglin, Senior Program Officer
Craig Drinkard, Senior Program Officer
Chiu Chan, Grants Manager

Desire is to help individuals in need reach their potential remains. Provides emergency coal for needy families and treated rheumatic fever in children.

New Mexico

2842 Arc of New Mexico
3655 Carlisle NE
Albuquerque, NM 87110-1644 505-883-4630
800-358-6493
FAX: 505-883-5564
e-mail: rcostales@arcnm.org
arcnm.org

Randy Costales, Executive Director
Dinah Harvey, Director of Operations/ Human Resources
Doris Husted, Director for Public Policy
Irene Sanchez, Finance Manager

Our mission is to improve the quality of life for individuals with developmental disabilities of all ages by advocating for equal opportunities and choices in where and how they learn, live, work, play and socialize. The Arc of New Mexico promotes self-determination, healthy families, effective community support systems and partnerships.

2843 Frost Foundation
511 Armijo St
Suite A
Santa Fe, NM 87501-2899 505-986-0208
e-mail: info@frostfound.org
frostfound.org
Mary Amelia Whited-Howell, President
Philip B. Howell, Executive Vice President
Taylor F. Moore, Secretary/Treasurer
Ann Rogers Gerber, Board Member
The Frost Foundation was created to be operated excusively for educational, charitable, and religious purposes.

2844 McCune Charitable Foundation
345 E Alameda St
Santa Fe, NM 87501-2229 505-983-8300
FAX: 505-983-7887
e-mail: mccune@nmmccune.org
nmmccune.org
Wendy Lewis, Executive Director
Henry Rael, Program Director
Carla Romero, Administrative Director
Jacquelyn Gutierrez, Grants Program Coordinator
Dedicated to enriching the health, education, environment, and cultural and spiritual life of New Mexicans.

2845 Santa Fe Community Foundation
PO Box 1827
501 Halona Street
Santa Fe, NM 87505 505-988-9715
FAX: 505-988-1829
e-mail: foundation@santafecf.org
www.santafecf.org
Jerry G. Jones, Interim President and CEO
Christa Coggins, Vice President for Community Philanthropy
Sarah A. Sawtell, CPA, Vice President for Finance and Operations
Yolanda Cruz, Health Councils and Community Coordinator

New York

2846 AT&T Foundation
32 Avenue of the Americas
24th Floor
New York, NY 10013-2473 212-226-2216
FAX: 212-387-5097
e-mail: info@att.com
www.att.com
Randall L Stephenson, Chairman, Chief Executive Officer and President
John T. Stanky, Group President and Chief Strategy Officer
Wayne Watts, Senior Executive Vice President and General Counsel
John Stephens, Senior Executive Vice President and Chief Financial Officer
Committed to advancing education, strengthening communities and improving lives.

2847 Altman Foundation
521 5th Ave
Fl 35
New York, NY 10175-3500 212-682-0970
e-mail: info@altman.org
altmanfoundation.org
Jane B O'Connell, President
Karen L. Rosa, Vice President & Executive Direc
Jeremy Tennenbaum, CFO
Megan McAllister, Program Officer
For the benefit of such charitable and educational institutions in the City of New York as said directors shall approve. Foundation grants support programs and institutions that enrich the quality of life in the city, with a particular focus on initiatives that help individuals, families and communities benefit from the services and opportunities that will enable them to achieve their full potential.

2848 Ambrose Monell Foundation
1 Rockefeller Plz
Suite 301
New York, NY 10020-2002 212-586-0700
FAX: 212-245-1863
e-mail: info@monellvetlesen.org
www.monellvetlesen.org
George Rowe Jr., President, Treasurer and Director
Ambrose K. Monell, Vice-President and Director
Eugene P. Grisanti, Vice-President and Director
Gary K. Beauchamp, Director
Voluntary aiding and contributing to religious, charitable, scientific, literary, and educational uses and purposes, in New York, elsewhere in the US and throughout the world.

2849 American Chai Trust
41 Madison Ave
Suite 400
New York, NY 10010-2202 212-889-0575
FAX: 212-743-8120
e-mail: info@perlmanandperlman.com
www.perlmanandperlman.com

2850 American Express Foundation
P.O. Box 981540
El Paso, TX 79998-1540 800-528-4800
TTY:800-221-9950
americanexpress.com
Kenneth I Chenault, Chairman and Chief Executive Officer
L. Kevin Cox, Chief Human Resources Officer
Marc D. Gordon, Executive Vice President and Chief Information Officer
John D. Hayes, Executive Vice President and Chief Marketing Officer
Grants are awarded in the three program areas: Community Service, Cultural Heritage, and Economic Independence. Most grants are made for projects operating where the company has a major employee or market presence.

2851 American Foundation for the Blind
2 Penn Plaza
Suite 1102
New York, NY 10001-2018 212-502-7600
200-232-5463
FAX: 888-545-8331
e-mail: afbinfo@afb.net
afb.org
Carl Augusto, President/ CEO
Kelly Bleach, Chief Administrative Officer
Rick Bozeman, Chief Financial Officer
Adrianna Montague-Devaud, Chief Communications and Marketing Officer
Dedicated to addressing issues of literacy, independent living, employment, and access through technology for the ten million Americans who are blind or visually impaired.

2852 Arthur Ross Foundation
20 E 74th St
Ste 4c
New York, NY 10021-2654 212-737-7311
FAX: 212-650-0332
Arthur Ross, President

2853 Artists Fellowship
47 5th Ave
New York, NY 10003-4303 212-255-7740
e-mail: info@artistsfellowship.org
www.artistsfellowship.org
Babette Bloch, President
Private, charitable foundation that assists professional fine arts and their families in times of emergency, disability, or bereavement.

2854 **Bodman Foundation**
767 3rd Ave
Fl 4
New York, NY 10017-9029 212-644-0322
FAX: 212-759-6510
e-mail: main@achelis-bodman-fnds.org
www.achelis-bodman-fnds.org

John B. Krieger, Executive Director
John N. Irwin III, Chairman
Russell P. Pennoyer, President
Peter Frelinghuysen, Vice President
Foundation concentrates their grant programs in New York City, but foundation also makes some grants in Northern New Jersey. Funding is concentrated in six program areas: Arts & Culture, Education, Employment, Health, Public Policy and Youth and Families.

2855 **Brooklyn Home for Aged Men**
P.O.Box 280062
Brooklyn, NY 11228 718-745-1638
FAX: 718-745-0813
www.brooklynhome.org

Catherine M. Birdseye, Co-President
William E. Spaulding, Co-President
Andelusia Wheeler, Co-President
Edwin A. Ames, Co-President
The Brooklyn Home For Aged Men has served the community for more than one hundred years. Although originally set up as a residence for men, it later accepted women and couples as well.

2856 **Cancer Care**
275 7th Avenue
22nd Floor
New York, NY 10001-6754 212-712-8400
800-813-4673
FAX: 212-712-8495
e-mail: info@cancercare.org
www.cancercare.org

Patricia J. Goldsmith, CEO
John Rutigliano, COO
Jan McDavitt, Chief Development Officer
Brian Tomlinson, MPA, BSW, Chief Program and Communications Officer
A national non-profit organization that provides free, professional support services to anyone affected by cancer: people with cancer, caregivers, children, loved ones, and the bereaved.

2857 **Children's Tumor Foundation**
120 Wall Street
16th Floor
New York, NY 10005-3904 212-344-6633
800-323-7938
FAX: 212-747-0004
e-mail: info@ctf.org
ctf.org

Annette Bakker, PhD, President and Chief Scientific Officer
Judi Swartout, CPA, CFO
John Heropoulos, Vice President
Simon Vukelj, Communications Director
A nonprofit 501 (c)(3) medical foundation, dedicated to improving the health and well-being of individuals and families affected by neurofibromatosis. The Foundation sponsors medical research, clinical services, public education programs and patient support services. It is the central source for up-to-date and accurate information about NF. It also assists patients and families with referrals to NF clinics and healthcare professionals specializing in NF. The goal is to find a cure for NF.

2858 **Commonwealth Fund**
1 E 75th St
New York, NY 10021-2692 212-606-3800
FAX: 212-606-3500
e-mail: info@cmwf.org
www.commonwealthfund.org

David Blumenthal, M.D., President
John E. Craig, Jr., Executive Vice President and Chief Operating Officer
Donald Moulds, Executive Vice President for Programs
Barry Scholl, Senior Vice President for Communications and Publishing
A private foundation with the broad charge to enhance the common good. Carries out this mandate by supporting efforts that help people live healthy and productive lives, and by assisting certain groups with serious and neglected problems. Supports independent research on health and social issues and makes grants to improve heathcare practice and policy.

2859 **Community Foundation for Greater Buffalo**
726 Exchange Street,
Suite 525
Buffalo, NY 14202 716-852-2857
FAX: 716-852-2861
e-mail: mail@cfgb.org
cfgb.org

Clotilde Per Dedecker, President/CEO
Betsy Constantine, Vice President, Giving Strategies
Kate Masiello, Director, Client Relations
Jane Mogavero, Esq., Director, Client Relations
Mission is connecting people, ideas, and resources to improve lives in Western New York

2860 **Community Foundation of Herkimer & Oneida Counties**
1222 State St
Utica, NY 13502-4728 315-735-8212
FAX: 315-735-9363
e-mail: info@foundationhoc.org
foundationhoc.org

Peggy O'Shea, President/CEO
Gilles Lauzon, Director of Finance
Elayne Johnson, Director of Fund Administration
Barbara Henderson, Vice President for Programs and Community Initiatives
Mission of the foundation is to improve the lives of the residents of Herkimer and Oneida Counties.

2861 **Community Foundation of the Capitol Region**
Six Tower Place
Albany, NY 12203-3749 518-446-9638
FAX: 518-446-9708
e-mail: info@cfgcr.org
www.cfgcr.org

Karen Bilowith, President/CEO
Mindy Derosia, Development Officer
Tom Hudy, Director of Finance
Jackie Mahoney, Vice President of Programs
Mission is to strengthen our community by attracting charitable endowments both large and small, maximizing benefits to donors, making effective gtants, and providing leadership to address community needs.

2862 **Comsearch: Broad Topics**
Foundation Center
79 5th Ave
New York, NY 10003-3034 212-620-4230
800-424-9836
FAX: 212-807-3677
e-mail: communications@foundationcenter.org
www.fdncenter.org

Bradford K. Smith, President
Lisa Philip, Vice President for Strategic Philanthropy
R. Nancy Albilal, Vice President for Development
Robert Yaeger, Vice President for Finance and Administration
Subset publications of The Foundation Grants Index, are printouts of actual foundation grants, covering 26 key areas of grantmaking. This tool is designed for fundraisers who wish to

examine grantmaking activities in a broad field of interest. *$55.00*

2863 DE French Foundation
Ste 503
120 Genesee St
Auburn, NY 13021-3672 315-252-3634

Walter Lowe, Owner

2864 Dana Foundation
Dana Alliance for Brain Initiatives
505 Fifth Avenue
6th floor
New York, NY 10017 212-223-4040
FAX: 212-317-8721
e-mail: danainfo@dana.org
www.dana.org

Edward F Rover, President /Chairman
Burton M. Mirsky, Executive Vice President, Finance
Barbara Rich, Ed.D., EVP, Communications; Assistant Secretary
Rosemary Shields, Director of Office Administration
A private philanthropy with principal interests in brain science, immunology, and arts education.

2865 David J Green Foundation
Ste 12
599 Lexington Ave
New York, NY 10022-6030 212-317-8820
FAX: 212-371-5099
www.djgreene.com

Valerie Ventolora, Manager
Michael Greene, Manager

2866 Easter Seals New York
40 W 37th St
Suite 503
New York, NY 10018-7907 212-220-2290
800-727-8785
FAX: 212-695-4807
e-mail: jmcgrath@eastersealsny.org
www.easterseals.com/newyork

John W. McGrath, MPA, Chief Executive Director
Aris Pavlides, Senior Vice President Development
Thomas Renart, M.A., M.S., Senior Vice-President Program Services
Kevin Carey, Director of Finance
Offers resources and expertise that allow children and adults with disabilities to live with dignity and independence. A long standing commitment to serve those for whom no other resources exist. Statewide, provides innovative solutions that enhance the lives of people with disabilities, while heightening community awareness and acceptance.

2867 Edna McConnel Clark Foundation
415 Madison Ave
Tenth Floor
New York, NY 10017-7949 212-551-9100
FAX: 212-421-9325
e-mail: info@emcf.org
emcf.org

Nancy Roob, President
Woodrow C. McCutchen, Vice President, Senior Portfolio Manager
Kelly Fitzsimmons, Vice President, Chief Program and Strategy Officer
Helps young people, ages 9-24, from low-income backgrounds become independent, productive adults.

2868 Edward John Noble Foundation
Fl 19
32 E 57th St
New York, NY 10022-8562 212-759-4212
FAX: 212-888-4531

June Noble Larkin, Owner
June Larkin, Owner

2869 Epilepsy Foundation of Long Island
506 Stewart Ave
Garden City, NY 11530-4706 516-739-7733
888-672-7154
FAX: 516-739-1860
e-mail: jlpsky@epil.org
www.epil.org

Paul Giotis, Executive Director
Provides education, counseling and residential care to Long Island residents with epilepsy and related conditions.

2870 Episcopal Charities
1047 Amsterdam Ave
New York, NY 10025-1747 212-316-7575

e-mail: episcopalcharities@dioceseny.org
episcopalcharities-newyork.org

John Talty, President
Lorraine A. LaHuta, Vice President
Susan Jansen, Treasurer
Evan A. Davis, Secretary
Provides funding and support to a broad range of community-based human service programs throughout the Diocese of New York. These programs, sponsored by Episcopal congregations, serve disadvantaged individuals, youth and families on a non-sectarian basis.

2871 Esther A & Joseph Klingenstein Fund
125 Park Avenue
Suite 1700
New York, NY 10017-5529 212-492-6195

e-mail: kathleen.pomerantz@klingenstein.com
www.klingfund.org

Charles D. Gilbert, Chairman
John Klingenstein, President
Kathleen Pomerantz, Vice President
Supports young investigators engaged in basic or clinical research that may lead to a better understanding of epilepsy

2872 Fay J Lindner Foundation
189 Wheatley Road
Brookville, NY 11545 516-686-4440

www.fayjlindnercenter.org

Terrence Ullrich, President
Dr. Robert Steinberger, Vice President
Thomas F. Moore, Treasurer
Frederick Sterbenz, Secretary

2873 Ford Foundation
320 E 43rd St
New York, NY 10017-4890 212-573-5000
FAX: 212-351-3677
e-mail: office-of-communications@fordfoundation.org
www.fordfound.org

Darren Walker, President
Rricardo A. Castro, Vice President, Secretary and General Counsel
Marta L. Tellado, Vice President/Communications
Nicholas M. Gabriel, Vice President, Treasurer and Chief Financial Officer
A resource for innovative people and institutions worldwide. Goals are to: strenghthen democratic values; reduce poverty and injustice; promote international cooperation; and advance human achievement. While not specific to disabilities, the Ford Foundation operates on several levels that indirectly assist and support those with disabilities through human and civil rights issues, social justice support, economic fairness and opportunity, and access to education involvements.

2874 Fortis Foundation
1 Chase Manhattan Plz
New York, NY 10005-1401 212-859-7029
FAX: 212-859-7010
e-mail: Investor.Relations@assurant.com
ir.assurant.com

Melissa Kivett, Senior Vice President, Investor
Suzanne Shepherd, Director, Investor Relations

2875 Foundation Center
79 5th Ave
New York, NY 10003-3076 212-620-4230
800-424-9836
FAX: 212-807-3677
e-mail: communications@foundationcenter.org
foundationcenter.org

Bradford K Smith, President
Gabriela Fitz, Director of Knowledge Management Initiatives
Anjula Duggal, Vice President for Marketing and Communications
R. Nancy Albilal, Vice President for Development
The Foundation Center publishes Foundation Directory Online, with key facts on the US grantmakers and their grants.

2876 Foundation Center Library Services
Foundation Center
79 5th Ave
New York, NY 10003-3076 212-620-4230
800-424-9836
FAX: 212-807-3677
e-mail: communications@foundationcenter.org
foundationcenter.org

Bradford K Smith, President
Gabriela Fitz, Director of Knowledge Management Initiatives
Anjula Duggal, Vice President for Marketing and Communications
R. Nancy Albilal, Vice President for Development
The Center disseminates current information on foundation and corporate giving through our national collections in New York City and Washington D.C., our field offices in San Francisco and our network of over 180 cooperating libraries in all 50 states and abroad.

2877 Foundation for Advancement in Cancer Therapy
P.O.Box 1242
New York, NY 10113-1242 212-741-2790
www.fact-ltd.org

Ruth Sackman, President
A clearinghouse for information regarding alternative cancer therapies, emphasizing nutritional and metabolic approaches.

2878 Gebbie Foundation
215 Cherry St
Jamestown, NY 14701-5207 716-487-1062
FAX: 716-484-6401
e-mail: info@gebbie.org
www.gebbie.org

Gregory J Edwards, CEO
Andrea Magnuson, Associate Director
Jennifer C. Cresanti, Program Officer
Karla LoPresti, Administrative Assistant
Giving in Chautauqua County, and secondly, in neighboring areas of western New York. Giving is offered in other areas only when the project is consonant with program objectives that cannot be developed locally.

2879 Gladys Brooks Foundation
1055 Franklin Avenue
Suite 208
Garden City, NY 11530
e-mail: kathy@gladysbrooksfoundation.org
www.gladysbrooksfoundation.org

Jessica L Rutledge, Director
The purpose of this Foundation is to provide for the intellectual, moral and physical welfare of the people of this country by establishing and supporting nonprofit libraries, educational institutions, hospitals and clinics. The Foundation will make grants only to private, publicly supported, nonprofit, tax-exempt organizations.

2880 Glickenhaus Foundation
546 5th Ave
New York, NY 10036-5000 212-953-7800
e-mail: info@glickenhaus.com
glickenhaus.com

Seth M. Glickenhaus, Senior Partner and Chief Investm

2881 Guide Dog Foundation for the Blind
371 East Jericho Turnpike
Smithtown, NY 11787-2976 800-548-4337
FAX: 631-930-9009
e-mail: info@guidedog.org
guidedog.org

Wells B. Jones, FASAE, CFRE, CA, CEO
Laura English, CFO
Loretta Quis, Director of Administrative Services
Andrew Rubenstein, Director of Marketing
Providing mobility through the use of trained guide or service dogs to individuals who are blind or with other special needs.

2882 Hearst Foundations
300 W 57th St
Fl 26
New York, NY 10019-3741 212-649-2000
FAX: 212-887-6855
hearst.com

Steven R. Swartz, President and Chief Executive Officer
National philanthropic resources for organziations and institutions working in the fields of education, health, culture and social services. Our goal is to ensure that people of all backgrounds have the opportunity to build healthy, productive and inspiring lives.

2883 Henry and Lucy Moses Fund
405 Lexington Ave
New York, NY 10174-1299 212-554-7800
FAX: 212-554-7700
e-mail: klinhardt@mosessinger.com
www.mosessinger.com

Irving Sitnick, President
Provides legal services to many prominent industries, individuals and families in the New York City area.

2884 Herman Goldman Foundation
Fl 18
61 Broadway
New York, NY 10006-2708 212-797-9090
nlnfoundation.org

Alan Nisselson, President
A private nonoperating foundation.

2885 Kenneth & Evelyn Lipper Foundation
Fl 6
101 Park Ave
New York, NY 10178 212-883-6333

Kenneth Lipper, Director

2886 Long Island Alzheimer's Foundation
5 Channel Dr
Port Washington, NY 11050-2216 516-767-6856
FAX: 516-767-6864
e-mail: info@liaf.org
www.liaf.org

Fred Jenny, Executive Director
Sean Phillips, Director of Development
Tiffany Ewald, Program Assistant
Luiz Reyes, Maintenance

2887 Louis and Anne Abrons Foundation
First Manhattan Company
437 Madison Ave
New York, NY 10022-7001 212-756-3300
FAX: 212-832-6698
firstmanhattan.com
David Manischewitz, CEO

2888 Margaret L Wendt Foundation
Ste 277
40 Fountain Plz
Buffalo, NY 14202-2200 716-855-2146
FAX: 716-855-2149
Robert J Kresse, Manager

2889 Merrill Lynch & Company Foundation
250 Vesey St
New York, NY 10080 212-449-1000
FAX: 212-449-7969
ml.com
Brian T Moynihan, CEO
Ongoing support for the arts, health, human services, and civic issues. Merrill Lynch's philanthropic priority is a sustained investment in education. Q992

2890 Metzger-Price Fund
Ste 2300
230 Park Ave
New York, NY 10169 212-867-9500
FAX: 212-599-1759
Isaac A Saufer, Secretary/Treasurer

2891 Milbank Foundation for Rehabilitation
116 Village Boulevard
Suite 200
New York, NY 8540 609-951-2283
FAX: 609-951-2281
fdnweb.org/milbank
Carl Helstrom, Executive Director
Awarding grants from trust funds based on a competitive selection process or the preferences of the foundation managers and granters. The foundations mission is to integrate people with disabilities into all aspects of american life. Current priorities include, but are not limited to: consumer-focused initiatives that enable people with disablities to lead fulfilling,independent lives; innovative policy research and education on market-based approaches to health care and rehabilitation...

2892 Morgan Stanley Foundation
1585 Broadway
New York, NY 10036-8293 212-761-4000
FAX: 212-761-0086
e-mail: mediainquiries@morganstanley.com
morganstanley.com
James P. Gorman, Chairman and Chief Executive Officer
Thomas Nides, Vice Chairman
Jeff Brodsky, Chief Human Resources Officer
Jim Rosenthal, Chief Operating Officer
Our overachieving mission is threefold: build the potential of individuals and families, encourage and support our employees charitable efforts, and strengthen relationships with our communities.

2893 Mount Sinai Medical Center
1 Gustave L Levy Pl
New York, NY 10029-6574 212-241-3066
305-674-2777
www.msmcfoundation.org
Kenneth L. Davis, MD, Chief Executive Officer and President
Dennis S. Charney, MD, Executive Vice President
Mark Callahan, MD, Chief Executive Officer
Arthur Klein, MD, President
Autism Research

2894 National Foundation for Facial Reconstruction
333 East 30th Street
Lobby Unit
New York, NY 10016-4974 212-263-6656
FAX: 212-263-7534
e-mail: info@nffr.org
nffr.org
Carolyn Spector, J.D., LLM., Executive Director
Erin Johnson, Director of Development
Kirsten Selert, Development and Events Manager
Dina Zuckerberg, Director of Family Programs
A nonprofit organization whose major purposes are to provide facilities for the treatment and assistance of individuals who are unable to afford private reconstructive surgical care, to train and educate professionals in this surgery, to encourage research in the field and to carry on public education.

2895 National Hemophilia Foundation
116 W 32nd St
11th floor
New York, NY 10001-3212 212-328-3700
FAX: 212-328-3777
e-mail: webmaster@hemophilia.org
hemophilia.org
Val D. Bias, CEO
Neil Frick, Vice President for Research and Medical Information
John Indence, Vice President for Marketing & Communications
Joseph Kleiber, Senior Vice President for Chapter Services
Dedicated to finding better treatments and cures for bleeding and clotting disorders to preventing the complications of these disorders through education, advocacy and research.

2896 Neisloss Family Foundation
Ste 7
1737 Veterans Hwy
Central Islip, NY 11749-1533 631-234-1600
FAX: 631-234-1066
Stanley Neisloss, President/Owner

2897 New York Community Trust
909 3rd Ave
22nd Floor
New York, NY 10022-4752 212-686-0010
FAX: 212-532-8528
e-mail: info@nycommunitytrust.org
nycommunitytrust.org
Lorie A Slutsky, President
Alan Holzer, CFO
Mary Z. Greenebaum, Chief Investment Officer
Eileen Casey, Director of Investment Reporting
Our goal is to out charitable money to work, making grants to the city's nonprofit community and building an endowment to tackle future problems.

2898 New York Foundation
10 E 34th St
10th Floor
New York, NY 10016-4327 212-594-8009
e-mail: info@nyf.org
nyf.org
Maria Mottola, Executive Director
Kevin Ryan, Program Director
Isabel Rivera, Grants Manager
Melissa Hall, Operations Manager
Grants are given that involve New York City or a particular neighborhood of the city. Emphasize advocacy and community organizing. Address a critical need or disadvantaged population, particularly youth or the elderly. Are strongly identified with a particular community. Require an amount of funding to which a Foundation grant would make a substantial contribution. And can show a clear role for the Foundation's funds.

2899 Northern New York Community Foundation
120 Washington St
Suite 400
Watertown, NY 13601-3376
315-782-7110
FAX: 315-782-0047
e-mail: info@nnycf.org
www.nnycf.org

Rande S. Richardson, Executive Director
Raises, manages and administers an endowment and collection of funds for the benefit of the community

2900 Parkinson's Disease Foundation
1359 Broadway
Room 1509
New York, NY 10018-7867
212-923-4700
800-457-6676
FAX: 212-923-4778
e-mail: info@pdf.org
www.pdf.org

Robin Athony Elliott, President
James Beck, Ph.D., Vice President, Scientific Affairs
Melissa Barry, Director of Communications
Christiana Evers, Vice President, Communications
The Parkinson's Disease Foundation is a leading national presence in Parkinson's disease research, education and public advocacy. We are working for the nearly one million people in the US who live with Parkinson's by funding promising scientific research to find the causes of and a cure for Parkinson's while supporting people with Parkinson's, their families and caregivers through educational programs and support services.

2901 Reader's Digest Foundation
Readers Digest Association
Readers Digest Rd
Pleasantville, NY 10570
914-238-1000
FAX: 914-238-4559
e-mail: letters@rd.com
rd.com

Mary G Berner, CEO
Dedicated to creating opportunities and promoting efforts that encourage individuals to make a positive difference in their communities, and to supporting programs designed to help young people learn, grow and enrich their lives.

2902 Research to Prevent Blindness
645 Madison Ave
Floor 21
New York, NY 10022-1010
212-752-4333
800-621-0026
FAX: 212-688-6231
e-mail: inforequest@rpbusa.org
www.rpbusa.org

Diane S. Swift, Chair
Brian F. Hofland PhD, President
David Brenner, Vice President and Secretary
Richard E. Baker, Treasurer and Assistant Secretary
National voluntary health foundation supported by foundations, corporations and voluntary gifts and bequests from individuals. Established to stimulate basic and applied research into the causes, prevention and treatment of blinding eye diseases.

2903 Rita J and Stanley H Kaplan Foundation
Rm 306
866 United Nations Plz
New York, NY 10017-1822
212-688-1047
FAX: 212-688-6907
www.kaplanfoundation.org

Susan B. Kaplan, President
Rita J. Kaplan, Vice Preisident
Nancy Kaplan Belsky, Vice Preisident
Scott Kaplan Belsky, Secretary & Treasurer

2904 Robert Sterling Clark Foundation
135 E 64th St
New York, NY 10065-7045
212-288-8900
FAX: 212-288-1033
e-mail: rscf@rsclark.org
rsclark.org

James Allen Smith, President
Clara Miller, Treasurer
Joanna D. Underwood, Secretary
Laura Wolff, Acting Executive Director
Giving primarily in New York with emphasis on advocacy, research, and public education aimed at informing New York City of state policies.

2905 Skadden Fellowship Foundation
4 Times Sq
New York, NY 10036-6518
212-735-3000
FAX: 212-735-2000
e-mail: info@skadden.com
www.skadden.com

Alan C Myers, Director
The aim of the Foundation is to give Fellows the freedom to pursue public intrest work, thus the Fellows create their own projects at public interest organizations with at least 2 lawyers on staff before they apply.

2906 St George's Society of New York
216 E 45th St
Suite 901
New York, NY 10017-3304
212-682-6110
FAX: 212-682-3465
e-mail: info@stgeorgessociety.org
stgeorgessociety.org

John Shannon, Almoner
Anna Titley, Director of Operations and Communications
Samantha Hamilton, Director of Development and Membership
Daisy Rowan, Operations Executive
St George's Society provides monthly stipends to the elderly and the handicapped.

2907 Stanley W Metcalf Foundation
Ste 503
120 Genesee St
Auburn, NY 13021-3672
315-252-3634

Walter Lowe, Owner

2908 Stonewall Community Foundation
446 West 33rd Street
New York, NY 10001-1913
212-367-1155
FAX: 212-367-1157
e-mail: stonewall@stonewallfoundation.org
www.stonewallfoundation.org

Paula Ettelbrick, Executive Director
Mission is to promote the well being of lesbian, gay, bisexual, and transgender (LGBT) individuals and strengthen the LGBT community. We do this by increasing resources; targeting those resources strategically to areas of greatest need; and by serving as a catalyst and clearinghouse for ideas and solutions. Through grant-making donor-advised funds, endowment funds and charitable education, Stonewall supports LGBT organizations and helps donors realize their philanthropic goals.

2909 Surdna Foundation
330 Madison Ave
30th Floor
New York, NY 10017-5016
212-557-0010

e-mail: grants@surdna.org
surdna.org

Sharon L. Alpert, Vice President, Programs and Strategic Initiatives
Marc de Venoge, Vice President, Finance and Administration
George Soule, Director of Communications
Jonathan Goldberg, Director of Grants Management, Learning and Information

The Foundation makes grants in the areas of environment, community revitalization, effective citizenry, the arts and the nonprofit sector.

2910 Tisch Foundation
Fl 19
655 Madison Ave
New York, NY 10065-8043 212-521-2930
FAX: 212-521-2983

Mark J Krinsky, VP

2911 Van Ameringen Foundation
509 Madison Ave
New York, NY 10022-5501 212-758-6221
FAX: 212-688-2105
e-mail: info@vanamfound.org
www.vanamfound.org

Kenneth A. Kind, President / Treasurer
Steadman Westergaard, Vice President and Secretary
Eleanor Sypher, Executive Director
Helaine Williams, Office Manager
From its beginning the Foundation has sought to stimulate prevention, education, and direct care in the mental health field with an emphasis on those individuals and populations having an impoverished background and few opportunities, for whom appropriate intervention would produce positive change.

2912 Verizon Foundation
1 Verizon Way
Basking Ridge, NJ 07920-1097 866-247-2687
FAX: 908-630-2660
e-mail: verizonfoundation@verizon.com
www.verizonfoundation.org

Binta Vann-Joseph, Director of Marketing Strategy
Mission is to improve education, literacy, family safety and healthcare by supporting Verizon's commitment to deliver technology that touches life. We focus our philanthropic efforts on 3 areas: Education, Safety and Health. & Volunteerism.

2913 Western New York Foundation
11 Summer St
Third Floor
Buffalo, NY 14209-2256 716-839-4425
FAX: 716-N99-8883
e-mail: bgosch@wnyfoundation.org
www.wnyfoundation.org

Jennifer S. Johnson, Chairman
James A. W. McLeod, President
John N. W. Walsh III, Vice President
Theodore V. Buerger, Treasurer
The Western New York Foundation makes grants in the seven counties of Western New York State: Erie, Niagra, Genesee, Wyoming, Allegany, Cattaraugus and Chautauqua

2914 William T Grant Foundation
570 Lexington Ave
18th Floor
New York, NY 10022-6837 212-752-0071
FAX: 212-752-1398
e-mail: info@wtgrantfdn.org
wtgrantfoundation.org

Adam Gamoran, President
Vivian Tseng, Vice President, Program
Deborah McGinn, Vice President, Finance and Administration
Vivian Louie, Program Officer
Purpose is to further the understanding of human behavior through research. The mission focuses on improving the lives of youth ages 8 to 25 in the United States.

North Carolina

2915 Arc of North Carolina
343 East Six Forks Rd.
Suite 320
Raleigh, NC 27609 919-782-4632
800-662-8706
FAX: 919-782-4634
e-mail: arcofnc@arcnc.org
www.arcnc.org

John Nash, Executive Director
Lisa Poteat, Senior Director
Holly Hunnicutt, Director of Employer of Record Services
Ben Akroyd, Assistant Director of Communications
Committed to securing for all people with mental retardation and other developmental disabilities the opportunity to choose and realize their goals of where and how they learn, live, work, and play.

2916 Bob & Kay Timberlake Foundation
1660 E Center Street Ext
Lexington, NC 27292-1309 336-243-7777
800-776-0822
FAX: 336-249-2469
bobtimberlake.com

Daniel Timberlake, President

2917 Duke Endowment
100 N Tryon St
Suite 3500
Charlotte, NC 28202-4012 704-376-0291
FAX: 704-376-9336
e-mail: info@tde.org
dukeendowment.org

Eugene W. Cochrane Jr., President
Arthur E. Morehead IV, Vice President/General Counsel
Susan L. McConnell, Director of Higher Education / Director of Human Resources
Terri W. Honeycutt, Corporate Secretary
Mission is to serve the people of North Carolina and South Carolina by supporting selected programs of higher education, health care, children's welfare, and spiritual life.

2918 First Union Foundation
301 S College St
Charlotte, NC 28288 704-383-0525
FAX: 704-374-2484

Judy Allison, Director

2919 Foundation for the Carolinas
220 N. Tryon Street
Charlotte, NC 28202 704-973-4500
800-973-7244
FAX: 704-973-4599
e-mail: mmarsicano@fftc.org
fftc.org

Michael Marsicano, Ph.D., President & CEO
Laura Smith, Executive Vice President
Debra S. Watt, SVP, Information Technology & Human Resources
Brian Collier, Executive Vice President
Giving primarily to organizations serving the citizens of North and South Carolina.

2920 Kate B Reynolds Charitable Trust
128 Reynolda Vlg
Winston Salem, NC 27106-5123 336-397-5500
800-485-9080
FAX: 336-723-7765
e-mail: joyce@kbr.org
kbr.org

Karen McNeil-Miller,, President
Lori Fuller, Director, Evaluation and Learning
Joel Beeson, Director, Operations
Nora Ferrell, Director, Communications

Mission is to improve the quality of life and quality of health for the financially needy of North Carolina. Grants resricted to the state of North Carolina only.

2921 Mary Reynolds Babcock Foundation
2920 Reynolda Rd
Winston Salem, NC 27106-3016
336-748-9222
FAX: 336-777-0095
e-mail: info@mrbf.org
mrbf.org

Jennifer Barksdale, Finance Officer
Toshawia Bruner, Office Assistant
Lavastian Glenn, Program Officer
Sandra Mikush, Interim Executive Director

For 1994, this foundation is committed to an extensive educational and planning process to better understand the Southeast and to articulate the role the foundation seeks to play in the region into the twenty-first century.

2922 Triangle Community Foundation
324 Blackwell St
Suite 1220
Durham, NC 27701-3690
919-474-8370
FAX: 919-941-9208
e-mail: info@trianglecf.org
trianglecf.org

Lori O'Keefe, President
Jovon Packard, Technology Officer
Ruth Peoples, Executive Assistant
Jessica Banks Gilmour Aylor, Director of Development & Community Partnerships

Triangle Community Foundation connects philanthropic resources with community needs, creates opportunity for enlightned change and encourages philanthropy as a way of life.

North Dakota

2923 Alex Stern Family Foundation
4152 30th Ave S
Suite 102
Fargo, ND 58104-8403
701-271-0263
FAX: 701-271-0408
alexsternfamilyfoundation.org

D L Scott, Executive Director

The Foundation supports the arts, social welfare/human services, education, youth recreation, civic projects and health issues for the benefit of the greater Fargo-Moorhead area.

2924 Arc of North Dakota
2500 DeMers Avenue
Grand Forks, ND 58208-2420
701-772-6191
877-250-2022
FAX: 701-772-2195
e-mail: thearc@arcuv.com
www.thearcuppervalley.com

Peggy Johnson, President
Joan Karpenko, First Vice President
Ruth Jenny, Secretary
Virginia Esslinger, Treasurer

Mission is to work in partnership with our constituents, members and affiliated chapters to ensure that children and adults with intellectual and developmental disabilities have the supports, benefits, and services they need, and are accepted, respected and fully included in their communities.

2925 North Dakota Community Foundation
309 N Mandan Street
P.O.Box 387
309 N Mandan Street, Suite 2
Bismarck, ND 58502-0387
701-222-8349
e-mail: kdvorak@ndcf.net
www.ndcf.net

Kevin Dvorak, CFP, President & CEO
Amy N. Warnke, CFRE, Development Director East
Kara L. Geiger, Development Director West
Jordan J. Neufeld, CPA, Chief Financial Officer

The mission of the North Dakota Community Foundation is to improve the quality of life for North Dakota's citizens through charitable giving and promothing philanthropy.

Ohio

2926 Akron Community Foundation
345 W Cedar St
Akron, OH 44307-2407
330-376-8522
FAX: 330-376-0202
e-mail: jpetures@akroncf.org
www.akroncommunityfdn.org

John T. Petures, Jr., President and CEO
Margaret Medzie, Vice President, Development & Donor Engagement
Laura Fink, Director of Development
Diane Schumaker, Development & Donor Engagement Officer

Mission is to improve the quality of life in the Greater Akron area by building permanent endowments, and providing philanthropic leadership that enables donors to make lasting investments in the community.

2927 Albert G and Olive H Schlink Foundation
49 Benedict Avenue, Suite C
Norwalk, OH 44857
e-mail: curtis@hwak.com
www.schlinkfoundation.org

2928 American Foundation Corporation
4518 North 32nd Street
Phoenix, AZ 85018
602-955-4770
FAX: 602-955-4707
e-mail: info@americanfoundation.org
www.americanfoundation.org

Ben L. Schaub, Founder and CEO

The American Foundation can be your sponsor, and help your company set up a corporate foundation in a "public charity" or "support organization" format.

2929 Arc of Ohio
1335 Dublin Rd
Suite 100-A
Columbus, OH 43215-7037
614-487-4720
800-875-2723
FAX: 614-487-4725
e-mail: info@thearcofohio.org
thearcofohio.org

Gary Tonks, Executive Director
John Hannah, President
Connie Calhoun, Vice President
Josh Ebling, Treasurer

The mission of The Arc of Ohio is to advocacte for human rights, personal dignity and community participation of individuals with mental retardation and other developmental disabilities, through legislative and social action, information and education, local chapter support and family involvement.

2930 Bahmann Foundation
8041 Hosbrook Rd
Suite 210
Cincinnati, OH 45236-2909 513-891-3799
FAX: 513-891-3722
e-mail: info@bahmann.org
www.bahmann.org

John Gatch, Executive Director
The mission of the Bahmann Foundation is to reduce isolation of low-income older adults through technology.

2931 Cleveland Foundation
1422 Euclid Ave
Suite 1300
Cleveland, OH 44115-2063 216-861-3810
FAX: 216-861-1729
e-mail: info@ClevelandFoundation.org
clevelandfoundation.org

Ronald B Richard, President and Chief Executive Officer
Sylvia E. Perez, Chief of Staff and Manager for Gov and International Affairs
Kimberly Sabo, Executive Assistant to the President and CEO
Cindy Naegele, Director of Principal Gifts
In general, grants are made in (but not restriced to) the areas of arts and culture, community development, economic development, education, environment, health and human services.

2932 Columbus Foundation and Affiliated Organizations
1234 E Broad St
Columbus, OH 43205-1453 614-251-4000
FAX: 614-251-4009
e-mail: info@columbusfoundation.org
columbusfoundation.org

Doug F. Kridler, President & CEO
Raymond J. Biddiscombe, CPA, Senior Vice President - Finance & Administration / CFO
Lisa Schweitzer Courtice, P, EVP - Community Research and Grants Management
Alicia Szempruch, Scholarship Manager
The Columbus Foundation offers a range of charitable fund types that can be used for individuals, families and businesses.

2933 Eleanora CU Alms Trust
Fifth Third Bank
Department 00864
9990 Montgomery Rd
Cincinnati, OH 45263 513-793-2200

Robert W Laclair, President
Giving is limited to Cincinnati, OH.

2934 Eva L And Joseph M Bruening Foundation
Foundation Management Services
1422 Euclid Ave
Suite 966
Cleveland, OH 44115-1952 216-621-2901
FAX: 216-621-8198
e-mail: cstarkey@fmscleaveland.com
www.fmscleveland.com

Janet E. Narten, Founder
Cristin N. Slesh, President
Susan O. Althans, Senior Associate
Kara L. McCullough, Manager, Grants and Office Operations
Charitable foundation providing grants to noprofit organizations located inCuyahoga county Ohio. No grant are awarded to invividuals.

2935 Fred & Lillian Deeks Memorial Foundation
P.O.Box 1118
Cincinnati, OH 45201-1118 937-339-2329
FAX: 937-339-1861

2936 GAR Foundation
277 East Mill Street
Akron, OH 44308 330-576-2926
FAX: 330-294-5315
e-mail: info@garfdn.org
www.garfdn.org

Christine Amer Mayer, President
Kirstin S. Toth, Senior Vice President
Candace Campbell Jackson, Consulting Program Officer
Brittany G. Zaehringer, Senior Program Officer
The mission of the Foundation is to strengthen communities in our region through discerning and creative support of worthy organizations.

2937 George Gund Foundation
Ste 1845
45 Prospect Avenue, West
Cleveland, OH 44115- 1008 216-241-3114
FAX: 216-241-6560
e-mail: info@gundfdn.org
gundfoundation.org

David T. Abbott, Executive Director
Marcia Egbert, Senior Program Officer (human services)
Deena M. Epstein, Senior Program Officer (arts)
Ann K. Mullin, Senior Program Officer (education)
The George Gund Foundation was established in 1952 as a private, nonprofit institution with the sole purpose of contributing to human well-being and the progress of society.

2938 Greater Cincinnati Foundation
200 W 4th St
Cincinnati, OH 45202-2775 513-241-2880
FAX: 513-852-6886
e-mail: info@gcfdn.org
greatercincinnatifdn.org

Kathryn e. Merchant, President/CEO
Terri Masur, Executive Assistant
Elizabeth Reiter Benson, APR, Vice President for Communications & Marketing
Shiloh Turner, Vice President for Community Investment
Offers a wide variety of giving tools to help people achieve their charitable goals and create lasting good work in their communities.

2939 HCR Manor Care Foundation
P.O.Box 10086
Toledo, OH 43699-0086 419-252-5500
FAX: 419-252-6404
e-mail: foundation@hcr-manorcare.com
hcr-manorcare.com

Paul A Ormond, Chairman, President and CEO
An independent, not-for-profit corporation that provides funding for organizations and programs that address the needs of the elderly and individuals requiring post-acute care services.

2940 Harry C Moores Foundation
100 S 3rd St
Columbus, OH 43215-4236 614-227-8884
bricker.com

Katherine Murphy, Chief Operating Officer
Ahmad Sino, Chief Information Officer
Steve Odum, Chief Financial Officer
Betsy Wetherby, Chief Human Resources Officer

2941 Helen Steiner Rice Foundation
1301 Western Ave.
Cincinnati, OH 45203 513-287-7022
800-877-2665
e-mail: hrice@cincymuseum.org
helensteinerrice.com

Virginia J. Ruehlmann, Creative Consultant
Dorothy C. Lingg, Office Manager
Willis D. Gradison, Jr., Board of Trustee
Gregory Ionna, Board of Trustee

Non-profit corporation whose purpose is to award grants to worthy charitable programs that aid the poor, the needy, and the elderly.

2942 Herbert W Hoover Foundation
220 Market Ave S
Canton, OH 44702-2180 330-453-5555
FAX: 330-453-5622
e-mail: contacthwh@hwhfoundation.org
www.hwhfoundation.org

Mark Butterworth, Ohio Director
Lynn Davidson, Program Director
Elizabeth Lacey Hoover, Chair
Colton Hoover Chase, Member of Trust Committee
The Herbert W Hoover Foundation will take a leadership role in funding unique opportunities that provide solutions to issues relater to the Community, Education, and the Environment.

2943 Nationwide Foundation
1 W Nationwide Blvd
Columbus, OH 43215-2239 614-249-7111
877-669-6877
FAX: 614-249-5721
www.nationwide.com

Kirt A. Walker, President and COO Nationwide Financial
Mark A. Pizzi, President and Chief Operating Officer, Nationwide Insurance
Stephen S. Rasmussen, Chief Executive Officer, Nationwide Mutual Insurance Company
W. Kim Austen, President and COO, Allied Group, Nationwide
The Nationwide Foundation is an independent corporation funded by Nationwide Companies to help positively impact the quality of life in communities where our associates, agents and their families live and work.

2944 Nordson Corporate Giving Program
28601 Clemens Rd
Westlake, OH 44145-1148 440-892-1580
FAX: 440-892-9507
e-mail: kladiner@nordson.com
nordson.com

Michael F. Hilton, President and Chief Executive Officer
Gregory A. Thaxton, Senior Vice President, Chief Financial Officer
John J. Keane, Senior Vice President, Advanced Technology Systems
Gregory P. Merk, Senior Vice President, Adhesive Dispensing Systems
Nordson Corporation encourages individual financial support of nonprofit organizations, colleges, and universities

2945 Parker-Hannifin Foundation
6035 Parkland Blvd
Cleveland, OH 44124-4141 216-896-3000
800-272-7537
FAX: 216-896-4000
parker.com

Donald E. Washkewicz, Chairman, Chief Executive Office
Lee C. Banks, Executive Vice President and Ope
Robert P. Barker, Executive Vice President, Operat
Jon P. Marten, Executive Vice President - Finan
To be a leading worldwide manufacturer of components and systems for the builders and users of durable goods.

2946 Reinberger Foundation
30000 Chagrin Blvd.
#300
Cleveland, OH 44124-4439 216-292-2790
FAX: 216-292-4466
e-mail: info@reinbergerfoundation.org
www.reinbergerfoundation.org

Karen R. Hooser, President
Sally R. Dyer, Trustee
Richard H. Oman, Trustee
William C. Reinberger, Trustee
Committed to enhancing the quality of life for individuals from all walks of life. To achieve this goal, proposals in the areas of the arts, education, healthcare, and social service are favored.

2947 Robert Campeau Family Foundation
7 W 7th St
Cincinnati, OH 45202-2424 513-579-7000
FAX: 513-579-7555
federated-fds.com
Terry J Lundgren, Chairman and Chief Executive Officer

2948 Sisler McFawn Foundation
P.O.Box 149
Akron, OH 44309 330-849-8887
FAX: 330-996-6215
Charlotte M Stanley, Grants Manager
Our trust restricts giving to certain programs and types of organizations. You can see recent giving has been by referring to the list of grants approved and paid during the past year. Call foundation office to request a guidelines brochure and list.

2949 Stark Community Foundation
400 Market Ave N
Suite 200
Canton, OH 44702-1557 330-454-3426
FAX: 330-454-5855
e-mail: info@starkcf.org
www.starkcommunityfoundation.org

Mark Samolczyk, President
Patricia Quick, Vice President and Chief Financial Officer
Carol Hawk, Director of Marketing and Communications
Jackie Gilin, Donor Services and Program Officer
Stark Community Foundation is dedicated to promoting the betterment of Stark County and enhancing the quality of life of all its citizens.

2950 Stocker Foundation
201 Burns Road
Lorain, OH 44035 440-366-4884
FAX: 440-366-4656
e-mail: contact@stockerfoundation.org
stockerfoundation.org

Brenda Norton, President
Dawn Dobras, Treasurer
Patricia O'Brien, Executive Director
Melanie R Wilson, Office Manager
The Stocker Foundation seeks creative ideas and projects that are catalysts for constructive change in the community through arts and culture, community needs, education, health social services and women's issues.

2951 Toledo Community Foundation
300 Madison Ave
Suite 1300
Toledo, OH 43604-1583 419-241-5049
FAX: 419-242-5549
e-mail: toledocf@toledocf.org
www.toledocf.org

Keith Burwell, CEO
Kim Cryan, Chief Financial Officer
Joanne Olnhausen, Communications and Scholarship Officer
Kenneth C. Frisch, ACFRE, Senior Philanthropic Services Officer
The Toledo Community Foundation is a public, charitable foundation which exists to improve the quality of life in the region.

2952 William J and Dorothy K O'Neill Foundation
7575 Northcliff Ave.
Suite 205
Cleveland, OH 44144 216-831-4134
FAX: 216-378-0594
e-mail: info@oneill-foundation.org
www.oneillfdn.org

Leah S Gary, President & CEO
Symone McClain, Manager of Grants & Office Operations
Timothy M. McCue, MPH, Senior Program Officer

2953 **Youngstown Foundation**
P.O.Box 1162
Youngstown, OH 44501-1162 330-744-0320
FAX: 330-744-0344
e-mail: Jan@youngstownfoundation.org
www.youngstownfoundation.org
Jan Strasfeld, Executive Director
Crissi Jenkins, Program Coordinator
Rena Colarossi, Admin. Assistant
Funds proposals that provide direct services to children with medically diagnosed disabilities. Grants are awarded to Ohio non-profit agencies that are qualified under the Internal Revenue Service Code 501 (c) (3) for the care of such children in the greater Youngstown Area.

Oklahoma

2954 **Anne and Henry Zarrow Foundation**
401 S Boston Ave
Suite 900
Tulsa, OK 74103-4012 918-295-8004
FAX: 918-295-8049
e-mail: bmajor@zarrow.com
www.zarrow.com

2955 **Sarkeys Foundation**
530 E Main St
Norman, OK 73071-5823 405-364-3703
FAX: 405-364-8191
e-mail: angela@sarkeys.org
sarkeys.org
Kim Henry, Executive Director
Llinda English Weeks, Senior Program Officer & Legal Counsel
Angella Holladay, Director of Grants Management
Susan C. Frantz, Senior Program Officer
Improves the quality of life in Oklahoma. Offers contributions in the areas of social services, arts and cultural programs, educational funding and health care and medical research. Funding only in agencies in the state of Oklahoma.

Oregon

2956 **Arc of Oregon**
2405 Front Street NE
Suite 120
Salem, OR 97301-4342 503-581-2726
877-581-2726
FAX: 503-363-7168
e-mail: info@arcoregon.org
arcoregon.org
Marcie Ingledue, Executive Director
Tiffany Tombleson, Administrative Assistant
Paula Boga, OSNT Program Director
Cici Gaynor, OSNT Administrative Assistant
Guardianship, Advocacy and Planning Services. Oregon special needs trust; information and referral.

2957 **Chiles Foundation**
1614 Mahan Center Boulevard
Suite 104
Tallahassee, Fl 32308 805-385-7800
FAX: 805-385-7808
e-mail: kchiles@lawtonchiles.org
chilesfoundation.org
Kitty Chiles, Executive Director
Todd Abernethy, Chief Financial Officer
Giving in Oregon, with emphasis on Portland, and the Pacific Northwest.

2958 **Jackson Foundation**
P.O.Box 3168
Portland, OR 97208-3168 503-275-4414
e-mail: march.voyles@usbank.com
www.thejacksonfoundation.com
Robert H Depew, Vice President & Senior Trust Officer
Libby Voyles, Trust Relationship Associate
Purpose is to respond to the requests deemed appropriate to promote the welfare of the public of the city of Portland or the State of Oregon or both.

2959 **Leslie G Ehmann Trust**
P.O.Box 3168
Portland, OR 97208-3168 503-275-5929
800-522-9100
FAX: 503-275-4117
e-mail: william.dollan@usbank.com
William Dolan, Trustee

Pennsylvania

2960 **Air Products Foundation**
7201 Hamilton Blvd
Allentown, PA 18195-9642 610-481-4911
FAX: 610-481-5900
e-mail: gigmrktg@airproducts.com
www.airproducts.com
Seifi Ghasemi, Chairman & CEO
M. Scott Crocco, Senior Vice President and Chief Financial Officer
Patricia A. Mattimore, Senior Vice President-Supply Chain
Mary T. Afflerbach, Corporate Secretary and Chief Governance Officer
Giving primarily in areas of company operations throughout the US.

2961 **Arc of Pennsylvania**
301 Chestnut Street
Suite 403
Harrisburg, PA 17101-2535 717-234-2621
800-692-7258
FAX: 717-234-2622
e-mail: info@thearcpa.org
thearcpa.org
Maureen Cronin, Executive Director
Pam Klipa, Government Relations Director
Gwen Adams, Operations Director
Ashlinn Masland-Sarani, Policy and Development Director
The Arc's mission is to work to include all children and adults with cognitive, intellectual, and developmental disabilities in every community. We promote active citizenship and inclusion in every community.

2962 **Arcadia Foundation**
105 E Logan St
Norristown, PA 19401-3058 202-747-0876
arcadiafoundation.org
Marilyn L Steinbright, President

2963 **Brachial Plexus Palsy Foundation**
210 Springhaven Cir
Royersford, PA 19468-1178
e-mail: contact@brachialplexuspalsyfoundation.org
www.brachialplexuspalsyfoundation.org

2964 **Columbia Gas of Pennsylvania Corporate Giving**
650 Washington Rd
Pittsburgh, PA 15228-2702 412-572-7104
FAX: 412-572-7140
e-mail: info@columbiaenergygroup.com
www.columbiagaspamd.com/html/
Rosemary Martinelli, Manager Corporation

2965 **Connelly Foundation**
1 Tower Brg
100 Front Street, Suite 1450
West Conshohocken, PA 19428-2873 610-834-3222
FAX: 610-834-0866
e-mail: info@connellyfdn.org
connellyfdn.org

Josephine C. Mandeville, Chair & President
Emily C Riley, Executive Vice President
Lewis W Bluemle, Senior Vice President
Stephen Connelly, Associate
Seeks to foster learning and to improve the quality of life in the Greater Philadelphia area. The Foundation supports local non-profit organizations in the fields of education, health and human services, arts and culture and civic enterprise.

2966 **Dolfinger-McMahon Foundation**
30 South 17th Street
Philadelphia, PA 19103-4196 215-979-1768
www.dolfingermcmahonfoundation.org

Sheldon M. Bonovitz, Trustee
David E. Loder, Trustee
Frank G. Cooper, Counsel
Sharon M. Renz, Executive Secretary

2967 **Heinz Endowments**
Howard Heinz Endowment
625 Liberty Ave
30 Dominion Tower
Pittsburgh, PA 15222- 3115 412-281-5777
FAX: 412-281-5788
e-mail: bobbyvagt@heinz.org
heinz.org

Grant Oliphant, President
Edward Kolano, Vice President Finance and Administration / Chief Investment
Stuart Redshaw, Director, Human Resources
Donna Evans Sebastian, Executive Assistant
Mission is to help our region thrive as a whole community-economically, ecologically, educationaly, and culturaly while advancing the state of knowledge and practice in the fields in which we work.

2968 **Henry L Hillman Foundation**
310 Grant Street
Suite 2000
Pittsburgh, PA 15219 412-338-3466
e-mail: foundation@hillmanfo.com
hillmanfamilyfoundations.org

David K Roger, President
Lisa R Johns, Treasurer and Senior Program Officer
Lauri K. Fink, Senior Program Officer
D.Tyler Gourley, Program Officer
Established with a broad purpose to improve the quality of life in Pittsburgh and southwestern Pennsylvania.

2969 **Jewish Healthcare Foundation of Pittsburgh**
650 Smithfield St
Suite 2400
Pittsburgh, PA 15222-3915 412-594-2550
FAX: 412-232-6240
e-mail: info@jhf.org
jhf.org

Karen Wolk Feinstein, PhD, President and Chief Executive Officer
The mission of the JHF is to support and foster the provision of healthcare services, healthcare education, and, when appropriate, medical and scientific research, and to respond to the health-related needs of elderly, underprivileged, indigent, and undeserved persons in both the Jewish and general community throughout Western Pennsylvania. .

2970 **Juliet L Hillman Simonds Foundation**
310 Grant Street
Suite 2000
Pittsburgh, PA 15219 412-338-3466
FAX: 412-338-3520
e-mail: foundation@hillmanfo.com
hillmanfamilyfoundations.org/foundations/juli

David K. Roger, President
Lisa R. Johns, Treasurer and Senior Program Officer
Lauri K. Fink, Senior Program Officer
D.Tyler Gourley, Program Officer

2971 **Oberkotter Foundation**
1600 Market St
Suite 3600
Philadelphia, PA 19103-7212 215-751-2601
FAX: 215-751-2678
e-mail: info@oberkotterfoundation.org
oraldeafed.org

George H Nofer, Executive Director
Mildred L. Oberkotter, M.S.W., Trustee
Bruce A. Rosenfield, J.D., Trustee
David A. Pierson, Ph.D., Trustee

2972 **PECO Energy Company Contributions Program**
Fl 7toorh
2301 Market St
Philadelphia, PA 19103-1338 215-841-4000
FAX: 215-841-6830
exceloncorp.com

Denis P O'Brien, CEO

2973 **PNC Bank Foundation**
249 5th Ave
Pittsburgh, PA 15222-2707 412-762-2000
FAX: 412-762-7829
e-mail: marianna.hallett@pnc.com
www.pncbank.com

Samuel R Patterson, Senior VP
The PNC Foundation's priority is to form partnerships with community-based nonprofit organizations within the markets PNC serves in order to enhance educational opportunities for children, particularly underserved pre-K children though our signature, PNC Grow Uo Great Program, and to promote the growth of targeted communities through economic development initiatives.

2974 **Philadelphia Foundation**
1234 Market St
Suite 1800
Philadelphia, PA 19107-3704 215-563-6417
FAX: 215-563-6882
e-mail: EOConnell@philafound.org
philafound.org

R Andrew Swinney, President
Pat Meller, Vice President for Finance & Administration
Andrea Congo, Executive Assistant
Betsy Anderson, Communications Director
The Philadelphia Foundation improves our community by advancing change, leading on issues of importance, forging meaningful relationships and providing knowledge, resources and stewardship.

2975 **Pittsburgh Foundation**
Five PPG Place
Suite 250
Pittsburgh, PA 15222-5405 412-391-5122
FAX: 412-391-7259
e-mail: oliphantg@pghfdn.org
pittsburghfoundation.org

Molly Beerman, Interim President and CEO
Jonathan Brelsford, Vice President of Investments
Marianne Cola, Executive Secretary
Christopher Whitlatch, Manager of Marketing and Communications

The Pittsburgh Foundation works to improve the quality of life in the Pittsburgh region by evaluating and addressing community issues, promoting responsible philanthropy, and connecting donors to the critical needs of the community.

2976 Shenango Valley Foundation
7 West State Street
Suite 301
Sharon, PA 16146-2713
724-981-5882
866-901-7204
FAX: 724-983-9044
e-mail: info@comm-foundation.com
www.sv-foundation.org

Lawrence E. Haynes, Executive Director
Amy Atkinson, Associate Director
Shelly Mason, Chief Financial Officer
Tristan Rice, Development Coordinator

Mission is to promote the betterment of our region and enhancement of the quality of life for all of its citizens.

2977 Staunton Farm Foundation
650 Smithfield St
Suite 210
Pittsburgh, PA 15222-3907
412-281-8020
FAX: 844-281-8020
e-mail: office@stauntonfarm.org
stauntonfarm.org

Joni S. Schwager, Executive Director
Bethany Hemingway, Program Officer
Liz Veri, Operations Manager
Robert Musca, Financial Manager

Dedicated to improving the lives of people who live with mental illness.

2978 Stewart Huston Charitable Trust
50 S 1st Ave
Coatesville, PA 19320-3418
610-384-2666
FAX: 610-384-3396
e-mail: admin@stewarthuston.org
stewarthuston.org

Scott G. Huston, Executive Director
Charles L. Huston III, Trustee
Samuel A. Cann, Esq., Trustee
Alex L. Cann Sr., Trustee

The purpose of the Trust is to provide funds, technical assistance and collaboration on behalf of non-profit organizations engaged exclusively in religious, charitable or educational work; to extend opportunities to deserving needs persons and, in general, to promote any of the above causes.

2979 Teleflex Foundation
155 S Limerick Rd
Limerick, PA 19468-1603
610-948-5100
FAX: 610-948-5101
teleflex.com

Jeffrey P Black, CEO

The Teleflex Foundation strives to create an impact on the quality of life in Teleflex communities and build supportive relationships among our stakeholders. The Foundation places a priority on progrmas that have the commitmenet and volunteer involvement of Teleflex communities.

2980 USX Foundation
600 Grant St
Pittsburgh, PA 15219-2702
412-433-1121
FAX: 412-433-6847
www.ussteel.com

CD Mallick, General Manager
Patricia Funaro, Program Manager

Giving primarily in areas of company operations located within the United States.

2981 William B Dietrich Foundation
Duane Morrs Llt
30 S 17th St
Philadelphia, PA 19103-4001
215-979-1000
FAX: 215-979-1020
www.duanemorrs.com

William B Dietrich, President

2982 William Talbott Hillman Foundation
310 Grant Street
Suite 2000
Pittsburgh, PA 15219
412-338-3466
FAX: 212-792-2677
e-mail: foundation@hillmanfo.com
hillmanfamilyfoundations.org/foundations/will

David K. Roger, President
Lisa R. Johns, Treasurer and Senior Program Officer
Lauri K. Fink, Senior Program Officer
D.Tyler Gourley, Program Officer

2983 William V and Catherine A McKinney Charitable Foundation
20 Stanwix St
Pittsburgh, PA 15222-4802
412-644-8332
FAX: 412-644-6058
verizon.com

William M Schmidt, Senior Vice President

Rhode Island

2984 Arc South County Chapter
2 Barber Avenue
Warwick, RI 02886-3549
401-480-9355
e-mail: paul@pence.com
www.riroads.com

2985 Arc of Blackstone Valley
500 Prospect St.
Wing B, Suite 203
Pawtucket, RI 02861- 4332
401-727-0150
800-257-6092
FAX: 401-727-1545
e-mail: contact@bvcriarc.org
www.bvcriarc.org

Kathleen O'Neill, President
Thomas E. Hodge, Vice President
John J. Padien III, Chief Executive Officer
Katherine S. Hunt, Chief Operating Officer

A private nonprofit organization providing residential, developmental, employment and recreational programs and services to more then 400 individuals with intellectual and related disabilities

2986 Arc of Northern Rhode Island
The Homestead Group Administrative Offices
68 Cumberland St
Suite 200
Woonsocket, RI 02895-3323
401-765-3700
FAX: 401-765-1124
e-mail: info@thgri.org
arcofnri.org

2987 Champlin Foundations
2000 Chapel View Boulevard
Suite 350
Cranston, RI 02920
401-944-9200
FAX: 401-944-9299
www.champlinfoundations.org

2988 CranstonArc
The Keystone Group
PO Box 20130
Cranston, RI 02920-942
401-941-1112
FAX: 401-383-8751
e-mail: CranstonArc.org
www.cranstonArc.org

Thomas Kane, President & CEO

Mission is to empower persons with differing ablilites to claim and enjoy their right to dignity and respect through their lives.

2989 Down Syndrome Society of Rhode Island
99 Bald Hill Rd
Cranston, RI 02920-2648
401-463-5751
FAX: 401-463-5337
TTY:800-745-5555
dssri.org

Joanne Burger
Marilyn Blanche
Jeff DiMillio
Gail Doyle

The Down Syndrome Society of Rhode Island (DSSRI) is dedicated to promoting the rights, dignity and potential of all individuals with Down syndrome through advocacy, education, public awareness, and support.

2990 Frank Olean Center
93 Airport Rd
Westerly, RI 02891-3420
401-596-2091
FAX: 401-596-3945
e-mail: info@oleancenter.org
oleancenter.org

Joan Gradilone, President
Tony Vellucci, Executive Director
Bob Mastrofino, CPA, CGMA, Finance Director
Tina Cherenzia, Director of Human Resources

A non-profit organization representing and providing services and supports to persons with developmental disabilities and their families throughout Southern Rhode Island and Southeastern Connecticut.

2991 Horace A Kimball and S Ella Kimball Foundation
23 Broad Street
Westerly, RI 02891-1879
401-348-1238
FAX: 401-364-3565
www.hkimballfoundation.org

Thomas F Black III, President
Norman D. Baker, Jr., Secretary and Treasurer

Makes grants almost exclusively to Rhode Island operatives (charities) or those benefitting Rhode Island residents and causes.

2992 James L. Maher Center
PO Box 4390
Middletown, RI 02842
401-846-4600
FAX: 401-849-4267
www.mahercenter.org

Bill Maraziti, Executive Director
Bill Rush, Finance Director
Den DeMarinis, Jr., Director of Development & Communications
Debbie Shears, Director Early Intervention

The mission is to advance independence and opportunity for children and adults with developmental disabilities and their families.

2993 Kent County Arc
3445 Post Rd
Warwick, RI 02886-7147
401-739-2700
FAX: 401-737-8907
e-mail: mmadden@kentcountyarc.org
www.kentcountyarc.org

Mary Madden, CEO

Providing individuals with disabilties meaningful opportunities throughout their communities.

2994 Rhode Island Arc
99 Bald Hill Rd
Cranston, RI 02920-2647
401-463-9191
FAX: 401-463-9244
e-mail: riarc@compuserve.com
riarc@compuserve.com

Mary Lou Mc Caffray, Executive Director

2995 Rhode Island Foundation
One Union Station
Providence, RI 02903-1758
401-274-4564
FAX: 401-331-8085
rifoundation.org

Neil Steinberg, President & CEO
Wendi DeClercq, Executive Assistant
James S. Sanzi, Esq., Vice President of Development
Pamela Tesler Howitt, Senior Development Officer

The Rhode Island Foundation works to build a better Rhode Island as a philanthropic resource, for people, communities, organizations, and programs.

South Carolina

2996 Arc of South Carolina
1202 12th Street
Cayce, SC 29033
803-748-5020
FAX: 803-445-1026
e-mail: TheArc@ArcSC.org
www.arcsc.org

Margie Williamson, Executive Director
Christie Fleming, Program Director
Cindy Tomlinson, Case Manager
Holly Spargo-Hicks, Program Director

The Arc of South Carolina advocates for and alongside people with cognitive, intellectual and developmental disabilities and their families.

2997 Center for Disability Resources
University of South Carolina
8301 Farrow Rd
Columbia, SC 29208-1
803-935-5231
FAX: 803-935-5059
e-mail: Joyce.Tensley@uscmed.sc.edu
www.usmc.med.edu/cdrhome

Dr. David A. Rotholz, Director

A University Affiliated Program which develops model programs designed to serve persons with disabilities and to train students in fields related to disabilities.

2998 Colonial Life and Accident Insurance Company Contributions Program
1200 Colonial Life Blvd W
Columbia, SC 29210-7670
803-798-7000
FAX: 803-731-2618

Randy Horn, President and Chief Executive Officer
Bill Deeham, Senior Vice President of Sales
Tim Arnold, Senior Vice President of Sales and Marketing
John Garrison, Vice President, General Counsel

Tennessee

2999 Arc of Anderson County
P.O.Box 4823
Oak Ridge, TN 37831-4823
865-481-0550
e-mail: arc@arcaid.org
www.arcaid.org

Sally Browning, President
Dennis Eldred, Executive Director

The Arc of Anderson County provides support and advocacy to people with cognitive, intellectual and developmental disabilities. The Arc provides support, information and training for families and caregivers of adults and children with these disabilities.

3000 Arc of Davidson County
111 N Wilson Blvd
Nashville, TN 37205-2411 615-248-4112
e-mail: arc@arcdc.org
arcdc.org

Jim Harris, President
Kate Deitzer, Vice President
Thom Druffel, Treasurer
Falon Veit Scott, Secretary
Provides services to adults and children with intellectual and developmental disabilities through a contract with the Tennesee Department of Mental Retardation Services Medicaid Waiver Program.

3001 Arc of Hamilton County
4613 Brainerd Rd
Chattanooga, TN 37411-3826 423-624-6887
800-624-6887
FAX: 423-624-3974
e-mail: arcofhamilton@aol.com
thearchc.org

Shawn Ellis, Executive Director
Provides assistance to individuals and families with mental retardation and related disabilities, in the form of advocacy, information, and support coordination

3002 Arc of Tennessee
151 Athens Way
Suite 100
Nashville, TN 37228-1367 615-248-5878
800-835-7077
FAX: 615-248-5879
e-mail: wrogers@thearctn.org
thearctn.org

Carrie Hobbs Guiden, Executive Director
Peggy Cooper, Membership, Chapter and Communications Manager
Nicole Davidson, Business Manager
Advocacy, information, referral and support for people with intellectual and developmental disabilities and their families.

3003 Arc of Washington County
110 East Mountcastle Drive
Johnson City, TN 37601-7557 423-928-9362
FAX: 423-928-7431
e-mail: kim@arcwc.org
www.arcwc.org

Malessa Fleenor, Executive Director
Kim Reid, Human Resources, Quality Assurance/Marketing Coordinator
Kim Wheeler, Respite Coordinator
Linda Tilson, Family Support Program Manager
Is a non-profit organization that serves individuals with disabilities and their families. They have an independent support coordination service, as well as, early intervention, family support and respite services.

3004 Arc of Williamson County
Ste 151
129 W Fowlkes St
Franklin, TN 37064-3562 615-791-0042
disabilitywilliamson.org

Sharon Bottorff, Executive Director
The Arc is a family-based organization committed to securing for all people with intellectual, developmental, or other disabilities the opportunity to choose and realize their goals of where and how they live, learn, work, and play.

3005 Arc-Diversified
453 Gould Dr
Cookeville, TN 38506 931-432-5981
800-239-9029
FAX: 931-432-5987
www.arcdiversified.com

3006 Benwood Foundation
736 Market St
Suite 1600
Chattanooga, TN 37402-4812 423-267-4311
FAX: 423-267-9049
e-mail: callen@benwood.org
benwood.org

Sarah Morgan, President
Kristy Huntley, Program & Financial Officer
Connie Perrin, Accounting & Grants Manager
Jeff Pfitzer, Program Officer
Benwood Foundation seeks to stimulate creative and innovative efforts to build and strengthen the Chattanooga community.

3007 Community Foundation of Greater Chattanooga
1270 Market St
Chattanooga, TN 37402-2713 423-265-0586
FAX: 423-265-0587
e-mail: info2@cfgc.org
cfgc.org

Peter T. Cooper, President
Rebecca Underwood, Vice President, Finance & Administration
Marty Robinson, Vice President, Donor Relations
Rebecca Smith, Director of Scholarships
A non-profit organization which receives, holds, invests and distributes assets contributed by individuals and organizations for the benefit of Chattanooga, its citizens and its institutions.

3008 Education and Auditory Research Foundation
PO Box 330867
Nashville, TN 37203-7506 615-627-2724
800-545-4327
FAX: 615-627-2728
e-mail: info@earfoundation.org
www.earfoundation.org

Michael Glasscock, President
Provides the general public support services promoting the integration of the hearing and balance impaired into mainstream society; to provide practicing ear specialists continuing medical education courses and related programs specifically regarding rehabilitation and hearing preservation; to educate young people and adults about hearing preservation and early detection of hearing loss, enabling them to prevent at an early age hearing and balance disorders.

3009 International Paper Company Foundation
6400 Poplar Ave
Memphis, TN 38197 901-419-9000
800-207-4003
FAX: 901-419-4439
e-mail: internationalpaper.comm@ipaper.com
internationalpaper.com

John V Faraci, Chairman & CEO
Mark S. Sutton, President & Chief Operating Officer
C. Cato Ealy, Senior Vice President, Corporate Development
William P. Hoel, Senior Vice President
The Foundation's primary focus is education-specifically environmental education, iliteracy programs for young children and minority career development opportunities for college bound youth.

3010 Montgomery County Arc
1825 K Street
NW, Suite 1200
Washington, DC 20006-2145 202-534-3700
800-433-5255
FAX: 202-534-3731
e-mail: info@thearc.org
www.thearc.org

Mohan Mehra, President
Nancy Webster, Vice President

Organization works to ensure that the estimated 7.2 million Americans with intellectual and developmental disabilities have the services and supports they need to grow, develop and live in communities across the nation.

Texas

3011 AFB Center on Vision Loss
American Foundation for the Blind
2 Penn Plaza
Suite 1102
New York, NY 10121-4524
212-502-7600
FAX: 888-545-8331
e-mail: afbinfo@afb.net
afb.org

Carl Augusto, President & CEO
Kelly Bleach, Chief Administrative Officer
Rick Bozeman, Chief Financial Officer
Paul Schroeder, Vice President, Programs and Policy
National nonprofit organization that expands possibilities for people with vision loss.

3012 Abell-Hangar Foundation
P.O.Box 430
Midland, TX 79702
432-684-6655
FAX: 432-684-4474
abell-hanger.org

David L Smith, Executive Director
The Foundation makes grants to nonprofit organizations, which are involved in such undertakings for public welfare, including but not limited to, education, health services, human services, arts and cultural activities and community or social benefit.

3013 Albert & Bessie Mae Kronkosky Charitable Foundation
112 E Pecan St
Suite 830
San Antonio, TX 78205-1574
210-475-9000
888-309-9001
FAX: 210-354-2204
e-mail: kronfndn@kronkosky.org
kronkosky.org

Palmer Moe, Managing Director
Mission is to produce profound good that is tangible and measurable in Bandera, Bexar, Comal, and Kendall counties in Texas by implimenting the Kronkosky's charitable purposes.

3014 Arc of Texas, The
8001 Centre Park Dr
Suite 100
Austin, TX 78754-5118
512-454-6694
800-252-9729
FAX: 512-454-4956
www.thearcoftexas.org

Amy Mizcles, Executive Director
The Arc of Texas creates opportunities for all people with intellectual and developmental disabilities to actively participate in their communities and make the choices that affect their lives in a positive manner.

3015 BA and Elinor Steinhagen Benevolent Trust
Chase Bank of Texas
700 North St.
Suite D
Beaumont, TX 77701-3928
409-832-6565
FAX: 409-832-7532
e-mail: cjourdan@setxnonprofit.org
www.setxnonprofit.org

Jean Moncla, CTFA, President
Ivy Pate, Treasurer
Chester Jourdan, Executive Director
Kristi Stott, Administrative Assistant

3016 Brown Foundation
P.O.Box 130646
Houston, TX 77219
713-523-6867
FAX: 713-523-2917
e-mail: bfi@brownfoundation.org
brownfoundation.org

Nancy Pittman, Executive Director
The purpose of the Brown Foundation is to distribute funds for public charitable purposes, principally for support, encouragement and assistance to education, the arts and community service.

3017 Burnett Foundation
P.O. Box 633
Northfield, MN 55057-6881
817-877-3344
e-mail: tomburnettfamilyfoundation@msn.com
www.tomburnettfoundation.org

V Neils Agather, Executive Director

3018 CH Foundation
P.O.Box 94038
Lubbock, TX 79493-4038
806-792-0448
FAX: 806-792-7824
e-mail: ksanford@chfoundation.com
www.chfoundationlubbock.com

Kay Sanford, Executive Director
Heather Hocker, Grants Administrator
Cheryl Sanford, Administrative Assistant
Mission of the CH foundation is to significantly improve human services and cultural and educational opportunities for the residents of the South Plain of Texas.

3019 Cockrell Foundation
1000 Main St
Suite 3250
Houston, TX 77002-6338
713-209-7500
e-mail: foundation@cockrell.com
www.cockrell.com

Ernest H. Cockrell, President
Nancy Williams, Executive Vice President
Purpose is for giving for higher education at the University of Texas at Austin; support also for cultural programs, social services, youth services and health care. Limitations are giving in Houston, Texas and no grants are awarded to individuals.

3020 Communities Foundation of Texas
5500 Caruth Haven Ln
Dallas, TX 75225-8146
214-750-4222
FAX: 214-750-4210
e-mail: jsmith@cftexas.org
cftexas.org
Brent E. Chrisopher, President and Chief Executive Officer
Elizabeth W. Bull, Senior Vice President and Chief Financial Officer
Jeverley R. Cook, Ph.D., Executive Director, W.W. Caruth, Jr. Foundation
John Fitzpatrick, Executive Director
Mission is to improve lives, we serve the community by investing wisely and making effective charitable grants.

3021 Community Foundation of North Texas
306 W 7th St
Suite 1045
Fort Worth, TX 76102-4906
817-877-0702
FAX: 817-632-8711
cfntx.org

Nancy E. Jones, President
Rob Miller, Director of Finance
Vicki Andrews, Director of Operations/Donor Services
Rose Bradshaw, Director of Grants and Community Engagement
Community Foundation is a tax exempt organization that provides stewardship for many individual charitable funds. With its specialized services, Community Foundation of North Texas gives donors efficient charitable fund administration.

3022 **Cullen Foundation**
601 Jefferson St
40th Floor
Houston, TX 77002-7900
713-651-8837
FAX: 713-651-2374
cullenfdn.org
Alan M. Stewart, Executive Director
Sue A Alexander, Grant administrator
Victor L. Mendoza, Accountant
Grants are restricted to Texas-based organizations for programs in Texas, primarily in the Houston area.

3023 **Curtis & Doris K Hankamer Foundation**
Ste 530
9039 Katy Fwy
Houston, TX 77024-1656
713-461-8140
Gregory A Herbst, Manager

3024 **Dallas Foundation**
3963 Maple Avenue
Ste. 390
Dallas, TX 75219-4447
214-741-9898
FAX: 214-741-9848
e-mail: info@dallasfoundation.org
dallasfoundation.org
Mary M Jalonick, President
Gary W. Garcia, Director of External Relations
Melinda Guravich, Director of Marketing & Communications
William T. Solomon, Jr., Chief Financial Officer
Serves as a leader, catalyst and resource for philanthropy by providing donors with a flexible means of making gifts to charitable causes that enhance our community.

3025 **David D & Nona S Payne Foundation**
P.O.Box 174
Pampa, TX 79066-174
806-665-0063
www.davidandnonapaynefoundation.com
Vanessa G Buzzard, Director
The David & Nona S Payne Foundation was established in August 1980. Mrs Payne established the foundation and did much of her charitable giving in honor of her late husband.

3026 **El Paso Natural Gas Foundation**
P.O.Box 2511
Houston, TX 77252-2511
713-420-2600
FAX: 713-420-5312
e-mail: foundation@elpaso.com
elpaso.com
Douglas Foshee, CEO
Focuses on the areas in locations where we have significant facilities or concentrated employees. Primary area of focus is Civic and Community, Education and Health and Human Services. Secondary area of focus is Arts and Culture and Environment.

3027 **Epilepsy Foundation of Southeast Texas**
8301 Professional Place
Landover, MD 20785-7608
866-330-2718
800-332-1000
FAX: 877-687-4878
e-mail: ContactUs@efa.org
www.epilepsyfoundation.org
Warren Lammert, Chair
Roger Heldman, Treasurer
May J. Liang, Secretary
Joyce A. Bender, Board Member
The Epilepsy Foundation of Southeast Texas is a non-profit organization to improve the lives of almost 100,000 adultsand children with epilepsy in the counties of north and southeast Texas.

3028 **Epilepsy Foundation: Central and South Texas**
10615 Perrin Beitel Rd
Ste 602
San Antonio, TX 78217- 3142
210-653-5353
888-606-5353
FAX: 210-653-5355
e-mail: staff@efcst.org
www.efcst.org
Anna Amos, President
Todd Drexler, Vice President
The Epilepsy Foundation of Central & South Texas is a voluntary health organization. We value all people with epilepsy. We commit our resources to empowering their independence and inspiring productive lives.

3029 **Harris and Eliza Kempner Fund**
P.O. Box 119
2201 Market St
Galveston, TX 77553-1529
409-765-6671
FAX: 409-765-9098
e-mail: information@kemperfund.org
kempnercapital.com
Diana L. Bartula, Vice President, Chief Compliance Officer, Treasurer
V. Delynn Greene, Vice President, Head Trader, Operations
Mission is to further the vision and heritage of the Kemper Family's commitment to philanthropy and sense of responsibility to society.

3030 **Hillcrest Foundation**
Bank of America
P.O.Box 830241
Dallas, TX 75283
214-209-1965
Daniel Kelly, VP

3031 **Hoblitzelle Foundation**
5556 Caruth Haven Lane
Suite 200
Dallas, TX 75225-8020
214-373-0462
e-mail: pharris@hoblitzelle.org
www.hoblitzelle.org
William T Solomon, Chairman
Paul W. Harris, President & CEO
Caren H. Prothro, Vice Chairman
J. McDonald Williams, Treasurer
Grants made by the directors are usually focused on specific, non-recurring needs of the educational, social service, medical, cultural, and civic organizations in Texas, particularly in the Dallas area.

3032 **Houston Endowment**
600 Travis St
Suite 6400
Houston, TX 77002-3003
713-238-8100
FAX: 713-238-8101
e-mail: info@houstonendowment.org
houstonendowment.org
Ann B Stern, President
Sheryl L Johns, Vice President for Administration
F. Xavier Pe�a, Vice President for Finance and General Counsel
Lisa A. Hall, Vice President for-Programs
A private philanthropic foundation that improves life for people of the greater Houston area through its contributions to charitable organizations and educational institutions.

3033 **John G & Marie Stella Kennedy Memorial Foundation**
555 N Carancahua
Suite 1700, Tower II
Corpus Christi, TX 78401
361-887-6565
FAX: 361-887-6582
www.kenedy.org
Judge J. A. Garcia, President and Director
Marc A. Cisneros, Chief Executive Officer, Executive Vice President
Ricardo Hinojosa, Vice-President and Director
Gloria Hicks, Secretary and Director

To advance and nurture activities that contribute to the foundation's core, Catholic values.

3034 John S Dunn Research Foundation
3355 W Alabama St
Suite 990
Houston, TX 77098-1722
713-626-0368
FAX: 713-626-3866
e-mail: jsdrf@swbell.net
johnsdunnfoundation.org

J. Dickson Rogers, President
John S Dunn, Jr, Vice President, Secretary and Treasurer
Dan S Wilford, First Vice President
John R. Wallace, Vice President

3035 Lola Wright Foundation
515 Congress Avenue
10th Floor
Austin, TX 78701
512-397-2001
e-mail: amber.carden@ustrust.com
fdnweb.org/lolawright

Wilford Flowers, President and Director
Paul Hilgers, Vice-President and Director
Ron Oliveira, Secretary and Director
Jay Stewart, Director

3036 Meadows Foundation
3003 Swiss Ave
Dallas, TX 75204-6049
214-826-9431
800-826-9431
e-mail: grants@mfi.org
www.mfi.org

Linda P Evans, President and CEO
Tom Gale, Vice President and Chief Investment Officer
Paula Herring, Vice President and Treasurer
Bruce H. Esterline, Vice President for Grants
The Meadows Foundation exists to assist people and institutions of Texas improve the quality and circumstances of life for themselves and future generations.

3037 Moody Foundation
2302 Post Office St
Suite 704
Galveston, TX 77550-1994
409-797-1500
e-mail: colleent@moodyf.org
moodyf.org

Frances Moody-Dahlderg, Executive Director
Jamie G. Williams, Human Resources Director
Garrik Addison, Chief Financial Officer
Samantha Seale, Scholarship Administrator
Created for the perpetual benefit of present and future generations.

3038 Pearle Vision Foundation
2534 Royal Ln
Dallas, TX 75229-3884
214-821-7770
www.pearlevision.com

Leo Priolo Jr, Owner
Organization dedicated to sight preservation through vision research and education.

3039 San Antonio Area Foundation
303 Pearl Parkway
Suite 114
San Antonio, TX 78215
210-225-2243
FAX: 210-225-1980
e-mail: info@saafdn.org
saafdn.org

Dennis E. Noll, President & CEO
Carrie A. Gray, Vice President, Development & Donor Services
Kathleen Finck, Director of Gift Planning
Rashanea Shakir, Community Outreach Manager
The San Antonio Area Foundation aspires to significantly enhance the quality of life in our community by providing outstanding service to donors, producting significant asset growth, strengthning community collaboration and managing an exemplary grants program.

3040 Shell Oil Company Foundation
P.O.Box 2463
Houston, TX 77252-2463
281-544-7171
FAX: 713-241-3329
e-mail: info@shellfoundation.org
www.shellfoundation.org

Robert Hummel, Plant Manager
A not-for-profit foundation funded by donations from Shell Oil Company and other participating Shell companies and subsidiaries.

3041 South Texas Charitable Foundation
P.O.Box 2459
Victoria, TX 77902
512-573-4383

Rayford L Keller, Secretary

3042 Sterling-Turner Foundation
815 Walker St
Suite 1543
Houston, TX 77002-5724
713-237-1117
FAX: 713-223-4638
e-mail: jeannie.arnold@stfdn.org
www.sterlingturnerfoundation.org

3043 TLL Temple Foundation
109 Temple Blvd
Lufkin, TX 75901-7321
936-639-5197
e-mail: wcorley@tlltf.com

Wayne Corley, Executive Director

3044 William Stamps Farish Fund
Ste 1250
1100 Louisiana St
Houston, TX 77002-5232
713-757-7313

Terry Ward, Manager

Utah

3045 Arc of Utah
P.O.Box 2786
Salt Lake City, UT 84110-2786
801-364-5060
800-371-3060
FAX: 801-364-6030
e-mail: gacosta@dunndunn.com
arcutah.org

Kathy Scott, Executive Director
The Arc of Utah advocates for and with cognitive, intellectual and developmental disabilities and their families through awareness, outreach, education, support and public policy.

3046 Marriner S Eccles Foundation
79 S Main St
Salt Lake City, UT 84111-1929
801-532-0934

Shannon K Toronto

3047 Questar Corporation Contributions Program
P.O.Box 45433
333 South State Street
Salt Lake City, UT 84111 801-324-5000
questarcorp.com

Ronald W Jibson, CEO
R. Allan Bradley, Executive vice president,
James R. Livsey, Executive vice president
Craig C. Wagstaff, Executive vice president, COO-Questar Gas
Focuses on promoting a healthy environment by investing in and fulfilling its corporate responsibility to support the well-being of communitites where Questar and its subsidiaries conduct business.

Vermont

3048 Vermont Community Foundation
3 Court Street
Middlebury, VT 05753 802-388-3355
FAX: 802-388-3398
e-mail: info@vermontcf.org
www.vermontcf.org

Stuart Comstock-Gay, President
Nina McDonnell, Grants Administrator
Janet McLaughlin, Special Projects Director
Jen Peterson, Vice President for Program and Grants
Helps build and manage charitable funds created by individuals, families, groups, organizations, and institutions to improve the quality of life in Vermont.

Virginia

3049 Arc of Virginia
2147 Staples Mill Road
Richmond, VA 23230 804-649-8481
FAX: 804-649-3585
e-mail: thearc@arcofva.org
www.thearcofva.org

Howard Cullum, President
Shareen Young-Chavez, President-Elect
Marisa Laios, Vice President
Donalda Lovelace, Secretary
The Arc of Virginia advocactes for individuals with mental retardation and developmental disabilities and their families, so they may all lead productive and fulfilling lives.

3050 Camp Foundation
P.O.Box 813
Franklin, VA 23851 757-562-3439

Bobby B Worrell, CEO

3051 Community Foundation of Richmond & Central Virginia
7501 Boulder View Dr
Suite 110
Richmond, VA 23225-4047 804-330-7400
FAX: 804-330-5992
e-mail: info@tcfrichmond.org
tcfrichmond.org

Darcy Oman, President
Bobby Thalhimer, Senior Vice President
Molly Dean Bittner, Vice President, Philanthropic Services
Lisa Pratt O'Mara, Vice President, Donor Engagement
The Community Foundation provides effective stewardship of philanthropic assets entrusted to its care by donors who wish to enhance the quality of community life.

3052 John Randolph Foundation
112 North Main Street
P.O.Box 1606
Hopewell, VA 23860- 1161 804-458-2239
FAX: 804-458-3754
e-mail: lsharpe@johnrandolphfoundation.org
www.johnrandolphfoundation.org

Lisa H. Sharpe, Executive Director
M. Stephen Cates, Director of Finance and Accounting
Brandon P. Butterworth, Development Program Officer
Tammy E. McCollum, Administrative Associate
The John Randolph Foundation is a community-based Foundation working to improve the health and quality of life for residents of Hopewell and surrounding areas through Grants and Scholarships.

3053 Norfolk Foundation
101 W. Main Street,
Suite 4500
Norfolk, VA 23510-2103 757-622-7951
FAX: 757-622-1751
e-mail: mbrunson@hamptonroadscf.org
www.hamptonroadscf.org

Deborah M DiCroce, Ed.D., President and CEO
Tim McCarthy, Chief Financial Officer
Kay A. Stine, CFRE, Vice President for Development
Lynn Watson Neumann, Director of Gift Planning
The mission of the Norfolk Foundation is to inspire philanthropy and transform the quality of life in southeastern Virginia.

3054 Robey W Estes Family Foundation
Robey W Estes Jr
3901 West Broad Street
Richmond, VA 23230-5612 866-378-3748
estes-express.com

Robey W Estes Jr, President and CEO

3055 Virginia Beach Foundation
Suite 4500
101 W. Main Street,
Virginia Beach, VA 23454 757-422-5249
FAX: 757-422-1849
e-mail: mbrunson@hamptonroadscf.org
www.hamptonroadscf.org

Deborah M DiCroce, President
Tim McCarthy, Chief Financial Officer
Mission is to stimulate the establishment of endowments to serve the people of Virgina Beach now and in the future. Respond to changing, emerging, community needs. Provide a vehicle and a service for donors with varied interests. Serve as a resource, broker, catalyst and leader in the community.

Washington

3056 Arc of Washington State
2638 State Ave NE
Olympia, WA 98506-4880 360-357-5596
FAX: 360-357-3279
e-mail: info@arcwa.org
arcwa.org

Cindy O'Neill, President
Nancy Stark, Vice President
Martha Schulte, Secretary
Peggy Blowers, Treasurer
Mission is to advocacte for the rights and full participation of all people with developmental disabilities.

3057 Ben B Cheney Foundation
3110 Ruston Way
Suite A
Tacoma, WA 98402-5308 253-572-2442
e-mail: Info@benbcheneyfoundation.org
benbcheneyfoundation.org
Bradbury F. Cheney, President
Piper Cheney, Vice President
Carolyn J. Cheney, Secretary Treasurer
Allan L. Undem, Board Member
The Foundation makes grants in communities where the Cheney Lumber Company was active. The Foundation's goal is to improve the quality of life in those communities by making grants to a wide range of activities.

3058 Community Foundation of North Central Washington
9 South Wenatchee Ave
Wenatchee, WA 98801-3332 509-663-7716
FAX: 888-317-8314
e-mail: beth@cfncw.org
www.cfncw.org
Beth Stipe, Executive Director
Judy A. Cleveland, CPA, Controller
Lila R. Edlund, Director of Administration
Jennifer Dolge, Director of Donor Services and Communications
Assists donors by helping identify their specific charitable and goals and provide grants and scholarships that help groups and people address critical issues in North Central Washington

3059 Glaser Progress Foundation
1601 Second Avenue
Suite 1080
Seattle, WA 98101-9223 206-728-1050
FAX: 206-728-1123
e-mail: martin@glaserfoundation.org
www.glaserfoundation.org
Martin Collier, Executive Director
Mitchell Fox, Program Officer
Melessa Rogers, Operations Manager
The Glaser Prograss Foundation focuses on four program areas: measuring progress, animal advocacy, independent media and global HIV/AIDS.

3060 Greater Tacoma Community Foundation
950 Pacific Ave
Suite 1100
Tacoma, WA 98402-4423 253-383-5622
FAX: 253-272-8099
e-mail: info@gtcf.org
www.gtcf.org
Rose Lincoln Hamilton, President and CEO
Shirley Brockmann, CPA, Vice President Finance & Administration
Elyse Rowe, Chief of Strategy and Community Relations
Gina Anstey, Director of Grants & Initiatives
Mission is fostering generosity by connecting people who care with causes that matter, forever enriching our community.

3061 Inland Northwest Community Foundation
421 West Riverside Avenue
Suite 606
Spokane, WA 99201- 5102 509-624-2606
888-267-5606
FAX: 509-624-2608
e-mail: admin@inwcf.org
www.inwcf.org
Mark Hurtubise, Ph.D., J.D., President and CEO
Troy Braga, CPA, Controller
P J Watters, Director of Gift Planning
Molly Sanchez, Director of Community Engagement
Serving 20 counties throughout Eastern Washington and Northern Idaho, mission is to foster vibrant and sustainable communities in the Inland Northwest.

3062 Medina Foundation
801 2nd Ave
Suite 1300
Seattle, WA 98104-1517 206-652-8791
FAX: 206-264-3007
e-mail: info@medinafoundation.org
www.medinafoundation.org
Jennifer Teunon, Executive Director
Jessica Case, Program Officer
Aana Lauckhart, Program Officer
Caroline Miceli, Grants Administrator
A family foundation that works to foster positive change in the Greater Puget Sound area. The Foundation strives to improve the human condition by supporting organizations that provide critical services to those in need.

3063 Norcliffe Foundation
999 3rd Ave
Suite 1006
Seattle, WA 98104-4001 206-682-4820
FAX: 206-682-4821
e-mail: arline@thenorcliffefoundation.com
www.thenorcliffefoundation.com
Arline Hefferline, Foundation Manager
Dana Pigott, President
Geographic area of funding limited to the Puget Sound Region in and around Seattle, Washington.

3064 Stewardship Foundation
1145 Broadway
Suite 1500
Tacoma, WA 98402-1278 253-620-1340
FAX: 253-572-2721
e-mail: info@stewardshipfdn.org
www.stewardshipfdn.org
Cary A. Paine, J.D., Ph.D., President
Amy Alva, Grants Manager
Zoe Malley, Office Manager
Christian, evangelical organizations - national or international impact.

3065 Weyerhaeuser Company Foundation
33663 Weyerhaeuser Way South
Federal Way, WA 98003 253-924-2345
800-525-5440
www.weyerhaeuser.com
Daniel S Fulton, President & CEO
Patricia M Bedient, EVP & CFO
Sandy D McDade, SVP & General Counsel
John A Hooper, SVP, Human Resources
Although the foundation does fund programs for disabled persons from time to time, it is not a specific priority for the foundation. Since it was formed in 1948, the foundation has given more than $81.1 million to nonprofit organizations and is one of the oldest funds for corporate philanthropy in the country. Nearly all of its contributions have been made within the communities where Weyerhaeuser employees live and work and awards approximately 600 grants annually.

West Virginia

3066 Bernard McDonough Foundation
311 4th St
Parkersburg, WV 26101-5315 304-424-6280
FAX: 304-424-6281
www.mcdonoughfoundation.org
Robert W Stephens, Ed.D., President
Mary Riccobene, Vice President
Francis C. McCusker, Treasurer
Katrina Valentine, Corporate Secretary
Directors and officers continue the legacy of the McDonoughs by providing grants that create a healthier, more educated and culturally appreciative citizenry.

3067 The Arc Of West Virginia
912 Market Street
Parkersburg, WV 26101-4737
304-422-3151
e-mail: christina.smith@arcwd.org
www.thearcwv.org

Wisconsin

3068 Arc of Dunn County
2602 Hils Court
Menomonie, WI 54751-4160
715-235-7373
FAX: 715-233-3565
e-mail: rebecca@arcofdunncounty.org
www.arcofdunncounty.org

Rebecca Cooper, Executive Director
Kathy Lausted, Guardianship Director
Advocating for the rights of citizens with disabilities.

3069 Arc of Eau Claire
4800 Golf Road
Suite 450
Eau Claire, WI 54701-6130
715-833-1735
FAX: 715-833-1215
e-mail: frcec@frcec.org
www.frcec.org

Brook Steele, President
Dave Swan, Vice President
Dr. Jennifer Eddy, Secretary
Dr. Emily Smith-Nguyen, Treasurer
Mission is to provide programs and services that build on family strengths through prevention, education, support and networking in collaboration with other resources in the community.

3070 Arc of Fox Cities
211 E. Franklin St.
Suite A
Appleton, WI 54911
920-735-0943
FAX: 920-725-1531
e-mail: info@arcfoxcities.com
arcfoxcities.com

Sonia Barham, Executive Director
Lori Allman, Director of Development
Diana Rehbein, Financial Administrator
Diana Quella, Administrative Assistant
Mission statement is to utilize advocacy, respect and concern to empower all people with disabilities to have the opportunity to choose and realize their goal of a full life and a secure future.

3071 Arc of Racine County
1220 Mound Ave
Suite 319
Racine, WI 53404-3350
262-634-6303
e-mail: sengle@thearcofracine.org
www.thearcofracine.org

Peggy Foreman, Executive Director
Alison Henry, Program Manager
Ross Gietzel, Program Assistant
The Arc of Racine's mission is to advocate for and provide information and services to improve lives.

3072 Arc of Wisconsin Disability Association
2800 Royal Ave
Suite 202
Monona, WI 53713-1518
608-222-8907
877-272-8400
FAX: 608-222-8908
e-mail: arcw@att.net
www.arc-wisconsin.org

John Beisbier, President
Donna Auchue, Vice President
Tina Beauprey, Secretary
The Arc-Wisconsin strives to be a major force in advocating and promoting self-determined quality of life opportunities for people with developmental and related disabilities and their families.

3073 Arc-Dane County
6602 Grand Teton Plz
Madison, WI 53719-1091
608-833-1199
FAX: 608-833-1307
e-mail: arcdane@chorus.net
arcdanecounty.org

Paul Yochum, Executive Director
The Arc-Dane County is a non-profit organization whose primary objective is to support children and adults with developmental disabilities and their families through advocacy to assure these individuals are offered the same opportunities and have the rights due all people. The Arc-Dane County provides numerous services through education, overall support, and legislation that assists those individuals with developmental disabilities be it within their homes, communities, or at work.

3074 Faye McBeath Foundation
101 W. Pleasant Street #210
Milwaukee, WI 53212-3157
414-272-2626
FAX: 414-272-6235
e-mail: info@fayemcbeath.org
www.fayemcbeath.org

Scott Gelzer, Executive Director
A private independent foundation providing grants to tax exempt nonprofit organizations principally the metropolitan Milwaukee area.

3075 Helen Bader Foundation
233 N Water St
4th Floor
Milwaukee, WI 53202-5761
414-224-6464
FAX: 414-224-1441
e-mail: info@hbf.org
www.hbf.org

Daniel J. Bader, President/CEO
Lisa G. Hiller, VP, Administration
Maria Lopez Vento, VP, Programs and Partnerships
Robert Tobon, Communications Director
Strives to be a philanthropic leader in improving the quality of life of the diverse communities in which it works. The Foundation makes grants, convenes partners, and shares knowledge to affect emerging issues in key areas.

3076 Johnson Controls Foundation
5757 N Green Bay Ave
P.O. Box 591
Milwaukee, WI 53201- 4408
414-524-1200
800-333-2222
FAX: 414-524-2077
johnsoncontrols.com

Stephen A Molinaroli, Chairman, President and CEO
Dr. Breda Bolzenius, Vice President, Vice Chairman
Kim Metcalf-Kupres, Vice President and Chief Marketing Officer
R. Bruce McDonald, Executive Vice President and CFO
Organized and directed to be operated for charitable purposes which include the distribution and application of financial support to soundly managed and operated organizations or causes which are fundamentally philanthropic.

3077 Lynde and Harry Bradley Foundation
1241 N Franklin Pl
Milwaukee, WI 53202-2901
414-291-9915
FAX: 414-291-9991
www.bradleyfdn.org

Michael W. Grebbe, President and CEO
Daniel P. Schmidt, Vice President for Program
Michael E. Hartmann, Director of Research and Evaluation
Janet F. Riordan, Director of Community Programs
The Foundation's programs support limited, competent government; a dynamic marketplace for economic, intellectual and cultural activity; a vigorous defense at home and abroad, of American ideas and institutions; and scholarly studies and academic achievement.

3078 **Milwaukee Foundation**
101 W Pleasant St
Suite 210
Milwaukee, WI 53212-3963 414-272-5805
FAX: 414-272-6235
e-mail: info@greatermilwaukeefoundation.org
www.greatermilwaukeefoundation.org
Ellen M Gilligan, President and CEO
Marcus White, Vice President
Kathryn J. Dunn, Vice President
Patti Dew, Vice President & CFO
Guided by three tenets- helping donors create personal legacies of giving that last beyond their lifetimes, investing donor funds for maximum return with minimal risk, and playing a leadership role tackling the communities most challenging needs.

3079 **Northwestern Mutual Life Foundation**
720 E Wisconsin Ave
Milwaukee, WI 53202-4703 414-271-1444
www.northwesternmutual.com
John E Schlifske, Chairman and CEO
Gregory C. Oberland, President
Michael G. Carter, Executive Vice President and CFO
Joann M. Eisenhart, Senior Vice President - Human Resources

3080 **Patrick and Anna M Cudahy Fund**
333 N. Michigan Ave.
Suite 510
Chicago, Il 60601 312-422-1442
FAX: 312-641-5736
e-mail: laurenkrieg@cudahyfund.org
cudahyfund.org
Janet S Cudahy MD, President
A general purpose foundation which primarily supports organizations in Wisconsin and the metropolitan Chicago area. Interests are social service, youth, and education with some giving for the arts, and other areas.

3081 **SB Waterman & E Blade Charitable Foundation**
Marshall & Ilsley Trust Company
111 E. Kilbourn Ave.,
Milwaukee, WI 53202-2980 414-287-8700
FAX: 414-765-8200
www.mitrust.com
Thomas C Boettcher, Director
Giving primarily to health associations. Geographical focus is Wisconsin.

Wyoming

3082 **Arc of Natrona County**
P.O. Box 393
Casper, WY 82601 307-577-4913
800-433-5255
FAX: 307-577-4014
e-mail: info@thearc.org
arcofnatronacounty.org
Beau Covert, President
Brooke Upmhlett, Vice President
Denise Bressler, Treasurer
Colbi Maddox, Secretary
Organization works to ensure that the estimated 7.2 million Americans with intellectual and developmental disabilities have the services and supports they need to grow, develop and live in communities across the nation.

Funding Directories

3083 **Chronicle Guide to Grants**
Ste 700
1255 23rd St NW
Washington, DC 20037-1146 202-466-1200
800-287-6072
FAX: 202-452-1033
e-mail: help@philanthropy.com
heideninc.com
Phil Semas, Manager
A computerized research tool, on floppy disks or a CD-ROM, for immediate use on any IBM compatible personal computer. Offers electronic listings of 10,000 grants from hundreds of foundations, with a subscription that offers 1,000 plus new listings every two months. Each listing offers grant information as well as names, addresses and phone numbers of the grant-making organizations. *$295.00*

3084 **College Student's Guide to Merit and Other No-Need Funding**
Reference Service Press
5000 Windplay Dr
Suite 4
El Dorado Hills, CA 95762-9319 916-939-9620
FAX: 916-939-9626
e-mail: info@rspfunding.com
www.rspfunding.com
Gail Schlachter, Founder
R. David Weber, Editor
Sandy Hirsh, Editor
Sandy Perez, Funding Finder
More than 1,200 funding opportunities for currently-enrolled or returning college students are described in this directory. *$32.50*
450 pages
ISBN 1-588410-41-2

3085 **Community Health Funding Report**
CD Publications
8204 Fenton St
Silver Spring, MD 20910-4502 301-588-6380
800-666-6380
FAX: 301-588-6385
e-mail: subscriptions@cdpublications.com
www.cdpublications.com
Michael Gerecht, President
The once twice-monthly report is now web-based to allow for breaking news updates and up the the minute information about funding, including: public and private grant announcements; reports on successful health programs nationwide; interviews with grant officials; plus national news on health policy topics affecting various organizations. *$439.00*
Web-based

3086 **Directory of Financial Aids for Women**
Reference Service Press
5000 Windplay Dr
Suite 4
El Dorado Hills, CA 95762-9319 916-939-9620
FAX: 916-939-9626
e-mail: info@rspfunding.com
www.rspfunding.com
Gail Schlachter, Founder
R. David Weber, Editor
Sandy Hirsh, Editor
Sandy Perez, Funding Finder
Funding programs listed support study, research, travel, training, career development, or innovative effort at any level; descriptions of more than 1,700 funding programs - representing billions of dollars in financial aid set aside for women; also an annotated bibliography of 60 key directories that identify even more financial aid opportunities and a set of indexes that let you search the directory by title, sponser, researching, tenability, subject, and deadline. *$45.00*
578 pages Biennial
ISBN 1-588410-00-5

3087 Disability Funding News
8204 Fenton St
Silver Spring, MD 20910-4502
301-588-6380
800-666-6380
FAX: 301-588-6385
e-mail: subscriptions@cdpublications.com
www.cdpublications.com

Michael Gerecht, President

3088 FC Search
Foundation Center
79 5th Ave
New York, NY 10003-3034
212-620-4230
800-424-9836
FAX: 212-807-3677
e-mail: order@foundationcenter.org
foundationcenter.org

Bradford K Smith, President
Lisa Philip, Vice President for Strategic Philanthropy
Jen Bokoff, Director of GrantCraft
Lawrence T. McGill, Vice President for Research

Provides access to the Foundation Center's comprehensive database of funders in a convenient CD-ROM format. *$1845.00*

3089 Federal Grants & Contracts Weekly
LRP Publications
360 Hiatt Drive
Palm Beach Gardens, FL 33418-1718
800-341-7874
FAX: 561-622-2423
e-mail: custserve@lrp.com
www.lrp.com

Kelly Sullivan, Editor
Kenneth F. Kahn, President

The latest funding announcements of federal grants for project opportunities in research, training and services. Provides profiles of key programs, tips on seeking grants, updates on legislation and regulations, budget developments and early alerts to upcoming funding opportunities. *$340.00*
Weekly

3090 Financial Aid for Asian Americans
Reference Service Press
5000 Windplay Dr
Suite 4
El Dorado Hills, CA 95762-9319
916-939-9620
FAX: 916-939-9626
e-mail: info@rspfunding.com
www.rspfunding.com

Gail Schlachter, Founder
R. David Weber, Editor
Sandy Hirsh, Editor
Sandy Perez, Funding Finder

This is the source to use if you are looking for financial aid for Asian Americans; nearly 1,000 funding opportunities are described. *$35.00*
336 pages
ISBN 1-588410-02-1

3091 Financial Aid for Hispanic Americans
Reference Service Press
5000 Windplay Dr
Suite 4
El Dorado Hills, CA 95762-9319
916-939-9620
FAX: 916-939-9626
e-mail: info@rspfunding.com
www.rspfunding.com

Gail Schlachter, Founder
R. David Weber, Editor
Sandy Hirsh, Editor
Sandy Perez, Funding Finder

Nearly 1,300 funding programs open to Americans of Mexican, Puerto Rican, Central American, or other Latin American heritage are described here. *$37.50*
472 pages
ISBN 1-588410-03-X

3092 Financial Aid for Native Americans
Reference Service Press
5000 Windplay Dr
Suite 4
El Dorado Hills, CA 95762-9319
916-939-9620
FAX: 916-939-9626
e-mail: info@rspfunding.com
www.rspfunding.com

Gail Schlachter, Founder
R. David Weber, Editor
Sandy Hirsh, Editor
Sandy Perez, Funding Finder

Detailed information is provided on 1,500 funding opportunities open to American Indians, Native Alaskans, and Native Pacific Islanders. *$37.50*
562 pages
ISBN 1-588410-04-8

3093 Financial Aid for Research and Creative Activities Abroad
Reference Service Press
5000 Windplay Dr
Suite 4
El Dorado Hills, CA 95762-9319
916-939-9620
FAX: 916-939-9626
e-mail: info@rspfunding.com
www.rspfunding.com

Gail Schlachter, Founder
R. David Weber, Editor
Sandy Hirsh, Editor
Sandy Perez, Funding Finder

Described here are 1,200 funding programs (scholarships, fellowships, grants, etc.) available to support research, professional, or creative activities abroad. *$45.00*
378 pages
ISBN 1-588410-82-5

3094 Financial Aid for Veterans, Military Personnel and their Dependents
Reference Service Press
5000 Windplay Dr
Suite 4
El Dorado Hills, CA 95762-9319
916-939-9620
FAX: 916-939-9626
e-mail: info@rspfunding.com
www.rspfunding.com

Gail Schlachter, Founder
R. David Weber, Editor
Sandy Hirsh, Editor
Sandy Perez, Funding Finder

According to Reference Book Review, this directory (with its 1,100 entries) is the most comprehensive guide available on the subject. *$40.00*
392 pages
ISBN 1-588410-43-9

3095 Financial Aid for the Disabled and Their Families
Reference Service Press
5000 Windplay Dr
Suite 4
El Dorado Hills, CA 95762-9319
916-939-9620
FAX: 916-939-9626
e-mail: info@rspfunding.com
www.rspfunding.com

Sandy Hirsh, Editor

This directory, which Children's Bookwatch calls invaluable describes more than 1,100 financial aid opportunities available to support persons with disabilities and members of their families. Updated every 2 years. *$37.50*
508 pages Every other yr.
ISBN 1-588410-01-3

3096 Foundation & Corporate Grants Alert
LRP Publications
360 Hiatt Drive
Palm Beach Gardens, FL 33418-1718
800-341-7874
FAX: 561-622-2423
e-mail: custserve@lrp.com
www.lrp.com

Kelly Sullivan, Editor
Kenneth F. Kahn, President
A complete guide to foundation and corporate grant opportunities for nonprofit organizations. Tracks developments and trends in funding and provides notification of changes in foundations' funding priorities. *$245.00*
Monthly
ISSN 1062-46 6

3097 Foundation 1000
Foundation Center
79 5th Ave
New York, NY 10003-3034
212-620-4230
800-424-9836
FAX: 212-807-3677
e-mail: order@foundationcenter.org
www.foundationcenter.org

Bradford K Smith, President
Lisa Philip, Vice President for Strategic Philanthropy
Jen Bokoff, Director of GrantCraft
Lawrence T. McGill, Vice President for Research
Offers comprehensive information on the 1000 largest foundations in the US. *$195.00*

3098 Foundation Directories
Foundation Center
79 5th Ave
New York, NY 10003-3034
212-620-4230
800-424-9836
FAX: 212-807-3677
e-mail: order@foundationcenter.org
foundationcenter.org

Bradford K Smith, President
Lisa Philip, Vice President for Strategic Philanthropy
Jen Bokoff, Director of GrantCraft
Lawrence T. McGill, Vice President for Research
Lists key facts on the top 20,000 US foundations. *$ 125.00*
ISBN 0-87954 -36-1

3099 Foundation Grants to Individuals
Foundation Center
79 5th Ave
New York, NY 10003-3034
212-620-4230
800-424-9836
FAX: 212-807-3677
e-mail: order@foundationcenter.org
foundationcenter.org

Bradford K Smith, President
Lisa Philip, Vice President for Strategic Philanthropy
Jen Bokoff, Director of GrantCraft
Lawrence T. McGill, Vice President for Research
The only publication that provides extensive coverage of foundation funding prospects for individual grantseekers. *$40.00*
Biennially

3100 From the State Capitals: Public Health
Wakeman/Walworth
P.O.Box 7376
Alexandria, VA 22307-376
703-768-9600
FAX: 703-768-9690
e-mail: newsletters@statecapitals.com
www.statecapitals.com

Mark Willen, Editor
Digest of state and municipal health care financing and cost containment measures, includes medical legislation, disease control, etc. *$245.00*
6 pages

3101 Grant Guides
Foundation Center
79 5th Ave
New York, NY 10003-3034
212-620-4230
800-424-9836
FAX: 212-807-3677
e-mail: order@foundationcenter.org
foundationcenter.org

Bradford K Smith, President
Lisa Philip, Vice President for Strategic Philanthropy
Jen Bokoff, Director of GrantCraft
Lawrence T. McGill, Vice President for Research
Provides descriptions of actual foundation grants awarded in various subject fields. *$35.00*
ISBN 0-87954 -90-6

3102 Guide to Funding for International and Foreign Programs
79 5th Ave
New York, NY 10003-3034
212-620-4230
800-424-9836
FAX: 212-807-3677
e-mail: order@foundationcenter.org
foundationcenter.org

Bradford K Smith, President
Lisa Philip, Vice President for Strategic Philanthropy
Jen Bokoff, Director of GrantCraft
Lawrence T. McGill, Vice President for Research
Grantmakers featured in this guide provide funding for international relief, disaster assistance, human rights, civil liberties, community development, conferences, and education. *$190.00*

3103 Guide to US Foundations their Trustees, Officers and Donors
Foundation Center
79 5th Ave
New York, NY 10003-3034
212-620-4230
800-424-9836
FAX: 212-807-3677
e-mail: order@foundationcenter.org
foundationcenter.org

Bradford K Smith, President
Lisa Philip, Vice President for Strategic Philanthropy
Jen Bokoff, Director of GrantCraft
Lawrence T. McGill, Vice President for Research
Provides crucial facts on grantmaking. Each entry includes contact information, current assets, annual contributions, officers, donors and more. *$135.00*

3104 High School Senior's Guide to Merit and Other No-Need Funding
Reference Service Press
5000 Windplay Dr
Suite 4
El Dorado Hills, CA 95762-9319
916-939-9620
FAX: 916-939-9626
e-mail: info@rspfunding.com
www.rspfunding.com

Gail Schlachter, Founder
R. David Weber, Editor
Sandy Hirsh, Editor
Sandy Perez, Funding Finder
Here's your guide to 1,100 funding programs that never look at income level when making awards to college bound high school seniors. *$29.95*
400 pages
ISBN 1-588410-44-X

3105 How to Pay for Your Degree in Business & Related Fields

Reference Service Press
5000 Windplay Dr
Suite 4
El Dorado Hills, CA 95762-9319
916-939-9620
FAX: 916-939-9626
e-mail: info@rspfunding.com
www.rspfunding.com

Gail Schlachter, Founder
R. David Weber, Editor
Sandy Hirsh, Editor
Sandy Perez, Funding Finder

If you need funding for an undergraduate or graduate degree in business or related fields, this is the directory to use (500+ funding programs described). *$30.00*

290 pages
ISBN 1-588411-45-1

3106 How to Pay for Your Degree in Education& Related Fields

Reference Service Press
5000 Windplay Dr
Suite 4
El Dorado Hills, CA 95762-9319
916-939-9620
FAX: 916-939-9626
e-mail: info@rspfunding.com
www.rspfunding.com

Gail Schlachter, Founder
R. David Weber, Editor
Sandy Hirsh, Editor
Sandy Perez, Funding Finder

Here's hundreds of funding opportunities available to support undergraduate and graduate students preparing for a career in education, guidance etc. *$30.00*

250 pages
ISBN 1-588411-46-x

3107 National Directory of Corporate Giving

Foundation Center
79 5th Ave
New York, NY 10003-3034
212-620-4230
800-424-9836
FAX: 212-807-3677
e-mail: order@foundationcenter.org
foundationcenter.org

Bradford K Smith, President
Lisa Philip, Vice President for Strategic Philanthropy
Jen Bokoff, Director of GrantCraft
Lawrence T. McGill, Vice President for Research

Offers over 2,000 corporate funders, current giving reviews and profiles of sponsoring companies. *$195.00*

3108 Older Americans Report

Business Publishers
2222 Sedwick Drive
Durham, NC 27713-1995
240-514-0600
800-223-8720
FAX: 800-508-2592
e-mail: custserv@bpinews.com
www.bpinews.com

Leonard Eiser, Publisher

Follows all programs and funding sources in education, housing, job training, therapy, Social Security Supplemental Security Income, Medicare, Medicaid and more of importance to persons with disabilities. Also covers the latest on the Americans with Disabilities Act. Publishes a newsletter. *$327.00*

3109 Student Guide

US Department of Education
400 Maryland Ave SW
Washington, DC 20202
202-401-2000
800-872-5327
FAX: 202-401-0689
TTY: 800-437-0833
e-mail: customerservice@inet.ed.gov
ed.gov

Arne Duncan, Secretary of Education
Jim Shelton, Deputy Secretary
Ted Mitchell, Under Secretary

Describes the major student aid programs the US Department of Education administers and gives detailed information about program procedures.

74 pages

Government Agencies

Federal

3110 **Administration on Aging**
One Massachusetts Ave NW
Washington, DC 20001 202-401-4634
FAX: 202-357-3555
e-mail: aclinfo@acl.hhs.gov
aoa.gov
Kathy Greenlee, Administrator
Sharon Lewis, Principal Deputy Administrator
Aaron Bishop, Commissioner
John Wren, Deputy Administrator
Administers the Older Americans Act of 1965 to assist states and local communities to develop programs for older persons.

3111 **Administration on Children, Youth and Families**
370 L Enfant Promenade SW
Washington, DC 20447 202-401-4634
800-422-4453
TTY:800-787-3224
www.acf.hhs.gov
William H. Bentley, Associate Commissioner
Jeannie Chaffin, Director
Eskinder Negash?, Director
Mathew McKearn?, Director
Responsible for federal programs that promote the economic and social well-being of families, children, individuals and communities.

3112 **Administration on Developmental Disabilities**
U S Department of Health and Human Services
370 L Enfant Promenade SW
Washington, DC 20447 202-401-4634
800-422-4453
TTY:800-787-3224
www.acf.hhs.gov/programs/add
William H. Bentley, Associate Commissioner
Jeannie Chaffin, Director
Eskinder Negash?, Director
Mathew McKearn?, Director
Ensures that individuals with developmental disabilities and their families participate in the design of and have access to culturally competent services, supports, and other assistance and opportunities that promote independence, productivity, and integration and inclusion into the community.

3113 **Americans with Disabilities Act Informationn**
US Department of Justice
950 Pennsylvania Ave NW
Washington, DC 20530 202-282-8000
800-514-0301
FAX: 202-307-1197
TTY: 800-514-0383
www.ada.gov
Gregory B. Friel, Chief
The ADA assures that Americans with disabilities have the same opportunities as all Americans. To this end, the Justice Department produces publications and conducts programs to increase compliance of the ADA nationwide.

3114 **Civil Rights Division/Disability Rights Section**
US Department Of Justice
950 Pennsylvania Ave NW
Washington, DC 20530 202-282-8000
800-514-0301
FAX: 202-307-1197
TTY: 800-514-0383
www.ada.gov
Gregory B. Friel, Chief
The US Department of Justice answers questions about the American Disabilities Act (ADA) and provides free publications by mail and fax through its ADA Information Line.

3115 **Committee for Purchase from People Who Are Blind or Severely Disabled**
1401 S. Clark Street
Ste 10800
Arlington, VA 22202-3259 703-603-7740
800-999-5963
FAX: 703-603-0655
e-mail: info@abilityone.gov
www.abilityone.gov
Tina Ballard, Executive Director & CEO
J Anthony Poleo, Chairperson
Kimberly Zeich, Deputy Executive Director & Chief Operating Officer
Angela Phifer, Chief of Staff
A federal agency that administers the Javits-Wagner-O'Day Program, directing federal agencies to purchase products and services from nonprofit agencies that employ people who are blind or have other severe disabilities. Provides a wide range of vocational options to individuals with severe disabilities.

3116 **Equal Opportunity Employment Commission**
131 M St NE
Washington, DC 20507-100 202-663-4599
800-669-4000
FAX: 202-419-0739
e-mail: info@eeoc.gov
www.eeoc.gov
Jacgueline Berrien, Chair
Constance S Baker, Commissioner
Milton A. Mayo Jr., Inspector General
This agency is responsible for drafting and implementing the regulations of Title I of the ADA.

3117 **Federal Communications Commission**
445 12th St SW
Washington, DC 20554 888-225-5322
888-835-5322
FAX: 866-418-0232
e-mail: fccinfo@fcc.gov
fcc.gov
Tom Wheeler, Chairman
Mignon Clyburn, Commissioner
Jessica Rosenworcel, Commissioner
Ajit Pai, Commissioner
Enforces ADA telecommunications provisions which require that companies offering telephone service to the general public must offer telephone relay services to individuals who use text telephones or similar devices. Also enforces closed captioning rules, hearing compatibility and access to equipment and services for people with disabilities.

3118 **Health Care Financing Administration**
200 Independence Ave SW
Washington, DC 20201-4 202-690-6726
FAX: 202-690-6262
William Roper, Administrator
Thomas Scully, President
Through the Social Security administration, it administers the Medicare program under Title XVIII of the Social Security Act. Administers grants to the states for Medicaid under Title XIX of the Social Security Act for individuals who are medically indigent.

3119 **National Coalition of Federal Aviation Employees with Disabilities**
Federal Aviation Administration
800 Independence Avenue, SW
Washington, DC 20594 405-954-4709
866-835-5322
FAX: 405-954-4490
TTY: 405-954-4587
www.faa.gov/acr/ncfaed.htm
Becky Pritchett, Treasurer
Alan Jones, President of Aeronautical Center
NCFAED is working on: 1) improvement of work conditions for employees; 2) expansion on National Coalition to serve all FAA employees; 3) promote equal opportunity for people with disabilities in the FAA workplace; 4) assist the FAA in its commitment to

remove physical and attudinal barriers which inhibit opportunities for people with disabilities; 5) align with internal and external organizations to attract future generations of people with disabilities to the FAA as employees.

3120 National Council on Disability
1331 F Street Northwest
Suite 850
Washington, DC 20004- 1138 202-272-2004
FAX: 202-272-2022
TTY:202-272-2074
www.ncd.gov

3121 National Division of the Blind and Visually Impaired
330 C St NW
Washington, DC 20001 202-205-8520

Chester Avery, Director
Develops methods, standards and procedures to assist state agencies in the rehabilitation of blind persons. Administers the Randolph-Sheppard Act, which assures priority for blind persons in the operation of vending facilities on federal property and serves as a program manager for the Helen Keller National Center for Youth who are deaf-blind.

3122 National Institutes of Health: National Eye Institute
31 Center Drive MSC 2510
Bethesda, MD 20892-2510 301-496-5248
e-mail: kcl@nei.nih.gov
www.nei.nih.gov

Paul A Sieving MD PhD, Director
Finances intramural and extramural research on eye diseases and vision disorders. Supports training of eye researchers.

3123 Office of Policy
Social Security Administration
1100 West High Rise
6401 Security Blvd
Baltimore, MD 21235 202-293-9138
800-772-1213
TTY:800-325-0778
e-mail: concepcion.mcneace@ssa.gov
www.ssa.gov/policy

Michael J Astrue, Commissioner
Edward Demarco, Assitant Deputy Commissioner
Serge Harrison, Executive Officer
Administers grants to the states for social services under Title XX of the Social Security Act to welfare recipients and others likely to become them.

3124 Office of Special Education Programs: Department of Education
400 Maryland Ave SW
Washington, DC 20202-7100 202-401-2000
800-872-5327
FAX: 202-401-0689
TTY: 800-437-0833
e-mail: customerservice@inet.ed.gov
www2.ed.gov/about/offices/list/osers/osep

Arne Duncan, Secretary of Education
Jim Shelton, Deputy Secretary
Ted Mitchell, Under Secretary
The Office of Special Education Programs (OSEP) is dedicated to improving results for infants, toddlers, children and youth with disabilities ages birth through 21 by providing leadership and financial support to assist states and local districts.

3125 President's Committee on People with Intellecutual Disabilities
370 L Enfant Promenade SW
Washington, DC 20447 202-619-0364
800-422-4453
TTY:800-787-3224
www.acf.hhs.gov

George Sheldon, Acting Assistant Secretary
Laverdia Roach, Acting Executive Director
Formerly the President's Committee on Mental Retardation, a federal advisory committee, estalished by the presidential executive order to adivse the President of the United States and the Secretary of the Department of Health and Human Services on issues concerning citizens with intellectual disabilities, coordinate activities between different federal agencies and assess the impact of their policies upon the lives of citizens with intellectual disabilities and their families.

3126 Rehabilitative Services Administration
400 Maryland Ave SW
Washington, DC 20202-7100 202-401-2000
800-872-5327
FAX: 202-401-0689
TTY: 800-437-0833
e-mail: customerservice@inet.ed.gov
www2.ed.gov

Arne Duncan, Secretary of Education
Jim Shelton, Deputy Secretary
Ted Mitchell, Under Secretary
The Rehabilitation Services Administration (RSA) oversees formula and discretionary grant programs that help individuals with physical or mental disabilities to obtain employment and live more independently through the provision of such supports as counseling, medical and psychological services, job training and other individualized services.

3127 Social Security Administration
5 Parks Center Court
Ste 100
Owing Mills, MD 21175 410-965-6114
800-772-1213
FAX: 410-966-2027
www.ssa.gov

Bill Vitek, Manager
Administers old age, survivors, and disability insurance programs under Title II of the Social Security Act. Also administers the federal income maintenance program under Title XVI of the Social Security Act. Maintains network of local/regional offices nationwide.

3128 US Department of Education: Office of Civil Rights
400 Maryland Ave SW
Washington, DC 20202-7100 202-401-2000
800-872-5327
FAX: 202-401-0689
TTY: 800-437-0833
e-mail: customerservice@inet.ed.gov
www2.ed/gov/about/offices/list/ocr

Arne Duncan, Secretary of Education
Jim Shelton, Deputy Secretary
Ted Mitchell, Under Secretary
Prohibits discrimination on the basis of disability in programs and activities funded by the Department of Education. Investigates complaints and provides technical assistance to individuals and entities with rights and responsibilities under Section 504.

3129 US Department of Labor: Office of Federal Contract Programs
200 Constitution Ave NW
Washington, DC 20210 866-487-2365
TTY:877-889-5627
e-mail: webmaster@dol.gov
www.dol.gov/ofccp

Thomas E. Perez, Secretary of Labor
Christopher Lu, Deputy Secretary of Labor
Mathew Colangelo, Chief of Staff
James Moore, Deputy Assistant Secretary
Prohibits discrimination on the basis of disability and requires federal contractors and sub-contractors with contracts of $2,500 or more to take affirmative action to employ and advance individuals with disabilities.

3130 US Department of Transportation
1200 New Jersey Ave SE
Washington, DC 20590
202-366-4000
855-368-4200
TTY:800-877-8339
www.dot.gov

Anthony Foxx, Secretary of Transportation
Peter Rogoff, Acting Under Secretary for Policy
Kathryn Thomson, General Counsel
Greg Winfree, Assistant Secretary for Research and Technology
Enforces ADA provisions that require nondiscrimination in public and private mass transportation systems and services.

3131 US Office of Personnel Management
1900 E St NW
Washington, DC 20415
202-606-1800
FAX: 202-606-0909
TTY:202-606-2532
e-mail: Informationquality@opm.gov
opm.gov

Katherine Archuleta, Director
Ann Marie Habershaw, Chief of Staff & Director External Affairs
Angela Bailey, Chief Operating Officer
Jen Mason, Director, Office of Public Engagement
Establishes policies for employment of the handicapped within the federal service. Administers a merit system for the federal employment that includes recruiting, examining, training, and promoting people on the basis of knowledge and skills, regardless of sex, race, religion or other factors.

Alabama

3132 Alabama Council For Developmental Disabilities
RSA Union Building
100 N Union St
PO Box 301410
Montgomery, AL 36130-1410
334-242-3973
800-232-2158
FAX: 334-242-0797
e-mail: Myra.Jones@mh.alabama.gov
www.acdd.org

Stefan Eisen, Jr., Chair
Sophia Whitted, Fiscal Manager
Elmyra Jones-Banks, Executive Director
Shungulla Moorey, Office Manager
Serves as an advocate for Alabama's citizens with developmental disabilities and their families; to empower them with the knowledge and opportunity to make informed choices and exercise control over their own lives; and to create a climate for positive socialchange to enable them to be respected, independent and productive integrated members of society.

3133 Alabama Department of Public Health
RSA Tower, 201 Monroe St
PO Box 303017
Montgomery, AL 36104-3017
334-206-5300
800-ALA-1818
www.adph.org

Kathy Vincent, Staff Assistant
Donald Williamson, Administrator
Provides professional services for the improvement and protection of the public's health through disease prevention and the assurance of public health services to resident and transient populations of the state regardless of social circumstances or the ability to pay.

3134 Alabama Department of Rehabilitation Services
602 S Lawrence St
Montgomery, AL 36104
334-293-7500
800-441-7607
FAX: 334-293-7383
e-mail: cary.boswell@rehab.alabama.gov
www.rehab.alabama.gov

Cary F Boswell, Commissioner
Jim Carden, Deputy Commissioner
Jim Harris Iii, Assistant Commissioner
Winona Nelson, Cheif Financial Officer
To enable Alabama's children and adults with disabilities to achieve their maximum potential.

3135 Alabama Department of Senior Services
201 Monroe Street
RSA Tower Suite 350
Montgomery, AL 36130
334-242-5743
877-425-2243
FAX: 334-242-5594
e-mail: ageline@adss.state.al.us
www.adss.alabama.gov

Irene Collins, Executive Director

3136 Alabama Disabilities Advocacy Program
University of Alabama
P.O.Box 870395
Tuscaloosa, AL 35487
205-348-4928
800-826-1675
FAX: 205-348-3909
e-mail: adap@adap.ua.edu
www.adap.net

Anita Davidson, Legal Assistant
Janet Owens, Accounting Specialist
James Tucker, Director
Rosemary Beck, Information Systems Administrator
The federally mandate statewide protection and advocacy system serving eligible individuals with disabilities in Alabama. ADAP has five program components: Protection and Advocacy for persons with developmental disabilities (PADD), Protection and Advocacy for Individuals with Mental Illness (PAIMT), Protection and Advocacy of Individual Rights (PAIR), Protection and Advocacy for Assistive Technology (PAAT) and Protection & Advocacy For Beneficiaries of Social Security (PABSS).

3137 Alabama Division of Rehabilitation and Crippled Children
602 S Lawrence Street
Montgomery, AL 36104
334-293-7500
800-441-7607
FAX: 334-293-7383
e-mail: sshiver@rehab.state.al.us
www.rehab.state.al.us

Cary F Boswell, Commissioner
Steven Kayes, Board Member
Jimmie Varnado, Board Member

3138 Alabama Governor's Committee on Employment of Persons with Disabilities
602 S Lawrence St
Montgomery, AL 36104
334-293-7500
800-441-7607
FAX: 334-293-7383
www.rehab.state.al.us

Jimmie Varnado, assistant vice president
Cary F Boswell, Commissioner

3139 Alabama State Department of Human Resources
Childcare Services Division
50 North Ripley St
Montgomery, AL 36130
334-242-1310
FAX: 334-353-1115
e-mail: barry.spear@dhr.alabama.gov
www.dhr.state.al.us

Nancy T. Buckner, Commissioner
Nancy Jinright, Chief of Staff/Ethics Officer
John Hardy, Communications
Conitha King, Finance

Partners with communities to promtoe family stability and provide for the safety and self-sufficiency of vulnerable Alabamians.

3140 Client Assistance Program: Alabama
400 S Union St
Ste 465
Montgomery, AL 36104
334-263-2749
800-288-3231
FAX: 334-230-9765
e-mail: rachel.hughes@rehab.alabama.gov
www.sacap.alabama.gov

Rachel Hughes, Director/Advocate

3141 Disability Determination Service: Birmingham
P.O.Box 830300
Birmingham, AL 35283
205-989-2100
FAX: 205-989-2295
ssa.gov

Tommy Warren, Executive Director
Janet Cox, Owner

3142 Social Security: Mobile Disability Determination Services
PO Box 2371
Mobile, AL 36652-2371
251-433-2820
800-292-6743
FAX: 251-436-0599
www.ssa.gov

Tommy Warren, Executive Director
Jack Miller, Office Manager

3143 Workers Compensation Board Alabama
649 Monroe St
Montgomery, AL 36131
334-242-2868
800-528-5166
FAX: 334-353-8262
e-mail: webmaster@labor.alabama.gov
labor.alabama.gov/wc

Charles DeLamar, Director
Al Pelham, Supervisor
Sandy Hallmark, Supervisor
Peggy Barton, Supervisor

Alaska

3144 ATLA
2217 E Tudor Rd
Ste 4
Anchorage, AK 99507-1068
907-563-2599
800-723-2852
FAX: 907-563-0699
e-mail: atla@atla.biz
www.atla.biz

Kathy Privratsky, Executive Director
Mystie Rail, Commissioner
Margaret Cisco, AT Specialist

Assistive Technology sales and services. ATLA is Alaska's only assistive technology resource center.

3145 Alaska Commission on Aging
150 Third Street
PO Box 110693
Juneau, AK 99811
907-465-3250
FAX: 970-465-1398
e-mail: hss.acoa@alaska.gov
dhss.alaska.gov/acoa

Denise Daniello, Executive Director
Jon Erickson, Planner II
Sherice Cole, Administrative Assistant II
Lesley Thompson, H&SS Planner I

3146 Alaska Department of Handicapped Children
Ste 314
1231 Gambell St
Anchorage, AK 99501-4664
907-346-1995

Gregory Lee, CEO

3147 Alaska Division of Vocational Rehabilitation:
PO Box 111149
Juneau, AK 99811-1878
907-465-2700
FAX: 907-465-2784
e-mail: dawn.duval@alaska.gov
labor.state.ak.us

Dianne Blummer, Commissioner
David G Stone, Deputy commissioner

Provides comprehensive services to people with disabilities to assist in achieving an employment outcome.

3148 Client Assistance Program: Alaska
2900 Boniface Pkwy
Ste 100
Anchorage, AK 99504-3132
907-333-2211
800-478-0047
FAX: 907-333-1186
e-mail: akcap@alaska.com
www.home.gci.net/~alaskacap

Pam Stratton, Executive Director

We provide informatory referral to other programs in Alaska that are funded under the Rehabilitation Act of 1973 as amended; Individual assistance or advocacy, if an individual with disability has applied for or received services from an agency funded under the Rehabilitation Act and has concerns or questions we will work with them to help resolve their concerns with the agency.

3149 Department Of Health& Social ServicesDivision Of Behaviorial Health
350 Main St
Juneau, AK 99801-1149
907-465-3370
800-465-4828
FAX: 907-465-2668
www.alaska.gov

Walter Majors, Director

The division plans for and provides appropriate prevention, treatment and support for families impacted by mental disorders or developmental disabilities while maximizing self-determination. Community based services are provided by grantees. Inpatient services are provided in two division operated facilities.

3150 Governor's Committee on Employment and Rehabilitation of People with Disabilities
Division of Vocational Rehabilitation (DVR)
801 W 10 St
Ste A
Juneau, AK 99801-1878
907-465-2814
800-478-2815
FAX: 907-465-2815
e-mail: dawn.duval@alaska.gov
www.labor.state.ak.us/dvr

Cheryl Walsh, Executive Director

Carries on a continuing program to promote the employment and rehabilitation of citizens with disabilities in the State of Alaska. Advocates for a comprehensive statewide system for access to assistive technology. Obtains and maintains cooperation with public and private groups and individuals in this field.

3151 Governor's Council on Disabilities and Special Education
201 C St
Ste 740
Anchorage, AK 99503
907-269-8990
888-269-8990
FAX: 907-269-8995
e-mail: sheryl.cobb@alaska.gov
www.hss.state.ak.us/gcdse/

Millie Ryan, Executive Director
Teresa Jones, Operations Director
Patrick Reinhart, Project Coordinator

3152 Protection & Advocacy System: Alaska
Disability Law Center of Alaska
3330 Arctic Blvd
Ste 103
Anchorage, AK 99503-4580
907-565-1002
800-478-1234
FAX: 907-565-1000
e-mail: akpa@dlcak.org
dlcak.org

Deborah Smith, President
James M Shine Sr

Deals with rights of the disabled. Works in conjunction with agencies, law offices and family members.

3153 Protection & Advocacy for Persons with Developmental Disabilities: Alaska
Advocacy Services of Alaska
Ste 101
615 E 82nd Ave
Anchorage, AK 99518-3100
907-222-2652
866-275-7273
FAX: 907-677-8777
TTY: 866-232-4525
e-mail: rtessardore@dlcakelcak.org

Greg Schomaker, Manager

3154 Workers Compensation Division
Department of Labor & Workforce Development
PO Box 115512
Juneau, AK 99811-5512
907-465-2790
FAX: 907-465-2797
e-mail: workerscomp@alaska.gov
www.labor.state.ak.us/wc

Clark Bishop, Commissioner
Trena Heikes, Division Director
Michael Monagle, Director

Arizona

3155 Arizona Department of Economic Security
1717 W Jefferson St
Phoenix, AZ 85007-3295
602-542-4719
FAX: 602-542-5320
www.azdes.gov

Neal Young, Director
Lynne Smith, Chief Exeecutive Officer
Will Humble, Director
Rex Critchfield, Manager

The Department of Economic Security is a human service agency providing services in six areas: Aging and Community Services, Benefits and Medical Eligibility, Child Support Enforcement, Children and Family Services, Developmental Disabilities and Employment and Rehabilitation Services.

3156 Arizona Department of Health Services
150 N 18th Ave
Ste 330
Phoenix, AZ 85007-3243
602-542-1025
FAX: 602-542-0883
www.azdhs.gov

Will Humble, Director
Neal Young, Director
Lynne Smith, Chief Exeecutive Officer
Rex Critchfield, Manager

The mission of Children's Rehabilitative Services is to improve the quality of life for children by providing family-centered medical treatment, rehabilitation, and related support services to enrolled individuals who have certain medical, handicapping, or potentially handicapping conditions.

3157 Arizona Division of Aging and Adult Services
1789 W Jefferson St
Phoenix, AZ 85007-3202
602-542-4446
FAX: 602-364-6575
www.azdes.gov

Rex Critchfield, Manager
Neal Young, Director
Lynne Smith, Chief Exeecutive Officer
Will Humble, Director

3158 Arizona Rehabilitation State Services for the Blind and Visually Impaired
4620 N 16th St, B-106
Ste 100
Phoenix, AZ 85016-5121
602-266-9579
FAX: 602-264-7819
www.azdes.gov

Paul Howell, Vocational Rehab Supervisor
Suzanne Sayre f, Rehab Counselor for Blind

Offers clients a conservation program, eye examinations, treatments, counseling, social work, psychological testing and evaluation, professional training, computer training and more for the visually impaired. The staff includes 56 full time employees.

3159 Developmental Disability Council: Arizona
2828 N Country Club Rd
Ste 100
Tucson, AZ 85716-3202
602-542-4049
800-889-5893
FAX: 602-542-5320
e-mail: valeria.hill@mail.de.state.az.us
www.cpes.com

David A Berns, Manager
Nebal Chavez, Executive Director
Susan Madison, Manager

The mission of the GovernorOs Council on Developmental Disabilities is to bring together persons with disabilities representing Arizona cultural diversity and their families and other community members, to protect rights, eliminate barriers, and jointly promote equal opportunities

3160 Governor's Council on Developmental Disabilities
1740 W Adams
Suite 201
Phoenix, AZ 85007
520-325-9688
877-665-3176
FAX: 520-325-3561
e-mail: lclausen@azdes.gov
azgovernor.gov/DDPC/

Larry Clausen, Executive Director
Shelly Adams, Executive Secretary

The purpose of the council is to advocate for and assure that individuals with developmental disabilities and their families participate in the design of and have access to culturally competent services, supports and provides opportunities to become integrated and included in the community.

3161 **International Dyslexia Association: Arizona Branch**
PO Box 6284
Scottsdale, AZ 85261-6284 480-941-0308
e-mail: arizona.ida@gmail.com
www.dyslexia-az.org
Meredith Puls, President
Yvonne Gill, Vice President
Melissa A. L. Pallister, Treasurer
Sue Noel, Secretary
Provides free information and referral services for diagnosis and tutoring for parents, educators, physicians, and individuals with dyslexia. The voice of our membership is heard in 48 countries. Membership includes yearly journal and quarterly newsletter. Call for conference dates.

3162 **Protection & Advocacy for Persons with Disabilities: Arizona**
Arizona Center for Disability Law
5025 E Washington St
Ste 202
Phoenix, AZ 85034 602-274-6287
800-927-2260
FAX: 520-884-0992
TTY: 602-274-6287
e-mail: center@azdisabilitylaw.org
www.azdisabilitylaw.org
Cathy Hunt, President
Loretta Cheeks, Vice President
J. J. Rico, Interim Executive Director
The Center provides disability-related legal information and advice to individuals who need their services and assistance. In addition to limited legal representation, their goal is to provide efficient, streamlined services to educate people with disabilities and their support on how to enforce their legal rights through self-advocacy. Guides and documents are available online by selecting Self-Advocacy Materials button on the homepage.

3163 **Social Security: Phoenix Disability Determination Services**
Social Security Admission
250 Seventh Avenue
Suite 100
Phoenix, AZ 85007 800-772-1213
TTY:800-325-0778
www.socialsecurity-disability.org/social-secu

3164 **Social Security: Tucson Disability Determination Services**
3500 N Campbell Ave
Tucson, AZ 85719-2030 520-670-5890
800-772-1213
TTY:800-325-0778
www.socialsecurity-disability.org/social-secu

Arkansas

3165 **Arkansas Assistive Technology Projects**
Increasing Capabilities Access
26 Corporate Hill Dr
Little Rock, AR 72205-4538 501-666-8868
800-828-2799
FAX: 501-666-5319
e-mail: info@ar-ican.org
www.arkansas-ican.org
Eddie Schmeckenbecher, Supervisor
Essie Hardin, Secretary
A consumer responsive ,statewide program promoting assistive technology devices and sources for persons of all ages with all disabilities. Referral and information services provide information about devices, where to obtain them and their cost.

3166 **Arkansas Division of Aging & Adult Services**
Department of Human Services
PO Box 1437
Little Rock, AR 72203-1437 501-682-2441
FAX: 501-682-8155
e-mail: aging.services@arkansas.gov
www.state.ar.us/dhs/aging
Herb Sanderson, Director
Coney Parker, Assistant Director
Sandra Barrett, Assistant Director
Eileen Dozier, Administrative Assistant
The division provides services geared for adults and the elderly including supervised living, home delivered meals, adult day care, senior centers, personal care, household chores, and adult protective services.

3167 **Arkansas Division of Developmental Disabilities Services**
Donaghey Plaza
PO Box 1437
Little Rock, AR 72203-1437 501-682-1001
FAX: 501-682-8820
humanservices.arkansas.gov/ddds/Pages/default
Charlie Green, Manager
State agency to assist persons with developmental disabilities and their family in obtaining appropriate assistance and services.

3168 **Arkansas Division of Services for the Blind**
Department Of Health and Human Services
700 Main St
Little Rock, AR 72201-4608 501-682-1001
800-960-9270
FAX: 501-682-0366
TTY: 800-285-1131
e-mail: donnabirdwell@arkansas.gov
www.state.ar.us/dhs/dsd/newdsb/index.html
Katy Morris, Manager
State program which offers services in the areas of health, counseling, social work, self help and education for the visually and multihandicapped. The staff includes 4 full time and 13 part time members including mobility specialists and rehabilitation teachers.

3169 **Arkansas Governor's Developmental Disabilities Council**
5800 W 10 Street
Suite 805
Little Rock, AR 72204-1763 501-661-2589
800-462-0599
FAX: 501-661-2399
e-mail: Regina.L.Wilson@arkansas.gov
ddcouncil.org
Regina Wilson, Executive Director
Brenda Mercer, Family Services Coordinator
Lee Russell, Information Oficer
Lacey Wynes, Administrative Assistant
A federally-funded state agency established to bring the perspective of individuals with developmental disabilities and his or her family or natural support system to policy makers and make improvements to the service system.

3170 **Baptist Health Rehabilitation Institute**
Baptist Heath
9601 Interstate 630 Exit 7
Little Rock, AR 72205-7299 501-202-2000
800-991-0888
FAX: 501-202-1115
www.baptist-health.com
Ellen Callaway, Director, Rehabilition Therapy
Jerry Baugh, Vice President
Russell Harrington, President
Acute rehab facility serving patients with ortho, spinal cord injury, brain injury, CVA, arthritis, cardiac and generalized weakness; JCAHO and CARF accredited; 17 outpatient therapy centers throughout central Arkansas.

3171 Children's Medical Services
P.O.Box 1437
Little Rock, AR 72203-1437
501-682-8207
800-482-5850
FAX: 501-682-8247
www.cms-kids.com

Nancy Holder, Program Director
Iris Fehr, Nursing Director
Rodney Farley, Parent Activities Coordinator

3172 President's Committee on People with Disabilities: Arkansas
7th & Main St
Little Rock, AR 72203

3173 Social Security: Arkansas Disability Determination Services
701 S Pulaski St
Little Rock, AR 72201-3990
501-682-3030
800-772-1213
FAX: 501-682-7553
www.socialsecurity.gov

Arthur Boutiette, COO

California

3174 California Department of Aging
1300 National Drive
Suite 200
Sacramento, CA 95834-1992
916-419-7500
FAX: 916-928-2267
TTY:800-735-2929
e-mail: webmaster@aging.ca.gov
aging.ca.gov

Lynn Daucher, Manager
David Supkofl, Manager
The Department contracts with the network of Area Agencies on Aging, who directly manage a wide array of federal and state-funded services that help older adults find employment; support older and disabled individuals to live as independently as possible in the community; promote healthy aging and community involvement; and assist family members in their vital care giving role

3175 California Department of Handicapped Children
714 P Street
Rm 323
Sacramento, CA 95814-6401
916-445-4171

Maridee Gregory
Diana Bonta, Chief Executive Officer

3176 California Department of Rehabilitation
830 K St
Sacramento, CA 95814-3510
916-445-4171
TTY:916-445-3971
e-mail: doroa.bpremo@hwl.cahwnet.gov

Brenda Premo, Director
David Supkofl, Manager
Assists people with disabilities, particularly those with severe disabilities, in obtaining and retaining meaningful employment and living independently in their communities. The department develops, purchases, provides and advocates for programs and services in vocational rehabilitation, habilitation and independent living with a priority on serving persons with all disabilities, especially those with the most severe disabilities.

3177 California Governor's Committee on Employment of People with Disabilities
Employment Development Department
800 Capitol Mall
PO Box 826880
Sacramento, CA 94280-0001
916-654-8055
800-695-0350
FAX: 916-654-9821
TTY: 916-654-9820
www.edd.ca.gov

Charlie Kaplan, Staff Director
GCEPD works to eliminate the barriers that preclude equal consideration for employment opportunities for people with disabilities. The Governor's Committee is responsible for providing leadership to increase the numbers of people with disabilities in the California workforce.

3178 California Protection & Advocacy: (PAI) A Nonprofit Organization
Protection and Advocacy (PA I)
1831 K Street
Sacramento, CA 95811-4114
916-504-5800
800-776-5746
FAX: 916-504-5802
e-mail: SERVICES@DISABILITYRIGHTSCA.ORG
www.disabilityrightsca.org

Catherine Blakemore, Executive Director
Andrew Mudryk, Deputy Director
Cara Armstrong, Manager
Advancing the human and legal rights of people with disabilities.

3179 California State Council on Developmental Disabilities
1507 21st Street
Suite 210
Sacramento, CA 95811-5297
916-322-8481
866-802-0514
FAX: 916-443-4957
e-mail: council@scdd.ca.gov
www.scdd.ca.gov

Carol Risley, Executive Director
Tammy Eudy, Office Assistant
Robin Maitino, Executive Assistant
The State Council on Developmental Disabilities (SCDD) is established by state and federal law as an independent state agency to ensure that people with developmental disabilities and their families receive the services and supports they need.

3180 Client Assistance Program: California
CA Health and Human Services Agency Dept of Rehab
721 Capitol Mall
PO Box 944222
Sacramento, CA 95814
916-324-1313
800-952-5544
FAX: 916-558-5391
TTY:916- 558-580
e-mail: capinfo@dor.ca.gov
www.dor.ca.gov

Tony P Sauer, Director
We have a three-pronged mission to provide services and advocacy that assist people with disabilities to live independently, become employed and have equality in the communities in which they live and work.

3181 International Dyslexia Association: Central California Branch
4594 E Michigan Ave
Fresno, CA 93703-1556
559-251-9385
800-222-3123
FAX: 599-252-1216
e-mail: dyslexias@attbi.com
www.interdys.org

Joy Moody, President
Provides free information and referral services for diagnosis and tutoring for parents, educators, physicians, and individuals with dyslexia. The voice of our membership is heard in 48 countries. Membership includes yearly journal and quarterly newsletter. Call for conference dates. Other locations also available in California.

3182 **Long Beach Department of Health and Human Services**
2525 Grand Ave
Long Beach, CA 90815-1765
562-570-4000
FAX: 562-570-4049
e-mail: info@ci.long-beach.ca.us/health
www.longbeach.gov/health/
Ron Arias, Executive Director
Michael Johnson, Manager

3183 **Los Angeles County Department of Health Services**
313 N Figueroa St
Los Angeles, CA 90012-2602
213-240-8101
800-427-8700
FAX: 213-250-4013
e-mail: webmaster@adhs.org
www.ladhs.org
Mitchell Katz, Director
John Schunhoff, Chief Deputy Director
Allan Wrecker, CFO
Los Angeles County Department of Health Services is one of the US's largest publicly supported health systems.The system is the main provider of health care for the area's poor and uninsured. It provides general medical and surgical care and is affiliated with the medical school at USC. The system also manages the Emergency Medical Services (EMS) Agency and the Community Health Plan HMO, a low-cost managed care plan for members of Medicaid and other state-funded programs.

3184 **Social Security: California Disability Determination Services**
3164 Garrity Way
Richmond, CA 94806-1983
800-772-1213
TTY:800-325-0778
www.ssa.gov
Sally Keen, San Francisco Regional PDF Coord

3185 **Social Security: Fresno Disability Determination Services**
Social Security
1052 C St
Fresno, CA 93706-3245
559-487-5391
800-772-1213
FAX: 510-970-2947
TTY: 800-325-0778
e-mail: sally.keen@ssa.gov
ssa.gov
Sally Keen, Regional PDF Coordinator

3186 **Social Security: Oakland Disability Determination Services**
238 11th St
Oakland, CA 94607-4490
800-772-1213
TTY:800-325-0778
www.ssa.gov

3187 **Social Security: Sacramento Disability Determination Services**
8351 Folsom Blvd
Suite A
Sacramento, CA 95826-3538
877-274-5419
800-772-1213
FAX: 916-263-5310
TTY: 916-381-9445
ssa.gov

3188 **Social Security: San Diego Disability Determination Services**
1333 Front St
San Diego, CA 92101-3603
800-772-1213
FAX: 619-278-4303
TTY:800-325-0778
e-mail: josesanbria@ssa.gov
www.ssa.gov

Colorado

3189 **Colorado Department of Aging & Adult Services**
1575 Sherman St
10th Floor
Denver, CO 80203-1702
303-866-5700
FAX: 303-620-2696
e-mail: cdhs.communications@state.co.us
www.cdhs.state.co.us/ADRS/AAS
Reggie Bicha, Executive Director
A department providing services to the elderly.

3190 **Colorado Developmental Disabilities Council**
1120 Lincoln
Suite 706
Denver, CO 80203
720-941-0176
FAX: 720-941-8490
e-mail: cdppc.email@state.co.us
coddc.org
Marcia Tewell, Manager
The mission is to advocate in collaboration with and on behalf of people with developmental disabilities for the establishment and implementation of public policy which will further their independence, productivity and integration.

3191 **Colorado Division of Mental Health**
3520 W Oxford Ave
Denver, CO 80236-3108
303-866-7857
FAX: 303-866-7048
colorado.gov
Keith Lagrenade, CEO
Administration of public health program

3192 **Colorado Health Care Program for Children with Special Needs**
4300 Cherry Creek South Dr
Denver, CO 80246-1530
303-692-2000
800-886-7689
FAX: 303-839-8068
e-mail: cdphe.information@state.co.us
www.state.cdphe.co.us
Arlene Miles, President
Christopher Urbina MD, Executive Director, Chief Medica
Rosalind Bedell, COO
Joni Reynolds, Public Health Program Director
Provides information and state aid to children with disabilities.

3193 **Division of Workers' Compensation Dapartment of Labor & Employment**
633 17th Street
Suite 201
Denver, CO 80202-3660
303-318-8700
800-388-5515
888-390-7936
FAX: 303-575-8882
www.coworkforce.com/dwc/
Ellen Golombek, Executive Director
Infomation regarding Division Rules and procedures for Claimants, Employers, Adjusters, and parties to claim.

3194 **Eastern Colorado Services for the Disabled**
P. O. Box 1682
617 South 10th Avenue
Sterling, CO 80751-3168
970-522-7121
FAX: 970-522-1173
e-mail: peggyb@ecsdd.org
www.easterncoloradoservices.org
Judy Fehringer, Executive Director
Traci Schrade, Finance Director
Beky Kizer, Case Management
Case coordination, infant stimulation, family support, residential and vocational programs.

3195 **International Dyslexia Association: Rocky Mountain Branch**
P.O.Box 461010
Glendale, CO 80246-5010
303-721-9425
800-222-3123
FAX: 303-721-9425
e-mail: ida_rmb@yahoo.com
www.dyslexia-rmbida.org

Elenn Steinberg, President
Debra Coultas, Vice President
Sally Pistilli, Treasurer
Katie Johansen, Recording Secretary

Provides free information and referral services for diagnosis and tutoring for parents, educators, physicians, and individuals with dyslexia in Utah, Colorado and Wyoming. The voice of our membership is heard in 48 countries. Membership includes yearly journal and quarterly newsletter. Call for conference dates.

3196 **Legal Center for People with Disabilities& Older People**
455 Shernan Street
Suite 130
Denver, CO 80203-4403
303-722-0300
800-288-1376
FAX: 303-722-0720
TTY: 303-722-3619
e-mail: tlcmail@thelegalcenter.org
thelegalcenter.org

Todd Blakely, President
Peter Lindquist, Vice President
Nancy Tucker, Secretary
John Paul Anderson, Treasurer

Uses the legal system to protect and promote the rights of people with disabilities and older people in Colorado through direct legal representation, advocacy, education and legislative analysis. The Legal Center is Colorado's Protection and Advocacy System. We are also the State Ombudsman for nursing homes and assisted living facilities. Call for a free publications and products list.

Connecticut

3197 **Connecticut Board of Education and Servicefor the Blind**
184 Windsor Ave
Windsor, CT 06095-4536
860-602-4000
800-842-4510
FAX: 860-602-4020
TTY: 860-602-4221
e-mail: brian.sigman@CT.GOV
www.ct.gov/besb/site/default.asp

Amy Porter, Commissioner

Offers rehabilitative services and information for persons with legal blindness and childrenwhonare visually impaired that are residents of Connecticut.

3198 **Connecticut Commission on Aging**
210 Capitol Ave
Hartford, CT 6106
860-240-5200
FAX: 860-240-5204
e-mail: coa@cga.ct.gov
www.cga.ct.gov/coa

Julie Evans Starr, Executive Director
Robert J Norton, Communications Director

Advocates on beha;f of elderly persons in Connecticut by regularly monitoring their status, assessing the impact of current and propsed initiatives, and conducting activities which promote the interests of these individuals and report to the Governor and the Legislature.

3199 **Connecticut Department of Children and Youth Services**
505 Hudson St
Hartford, CT 6106
860-550-6300
FAX: 860-724-2001
e-mail: Commissioner.dcf@ct.gov
www.ct.gov

Gary Scappini, Manager
Bruce Douglas, Executive Director

3200 **Connecticut Developmental Disabilities Council**
263 Farmington Avenue
Farmington, CT 6030
860-679-1561
800-653-1134
FAX: 860-679-1571
TTY: 860-679-1502
ctkasa.org

Ed Preneta, Executive Director

Kids As Self Advocates (KASA) is a national grassroots network that helps youth with special needs and their friends become self-advocates, helps other people in the community understand what it's like to live with special health care needs.

3201 **Connecticut Office of Protection and Advocacy for Persons with Disabilities**
60 Weston Street
Suite B
Hartford, CT 06120-1551
860-297-4300
800-842-7303
FAX: 860-566-8714
TTY: 860-297-4320
e-mail: OPA-Information@po.state.ct.us
www.ct.gov/opapd

James Mc Gaughey, Executive Director
Gretchen Knaff, Assistant Director
Linda Mizzi, Assistant Program Director

Provides information, referrals, advocacy assistance & limited legal services to people with disabilities in the state of Connecticut whose civil rights have been violated or who are experiencing the difficulty securing relevant support services. P & A supports the development of community advocacy groups by providing training & technical assistance. P & A is responsible for investigating abuse & neglect of all individuals with intellectual disability ages 18-59.

3202 **Social Security: Hartford Area Office**
960 Main Street
2nd Floor
Hartford, CT 6103-1228
877-619-2851
800-772-1213
FAX: 860-566-1795
TTY: 860-525-4967
www.ssa.gov

Jan Gilbert, Professional Relations Coord.

Delaware

3203 **Delaware Assistive Technology Initiative(DATI)**
461 Wyoming Road
Newark, DE 19716-0269
302-831-0354
FAX: 302-831-4690
TTY:800-870-3284
e-mail: dati@asel.udel.edu
www.dati.org

Beth Mineo, Project Director
Joann McCafferty, Staff Assistant

The Delaware Assistive Technology Initiative (DATI) connects Delawareans who have disabilities with the tools they need in order to learn, work, play and participate in community life safely and independently. DATI services include: Equipment demonstration centers in each county; no-cost, short-term equipment loans that let you try before you buy; Equipment Exchange Program; AT workshops and other training sessions; advocacy for improved AT access policies and funing and several more.

3204 **Delaware Client Assistance Program**
United Cerebral Palsy Association
254 E Camden Wyoming Ave
Camden, DE 19934-1303
302-698-9336
800-640-9336
FAX: 302-698-9338
e-mail: capucp@magpage.com
www.icdri.org

Melissa Shahan, Executive Director

Provides advocacy services for persons involved with programs covered under the Rehabilitation Act of 1973 as amended, information and referrals on ADA, Title I.

3205 **Delaware Department of Health and Social Services**
Administration Building D HS S Campus
1901 N Dupont Hwy
Main Building
New Castle, DE 19720- 1160 302-255-9040
800-464-4357
FAX: 302-255-4429
TTY: 302-744-4556
e-mail: dhssinfo@state.de.us
www.dhss.delaware.gov
Rita Landgraf, Cabinet Secretary
Provides most of the human services available through Delaware State Government, including Medicaid, the Children's Health Insurance Program, food stamps, welfare-to-work, vaccines for children, child support enforcement, public health programs, and general services for the aging. Also for individuals with developmental and physical disabilities, visual impairements, mental illness and other vulnerable populations.

3206 **Delaware Department of Public Instructing**
PO Box 1402
Dover, DE 19903-1402 302-739-4686
800-433-5292
FAX: 302-739-3092
Dr. Pascal D Forgione Jr, Superintendent
A publicly funded, state agency that gives information about local facilities and administers supplemental funds for visually handicapped students in local schools. It also maintains special teachers of sight conservation and braille programs for both children and adults.

3207 **Delaware Developmental Disability Council**
410 Federal St
Suite 2
Dover, DE 19901-3640 302-739-2232
800-464-4357
e-mail: pat.maichle@state.de.us
www.ddc.delaware.gov
Diann Jones, Council Chair
Patricia L. Maichle, Council Staff
Kristin Cosden, Social Service Administrator
Stefanie Lancaster, Administrative Officer

3208 **Delaware Division for the Visually Impaired**
1901 N Dupont Hwy
New Castle, DE 19720-1160 302-255-9040
FAX: 302-255-4429
e-mail: dhssinfo@state.de.us
www.dhss.delaware.gov/dvi/
Rita Landgraf, Secretary
Henry Smith, Deputy Secretary
Betsy Deldeo, Office Manager
State agency serving the visually impaired persons from birth, with or without other handicaps. Services offered include vocational rehabilitation, independent living, orientation and mobility, technology assessment, transition from school to work.

3209 **Delaware Industries for the Blind**
1901 N Dupont Hwy
New Castle, DE 19720-1160 302-255-9855
FAX: 302-255-4442
e-mail: awingrove@state.de.us
www.promoplace.com/dib
Alan Wingrove, Manager
Delaware Industries for the Blind is a multi-faceted company that specializes in creating employment opportunities for Delaware citizens who are blind and visually impaired. DIB accomplishes this by providing quality goods and guaranteed services under contracts from Federal, State and Local Agencies and Industries.

3210 **Delaware Protection & Advocacy for Persons with Disabilities**
Arc of Delaware
144 E Market St
Georgetown, DE 19947-1411 302-856-6019
FAX: 302-856-6133
e-mail: challdover@aol.com
Becky Allen, Executive Director

3211 **Delaware Workers Compensation Board**
Industrial Accident Board de dept
4425 N Market St
Wilmington, DE 19802-1307 302-761-8085
FAX: 302-761-6601
www.delawareworks.com
James Cagle, Manager

3212 **Social Security: Wilmington Disability Determination**
U S Department of Health and Human Services
1528 S 16th Street
Wilmington, NC 28401-3908 866-964-6227
800-772-1213
FAX: 910-254-3444
TTY: 910-815-4695
www.socialsecurity.gov
J Allen Murphy, Founder
Vickie O'Brien, Manager

District of Columbia

3213 **District of Columbia Department of Handicapped Children**
D C General Hospital
Bldg 10
1900 Massachusetts Ave SE
Washington, DC 20003- 2542 202-541-6337
FAX: 202-675-7694
Jacqueline Mcmorris, Acting Chief
Nayab Ali, MD

3214 **District of Columbia Office on Aging**
441 4th St SW
Suite 900
Washington, DC 20001-2714 202-724-5622
FAX: 202-724-4979
TTY:202-724-8925
e-mail: dcoa@dc.gov
dcoa.dc.gov
John Thompson, Executive Director
Serves the District of Columbia residents 60 years of age and older. Contact the Information and Assistance Unit for more information about innovative programs and services offered by the Office.

3215 **Information, Protection & Advocacy for Persons with Disabilities**
IPACHI
220 I Street, N.E.
Suite 130
Washington, DC 20002 202-547-0198
FAX: 202-547-2083
e-mail: jbrown@uls-dc.org
www.acf.hhs.gov/programs/add/states/pas.html
Jane Brown, Executive Director
Ronald Tyson, Information/Referral
Offers services and support for persons with disabilities in the Washington, DC area.

3216 Information, Protection and Advocacy Center for Handicapped Individuals
220 I Street, N.E.
Suite 130
Washington, DC 20002-2340
202-547-0198
FAX: 202-547-2083
e-mail: jbrown@uls-dc.org
www.acf.hhs.gov/programs/add/states/pas.html
Jane Brown, Executive Director
Serves all persons with disabilities in the DC, Maryland and Virginia areas offering them legal representation and advocacy, information and referrals and several publications.

3217 International Dyslexia Association of DC
40 York Rd., 4th Floor
Baltimore, MD 21204-1016
410-29- 023
800-222-3123
FAX: 410-321-5069
e-mail: info@interdys.org
www.interdys.org
Ruth R Tifford LCSW, President
The DC Capital Area Branch, provides support for individuals with dyslexia and their families in the Washington, DC metropolitan area, including parts of Maryland, Virginia and West Virginia. Our conferences, book sales and online information resources are designed to further the understanding of dyslexia and encourage the use of systematic, multisensory teaching methods enabling children and adults to reach their educational potential.

3218 Wage and Hour Division of the Employment Standards Administration
US Department of Labor
200 Constitution Ave NW
Washington, DC 20210-1
202-693-5000
866-487-2365
FAX: 202-219-8822
TTY: 877-889-5627
www.dol.gov
Hilda Solis, Secretary of Labor
Seth Harris, Deputy Secretary
Elizabeth Kim, Executive Secretariat Director
Betsey Stevenson, Chief Economist
Administers regulations governing the employment of individuals with disabilities in sheltered workshops and the disabled workers industries.

3219 Washington Hearing and Speech Society
2150 N 107th St, Ste 205
Seattle, WA 98133-2633
202-537-4010
FAX: 202-243-5255
e-mail: support@dcsha.org
www.wslha.org
Karen Simpson, President
Judith Burnier, Secretary
Julie Leonardo, Treasurer
Offers individuals with hearing or speech impairments, in the DC area, speech, reading classes, audiological services and new aids.

3220 Well Mind Association of Greater Washington
18606 New Hampshire Ave
Ashton, MD 20861-9789
301-774-6617
FAX: 301-946-1402

3221 Workers Compensation Board: District of Columbia
1200 Upshur St NW
Washington, DC 20011-5626

Florida

3222 ARC Gateway
3932 N 10th Ave
Pensacola, FL 32503-2807
850-434-2638
FAX: 850-438-2180
e-mail: info@arc-gateway.org
www.arc-gateway.org
Peter Mougey, President
Patricia Young, Vice President
Lynn Erickson, Secretary
Donna Fassett, Executive Director
ARC Gateway is a non-profit organization that serves children who have or are at risk of developmental disabilities as well as adults with developmental disabilitie

3223 Advocacy Center for Persons with Disabilities
2728 Centerview Drive
Suite 102
Tallahassee, FL 32301- 5020
850-488-9071
800-342-0823
FAX: 850-488-8640
TTY: 800-346-4127
e-mail: info@advocacy.org
advocacycenter.org
Bob Whitley, Executive Director
Paige Morgan, Executive Assistant
Peter Schoemann, Chair
Catherine Piecora, Vice Chair
Disability Rights Florida is the designated protection and advocacy system for individuals with disabilities in the State of Florida.

3224 Assistive Technology Educational Network of Florida
1207 S Mellonville Ave
Sanford, FL 32771-2240
800-328-3678
FAX: 407-688-4593
e-mail: diane_penn@scps.k12.fl.us
www.aten.scps.k12.fl.us
Dee Wright, Executive Secretary
Diane Penn, MA, Technology Specialist
Provides state-wide information, awareness and training for students, family members, teachers and other professionals in the area of assisted technology; a quarterly newsletter and a network of specialists (Local Assistive Technology Specialists) trained by ATEN to provide support at the district level.

3225 Bureau Of Exceptional Education And Student Services
325 West Gaines Street Suite 614
Tallahassee, FL 32399
850-245-0475
FAX: 850-245-0953
e-mail: Monica.Verra-Tirado@fldoe.org
www.fldoe.org
Pam Stewart, Education Commissioner
Provides consultative services for the establishment and operation of school programs for visually impaired students. Provides assistance for in-service teacher training through state or regional workshops or technical assistance to individual programs.

3226 Department of Health & Rehabilitative Services
1317 Winewood Blvd
Building 1
Tallahassee, FL 32399-700
850-487-1111
FAX: 850-922-2993
www.dcf.state.fl.us
David Wilkins, Secretary
Ramin Kouzehkanani, Deputy Secretary
John Bryant, Manager
The Florida Department of Children and Families has adopted an integrated approach to programs and services as we work to help improve the lives of individuals and families.

3227 Division of Workers Compensation
200 East Gaines Street
Tallahassee, FL 32399-6583
850-413-3098
877-693-5236
FAX: 850-413-2950
www.fldfs.com

Robert Kneip, PhD, Chief of Staff
Stephanie Iliff, Director
Terry Kester, Chief Information Officer

3228 Florida Adult Services
1317 Winewood Blvd
Building 1
Tallahassee, FL 32399-700
850-487-1111
FAX: 850-922-2993
www.dcf.state.fl.us

David Wilkins, Secretary
Ramin Kouzehkanani, Deputy Secretary
The Florida Department of Children and Families has adopted an integrated approach to programs and services as we work to help improve the lives of individuals and families.

3229 Florida Department of Handicapped Children
4030 Esplanade Way
Suite 380
Tallahassee, FL 32399-7016
850-488-4257
866-273-2273
FAX: 850-245-1075
e-mail: apd_info@apd.state.fl.us
www.apd.myflorida.com

Mike Gresham, Executive Director
John Bryant, Manager
The APD works in partnership with local communities and private providers to assist people who have developmental disabilities and their families.

3230 Florida Department of Mental Health and Rehabilitative Services
1317 Winewood Blvd
Building 1
Tallahassee, FL 32399-700
850-487-1111
FAX: 850-922-2993
www.dcf.state.fl.us

David Wilkins, Secretary
Ramin Kouzehkanani, Deputy Secretary

3231 Florida Developmental Disabilities Council
124 Marriot Drive
Suite 203
Tallahassee, FL 32301-2981
850-488-4180
800-580-7801
FAX: 850-922-6702
TTY: 888-488-863
e-mail: fddc@fddc.org
fddc.org

Debra Dowds, Executive Director
Mike Capp, Program Manager
Vanda Bowman, Staff Assistant
To advocate and promote meaningful participation in all aspects of life for Floridians with developmental disabilities.

3232 Florida Division of Vocational Rehabilitation
2002 Old Saint Augustine Road
Building 1
Tallahassee, FL 32301-4862
850-245-3399
800-451-4327
FAX: 850-245-3316
TTY: 850-488-2867
e-mail: costin@vr.doe.state.fl.us
rehabworks.org

Bill Palmer, Manager
Linda Parnell, Manager
State agency serving individuals with physical or mental disabilities that interfere with them keeping or maintaining employment.

3233 Florida's Protection and Advocacy Programs for Persons with Disabilities
2928 Center View Drive
Suite 102
Tallahassee, FL 32301
850-488-9071
800-342-0823
FAX: 850-488-8640
TTY: 800-346-4127
www.advocacycenter.org

Robert Whitney, Executive Director
The Center is a non-profit organization providing protection and advocacy services in the State of Florida. The Center's mission is to advance the dignity, equality, self-determination and expressed choices of individuals with disabilities.

3234 International Dyslexia Association: Florida Branch
40 York Rd., 4th Floor
Baltimore, MD 21204-3896
410-296-0232
800-222-3123
FAX: 410-321-5069
e-mail: ear228@aol.com
www.interdys.org

Kristen Penczek, Executive Director
David Holste, Director Of Operations
Stacy Friedman, Manager of Operation
Cyndi Powers, Office Manager
The Florida Branch is a non-p;rofit, scientific, educational organization committed to the study, prevention and treatment of language-based learning disabilities (dyslexia) for those in Florida and Puerto Rico. It is specifically concerned with the many children and adults with average or superior intelligence who experience difficulty in learning skills such as speaking, reading, writing, spelling and math.

3235 Social Security Administration
2002 Old Saint Augustine Rd
Suite B12
Tallahassee, FL 32301-4861
850-942-8978
800-772-1213
FAX: 850-942-8980
ssa.gov

Carrie Tucker, Operations Supervisor
Sheila Lee, Management Support Specialist
Administers the Title II and Title XVII disability programs. To be insured for Title II benefits, applicants must have worked in covered employment for at least five of the last ten years prior to becoming disabled. To be eligible for Title XVII disability benefits, applicants must meet an income and resource test.

3236 Social Security: Miami Disability Determination
Social Security
11401 W Flagler St
Miami, FL 33174-1023
305-226-0449
800-772-1213
FAX: 800-325-0778
www.ssa.gov

Robert L Meekins, Deputy General for Executive Ope

3237 Social Security: Orlando Disability Determination
Social Security
80 N Hughey Ave
Orlando, FL 32801-2231
407-648-6673
800-342-2065
TTY:407-245-7057
www.ssa.gov

John C Massolio Jr, Founder
Neil Bush, President

3238 Social Security: Tampa Disability Determination
Social Security Administration
PO Box 340572
Tampa, FL 33694-572
813-878-2906
800-772-1213
e-mail: info@dbstampabay.org
www.dbsatampabay.org
Gina B. Burford, President
Neil Bush, 1st Vice President
John Balcomb, 2nd Vice President
Carol Yaros, Treasurer
The Depression and Bipolar Support Alliance Tampa Bay, is a nonprofit and all volunteer organization for individuals, family and friends of those who have been diagnosed with bipolar disorder, depression and other affective disorders.

Georgia

3239 ADA Technical Assistance Program
Southeast Disability & Business Technical Assist.
1419 Mayson Street
Atlanta, GA 30324
404-541-9001
800- 94- 42
FAX: 404-541-9002
e-mail: ADAsoutheast.org
www.sedbtac.org
Amy Oliveras, Administrative Assistant
Shelley Kaplan, Director
Pam Williamson, Assistant Director
One of ten regional centers funded by NIDRR, to provide information and technical assistance to assist in voluntary compliance with the Americans with Disabilities Act, and accessible education-based information technology.

3240 Division of Birth Defects and Developmental Disabilities
1600 Clifton Rd.
Atlanta, GA 30333
404-498-3800
800-232-4636
TTY:888-232-6348
e-mail: cdcinfo@cdc.gov
www.cdc.gov
Thomas Frieden MD, Director

3241 Georgia Advocacy Office
150 E Ponce De Leon Ave
Suite 430
Decatur, GA 30030- 2547
404-885-1234
800-537-2329
FAX: 404-378-0031
e-mail: info@thegao.org
thegao.org
Ruby Moore, Executive Director
Crystal Beelner, Program Manager
Jennifer Puestow, Program Director
Protection and advocacy services for Georgians with disabilities.

3242 Georgia Client Assistance Program
Division of Rehabilitation Services
2 Peachtree Street NW
Suite 29-250
Atlanta, GA 30303- 3141
404-656-4507
800-822-9727
FAX: 404-651-6880
e-mail: connect.georgia.gov
dhs.georgia.gov/
Mark Trail, Manager
Helps eligible persons with complaints, appeals and understanding available benefits under the 1992 Rehabilitation Act Amendments and Title I of the Americans with Disabilities Act, CAP investigates complaints, mediates conflict, represents complainants in appeals, provides legal services if warranted, advocates for due process, identifies and recommends solutions to system problems, advises of benefits available under the 1992 Rehab Act Amendments and Americans with Disabilities Act.

3243 Georgia Council On Developmental Disabilities
2 Peachtree St N.W.
26th Floor, Suite 246
Atlanta, GA 30303-3141
404-657-2126
888-275-4233
FAX: 404-657-2132
TTY:404-657-2133
e-mail: eejacobson@dhr.state.ga.us
www.gcdd.org
Eric Jacobson, Executive Director
Caitlin Childs, Organizing Director
Dottie Adams, Family/Individual Support Dir.
Valerie Meadows Suber, Public Information Director
The Georgia Council on Developmental Disabilities collaborates with Georgia's citizens, public and private advocacy organizations and policymakers to positively influence public policies that enhance the quality of life for people with disabilities and their families. GCDD provides this through education and advocacy activities, program implementation, funding and public policy analysis and research.
Quartlery

3244 Georgia Department of Aging
2 Peachtree Street NW
Suite 29-250
Atlanta, GA 30309- 3933
404-656-4507
FAX: 404-223-2299
e-mail: connect.georgia.gov
dhs.georgia.gov/
Stephen Dolinger, President
Andrea Fuller-Ruffin, Administrator

3245 Georgia Department of Handicapped Children
2600 Skyland Dr NE
Atlanta, GA 30319-3640
404-679-1625
FAX: 404-679-1630
Ron Jackson, Manager
Frank Koues, Auditor

3246 Georgia Division of Mental Health, Developmental Disabilities & Addictive Diseases
Two Peachtree Drive NW
24th Floor
Atlanta, GA 30303-3142
404-657-2252
800-715-4225
FAX: 404-657-2310
e-mail: srhall1@dhr.ga.gov
mhddad.dhr.georgia.gov
Frank Schelp MD, Commissioner
MHDDAD provides treatment and support services to people with mental illnesses and addictive diseases, and support to people with mental retardation and related developmental disabilities. MHDDAD serves people of all ages with the most severe and likely to be long-term conditions.

3247 Georgia State Board of Workers' Compensation
270 Peachtree St NW
Atlanta, GA 30303-1299
404-656-3875
800-533-0682
FAX: 404-657-1767
sbwc.georgia.gov
Judge Frank Mckay, President
Judge Elizab Gobeil, Director
Judge Hal Dawkins, Director

3248 **International Dyslexia Association: Georgia Branch**
40 York Rd., 4th Floor
Baltimore, GA 21204-2622
410-296-0232
800-222-3123
FAX: 410-321-5069
e-mail: info@idaga.org
www.interdys.org

Guinevere Eden, President
Eric Tridas, President Elect
Suzanne Carreker PhD, CALT-QI Vice President
Cinthia Coletti Haan, Vice President
The Georgi Branch was formed to increase public awareness about dyslexia in the State of Georgia. In addition, the Branch encourages teachers to train in multisensory language instruction. The Branch also provides a network for individuals with dyslexia, their families and professionals in the educational and medical fields.

3249 **Social Security: Atlanta Disability Determination**
401 W Peachtree St NW
Suite 2860
Atlanta, GA 30308-3538
800-772-1213
TTY:800-325-0778
www.socialsecurity.gov

3250 **Social Security: Decatur Disability Determination**
2853 Candler Rd
Suite 8
Decatur, GA 30034-1421
800-772-1213
TTY:800-325-0778
ssa.gov

Hawaii

3251 **Assistive Technology Resource Centers of Hawaii**
414 Kuwilli Street
Suite 104
Honolulu, HI 96817-5362
808-532-7110
800-645-3007
FAX: 808-532-7120
TTY: 808-532-7113
e-mail: barbara@atrc.org
www.atrc.org

Barbara Fischlowitz-Leong, Executive Director
Provides information and referral to anyone interested in assistive technology devices and services. Operates equipment loan. Bank Provides training to consumer and professional groups including self-advocacy skills for consumers and family members. Works to ensure that schools, vocational rehabilitation agencies and health insurers provide assessments, funding and training in the use of assistive technology devices and services for their clients. Low-interest loan programs available.

3252 **Diabetes Network of East Hawaii**
1221 Kilauea Ave
Suite 70
Hilo, HI 96720-4264
808-935-1673
FAX: 808-935-6760

Steve Fukunada, Manager

3253 **Disability and Communication Access Board**
919 Ala Moana Blvd
Ste 101
Honolulu, HI 96814-4920
808-586-8121
FAX: 808-586-8129
e-mail: dcab@doh.hawaii.gov
hawaii.gov/health/dcab

Francine Wai, Executive Director
Charlotte Townsend, Coordinator Programs/Policy Dev
Debbra Jackson, Planner/ADA Coordinator
Curtis Motoyama, Coordinator Facility Access Unit
Provides ADA coordination for state & county government; reviews state & county construction documents to appropriate federal & state accessibility guidelines; credentials american sign language interpreters; coordinates parking for persons with disabilites; coordinates information & referral for consumers, parents and others seeking disability related information.

3254 **Hawaii Assistive Technology Training and**
414 Kuwilli Street
Suite 104
Honolulu, HI 96817-5362
808-532-7110
e-mail: barbara@atrc.org
www.atrc.org

Barbara Fischlowitz-Leong, Executive Director

3255 **Hawaii Department for Children With Special Needs**
Department of Health
741a Sunset Ave
Honolulu, HI 96816-2343
808-733-9055
FAX: 808-733-9068
hawaii.gov

Patricia Heu, Manager
Karen Mak, Manager

3256 **Hawaii Department of Health, Adult Mental Health Division**
P.O.Box 3378
Honolulu, HI 96801-3378
808-586-4686
FAX: 808-586-4745
www.amhd.org

3257 **Hawaii Department of Human Services**
Hawaii Department of Human Serv
1901 Bachelot St
Honolulu, HI 96817-2432
808-941-3894
FAX: 808-941-3894
hawaiianswers.com

Linda Lingel, Governor
Lillian Koller, Director
Provides services to blind and visually impaired persons in adjustment to blindness, vocational rehabilitation, low vision evaluation and assistance. Work Evaluation, operates Work Activities Center, Vending training and the Ho'opono Workshop, a sheltered workshop program for the blind and visually impaired persons.

3258 **Hawaii Disability Compensation Division Department of Labor and Industrial Relations**
Rm 211
830 Punchbowl St
Honolulu, HI 96813-5095
808-586-9200
FAX: 808-586-9219
hawaii.gov/labor

Walter Kawamura, Administrator
Clyde Imada, Workers Comp Chief
Administers Hawaii's Workers' Compensation Program.

3259 **Hawaii Disability Rights Center**
1132 Bishop Street
Suite 2102
Honolulu, HI 96813-3701
808-949-2922
800-882-1052
FAX: 808-949-2928
e-mail: info@hawaiidisabilityrights.org
hawaiidisabilityrights.org

John Dellera, Executive Director
Ann Collins, Director Of Operations

3260 **Hawaii Executive Office on Aging**
250 S Hotel Street
Suite 406
Honolulu, HI 96813-2831
808-586-0100
800-468-4644
FAX: 808-586-0185
e-mail: eoa@mail.health.state.hi.us
hawaii.gov/health/eoa

Noemi Pendleton, Manager

State unit on aging responsible for policy formulation, program development, planning, information dissemination, advocacy and other activities, for persons age 60 and over.

3261 Hawaii State Council on Developmental Disabilities
919 Ala Moana Blvd
Room 113
Honolulu, HI 96814-4920 808-586-8100
FAX: 808-586-7543
e-mail: plan@hiddc.org
www.hiddc.org

Waynette K Y Cabral, Executive Administrator

The mission of the council is to support people with developmental disabilities to control their own destiny and determine the quality of life they desire. The Council: engages in analysis and policy development; provides training in legislative advocacy and leadership development for individuals with disabilities and their families; demonstrates new approaches to services and supports; informs policymakers about developmental disability issues; and fosters interagency collaboration.

3262 International Dyslexia Association: Hawaii Branch
P.O.Box 61610
Honolulu, HI 96839-1610 808-538-7007
FAX: 808-566-6837
e-mail: hida@dyslexia-hawaii.org
dyslexia-hawaii.org

Margaret Higa, Manager

Provides free information and referral services for diagnosis and tutoring for parents, educators, physicians, and individuals with dyslexia. The voice of our membership is heard in 48 countries. Membership includes yearly journal and quarterly newsletter. Call for conference dates.

3263 Social Security: Honolulu Disability Determination
Social Security
300 Ala Moana Blvd
Honolulu, HI 96850-1 808-541-3600
800-772-1213
FAX: 800-825-0778
e-mail: hivrsbd@kestrok.com
www.ssa.gov

Neil Shim, Administrator

3264 State Planning Council on Developmental Disabilities
919 Ala Moana Blvd
Room 101
Honolulu, HI 96814-4920 808-586-8121
FAX: 808-586-8129
TTY:808-586-8121
e-mail: tiza100w@wonder.cm.cdc.gov
hawaii.gov/health/dcab

Francine Wai, Executive Director

Consists of 25 Hawaii residents appointed by the governor. The council addresses the needs of the people with developmental disabilities: specifically, develops a state plan that sets the priorities for persons with developmental disabilities.

Idaho

3265 Idaho Commission on Aging
341 W Washington
Boise, ID 83702-1 208-334-3833
800-926-2588
FAX: 208-334-3033
e-mail: icoa@aging.idaho.gov
www.idahoaging.com

Kim Torianski, Manager
Cathy Hart, State Ombudsman

3266 Idaho Council on Developmental Disabilities
Health and Wellfare
700 W. State Street, 1st Floor
Boise, ID 83702-5848 208-334-2178
800-544-2433
FAX: 208-334-3417
e-mail: info@icdd.idaho.gov
www.state.id.us/icdd

Marilyn B Sword, Manager

3267 Idaho Department of Handicapped Children
Statehouse
Boise, ID 83720-1 208-334-8000

Thomas Bruck, Chief
Sandy Frazier, Manager

3268 Idaho Disability Determinations Service
PO Box 21
Boise, ID 83707-21 208-327-7333
800-626-2681
FAX: 208-327-7331
TTY: 800-377-3529
labor.idaho.gov

Roger B Madsen, Director
Rogelio Valdez, Executive Director

Under contract with the Social Security Administration, makes determinations of medical eligibility for disability benefits.

3269 Idaho Industrial Commission
700 S Clearwater Lane
Boise, ID 83712 208-334-6000
800-950-2110
FAX: 208-334-2321
e-mail: mholbrook@iic.idaho.gov
www.iic.idaho.gov

Mindy Montgomery, Manager

Free rehabilitation services to workers' who have suffered on the job injuries in Idaho. Field offices throughout the state.

3270 Idaho Mental Health Center
1720 N Westgate Dr
Boise, ID 83704-7164 208-334-0808
800-926-2588
FAX: 208-334-0828
healthandwelfare.idaho.gov

Richard Armstrong, Director
Pat Fitzpatrick, Manager

Illinois

3271 Attorney General's Office: Disability Rights Bureau & Health Care Bureau
100 W Randolph St
Chicago, IL 60601-3218 312-814-3000
877-305-5145
FAX: 312-793-0802
TTY: 800-964-5145
illinoisattorneygeneral.gov

Lisa Madigan, Manager
Raymond Throlkeld, Chief Health Care Bureau

Information on Illinois' Comprehensive Health Insurance Plan and architectural accessibility. Enforcement of Illinois' access law and standards and other disability rights laws. Information on initiatives such as: Opening the Courthouse Doors to People with Disabilities; the abuse, neglect or financial exploitation of people with disabilities and voter accessibility. Other information and referrals.

3272 Client Assistance Program (CAP)
Illinois State Board of Education
100 N 1st St
1st Floor
Springfield, IL 62777-1
217-782-4321
800-641-3929
866-262-6663
FAX: 217-524-1790
TTY:217-782-1900
www.isbe.state.il.us/

Dr. Christop Koch, State Superintendent

3273 Equip for Equality
20 N Michigan Ave
Suite 300
Chicago, IL 60602-4861
312-341-0022
800-537-2632
FAX: 312-541-7544
TTY: 800-610-2779
e-mail: contactus@equipforequality.org
equipforequality.org

Zena Naiditch, President/CEO
Barry C Taylor, Legal Advocacy Director
Equip for equality is an independent, private, not-for-profit organization designated by the Governor in 1985 to implement the federally mandated Protection and Advocacy (P&A) System in Illinois. The mission of Equip for Equality is to advance the human and civil rights of children and adults with disabilities in Illinois.

3274 Equip for Equality - Carbondale Office
300 East Main St
Suite 18
Carbondale, IL 62901
618-457-7930
800-758-0559
FAX: 618-457-7985
TTY: 800-610-2779
e-mail: contactus@equipforequality.org
equipforequality.org

Zena Naiditch, President/CEO
Barry C Taylor, Legal Advocacy Director
Equip for equality is an independent, private, not-for-profit organization designated by the Governor in 1985 to implement the federally mandated Protection and Advocacy (P&A) System in Illinois. The mission of Equip for Equality is to advance the human and civil rights of children and adults with disabilities in Illinois.

3275 Equip for Equality - Moline Office
1515 Fifth Ave
Suite 420
Moline, IL 61265
309-786-6868
800-758-6869
FAX: 309-797-8710
TTY: 800-610-2779
e-mail: contactus@equipforequality.org
equipforequality.org

Zena Naiditch, President/CEO
Barry C Taylor, Legal Advocacy Director
Equip for equality is an independent, private, not-for-profit organization designated by the Governor in 1985 to implement the federally mandated Protection and Advocacy (P&A) System in Illinois. The mission of Equip for Equality is to advance the human and civil rights of children and adults with disabilities in Illinois.

3276 Equip for Equality - Springfield Office
235 South Fifth Street
Springfield, IL 62701
217-544-0464
800-758-0464
FAX: 217-523-0720
TTY: 800-610-2779
e-mail: contactus@equipforequality.org
equipforequality.org

Zena Naiditch, President/CEO
Barry C Taylor, Legal Advocacy Director
Equip for equality is an independent, private, not-for-profit organization designated by the Governor in 1985 to implement the federally mandated Protection and Advocacy (P&A) System in Illinois. The mission of Equip for Equality is to advance the human and civil rights of children and adults with disabilities in Illinois.

3277 Illinois Assistive Technology Project
1 W Old State Capitol Plz
Suite 100
Springfield, IL 62701-1200
217-522-7985
800-852-5110
FAX: 217-522-8067
TTY: 217-522-9966
e-mail: iatp@iltech.org
iltech.org

Wilhelmina Gunther, Executive Director
Barbara Howell, Administration
Directed by and for people with disabilities and their family members. As a federally mandated program, IATP strives to break down barriers and change policies that make getting and using technology difficult. IATP offers solutions to help people find what is available in products and services that will best meet their needs, where to find it, and how to get it.

3278 Illinois Council on Developmental Disability
State of Illinois Center
100 W Randolph St
16-100
Chicago, IL 60601-3218
312-814-2121
800-843-6154
FAX: 312-814-7441
e-mail: drs@dhs.state.il.us
www.state.il.us/agency/icdd/

Sheila Romano, Executive Director
Dennis Sienko, Manager

3279 Illinois Department of Mental Health and Developmental Disabilities
Suite 3b
314 E Madison
Springfield, IL 62701
217-782-6680
FAX: 217-524-3834

Karen Perrin, Manager
Lori Stone, Director

3280 Illinois Department of Rehabilitation
100 South Grand Avenue East
Springfield, IL 62762-1304
217-782-6680
800-843-6154
FAX: 217-524-3834
TTY: 800-447-6404
e-mail: DHS.ORS@illinois.gov
www.dhs.state.il.us/page.aspx?item=29736
Robert Kilbury, Director
Timothy Martin, Manager

3281 Illinois Department on Aging
One Natural Resources Way #100
Springfield, IL 62702-1271
217-785-2870
800-252-8966
FAX: 217-785-4477
TTY: 888-206-1327
e-mail: ilsenior@illinois.gov
www.state.il.us/aging

Charles D Johnson, Executive Director

3282 **International Dyslexia Association: Illinois Branch**
40 York Rd., 4th Floor
Baltimore, MD 21204-3896 410-296-0232
800-222-3123
FAX: 410-321-5069
e-mail: info@readibida.org
www.interdys.org
Susan Hall, President
Maria Leibold, Executive Director
Gail Oliphant, Manager
Provides free information and referral services for diagnosis and tutoring for parents, educators, physicians, and individuals with dyslexia in Illinois and Missouri. The voice of our membership is heard in 48 countries. Membership includes yearly journal and quarterly newsletter. Call for conference dates.

3283 **Social Security: Springfield Disability Determination**
2715 W Monroe St
Springfield, IL 62704-1323 217-862-6651
800-772-1213
TTY:217-862-6681
ssa.gov

3284 **Workers Compensation Board Illinois**
100 W Randolph St
Ste 8-200
Chicago, IL 60601-3227 312-814-6611
866-352-3033
FAX: 312-814-6523
e-mail: infoquestions.wcc@illinois.gov
www.state.il.us/agency/iic/
Dennis Ruth, Manager

Indiana

3285 **Indiana Client Assistance Program**
4701 Keystone Avenue
Suite 222
Indianapolis, IN 46204- 1191 317-860-2876
800-622-4845
FAX: 317-722-5564
TTY: 317-722-5555
e-mail: tgallagher@ipas.state.in.us
www.icdri.org/legal/IndianaCAP.htm
Michael Burks, Chairman
Wen Lu, Secretary and Treasurer

3286 **Indiana Developmental Disability Council**
150 West Market Street
Suite 628
Indianapolis, IN 46204-2801 317-232-7770
FAX: 317-233-3712
e-mail: gpcpd@gpcpd.org
www.acf.hhs.gov
Mike Flores, Manager

3287 **Indiana Protection & Advocacy Services Commission**
4701 N. Keystone Avenue
Suite 222
Indianapolis, IN 46205-1561 317-722-5555
800-622-4845
FAX: 317-722-5564
e-mail: tgallagher@ipas.in.gov
www.in.gov/ipas
Thomas Gallagher, Executive Director
Milo Gray, Client & Legal Services Director
Gary Richter, Support Services Director
Karen Pedevilla, Education/Training Director
An independent state agency established to protect and promote the rights of individuals with disabilities through empowerment and advocacy.

3288 **Indiana State Commission for the Handicapped**
P.O.Box 1964
Indianapolis, IN 46206 317-233-1292

3289 **International Dyslexia Association: Indiana Branch**
7944 Destry Place
Fisher, IN 46038 317-926-1450
800-222-3123
FAX: 317-926-1450
e-mail: gcrahen@sbcglobal.net
www.interdys.org
Tracey Horth-Kreuger, Executive Director
The Indiana Branch was formed to help the members of the learning disabilities community in Indiana. Promotes understanding and facilitate treatment of the Specific Language Disability (Dyslexia) in children and adults, promotes teacher training and educational intervention strategies for dyslexic students and to foster effective teaching, supports research in the field and early identification of dyslexia, serves as a clearinghouse for information and to actively disseminate knowledge.

Iowa

3290 **Governor's Developmental Disability Council**
617 East Second Street
Des Moines, IA 50309-1831 515-281-9082
800-452-1936
FAX: 515-281-9087
e-mail: fmorris@dhs.state.ia.us
http://idaction.com/
Becky Harker, Executive Director
Rik Shannon, Public Policy Manager
Janet Shoeman, Program Planner/Contract Manager
Fran Morris, Council Secretary
The Council identifies, develops and promotes public policy and support practices through capacity building, advocacy, and systems change activities. The purpose is to ensure that people with developmental disabilities and their families are included in planning, decision making, and development of policy related to services and supports that affect their quality of life and full participation in communities of their choice.

3291 **International Dyslexia Association: Iowa Branch**
40 York Rd., 4th Floor
Baltimore, MD 21204-3896 410-296-0232
800-222-3123
FAX: 410-321-5069
e-mail: og-ida_tmjp@earthlink.net
www.interdys.org
Terri Peterson, President
The purpose of the Iowa Branch of IDA (IDA-IA) is to increase awareness of dyslexia and promote services that address the importance of diagnosis and remediation for those not meeting their reading potential. Our goal is to provide services and assistance in a way that promotes unity, support, and cooperation among those who work with these individuals so that all communities in Iowa benefit from the skills and talents of its citizens.

3292 **Iowa Child Health Specialty Clinics**
100 Hawkins Dr
Room 247 CDD
Iowa City, IA 52242-1016 319-356-1117
866-219-9119
FAX: 319-356-3715
e-mail: kathy-colbert@uiowa.edu
www.uihealthcare.com/chsc
Jeffrey Lobas, Director
Brian Wilkes, Director Of Operations
Child Health Specialty Clinics has a mission to improve the health, development, and well-being of Iowa's children and youth with special health care needs in partnership with families, service providers, and communities.

3293 **Iowa Commission of Persons with Disabilities**
Department of Human Rights
321 E 12th St
Des Moines, IA 50319-2006
515-242-6171
888-219-0471
FAX: 515-242-6119
TTY: 888-219-0471
e-mail: dhr.disabilities@dhr.state.ia.us
www.state.ia.us/dhr/pd

Jill Fulitano-Avery, Administrator

3294 **Iowa Compass**
Center for Disabilities and Development
100 Hawkins Dr
#S295
Iowa City, IA 52242-1011
319-353-6900
800-779-2001
FAX: 319-356-1343
TTY: 877-686-0032
e-mail: iowa-compass@uiowa.edu
www.iowacompass.org/

Jane Gay, Project Director
David Sorton, President
Mark Moser, Administrator

A statewide program provides free information and referral about disability related services and resources: advocacy, assistive technology, community services, early intervention, education, financial support, healthcare, legal aid, residential services and transportation.
BiMonthly

3295 **Iowa Department for the Blind**
State Of Iowa
524 4th Street
Des Moines, IA 50309-2364
515-281-1333
800-362-2587
FAX: 515-281-1263
TTY: 515-281-1355
e-mail: information@blind.state.ia.us
www.IDBonline.org

Richard Sorey, Director
Jodi Aldini, Library Support Staff
Julie Aufdenkamp, Transition Specialist, Transition Program
Jessica Badding, Vocational Rehabilitation Counselor

Mission is to be the means for persons who are blind to obtain univeral access and full participation as citizens in whatever roles they may choose.

3296 **Iowa Department of Human Services**
1305 E Walnut St
Des Moines, IA 50319-114
515-242-6510
800-972-2017
FAX: 515-281-4597
e-mail: mfinkel@dhs.state.ia.us
www.dhs.state.ia.us

M. Finkelstein, Compliance Officer

Help individuals and families to achieve stable and healthy lives.

3297 **Iowa Department on Aging**
510 E 12th Street, Suite 2
Des Moines, IA 50319-9025
515-725-3333
800-532-3213
FAX: 866-236-1430
www.aging.iowa.gov

Donna K. Harvey, Director
Danika Welch, Executive Secretary
Joel Wulf, Administartor
Jeanne Yordi, State Long Term Care Ombudsman

3298 **Iowa Protection & Advocacy for the Disabled**
400 East Court
Suite 300
Des Moines, IA 50309
515-278-2502
800-779-2502
FAX: 515-278-0539
e-mail: info@disabilityrightsiowa.org
ipna.org

Sylvia Piper, Executive Director

3299 **Social Security: Des Moines Disability Determination**
Social Security Administration
Riverpoint Office Complex
455 SW 5TH ST STE F
Des Moines, IA 50309-2115
515-284-4260
800-772-1213
FAX: 515-284-4394
TTY: 800-325-0778
ssa.gov

Leroy Brown, Manager

3300 **Workers Compensation Board Iowa**
1000 E Grand Ave
Des Moines, IA 50319-1020
515-281-5387
FAX: 515-281-6501
iowaworks.org

Kansas

3301 **Beach Center on Families and Disability**
University of Kansas
1200 Sunnyside Ave
Room 3136
Lawrence, KS 66045-7600
785-864-7600
FAX: 785-864-7605
e-mail: beachcenter@ku.edu
www.beachcenter.org

HR Turnbull, Director
Ann Turnbull, Co-Director
Robert Hemenway, CEO

A federally funded center that conducts research and training in the factors that contribute to the successful functioning of families with members who have disabilities.

3302 **International Dyslexia Association: Kansas/West Missouri Branch**
430 E Blue Ridge Blvd
Kansas City, MO 64145-1422
816-942-6808
FAX: 816-942-6898
e-mail: info@AppliedLearningProcesses.com
appliedlearningprocesses.com

Billie Calvery, Owner
Arden Murilo, VP

IDA members in Kansas and Missouri work to establish and maintain a presence for IDA with parents, schools, and teachers in order to help individuals with dyslexia. We maintain a list of individuals in Kansas and Missouri who have specialized training and who are available for diagnosis and remediation of reading, writing, and spelling problems, information for parents, information for teachers, an annual spring conference, newsletter dealing with state and local issues.

3303 **Kansas Advocacy and Protective Services**
635 S.W. Harrison Street
Suite 100
Topeka, KS 66603-3726
785-273-9661
877-776-1541
FAX: 785-273-9414
TTY: 877-335-3725
e-mail: michelle@ksadv.org
www.drckansas.org/

Kevin Oneslager, Owner
Tim Voth, Attorney
Michelle Rola, Director Operations

Protection and advocacy for persons with disabilities.

3304 **Kansas Client Assistance Program**
635 SW Harrison
Suite 100
Topeka, KS 66603
785-273-9661
877-776-1541
FAX: 785-273-9414
TTY: 877-335-3725
e-mail: rocky@drckansas.org
www.icdri.org/legal/KansasCAP.htm

3305 **Kansas Commission on Disability Concerns**
900 SW Jackson
Room 100
Topeka, KS 66612-1246
785-296-1722
800-295-5232
FAX: 785-296-1795
e-mail: mgabehart@kcdcinfo.com
www.kcdcinfo.com

Martha Gabehart, Executive Director
Kerrie Bacon, Employment/Training Liaison
Kerrie Bacon, Legislative Liasion
KCDC believes that all people with disabilities are entitled to be equal citizens and partners in Kansas society. The purpose is to involve all segments of the Kansas Community through legislative advocacy, education and resource networking to ensure full and equal citizenship for all Kansans with disabilities.

3306 **Kansas Department on Aging**
503 S Kansas Ave
Topeka, KS 66603-3404
785-296-4986
800-432-3535
FAX: 785-296-0256
e-mail: wwwmail@aging.ks.us
agingkansas.org

Kathy Greenlee, Manager
Barbara Conant, Public Information Officer
Services and information for Kansas seniors, over age 60.

3307 **Kansas Developmental Disability Council**
Disability Rights Center of Kansas
1717 SW Topeka Blvd
Topeka, KS 66612-3726
785-431-7200
877-776-1541
FAX: 785-296-2608
TTY: 877-335-3725
e-mail: info@drckansas.org
www.kcdd.org/

Jane Rhys PhD, Executive Director
Charline Cobbs, Senior Administrative Assistant
To protect children and promote adult self-sufficiency.

Kentucky

3308 **Kentucky Council on Developmental Disability**
275 E. Main St.
1E-B
Frankfort, KY 40621
502-564-5497
800-372-2973
FAX: 502-564-9523
e-mail: David.Boswell@ky.gov
www.kcdd.ky.gov

John Burt, Manager
Implementation of Developmental Disabilities Planning Council responsible under P.L. 101-496.

3309 **Kentucky Department for Mental Health and Mental Retardation Services**
275 E. Main St.,
1E-B
Frankfort, KY 40621
502-564-5497
FAX: 502-564-9523
chfs.ky.gov

John Burt, Manager
Deborah Anderson, Staff Assistant
The Department for Mental Health and Mental Retardation Services contracts with fourteen regional community mental health and mental broads to provide an array of community based mental health services; operates three psychiatric hospitals and contracts with two additional hospitals; operates or contracts for 10 ICFs/MR; also operates two nursing facilities.

3310 **Kentucky Department for Mental Health:**
275 E. Main St.,
1E-B
Frankfort, KY 40621
502-564-5497
FAX: 502-564-9523
chfs.ky.gov

John Burt, Manager
Deborah Anderson, Staff Assistant
The Department for Mental Health and Mental Retardation Services contracts with fourteen regional community mental health and mental broads to provide an array of community based mental health services; operates three psychiatric hospitals and contracts with two additional hospitals; operates or contracts for 10 ICFs/MR; also operates two nursing facilities.

3311 **Kentucky Department for the Blind**
275 East Main Street
Frankfort, KY 40601
502-782-3414
800-321-6668
FAX: 502-564-2951
TTY: 502-564-2929
e-mail: Wayne.Thompson@ky.gov
http://blind.ky.gov

Beth Cross, Executive Director
Provides career services and assistance to adults with severe visual handicaps who want to become productive in the home or work force. Also provides the Client Assistance Program established to provide advice, assistance and information available from rehabilitation programs to persons with handicaps.

3312 **Kentucky Office of Aging Services**
Cabinet for Health Services
275 East Main Street
Suite 1E-B
Frankfort, KY 40621
502-564-5497
FAX: 502-564-9523
e-mail: David.Boswell@ky.gov
www.kcdd.ky.gov

Jerry Whitley, Manager
The Kentucky Office of Aging Services is the state agency directly responsible for programs and services for people with disabilities. Efforts are made to fully integrate the service response information that considers broad farmiliar implications.

3313 **Kentucky Protection & Advocacy**
100 Fair Oaks Ln 3rd Fl
Frankfort, KY 40601-1108
502-564-2967
800-372-2988
FAX: 502-564-0848
e-mail: info@kypa.net
kypa.net

Marsha Hockensmith, Executive Director
Protection and advocacy, Kentucky's federally-mandated protection and advocacy system, protects & promotes the disability rights of individuals through free legally-based advocacy, technical assistance, and education.

3314 **Social Security: Frankfort Disability Determination**
Social Security
140 Flynn Avenue
Frankfort, KY 40601
502-875-2232
800-772-1213
866-964-1724
FAX: 502-226-4519
TTY:502-226-4519
www.ssa.gov

Stephen Jones, Director
Burton Sisk, Manager

3315 Social Security: Louisville Disability Determination
Social Security
601 W Broadway
Room 101
Louisville, KY 40202-2227 502-582-6690
800-772-1213
866-716-9671
TTY:502-582-5517
ssa.gov

Louisiana

3316 Advocacy Center
8325 Oak Street
New Orleans, LA 70118 504-237-2337
800-960-7705
FAX: 504-522-5507
TTY: 855-861-3577
e-mail: advocacycenter@advocacyla.org
advocacyla.org

Lois Simpson, Executive Director
The Advocacy Center is Louisiana's protection and advocacy system. AC provides free legal services to people with disabilities in designated priority areas. In addition, AC also provides legal assistance to people residing in nursing homes in Louisiana and people over 60 in Orleans, Plaquemines and St. Tammany parishes. AC ombudsmen advocate for the rights of group home and nursing home residents. Benefits specialists help people who receive public benefits to return to work or go to work.

3317 Louisiana Assistive Technology Access Network
3042 Old Forge Dr.
P O Box 14115
Baton Rouge, LA 70898 225-925-9500
800-270-6185
FAX: 225-925-9560
e-mail: cporciau@latan.org
www.latan.org/

Jim Parks, President & CEO
Sandee Winchell, Executive Director
An information and training resource on Assistive Technology for the State of Louisiana. LATAN operates three regional centers to provide better access for consumers.

3318 Louisiana Center for Dyslexia and Related Learning Disorders
PO Box 2050
Thibodaux, LA 70310-1 985-448-4214
FAX: 985-448-4423
www.nicholls.edu

Karen Chauvin, Director
Rhonda Zerinque, Administrative Secretary
Provides free information and referral services for diagnosis and tutoring for parents, educators, physicians and individuals with dyslexia. The voice of our membership is heard in 48 countries. Membership includes yearly journal and quarterly newsletter. Call for conference dates.

3319 Louisiana Department of Aging
Office of Elderly Affairs
PO Box 629
Baton Rouge, LA 70821-629 225-342-9500
FAX: 225-342-5568
e-mail: dhhwebinfo@la.gov
new.dhh.louisiana.gov/

David Elder, Manager
Ronald Blereau, Deputy Assistant Secretary
Serves as a focal point for Louisiana's senior citizens and administers a broad range of home and community based services through a network of 37 Area Agencies on Aging. Serve as the focal point for the development, implementation, and administration of the public policy for the state of Louisiana, and address the needs of the state's elderly citizens.

3320 Louisiana Developmental Disability Council
PO Box 3455
Baton Rouge, LA 70821-3455 225-342-6804
800-450-8108
FAX: 225-342-1970
e-mail: shawn.fleming@la.gov
www.laddc.org

Sandee Winchell, Executive Director

3321 Louisiana Division of Mental Health
PO Box 629
Baton Rouge, LA 70821-4049 225-342-9500
FAX: 225-342-5568
e-mail: dhhwebinfo@la.gov
new.dhh.louisiana.gov/index.cfm/directory/det

Dr. Rochelle Head-Dunham, Director
William Payne, Manager

3322 Louisiana Learning Resources System
2525 Wyandotte St
Baton Rouge, LA 70805-6464 225-355-6197
FAX: 225-357-3508

Bobbie Robertson, Administrator
Provides consultation on educational seOrvices for local schools, offers psychological testing and evaluation, maintains resource rooms in district schools and more for the blind and handicapped throughout the state.

3323 Social Security: Baton Rouge Disability Determination
Department of Social Services
Rm 328
755 N 3rd St
Baton Rouge, LA 70802-5233 225-342-0286
800-772-1213
FAX: 225-219-9399
e-mail: adren.wilson@dss.state.la.us
www.ssa.gov

Shirley Williams, Director
Ann Williamson, Manager

3324 Workers Compensation Board Louisiana
1001 North 23rd Street
Post Office Box 94094
Baton Rouge, LA 70804-9094 225-342-3111
800-259-5154
FAX: 225-342-7960
e-mail: owd@lwc.la.gov
www.laworks.net

Maine

3325 Maine Assistive Technology Projects
University of Maine at Augusta
University Hts
490 Tenth Street
Atlanta, GA 30332 404-894-4960
FAX: 404-894-9320
e-mail: catea@coa.gatech.edu
assistivetech.net

3326 Maine Bureau of Elder and Adult Services
1 State House Station
Augusta, ME 04333 207-287-3531
FAX: 207-287-1034
www.maine.gov

Diana Scully, Administrator

3327 Maine Department of Health and Human Services
221 State Street
Augusta, ME 04333
207-287-3707
FAX: 207-287-3005
e-mail: brenda.harvey@maine.gov
www.maine.gov/dhhs

Brenda Harvey, Commissioner
Christopher Pierce, Deputy Commissioner, Financial
William Boeschenstein, Chief Operating Officer
Stephanie Nadeau, Director, MaineCare Service

Provision of an array of services to people with nental illness, substance abuse issues, children with special needs and people with developmental disabilities.

3328 Maine Developmental Disabilities Council
295 Water Street, Ste 5
Augusta, ME 04330
207-287-4213
800-244-3990
FAX: 207-287-8001
e-mail: jbell@maineddc.org
www.maineddc.org

Nancy Cronin, Executive Director
Rachel Dyer, Policy and Planning Specialist
Erin Howes, Office Manager

The MDDC is a partnership of people with disabilities, their families, and agencies which identifies barriers to community inclusion, self-determination, and independence, and acts to effect positive change.

3329 Maine Division for the Blind and Visually Impaired
2 Anthony Avenue
Augusta, ME 04333
207-624-5120
800-760-1573
FAX: 207-624-5133
TTY: 800-633-0770
e-mail: mdol@maine.gov
www.maine.gov/rehab/dbvi

Harold Lewis, Director
Sandra Cavanaugh, Executive Director

Works to bring about full access to employment, independence and community integration for people with disabilities in Maine.

3330 Maine Office of Elder Services
State of Maine
11 State House Station
Augusta, ME 04333
207-287-9200
800-262-2232
FAX: 207-287-9229
TTY: 800-606-0215
e-mail: mdol@maine.gov
www.maine.gov/dhhs/oads/aging

Ricker Hamilton, Director
Elizabeth Gattine, Director Long Term Care
Romaine Turyn, Director Policy, Planning & Reso
Rick Mooers, Director Adult Protective Servic

The Office of Elder Services (OES), an Office within the Maine Department of Health and Human Services, promotes programs and services for older adults, their families and for people with disabilities.

3331 Maine Workers' Compensation Board
27 State House Sta
Augusta, ME 04333
207-287-3751
888-801-9087
FAX: 207-287-7198
TTY:877-832-5525
www.maine.gov/wcb

Paul H Sighinolfi, Executive Director
Mitchell Sammons, Management Representative
Gary Koocher, Management Representative
Ron Green, Labor Representative

The general mission of the Maine Workers' Compensation Board is to serve the employees and employers of the State fairly and expeditiously by ensuring compliance with the workers' compensation laws, ensuring the prompt delivery of benefits legally due, promoting the prevention of disputes, utilizing dispute resolution to reduce litigation and facilitating labor-management cooperation.

3332 Social Security: Maine Disability Determination
40 Western Ave
Augusta, ME 04330-6325
207-622-1451
800-772-1213
TTY:800-325-0778
ssa.gov

Louis Tepin, Manager

This office makes the medical determination about whether a consumer is disabled and, therefore, medically eligible for Social Security benefits. Legally, an individual is considered disabled if he or she is unable to do any substantial gainful work activity because of a medical condition (or conditions), that has lasted, or can be expected to last for at least 12 months, or that is expected to result in death.

Maryland

3333 Health Resources & Services Administration: State Bureau of Health
Federal Government
5600 Fishers Ln
Rockville, MD 20857
301-443-2216
888-275-4772
e-mail: ask@hrsa.gov
www.hrsa.gov

Marcia Brand, Deputy Administrator
Tina Cheatham, Senior Advisor
Mary Wakefield, Administrator

Through appropriated funds, supports education programs, credentialing analysis, and development of human resources needed to staff the U.S. health care system.

3334 International Dyslexia Association: Maryland Branch
International Dyslexia Association
40 York Rd 4th floor
Baltimore, MD 21204
410-296-0232
800-222-3123
FAX: 410-321-5069
e-mail: info@interdys.org
www.interdys.org

Hal Malchow, President
Eric Q. Tridas, M.D., Immediate Past President
Suzanne Carreker, Ph.D., CALT, Secretary
Ben Shifrin, M.Ed., Vice President

Nonprofit organization providing free information and referral services for diagnosis and tutoring for parents, educators, physicians, and individuals with dyslexia. The voice of our membership is heard in 48 countries. Membership includes yearly journal and quarterly newsletter. Call for conference dates.

3335 Maryland Client Assistance Program Division of Rehabilitation Services
2301 Argonne Dr
Baltimore, MD 21218-1628
410-554-9361
800-638-6243
FAX: 410-554-9362
TTY: 410-554-9360
e-mail: cap@dors.state.md.us
www.dors.state.md.us/dors/programservices/cap

Tom Laverty, Director,Client Assistance Progr

Helps individuals with disabilities understand the rehabilitation process and receives appropriate and quality services from the Division of Rehabilitation Services and other programs and facilities providing services under the Rehabilitation Act of 1973.

3336 Maryland Department of Aging
State Office Building
301 W Preston St
Suite 1007
Baltimore, MD 21201-2393
410-767-1100
877-634-6361
e-mail: drb@mail.ooa.state.md.us
www.mdoa.state.md.us/

Dakota Burgess, Senior Information Program Manag
Gloria Gary Lawlah, Secretary

3337 **Maryland Department of Handicapped Children**
201 W Preston St
Unit 50
Baltimore, MD 21201-2301 410-335-6470
www.msa.md.gov
Judson Force, Director
Children's Medical Services is a joint federal/state/local program which assists in obtaining specialized medical, surgical and related habilitative/rehabilitative evaluation and treatment services for children with special health care needs and their families. To be eligible for the program's services, an individual must be a resident of Maryland, younger than 22 years, have or be suspected of having an eligible medical condition and meet both medical and financial criteria.

3338 **Maryland Developmental Disabilities Council**
217 E Redwood St
Suite 1300
Baltimore, MD 21202-3313 410-767-3670
800-305-6441
FAX: 410-333-3686
www.md-council.org
Brian Cox, Executive Director
Catherine Lyle, Deputy Director
Rachel London, Director, Children & Family Policy
Angela Castillo-Epps, Director of Communications/Policy
A public policy organization comprised of people with disabilities and family members who are joined by state officials, service providers and other designated partners. The Council is an independent, self-governing organization that represents the interests of people with developmental disabilities and their families.

3339 **Maryland Division of Mental Health**
2301 Argonne Dr
Baltimore, MD 21218-1628 410-243-7495
FAX: 410-333-7482
www.dors.state.md.us/dors
Norma Pinette, Executive Director

3340 **National Maternal and Child Health Bureau**
Rm 1805
5600 Fishers Ln
Rockville, MD 20852-1750 301-443-2216
888-275-4772
e-mail: ask@hrsa.gov
hrsa.gov
Marcia Brand, Deputy Administrator
Tina Cheatham, Senior Advisor
Mary Wakefield, Administrator
Offers information, books and pamphlets to professionals, parents and children facing health issues or disabilities.

3341 **Social Security: Baltimore Disability Determination**
711 W 40th St
Baltimore, MD 21211-2120 800-772-1213
TTY:800-325-0778
ssa.gov

3342 **Workers Compensation Board Maryland**
10 E Baltimore St
Baltimore, MD 21202-1641 410-864-5100
800-492-0479
FAX: 410-333-8122
e-mail: info@wcc.state.md.us
www.wcc.state.md.us
R. Karl Aumann, Chairperson
Mary K. Ahearn, Chief Executive Officer
David E. Jones, Chief Financial Officer
Joyce McNemar, Chief Information Officer

Massachusetts

3343 **Center for Public Representation**
22 Green St
Northampton, MA 01060-3708 413-586-6024
FAX: 413-586-5711
e-mail: info@cpr-ma.org
centerforpublicrep.org
Bob Agoglia, President
Nickie Chandler, Clerk/Treasurer
Bob Riedel, Director
Neal Rosen, Esq., Director

3344 **International Dyslexia Association of New England**
40 York Rd 4th floor
Baltimore, MD 21204 410-296-0232
800-222-3123
FAX: 410-321-5069
e-mail: info@interdys.org
www.interdys.org
Hal Malchow, President
Eric Q. Tridas, M.D., Immediate Past President
Suzanne Carreker, Ph.D., CALT, Secretary
Ben Shifrin, M.Ed., Vice President
Provides free information and referral services for diagnosis and tutoring for parents, educators, physicians, and individuals with dyslexia in Connecticut, Maine, New Hampshire, Rhode Island, and Vermont. The voice of our membership is heard in 48 countries. Membership includes yearly journal and quarterly newsletter. Call for conference dates.

3345 **Massachusetts Assistive Technology Partnership**
Children s Hospital Boston
1295 Boylston St
Suite 310
Boston, MA 02215-3407 617-355-7820
800-848-8867
FAX: 617-355-6345
e-mail: info@matp.org
www.mass.gov/eohhs/gov/departments/dds/assist
Marylyn Howe, Project Director
Pat Hill, Training Coordinator
A statewide program promoting assistive technology devices and services for persons with all disabilities.

3346 **Massachusetts Client Assistance Program**
Massachusetts Office on Disability
1 Ashburton Pl
Suite 1305
Boston, MA 02108-1518 617-727-7440
800-322-2020
e-mail: james.aprea@state.ma.us
www.mass.gov/anf/employment-equal-access-disa
Barbara Lybarger, Assistant Director
Myra Berloff, Director
Michael Dumont, Assistant Director
Jeffrey Dougan, Assistant Director
Provides advocacy and information services.

3347 **Massachusetts Department of Mental Health**
25 Staniford St
Boston, MA 02114-2503 617-626-8000
800-221-0053
FAX: 617-727-9842
TTY:617-727-9842
e-mail: dmhinfo@dmh.state.ma.us
http://www.mass.gov/eohhs/gov/departments/dmh
Eileen Elias, Commissioner
Michele Anzaldi, Site Director
The Massachusetts Department of Mental Health (DMH) sets the standards for the operation of mental health facilities and community residential programs and provides clinical, rehabilitative and supportive services for adults with serious mental illness, and children and adolescents with serious mental illness or serious emotional disturbance.

3348 **Massachusetts Developmental Disabilities Council**
100 Hancock Street
Second Floor, Suite 201
Quincy, MA 02169-4398 617-770-7676
FAX: 617-770-1987
TTY:617-770-9499
e-mail: adelia.deltrecco@state.ma.us
www.state.ma.us/mddc/
Daniel Shannon, Executive Director
Faith Behum, Disability Policy Specialist
Kristin Britton, Director of Public Policy
Adelia DelTrecco, Member Services Coordinator
Group of citizens which analyzes needs of people with severe, lifelong disabilities and works to improve public policy. MDDC produces several publications and has committees and a grants program to study and advocate for changes in the service system.

3349 **Social Security: Boston Disability Determination**
1100 West High Rise
6401 Security Blvd.
Baltimore, MD 21235-1047 800-772-1213
TTY:800-325-0778
www.socialsecurity.gov
Michael F. Bertrand, Commissioner

3350 **Workers Compensation Board Massachusetts**
Rm 211
1 Ashburton Pl
Boston, MA 02108-1518 617-626-7122
FAX: 617-727-1090
www.state.ma.us/dia
Russell Gilfus, Manager
The Massachusetts Workers' Compensation system is in place to make sure that workers are protected by insurance if they are injured on the job or contract a work-related illness. Under this system, employers are required by Massachusetts General Laws c. 152, 25A to provide workers' compensation (WC) insurance coverage to all their employees.

Michigan

3351 **Department of Blind Rehabilitation**
Western Michigan University
1903 W Michigan Ave
Kalamazoo, MI 49008-5218 269-387-3455
FAX: 269-387-3567
e-mail: g.dennis@wmich.edu
www.wmich.edu/visionstudies
James Leja, Chair
Charles Adams, Faculty Specialist I
Gayle Dennis, Office Coordinator
Jeannyne Depoian, Office Associate
The Department of Blindness and Low Vision Studies at Western Michigan University is recognized internationally as the oldest, largest and best program of its kind. It originated in 1961 with a graduate degree in Orientation and Mobility, responding to the need for professionals to rehabilitate the many military personnel blinded during World War Two and the Korean War. Initially named the Department of Blind Rehabilitation, it prepared professionals to teach people who were blind to travel with

3352 **Michigan Association for Deaf and Hard of Hearing**
5236 Dumond Court
Suite C
Lansing, MI 48917-6001 517-487-0066
800-968-7327
FAX: 517-487-0202
TTY: 517-487-2586
e-mail: info@madhh.org
www.madhh.org
Nancy Asher, Executive Director
Pat Walton, Office Manager
MADHH is a statewide collaboration agency dedicated to improving the lives of people who are deaf and hard of hearing through leadership in education, advocacy & services. Interpreter IC print-out, assistive devices available.

3353 **Michigan Association for Deaf, and Hard of Hearing**
5236 Dumond Court
Suite C
Lansing, MI 48917-6001 517-487-0066
800-968-7327
FAX: 517-487-2586
e-mail: info@madhh.org
www.madhh.org
Nancy Asher, Executive Director
Pat Walton, Office Manager
MADHH is a statewide collaboration agency dedicated to improving the lives of people who are deaf and hard of hearing through leadership in education, advocacy and services.

3354 **Michigan Client Assistance Program**
4095 Legacy Pkwy
Ste 500
Lansing, MI 48911-4264 517-487-1755
800-288-5923
FAX: 517-487-0827
TTY: 800-288-5923
e-mail: molson@mpas.org
www.mpas.org
Kate Pew Wolters, President
Thomas Landry, Ist Vice President
John McCulloch, 2nd Vice President
Elmer L. Cerano, Executive Director
The Client Assistance Program (CAP) assists people who are seeking or receiving services from Michigan Rehabilitation Services, Consumer Choice Programs, Michigan Commission for the Blind, Centers for Independent Living, and Supported Employment and Transition Programs. The CAP program is part of Michigan Protection and Advocacy Service, Inc.

3355 **Michigan Coalition for Staff Development and School Improvement**
Ste C
530 W Ionia St
Lansing, MI 48933-1062 734-513-9080
800-444-2014
FAX: 517-371-1170

3356 **Michigan Commission for the Blind - Gaylord**
Ste 102
209 W 1st St
Gaylord, MI 49735-1386 989-732-2448
800-292-4200
FAX: 989-731-3587
www.michigan.gov
Judy Terwilliger, Manager
The mission of the Michigan Commission for the Blind (MCB) is to provide opportunity to individuals who are blind or visually impaired to achieve employability and/or function independently in society. The MCB vision is that someday it will be said that Michigan is a great place for blind people to live, learn, work, raise a family, and enjoy life

3357 **Michigan Commission for the Blind**
Michigan Dept Of Energy, Labor & Economic Growth
PO Box 30652
Lansing, MI 48909-8152 517-373-2062
800-292-4200
FAX: 517-335-5140
TTY: 517-373-4025
e-mail: turneys@michigan.gov
www.michigan.gov/mcb
Patrick Cannon, State Director
The Michigan Commision for the blind is a state government agency that provides state and federally funded training and other services to individuals who are legally blind (blind and visually impaired). Services are provided to people of all ages throughout the state of Michigan toward the goal of employment and/or independence.

3358 Michigan Commission for the Blind Training Center
PO Box 30652
Lansing, MI 48909
517-373-2062
800-292-4200
FAX: 517-335-5140
TTY: 517-373-4025
e-mail: mossc@michigan.gov
www.michigan.gov/mcb

Cheryl L Heibeck, Director
Bruce Schultz, Assistant Director

Residential facility that provides instruction to legally blind adults in braille, computer operation and assistive technology, handwriting, cane travel, cooking, personal management, industrial arts and also crafts. During training students will develop career plans which may include work experience, internships, volunteer opprtunities and even part-time paid employment.

3359 Michigan Commission for the Blind: Escanaba
305 Ludington St
State Office Bldg., 1st Floor
Escanaba, MI 49829-4029
906-786-8602
800-323-2535
FAX: 906-786-4638
michigan.gov/mcb

Bernie Kramer, Manager

The mission of the Michigan Commission for the Blind (MCB) is to provide opportunity to individuals who are blind or visually impaired to achieve employability and/or function independently in society. The MCB vision is that someday it will be said that Michigan is a great place for blind people to live, learn, work, raise a family, and enjoy life

3360 Michigan Commission for the Blind: Flint
125 E Union St
Fl 7
Flint, MI 48502-2041
810-760-2030
800-292-4200
FAX: 810-760-2032
www.dlcq.state.mi.us

Debbie Wilson, Manager

Vocational and Independent living skills training for individuals who are legally blind.

3361 Michigan Commission for the Blind: Grand Rapids
305 Ludington St
Escanaba, MI 49829-4029
906-786-8602
800-323-2535
FAX: 906-786-4638
michigan.gov/mcb

Bernie Kramer, Manager

The mission of the Michigan Commission for the Blind (MCB) is to provide opportunity to individuals who are blind or visually impaired to achieve employability and/or function independently in society. The MCB vision is that someday it will be said that Michigan is a great place for blind people to live, learn, work, raise a family, and enjoy life

3362 Michigan Council of the Blind and Visually Impaired (MCBVI)
Neal Freeling
350 Ottawa Ave NW
Grand Rapids, MI 49503-2316
616-356-0180
800-292-4200
FAX: 616-356-0199
michigan.gov/mcb

Bernie Kramer, Manager

MCBVI is a diverse group of very friendly people from around the state working together to improve the lives of all citizens who are blind or visually impaired.

3363 Michigan Department of Handicapped Children
3423 N Martin Luther King Jr Blvd
Lansing, MI 48906-2934
517-484-9312
FAX: 517-484-9836

Alan Curtiss, President
Bobbie Butler, Manager

3364 Michigan Developmental Disabilies Council
1033 S Washington Ave
Lansing, MI 48910-1646
517-334-6123
FAX: 517-334-7353
TTY:517-334-7354
e-mail: sharp@michigan.gov
www.michigan.gov/ddcouncil

Vendella Collins, Executive Director
Andre K Robinson, Chair
Mitzi Allen, Administrative
Yasmina Bouraoui, Deputy Director

The Michigan DD Council is a group of citizens from across the state. Its membership is made up of: people with developmental disabilities; people from families who have, among their members, people with developmental disabilities; and professionals from state and local agencies charged with assisting people with developmental disabilities.

3365 Michigan Office of Services to the Aging
P.O.Box 30676
Lansing, MI 48909-8176
517-373-8230
FAX: 517-373-4092
e-mail: lewisp3@michigan.gov
www.michigan.gov/osa

Wendi Middleton, Division Director
Kari Sederburg, Director
Carol Dye, Senior Executive Assistant
Annette Gamez, Executive Assistant

State unit on aging; allocates and monitors state and federal funds for the Older American Act services: nutrition, community services, administers home and community based waiver, develops programs through Area Agencies on Aging, advocates on behalf of seniors with legislature, governor, state departments, federal government, responsible for state planning of aging services, develops formula for distribution of state and federal funds.

3366 Michigan Protection & Advocacy Service
4095 Legacy Pkwy
Ste 500
Lansing, MI 48911-4264
517-487-1755
800-288-5923
FAX: 517-487-0827
e-mail: molson@mpas.org
mpas.org

Kate Pew Wolters, President
Thomas Landry, Ist Vice President
John McCulloch, 2nd Vice President
Elmer L. Cerano, Executive Director

People with disabilities have to deal with a wide variety of issues. TThey try to answer any questions you may have relating to disability. They have experience in the following areas: discrimination in education, employment, housing, and public places; abuse and neglect; Social Security benefits; Medicaid, Medicare and other insurance; housing; Vocational Rehabilitation; HIV/AIDS issues; and many other disability-related topics

3367 Michigan Rehabilitation Services
300 N. Washington Sq.
Lansing, MI 48913
517-335-4590
888-784-7328
FAX: 517-373-0059
TTY: 517-373-4035
e-mail: zimmermang@michigan.org
www.michigan.org

George Zimmermann, Vice President
Michelle Begnoche, Communications Specialist
Bonnie Fink, Travel Consultant Coordinator
David Lorenz, Public and Industry Relations Ma

A state and federally funded program that helps persons with disabilities prepare for and fund a job that matches their interests and abilities. Assistance is also available to workers with disabilities who are having difficulty keeping a job. A person is eligible for MRS services if he or she has a disability, is unemployed and needs vocational rehabilitation services to prepare for and find a job or independent living services.

3368 Social Security Administration
1100 West High Rise
6401 Security Blvd.
Baltimore, MD 21235-3878
517-393-3876
800-772-1213
FAX: 517-393-4686
TTY: 800-325-0778
e-mail: jennifer.bower@ssa.gov
ssa.gov

Tiffany L. Flick, Executive Secretary
Michael J. Astrue, Commissioner
Carolyn W. Colvin, Deputy Commissioner

We deliver services through a nationwide network of over 1,400 offices that include regional offices, field offices, card centers, teleservice centers, processing centers, hearing offices, the Appeals Council, and our State and territorial partners, the Disability Determination Services. We also have a presence in U.S. embassies around the globe. For the public, we are the "face of the government." The rich diversity of our employees mirrors the public we serve.

3369 State of Michigan Workers' Compensation Agency
PO Box 30016
Lansing, MI 48909-7516
888-396-5041
FAX: 517-322-1808
e-mail: wcinfo@michigan.gov
www.michigan.gov/wca/

Kevin A. Elsenheimer, Director
Jack A. Nolish, Deputy Director
Sue Bickel, Secretary
Ted Day, Division Manager

Michigan's injured workers and their employers are governed by the Workers' Disability Compensation Act. This Act was first adopted in 1912 and provides compensation to workers who suffer an injury on the job and protects employers' liability. The mission of the Workers' Compensation Agency is to efficiently administer the Act and provide prompt, courteous and impartial service to all customers.

Minnesota

3370 International Dyslexia Association: Minnesota Branch
International Dyslexia Association
5021 Vernon Ave S
Minneapolis, MN 55436-2102
612-486-4242
800-222-3123
FAX: 410-321-5069
e-mail: info@ida-umb.org
www.interdys.org

Eric Q. Tridas, M.D., President
Suzanne Carreker, Ph.D., CALT-, Vice President
Cinthia Coletti Haan, Vice President
Susan Lowell, M.A., B.C.E.T, Vice President

UMBIDA-the Upper Midwest Branch of the International Dyslexia Association (IDA-serves the residents of Minnesota, North Dakota, South Dakota, and Winnipeg, Canada and offers: local educational conferences about dyslexia and related subjects, Orton-Gillingham training for teachers, tutors, and parents, Quarterly speaker series, member discounts on conferences, information line, and tutor referral.

3371 Minnesota Assistive Technology Project
STAR
358 Centennial Office Building
658 Cedar Street
Saint Paul, MN 55155-1402
651-201-2640
888-234-1267
800-627-3529
FAX: 651-282-6671
e-mail: star.program@state.mn.us
mn.gov/star/about.htm

Chuck Rassbach, Program Director
Nancy Stark, Executive Secretary
Jennie Delisi, Program Staff
Joan Gillum, Program Staff

A statewide program promoting assistive technology devices and services for persons of all ages with all disabilities.

3372 Minnesota Board on Aging
P.O. Box 64976
Saint Paul, MN 55164-0976
651-431-2500
800-882-6262
800-333-2433
FAX: 651-431-7453
TTY:800-627-3529
e-mail: mba@sate.mn.us
www.mnaging.org

Don Samuelson, Chair
Jean Wood, Executive Director
Leonard Axelrod, Board Member
Tracy Keibler, Board Member

A state unit on aging for the state of Minnesota. Funds 14 area agencies on aging throughout the state that provide services at the local level. The mission is to keep older people in the homes or places of residence for as long as possible.

3373 Minnesota Children with Special Needs, Minnesota Department of Health
P.O.Box 64882
Saint Paul, MN 55164-0882
651-201-3650
888-345-0823
800-728-5420
FAX: 651-201-3655
TTY:651-201-5797
e-mail: health.cyshn@state.mn.us
www.health.state.mn.us/mcshn

Dr. Edward Ehlinger, Commissioner
James G. Koppel, Deputy Commissioner
Jeanne F. Ayers, Assistant Commissioner
Barb Dalbec, Director

Minnesota Children with Special Health Needs (MCSHN) provides leadership through partnerships with families and other key stakeholders to improve the access and quality of all systems impacting children and youth with special health care needs and their families.

3374 Minnesota Department of Labor & Industry Workers Compensation Division
443 Lafayette Rd N
Saint Paul, MN 55155-4301
651-284-5005
800-342-5354
TTY:651-297-4198
e-mail: dli.communications@state.mn.us
doli.state.mn.us

Ken Petersom, Commissioner
Kris Eiden, Deputy Commisioner
James Honerman, Communications
Gail Krieg, Human Resources

To reduce the impact of work related injuries for employees and employers. Advice is given and questions answered on the toll-free number.

3375 Minnesota Disability Law Center
430 1st Avenue North
Suite 300
Minneapolis, MN 55401- 1780
612-334-5970
800-292-4150
FAX: 612-334-5755
TTY: 612-332-4668
e-mail: website@mylegalaid.org
mylegalaid.org/about/our-work/disability-law

Mary L. Knoblauch, Chair
Cathy Haukedahl, Executive Director
Andrea Kaufman, Director of Development
Lisa Cohen, Deputy Director of Operations

Provides free, civil, legal assistance to Minnesotans with disabilities on issues related to their disability.

3376 Minnesota Governor's Council on Developmental Disabilities GCDD
370 Centennial Office Building
658 Cedar St
Saint Paul, MN 55155-1603 651-296-4018
877-348-0505
FAX: 651-297-7200
e-mail: admin.dd@state.mn.us
www.mncdd.org
Dan Reed, Chair
Colleen Wieck PhD, Executive Director
Mary O'Hara Anderson, Council Member
Ashley Bailey, Council Member
The mission of the Minnesota Governor's Council on Developmental Disabilities is to provide information, education, and training to build knowledge, develop skills, and change attitudes that will lead to increased independence, productivity, self determination, integration and inclusion (IPSII) for people with developmental disabilities and their families.

3377 Minnesota Mental Health Division
Human Services Building
444 Lafayette Rd N
Saint Paul, MN 55155-3802 651-431-2000
800-366-5411
TTY:800-627-3529
e-mail: dhs.info@state.mn.us
www.dhs.state.mn.us/Provider/faqs/mental_heal
Lucinda E. Jesson, Commissioner
Anne Barry, Deputy Commissioner
Nancy Johnston, Executive Director
Brownell E. Mack, Assistant Commissioner
Oversees the provision of services to people with mental illness in the state of Minnesota. Services are provided on the local level through a network of 87 county social service departments.

3378 Minnesota Protection & Advocacy for Persons with Disabilities
Minnesota Disability Law Center
2324 University Avenue W.
Suite 1018
Saint Paul, MN 55114-1742 651-228-9105
800-292-4150
FAX: 651-222-0745
e-mail: statesupport@mnlegalservices.org
www.mnlegalservices.org/mdlc
Mary Kaczorek, Supervising Attorney
Anne Conroy, Office Manager
Elsa Marshall, Education for Justice Coordinator
Jessica Nault, Legal Project Manager

3379 Minnesota State Council on Disability(MSCOD)
121 7th Pl E
Suite 107
Saint Paul, MN 55101-2114 651-361-7800
800-945-8913
FAX: 651-296-5935
e-mail: council.disability@state.mn.us
www.disability.state.mn.us
Joan Willshire, Executive Director
Linda Gremillion, Business Operations Manager
Margot Imdieke Cross, Accessibility Specialist
George Shardlow, Public Policy Intern
The MSCOD collaborates, advocates, advises and provide technical information to expand opportunities, increase the quality of life and empower all persons with disabilities. This mission is accomplished by: providing information, referral and technical assistance to thousands of individuals every year via email, letter or telephone; through trainings on a variety of disability related topics; through publications and its web site; and through its advocacy and advisory work.

3380 Minnesota State Services for the Blind
2200 University Avenue West
Suite 240
Saint Paul, MN 55114-1840 651-642-0500
800-652-9000
FAX: 651-649-5927
TTY: 651-642-0506
e-mail: star.program@state.mn.us
http://mn.gov/deed/job-seekers/blind-visual-i
Richard Strong, Executive Director
Kenneth Trebelhorn, Council Member
Jan Bailey, Chair
Steve Jacobson, Council Member
State agency serving blind and visually impaired persons with rehabilitation, information access, assistive technology, training and job placement services. Extensive older blind program.

3381 Social Security: St. Paul Disability Determination
5210 Perry Robinson Cir
Lansing, MI 48911-3878 517-393-3876
800-772-1213
FAX: 517-393-4686
TTY: 800-325-0778
e-mail: jennifer.bower@ssa.gov
www.ssa.gov
Karena L. Kilgore, Executive Secretary
Carolyn W. Colvin, Commissioner
Carolyn W. Colvin, Deputy Commissioner
James A. Kissko, Chief of Staff
We deliver services through a nationwide network of over 1,400 offices that include regional offices, field offices, card centers, teleservice centers, processing centers, hearing offices, the Appeals Council, and our State and territorial partners, the Disability Determination Services. We also have a presence in U.S. embassies around the globe. For the public, we are the "face of the government." The rich diversity of our employees mirrors the public we serve.

Mississippi

3382 International Dyslexia Association: Mississippi Branch
1997 Atkins Rd.
Ruston, LA 71270 985-414-2575
800-222-3123
FAX: 410-321-5069
e-mail: alicehiginbotham@hotmail.com
http://www.ladyslexia.com/LaBIDA/Welcome.ht ml
Alice Higginbotham, President
Maureen Landry, Vice President/Chair of Public
Becky Clingman, Branch Council Rep
Dawn Amy, Director/Chair Education
It is the mission of the Louisiana Branch to provide information and resources to parents, educators, students and the community in a way that creates a clear and positive understanding of dyslexia and related language learning needs so that every individual has the opportunity to lead a productive and fulfilling life for the benefit of society.

3383 Mississippi Assistive Technology Division
1281 Highway 51
PO Box 1698
Jackson, MS 39215-1698 601-853-5160
800-443-1000
FAX: 601-853-5158
www.mdrs.state.ms.us
Kris Geroux, Coordinator
Marie Gaddis, Administrative Assistant
A statewide program promoting assistive technology devices and services for persons of all ages with all disabilities.

3384 Mississippi Bureau of Mental Retardation
1101 Robert E Lee Bldg
239 North Lamar Street
Jackson, MS 39201
601-359-1288
877-240-8513
FAX: 601-359-6295
TTY: 601-359-6230
e-mail: ed.legrand@dmh.state.ms.us
www.dmh.state.ms.us

Sampat Shivengi, M.D., Chair
George N. Harrison, Vice Chair
Edwin C. Legrand, Executive Director
Kris Jones, Bureau Director of Quality Manag

Since its inception in 1974, the Mississippi Department of Mental Health has endeavored to provide services of the highest quality through a statewide service delivery system. As one of the major state agencies in Mississippi, the Department of Mental Health provides a network of services to persons who experience problems with mental illness, alcohol and/or drug abuse/dependence, or who have intellectual and developmental disabilities. Services are provided through an array of facilities and ag

3385 Mississippi Client Assistance Program
Mississippi Department of Rehabilitation Services
500-G East Woodrow Wilson Drive
P.O. Box 4958
Jackson, MS 39296
601-982-7051
FAX: 601-982-1951
www.msdisabilities.com

Ken Cleveland, President
Presley Posey, Executive Director
Dr. Michael Ogburn, Executive Director
David Cleland, Executive Director

Advocacy program for clients/client applicants for state of MS vocational services.

3386 Mississippi Department of Mental Health
1101 Robert E Lee Bldg
239 North Lamar Street
Jackson, MS 39201
601-359-1288
877-240-8513
FAX: 601-359-6295
TTY: 601-359-6230
e-mail: ed.legrand@dmh.state.ms.us
dmh.state.ms.us

Sampat Shivengi, M.D., Chair
George N. Harrison, Vice Chair
Edwin C. Legrand, Executive Director
Kris Jones, Bureau Director of Quality Manag

Administers Mississippi's public programs of serving persons with mental illness, mental retardation, alcohol and substance abuse problems, and alzheimer's disease and related dementia.

3387 Mississippi Division of Aging and Adult Services
Mississippi Department Of Human Services
750 North State Street
Jackson, MS 39202-3033
601-355-5536
800-345-6347
877-882-4916
FAX: 601-359-3664
e-mail: webspinner@mdhs.state.ms.us
www.mdhs.state.ms.us/

Donald R. Taylor, Executive Director
Julia M. Todd, Director
Judy Collins, Director
Mary Scott, Director

Protects the rights of older citizens while expanding their opportunities and access to quality services.

3388 Mississippi State Department of Health
Children s Medical Program
4777 Medgar Evrs Blvd
Jackson, MS 39213-1700
601-362-9892
866-458-4948
FAX: 601-364-7447
e-mail: web@HealthyMS.com
www.msdh.state.ms.us

Larry Clark, Director
Vickey Berryman, Director, Bureau of Licensure
Jim Craig, Director, Office of Health Pro
Tim Darnell, Director, MSDH Field Services

Financial assistance to families of children with physical handicaps. Rehabilitative in nature and has as its goal the correction or reduction of physical handicaps. Eligibility determined by diagnosis and provided to children from birth to age twenty-one. Financial eligibility is determined by factors of family income, family size, estimated cost of treatment and family liabilities. Categories include, but are not limited to: orthopedic, congenital heart defects, cerebral palsy, etc.

3389 Mississippi: Workers Compensation Commission
1428 Lakeland Dr
P.O. Box 5300, 39296-5300
Jackson, MS 39216-4718
601-987-4200
866-473-6922
FAX: 601-987-4220
e-mail: mwcc.state.ms.us
www.mwcc.state.ms.us

Liles Williams, Chairman
John Junkin, Commissioner
Debra Gibbs, Commissioner
Cindy Polk Wilson, Administrative Judge

Our goal is to provide the public with useful information regarding Workers' Compensation in the state of Mississippi.

Missouri

3390 Institute for Human Development
University of Missouri-Kansas City
215 W. Pershing Road
6th floor
Kansas City, MO 64108- 2639
816-235-1770
800-444-0821
FAX: 888-503-3107
TTY: 800-452-1185
e-mail: beckmanncc@umkc.edu
www.ihd.umkc.edu

Carl F. Calkins, Ph.D., Director
Kay Conklin, Training Director
Cindy Beckmann, Assistant to the Director
Kathy Fuger, Director, Early Childhood and Yo

A statewide program promoting person-centered planning and services for persons of all ages with all disabilities.

3391 Missouri Division Of Developmental Disabilities
Missouri Department Of Mental Health
1706 E. Elm St.
P.O.Box 687
Jefferson City, MO 65102
573-751-4054
800-364-9687
FAX: 573-751-9207
e-mail: ddmail@dmh.mo.gov
www.dmh.mo.gov

Jay Nixon, Governor
Keith Schafer, Ed.D., Director
Bob Bax, Deputy Director
Rikki J. Wright, J.D., General Counsel

The Missouri Department of Mental Health was first established as a cabinet-level state agency by the Omnibus State Government Reorganization Act, effective July 1, 1974. State law provides three principal missions for the department: (1) the prevention of mental disorders, developmental disabilities, substance abuse, and compulsive gambling; (2) the treatment, habilitation, and rehabilitation of Missourians who have those conditions; and (3) the improvement of public understanding and attitudes

3392 Missouri Protection & Advocacy Services
925 S Country Club Dr
Jefferson City, MO 65109-4510 573-893-3333
800-392-8667
FAX: 573-893-4231
TTY: 800-735-2966
e-mail: mopasjc@embarqmail.com
moadvocacy.org

Joe Wrinkle, Chair
Barbara H. French, Vice Chair
Shawn De Loyola, Executive Director
Susan Pritchard-Green, Secretary/Treasurer

MO P&A potects the rights of individuals with disabilities by providing advocacy and legal services for disability related issues. As Missouri's Protection and Advocacy system, Mo P&A investigates allegations of abuse, neglect, death, and violations of rights against individuals with disabilities. Those who contact Mo P&A can receive information, referrals, advocacy services or legal counsel provided through one of nine federally-funded programs.

3393 Missouri Rehabilitation Services for the Blind
615 Howerton Court
PO Box 2320
Jefferson City, MO 65102-2320 573-751-4249
800-592-6004
FAX: 573-751-4984
e-mail: askrsb@dss.mo.gov
www.dss.mo.gov/fsd/rsb/

Mark Laird, Executive Director
Ronald J. Levy, Director
Brian Kinkade, Deputy Director
Jennifer Tidball, Division Director

Offers services for the totally blind, legally blind, visually impaired, including counseling, educational, recreational, rehabilitation, computer training and professional training services.

3394 Social Security: Jefferson City Disability Determination
129 SCOTT STATION ROAD
Jefferson City, MO 65101-4421 877-405-9803
800-772-1213
FAX: 517-393-4686
TTY: 800-325-0778
e-mail: jennifer.bower@ssa.gov
www.ssa.gov

Karena L. Kilgore, Executive Secretary
Carolyn W. Colvin, Commissioner
Carolyn W. Colvin, Deputy Commissioner
James A. Kissko, Chief of Staff

We deliver services through a nationwide network of over 1,400 offices that include regional offices, field offices, card centers, teleservice centers, processing centers, hearing offices, the Appeals Council, and our State and territorial partners, the Disability Determination Services. We also have a presence in U.S. embassies around the globe. For the public, we are the "face of the government." The rich diversity of our employees mirrors the public we serve.

3395 Workers Compensation Board Missouri
Department of Labor and Industrial Realtions
421 East Dunkin Street
P.O. Box 59
Jefferson City, MO 65102-0059 573-751-3251
800-775-2667
800-320-2519
FAX: 573-751-4945
e-mail: appealstribunal@labor.mo.gov
labor.mo.gov/DWC/

John J. Larsen,Jr., Chairman
James Avery, Commissioner
Curtis E. Chick, Commissioner
Ryan McKenna, Department Director

The Missouri Division of Workers' Compensation administers the programs providing services to all stake holders including workers who have been injured on the job or been exposed to occupational disease arising out of and in the course of employment. The Division makes sure that an injured worker receives benefits that he/she is entitled to under the Missouri Workers' Compensation law. The Division's Administrative Law Judges have the authority to approve settlements or issue awards after a hear

Montana

3396 Addictive & Mental Disorders Division
555 Fuller Ave
PO Box 202905
Helena, MT 59620-2905 406-444-3964
FAX: 406-444-4435
e-mail: lothompson@mt.gov
http://www.dphhs.mt.gov/amdd/

Lou Thompson, Administrator
Joan Cassidy, Chemical Dependency Bureau Chief
E. Lee Simes, Medical Director
Deb Matteucci, Behavioral Health Program Facili

The mission of the Addictive and Mental Disorders Division (AMDD) of the Montana Department of Public Health and Human Services is to implement and improve an appropriate statewide system of prevention, treatment, care, and rehabilitation for Montanans with mental disorders or addictions to drugs or alcohol.

3397 Disability Rights Montana
1022 Chestnut Street
Helena, MT 59601-890 406-449-2344
800-245-4743
FAX: 406-449-2418
TTY: 406-449-2344
e-mail: advocate@disabilityrightsmt.org
www.disabilityrightsmt.org/janda3/

Bernadette Franks-Ongoy, Executive Director
Kelli Kaufman, Director of Finance & Administra
Steve Heaverlo, Director of Programs/Advocacy Sp
Laurie t Danforth, Paralegal/Executive Suppor

Protects and advocates the human and legal rights of Montanans with mental and physical disabilities while advancing dignity, equality, and self-determination. Designated federal P&A, with AT, CAP, PADD, PAIMI and PAIR programs. Advocacy and legal services for abuse, neglect, rights violations, access, discrimination in employment, accommodations and housing, and assistance with vocational rehabilitation/visual services.

3398 MonTECH
700 SW Higgins Ave.
Suite 250
Missoula, MT 59803 406-243-5751
877-243-5511
FAX: 406-243-4730
e-mail: montech@ruralinstitute.umt.edu
www.montech.ruralinstitute.umt.edu

Kathleen Laurin, Program Director
Chris Clasby, Program Coordinator
Leslie Mullette

Specializing in Assistive Technology and oversee a variety of AT related grants and contracts. The overall goal is to develop a comprehensive, statewide system of assistive technology related assistance. Striving to ensure that all people in Montana with disabilities have equitable access to assistive technology devices and services in order to enhance their independence, productivity and quality of life.

3399 Montana Blind & Low Vision Services
111 N Last Chance Gulch, Suite 4C
PO Box 4210
Helena, MT 59604-4210 406-444-2590
877-296-1197
FAX: 406-444-3632
e-mail: lothompson@mt.gov
http://www.dphhs.mt.gov/vocrehab/blvs/

Lou Thompson, Administrator
Joan Cassidy, Chemical Dependency Bureau Chief
E. Lee Simes, Medical Director
Deb Matteucci, Behavioral Health Program Facili

Mission: promoting work and independence for Montanans with disabilities.

3400 Montana Council on Developmental Disabilities
2714 Billings Ave
Helena, MT 59601-9767
406-443-4332
866-443-4332
FAX: 406-443-4192
e-mail: deborah@mtcdd.or
www.mtcdd.org

Deborah Swingley, CEO/Executive Director
Dee Burrell, Contract Manager

The Council is made up of Montanans both with and without developmental disabilities, who believe in improving the lives of Montana's citizens who have a disability. We concentrate on issues related to self-determination, education, employment, transportation, housing, recreation, health care, community inclusion and the overall quality of life of people with developmental disabilities. As a Council we are committed to both question, and action as we work to discover and promote creative ways t

3401 Montana Department of Aging
Room 219
Capitol Sta
Helena, MT 59620
406-444-7734
FAX: 406-444-3465

Keith Messmer, Manager
Jeff Sturm, President

3402 Montana Department of Handicapped Children
Cogswell Building
Helena, MT 59620
406-444-7734
FAX: 406-444-3465

Keith Messmer, Manager

3403 Montana Protection & Advocacy for Persons with Disabilities
1022 Chestnut Street
Helena, MT 59601-890
406-449-2344
800-245-4743
FAX: 406-449-2418
TTY: 406-449-2344
e-mail: advocate@disabilityrightsmt.org
www.disabilityrightsmt.org/janda3/

Susie McIntyre, President
Will Warberg, Sales and Marketing Manager
Bernadette Franks-Ongoy, Executive Director
Kelli Kaufman, Director of Finance & Administra

Disability Rights Montana is the federally-mandated civil rights protection and advocacy system for Montana. We have the legal authority to represent almost any person with a disability.

3404 Montana State Fund
P.O.Box 4759
Helena, MT 59604-4759
406-495-5000
800-332-6102
FAX: 406-495-5020
TTY: 406-495-5030
www.montanastatefund.com

Elizabeth Best, Chairman

Montana State Fund is committed to the health and economic prosperity of Montana through superior service, leadership and caring individuals, working in an environment of teamwork, creativity and trust.

3405 Social Security: Helena Disability Determination
10 W 15th St
Ste 1600
Helena, MT 59626-9704
406-441-1270
800-772-1213
TTY:406-441-1278
www.socialsecurity.gov

Karena L. Kilgore, Executive Secretary
Carolyn W. Colvin, Commissioner
Carolyn W. Colvin, Deputy Commissioner
James A. Kissko, Chief of Staff

Social Security offers online information and services to third parties who do business with them.

Nebraska

3406 International Dyslexia Association: Nebraska Branch
40 York Rd.
4th Floor
Baltimore, MD 21204
410-296-0232
800-222-3123
FAX: 410-321-5069
e-mail: carolyn.brandle@ne-ida.com
www.interdys.org

Hal Malchow, President
Elsa Cardenas-Hagan, Vice President
Ben Shifrin, Vice President
Kristen Penczek, Interim Executive Director

The Nebraska Branch of the International Dyslexia Association is a 501(c)(3), non-profit organization dedicated to the study and treatment of dyslexia and related learning differences. This Branch was formed in 1981 to increase public awareness of dyslexia throughout Nebraska, and to serve individuals with dyslexia and their families. The organization includes professionals in the area of learning disabilities education, counseling and medicine as well as dylexics and their families and friends.

3407 Nebraska Advocacy Services
134 S 13th St
Suite 600
Lincoln, NE 68508-1930
402-474-3183
800-422-6691
FAX: 402-474-3274
e-mail: info@disabilityrightsnebraska.org
www.disabilityrightsnebraska.org

Jill Flagel, Chairperson
Mary Angus, Vice-Chairperson
Timothy F. Shaw, Chief Executive Officer
Eric Evans, Chief Operating Officer

Offers protection and advocacy services to people with developmental disabilities or mental illness. Direct assistance provided if issue within broad case priorities. Sliding scale fee. Information and referral at no cost.

3408 Nebraska Client Assistance Program
301 Centennial Mall South
P. O. Box 94987
Lincoln, NE 68509-4987
402-471-3656
800-742-7594
FAX: 402-471-3656
e-mail: victoria.rasmussen@nebraska.gov
www.cap.state.ne.us/

3409 Nebraska Commission for the Blind & Visually Impaired
4600 Valley Rd
Suite 100
Lincoln, NE 68510-4844
402-471-2891
877-809-2419
FAX: 402-471-3009
e-mail: kathy.stephens@nebraska.gov
ncbvi.state.ne.us

Pearl Van zandt, Executive Director
Carlos Servan, Deputy Director
Bob Deaton, Deputy Director
Barbara Loos, Chairman

Offers services for the totally blind, legally blind, visually impaired, mentally retarded blind and more with health, counseling, educational, recreational, rehabilitation, computer training and professional training services.

3410 Nebraska Department of Health & Human Services of Medically Handicapped Children's Prgm
301 Centennial Mall S
5TH Floor
Lincoln, NE 68508-2529
402-471-3121
800-383-4278
FAX: 402-471-3577
e-mail: mary.gordon@nebraska.gov
dhhs.ne.gov

Kerry Winterer, Chief Executive Officer
Amy Borer, Admininstrative Assistant,Divisi
Dan Howell, CEO,Beatrice State Developmental

Maternal and child health, Title V, children with special health care needs; community based, statewide programs to facilitate diagnoses and care of children with disabilities and chronic medical conditions.

3411 Nebraska Department of Health and Human Services, Division of Aging Services
P.O.Box 95026
Lincoln, NE 68509-5026
402-471-2115
800-942-7830
FAX: 402-471-3577
e-mail: mary.gordon@nebraska.gov
dhhs.ne.gov

Kerry Winterer, Chief Executive Officer
Amy Borer, Admininstrative Assistant,Divisi
Dan Howell, CEO,Beatrice State Developmental

The Council focuses on persons who experience a severe disability that occurs before the individual attains the age of 22, which includes persons with physical disabilities, mental/behavioral health conditions and persons that are served by the current state developmental disabilities system.

3412 Nebraska Department of Mental Health
4545 South 86th Street
Lincoln, NE 68526-2529
402-483-6990
888-210-8064
FAX: 402-483-7045
www.nmhc-clinics.com

Jill Zlomke McPherson, Executive Director
Thomas I. McPherson, Technical Coordinator
Lee Zlomke, Clinical Director
Lisa Logsden, Staff Psychologist

Nebraska Mental Health Centers is a family mental health clinic for people from all walks of life. Among the many services we provide are psychological evaluations, individual and group counseling, substance abuse care, neuropsychological services, domestic violence group intervention and help for victims of domestic violence, treatment for eating disorders, an ADHD clinic, Women's Counseling and much more.

3413 Nebraska Planning Council on Developmental Disabilities
Department of Health and Human Services
P.O.Box 95026
Lincoln, NE 68509-5026
402-471-2115
FAX: 402-471-3577
TTY:402-471-9570
e-mail: mary.gordon@nebraska.gov
dhhs.ne.gov/developmental_disabilities/Pages/

Mary Gordon, Executive Director
Kerry Winterer, Chief Executive Officer
Amy Borer, Admininstrative Assistant,Divisi
Dan Howell, CEO,Beatrice State Developmental

The Council focuses on persons who experience a severe disability that occurs before the individual attains the age of 22, which includes persons with physical disabilities, mental/behavioral health conditions and persons that are served by the current state developmental disabilities system.

3414 Nebraska Workers' Compensation Court
State of Nebraska
P.O.Box 98908
Lincoln, NE 68509-8908
402-471-6468
800-599-5155
FAX: 402-471-8231
www.wcc.ne.gov/

Glenn W. Morton, Administrator
Susan K. Davis, Public Information Manager
Jacqueline J Boesen, General Counsel
Randall Cecrle, Information Technology Manager

It is the web site of the Nebraska Workers' Compensation Court. The court maintains this web site to enhance public access and provide general information regarding workers' compensation in Nebraska.

3415 Social Security: Lincoln Disability Determination
Department of Education
P.O.Box 94987
Lincoln, NE 68509-4987
402-471-2295
800-772-1213
TTY:402-471-3659
e-mail: flloyd@nde4.nde.state.ne.us
www.socialsecurity.gov

Karena L. Kilgore, Executive Secretary
Carolyn W. Colvin, Commissioner
Carolyn W. Colvin, Deputy Commissioner
James A. Kissko, Chief of Staff

Social Security offers online information and services to third parties who do business with them.

Nevada

3416 Aging and Disability Services Division
3416 Goni Rd
Suite D 132
Carson City, NV 89706-8008
775-687-4210
800-992-0900
FAX: 775-687-0574
e-mail: adsd@adsd.nv.gov
adsd.nv.gov

Jane Gruner, Administrator
Tina Gerber-Winn, Deputy Administrator
Michele Ferral, Deputy Administrator

Provides services for seniors in Nevada including community based care. advocacy and volunteer programs. Call write or e-mail for more information.

3417 Nevada Assistive Technology Project
Ste 32
3656 Research Way
Carson City, NV 89706-7932
775-687-4452
888-337-3839
FAX: 775-687-3292
www.hr.state.nv.us

Todd Butterworth, Manager

Serves all ages and all disabilities through partnerships with community organizations. The NATP provides training, advocacy, funding, information and referral services, a newsletter and weekly television show.

3418 Nevada Bureau of Vocational Rehabilitation
1933 N Carson St
Carson City, NV 89703
775-684-0400
FAX: 775-684-4184
TTY:775-684-0360
detr.state.nv.us

Maureen Cole, Administrator
Melaine Mason, Deputy Administrator, Operations
Janice John, Deputy Administrator, Programs
Mechelle Merrill, Rehabilitation Chief II

Bureau of Vocational Rehabilitation is a state and federally funded program designed to help people with disabilities become employed and to help those already employed perform more successfully through training, counseling and other support methods.

3419 Nevada Community Enrichment Program (NCEP)
2550 University Avenue
Suite 330N
Saint Paul, MN 55114
651-645-7271
800-466-7722
FAX: 651-645-0541
TTY: 800-627-352
e-mail: info@accessiblespace.org
accessiblespace.org

Kay Knutson, Vice Chairman
Maynard Bostrom, Board Member
Patrick C. Horan, Board Member
Mary Lindgren, Board Member
Comprehensive neurological rehabilitation and life skills training.

3420 Nevada Developmental Disability Council
896 W. Nye Ln.
Suite 202
Carson City, NV 89703
775-687-8619
FAX: 775-684-8626
e-mail: smanning@dhhs.nv.gov
www.nevadaddcouncil.org

Lisa Antram, Chairman
Santa Perez, Vice Chairman
Sherry Manning, Executive Director
Kari Horn, Project Manager
The mission of the Nevada Developmental Disabilities Council is to provide resources at the community level which promote equal opportunity and life choices for people with disabilities through which they may positively contribute to Nevada society.

3421 Nevada Disability Advocacy and Law Center -Sparks/Reno Office
6039 Eldora Ave
#C-3
Las Vegas, NV 89146
702-257-8150
888-349-3843
FAX: 702-257-8170
e-mail: lasvegas@ndalc.org
www.ndalc.org

Reggie Bennettr, Secretary/Treasurer
Jana Spoor, President
John Miller, Vice President
Bob Bennett, Chairman
Nevada's protection and advocacy system for the human legal and service rights of individuals with disabilities. NDALC has offices in Reno/Sparks and Las Vegas, with services provided statewide.

3422 Nevada Division for Aging: Las Vegas
100 Liberty Way
Dover, NH 03820
888-398-8924
libertymutual.com
Michael J. Babcockrs, Director
Marian L. Heard, Director
Martn P. Slark, Director
Develops, coordinates and delivers a comprehensive support service system in order for Nevada' senior citizens to lead independent, meaningful and dignified lives.

3423 Nevada Division of Mental Health and Developmental Services
5865 Lakeshore Road
Buford, GA 30518
770-945-4441
FAX: 678-482-1965
e-mail: info@mhds.net
mhds.com

Keith Mixon, CEO/President
Offers treatment, prevention, education, habitation and rehabilitation for mental disorders. Works with advocacy groups, families, agencies and the community.

3424 Social Security: Carson City Disability Determination
1170 Harvard Way
Reno, NV 89502-2107
775-784-5221
800-772-1213
FAX: 775-784-5501
TTY: 800-325-0778
www.socialsecurity.gov

Karena L. Kilgore, Executive Secretary
Carolyn W. Colvin, Commissioner
Carolyn W. Colvin, Deputy Commissioner
James A. Kissko, Chief of Staff
Social Security offers online information and services to third parties who do business with them.

3425 State of Nevada Client Assistance Program
2450 Wrondel Way
Suite E
Reno, NV 89502-3767
775-688-1440
800-633-9879
800-633-9879
FAX: 775-688-1627
TTY:800-633-9879
e-mail: webauer@nvdetr.org
www.eelders.org

3426 Workers Compensation Board Nevada
6515 E Musser St
Carson City, NV 89714
775-684-7270
FAX: 775-687-6305

New Hampshire

3427 New Hampshire Workers Compensation Board
46 Donovan St
Concord, NH 03301-2624
603-225-2841
800-698-2364
FAX: 603-226-6903
www.nhprimex.org

Ty Gagne, CEO
Jonathan Kipp, Operations Manager
Julie Converse, Director of Finance
Carl Weber, Director of Member Services
Primex3 stands ready to provide our school, municipal, and county government members with the most comprehensive coverages and services available to New Hampshire local government.

3428 New Hampshire Assistive Technology Partnership Project
Department of Education
State of New Hampshire
Concord, NH 03824
603-862-2260
FAX: 603-228-2468
Jan Nisbet, Director
Mary Schuh, Associate Director
Eve Fralick, Associate Director
The goal of the New Hampshire Assistive Technology Partnership Project is to increase access to assistive technology through the creation and support of consumer driven systems for the provision of state-of-the-art assistive technology products and services for citizens with disabilities in the state of New Hampshire.

3429 New Hampshire Bureau of Developmental Services
Department of Health and Human Services
129 Pleasant St
Concord, NH 03301-3852
603-271-5034
FAX: 603-271-5166
e-mail: mertas@dhhs.state.nh.us
www.dhhs.nh.gov

Matthew Ertas, Director
Peggy Sue Greenwood, Administrative Assistant
Developmental Services promotes opportunities for normal life experiences for persons with developmental disabilities and aquired brain disorders in all areas of community life: employment, housing, recreation, social relationships and community association. Services and supports are organized throught a central state office and ten private nonprofit community area agen-

cies. Family support is provided to families of children with chronic health conditions or are developmentally disabled.

3430 New Hampshire Client Assistance Program
57 Regional Dr
Concord, NH 03301-8518 603-271-2773
800-852-3405
FAX: 603-271-2837
e-mail: Disability@nh.gov
www.state.nh.us/disability/caphomepage.html

Bill Hagy, Ombudsman
John Richards, Executive Director
Jillian Shedd, Accessibility Coordinator
Gayle Baird, Accountant

The Commission's goal is to remove the barriers, architectural, attitudinal or programmatic, that bar persons with disabilities from participating in the mainstream of society.

3431 New Hampshire Commission for Human Rights
2 Chenell Dr
Concord, NH 03301-8501 603-225-3431
800-735-2964
FAX: 603-224-3766
e-mail: webmaster@nh.gov
www.nh.gov

Peggy Mc Allister, Executive Director

Enforces New Hampshire law against discrimination in housing, employment or public accomodations. Disability discrimination is prohibited under New Hampshire law. Takes formal charges and investigates them.

3432 New Hampshire Department of Mental Health
State Office Park S
Concord, NH 03301 603-226-0111
FAX: 603-271-5058

Donald Shumway, Director
Paul Garmon
Tim Rourke, Religious Leader

3433 New Hampshire Developmental Disabilities Council
Suite 22
21 Fruit Street
Concord, NH 03301 603-271-3236
800-852-3345
800-852-3236
FAX: 603-271-1156
TTY:800-735-2964
nhddc.org

Sue Fox, Chairman
Peter Fleming, Co-Vice Chairman
Carol Stamatakis, Executive Director
David Ouellette, Project Director

Offers information, referral and support services to disabled persons. A federally funded state agency.

3434 New Hampshire Division of Elderly and Adult Services
Bureau of Elderly & Adult Services
129 Pleasant St
Concord, NH 03301-3852 603-271-4680
800-351-1888
FAX: 603-271-4643
e-mail: pio@dhhs.state.nh.us
www.dhhs.state.nh.us

Nicholas A. Toumpas, Comissioner
Mary Maggioncaida, Administrator
Marilee Nihan, Deputy Commissioner
Sheri Rockburn, Chief Financial Officer

The Bureau of Elderly and Adult Services provides a variety of social and long-term supports to adults age 60 and older and to adults between the ages of 18 and 60 who have a chronic illness or disability. These services range from home care, meals on wheels, care management, transportation assistance and assisted living to nursing home care.

3435 New Hampshire Governor's Commission on Disability
121 South FruitStreet
Suite 101
Concord, NH 03301-8518 603-271-2773
800-852-3405
FAX: 603-271-2837
e-mail: Disability@nh.gov
www.nh.gov/disability

Paul Van Blarigan, Chairman
Charles J. Saia, Executive Director
Michael Coe, Accessibility Coordinator
Carol Conforti-Adams, Information and Referral Special

The Commission's goal is to remove the barriers, architectural, attitudinal or programmatic, that bar persons with disabilities from participating in the mainstream of socie

3436 New Hampshire Protection & Advocacy for Persons with Disabilities
Disabilities Rights Center, Inc
64 North Main Street
Suite 2
Concord, NH 03301-4971 603-228-0432
800-834-1721
FAX: 603-225-2077
TTY: 800-834-1721
e-mail: advocacy@drcnh.org
drcnh.org

Paul Levy, President
Joanne Malloy, Vice President
Richard Cohen, Executive Director
Aaron Ginsberg, Staff Attorney

Legal services for individuals with disabilities; I & R.

3437 Social Security: Concord Disability Determination
Ste 100
70 Commercial St
Concord, NH 03301-5005 603-224-1939
800-772-1213
TTY:800-325-0778
www.ssa.gov

Karena L. Kilgore, Executive Secretary
Carolyn W. Colvin, Commissioner
Carolyn W. Colvin, Deputy Commissioner
James A. Kissko, Chief of Staff

Social Security offers online information and services to third parties who do business with them.

3438 Workers Compensation Board New Hampshire
PO Box 2076
Concord, NH 03302 603-271-3176
800-272-4353
FAX: 603-271-2668
e-mail: workerscomp@labor.state.nh.us
www.nh.gov/labor

Kathryn J. Barger, Director, Workers' Compensation
George N. Copadis, Commissioner of Labor
David M. Wihby, Deputy Commissioner

The Department of Labor monitors Employers, Workers Compensation, and Insurance Carriers to insure that they are in compliance with NH Labor laws. These laws range from minimum wage, overtime, safety issues and workers compensation.

New Jersey

3439 Division of Developmental Disabilities
210 South Broad Street
3rd Floor
Trenton, NJ 08608 609-292-9742
800-922-7233
FAX: 609-777-0187
TTY: 609-633-7106
e-mail: advocate@drnj.org
www.njpanda.org

James W Smith Jr, Executive Director

New Jersey's designated protection and advocacy system for poeple with disabilities and provides legal, nonlegal individual and systems advocacy.

3440 International Dyslexia Association: New Jersey Branch
P.O.Box 32
Long Valley, NJ 07853 908-879-1179
e-mail: njida@msn.com
www.interdys.org

Hal Malchow, President
Elsa Cardenas-Hagan, Ed.D.,, Vice President
Ben Shifrin, M.Ed., Vice President
Kristen Penczek, Interim Executive Director

The New Jersey Branch of The International Dyslexia Association is a 501(c)(3) non-profit, scientific and educational organization which was formed to increase public awareness of dyslexia in New Jersey. We have been serving individuals with dyslexia, their families, and professionals in the field in this community for more than 25 years.

3441 New Jersey Commission for the Blind and Visually Impaired
153 Halsey St, Fl 6
PO Box 47017
Newark, NJ 7101-4701 973-648-3333
877-685-8878
FAX: 973-693-5046
e-mail: Vito.DeSantis@dhs.state.nj.us
www.state.nj.us/humanservices/cbvi

Patricia Dunn, Manager
James W Smith, Jr, Acting Commissioner
Jose Morales, Manager

The mission of the New Jersey Commission for the Blind and Visually Impaired is to promote and provide services in the areas of education, employment, independence and eye health through informed choice and partnership with persons who are blind or visually impaired, their families and the community. Serves Bergen, Essex, Hudson, Morris, Passaic, Sussex and Warren Counties.

3442 New Jersey Department of Aging
210 South Broad Street
3rd Floor
Trenton, NJ 08608 609-292-9742
800-922-7233
FAX: 609-777-0187
TTY: 609-633-7106
e-mail: advocate@drnj.org
www.drnj.org

Walter Anthony Woodberry, Chairman
Andrew McGeady, Vice Chairman
Linda K. Soley, Treasurer
Leah Ziskin, Secretary

3443 New Jersey Department of Health/Special Child Health Services
New Jersey Department of Health and Senior Service
P.O.Box 360
Trenton, NJ 08625-0360 609-777-7778
FAX: 609-292-3580
e-mail: plisciotto@doh.state.nj.us
www.nj.gov/health/fhs/sch/

Jennifer Velez, ESQ, Commissioner

Provides services for New Jersey children that will prevent or reduce the effects of a developmental delay, chronic illness or behavioral disorder.

3444 New Jersey Division of Mental Health Services
Department Human Services
222 South Warren Street
P.O. Box 700
Trenton, NJ 8625- 700 609-292-3717
800-382-6717
FAX: 609-341-3333
www.state.nj.us/humanservices

Jennifer Velez, ESQ, Commissioner
Lynn A. Kovich, Assistant Commissioner

Oversees the public mental health system for the state of New Jersey. Operates six regional and specialty psychiatric hospitals, and contracts with over 125 not-for-profit agencies to provide a comprehensive system of community mental health services throughout all counties in the state.

3445 New Jersey Governor's Liaison to the Office of Disability Employment Policy
1 John Fitch Plaza
P. O.Box 110
Trenton, NJ 08625-110 609-659-9045
FAX: 609-633-9271
e-mail: Constituent.Relations@dol.state.nj.us
lwd.state.nj.us/labor

Harold J. Wriths, Commissioner
Frederick J. Zavaglia, Chief of Staff
Aaron R. Fichtner, Ph.D., Deputy Commissioner
Brian T. Murray, Director of Communications & Mar

The Division of Vocational Rehabilitation Services provides vocational rehabilitation services to prepare and place in employment eligilbe individuals with disabilities who, because of their disabling conditions, would otherwise be unable to secure and/or mantain employment

3446 New Jersey Protection & Advocacy for Persons with Disabilities
210 South Broad Street
3rd Floor
Trenton, NJ 08608 609-292-9742
800-922-7233
FAX: 609-777-0187
TTY: 609-633-7106
e-mail: advocate@drnj.org
www.drnj.org

Walter Anthony Woodberry, Chairman
Andrew McGeady, Vice Chairman
Linda K. Soley, Treasurer
Leah Ziskin, Secretary

3447 Regional ADA Technical Assistance Center
United Cerebral Palsy Associations of New Jersey
201 Dolgen Hall
Ithaca, NY 14853 607-255-6686
800-949-4232
FAX: 607-255-2763
e-mail: northeastada@cornell.edu
www.northeastada.org

LaWanda H. Cook, Ph.D., Extension Associate/Training Spe
Hannah Rudstam, Ph.D., Director of Training
Erin Sember-Chase, Project Coordinator and Technic
Luz Semeah, Technical Assistance

3448 Social Security Administration
1100 West High Rise
6401 Security Blvd.
Baltimore, MD 21235 800-772-1213
TTY:800-325-0778
www.ssa.gov

Karena L. Kilgore, Executive Secretary
Carolyn W. Colvin, Commissioner
Carolyn W. Colvin, Deputy Commissioner
James A. Kissko, Chief of Staff

Social Security disability is a social insurance program that workers and employers pay for with their Social Security taxes. Eligibility is based on your work history, and the amount of your benefit is based on your earnings. Social Security also has a disability program for people with limited income and resources- the Supplemental Security Income (SSI) program. For more information on these federal programs, please call our nationwide toll-free number.

New Mexico

3449 New Mexico Aging and Long-Term Services Department
2550 Cerrillos Rd
Santa Fe, NM 87505-3260
505-476-4799
866-451-2901
FAX: 505-476-4836
www.nmaging.state.nm.us

Miles Copeland, Deputy Secretary
Retta Ward, Secretary
Jason Sanchez, Administrative Services Division
Greg Rockstroh, IT Manager

Information and services for seniors, people with disabilities and their families.

3450 New Mexico Client Assistance Program
1720 Louisiana Blvd NE
Site 204
Albuquerque, NM 87110- 7070
505-256-3100
800-432-4682
FAX: 505-256-3184
e-mail: info@drnm.org
www.drnm.org

Brenda Crocker, Chairperson
Cyndy Costanza, Vice Chairperson
Adam Carrasco, President
Deanna DeVore, Vice President

The mission of Disability Rights New Mexico (DRNM) is to protect, promote and expand the legal and civil rights of persons with disabilities. DRNM is an independent, private nonprofit agency operating federally mandated and other advocacy programs in pursuit of this mission.

3451 New Mexico Commission for the Blind
2905 Rodeo Park Dr E
Bldg 4, Suite 100
Santa Fe, NM 87505-6342
505-476-4479
888-513-7968
FAX: 505-476-4475
e-mail: greg.trapp@state.nm.us
www.cfb.state.nm.us/

Arthur A. Schreiber, Chairman
Jim Babb, Commissioner
Dallas Allen, Commissioner
Greg Trapp, Executive Director

Offers services for the totally blind, legally blind, visually impaired, mentally retarded blind and more with health, counseling, educational, recreational, rehabilitation, computer training and professional training services.

3452 New Mexico Department of Health: Children's Medical Services
1190 S Saint Francis Dr
Santa Fe, NM 87505-4173
505-827-2613
877-890-4692
FAX: 505-827-2530
e-mail: lchristiansen@doh.state.nm
nmhealth.org/phd/cms.shtml

Gloria Bonner, Program Manager
Susan Baum, Medical Director
Freida Adams, Nurse Coordinator
Kim Love, Operations Manager

Title V MCH Program for children with special health care needs from birth to age 21 years. Services provided include: diagnosis, medical intervention, clinics and service coordination.

3453 New Mexico Governor's Committee on Concerns of the Handicapped
491 Old Santa Fe Trl
Santa Fe, NM 87501-2753
505-476-0412
877-696-1470
FAX: 505-827-6328
e-mail: gcd@state.nm.us
www.gcd.state.nm.us/

James Hay, Chair
Susan Gray, Vice Chair
Jim Parker, Director
Karen Courtney-Peterson, Chief Financial Officer

3454 New Mexico Protection & Advocacy for Persons with Disabilities
1720 Louisiana Blvd NE
Site 204
Albuquerque, NM 87110- 7070
505-256-3100
800-432-4682
FAX: 505-256-3184
e-mail: info@drnm.org
www.drnm.org

Brenda Crocker, Chairperson
Cyndy Costanza, Vice Chairperson
Adam Carrasco, President
Deanna DeVore, Vice President

The mission of Disability Rights New Mexico (DRNM) is to protect, promote and expand the legal and civil rights of persons with disabilities. DRNM is an independent, private nonprofit agency operating federally mandated and other advocacy programs in pursuit of this mission.

3455 New Mexico Technology Assistance Program
435 Saint Michaels Dr
Ste D
Santa Fe, NM 87505-7679
505-827-8535
800-866-2253
FAX: 505-954-8608
TTY: 800-659-4915
e-mail: julie.martinez@state.nm.us
www.nmtap.com

Julie Martinez, Program Director

Examines and works to eliminate barriers to obtaining assistive technology in New Mexico. Has established a statewide program for coordinating assistive technology services; is designed to assist people with disabilities to locate, secure, and maintain assistive technology.

3456 New Mexico Workers Compensation Administration
2410CentreAvenue SE
P.O.Box 27198
Albuquerque, NM 87125-7198
505-841-6000
800-255-7965
FAX: 505-841-6009
www.workerscomp.state.nm.us/

Ned S. Fuller, Director
Robert E. Doucette, Executive Deputy Director
Darin A. Childers, General Counsel
Thomas E. Dow, Executive Deputy Director

Regulates workers' compensation in New Mexico.

3457 Social Security: Santa Fe Disability Determination
6401 Security Blvd.
Baltimore, MD 21235
800-772-1213
TTY:800-325-0778
www.socialsecurity.gov

Karena L. Kilgore, Executive Secretary
Carolyn W. Colvin, Commissioner
Carolyn W. Colvin, Deputy Commissioner
James A. Kissko, Chief of Staff

3458 Southwest Branch of the International Dyslexia Association
International Dyslexia Association
3915 Carlisle Blvd. NE
Albuquerque, NM 87107
505-255-8234
800-222-3123
FAX: 505-262-8547
e-mail: swida@southwestida.org
southwestida.com

Montine Gibbons, President
Cathleen Tomlinson, Vice President
Erin Brown, Recording Secretary
Mary Poirier Gilroy, Corresponding Secretary

Provides free information and referral services for diagnosis and tutoring for parents, educators, physicians, and individuals with dyslexia. The voice of our membership is heard in 48 countries. Membership includes yearly journal and quarterly newsletter. Call for conference dates.

3459 Workers Compensation Board New Mexico
2410CentreAvenue SE
P.O.Box 27198
Albuquerque, NM 87125-7198
505-841-6000
800-255-7965
FAX: 505-841-6009
www.workerscomp.state.nm.us/

Ned S. Fuller, Director
Robert E. Doucette, Executive Deputy Director
Darin A. Childers, General Counsel
Thomas E. Dow, Executive Deputy Director

Regulates workers' compensation in New Mexico.

New York

3460 Albany County Department for Aging and Albany Social Services
162 Washington Ave
Albany, NY 12210-2304
518-447-7177
FAX: 518-447-7188
e-mail: aging@albanycounty.com
albanycounty.com

George Brown, Commissioner
Judy L. Coyne, Commissioner
Kathleen M. Dalton, Ph.D., Commissioner

The Point of Entry access line provides information and assistance and comprehensive referrals, and or assessments for the elderly, adults and children with disabilities, their family, or service providers.

3461 International Dyslexia Association of NY: Buffalo Branch
2491 Emery Rd
South Wales, NY 14139-9408
716-687-2030
800-222-3123
e-mail: bufida@gow.org
www.interdys.org

Hal Malchow, President
Elsa Cardenas-Hagan, Vice President
Ben Shifrin, Vice President
Kristen Penczek, Interim Executive Director

3462 Jawonio
260 N Little Tor Road
New City, NY 10956-2627
845-708-2000
FAX: 845-634-7731
TTY:845-639-3521
www.jawonio.org

Jill A. Warner, Executive Director & CEO
Matthew Shelly, Chief Program Officer
Diana Hess, Chief Communications Officer
Joseph Bloss, Chief Financial Officer

A dedicated community resource providing services to more than 500 children and adults annually. Provide early intervention, day care and pre-school special ed to our children. Job training, day habilitation, recreation, medical and service coordination for adults.

3463 Jawonio Vocational Center
260 N Little Tor Rd
New City, NY 10956-2627
845-708-2000
FAX: 845-634-7731
TTY:845-639-3521
jawonio.org

Jill A. Warner, Executive Director & CEO
Matthew Shelly, Chief Program Officer
Diana Hess, Chief Communications Officer
Joseph Bloss, Chief Financial Officer

A dedicated community resource providing services to more than 500 children and adults annually. Provide early intervention, day care and pre-school special ed to our children. Job training, day habilitation, recreation, medical and service coordination for adults.

3464 NYS Commission on Quality of Care & Advocacy for Persons with Disabilities
401 State St
Schenectady, NY 12305-2300
518-388-2892
FAX: 518-388-2890
e-mail: marcelc@cqc.state.ny.us
www.cqcapd.state.ny.us

Andrew M. Cuomo, Governor
Roger Bearden, Chair
Bruce Blower, Member
Patricia Okoniewski, Member

3465 NYSARC
393 Delaware Ave
Delmar, NY 12054-3094
518-439-8311
800-724-2094
FAX: 518-439-1893
e-mail: info@nysarc.org
nysarc.org

John A. Schuppenhauer, President
Laura Kennedy, Senior Vice President
Patricia Campanella, Vice President
Marc N. Brandt, Executive Director

3466 National Alliance on Mental Illness of New York State
99 Pine Street
Suite 302
Albany, NY 12207-1336
518-462-2000
800-950-3228
FAX: 518-462-3811
e-mail: info@naminys.org
www.naminys.org

Sherry Grenz, President
Donald Capone, Executive Director
Sharon Clairmont, Finance & Business Office Dir.
Matthew Shapiro, Development/Events Coordinator

3467 New State Office of Mental Health Agency
Office of Mental Health
44 Holland Ave
Albany, NY 12229
518-474-4403
800-597-8481
FAX: 518-474-2149
www.omh.ny.gov

Mike Hogan, Commissioner

Promoting the mental health of all New Yorkers with a particular focus on providing hope and recovery for adults with serious mental illness and children with serious emotional disturbances.

3468 New York Client Assistance Program
855 Central Avenue
Suite 110
Albany, NY 12206
518-459-6422
FAX: 518-459-7847
TTY:518-459-6422
www.nls.org/caplist.htm

3469 New York Department of Handicapped Children
Department of Heath Education
Corning Tower
Empire State Plaza
Albany, NY 12237 518-456-0665
866-881-2809
FAX: 518-456-1126
e-mail: jcrucetti@albanycounty.com
www.health.ny.gov

Andrew M. Cuomo, Governor
Dr James B. Crucetti, MD, MPH, Commisioner
Howard Zucker, Acting Commissioner

3470 New York State Commission for the Blind
52 Washington St
Rensselaer, NY 12144-2796 518-473-1774
866-871-3000
FAX: 518-486-7550
www.ocfs.state.ny.us

Madeline Raciti, Manager
Offers services for the totally blind, legally blind, visually impaired, mentally retarded blind and more with health, counseling, educational, recreational, rehabilitation, computer training and professional training services.

3471 New York State Commission on Quality of Care
401 State St
Schenectady, NY 12305-2300 518-388-2892
FAX: 518-388-2890
e-mail: marcelc@cqc.state.ny.us
www.cqc.state.ny.us

Andrew M. Cuomo, Governor
Roger Bearden, Chair
Bruce Blower, Member
Patricia Okoniewski, Member

3472 New York State Congress of Parents and Teachers
1 Wembley Ct
Albany, NY 12205-6258 518-452-8808
877-569-7782
FAX:518-452-8105
e-mail: pta.office@nyspta.org
nyspta.org

Lana Ajemain, President
Janet Meyerson, First Vice President
Bonnie Russell, Vice President
Penny Hollister, Vice President
Parent Teacher Association and PTA are registered service marks of the National Congress of Parents and Teachers (National PTA). Only those groups chartered by the New York State PTA are entitled to use the name PTA. Any other use constitutes trademark infringement.

3473 New York State Office of Advocates for Persons with Disabilities
Ste 1001
1 Empire State Plz
Albany, NY 12223-1100 518-449-7860
800-522-4369
FAX: 518-473-6005
e-mail: oapwdinfo@oapwd.org
www.oapwd.org

Gary O'Brien, Chair Commissioner
Provides information and referral services; administers NYS Tech Art Project; promotes implementation of disability-related laws.

3474 New York State Office of Mental Health
44 Holland Ave
Albany, NY 12229-1 518-474-4403
800-597-8481
FAX: 518-474-2149
www.omh.state.ny.gov in

Michael Hogan, Ph.D.
Promoting the mental health of all New Yorkers with a particular focus on providing hope and recovery for adults with serious mental illness and children with serious emotional disturbances.

3475 New York State TRAID Project
New York State Commisionon Qualityof Careand Advoc
Ste 1001
1 Empire State Plz
Albany, NY 12223-1100 518-449-7860
800-522-4369
FAX: 518-473-6005
www.oatwd.org

Cliff Sigfride, Manager

3476 Parent to Parent of New York State
500 Balltown Rd
Schenectady, NY 12304-2247 518-381-4350
800-305-8817
FAX: 518-393-9607
e-mail: mjuda@ptopnys.org
parenttoparentnys.org

Linda Coull, President
Louise Nitto, Vice President
Jim Costello, Secretary
Michele Juda, Executive Director
Parent to Parent of NYS, which began in 1994, is a statewide not for profit organization established to support and connect families of individuals with special needs. The 13 offices, located throughout NYS, are staffed by Regional Coordinators, who are parents or close relatives of individuals with special needs.

3477 Protection and Advocacy Agency of NY
401 State St
Schenectady, NY 12305-2303 518-388-2892
FAX: 518-388-2890
e-mail: marcelc@cqc.state.ny.us
www.cqc.state.ny.us

Andrew M. Cuomo, Governor
Roger Bearden, Chair
Bruce Blower, Member
Patricia Okoniewski, Member

3478 Regional Early Childhood Director Center
89 Washington Ave.
Room 580 EBA
Albany, NY 12234 518-474-2925
800-222-5627
e-mail: accesadm@mail.nysed.gov
www.acces.nysed.gov

3479 Schools And Services For Children With Autism Spectrum Disorders.
116 E 16th St
5th Floor
New York, NY 10003-2164 212-677-4650
FAX: 212-254-4070
e-mail: info@resourcesnyc.org
www.resourcesnyc.org

Ellen Miller-Wachtel, Chairman
Shon E. Glusky, President
Owen P. J. King, Treasurer
Rachel Howard, Executive Director
This publication fun resource for children provides extreme coverage of services for children with autism, asbergez syndrome, and/or PDD.

3480 Singeria/Metropolitan Parent Center
2082 Lexington Ave.
4th Floor
New York, NY 10035
212-643-2840
866-867-9665
FAX: 212-496-5608
e-mail: intake@sinergiany.org
sinergiany.org

Len Torres, President
Johnny C. Rivera, Vice President
Paola Jordan, Treasurer
Myrta Cuadra-Lash, Executive Director

3481 Social Security: Albany Disability Determination
1 Clinton Ave
Albany, NY 12207
518-431-4051
800-772-1213
TTY:518-431-4050
www.ssa.gov

Karena L. Kilgore, Executive Secretary
Carolyn W. Colvin, Commissioner
Carolyn W. Colvin, Deputy Commissioner
James A. Kissko, Chief of Staff

3482 State Agency for the Blind and Visually Impaired
52 Washington St
Rensselaer, NY 12144-2834
518-473-7793
866-871-3000
FAX: 518-486-7550
e-mail: info@ocfs.state.ny.us
www.ocfs.state.ny.us

3483 State Education Agency Rural Representative
89 Washington Avenue
Albany, NY 12234
518-474-3852
FAX: 518-473-2860
e-mail: RegentsOffice@mail.nysed.gov
www.nysed.gov

Merryl H. Tisch, Chancellor
Anthony S. Bottar, Vice Chancellor

3484 State Mental Health Representative for Children and Youth
44 Holland Ave
Albany, NY 12229
518-473-6328
e-mail: cocompz@omh.state.ny.us

David Woodlock, Deputy Commissioner

3485 State Mental Retardation Program
44 Holland Ave
Albany, NY 12229
518-474-6601
FAX: 518-473-1271
omr.state.ny.us

Diana Ritter, Manager

3486 United We Stand of New York
98 Moore St
Brooklyn, NY 11206-3326
718-302-4313
FAX: 718-302-4315
e-mail: uwsofny@aol.com
www.uwsony.org

Lourdes Rivera-Putz, Executive Director
Lourdes Figueroa, Intake/Receptionist
Carmen Soltero, Outreach/Trainer
Martha Vizcarrondo, Family Support Associate
Assists families with improving the quality of life for all individuals with disabilities.

3487 University Afiliated Program/Rose F Kennedy Center
1971
1300 Morris Park Avenue
Bronx, NY 10461
718-430-2000
e-mail: information@einstein.yu.edu
www.einstein.yu.edu

Maris D. Rosenberg, Interim Director
Christine M. Baric, Assistant Director
John J. Foxe, Director
Robert W. Marion, Director

3488 University of Rochester Medical Center
601 Elmwood Ave
Rochester, NY 14627
585-275-8762
FAX: 585-275-3366
e-mail: phil_davidson@urmc.rochester.edu
www.rochester.edu

Brad Berk, MD, PhD, CEO

3489 VESID
New York State Education Department
89 Washington Ave.
Room 580 EBA
Albany, NY 12234
800-222-5627
FAX: 518-474-8802
e-mail: accesadm@mail.nysed.gov
www.acces.nysed.gov/vr/

Dr Rebecca Cort, Deputy Commissioner
Vocational and educational services for individuals with disabilities.

3490 VSA Arts of New York City
2700 F Street, NW
Washington, DC 20566
202-467-4600
800-444-1324
FAX: 717-225-6305
e-mail: bbvsanyc@msn.com
www.vsarts.org

David M. Rubenstein, Chairman
Michael M. Kaiser, President
Christoph Eschenbach, Music Director
Provides art, educational and creative expression experiences to thousands of children, youth, and adults with disabilities who reside in the five boroughs of New York City. It provides opportunities for people with disabilities to demonstrate their accomplishments in the arts and foster increased understanding and acceptance.

3491 Westchester Institute for Human Development
Cedarwood Hall
Valhalla, NY 10595
914-493-8150
e-mail: info@WIHD.org
www.wihd.org

Susan Koehn Habermann, Chairman
William H. Bave, Vice Chairman
Ansley Bacon PhD, President/CEO
David O'Hara PhD, COO
WIHD advances policies and practices that foster the healthy development and ensure the safety of all children, strengthen families and communities, and promote health and well-being among people of all ages with disabilities and special health care needs.

3492 Workers Compensation Board New York
PO Box 5205
Binghamton, NY 13902-5205
518-462-8880
877-533-0337
FAX: 518-473-1415
e-mail: general_information@wcb.ny.gov
www.wcb.ny.gov

Andrew M. Cuomo, Governor
Robert E. Beloten, Chairman
Richard A. Bell, Commissioner

North Carolina

3493 Developmental Disability Services Section
Building 325n
Albemarle
Raleigh, NC 27699
919-420-7901
FAX: 919-420-7917
www.dhhs.state.nc.us/mhddsas/

Diana Simmons, Human Resources Manager
Ureh N. Lekwauwa, Chief, Clinical Policy
Courtney Cantrell, Acting Director
Jim Jarrard, Deputy Director

Makes policies and monitors public services and supports to people with mental illness, developmental disabilities and substance abuse throughout North Carolina.

3494 International Dyslexia Association: North Carolina Branch
40 York Rd.
4th Floor
Baltimore, MD 21204
410-296-0232
FAX: 410-321-5069
www.interdys.org

Hal Malchow, President
Elsa Cardenas-Hagan, Vice President
Ben Shifrin, Vice President
Kristen Penczek, Interim Executive Director

The North Carolina Branch of The International Dyslexia Association (NCIDA) is a 501 (c)(3) non-profit, scientific and organization dedicated to educating the public about the learning disability, dyslexia. The North Carolina Branch has four objectives: to increase awareness in the dyslexic and general community; to network with other learning disability groups and legislators in education;to increase membership and provide services that will strengthen members presence in their communities

3495 North Carolina Workers Compensation Board
4340 Mail Service Center
Raleigh, NC 27699-4340
919-807-2501
800-688-8349
FAX: 919-508-8210
e-mail: infospec@ic.nc.gov
www.ic.nc.gov

Julian Bunn, Owner

3496 North Carolina Assistive Technology Project
1110 Navaho Dr
Suite 101
Raleigh, NC 27609-7322
919-872-2298
FAX: 919-850-2792
e-mail: ncatp@minespring.com
ncatp.org

Ricki Cook, Project Director
Annette Lauber, Funding Specialist
Jacquelyne Gordon, Consumer Resource Specialist
Tony Hiatt, Executive Director

The North Carolina Assistive Technology Project exists to create a statewide, consumer-responsive system of assistive technology services for all North Carolinians with disabilities. The project's activities impact children and adults with disabilities across all aspects of their lives.

3497 North Carolina Children & Youth Branch
North Carolina Publc of Health
1928 Mail Service Ctr
Raleigh, NC 27699-1900
919-839-6262
FAX: 919-733-8034
e-mail: cathy.kluttz@nemail.net
www.nchealthychildren.com

Lawrence J Wheeler, Manager
Cathy Kluttz, Unit Manager Special Service
Dianne Tyson, Help Line Manager
Ran Coble, Executive Director

3498 North Carolina Client Assistance Program
2806 Mail Service Ctr
Raleigh, NC 27699-2800
919-855-3600
800-215-7227
FAX: 919-715-2456
e-mail: nccap@dhhs.nc.gov
cap.state.nc.us

Kathy Brack, Director
Diane Rawdarowicz, Client Advocate
Sharon Wisner, Client Advocate

A federally funded program designed to assist individuals with disabilities in understanding and using rehabilitation services. CAP serves as an integral part of the rehabilitation system by advising and informing individuals of all services and benefits available to them through programs authorized under both the Rehabilitation Act and Title 1 of the Americans with Disabilities Act.

3499 North Carolina Developmental Disabilities
Ste Gl103
1001 Navaho Dr
Raleigh, NC 27609-7368
919-821-2777
800-357-6916
FAX: 919-821-4778
e-mail: Holly.Riddle@ncmail.net
www.nc-ddc.org

Caroline Valand, Executive Director

A planning council established to assure that individuals with developmental disabilities and their families participate in the planning of and have access to culturally competent services, supports, and other assistance and opportunities that promote independence, productivity, and integration and inclusion into the community; and to promote, through systemic change, capacity building and advocacy activities, a consumer and family-centered comprehensive system.

3500 North Carolina Division of Aging
2101 Mail Service Ctr
Raleigh, NC 27699-2001
919-855-4800
FAX: 919-733-0443
ncdhhs.gov

Dennis Streets, Manager
Jim Slate, Director
Laketha Miller, Controller
Emery Edwards Milliken, General Counsel

3501 North Carolina Industrial Commission
4340 Mail Service Center
Raleigh, NC 27699-4340
919-807-2501
800-688-8349
FAX: 919-508-8210
e-mail: infospec@ic.nc.gov
www.ic.nc.gov

J Howard Bunn Jr, Chairman
Peg Dorer, Executive Director

3502 Social Security Administration
4701 Old Wake Forest Rd
Raleigh, NC 27609-4919
877-803-6311
800-772-1213
800-325-0778
FAX: 919-790-2860
TTY:919-790-2773
e-mail: www.socialsecurity.gov
www.socialsecurity.gov

Karena L. Kilgore, Executive Secretary
Carolyn W. Colvin, Commissioner
Carolyn W. Colvin, Deputy Commissioner
James A. Kissko, Chief of Staff

Provides information on how to obtain social security through a disability.

North Dakota

3503 Division of Mental Health and Substance Abuse
600 EastBoulevardAvenue
Dept 325
Bismarck, ND 58505- 0250
701-328-2310
800-472-2622
FAX: 701-328-2359
e-mail: dhseo@nd.gov
www.nd.gov/humanservices

Dennis Goetz, Executive Diretor
Kerry Wicks, Executive Diretor
Andrew J. McLean, Medical Director
Alex Schweitzer, Superitendent

The Department of Human Services' Mental Health and Substance Abuse Services Division provides leadership for the planning, development, and oversight of a system of care for children, adults, and families with severe emotional disorders, mental illness, and/or substance abuse issues.

3504 North Dakota Workers Compensation Board
50 E Front Ave
Bismarck, ND 58504
701-328-3800
800-777-5033
FAX: 701-329-9911
TTY: 701-328-3786
www.ndworkerscomp.com

Brent Edison, Director

3505 North Dakota Client Assistance Program
400 East Broadway
Suite 409
Bismarck, ND 58501-4071
701-328-2950
800-472-2670
FAX: 701-328-3934
e-mail: panda@nd.gov
www.ndpanda.org/cap

Dennis Lyon, CEO
Janelle Olson, Advocate
Paula Rustad, Office Assistant
Angie Dubovoy, Advocate

CAP assists clients and client applicants of North Dakota Vocational Rehabilitation services, Tribal Vocational Rehabilitation, or Independent Living services.

3506 North Dakota Department of Human Resources
1237 W Divide Ave
Suite 6
Bismarck, ND 58501-1208
701-328-5300
800-451-8693
FAX: 701-328-5320
e-mail: dhsaging@nd.gov
www.nd.gov

Shane Goettle, Manager

3507 North Dakota Department of Human Services
600 E Boulevard Ave
Dept 325
Bismarck, ND 58505-0250
701-328-2310
800-472-2622
FAX: 701-328-2359
e-mail: dhseo@nd.gov
www.nd.gov/dhs

Carol K Olson, Executive Director
Dennis Goetz, Executive Diretor
Kerry Wicks, Executive Diretor
Andrew J. McLean, Medical Director

Provides services that help vulnerable North Dakotans of all ages to maintain or enhance their quality of life, which may be threatened by lack of financial resources, emotional crises, disabling conditions, or an inability to protect themselves.

3508 Protection & Advocacy Project
1984
400 East Broadway
Suite 409
Bismarck, ND 58501-4071
701-328-2950
800-472-2670
FAX: 701-328-3934
e-mail: panda@nd.gov
ndpanda.org

Teresa Larsen, Executive Director
Janelle Olson, Advocate
Paula Rustad, Office Assistant
Angie Dubovoy, Advocate

The Protection and Advocacy is a state agency whose purpose is to advocate for and protect the rights of people with disabilities. The Protection and Advocacy Project has programs to serve people with developmental disabilities, mental illnesses and other types of disabilities. The projects programs and services are free to eligible individuals.

3509 Social Security: Bismarck Disability Determination
1680 E Capitol Ave
Bismarck, ND 58501-5603
701-250-4200
800-772-1213
TTY:701-250-4620
ssa.gov

Karena L. Kilgore, Executive Secretary
Carolyn W. Colvin, Commissioner
Carolyn W. Colvin, Deputy Commissioner
James A. Kissko, Chief of Staff

3510 Workers Compensation Board North Dakota
4007 State St
Bismarck, ND 58503-689
701-328-3800
FAX: 701-328-3820

Sandy Blunt, CEO

Ohio

3511 Epilepsy Council of Greater Cincinnati
Ste 550
895 Central Ave
Cincinnati, OH 45202-5700
513-721-2905
877-804-2241
FAX: 513-721-0799
e-mail: ecgc@fuse.net
ecgc-ohnky.net

Kathy Stewart, Executive Director

3512 International Dyslexia Association: Central Ohio Branch
40 York Rd.
4th Floor
Baltimore, MD 21204
410-296-0232
FAX: 410-321-5069
e-mail: cybdischultz@columbus.rr.com
www.interdys.org

Hal Malchow, President
Elsa Cardenas-Hagan, Vice President
Ben Shifrin, Vice President
Lee Grossman, Executive Director

Provides free information and referral services for diagnosis and tutoring for parents, educators, physicians, and individuals with dyslexia. The voice of our membership is heard in 48 countries. Membership includes yearly journal and quarterly newsletter. Call for conference dates. Other locations available in Ohio state.

3513 Ohio Bureau for Children with Medical Handicaps
Ohio Department of Health
246 N. High St
P.O.Box 1603
Columbus, OH 43215-1603
614-466-3543
800-755-4769
FAX: 614-728-3616
e-mail: bcmh@odh.ohio.gov
www.odh.ohio.gov

John R. Kasich, Governor
James Bryant Md, Bureau Chief
Alvin Jackson, MD, Director
Lance D. Himes, Interim Director

Provides funding for the diagnosis, treatment and coordination of services for eligible Ohio children, under age 21, with medical handicaps; conducts quality assurance activities to establish standards of care and determine unmet needs of children with handicaps and their families; collaborates with public health nurses to increase access to care; and assists families to access and use third party resources. Conducts a separate program for adults with cystic fibrosis.

3514 Ohio Bureau of Worker's Compensation
30 W Spring St
Columbus, OH 43215-2256
800-335-0996
FAX: 877-321-9481
TTY:800-292-4833
e-mail: ombudsperson@bwc.state.oh.us
ohiobwc.com

Stephen Buehrer, Administrator/CEO
Dale Hamilton, Chief Operating Officer (COO)
Kevin Abrams, Chief of Employers Services
Toni Brokaw, Chief of Human Resources

To provide a quality, customer-focused workers' compensation insurance system for Ohio's employers and employees.

3515 Ohio Client Assistance Program
50 W. Broad St.
Suite 1400
Columbus, OH 43215-5923
614-466-7264
800-282-9181
FAX: 614-752-4197
TTY: 614-728-2553
www.olrs.ohio.gov

Donald Bishop, Executive Director

3516 Ohio Department of Aging
1982
50 W Broad St
Fl 9
Columbus, OH 43215-3363
614-466-5500
866-243-5678
888-243-5678
FAX: 614-466-5741
TTY:614-466-6191
www.aging.ohio.gov

Bonnie Kantor-Burman, Director
John Ratliff, Public Information Officer

The department serves and represents about 2 million Ohioans age 60 & older. They advocate for the needs of all older citizens with emphasis on improving the quality of life, helping senior citizens live active, healthy, & independent lives, & promoting positive attitudes toward aging & older people. Committed to helping the frail elderly who choose to remain at home by providing home & community based services, their goal is to promote the level of choice, independence & self-care.

3517 Ohio Department of Mental Health
30 E Broad St
8th Floor
Columbus, OH 43215-3414
614-466-4775
877-275-6364
FAX: 614-752-8410
e-mail: uhricks@mh.state.oh.us
mh.state.oh.us

Michael Hogan, Director
Christine Vincenty, Manager

3518 Ohio Developmental Disabilities Council
899 E Broad St, Ste 203
Columbus, OH 43205
614-466-5205
800-766-7426
FAX: 614-466-0298
e-mail: carla.sykes@dmr.state.oh.us
www.ddc.ohio.gov

Carolyn Knight, Executive Director

The Ohio Developmental Disabilities Council is one of 55 councils found in all states and territories which provides funding for systems change grant projects. The DD Council is a planning and advocacy agency that seeks to improve the lives of Ohioans with disabilities.

3519 Ohio Developmental Disability Council (ODDC)
899 E Broad St, Ste 203
Columbus, OH 43205
614-466-5205
800-766-7426
FAX: 614-466-0298
www.ddc.ohio.gov

Carolyn Knight, Executive Director

3520 Ohio Governor's Council on People with Disabilities
400 E Campus View Blvd
Columbus, OH 43235-4685
614-438-1200
800-282-4536
e-mail: RSC.Webmaster@rsc.state.oh.us
gcpd.ohio.gov

Jacqueline Romer-Sensky, Chairman
Jack Licate, Vice Chairman
Kevin Miller, Executive Director
Bill Bishilany, Assistant Executive Director

The Governor's Council on People with Disabilities exists to: Advise the Governor and General Assembly on statewide disability issues, promote the value of diversity, dignity and the quality of life for people with disabilities, be a catalyst to create systemic change promoting awareness of disability-related issues that will ultimately benefit all citizens of Ohio, Educate and advocate for: partnerships at the local, state and national level, promotion of equality, access and independence.

3521 Ohio Rehabilitation Services Commission
400 E Campus View Blvd
Columbus, OH 43235-4604
614-438-1200
800-282-4536
e-mail: RSC.Webmaster@rsc.state.oh.us
ohio.gov

Kevin Miller, Executive Director

RSC is Ohio's state agency that provides vocational rehabilitation (VR) services to help people with disabilities become employed and independent. We also offer a variety of services to Ohio businesses, resulting in quality jobs for individuals who have disabilities.

3522 Ohio Women, Infants, & Children ProgramOhio Department of Health
246 N High St
Columbus, OH 43215-2406
614-644-8006
FAX: 614-564-2470
odh.ohio.gov

Michele Frizzell, Chief, Bureau of Nutrition Svcs.

3523 Social Security: Columbus Disability Determination
90 E Washington Bridge Rd
Suite 140
Worthington, OH 43085
614-888-5339
800-772-1213
TTY:614-288-0226
www.socialsecurity.gov

Karena L. Kilgore, Executive Secretary
Carolyn W. Colvin, Commissioner
Carolyn W. Colvin, Deputy Commissioner
James A. Kissko, Chief of Staff

Oklahoma

3524 **Oklahoma Workers Compensation Board**
Department of Labor
3017 N. Stiles, Suite 100
Oklahoma City, OK 73105 405-521-6100
888-269-5353
FAX: 405-521-6018
www.ok.gov/odol

Jim Marshall, Chief of Staff
Mark Costello, Commissioner of Labor
Lizzette McNeill, Communications Director
Stacy Bonner, Deputy Commissioner

3525 **Oklahoma Client Assistance Program/Office of Disability Concerns**
2401 NW 23rd Street
Suite 90
Oklahoma City, OK 73107- 2431 405-521-3756
800-522-8224
FAX: 405-522-6695
www.ok.gov

Todd Lamb, Governor
Gary Jones, Auditor and Inspector
E. Scott Pruitt, Attorney General
Ken Miller, Treasurer
CAP informs and advises applicants and consumers about the vocational rehabilitation process and services available under the Federal Rehabilitation Act, including services provided by DVR and DVS. CAP staff can help you communicate concerns to the DVR/DVS and assist you with administrative, mediation, fair hearing, legal and other solutions

3526 **Oklahoma Department of Human Services Aging Services Division**
25 Sigourney Street, 10th Floor
Hartford, CT 06106 405-521-3646
866-218-6621
800-522-7233
FAX: 860-424-5301
okdhs.org

Margaret Ger Murkette, MSW, Director
Ed Lake, Director

3527 **Oklahoma Department of Labor**
3017 N. Stiles
Suite 100
Oklahoma City, OK 73105-5206 405-521-6100
888-269-5353
FAX: 405-521-6018
www.labor.ok.gov

Mark Castello, Commissioner
Jim Marshall, Chief of Staff
Stacy Bonner, Deputy Commissioner
Don Schooler, General Counsel

3528 **Oklahoma Department of Mental Health & Substance Abuse Services**
1200 NE 13thStreet
P.O.Box 53277
Oklahoma City, OK 73152-3277 405-522-3908
800-522-9054
FAX: 405-522-3650
TTY: 405-522-3851
www.odmhsas.org

J. Andy Sullivan, Chairperson
Gail Henderson, Vice-Chair
Terri White, Comissioner
Durand Crosby, Chief Operating Officer
State agency providing mental helath, substance abuse and domestic violence services.

3529 **Oklahoma Department of Rehabilitation Services**
3535 NW 58th St
Suite 500
Oklahoma City, OK 73112-4824 405-951-3400
800-845-8476
FAX: 405-951-3529
TTY: 405-951-3400
e-mail: jharlan@okdrs.gov
www.okdrs.gov

Michael O'Brien, Director
Jody Harlan, Public Information Administrator
David Ligon, Chief Of Staff
The Oklahoma Department of Rehabilitation Services (DRS) provides assistance to Oklahomans with disabilities through vocational rehabilitation, employment, independent living, residential and outreach programs, and the determination of medical eligibility for disability benefits.

3530 **Workers Compensation Board Oklahoma**
1915 N Stiles Ave
Oklahoma City, OK 73105-4918 405-522-8600
800-522-8210
owcc.state.ok.us

Leroy E Young, D.O., Chairman
Joyce Sanders, Supervisor
Michael J. Harkey, Vice Presiding Judge
Katrina Stephenson, Assistant Court Clerk

Oregon

3531 **International Dyslexia Association: Oregon Branch**
International Dyslexia Association
PO Box 2609
Portland, OR 97208-2609 503-228-4455
800-530-2234
FAX: 410-321-5609
e-mail: info@orbida.org
www.orbida.org

Karen Brown, President
Provides free information and referral services for diagnosis and tutoring for parents, educators, physicians, and individuals with dyslexia. The voice of our membership is heard in 48 countries. Membership includes yearly journal and quarterly newsletter. Call for conference dates.

3532 **Office of Vocational Rehabilitation Services (OVRS)**
500 Summer St NE
Salem, OR 97301-1063 503-945-5944
FAX: 503-378-2897
TTY:503-945-6214
www.oregon.gov/dhs/index.shtml

Erinn Kelley-Siel, Director
Gene Evans, Communication Director
Eric Moore, Chief Financial Officer
Jim Scherzinger, Chief Operating Officer
The mission of OVRS to assist Oregonians with disabilities to achieve and maintain employment and independence.

3533 **Oregon Advocacy Center**
620 SW 5th Ave
5th Floor
Portland, OR 97204-1428 503-243-2081
800-452-6094
FAX: 503-243-1738
TTY: 800-556-5351
e-mail: welcome@oradvocacy.org
oradvocacy.org

Robert Joondeph, Executive Director
Barbara Herget, Operations Director
The protection and advocacy system for Oregon.

3534 **Oregon Client Assistance Program**
620 SW 5th Ave
5th Floor
Portland, OR 97204-1420
503-243-2081
FAX: 503-243-1738
TTY:800-556-5351
e-mail: welcome@oradvocacy.org
oradvocacy.org

Robert Joondeph, Executive Director

3535 **Oregon Commission for the Blind**
535 SE 12th Ave
Portland, OR 97214-2408
971-673-1588
888-202-5463
FAX: 503-234-7468
TTY: 971-673-1577
e-mail: ocb.mail@state.or.us
www.oregon.gov/blind

Jodi C. Roth, Chairman
Dacia Johnson, Executive Director
Angel Hale, Director of Rehabilitation Services
Richard Turner, Director

3536 **Oregon Department of Mental Health**
500 Summer St NE
Salem, OR 97301-1063
503-945-5944
FAX: 503-378-2897
TTY:503-945-6214
www.oregon.gov/DHS

Erinn Kelley-Siel, Director
Gene Evans, Communication Director
Eric Moore, Chief Financial Officer
Jim Scherzinger, Chief Operating Officer
Sets out the purpose and guides the activities of our large, complex organization. Vision is for better outcomes for clients and communities through collaboration, integration and shared responsibility.

3537 **Oregon Technology Access for Life**
2225LancasterDrive NE
Salem, OR 97305-1396
503-361-1201
800-677-7512
FAX: 503-370-4530
TTY: 503-361-1201
e-mail: info@accesstechnologiesinnc.com
www.accesstechnologiesinc.org

Laurie Brooks, President
A statewide program promoting assistive technology devices and services for persons of all ages with all disabilities.

3538 **Social Security: Salem Disability Determination**
90 E Washington Bridge Rd
Suite 140
Worthington, OH 43085-3772
614-888-5339
800-722-1213
TTY:614-288-0226
www.socialsecurity.gov

Karena L. Kilgore, Executive Secretary
Carolyn W. Colvin, Commissioner
Carolyn W. Colvin, Deputy Commissioner
James A. Kissko, Chief of Staff

3539 **Washington County Disability, Aging and Veteran Services**
Ste 208
180 E Main St
Hillsboro, OR 97123-4054
503-640-3489
FAX: 503-693-6124
www.co.washington.or.us/aging

Jeff Hill, Director
Janet Long, Support Staff
Provides services to individuals through the Older Americans Act, state in home care services and represent, veterans in benefit claims process with Federal VA.

Pennsylvania

3540 **International Dyslexia Association: Pennsylvania Branch**
1062 E. Lancaster Avenue, 15A
Rosemont, PA 19010-251
610-527-1548
FAX: 610-527-5011
e-mail: dyslexia@pbida.org
www.pbida.org

Eugenie Flaherty PhD, President
Tracy Bowes, Office Manager
Provides free information and referral services for diagnosis and tutoring for parents, educators, physicians, and individuals with dyslexia. The voice of membership is heard in 48 countries. Membership includes yearly journal and quarterly newsletter, and Pennsylvania newsletter; discounts to conferences and events.

3541 **Mental Health Association in Pennysylvania**
1414 N Cameron St
1st Floor
Harrisburg, PA 17103-1049
717-346-0549
866-578-3659
FAX: 717-236-0192
e-mail: mfo@mhapa.org
www.mhapa.org

Jack Boyle, President
Sue Waither, Executive Director
Madelyn Roman-Scott, Youth Advocate
Carl Onufer, Treasurer

3542 **Pennsylvania Workers Compensation Board**
651 Boas Street
Room 1700
Harrisburg, PA 17121-2510
717-787-5279
FAX: 717-772-0342
dli.state.pa.us

Joseph Brimmeier, CEO

3543 **Pennsylvania Bureau of Blindness & VisualServices**
Department of Pennsylvania
1521 N 6th St
Harrisburg, PA 17102
717-787-3201
800-622-2842
FAX: 717-787-3210
www.dli.state.pa.us

David Denotaris, Director
Jennifer Cave, Clerk Typist 3
Offers services for the totally blind, legally blind, visually impaired, mentally retarded blind and more with health, counseling, educational, recreational, rehabilitation, computer training and professional training services.

3544 **Pennsylvania Client Assistance Program**
1515 Market Street
Suite 1300
Philadelphia, PA 19102- 1819
215-557-7112
888-745-2357
FAX: 215-557-7602
e-mail: info@equalemployment.org
www.equalemployment.org

Stephen S. Pennington, Executive Director
Jamie C Ray, Assistant Director
Margaret Passio-McKenna, Senior Advocate
Lee Lippi, Advocate
The Pennsylvania Client Assistance Program is dedicated to ensuring that the rehabilitation system in Pennsylvania is open and responsive to your needs. CAP help is provided to you at no charge, regardless of income. CAP helps people who are seeking services from the Office of Vocational Rehabilitation, Blindness and Visual Services, Centers for Independent Living and other programs funded under federal law.

3545 Pennsylvania Department of Aging
555 Walnut St
5th Floor
Harrisburg, PA 17101-1919
717-783-1550
FAX: 717-783-6842
e-mail: aging@pa.gov
www.aging.state.pa.us

Nora Eisenhower, Manager

3546 Pennsylvania Department of Children with Disabilities
P.O. Box 2675
Harrisburg, PA 17105-2675
717-787-2600
FAX: 717-772-0323
www.pachildren.state.pa.US

Tom Corbett, Governor
Shelly Yanoff, Commission Chair

3547 Pennsylvania Developmental Disabilities Council
569 Forum Building
Harrisburg, PA 17120
717-789-6057
877-685-4452
TTY:717-705-0819
www.paddc.org

Amy High, Vice Chairperson
Graham Mulholland, Executive Director
Sandra Amador Dusek, Deputy Director

3548 Pennsylvania Protection & Advocacy for Persons with Disabilities
1414 N Cameron St
2nd Floor
Harrisburg, PA 17103-1049
717-236-8110
800-692-7443
FAX: 717-236-0192
TTY: 877-375-7139
e-mail: ldo@drnpa.org
drnpa.org

Ken Oakes, Chairman
Nicole Turman, Vice Chairman
Peri Jude Radecic, CEO
Judy Banks, Deputy Director
Provide advocacy, information and referral for persons with disabilities and mental illness issues.

3549 Public Interest Law Center of Philadelphia
United Way Building, 2nd Floor
1709 Benjamin Franklin Parkway
Philadelphia, PA 19103-5153
215-627-7100
FAX: 215-627-3183
e-mail: general@pilcop.org
pilcop.org

Eric J. Rothschild, Chair
Brian T. Feeney, Vice Chair
Jennifer R. Clarke, Executive Director
Latrice Brooks, Director of Administration
A non-profit, public interest law firm with a Disabilities Project specializing in class action suits brought by individuals and organizations.

3550 Social Security: Harrisburg Disability Determination
Suite 160
90 E Washington Bridge Rd
Worthington, OH 17101-1925
614-888-5339
800-722-1213
TTY:614-288-0226
ssa.gov

Karena L. Kilgore, Executive Secretary
Carolyn W. Colvin, Commissioner
Carolyn W. Colvin, Deputy Commissioner
James A. Kissko, Chief of Staff

3551 Workers Compensation Board Pennsylvania
651 Boas Street
Room 1700
Harrisburg, PA 17121-2510
717-787-5279
FAX: 717-772-0342
www.dli.state.pa.us

Tom Corbett, Governor
Julia K. Hearthway, Secretary
Joseph Brimmeier, CEO

Rhode Island

3552 Department of Mental Health, Retardation and Hospitals of Rhode Island
Goverment of Rhode Isalnd
14 Harrington Rd
Cranston, RI 02920-3080
401-462-2339
FAX: 401-462-3204
e-mail: Craig.Stenning@bhddh.ri.gov
www.bhddh.ri.gov/

Craig S. Stenning, Director
Ellen Nelson, Manager
Kathleen Spangler, Manager
State department responsible for creating and administering systems of care for individuals with disabilities, specifically focused on mental health and mental illness; developmental disabilities, substance abuse and long term hospital care.

3553 Rhode Island Department Health
3 Capitol Hl
Providence, RI 02908-5097
401-222-3855
FAX: 401-222-6548
e-mail: library@doh.state.ri.us
gotasthma.com

Mary Salerno, Manager
Patricia Nolan, Executive Director
Pamela Corcoran, Disability Health Program

3554 Rhode Island Department of Elderly Affairs
74 West Road
Hazard Bldg, 2nd Floor
Cranston, RI 02920- 3001
401-462-3000
FAX: 401-462-0503
e-mail: larry@dea.state.ri.us
www.dea.state.ri.us

Corrine Russo, Manager

3555 Rhode Island Department of Mental Health
Cottage 405 Court B
Cranston, RI 02920
401-462-2003
FAX: 401-462-2008
www.butler.org

George W. Shuster, Chairman
Dennis D. Keefe, President & CEO
Reed Cosper, Manager

3556 Rhode Island Developmental Disabilities Council
400 Bald Hill Rd
Suite 515
Warwick, RI 02886-1692
401-737-1238
FAX: 401-737-3395
TTY:401-737-1238
e-mail: riddc@riddc.org
www.riddc.org

Charles Zawacki, Chairperson, Individual & Family
John Susa, Chairperson, Executive Committee
Anne Frank, Chairperson, Individual & Family
Mary Okero, Executive Director
The Rhode Island Developmental Disabilities Council works to make Rhode Island a better place for people with developmental disabilities to live, work, go to school, and be part of their community.

3557 Rhode Island Governor's Commission on Disabilities
John O Pastore Center
Warwick City Hall
3275 Post Road
Warwick, RI 02920- 3049
401-738-2000
FAX: 401-462-0106
e-mail: disabilities@gcd.state.ri.gov
www.warwickri.gov

Bob Cooper, Executive Secretary

The Commision is responsible for: coordinating compliance by state agencies with federal and state disablity right laws; approving or modifying state and local goverment agency's open meeting accessibility for persons with disabilities transition plans; assisting local boards of canvassers to ensure accessible polling places locations; aproving or rejecting requests to waive the state building code's standards for accessibility at facilities to be leased by state agencies...

3558 Rhode Island Parent Information Network
1210 Pontiac Avenue
Cranston, RI 02920
401-270-0101
800-464-3399
FAX: 401-270-7049
e-mail: info@ripin.org
ripin.org

Kathleen DiChiara, Chairman
Ammala Douangsavanh, Vice Chairman
Stephen Brunero, Executive Director
Matthew Cox, Associate Exeutive Director

A nonprofit organization established by parents and concerned professionals providing culturally appropriate information, training and support for families and professionals designed to improve educational and life outcomes for all children. Serving the State of Rhode Island.

3559 Rhode Island Protection & Advocacy for Persons with Disabilities
Rhode Island Disability Law Center
275 Westminster Street
Suite 401
Providence, RI 02903- 3434
401-831-3150
800-733-5332
FAX: 401-274-5568
TTY: 401-831-5335
e-mail: info@ridlc.org
www.ridlc.org

Raymond Bandusky, Executive Director

Rhode Island Disability Law Center (RIDLC) provides free legal assistance to persons with disabilities. Services include individual representation to protect rights or to secure benefits and services; self-help information; educational programs; and administrative and legislative advocacy. The agency administers eight federally funded advocacy programs, each of which has its own eligibility criteria.

3560 Rhode Island Services for the Blind and Visually Impaired
40 Fountain St
Providence, RI 02903-1830
401-421-7005
800-752-8088
FAX: 401-421-9259
TTY: 401-421-7016
e-mail: thompson@ors.state.ri.us
www.ors.ri.gov

John Microulis, Administrator
Kathleen Grygiel, Deputy Administrator
Ronald Racine, Acting Associate Director
Roberta Greene-Whittemore, Assistant Administrator of VR

Offers services for the totally blind, legally blind, visually impaired, mentally retarded blind and more with health, counseling, educational, recreational, rehabilitation, computer training and professional training services.

3561 Services for the Blind and Visually Impaired
40 Fountain St
Providence, RI 02903-1830
401-421-7005
FAX: 401-222-1328
TTY:401-421-7016
www.ors.ri.gov

John Microulis, Administrator
Kathleen Grygiel, Deputy Administrator
Ronald Racine, Acting Associate Director
Roberta Greene-Whittemore, Assistant Administrator of VR

Offers services for the blind and visually impaired.

3562 Social Security: Providence Disability Determination
Social Security
40 Fountain Street
6th Floor
Providence, RI 02903-3246
401-222-3182
800-772-1213
FAX: 401-222-3868
TTY: 401-273-6648
e-mail: Deborah.A.Cannon@ssa.gov
www.ssa.gov

Karena L. Kilgore, Executive Secretary
Carolyn W. Colvin, Commissioner
Carolyn W. Colvin, Deputy Commissioner
James A. Kissko, Chief of Staff

We deliver services through a nationwide network of over 1,400 offices that include regional offices, field offices, card centers, teleservice centers, processing centers, hearing offices, the Appeals Council, and our State and territorial partners, the Disability Determination Services. We also have a presence in U.S. embassies around the globe. For the public, we are the "face of the government." The rich diversity of our employees mirrors the public we serve.

3563 Workers Compensation Board Rhode Island
1 Dorrance Plz
Providence, RI 02903-3973
401-458-5000
FAX: 401-222-3121
courts.ri.gov

George E Healy Jr, Manager
George Healy Jr, Manager

South Carolina

3564 Protection & Advocacy for People with Disabilities
Ste 208
3710 Landmark Dr
Columbia, SC 29204-4034
803-782-0639
866-275-7273
FAX: 803-790-1946
TTY: 866-232-4525
e-mail: info@pandasc.org
protectionandadvocacy-sc.org

Gloria Prevost, Executive Director
Anne Trice, Director of Administration
J. Ashley Twombley, Chair
Sherry Williams, Vice-Chair

An independent, nonprofit organization responsible for safe guarding rights of South Carolinians with disabilities and other handicapped individuals without regard to age, income, severity of disability, sex, race, or religion.

3565 Social Security: West Columbia Disability Determination
P.O. Box 60
Columbia, SC 29171-0060
803-896-6400
800-772-1213
FAX: 803-822-4318
TTY: 800-325-0078
e-mail: Kenneth.Norris@ssa.gov
www.socialsecurity.gov

Karena L. Kilgore, Executive Secretary
Carolyn W. Colvin, Commissioner
Carolyn W. Colvin, Deputy Commissioner
James A. Kissko, Chief of Staff

We deliver services through a nationwide network of over 1,400 offices that include regional offices, field offices, card centers, teleservice centers, processing centers, hearing offices, the Appeals Council, and our State and territorial partners, the Disability Determination Services. We also have a presence in U.S. embassies around the globe. For the public, we are the "face of the government." The rich diversity of our employees mirrors the public we serve.

3566 South Carolina Assistive Technology Project
Midlands Center
8301 Farrow Road
Columbia, SC 29203
803-935-5263
800-915-4522
FAX: 803-935-5342
TTY: 803-935-5263
e-mail: jjendron@usit.net
www.sc.edu/scatp/

Carol Page, Ph.D, CCC-SLP, A, Program Director
Janet Jendron, Program Coordinator
Mary Alice Bechtler, Program Coordinator
Lydia Durham, Administrative Assistant

A statewide program promoting assistive technology devices and services for persons of all ages with all disabilities. Recently a statewide AT resource, demonstrations and equipment loan center and lab annual expo and training and workshops on a variety of disabilities and technology topics.

3567 South Carolina Client Assistance Program
Governor's Office oe Executive Policy & Programs
1205 Pendleton St
Columbia, SC 29201-3756
803-734-0285
800-868-0040
FAX: 803-734-0546
TTY: 803-734-1147
e-mail: cap@oepp.sc.gov
www.govoepp.state.sc.us/cap

Denise Riley Pensmith,MSW, Executive Director
Cindy Popenhagen, Administrative Assistant

The Client Assistance Program (CAP) helps citizens of the State by acting as advocates regarding services provided by the Vocational Rehabilitation Department (VR), Commission for the Blind, and all Independent Living programs and projects funded under the Rehabilitation Act of 1973. As advocates, CAP staff can investigate, negotiate, mediate, and pursue administrative, and other remedies to ensure that clients' rights are protected.

3568 South Carolina Commission for the Blind
1430 Confederate Avenue
P. O. Box 2467
Columbia, SC 29202-79
803-898-8731
800-922-2222
888-335-5951
FAX: 803-898-8800
e-mail: publicinfo@sccb.sc.gov
www.sccb.state.sc.us

James Kirby, Commissioner
Peter Smith, Board Member
Dr. Julianne Kleckley, Board Member
Dr. Julia Barnes, Board Member

Offers services for the totally blind, legally blind, visually impaired, mentally retarded blind and more with health, counseling, educational, recreational, rehabilitation, computer training and professional training services.

3569 South Carolina Department of Children with Disabilities
2600 Bull St
Columbia, SC 29201-1708
803-434-4260

Miroslav Cuturic, Director
Peter Getz, Administrator

3570 South Carolina Department of Mental Healthand Mental Retardation
Administration Building
2414 Bull Streets
Columbia, SC 29202-485
803-898-8581
800-273-8255
FAX: 864-297-5130
e-mail: webmaster@scdmh.org
www.state.sc.us/dmh

John H. Magill, State Director
Mark Binkley, Deputy Director
David Schaefer, Director
Eleanor Odom, Director

The S.C. Department of Mental Health gives priority to adults, children, and their families affected by serious mental illnesses and significant emotional disorders. We are committed to eliminating stigma and promoting the philosophy of recovery, to achieving our goals in collaboration with all stakeholders, and to assuring the highest quality of culturally competent services possible.

3571 South Carolina Developmental Disabilities Council
Office of the Governor
1205 Pendleton St
Suite 461
Columbia, SC 29201-3756
803-734-0465
FAX: 803-734-1409
TTY:803-734-1147
e-mail: jvancleave@oepp.sc.gov
www.scddc.state.sc.us

Valarie Bishop, Executive Director
Cheryl English, Program Information Coordinator
Kimberly Johnson Fontanez, Grants Administrator
Esther Williams, Administrative Support Specialis

The mission of the South Carolina Developmental Disabilities Council is to provide leadership in advocating, funding and implementing initiatives which recognize the inherent dignity of each individual, and promote independence, productivity, respect and inclusion for all persons with disabilities and their families.

3572 Workers Compensation Board: South Carolina
PO Box 1715
Columbia, SC 29202-1715
803-737-5700
FAX: 803-737-5768
www.state.sc.us/wcc

Gary Cannon, Executive Director
Kim Balleutine, Admin. Assistant

South Dakota

3573 Children's Special Health Services Program
600 E Capitol Ave
Pierre, SD 57501-2536
605-773-3361
800-738-2301
FAX: 605-773-5683
e-mail: DOH.info@state.sd.us
www.doh.sd.gov

Dianne Weyer, Manager
Barb Hemmelman, Program Manager

Health KiCC is a program, funded through federal and state monies, that provides financial assistance for medical appointments, procedures, treatments, medications and travel reimbursement for children with certain chronic health conditions.

3574 **Division of Labor and Management**
South Dakota Department of Labor
700 Governors Dr
Pierre, SD 57501-2291
605-773-3101
FAX: 605-773-6184
e-mail: jamesmarsh@state.sd.us
dlr.sd.gov
Sara Minton, Executive Director
Pamela S Roberts, Secretary
Marcia Hultman, Deputy Secretary of Labor and D
Lyle Harter, Director of Administrative Servi
Our mission is to promote economic opportunity and financial security for individuals and businesses through quality, responsive and expert services; fair and equitable employment solutions; and safe and sound business practices.

3575 **Health KiCC**
South Dakota Department of Health
600 E Capitol Ave
Pierre, SD 57501-2536
605-773-3361
800-738-2301
FAX: 605-773-5683
e-mail: DOH.info@state.sd.us
www.doh.sd.gov
Dianne Weyer, Manager
Health KiCC is a program, funded through federal and state monies, that provides financial assistance for medical appointments, procedures, treatments, medications and travel reimbursement for children with certain chronic health conditions.

3576 **South Dakota Advocacy Services**
221 S Central Ave
Ste. 38
Pierre, SD 57501-2479
605-224-8294
800-658-4782
FAX: 605-224-5125
e-mail: sdas@sdadvocacy.com
sdadvocacy.com
Sandy Stocklin Hook, Partners Coordinator
Designated protection and advocacy progam for South Dakota providing legal, administrative, mediation and other services to elgible persons with disabilities in the state.

3577 **South Dakota Department of Aging**
700 Governors Dr
Pierre, SD 57501-2291
605-773-3656
866-854-5465
FAX: 605-773-4085
e-mail: ASA@state.sd.us
pierre.sd.welfareinfo.org
Marilyn Kinsman, Division Director
Lynne Valenti, Deputy Secretary
Amy Iversen-Pollreisz, Deputy Secretary
Kristin Kellar, Communications Director
The Division of Adult Services and Aging (ASA) provides home and community service options to individuals 60 years of age and older and 18 years of age and older with physical disabilities, regardless of income.

3578 **South Dakota Department of Human Services Division of Community Behavioral Health**
South Dakota of Human Services
700 Governors Drive
Hillsview Properties Plaza
Pierre, SD 57501-5007
605-773-3165
800-265-9684
FAX: 605-773-7076
e-mail: infoMH@state.sd.us
http://dss.sd.gov/behavioralhealthservices
Shawna Fullerton, Division Director
South Dakota's state mental health authority.

3579 **South Dakota Developmental Disability Council**
Hillsview Plaza 3800 E Highway 34
c/o 500 East Capital Avenue
Pierre, SD 57501
605-773-5990
800-265-9684
FAX: 605-773-5483
TTY: 605-773-6412
e-mail: infodhs@state.sd.us
www.state.sd.us/dhs/ddc
Dan Lusk, Director
Laurie R. Gill, Secretary
Carol Ruen, Assistant Director
Lindsay Dummer, Program Specialist II
To assist individuals with developmental disabilities to control their own destiny and to achieve the quality of life they desire.

3580 **South Dakota Division of Rehabilitation**
700 Governors Dr
Pierre, SD 57501-2291
605-773-3101
FAX: 605-773-6184
e-mail: jamesmarsh@state.sd.us
www.sdjobs.org
Sara Minton, Executive Director
Pamela S . Roberts, Secretary
Marcia Hultman, Deputy Secretary of Labor and Director of Workforce Service
Lyle Harter, Director of Administrative Services
Offers diagnosis, evaluation and physical restoration services, counseling, social work, educational and professional training, employment and rehabilitation services for the disabled.

3581 **Workers Compensation Board: South Dakota**
700 Governors Dr
Pierre, SD 57501-2291
605-773-3101
FAX: 605-773-6184
e-mail: jamesmarsh@state.sd.us
www.sdjobs.org
Sara Minton, Executive Director
Marcia Hultman, Secretary
Lyle Harter, Director ofAdministrative Services
Bret Afdahi, Director of theDivision of Banking
Our mission is to promote economic opportunity and financial security for individuals and businesses through quality, responsive and expert services; fair and equitable employment solutions; and safe and sound business practices.

Tennessee

3582 **International Dyslexia Association: Tennessee Branch**
TTU Box 5074
Cookeville, TN 37931-2311
800-222-3123
877-836-6432
FAX: 865-693-3653
e-mail: htdainty@gmail.com.
www.tnida.org
Emily Dempster, President
Erin Alexander, Senior Vice President
Shannon Polk, Secretary
Jean Hutchinson, Treasurer
The Tennessee Branch of the International Dyslexia Association (TN-IDA) was formed to increase awareness about Dyslexia in the state of Tennessee. TN-IDA supports efforts to provide information regarding appropriate language arts instruction to those involved with language-based learning differences and to encourage the identity of these individuals at-risk for such disorders as soon as possible.

3583 Social Security: Nashville Disability Determination
Social Security
P.O. Box 77
Nashville, TN 37202-4732
615-743-7774
800-772-1213
800-342-1117
FAX: 615-253-1840
e-mail: Betty.J.Hood@ssa.gov
ssa.gov

Karena L. Kilgore, Executive Secretary
Carolyn W. Colvin, Commissioner
Carolyn W. Colvin, Deputy Commissioner
James A. Kissko, Chief of Staff

We deliver services through a nationwide network of over 1,400 offices that include regional offices, field offices, card centers, teleservice centers, processing centers, hearing offices, the Appeals Council, and our State and territorial partners, the Disability Determination Services. We also have a presence in U.S. embassies around the globe. For the public, we are the "face of the government." The rich diversity of our employees mirrors the public we serve.

3584 Tennessee Assistive Technology Projects
Citizens Plaza State Office Buildin
511 Union St.
Nashville, TN 37219-1403
615-313-5183
800-732-5059
TTY:615-313-5695
e-mail: TN.TTAP@tn.gov
www.tn.gov

Bill Haslam, Governor
Raquel Hatter, Commissioner
Beth White, Manager
Julie Oden, Manager

A statewide program promoting assistive technology devices and services for persons of all ages with all disabilities.

3585 Tennessee Client Assistance Program
Tennessee Protection and Advocacy
P.O.Box 121257
Nashville, TN 37212-1257
615-298-1080
800-342-1660
FAX: 615-298-2046
e-mail: gethelp@tpainc.org
www.tpainc.org

Shirley Shea, Executive Director
Doris Lopez, Assistant Executive Director

3586 Tennessee Commission on Aging and Disability
161 Rosa L. Parks Boulevard
3rd Floor
Nashville, TN 37243-860
615-741-2056
FAX: 615-741-3309
e-mail: cindy.warf@tn.gov
www.tn.gov/comaging

Richard M. Honn, Executive Director
Ryan Ellis, Aging Info. & Data Director
Kathy Zamata, Aging Program Director
Richard Presler, Fiscal Director

3587 Tennessee Council on Developmental Disabilities
404 James Robertson Pkwy
Parkway Towers, Suite 130
Nashville, TN 37243
615-532-6615
FAX: 615-532-6964
e-mail: tnddc@tn.gov
www.state.tn.us/odd

Wanda Willis, Executive Director
Bill Haslam, Governor
Alicia Cone, Coordinator, Project Research an
William Edington, Public Policy Director

Provides leadership to ensure independence, productivity, integration and inclusion of individuals with disabilities in the community through promotion of systems change. The council works with members of the community, including public and private aencies, business, legislators and policymakers, to create a future in which; people with disabilities are full included in the community and experience no barriers related to attitudes about their disabilities as they persue their goals.

3588 Tennessee Department of Children with Disabilities
511 Union St.
Nashville, TN 37219-9004
615-741-9701
800-861-1935
FAX: 615-253-5216
e-mail: dcs.email@tn.gov
www.tn.gov

Ruth S Letson, Manager
Haticile Buchanan, Manager
Mary Beth Franklyn, CS Program Director
Kristi Faulkner, Special Counsel to the Commissio

Tennessee's children thrive in safe, healthy and stable families. Families thrive in healthy, safe and strong communities. Tennessee's citizens benefit from the best child welfare and juvenile justice agency in the country.

3589 Tennessee Department of Mental Health
425 5th Ave N
Nashville, TN 37243-3400
615-741-7213
800-560-5767
FAX: 615-532-6514
e-mail: oc.tdmh@tn.gov
www.state.tn.us/mental

Doug Varney, Commissioner
Grant Lawrence, Director Office of Communication
Bob Grunow, Deputy Commissioner
Howard Burley, Asst Commissioner Clinical Ldrsp

TDMH is the state's mental health and substance abuse authority. Its mission is to plan for and promote the availability of a comprehensive array of quality prevention, early intervention, treatment, habilitation, and rehabilitation services and supports based on the needs and choices of individuals and families served. Responsible for policy, and oversight, and for advocacy of the consumer within the state.

3590 Tennessee Division of Rehabilitation
400 Deaderick St
Nashville, TN 37243-1403
615-313-4700
800-270-1349
TTY:615-313-5695
e-mail: connie.phillips@tn.gov
http://www.tn.gov

Patsy Matthews, Commissioner
Randall Beasley, Manager
Raquel Hatter, Commissioner
Bill Haslam, Givernor

Offers rehabilitation, medical and therapeutic information and referrals to the disabled.

3591 Workers Compensation Division Tennessee
Dept of Labor & Workforce Development
220 French Landing Drive
1st Floor
Nashville, TN 37243- 1002
615-741-6642
800-332-2667
FAX: 615-532-1468
e-mail: wc.info@tn.gov
www.tn.gov/labor-wfd/wcomp.html

Karla Davis, Commissioner
Alisa Malone, Deputy Commissioner
Stephanie Mitchell, General Counsel
Ron Jones, Administrator of Fiscal Services

We administer the workers' compensation system and promote a better understanding of the program's benefits by informing employees and employers of their rights and responsibilities. Workers' Compenstation administers a mediation program for disputed claims, encourage workplace safety, participate in a public awareness campaign concerning fraud, and oversee an information awareness program for educating the public on laws and regulations which define workers' compensation requirements. We ensure

Texas

3592 Disability Policy Consortium
2222 West Braker Lane
Austin, TX 78758-1024
512-454-4816
800-252-9108
FAX: 512-323-0902
e-mail: dpctexas@advocacyinc.org
www.disabilityrightstx.org
Mary Faithful, Executive Director
Roberta Rosenberg-Roque, Manager
An independent group of statewide advocacy organizations that strives to achieve the development and full implementation of public policy that promotes and supports the rights, inclusion, integration and independence of Texans with disabilities.

3593 Division of Special Education
1701 Congress Ave
Austin, TX 78701-1402
512-463-9734
FAX: 512-463-9838
e-mail: teainfo@tea.state.tx.us
www.tea.state.tx.us
Bill Abasolo, Federal & State Education Policy
Robert Scott, Commissioner of Education
Lizzette Gonzalez Reynolds, Deputy Commissioner, Policy & Pr
Anita Givens, Associate Commissioner, Standard
The Texas public school system is a $46 billion a year enterprise. Running a school district requires superintendents to operate one of the largest, if not the largest, business in their community. This website attempts to provide administrators with easy access to information they need to successfully carry out their duties.

3594 Easter Seal of Greater Dallas, TX
233 South Wacker Drive
Suite 2400
Chicago, IL 60606-4743
972-394-8900
800-580-4718
800-221-6827
FAX: 972-394-6266
e-mail: wjohnson@dallas.easterseals.com
easterseals.com
Richard W. Davidson, Chairman
Sandra L. Bouwman, 1st Vice Chairman
Joseph G. Kern, 2nd Vice Chairman
Bennett Leventhal, M.D., President
Easter Seals has a longstanding history in our community of providing a wealth of unique programs and services for individual with a wide variety of disabilities, including Autism Spectrum Disorder, Alzheimer's disease, Down syndrome, Cerebral Palsy, Mental and Developmental Delays, and a wealth of other disabilities. We provide programs and services, education, outreach, and advocacy so that people living with disabilities can live, learn, work and play in our communities.

3595 Easter Seals Greater NW Texas
2100 Circle Dr
Fort Worth, TX 76119-8130
817-332-717
888-617-7171
FAX: 817-332-7601
e-mail: wjohnson@dallas.easterseals.com
Donna Dempsey, President and Chief Executive Of
Nancy Robinson, Executive Vice President & Chief
Nancy Swartz, Vice President of Development an
Lenee Bassham, Vice President Community Living
Easter Seals has a longstanding history in our community of providing a wealth of unique programs and services for individual with a wide variety of disabilities, including Autism Spectrum Disorder, Alzheimer's disease, Down syndrome, Cerebral Palsy, Mental and Developmental Delays, and a wealth of other disabilities. We provide programs and services, education, outreach, and advocacy so that people living with disabilities can live, learn, work and play in our communities.

3596 El Valle Community Parent Resource Center
Ste J
530 S Texas Blvd
Weslaco, TX 78596-6262
956-969-0215
800-680-0255
FAX: 956-968-7102
e-mail: texasfiestaedu.org
www.tfepodder.org
Robert Garza, Owner

3597 Grassroots Consortium
Greenroots Consortium
6202 Belmark St
Houston, TX 77087-6324
713-643-9576
FAX: 713-643-6291
Speckids@aol.com
Agnes A Johnson, Director

3598 International Dyslexia Association: Austin Branch
P.O.Box 92604
Austin, TX 78709-2604
512-452-7658
800-222-3123
e-mail: info@interdys.org
www.interdys.org
Hal Malchow, President
Elsa Cardenas-Hagan, Vice President
Ben Shifrin, Vice President
Lee Grossman, Executive Director
The Austin Area Branch of the International Dyslexia Association is a 501(c)(3) non profit organization dedicated to promoting reading excellence for all children through early identification of dyslexia, effective literacy education for adults and children with dyslexia, and teacher training.

3599 NAMI Texas
FOUNTAINPark Plaza III
2800 S. I-35,SUITE140
Austin, TX 78704-5700
512-693-2000
800-633-3760
FAX: 512-693-8000
e-mail: namitexas@texami.org
namitexas.org
Andrea Hazlitt, President
Ed Dickey, Vice President
Chris Scroggin, Executive Director
Kelly Jeschke, Membership Coordinator
NAMI Texas has a variety of programs directed to mental health consumers, family members, friends, professionals, other stake holders and the community at large to address the mental health needs of Texans. NAMI Texas works to inform the public about mental illness by distributing information about mental illness through every means of communication. Interviews are produced on television, stories are featured in newspapers, brochures are distributed, referrals are provided and more.

3600 Parent Connection
1020 Riverwood Ct
Conroe, TX 77304-2811
936-756-8321
800-839-8876
e-mail: parentCNCT@aol.com
http://www.parentingaspergerscommunity.com/pu
Dave Angel, Founder
Includes parenting help and Aspergers advice, including parenting tips, tricks and techniques to help your child with Aspergers. Our worldwide membership base is helping parents to understand their child with Aspergers better and make their home & family life a better place to be.

3601 Parents Supporting Parents Network
8001 Centre Park Drive
Suite 100
Austin, TX 78754
512-454-6694
800-252-9729
FAX: 512-454-4956
e-mail: secretary@thearcoftexas.org
www.thearcoftexas.org

Clay Boatrigh, President
Carol Maxwell, Vice-President
Lucio Mendoza, Treasurer
Charlie Huber, Secretary
Since our founding in 1950 by a group of parents of children with intellectual and developmental disabilities, The Arc at the local, state and national level has been instrumental in the creation of virtually every program, service, right, and benefit that is now available to more than half a million Texans with intellectual and developmental disabilities. Today, The Arc continues to advocate for including people with intellectual and developmental disabilities in all aspects of society.

3602 Partners Resource Network
Ste B
1090 Longfellow Dr
Beaumont, TX 77706-4819
409-898-4684
800-866-4726
FAX: 409-898-4869
e-mail: partnersresource@sbcglobal.net
partnerstx.org

Janice Meyer, Executive Director
Statewide network of three parent training and information centers.

3603 Social Security: Austin Disability Determination
P.O. Box 149198
Austin, TX 78714-9198
512-437-8311
800-772-1213
800-252-9627
FAX: 512-437-8595
TTY:512-916-5958
e-mail: dan.tippit@ssa.gov
www.ssa.gov

Karena L. Kilgore, Executive Secretary
Carolyn W. Colvin, Commissioner
Carolyn W. Colvin, Deputy Commissioner
James A. Kissko, Chief of Staff
We deliver services through a nationwide network of over 1,400 offices that include regional offices, field offices, card centers, teleservice centers, processing centers, hearing offices, the Appeals Council, and our State and territorial partners, the Disability Determination Services. We also have a presence in U.S. embassies around the globe. The rich diversity of our employees mirrors the public we serve.

3604 Statewide Information at Texas School for the Deaf
1102 S Congress Ave
Austin, TX 78704-1728
512-462-5353
FAX: 512-462-5353
e-mail: webmaster@tsd.state.tx.us
www.tsd.state.tx.us
Sonia Karimi Bridges, Video Communication Specialist
Avonne Brooker-Rutowski, Program Specialist
David Coco, Program Specialist
Lisa Crawford, Parent Liason
Welcome to Texas School for the Deaf, a place where students who are deaf or hard of hearing including those with additional disabilities, have the opportunity to learn, grow and belong in a culture that optimizes individual potential and provides accessible language and communication across the curriculum. Our educational philosophy is grounded in the belief that all children who are deaf and hard of hearing deserve a quality language and communication-driven program that provides education tog

3605 Texas Advocates Supporting Kids with Disabilities
P.O.Box 162685
Austin, TX 78716-2685
512-310-2102
FAX: 512-310-2102
e-mail: ASKTASK@aol.com
www.main.org/task/

3606 Texas Commission for the Blind
P.O.Box 12866
Austin, TX 78711-2866
512-459-8575
800-252-5204
FAX: 512-459-0200

Canzata Crowder, Manager
Offers services for the totally blind, legally blind, and visually impaired, with counseling, educational, recreational, rehabilitation, computer training and professional training services.

3607 Texas Commission for the Deaf and Hard of Hearing
D AR S
P.O. Box 149198
Austin, TX 78714-9198
512-407-3250
800-628-5115
FAX: 512-407-3299
TTY: 512-407-3251
e-mail: DARS.Inquiries@dars.state.tx.us
www.dars.state.tx.us

Veronda L. Durden, Commissioner
Glenn Neal, Deputy Commissioner
David Myers, Executive Director
Daniel Bravo, Chief Operating Officer

3608 Texas Council for Developmental Disabilities
6201 E Oltorf St
Suite 600
Austin, TX 78741-7509
512-437-5432
800-262-0334
FAX: 512-437-5434
TTY: 512-437-5431
e-mail: tcdd@tcdd.texas.gov
txddc.state.tx.us

Mary Durheim, Chairman
Andrew D. Crim, Vice Chairman
Roger Webb, Executive Director
Koren Vogel, Executive Assistant
The Texas Council for Developmental Disabilities is a 27-member board dedicated to ensuring that all Texans with developmental disabilities, about 411,479 individuals, have the opportunity to be independent, productive and valued members of their communities. The mission of the Texas Council for Developmental Disabilities is to create change so that all people with disabilities are fully included in their communities and exercise control over their own lives.

3609 Texas Department of Human Services
701 W 51st St
P.O. Box 149030
Austin, TX 78751-2312
512-438-3011
888-834-7406
FAX: 512-472-0603
TTY: 888-425-6889
e-mail: mail@dads.state.tx.us
www.dads.state.tx.us

Jon Weizenbaum, Commissioner
Kristi Jordan, Associate Commissioner
Chris Adams, Deputy Commissioner
Elisa J. Garza, Assistant Commissioner for Access and Intake

3610 Texas Department of Mental Health & Mental Retardation
P.O.Box 12668
Austin, TX 78711-2668
512-472-4138
FAX: 512-472-0603
www.mhmr.state.tx.us

Bill West, Manager
Randy Fritz, Chief Operating Officer

3611 Texas Department on Aging
701 W 51st St
P.O. Box 149030
Austin, TX 78751-2312
512-438-3011
800-252-9240
e-mail: mail@tdoa.state.tx.us
www.dads.state.tx.us

Jon Weizenbaum, Commissioner
Kristi Jordan, Associate Commissioner
Chris Adams, Deputy Commissioner
Elisa J. Garza, Assistant Commissioner for Access and Intake

3612 Texas Federation of Families for Children's Mental Health
Ste 505
7701 N Lamar Blvd
Austin, TX 78752-1000
512-407-8844
866-893-3264
FAX: 512-407-8266
e-mail: info@txffcmh.org
www.txffcmh.org

Patti Derr, Executive Director
Pat Calley, Chairperson
S Barron, Operations Director

3613 Texas Governor's Committee on People with Disabilities
1100 San Jacinto Blvd
P.O. Box 12428
Austin, TX 78701- 1935
512-463-2000
FAX: 513-463-5745
e-mail: CPD@gov.texas.gov
www.governor.state.tx.us/disabilities

Angela English, LPC, LMFT, Executive Director
Erin Lawler, JD, MS, Accessibility and Disability Rig
Nancy Van Loan, Executive Assistant
Jo Virgil, MS, Community Outreach and Informati

The Governor's Committee on People with Disabilities is within the office of the Governor. The committee's mission is to further opportunities for persons with disabilities to enjoy full and equal access to lives of independence, productivity, and self-determination. The committee is composed of 12 members appointed by the governor and of nonvoting ex officio members.

3614 Texas Protection & Advocacy Services for Disabled Persons
Advocacy
2222 West Braker Lane
Austin, TX 78758-1024
512-454-4816
800-252-9108
800-315-3876
FAX: 512-323-0902
e-mail: dpctexas@advocacyinc.org
www.disabilityrightstx.org

Mary Faithful, Executive Director
Roberta Rosenberg-Roque, Manager

A federally funded, independent, nonprofit agency that advocates for the legal, human and service rights of persons with disabilities. Publishes 'Special Edition' newsletter, at a small fee and 'It's a Good Idea!' a parent manual for $10, plus many other handouts free of charge.

3615 Texas Respite Resource Network
P.O.Box 7330
San Antonio, TX 78207-330
512-228-2794
e-mail: elizabethnewhouse@srhcc.org

Jennifer Cernoch, Director
Liz Newhouse, Assistant Director

A state clearinghouse and technical assistance network for respite in Texas. TRRN identifies, initiates and improves respite options for families caring for individuals with disabilities on the local, state and national levels. TRRN provides training/technical assistance to programs/groups wanting to establish respite services.

3616 Texas Technology Access Project
Center for Disabilities Studies
10100 Burnet Rd
Austin, TX 78758-4445
512-232-0740
800-828-7839
FAX: 512-232-0761
TTY: 512-232-0762
e-mail: rogerlevy@austin.utexas.edu
techaccess.edb.utexas.edu

Roger Levy, Program Director
Darlene West, Assistive Technology Coordinator
Steve Thomas, Operations and External Relation
Darlene West, Assistive Technology Specialist

Their mission is to increase access for people with disabilities to assistive technology that provides them more control over their immediate environments and an enhanced ability to function independently.

3617 Texas UAP for Developmental Disabilities
University of Texas
1 University Station
Austin, TX 78712
512-471-3434
800-828-7839
e-mail: hello@utexas.edu
www.utexas.edu

William Powers Jr., President
Steven Leslie, Executive Vice President and Pr
Penny Seay, Executive Director
Bob Harkins, Manager

Welcome to The University of Texas at Austin. Founded in 1883, UT is one of the largest and most respected universities in the nation. Ours is a diverse learning community, with students from every state and more than 100 countries. We're a university with world talent and Texas traditions. Discover more about us online and come visit our beautiful campus in person.

3618 Texas Workers Compensation Commission
7551 Metro Center Drive
Suite 100
Austin, TX 78744-1645
512-804-4000
800-372-7713
800-252-3439
FAX: 512-804-4401
TTY:512-322-4238
e-mail: WebStaff@tdi.state.tx.us
www.tdi.texas.gov

Robert Shipe, Executive Director
Rod Bordelon, Commissioner

Workers' compensation is a state-regulated insurance program that pays medical bills and replaces some lost wages for employees who are injured at work or who have work-related diseases or illnesses.

3619 United Cerebral Palsy of Texas
National Cerebral Palsy of American
Ste 145
1016 La Posada Dr
Austin, TX 78752-3828
512-472-8696
800-798-1492
FAX: 512-472-8026
e-mail: info@ucptexas.org
ucptexas.org

Jean Langendorf, Executive Director

Offers a unique array of programs and services designed for one specific purpose: to ensure that people with cerebral palsy and similar disabilities have the opportunity to participate fully and equally in every aspect of our society.

Utah

3620 Access Utah Network
Ste 100
155 S 300 W
Salt Lake City, UT 84101-1288
801-533-4636
800-333-8824
FAX: 801-533-3968
e-mail: access@utah.gov
accessut.org

Mark L. Smith, Information Specialist
Access Utah Network is Utah's prime source for information and referral for individuals with disabilities and their caregivers since 1990. Our operators can provide you with the information you need to find accessible housing, assistive technology and financial and social supports needed to live independently with a disability. Call us or explore our web site today to see how Access Utah Network can help you become more independent.

3621 Social Security: Salt Lake City Disability Determination
Social Security
P.O. Box 144032
Salt Lake City, UT 84111-4032
801-321-6500
800-772-1213
800-221-3493
FAX: 801-321-6599
TTY:801-524-5047
e-mail: Dave.Carlson@ssa.gov
www.ssa.gov

Karena L. Kilgore, Executive Secretary
Carolyn W. Colvin, Commissioner
Carolyn W. Colvin, Deputy Commissioner
James A. Kissko, Chief of Staff
We deliver services through a nationwide network of over 1,400 offices that include regional offices, field offices, card centers, teleservice centers, processing centers, hearing offices, the Appeals Council, and our State and territorial partners, the Disability Determination Services. We also have a presence in U.S. embassies around the globe. The rich diversity of our employees mirrors the public we serve.

3622 Utah Assistive Technology Projects
Utah State University
6855 Old Main Hl
Logan, UT 84322-6855
435-797-3824
800-524-5152
TTY:435-797-2355
www.uatpat.org

Sachin Pavithran, Program Director
Alma Burgess, CReATE Program Coordinator
Clay Christensen, Lab Coordinator
Marilyn ' Hammond, Executive Director
A statewide program promoting assistive technology devices and services for persons of all ages with all disabilities.

3623 Utah Client Assistance Program
205 N 400 W
Salt Lake City, UT 84103-1125
801-363-1347
800-662-9080
FAX: 801-363-1437
www.disabilitylawcenter.org

Bryce Fifield Ph.D, President
Jared Fields, Vice President
Barbara M. Campbell, Treasurer
Kevin Murphy, Board Member
Since 1979, the Disability Law Center (DLC) has helped thousands of Utahns with disabilities and their families. The DLC has broad statutory powers to safeguard the human and civil rights of persons with disabilities. We provide self-advocacy assistance, legal services, disability rights education, and public policy advocacy on behalf of the more than 400,000 Utah residents with disabilities. Our services are available statewide and without regard for ability to pay.

3624 Utah Department of Aging
195 North 1950 West
Salt Lake City, UT 84116
801-538-3910
877-424-4640
FAX: 801-538-4395
e-mail: debooth@utah.gov
www.hsdaas.utah.gov

Nels Holmgren, Director
Michael S. Styles, Assistant Director
Michelle Benson, Director
Sarah Brenna, Director
We administer a wide variety of home and community-based services for Utah residents who are 60 or older. Programs and services are primarily delivered by a network of 12 Area Agencies on Aging which reach all geographic areas of the state. Our goal is to provide services that allow people to remain independent.

3625 Utah Department of Human Services: Division of Services for People with Disabilities
Utah Department of Human Services
195 North 1950 West
Salt Lake City, UT 84116
801-538-3910
877-424-4640
FAX: 801-538-4395
e-mail: debooth@utah.gov
www.hsdspd.utah.gov

Paul T. Smith, Division Director
Clay Hiatt, Fiscal Management
Information and referral services for people with disabilities, including DD/MR, brain injury and physical disabilities throughout the state of Utah.

3626 Utah Division Of Substance Abuse & MentalHealth
Utah Department of Human Services
195 No. 1950 West
Salt Lake City, UT 84103-1550
801-538-4171
FAX: 801-538-4016
WWW.DHS.UTAH.GOV

Lana Stohl, Executive Director

3627 Utah Division of Services for the Disabled
195 North 1950 West
Salt Lake City, UT 84116
801-538-4200
800-837-6811
FAX: 801-538-4279
e-mail: dirdhs@utah.gov
www.hsdspd.utah.gov

Paul T. Smith, Division Director
Clay Hiatt, Fiscal Management
Offers services for the totally blind, legally blind, visually impaired, mentally retarded blind and more with health, counseling, educational, recreational, rehabilitation, computer training and professional training services.

3628 Utah Governor's Council for People with Disabilities
155 S 300 W
Suite 100
Salt Lake City, UT 84101-1288
801-533-4636
FAX: 801-533-3968
e-mail: alozano@utah.gov
www.gcpd.org/

Mark Smith, Manager
Angela Allen, Administrative Secretary

3629 Utah Labor Commission
160 East 300 South, 3rd Floor
P.O.Box 146630
Salt Lake City, UT 84114-6600
801-530-6800
800-222-1238
FAX: 801-530-6390
e-mail: laborcom@utah.gov
www.laborcommission.utah.gov

Sherrie Hayashi, Commissioner and Department Director
Jaceson Maughan, Deputy Commisioner
Pete Hackford, Director
Ron Dressler, Director

Problems with employers not paying employees, employers not paying the minimum wage, the employment of minors and retaliation for wage complaints filed are handled by the Wage Claim Unit.

3630 Utah Protection & Advocacy Services for Persons with Disabilities
Disability Law Center
205 N 400 W
Salt Lake City, UT 84103-1125
801-363-1347
800-662-9080
FAX: 801-363-1437
www.disabilitylawcenter.org

Bryce Fifield Ph.D, President
Jared Fields, Vice President
Barbara M. Campbell, Treasurer
Kevin Murphy, Board Member

Since 1979, the Disability Law Center (DLC) has helped thousands of Utahns with disabilities and their families. The DLC has broad statutory powers to safeguard the human and civil rights of persons with disabilities. We provide self-advocacy assistance, legal services, disability rights education, and public policy advocacy on behalf of the more than 400,000 Utah residents with disabilities. Our services are available statewide and without regard for ability to pay.

Vermont

3631 Disability Law Project
57 N Main St
Rutland, VT 05701-3246
800-889-2047
FAX: 802-775-0022
e-mail: nbreiden@vtlegalaid.org
vtlegalaid.org

Nanci Smith, President
Jessica Porter, Vice President/Secretary
John Holme, Treasurer
Eric Avildsen, Executive Director

Legal services (protection and advocacy) for people with disabilities on legal issues arising from disability. Statewide. Adults and children. Employment, education, discrimination, housing, public benefits, health care.

3632 Disability Rights Vermont
141 Main Street
Suite 7
Montpelier, VT 05602-2916
802-229-1355
800-834-7890
FAX: 802-229-1359
TTY: 800-889-2047
e-mail: info@disabilityrightsvt.org
www.disabilityrightsvt.org

Sarah Wendell-Launderville, President
David Gallagher, Vice president
Ed Paquin, Executive Director
Donna Samson-Sprake, Business Manager

Advocacy and legal services for people with mental illness on legal issues arising, out of disabilities. Children and adults.

3633 Social Security: Vermont Disability Determination Services
Ste 6
93 Pilgrim Park Rd
Waterbury, VT 05676-1729
802-241-2463
800-734-2463
800-772-1213
FAX: 802-241-2492
e-mail: Deborah.Fennell@ssa.gov
www.ssa.gov

Karena L. Kilgore, Executive Secretary
Carolyn W. Colvin, Commissioner
Carolyn W. Colvin, Deputy Commissioner
James A. Kissko, Chief of Staff

We deliver services through a nationwide network of over 1,400 offices that include regional offices, field offices, card centers, teleservice centers, processing centers, hearing offices, the Appeals Council, and our State and territorial partners, the Disability Determination Services. We also have a presence in U.S. embassies around the globe. The rich diversity of our employees mirrors the public we serve.

3634 Vermont Assistive Technology Projects
103 S Main St
Weeks Building
Waterbury, VT 05671-2305
800-750-6355
800-750-6355
FAX: 802-871-3048
TTY: 802-241-1464
e-mail: amber.fulcher@state.vt.us
atp.vermont.gov

Amber Fulcher, Program Director
Sharon Alderman, Assistive Technology Reuse Coord
Emma Cobb, Assistive Technology Services Co
Dan Gilman, ATP, Assistive Technology Access Spec

Increase awareness and change policies to insure assistive technology (AT) is available to all Vermonters with disabilities. Our Commitment is to enable Vermonters with disabilities to have greater independence, productivity, and confidence. To provide them with a clear and direct avenue toward integration and inclusion within the work force and community.

3635 Vermont Client Assistance Program
57 N Main St
Rutland, VT 05701-3246
802-775-0021
800-769-7459
www.vocrehabvermont.org/html/clientassistance

Patrick Flood, Commissioner

The Client Assistance Program (CAP) is an independent advocacy program to help if you are applying for or receiving services from one of the following sources: Division of Vocational Rehabilitation (VR); Vermont Center for Independent Living (VCIL); Division for the Blind and Visually Impaired (DBVI); Vermont Association of Business, Industry & Rehabilitation (VABIR); Vermont Association for the Blind and Visually Impaired (VABVI); Supported Employment Programs; Transition Programs.

3636 Vermont Department of Aging
103 S Main St
Weeks Building
Waterbury, VT 05671-2305
802-871-3350
FAX: 802-871-3281
TTY:802-241-3557
e-mail: AHS-DAIL-DeptWebMaster@state.vt.us
dail.vermont.gov

Susan Wehry, Commissioner
Marybeth McCaffrey, Director
Linda Henzel, Executive Staff Assistant
Adele Edelman, Assistant Division Director

3637 Vermont Department of Developmental and
103 S Main St
Weeks Building
Waterbury, VT 05671-2305
802-871-3350
FAX: 802-871-3281
TTY:802-241-3557
dail.vermont.gov

Jonathan Wood, Manager

3638 Vermont Department of Disabilities, Aging and Independent Living
Aging and Disabilities
103 S Main St
Waterbury, VT 05671-9800
802-241-2401
FAX: 802-241-2325
dail.vermont.gov

Susan Wehry, Commissioner
Camille George, Deputy Commissioner

3639 **Vermont Department of Health: Children with Special Health Needs**
Vermont Department Of Health
108 Cherry Street
Burlington, VT 05402-70
802-863-7200
800-464-4343
FAX: 802-865-7754
healthvermont.gov

Harry Chen, M.D., Commissioner
Barbara Cimaglio, Deputy Commissioner for Alcohol
Tracy Dolan, Deputy Commissioner for Public H
Dixie Henry, Esq., Senior Policy and Legal Advisor

Multidisciplinary clinics and family support for children with chronic conditions, birth to age 21 years.

3640 **Vermont Developmental Disabilities Council**
103 S Main St
Waterbury, VT 05671-9800
082-241-2220
e-mail: vtddc@upgate1.ahs.state.vt.us
www.ahs.state.vt.us/vtddc

Cynthia D LaWare, Secretary

The mission of VTDDC is to facilitate connections and to promote supports that bring people with developmental disabilities into the heart of Vermont Communities.

3641 **Vermont Division for the Blind & Visually Impaired**
Agency of Human Svcs Dept Disabilities, Aging & IL
103 S Main St
Weeks Building
Waterbury, VT 5671-2304
802-871-3038
800-405-5005
888-405-5005
FAX: 802-871-3048
e-mail: DBVI-Info@state.vt.us
www.dbvi.vermont.gov

Fred Jones, Director
Scott Langley, Counselor
Heather Allen, Administrative Assistant
Paul Putnam, Rehabilitation Associate

Offers services for the totally blind, legally blind, visually impaired, mentally retarded blind and more with health, counseling, educational, recreational, rehabilitation, computer training and professional training services.

3642 **Vermont Division of Disability & Aging Services**
103 S Main St
Weeks Building
Waterbury, VT 05671-2305
802-871-3350
FAX: 802-871-3281
TTY:802-241-3557
e-mail: AHS-DAIL-DeptWebMaster@state.vt.us
www.dail.vermont.gov

Susan Wehry, Commissioner
Marybeth McCaffrey, Director
Linda Henzel, Executive Staff Assistant
Adele Edelman, Assistant Division Director

Provides services to adults and children with developmental disabilities all to the aging.

3643 **Workers Compensation Board Vermont**
Department of Labor
5 Green Mountain Drive
PO Box 488
Montpelier, VT 05601- 0488
802-828-4301
FAX: 802-828-2195
e-mail: labor-wccomp@state.vt.us
labor.vermont.gov

Deborah Bruce, Human Resource Administrator
Allen Evans, Executive Director Workforce Dev
Annie Noonan, Commissioner
Erika Wolf?ng, Principal Assistant

Welcome to the Vermont Department of Labor's website. VDOL's primary focus is to provide services that assist businesses, workers, and job seekers.

Virginia

3644 **International Dyslexia Association: Virginia Branch**
804 Industrial Avenue
Suite I
Chesapeake, VA 23324
866-893-0583
800-988-8336
FAX: 804-285-1946
e-mail: info@vbida.org
www.interdys.org

Hal Malchow, President
Elsa Cardenas-Hagan, Vice President
Ben Shifrin, Vice President
Lee Grossman, Executive Director

The Virginia Branch of The International Dyslexia Association (VBIDA) is a 501(c)(3) non-profit, scientific and educational organization dedicated to the study and treatment of the learning disability, dyslexia. This Branch was formed to increase public awareness of dyslexia in the State of Virginia. We serve the entire state, with the exception of Northern Virginia, which is part of the DC-Capital Branch in Washington, DC. We have been serving individuals with dyslexia, their families.

3645 **Virginia Department for the Blind and Vision Impaired**
397 Azalea Ave
Richmond, VA 23227-3623
804-371-3140
800-622-2155
FAX: 804-371-3351
e-mail: Kimberley.Jennings@dbvi.virginia.gov
www.vdbvi.org

Robert S. Dendy, Chair
Raymond E. Hopkins, Commissioner
Dr. Rick L. Mitchell, Deputy Commissioner
James R. Meehan, Deputy Commissioner

Offers services for the totally blind, legally blind, visually impaired, mentally retarded blind and more with health, counseling, educational, recreational, rehabilitation, computer training and professional training services.

3646 **Virginia Department of Mental Health**
P.O.Box 1797
Richmond, VA 23218-1797
804-786-3921
FAX: 804-371-6638
TTY:804-371-8977
e-mail: jim.stewart@dbhds.virginia.gov?subject=(E-mai
www.dbhds.virginia.gov

Debra Ferquson, Commissioner
John Pezzoli, Deputy Commissioner
Daniel Herr, Assistant Commissioner of Behavioral Health Services
Connie Cochran, Assistant Commissioner of Developmental Services

Available to citizens statewide, Virginia's public mental health, intellectual disability and substance abuse services system is comprised of 16 state facilities and 40 locally-run community services boards (CSBs) The CSBs and facilities serve children and adults who have or who are at risk of mental illness, serious emotional disturbance, intellectual disabilities, or substance abuse disorders.

3647 **Virginia Developmental Disability Council**
103 S Main St
Waterbury, VT 05671-9800
082-241-2220
e-mail: vtddc@upgate1.ahs.state.vt.us
www.ahs.state.vt.us/vtddc

Cynthia D LaWare, Secretary

The mission of VTDDC is to facilitate connections and to promote supports that bring people with developmental disabilities into the heart of Vermont Communities.

3648 Virginia Office Protection and Advocacy for People with Disabilities
1910 Byrd Ave, Ste 5
Richmond, VA 23230-3034 804-225-2042
800-552-3962
FAX: 804-662-7431
e-mail: general.vopa@vopa.virginia.gov
disabilitylawva.org
Coleen Miller, Executive Director
Through zealous and effective advocacy and legal representation to: protect and advance legal, human, and civil rights of persons with disabilities; combat and prevent abuse, neglect, and discrimination; and promote independence, choice, and self-determination by persons with disabilities.

3649 Virginia Office for Protection & Advocacy
1910 Byrd Ave
Suite 5
Richmond, VA 23230-3034 804-225-2042
800-552-3962
FAX: 804-662-7057
e-mail: info@dLCV.org
vopa.state.va.us
V Coleen Miller, Executive Director
Rusty Hill, Administrative Assistant
LaToya Blizzard, Deputy Director for Fiscal and Operations
Mickie Chapman, Information Technology Specialist
An independent state agency that helps ensure that the rights of persons with disabiltiies in the Commonwealth are protected. The mission of DRVD is to provide zealous and effective advocacy and legal representation to protect and advance legal, human and civil rights of persons with disabilities, combat and prevent abuse, neglect and discrimination, and promote independence, choice and self-determination by persons with disabilities.

3650 Virginia Office for Protection and Advocacy
1910 Byrd Ave
Suite 5
Richmond, VA 23230-3034 804-225-2042
800-552-3962
FAX: 804-662-7057
e-mail: info@dLCV.org
vopa.state.va.us
V Coleen Miller, Executive Director
Rusty Hill, Administrative Assistant
LaToya Blizzard, Deputy Director for Fiscal and Operations
Mickie Chapman, Information Technology Specialist
An independent state agency that helps ensure that the rights of persons with disabiltiies in the Commonwealth are protected. The mission of DRVD is to provide zealous and effective advocacy and legal representation to protect and advance legal, human and civil rights of persons with disabilities, combat and prevent abuse, neglect and discrimination, and promote independence, choice and self-determination by persons with disabilities.

3651 Virginia's Developmental Disabilities Planning Council
Stae Agency
1100 Bank Street
7th Floor
Richmond, VA 23219-3426 804-786-0016
800-846-4464
FAX: 804-662-7662
TTY: 800-811-7893
e-mail: info@vbpd.virginia.gov
www.vaboard.org
Korinda Rusinyak, Chairman
Charles Meacham, Vice Chairman
Dennis Manning, Secretary
Heidi L. Lawyer, Executive Director
To create a Commonwealth that advances opportunities for independence, personal decision-making and full participation in community life for individuals with developmental disabilities.

Washington

3652 DSHS/Aging & Adult Disability Services Administration
P.O.Box 45130
Olympia, WA 98504-5130 360-902-7797
800-737-0617
FAX: 360-902-7848
TTY: 800-737-7931
aasa.dshs.wa.gov
Dan Murphy, Director
Bea Rector, Project Director
Tamarra Paradee, Executive Secretary
Bill Moss, Director
The Aging and Disability Services Administration assists children and adults with developmental delays or disabilities, cognitive impairment, chronic illness and related functional disabilities to gain access to needed services and supports by managing a system of long-term care and supportive services that are high quality, cost effective, and responsive to individual needs and preferences.

3653 Disability Rights: Washington
315 5th Avenue South
Suite 850
Seattle, WA 98104-2691 206-324-1521
800-562-2702
FAX: 206-957-0729
TTY: 206-957-0728
e-mail: info@dr-wa.org
www.disabilityrightswa.org
Mark Stroh, Executive Director
David Carison, Director of Legal Advocacy
Emily Cooper, Staff Attorney
Charlotte Cunningham, Staff Attorney
WPAS is a private, non-profit right protection agency for persons with disabilities residin in Washington state. Our advocacy services include information referral, technical assistance, training, publications and systemic advocacy.

3654 International Dyslexia Association: Washington State Branch
P.O.Box 27435
Seattle, WA 98165 206-382-1020
800-222-3123
e-mail: info@wabida.org
www.wabita.org
Kay Nelson, President
Kathleen Conklin, Secretary
Bev Wolf, Treasurer
Janet Miller, Managing Director
Provides free information and referral services for diagnosis and tutoring for parents, educators, physicians, and individuals with dyslexia in Arkansas, Idaho, Montana and Washington state. The voice of our membership is heard in 48 countries. Membership includes yearly journal and quarterly newsletter. Call for conference dates.

3655 Social Security: Olympia Disability Determination
Social Security
P.O. Box 9303-MS-45550
Olympia, WA 98507 360-664-7356
800-772-1213
800-562-6074
FAX: 360-586-0851
TTY:800-325-0778
e-mail: Jennifer.Elsen@ssa.gov
www.ssa.gov
Karena L. Kilgore, Executive Secretary
Carolyn W. Colvin, Commissioner
Carolyn W. Colvin, Deputy Commissioner
James A. Kissko, Chief of Staff
We deliver services through a nationwide network of over 1,400 offices that include regional offices, field offices, card centers, teleservice centers, processing centers, hearing offices, the Appeals Council, and our State and territorial partners, the Disability Determination Services. We also have a presence in U.S.

embassies around the globe. The rich diversity of our employees mirrors the public we serve.

3656 WA Department of Services for the Blind
4565 7th Avenue SE
PO Box 40933
Lacey, WA 98503
360-725-3830
800-552-7103
FAX: 360-407-0679
e-mail: info@dsb.wa.gov
www.dsb.wa.gov

Sue Ammeter, council chair
Nancy Kim
Veronica Baca, Council Member
Michael Cunningham, Council Member
Vocational rehabilitation for the blind.

3657 Washington Client Assistance Program
2531 Rainier Ave S
Seattle, WA 98144-5328
206-721-5999
800-544-2121
888-721-6072
FAX: 206-721-4537
TTY:206-721-6072
e-mail: info@washingtoncap.org
www.washingtoncap.org

Jerry Johnson, Executive Director
Bob Huven, rehabilitation coordinator
Advocacy and information assistance for persons of disability seeking services through vocational rehabilitation or other program under the 1973 Rehabilitation Act as commented. We provide counseling.

3658 Washington Department of Mental Health
Department of Social and Health Services
P.O.Box 45330
Olympia, WA 98504-5330
360-725-3700
800-446-0259
FAX: 360-902-7691
TTY: 800-833-6384
e-mail: adsahelpdesk@dshs.wa.gov
www.dshs.wa.gov

Chris Imhoff, DBHR Director
David Albert, Sr. Planner and Policy Analyst,
Debbie Arthur, Fiscal Program Manager
Stephanie Atherton,, Prevention Systems Manager
In July 2009 the DSHS Division of Alcohol and Substance Abuse and the Mental Health Division merged to become the Division of Behavioral Health and Recovery (DBHR). Through this integration, we are in a better position to both assess and treat patients with co-occurring mental health and substance use disorders. Our longer term vision calls for the fullest possible integration of behavioral health and primary care services under health reform, creating a person-centered health care home for al

3659 Washington Developmental Disability
2600 Martin Way E
Suite F
Olympia, WA 98506-4974
360-586-3560
800-634-4473
FAX: 360-586-2424
e-mail: Ed.Holen@ddc.wa.gov
www.ddc.wa.gov

Diana Zottman, Chairman
Ed Holen, Executive Director
Brain Dahl, Support Coordinator
Laurie Bahr, Budget & Fiscal Director
Developmental Disabilities Council members are appointed by the Governor to plan comprehensive services for the State of Washington's citizens with developmental disabilities.

3660 Washington Governor's Committee on Disability Issues & Employment
605 Woodland Square Loop SE
Lacey, WA 98503
360-438-3168
FAX: 360-438-3208
e-mail: gcdetz@gmail.com
www.gcde.org

Martin Haule, Director
Toby Olson, Manager

3661 Washington Office of Superintendent of Public Instruction
600 Washington St. S.E.
P. O. Box 47200
Olympia, WA 98504-7200
360-725-6000
TTY:360-644-3631
e-mail: webmaster@ospi.wednet.edu
www.k12.wa.us

Randy Dorn, State Superintendent
Alan Burke, Deputy Superintendent
Robert Butts, Assistant Superintendent
Ken Kanikeberg, Chief of Staff
The Office of Superintendent of Public Instruction (OSPI) is the primary agency charged with overseeing K-12 education in Washington state. OSPI works with the state's 296 school districts to administer basic education programs and implement education reform on behalf of more than one million public school students.

3662 Washington State Developmental Disabilities Council
2600 Martin Way E
Suite F
Olympia, WA 98506-4974
360-586-3560
800-634-4473
FAX: 360-586-2424
e-mail: Ed.Holen@ddc.wa.gov
www.ddc.wa.gov

Diana Zottman, Chairman
Ed Holen, Executive Director
Brain Dahl, Support Coordinator
Laurie Bahr, Budget & Fiscal Director
Developmental Disabilities Council members are appointed by the Governor to plan comprehensive services for the State of Washington's citizens with developmental disabilities.

3663 Workers Compensation Board Washington
State of Washington
7273 Linderson Way SW
Tumwater, WA 98501-5414
360-902-5800
800-547-8367
FAX: 360-902-5798
TTY: 360-902-5797
www.lni.wa.gov

Judy Schurke, Director
Lisa Rodriguez, Executive Assistant
Vickie Kennedy, Special Assistant
Tamara Jones, Dir of Government Relations
&I is a diverse state agency dedicated to the safety, health and security of Washington's 3.2 million workers. We help employers meet safety and health standards and we inspect workplaces when alerted to hazards. As administrators of the state's workers' compensation system, we are similar to a large insurance company, providing medical and limited wage-replacement coverage to workers who suffer job-related injuries and illness. Our rules and enforcement programs also help ensure workers are pai

West Virginia

3664 Bureau of Employment Programs Division of Workers' Compensation
State of West Virginia
409 Virginia St E
Charleston, WV 25301-2531
304-357-0101
800-628-4265
FAX: 304-357-0788
e-mail: helpdesk@kanawha.us
kanawha.us
Patricia Starkey, Manager
Vern Cormick, Manager
Michael ' Campbell, Director of IT
Larry McDonnell, Chief Webmaster
Kanawha County today is an exciting technology center that is earning recognition in information technology, medical research, chemical synthesis research, and telecommunications.

3665 Disability Determination Section
Ste 500
500 Quarrier St
Charleston, WV 25301-2913
304-343-5055
800-772-1213
800-344-5033
FAX: 304-353-4212
e-mail: Kenneth.Lim@ssa.gov
www.ssa.gov
Karena L. Kilgore, Executive Secretary
Carolyn W. Colvin, Commissioner
Carolyn W. Colvin, Deputy Commissioner
James A. Kissko, Chief of Staff
We deliver services through a nationwide network of over 1,400 offices that include regional offices, field offices, card centers, teleservice centers, processing centers, hearing offices, the Appeals Council, and our State and territorial partners, the Disability Determination Services. We also have a presence in U.S. embassies around the globe. The rich diversity of our employees mirrors the public we serve.

3666 Social Security: Charleston Disability Determination
Social Security
500 Quarrier Street
Suite 500
Charleston, WV 25301-2913
304-343-5055
800-772-1213
800-344-5033
FAX: 304-353-4212
e-mail: Kenneth.Lim@ssa.gov
www.ssa.gov
Karena L. Kilgore, Executive Secretary
Carolyn W. Colvin, Commissioner
Carolyn W. Colvin, Deputy Commissioner
James A. Kissko, Chief of Staff
We deliver services through a nationwide network of over 1,400 offices that include regional offices, field offices, card centers, teleservice centers, processing centers, hearing offices, the Appeals Council, and our State and territorial partners, the Disability Determination Services. We also have a presence in U.S. embassies around the globe. The rich diversity of our employees mirrors the public we serve.

3667 West Virginia Advocates
1207 Quarrier St
Suite 400
Charleston, WV 25301-1826
304-346-0847
800-950-5250
FAX: 304-346-0867
e-mail: kellie.l.aikman@wv.gov
wvadvocates.org
Terry Dilcher, President
John Galloway, Treasurer
Don Neurman, Secretary
Clarice Hausch, Executive Director
West Virginia Advocates, Inc. (WVA) is the federally mandated protection and advocacy system for people with disabilities in West Virginia. WVA is a private, nonprofit agency. Our services are confidential and free of charge.

3668 West Virginia Client Assistance Program
West Virginia Advocates
1900 Kanawha Blvd E
Room 9
Charleston, WV 25305-1
304-558-3780
FAX: 304-558-4092
e-mail: vhuffman@access.k12.wv.us
legis.state.wv.us
Clarice Hausch, Executive Director

3669 West Virginia Department of Aging
1900 Kanawha Blvd. East
Charleston, WV 25305
304-558-3317
877-987-3646
FAX: 304-558-5609
e-mail: hollygrove@juno.com
www.wvseniorservices.gov
Robert E. Roswall, Commissioner
Nel Kimble
The information we offer is tailored to those who are seeking to locate programs and services for themselves or their loved ones and also for professionals who may be looking for up-to-date information relating to the field of aging.

3670 West Virginia Department of Children with Disabilities
Children with Special Health Care Needs
One Davis Square
Suite 100 East
Charleston, WV 25301- 1757
304-558-0684
FAX: 304-558-1130
e-mail: DHHRSecretary@wv.gov
www.dhhr.wv.gov
Douglas M. Robinson, Deputy Commissioner
Virginia Mahan, Executive Secretary
Karen Villanueva-Matkovich, General Counsel
Melissa Rosen, CFO
The Bureau for Public Health directs public health activities at all levels within the state to fulfill the core functions of public health: the assessment of community health status and available resources; policy development resulting in proposals to support and encourage better health; and assurance that needed services are available, accessible, and of acceptable quality.

3671 West Virginia Department of Health
One Davis Square
Suite 100 East
Charleston, WV 25301
304-558-0684
FAX: 304-558-1130
e-mail: DHHRSecretary@wv.gov
www.dhhr.wv.gov
Douglas M. Robinson, Deputy Commissioner
Virginia Mahan, Executive Secretary
Karen Villanueva-Matkovich, General Counsel
Melissa Rosen, CFO
The Bureau for Public Health directs public health activities at all levels within the state to fulfill the core functions of public health: the assessment of community health status and available resources; policy development resulting in proposals to support and encourage better health; and assurance that needed services are available, accessible, and of acceptable quality.

3672 West Virginia Developmental Disabilities Council
110 Stockton St
Charleston, WV 25387
304-558-0416
FAX: 304-558-0941
TTY:304-558-2376
e-mail: dhhrwvddc@wv.gov
www.ddc.wv.gov
Diana Zottman, Chairman
Ed Holen, Executive Director
Brain Dahl, Support Coordinator
Laurie Bahr, Budget & Fiscal Director
Working to assure that West Virginians with developmental disabilities receive the services, supports, and other forms of assis-

tance they need to exercise self-determination and achieve independence, productivity, integration, and inclusion in the community.
6-8 pages Quarterly Newsl

3673 West Virginia Division of Rehabilitation Services
107 Capitol Street
Charleston, WV 25301-2609
304-356-2060
800-642-8207
www.wvdrs.org
Donna L. Ashworth, Acting Director
Kay Goodwin, Cabinet Secretary
DRS' mission is to enable and empower individuals with disabilities to work and to live independently.

Wisconsin

3674 Disability Rights Wisconsin: Milwaukee Office
Ste 3230
6737 W Washington St
Milwaukee, WI 53214-5651
414-773-4646
800-708-3034
FAX: 414-773-4647
TTY: 888-758-6049
e-mail: info@drwi.org
disabilityrightswi.org
Tom Masseau, Executive Director
Linda Apple, Office Manager
Molly Bandt, Managing Attorney
Kristine Beck, Administrative Specialist
The protection and advocacy agency for people with disabilities in Wisconsin. DRW provides guidance, advice, investigation, negotiation and in some cases legal representation to people with disabilities and their families. Local and state level systems advocacy and training are also provided.

3675 International Dyslexia Association: Wisconsin Branch
133 W. Ellsworth Lane Bayside
Baraboo, WI 53217
608-355-0911
800-222-3123
e-mail: wibida@gmail.com.
www.wibida.org
Tammy Tillotson, President
Kimberly Chan, Treasurer
Connie Day, Director
Darlene Larson, Director
The International Dyslexia Association actively promotes effective teaching approaches and related clinical educational intervention strategies for dyslexics. We support and encourage interdisciplinary study and research. We facilitate the exploration of the causes and early identification of dyslexia and are committed to the responsible and wide dissemination of research-based knowledge.

3676 Social Security: Madison Field Office
6011 Odana Rd
Madison, WI 53719-1101
866-770-2262
800-772-1213
FAX: 608-270-1021
TTY: 800-325-0778
e-mail: wi.fo.madison@ssa.gov
www.ssa.gov

3677 West Virginia Department of Health
One Davis Square
Suite 100 East
Charleston, WV 25301
304-558-0684
800-441-4576
FAX: 304-558-1130
e-mail: DHHRSecretary@wv.gov
www.dhhr.wv.gov
Rocco S. Fucillo, Cabinet Secretary
Susan Shelton Perry, Deputy Secretary for Legal Servi
Ellen Cannon, Privacy Officer
Virginia Mahan, Executive Secretary
The Department of Health and Family Services operates the federal Title V Maternal and Child Health Block Grant Program for Children with Special Health Care Needs. The program provides program monitoring, consultation and technical assistance to five regional CSHCN centers throughout Wisconsin; a Birth Defects Monitoring and Surveillance Program and a Universal Newborn Hearing Screening Program.

3678 Wisconsin Board for People with Developmental Disabilities (WBPDD)
201 W Washington Ave
Suite 111
Madison, WI 53703-2796
608-266-7826
888-332-1677
FAX: 608-267-3906
TTY:608-266-6660
e-mail: bpddhelp@wcdd.org
wcdd.org
Jennifer Ondrejka, Manager
Joshua Ryf, Office Manager
Statewide systems advocacy group for people with developmental disabilities in Wisconsin.

3679 Wisconsin Bureau of Aging
State Office of Wisconsin
1 West Wilson Street
Madison, WI 53703
608-266-1865
FAX: 608-267-3203
TTY:888-701-1251
e-mail: DHSwebmaster@wisconsin.gov
www.dhfs.state.wi.us/aging
Donna Mc Dowell, Executive Director
Gail Schwersenska, Section Chief
Dennis G. Smith, Secreatary
Keeps and updates information and printed materials on senior housing directories, nursing home listings, and home care agencies.

3680 Wisconsin Coalition for Advocacy: Madison Office
16 N Carroll St
Suite 400
Madison, WI 53703-2762
608-267-0214
800-928-8778
FAX: 608-267-0368
www.w-c-a.org
Kim Hogan, Intake Specialist
Mr Lynn Breedlove, Executive Director
The protection and advocacy agency for people with disabilities in Wisconsin. WCA provides guidance, advice, investigation, negotiation and in some cases legal representation to people with disabilities and their families. Local and state level systems advocacy and training are also provided.

3681 Wisconsin Governor's Committee for People with Disabilities
1 West Wilson Street
Madison, WI 53703
608-266-1865
877-865-3432
FAX: 608-266-3386
TTY: 888-701-1251
e-mail: DHSwebmaster@wisconsin.gov
www.dhfs.state.wi.us
Donna Mc Dowell, Executive Director
Gail Schwersenska, Section Chief
Dennis G. Smith, Secreatary
To advise the Governor and state agencies on problems faced by people with disabilities; to review legislation affecting people with disabilities; to promote effective operation of publicly-administered or supported programs serving people with disabilities; to promote the collection, dissemination and incorporation of adequate information about persons with disabilities for purposes of public planning at all levels of government.

3682 Workers Compensation Board Wisconsin
Room C100, 201 E. Washington Avenue
P. O. Box 7901
Madison, WI 53707-7901
608-266-1340
FAX: 608-267-0394
dwd.wisconsin.gov/wc

Reggie Newson, Secretary
Jonathan Barry, Deputy Secretary
John Metcalf, Division Administrator
Brain Krueger, Deputy Administrator

The Worker's Compensation Division administers programs designed to ensure that injured workers receive required benefits from insurers or self-insured employers; encourage rehabilitation and reemployment for injured workers; and promote the reduction of work-related injuries, illnesses, and deaths.

Wyoming

3683 Social Security: Cheyenne Disability Determination
Social Security
821 W Pershing Blvd
Cheyenne, WY 82002-1
307-777-7341
800-438-5788
FAX: 307-637-0247
e-mail: Jeff.Graham@ssa.gov
ssa.gov

Karena L. Kilgore, Executive Secretary
Carolyn W. Colvin, Commissioner
Carolyn W. Colvin, Deputy Commissioner
James A. Kissko, Chief of Staff

We deliver services through a nationwide network of over 1,400 offices that include regional offices, field offices, card centers, teleservice centers, processing centers, hearing offices, the Appeals Council, and our State and territorial partners, the Disability Determination Services. We also have a presence in U.S. embassies around the globe. The rich diversity of our employees mirrors the public we serve.

3684 WY Department of Health: Mental Health and Substance Abuse Service Division
401HathawayBuilding
Cheyenne, WY 82002-1
307-777-7656
800-535-4006
FAX: 307-777-7439
TTY: 307-777-5581
e-mail: wdh@state.wy.us
www.health.wyo.gov

Thomas O. Forslund, Director
Lee Clabots, Deputy Director
Bob Peck, Chief Financial Officer
Heather Babbitt, Senior Administartor

State office responsible for purchase of service and program development policy.

3685 Workers Compensation Board Wyoming
350 South Washington Street
PO Box 1068
Afton, WY 83110-3004
307-886-9260
FAX: 307-886-9269
wyomingworkforce.or

3686 Wyoming Client Assistance Program
Protection and Advocacy System
2nd Fl
320 W 25th St
Cheyenne, WY 82001-3069
307-632-2682
877-854-5041
FAX: 307-638-0815
e-mail: wypanda@vcn.com
ap.org

Jeanne Thobro, Manager
Jeanne A Thobro, Executive Director

3687 Wyoming Department of Aging
State Department of Wyoming
401HathawayBuilding
Cheyenne, WY 82002-1
307-777-7656
800-442-2766
FAX: 307-777-7439
e-mail: wyaging@wyo.gov
health.wyo.gov

Thomas O. Forslund, Director
Lee Clabots, Deputy Director
Bob Peck, Chief Financial Officer
Heather Babbitt, Senior Administartor

The Wyoming Department of Health's Aging Division is committed to providing care, ensuring safety and and promoting independent choices for Wyoming's older adults

3688 Wyoming Developmental Disability Council
122 W 25th St
1st. Fl. West, Herschler Building,
Cheyenne, WY 82002
307-777-7230
800-438-5791
FAX: 307-777-5690
e-mail: wgcdd@wyo.gov
ddcouncil.state.wy.u

Shannon Buller, Executive Director
Von Maul, Administrative Assistant
Sam Janney, Public Information Officer
Calob Taylor, Grants & Policy Analyst

Our purpose is to assure that individuals with developmental disabilities and their families participate in and have access to needed community services, individualized supports and other forms of assistance that promote independence, productivity, integration and inclusion in all facets of community life.

3689 Wyoming Protection & Advocacy for Persons with Disabilities
7344 Stockman Street
Cheyenne, WY 82009
307-632-3496
FAX: 307-638-0815
e-mail: wypanda@wypanda.com
wypanda.com

Tori Rosenthal, President
Jeanne A Thobro, Executive Director

Wyoming Protection & Advocacy System, Inc. (P&A), established in 1977, is the official non-profit corporation authorized to implement certain mandates of several federal laws. Enacted by Congress, these laws provide various protection and advocacy services.

Independent Living Centers

Alabama

3690 **Birdie Thornton Center**
2350 Hine Street
Athens, AL 35611
256-232-0366
FAX: 256-230-9398
www.birdiethorntoncenter.com

Kristy Allen King, Program Director
Heather Mereidth, Program Professional, QMRP
Rabieb Clem, Senior Aid
Kay Green, Training Specialist

The Birdie Thornton Center is devoted to providing care, education, and training to adults with developmental delays and disabilities.

3691 **Independent Living Center of Mobile**
5301 Moffett Rd
Suite 110
Mobile, AL 36618-2926
251-460-0301
FAX: 251-341-1267
TTY:251-460-2872
e-mail: Michaeld@ilcmobile.org
ilcmobile.org

Michael Davis, Executive Director
Darmita Flood, Administrative Assistant
Barbara Hattier, ILS/Transportation Coordinator
James Flora, ILS/Outreach Specialist

Helping people with disabilities become independent.

3692 **Independent Living Resources Of Greater Birmingham: Alabaster**
120 Plaza Cir, Suite C
P. O. Box 2048
Alabaster, AL 35007-7034
205-685-0570
FAX: 205-251-0605
TTY:205-685-0570
e-mail: gwen.brown@drradvocates.org
www.ilrgb.org

Graham Sisson, President
Elizabeth Ray, Vice President
Susan Parker, Secretary
Phil Klebine, Treasurer

The mission of this Independent Living Center is to empower people with disabilities to fully participate in the community.

3693 **Independent Living Resources of Greater Birmingham: Jasper**
300 Birmingham Ave
PO Box 434
Jasper, AL 35501-3811
205-387-0159
FAX: 205-387-0162
TTY:205-387-0159
e-mail: vickie.stovall@drradvocates.org
www.ilrgb.org

Graham Sisson, President
Elizabeth Ray, Vice President
Susan Parker, Secretary
Phil Klebine, Treasurer

The purpose of this Independent Living Center is to empower people with disabilities to fully participate in the community.

3694 **Independent Living Resources of Greater Birmingham**
1418 6th Avenue North
Birmingham, AL 35203-1317
205-251-2223
FAX: 205-251-0605
TTY:205-251-2223
e-mail: judy.roy@drradvocates.org
www.ilrgb.org

Graham Sisson, President
Elizabeth Ray, Vice President
Susan Parker, Secretary
Phil Klebine, Treasurer

The mission of this Independent Living Center is to empower people with disabilities to fully participate in the community.

3695 **Montgomery Center for Independent Living**
600 S Court St
Montgomery, AL 36104-4106
334-240-2520
FAX: 334-240-6869
TTY:334-240-2520
e-mail: mcil@bellsouth.net
www.montgomerycil.org

Scott Renner, Executive Director
Barbara F. Crozier, President
Kenneth Marshall, Vice President
Vickie P. FitzGerald, Secretary

Encourgaes people with disabilities to support one another in reaching their own independent living goals.

Alaska

3696 **Access Alaska: ADA Partners Project**
1217 East 10th Ave
Suite 105
Anchorage, AK 99501-2044
907-248-4777
800-770-4488
888-462-1444
FAX: 907-263-1942
TTY:907-248-8799
e-mail: info@accessalaska.org
accessalaska.org

Lorali Simon, President
Mike O'Neill, Vice President
Jim Duffield, Treasurer
Eric Spangler, Member

Assisting Alaskans with disabilities to live independently in the community of their choice.

3697 **Access Alaska: Fairbanks**
526 Gaffney Rd
Suite 100
Fairbanks, AK 99701-4914
907-479-7940
800-770-7940
FAX: 907-474-4052
TTY: 907-474-8619
e-mail: info@accessalaska.org
accessalaska.org

Mike O'Neill, President
Lorali Simon, Vice President
Jim Babb, Secretary

A local non profit agency using its resources to actively promote a society where persons with disabilities can live and work independently in the community of their choice.

3698 **Access Alaska: Mat-Su**
1075 Check St,
Suite 109
Wasilla, AK 99654-6937
907-357-2588
800-770-0228
FAX: 907-357-5585
e-mail: info@accessalaska.org
accessalaska.org

Lorali Simon, President
Mike O'Neill, Vice President
Jim Duffield, Treasurer
Eric Spangler, Member

Provides independent living services to persons with significant disabilities. Mission is to encourage and promote the total integration of persons with disabilities into the community of their choice. Services include independent living skills training, information and referral, advocacy, peer support, and at home modifications.

3699 Alaska SILC
Ste 206
1057 W Fireweed Ln
Anchorage, AK 99503-1760
907-263-2011
888-294-7452
FAX: 907-263-2012
e-mail: nationsa.silc@gmail.com
www.alaskasilc.org

Andi Nations, Executive Director

The Alaska Statewide Independent Living is committed to promoting a philosophy of consumer control, peer support, self help, self determination, equal access, and individual and systems advocacy, in order to maximize leadership, empowerment, independence, productivity, and to support full inclusion and integration of individuals with disabilities into the mainstream of American society.

3700 Arctic Access
P.O.Box 930
Kotzebue, AK 99752-930
907-412-0695
877-442-2393
TTY:907-442-2393
e-mail: arcticaccesskotz@gci.net
arcticaccesscil.org

Roger Wright Jr, Executive Director
Russell Williams, Jr,, Elder & Disability Resource Coor
Audrey Aanes

The Arctic Access Independent Living Center provides services and opportunities for elders and others with disabilities so they may remain in their village and be as active as possible with their families and commuities in the North West Arctic and Bering Straits Regions of Alaska.

3701 Hope Community Resources
540 W Intl Airport Rd
Anchorage, AK 99518-1105
907-561-5335
800-478-0078
FAX: 907-564-7429
e-mail: info@hopealaska.org
hopealaska.org

Robert Owens, President
John Dittrich, Vice President
Eugene 'Gene' Bates, Treasurer
Stephen P. Lesko, Executive Director

Provider of services to individuals who experience a disability.

3702 Kenai Peninsula Independent Living Center
265 E. Pioneer Suite 201
P.O.Box 2474
Homer, AK 99603- 2474
907-235-7911
800-770-7911
FAX: 907-235-6236
e-mail: info@peninsulailc.org
peninsulailc.org

Joyanna Geisler, Executive Director

Offers peer counseling, disability education and awareness, attendant care registry and information on accessible housing.

3703 Kenai Peninsula Independent Living Center: Seward
201 Third Avenue, Suite 101Bs
P. O. Box 3523
Seward, AK 99664-3523
907-224-8711
FAX: 907-224-7793
e-mail: info@peninsulailc.org
www.peninsulailc.org

Joyanna Geisler, Executive Director

Offers peer counseling, disability, education and awareness, attendant care registry and information on accessible housing.

3704 Keni Peninsula Independent Living Center: Central Peninsula
47255 Princeton Avenue
Suite 8
Soldotna, AK 99669
907-262-6333
FAX: 907-260-4495
e-mail: info@peninsulailc.org
www.peninsulailc.org

Joyanna Geisler, Executive Director

Offers peer counseling, disability education and awareness, attendant care registry and information on accessible housing.

3705 Southeast Alaska Independent Living
3225 Hospital Drive
Suite 300
Juneau, AK 99801-7863
907-586-4920
800-478-7245
FAX: 907-586-4980
TTY: 907-523-5285
e-mail: info@sailinc.org
sailinc.org

Robert Purvis, President
Jeff Irwin, Vice President
Joan O'Keefe, Executive Director
Jorden Nigro, Deputy Director

To empower consumers with disabilities by providing services and information to support them in making choices that will positively affect their independence and productivity in society.

3706 Southeast Alaska Independent Living: Ketchikan
602 Dock St
Suite 107
Ketchikan, AK 99901-6574
907-225-4735
888-452-7245
FAX: 907-247-4735
e-mail: ketchikan@sailinc.org
www.sailinc.org

Robert Purvis, President
Jeff Irwin, Vice President
Joan O'Keefe, Executive Director
Jorden Nigro, Deputy Director

To empower consumers with disabilities by providing services and information to support them in making choices that will positively affect their independence and productivity in society.

3707 Southeast Alaska Independent Living: Sitka
514 Lake St
Suite C
Sitka, AK 99835-7405
907-747-6859
888-500-7245
FAX: 907-747-6783
e-mail: sitka@sailinc.org
www.sailinc.org

Robert Purvis, President
Jeff Irwin, Vice President
Joan O'Keefe, Executive Director
Jorden Nigro, Deputy Director

To empower consumers with disabilities by providing services and information to support them in making choices that will positively affect their independence and productivity in society.

Arizona

3708 ASSIST! to Independence
P.O.Box 4133
Tuba City, AZ 86045-4133
928-283-6261
888-848-1449
FAX: 928-283-6284
TTY: 928-283-6672
e-mail: assist01@frontiernet.net
www.assisttoindependence.org

Michael Blatchford, Executive Director
Priscilla Lane, IL Services Coordinator/Dep Dir

A community based, American Indian owned and operated non-profit agency that was established by and for people with disabilities and chronic health conditions to help fill some of the gaps in service delivery.

3709 Arizona Bridge to Independent Living
5025 E Washington St
Suite 200
Phoenix, AZ 85034-7439
602-256-2245
800-280-2245
FAX: 602-254-6407
e-mail: boardofdirectors@abil.org
www.abil.org

Lynn Larson, Chairman
Mary Slaughter, Vice Chairman
Phil Pangrazio, President & CEO
Regina Mitzel, V. P. & Chief Administrative Officer

ABIL offers and promotes programs designed to empower people with disabilities to take personal responsibility so they may achieve or continue independent lifestyles within the community.

3710 Arizona Bridge to Independent Living: Phoenix
1229 E.Washington St.
Suite D405
Phoenix, AZ 85034
602-296-0551
800-280-2245
FAX: 602-256-0184
TTY: 602-296-0591
e-mail: boardofdirectors@abil.org
www.abil.org

Lynn Larson, Chairman
Mary Slaughter, Vice Chairman
Phil Pangrazio, President & CEO
Regina Mitzel, V. P. & Chief Administrative Officer

ABIL offers and promotes programs designed to empower people with disabilities to take personal responsibility so they may achieve or continue independent lifestyles within the community.

3711 Arizona Bridge to Independent Living: Mesa
2150 S Country Club Dr
Suite 10
Mesa, AZ 85210-6879
480-655-9750
800-280-2245
FAX: 480-655-9751
TTY: 480-655-9750
e-mail: boardofdirectors@abil.org
www.abil.org

Lynn Larson, Chairman
Mary Slaughter, Vice Chairman
Phil Pangrazio, President & CEO
Regina Mitzel, V. P. & Chief Administrative Officer

ABIL offers and promotes programs designed to empower people with disabilities to take personal responsibility so they may achieve or continue independent lifestyles within the community.

3712 Community Outreach Program for the Deaf
268 W Adams St
Tucson, AZ 85705-6534
520-792-1906
FAX: 520-770-8554
TTY:520-792-1906
e-mail: request@copdaz.org
copdaz.org

Anne Levy, Executive Director

A non-profit organization, which has been serving the needs of people in Southern Arizona who are deaf or hard of hearing.

3713 DIRECT Center for Independence
1023 N Tyndall Ave
Tucson, AZ 85719-4446
520-624-6452
800-342-1853
FAX: 520-792-1438
TTY: 520-624-6452
e-mail: direct@directilc.org
www.directilc.org

Ron Trozzi, President
Marrill Eisenberg, Vice President
Steve Fristoe, Treasurer
Loretta Alvarez, Secretary

A non-consumer directed, community-based advocacy organization, that promotes independent living and offers a variety of programs for all people with disabilities which encourage them to achieve their full potential and to participate in the community.

3714 New Horizons Independent Living Center: Prescott Valley
8085 E Manley Dr
Prescott Valley, AZ 86314-6154
928-772-1266
800-406-2377
FAX: 928-772-3808
TTY: 928-772-1266
e-mail: ltoone@newhorizonsilc.org
www.newhorizonsilc.org

Deborah Henderson, Adminstrative Assistant
Liz Toone, Executive Director

To provide services and advocacy which empower and enable people with disabilities to self-determine the goals and activities of their lives.

3715 Services Maximizing Independent Living and Empowerment (SMILE)
1931 South Arizona Ave
Suite 4
Yuma, AZ 85364-5721
928-329-6681
855-209-6715
FAX: 928-329-6715
TTY: 928-782-7458
e-mail: info@smile-az.org
www.smile-az.org

Laura Duval, Executive Director
Brenda Howard, Finance Manager/ Admin Assistant
Shawnnita Miranda, Advocate/ Home modification Mana
Brandon Howard, Outreach Coordinator, Technology

SMILE continually advocates for the Independent Living Philosophy, both individually and system wide. The Board and staff constantly strives to improve the system by writing letters, training staff, providing services, and creating public awareness as to the services and opportunities open to people who have disabilities.

3716 Sterling Ranch: Residence for Special Women
Sterling Ranch
P.O.Box 36
Skull Valley, AZ 86338-36
928-442-3289
FAX: 928-442-9272
e-mail: director@sterlingranch.info
www.sterlingranch.info

Russell Dryer, Executive Director
Trent Nichel, Manager

A nonprofit residence for women with developmental disabilities which has been in operation since 1947. As a small facility (19 residents) the orientation is personal and family-like. Offers activities that range from gardening, quilting, academics, sign-language, crafts and a myriad of field trips and excursions. Private rooms and spacious living on 4 1/2 acres.

Arkansas

3717 Arkansas Independent Living Council
11324 Arcade Drive
Suite 7
Little Rock, AR 72212
501-372-0607
800-772-0607
FAX: 501-372-0598
e-mail: arkansasilc@att.net
www.ar-ilc.org

Katy Morris, Director
Cheryl, Director
Brenda Stinebuck, Chair
Liz Adams, Vice Chair

A non-profit organization promoting independent living for people with disabilities.

3718 **Delta Resource Center for Independent Living**
3131 West 28th Avenue
Pine Bluff, AR 71603-6249 870-535-2222
FAX: 800-824-0009
e-mail: drcilar@yahoo.com
www.ar-ilc.org

Lynne McAllester, Director
Katy Morris, Director
Cheryl, Director
Brenda Stinebuck, Chair

Provides services, support, and advocacy which enables people with severe disabilities to live as independently as possible within their family and community.

3719 **Mainstream**
300 S Rodney Parham Rd
Suite 5
Little Rock, AR 72205- 4774 501-280-0012
800-371-9026
FAX: 501-280-9267
TTY: 501-280-9262
e-mail: mainstreamlrc@earthlink.net
mainstreamilrc.com

Rita Byers, Executive Director
Vincent McKinney
Vincent Acklin
Debbie Gillespie

A non residential, consumer driven independent living resource center for persons with disabilities. Mainstream operates with conviction that people with disabilities have the right and responsibility to make choices, to control their lives and to participate fully and equally in the community.

3720 **Our Way: The Cottage Apt Homes**
10434 W 36th St
Little Rock, AR 72204-6616 501-225-5030
FAX: 501-225-5190

Katrina Williams, Manager
Crystal Brown, Assistant Manager

Advocacy and information services. One bedroom apartments for mobility impaired and elderly 62 years or older persons.
Based on income

3721 **Sources for Community IL Services**
1918 N Birch Ave
Fayetteville, AR 72703-2408 479-442-5600
888-284-7521
FAX: 479-442-5192
TTY: 479-251-1378
e-mail: jmather@arsources.org
www.arsources.org

Brent Williams, PhD, President
Elise Burt, Treasurer
Burke Fanari, Secretary
Jim Mather, Executive Director

Provides services, support, and advocacy for individuals with disabilities, their families and the community.

3722 **Spa Area Independent Living Services**
621AlbertPike
Hot Springs, AR 71913 501-624-7710
800-255-7549
FAX: 501-624-7003
e-mail: info@restsearch.com
www.ar-sails.org

Dejan S. Vojnovic, President
Joseph E. Anderson, Vice President - Real Estate
Bryan S. Cox, Vice President - Technology
Brenda Stinebuck, Executive Director

Provides services and advocacy by and for persons with all types of disabilities. The goal is to assist individuals with disabilities to achieve thier maximum potential within their families and communities.

California

3723 **Access Center of San Diego**
8885 Rio San Diego Dr
Suite 131
San Diego, CA 92108-1625 619-293-3500
800-300-4326
FAX: 619-293-3508
TTY: 619-293-7757
e-mail: info@a2isd.org
www.a2isd.org

Louis Frick, Executive Director
Deirdre DuPlessis, Director of Administration
Amy Kalivas, Program Manager
Leticia Vizcarra, Program Manager

Access to Independence is an independent living center (ILC), a nonresidential, cross-disability, non-profit corporations that provide services to people with disabilities to help maximize their independence and fully integrate into their communities. Access to Independence is one of 391 ILCs across the country and one of 29 serving Californians. Like all ILCs, Access to Independence offers required federal and state programs and services to people of all disability types and ages at no charge.

3724 **Access to Independence**
8885 Rio San Diego Drive
Suite 131
San Diego, CA 92108- 1625 619-293-3500
800-300-4326
FAX: 619-293-3508
TTY: 619-293-7757
e-mail: info@a2isd.org
www.a2isd.org

Louis Frick, Executive Director
Deirdre DuPlessis, Director of Administration
Amy Kalivas, Program Manager
Leticia Vizcarra, Program Manager

A community resource for people with disabilities to lead independent lives.

3725 **Access to Independence of Imperial Valley**
101 Hacienda Drive
Suite 13
Calexico, CA 92231-2875 760-768-2044
866-976-3515
FAX: 760-768-4977
TTY: 619-293-7757
e-mail: info@a2isd.org
www.a2sid.org

Louis Frick, Executive Director
Deirdre DuPlessis, Director of Administration
Amy Kalivas, Program Manager
Leticia Vizcarra, Program Manager

A community resource for people with disabilities to lead independent lives.

3726 **Access to Independence of North County**
209 E Broadway
Vista, CA 92084-6005 760-643-0447
FAX: 760-435-9206
e-mail: info@a2isd.org
www.a2sid.org

Louis Frick, Executive Director
Deirdre DuPlessis, Director of Administration
Amy Kalivas, Program Manager
Leticia Vizcarra, Program Manager

A community resource for people with disabilities to lead independent lives.

3727 **Beaumont Senior Center: Community Access Center**
1310 Oak Valley Parkway
Beaumont, CA 92223-2218 951-769-8539
FAX: 951-769-1372
TTY:909-769-2794
e-mail: ilser5@ilcac.org

Laurie Hoirup, Director

A non profit organization; one of 29 similar programs throughout the state of California CAC is a community resource, advocate, and educator for Riverside County residents with disabilities.

3728 California Foundation For Independent Living Centers
1234 H Street
Suite 100
Sacramento, CA 95814-1912
916-325-1690
FAX: 916-325-1699
TTY:916-325-1695
e-mail: cfilc@cfilc.org
www.cfilc.org

Robert Hand, Chairperson
Ana Acton, Vice Chairperson
Tink Miller, Executive Director
Kim Cantrell, Program Director
Community Rehabilitation Services, Inc. (CRS) is a private, non-profit agency established in 1974 to assist persons with disabilities within the East/North East areas of Los Angeles County to enhance their options for living independently. Any person who is 18 yrs of age or more with physical, sensory, mental/emotional or developmental disabilities can work with us to become more self-sufficient. Our intake procedures provide an orientation to the staff, facilities and services at CRS.

3729 California Foundation for Independent Living Centers
1235 H Street
Suite 100
Sacramento, CA 95814-1913
916-325-1690
FAX: 916-325-1699
TTY:916-325-1695
e-mail: cfilc@cfilc.org
www.cfilc.org

Robert Hand, Chairperson
Ana Acton, Vice Chairperson
Tink Miller, Executive Director
Kim Cantrell, Program Director
CFILC's mission is to support independent living centers in their local communities through advocating for systems change and promoting access and integration for people with disabilities.

3730 California State Independent Living Council (SILC)
1600 K St
Suite 100
Sacramento, CA 95814-4010
916-445-0142
866-866-7452
FAX: 916-445-5973
TTY: 866-745-2889
e-mail: neal@calsilc.org
www.calsilc.org

Susan M. Madison, Chairman
Eli Gelardin, Vice Chairman
Liz Pazdral, Executive Director
Caroline Kuhn, Staff Services Analyst
To maximize options for independence for persons with disabilities

3731 Center for Independence of the Disabled
Ste 400
1515 S El Camino Real
San Mateo, CA 94402-3062
650-645-1780
FAX: 650-645-1785
TTY:650-522-9313
e-mail: info@cidbelmont.org
http://www.cidsanmateo.org

Brad Friedman, Co-President
Laura Whitsitt Hillyard, Co-President
Thomas J. Devine, Vice President
John Horgan, Secretary
Increase the social, educational, and economic participation of persons with disabilities in San Mateo County, and to encourage, support, and provide options for self determination, equal access and freedom of choice.

3732 Center for Independence of the Disabled- Daly City
Ste 256
355 Gellert Blvd
Daly City, CA 94015-2675
650-991-5124
FAX: 650-757-2075
TTY:650-991-5182
e-mail: dalycity5@aol.com
www.cidbelmont.org

Kent Mickelson, Director
The Daly City Branch office fulfills its mission by serving disabled consumers in Brisbane, Colma, Daly City, El Granada, Half Moon Bay, Montara, Moss Beach, Pacifica, Pescadero, Princeton and South San Francisco. Our mission is to increase the social, educational, economic, social and political participants of persons with disabilities in San Mateo county, California.

3733 Center for Independent Living
3075 Adeline Street, Suite 100
Berkeley, CA 94703
510-841-4776
FAX: 510-841-6168
TTY:510-848-3101
e-mail: ywrong@cilberkeley.org
cilberkeley.org

Yomi Wrong, Executive Director
Makr Burns, Deputy Director
The Center for Independent Living, Inc (CIL) is a national leader in helping people with disabilities live independently and become productive members of society. Founded in 1972, CIL is a pioneer advocating for greater accessibility in communities, designing techniques in independent living and providing direct services to people with disabilities. A partial list of services includes Information and Referral, Personal Assistance Services, Independent Living Skills Training and Peer Counseling.

3734 Center for Independent Living: East Oakland
Ste 9a
7200 Bancroft Ave
Oakland, CA 94605-2403
510-635-4920
FAX: 510-635-4261
e-mail: cwood@cilberkeley.org

Theo Polk, Manager
A national leader in helping people with disabilities live independently and become productive, fully participating members of society.

3735 Center for Independent Living: Oakland
1904 Franklin Street
Ste 320
Oakland, CA 94612-1285
510-763-9999
FAX: 510-763-4910
TTY:510-444-1837
e-mail: info@cilberkeley.org
cilberkeley.org

Henry Leng, President
Hank Stratford, Treasurer
Yomi Wrong, Executive Director
Ted Dienstfrey, Finance Committee
A national leader in supporting disabled people in their efforts to lead independent lives.

3736 Center for Independent Living: Tri-County
2822 Harris Street
Eureka, CA 95503
707-445-8404
877-576-5000
FAX: 707-445-9751
TTY: 707-445-8405
e-mail: aa@tilinet.org
www.tilinet.org

Gail Pascoe, President
Linda Arnold, Vice President
Kevin O'Brien, Tresurer
Chris Jones, Executive Director

3737 **Center for Independent Living:Fresno**
3475 Wesy Shaw Ave
Suite 101
Fresno, CA 93711 559-276-6777
FAX: 559-276-6778
TTY:559-276-6779
e-mail: execdirector@cil-fresno.org
www.cil-fresno.org

Bob Hand, Manager

3738 **Center for Independent Living; Oakland**
1904FranklinStreet
Suite 320
Oakland, CA 94601-2324 510-763-9990
FAX: 510-763-4910
TTY:510-536-2271
e-mail: info@cilberkeley.org
cilberkeley.org

Henry Leng, President
Hank Stratford, Treasurer
Paul Hippolitus, Member of Program
Ted Dienstfrey, Finance Committee
Independent living center to maximise the options for independence for persons with disabilities.

3739 **Center of Independent Living: Visalia**
121 E Main
Suite 101
Visalia, CA 93291-6262 559-622-9276
FAX: 559-622-9638
e-mail: f_phillips@cil-fresno.org
www.cil-fresno.org

Fran Phillips, Executive Directorram Manager
Renee Ezelle, Manager

3740 **Central Coast Center for IL: San Benito**
1235 H Street
Suite 100
Sacramento, CA 95814-1914 916-325-1690
FAX: 916-325-1699
TTY:916-325-1695
e-mail: cfile@cfilc.org
www.cfilc.org

Robert Hand, Chairperson
Ana Acton, Vice Chairperson
Tink Miller, Executive Director
Kim Cantrell, Program Director
To advocate for barrier-free access and equal opportunity for people with disabilities to participate in the community life by increasing the capacity of Independent Living Centers to achieve their missions.

3741 **Central Coast Center for Independent Living**
318 Cayuga St.
Suite 208
Salinas, CA 93901-2600 831-757-2968
FAX: 831-757-5549
TTY:831-757-3949
e-mail: cccil@cccil.org
cccil.org

Jennifer L. Williams, President
Elsa Quezada, Executive Director
Brenda Cardoza, Information and Referral Specialist
Gabriel Garcia, Independent Living Specialist
CCCIL promotes the independence of people with disabilities by supporting their equal and full participation in community life. CCCIL provides advocacy, education and support to all people with disabilities, their families and the community.

3742 **Central Coast Center: Independent Living - Santa Cruz Office**
350 - 41st Avenue
Suite 101
Capitola, CA 95010-3930 831-462-8720
FAX: 831-462-8727
TTY:831-462-8729
e-mail: cccil@cccil.org
www.cccil.org

Jennifer L. Williams, President
Elsa Quezada, Executive Director
Brenda Cardoza, Information and Referral Specialist
Gabriel Garcia, Independent Living Specialist
CCCIL promotes the independence of people with disabilities by supporting their equal and full participation in community life. CCCIL provides advocacy, education and support to all people with disabilities, their families and the community.

3743 **Central Coast for Independent Living**
1111 San Felipe Rd
Suite 107
Hollister, CA 95023-2814 831-636-5196
FAX: 831-637-0478
TTY:831-637-6235
e-mail: cccil@cccil.org
www.cccil.org

Jennifer L. Williams, President
Elsa Quezada, Executive Director
Brenda Cardoza, Information and Referral Specialist
Gabriel Garcia, Independent Living Specialist
CCCIL promotes the independence of people with disabilities by supporting their equal and full particpation in community life. CCCIL provides advocacy, education and support to all people with disabilities, their families and the community.

3744 **Central Coast for Independent Living: Watsonville**
18 W. Beach St.
Suite Y
Watsonville, CA 95076-4371 831-724-2997
FAX: 831-724-2915
TTY:831-786-0915
e-mail: cccil@cccil.org
www.cccil.org

Jennifer L. Williams, President
Elsa Quezada, Executive Director
Brenda Cardoza, Information and Referral Specialist
Gabriel Garcia, Independent Living Specialist
An advocacy and information center organized by and for people with disabilities that strives to make our communities more accessible and to empower people with disabilities with information and skills to live fulfilling lives in our communities.

3745 **Communities Actively Living Independent and Free**
634 S Spring St
2nd Floor
Los Angeles, CA 90014-3921 213-627-0477
FAX: 213-627-0535
TTY:213-623-9502
e-mail: info@calif-ilc.org
califilc1.wix.com

Lillibeth Navarro, Founder & Executive Director
Alex San Martin, Temporary Chair
Fernando Roldan, Board Secretary
Joseph Wander, Board Member
Envisions a culturally diverse independent living center designed to empower the Disability Community.

3746 Community Access Center
6848 Magnolia Ave
Suite 150
Riverside, CA 92506-2858
951-274-0358
FAX: 951-274-0833
TTY:951-274-0834
e-mail: execdir@ilcac.org
ilcac.org

Mark Dyer, President
Janet Newcomer, Vice President
Perry Halteman, Secretary
Chuck Reutter, Treasurer

A non-profit organization; one of 29 similar programs throughout the state of California. CAC is a community resource, advocate, and educator for Riverside County residents with disabilities.

3747 Community Access Center: Indio Branch
83233 Indio Blvd
Indio, CA 92201-4748
760-347-4888
FAX: 760-347-0722
TTY:760-347-6802
e-mail: pmgr3@ilcac.org
www.ilcac.org

Mark Dyer, President
Janet Newcomer, Vice President
Perry Halteman, Secretary
Chuck Reutter, Treasurer

To empower persons with disabilities to control their own lives, create an accessible community and advocate to achieve complete social, economic, and political integration. We implement this vision by providing information, supportive services and independent living skills training.

3748 Community Access Center: Perris
371 Wilkerson Ave
Perris, CA 92570-2241
951-443-1158
FAX: 951-443-2608
TTY:951-443-1158
e-mail: spmgr@ilcac.org
www.ilcac.org

Mark Dyer, President
Janet Newcomer, Vice President
Perry Halteman, Secretary
Chuck Reutter, Treasurer

Community Access Center empowers persons with disabilities to control their own lives, create an accessible community and advocate to achieve complete social, economic, and political integration. CAC also implements this vision by providing information, suportive services and independent living skills training.

3749 Community Rehabilitation Services
844 E. Mission Road
Suite A & B
San Gabriel, CA 91776- 2759
323-266-0453
FAX: 626-614-1590
TTY:323-266-3016
e-mail: executivedirector@crs-ilc.org
www.crs-ilc.org

Frances Garcia, Executive Director

CRS is an independent living center that provides free services to persons with disabilities in the areas of advocacy, housing and independent living skills; assistive technology, employment, personal assistant services, peer counseling and information and referral.

3750 Community Resources for Independence: Mendocino/Lake Branch
Ste B
415 Talmage Rd
Ukiah, CA 95482-7486
707-463-8875
FAX: 707-463-8878
TTY:707-463-4498
www.cri-dove.org

Tanner Silva, Manager

A non-profit corporation established by a group of disabled and non-disabled individuals to advance the rights of persons with disabilities to equal justice, access, opportunity and participation in the communities.

3751 Community Resources for Independence: Napa
Ste 208
1040 Main St
Napa, CA 94559-2605
707-258-0270
FAX: 707-258-0275
TTY:707-257-0274
cri-dove.org

Tyler Stanley, Manager
Matthew Shultz, Independent Living Advocate

A non-profit corporation established by a group of disabled and non-disabled individuals to advance the rights of persons with disabilities to equal justice, access, opportunity and participation in the communities.

3752 Community Resources for Independent Living: Hayward
3311 Pacific Ave
Livermore, CA 94550-5013
925-371-1531
FAX: 925-373-5034
TTY:925-371-1533
e-mail: info@cril-online.org
cril-online.org

Sheri Burns, Executive Director

CRIL offers independent living services at no charge to persons with disabilities living in southern and eastern Alameda county. CRIL is also a resource for disability awareness education and training, advocacy and technical advice.

3753 Community Resources for Independent Living
39155 Liberty St
Suite A100
Fremont, CA 94538-1503
510-794-5735
e-mail: info@cril-online.org
crilhayward.org

Sheri Burns, Executive Director
Michael Galvan, PhD., Program Director
April Monroe, Finance Director
Esperanza Diaz-Alvarez, PAS Coordinator/Benefits Advocat

Community Resources for Independent Living is a peer-based disability organization that advocates and provides resources for people with disabilities to improve lives and make communities fully accessible.

3754 DRAIL (Disability Resource Agency for Independent Living)
501 W Weber Ave
Ste 200-A
Stockton, CA 95203-6239
209-477-8143
FAX: 209-477-7730
TTY:209-465-5643
e-mail: barry@drail.org
www.drail.org

Terry Gray, President
Michael Kim Cornelius, Treasurer
Adeline Bagwell, Secretary
Barry Smith, Executive Director

A non-profit corporation that is community based, consumer controlled, consumer choice, cross disability center for independent living.

3755 Dayle McIntosh Center: Laguna Niguel
24031 El Toro Road
Suite 300
Laguna Hills, CA 92653-3632
949-460-7784
FAX: 949-855-8742
TTY:714-663-2087
www.daylemc.org

Libby Partain, President
Cindy McLeroy, Vice President
Eva Casas-Sarmiento, Secretary
Michael Ryan, Treasurer

DMC advances empowerment and inclusion of all persons with disabilities. DMC is the largest Independent Living Center in California, and was named in memory of a young woman with a severe physical disability who worked to found the center.

3756 Disability Resource Agency for Independent Living: Modesto
920-12th Street
Modesto, CA 95354-543
209-521-7260
FAX: 209-521-4763
TTY:209-576-2409
e-mail: larry@drail.org
www.drail.org

Barry Smith, Executive Director
Leng Power, Program Manager
Kris Rowe, Assistive Technology Advocat

A non-profit corporation that is community based, consumer controlled, consumer choice, cross disability center for independent living.

3757 Disability Services & Legal Center
521 Mendocino Ave.
Santa Rosa, CA 95401-1649
707-528-2745
FAX: 707-528-9477
TTY:707-528-2151
e-mail: dawsons@sonic.net
www.disabilityserviceandlegal.org

Adam Brown, Chairman
Shirley Johnson-Foell, Board President
Jack Geary, Board Member
Ben Karpilow, Board Secretary

A non-profit corporation established by a group of disabled and non-disabled individuals to advance the rights of persons with disabilities to equal justice, access, opportunity and participation in the communities.

3758 Disabled Resources Center
2750 E Spring St
Suite 100
Long Beach, CA 90806-2263
562-427-1000
FAX: 562-427-2027
TTY:562-427-1366
e-mail: info@drcinc.org
drcinc.org

C.Timothy Lashlee, President
Dora Hogan, Vice President
Finola Campbell, Treasurer
Dolores Nason, Executive Director

To empower people with disabilities to live independently in the community, to make their own decisions about their lives and to advocate on their own behalf.

3759 FREED Center for Independent Living
2059NevadaCity Hwy
Suite 102
GrassValley, CA 95945- 3227
530-477-3333
800-655-7732
FAX: 530-477-8184
TTY: 530-477-8194
e-mail: contact-04@freed.org
freed.org

Ana Acton, Executive Director

To eliminate barriers to full equality for people with disabilities through programs which promote independent living.

3760 FREED Center for Independent Living: Marysville
508 J St
Marysville, CA 95901-5636
530-742-4476
TTY:530-742-4474
e-mail: contact-04@freed.org
freed.org

Claudia Hallis, Manager

To eliminate barriers to full equality for people with disabilities through programs which promote independent living.

3761 First Step Independent Living
1174 Nevada St
Redlands, CA 92374-2893
800-362-0312
e-mail: cvsfs@deltanet.com

3762 Independent Living Center of Kern County
5251 Office Park Dr
Suite 200
Bakersfield, CA 93309
661-325-1063
877-688-2079
800-529-9541
FAX: 661-325-6702
TTY:661-325-6702
e-mail: info@ilcofkerncounty.org
www.ilcofkerncounty.org

Jimmie Soto, Executive Director
Tammy Hartsch, Finance Manager
Harvey Clowers, Special Projects and AT Coordina
Olivia Kent, Systems Change Advocate

A consumer-based consumer-directed non-profit agency assisting persons with disabilities to live independently in their community. The ILCKC presently offers a wide range of services to a growing population of persons with disabilities.

3763 Independent Living Center of Lancaster
606 East Avenue K4
Lancaster, CA 93535-2844
661-942-9726
FAX: 661-945-5690
TTY:661-723-2509
e-mail: ilcsclanc@ilcsc.org
www.ilcsc.org

Taura Jacob, Manager
Marcy Hernandez
Niyanta Dave

ILCSC is a non-profit, consumer based, non-residential agency providing a wide range of services to a growing population of people with disabilities. ILCSC is dedicated to empowering persons with disabilities to exercise indpendence-pofessionally, personally and creatively-while striving to educate the community on their needs.

3764 Independent Living Resource Center
7425 El Camino Real
Suite R
Atascadero, CA 93422-4656
805-464-3203
FAX: 805-462-1166
TTY:805-462-1162
e-mail: info@ilrc-trico.org
www.ilrc-trico.org

Dondra Lopez, M.A., President
Kathy McMillion, Vice President
Jo Black, Executive Director
Jennifer Griffin, Business Manager

To assist and encourage individuals to achieve their optimal level of self-sufficiency while eliminating the architectural, communication and attitudinal barriers which prevent them from full participation in the community.

3765 Independent Living Resource Center: Santa Barbara
423 W Victoria St
Santa Barbara, CA 93101-3619
805-284-9051
FAX: 805-963-1350
TTY:805-963-0595
e-mail: info@ilrc-trico.org
ilrc-trico.org

Dondra Lopez, M.A., President
Kathy McMillion, Vice President
Jo Black, Executive Director
Jennifer Griffin, Business Manager

To assist and encourage individuals to achieve their optimal level of self-sufficiency while eliminating the architectural, communication and attitudinal barriers which prevent them from full participation in the community.

3766 Independent Living Resource Center: San Francisco
Fl 3
649 Mission St
San Francisco, CA 94105-4128
415-543-6222
FAX: 415-543-6318
TTY:415-543-6698
e-mail: info@ilrcsf.org
ilrcsf.org

Jessie Lorenz, Executive Director

To ensure that people with disabilities are full social and economic partners, both within their families and in a fully accessible community.

3767 Independent Living Resource Center: Santa Maria Office
327 East Plaza Dr
Suite 3A
Santa Maria, CA 93454-6930 805-354-5948
FAX: 805-349-2416
TTY:805-925-0015
e-mail: info@ilrc-trico.org
www.ilrc-trico.org

Dondra Lopez, M.A., President
Kathy McMillion, Vice President
Jo Black, Executive Director
Jennifer Griffin, Business Manager
To assist and encourage individuals to achieve their optimal level of self-sufficiency while eliminating the architectural, communication and attitudinal barriers which prevent them from full participation in the community.

3768 Independent Living Resource Center: Ventura
1802 Eastman Ave
Suite 112
Ventura, CA 93003-5759 805-256-1036
FAX: 805-650-9278
TTY:805-650-5993
e-mail: info@ilrc-trico.org
www.ilrc-trico.org
Dondra Lopez, M.A., President
Kathy McMillion, Vice President
Jo Black, Executive Director
Jennifer Griffin, Business Manager
An organization of, by and for persons with disabilities who reside or work in the service area. Purpose is to assist and encourage individuals to achieve their optimal level of self-sufficiency while eliminating the architectural, communication and attitudinal barriers which prevent them from full participation in the community.

3769 Independent Living Resource of Contra Coast
1850 Gateway Blvd
Suite 120
Concord, CA 94520-3293 925-363-7293
FAX: 925-363-7296
ilrccc.org
Sarah BirdwelL, Board President
Kathy Mitsopoulos, Board Vice President
Teri Ruggiero, Board Secretary
Susan Rotchy, Executive Director
Offers workshops, services are accessible to individuals with cognitive disabilities, physical disabilities, deaf and hard of hearing, emotional disabilities, visual impairments, learing disabilities and seniors.

3770 Independent Living Resource of Fairfield
470 Chadbourn Rd
Ste. B
Fairfield, CA 94534 707-435-8174
FAX: 707-435-8177
e-mail: susanr@ilrcoco-sol.org
www.ilrccc.org
Sarah BirdwelL, Board President
Kathy Mitsopoulos, Board Vice President
Teri Ruggiero, Board Secretary
Susan Rotchy, Executive Director
To empower people with disabilities to: control their own lives, provide advocacy and support for individuals with disabilities to live independently, create an accessible community free of physical and attitudinal barriers.

3771 Independent Living Resource: Antioch
3727SunsetLane
#103
Antioch, CA 94509-1761 925-754-0539
TTY:925-755-0934
www.ilrccc.org
Sarah BirdwelL, Board President
Kathy Mitsopoulos, Board Vice President
Teri Ruggiero, Board Secretary
Susan Rotchy, Executive Director
Non-profit organizations run and controlled by persons with disabilities. They are non-residential, community-based centers where people with disabilities can receive assistance with a variety of daily living issues and learn the skills they need to take controll of their lives from people who have had similar experiences living with a disability.

3772 Independent Living Resource: Concord
1850 Gateway Blvd
Suite 120
Concord, CA 94520-3293 925-363-7293
FAX: 925-363-7296
e-mail: gilc@ilrccc.org
www.ilrccc.org
Bryan Balch, Executive Director
To empower people with disabilities to: control their own lives, provide advocacy and support for individuals with disabilities to live independently, create an accessible community free of physical and attitudinized barriers.

3773 Independent Living Resources (ILR)
Bldg 2a
101 Broadway
Richmond, CA 94804-1945 510-233-7400
e-mail: info@ilrccc.org
Marvin Dyson, Manager
Provides services to meet the diverse needs of people who have a variety of disabilities in all age groups.

3774 Independent Living Service Northern California: Redding Office
169 Hartnell Ave
Suite 128
Redding, CA 96002-1849 530-242-8550
800-464-8527
FAX: 530-241-1454
TTY: 530-242-8550
e-mail: info@ilsnc.org
www.ilsnc.org
Lauri Evans, President
Frank Smith, Vice President
Evan Levang, Executive Director
Tracy Barker, Program Manager
Independent Living Services of Northern California is a private non profit organization that provides support services to help empower community members with disabilities.

3775 Independent Living Services of Northern California
Jennifer Roberts Building
1161 East Ave
Chico, CA 95926-1018 530-893-8527
800-464-8527
FAX: 530-893-8574
TTY: 530-893-8527
e-mail: info@ilsnc.org
ilsnc.org
Lauri Evans, President
Frank Smith, Vice President
Evan Levang, Executive Director
Tracy Barker, Program Manager
Independent Living Services of Northern California is a private, non profit organization that provides support services to help empower community members with disabilities.

3776 Marin Center for Independent Living
710 4th St
San Rafael, CA 94901-3213
415-459-6245
FAX: 415-459-7047
TTY:415-459-7027
marincil.org

Chris Schultz, President
Joe Brnnett, Vice President
Eli Gelardin, Executive Director
Susan Malardino, Deputy Director

A non-profit organization that provides advocacy and services for seniors and persons with disabilities.

3777 Mother Lode Independent Living Center(DRAIL: Disability Resource Agency for Independent
Living)
67 Linoberg St
Suite A.
Sonora, CA 95370-4646
209-532-0963
FAX: 209-532-1591
TTY:209-288-3309
e-mail: barry@drail.org
www.drail.org

Terry Gray, President
Michael Kim Cornelius, Treasurer
Adeline Bagwell, Secretary
Barry Smith, Executive Director

DRAIL is a non-profit, community based, consumer controlled, cross disability center for independent living.

3778 Placer Independent Resource Services
11768 Atwood Road
Suite 29wood Rd
Auburn, CA 95603-9074
530-885-6100
800-833-3453
FAX: 530-885-3032
TTY: 530-885-0326
e-mail: tmiller@pirs.org
pirs.org

Susan Miller, Executive Director

A non profit independent living center whose mission is to advocate, empower, educate and provide services for people with disabilities enabling them to control their alternatives for independent living.

3779 Resources for Independent Living
420 i St, Level B.
Suite 3
Sacramento, CA 95814-2319
916-446-3074
FAX: 916-446-2443
e-mail: leonc@ril-sacramento.org
www.ril-sacramento.org

Ramona Garcia, Board Chairperson
Francisco Godoy, Vice Chairperson
Joanne Bodine, Treasurer
Frances Gracechild, Executive Director

Promoting the socio-economic independence of persons with disabilities by providing peer-supported, consumer-directed independent living services and advocacy.

3780 Rolling Start
570 W 4th St
Suite 107
San Bernardino, CA 92401-1438
909-884-2129
FAX: 909-386-7446
TTY:909-884-7396
e-mail: support@rollingstart.com
www.rollingstart.org

John Anaya, Chairperson
Kathi Pryor, Treasurer
Francis Bates, Executive Director
Tony Chavez, Deputy Director

Empowers and educates people with disabilities to achieve the independent life of their choice.

3781 Rolling Start: Victorville
17330 Bear Valley Road
Suite A102
Victorville, CA 92395
760-843-7959
FAX: 760-843-7977
TTY:760-951-8175
e-mail: Patty@rollingstart.com
www.rollingstart.org

John Anaya, Chairperson
Kathi Pryor, Treasurer
Francis Bates, Executive Director
Tony Chavez, Deputy Director

Empowers and educates people with disabilities to achieve the independent life of their choice.

3782 Services Center For Independent Living
107 S Spring Street
Claremont, CA 91711-549
909-621-6722
800-491-6722
FAX: 909-445-0727
TTY: 949-445-0726
e-mail: janice@scil-ilc.org
www.scil-ilc.org

Larry Grable, Executive Director
Janice Ornelas, Independent Living Specialist
Angela Nwokike, System Change Advocate
Albert Gonzales, Benefits Specialist

Dedicated to expanding access, information and resources to help increase independence and enhance the quality of life for the East San Gabriel Valley residents with disabilities.

3783 Silicon Valley Independent Living Center
2202 N. First St.
San Jose, CA 95131-1115
408-894-9041
FAX: 408-894-9050
TTY:408-894-9012
e-mail: info@svilc.org
svilc.org

Patricia Kokes, President
Richard A. Wentz, Vice President
Gabe Lopez, Treasurer
Nayana Shah, Executive Director

A private, consumer-driven, nonprofit corporation that offers quality services to individuals with disabilities in Silicon Valley.

3784 Silicon Valley Independent Living Center: South County Branch
7800 Arroyo Cir
Suite A
Gilroy, CA 95020-7346
408-846-1480
FAX: 408-842-2321
TTY:408-842-2591
e-mail: info@svilc.org
www.svilc.org

Patricia Kokes, President
Richard A. Wentz, Vice President
Gabe Lopez, Treasurer
Nayana Shah, Executive Director

A private, consumer-driven, non-profit corporation that offers quality services to individuals with disabilities in Silicon Valley.

3785 Southern California Rehabilitation Services
7830 Quill Dr
Suite D
Downey, CA 90242-3440
562-862-6531
FAX: 562-923-5274
TTY:562-869-0931
e-mail: scrs@scrs-ilc.org
scrs-ilc.org

Lisa Hayes, President
Michael Strong, Vice President
Carol Trees, Secretary/Treasurer
Chad Williams, Board Member

Empowers persons with disabilities to achieve their personalized goals through community education and individualized services that provide the knowledge, skills, and confidence building to maximize their quality of life.

3786 **Through the Looking Glass**
3075 Adeline St.
Ste. 120
Berkeley, CA 94703
510-848-1112
800-644-2666
FAX: 510-848-4445
TTY: 510-848-1005
e-mail: tlg@lookingglass.org
www.lookingglass.org

Maureen Block, J.D., Board President
Thomas Spalding, Board Treasurer
Alice Nemon, D.S.W., Board Secretary
Karen Fessel, Ph.D., Executive Director
To create, demonstrate and encourage non-pathological and empowering reesources and model early intervention services for families with disability issues in parent or child which integrate expertise derived from personal disability experience and disability culture.

3787 **Tri-County Independent Living Center**
2822 Harris Street
Eureka, CA 95503
707-445-8404
877-576-5000
FAX: 707-445-9751
TTY: 707-445-8405
e-mail: aa@tilinet.org
www.tilinet.org
Gail Pascoe, President
Linda Arnold, Vice President
Kevin O'Brien, Treasurer
Chris Jones, Executive Director
Promotes the philosophy of independent living, to connect individuals to services, and to create and accessible community, so that people with disabilities can have control over their lives and full access to the communities in which they live.

3788 **Westside Center for Independent Living**
12901 Venice Blvd
Los Angeles, CA 90066-3509
310-390-3611
888-851-9245
FAX: 310-390-4906
TTY: 310-398-9204
e-mail: development@wcil.org
www.wcil.org
Jorge Sandoval, President
Chris Knauf, 1st Vice President
Brenda Green, Secretary
Aliza Barzilay, Executive Director
The Westside Center for Independent Living (WCIL) helps people living with disabilities maintain self-sufficient and productive lives through non-residential peer support services and training programs. Independent Living promotes self-determination, community living, full participation in community life and access to the same opportunities and resources available to people without disabilities.

Colorado

3789 **Atlantis Community**
201 S Cherokee St
Denver, CO 80223-1836
303-733-7719
FAX: 303-733-6211
TTY:303-733-0047
e-mail: adaptbabs@earthlink.net
www.atlantiscommunity.net

David Hays, Manager
Provide direct services, and to empower people with disabilities integrating, with full and equal rights, into all parts of society including employment, affordable, accessible, housing, transportation, recreation, communication, education, and public places while exercising and exerting choice and self determination.

3790 **Center for Independence**
740 Gunnison Ave
Grand Junction, CO 81501-3222
708-588-0833
FAX: 708-588-0406
center-for-independence.org
Linda Taylor, Executive Director
The Center for Independence works to promote community solutions and to empower individuals with disabilities to live independently.

3791 **Center for People with Disabilities**
615 Main St
Longmont, CO 80501-4983
303-772-3250
FAX: 303-772-5125
TTY:303-772-3250
e-mail: info@cpwd.org
www.cpwd-ilc.org

Dale Gaar, Board President
Deborah.A Conley, Board Vice President
Nancy Phares-Zook, Board Secretary
Ruth Arnold, Board Treasurer
Provides resources, information, and advocacy to assist people with disabilities in overcoming barriers to independent living.

3792 **Center for People with Disabilities: Pueblo**
1304 Berkley Ave
Pueblo, CO 81004-3002
719-546-1271
800-659-3656
FAX: 719-546-1374
e-mail: ivaleneamidei@yahoo.com
www.du.edu/~bfox2/ilcpueblo

Larry Williams, Executive Director
One of the 10 centers for independent living in Colorado founded under Title VII of the Rehabilitation Act of 1973 as amended in 1978. All new centers under this Independent Living (CIL) Title of the Act received initial and ongoing grants through this new Federal Program created by the Act.

3793 **Center for People with Disabilities: Boulder**
1675 Range St
Boulder, CO 80301-2722
303-442-8662
888-929-5519
FAX: 303-442-0502
e-mail: info@cpwd.org
www.cpwd.org
Dale Gaar, Board President
Deborah.A Conley, Board Vice President
Nancy Phares-Zook, Board Secretary
Ruth Arnold, Board Treasurer
Providing resources, information and advocacy to people with disabilities. Assist people with disabilities in transitioning from nursing homes to independent living in the community. Also provide personal assistance services.

3794 **Colorado Springs Independence Center**
729 South Tejon Street
Colorado Springs, CO 80903
719-471-8181
FAX: 719-471-7829
TTY:719-471-2076
e-mail: info@csicindliving.org
www.csicindliving.org

Vicki Skoog, Executive Director
To empower persons with disabilities to maximize their independence within the community and to remove barriers which impact their quality of life, while encouraging them to live independently in their community.

3795 **Connections for Independent Living**
Ste E
1024 9th Ave
Greeley, CO 80631-4027
970-352-8682
800-887-5828
FAX: 970-353-8058
TTY: 970-352-8682
e-mail: pattid4z@yahoo.com
Beth Danielson, Executive Director

Certified IL Center, I and R advocacy, peer support, skills training, sign language interpretations, reader services, housing. Cross-disability, all ages.

3796 Denver CIL
Ste 100
777 Grant St
Denver, CO 80203-3501 303-837-1020
FAX: 303-837-0859

Greg Beran, Owner
Provides resources, information, and advocacy to assist people with disabilities in overcoming barriers to independent living.

3797 Disability Center for Independent Living
4821 East 38th Avenue
Denver, CO 80207-1232 303-320-1345
FAX: 303-320-1345
TTY:303-322-2330
e-mail: avillasenor.dcil@gmil.com
www.accil.net

Larry Williams, Executive Director
John Wooster, Consultant
Anthony Gonzales, Housing Coordinator
Jenna Emery, OBI Specialist
Independent living center providing quality services for people with disabilities.

3798 Disabled Resource Services
1017 Robertson Street
Unit B
Fort Collins, CO 80524-3915 970-482-2700
FAX: 970-449-6972
TTY:970-407-7060
e-mail: drs@frii.com
www.fortnet.org/drs

George Tremblay, Chairman
John Weins, Vice Chairman
Nancy Jackson, Executive Director
Marj Grell, Office Manager
To empower individuals with disabilities to achieve their maximum level of independence and to gain personal dignity within society. Disabled Resource Services, as a private non-profit state certified center for independent living, is dedicated to working with individuals with all types of disabilities in Larimer County to promote their independence and equality through services which support advocacy, awareness and access to their community.

3799 Disbled Resource Services
640 E Eisenhower Blvd
Loveland, CO 80537-3954 970-667-0816
FAX: 970-593-6582
e-mail: drs@frii.com
www.fortnet.org/drs

George Tremblay, Chairman
John Weins, Vice Chairman
Nancy Jackson, Executive Director
Marj Grell, Office Manager
To empower individuals with disabilities to achieve their maximum level of independence and to gain personal dignity within society.

3800 Greeley Center for Independence
2780 28th Ave
Greeley, CO 80634-7803 970-339-2444
800-748-1012
FAX: 970-339-0033
e-mail: gciinc@gciinc.org
www.gciinc.org

Chari Armagost, Chief Financial Officer
Sarita Reddy, PH. D, Executive Director
Rob Rabe, Director of Outpatient Service
Judy Weimer, R.N., Director of Nursing
Provides places of growth, transition and encouragement, where people with temporary and permanent disabilities can reach toward their maximum potential of personal independence and wellness.

3801 Independent Life Center
P.O.Box 612
Craig, CO 81626-612 970-826-0833
888-526-0833
FAX: 970-826-0832
TTY: 970-826-0833
e-mail: info@indlife.org
www.accil.net

Larry Williams, Executive Director
John Wooster, Consultant
Anthony Gonzales, Housing Coordinator
Jenna Emery, OBI Specialist
Provides resources, information, and advocacy to assist people with disabilities in overcoming barriers to independent living.

3802 Pueblo Goodwill Industries
15810 Indianola Drive
Rockville, MD 20855 240-333-5590
800-GOO-WILL
e-mail: contactus@goodwill.org
www.goodwill.org

Debi Diaz, CEO
Lauren Lawson-Zilai, Director of Public Relations
Charlene Sarmiento, Senior Specialist, Public Relati
PGoodwill works to enhance the dignity and quality of life of individuals and families by strengthening communities, eliminating barriers to opportunity, and helping people in need reach their full potential through learning and the power of work.

3803 Southwest Center for Independence
835 E 2nd Ave
Suite 200
Durango, CO 81301-5474 970-259-1672
866-962-2158
FAX: 970-259-0947
TTY: 970-259-1672
e-mail: director@swcidur.org
www.swcidur.org

Martha Mason, Executive Director
Susan Kimbler, Chair
Carol Lynn Rising, Vice-President
Jason Armstrong, Treasurer
Empowering individuals with disabilities and their families to achieve their maximum level of independence in work, play and other areas of life.

3804 Southwest Center for Independence: Cortez
2409 EastEmpireStreet
PO Box 640
Cortez, CO 81321-9164 970-570-8001
866-962-2158
FAX: 970-565-7169
e-mail: director@swilc.org
www.swilc.org

Mariellen Walz, Chair
Johnny Bulson, Vice Chair
Jason Armstrong, Treasurer
Martha Mason, Executive Director
Empowers individuals with disabilities and their families to achieve their maximum level of independence in work, play and other areas of life.

Connecticut

3805 Center for Disability Rights
764-BCampbellAve
764 Campbell Ave
W Haven, CT 06516- 3786 203-934-7077
FAX: 203-934-7078
TTY:203-934-7079
e-mail: info@cdr-ct.org
cdr-ct.org

Marc Gallucci, Executive Director
Chris Zurcher, Consumer Relations
Dana Canevari, I&R Specialist
Susan St. John, Administrative Assistant

Resources, information, and advocacy to assist people with disabilities in overcoming barriers to independent living.

3806 Center for Independent Living SC
26 Palmers Hill Rd
Stamford, CT 06902-2113
203-353-8550
FAX: 203-353-1423
TTY:203-353-8550

Dana Canevari, Director
Provides resources, information, and advocacy to assist people with disabilities in overcoming barriers to independent living.

3807 Chapel Haven
1040 Whalley Ave
New Haven, CT 06515-1740
203-397-1714
FAX: 203-937-2466
e-mail: admissions@chapelhaven.org
chapelhaven.org

Michael Storz, President
The only combined state-accredited special education facility and independent living facility for adults with cognitive disabilities.

3808 Disabilities Network of Eastern Connecticut
19 Ohio Avenue
Suite 2
Norwich, CT 06360-2111
860-823-1898
FAX: 860-886-2316
e-mail: CFerry@dnec.org
dnec.org

Katherine Pellerin, President
Robert Davidson, Vice President
Jane O'Friel, Secretary/Treasurer
Cathy Ferry, Executive Director
Dedicated to supporting and advancing the rights of individuals with disabilities. The goal is to creat a completely inclusive society where people live together in communities regardless of their abilities.

3809 Disability Resource Center of Fairfield County
80 Ferry Blvd
Suite 205
Stratford, CT 06615-6079
203-378-6977
FAX: 203-375-2748
TTY:203-378-3248
e-mail: info@drcfc.org
www.accessinct.org

Ethel M R, President
Thomas D, Vice-President
Anthony Lacava, Executive Director
Glenn Calaffin, Program Director
A crosss-disability resource and advocacy organization for people with disabilities that has provided unique, consumer-directed services both for individuals and for the communities of Fairfield County.

3810 Independence Northwest Center for Independent Living
1183 New Haven Rd
Suite 200
Naugatuck, CT 06770-5033
203-729-3299
FAX: 203-729-2839
TTY:203-729-1281
e-mail: info@independencenorthwest.org
www.independencenorthwest.org

Maureen Mayo, President
Tom Ford, Vice President
Charles Marino, Treasurer
Jaff Laliberte, Secretary
Provides services in such areas as peer counseling, advocacy, independent living skills training and information and referral.

3811 Independence Unlimited
151 New Park Ave
Suite D
Hartford, CT 06106-2170
860-523-0126
FAX: 860-523-5603
e-mail: info@ctsilc.org
ctsilc.org

Eileen Heall, President
Shirley Ricart, Vice President
Kartherine Pellerin, Secretary
Keith Mullinar, Treasurer
Center for independent living that provides skills training, peer counseling, advocacy, transition from institutions to the community and a variety of other services.

3812 New Horizons Village
37 Bliss Rd
Unionville, CT 06085
860-673-8893
FAX: 860-675-4369
e-mail: Michael.Shaw@NewHorizonsVillage.com
newhorizonsvillage.com

Carolyn Fields, Administrator
A 68 unit apartment complex designed for people who have severe physical disabilities.

Delaware

3813 Freedom Center for Independent Living
400 N Broad St
Middletown, DE 19709-1089
302-376-4399
866-687-3245
FAX: 302-376-4395
TTY: 302-376-4397
e-mail: info@fcilde.org
fcilde.org

Hersernest Cole, Executive Director
Lillian Evans, Independent Living Specialist
Protects the Civil Rights and promote the empowerment of persons with disabilities and their families through our independent living philosophy.

3814 Independent Living
Apt 210
1800 N Broom St
Wilmington, DE 19802-3854
302-429-6693
FAX: 302-429-8031
TTY:302-429-8034

Susan Cycyk, Executive Director
Providing skilled support and caring guidance to adults with disabilities. Our case management services include: daily living skills training, medical coordination, transportation assistance, financial management, housing assistance, and vocational/educational planning.

3815 Independent Resource Georgetown
Ste 37
410 S Bedford St
Georgetown, DE 19947-1850
302-854-9330
FAX: 302-854-9408
TTY:302-854-9340
e-mail: pboyd@independentresource.org

Larry Henderson, Director
Pat Boyd, Manager
Provides independent living services to persons who experience a significant disability. Offers skills training, individually and in small groups, peer support/peer counseling and information and referral services. Strives to remove the architectural and attitudnal barriers through individual and systems advocacy.

3816 Independent Resources: Dover
154 South Governor's Avenue
Dover, DE 19904-7311
302-735-4599
FAX: 302-735-5623
TTY:302-735-5629
e-mail: lhenderson@independentresources.org
www.iri-de.org

Tes DelTufo, Office Director
Carolyn Miller, IL Specialist
Debbie Justice, IL Specialist
Barty Rochester, Peer Support Coordinator

Private, non-profit, consumer-controlled, community based organization providing services and advocacy by and for persons with all types of disabilities. Their goal is to assist individuals with disabilities to achieve their maximum potential within their families and communities.

3817 Independent Resources: Wilmington
6 Denny Rd
Suite 101
Wilmington, DE 19809-3444
302-765-0191
FAX: 302-765-0195
TTY:302-765-0194
e-mail: fox205007@aol.com
www.iri-de.org

Larry D Henderson, Executive Director
Phyllis Farrare, Director of Operations

Private, non-profit, consumer-controlled, community based organization providing services and advocacy by and for persons with all types of disabilities. Their goal is to assist individuals with disabilities to achieve their maximum potential within their families and communities.

3818 Mosaic Of De
4980 S. 118TH ST
Omaha, NE 68137
302-456-5995
877-366-7242
FAX: 402-896-1511
e-mail: info@mosaic.org
mosaicinfo.org

Terry Olson, Executive Director

Provides services to adults with developmental disabilities who reside in homes and apartments. Services are designed to provide them with opportunities for choices and participation in the life of their communities. Supports are geared to assist each individual in becoming more independent in activities of daily living, vocational skills, community mobility and transportation, and recreation and leisure activities.

District of Columbia

3819 District of Columbia Center for Independent Living
1400 Florida Ave NE
Washington, DC 20002-5032
202-388-0033
FAX: 202-398-3018
e-mail: info@dccil.org
dccil.org

Rev. Patric Hailes Fears, President
Dr. John Thompson, Vice President
Carl Bartels, Treasurer
Angela Washington, Secretary

Mission is to maximize the leadership, empowerment, independence, and productivity of individuals with disabilities, and to integrate these individuals into the mainstream of American society.

3820 National Council on Independent Living
2013 H St. NW
6th Floor
Washington, DC 20006-3007
202-207-0334
877-525-3400
FAX: 202-207-0341
TTY: 202-207-0340
e-mail: ncil@ncil.org
www.ncil.org

Kelly Buckland, Executive Director
Tim Fuchs, Operations Director
Jorge Pineda, Accountant
Denise Law, Member Services Associate

As a membership organization, NCIL advances independent living and the rights of people with disabilities through consumer-driven advocacy.

Florida

3821 Ability 1st
1300 E. Green Street
Pasadena, CA 91106
626-396-1010
877-768-4600
FAX: 626-396-1021
e-mail: info@abilityfirst.org
abilityfirst.org

Steve Brockmeyer, Chairman
John Kelly, Vice Chairman
Lori.E Gangemi, President
Steve.S Schultz, CFO

To empower persons with disabilities to live independently and participate actively in their community.

3822 Adult Day Training
Goodwill Industries - Suncoast
10596 Gandy Blvd N
St Petersburg, FL 33702-1422
727-523-1512
888-279-1988
FAX: 727-563-9300
TTY:727-579-1068
e-mail: gw.marketing@goodwill-suncoast.com
www.goodwill-suncoast.org

Oscar J. Horton, Chairman
Martin W. Gladysz, Vice Chairman
Heather Ceresoli, Vice Chairman
Deborah.A Passerini, President

An innovative program which uses job skills to teach self-help, daily living, communication, mobility, travel, decision-making, behavioral and social skills. This focus provides concrete, transferable experiences to help prepare individuals for greater community inclusion by achieving the highest possible degree of independence in their daily life, increasing their confidence and supporting their successful transitions to less structured, self-sufficient environments.

3823 CIL of Central Florida
720 N Denning Dr
Winter Park, FL 32789-3020
407-623-1070
FAX: 407-623-1390
e-mail: info@cilorlando.org
cilorlando.org

Jason Vennings, Manager
Allison Gould, Volunteering Department

A private, non-profit organization dedicated to helping people with disabilities achieve their self-determined goals for independent living.

3824 Caring and Sharing Center for Independent Living
12552 Belcher Rd S
Largo, FL 33773-3014
727-539-7550
866-539-7550
FAX: 727-539-7588
e-mail: cascil@cascil.org
cascil.org

Barbara Dandro, Treasurer
Mary Bucca, Secretary
Patricia Bell, Director
Dennis Shelt, Director
Empowering people with disabilities.

3825 Caring and Sharing Center: Pasco County
12552 Belcher Rd S
Largo, FL 33773-3014
727-539-7550
866-539-7550
FAX: 727-539-7588
e-mail: cascil@cascil.org
www.cascil.org

Barbara Dandro, Treasurer
Mary Bucca, Secretary
Patricia Bell, Director
Dennis Shelt, Director
Empowering people with disabilities.

3826 Center for Independent Living in Central Florida
720 N Denning Dr
Winter Park, FL 32789-3095
407-623-1070
FAX: 407-623-1390
e-mail: info@cilorlando.org
cilorlando.org

Jason Vennings, Manager
Allison Gould, Volunteering Department
In partnership with the community, promotes personal right snad responsiblities among people with all disabilities.

3827 Center for Independent Living of Broward
4800 N State Road 7
Suite 102
Lauderdale Lakes, FL 33319-5811
954-722-6400
888-722-6400
FAX: 954-735-1958
e-mail: cilb@cilbroward.org
www.cilbroward.org

Craig Lilienthal, President
Christopher Sharp, VP
Shea Smith, Treasurer
Laurie Menekou, Secretary
Offers assistance to people with disabilities in fulfilling the goals of independence and self-sufficiency.

3828 Center for Independent Living of Florida Keys
103400 Overseas Hwy
Suite 243
Key Largo, FL 33037-2849
305-453-3491
877-335-0187
FAX: 305-453-3488
TTY: 305-453-3491
e-mail: cilkeys@cilkeys.org
www.cilofthekeys.org

Brenda K Pierce, Executive Director
Offers assistance to persons with disabilities in acquiring independent living and self-advocacy skills in order to obtain and maintain independence and self-sufficiency.

3829 Center for Independent Living of N Florida
1823 Buford Ct
Tallahassee, FL 32308-4465
850-575-9621
FAX: 850-575-5740
TTY:850-575-5245
e-mail: cilnf@nettally.com
www.ability1st.info/about-us

Judith Barrett, Executive Director
Offers assistance to persons with disabilities in acquiring independent living and self-advocacy skills in order to obtain and maintain independence and self-sufficiency

3830 Center for Independent Living of NW Florida
3600 N Pace Blvd
Pensacola, FL 32505-4240
850-595-5566
877-245-2457
FAX: 850-595-5560
e-mail: cil-drc@cil-drc.org
cil-drc.org

James Hicks, President
Kathleen Wilks, Secretary
John Bouchard, Treasurer
Frank Cherry, Executive Director
Provides services such as information and referral, peer counseling, housing, advocacy, training, independent living skills training, free wheelchairs, loan locker, assistive technology.

3831 Center for Independent Living of North Central Florida
3774 W Gulf To Lake Hwy
Lecanto, FL 34461-9214
352-527-8399
877-232-8261
FAX: 352-527-9511
www.cilncf.org

Joe Dyke, President
Robert Miller, Vice President
David Christie, Treasurer
Jim Gorske, Secretary
Empowers people with disabilities to exert their individual rights to live as independently as possible, make personal life choices and achieve full community inclusion.

3832 Center for Independent Living of North Central Florida
222 SW 36th Ter
Gainesville, FL 32607-2863
352-378-7474
800-265-5724
FAX: 352-378-5582
TTY: 352-372-3443
www.cilncf.org

Joe Dyke, President
Robert Miller, Vice President
David Christie, Treasurer
Jim Gorske, Secretary
Empowering people with disabilities to exert their individual rights to live as independently as possible, make personal life choices and achieve full community inclusion.

3833 Center for Independent Living of S Florida
6660 Biscayne Blvd
Miami, FL 33138-6285
305-751-8025
FAX: 305-751-8944
TTY:305-751-8891
e-mail: info@soflacil.org
soflacil.org

Alvin W. Roberts, President
Gregg Goldfarb, Vice President
Timothy Werner, Ph.D, Secretary
Jay Weiss, M.B.A., Treasurer
A community based non for profit, independent living center serving people of all ages with any type of disability. Services: Basic education, GED preperation, American sign language advocacy, peer support, information and referral, independent living skills training, housing assistance, transportation assistance, home modiifications, transition from nursing facility to the community assisatnace filing ADA complaints, accessibility surveys, diability awareness traing.

3834 Center for Independent Living of SW Florida
2321 Bruner Ln
Fort Myers, FL 33912-1904
239-277-1447
800-435-7352
FAX: 239-277-1647
www.cilfl.org

Ronald J Muschong, Interim Executive Director
Helping people with disabilities achieve independence and self-determination in their lives.

3835 **Coalition for IndependentLiving Options: Okeechobee**
TD Bank Building
8000 South US Hwy 1, Suite 304
Port St. Lucie, FL 34952 772-878-3500
FAX: 772-878-3344
www.cilo.org

Scott Shoemaker, President
Sharon D'Eusanio, Vice President
Joseph Fields Jr., Esquire, Secretary
Genevieve Cousminer,Esq, Executive Director

Private non-profit promoting independences for people with disabilities in Palm Beach, Martin, St. Lucie & Okeechobee Counties. Services include advocacy, independent living skills & training, peer support, after school & summer programs for teens, crime victim support services, and veterans transition services.

3836 **Coalition for Independent Living Options: Fort Pierce**
6800 Forest HIll Boulevard
West Palm Beach, FL 33413 561-966-4288
FAX: 561-641-6619
www.cilo.org

Scott Shoemaker, President
Sharon D'Eusanio, Vice President
Joseph Fields Jr., Esquire, Secretary
Genevieve Cousminer,Esq, Executive Director

Private non-profit promoting independences for people with disabilities in Palm Beach, Martin, St. Lucie & Okeechobee Counties. Services include advocacy, independent living skills & training, peer support, after school & summer programs for teens, crime victim support services, and verterans transition services.

3837 **Coalition for Independent Living Options**
6800 Forest Hill Blvd
Greenacres, FL 33413-3310 561-966-4288
FAX: 561-641-6619
www.cilo.org

Scott Shoemaker, President
Sharon D'Eusanio, Vice President
Joseph Fields Jr., Esquire, Secretary
Genevieve Cousminer,Esq, Executive Director

Private non-profit promoting independences for people with disabilities in Palm Beach, Martin, St. Lucie & Okeechobee Counties. Services include advocacy, independent living skills & training, peer support, after school & summer programs for teens, crime victim support services, and veterans transition services.

3838 **Coalition for Independent Living Options: Stuart**
850 NW Federal Hwy
Unit 104
Stuart, FL 34994-1056 772-233-4301
FAX: 772-233-4302
www.cilo.org

Scott Shoemaker, President
Sharon D'Eusanio, Vice President
Joseph Fields Jr., Esquire, Secretary
Genevieve Cousminer,Esq, Executive Director

Private non-profit promoting independences for people with disabilities in Palm Beach, Martin, St. Lucie & Okeechobee Counties. Services include advocacy, independent living skills & training, peer support, after school & summer programs for teens, crime victim support services, and veterans transition services.

3839 **Disability Resource Center**
300 W. 5th St.
Panama City, FL 32401-4704 850-769-6890
FAX: 850-769-6891
e-mail: outreach@drcpc.org
www.drcpc.org

Robert Cox, Executive Director
Becky Cadwell, Independent Living Specialist

They are commiteed to collaborating with other disability/consumer-focused organizations in their community

3840 **Lakeland Adult Day Training**
3033 Drane Field Rd
Suite 5
Lakeland, FL 33811-3305 863-701-1351
TTY:863-701-1356
e-mail: gw.marketing@goodwill-suncoast.com
www.goodwill-suncoast.org

Oscar J. Horton, Chairman
Martin W. Gladysz, Vice Chairman
Heather Ceresoli, Vice Chairman
Deborah.A Passerini, President

An innovative program which uses job skills to teach self-help, daily living, communication, mobility, travel, decision-making, behavioral and social skills. This focus provides concrete, transferable experiences to help prepare individuals for greater community inclusion by achieving the highest possible degree of independence in their daily life, increasing their confidence and supporting their successful transitions to less structured, self-sufficient environments.

3841 **Lighthouse Central Florida**
215 E New Hampshire St
Orlando, FL 32804-6403 407-898-2483
FAX: 407-895-5255
e-mail: lvaneepoel@lcf-fl.org
lighthousecentralflorida.com

Lee Nasehi, President,CEO
Lee Van Eepoel, Program Service Director
Donna Esbensen,CPA, MBA, Vice President,Chief Financial O
Kimberley Pawling,PhD, Director of Education & Rehabili

Promote the independence and success of people living with vision impairment.

3842 **Miami-Dade County Disability Services and Independent Living (DSAIL)**
1335 NW 14th St
Miami, FL 33125-1647 305-547-5444
FAX: 305-547-7355
e-mail: morrina@miamidade.gov
http://www.miamidade.gov/dhs/elderly_disabili

Michael Moxam, Manager

Offers information and referral services serving all types of disabilities with the goal of assisting the disabled acquiring independence and control over their lives. Teaches independent living skills, job readiness and placement, home health care, sensitivity training, training in ASL and Braille, counsel people with disabilities or wide range of problems.

3843 **Ocala Adult Day Training**
2920 W Silver Springs Blvd
Ocala, FL 34475-5654 352-629-0456
TTY:352-629-0874
e-mail: gw.marketing@goodwill-suncoast.com
www.goodwill-suncoast.org

Oscar J. Horton, Chairman
Martin W. Gladysz, Vice Chairman
Heather Ceresoli, Vice Chairman
Deborah.A Passerini, President

An innovative program which uses job skills to teach self-help, daily living, communication, mobility, travel, decision-making, behavioral and social skills. This focus provides concrete, transferable experiences to help prepare individuals for greater community inclusion by achieving the highest possible degree of independence in their daily life, increasing their confidence and supporting their successful transitions to less structured, self-sufficient environments.

3844 **Pinellas Park Adult Day Training**
7601 Park Blvd
Pinellas Park, FL 33781-3704 727-541-6205
TTY:727-544-5835
e-mail: gw.marketing@goodwill-suncoast.com
www.goodwill-suncoast.org

Oscar J. Horton, Chairman
Martin W. Gladysz, Vice Chairman
Heather Ceresoli, Vice Chairman
Deborah.A Passerini, President

An innovative program which uses job skills to teach self-help, daily living, communication, mobility, travel, decision-making, behavioral and social skills. This focus provides concrete, transferable experiences to help prepare individuals for greater community inclusion by achieving the highest possible degree of independence in their daily life, increasing their confidence and supporting their successful transitions to less structured, self-sufficient environments.

3845 SCCIL at Titusville
725 S Deleon Ave
Titusville, FL 32780-4115
407-268-2244
FAX: 706-724-6729
TTY:706-724-6324
e-mail: kswoil@csranet.com
www.virtualcil.net

Gerri Martin, Executive Director
Directory of Independent Living Centers throughout the United States.

3846 Self Reliance
8901 N Armenia Ave
Tampa, FL 33604-1041
813-375-3965
FAX: 813-375-3970
TTY:813-375-3972
e-mail: bruehl@self-reliance.org
www.self-reliance.org

Brenda Ruehl, Executive Director
Liz Fields, Director of Finance & Operations
A cross disability agency providing services to both children and adults with disabilities to identify and overcome barriers to independence in their lives. Self Reliance also promotes independence through empowering persons with disabilities and improving the communities in which they live.

3847 Space Coast Center for Independent Living
571 Haverty Court, Suite W.
Rockledge, FL 32955
321-633-6011
FAX: 321-633-6472
http://spacecoastcil.org

Michael Lavoie, President
Howard Fetes, VP
Jason Miller, Treasurer/Secretary
Provides overall services for individuals with al types of disabilities. Offers peer support, advocacy, skills training, accessibility surveys, support groups, transportation, specialized equipment and sign language interpreter referral services and home modifications.

3848 Suncoast Center for Independent Living, Inc.
3281 17th Street
Sarasota, FL 34235
941-351-9545
FAX: 941-316-9320
e-mail: Info@scil4u.org
www.scil4u.org

Candy Partee, Chair
Fredd Atkins, Vice Chair
Vicke Mack, Treasurer
Scott Biehler, Secretary
Helping people with disabilities live independently.

3849 disAbility Solutions for Independent Living
119 S Palmetto Ave
Suite 180
Daytona Beach, FL 32114- 4369
386-255-1812
866-310-1039
FAX: 386-255-1814
TTY: 386-252-6222
e-mail: info@dsil.org
www.dsil.org

Julie M Shaw, Executive Director
To maximize the leadership, empowerment, independence and productivity of individuals with disabilities, to promote and attain integration and full inclusion of individuals with disabilities in all aspects of our society; accomplished through consumer control, peer support, education, self-determination, equal access and individual and systems advocacy

Georgia

3850 Arms Wide Open
3013 Rainbow Dr
Suite 124
Decatur, GA 30034-1677
770-413-2241
FAX: 770-498-2778
e-mail: kenmorris@armswideopen.org
www.armswideopen.org

Ken Morris, Director
Arms Wide Open operates a durable medical equipment loan program and a life care program. The mission of Arms Wide Open is to provide support services to the aged, disabled and chronically ill for the purpose of helping them to avoid institutional placement.

3851 Bain, Inc. Center For Independent Living
316 W Shotwell St
Bainbridge, GA 39819-3906
229-246-0150
888-830-1530
FAX: 229-246-1715
TTY: 888-830-1530
e-mail: bain@surfsouth.com
www.baincil.org

Virginia Harris, Executive Director
Malissa Thompson, Program Manager
Tomonia Becon, Nursing Home Transition Coordina
Julie Harris, Independent Living Specialist
A non-residential Center for Independent Living serving eleven counties throughout Southwest. BAIN is a non-profit, community based resource and advocacy center run by and for individuals with disabilities.

3852 Disability Connections
170 College St
Macon, GA 31201-1656
478-741-1425
800-743-2117
FAX: 478-755-1571
e-mail: dcinfo@disabilityconnections.com
disabilityconnections.com

Jerilyn Leverett, Executive Director
A private non-profit organization that looks to enable all people with disabilities to attain and have access to all opportunities in life.

3853 Division of Rehabilitation Services
Georgia Department of Labor
410 Mall Blvd
Suite B
Savannah, GA 31406-4869
912-356-2226
FAX: 912-356-2875
TTY:912-356-2940
e-mail: www.dol.state.ga.us
dol.state.ga.us

Mark Bultler, Commissioner
Jody Lane, Manager
George Foley, Manager
Vocational rehabilitation services.

3854 Living Independence for Everyone (LIFE)
5105 Paulsen Street
Suite 143-B
Savannah, GA 31405
912-920-2414
800-948-4824
FAX: 912-920-0007
e-mail: info@lifecil.com
www.lifecil.com

John Paul Berlon, President
Jason Wilson, Vice President
Kim Harrison, Secretary
Mark Schreiber, Treasurer
The Southeast's Regional disability resource center that offers a wide range of resources, education, and advocacy to the community to help level the playing field for people with disabilities to create a world in which everyone can fully participate.

3855 **Multiple Choices Center for Independent Living**
850 Gaines School Rd
Athens, GA 30605-3133 706-549-3131
e-mail: info@multiplechoices.us
www.multiplechoices.us
Doug Hatch, President
Donald Veater, VP
Elllen Des Jardines, Secretary
William Holley, Executive Director
To break down all barriers to inclusion by enhancing the equality of life and empowering people with disabilities through advocacy, education and training.

3856 **North District Independent Living Program**
Ste 209
311 Green St NW
Gainesville, GA 30501-3364 770-535-5930
Sharon McCurry, Coordinator
Cindy Hanna, Executive Director
Information and referral, advocacy, peer counseling, service coordination and ADA consultation.

3857 **Southwest District Independent Living Program**
P.O.Box 1606
Albany, GA 31702-1606 229-430-4170
FAX: 229-430-4466
Bill Layton, Director
Diane Davis, Executive Director
Offers peer counseling, disability education and awareness, attendant care registry, and information on accessible home for the disabled.

3858 **Statewide Independent Living Council of Georgia**
315 West Ponce de Leon Avenue
Suite 600
Decatur, GA 30030-2617 770-270-6860
888-288-9780
FAX: 770-270-5957
e-mail: shellys5@hotmail.com
silcga.org
Steve Oldaker, President
Angela Denise Davis, Vice President
Mark Schreiber, Treasurer
Scott Osborne, Secretary
Founded to ensure that people with disabilities have opportunities to live as independently as possible.

3859 **Walton Options for Independent Living**
948 Walton Way
Augusta, GA 30901-519 706-724-6262
877-821-8400
FAX: 706-724-6729
TTY: 706-724-6262
e-mail: tjohnston@waltonoptions.org
www.waltonoptions.org
Tiffany Cilford, Executive Director
Judy Bartee, Director
Robert Bryant, Peer Support Coordinator
Brian Mosley, Employment Services
Services include individual and systems advocacy, peer support, skills training (including basic computer and return to work skills), information and referral services and transition from institutions back to the community.

3860 **disABILITY LINK: Rome**
755 Commerce Drive
Suite 105
Decatur, GA 30030 404-687-8890
FAX: 404-687-8298
e-mail: info@disabilitylink.org
disabilitylink.org
Kim Gibson, Executive Director
Barbara Adle, Health, Wellness and Resource Specialist
Larry Brown, Finance Director
Hillary Elliott, Independent Living Services Program Director
Committed to promoting the rights of all people with disabilities.

Hawaii

3861 **Center For Independent Living- Kauai**
State Office Building 3060 Eiwa Str
Lihue, HI 96766-6529 808-274-3484
FAX: 808-245-3485
e-mail: kauaiddc@pixi.com
www.hiddc.org/kauai
Humberto Blanco, Administrator
Teri Yamashiro, IL Specialist
Offers peer counseling, disability education, attendant care registry, outreach services and advocacy.

3862 **Hawaii Center For Independent Living**
1055 Kinoole Street
Suite 105le St
Hilo, HI 96720-3872 808-935-3777
800-420-6928
TTY:808-935-7888
e-mail: info@pacificil.org
www.cil-hawaii.org
Gordon Fuller, Executive Director
Provides an array of support services for people with all types of disabilities of any age.

3863 **Hawaii Center for Independent Living-Maui**
220 Imi Kala Street
Suite 103
Wailuku, HI 96793-1209 808-242-4966
866-303-4245
800-420-6928
FAX: 808-244-6978
TTY:808-242-4968
e-mail: mcilogg@gte.net/ clytien@pacificil.org
www.cil-hawaii.org
Clytie Nishihara, Manager
T Lay, Administrative Assistant
Offers disability education and awareness, advocacy and counseling.

3864 **Hawaii Centers for Independent Living**
200 N. Vineyard Blvd Bldg. A501
Honolulu, HI 96817-3950 808-522-5400
800-420-6928
FAX: 808-522-5427
e-mail: info@pacificil.org
www.cil-hawaii.org
Cheryl Mizusaawa, Executive Director
M.J. (Kimo) Keawe, COO & Executive Director
Our staff and Board of directors are excellent advocates with the disabled community. We will connect you with resources to make your own choices for housing, employment, and personal care and to find assistive devices and technology to improve quality of life. On both the islands of Oahu and Hawaii, we have an independent living specialist who is fluent in American sign language and is well known in the deaf community.

3865 **Kauai Center for Independent Living**
4340 Nawiliwili Rd.
Lihue, HI 96766-6529 808-246-4800
800-420-6928
FAX: 808-245-7218
e-mail: kcil@mail.aloha.net
www.cil-hawaii.org
Laurao Tobosa, Program Coordinator
Provides a variety of support services for people with all types of disabilities.

Idaho

3866 **American Falls Office: Living Independently for Everyone (LIFE)**
250 S. Skyline
Idaho Falls, ID 83402-4508
208-529-8610
FAX: 208-529-6804
e-mail: diane@idlife.org
www.idlife.org

Dean Nilson, Executive Director
Tina Noreen, Programs Coordinator
Enables people with disabilities to manage their own lives, make their own choices, and give information and knowledge to assist in living with dignity and bravado.

3867 **Dawn Enterprises**
280 Cedar Street P.O.Box 388
Blackfoot, ID 83221-388
208-785-5890
FAX: 208-785-3095
www.orgsites.com/id/dawnent

Donna Butler, Executive Director
Teresa Oakes, Assistant Director/Fiscal Coordi
To assist individuals of Southeastern Idaho with mental, physical or social disabilities in achieving independence through employment training, skill training, social development, or living enhancements up to each individual's maximum capability.

3868 **Disability Action Center NW**
505 N Main St
Moscow, ID 83843-2615
208-883-0523
800-475-0070
FAX: 208-883-0524
e-mail: moscow@dacnw.org
www.dacnw.org

Larry Topp, President
Jean Coil, Vice President
Mark Leeper, CEO
Karl Johanson, Treasurer
A non-profit community partnership working to promote the independence and equality of all individuals with disabilities in all aspects of society. *$45.00*

3869 **Disability Action Center NW: Coeur D'Alene**
7560 N Government Way
Suite 1
Coeur D Alene, ID 83815- 4069
208-664-9896
800-854-9500
FAX: 208-666-1362
e-mail: cda@dacnw.org
www.dacnw.org

Larry Topp, President
Jean Coil, Vice President
Mark Leeper, CEO
Karl Johanson, Treasurer
A non-profit community partnership working to promote the independence and equality of all individuals with disabilities in all aspects of society.

3870 **Disability Action Center NW: Lewiston**
330 5th Street
Suite A1
Lewiston, ID 83501-2086
208-746-9033
800-746-9033
FAX: 208-746-1004
e-mail: lewiston@dacnw.org
www.dacnw.org

Larry Topp, President
Jean Coil, Vice President
Mark Leeper, CEO
Karl Johanson, Treasurer
A non-profit community partnership working to promote the independence and equality of all individuals with disabilities in all aspects of society.

3871 **Idaho Falls Office: Living Independently for Everyone (LIFE)**
250 S. Skyline
Idaho Falls, ID 83402-3702
208-529-8610
800-631-2747
FAX: 208-232-2753
e-mail: diane@idlife.org
www.idlife.org

Dean Nielson, Executive Director
Tina Noreen, Programs Coordinator
Mickey Palmer, Fiscal Intermediary Manager
Enables people with disabilities to manage their own lives, make their own choices, and give information and knowledge to assist in living with dignity and bravado.

3872 **LIFE: Fort Hall**
2323 S. Shepherd, Suite 1000
Houston, TX 77019
713-520-0232
FAX: 71- 52- 578
TTY:713-520-0232
e-mail: ilro@ilro.org
www.ilru.org

Wnedy Parker, Director
Enables people with disabilities to manage their own lives, make thier own choices, and give information and knowledge to assist in living with dignity and bravado.

3873 **Living Independence Network Corporation**
1878 W Overland Rd
Boise, ID 83705-3142
208-336-3335
FAX: 208-384-5037
e-mail: info@lincidaho.org
lincidaho.org

Roger Howard, Executive Director
A non-profit organization empowering people with disabilities to achieve their desired level of independence.

3874 **Living Independence Network Corporation: Twin Falls**
1182 Eastland Dr North
Suite C
Twin Falls, ID 83301-8972
208-733-1712
FAX: 208-733-7711
e-mail: info@lincidaho.org
www.lincidaho.org

Melva Heinrich, Executive Director
A non-profit organization empowering people with disabilities to achieve their desired level of independence.

3875 **Living Independence Network Corporation: Caldwell**
1609 Kimball Ave
Ste. 201
Caldwell, ID 83605-6965
208-454-5511
FAX: 208-454-5515
TTY:208-454-5511
e-mail: info@lincidaho.org
www.lincidaho.org

Heidi Caldwell, Executive Director
A non-profit organization empowering people with disabilities to achieve their desired level of independence.

3876 **Living Independent for Everyone (LIFE): Pocatello Office**
640 Pershing Ave
PO Box 4185
Pocatello, ID 83201-3702
208-232-2747
800-631-2747
FAX: 208-232-2753
TTY: 208-232-2747
e-mail: tracy@idlife.org
www.idlife.org

Dean Nielson, Executive Director
Mickey Palmer, Fiscal Intermediary Manager
Enables people with disabilities to manage thier own lives, make their own choices, and give information and knowledge to assist in living with dignity and bravado.

3877 **Living Independently for Everyone (LIFE): Blackfoot Office**
Living Independently for Everyone (LIFE): Pocate
570 W. Pacific
P.O.Box 86
Blackfoot, ID 83221-86
208-785-9648
FAX: 208-785-2398
e-mail: lori@idlife.org
www.idlife.org

Dean Nielson, Executive Director
Lori Galvan, Independent Living Advisor
Mickey Palmer, Fiscal Intermediary Manager
Enable people with disabilities to manage their own lives, make their own choices, and give information and knowledge to assist in living with dignity and bravado.

3878 **Living Independently for Everyone: Burley**
2311 Park Ave
Suite 7
Burley, ID 83318-2170
208-678-7705
FAX: 208-678-7771
e-mail: hotwheels@idlife.org
www.idlife.org

Dean Nielson, Executive Director
Mickey Palmer, Fiscal Intermediary Manager
Sandra Dressel, Manager
Enables people with disabilities to manage their own lives, make their own choices, and give information and knowledge to assist in living with dignity and bravado.

3879 **Southwestern Idaho Housing Authority**
1108 W Finch Dr
Nampa, ID 83651-1732
208-467-7461
FAX: 208-463-1772
David W Patten, Manager
Offers housing for rent and section/8

Illinois

3880 **Access Living of Metropolitan Chicago**
115 W Chicago Ave
Chicago, IL 60654-3209
312-640-2100
800-613-8549
FAX: 312-640-2101
TTY: 312-640-2102
e-mail: info@accessliving.org
accessliving.org

Marca Bristo, CEO
Bhuttu Mathews, Disability Resources Coordinator
Gary Arnold, Public Relations Coordinator
Established in 1980,access living is a change agent commited to fostering an incusive society that enables Chicagoans with disabilities to live fully engaged and self-directed lives. Nationally recognized as a leading force in the disability community. Access Living challenges stereotypes, protects civil rights, and champions social reform.

3881 **Center on Deafness**
3444 Dundee Rd
Northbrook, IL 60062-2258
847-559-0110
FAX: 847-559-8199
TTY:847-559-9493
e-mail: centerondeafness.org
www.centerondeafness.org

Bonnie Simon, Executive Director
Donna Gomez, Residential Services/ Adult Plac
Brandi Buie, School Intake
David Wood, Coordinator
COD is dedicated to providing quality services for persons who are deaf or hard of hearing and their families, through educational, vocational, and residential services in a therapuetic, community-based environment

3882 **Community Residential Alternative**
Coleman Tri- County Services
22VeteransDrive, ST. A
P.O. Box 869
Harrisburg, IL 62946-2017
618-252-0275
FAX: 618-252-2389
TTY:618-269-4211
e-mail: cts.62946@frontier.com
colemantricounty.tripod.com

Samantha Austin, Executive Director
Six bed group home that provides a residential alternative for the developmentally disabled adult. This program is designed to promote independence in daily living skills, economic self-sufficiency, and integration into the community.

3883 **Division of Rehabilitation Services**
Department of Human Services
100 South Grand Avenue East
Springfield, IL 62762-2625
217-782-2093
800-843-6154
FAX: 217-524-2471
e-mail: DHS.WebBits@illinois.gov
www.dhs.state.il.us

Carol Adams, President
Provides medical, therapeutic and counseling services for the disabled, as well as employment services.

3884 **DuPage Center for Independent Living**
739 Roosevelt Rd
Bldg 8
Glen Ellyn, IL 60137-5877
630-469-2300
FAX: 630-469-2606
TTY:630-469-2300
e-mail: dcil@mcs.com
www.dupagecil.org

Charles Stack, Board President
Bette Lawrence Water, Vice President
John Lausas, Treasurer
Jeff Gullang, Secretary
A non residential, community based, not for profit agency wich provides advocacy and services to persons with disabilities in DuPage County.

3885 **Fite Center for Independent Living**
1230 Larkin Ave
Elgin, IL 60123-6200
847-695-5818
FAX: 847-695-5892
e-mail: info@fitecil.org
www.fitecil.org

Linda Bradford-Foster, Chairman, Board Treasurer
Gracia Bittner, Board Secretary
Provides services to people with disabilities in Kane, Kendall and McHenry counties. Our non-residential agency provides independent living skills training, advocacy, systemic + individual peer counseling, information and referral and housing services. Also provides technical assistance to businesses and agencies to work with people with disabilities. Locations in Elgin and Aurora. Please call for further details.

3886 **Illinois Department of Rehab Services**
Department of Human Services
100 South Grand Avenue East
Springfield, IL 62762-1
217-782-2093
800-843-6154
FAX: 217-524-2471
e-mail: DHS.WebBits@illinois.gov
www.dhs.state.il.us

Carol Adams, President
Karen Perrin, Manager
The state's lead agency serving individuals with disabilities. DRS works in partnership with people with disabilities and their families to assist them in making informed choices to achieve full community participation through employment, education, and independent living opportunities.

3887 Illinois Valley Center for Independent Living
18 Gunia Dr
La Salle, IL 61301-9780
815-224-3126
800-822-3246
FAX: 815-224-3576
e-mail: ivcil@ivcil.com
ivcil.com

John Hurst, President
Gary Rydleski, Vice President
Rachael Mellen, Executive Director
Laura Sutton, Secretary
A nonprofit service and advocacy organization that assists persons with disabilities in opening doors to their independence.

3888 Illinois and Iowa Center for Independent Living
501 11th St.
PO Box 6156
Rock Island, IL 61231-6156
309-793-0090
877-541-2505
855-744-8918
FAX: 309-793-5198
e-mail: iicil@iicil.com
www.iicil.com

Liz Sherwin, Executive Director
Alfonso Ayew-Ew, Blind Independent Living Skill Specialist
Eddie Williams, CommunityReintegration Advocate
Hershel Jackson, Deaf & Hard of Hearing Advocate
To create and maintain independence options for people with disabilities by advocating for civil rights, providing services, and promoting full participation of disabled individuals in all aspects of the community.

3889 Impact Center for Independent Living
2735 E Broadway
Alton, IL 62002-1859
618-462-1411
888-616-4261
FAX: 618-474-5309
e-mail: staff@impactcil.org
impactcil.org

Susy Woods, President
Judy O'Malley, Vice President
Jeffrey Owen, Treasurer
Cathy Contarino, Executive Director
Promotes pride and respect for people with disabilities by sharing the tools that are necessary to take control of one's own life.

3890 Jacksonville Area CIL: Havana
220 W Main St
Havana, IL 62644-1138
309-543-6680
877-759-2187
FAX: 309-543-6711
e-mail: info@jacil.org
www.jacil.org

Vicki Mullis, President
Phil Foxworth, Vice President
Ruth Linear, Secretary
Mark Arnold, Treasurer
Committed to enabling persons with disabilities to gain effective control and director of their own lives in the home, in the workplace and in the community.

3891 Jacksonville Area Center for Independent Living
15 Permac Road
Jacksonville, IL 62650-2071
217-245-8371
FAX: 217-245-1872
TTY:217-245-8371
e-mail: info@jacil.org
www.jacil.org

Becky Mc Ginnis, Executive Director
Committed to enabling persons with disabilities to gain effective control and direction of their own lives in the home, in the workplace and in the community.

3892 LIFE Center for Independent Living
Ste 1
2201 Eastland Dr
Bloomington, IL 61704-7923
309-663-5433
888-543-3245
FAX: 309-663-7024
TTY:309-663-5433
e-mail: gail@lifecil.org
lifecil.org

Gail Kear, Executive Director
A community-based, not-for-profit, non-residential organization that promotes disability rights, equal access, and full community participation for persons with disabilities.

3893 LINC-Monroe Randolph Center
Ste 4
1514 S Main St
Red Bud, IL 62278-1382
618-282-3700
FAX: 618-282-2740
TTY:618-282-3700

Violete Nast, Manager

3894 Lake County Center for Independent Living
377 N Seymour Ave
Mundelein, IL 60060-2322
847-949-4440
FAX: 847-949-4445
TTY:847-949-0641
e-mail: lindsey@lccil.org
www.lccil.org

Kelli Brooks, Executive Director
Lindsay Schultz, Information & Referral Advocate
Lake County Center for Indepdendent Living is a disability rights organization governed and staffed by a majority of people with disabilities. LCCIL offers services and advocacy that promote a fully accessible society, which expects participation by persons with disabilities.

3895 Life Center for Independent Living: Pontiac
318 West Madison Street
Pontiac, IL 61764-1785
815-844-1132
FAX: 815-844-1148
e-mail: lifecil@lifecil.org
www.lifecil.org

John Evans, President
George Meisenbach, Vice President
Jim Martin, Treasurer
Donna Evans, Secretary
A community-based, not-for-profit, non-residential organization that promotes disability rights, equal access, and full community participation for persons with disabilities.

3896 Living Independently Now Center (LINC)
120 E a St
Belleville, IL 62220-1401
618-235-9988
FAX: 618-233-3729
TTY:618-235-9988
e-mail: info@lincinc.org
lincinc.org

Erica Edwards, Executive Director
Empowers persons with disabilities to live independently and to promote accessibility and inclusion in all areas.

3897 Living Independently Now Center: Sparta
Western Egyptian Building
207 West 4th Street
Waterloo, IL 62298
618-317-4028
e-mail: info@lincinc.org
www.lincinc.org

Linda Conley, President
Rebecca Ray, Vice-President
Lynn Jarman, Executive Director
Ron Tialdo, Treasurer
Empowers persons with disabilities to live independently and to promote accessibility and inclusion in all areas.

3898 Living Independently Now Center: Waterloo
Western Egyptian Building
207 West 4th Street
Waterloo, IL 62298-1336
618-317-4028
e-mail: info@lincinc.org
www.lincinc.org
Linda Conley, President
Rebecca Ray, Vice-President
Lynn Jarman, Executive Director
Ron Tialdo, Treasurer
Empowers persons with disabilities to live independently and to promote accessibility and inclusion in all areas.

3899 Mosaic: Pontiac
725 W Madison St
Pontiac, IL 61764-1621
815-842-4166
FAX: 815-842-4053
mosaicinfo.org
Max Miller, Chairperson
James Zis, Vice Chairperson
Lisa Negstad, 2nd Vice Chairperson
Kathy Patrick, Secretary
A faith-based organization serving people with developmental disabilities.

3900 Opportunities for Access: A Center for Independent Living
4206 Williamson Pl
Suite 3
Mount Vernon, IL 62864-6705
618-244-9212
FAX: 618-244-9310
TTY:618-244-9575
e-mail: spud@ofacil.org
ofacil.org
Michael Egbert, Executive Director
Serves, trains and provides information to persons with disabilities, family members and significant others and service providers. Services include: advocacy, information and referral, peer support, skills training, volunteer programs and other related services. Services are free. A cross disability community based, non-residential, nonprofit organization serving Clay, Clinton, Edwards, Effingham, Fayette, Hamilton, Jasper, Jefferson, Marion, Wabash, Washington, Wayne and White Counties.

3901 Options Center for Independent Living: Bourbonnais
22 Heritage Dr
Suite 107
Bourbonnais, IL 60914-2510
815-936-0100
FAX: 815-936-0117
TTY:815-936-0132
e-mail: optionscil@optionscil.com
optionscil.com
Mark Mountain, President
Ronald D. Smith, Vice President
Dina Raymond, Co-Secretary
Daniel Brough, Treasurer
A non-residential, not-for-profit, community-based organization that promotes independent living for people with disabilities.

3902 Options Center for Independent Living: Watseka
103 Laird Ln
Suite 103
Watseka, IL 60970
815-432-1332
FAX: 815-432-1360
TTY:815-432-1361
e-mail: optionscil@optionscil.com
www.optionscil.com
Mark Mountain, President
Ronald D. Smith, Vice President
Dina Raymond, Co-Secretary
Daniel Brough, Treasurer
A non-residential, not-for-profit, community-based organization that promotes independent living for people with disabilities.

3903 PACE Center for Independent Living
1317 E Florida Ave
Urbana, IL 61801-6007
217-344-5433
FAX: 217-344-2414
TTY:217-344-5024
e-mail: info@pacecil.org
pacecil.org
Evelyn Brown, President
Fred Neubert, Vice President
Nancy McClellan-Hickey, Executive Director
Arland Stratton, Treasurer
Promotes the full participation of people with disabilities in the rights and responsibilities of society. Provides services, which assist people with disabilities in achieving or maintaining independence.

3904 Progress Center for Independent Living
7521 Madison St
Forest Park, IL 60130-1407
708-209-1500
FAX: 708-209-1735
TTY:708-209-1826
e-mail: info@progresscil.org
www.progresscil.org
Anne Gunter, Independent Living Advocate
Kim Liddell, Independent Living Advocate
Osbaldo Flores, Independent Living Advocate
Art Johnson, Home Services Team Coordinator
A community-based, non-profit, non-residential, service and advocacy organization operated for people with disabilities, by people with disabilities.

3905 Progress Center for Independent Living: Blue Island
12940 Western Ave
Blue Island, IL 60406-3766
708-388-5011
FAX: 708-388-5016
TTY:708-389-8250
e-mail: info@progresscil.org
www.progresscil.org
Horacio Esparza, Executive Director
Anne Gunter, Independent Living Advocate
Kim Liddell, Independent Living Advocate
Art Johnson, Home Services Team Coordinator
A community-based, non-profit, non residential, service and advocacy organization operated for people with disabilities, by people with disabilities.

3906 Regional Access & Mobilization Project
202 Market St
Rockford, IL 61107-3954
815-968-7467
FAX: 815-968-7612
TTY:815-968-2401
www.rampcil.org
Shari Snyder, President
Tina Kaatz, Vice President
Craig Fetty, Secretary
Sharon Wyland, Treasurer
To promote an accessible society that allows and expects full participation by people with disabilities.

3907 Regional Access & Mobilization Project: Belvidere
530 S State St
Suite 103
Belvidere, IL 61008-3711
815-544-8404
FAX: 815-544-1896
TTY:815-544-8404
www.rampcil.org
Shari Snyder, President
Tina Kaatz, Vice President
Craig Fetty, Secretary
Sharon Wyland, Treasurer
Promote an accessible society that allows and expects full participation by people with disabilities.

3908 **Regional Access & Mobilization Project: De Kalb**
115 N First Street
Dekalb, IL 60115-3055
815-756-3202
FAX: 815-756-3556
TTY:815-756-4263
www.rampcil.org

Shari Snyder, President
Tina Kaatz, Vice President
Craig Fetty, Secretary
Sharon Wyland, Treasurer
Promotes an accessible society that allows and expects full partiipation by persons with disabilities.

3909 **Regional Access & Mobilization Project: Freeport**
2155 W Galena Ave
Freeport, IL 61032-3013
815-233-1128
FAX: 815-233-0743
TTY:815-233-1128
rampcil.org

Shari Snyder, President
Tina Kaatz, Vice President
Craig Fetty, Secretary
Sharon Wyland, Treasurer
Promotes an accessible society that allows and expects full partiipation by persons with disabilities.

3910 **Soyland Access to Independent Living(SAIL)**
2449 E Federal Dr
Decatur, IL 62526-2160
217-876-8888
800-358-8080
FAX: 217-876-7245
TTY: 217-876-8888
e-mail: sail@decatursail.com
www.decatursail.com

Jeri J Wooters, Executive Director
A community-based, non-residential Center for Independent Living whose purpose is to promote and practice independent living for all people with disabilities.

3911 **Soyland Access to Independent Living: Charleston**
757 Windsor Rd
Charleston, IL 61920-7474
217-345-7245
FAX: 217-345-7226
TTY:217-345-7245
e-mail: triplec@consolidated.net
www.decatursail.com

Matthew Hutti, Manager
Jeri J Wooters, Executive Director
A community-based, non-residential Center for Independent Living whose purpose is to promote and practice independent living for all people iwth disabilities.

3912 **Soyland Access to Independent Living: Shelbyville**
1810 W.S. 3rd ST P.O.Box 650
Shelbyville, IL 62565-650
217-774-4322
FAX: 217-774-4368
TTY:217-774-4322
e-mail: sailsel@consolidated.net
www.decatursail.com

Jeri J Wooters, Executive Director
Betty Watkins, Rural Outreach Coordinator
A community-based, non-residential Center for Independent Living whose purpose is to promote and practice independent living for all people with disabilities.

3913 **Soyland Access to Independent Living: Sullivan**
1102 W Jackson St
Sullivan, IL 61951-1067
217-728-3186
FAX: 217-728-2299
TTY:217-728-3186
e-mail: sulsail@wireless111.com
www.decatursail.com

Lou Anne Banks, Manager
Jeri J Wooters, Executive Director
Betty Watkins, Rural Outreach Coordinator
A community-based, non-residential Center for Independent Living whose purpose is to promote and practice independent living for all people with disabilities.

3914 **Springfield Center for Independent Living**
330 South Grand Ave W
Springfield, IL 62704-3716
217-523-4032
800-447-4221
FAX: 217-523-0427
TTY: 217-523-4032
e-mail: scil@scil.org
scil.org

Pete Roberts, Executive Director
Susan Coopers, Program Director
Robin Ashton-Hale, Reintegration Coordinator
Kathryn Cline, Business Manager
To increase opportunities for equality, integration and independence for all persons with disabilities through advocacy, services, and public education.

3915 **Stone-Hayes Center for Independent Living**
39 N Prairie St
Galesburg, IL 61401-4613
309-344-1306
888-347-4245
FAX: 309-344-1305
TTY: 309-344-1306
e-mail: stonehayes@misslink.net
stone-hayes.org

Vanya Peterson, Executive Director
Michael Bohnenkamp, Associate Director
John Hunigan, Office Manager
Lynn Voeller, Independent Living Associate
The purpose of INCIL is to facilitate the collaboration of all Centers for Independent Living in Illinois for promoting, through the Independent Living Movement, equal opportunities and civil rights for all persons with disabilities.

3916 **West Central Illinois Center for Independent Living**
639 York St.
Suite 204
Quincy, IL 62301-1065
217-223-0400
FAX: 217-223-0479
TTY:217-223-0475
e-mail: info@wcicil.org
www.wcicil.org

Glenda Hackemack, Executive Director
Dale Winner, Information & Referral Coordinat
Dustin Gorde Director of Community, Jenny
Kelly Transition Co-Ordinato
A not-for-profit advocacy center funded by state and federal grants to provide services to people with disabilities.

3917 **West Central Illinois Center for Independent Living: Macomb**
440 N Lafayette St
Macomb, IL 61455-1512
309-833-5766
FAX: 309-833-4690
TTY:217-223-0475
e-mail: info@wcicil.org
www.wcicil.org

Glenda Hackemack, Executive Director
Dale Winner, Information & Referral Coordinat
Dustin Gorde Director of Community, Jenny
Kelly Transition Co-Ordinato
A not-for-profit advocacy center funded by state and federal grants to provide services to people with disabilities.

3918 **Will Grundy Center for Independent Living**
2415 W Jefferson St
Suite A
Joliet, IL 60435-6464
815-729-0162
FAX: 815-729-3697
TTY:815-729-2085
e-mail: pamwgcil@sbcglobal.net
will-grundycil.org

Robert Smith, President
Jim Albritton, Vice President
Donald Cordano, Treasurer
Elaine Sommer, Secretary

A cross-disability, community based organization that strives for equalityand empowerment of persons with disabilities in the Will and Grundy County areas.

Indiana

3919 **Assistive Technology Training and Information Center (ATTIC)**
1721 Washington Ave
Vincennes, IN 47591-4823
812-886-0575
877-96A-8842
FAX: 812-886-1128
e-mail: inbox@atticindiana.org
www.atticindiana.org

Patricia Stewart, Executive Director
Rebecca Anderson, Assistant Director
Mark Schmitt, Fiscal Controller
Jackie Evans, Independent Living Coordinator

ATTIC provides support, information and education for individuals with disabilities and for families of children with special needs, and the professionals who assist these families. All disabilities, all ages.

3920 **DAMAR Services**
6067 Decatur Blvd.
Indianapolis, IN 46241
317-856-5201
FAX: 317-856-2333
e-mail: info@damar.org
damar.org

Gail Shiel, Chairman
Rick Torbeck, Cice Chairman
Jim Dalton, Psy.D., HSPP, President and CEO
Richard L. Harcourt, Vice President & CFO

Builds better futures for children and adults facing life's greatest developmental and behavioral challenges.

3921 **Everybody Counts Center for Independent Living**
9120 Connecticut Dr.
Suite E
Merrillville, IN 46410-7097
219-769-5055
888-769-3636
FAX: 219-769-5326
TTY:219-756-3323
e-mail: info@everybodycounts.org
everybodycounts.org

Teresa Torres, Executive Director
Emma Lewis Sullivan, On Loan Consultant
Mark Torres, Systems Manager
Jodi Hawn, Administrative Assistant

A nonprofit corporation dedicated to the achievement of maximum independence and enhanced quality of life for persons with disabilities.

3922 **Four Rivers Resource Services**
Hwy. 59 South
P.O. Box 249
Linton, IN 47441-249
812-847-2231
FAX: 812-847-8836
e-mail: fourrivers@frrs.org
frrs.org

Stephen Sacksteder, Executive Director
Robin Duncan, Chief Financial Officer
Dean Dorrell, Information Systems Director
Jessica Davis, Development Coordinator

FRRS is established to enable individuals with disabilities and other challenges to attain self independence and natural interdependence, inclusion in normal life experiences and opportunities, and general life enrichment, by working in partnership with them, their families and the communities in and around Greene, Sullivan, Daviess, and Martin Counties.

3923 **Future Choices Independent Living Center**
309 N High St
Muncie, IN 47305-1618
765-741-8332
866-741-3444
FAX: 765-741-8333
futurechoices.org

Beth Y. Quarles, President

Provides unlimited options for minorities, youth, and Hoosiers with disabilities.

3924 **Independent Living Center of Eastern Indiana (ILCEIN)**
1818 W Main St
Richmond, IN 47374-3822
765-939-9226
877-939-9226
FAX: 765-935-2215
www.ilcein.org

Jim McCormick, Executive Director
Dean Turner, Administrative Director
Ann Barnhart, Compliance Manager
Michelle Satterfield, Service Coordinator

Serving Fayette, Franklin, Henry, Decatur, Rush, Union and Wayne Counties.

3925 **Indianapolis Resource Center for Independent Living**
5302 East Washington Street
Indianapolis, IN 46219
317-926-1660
866-794-7245
FAX: 317-926-1687
e-mail: info@abilityindiana.org
ircil.org

Judy Townsend, President
Dave Trulock, Vice President
Jacqueline Troy, Treasurer
Don Lane, Secretary

Provides services, support and information to people with disabilities to help insure equal access to all aspects of community life.

3926 **League for the Blind and Disabled**
5821 S Anthony Blvd
Fort Wayne, IN 46816-3701
260-441-0551
800-889-3443
FAX: 260-441-7760
TTY: 800-889-3443
e-mail: the-league@the-league.org
the-league.org

David A. Nelson, CEO/President
Nancy Gasparini, Director Independent Living Serv
Anne Palmer, Administrative Assistant
Kevin Showalter, Youth Services Coordinator

To provide and promote opportunities that empower people with disabilities to achieve their potential.

3927 **Martin Luther Homes of Indiana**
Mosaic
26 N Brown Ave
Terre Haute, IN 47803-1523
812-235-3399
FAX: 812-235-1590
e-mail: abean@mlhs.com

3928 **Ruben Center for Independent Living**
5302 East Washington Street
Indianapolis, IN 46219-3227
317-926-1660
FAX: 317-926-1687
TTY:219-397-6496
www.abilityindiana.org

Judy Townsend, President
Dave Trulock, Vice President
Jacqueline Troy, Treasurer
Don Lane, Secretary

An independent living center providing support, information and education.

3929 **SILC, Indiana Council on Independent Living (ICOIL)**
P.O.Box 7083
Indianapolis, IN 46207-7083
317-232-1303
800-545-7763
FAX: 317-232-6478
e-mail: nancy.young@fssa.in.gov
Nancy Young, Program Director
Richard Simers, SILC Chairperson

3930 **Southern Indiana Center for Independent Living**
1494 W. Main Street
PO Box 308
Mitchell, IN 47446-1943
812-277-9626
800-845-6914
FAX: 812-277-9628
sicilindiana.org
Al Tolbert, Executive Director
Darlene Webster, Independent Living Center Direct
SICIL is a consumer controlled, community based, cross-disability, non-residential and not for profit organization that promotes and practices the philosophy of independent living: consumer control, peer support, self-help, self-determination, equal access, and individual and community advocacy. SICIL also promotes accesible and affordable housing, recreation and transportation.

3931 **Wabash Independent Living Center & Learning Center (WILL)**
1 Dreiser Square
Terre Haute, IN 47807
812-298-9455
877-915-9455
FAX: 812-299-9061
TTY: 877-915-9455
e-mail: info@thewillcenter.org
www.thewillcenter.org
Don Rogers, Chairman
Jody Pomfret, Vice Chairman
Kevin Burke, Treasurer
Peter Ciancone, Secretary-Executive Director
To empower people with disabilities to ensure that they have full and complete access to community resources to promote their independence

Iowa

3932 **Black Hawk Center for Independent Living**
2800 Falls Ave.
P.O. Box 2275
Waterloo, IA 50701-2275
319-291-7755
888-291-7754
FAX: 319-291-7781
TTY:800-735-2942
www.blackhawkcenter.org

3933 **Central Iowa Center for Independent Living**
655 Walnut St
Suite 131
Des Moines, IA 50309-3930
515-243-1742
888-503-2287
FAX: 515-243-5385
e-mail: ctoman@centraliowacil.com
www.centraliowacil.com
Bob Jeppesen, Executive Director
Frank Strong, Associate Director
Crystal Toman, Office Coordinator
Dee Howard, Independent Living Specialist
CICIL is a community based, non-profit, non-residential program serving persons with disabilities. CICIL assists all persons, regardless of disability in making choices about their own lives and in experiencing success in achieving independence.

3934 **Evert Conner Rights & Resources CIL**
730 S Dubuque St
Iowa City, IA 52240-4202
319-338-3870
800-982-0272
FAX: 319-354-1799
e-mail: info@ownersvoices.com
www.ownersvoices.com
Scott Gill, Executive Director
Provides community services like disability awareness training and classroom presentations. Individual services include independent living skills training and peer counseling. All services are custom designed to support the independence of people with disabilities in their own community.

3935 **Hope Haven**
1800 19th St
PO Box 70
Rock Valley, IA 51247-1098
712-476-2737
FAX: 712-476-3110
hopehaven.org
Dr. Kent Eric Eknes, President
Howard John Beernink, Vice President
David Vanningen, Executive Director
Calvin Helmus, Chief Operating Officer
Unleashes the potential in people through work and life skills so that they may enjoy a productive life in their community.

3936 **League of Human Dignity, Center for Independent Living**
1520 Avenue M
Council Bluffs, IA 51501-1185
712-323-6863
FAX: 712-323-6811
e-mail: Cinfo@leagueofhumandignity.com
www.leagueofhumandignity.com
Carrie England, Director
League of Human Dignity actively promotes the full integration of individuals with disabilities into society. To this end, the League will advocate their needs and rights, and provide quality services to involve these persons in becoming and remaining independent citizens.

3937 **Martin Luther Homes of Iowa**
P.O.Box 15
Waukon, IA 52172-0015
563-568-3992
FAX: 563-568-3992
www.rwjf.org
Mary Lynn ReVoir, Project Director
Fred Naumann III, Communications
Richard Wicks, Executive Director
.

3938 **South Central Iowa Center for Independent Living**
117 1st Ave W
Oskaloosa, IA 52577-3243
641-672-1867
800-651-7911
FAX: 641-672-1867
e-mail: oskyscicil@mahaska.org
Deb Philpot, Executive Director
Provides services, support, information and referral to people with disabilities to help insure equal access to all aspects of community life.

3939 **Three Rivers Center for Independent Living**
900 Rebecca Avenue
Pittsburgh, PA 15221-2938
412-371-7700
800-633-4588
FAX: 412-371-9430
TTY: 412-371-6230
e-mail: sholbrook@trcil.org
trcil.myfastsite.net
Stanley A. Holbrook, President & Executive Director
Erin Ryan, SR. Program Manager
Roxanne Huss, Director of Waiver Services
Charles Keenan, TRCIL Real Properties Board
Providing a wide array of services to assist individuals and families in achieving positive life goals.

Kansas

3940 **Advocates for Better Living For Everyone(A.B.L.E.)**
Ste C
521 Commercial St
Atchison, KS 66002
913-367-1830
888-845-2879
FAX: 913-367-1830
www.ableks.org
Ken Gifford, President & CEO
A not for profit agency providing services within the State of Kansas. ABLE looks to assist people with disabilities as well as any other member of the community to live an integrated, quality life with dignity, respect, and independence.

3941 **Center for Independent Living SW Kansas: Liberal**
1023 N Kansas Ave
Suite 2
Liberal, KS 67901-2655
620-624-5500
800-327-4048
FAX: 620-624-6576
TTY: 620-624-5500
www.cilswks.org
Victor Otero, Manager
Crystal Tharp, Independent Living Advocate
Dedicated to helping people achieve full participation in society.

3942 **Center for Independent Living Southwest Kansas**
P.O.Box 2090
Garden City, KS 67846-2090
620-276-1900
800-736-9443
FAX: 620-271-0200
e-mail: info@cilswks.org
cilswks.org
Troy Horton, Executive Director
Dedicated to helping people achieve full participation in society.

3943 **Center for Independent Living Southwest Kansas: Dodge City**
2601 Central Ave
Dodge City, KS 67801-6200
620-227-6660
800-326-1366
FAX: 620-227-8185
TTY: 620-227-6660
www.cilswks.org
Mary Jane Sandoval, Independent Living Advocate
Dedicated to helping people achieve full participation in society

3944 **Coalition for Independence**
4911 State Ave
Kansas City, KS 66102-1749
913-321-5140
866-201-3829
FAX: 913-321-5182
TTY: 913-321-5216
cfi-kc.org
Clarence Smith, Executive Director
Laarni Sison, Executive Assistant
Claire Marr, Lead Independent Living Speciali
Shauna Garrett, Lead Accountant
Facilitates positive and responsible independence for all people with disabilities by acting as an advocate for individuals with disabilities, providing services, and promoting accessibility and acceptance.

3945 **Cowley County Developmental Services**
P.O.Box 618
Arkansas City, KS 67005-618
620-442-5270
866-442-5270
FAX: 620-442-5623
www.ccds-cddo.org
Bill Brooks, Executive Director
Provides services for persons with developmental disabilities in Cowley County..

3946 **Independence**
2001 Haskell Ave
Lawrence, KS 66046-3249
785-841-0333
888-824-7277
FAX: 785-841-1094
e-mail: comment@independenceinc.org
independenceinc.org
Edward Canda, President
Mary Chappell, Vice President
Clark Cropp, Treasurer
Athena Johnson, Secretary
Provides advocacy, services, and education for people with disabilities and our communities.

3947 **Independent Connection**
1710 W. Schilling Road
P.O.Box 1160
Salina, KS 67402- 1160
785-827-9383
800-526-9731
FAX: 785-823-2015
TTY: 785-827-9383
www.occk.com
Shelia Nelson-Stout, President/CEO
Deanna L. Lamer, Senior Director,Human Resources
Tasha Suppes, Human Resources Coordinator
Dedicated to helping people with physical or mental disabilities remove barriers to employment, independent living, and full participation in their communities.

3948 **Independent Connection: Abilene**
Suite 221
300 N. Cedar St.
Abilene, KS 67410
785-263-2208
FAX: 785-263-3795
TTY:785-263-2208
www.occk.com
Shelia Nelson-Stout, President/CEO
Deanna L. Lamer, Senior Director,Human Resources
Tasha Suppes, Human Resources Coordinator
Dedicated to helping people with physical or mental disabilities remove barriers to employment, independent living, and full participation in their communities.

3949 **Independent Connection: Beloit**
501 W 7th St
Beloit, KS 67420-2107
785-738-5423
FAX: 785-738-3320
TTY:785-738-5423
www.occk.com
Shelia Nelson-Stout, President/CEO
Deanna L. Lamer, Senior Director,Human Resources
Tasha Suppes, Human Resources Coordinator
Dedicated to helping people with physical or mental disabilities remove barriers to employment, independent living, and full participation in their communities.

3950 **Independent Connection: Concordia**
1502 Lincoln St
Concordia, KS 66901-4830
785-243-1977
FAX: 785-243-4524
TTY:785-243-1977
www.occk.com
Shelia Nelson-Stout, President/CEO
Dedicated to helping people with physical or mental disabilities remove barriers to employment, independent living, and full participation in their communities.

3951 **Independent Living Resource Center**
3033 W 2nd St N
Wichita, KS 67203-5357
316-942-6300
800-479-6861
FAX: 316-942-2078
ilrcks.org
James Thayer, President
John Brennan, Vice Chairman
Jane Mobley, Secretary/Treasurer
TraceAnn Adkins, Human Resources Manager

Empower people with disabilities to lead independent lives by providing advocacy, education and direct services. Serve people with all types of disabilities; permanent or temporary, physical disabilities, mental disabilities, and developmental disabilities.

3952 Kansas Services for the Blind & Visually Impaired
2601 SW East Circle Dr N
Topeka, KS 66606-2445
785-296-3738
800-547-5789
FAX: 785-291-3138
e-mail: rehab@srskansas.org
srskansas.org

Dennis Ford, Manager
Michael Donnelly, Director

Helps persons who are blind or visually to improve their quality of life. KSBVI provides people with an array of services and experiences aimed at overcoming not only the physical difficulties brought on by the loss of vision, but also the fear of change associated with vision loss. KSBVI can also help with job search and retention activities; life skills training; access to medical services; and technical assistance..

3953 LINK: Colby
505 N Franklin Ave
Suite G
Colby, KS 67701-2342
785-462-7600
800-736-9418
TTY:785-462-7600
www.linkinc.org

Brian Atwell, Executive Director

Promotes and supports the civil rights of people with disabilities and empowers them to achieve a life of independence and equality..

3954 Living Independently in Northwest Kansas: Hays
2401 E 13th St
Hays, KS 67601-2663
785-625-6942
800-596-5926
FAX: 785-625-2334
TTY: 785-625-6942
linkinc.org

Brian Atwell, Executive Director

Promotes and supports the civil rights of people with disabilities and empowers them to achieve a life of independence and equality.

3955 Prairie IL Resource Center
103 W 2nd St
Pratt, KS 67124-2644
620-672-9600
FAX: 620-672-9601
e-mail: info@pilr.org
www.pilr.org

Dave Mullins, President
Stephanie Guthrie, Vice President
Chris Owens, Executive Director
Roger Frischenmeyer, Independent Living Specialist

To achieve the full inclusion and acceptance of people with disabilities through education and advocacy

3956 Prairie Independent Living Resource Center
17th S Main St
Hutchinson, KS 67501
620-663-3989
888-715-6818
FAX: 620-663-4711
TTY:620-663-9920
e-mail: info@pilr.org
pilr.org

Dave Mullins, President
Stephanie Guthrie, Vice President
Chris Owens, Executive Director
Roger Frischenmeyer, Independent Living Specialist

To achieve the full conclusion and acceptance of people with disabilities through education and advocacy

3957 Resource Center for Independent Living
726 W Patterson Ave
Iola, KS 66749-8805
620-365-8144
877-944-8144
FAX: 620-365-7726
www.rcilinc.org

Chad Wilkins, Executive Director

Committed to working with individuals, families, and communities to promote independent living and individual choice to persons with disabilities.

3958 Resource Center for Independent Living, Inc. (RCIL)
409 Columbia St.
Utica, NY 13503-210
315-797-4642
800-580-7245
FAX: 315-797-4747
TTY: 315-797-5837
www.rcilinc.org

Chad Wilkins, Executive Director

Committed to working with individuals, families, and communities to promote independent living and individual choice to persons with disabilities. As a center for independent living in Kansas, we provide advocacy, peer counseling, information and referral, independent living skills training and deinstitutionalization. In addition to these services, we also provide HOBS payroll services and a variety of programs benefiting individuals with disabilities.

3959 Resource Center for Independent Living: Emporia
215 West Sixth Avenue
Suite 202
Emporia, KS 66801-2886
620-342-1648
888-261-4024
FAX: 620-342-1821
e-mail: info@rcilinc.org
www.rcilinc.org

Deone Wilson, Executive Director
Beth Combes, Information & Outreach Coordinat
Amy Richardson, Targeted Case Manager
Trevor Larson, Office Assistant

Committed to working with individuals, families, and communities to promote independent living and individual choice to persons with disabilities.

3960 Resource Center for Independent Living: Arkansas City
P.O. Box 257
1137 Laing
Osage City, KS 66523
785-528-3105
800-580-7245
FAX: 785-528-3665
TTY: 785-528-3106
e-mail: info@rcilinc.org
www.rcilinc.org

Deone Wilson, Executive Director
Tania Harrington, Director of Quality Assurance
Adam Burnett, Director of Core Services
Mike Pitts, Finance Committee Chairperson

Committed to working with individuals, families, and communities to promote independent living and individual choice to persons with disabilities.

3961 Resource Center for Independent Living: Burlington
P.O. Box 257
1137 Laing
Osage City, KS 66523
785-528-3105
800-580-7245
FAX: 785-528-3665
TTY: 785-528-3106
e-mail: info@rcilinc.org
www.rcilinc.org

Deone Wilson, Executive Director
Tania Harrington, Director of Quality Assurance
Adam Burnett, Director of Core Services
Mike Pitts, Finance Committee Chairperson

Committed to working with individuals, families, and communities to promote independent living and individual choice to persons with disabilities.

3962 Resource Center for Independent Living: Coffeyville
P.O. Box 257
1137 Laing
Osage City, KS 66523
785-528-3105
800-580-7245
FAX: 785-528-3665
TTY: 785-528-3106
e-mail: info@rcilinc.org
www.rcilinc.org

Deone Wilson, Executive Director
Tania Harrington, Director of Quality Assurance
Adam Burnett, Director of Core Services
Mike Pitts, Finance Committee Chairperson

Committed to working with individuals, families, and communities to promote independent living and individual choice to persons with disabilities.

3963 Resource Center for Independent Living: El Dorado
615 1/2 N Main St
El Dorado, KS 67042-2027
316-322-7853
800-960-7853
FAX: 316-322-7888
e-mail: info@rcilinc.org
www.rcilinc.org

Macy Gaines, Independent Living Specialist
Doris Hammons, Targeted Case Manager
Shirley Mullin, Targeted Case Manager
Barbara Ehret, Office Assistant

Committed to working with individuals, families, and communities to promote independent living and individual choice to persons with disabilities.

3964 Resource Center for Independent Living: Ft Scott
P.O. Box 257
1137 Laing
Osage City, KS 66523
785-528-3105
800-580-7245
FAX: 785-528-3665
TTY: 785-528-3106
e-mail: info@rcilinc.org
www.rcilinc.org

Deone Wilson, Executive Director
Tania Harrington, Director of Quality Assurance
Adam Burnett, Director of Core Services
Mike Pitts, Finance Committee Chairperson

Committed to working with individuals, families, and communities to promote independent living and individual choice to persons with disabilities.

3965 Resource Center for Independent Living: Ottawa
233 W 23rd Street
Ottawa, KS 66067-3533
785-242-1805
800-995-1805
FAX: 785-242-1448
www.rcilinc.org

Chad Wilkins, Executive Director

Committed to working with individuals, families, and communities to promote independent living and individual choice to persons with disabilities.

3966 Resource Center for Independent Living: Overland Park
Ste 100
10200 W 75th St
Shawnee Mission, KS 66204-2242
913-362-6618
877-439-2847
FAX: 913-677-2742
www.rcilinc.org

Chad Wilkins, Executive Director

RCIL is committed to working with individuals, families, and communities to promote independent living and individual choice to persons with disabilities.

3967 Resource Center for Independent Living: Topeka
1507 S.W. 21stStreet
Suite 203
Topeka, KS 66604-2356
785-267-1717
877-719-1717
FAX: 785-267-1711
e-mail: info@rcilinc.org
rcilinc.org

Rosie Cooper, Director of Independent Living S
Stuart Jones, Assistive Technology Specialist
Mikel McCary, Assistive Technology Specialist
Mandy Smith, Finance Committee Chairperson

Committed to working with individuals, families, and communities to promote independent living and individual choice to persons with disabilities.

3968 Southeast Kansas Independent Living (SKIL)
1801 Main
P.O. Box 957
Parsons, KS 67357-957
620-421-5502
800-688-5616
FAX: 620-421-3705
TTY: 620-421-0983
e-mail: skil@skilonline.com
www.skilonline.com

Nancy Varner, Chairman
Janet Spillman, Vice Chairman
Shari Coatney, CEO/President
Olivia Lyons, Secretary/Treasurer

To empower, integrate and maximize independence for all persons with disabilities.

3969 Southeast Kansas Independent Living: Independence
107 East Main
P.O.Box 944
Independence, KS 67301-944
620-331-1006
866-927-1006
FAX: 620-331-1257
TTY: 620-331-1006
e-mail: skilindy@skilonline.com
www.skilonline.com

Nancy Varner, Chairman
Janet Spillman, Vice Chairman
Shari Coatney, CEO/President
Olivia Lyons, Secretary/Treasurer

To empower, integrate and maximize independence for all persons with disabilities.

3970 Southeast Kansas Independent Living: Chanute
2 W. Main
P.O.Box 645
Chanute, KS 66720-645
620-431-0757
866-927-0757
FAX: 620-431-7274
TTY: 620-431-0757
e-mail: skilchanute@skilonline.com
www.skilonline.com

Nancy Varner, Chairman
Janet Spillman, Vice Chairman
Shari Coatney, CEO/President
Olivia Lyons, Secretary/Treasurer

To empower, integrate and maximize independence for all persons with disabilities.

3971 Southeast Kansas Independent Living: Columbus
125 East Maple
P.O. Box 478
Columbus, KS 66725-1801
620-429-3600
866-927-3600
FAX: 620-429-1027
e-mail: skilcolumbus@skilonline.com
skilonline.com

Nancy Varner, Chairman
Janet Spillman, Vice Chairman
Shari Coatney, CEO/President
Olivia Lyons, Secretary/Treasurer

To empower, integrate and maximize independence for all persons with disabilities.

3972 Southeast Kansas Independent Living: Fredonia
623 Monroe
P.O.Box 448
Fredonia, KS 66736-448
620-378-4881
866-927-4881
FAX: 620-378-4851
TTY: 620-378-4881
e-mail: skilfredonia@skilonline.com
www.skilonline.com

Nancy Varner, Chairman
Janet Spillman, Vice Chairman
Shari Coatney, CEO/President
Olivia Lyons, Secretary/Treasurer
To empower, integrate and maximize independence for all persons with disabilities.

3973 Southeast Kansas Independent Living: Hays
510 W. 29thStreet, Suite A
PO Box 366
Hays, KS 67601- 366
785-628-8019
800-316-8019
FAX: 785-628-3116
TTY: 785-628-3128
e-mail: skilhays@skilonline.com
www.skilonline.com

Nancy Varner, Chairman
Janet Spillman, Vice Chairman
Shari Coatney, CEO/President
Olivia Lyons, Secretary/Treasurer
To empower, integrate and maximize independence for all persons with disabilities.

3974 Southeast Kansas Independent Living: Pittsburg
1403 N. Broadway
P.O.Box 1706
Pittsburg, KS 66762-1706
620-231-6780
866-927-6780
FAX: 620-232-9915
TTY: 620-231-6780
e-mail: skilpittsburg@skilonline.com
skilonline.com

Nancy Varner, Chairman
Janet Spillman, Vice Chairman
Shari Coatney, CEO/President
Olivia Lyons, Secretary/Treasurer
To empower, integrate and maximize independence for all persons with disabilities.

3975 Southeast Kansas Independent Living: Sedan
113 West Main
P.O.Box 340
Sedan, KS 67361-340
620-725-3990
866-906-3990
FAX: 620-725-3942
TTY: 620-725-3990
e-mail: skilsedan@skilonline.com
www.skilonline.com

Nancy Varner, Chairman
Janet Spillman, Vice Chairman
Shari Coatney, CEO/President
Olivia Lyons, Secretary/Treasurer
To empower, integrate and maximize independence for all persons with disabilities.

3976 Southeast Kansas Independent Living: Yates Center
119 W. Butler
P.O.Box 129
Yates Center, KS 66783-129
620-625-2818
866-927-2818
FAX: 620-625-2585
e-mail: skilyc@skilonline.com
www.skilonline.com

Nancy Varner, Chairman
Janet Spillman, Vice Chairman
Shari Coatney, CEO/President
Olivia Lyons, Secretary/Treasurer
To empower, integrate and maximize independence for all persons with disabilities.

3977 The Whole Person: Nortonville
7301 Mission Road
Suite 135
Prairie Village, KS 66208- 3006
913-262-1294
877-767-8896
FAX: 913-262-2392
e-mail: info@thewholeperson.org
www.thewholeperson.org

Brian Ellefson, President
Rick O'Neal, Vice President
Donna Bradford, Interim Chief Executive Officer
Mike Wiley, Chief Operating Officer
Assists people with disabilities to live independently and encourages change within the community to expand opportunities for independent living.

3978 The Whole Person: Prairie Village
7301 Mission Road
Suite 135
Prairie Village, KS 66208- 3006
913-262-1294
877-767-8896
FAX: 913-262-2392
e-mail: info@thewholeperson.org
www.thewholeperson.org

Brian Ellefson, President
Rick O'Neal, Vice President
Donna Bradford, Interim Chief Executive Officer
Mike Wiley, Chief Operating Officer
Assists people with disabilities to live independently and encourages change within the community to expand opportunities for independent living.

3979 Three Rivers Independent Living Center
504 Miller Drive
P.O.Box 408
Wamego, KS 66547-0408
785-456-9915
800-555-3994
FAX: 785-456-9923
TTY: 785-456-9915
e-mail: reception@threeriversinc.org
threeriversinc.org

Audrey Schremmer-Philips, Executive Director
Sandy Simmer, Finance Manager
Barbara Feldkamp, IL Specialist
Rebel Eichelberger, Accounting Assistant
A nonprofit organization promoting the self reliance of individuals with disabilities through education, advocacy, training and support.

3980 Three Rivers Independent Living Center: Clay
719 5th Street
P.O.Box 33
Clay Center, KS 67432-0033
785-632-6117
FAX: 785-632-6117
TTY:785-632-6117
e-mail: reception@threeriversinc.org
www.threeriversinc.org

Rose Scott, Manager
Audrey Schremmer-Philips, Executive Director
Sandy Simmer, Finance Manager
Rebel Eichelberger, Accounting Assistant
A non-profit organization promoting the self reliance of individuals with disabilities through, education, advocacy, training and support.

3981 Three Rivers Independent Living Center: Manhattan
401 Houston St.
Manhattan, KS 66502
785-776-9294
800-432-2703
FAX: 785-776-9479
e-mail: reception@threeriversinc.org
www.threeriversinc.org

Audrey Schremmer-Philips, Executive Director
Sandy Simmer, Finance Manager
Elizabeth Moore, IL Specialist
Rebel Eichelberger, Accounting Assistant

A non profit organization promoting the self reliance of individuals with disabilities through education, advocacy, training and support.

3982 Three Rivers Independent Living Center: Seneca
416 Main St
Seneca, KS 66538-1926
785-336-0222
FAX: 785-336-0288
e-mail: reception@threeriversinc.org
www.threeriversinc.org

Lynn Neihaus, Manager
Audrey Schremmer-Philips, Executive Director
Sandy Simmer, Finance Manager
Rebel Eichelberger, Accounting Assistant

A non profit organization promoting the self reliance of individuals with disabilities through education, advocacy, training and support.

3983 Three Rivers Independent Living Center: Topeka
P.O.Box 4152
Topeka, KS 66604-4152
785-273-0249
FAX: 785-273-0249
e-mail: reception@threeriversinc.org
www.threeriversinc.org

Audrey Schremmer-Philips, Executive Director
Sandy Simmer, Finance Manager
Dave Reed, Recreation Specialist
Rebel Eichelberger, Accounting Assistant

A non profit organization promoting the self reliance of individuals with disabilities through education, advocacy, training and support.

3984 Topeka Independent Living Resource Center
501 SW Jackson St
Suite 100
Topeka, KS 66603-3300
785-233-4572
FAX: 785-233-1561
TTY:785-233-4572
e-mail: tilrcweb@tilrc.org
tilrc.org

Mike Oxford, Executive Director
Evan Korynta, Operations Manager
Angie Harter, Independent Living Advocacy Staf
Carol Doss, Independent Living Advocacy Staf

A civil and human rights organization that advocates for justice, equality and essential services for a fully integrated and accessible society for all people with disabilities.

3985 Whole Person: Nortonville
7301 Mission Road
Suite 135
Prairie Village, KS 66208- 3006
913-262-1294
877-767-8896
FAX: 913-262-2392
e-mail: info@thewholeperson.org
www.thewholeperson.org

Brian Ellefson, President
Rick O'Neal, Vice President
Donna Bradford, Interim Chief Executive Officer
Mike Wiley, Chief Operating Officer

Assists people with disabilities to live independently and encourages change within the community to expand opportunities for independent living.

3986 Whole Person: Prairie Village
7301 Mission Rd
Prairie Village, KS 66208-3006
913-262-1294
FAX: 913-262-2392
e-mail: info@thewholeperson.org
www.thewholeperson.org

Brian Ellefson, President
Rick O'Neal, Vice President
Donna Bradford, Interim Chief Executive Officer
Mike Wiley, Chief Operating Officer

Assists people with disabilities to live independently and encourages change within the community to expand opportunities for independent living.

3987 Whole Person: Tonganoxie
7301 Mission Road
Suite 135
Prairie Village, KS 66208- 3006
913-262-1294
877-767-8896
FAX: 913-262-2392
e-mail: info@thewholeperson.org
www.thewholeperson.org

Brian Ellefson, President
Rick O'Neal, Vice President
Donna Bradford, Interim Chief Executive Officer
Mike Wiley, Chief Operating Officer

Assists people with disabilities to live independently and encourages change within the community to expand opportunities for independent living.

Kentucky

3988 Center for Accessible Living
501 S. 2nd Street
Ste 200
Louisville, KY 40202-2121
502-589-6620
888-813-8497
FAX: 502-589-3980
TTY:502-589-6690
e-mail: info@calky.org
calky.org

Jan Day, CEO
Michael Markiewicz, Chief Financial Officer
Jeanne M. Gallimore, Branch Director
Susan Tharpe, Independent Living Specialist

To assist the individuals with disabilities who seek to live independently.

3989 Center for Accessible Living: Murray
1051 N 16th St
Suite C
Murray, KY 42071-8511
270-753-7676
888-261-6194
FAX: 270-753-7729
TTY:270-767-0549
e-mail: info@calky.org
www.calky.org

Jeanne M. Gallimore, Branch Director
Susan Tharpe, Independent Living Specialist
Jan Day, CEO
Michael Markiewicz, Chief Financial Officer

To assist the individuals with disabilities who seek to live independently.

3990 Center for Independent Living: Kentucky Department for the Blind
Independent Living Office
Rear
409 N Miles St
Elizabethtown, KY 42701-1834
270-766-5126
e-mail: buel.stalls@mail.state.ky.us

Buel E Stalls Jr, Office Manager and IL Specialist
Nancy Bachuss, Manager

Offers peer counseling, attendant care registry and other services to the community as they relate to the blind community. The Murray office is an independent living regional office which covers 20 far western counties of Kentucky..

3991 Disability Coalition of Northern Kentucky
Ste 219
525 W 5th St
Covington, KY 41011-1293
859-431-7668
FAX: 859-431-7688
TTY:800-648-6057
e-mail: dcnky@fuse.net

Kitt Heeg, Executive Director

Empowering people with disabilities through education, networking, and positive attitudes..

3992 Disability Resource Initiative
624 Eastwood St
Bowling Green, KY 42103-1602
270-796-5992
877-437-5045
FAX: 270-796-6630
www.dri-ky.org

Marilyn Mitchell, Executive Director
Tracy Cole, Independent Living Specialist
Steve Burchett, IT Specialist
Jenny McCallister, Administrative Assistant

One of the most important premises in Independent Living is that people with disabilities are the most knowledgable about their own needs. Because of this all of their services are designed to be consumer-driven. Within each service, Center Staff work with both participant and provider to achieve and maintain an Independent Lifestyle.

3993 Independence Place
1093 S. Broadway
Suite 1218
Lexington, KY 40504-1787
859-266-2807
877-266-2807
FAX: 859-335-0627
TTY: 800-648-6056
e-mail: info@independenceplaceky.org
www.independenceplaceky.org

Michael Fein, Chairman
Carla Webster, Vice Chairwoman
Pamela Roark-Glisson, Executive Director
Orissa Mason, Consumer Services Coordinator

To assist people with disabilities to achieve their full potential for community inclusion through improving access, choice and equal opportunity.

3994 Pathfinders for Independent Living
105 E Mound St
Harlan, KY 40831-2355
606-573-5777
877-340-PATH
FAX: 606-573-5739
TTY: 606-573-5777
www.pahtfindersilc.org

Sandra Goodwyn, Executive Director
Andrew Saylor, Director of IT (Internal) and Fi
Stacy Marple, Director of IT (External)
Ron Walker, Public Affairs Specialist

They publish a newsletter called LifeLine 4-5 times a year. Most articles are written by Sandra Goodwyn. Editor is Andrew Saylor. Serves people with disabilities to maintain as much independence as they desire

3995 SILC Department of Vocational Rehabilitation
209 Saint Clair St
Frankfort, KY 40601-1817
502-564-4440
800-372-7172
FAX: 502-564-6745
e-mail: sarahf.richardson@ky.gov
www.ovr.ky.org

Sarah Richardson, SILC Liaison

We recognize and respect the contributions of all individuals as a necessary and vital part of a productive society..

Louisiana

3996 New Horizons: Central Louisiana
Ste 18
2406 Ferrand St
Monroe, LA 71201-3236
318-323-4374
800-428-5505
FAX: 318-323-5445
www.nhilc.org

3997 New Horizons: Northeast Louisiana
Ste A
3400 Jackson St
Alexandria, LA 71301-4037
318-484-3596
888-361-3596
FAX: 318-484-3640
e-mail: nhilc@nhilc.org
www.nhilc.org

Dimple Hughes, Executive Director

A private, non-profit, non-residential, consumer controlled, community based organization that enables people with disabilities to live independently.

3998 New Horizons: Northwest Louisiana
Ste D
8508 Line Ave
Shreveport, LA 71106-6144
318-671-8131
877-219-7327
FAX: 318-688-7823
e-mail: nhilc@nhilc.org
nhilc.org

Gale Dean, Manager

A private, non-profit, non-residential, consumer-controlled, community based organization that enables people with disabilities to live independently.

3999 Resources for Independent Living: Baton Rouge
New Orleans Resources for Independent Living
3233 South Sherwood Forest Blvd.
Suite 101A
Baton Rouge, LA 70816
225-753-4772
877-505-2260
FAX: 225-753-4831
e-mail: contact@noril.org
www.noril.org

Yavonka G. Archaga, Executive Director
Alisha S. Hammond, Assistant Director
Rosie Calvin, Program Manager
Deonne T. Bailey, Core Service Manager

RIL provides quality services to individuals with disabilities to assist with living independent. RIL also offers services to inculde information and referral, advocacy, peer support and independent living skills training.

4000 Resources for Independent Living: Metairie
2001 21st Street Kenner
Kenner, LA 70062
504-522-1955
877-505-2260
FAX: 504-522-1954
e-mail: contact@noril.org
noril.org

Yavonka G. Archaga, Executive Director
Alisha S. Hammond, Assistant Director
Rosie Calvin, Program Manager
Deonne T. Bailey, Core Service Manager

RIL provides quality services to individuals with disabilities to assist with living independently. RIL also offers an array of services to include information and referral, advocacy, peer support and independent living skills training.

4001 Southwest Louisiana Independence Center: Lake Charles
2016 Oak Park Boulevard
Lake Charles, LA 70601-5391
337-477-7198
888-403-1062
FAX: 337-477-7198
TTY: 337-477-7198
slic.org

4002 Southwest Louisians Independence Center: Lafayette
850 Kaliste Saloom Rd
Suite 118
Lafayette, LA 70508-4230
337-269-0027
888-516-5009
FAX: 337-233-7660
www.slic-la.org

4003 Volunteers of America of Greater New Orleans
4152 Canal St.
New Orleans, LA 70119
504-482-2130
FAX: 504-482-1922
voagno.org

Robert C. Rhoden, Chair
Wayne M. Baquet, Chair Elect
James M. Le Blanc, President/CEO
Geoffrey C. Artigues, Treasurer

Volunteers of America Greater New Orleans offers many services that aim to improve the lives of children, youth, and families.

4004 W Troy Cole Independent Living Specialist
Ste H
1900 Lamy Ln
Monroe, LA 71201-9200
318-323-4374

Katherine Carnell, Manager

Maine

4005 Alpha One: Bangar
Suite 302
2937 SW 27th Avenue
Miami, FL 33133
305-567-9888
877-228-7321
FAX: 305-567-1317
www.alphaone.org

John W. Walsh, President & CEO, Co-founder
Marcia F. Ritchie, Vice President & Chief Operatin
Marsha A. Carnes, Director of Program Evaluation
Robert Campbell, Communications Manager

Committed to being a leading enterprise providing the community with information, services and products that create opportunities for people with disabilities to live independently. Provides many services including adaptive and mobility equipment selection, peer support, advocacy, information and referral services, adapted drive evaluation and training, and consumer directed personal assistance.

4006 Alpha One: South Portland
127 Main St
South Portland, ME 04106-2647
207-767-2189
800-640-7200
FAX: 207-799-8346
TTY: 207-767-5387
www.alphaonenow.com

Dennis Stubbs, Chairman
Bob McPhee, Vice-Chairman
Darlene Stewart, Independent Living Specialist
Ketra S Crosson, Aroostook County Coordinator

Committed to being a leading enterprise providing the community with information, services and products that create opportunities for people with disabilities to live independently. Offers adaptive equipment loan program, independent living skills instruction, adapted driver evaluation and training, information and referral services, peer support, advocacy, access design consultation, and more.

4007 Motivational Services
71 Hospital Street
P.O.Box 229
Augusta, ME 04332-0229
207-626-3465
FAX: 207-626-3469
TTY:207-621-2542
e-mail: information@mocomaine.com
www.mocomaine.com

Connie Dunn, President
Grace Leonard, Vice President/Secretary
Faith Madore, Treasurer
Richard Weiss, Executive Director

Improving the lives of people with disabilities through housing, employment and community support.

4008 Shalom House
106 Gilman St
Portland, ME 04102-3034
207-874-1080
FAX: 207-874-1077
TTY:207-842-6888
e-mail: generalmail@shalomhouseinc.org
shalomhouseinc.org

Megan Lewis, Human Resources Manager
Mary Haynes-Rodgers, Executive Director
Kristine Lausier, Quality Assurance Administrator
Jane Collette, Accounting Manager

Offers hope for adults living with severe mental illness by providing a choice of quality housing and support services that help people lead stable and fulfilling lives in the community.

Maryland

4009 Broadmead
13801 York Rd
Cockeysville, MD 21030-1899
410-527-1900
877-STA-HOME
www.broadmead.org

Ann H. Heaton, Chair
John E. Howl, Chief Executive Officer
Patricia Gordon, Chief Financial Officer/Treasurer
Douglas Bareis, Director of Support Services

To provide continuing care services to a diverse group of seniors in a warm, congenial community founded and operated in the spirit of the Religious Society of Friends.

4010 Eastern Shore Center for Independent Living
309 Sunburst Highway
Suite 9
Cambridge, MD 21613-2050
410-221-7701
800-705-7944
FAX: 410-221-7714
TTY: 410-221-4150
e-mail: escil@escil.org
www.escil.org

Shirley Tarbox, Executive Director
Steven Melvin, Program Director
Betsy B. Jones, Executive Assistant
Doretha Luke, Administrative Assistant

ESCIL provides services to people with all disabilities regardless of age, religion, gender, ethnicity, race or national origin. In addition to the core services of information and referral, skills training, peer support and advocacy, ESCIL also offers assistance with accessibility modifications, Americans with Disabilities Act education and training, housing referrals and counseling, transportation referral and information, Brailling capabilities, Personal Attendent Services referral, and more.

4011 Freedom Center
14 W. Patrick Street
Suite 10
Frederick, MD 21701
301-846-7811
FAX: 301-846-9070
e-mail: advocate@thefreedomcenter-md.org
thefreedomcenter-md.org

Jamey George, Executive Director
Russell Holt, President
Patrick Mcmurtray, Vice-President
Craig Shafer, Treasurer

A walk in center for independent living, provides services and supports to empower individuals with disabilities to lead self-directed, independent, and productive lives in a barrier-free community.

4012 Housing Unlimited
Ste G1
1398 Lamberton Dr
Silver Spring, MD 20902-3435 301-592-9314
FAX: 301-592-9318
e-mail: information@housingunlimited.org
www.housingunlimited.org

Nancy Cohen, President Emerita
Russell Phillips, President
Robyn S. Raysor, Vice President
Johnnie Mae Armstrong, Treasurer

To address the housing crisis for adults with psychiatric disabilities who reside in Montgomery County, Maryland.

4013 Independence Now
Ste 101
12301 Old Columbia Pike
Silver Spring, MD 20904-1656 301-277-2839
FAX: 301-625-9777
e-mail: info@innow.org
innow.org

Sarah Sorensen, Executive Director
Trish Foley, Director of Community Services
Todd Thorpe, Director of Operations
Mike Polits, Director Finance

A nonprofit organization created by people with disabilities and provides services that promote independence and the inclusion of people with disabilities in their communities.

4014 Independence Now: Silver Spring
Ste 101
12301 Old Columbia Pike
Silver Spring, MD 20904-1659 301-277-2839
FAX: 301-625-9777
e-mail: info@innow.org
innow.org

Sarah Sorensen, Executive Director
Trish Foley, Director of Community Services
Todd Thorpe, Director of Operations
Mike Polits, Director Finance

A nonprofit organization created by people with disabilities that provides services that promotes independence and the inclusion of people with disabilities in their communities.

4015 Making Choices for Independent Living
Ste 202
1118 Light St
Baltimore, MD 21230-4152 410-234-8195
888-560-2221
e-mail: andreab@mcil-md.org
www.mcil-md.org

Jimmie Joku Cooper, Owner

Provides services to help empower people with disabilities to lead self-directed, independent and productive lives in the community and protect their civil rights.OUTOF ORDER.

4016 Resources for Independence
30 N. Mechanic Street
Unit B
Cumberland, MD 21502-2705 301-784-1774
800-371-1986
FAX: 301-784-1776
www.rficil.org

Lori Magruder, Executive Director
John Michaels, Assistant Director
Robert Cannon, Resource Developer
Sherry Williams, Finance Director

Private, non-profit, consumer-controlled, community-based organization providing services and advocacy by and for persons with all type of disabilities. Their goal is to create opportunities for independence, and to assist individuals with disabilities to achieve their maximum level of independent functioning within their families and communities.

4017 Southern Maryland Center for LIFE
P.O.Box 657
Charlotte Hall, MD 20622-657 301-884-4498
FAX: 301-884-6099
e-mail: cflife@eartlink.net
www.somd.com

Marie Robinson, Executive Director
Carrie Lanthier, Administrative Assistant

A non-profit community based organization which provides services to disabled people who live or work in the tri-county area. Our mission is to empower people with disabilities to lead self-directed, independent, and productive lives in their community.

Massachusetts

4018 Adlib
215 North St
Pittsfield, MA 01201-4644 413-442-7047
800-232-7047
FAX: 413-443-4338
e-mail: adlib@adlibcil.org
adlibcil.org

Linda Febles, President
Michael Hinkley, Vice President
Allison Bedard, Treasurer
Shannon Miller, Secretary/Clerk

Offers information and referral services, independent living skills training, peer counseling, individual and group advocacy services available to all people with disabilities. Access consultation provided to businesses, agencies and institutions in accordance to the Americans with Disabilities Act.

4019 Arc of Cape Cod
P.O.Box 428
171 Main Street
Hyannis, MA 02601-428 508-790-3667
FAX: 508-775-5233
e-mail: info@arcofcapecod.org
www.arcofcapecod.org

4020 Boston Center for Independent Living
5th Floor
60 Temple Place
Boston, MA 02111-1324 617-338-6665
FAX: 617-338-6661
TTY:617-338-6662
e-mail: info@bostoncil.org
www.bostoncil.org

Sergio Goncalves, Chairman
Linda Landry, Vice Chairman
Stacey Zelbow, Treasurer
Bill Henning, Executive Director

A frontline civil rights organization led by people with disabilities that advocates to eliminate discrimination, isolation and segregation by providing advocacy, information and referral, peer support, skills training, and PCA services in order to enhance the independence of people with disabilities.

4021 Cape Organization for Rights of the Disabled (CORD)
106 Bassett Lane
Hyannis, MA 2601 508-775-8300
800-541-0282
FAX: 508-775-7022
TTY: 800-541-0282
e-mail: cordinfo@cilcapecod.org
www.cilcapecod.org

Coreen Brinkerhoff, Executive Director

The Cape Organization for the Rights of the Disabled (CORD) has been aggresively working since 1984 to advance the independence, productivity, and integration of people with disabilities into mainstream society. CORD is the Center for Independent Living (CIL) and is a member of the Aging and Disability Resources Consortium (ADRC) servinf Cape Cod and the Islands.

4022 Center for Living & Working: Fitchburg
76 Summer Street
Suite 110
Fitchburg, MA 01420-5785
978-345-1568
TTY:978-345-1568
e-mail: centerlwA@centerlw.org
www.centerlw.org

Cindy Purcell, Board President
Mary Ann Donovan, Treasurer
Ed Roth, Secretary
Jim O'Day, Advisor to CLW Board of Director

The Center for Living and Working is a non-profit Independent Living Center which takes its direction from persons with disabilities. The Center advocates to empower persons with disabilities to take active roles in their lives and in their community in which they live. Also provides comprehensive and innovative programs and services in order to maximize individual independence and opportunities.

4023 Center for Living & Working: Framingham
484 Main St
Suite 345
Worcester, MA 01608-1824
508-798-0350
FAX: 508-797-4015
TTY:508-755-1003
e-mail: opsearch@centerlw.org
www.centerlw.org

Cindy Purcell, Board President
Mary Ann Donovan, Treasurer
Ed Roth, Secretary
Jim O'Day, Advisor to CLW Board of Director

The Center for Living and Working is a non-profit Independent Living Center which takes its direction from persons with disabilities. The Center advocates to empower persons with disabilities to take active roles in their lives and in their community in which they live. Also provides comprehensive and innovative programs and services in order to maximize individual independence and opportunities.

4024 Center for Living & Working: Worcester
484 Main St
Suite 345
Worcester, MA 01608-1824
508-798-0350
FAX: 508-797-4015
TTY:508-755-1003
e-mail: opsearch@centerlw.org
centerlw.org

Cindy Purcell, Board President
Mary Ann Donovan, Treasurer
Ed Roth, Clerk/Secretary
Jim O'Day, Advisor to CLW Board of Director

The Center for Living and Working is a non-profit Independent Living Center which takes its direction from persons with disabilities. The Center advocates to empower persons with disabilities to take active roles in their lives and in their community in which they live. Also provides comprehensive and innovative programs and services in order to maximize individual independence and opportunities.

4025 Developmental Evaluation and Adjustment Facilities
215 Brighton Ave
Allston, MA 02134-2013
617-254-4041
800-886-5195
FAX: 617-254-7091
e-mail: info@deafinconline.org
deafinconline.org

Sharon L. Applegate, Executive Director
Thomas Keydel, President
Jonathan Medeiros, Treasurer
Kendra Timko-Hochkeppel, Vice President

Encourages and empowers deaf, hard of hearing, deafblind and late-deafened individuals to lead independent and productive lives.

4026 Independence Associates
141 Main St
1st Floor
Brockton, MA 02301-4012
508-583-2166
800-649-5568
FAX: 508-583-2165
e-mail: info@iacil.org
iacil.org

Mark Lewis, President
James Clark, Treasurer
Anita Ashdon, Secretary
Steven Higgins, Executive Director

Provides comprehensive services which will enhance the range of acceptable options available to the consumer and improve the quality of life of persons with disabilities; to work on behalf of the objective of the disablility rights and independent living movement.

4027 Independent Living Center of Stavros: Greenfield
55 Federal St
Greenfield, MA 01301-2546
413-774-3001
www.stavros.org

Glenn Hartmann, President
Nancy Bazanchuk, Vice President
Donna M. Bliznak, Treasurer
Greta Biagi, Clerk

Promoting independence and access in the communities for persons with disabilities and deaf people.

4028 Independent Living Center of Stavros: Springfield
210 Old Farm Road
Amherst, MA 01002-2704
413-256-0473
800-804-1899
FAX: 413-256-0190
stavros.org

Glenn Hartmann, President
Nancy Bazanchuk, Vice President
Donna M. Bliznak, Treasurer
James Kruidenier, Executive Director

Promoting independence and access in the communities for persons with disabilities and deaf people.

4029 Independent Living Center of the North Shore & Cape Ann
27 Congress St
Suite 107
Salem, MA 01970-5577
978-741-0077
888-751-0077
FAX: 978-741-1133
e-mail: information@ilcnsca.org
ilcnsca.org

Mary Margaret Moore, Executive Director
Marion A Dawicki, President
Patricia Cox, Vice President
Stephen C. Turner, Treasurer

A service and advocacy center run by and for people with disabilities that supports the struggle of people who have all types of disabilities to live independently and participate fully in community life.

4030 MetroWest Center for Independent Living
280 Irving Street
Framingham, MA 01702-7306
508-875-7853
FAX: 508-875-8359
TTY:508-875-7853
e-mail: info@mwcil.org
mwcil.org

Youcef J. Bellil, President
Michael Kennedy, Vice President
Edward J. Carr, Treasurer
Penny Kelley, Secretary

To help individuals with disabilities become productive and contributing members of the community and to eliminate barriers within the community that impede this process.

4031 **Multi-Cultural Independent Living Center of Boston**
329 Centre Street
Jamaica Plain, MA 02130-1232 617-942-8060
FAX: 617-942-8630
TTY:617-288-2707
e-mail: info@milcb.org
milcb.org

Derrick Dominique, Executive Director
Ana Ortiz, Director of Services
Eleanor Slaughter, Senior IL Advocate
Louise Beach, Community Outreach Coordinator

Seeks to create opportunities for people with disabilities and their families in unserved/under-served populations and cultures who reside in Boston's inner city.

4032 **Northeast Independent Living Program**
20 Ballard Rd
Lawrence, MA 01843-1018 978-687-4288
FAX: 978-689-4488
TTY:978-687-4288
e-mail: help@nilp.org
nilp.org

June Cowen, Executive Director
Nanette Goodwin, Assistant Director
Lisa DiGiuseppe, Director of Finance
Jim Lyons, Director, Community Development

A consumer controlled Independent Living Center providing Advocacy and Services to people with all disabilities in the greater Merrimack Valley who wish to live as independently as possible in the community.

4033 **Renaissance Clubhouse**
176 Walker St
2nd Floor
Lowell, MA 01854-3126 978-454-7944
FAX: 978-937-7867
e-mail: renclub1@gmail.com
www.renclublowell.org

Elaine Walker, Executive Director
Pammy Sadoie, Assistant Director

Offers daily structure, assistance wtih jobs, retirement, and housing.

4034 **Southeast Center for Independent Living**
66 Troy Street
Suite 3
Fall River, MA 02720-3023 508-679-9210
FAX: 508-677-2377
TTY:508-679-9210
e-mail: scil@secil.org
secil.org

Lisa M Pitta, Executive Director
Damase Cote, President
Paul Remy, Vice President
Debbie Pacheco, Treasurer / Secretary

The Philosophy of Independent Living, maintains that individuals with disabilities have the right to choose services and make decisions for themselves. This belief is the foundation and guiding principle of all of SCIL's policies and operations. SCIL provides training, information and support to help consumers achieve individual goals, experience personal growth and participate fully in community life.

4035 **Student Independent Living Experience Massachusetts Hospital School**
560 Harrison Avenue
Suite 600
Boston, MA 02118-2447 617-338-6409
800-843-5879
TTY:800-328-3202
e-mail: JurorHelp@jud.state.ma.us.
www.mass.gov

Michigan

4036 **Ann Arbor Center for Independent Living**
3941 Research Park Drive
Ann Arbor, MI 48108-6852 734-971-0277
FAX: 734-971-0826
www.aacil.org

Glen Ashlock, Program Manager
Chris Baty, Theater Coordinator
Bryan Wilkinson, Director of Operations and Sales
Shirley Coombs, Chief Financial Officer

AACIL assists people with disabilities and their families in living full and productive lives. AACIL assures the equality of opportunity, full participation, independent living and economic self-sufficiency of people with disabilities in the community.

4037 **Arc Michigan**
1325 S Washington Ave
Lansing, MI 48910-1652 517-487-5426
800-292-7851
FAX: 517-487-0303
e-mail: dhoyle@arcmi.org
arcmi.org

Donald Teegarden, President
Laurel Robb, Vice President
Paul White, Secretary
Shari Fitzpatrick, Treasurer

Exists to empower local chapters of The ARC to assure that citizens with developmental disabilities are valued and that they and their families can participate fully in and contribute to the life of their community.

4038 **Arc/Muskegon**
1145 Wesley Ave
Muskegon, MI 49442-2197 231-777-2006
FAX: 231-777-3507
e-mail: info@arcmuskegon.org
www.arcmuskegon.org

Margaret O'Toole, Executive Director
Mikki Rosema, Administrative Assistant
Karen L. Bowne, CLS Program Coordinator
Tim Michalski, Director

Offers information and referral, advocacy services and peer counseling.

4039 **Bad Axe: Blue Water Center for Independent Living**
614 N Port Crescent Street
P.O. Box 29
Bad Axe, MI 48413-1207 989-269-5421
FAX: 989-269-5422
e-mail: info@bwcil.org
www.bwcil.org

Toni Mazure, Independent Living Specialist
Karen Massaro-Mundt, President
Chuck Wanninger, Treasurer
Ann Chapaton, Manager

A non-profit, consumer-based organization that advocates, informs and supports persons with disabilities in the community.

4040 **Bay Area Coalition for Independent Living**
Ste 17
701 S Elmwood Ave
Traverse City, MI 49684-3185 231-929-4865
FAX: 231-929-4896
e-mail: steve@bacil.org

Steve Wade, Director

4041 Capital Area Center for Independent Living
2812 N. Martin Luther King Jr. Blvd
Lansing, MI 48906
517-999-2760
FAX: 517-999-2767
TTY:800-649-3777
e-mail: info@cacil.org
www.cacil.org

Mark Pierce, Executive Director
Jeffrey Gass, Financial Manager
Jean Harris, Independent Living Specialist
Laurie Parker, VA Programs and IT Services Director

CACIL provide training, mentoring, and referrals to help people with disabilities and their families live productive lives.

4042 Caro: Blue Water Center for Independent Living
1184 Cleaver Rd
Caro, MI 48723-1143
989-673-3678
FAX: 989-673-3656
e-mail: info@bwcil.org
www.bwcil.org

Alex Busch, Independent Living Specialist
Karen Massaro-Mundt, President
Chuck Wanninger, Treasurer
Ann Chapaton, Manager

A non-profit, consumer-based organization that advocates, informs and supports persons with disabilities in the community.

4043 Center for Independent Living of Mid-Michigan
3941 Research Park Drive
Ann Arbor, MI 48108-6832
734-971-0277
FAX: 734-971-0826
www.annarborcil.org

Glen Ashlock, Program Manager
Chris Baty, Theater Coordinator
Bryan Wilkinson, Director of Operations and Sales
Shirley Coombs, Chief Financial Officer

Comprised of over 51 percent of people with disabilities, and advocates for the rights of people with disabilities in the Mid-Michigan area. Call for information on disability issues or for assistance in obtaining services, within your community..

4044 Community Connections of Southwest Michigan
Ste 2
133 E Napier Ave
Benton Harbor, MI 49022
269-925-6422
800-578-4245
FAX: 269-925-7141
e-mail: kellis@miconnect.org
www.miconnect.org

Kathy Ellis, Director

An advocacy organization that teaches and empowers people with disabilities to make choices about living life to the fullest, controlling and directing their own lives and asserting their rights and responsibilites within their Berrien County communities..

4045 Cristo Rey Handicappers Program
1717 N High St
Lansing, MI 48906-4529
517-372-4700
FAX: 517-372-8499
e-mail: info@cristo-rey.org
www.cristo-rey.org

Marlene M Berens, Manager

To care for the spiritual and social needs of individuals and families by offering services that encourage self-sufficiency and recognize the dignity of the human person..

4046 Detroit Center for Independent Living
1042 Griswold
Suite 2
Port Huron, MI 48060
810-987-9337
FAX: 810-987-9548
e-mail: info@bwcil.org
www.bwcil.org

Angela Hoff, Executive Director
Karen Massaro-Mundt, President
Chuck Wanninger, Treasurer
Ann Chapaton, Manager

BWCIL is a consumer-based organization designed to serve persons with disabilities who have physical, psychiatric, sendory, cognitive, and multiple disabilities through the provision of advocacy, information and referral, service provision, and the promotion of needed services so to maximize the individual's optimal level of independence.

4047 Disability Advocates of Kent County
3600 Camelot Drive SE
Grand Rapids, MI 49546-8103
616-949-1100
FAX: 616-949-7865
e-mail: contact@dakc.us
disabilityadvocates.us

David Bulkowski, JD, Executive Director
Denise Borges, Employment Specialist
Kim M Frost, Access Coordinator
Bonnie Miller, Independent Living Specialist

Exists to advocate, assist, educate and inform on independent living options for persons with disabilities and to create a barrier-free society for all.

4048 Disability Connection
27 E. Clay Avenue
Muskegon, MI 49442
231-722-0088
866-322-4501
FAX: 231-722-0066
dcilmi.org

Susan Cloutier-Myers, Executive Director
John Wahlberg, President
Michael Hamm, Vice President
Thomas Grein, Treasurer

To advocate, educate, empower, and provide resources for persons with disabilities and promote accessible communities.

4049 Disability Network Southwest Michigan
517 E Crosstown Pkwy
Kalamazoo, MI 49001-2867
269-345-1516
FAX: 269-345-0229
e-mail: info@dnswm.org
www.dnswm.org

Robyn Hill, Chair
Eric Large, Vice Chair
Joel W Cooper, President
Jeff Visser, Treasurer

To educate and empower people with disabilities to create change intheir own lives, and to advocate for social change to create inclusive communities. As a center for independent living, they are part of the disability rights movement.

4050 Disability Network of Mid-Michigan
1705 S. Saginaw Road
Midland, MI 48640-6825
989-835-4041
800-782-4160
FAX: 989-835-8121
e-mail: info@dnmm.org
dnmm.org

David Emmel, Executive Director
Jerry Pritchett, President
Teresa Oliver, Vice President
Bill Bateman, Treasurer

To promote and encourage independence for all people with disabilities.

4051 Disability Network of Oakland & Macomb
16645 15 Mile Rd
Clinton Township, MI 48035-2206
586-268-4160
800-284-2457
FAX: 586-285-9942
e-mail: info@dnom.org
dnom.org

Andrew Maurer, Chairperson
Randy Charon, Vice Chairperson
Kellie Boyd, Executive Director
Mark Cronmiller, Secretary

Commited to advancing personal choice, independence, and positive social change for persons with disabilities through advocacy, education and outreach.

4052 Disability Network/Lakeshore
426 Century Lane
Holland, MI 49423-2200
616-396-5326
800-656-5245
FAX: 616-396-3220
TTY: 616-396-5326
e-mail: info@dnlakeshore.org
dnlakeshore.org

Todd Whiteman, Executive Director
Michelle Chaney, President
Amber Marcy, Vice President
Brian Dykhuis, Treasurer
A cross-disability, community-based organization providing advocacy, education, and information and referral to persons with disabilities in Ottawa and Allegan counties.

4053 Grand Traverse Area Community Living Management Corporation
935 Barlow St
Traverse City, MI 49686-4250
231-932-9030
e-mail: mmacy@GTACLMC.com
www.gtaclmc.org

Mary Jean Brick, Administrative Director
We are a training home for individuals with developmental disabilities over the age of 18

4054 Great Lakes/Macomb Rehabilitation Group
Apt 104
4 E Alexandrine St
Detroit, MI 48201-2032
313-832-3371
FAX: 313-832-3850
e-mail: jlcil@home.msen.com
Jeannie Meece-Brooks, Contact
Independent living center. .

4055 JARC
30301 Northwestern Hwy
Suite 100
Farmington Hills, MI 48334-3277
248-538-6611
877-767-7781
FAX: 248-538-6615
e-mail: jarc@jarc.org
jarc.org

Ronald Applebaum, President
Richard A. Loewenstein, Chief Executive Officer
Randy P. Baxter, Chief Financial Officer
Rena Friedberg, CFRE, Chief Development Officer
A nonprofit, nonsecretarian agency dedicated to enabling people with disabilities to live full, dignified lives in the community, and to providing support and advocacy for their families.

4056 Lapeer: Blue Water Center for Independent Living
392 West Nepessing Street
Lapeer, MI 48446-2192
810-664-9098
FAX: 810-664-0937
e-mail: info@bwcil.org
www.bwcil.org

Karen Massaro-Mundt, President
Chuck Wanninger, Treasurer
Christine Cook, Housing Specialist
Karen Cook, Transition Specialist
A non-profit, consumer-based organization that advocates, informs and supports persons with disabilities in the community.

4057 Livingston Center for Independent Living
3075 E Grand River Ave
Suite 108
Howell, MI 48843-6585
517-545-1741
FAX: 517-548-1751
e-mail: gsims@aacil.org
www.virtualcil.net

Dan Durci, Director
Independent living skills training and empowerment training for persons with disabilities..

4058 Michigan Commission for the Blind: Independent Living Rehabilitation Program
411 E Genesee Ave
Saginaw, MI 48607-1254
989-758-1765
800-292-4200
FAX: 989-758-1405
www.mfia.state.mi.us

Debbie Wilson, Manager
Patrick Cannon, Agency Director
Rehabilitation teaching, independent living skills for persons over 55 with severe vision loss.

4059 Michigan Commission for the Blind: Detroit
Ste 4-450
3038 W Grand Blvd
Detroit, MI 48202-6012
313-456-1646
FAX: 313-456-1645
e-mail: mcnealg@michigan.gov

Gwen McNeal, Supervisor
Shawnese Laury-Johnson, Assistant East Region Manager
Promotes the inclusion of people with legal blindness into our communities on a full and equal basis through empowerment, education, participation, and choice..

4060 Monroe Center for Independent Living
1285 N Telegraph Rd
Monroe, MI 48162-3368
734-242-5919
e-mail: mrawlings@aacil.org
monroecil.tripod.com

Linda Maier, Manager
To act as a catalyst for personal and social change through the empowerment of people with disabilities; and, to replace the perception of disability as tragic with a disability culture promoting pride, power and personal style.

4061 Port Huron: Blue Water Center for Independent Living
1042 Griswold St
Suite 2
Port Huron, MI 48060-5431
810-987-9337
FAX: 810-987-9548
e-mail: info@bwcil.org
bwcil.org

Angela Hoff, Executive Director
A non-profit, consumer-based organization that advocates, informs and supports persons with disabilities in the community.

4062 Sandusky: Blue Water Center for Independent Living
103 East Sanilac Road
Suite 3
Sandusky, MI 48471-1615
810-648-2555
FAX: 810-648-2583
e-mail: info@bwcil.org
www.bwcil.org

Karen Massaro-Mundt, President
Chuck Wanninger, Treasurer
Ann Chapaton, Manager
Lynda Freitag, Independent Living Specialist
A non-profit, consumer-based organization that advocates, informs and supports persons with disabilities in the community.

4063 Southeastern Michigan Commission for the Blind
4450 Grandy St
Detroit, MI 48207
313-456-0334
877-932-6424
FAX: 313-456-1645
www.michigan.gov

Patrick Cannon, Executive Director
Pat Bragg, Manager
Vocational rehabilitation agency. Personal adjustment vocational assessment and training, job placement and follow-up services. .

4064 **Superior Alliance for Independent Living(SAIL)**
1200 Wright Street
Suite 3
Marquette, MI 49855
906-228-5744
800-379-7245
FAX: 906-228-5573
TTY: 906-228-5744
www.upsail.com

Amy Maes, Executive Director
Judy Vivian, Finance Director
Emily Gregorich, Independent Living Advocate
Sarah Peura, Associate Director

Promotes the inclusion of people with disabilities into our communities on a full and equal basis through empowerment, education, participation and choice.

4065 **disAbility Connections**
409 Linden Ave
Jackson, MI 49203-4065
517-782-6054
FAX: 517-782-3118
e-mail: lesia@disabilityconnect.org
www.disabilityconnect.org

Lesia Pikaart, Executive Director
JoAnn Lucas, Associate Director
Brenda Bobon, Independent Living Counselor
Jim Cyphers, Independent Living Specialist

Supporting Jackson County residents in their efforts to lead independent, fulfilling, productive lives.

Minnesota

4066 **Accessible Space, Inc.**
2550 University Avenue West
Suite 330N
Saint Paul, MN 55114-1085
651-645-7271
800-466-7722
FAX: 651-645-0541
TTY: 800-627-3529
e-mail: info@accessiblespace.org
www.accessiblespace.org

Mark E. Hamel, Esq., Chairman
Kay Knutson, Vice Chairman
Steve Schugel, Treasurer
John W. Adams, Secretary

Accessible, rent-subsidized apartments for very low-income adults with qualifying physical disabilities as well as seniors. Accessible Space, Inc., sponsors, develops and manages housing & ASI apartments are rent based on income and are located across the country.

4067 **Accessnorth CIL of Northeastern MN: Aitkin**
1309 East 40th Street
Hibbing, MN 55746-1821
218-262-6675
800-390-3681
FAX: 218-262-6677
TTY: 218-262-6675
e-mail: info@accessnorth.net
www.accessnorth.net

Mary Ribich, Chair
David Hohl, Vice-Chair
Judith Bonelli, Treasurer
Kathy Husmann, Secretary

Assists individuals to live independently, pursue meaningful goals, and have equal opportunities and choices.

4068 **Accessnorth CIL of Northeastern MN: Duluth**
118 East Superior Street
Duluth, MN 55802-2155
218-625-1400
888-625-1401
FAX: 218-625-1401
e-mail: info@accessnorth.net
www.accessnorth.net

Mary Ribich, Chair
David Hohl, Vice-Chair
Judith Bonelli, Treasurer
Kathy Husmann, Secretary

Assisting individuals with disabilities to live independently, puruse meaningful goals, and have equal opportunities and choices.

4069 **Center for Independent Living of NE Minnesota**
1309 East 40th Street
Hibbing, MN 55746-1821
218-262-6675
800-390-3681
FAX: 218-262-6677
TTY: 218-262-6675
e-mail: info@accessnorth.net
accessnorth.net

Mary Ribich, Chair
David Hohl, Vice-Chair
Judith Bonelli, Treasurer
Kathy Husmann, Secretary

Assisting individuals with disabilities to live independently, pursue meaningful goals, and have an equal opportunities and choices

4070 **Courage Center**
3915 Golden Valley Rd
Minneapolis, MN 55422-4298
763-588-0811
888-846-8253
FAX: 763-520-0577
TTY:763-520-0245
e-mail: couragekenny@allina.com
www.couragecenter.org

Jan Malcolm, CEO
Alice Johnson, Chief Financial Officer
Stephen Bariteau, Chief Development Officer
Pamela J. Lindemoen, Executive Vice President of Oper

A nonprofit rehabilitation and resource center that advances the lives of children and adults experiencing barriers to health and independence. Specialize in treating brain injury, spinal cord injury, stroke, chronic pain, autism and disabilities experienced since birth.

4071 **Freedom Resource Center for Independent Living: Fergus Falls**
125 W Lincoln Avenue
Suite 17
Fergus Falls, MN 56537- 2152
218-998-1799
800-450-0459
FAX: 218-998-1798
e-mail: freedom@freedomrc.org
www.freedomrc.org

Nate Aalgaard, Executive Director
Angie Bosch, Office Coordinator
Mark Mark Bourdon Bourdon, Program Director
Andrea Nelson, Independent Living Advocate

Freedom Resource Center assists people in working towards goals they establish for themselves.

4072 **Metropolitan Center for Independent Living**
Ste 16
1600 University Ave W
Saint Paul, MN 55104-3825
651-646-8342
FAX: 651-603-2006
TTY:651-603-2001
e-mail: homeramps@gmail.com
www.klownwerkz.com

4073 **Minnesota Association of Centers for Independent Living**
215 North Benton Drive
Sauk Rapids, MN 56379
320-529-9000
888-529-0747
FAX: 320-529-0747
e-mail: ilicil@independentlifestyles.org
independentlifestyles.org

Cara Ruff, Executive Director
Jay Keller, Board Chairman
Pamela Kotzenmacher, Treasurer
Autumn Gould, Attorney

A non-profit organization whose purpose is to advocate for the independent living needs of people with disabilities who are citizens of the State of Minnesota

4074 OPTIONS
Ste B
123 S Main St
Crookston, MN 56716-1970 218-281-5722
FAX: 218-281-5722
TTY:218-281-5722
e-mail: options3@rrv.net

Gordie Haug, Manager
Provides people with disabilities advocacy, information, skills training and peer mentoring relationships to help them achieve their personal goals of how and where they live their lives.

4075 Options Interstate Resource Center for Independent Living
318 3rd St NW
East Grand Forks, MN 56721-1887 218-773-6100
800-726-3692
FAX: 218-773-7119
TTY: 218-773-6100
e-mail: options@myoptions.info
www.macil.org/options.html

Randy Sorensen, Executive Director
Located in Minnesota, but also serves North Dakota..

4076 Perry River Home Care
330 High Way Pen S
Saint Cloud, MN 56304 320-255-1882
FAX: 320-255-5137

Berna Florentine, CEO
Ken Figge, President
Courtney Salzi, Administrator
Offers skilled nursing services RN, LPN, TV Therapy, Pediatrics, Rehabilitation Services, PT, OT, ST, Paraprofessional staff, Home Health Aides, Homemakers, Personal Care Attendents, Companions, Live-ins, Sleep overs, Respite care, Extended hours.

4077 SMILES
Ste 1
820 Winnebago Ave
Fairmont, MN 56031-3619 507-345-7139
888-676-6498
FAX: 507-235-3488
www.smilescil.org

Alan Augustin, Executive Director
David Cunningham, Administrative Assistant
Anne Murray, Education and communication Mana
Doug Miller, Operations Manager
A nonprofit organization committed to providing a wide array of services that assist individuals with disabilities that live independently, pursue meaningful goals, and enjoy the same opportunities and choices as all persons.

4078 SMILES: Mankato
709 S. Front Street
Suite 7
Mankato, MN 56001-3887 507-345-7139
888-676-6498
FAX: 507-345-8429
e-mail: smiles@smilescil.org
smilescil.org

Alan Augustin, Executive Director
Doug Miller, Operations Manager
Anne Murray, Community Education Manager
A nonprofit organization committed to providing a wide array of services that assist individuals with disabilities that live independently, pursue meaningful goals, and enjoy the same oportunities and choices as all persons.

4079 Southeastern Minnesota Center for Independent Living: Red Wing
2200 2nd Street SW
Rochester, MN 55902 507-285-1815
888-460-1815
FAX: 507-288-8070
e-mail: semcil@semcil.org
www.semcil.org

Brian Koch, President
Becky Noble, MemberSales
Jay Toogood, Member Systems Advisor
Marie Peterson, Member Enrollment Counselor
Non profit organization that assists people with disabilities to become independent and productive community members.

4080 Southeastern Minnesota Center for Independent Living: Rochester
2200 Second Street SW
Rochester, MN 55906-3980 507-285-1815
888-460-1815
FAX: 507-288-8070
e-mail: semcil@semcil.org
www.semcil.org

Vicki Dalle Molle, Executive Director
A non profit organization that assists people with disabilities to become independent and productive community members.

4081 Southwestern Center for Independent Living
109 South Fifth Street
SUITE #700
Marshall, MN 56258- 1298 507-532-2221
800-422-1485
FAX: 507-532-2222
TTY: 507-532-2221
e-mail: swcil@swcil.com
www.swcil.org

Steve Thovson, Executive Director
SWCIl is a private, non-profit consumer controlled, non-residential, cross-disability, community-based organization providing independent living services to assist people with disabilities in obtaining and maintaining the greatest control over their lives. Services are available in southwestern Minnesota to persons of all ages, with all disability without regard to income.

4082 Vinland Center Lake Independence
3675 Ihduhapi Road
Loretto, MN 55357-308 763-479-3555
866-956-7612
FAX: 763-479-2605
e-mail: vinland@vinlandcenter.org
www.vinlandcenter.org

Duane Reynolds, Associate Director
Mary Roehl, Operations Director
A Minnesota based rehabilitation center which offers services in three distinct service areas: vocational rehabilitation; inclusive community programs; and for people with cognitive disabilities, specially adapted chemical dependency treatment.

Mississippi

4083 Alpha Home Royal Maid Association for the Blind
PO Drawer 30
Hazlehurst, MS 39083-30 601-894-1771
FAX: 601-894-2993
e-mail: sigworks@teclink.net

Howard Becker, Director
Offers attendant care registry, information on accessible housing and referrals.

4084 Gulf Coast Independent Living Center
18 JM Tatum Industrial Drive
Hattiesburg, MS 39401-8341 601-544-4860
FAX: 601-582-2544

Albert Holifield, Executive Director
Independent living center.

4085 **Jackson Independent Living Center**
1981 Hollywood Dr
Jackson, TN 38305-2131
601-961-4140
FAX: 601-354-6678
TTY:601-351-1585
e-mail: information@jcil.tn.org
www.j-cil.com/contact-us.html
Denea Smith, Director
Timothy Jackson
Provides services to consumers with severe disabilities.

4086 **LIFE of Mississippi**
1304 Vine St
Jackson, MS 39202-3429
601-969-4009
800-748-9398
FAX: 601-969-1662
TTY: 800-748-9398
www.lifeofms.com
Christy Dunaway, Executive Director
Augusta Smith, Asst. Director
To empower people wit significant disabilities to be as independent and as fully involved in their communities as they can and want to be.

4087 **LIFE of Mississippi: Biloxi**
2030 Pass Road
Suite C
Biloxi, MS 39531
228-388-2401
FAX: 228-338-2413
www.lifeofms.com
Terri Redding, Manager
To empower people with significant disabilities to be as independent and as fully involved in their communities as they can and want to be.

4088 **LIFE of Mississippi: Greenwood**
502a W Park Ave
Greenwood, MS 38930-2906
662-453-9940
FAX: 662-453-9934
www.lifeofms.com
Pamela Wraggs, Manager
To empower people with significant disabilities to be as independent and as fully involved in their communities as they can and want to be.

4089 **LIFE of Mississippi: Hattiesburg**
710 Katie Ave
Hattiesburg, MS 39401-4377
601-583-2108
www.lifeofms.com
Susan Hanks, Executive Director
To empower people with significant disabilities to be as independent and as fully involved in their communities as they can and want to be.

4090 **LIFE of Mississippi: McComb**
915-A S. Locust Street
McComb, MS 39648-4817
601-684-3079
www.lifeofms.com
Alida Moncilva, Owner
To empower people with significant disabilities to be as independent and as fully involved in their communities as they can and want to be.

4091 **LIFE of Mississippi: Meridian**
Ste 103a
2440 N Hills St
Meridian, MS 39305-2653
601-485-7999
www.lifeofms.com
Sharon Burt, Independent Living Specialist
To empower people with significant disabilities to be as independent and as fully involved in their communities as they can and want to be.

4092 **LIFE of Mississippi: Oxford**
Ste 5
404 Galleria Dr
Oxford, MS 38655-4383
662-234-7010
www.lifeofms.com
Judy Pettit, Independent Living Specialist
To empower people with significant disabilities to be as independent and as fully involved in their communities as they can and want to be.

4093 **LIFE of Mississippi: Tupelo**
1051 Cliff Gookin Blvd
Tupelo, MS 38801-6739
662-844-6633
FAX: 662-844-6803
www.lifeofms.com
Michael Sullivan, Regional Coordinator
To empower people with significant disabilities to be as independent and as fully involved in their communities as they can and want to be.

Missouri

4094 **Access II Independent Living Center**
101 Industrial Parkway
Gallatin, MO 64640-1280
660-663-2423
888-663-2423
FAX: 660-663-2517
e-mail: access@accessii.org
www.accessii.org
Heather Swymeler, Executive Director
Deanna Brown, Program Director
The mission of Access II is to remove architectural and attitudinal barriers that limit the independence of persons with disabilities, promote a positive change in attitudes about disability and persons with disabilities, and encourage greater independence for persons with disabilities within our communities. As a Center for Independent Living, Access II is comitted to the provision of a full range of independent living services.

4095 **Bootheel Area Independent Living Services**
PO Box 326
Kennett, MO 63857-326
573-888-0002
888-449-0949
FAX: 573-888-0708
TTY:573-888-0002
e-mail: tshaw@bails.org
www.bails.org
Tim Shaw, Executive Director
BAILS goal is to foster an open, barrier free society flor all people regardless of their disability. BAILS service area is predominantly rural and includes the Southeast Missouri counties of: Dunklin, New Madrid, Pemiscot and Stoddard.

4096 **Coalition for Independence: Missouri Branch Office**
6724 Troost Ave
Ste. 408
Kansas City, MO 66131
816-822-7432
FAX: 816-363-3469
TTY:913-321-5126
e-mail: csmith@cfi-kc.org
www.cfi-kc.com
Clarenece Smith, Executive Director
Coalition For Independence (CFI) is to facilitate positive and responsible independence for all people with disabilities by acting as an advocate for individuals with disabilities, providing services, and promoting accessibility and acceptance.

4097 Delta Center for Independent Living
5933 S Highway 94
Suite #107
Weldon Spring, MO 63304- 5608 636-926-8761
866-727-3245
FAX: 636-447-0341
e-mail: info@dcil.org
www.dcil.org

Nancy Murphy, Executive Director

A non profit corporation which assists people with significant disabilities who want to live more independently.

4098 Disability Resource Association
130 Brandon Wallace Way
Festus, MO 63028-1726 636-931-7696
FAX: 636-931-4863
TTY:636-937-9016
e-mail: dra@disabilityresourceassociation.org
www.disabilityresourceassociation. org

Craig Henning, Executive Director
Nancy Pope, Assistant Director
Suzan Weller, Director/Resource Developer

Independent Living Cener.

4099 Independent Living Center of Southeast Missouri
511 Cedar St
Poplar Bluff, MO 63901-7301 573-686-2333
888-890-2333
FAX: 573-686-0733
TTY:573-776-1178
e-mail: bruce.lynch@ilcsemo.org
www.ilcsemo.org

Bruce Lynch, Executive Director
Debbie Hardin, Independent Living Director

To make Southeast Missouri barrier free for all persons with disabilities, enabling them to live more independently, extending their rights to control and direct their own lives and empowering them to live more producitve lives.

4100 Life Skills Foundation
10176 Corporate Square Drive
Suite #100
Saint Louis, MO 63132-2935 314-567-7705
FAX: 314-567-6539
TTY:314-802-5299
e-mail: intake@lifeskills-stl.org
www.lifeskills-stl.org

Wendy Sullivan, President
Katie Smallen, VP of Operations

Assists people with disabilities live and work with dignity in the community.

4101 Midland Empire Resources for Independent Living (MERIL)
4420 South 40th St
Saint Joseph, MO 64503-2157 816-279-8558
800-637-4548
FAX: 816-279-1550
TTY: 816-279-4943
www.meril.org

Dr. Robert Bush, Chair
Jaren Pippitt, Vice Chair
Wayne Crawford, Secretary
J. Robert Brown, Treasurer

Designed to promote independent living and to enhance the quality of life for persons with disabilities by empowering them to control and direct their lives.

4102 Northeast Independent Living Services
909 Broadway
Suite 350
Hannibal, MO 63401 573-221-8282
877-713-7900
FAX: 573-221-9445
www.neilscenter.org

Brooke Kendrick, Executive Director
Rose McNally, President
Dawn Davis, Vice President
Kendra Adams, Kendra Adams

To empower persons with disabilities to live as full and productive members of society.

4103 On My Own
428 E Highland Ave
Nevada, MO 64772-2609 417-667-7007
800-362-8852
FAX: 417-667-6262
e-mail: onmyowngundy@softnet.net
onmyowninc.com

Jennifer Gundy, Executive Director

A non profit independent living center.

4104 Ozark Independent Living
109 Aid Ave
West Plains, MO 65775-3529 417-667-7007
888-440-7500
FAX: 417-257-2380
TTY: 888-440-7500
e-mail: info@ozarkcil.com
www.ozarkcil.org

Cindy Moore, Executive Director

OIL?was created to provide independent living services to persons with disabilities who reside in the following counties in Missouri: Oregon Ozark, Shannon, Wright, Howell, Texas, and Douglas. OIL is non-profit, on-residential supported by grants, donations, and volunteers

4105 Paraquad
5240 Oakland Ave
Saint Louis, MO 63110-1436 314-289-4200
FAX: 314-289-4201
TTY:314-289-4252
e-mail: contactus@paraquad.org
www.paraquad.org

Robert Funk, Executive Director

Paraquad works to empower people with disabilities to increase their independence through choice and opportunity.

4106 Places for People
4130 Lindell Blvd
Saint Louis, MO 63108-2914 314-535-5600
FAX: 314-535-6037
e-mail: contact@placesforpeople.org
www.placesforpeople.org

Joe Yancey, Executive Director

Places for People provides individualized, high quality and effective services to adults with serious and persistent mental disorders to assist them in living, working and socializing responsibility to serve those individuals who rely on public funding.

4107 RAIL
3024 Dupont Circle
Jefferson City, MO 65109 573-526-7039
877-222-8963
888-667-2117
FAX: 573-751-1441
e-mail: mo.silc@vr.dese.mo.gov
www.mosilc.org

Chris Camene, Chairperson
Jessica Hatfield, Vice-Chairperson
Barrnie Cooper, Secretary/Treasurer
Teresa Myers, Executive Director

RAIL is an Independent Living Center, one of twenty-two in the State of Missouri, RAIL's Mission is to assist persons with disabilities to live as independently as they choose within the communities of their choice. RAIL offers four core services which are: Advocacy, Peer Support, Information & Referral, and Independent Living Skills Training. RAIL is a Consumer Services Directed Program vendor

4108 SEMO Alliance for Disability Independence
1913 Rusmar St
Cape Girardeau, MO 63701-7623 573-651-6464
800-898-7234
FAX: 573-651-6565
TTY: 573-651-6464
e-mail: miki@mail.sadi.org
www.sadi.org

A. Wayne Wallingford Jr., President
Vicki Abernathy, Vice-President
A community based, non-profit, nonresidential center for independent living that is committed to providing services to persons with disabilities to enable them to remain in their own home and community, not an institution.

4109 Services for Independent Living
1401 Hathman Place
Columbia, MO 65201-5552 573-874-1646
800-766-3619
FAX: 573-874-3564
TTY: 573-874-4121
e-mail: sil@silcolumbia.org
www.silcolumbia.org

Jim Crane, Manager
Leslie Anderson, Program Manager
A non-residential, community-based center for independent living. Provides individualized and group services to persons with severe disabilities in the Mid-Missouri area; works to help people with disabilities achieve their highest potential in independent living and community life.

4110 Southwest Center for Independent Living (S CIL)
2864 S Nettleton Ave
Springfield, MO 65807-5970 417-886-3619
800-676-7245
FAX: 417-886-3619
TTY: 417-886-1188
e-mail: scil@swcil.org
www.swcil.org

Gary Maddox, Executive Director
Provides services, advocacy, and resources for people with any disability in Christian, Dallas, Greene, Lawrence, Polk, Stone, Taney and Webster Counties of Southwest Missouri.

4111 The Whole Person
3710 Main Street
Kansas City, MO 64111-7501 816-561-0304
800-878-3037
FAX: 816-931-0529
TTY: 816-561-0304
e-mail: info@thewholeperson.org
thewholeperson.org

David Robinson, CEO
The Whole Person, assists people with disabilities to live independently and encourages change within the community to expand opportunities for independent living.

4112 Tri-County Center for Independent Living
1420 HWY 72 East
Rolla, MO 65401 573-368-5933
FAX: 573-368-5991
TTY:573-368-5933
e-mail: vevans@fidnet.com
www.tricountycenter.com

Victoria Evans, Executive Director
Mission is to eliminate physical and attitudinal barriers through the power of advocacy, enlightenment, and reformation.

4113 West Central Independent Living Solutions
610 N Ridgeview Dr
Suite B
Warrensburg, MO 64093-9323 660-422-7883
800-236-5175
FAX: 660-422-7895
TTY: 660-422-7894
e-mail: info@w-ils.org
www.w-ils.org

Martha Fiene, Executive Director
Works to empower people with disabilities to become more independent by providing independent living skills training, peer support, information and referral and advocacy. West Central Independent Living Solutions now has satellite offices in Sedalia, MO and Lexington.

4114 Whole Person: Kansas City
3710 Main Street
Kansas City, MO 64111-7501 816-561-0304
800-878-3037
FAX: 816-931-0529
TTY: 816-627-2202
e-mail: info@thewholeperson.org
thewholeperson.org

David Robinson, CEO
Assists people with disabilities to live independently and encourages change within the community to expand opportunities for independent living.

Montana

4115 Living Independently for Today and Tomorrow
1201 Grand Avenue #1
Billings, MT 59102-2033 406-259-5181
800-669-6319
FAX: 406-259-5259
TTY: 406-245-1225
e-mail: beckerb@midrivers.com
www.liftt.org

Bobbie Becker, Executive Director
Martha Carstensen, Program Director
LIFTT's Independent living program works with people with disabilities so they can live independently and have access to the community. LIFTT staff, most of whom have disabilities, serve as mentors to people as they work to achieve the goals they have set for themselves.

4116 Montana Independent Living Project, Inc.
825 Great Northern Blvd
Suite 105
Helena, MT 59601-4715 406-442-5755
800-735-6457
FAX: 406-442-1612
TTY: 406-442-5755
e-mail: bmaffit@milp.us
www.milp.us

Bob Maffit, Executive Director
Les Clark, Independent Living Specialist
Charlene White, Financial Manager
Marie Largent, Office Manager
A not-for-profit agency that provides services that promote independence for people with disabilities.

4117 North Central Independent Living Services
1120 25th Ave
Black Eagle, MT 59414-1037 406-452-9834
800-823-6245
FAX: 406-453-3940
e-mail: ncils.osborn@sofast.net

Tom Osborn, Executive Director
North Central Independent Living Services is located in Great Falls and provides services from Glacier County across the Hi-Line to the North Dakota border. A satellite office is set up in Glasgow.

4118 **Summit Independent Living Center: Kalipsell**
1203 Highway 2 W.
Suite #35
Kalispell, MT 59901-6020
406-257-0048
800-995-0029
TTY:406-257-0048
e-mail: webmaster@bils.org
www.summitilc.org
Flo Kiewel, Manager
To promote community awareness, equal access, and the independence of people with disabilities through advocacy, education, and the advancement of civil rights.

4119 **Summit Independent Living Center: Hamilton**
316 North 3rd St
Suite #113
Hamilton, MT 59840-2479
406-363-5242
800-398-9013
e-mail: webmaster@bils.org
www.summitilc.org
Joanne Berwolf, Manager
To promote community awareness, equal access, and the independence of people with disabilities through advocacy, education, and the advancement of civil rights.

4120 **Summit Independent Living Center: Missoula**
700 SW Higgins Ave
Suite #101
Missoula, MT 59803-1489
406-728-1630
800-398-9002
FAX: 406-829-3309
e-mail: missoula@summitilc.org
www.summitilc.org
Mike Mayer, Executive Director
Kathy Boyer, Secretary
To promote community awareness, equal access, and the independence of people with disabilities through advocacy, education, and the advancement of civil rights.

4121 **Summit Independent Living Center: Ronan**
111 2nd Ave SW
Ronan, MT 59864-2718
406-676-0190
800-230-6936
FAX: 406-676-0191
e-mail: ronan@summitilc.org
www.summitilc.org
Gary Stevens, Manager
Scott Williamson, Co-County Coordinator
Michelle Williamson, Co-County Coordinator
To promote community awareness, equal access, and the independence of people with disabilities through advocacy, education, and the advancement of civil rights.

Nebraska

4122 **Center for Independent Living of Central Nebraska**
3204 College St
Grand Island, NE 68803-1730
308-382-9255
877-400-1004
FAX: 308-384-7832
TTY: 308-382-9255
e-mail: jthomas@cilne.org
www.cilne.org
Joni Thomas, Executive Director
Irene Britt, Western Program Manager
Deanna Church, Executive Assistant/IL Specialist
Mike Niece, Driving Program Coordinator
Offers independent living skills training, peer sharing, information and referral, housing counseling and referral, accessibility and barrier removal consultation including ADA training and technical assistance, driver education and training, assistive technology services including demonstration and equipment loan, and a free lending library of adapted toys and ability switches for children with severe disabilities. Serves all diabilities and all ages.

4123 **League of Human Dignity: Lincoln**
1701 P St
Lincoln, NE 68508-1799
402-441-7871
888-508-4758
FAX: 402-441-7650
TTY:402-441-7871
e-mail: info@leagueofhumandignity.com
www.leagueofhumandignity.com
Mike Schafer, CEO
The mission of the League of Human Dignity is to actively promote the full integration of individuals with disabilities into society. To this end, we will advocate their needs and rights, and provide quality services to involve these persons in becoming and remaining independent citizens.

4124 **League of Human Dignity: Norfolk**
400 Elm Ave
Norfolk, NE 68701-4033
402-371-4475
800-843-5785
FAX: 402-371-4625
TTY: 402-371-4475
e-mail: ninfo@leagueofhumandignity.com
leagueofhumandignity.com
Mike Shafer, CEO
Jean M. Kloppenborg, Norfolk CIL Director
The mission of the League of Human Dignity is to actively promote the full integration of individuals with disabilities into society. To this end, we will advocate their needs and rights, and provide quality services to involve these persons in becoming and remaining independent citizens.

4125 **League of Human Dignity: Omaha**
5513 Center St
Omaha, NE 68106-3001
402-595-1256
800-843-5784
FAX: 402-595-1410
e-mail: oinfo@leagueofhumandignity.com
www.leagueofhumandignity.com
Mike Schafer, CEO
Bob Gomez, Executive Director
The mission of the League of Human Dignity is to actively promote the full integration of individuals with disabilities into society. To this end, we will advocate their needs and rights, and provide quality services to involve these persons in becoming and remaining independent citizens.

4126 **Mosaic of Axtell Bethpage Village**
1044 23rd Rd.
PO Box 67
Axtell, NE 68924-67
308-743-2401
FAX: 308-743-2659
www.mosaicinfo.org/axtell
Linda Timmons, President and Chief Executive Officer
Raul Saldivar, Chief Operating Officer and Chief Integrity Officer
Cindy Schroeder, Chief Financial Officer
Donna Werner, Senior Vice President of Organizational Development
Provides services that respect the human diginity and rights of each person. An interdisciplinary team of family, staffmembers and professional consultatns support individuals served in developing personal goals and programs, helping them to fully participate in Axtell's community life. Mosaic at Axtell offers residential and community services.

4127 **Mosaic of Beatrice**
722 S. 12th St.
PO Box 607
Beatrice, NE 68310-607
402-223-4066
FAX: 402-223-4951
e-mail: jerry.campbell@mosaicinfo.org
www.mosaicinfo.org/beatrice
Linda Timmons, President and Chief Executive Officer
Raul Saldivar, Chief Operating Officer and Chief Integrity Officer
Cindy Schroeder, Chief Financial Officer
Donna Werner, Senior Vice President of Organizational Development
Provides individualized services, living options, work choices, spiritual nurture and advocacy to people with disabilities in more

than 250 communities across 14 states and Great Britain through the work of 4,800 employees.

4128 Mosiac: York
220 W South 21st St
York, NE 68467-9316
402-362-2180
FAX: 402-362-2961
www.mosaicinfo.org
Linda Timmons, President and Chief Executive Officer
Raul Saldivar, Chief Operating Officer and Chief Integrity Officer
Cindy Schroeder, Chief Financial Officer
Donna Werner, Senior Vice President of Organizational Development
Providing a wide array of services to assist individuals and families in achieving positive life goals. Services to persons with disabilities and other special needs include community living options, training and employment options, spiritual growth and development options, training and counseling support.

Nevada

4129 Carson City Center for Independent Living
900 Mallory Way
Carson City, NV 89701
775-841-2580
Sandra Coyle, Owner
Helps consumers continue to live independently in the community through a variety of individual and community services.

4130 Northern Nevada Center for Independent Living: Fallon
1919 Grimes St
Suite B
Fallon, NV 89406-3100
775-423-4900
800-885-3712
FAX: 775-423-1399
TTY: 775-423-4900
e-mail: nncilf@cccomm.net
www.nncil.org
Lisa Bonie, Executive Director
Hilda Velasco, Operations Manager
Joni Inglis, Independent Living Advocate
Hentjie Apag, Community and Home Access Program Manager
Independent Living Center.

4131 Rural Center for Independent Living
1895 E Long St
Carson City, NV 89706-3214
775-841-2580
FAX: 775-841-2580
e-mail: ruralcil@yahoo.com
Dee Dee Foremaster, Executive Director
Advocacy, Benefit Assistance, social security assistance, peer support, housing information and home-less day drop-in center for individuals with disabilities.

4132 Southern Nevada Center for Independent Living: North Las Vegas
3100 E Lake Mead Blvd
North Las Vegas, NV 89030-7380
702-649-3822
800-398-0760
FAX: 702-649-5022
TTY: 702-649-3822
e-mail: sncilnv@aol.com
www.sncil.org
Connie Kratky, President
Pamela Rake, Secretary
Elliot Yug, Vice - President
Pamela Rake, Secretary
SNCIL is committed to removing barriers preventing indpendent living by providing services designed to empower people with disabilities.

4133 Southern Nevada Center for Independent Living: Las Vegas
6039 Eldora Avenue
Suite H-8
Las Vegas, NV 89146-5611
702-889-4216
800-870-7003
FAX: 702-889-4574
TTY: 702-889-4216
e-mail: sncil2@aol.com
www.sncil.org
Connie Kratky, President
Pamela Rake, Secretary
Elliot Yug, Vice - President
Pamela Rake, Secretary
SNCIL is committed to removing barriers preventing Independent Living by providing services designed to empower people with disabilities.

New Hampshire

4134 Granite State Independent Living Foundation
76 Main St
Littleton, NH 3561-4079
603-228-9680
800-826-3700
FAX: 603-444-3128
TTY: 603-228-9680
e-mail: info@gsil.org
www.gsil.org
Clyde E. Terry, JD, Chief Executive Officer
Debora Krider, Ed.D, Chief Operating Officer
Peter Darling, Vice President of Community Economic Development
Jerry Grantham, Vice President of Resource Development
GSIL is a statewide non-profit that recognizes the fact that all of us will need some type of support in the course of the lives. GSIL offers tools and resources so that individuals can participate as fully as the choose in their lives, families and communities. Contact the Independent Living Foundation for referrals to living situations.

New Jersey

4135 Alliance Center for Independance
Alliance for Disabled in Action
629 Amboy Ave, First Floor
Edison, NJ 08837-3579
732-738-4388
FAX: 732-738-4416
TTY:732-738-9644
e-mail: adacil@adacil.org
www.adacil.org
Carole Tonks, Executive Director
Colleen Roche, Board Chair
Bruce Bentz, Vice Chairperson
Bernard Zuckerman, Treasurer
Alliance for Disabled in Action is a private, not-for-profit center for independent living serving people in Middlesex, Somerset and Union Counties of New Jersey. ADA's mission is to support and promote choice, self-direction and independent living in the lives of people with disabilities, with the right of individuals to inclusion in the community as the primary goal.

4136 Camden City Independent Living Center
2600 Mount Ephraim Ave
Camden, NJ 8104-3236
856-966-0800
FAX: 856-966-0832
TTY:856-966-0830
e-mail: vedasmithccilc@aol.com
www.camdencityilc.org
Veda Smith, Executive Director
Kathleen Zehnder, Chair Person
John Quann, Treasurer
Bruce Smith, Secretary
Provides services designed to empower people with disabilities. To provide services to individuals with significant disabilities. Services include information referral, advocacy, peer support,

and independent living skills training. CCILC services individuals in Camden City

4137 **Center for Independent Living: Long Branch**
279 Broadway
Suite #201
Long Branch, NJ 7740-6940
732-571-4884
FAX: 732-571-4003
TTY:732-571-4878
www.moceanscil.org

Joanne Goff, Executive Director
Elizabeth Reyes, PASP Coordinator
Stan Soden, Director IL Services
Susan Pniewski, IL Transition Specialist

Offers peer support, disability education and personal assistant services. Serving Monmouth and Ocean Counties with information and referrals, advocacy, peer support and independent living instructions.

4138 **Center for Independent Living: South Jersey**
1150 Delsea Drive
Suite #1
Westville, NJ 8093-2251
856-853-6490
800-413-3791
FAX: 856-853-1466
TTY: 856-853-7602
e-mail: cilsj@verizon.net
www.cilsj.org

Hazel Lee-Briggs, Executive Director
Danuta Debicki, Program Manager
Terryama Davis, Independent Living Specialist

Dedicated to providing people with disabilities in Gloucester and Camden counties the opportunity to actively participate in society, to provide freedom of choice, to work, to own a home, raise a family and in general, to participate to the fullest extent in day-to-day activities. The center provides information and referrals, advocacy, peer support, and independent living skills training.

4139 **DAWN Center for Independent Living**
30 Broad Street
Suite #5
Denville, NJ 7834-1235
973-625-1940
888-383-3296
FAX: 973-625-1942
TTY: 973-625-1932
e-mail: info@dawncil.org
www.dawncil.org

Carmela Slivinski, Executive Director
Elizabeth Lehmann, Board President
Lydia Kirschenbaum, Board Vice President
Ken Brucato, Board Treasurer

DAWN is the Center for Independent Living serving Morris, Sussex and Warren counties. DAWN empowers people with disabilities to strive for equality and to take control of their own lives by providing the tools that encourage independence and self-advocacy, promoting public awareness of the needs, desires and rights to individuals living with disabilities, and offering community activities that create new experiences and opportunities.

4140 **Dial: Disabled Information Awareness & Living**
2 Prospect Village Plaza
Floor 1
Clifton, NJ 7013-1918
973-470-8090
866-277-1733
FAX: 973-470-8171
TTY: 973-470-2521
e-mail: info@dial-cil.org
www.dial-cil.org

John Petix, Executive Director
Cynthia DeSouza, President
Anthony Gianduso, Vice President
Tim Burns, Secretary

Promotes the full inclusion of all people living with disabilities into society and encourage the consumers and the community at large to seek involvement in this self-governing organization to the fullest extent.

4141 **Disability Rights New Jersey**
New Jersey Protection and Advocacy
210 S. Broad Street
Floor 3
Trenton, NJ 08608-2407
609-292-9742
800-922-7233
FAX: 609-777-0187
TTY: 609-633-7106
e-mail: advocate@drnj.org
www.drnj.org

Walter Anthony Woodberry, Chair
Kathleen F. Wood, Vice Chair
Mitchell P. Friedman, Treasurer
Andrew McGeady, Secretary

Assistive Technology Advocacy Center provides assistance to personswith disabilities in helping them to obtain assistive technology devices and/or services.

4142 **Family Resource Associates**
35 Haddon Ave
Shrewsbury, NJ 7702-4007
732-747-5310
FAX: 732-747-1896
e-mail: info@frainc.org
www.frainc.org

Nancy Phalanukorn, Executive Director
Sue Levine, Early Intervention/Programs
Michael Bell, President
Bill Sheeser, Vice President

FRA is dedicated to helping children, adolescents and people of all ages with disabilities to reach their fullest potential. FRA also connects individuals to independence through modern therapies and advanced technology. FRA provides direct services to those in the greater Nonmouth/Ocean County area.

4143 **Heightened Independence and Progress: Hackensack**
131 Main St
Suite #120
Hackensack, NJ 7601-7182
201-996-9100
FAX: 201-996-9422
TTY:201-966-9424
e-mail: ber@hipcil.org
www.hipcil.org

Eileen Goff, Executive Director

Empowers people with disabilities to achieve independent living through outreach, advocacy and education.

4144 **Heightened Independence and Progress: Jersey City**
35 Journal Square
Suite #703
Jersey City, NJ 7306-4105
201-533-4407
FAX: 201-533-4421
TTY:201-533-4409
e-mail: hud@hipcil.org
www.hipcil.org

Jean Csaposs, Board Chair
Lottie Esteban, First Vice Chair
Eileen Goff, President/CEO
Trish Carney, Finance and Development Director

Empowering People with Disabilities to Achieve Independent Living through Outreach, Advocacy, and Education.

4145 **Progressive Center for Independent Living**
1262 Whitehorse-Hamilton Square Rd
Suite 102 Bldg A
Hamilton, NJ 8690-3710
609-581-4500
877-917-4500
FAX: 609-581-4555
TTY: 609-581-4550
e-mail: info@pcil.org
www.pcil.org

Scott Elliott, Executive Director
Jerry Carbone, Training Coordinator
Scott Ellis, Emergency Preparedness Coordinator
Renee Pfaff, Student Transition Specialist

Advocates for the rights of people with disabilities to achieve and maintain independent lifestyles. The Center has programs to assist with employment, transition from school to adult life, and emergency preparedness.

4146 **Progressive Center for Independent Living: Flemington**
Ste 410
4 Walter E Foran Blvd
Flemington, NJ 8822-4669
908-782-1055
877-376-9174
FAX: 908-782-6025
TTY: 908-782-1081
e-mail: info@pcil.org
pcil.org

Scott Elliott, Executive Director
Jerry Carbone, Training Coordinator
Scott Ellis, Emergency Preparedness Coordinator
Renee Pfaff, Student Transition Specialist

Advocates for the rights of people with disabilities to achieve and maintain independent lifestyles.

4147 **Project Freedom**
223 Hutchinson Rd
Robbinsville, NJ 8691-3457
609-448-2998
FAX: 609-448-7293
e-mail: ProjectFreedom1@aol.com
www.projectfreedom.org

Tim Doherty, Executive Director
Norman A. Smith, Assoc Ex Director
Elizabeth Maxwell, Office Manager
Paul Campanella, Property Manager

Dedicated to developing, supporting, and advocating opportunities for independent living persons with disabilities.

4148 **Project Freedom: Hamilton**
715 Kuser Rd
Hamilton, NJ 8619-3924
609-588-9919
FAX: 609-588-8831
e-mail: cfunk@projectfreedom.org
www.projectfreedom.org

Cecilia Funk, Social Service Coordinator
Judy Wilkinson, Office Manager
Paul Campanella, Property Manager

Dedicated to developing, supporting, and advocating opportunities for independent living persons with disabilities.

4149 **Project Freedom: Lawrence**
1 Freedom Blvd
Lawrence, NJ 8648-4531
609-278-0075
FAX: 609-278-1250
e-mail: jelsowiny@projectfreedom.org
www.projectfreedom.org

Jacklene Elsowiny, Social Serv Coordinator
Tim Doherty, Executive Director
Stephen Schaefer, CFO
Tracee Battis, Director of Housing Development

Dedicated to developing, supporting, and advocating opportunities for independent living persons with disabilities.

4150 **Total Living Center**
6712 Washington Ave
Egg Harbor Township, NJ 8234-1999
609-645-9547
FAX: 609-813-2318
TTY:609-645-9593
e-mail: info@tlcenter.org
www.tlcenter.org

Jo Hudson, President
Cliff Anderson, Vice President
Cathy Shaner, Secretary
Julia Bonelli, Executive Director

Total Living Center is a non-profit organization whose mission is to empower individuals with significant disabilities to maximize their potential for independence and productivity, to live as fully as possible within the community, taking responsibility for themselves, and sharing this commitment with others.

New Mexico

4151 **Ability Center**
715 E. Idaho Ave
Building 3E
Las Cruces, NM 88001-4702
575-526-5016
800-376-4372
FAX: 575-526-1202
TTY: 505-526-5016
e-mail: freedom@theabilitycenter.org
www.theabilitycenter.org

Vincent Montano, Executive Director
Cesar Rodriguez, Vice-President
C. Neil Gibbs, Treasurer

The Ability Center is a private, nonresidential, nonprofit, New Mexico corporation. As a center for independent living (CIL) TACIL provides a variety of services to promote independence, self-reliance, and community integration. Our professional staff and active board of directors are dedicated to helping our consumers maintain their personal freedom at home, in the community, and throughout the state.

4152 **CASA Inc.**
116 West Baltimore Street
Hagerstown, MD 21740
301-739-4990
FAX: 301-790-0064
e-mail: casa4@myactv.net
www.casaabq.com

Sherry Donovan, President
Linda Davis, Vice-President
Melinda Marsden, Treasurer
Laura Allis, Secretary

Offers peer counseling and information and referral services.

4153 **CHOICES Center for Independent Living**
200 E 4th St.
Suite #200
Roswell, NM 88201-6237
575-627-6727
800-387-4572
FAX: 575-627-6754
TTY: 505-627-6727

Julia Calvert, Executive Director

Offers many core services including independent living skills training, peer support, information and referral, advocacy and transition.

4154 **New Mexico Technology Assistance Program**
491 Old Santa Fe Trail, Room 117
Santa Fe, NM 87501
505-476-0412
877-696-1470
FAX: 505-827-6328
TTY: 800-659-4915
e-mail: gcd@state.nm.us
www.tap.gcd.state.nm.us

Julie Martinez, Program Director

Examines and works to eliminate barriers to obtaining assistive technology in New Mexico. Has established a statewide program for coordinating assistive technology services; is designed to assist people with disabilities to locate, secure, and maintain assistive technology.

4155 **New Vistas**
1121 Alto St
Santa Fe, NM 87501-2483
505-988-3803
FAX: 505-989-8740
e-mail: info@newvistas.org
www.newvistas.org

Ronald I. Garcia, Executive Director
William A. Moffett, President
Victor Ortega, Vice-President
Gay Romero, Secretary/Treasurer

Partners with and supports people with disabilities and families of children with special needs to enrich their quality of life in New Mexico.

4156 **San Juan Center for Independence**
1204 San Juan Blvd
Farmington, NM 87401
505-566-5827
877-484-4500
FAX: 505-566-5842
TTY: 505-566-5827
e-mail: sjci@sjci.org
www.sjci.org

Patricia Ziegler, Executive Director
Tim Carver, CFO

SJCI is a New Mexico private non residential, nonprofit corporation that serves people with disabilities. The purpose of SJCI is to provide a variety of community based, consumer driven service to people with disablities to promote independence, self-residence and intergration into the community.

New York

4157 **AIM Independent Living Center: Corning**
271 E 1st St
Corning, NY 14830-2924
607-962-8225
FAX: 607-937-5125
TTY:607-962-8225
e-mail: troche@aimcil.com
www.aimcil.com

Rene Snyder, Executive Director
Sabrina Mineo-O'Connell, President
George Spisack, Vice President
Barbara Squires, Treasurer

AIM is a non-profit organization dedicated to people with disabilities, their families, friends, the businesses that serve them and those with an interest in disabilities. The mission of AIM is to support the individuals ability to make independent, self-directing choices through education, advocacy, information and referral.

4158 **AIM Independent Living Center: Elmira**
650 Baldwin St.
Elmira, NY 14901-2216
607-733-3718
FAX: 607-733-0180
TTY:607-733-7764
e-mail: troche@aimcil.com
www.aimcil.com

Rene Snyder, Executive Director
Sabrina Mineo-O'Connell, President
George Spisack, Vice President
Barbara Squires, Treasurer

AIM's goal is to enable the consumer to live an independent and comfortable lifestyle in the security of their home environment so they may feel dignity and pride in their achievements while controling their own care.

4159 **ARISE**
635 James St
Syracuse, NY 13203-2661
315-472-3171
FAX: 315-472-9252
TTY:315-479-6363
e-mail: info@ariseinc.org
www.ariseinc.org

Thomas Mc Keown, Executive Director
Tania Anderson, President
Sue Judge, Vice President
Michael Cook, Treasurer

Founded in 1979, ARISE's mission is to work with people of all abilities to create a fair and just community in which everyone can fully participate. As a center for independent living, ARISE is a non-profit organization run by and for individuals with disabilities. ARISE serves over 3,000 children and adults with disabilities each year through our programs and services in several broad areas including advocacy, employment, independent living/integrated recreation programs, and much more.

4160 **ARISE: Oneida**
131 Main St
Suite #107
Oneida, NY 13421-1644
315-363-4672
FAX: 315-363-4675
TTY:315-363-2364
e-mail: info@ariseinc.org
www.ariseinc.org

Tania Anderson, President
Matt Dadey, Vice President
Mitch Mitchell, Treasurer
Gary Forbes, Secretary

A consumer controlled, non-profit Independent Living Center that promotes the full inclusion of people with disabilities in the community.

4161 **ARISE: Oswego**
9 Fourth Avenue
Oswego, NY 13126-1803
315-342-4088
FAX: 315-342-4107
TTY:315-342-8696
e-mail: info@ariseinc.org
www.ariseinc.org

Tania Anderson, President
Matt Dadey, Vice President
Mitch Mitchell, Treasurer
Gary Forbes, Secretary

A consumer controlled, non-profit Independent Living Center that promotes the full inclusion of people with disabilities in the community.

4162 **ARISE: Pulaski**
2 Broad St
Pulaski, NY 13142-4446
315-298-5726
FAX: 315-298-5729
e-mail: info@ariseinc.org
www.ariseinc.org

Tania Anderson, President
Matt Dadey, Vice President
Mitch Mitchell, Treasurer
Gary Forbes, Secretary

A consumer controlled, non-profit Independent Living Center that promotes the full inclusion of people with disabilities in the community.

4163 **Access to Independence of Cortland County, Inc.**
26 N Main St
Cortland, NY 13045-2198
607-753-7363
FAX: 607-756-4884
e-mail: info@aticortland.org
www.aticortland.org

Mary E. Ewing, Executive Director
Chad W. Underwood, Chief Operating Officer
Lisa Perfetti, Chair
Larry Pfister, Vice Chair

Access to Independence is Cortland County's foremost disability resource. It empowers people to lead independent lives in their community and strives to open doors to full participation and access for all.

4164 **Action Toward Independence: Middletown**
130 Dolson Avenue
Suite 35
Middletown, NY 10940-6563
845-343-4284
FAX: 845-342-5269
e-mail: ati@warwick.net
actiontowardindependence.org

Stephen McLaughlin, Executive Director
Joann Hargabus, Services Director, Orange Cnty.
Gilles Malkine, Services Director, Sullivan Cnty
Cheryl Babcock, Fiscal Manager

Independent living center that serves Orange & Sullivan counties. Provides programs and services to individuals who have disabilities and to their families. These services include peer counseling, individual & systems advocacy, independent living, skills training, information and referral, benefits advisement, recreation and a drop in center. We are designed to enable people with disabilities to achieve independence, inclusion and participation in their communities.

4165 Action Toward Independence: Monticello
309 E Broadway
Suite A
Monticello, NY 12701-8810
845-794-4228
FAX: 845-794-4475
TTY:845-794-4228
e-mail: szecchini@atitoday.org
www.atitoday.org

Steve McLaughlin, Executive Director
Joann Hargabus, Director of Services

A not-for-profit, non residential, peer run, referral and advocacy agency for persons with disaiblities in Orange and Sullivan counties. Our services are aimed at promoting accessibility, community integration, and equal opportunity in all aspects of society for persons with all types of disabilities.

4166 Bronx Independent Living Services
4419 Thrid Avenue
Suite 2C
Bronx, NY 10457
718-515-2800
FAX: 718-515-2844
TTY:718-515-2803
e-mail: webmaster@bils.org
www.bils.org

Brett L. Eisenberg, Executive Director
Barbara Linn, President
Anita Richichi, Vice President
Sheldon Mann, Treasurer

BILS is a not-for-profit community agency serving people with all kinds of disabilities. The mission is to empower people with disabilities toward living independent lives. BILS assists individuals by providing advocacy, peer counseling, housing information, and independent living training/counseling.

4167 Brooklyn Center for Independence of the Disabled
27 Smith Street
Suite #200
Brooklyn, NY 11201
718-998-3000
FAX: 718-998-3743
TTY:718-998-7406
e-mail: advocate@bcid.org
www.bcid.org

Joan Peterss, Executive Director
Sandrina Kingston, Program Director
Princess Davis, Office Manager
Michael Godino, Director of Advocacy

Operated by a majority of people with disabilities, BCID is dedicated to guaranteeing the civil rights of people with disabilities. BCID exists to improve the quality of life of brooklyn residents with disabilities thgouh programs that empower them to gain greater control of their lives and achieve full and equal integration into society.

4168 Capital District Center for Independence
845 Central Ave
South 3
Albany, NY 12206-1342
518-459-6422
FAX: 518-459-7847
TTY:518-459-6422
e-mail: info@cdciweb.com
www.cdciweb.com

Laurel Kelley, Executive Director

One of 37 Independent Living Centers in New York State, the Center is a non-residential, community based organization, which primarily serves Albany and Schenetady Counties. The Center's mission is to assist people with disabilities to acquire self-advocacy skills and by teaching through example, consumers achieve greater control over the direction of their lives.

4169 Catskill Center for Independence
6104 State Highway 23
Oneonta, NY 13820
607-432-8000
FAX: 607-432-6907
TTY:607-432-8000
e-mail: ccfi@ccfi.us
www.ccfi.us

Chris Zachmeyer, Executive Director
Christine Worden, Assistant Director

One of 37 community-based independent living centers located throughout the state of New York. As an advocacy agency, we provide a vareity of services to people with disabilities, their friends and family members. In addition, we provide advocacy, training, and technical assistance to our community members, organizations, businesses and state and local governments in a variety of disability related areas. Serves Otsego, Delaware and Schoharie counties.

4170 Center for Community Alternatives
115 E Jefferson St
Suite #300
Syracuse, NY 13202-2018
315-422-5638
FAX: 315-471-4924
e-mail: cca@communityalternatives.org
www.communityalternatives.org

Marsha Weissman, Executive Director
Bonnie Catone, President
Susan R. Horn, Esq., Vice-President
Carole A. Eady, Secretary

Promotes reintegrative justice and a reduced reliance on incarceration through advocacy, services and public policy development in pursuit of civil and human rights.

4171 Center for Independence of the Disabled of New York
80-02 Kkew Garden Rd.
Suite 107
Kew Gardens, NY 11415
646-442-1520
FAX: 718-886-0428
TTY:718-886-0427
e-mail: info@cidny.org
www.cidny.org

Susan Dooha, Executive Director
Martin Eichel, President
Anne M. Davis, Vice President
John O'Neill, Vice President

To ensure full integration, independence and equal opportunity for all people with disabilities by removing barriers to the social, economic, cultural and civic life of the community.

4172 Center for Independence of the Disabled of New York
841 Broadway
Suite #301
New York, NY 10003-4708
212-674-2300
FAX: 212-254-5953
TTY:212-674-5619
e-mail: info@cidny.org
www.cidny.org

Susan Dooha, Executive Director
Martin Eichel, President
Anne M. Davis, Vice President
John O'Neill, Vice President

To ensure full integration, independence and equal opportunity for all people with disabilities by removing barriers to the social, economic, cultural and civic life of the community.

4173 DD Center/St Lukes: Roosevelt Hospital Center
St Lukes Roosevelt
1000 10th Ave
New York, NY 10019-1192
212-473-2045
FAX: 212-473-0501

Charles Raimondo, VP
Farooq Chaudry, MD

Independent living center that advocates for people with disabilities by assisting with the application process of housing, benefits, etc.

4174 Finger Lakes Independence Center
215 5th St
Ithaca, NY 14850-3403
607-272-2433
FAX: 607-272-0902
TTY:607-272-2433
e-mail: flic@fliconline.org
www.fliconline.org

Lenore Schwager, Executive Director

FLIC assists all people with disabilities, their families and friends to promote independence and make informed decisions in pursuit of their goals. The servides provided are free of charge, and services are primarily served to residents of Tompkins, Schyler counties.

4175 Harlem Independent Living Center
289 St. Nicholas Avenue
Suite #21
New York, NY 10027- 4805
212-222-7122
800-673-2371
FAX: 212-222-7199
e-mail: harlemilc@aol.com
www.hilc.org

Christina Curry, Executive Director
Edward Randolph, Resource Specialist
Dr. Herbert Thornhill, Emeritus
Vanessa J. Young, Chair

A non-profit agency that advocates for people with disabilities by assisting with the application process of housing, benefits, etc. Our services are free of charge.
Monthly

4176 Independent Living
5 Washington Terrace
Newburgh, NY 12550-5383
845-565-1162
FAX: 845-565-0567
TTY:845-565-0337
e-mail: info@myindependentliving.org
www.myindependentliving.org

Matthew Migliaccio, President
Charles Walwyn, III, Vice President
Douglas J. Hovey, Executive Director
Anne Miller, Director of Development

A consumer directed, cross-disability advocacy organization dedicated to enhancing quality of life for persons with disabilities.

4177 Long Island Center for Independent Living
3601 Hempstead Tpke
Suites 208 & 500
Levittown, NY 11756-1331
516-796-0144
FAX: 516-520-1247
TTY:516-796-0135
e-mail: licil@aol.com
www.licil.net

Patricia Moore, Executive Director

LICIL is committed to the empowerment of consumers with disabilities. LICIL staff functions as ambassadors to the belief that individuals with disabilities have a responsibility to take an active role in their own lives and self determined view of their futures.

4178 Massena Independent Living Center
156 Center St
Massena, NY 13662-1495
315-764-9442
877-397-9613
FAX: 315-764-9464
TTY: 315-764-9442
e-mail: mindepli@twcny.rr.com
www.milcinc.org

Jeff Reifensnyder, Executive Director

Provides a variety of non-residential direct services as well as educating the public through community awareness campaigns. Also seeks to address the current appropriate unmet needs of persons experiencing a disability - primarily in St Lawrence and Franklin Counties.

4179 NYS Independent Living Council
111 Washington Ave
Suite #101
Albany, NY 12210-2280
518-427-1060
877-397-4126
FAX: 518-427-1139
e-mail: bradw@nysilc.org
www.nysilc.org

Brad Williams, Executive Director
Patty Black, Administrative Assistant

Provides support and technical assistance to 37 independent living centers-community-based organizations directed by and for people with disabilities.

4180 Nassau County Office for the Physically Challenged
60 Charles Lindberg Blvd
Uniondale, NY 11553-4812
516-227-7399
www.nassaucountyny.gov

Edward P. Mangano, County Executive

This agency serves as the ADA compliance coordinating office for all Nassau County governmental facilities, programs and services. It also serves in an advisory capacity to local, regional and national policy-making organizations, planning committees and legislative bodies and conducts advocacy as well as direct programs and services to enhance inclusion by people with disabilities to employment, consumerism and transportation.

4181 North Country Center for Independent Living
80 Sharron Avenue
Plattsburgh, NY 12901-3827
518-563-9058
FAX: 518-563-0292
TTY:518-563-9058
e-mail: andrew@ncci-online.com
www.ncci-online.com

Deb Piper, CDPAP Coordinator
Greg Lyman, Radio Reading Service Coordinator
John Farley, Accessibilty Consultant
Judy Harris, AmeriCorps

To empower people with disabilities to live more independent and productive lives, and to promote beneficial policies and community understanding of disability issues.

4182 Northern Regional Center for Independent Living: Watertown
210 Court St
Suite #107
Watertown, NY 13601-4546
315-785-8703
800-585-8703
FAX: 315-785-8612
TTY: 315-785-8704
e-mail: nrcil@nrcil.net
www.nrcil.net

Ronald Griffin, President
Rebecca Shamey, Vice President
Alicia Kohler, Secretary
Brenda Campany, Executive Director

A disability rights and resource center that promotes community efforts to end discrimination, segregation, and prejudice against people with disabilities.

4183 Northern Regional Center for Independent Living: Lowville
7632 N State St
Lowville, NY 13367-1318
315-376-8696
FAX: 315-376-3404
TTY:315-376-8696
e-mail: karenb@nrcil.net
www.nrcil.net

Ronald Griffin, President
Rebecca Shamey, Vice President
Alicia Kohler, Secretary
Brenda Campany, Executive Director

A disability rights and resource center that promotes community efforts to end discrimination, segregation, and prejudice against people with disabilities.

4184 Options for Independence: Auburn
75 Genesee St
Auburn, NY 13021-3667
315-255-3447
FAX: 315-255-0836
e-mail: gguy@optionsforindependence.org
www.optionsforindependence.org

Greg Guy, Executive Director
Joyce McGlynn, MSC Consulting Supervisor
Sara Douglass, Youth Advocate
Felicia Thompson, Benefits Advisor/Rep. Payee

Options for Independence is an Independent Living Center which assists people with disabilities to gain opportunities, make their own decisions, pursue activities and become part of comunity life. Options provides a variety of services to all people with disabilities, their families, friends, and service providers in Cayuga and Seneca Counties.

4185 Putnam Independent Living Services
1961 Route 6
2nd Floor
Carmel, NY 10512-2324
845-228-7457
FAX: 845-228-7460
TTY:866-933-5390
e-mail: info@wilc.org
www.putnamils.org

Joe Bravo, Executive Director
Mildred Caballero-Ho, Deputy Executive Director
Margaret Valenzuela, Program Director, IL Services
Jessica Baumann, Program Director, Educational Advocacy Services

A non-profit, community-based advocacy and resource center that serves people with all types of disabilities.

4186 Regional Center for Independent Living
497 State St
Rochester, NY 14608-1642
585-442-6470
FAX: 585-271-8558
TTY:585-442-6470
e-mail: bdarling@rcil.org
www.rcil.org

Bruce E Darling, Executive Director
Chris Hilderbrant, Chief Operating Officer
Linda Taylor, Executive Assistant
Paul Akers, Director of Programs

To empower people with disabilities to self-advocate, to live independently and to enhance the quality of community life.

4187 Resource Center for Accessible Living
727 Ulster Ave
Kingston, NY 12401-1709
845-331-0541
FAX: 845-331-2076
TTY:845-331-4527
e-mail: rcal@hvc.rr.com
www.rcal.org

Paul Scarpati, President
Paula Kindos-Carberry, Co-Vice President
Bernadette Mueller, Co-Vice President
Susan Hoger, RCAL Executive Director

RCAL is a non-profit, community based service and advocacy run by and for people with any type of disability. RCAL is dedicated to assisting and empowering individuals, of all ages, to live independently and participate in all aspects of community life.

4188 Resource Center for Independent Living
347 W Main St
Amsterdam, NY 12010-2225
518-842-3561
FAX: 518-842-0905
TTY:518-842-3593
e-mail: bdanovitz@rcil.com
www.rcil.ocom

Burt Danovitz, Executive Director
Wendy Gagliardo, Chief Financial Officer
Joann Marshall, Chief Operating Officer
Miyoshi Collins, Senior Program Director

Peer counseling, advocacy, independent living skills training, information and referral services, self-advocacy training, ADA consultation, home and community based services, community education, benefits advisement and more. All programs and services are available in English and Spanish.

4189 Rockland Independent Living Center
873 Route 45
Suite 108
New City, NY 10956-2712
845-624-1366
FAX: 845-624-1369
TTY:845-624-0848
e-mail: info@rilc.org
www.rilc.org

Audrey Rosenfield, President
Myrna Wulfson, Vice President / Secretary
David Aron, CPA, Treasurer
George Hoehmann M.A., Executive Director

RILC serves all individuals with disabilities. We promote philosophy consumer empowerment and control. The services we provide include benefit and advisement information and referral and consumer directed personal assistants.

4190 Southern Adirondack Independent Living
418 Geyser Rd
Country Club Plaza
Ballston Spa, NY 12020-6002
518-584-8202
FAX: 518-584-1195
e-mail: sail@sail-center.org
www.sail-center.org

Karen Thayer, Executive Director
Anna Livingston, Assistant Director
Barbara Potvin, Executive Assistant
Michele Nicholson, Administrative Assistant

To assist individuals with disabilities to become independent empowered self-advocates.

4191 Southern Adirondack Independent Living Center
71 Glenwood Ave
Queensbury, NY 12804-1728
518-792-3537
FAX: 518-792-0979
TTY:518-792-0505
e-mail: sail@sail-center.org
www.sail-center.org

Karen Thayer, Executive Director
Anna Livingston, Assistant Director
Shirley Dumont, Director of Advocacy
Barbara Potvin, Executive Assistant

To assist individuals with disabilities to become independent empowered self-advocates.

4192 Southern Tier Independence Center
135 E Frederick St
Binghamton, NY 13904-1224
607-724-2111
FAX: 607-772-3600
TTY:607-724-2111
e-mail: stic@stic-cil.org
www.stic-cil.org

Maria Dibble, Executive Director
Frank Pennisi, Accessibility Services

STIC provides assistance and services to all people with disabilities of all ages to increase their independence in all aspects of integrated community life. STIC also serves their families and friends, and businesses, agencies, and goverments to enable them to better meet the needs of people with disabilities, and finally STIC educates and influences the community in pursuit of full inclusion of people with disabilities.

4193 Southwestern Independent Living Center
843 N Main St
Jamestown, NY 14701-3546
716-661-3010
FAX: 716-661-3011
TTY:716-661-3012
e-mail: info@ilc-jamestown-ny.org
ilc-jamestown-ny.org

Marie T Carrubba, Executive Director
Linda Rumbaugh, Independent Living Specialist
Christine Ahlstrom, Independent Living Specialist
Helen Kern, Independent Living Specialist

A non-residential, private, nonprofit agency established to provide services throughout Chautauqua County that will assist individuals with disabilities in reaching maximum independence and an enriched quality of life.

4194 **Staten Island Center for Independent Living, Inc.**
470 Castleton Ave
Staten Island, NY 10301 718-720-9016
FAX: 718-720-9664
TTY:718-720-9870
e-mail: ldesantis@siciliving.org
www.siciliving.org

Lorraine DeSantis, Executive Director
Claudia J. Stanton, Office Manager
Michelle Sabatino, Independent Living Specialist
John Mastellone, Community Consultant / Benefits Advisement / Computer Tech
Mission is to provide all individuals with disabilities the information, life skills training, and facilitative assistance which contributes to independence, individuality, and integration in the community and provides the skills and knowledge necessary to function in the least restrictive, personally fulfilling, most self reliant and productive manner.

4195 **Suffolk Independent Living Organization(SILO)**
2111 Lakeland Ave.
Suite A
Ronkonkoma, NY 11779 631-880-7929
FAX: 631-946-6377
TTY:631-946-6585
www.siloinc.org/?

Edward Ahern, Manager
Glenn Campbell, Co-Executive Director
A not-for-profit organization that helps the disabled become more independent and more involved in the community by providing them with information on referrals on Housing, Education, Employment and Benefits.

4196 **Taconic Resources for Independence**
82 Washington St
Suite #214
Poughkeepsie, NY 12601-2305 845-452-3913
866-948-1094
FAX: 845-485-3196
e-mail: tri@taconicresources.org
www.taconicresources.org

Cynthia L. Fiore, Executive Director
Patrick Muller, Program Director
Diane Barkstrom, Program Director/Staff Interpreter
Jeanine Byrnes, Coordinator of Deaf & Hard of Hearing Services
A center for independent living, benefits advisement information, and referral, advocacy, independent living skills, peer counseling, parent advocacy, sign language interpreters.

4197 **Westchester Disabled on the Move**
984 N. Broadway
Suite LL-10
Yonkers, NY 10701-1320 914-968-4717
FAX: 914-968-6137
e-mail: info@wdom.org
www.wdom.org

Gail Cartenuto Cohn, President
Mattie Trupia, Vice President
Sandra Dolman, Secretary
Chandra Sookdeo, Assistant Recording Secretary
WDOM empowers people with disabilities to control their own lives; advocates for civil rights and a barrier free society; encourages people with disabilities to participate in the political process; educates government, business, other entities, and a society as a whole to understand, accept, and accommodate people with disabilities; creates an environment that inspires self-respect

4198 **Westchester Independent Living Center**
200 Hamilton Avenue
2nd Floor
White Plains, NY 10601- 1809 914-682-3926
FAX: 914-682-8518
TTY:866-933-5390
e-mail: Contact@wilc.org
www.wilc.org

Joseph Bravo, Executive Director
A not-for-profit, community-based advocacy and resource center that serves people with all types of disabilities.

North Carolina

4199 **Disability Awareness Network**
609 Country Club Dr.
Suite C
Greenville, NC 27834-6210 252-353-5522
FAX: 252-353-5160
e-mail: DAWNpittco@aol.com
consolidatedmachines.com

Jackie Hansley, Owner
Information and referral for diabled persons; peer counseling for diabled persons; advocacy on ADA issues; independent living skills and training.

4200 **Disability Rights & Resources**
5801 Executive Center Dr.
Suite #101
Charlotte, NC 28212-8870 704-537-0550
800-755-5749
FAX: 704-566-0507
TTY: 704-537-0550
e-mail: mailto@disability-rights.org
www.disability-rights.org

Maura Chavez, President
Marta Fales, Vice President
Holly Howell, Secretary
Rick Griffiths, Treasurer
To guard the civil rights of people wtih disabilities by empowering ourselves and others to live as we choose.

4201 **Joy: A Shabazz Center for Independent Living**
235 N Greene St
Greensboro, NC 27401-2410 336-272-0501
FAX: 336-272-0575
TTY:336-272-0501
e-mail: aaron.shabazz@shabazzcenter.org
www.wangshuai.net

Aaron Shabazz, Executive Director
James Wells, President
Stephen Simpson, Vice-President
B. J. Gerald Covington, Secretary/Treasurer
A non-profit, consumer oriented, Center for Independent Living (CIL) providing advocacy, peer counseling and peer support, independent living skills, training, information and referrals, with other related services for persons with disabilites.

4202 **Live Independently Networking Center**
P.O.Box 1135
Newton, NC 28658-1135 828-464-0331
FAX: 828-464-7375
TTY:828-464-2838
e-mail: linc@twave.net
www.linconline.org

Donavon Kirby, Deputy Director
Private, nonprofit, federally funded center for independent living located in Western North Carolina.

4203 **Live Independently Networking Center: Hickory**
2830 16th St NE
Apt. 17
Hickory, NC 28601-8606 828-464-0331
FAX: 828-464-7375

4204 **Pathways for the Future Center for Independent Living**
525 Mineral Springs Dr
Sylva, NC 28779-9077
828-631-1167
FAX: 828-631-1169
TTY:828-631-1167
e-mail: bdavis@pathwayscil.org
www.pathwayscil.org

Barbara Davis, Executive Director

Dedicated to increasing independence, changing attitudes, promoting equal access and building a peer support network in western North Carolina through the use of community education, independent living services and advocacy.

4205 **Western Alliance Center for Independent Living**
30b London Rd
Asheville, NC 28803-2706
828-274-0444
FAX: 828-274-4461
e-mail: wacil@main.nc.us
westernalliance.org

Katy Hollingsworth, Manager
Jerry Brewton, Independent Living Specialist

4206 **Western Alliance for Independent Living**
108 New Leicester Highway
Asheville, NC 28806
828-298-1977
FAX: 828-298-0875
e-mail: khollingsworth@disabilitypartners.org
www.disabilitypartners.org

Kathy Hollingsworth, Associate Director
Rosemary Weaver, Independent Living Specialist
Mechelle Holt, Volunteer/Program Coordinator
Eva Reynolds, Emploment Network Coordinator

North Dakota

4207 **Dakota Center for Independent Living: Dickinson**
26-1st street East
Suite 103
Dickinson, ND 58601-5103
701- 48- 436
800-489-5013
FAX: 701- 48- 436
TTY: 800489501363
e-mail: dcil@ndsupernet.com
www.dakotacil.org

Robin Were, President
Claudia Ziegler, Vice president
Carol Mihulka, Secretary/Treasurer
Royce Schultze, Executive Director

Believes in self-determination for people with disabilities and creates the environment in which it is achieved.

4208 **Dakota Center for Independent Living: Bismarck**
3111 E Broadway Ave
Bismarck, ND 58501-5085
701-222-3636
800-489-5013
FAX: 701-222-0511
TTY: 701-222-3636
e-mail: maryr@dakotacil.org
www.dakotacil.org

Robin Were, President
Cladia Ziegler, Vice president
Carol Mihulka, Secretary/Treasurer
Royce Schultze, Executive Director

Believes in self-determination for people with disabilities and creates the environment in which it is achieved.

4209 **Fraser**
2902 University Drive South
Fargo, ND 58103-6053
701-232-3301
FAX: 701-237-5775
e-mail: fraser@fraserltd.org
fraserltd.org

Sandra Leyland, Executive Director
Mark Brodshaug, President
Michael Kirk, Vice President
David A. Laske, Treasurer

Private non-profit, federally funded center for independent living

4210 **Freedom Resource Center for Independent Living: Fargo**
2701 9th Ave S
Suite H
Fargo, ND 58103-8712
701-478-0459
800-450-0459
FAX: 701-478-0510
TTY: 701-478-0459
e-mail: freedom@freedomrc.org
www.freedomrc.org

Nate Aalgaard, Executive Director
Angie Bosch, Office Coordinator
Mark Mark Bourdon Bourdon, Program Director
Andrea Nelson, Independent Living Advocate

To work toward equality and inclusion for people with disabilities through programs of empowerment, community education, and systems change.

4211 **Resource Center for Independent Living: Minot**
300 3rd Ave SW
Suite F
Minot, ND 58701-4346
701-839-4724
800-377-5114
FAX: 701-838-1677
TTY: 701-839-4724
e-mail: independencecil@independencecil.org
www.independencecil.org/?

Susan Ogurek, Chair
Scott Burlingame, Executive Director
Dee Tischer, Senior Independent Living Specialist
Jamie Hardt, Youth Transition Specialist

A resource center for independent living. Mission is to advocate for the freedom of choice for individuals with disabilities to live independently through the removal of all barriers.

Ohio

4212 **Ability Center of Greater Toledo**
5605 Monroe St
Sylvania, OH 43560-2702
419-885-5733
866-885-5733
FAX: 419-882-4813
TTY: 419-885-5733
www.abilitycenter.org

Tim Harrington, Executive Director
Lisa Justice, Executive Assistant
Dale Abell, Director of Programme Development
Debbie Keller, Tomorrow Planning Specialist

To assist people with disabilities to live, work and socialize within a fully accessible community.

4213 **Ability Center of Greater Toledo: Defiance**
5605 Monroe St
Sylvania, OH 43560-2702
419-885-5733
866-885-5733
FAX: 419-882-4813
TTY: 419-885-5733
www.abilitycenter.org

Tim Harrington, Executive Director
Lisa Justice, Executive Assistant
Dale Abell, Director of Programme Development
Debbie Keller, Tomorrow Planning Specialist

To assist people with disabilities to live, work and socialize within a fully accessible community.

4214 **Ability Center of Greater Toledo: Port Clinton**
1848 East Perry Street
Suite #110
Port Clinton, OH 43452-1802
419-734-0330
877-734-0330
FAX: 419-732-6864
TTY: 419-734-0330
www.abilitycenter.org

Tim Harrington, Executive Director
Lisa Justice, Executive Assistant
Dale Abell, Director of Programme Development
Debbie Keller, Tomorrow Planning Specialist

To assist people with disabilities to live, work and socialize within a fully accessible community.

4215 **Access Center for Independent Living**
901 S Ludlow St
Dayton, OH 45402-2614
937-341-5202
FAX: 937-341-5217
TTY:937-341-5218
e-mail: info@acils.com
www.acils.com/?

Darrell Price, IL Team Co-Leader
Tonya Banther, IL Team Co-Leader
Melody Burba, Information & Referral Specialist
John Dixon, Information & Referral Specialist

Offers peer counseling, disability education and other services to the community.

4216 **Center for Independent Living Options**
2031 Auburn Avenue
Cincinnati, OH 45219-2436
513-241-2600
FAX: 513-241-1707
TTY:513-241-7170
e-mail: cilo@cilo.net.
cilo.net

Lin Laing, Executive Director
Justin Bifro, President
Brian Frazier, Vice-President
Ed Klene, Treasurer

The oldest center for independent living in Ohio serving individuals with disabilities in the Greater Cincinnati/Northern Kentucky region.

4217 **Fairfield Center for Disabilities and Cerebral Palsy**
681 E 6th Ave
Lancaster, OH 43130-2602
740-653-5501
FAX: 740-653-6046
e-mail: fcdcp@sbcglobal.net
www.fcdcp.org

David Macioci, President
David Welsh, Vice-President
Mary Snider, Treasurer
Edwin R. Payne, Secretary

Adult Day Program and Transportation. The mission of the Fairfield Center for disabilities and Cerebral Palsy, Inc, is to create a better future for people with a disability by increasing and enhancing their lifestyle opportunities.

4218 **Linking Employment, Abilities and Potential**
2545 Lorain Ave.
Cleveland, OH 44113-3102
216-696-2716
FAX: 216-687-1453
www.leapinfo.org

Charles Heindrichs, President
Brian Roof, Vice President
Vincent Shemo, Treasurer
Betsey Kamm, Secretary

Consumer-directed to ensure a society of equal opportunity for all persons, regardless of disability.

4219 **Mid-Ohio Board for an Independent Living Environment (MOBILE)**
690 S High St
Columbus, OH 43206-1016
614-443-5936
FAX: 614-443-5954
TTY:614-443-5957
e-mail: info@mobileonline.org
www.mobileonline.org

Darry Moore, President
Thomas Shapaka, Vice-President
Mark Morton, Treasurer
Warren King, Secretary

A non-profit Center for Independent Living directed by persons with disabilities. MOBILE was founded on principles that affirm the right of persons with disabilities to live their lives with a full measure of liberty and human dignity.

4220 **Ohio Statewide Independent Living Council**
670 Morrison Road
Suite 200
Gahanna, OH 43230-5324
614-892-0390
800-566-7788
FAX: 614-861-0392
www.ohiosilc.org

Kay Grier, Executive Director
Eugene Iacovetta, Special Projects Coordinator
Mary Butler, Systems Change Coordinator
Janae Miller, Office Manager

Committed to promoting a philosophy of consumer control, peer support, self-help, self-determination, equal acess, and individual and systems advocacy, in order to maximize leadership, empowerment, independence, productivity and to support full inclusion and integration of individuals with disabilities into the mainstream of American society.

4221 **Rehabilitation Service of North Central Ohio**
270 Sterkel Blvd
Mansfield, OH 44907-1508
419-756-1133
800-589-1133
FAX: 419-756-6544
e-mail: info@therehabcenter.org
www.therehabcenter.org

Veronica L. Groff, President/CEO
Susan Baker, Chairman
Dan Wiegand, Vice-Chairman
Scott Donnenwirth, Secretary

Private nonprofit organization providing coordinated, team-oriented comprehensive outpatient rehabilitation services to children and adults of all ages. Serves 8 counties in N/C Ohio. Four umbrella areas of service include medical rehabilitation services, vocational rehabilitation services, behavioral health service and drug and alcohol addiction services. Medical rehabilitation services include physical therapy, occupational therapy, speech therapy and audiology.

4222 **Samuel W Bell Home for Sightless**
3775 Muddy Creek Rd
Cincinnati, OH 45238-2055
513-241-0720
FAX: 513-241-1481
e-mail: swbellhome@fuse.net
www.samuelbell.org

: Timothy Lighthal, President
Kevin Kappa, Vice-President
:Miles L.Hoff, Treasurer
James Witte, Secretary

Offers a residential, independent living environment for blind and legally blind adults.

4223 **Services for Independent Living**
25100 Euclid Ave
Suite #105
Cleveland, OH 44117-2663
216-731-1529
FAX: 216-731-3083
TTY:216-731-1529
e-mail: sil@sil-oh.org
www.sil-oh.org

Lynn Hildebrand, Executive Director

Offers support ADA, consultation and education, advocacy, transitional education services, independent living skills training, information and referrals.

4224 Society for Equal Access: Independent Living Center
1458 5th St NW
New Philadelphia, OH 44663-1224
330-343-9292
888-213-4452
FAX: 330-602-7425
TTY:330-602-2557
e-mail: ilc@tusco.net
www.sealc.org

Scott Huston, President
Edna Fillinger, Vice-President
Victoria Eichel, Secretary
Twyla Mccartney, Treasurer
The Society works with individuals to become more independent. Our agency assists with peer support, advocacy, information and referral, independent living skills and transportation. Our goal is to move those with challenges in the direction ofn independence.

Oklahoma

4225 Ability Resources
823 S Detroit Ave
Suite #110
Tulsa, OK 74120-4223
918-592-1235
800-722-0886
FAX: 918-592-5651
e-mail: webadmin@ability-resources.org
www.ability-resources.org
Carla Lawson, Executive Director
To assist people with disabilities in attaining and maintaining their personal independence.

4226 Green County Independent Living Resource Center
4100 S.E. Adams Rd
Suite C-106
Bartlesville, OK 74006- 8409
918-335-1314
800-559-0567
FAX: 918-333-1814
TTY: 918-335-1314
Vicki Haws, Executive Director
Independent living skills training, information and referrals, advocacy, a loan library of adaptive equipment and books. Services available to all individuals with disabilities and their family members who reside in Northeastern Oklahoma.

4227 Oklahomans for Independent Living
601 East Carl Albert Parkway
McAlester, OK 74501-5410
918-426-6220
800-568-6821
FAX: 918-426-3245
TTY: 918-426-6263
e-mail: info@oilok.org
www.oilok.org
Pam Pulchny, Executive Director/ADAspecialist
Terry Yates, Administrative Assistant/Bookkeeper
Leanna Amos, Service Management Specialist
Stephen Strickland, Living Choice Coordinator
OIL encourages individuals of all ages, with all types of disabilities to increase: personal dependence; empowerment and self determiation; and ful integration and participation in their work, community, school and home activities.

4228 Progressive Independence
121 N Porter Avenue
Norman, OK 73071-5834
405-321-3203
800-801-3203
FAX: 405-321-7601
TTY: 405-321-2942
e-mail: heathera@progind.org
www.progind.org
Jeff Hughes, Executive Director
Josh Gray, Office Manager
Preovides four cores services of Information & Referral, Individaul& Systems Advocacy, Peer Counseling, and Skills Training; in addition, offers accessible computer lab, short term DME loans, ande benefits counseling for SSI/SSDI.

Oregon

4229 Abilitree
2680 NE Twin Knolls Dr.
Suite 150
Bend, OR 97701
541-388-8103
FAX: 541-389-2337
TTY:541-388-8103
e-mail: coril@coril.org
www.abilitree.org
Jim Lee, Executive Director
Mike Smith, Work Center Manager
CORIL empowers people with disabilities to maximize their independence, productivity and inclusio in community life. CORIL envisions a society where all people have the opportunity to develop their full capabilities with independence, productivity and more meaningful involvment in local community events and activities.

4230 Eastern Oregon Center for Independent Living
1021 SW 5th Ave
Ontario, OR 97914-3301
541-889-3119
866-248-8369
FAX: 541-889-4647
e-mail: eocil@eocil.org
www.eocil.org
Kirt Toombs, Executive Director
EOCIL is a nonprofit community based resource and advocacy center that promotes independent living and equal access for all persons with disabilities. EOCIL serves consumers in the counties of: Baker, Gilliam, Grant, harney, Malheur, Morrow, Umatilla, Union, Wallowa and Wheeler.

4231 HASL Independent Abilities Center
305 NE 'E' Street
Grants Pass, OR 97526
541-479-4275
800-758-4275
FAX: 541-479-7261
TTY: 541-479-3588
e-mail: haslstaff@yahoo.com
www.haslonline.org
Randy Samuelson, Executive Director
To promote public awareness of the special needs and legal rights of individuals with cross-disabilities; to facilitate their integration into society and provide support through advocacy, peer counseling, skills training and information and referral to encourage independence.

4232 Independent Living Resources
1839 NE Couch Street
Portland, OR 97232-5308
503-232-7411
FAX: 503-232-7480
TTY:503-232-8404
e-mail: info@ilr.org
www.ilr.org/?
Barry Fox-Quamme, Executive Director
May Altman, LCSW, Associate Director
Barbara Norris, Office Manager, Executive Assistant
Lina Bensel, Independent Living Specialist, Rent Well Trainer
ILR looks to promote the philosophy of Independent Living by creating opportunities, encouraging choices, advancing equal access, and furthering the level of independence for all people with disabilities

4233 **Laurel Hill Center**
2145 Centennial Plaza
Eugene, OR 97401-2474
541-485-6340
FAX: 541-984-3124
TTY:541-684-6822
e-mail: info@laurel.org
www.laurel.org

Tom Fauria, President
DAVE Burtner, Vice-President
EDUARDO Sifuentez, Secretary
Lt. Jennifer Bills, Special operations
Provides natoinall-recognized, recovery-focused rehabilitation services in Lane County, Oregon, for people with severe and persistent mental illnesses

4234 **Progressive Options**
611 S.W. Hurbert Street
Suite A
Newport, OR 97365-9678
541-265-4674
FAX: 541-574-4313
TTY:541-574-1927
e-mail: progop541@yahoo.com
www.progressive-options.org

Rhonda Walker, Executive Director
Progressive Options seeks to provide free services and support to people with disabilities of all kinds to help them achieve and maintain maximum independence and self-sufficiency in Lincoln County and surrounding areas in Oregon.

4235 **SPOKES Unlimited**
1006 Main St
Klamath Falls, OR 97601-6029
541-883-7547
FAX: 541-885-2469
TTY:541-883-7547
e-mail: info@spokesunlimited.org
www.spokesunlimited.org

Wendy Howard, Executive Director
Mission is to enhance the ability of people with disabilities to live more independently.

4236 **Umpqua Valley Disabilities Network**
736 SE Jackson Street
Roseburg, OR 97470-110
541-672-6336
FAX: 541-672-8606
TTY:541-440-2882
e-mail: uvdn@uvdn.org
www.uvdn.org

David Fricke, Executive Director
Heather Vialpando, Executive Assistant
UVDN's mission is to promote independent living and community inclusion for people with disabilities.

Pennsylvania

4237 **Abilities in Motion**
210 N 5th St
Reading, PA 19601-3304
610-376-0010
888-376-0120
FAX: 610-376-0021
TTY: 610-228-2301
e-mail: staff@abilitiesinmotion.org
www.abilitiesinmotion.org

Terry Graul, Board President
David Lerch, Vice-President
Bonnie Milke, Treasurer
Ralph Trainer, Executive Director
Dedicated to advancing the rights of persons with disabilities in orer to promote a full life in the community through the prevention and elimination of physical, psychological, social and attitudinal barriers which serve to deny them the rights and privileges common to the general public.

4238 **Anthracite Region Center for Independent Living**
Pennsylvania Council on Independent Living
8 West Broad St
Suite 228
Hazleton, PA 18201-6418
570-455-9800
800-777-9906
FAX: 570-455-1731
TTY: 570-455-9800
e-mail: dcorcoran@anthracitecil.org
www.anthracitecil.org

Irene Mordosky, President
Margo Madden, Vice-President
Rand Martin, Treasurer
Tracy Clark, Secretary
Enables individuals with disabilities to attain their highest possible level of independence.

4239 **Brian's House**
1300 S Concord Rd
West Chester, PA 19382-8531
610-399-1175
e-mail: ekihara@brianshouse.org
brianshouse.org

Lori Plunkettt, Executive Director
Diana L. Ramsay, MPP, OTR, FAOT, Resident and Chief Executive Officer
Peter M. Shubiak, MA, Executive Vice President and Chief Operating Officer
A non-profit organization that provides residential, vocational and recreational/respite programs for children and adults with intellectual and developmental disabilities.

4240 **Community Resources for Independence**
3410 W 12th St
Erie, PA 16505-3649
814-838-7222
800-530-5541
FAX: 814-838-8491
TTY: 814-838-8115
www.crinet.org

Timothy Finegan, Executive Director
William Essigmann, Administrative Program Manager
Carl Berry, Human Resources Director
Marty Pushchak, Controller
A community based, nonprofit, nonresidential organization that offers services and assistance to enable people with disabilities to expand their options, pursue their goals, and achieve and maintain self-sufficient and producitve lives in the community.

4241 **Community Resources for Independence, Inc., Bradford**
3410 West 12th Street
Erie, PA 16505
814-838-7222
800-530-5541
FAX: 814-838-8491
TTY: 814-838-8115
crinet.org

Timothy J. Finegan, Executive Director
William Essigmann, Administrative Program Manager
Carl Berry, Human Resources Director
Marty Pushchak, Controller
Community Resources for Independence, Inc is committed to preserve, enhance and enrich the quality of life for all people with disabilities.

4242 **Community Resources for Independence: Lewistown**
33 East Hale Street
Suite L
Lewistown, PA 17044-2160
717-248-8011
800-309-0989
FAX: 717-248-8029
www.crinet.org

Timothy Finegan, Executive Director
William Essigmann, Administrative Program Manager
Carl Berry, Human Resources Director
Marty Pushchak, Controller
A community based, nonprofit, nonresidential organization that offers services and assistance to enable people with disabilities to expand their options, pursue their goals, and achieve and maintain self-sufficient and producitve lives in the community.

4243 Community Resources for Independence: Altoona
1331 Twelth Ave
Suite #103
Altoona, PA 16601
814-994-2645
866-944-2645
FAX: 814-944-2683
www.crinet.org

Timothy Finegan, Executive Director
William Essigmann, Administrative Program Manager
Carl Berry, Human Resources Director
Marty Pushchak, Controller

A community based, nonprofit, nonresidential organization that offers services and assistance to enable people with disabilities to expand their options, pursue their goals, and achieve and maintain self-sufficient and producitve lives in the community.

4244 Community Resources for Independence: Clarion
1200 Eastwood Drive
Suite #1
Clarion, PA 16214-8824
814-297-7141
800-372-0140
FAX: 814-297-7161
www.crinet.org

Timothy J. Finegan, Executive Director
William Essigmann, Administrative Program Manager
Carl Berry, Human Resources Director
Marty Pushchak, Controller

A community based, nonprofit, nonresidential organization that offers services and assistance to enable people with disabilities to expand their options, pursue their goals, and achieve and maintain self-sufficient and producitve lives in the community.

4245 Community Resources for Independence: Clearfield
209 E Locust St
Clearfield, PA 16830-2422
814-765-6405
866-619-6405
FAX: 814-765-1269
www.crinet.org

Timothy Finegan, Executive Director
William Essigmann, Administrative Program Manager
Carl Berry, Human Resources Director
Marty Pushchak, Controller

A community based, nonprofit, nonresidential organization that offers services and assistance to enable people with disabilities to expand their options, pursue their goals, and achieve and maintain self-sufficient and producitve lives in the community.

4246 Community Resources for Independence: Hermitage
3875 East State St
Suite B
Hermitage, PA 16148-3415
724-347-4121
FAX: 724-347-5966
www.crinet.org

Timothy J. Finegan, Executive Director
William Essigmann, Administrative Program Manager
Carl Berry, Human Resources Director
Marty Pushchak, Controller

A community based, nonprofit, nonresidential organization that offers services and assistance to enable people with disabilities to expand their options, pursue their goals, and achieve and maintain self-sufficient and producitve lives in the community.

4247 Community Resources for Independence: Lewisburg
11 Reitz Blvd
Suite #105
Lewisburg, PA 17837-1493
570-524-4314
800-332-4135
FAX: 570-524-9236
www.crinet.org

Timothy J. Finegan, Executive Director
William Essigmann, Administrative Program Manager
Carl Berry, Human Resources Director
Marty Pushchak, Controller

A community based, nonprofit, nonresidential organization that offers services and assistance to enable people with disabilities to expand their options, pursue their goals, and achieve and maintain self-sufficient and producitve lives in the community.

4248 Community Resources for Independence: Oil City
250 Elm St
Oil City, PA 16301-1413
814-677-4655
866-209-3882
FAX: 814-677-4915
www.crinet.org

Tim Finegan, Executive Director
William Essigmann, Administrative Program Manager
Carl Berry, Human Resources Director
Marty Pushchak, Controller

A community based, nonprofit, nonresidential organization that offers services and assistance to enable people with disabilities to expand their options, pursue their goals, and achieve and maintain self-sufficient and producitve lives in the community.

4249 Community Resources for Independence: Warren
1003 Pennsylvania Ave W
Warren, PA 16365-1837
814-726-3404
866-579-3404
FAX: 814-726-3428
www.crinet.org

Timothy Finegan, Executive Director
William Essigmann, Administrative Program Manager
Carl Berry, Human Resources Director
Marty Pushchak, Controller

A community based, nonprofit, nonresidential organization that offers services and assistance to enable people with disabilities to expand their options, pursue their goals, and achieve and maintain self-sufficient and producitve lives in the community.

4250 Community Resources for Independence: Wellsboro
38 Plaza Ln
Wellsboro, PA 16901-1766
570-724-5852
866-401-7911
FAX: 570-724-3945
www.crinet.org

Timothy Finegan, Executive Director
William Essigmann, Administrative Program Manager
Carl Berry, Human Resources Director
Marty Pushchak, Controller

A community based, nonprofit, nonresidential organization that offers services and assistance to enable people with disabilities to expand their options, pursue their goals, and achieve and maintain self-sufficient and producitve lives in the community.

4251 Freedom Valley Disability Center
3607 Chapel Road
Suite B
Newtown Square, PA 19073-3602
610-353-6640
800-427-4754
FAX: 610-353-6753
TTY: 610-353-8900
fvdc.info

Ann Cope, Executive Director

Assists persons with disabilities in the achievement of independent living goals. Also promotes individual and community options to maximize independence for persons with disabilities. Serves people with disabilities in Chester, Delaware, and Montgomery Counties.

4252 Institute on Disabilities At Temple Univ.
Temple University
1755 N. 13th St
Student Center, Rm. 4115
Philadelphia, PA 19122-6099
215-204-1356
FAX: 215-204-6336
e-mail: iod@temple.edu
www.disabilities.temple.edu

James Earl Davis, Phd, Interim Executive Director
Celia Feinstein, Co-Executive- Director
Amy Goldman, Co-Executive- Director
Ann Marie White, Deputy- Director

Leads by example, creating connections and promoting networks within and among communitites so that people with disabilities are recognized as integral to the fabric of community life.

4253 Lehigh Valley Center for Independent Living
435 Allentown Drive
Allentown, PA 18109-9121
610-770-9781
800-495-8245
FAX: 610-770-9801
TTY: 610-770-9789
e-mail: info@lvcil.org
www.lvcil.org

Amy Beck, Executive Director
Cara Steidel, Fiscal Coordinator
Greg Bott, Development Coordinator
Rebecca Dubin, Administrative Assistant

Serves persons in Lehigh and Northampton Counties with any type of disability and/or his/her family.

4254 Liberty Resources
714 Market St
Suite #100
Philadelphia, PA 19106-2337
215-634-2000
888-634-2155
FAX: 215-634-6628
TTY:215-634-6630
e-mail: lrinc@libertyresources.org
www.libertyresources.org

Thomas Earle, CEO
Marsha Thrower, Chairman
Mary Ellen Caffrey, Vice-Chairman
Melissa Monser, Secretary

A non-profit, consumer driven organization that advocates and promotes Independent Living for persons with disabilities.

4255 Life and Independence for Today
503 E Arch St
Saint Marys, PA 15857-1779
814-781-3050
800-341-5438
FAX: 814-781-1917
TTY: 814-781-3050
e-mail: lift@liftcil.org
www.liftcil.org

Stephen DePrater, President
Linda McKinstry, Vice-President
Charles Williams, Treasurer
Larry Caggeso, Board Member

Offers services to enable people with disabilities to achieve new goals and broaden their horizons. It enables them to achieve and maintain self-sufficient and productive lives.

4256 Northeastern Pennsylvania Center for Independent Living
1142 Sanderson Ave
Suite #1
Scranton, PA 18509
570-344-7211
800-344-7211
FAX: 570-344-7218
TTY: 570-344-5275
e-mail: nepacilinfo@nepacil.org
www.nepacil.org

Robert Treptow, President
Michael Sporer, Secretary
Chris Armone,Esq, Treasurer

Established to assist in removing barriers and expanding independent living options available to people with disabilities.

4257 South Central Pennsylvania Center for Independence Living
1019 Logan Blvd
Altoona, PA 16602-2434
814-949-1905
800-237-9009
FAX: 814-949-1909
TTY: 814-949-1912
e-mail: cilscpa@cilscpa.org
www.cilscpa.org

Susan Estep, Executive Director

The missio of the Center for Independent Living of South Central PA is to empower people with disabilities to lead independent lives in their commnuitites. The Center covers Bedford, Blair, cambria, Fulton, Huntingdon, Indiana and Somerset counties.

4258 Three Rivers Center for Independent Living: New Castle
900 Rebecca Ave
Pittsburgh, PA 15221-9383
412-371-7700
800-633-4588
FAX: 412-371-9430
TTY: 412-371-6230
e-mail: sholbrook@trcil.org
www.trcil.myfastsite.net/

Stanley A Holbrook, President
Kourtney T. Diaz, Chairperson
Shanicka Kennedy, Esq, Vice-Chairperson
Roxanne Huss, Director of Waiver Services

To empower people with disabilities to enjoy self-directed, personally meaningful lives by providing outstanding consumer controlled services and by advocating for effective community college.

4259 Three Rivers Center for Independent Livi ng: Washington
900 Rebecca Ave
Pittsburgh, PA 15221-4425
412-371-7700
800-633-4588
FAX: 412-371-9430
TTY: 412-371-6230
e-mail: sholbrook@trcil.org
www.trcil.myfastsite.net/

Stanley A Holbrook, President
Kourtney T. Diaz, Chairperson
Shanicka Kennedy, Esq, Vice-Chairperson
Roxanne Huss, Director of Waiver Services

To empower people with disabilities to enjoy self-directed, personally meaningful lives by providing outstanding consumer controlled services and by advocating for effective community college.

4260 Three Rivers Center for Independent Living
900 Rebecca Ave
Pittsburgh, PA 15221-2938
412-371-7700
800-633-4588
FAX: 412-371-9430
TTY: 412-371-6230
e-mail: sholbrook@trcil.org
www.trcil.myfastsite.net/

Stanley A Holbrook, President
Kourtney T. Diaz, Chairperson
Shanicka Kennedy, Esq, Vice-Chairperson
Roxanne Huss, Director of Waiver Services

To empower people with disabilities to enjoy self-directed, personally meaningful lives by providing outstanding consumer controlled services and by advocating for effective community college.

4261 Tri-County Patriots for Independent Living
69 East Beau St
Washington, PA 15301-4711
724-223-5115
FAX: 724-223-5119
TTY:724-228-4028
www.tripil.com

Kathleen Kleinmann, Chief Executive Officer
Maxine Berton, Administrative Assistant
Jeffry D. Woods, Chief Information Officer
Jan Crockett, Chief Financial Officer

Brings together individuals who share common problems in equal access, education, housing, employment, attendant care, transportation, and access to technology.

4262 Voices for Independence
1107 Payne Ave
Erie, PA 16503-1741
814-874-0064
866-407-0064
FAX: 814-874-3497
TTY: 814-874-0064
e-mail: web@vficil.org
www.vficil.org

Edna Anabui, Executive Administrative Assistant
Bob Bach, Director of Development & Public Relations
Ron Bright, Bookkeeper
Waine Byrd, Personal Attendant Supervisor

To empower people with disabilities and promote independent living.

Rhode Island

4263 Arc of Blackstone
500 Prospect St.
Wing B, Suite 203
Pawtucket, RI 2860- 4396
401-727-0150
800-257-6092
FAX: 401-727-1545
e-mail: contact@bvcriarc.org
www.bvcriarc.org

Lester B. Keats, President
Kathleen O'Neill, Vice-President
A. Melanie Cherry, Treasurer
Constance B. Boisse, Secretary
Committed to supporting people with developmental disabilities secure the opportunity to choose and realize their goals of where and how they live, learn, work and play

4264 Franklin Court Assisted Living
180 Franklin St
Bristol, RI 2809-3352
401-253-3679
FAX: 401-253-5855
e-mail: mgargano@ebcdc.org
www.ebcdc.org

Jean Pierce, Administrator
Offers local seniors an affordable assisted living option with first-rate services and gracious accommodations.

4265 IN-SIGHT Independent Living
43 Jefferson Blvd
Warwick, RI 2888-1078
401-941-3322
FAX: 401-941-3356
e-mail: cbutler@in-sight.org
www.in-sight.org

James Hahn, Chairman
Robert Tyler, Vice-Chairman
Jean Saylor, Treasurer
Karl Sherry, Secretary
Creating opportunities and choices for people who are blind and visually impaired

4266 Ocean State Center for Independent Living
1944 Warwick Avenue
Warwick, RI 2889-2448
401-738-1013
866-857-1161
FAX: 401-738-1083
TTY: 401-738-1015
e-mail: info@oscil.org
www.oscil.org

Lorna Ricci, Executive Director
OSCIL is a consumer controlled, community based, nonprofit organization established to provide a range of independent living services to enhance, through self direction, the quality of life of Rhode Islander with significant disability and to promote integration into the community.

4267 Office of Rehabilitation Services
40 Fountain St
Suite #4B
Providence, RI 2903-1898
401-421-7005
FAX: 401-421-7016
www.ors.ri.gov

Steve Brunero, Acting Administrator ORD
Ron Racine, Deputy Administrator Blind
John Microulis, Deputy Administrator Disability
Their goal is to help individuals with physical and mental disabilities prepare for and obtain appropriate employment.

4268 PARI Independent Living Center
500 Prospect St
Pawtucket, RI 2860-6259
401-725-1966
FAX: 401-725-2104
TTY:401-725-1966
e-mail: info@pari-ilc.org
www.pari-ilc.org

Leo Canuel, Executive Director
Sue Bilodau, Program Director
Offers information and referral services, personal care attendant services, home modifications, advocacy services and peer counseling, independent living skills training, and recycled equipment.

South Carolina

4269 Columbia Disability Action Center
136 Stonemark Lane
Suite #100
Columbia, SC 29210
800-681-6805
FAX: 803-779-5114
TTY:803-779-0949
www.able-sc.org/

Leo Tissot, Interim Executive Director
Sara Marin, Director of Administration
Jerri Davison, Assistant Director
Kat Tracy, Area Co-ordinator
A non-profit consumer governed Center for Independent Living. Programs and services support persons with disaibilities in taking full advantage of community resources, enhancing personal opportunities, and determining the direction of their lives.

4270 Disability Action Center
330B Pelham Rd
Suite 100 A
Greenville, SC 29615-3116
864-235-1421
800-681-7715
FAX: 864-235-2056
TTY: 864-235-8798
e-mail: amayne@dacsc.org
www.able-sc.org/

Leo Tissot, Interim Executive Director
Sara Marin, Director of Administration
Jerri Davison, Assistant Director
Kat Tracy, Area Co-ordinator
Empowering people with disabilities to reach their highest level of independence.

4271 Graham Street Community Resources
306 Graham St
Florence, SC 29501-4735
843-665-6674
FAX: 843-665-6674

Faye Thompson, Manager
Promotes independent living and empowers people with disabilities to reach their highest level of independence.

4272 South Carolina Independent Living Council
136 Stonemark Lane
Suite #100
Columbia, SC 29210-7318
803-217-3209
800-994-4322
FAX: 803-731-1439
TTY: 803-217-3209
e-mail: scilc@scilconline.org
www.scsilc.com/

Mike Le Fever, President
Committed to equal opportunity, equal access, self determination, independence, and choice for all people with disabilities and pursues these goals by the means available.

4273 **Walton Options for Independent Living: North Augusta**
325 Georgia Ave
North Augusta, SC 29841-3848 803-279-9611
FAX: 803-279-9135
e-mail: tjohnston@waltonoptions.org
www.waltonoptions.org

Cynthia Anzek, Executive Director

Empowers persons of all ages with all types of disabilities to reach their highest level of independence, community inclusion and employment.

South Dakota

4274 **Adjustment Training Center**
607 N 4th St
Aberdeen, SD 57401-2733 605-229-0263
FAX: 605-225-3455
www.aspiresd.org

Jennifer Gray, Executive Dirtector
Arlette Keller, Director of Service Coordination/Quality Assurance
Janae Hamilton, Director of Community Living Services
Paul Schumacher, Director of Vocational Services

Offers peer counseling, attendant care registry and referrals.

4275 **Black Hills Workshop & Training Center**
Black Hills Workshop
PO Box 2104
Rapid City, SD 57709-2104 605-343-4550
FAX: 605-343-0879
TTY:800-877-1113
e-mail: drosby@bhws.com
www.bhws.com

Larry Meendering, Director of Vocational Services
Gayle Steiger, Director of Human Resources
JoAnne Schriver, Development Director
Marty Krause, VP Agency Operations

Offers job placement, housing options, case coordination, supported employment and supported living for all disability groups, as well as specialized services for brian injury victims.

4276 **Communication Service for the Deaf: Rapid City**
150 Knollwood Dr
Rapid City, SD 57701-694 605-496-0738
800-642-6410
FAX: 605-394-6609
TTY: 866-273-3323
e-mail: inquiry@c-s-d.org
www.c-s-d.org

Dr. Benjamin Soukup, Founder, Chairman & CEO
Christopher Soukup, President
Brad Hermes, Chief Financial Officer
Christina Kokenge, Vice President, Human Resources

A private, nonprofit organization dedicated to providing broad-based services, ensuring public accessibility and increasing public awareness of issues affecting deaf and hard of hearing inividuals.

4277 **Native American Advocacy Program for Persons with Disabilities**
P.O.Box 527
Winner, SD 57580-527 605-842-3977
800-303-3975
FAX: 605-842-3983
TTY: 605-842-3977
e-mail: officemgr@nativeamericanadvocacy.org
www.nativeamericanadvocacy.org

Marla Bull Bear, Executive Director
Charles Bull Bear, Specialist
Betty Farr, Il Specialist
Megan L. Garcia, Prevention Specialist

The mission is to encourage a healthy organization that assists Native Americans with disabilities, by providing prevention, education and training, advocacy, support, independent living skills and referrals.

4278 **Prairie Freedom Center for Independent Living: Sioux Falls**
301 S. Garfield Ave
Suite #9
Sioux Falls, SD 57104-3100 605-367-5630
FAX: 605-367-5639
e-mail: i-l-c@ilcchoices.org
www.pfcil.org

Matthew Cain, Executive Director
Steve Tripp, President
Cheri Raymond, Vice President
Laura Staebner, Treasurer

Established to provide basic skills so many of us take for granted: to take care of our own needs and to make our own decisions to be independent.

4279 **Prairie Freedom Center for Independent Li ving: Madison**
Ste 102
411 SE 10th St
Madison, SD 57042-3570 605-256-5070
FAX: 605-256-5071
e-mail: i-l-c@ilcchoices.org
www.pfcil.org

Matt Cain, Executive Director
Steve Tripp, President
Cheri Raymond, Vice President
Laura Staebner, Treasurer

Established to provide basic skills so many of us take for granted: to take care of our own needs and to make our own decisions to be independent.

4280 **Prairie Freedom Center for Independent Living: Yankton**
413 West 15th St
Suite #107
Yankton, SD 57078-2800 605-668-2940
FAX: 605-668-3060
TTY:605-668-3060
e-mail: i-l-c@ilcchoices.org
www.pfcil.org

Matt Cain, Executive Director
Steve Tripp, President
Cheri Raymond, Vice President
Laura Staebner, Treasurer

Established to provide basic skills so many of us take for granted: to take care of our own needs and to make our own decisions to be independent.

4281 **South Dakota Assistive Technology Project: DakotaLink**
1161 Deadwood Ave N
Suite #5
Rapid City, SD 57702-382 605-394-6742
800-645-0673
FAX: 605-394-6744
TTY: 605-394-6742
e-mail: info@dakotalink.net
dakotalink.tie.net

Pat Czerny, Manager
Patrick Czerny, Technical Services Coordinator
David Scherer, Program Coordinator

DakotaLink, the South Dakota Assistive Technology Program, provides resources and supports to individuals of all ages to ensure greater access to and acquisition of assistive technology devices and services.

4282 **Western Resources for dis-ABLED Independence**
405 East Omaha St
Suite D
Rapid City, SD 57701-2974 605-718-1930
888-434-4943
FAX: 605-718-1933
TTY: 605-718-1930
e-mail: ann@wrdi.org
www.wrdi.org

Jeff Wangen, President
Dennis Coull, Vice-President
Linda Lockner, Secretary
Mike Pendo, Treasurer

WRDI advocates for the rights of equal inclusion of people with disabilities in all aspects of community life. WRDI also strives to identify and promote access to existing resources and to advocate for the development of new resources, which may enable people with disabilities to live more independently.

Tennessee

4283 Center for Independent Living of Middle Tennessee
955 Woodland St
Nashville, TN 37206-3753
615-292-5803
866-992-4568
FAX: 615-383-1176
TTY: 615-292-7790
e-mail: cilmt@tndisability.org
www.cil-mt.org

Tom Hopton, Executive Director
Tria Bridgeman, Benefits Analyst-Jackson
Dylan Brown, Benefits Analyst-Nashville
Pattrick Gallaher, Employment Assistant-Nashville

CILMT provides persons with disabilities opportunities to be self advocates and make their own decisions regarding living arrangements, means of transportation, employment, social and recreational activities, as well as other aspects of everyday life. Serves Davidson, Cheatham, Wilson, Robertson, Rutherford, Sumner and Williamson Counties.

4284 DisAbility Resource Center: Knoxville
900 E Hill Ave
Suite #120
Knoxville, TN 37915-2567
865-637-3666
FAX: 865-637-5616
TTY:865-637-6976
e-mail: drc@drctn.org
www.drctn.org

Lillian Burch, Executive Director
Nicole Craig, Programme Director
Katherine Moore, Independent Living Specialist
Sam Moreno, Peer Mentor

DRCTN mission is to empower people with disabilities to fully integrate and participate in the community. DRC is a community-based non-residential program of services designed to assist people with disabilities to gain independence and to assist the community in eliminating barriers of independence.

4285 Jackson Center for Independent Living
1981 Hollywood Drive
Jackson, TN 38305-4388
731-668-2211
FAX: 731-668-0406
TTY:731-664-3970
e-mail: information@jcil.tn.org
www.j-cil.com

Glen Barr, Executive Director

JCIL works with people with significant disabilities and the Deaf Community in achieving their Independent Living Goals while assisting the community in eliminating barriers to Independent Living.

4286 Memphis Center for Independent Living
1633 Madison Ave
Memphis, TN 38104-2506
901-726-6404
800-848-0298
FAX: 901-726-6521
TTY: 901-726-6404
e-mail: mcil@mcil.org
www.mcil.org

Kevin Lofton, Chairman
Marvin Glenn Bailey, Vice-Chairman
Charles M. Weirich, Jr., Board Counsel

MCIL is a community based non-profit organization whose primary mission is to facilitate the full integration of persons with disabilities into all aspects of community life.

4287 Tennessee Technology Access Program (TTAP)
400 Deaderick St
14th Fl
Nashville, TN 37243-1403
615-313-5183
800-732-5059
FAX: 615-532-4685
TTY: 615-313-5695
e-mail: tn.ttap@state.tn.us
www.state.tn.us/humanserv/rehab/ttap.htm

Kevin Wright, Director

TTAP's mission is to maintain a statewide program of technology-rated assistance that is timely, comprehensive and consumer driven to ensure that all Tennesseans with disabilities have the information, services and deices that they need to make choices about where and how they spend their time as independently as possible. .

4288 Tri-State Resource and Advocacy Corporation
5708 Uptain Rd.
Suite 350
Chattanooga, TN 37411-5501
423-892-4774
800-868-8724
FAX: 423-892-9866
TTY: 423-892-4774
e-mail: 4trac@bellsouth.net
www.4trac.org

Mark Woofall, Executive Director

TRAC is dedicated to improving opportunities for individuals wuth disabilities.

Texas

4289 ABLE Center for Independent Living
3415 Brentwood Drive
Odessa, TX 79762-6906
432-580-3439
e-mail: info@ablecenterpb.org
www.ablecenterpd.org

Marilyn Hancock, Executive Director
Kathleen Story MA, Independent Living Specialist

To promote independent living for people with disabilities.

4290 Austin Resource Center for Independent Living
825 E. Rundberg Ln
Suite E6
Austin, TX 78753-4813
512-832-6349
800-414-6327
FAX: 512-832-1869
e-mail: arcil@arcil.com
www.arcil.com

Ross Davis, Chair
Linda Loach, Vice-Chair
Sylvia Davis, Secretary/Treasurer
Vonnye Gardner, Member

Serving people with disabilities, their families and communities throughout Travis and surrounding counties.

4291 Austin Resource Center: Round Rock
525 Round Rock West
Suite A120
Round Rock, TX 78681-5020
512-828-4624
FAX: 512-828-4625
e-mail: sally@arcil.com
www.arcil.com

Ross Davis, Chair
Linda Loach, Vice-Chair
Sylvia Davis, Secretary/Treasurer
Vonnye Gardner, Member

Serving peole with disabilities, their families and communities throughout Travis and surrounding counties.

4292 **Austin Resource Center: San Marcos**
618 South Guadalupe St
Suite #103
San Marcos, TX 78666- 6977
512-396-5790
800-572-2973
FAX: 512-396-5794
e-mail: sanmarcos@arcil.com
www.arcil.com

Ross Davis, Chair
Linda Loach, Vice-Chair
Sylvia Davis, Secretary/Treasurer
Vonnye Gardner, Member

Serving people with disabilities, their families and communities throughout Travis and surounding counties.

4293 **Brazoria County Center For Independent Living**
1104D East Mullberry Street
Suite D
Angleton, TX 77515- 3952
979-849-7060
888-872-7957
FAX: 979-849-8465
TTY: 979-849-7060
e-mail: bccil@neosoft.com
www.hcil.cc/

Chamane Barrow, Manager

To promote the full inclusion, equal opportunity and participation of persons with disabilities in every aspect of community life. We believe that people with disabilities have the right to make choices affecting their lives, a right to take risks, a right to fail, and a right to succeed.

4294 **Crockett Resource Center for Independent Living**
1020 Loop 304 East
Crockett, TX 75835-1806
936-544-2811
FAX: 936-544-7315
TTY:936-544-2811
e-mail: crcil@windstream.net
www.crockettresourcecenter.org

Sara Minton, Executive Director
Mary Killough, Chief Financial Officer
Tammy Dale, Information/Outreach Coordinator
Cathy Newsome, Program Director

Provides independent living services to cross-disability groups to increase their personal self-determination and minimize dependence on others. Maintain comprehensive information on availability of resources and provides referrals to such resources. Provides instruction to assist people with disabilities to gain skills that would empower them to live independently. Peer counseling, advocacy - both individual and community by assisting to obtain support services to make changes in society.

4295 **Houston Center for Independent Living**
6201 Bonhomme Rd
Ste 150
South Houston, TX 77036
713-974-4621
FAX: 713-974-6927
TTY:713-974-2703
e-mail: hcil@neosoft.com
coalitionforbarrierfreeliving.com

Sandra Bookman, Executive Director

Advocacy organization created by and for people with disabilities (PWD) to empower and protect their rights. Services include but not limited to: peer support, individual and systems advocacy, independent living skills training, information and referral, disability cultural awareness, ASL classes, ADA technical assistance, computer technology training, work incentive counseling, equipment loan program.

4296 **Independent Life Styles**
215 North Benton Drive
Sauk Rapids, MN 56379-1874
320-529-9000
888-529-0743
FAX: 320-529-0747
e-mail: ilicil@independentlifestyles.org
www.independentlifestyles.org

Peter Simmons, Director

Offers peer counseling, advocacy and other services to the community.

4297 **Independent Living Research Utilization Project**
Institute For Rehabilitation & Research
2323 S. Sheperd Dr
Suite #100
Houston, TX 77019-7031
713-520-0232
FAX: 713-520-5785
TTY:713-520-0232
e-mail: ilru@ilru.org
www.ilru.org

Lex Frieden, Manager
Linda CoVan, Grant Coordinator
Maria Del Bosque, Project Associate
Diego Demaya, Legal Specialist

ILRU is a national center for information, training, research and technical assistance in independent living. Its goal is to expand the body of knowledge in independent living and to improve utilization of results of research programs and demonstration projects in this field. ILRU is a program of The Institute for Rehabilitation and Research, a nationally recognized medical rehabilitation facility for persons with disabilities. TTY phone number: (713) 520-5136.

4298 **LIFE/ Run Centers for Independent Living**
8240 Boston Avenue
Lubbock, TX 79423-2342
806-795-5433
FAX: 806-795-5607
TTY:806-795-5433
e-mail: wilmacrain@yahoo.com
www.liferun.org

Michelle Crain, Executive Director

Committed to providing individuals with disabilities the information and skills necessary to become independent and to achieve full inclusion in every aspect of their life.

4299 **Office for Students with Disabilities, University of Texas at Arlington**
701 South Nedderman Drive
Arlington, TX 76019-1
817-272-3364
800-735-2989
FAX: 817-272-1447
TTY: 800-735-2989
e-mail: helpdesk@uta.edu
www.uta.edu/disability

Dianne Hengst, Director

Offers disability counseling and academic accomodation to UT Arlington community.

4300 **Palestine Resource Center for Independent Living**
421 Avenue a St
Palestine, TX 75801-2903
903-729-7505
888-326-5166
FAX: 903-729-7540
TTY:903-729-7505
e-mail: prcil@embarqmail.com
www.palestineresourcecenter.org/?

Sara Minton, Executive Director
Mary Killough, Chief Financial Officer
Susan Dorsey, Community/ Consumer Coordinator
Cathy Newsome, Program and Outreach Coordinator

Provides independent living services to cross-disability groups to increase their personal self-determination and minimize dependence on others. Maintain comprehensive information on availability of resources and provides referrals to such resources. Provides instruction to assist people with disabilities to gain skills that would empower them to live independently. Peer counseling, advocacy - both individual and community by assisting to obtain support services to make changes in society.

4301 Panhandle Action Center for Independent Living Skills
417 W. 10th Avenue
Amarillo, TX 79101-4316
806-374-1400
FAX: 806-374-4550
TTY:806-374-2774
e-mail: advocacy@nts-online.net
www.panhandleilc.org

Carl Mc Millen, Executive Director
Bart Hill, Employment Director
Joe Rogers, Development Director
Cynthia Hammett, Consumer Coordinator & Youth Transition

PILC is a non profit organization dedicated to the advancement of full participation in all aspects of life. PILC services are developed, directed, delivered, and governed primarily by individuals with disabilities.

4302 REACH of Dallas Resource Center on Independent Living
8625 King George Drive
Suite 210
Dallas, TX 75235-2286
214-630-4796
FAX: 214-630-6390
TTY:214-630-5995
e-mail: reachdallas@reachcils.org
reachcils.org

Charlotte A. Stewart, Executive Director
Kevan Johnson, Employment Consultant
Janie Peachee, Information & Referral Specialist
Kiowanda Jasso, Information & Referral Specialist

Information and referral, peer support/peer counseling, independent living skills training and advocacy assistance.

4303 REACH of Denton Resource Center on Independent Living
405 S. Elm St
Suite 202
Denton, TX 76201-6068
940-383-1062
FAX: 940-383-2742
e-mail: reachden@reachcils.org
www.reachcils.org

Charlotte A. Stewart, Executive Director
Missy Dickenson, Assistant Director
Murphy Hardinger, IL Skills Training & ADA Specialist
Becky Teal, Office Manager

To provide for people with disabilities so that they are enabled to lead self-directed lives and to educate the general public about disability-related topics in order to promote a barrier free community.

4304 REACH of Fort Worth Resource Center on Independent Living
1000 Macon Street
Suite 200
Fort Worth, TX 76102-4527
817-870-9082
FAX: 817-877-1622
TTY:817-870-9086
e-mail: reachftw@reachcils.org
www.reachcils.org

Charlotte A. Stewart, Executive Director
Missy Dickenson, Assistant Director
Murphy Hardinger, IL Skills Training & ADA Specialist
Becky Teal, Office Manager

To provide services for people with disabilities so that they are enabled to lead self-directed lives and to educate the general public about disability-related topics in order to promote a barrier free community.

4305 RISE-Resource: Information, Support and Empowerment
755 11th Street
Suite 101
Beaumont, TX 77701-3723
409-832-2599
FAX: 409-838-4499
TTY:409-832-2599
www.risecil.org

Jim Brocato, Executive Director
Amanda Powe, Relocation Services Specialist
Cheryl Bass, Program Director
Gracie Jackson, Independent Living Specialist

A non-profit center for independent living.

4306 SAILS
1028 S Alamo St
San Antonio, TX 78210-1170
210-281-1878
800-474-0295
FAX: 210-281-1759
TTY: 210-281-1878
e-mail: kbrietzke@sailstx.org
www.sailstx.org

Kitty Brietzke, Executive Director
Gloria Banik, Assistant Executive Director

SAILS advocates for the rights and empowerment of people with disabilities in San Antonio; as well as surrounding areas. Services are provided to people with disabilities in the following counties: Atacosa, Bandera, Bexar, Calhoun, Comal, DeWitt, Dimmit, Edwards, Frio, Gillespie, Goliad, Gonzalez, Guadalupe, Jackson, Karnes, La Salle, Kendall, Kerr, Kinney, Lavaca, Maverick, Medina, Real, Uvalde, Val Verde, Victoria, Wilson and Zavala.

4307 Texas Department of Assistive and Rehabilitative Services
4800 N. Lamar Blvd
Austin, TX 78756
512-472-4138
800-628-5115
FAX: 512-472-0603
TTY: 866-581-9328
e-mail: dars.inquiries@dars.state.tx.us
www.dars.state.tx.us

Bill West, Manager

Provides technical assistance and other support services to the state's Independent Living Council, Independent Living Centers and Independent Living Counseling programs.

4308 The Centre
3550 West Dallas Rd
Houston, TX 77019
713-525-8400
FAX: 713-525-8444
www.cri-usa.org

Brian J. Cohen, President
Bill Coorsh, Vice-President
Paul Franks, Secretary
Glen Shepherd, Treasurer

Provides services for more than 600 children and adults with mental retardation and other developmental disabilities. The Center also offers a wide array of programs including education, vocational training and job placement services, three different residential options representing both urban and rural living environments, special programs designed to meet the needs of older adults, and a variety of therapeutic support services.

4309 VOLAR Center for Independent Living
1220 Golden Key Circle
El Paso, TX 79925-5825
915-591-0800
800-591-0800
FAX: 915-591-3506
TTY: 915-591-0800
e-mail: volar@volarcil.org
www.volarcil.org

Luis Chew, Executive Director
Danny Monroe, Chief Financial Officer
Nena Garcia, Records Manager/ Bookkeeper
Thelma Hernandez, Office Manager

VOLAR is committed to providing independent living ervices and information and referral, and to developing community options for persons with cross disabilities to empower them to live the kind of lives they choose. VOLAR is an organization of and for people with disabilities, advocating human and civil rights, community options and empowering people to live the lives they choose. Newsletter available.

4310 Valley Association for Independent Living (VAIL)
P.O. Box 5035
McAllen, TX 78502-5035
956-668-8245
866-400-8245
FAX: 956-631-7914
e-mail: wjohnston@valleyassociation.org
www.valleyassociation.org

Woodie Johnston, Executive Director

Offers information and referral, peer couseling, MS supprt group, independent living skills training, and advocacy, work incentives planning and assistance, transitioning people with disabilities from the nursing home into the community.

4311 Valley Association for Independent Living: Harlingen
1824 W. Jefferson Ave
Suite B
Harlingen, TX 78550-5247
956-428-1126
866-400-8245
FAX: 956-428-4339
e-mail: smyers@valleyassociation.org
www.valleyassociation.org

Soledad Myers, Manager
Provides information and referral, peer counseling, support groups, independent living skills training, community rehab program and advocacy

Utah

4312 Active Re-Entry
10 S Fairgrounds Rd
Price, UT 84501
435-637-4950
FAX: 435-637-4952
TTY:435-637-4950
e-mail: active@arecil.org
arecil.org

Nancy Bentley, Executive Director
Active Re-Entry is a community based program which assists individuals with disabilities to acheive or maintain self-sufficient and productive live in their own communities. Active Re-Entry is committed to promoting the rights, dignity, and quality of life for all persons with disabilities.

4313 Active Re-Entry: Vernal
10 S Fairgrounds Rd
Price, UT 84501-9727
435-637-4950
FAX: 435-789-6090
TTY:435-789-4021
e-mail: active@arecil.org
www.arecil.org

Heather Moore, President
Active Re-Entry is a community based program which assists individuals with disabilities to achieve or maintain self-sufficient and productive lives in their own communities. We are committed to promoting the rights, dignity, and quality of life for all persons with disabilities.

4314 Central Utah Independent Living Center
3445 S Main St
Salt Lake City, UT 84115-2824
801-466-5565
877-421-4500
FAX: 801-466-2363
TTY: 801-373-5044
e-mail: uilc@uilc.org
www.uilc.org/

Debra Mair, Executive Director
Kim Meichle, Assistant Director
Patty Trent, Fiscal Manager
Shauna Brock, Independent Living Specialist
Empowers people with disabilities to reach their full potential in community settings through peer support, advocacy, and education.

4315 OPTIONS for Independence
Northern Utah Center for Independent Living
106 East 1120 N
Logan, UT 84341-2215
435-753-5353
FAX: 435-753-5390
TTY:435-753-5353
e-mail: jbiggs@optionind.org
www.optionsind.org

Cheryl Atwood, Executive Director
OPTIONS for Independence, the Northern Utah Center for Independent Living serves people of all ages with all types of disabilities. OPTIONS is a nonresidential Center that provides services to individuals with disabilities to facilitate their full participation in the community and raise the understanding of disability issues and access to the community. The Independent Living philosophy is strictly adhered to: consumer control and choice being the focus.

4316 OPTIONS for Independence: Brigham Satellite
106 East 1120 N
Logan, UT 84341-3379
435-753-5353
FAX: 435-753-5390
TTY:435-723-2171
e-mail: dcrockett@qwestoffice.net
www.optionsind.org

Cheryl Atwood, Executive Director
Deanna Crockett, Manager
OPTIONS is a nonresidential Independent Living Center where people with disabilities can learn skills to gain more control and independence over their lives. OPTIONS raises the vision and capability of the community at large to the point where people of all abilities will have equal access.

4317 Red Rock Center for Independence
515 W 300 N
Suite A
Saint George, UT 84770-4578
435-673-7501
800-649-2340
FAX: 435-673-8808
e-mail: rrci@rrci.org
www.rrci.org

Barbara Lefler, Executive Director
Sonjia Schugk, Human Resources and Fiscal Management
Kim Lister, Program Manager
Kelly Sharp, Independent Living Coordinator
Red Rock Center for Independence assists people with disabilities to live and participate independently.

4318 Tri-County Independent Living Center
P.O.Box 428
Ogden, UT 84402-428
801-612-3215
866-734-5678
FAX: 801-612-3732
TTY: 801-612-3215
www.tricountyilc.org

Andy Curry, Executive Director
The mission of the Tri-County ILC is to enhance independence for all people with disabilities. Serves Davis, Weber and Morgan Counties.

4319 Utah Assistive Technology Program (UTAP) Utah State University
6855 Old Main Hill
Logan, UT 84322-6855
435-797-3811
800-524-5152
FAX: 435-797-2355
www.uatpat.org

Sachin Pavithran, UATP Program Director
Marilyn Hammond, Utah Assistive Technology Foundation Executive Director
Lois Summers, UATP Staff Assistant/UATF Business Assistant
Alma Burgess, Citizens Reutilizing Assistive Technology Equipment (CReATE)
Provides expertise, resources, and a structure to enhance and expand AT services provided by private and public agencies in Utah. Occurs through monitoring, coordination, information dissemination, empowering individuals, the identification and removal of barriers, and expanding state resources.

4320 **Utah Independent Living Center**
3445 S Main St
Salt Lake City, UT 84115-4453 801-466-5565
800-355-2195
FAX: 801-466-2363
TTY: 801-466-5565
e-mail: uilc@uilc.org
www.uilc.org

Debra Mair, Executive Director
Kim Meichle, Assistant Director
Julie Beckstead, Program Coordinator
Patty Trent, Fiscal Manager
Offers information and referral services. To assist persons with disabilities achieve independence by providing services and activities which enhance independent living skillspromote the public's understanding, accomodation, and acceptance of their rights, needs and abilities.

4321 **Utah Independent Living Center: Minersville**
P.O.Box 168
Minersville, UT 84752-168 435-691-7724
e-mail: rrci@rrci.org
www.rrci.org

Gary Owens, Executive Director
To enhance independence for all people with disaibilities.

4322 **Utah Independent Living Center: Tooele**
42 S Main St
Tooele, UT 84074-2132 435-843-7353
FAX: 435-843-7359
TTY:435-843-7353
e-mail: angies@uilc.org
www.uilc.org

Debra Mair, Executive Director
Kim Meichle, Assistant Director
Julie Beckstead, Program Coordinator
Patty Trent, Fiscal Manager
Mission is to assist persons with disabilities achieve greater independence by providing services and activities which enhance independent living skills and promote the public's understanding, accomodation, and acceptance of their rights, needs and abilities.

Vermont

4323 **Vermont Assistive Technology Program**
Department of Aging and Independent Living
103 S Main St
Weeks Building
Waterbury, VT 5671-2305 802-871-3353
800-750-6355
FAX: 802-871-3048
TTY: 802-241-1464
e-mail: amber.fulcher@state.vt.us
www.atp.vermont.gov/tryout-centers

Julie Tucker, Program Director
David Punia ATP, Information/Education Specialist
Encompasses a state coordinating council for assistive technology issues, regional centers for demonstration, trial and technical support with computer and augmentative communication equipment and regional seating and positioning centers.

4324 **Vermont Center for Independent Living: Bennington**
602 Main St
Bennington, VT 5201-2875 802-447-0574
800-639-1522
e-mail: info@vcil.org
www.vcil.org

Colleen Arcodia, Peer Advocate Counselor
Denise Bailey, Direct Services Coordinator
Dhiresha Blose, Development Officer
Sue Booth, Business Office Coordinator
Believes that individuals with disabilities have the right to live with dignity and with appropriate support in their own homes, fully participate in their communities, and to control and make decisions about their lives.

4325 **Vermont Center for Independent Living: Chittenden**
145 Pine Haven Shores Rd
Suite 1137A
Shelburne, VT 5482-7703 802-985-9841
800-639-1522
TTY:802-985-9841
e-mail: vcil@vcil.org
www.vcil.com

Deborah Lisi-Baker, Executive Director
Believes that individuals with disabilities have the right to live with dignity and with appropriate support in their own homes, fully participate in their communities, and to control and make decisions about their lives.

4326 **Vermont Center for Independent Living: Montpelier**
11 E State St
Montpelier, VT 05602-3008 802-229-0501
800-639-1522
FAX: 802-229-0503
e-mail: info@vcil.org
vcil.org

Colleen Arcodia, Peer Advocate Counselor
Denise Bailey, Direct Services Coordinator
Dhiresha Blose, Development Officer
Sue Booth, Business Office Coordinator
Believes that individuals with disabilities have the right to live with dignity and with appropriate support in their own homes, fully participate in their communities, and to control and make decisions about their lives.

Virginia

4327 **Access Independence**
324 Hope Dr
Winchester, VA 22601-6800 540-662-4452
FAX: 540-662-4474
TTY:540-662-5556
e-mail: askai@accessindependence.org
www.accessindependence.org

Donald Price, Executive Director
Diane Starkey, Programs Manager
Joan Davis, Manager Operations/Rep Payee
Ana Ervin, Executive Administrative Assistant
Offers support services to persons with disabilities to assist in maintaining or increasing their independence and self-determination. Includes housing assistance, independent living skills training, information, referral services, assistance and representative payee and advocacy.

4328 **Appalachian Independence Center**
230 Charwood Dr
Abingdon, VA 24210-2566 276-628-2979
FAX: 276-628-4931
TTY:276-676-0920
e-mail: aicadmin@ntelos.net
aicadvocates.org

Greg Morrell, Executive Director
Donna Buckland, Development Director
Scarlett Cox, Operations Director
Mission is to advocate for and with people with disabilities to promote full participation in society

4329 **Blue Ridge Independent Living Center**
Ste B
1502 Williamson Rd NE
Roanoke, VA 24012-5100 540-342-1231
FAX: 540-342-9505
TTY:540-342-1231
e-mail: brilc@brilc.org
brilc.org

Karen Michalski-Karn, Executive Director
Dana Jackson, Program Services Director
Lottie Diomedi, Independent Living Coordinator
Sallee Ebbett, Finance Manager
BRILC assists people with disabilities to live independently. The Center also serves the community at large by helping to create and

environment that is accessible to all. BRILC offers a variety of services ranging from referrals to community resources, support services, and direct services. These include peer counseling, support groups, training and seminars, advocacy, education, support services, awareness, aid in obtaining specialized equipment, and much more.

4330 Blue Ridge Independent Living Center: Christianburg
210 Pepper Street S
Christiansburg, VA 24073-3571 540-381-8829
FAX: 540-381-8833
TTY:540-381-9149
e-mail: brilc@brilc.org
www.brilc.org

Karen Michalski-Karney, Executive Director
Dana Jackson, Program Services Director
Lottie Diomedi, Independent Living Coordinator
Sallee Ebbett, Finance Manager

Assists people with disabilities to live independently. The center also serves the community at large by helping to create an environment that is accessible to all.

4331 Blue Ridge Independent Living Center: Low Moor
P.O.Box 7
Low Moor, VA 24457-7 540-862-0252
FAX: 540-862-0252
TTY:540-862-0252
www.brilc.org

4332 Clinch Independent Living Services
1139C Plaza Drive
Grundy, VA 24614-6780 276-935-6088
800-597-2322
FAX: 276-935-6342
TTY: 276-935-6088
e-mail: cils@clinchindependent.org
www.cils-online.org

Betty Bevins, Executive Director

Nonprofit organization providing information and referral, peer counseling, advocacy and independent living skills training to persons with disabilities.

4333 Disability Resource Center
409 Progress St
Fredericksburg, VA 22401-3337 540-373-2559
800-648-6324
FAX: 540-373-8126
TTY: 540-373-5890
e-mail: drc@cildrc.org
www.cildrc.org

Debe Fults, Executive Director

Mission is to assist people with disabilities, those who support them, and the community, through information, education and resources, to achieve the highest potential and benefit of independent living.

4334 ENDependence Center of Northern Virginia
2300 Claredon Blvd.
Suite 3305
Arlington, VA 22201-3367 703-525-3268
866-849-3852
FAX: 703-525-3585
TTY: 703-525-3553
e-mail: info@ecnv.org
www.ecnv.org

Kimball Gray, Director of Community Services
Layo Oyewole, Director of Medicaid Programs
Doris Ray, Director of Advocacy and Outreach
Kathy Adams, Medicaid Programs Assistant

ECNV is a community-based resource and advocacy enter which is managed by and for people with disabilities. ENCV promotes independent living philosophy and equal access for all persons with disabilities and, like the nearly 400 centers for independent living across the country, ECNV grew from local disability rights and self-help movements.

4335 Equal Access Center for Independence
4031 University Drive
Suite #301
Fairfax, VA 22030-3409 703-934-2020
TTY:703-277-7730
e-mail: drc@patriot.net

David Sharp, Executive Director

Provides information and referral, peer counseling, advocacy and independent living skills training to persons with disabilities.

4336 Independence Empowerment Center
9001 Digges Road
Suite #103
Manassas, VA 20110-4414 703-257-5400
FAX: 703-257-5043
TTY:703-257-5400
e-mail: info@ieccil.org
www.ieccil.org

Mary D Lopez, Executive Director
Roberta McEachern, Program Director
Gary Allen, Independent Living Advocate
Alan Smiley, Service Facilitator

A non-profit Center for Independent Living. One of over 500 centers in the United States with roots in civil rights models of the 1960's.

4337 Independence Resource Center
815 Cherry Ave
Charlottesville, VA 22903-3448 434-971-9629
FAX: 434-971-8242
TTY:434-971-9629
e-mail: tvandever@ntelos.net
www.charlottesvilleirc.org

Tom Vandever, Executive Director
Brenda Gianniny, Administrator
Carolyn Berry, Participant Services Coordinator
Nate Brown, Senior Peer Advocate

Information and referral services.

4338 Independent Living Center Network: Department of the Visually Handicapped
Ste 300
1809 Staples Mill Rd
Richmond, VA 23230-3515 FAX: 804-355-9297
Robert W Partin, Director
Robert Kastenbaum, Partner

Information and referral services.

4339 Junction Center for Independent Living
P.O.Box 1210
Norton, VA 24273-913 276-679-5988
FAX: 276-679-6569
TTY:276-679-5988
e-mail: jcil1@junctioncenter.org
junctioncenter.org

Dennis Horton, Executive Director
Cindy Mefford, Assistant to the Executive Director
Joe Brady, Deaf and Hard of Hearing Coordinator
Brenda Cowden, Housing Specialist

To assist those who have significant disabilities so that they migh live independently in the least restrictive and most integrated environment possible.

4340 Junction Center for Independent Living: Duffield
P.O.Box 408
Duffield, VA 24244-408 276-431-1195
FAX: 276-431-1196
TTY:276-431-1195
e-mail: jcil1@junctioncenter.org
junctioncenter.org

Dennis Horton, Executive Director
Cindy Mefford, Assistant to the Executive Director
Joe Brady, Deaf and Hard of Hearing Coordinator
Brenda Cowden, Housing Specialist

To assist those who have significant disabilities so that they might live independently in the least restrictive and most integrated environment possbile.

4341 Lynchburg Area Center for Independent Living
500 Alleghany Ave
Suite #520
Lynchburg, VA 24501-2610 434-528-4971
FAX: 434-528-4976
TTY:434-528-4972
e-mail: lacil@lacil.org
www.lacil.org

Phil Theisen, Executive Director
LACIL is a private non-profit, non-residential consumer driven organization that promotes the efforts of persons with disabilities to live independently in the community and supports the efforts of the community to be open and accessible to all citizens.

4342 Peidmont Independent Living Center
Piedmont Living Center
601 S. Belvidere Street
Richmond, VA 23220 804-782-1986
800-828-1140
FAX: 877-VHD- 123
www.vhda.com

Kit Hale, Chairman
Timothy M. Chapman, Vice Chairman
Susan Dewey, Executive Director
Tammy Neale, Chief Learning Officer
Empowering indiviuals with disabilities to become self-sufficient and independent within their communities.

4343 Peninsula Center for Independent Living
2021-A Cunningham Drive
Suite #2
Hampton, VA 23666-3320 757-827-0275
FAX: 757-827-0655
TTY:757-827-8800
e-mail: rshelman@hvacil.org
www.hvacil.org

Ralph Shelman, Executive Director
IEPCIL is a private non-profit non-residential Agency established to provide services to people with disabilities. The Centers Philosophy is that people with a disability should play a major role in deciding their future.The center provides services to people with disabilities in the cities of Hampton, Newport News, Poquoson, Williamsburg, and counties of James City, York, and Gloucester.

4344 Piedmont Independent Living Center
1045 Main Street
Suite #2
Danville, VA 24541-1800 434-797-2530
FAX: 434-797-2568
TTY:434-797-2530

Clarence Dickerson, Executive Director
Jeanette King, ILS Coordinator/BPAD
Lori Penn, Office Manager
Empowering indiviuals with disabilities to become self-sufficient and independent within their communities.

4345 Resources for Independent Living
4009 Fitzhugh Ave
Richmond, VA 23230-3953 804-353-6503
FAX: 804-358-5606
TTY:804-353-6583
e-mail: info@ril-va.org
www.ril-va.org

Gerald O'Neill, Executive Director
Marcia Guardino, Program Manager
Kelly Hickok, Community Services Manager
Assisting persons who are severly disabled to live independently in the community and to encourage necessary change within the community so independent living is a possibility.

4346 Valley Associates for Independent Living (VAIL)
Shenandoah Valley Workforce Investment Board
P.O.Box 869
Harrisonburg, VA 22803-869 540-442-7134
FAX: 540-434-0803
TTY:800-828-1120
e-mail: svwib@valleyworkforce.com
www.govail.org

Marcia Du Bois, Executive Director
Bob Satterwhite, Executive Director
VAIL is a not-for-profit, private Center for Independent Living providing advocacy, information and referral, independent living skills training, supported employment, and peer counseling to individuals with disabilities in our planning district.

4347 Valley Associates for Independent Living: Lexington
205-B South Liberty St
Harrisonburg, VA 22801-3638 540-433-6513
888-242-8245
FAX: 540-433-6313
TTY:540-438-9265
e-mail: vail@govail.org
www.govail.org

Marcia Du Bois, Executive Director
Promoting self-direction among people with disabilities and removing barriers to independence in the community.

4348 Woodrow Wilson Rehabilitation Center Training Program
243 Woodrow Wilson Avenue
Fishersville, VA 22939-1500 540-332-7000
800-345-9972
FAX: 540-332-7132
TTY: 800-811-7893
e-mail: WWRCInfo@wwrc.virginia.gov
www.wwrc.net

Rick Sizemore, Executive Director
Information & referral services. Six week Virginia residential programs and evaluation services.

Washington

4349 Alliance for People with Disabilities: Seattle
1120 E. Terrace St
Suite 100
Seattle, WA 98122 206-545-7055
866-545-7055
FAX: 206-545-7059
TTY: 206-632-3456
e-mail: info@disabilitypride.org
www.disabilitypride.org

Lucille Walls, Executive Director
Ashica Demira, Executive Assistant and Program Staff Manager
Jerry Reed, Business Manager
Elizabeth Kennedy, Human Resources
The Alliance promotes equality and choice for people with disabilities. They provide advocacy, peer support, independent living skills training, information and referral, transition assistance for youth, civil rights legal aid, assistive technology, training and nursing home transition back into the community.

4350 Alliance of People with Disabilities: Redmond
East King County Office
16315 NE 87th St
Suite B-3
Redmond, WA 98052-3537 425-558-0993
800-216-3335
FAX: 425-558-4773
TTY: 425-861-4773
e-mail: info@disabilitypride.org
www.disabilitypride.org

Lucille Walls, Executive Director
Ashica Demira, Executive Assistant and Program Staff Manager
Jerry Reed, Business Manager
Elizabeth Kennedy, Human Resources

Services include: information and referral, independent living skills training, peer groups, disAbility law project (DLP), access reviews, health insurance advising, and systems advocacy.

4351 Coalition of Responsible Disabled
612 N Maple St
Spokane, WA 99201-1801
509-326-6355
877-606-2680
FAX: 509-327-2420
TTY: 509-326-6355
e-mail: contact@cordwa.info
www.cordwa.info

Charley Lane, Transition Manager
MaryAnn S., Supervisor
Holly M., BS, Representative Payee
Judy M., MBA, Representative Payee
To improve the self-determination and self-reliance of people with disabilities through systems and individual advocacy, education and independent living services.

4352 Community Services for the Blind and Partially Sighted Store: Sight Connection
9709 Third Ave NE
Suite #100
Seattle, WA 98115-2027
206-525-5556
800-458-4888
FAX: 206-525-0422
e-mail: info@sightconnection.org
www.sightconnection.org

Mary Lewis, Secretary
June Mansfield, President/CEO
Jill Braun, Vice President, Vision Rehabilitation
Michael Lee Craig, Vice President, Development & Marketing
Over 300 practical products for living with vision loss selected by certified vision rehabilitation specialists from Community Services for the Blind and Partially Sighted. Easy-to-use online store features large print, large photos, secure transactions, and links to other vision-related resources.

4353 DisAbility Resource Connection: Everett
607 SE Everett Mall Way
Suite 6C
Everett, WA 98208-3210
425-347-5768
800-315-3583
FAX: 425-710-0767
TTY: 425-347-5768
e-mail: drcservices@drconline.net
www.drconline.net

Charley Lane, Executive Director
disAbility Resource Connection is all about living your life as you choose. The staff is committed to assisting every individual to connect to resources, connect to skills, connect to life.

4354 Kitsap Community Resources
845 8th St
Bremerton, WA 98337-1517
360-478-2301
FAX: 360-415-2706
e-mail: info@kcr.org
www.kcr.org

Larry Eyer, Executive Director
Rick MacLennan, VP
Kitsap Community Resources is a local, non-profit organization dedicated to helping people in need. KCR creates hope and opportunity for low-income Kitsap County Residents by providing resources that promote self-sufficiency.

4355 Tacoma Area Coalition of Individuals with Disabilities
6315 S 19th St
Tacoma, WA 98466-6217
253-565-9000
877-538-2243
FAX: 253-565-5578
TTY: 253-565-3486
e-mail: tacid@tacid.org
www.tacid.org

Ken Gibson, Executive Director
Steve Pierce, CFO
Jo Ann Maxwell, Deputy Executive Director - Philanthropy, Partnerships, Mark
Marsha Doman-Masters, Executive Assistant - Administration, Philantropy & Accounti
Promotes the independence of individuals with disabilities.

West Virginia

4356 Appalachian Center for Independent Living
4710 Chimney Drive
Suite # C
Charleston, WV 25302-4841
304-965-0376
800-642-3003
FAX: 304-965-0377
TTY: 800-642-3003
e-mail: acil@yahoo.com
www.mtstcil.org

Larry E Paxton, Executive Director
A resource center for persons with disabilities and their communities. Serves Kanawha, Clay, Boone and Putnam counties.

4357 Appalachian Center for Independent Living: Spencer
811 Madison Avenue
Suite #106
Spencer, WV 25276-1900
304-927-4080
FAX: 304-927-4330
TTY:800-642-3003
e-mail: susanacil@yahoo.com
www.mtstcil.org

Todd Ramsey, Manager
A resource center for persons with disabilities and their communities. Serves Jackson, Roane, and Calhoun counties.

4358 Mountain State Center for Independent Living
329 Prince St
Beckley, WV 25801-4515
304-255-0122
FAX: 304-255-0157
TTY:304-255-0122
e-mail: aoweeks@mtstcil.org
www.mtstcil.org

Kevin Maynus, Manager
Anne Weeks, Chief Executive Officer
This office provides individual and systems advocacy, independent living skills development, information and referral, peer support, personal assistance services, housing referral and training, transportation. Serves Raleigh counties.

4359 Mountain State Center for Independent Living
821 Fourth Avenue
Huntington, WV 25701-1406
304-525-3324
866-687-8245
FAX: 304-525-3360
TTY: 304-525-3324
e-mail: aoweeks@mtstcil.org
www.mtstcil.org

Ann Weeks, Executive Director
John Gallaher, Manager
Services provided are: individual and systems advocacy, independent living skills development, information and referral, peer support, personal assistance services, supported employment, community integration program, housing referral and training, transportation. Serves Cabell and Wayne counties.

4360 **Northern West Virginia Center for Independent Living**
601-603 East Brockway
Suite A & B
Morgantown, WV 26501
304-296-6091
800-834-6408
FAX: 304-292-5217
TTY: 304-296-6091
e-mail: nwvcil@nwvcil.org
www.mtstcil.org

Jan Derry, Executive Director
NWVCIL is committed to the philosophy that all persons have equal access and unconditional value, that all individuals shall be respected for their uniqueness and shall have the right to live within the community of their choice, having equal access to participate in and contribute to that community.

Wisconsin

4361 **Center for Independent Living of Western Wisconsin**
2920 Schneider Avenue East
Menomonie, WI 54751-2331
715-233-1070
800-228-3287
FAX: 715-233-1083
TTY: 800-228-3287
e-mail: cilww@cilww.com
www.cilww.com

Tim Sheehan, Executive Director
Kay Sommerfeld, Assistant Director
Tammy Grage, Fiscal & HR Manager
Noelle Johnson, Resource Counselor Camp Quest
Advocates for the full participation in society of all persons with disabilities. Our goal is empwowering individuals to exercise choices to maintain or increase their indpendence. Our strategy is providing consumer-driven services at no cost to persons with disabilities in Western Wisconsin

4362 **Independence First**
540 South 1st Street
Milwaukee, WI 53204-1516
414-291-7520
FAX: 414-291-7525
TTY:414-297-7520
e-mail: lschulz@independencefirst.org
www.independencefirst.org

Lee Schulz, Executive Director
A non-profit agency directed by, and for the benefit of, persons with disabilities, primarily serving the four county metropolitan Milwaukee area.

4363 **Independence First: West Bend**
735 S Main St
West Bend, WI 53095-3965
262-306-6717
e-mail: lschulz@independencefirst.org
www.independencefirst.org
Lee Schulz, Executive Director
A non-profit agency directed by, and for the benefit of, persons with disabilities, primarily serving the four county Metropolitan Milwaukee area.

4364 **Inspiration Ministries**
N2270 State Road 67
Walworth, WI 53184-948
262-275-6131
FAX: 262-275-3355
e-mail: tschnake@inspirationministries.org
inspirationministries.org
Robin Knoll, President
Tim Schnake, VP Resident Services
Formerly known as Christian League for the Handicapped, Inspiration Ministries is a vibrant community of adults with disabilities engaged in living, working, leisure and faith activities designed to provide a complete living experience. The campus consists of a modern residential facility offering a range of living accomodations; a work center and resale shop; and Inspiration Center, a retreat/camping center designed to be 100% wheelchair accessible.

4365 **Mid-State Independent Living Consultants: Wausau**
415 Campus Dr
Wausau, WI 54401
715-675-7600
800-311-5044
FAX: 715-298-2335
TTY: 800-311-5044
e-mail: jkaetterhenry@milc-inc.org
www.milcinc.net

Tom Vandehey, President
Becky Paulson, Independent Living Consultant
Working for persons with disabilities towards empowerment to make informed choices.

4366 **Mid-state Independent Living Consultants: Stevens Point**
3262 Church Street
Suite #1
Stevens Point, WI 54481-5321
715-344-4210
800-382-8484
FAX: 715-344-4414
TTY: 800-382-8484
e-mail: milc@milc-inc.org
www.milcinc.net

Jenny Fasula, Executive Director
Karalyn Peterson, Resource Director
Committed to enhancing personal and community relationships, providing opportunities for growth, and helping people with varying abilities achieve their personal goals.

4367 **North Country Independent Living**
69 N 28th St.
Suite 28
Superior, WI 54880-5138
715-392-9118
800-924-1220
FAX: 715-392-4636
e-mail: john@northcountryil.org
northcountryil.com
John Nousaine, Executive Director
Gloria Hakkila-Johnson, Assistant Director
Jim Glaeser, Accountant
Russ Stover, Office Assistant
Empowers people with disabilities.

4368 **North Country Independent Living: Ashland**
422 3rd St. W.
Suite #114
Ashland, WI 54806-1553
715-682-5676
800-499-5676
FAX: 715-682-3144
TTY: 715-682-5676
e-mail: ncilstew@superior-nfp.org
www.northcountryil.com
John Nousaine, Director
Empowers people with disabilities.

4369 **Options for Independent Living**
555 Country Club Road
Green Bay, WI 54307-1967
920-490-0500
888-465-1515
FAX: 920-490-0700
TTY:920-490-0600
e-mail: info@optionsil.com
www.optionsil.com
Thomas Diedrick, Executive Director
Kathryn C. Barry, Assistant Director
Sandra L. Popp, Independent Living Coordinator
Vicky Lasch, Independent Living Coordinator
A non-profit organization committed to empowering people with disabilities to lead independent and productive lives in their community through advocacy, the provision of information, education, technology and related services.

4370 Options for Independent Living: Fox Valley
820 West College Ave
Suite #5
Appleton, WI 54914
920-997-9999
888-465-1515
FAX: 920-997-9381
TTY:920-490-0600
e-mail: info@optionsil.com
www.optionsil.com

Thomas Diedrick, Executive Director
Kathryn C. Barry, Assistant Director
Sandra L. Popp, Independent Living Coordinator
Vicky Lasch, Independent Living Coordinator

A non-profit organization committed to empowering people with disabilities to lead independent and productive lives in their community through advocacy, the provision of information, education, technology and related services.

4371 Society's Assets: Elkhorn
615 E Geneva St
Elkhorn, WI 53121-2301
262-723-8181
800-261-8181
FAX: 262-723-8184
TTY: 866-840-9763
e-mail: info@societysassets.org
www.societysassets.org

Bruce Nelson, Director
Jill Vigueres, Manager

To ensure the rights of all persons with disabilities to live and function as independently as possible in the community of their choice, through supporting individual's efforts to achieve control over their lives and become integrated into community life.

4372 Society's Assets: Kenosha
5455 Sheridan Road
Suite 101
Kenosha, WI 53140-4103
262-657-3999
800-317-3999
FAX: 262-657-1672
TTY: 866-840-9762
e-mail: info@societysassets.org
www.societysassets.org

Sue Liu, Manager
Bruce Nelsen, Executive Director

To ensure the rights of all persons with disabilities to live and function as independently as possible in the community of their choice, through supporting individuals efforts to achieve controll over their lives and become integrated into community life. Offers home care and independent living services.

4373 Society's Assets: Racine
5200 Washinton Ave
Suite #225
Racine, WI 53406-4238
262-637-9128
800-378-9128
FAX: 262-637-8646
TTY: 886-840-9761
e-mail: info@societysassets.org
www.societysassets.org

Deb Pitsch, Administrator
Karen Olufs, Director Independent Living
Jean Rumachik, Director Home Care Services

Society's Assets assists people with disabilities to live as independently as possible. A non-profit human services agency, Society's Assets provides information and referal, independent living skills training, peer support, advocacy, and supportive home care. Home health care is provided by SAI Home Health Care. The agency serves 5 counties in southeastern Wisconsin and also provides information about interpreters, employment, benefits, home modifications, assistive equipment and accessibility.

Fees vary

Wyoming

4374 RENEW: Gillette
623 N Commercial Dr
Gillette, WY 82716-2555
307-686-2125
888-253-4653
FAX: 307-686-8167
www.renew-wyo.com

Kris Blair, Manager

Empowering persons with disabilities to enrich their lives.

4375 RENEW: Rehabilitation Enterprises of North Eastern Wyoming
1969 S Sheridan Ave
Sheridan, WY 82801-6108
307-672-7481
888-309-2020
FAX: 307-674-5117
e-mail: pr@renew-wyo.com
www.renew-wyo.com

Larry Samson, CEO

Multi-disciplinary organization dedicated to the highest possible economic and social independence for persons with disabilities. Extensive referral service, specialized employment placement, occupational therapy, psychological services, evaluation services, and coordination of external services as needed to meet client plans and objectives.

4376 Rehabilitation Enterprises of North Eastern Wyoming: Newcastle
35 Fairgrounds Rd
Newcastle, WY 82701-2625
307-746-4733
888-693-9245
FAX: 307-746-9701
e-mail: pr@renew-wyo.com
www.renew-wyo.com

Dennis Birchacek, Manager

Empowering persons with disabilities to enrich their lives.

4377 Wyoming Services for Independent Living
1156 S 2nd St
Lander, WY 82520-3905
307-332-4889
800-266-3061
FAX: 307-332-2491
TTY: 307-332-7582
e-mail: sjuergens@wyoming.com
www.wysil.org

Stephen J. Juergens, Executive Director
Alan Ramage, Data and Program Director
Corey McGregor, Independent Living Program Manager
Kay Anderson, Consumer Directed Care Program Manager

Committed to enhancing personal and community relationships, providing opportunities for growth, and helping people with varying abilities achieve thier personal goals.

Law

Associations & Referral Agencies

4378 AIDS Legal Council of Chicago
180 N Michigan Ave
Ste 2110
Chicago, IL 60601
312-427-8990
866-506-3038
FAX: 312-427-8419
e-mail: info@aidslegal.com
aidslegal.com

Tom Yates, Executive Director
D. Matthew Feldhaus, Esq., President
Mike Sullivan, Esq., Vice-President
Andrew Skiba, CRSP, Treasurer
Legal assistance for people with HIV/AIDS related issues. Greater Chicago area.

4379 AIDSLAW of Louisiana
3801 Canal Street
New Orleans, LA 70119
504-568-1631
800-375-5035
e-mail: info@aidslaw.org
www.aidslaw.org

Don Paul Landry, Executive Director
Stacy Morris, Deputy Executive Director
Joshua Holmes, Full-time Staff Attorney
Louise Bienvenu, Supervising Attorney
The mission of AIDSLaw is to provide excellent, specialized legal services for people living with HIV/AIDS in Louisiana, to improve their quality of life and access to health care, related to their HIV/AIDS status.
1989

4380 Center for Disability and Elder Law, Inc.
79 West Monroe Street
Suite 919
Chicago, IL 60603-4908
312-376-1880
866-519-2413
FAX: 312-376-1885
e-mail: info@cdelaw.org
www.cdelaw.org

Michael Roth, Executive Director
M. Catherine Taylor, Associate Director
Thomas Wendt, Chief Legal Officer
A not-for-profit, 501(c)(3) legal services organization which provids legal services to low income persons residing in Chicago and Cook County, Il., who are either elderly and/or persons with disabilities. CDEL provides legal services by matching qualified candidates with volunteer attorneys who represent them, pro bono, in a wide range of civil legal matters;and (2) through special initiatives including the Senior Center Initiative (SCI) and the Senior Tax Opportunity program (STOP).

4381 Chicago Lawyers' Committee for Civil Rights Under Law
100 N Lasalle Street
Suite 600
Chicago, IL 60602-2403
312-630-9744
FAX: 312-630-1127
e-mail: opportunities@clccrul.org.
www.clccrul.org

Jay Readey, Executive Director
Promotes and protects civil rights, particularly the civil rights of poor, minority, and disadvantaged people in the social, economic, and political systems of the nation.

4382 DNA People's Legal Services
PO Box 306
Window Rock, AZ 86515
928-871-4151
800-789-7287
FAX: 928-871-5036
www.dnalegalservices.org

Kathy Gallagher, Development Director
Tom Parker, Development Assistant
A nonprofit legal aid organization working to protect civil rights, promote tribal sovereignty and alleviate civil legal problems for people who live in poverty in the Southwestern United States.
1967

4383 Disability Rights Education and Defense Fund
3075 Adeline Street
#210
Berkeley, CA 94703-2219
510-644-2555
800-348-4232
FAX: 510-841-8645
e-mail: info@dredf.org
dredf.org

Sue Henderson, Executive Director
Nonprofit organization dedicated to advancing the civil rights of individuals with disabilities through legislation, litigation, informal and formal advocacy and education and training of lawyers, advocates and clients with respect to disability issues. DREDF also provides training, advocacy, technical assistance and referrals for parents of disabled children.

4384 Disability Rights Texas
2222 West Braker Lane
Austin, TX 78758-1024
512-454-4816
FAX: 512-302-4936
www.disabilityrightstx.org

Mary Faithfull, Executive Director
The federally designated legal protection and advocacy agency (P&A) for people with disabilities in Texas. Helps people with disabilities understand and exercise their rights under the law, ensuring their full and equal participation in society.

4385 Equal Employment Advisory Council
1501 M Street NW
Suite 400
Washington, DC 20005
202-629-5650
FAX: 202-629-5651
e-mail: info@eeac.org
www.eeac.org

Jeffrey A Norris, President
Nicole McDuffie, Administrator
Nonprofit employer association founded in 1976 to provide guidance to its member companies on understanding and complying with their EEO and affirmative action obligations.

4386 Guardianship Services Associates
41A South Blvd
Oak Park, IL 60302-2777
708-386-5398
FAX: 708-386-5970
e-mail: GSAoakpark@sbcglobal.net

Robert R. Wohlgemuth, Owner
Information and counseling on guardianship and its alternatives. Can provide direct assistance in obtaining guardianship for disabled adults in Cook County. Also provides information and direct assistance on durable powers of attorney. Can assume appointment as guardian in selected cases.

4387 Independence Council for Economic Development
201 N Forest Avenue
Suite 120
Independence, MO 64050- 2753
816-252-5777
FAX: 816-254-1641
e-mail: tlesnak@inedc.biz
www.iced.org

Tom Lesnak, President
A non-profit, public/private partnership established for the purpose of supporting and enhancing the economic growth of independence.

4388 Judge David L Bazelon Center for Mental Health Law
1101 15th Street NW
Suite 1212
Washington, DC 20005
202-467-5730
FAX: 202-223-0409
TTY:202-467-4232
e-mail: communications@bazelon.org
www.bazelon.org

Robert Berstein, Executive Director
A nonprofit organization devoted to improving the lives of people with mental illnesses through changes in policy and law.

4389 Legal Action Center
236 Massachusetts Avenue NE
Suite 505
Washington, DC 20002-4980
202-544-5478
FAX: 202-544-5712
e-mail: lacdc@lac.org
www.lac.org

Paul N Samuels, Director/President
The only non-profit law and policy organization in the United States whose sole mission is to fight discrimination against people with histories of addiction, HIV/AIDS, or criminal records, and to advocate for sound public policies in these areas.

4390 Legal Center for People with Disabilities& Older People
455 Sherman Street
Suite 130
Denver, CO 80203
303-722-0300
FAX: 303-722-0720
e-mail: tlcmail@thelegalcenter.org
www.thelegalcenter.org

Peter Lindquist, Esq., President
Protects and promotes the rights of people with disabilities and older people in Colorado through direct legal representation, advocacy, education and legislative analysis.

4391 Legislative Handbook for Parents
NAPVI
1 North Lexington Avenue
8th Floor
White Plains, NY 10601
617-972-7441
800-562-6265
FAX: 617-972-7444
e-mail: napvi@guildhealth.org
www.napvi.org

Susan LaVenture, Executive Director
Julie Urban, President
Venetia Hayden, Vice President
Randi Sher, Secretary
A helpful publication for parents who make direct contact with public officials on behalf of their children. Sample letters, do's-and-dont's, and a glossary of legislative terms are some of the useful topics that are contained in this manual. *$5.50*
24 pages Paperback

4392 NHeLP
3701 Wilshire Blvd
Suite 750
Los Angeles, CA 90010
310-204-6010
FAX: 213-368-0774
e-mail: nhelp@healthlaw.org
www.healthlaw.org

Abbi Coursolle, Staff Attorney
Kimberly Lewis, Managing Attorney
A national public interest law firm that seeks to improve health care for America's working and unemployed poor, minorities, the elderly and people with disabilities. NHeLP serves legal services programs, community-based organizations, the private bar, providers and individuals who work to preserve a health care safety net for the millions of uninsured or underinsured low-income people.
1970

4393 National Right to Work Legal Defense and Education Foundation
8001 Braddock Rd, Ste 600
Springfield, VA 22160-1
703-321-8510
800-336-3600
FAX: 703-321-9319
e-mail: legal@nrtw.org
nrtw.org

Raymond LaJeunesse, Director
Provides free legal aid to employees whose human and civil rights are being violated by compulsory unionism abuses.

4394 Pocket Guide to the ADA: Accessibility Guidelines for Buildings and Facilities
Wiley Publishing
111 River St
Hoboken, NJ 07030-5774
201-748-6000
FAX: 201-748-6088
e-mail: info@wiley.com
www.wiley.com

Evan Terry, Editor
Helps readers understand the facilities requirements of the Americans with Disabilities Act Accessibility Guidelines. Presents the technical requirements for accessible elements and spaces in new construction, alterations and additions. *$30.00*
198 pages Paperback
ISBN 0-470108-70-3

4395 Public Law 101-336
US Department of Justice
950 Pennsylvania Ave NW
Washington, DC 20530-9
202-307-0663
800-514-0301
FAX: 202-307-1197
TTY: 800-514-0383
www.ada.gov

Rebecca B. Bond, Chief
Zita Johnson Betts, Deputy Chief
Sally Conway, Deputy Chief
James Bostrom, Deputy Chief
Text of the Americans with Disabilities Act, as enacted on July 26, 1990.

4396 Questions and Answers: The ADA and Hiring Police Officers
US Department of Justice
950 Pennsylvania Ave NW
Washington, DC 20530
202-307-0663
800-574-0301
FAX: 202-307-1197
www.ada.gov

Rebecca B. Bond, Chief
Zita Johnson Betts, Deputy Chiefs
James Bostrom, Deputy Chiefs
Sally Conway, Deputy Chiefs
Provides information on ADA requirements for interviewing and hiring police officers.
5 pages

4397 REACH/Resource Centers on Independent Living
1000 Macon Street
Suite 200
Fort Worth, TX 76102-4527
817-870-9082
FAX: 817-877-1622
TTY:817-870-9086
e-mail: reachfwt@reachcils.org
www.reachcils.org

Charlotte A Stewart, Executive Director
Missy Dickenson, Assistant Director
Murphy Hardinger, IL Skills Training & ADA Specialist
Becky Teal, Office Manager
Providing services for people with disabilities so that they are empowered to lead self-directed lives and educating the general public on disability-related topics in order to promote a barrier-free community.

4398 Strengthening the Roles of Independent Living Centers Through Implementing Legal Service
Independent Living Research Utilization ILRU
1333 Moursund
Houston, TX 77030-7031 713-520-0232
FAX: 713-520-5785
TTY:713-520-0232
e-mail: ilru@ilru.org
ilru.org

Lex Frieden, Director
Jacquie Brennan, Legal Specialist
Linda CoVan, Grant Coordinator
Maria Del Bosque, Project Associate
Featuring the Disability Law Clinic at Community Resources for Independence (CRI) in Northern California.
10 pages

4399 Summaries of Legal Precedents & Law Review
Through the Looking Glass
3075 Adeline Street
Suite 120
Berkeley, CA 94703 510-848-1005
800-644-2666
FAX: 510-848-4445
e-mail: TLG@lookingglass.org
www.lookingglass.org

Stephanie Miyashiro, Board President
Thomas Spalding, Board Treasurer
Alice Nemon, Board Secretary
Christina Jopes, Board Member
Summarized legal precedents and law review articles relevant to marital custody and child protection situations of parents with diverse disabilities. *$25.00*
24 pages

4400 TASH Connections
1001 Connecticut Avenue NW
Suite 325
Washington, DC 20036 202-540-9020
FAX: 202-540-9019
e-mail: info@tash.org
www.tash.org

Barbara Trader, Executive Director
Jonathan Riethmaier, Advocacy Communications Manager
Haley Kimmet, Program Manager
Patrick Allen, Program Assistant
Received as a member benefit that keeps readers informed on best practices, family concerns, advocacy events and policy changes.
Quarterly

Resources for the Disabled

4401 ABDA/ABMPP Annual Conference
American Board of Disability Analysts
4525 Harding Road
2nd Floor
Nashville, TN 37205 615-327-2984
FAX: 615-327-9235
e-mail: americanbd@aol.com
www.americandisability.org

Alexander E. Horowitz, Executive Officer Emeritus
Kenneth N. Anchor, Administrative Officer/Editor
Gabriel Sella, Education Coordinator
Lela Boggs, Business Manager
February workshop. Workshop leader: Dr. William Tsushima.

4402 Americans with Disabilities Act Manual
US Department of Justice
950 Pennsylvania Ave NW
Washington, DC 20530-9 202-307-0663
800-514-0301
FAX: 202-307-1197
TTY: 800-514-0383
www.ada.gov

Rebecca B. Bond, Chief
Zita Johnson Betts, Deputy Chief
Sally Conway, Deputy Chief
James Bostrom, Deputy Chief
An in-depth analysis of the legal and practical implications of the ADA using non-technical language. *$20.00*

4403 Americans with Disabilities Act: Selected Resources for Deaf
Gallaudet University Bookstore
800 Florida Avenue NE
Washington, DC 20002-3695 202-651-5000
800-621-2736
FAX: 202-651-5508
e-mail: clerc.center@gallaudet.edu
www.gallaudet.edu

Priscilla O'Donnell, Bookstore Manager
Iva Williams, Bookstore Secretary
Elaine Vance, Human Resources Director
Marteal Pitts, Circulation Coordinator
This resource identifies programs and publications specific to the ADA and deafness and also lists ADA materials and programs for people with any disability.

4404 Approaching Equality
T J Publishers
Ste 108
2544 Tarpley Rd
Carrollton, TX 75006-2288 972-416-0800
800-999-1168
FAX: 301-585-5930
e-mail: TJPubinc@aol.com

Frank Bowe, Author
Public education laws guarantee special education for all deaf children, but may find the special education system confusing, or are unsure of their rights under current laws. For anyone with an interest in education, advocacy and the deaf community, this book reviews dramatic developments in education of deaf children, youth and adults since COED's 1988 report, Toward Equality.. *$12.95*
112 pages
ISBN 0-93266 -39-6

4405 Assessment of the Feasibility of Contracting with a Nominee Agency
Mississippi State University
PO Drawer 6189
Mississippi State, MS 39762 662-325-2001
FAX: 662-325-8989
e-mail: rrtc@colled.msstate.edu
www.blind.msstate.edu

Michelle Capella McDonnall, Interim Director
Stephanie Hall, Business Manager
Douglas Bedsaul, Research and Training Coordinator
Jacqui Bybee, Research Associate II
Only five State Licensing Agencies currently utilize nominee agreements. This study compared the Pennsylvania BE program with four states that utilize nominee agencies and four states that do not. *$20.00*
152 pages Paperback

4406 Bluebook: Explanation of the Contents of the ADA
Disability Rights Education and Defense Fn
3075 Adeline Street
Suite 210
Berkeley, CA 94703
510-644-2555
800-348-4232
FAX: 510-841-8645
TTY: 510-841-8645
e-mail: info@dredf.org
dredf.org

Claudia Center, President and Chair
Ann Cupolo Freeman, Secretary and Treasurer
Susan Henderson, Executive Director
Arlene B. Mayerson, Directing Attorney

Written in narrative form for both professionals and lay people, DREDF's bluebook offers detailed, thorough analysis of all of the law's provisions, encompassing ADA legislative history, the statute and regulations. Available in alternative formats. *$100.00*
214 pages

4407 Can America Afford to Grow Old?
Brookings Institution
1775 Massachusetts Ave NW
Washington, DC 20036-2103
202-797-6000
FAX: 202-797-6004
e-mail: bibooks@brookings.edu
www.brookings.edu

William Antholis, Managing Director
Steven Bennett, Vice President and Chief Operating Officer
Kimberly Churches, Vice President for Development
Kemal Dervis, Vice President and Director, Global Economy and Development

Social security laws and regulations. *$8.95*
144 pages Paperback
ISBN 0-815700-43-1

4408 Childcare and the ADA
Eastern Washington University
Rm 223
705 W 1st Ave
Spokane, WA 99201-3909
509-623-4200
FAX: 509-623-4230
e-mail: susan.vanmeter@mail.ewu.edu

Nancy Ashworth, Director Child Development
Allen Barrom, Manager

Provides information on how childcare providers must comply with the ADA. Eight videotapes plus an instructional manual with examples of situations and problems.. *$85.00*
Set

4409 Common ADA Errors and Omissions in New Construction and Alterations
US Department of Justice
950 Pennsylvania Ave NW
Washington, DC 20530
202-307-0663
800-574-0301
FAX: 202-307-1197
www.ada.gov

Rebecca B. Bond, Chief
Zita Johnson Betts, Deputy Chiefs
James Bostrom, Deputy Chiefs
Sally Conway, Deputy Chiefs

Lists a sampling of common accessibility errors or omissions that have been identified through the Department of Justice's ongoing enforcement efforts.
13 pages

4410 Commonly Asked Questions About Child Care Centers and the Americans with Disabilities Act
US Department of Justice
950 Pennsylvania Ave NW
Washington, DC 20530
202-307-0663
800-574-0301
FAX: 202-307-1197
www.ada.gov

Rebecca B. Bond, Chief
Zita Johnson Betts, Deputy Chiefs
James Bostrom, Deputy Chiefs
Sally Conway, Deputy Chiefs

Explains how the requirements of the ADA apply to Child Care Centers. Also describes some of the Department of justice's ongoing enformcement efforts in the child care area and it provides a resource list on sources of information on the ADA.
13 pages

4411 Commonly Asked Questions About Title III of the ADA
US Department of Justice
950 Pennsylvania Ave NW
Washington, DC 20530-9
202-307-0663
800-574-0301
FAX: 202-307-1197
TTY: 800-514-0383
www.ada.gov

Rebecca B. Bond, Chief
Zita Johnson Betts, Deputy Chief
Sally Conway, Deputy Chief
James Bostrom, Deputy Chief

A 6-page publication providing information for state and local governments about ADA requirements for ensuring that people with disabilities receive the same services and benefits as provided to others.
on-line

4412 Commonly Asked Questions About the ADA and Law Enforcement
US Department of Justice
950 Pennsylvania Ave NW
Washington, DC 20530-9
202-307-0663
800-574-0301
FAX: 202-307-1197
TTY: 800-514-0383
www.ada.gov

Rebecca B. Bond, Chief
Zita Johnson Betts, Deputy Chief
Sally Conway, Deputy Chief
James Bostrom, Deputy Chief

A publication explaining ADA requirements for ensuring that people with disabilities receive the same law enforcement services and protections as provided to others.
13 pages on-line

4413 Complying with the Americans with Disabilis Act
Greenwood Publishing Group
130 Cremona Drive
Santa Barbara, CA 93117
805-968-1911
800-368-6868
FAX: 866-270-3856
e-mail: CustomerService@abc-clio.com
www.greenwood.com

Don Fresh, Author
Peter W Thomas, Co-Author
John Gosden, Library Resource Consultants
Lina Gosden, Library Resource Consultants

A guidebook for management and people with disabilities. This unique guidebook presents a comprehensive analysis of the new Americans with Disabilities Act (ADA), the most significant federal civil rights law in almost 30 years, and its impact on over four million American businesses, state and local governments, nonprofit associations, 87 percent of American's private sector jobs, and 22.7 million working-age people with disabilities. *$117.95*
280 pages Hardcover
ISBN 0-899307-14-0

4414 Court-Related Needs of the Elderly and Persons with Disabilities
Mental Health Commission
2700 Martin Luther King Jr Ave SE
Washington, DC 20032- 2601
202-282-0027
FAX: 202-373-7982

276 pages

4415 Criminal Law Handbook on Psychiatric & Psychological Evidence & Testimony
New York City Bar
42 West 44th Street
New York, NY 10036-6604
212-382-6600
FAX: 212-768-8116
e-mail: phynes@nycbar.org
www.nycbar.org

Bret Parker, Executive Director
Debra Raskin, President
Alan Rothstein, General Counsel
Maria Cilenti, Director Legislative Affairs

The Criminal Law Handbook provides lawyers, judges and forensic experts with comprehensive, in-depth treatment of admissibility (and limitations on admissibility) of psychiatric and psychological evidence and testimony pertaining to key criminal mental health law standards. *$47.00*

4416 Department of Justice ADA Mediation Program
US Department of Justice
950 Pennsylvania Ave NW
Washington, DC 20530
202-307-0663
800-574-0301
FAX: 202-307-1197
TTY: 800-514-0383
www.ada.gov

Rebecca B. Bond, Chief
Zita Johnson Betts, Deputy Chiefs
James Bostrom, Deputy Chiefs
Sally Conway, Deputy Chiefs

Provides an overview of the Department's Mediation Program and examples of successfully mediated cases.
6 pages

4417 Dimensions of State Mental Health Policy
Greenwood Publishing Group
130 Cremona Drive
Santa Barbara, CA 93117
805-968-1911
800-368-6868
FAX: 866-270-3856
e-mail: CustomerService@abc-clio.com
www.greenwood.com

Christopher Hudson, Author
Arthur J Cox, Co-Author
John Gosden, Library Resource Consultants
Lina Gosden, Library Resource Consultants

Introduces students to the emerging field of state mental health policy, its history, current policies, organizational models and required programming knowledge. *$86.95*
320 pages Hardcover
ISBN 0-275932-52-7

4418 Disability Compliance for Higher Education
LRP Publications
360 Hiatt Dr
Palm Beach Gardens, FL 33418
561-622-6520
800-341-7874
FAX: 561-622-0757
e-mail: lrpitvp@lrp.com
www.lrp.com

Kenneth Kahn, CEO

Gives guidance on the most difficult issues faced, such as supporting students with psychological disabilities, ensuring accessibility, understanding OCR rulings, and more. *$57.29*
300 pages

4419 Disability Discrimination Law, Evidence and Testimony
ABA Commission on Mental & Physical Disability Law
1050 Connecticut Ave. N.W.
Suite 400
Washington, DC 20036
202-662-1000
800-285-2221
FAX: 202-442-3439
e-mail: cmpdl@americanbar.org
www.americanbar.org

John W Parry JD, Author

Explains and analyzes key aspects of disability discriminiation law from several different perspectives to guide you through the myriad federal and state statutes, court cases, and regulations.
$105.00
694 pages Paperback
ISBN 1-604420-12-8

4420 Disability Law in the United States
William Hein & Company
2350 North Forest Rd.
Getzville, NY 14068-1296
716-882-2600
800-828-7571
FAX: 716-883-8100
e-mail: mail@wshein.com
www.wshein.com

Dr Bernard D Reams Jr, Author
Peter J McGovern, Co-Author
Jon S Schultz, Co-Author

Offers thousands of pages of information on the laws and legislation affecting the disabled in the United States. Its purpose is to provide a clear and comprehensive mandate to end discrimination against individuals with disabilities and to bring disabled persons into the economic and social midstream of American Life.
$675.00
5750 pages
ISBN 0-899417-97-3

4421 Disability Rights Now
Disability Rights Education and Defense Fund
3075 Adeline Street
Suite 210
Berkeley, CA 94703
510-644-2555
800-348-4232
FAX: 510-841-8645
TTY: 510-841-8645
e-mail: info@dredf.org
dredf.org

Claudia Center, President and Chair
Ann Cupolo Freeman, Secretary and Treasurer
Susan Henderson, Executive Director
Arlene B. Mayerson, Directing Attorney

Free quarterly publication describing the activities of the Disability Rights Education and Defense Fund, available in alternative formats.
Quarterly

4422 Disability Under the Fair Employment & Housing Act: What You Should Know About the Law
California Department of Fair Employment & Housing
2218 Kausen Drive
Suite 100
Elk Grove, CA 95758
916-478-7251
800-884-1684
FAX: 916-227-2870
e-mail: contact.center@dfeh.ca.gov
www.dfeh.ca.gov

Phyllis W Cheng, Director

Intended to highlight and summarize workplace disability laws enforced by the California Department of Fair Employment and Housing. It will familiarize people with the content of these laws, including recent changes and amendments to state statutes and attendent accommodation responsibilities.

4423 Discrimination is Against the Law
California Department of Fair Employment & Housing
2218 Kausen Drive
Suite 100
Elk Grove, CA 95758
916-478-7251
800-884-1684
FAX: 916-227-2870
e-mail: contact.center@dfeh.ca.gov
www.dfeh.ca.gov
Phyllis Cheng, Director
Enforces California state laws that prohibit harassment and discrimination in employment, housing, and public accomodations and that provide for pregnancy leave and family and personal leave.

4424 Education of the Handicapped: Laws, Legislative Histories and Administrative Document
William S Hein & Co Inc
2350 North Forest Rd.
Getzville, NY 14068-1296
716-882-2600
800-828-7571
FAX: 716-883-8100
e-mail: mail@wshein.com
www.wshein.com
Bernard D Reams Jr, Editor
Focuses upon Elementary and Secondary Education Act of 1965 and its amendment, Education For All Handicapped Children Act of 1975 and its amendments and acts providing services for the blind, deaf, mentally retarded, etc. *$2950.00*
55 volumes
ISBN 0-899411-57-6

4425 ElderLawAnswers.com
150 Chestnut Street
4th Floor, Box 15
Providence, RI 02903
617-267-9700
866-267-0947
e-mail: support@elderlawanswers.com
www.elderlawanswers.com
Harry S Margolis, Founder/President
Mark Miller, Director of Product and Business Development
Ken Coughlin, Managing Editor
Supports seniors, their families and their attorneys in achieving their goals by providing

4426 Employment Discrimination Based on Disability
California Department of Fair Employment & Housing
2218 Kausen Drive
Suite 100
Elk Grove, CA 95758
916-478-7251
800-884-1684
FAX: 916-227-2870
e-mail: contact.center@dfeh.ca.gov
www.dfeh.ca.gov
Phyllis W Cheng, Director
Prohibits employment discrimination and harassment based on a person's disability or perceived disability. Also requires employers to reasonably accommodate individuals with mental or physical disabilities unless the employer can show that to do so would cause an undue hardship.

4427 Employment Standards Administration Department of Labor (ESA)
200 Constitution Ave NW
Washington, DC 20210-1
800-321-6742
TTY:877-889-5627
osha.gov
David Michaels, Assistant Secretary
Jordan Barab, Deputy Assistant Secretary
Richard Fairfax, Deputy Assistant Secretary
Deborah Berkowitz, Chief of Staff
Monitors compliance with sub-minimum wage requirements for handicapped workers in sheltered workshops, competitive industry and hospitals and institutions under Section 14 of the Fair Labor Standards Act of 1938.

4428 Enforcing the ADA: A Status Report from the Department of Justice
US Department of Justice
950 Pennsylvania Ave NW
Washington, DC 20530
202-307-0663
800-514-0301
FAX: 203-307-1197
www.ada.gov
Rebecca B. Bond, Chief
Zita Johnson Betts, Deputy Chiefs
James Bostrom, Deputy Chiefs
Sally Conway, Deputy Chiefs
A brief report issued by the Justice Department each quarter providing timely information about ADA cases and settlements, building codes that meet ADA accessibility standards, and ADA technical assistance activities.

4429 Federal Laws of the Mentally Handicapped: Laws, Legislative Histories and Admin. Documents
William Hein & Company
2350 North Forest Rd.
Getzville, NY 14068-1296
716-882-2600
800-828-7571
FAX: 716-883-8100
e-mail: mail@wshein.com
www.wshein.com
Bernard D Reams Jr, Editor
Chronological compilation of all relevant federal laws dealing with the mentally handicapped along with supporting documentation necessary to create a complete legislative history. *$3500.00*
42 Volume/Set
ISBN 0-899411-06-1

4430 Formed Families: Adoption of Children with Handicaps
Haworth Press
711 Third Avenue
New York, NY 10017
212-216-7800
800-354-1420
FAX: 212-244-1563
e-mail: subscriptions@tandf.co.uk.
www.haworthpress.com
William Cohen, Owner
Provides broad coverage of the issues relating to the adoption of children with handicaps. Concerned professionals can find here all the answers about clinical programs, legal issues, estimates of frequency, and important factors related to positive and negative outcomes of these adoptions. *$74.95*
242 pages Hardcover
ISBN 0-866569-14-6

4431 Free Appropriate Public Education: The Law and Children with Disabilities
Love Publishing Company
9101 E Kenyon Avenue
Suite 2200
Denver, CO 80237
303-221-7333
FAX: 303-221-7444
e-mail: lpc@lovepublishing.com
www.lovepublishing.com
H Rutherford Turnbull III, Author
Matthew J Stowe, Co-Author
Nancy E Huerta, Co-Author
Includes the 2004 IDEA reauthorization and the proposed regulations. This up-to-the-minute resource brings you the most recent developments in legislation, case law techniques, due process, parent participation and much, much more. *$78.00*
448 pages Hardcover
ISBN 0-891083-25-2

4432 Health Care Quality Improvement Act of 1986
William Hein & Company
2350 North Forest Rd.
Getzville, NY 14068-1296
716-882-2600
800-828-7571
FAX: 716-883-8100
e-mail: mail@wshein.com
www.wshein.com

Bernard D Reams Jr, Editor

In order to encourage more stringent peer review by doctors and hospitals, and to protect reporting physicians and institutions from retaliatory lawsuits, Congress enacted The Health Care Quality Improvement Act. The Act was also intended to address the increasing incidence of medical malpractice and to prevent the ease with which incompetent practitioners moved from state to state. Hardcover. *$125.00*

721 pages
ISBN 0-899416-93-4

4433 Housing and Transportation of the Handicapped
William Hein & Company
2350 North Forest Rd.
Getzville, NY 14068-1296
716-882-2600
800-828-7571
FAX: 716-883-8100
e-mail: mail@wshein.com
www.wshein.com

Bernard D Reams Jr, Editor

National laws, recognizing the problems encountered by the handicapped in the areas of Housing and Transportation and providing assistance in an effort to surmount those problems, span more than half a century. *$1552.50*

30000 pages 250 documents
ISBN 0-899412-47-5

4434 Human Resource Management and the Americans with Disabilities Act
Greenwood Publishing Group
130 Cremona Drive
Santa Barbara, CA 93117
805-968-1911
800-368-6868
FAX: 866-270-3856
e-mail: CustomerService@abc-clio.com
www.greenwood.com

John G Veres, Author
Ronald R Sims, Co-Author
John Gosden, Library Resource Consultants
Lina Gosden, Library Resource Consultants

Concrete advice for human resource professionals on how to cope with the vague, often obscure provisions of the Americans with Disabilities Act. *$107.95*

232 pages Hardcover
ISBN 0-899308-57-9

4435 International Handbook on Mental Health Policy
Greenwood Publishing Group
130 Cremona Drive
Santa Barbara, CA 93117
805-968-1911
800-368-6868
FAX: 866-270-3856
e-mail: CustomerService@abc-clio.com
www.greenwood.com

John Gosden, Library Resource Consultants
Lina Gosden, Library Resource Consultants
Steve Pearson, Library Resource Consultants
Lou Pingitore, Library Resource Consultants

The first major reference book for academics and practitioners that provides a systematic survey and analysis of mental health policies in twenty representative countries. *$179.95*

512 pages Hardcover
ISBN 0-313275-67-8

4436 Knowing Your Rights
A AR P Fulfillment
601 E St NW
Washington, DC 20049-1
202-434-3525
800-687-2277
FAX: 202-434-3443
TTY: 877-434-7598
e-mail: member@aarp.org
www.aarp.org

William D. Novelli, CEO
Lynn Smith, Director of Human Resources

Describes how changes in Medicare's reimbursement policies are designed to reduce health care costs and suggests steps that Medicare beneficiaries, their families and friends can take to assure that they continue to receive quality care under the Prospective Payment System.

19 pages

4437 Law Center Newsletter
Public Interest Law Center of Philadelphia
1709 Benjamin Franklin Parkway
United Way Building
Philadelphia, PA 19103
215-627-7100
FAX: 215-627-3183
e-mail: general@pilcop.org
www.pilcop.org

Eric J Rothschild, Chair
Brian T Feeney, Vice Chair
Jennifer R. Clarke, Executive Director
Ellen S Friedell, Treasurer

Information on mental health, foster care and public education. Provides all updates concerning the law in these areas.

4438 Legal Center for People with Disabilities& Older People
455 Sherman St
Suite 130
Denver, CO 80203
303-722-0300
800-288-1376
FAX: 303-722-0720
TTY: 303-722-3619
e-mail: tlcmail@thelegalcenter.org
www.thelegalcenter.org

Mary Anne Harvey, Executive Director
John R. Posthumus, President
Stephen P. Rickles, Vice President
John Paul Anderson, Treasurer

Uses the legal system to protect and promote the rights of people with disabilities and older people in Colorado through direct legal representation, advocacy, education and legislative analysis. The Legal Center is Colorado's Protection and Advocacy System. We are also the State Ombudsman for nursing homes and assisted living facilities. Call for a free publications and products list.

4439 Legal Right: The Guide for Deaf and Hard of Hearing People
National Association of the Deaf
8630 Fenton Street
Suite 820
Silver Spring, MD 20910- 3819
301-587-1789
FAX: 301-587-1791
TTY:301-587-1789
www.nad.org

Christopher Wagner, Board Chair
Howard A. Rosenblum, Chief Executive Officer
Marc P. Charmatz, Staff Attorney
Lizzie Sorkin, Director of Communications

This revised fifth edition is in easy-to-understand language, offering the latest state and federal statues and administrative procedures that prohibit discrimination against the deaf, hard of hearing and other physically challenged people. *$32.50*

264 pages Paperback
ISBN 1-563680-00-9

4440 Legal Rights of Persons with Disabilities
LRP Publications
360 Hiatt Dr
Palm Beach Gardens, FL 33418-7106 561-622-6520
800-341-7874
FAX: 561-622-0757
e-mail: lrpitvp@lrp.com
www.lrp.com
Kenneth Kahn, CEO
Shows what is required, permitted and guaranteed by federal disability laws-including the ADA, Section 504 of the Rehabilitation Act and the IDEA. Explores the boundaries of accceptable behavior under disability laws and provides guidelines to help clients fulfill their legal obligations. *$365.00*
2722 pages

4441 Legislative Network for Nurses
Business Publishers
2222 Sedwick Drive
Durham, NC 27713 800-223-8720
FAX: 800-508-2592
e-mail: custserv@bpinews.com
www.bpinews.com
8 pages Newsl./BiMonthly

4442 Loving Justice
Exceptional Parent Library
P.O.Box 1807
Englewood Cliffs, NJ 7632-1207 201-947-6000
800-535-1910
FAX: 201-947-9376
e-mail: eplibrary@aol.com
www.eplibrary.com

4443 Making News: How to Get News Coverage of Disability Rights Issues
Advocado Press
PO Box 406781
Louisville, KY 40204 888-739-1920
FAX: 502-899-9562
e-mail: contact145@avocadopress.org
www.advocadopress.org
Tari Susan Hartman, Author
Mary Johnson, Co-Author
This book gives examples and tips on how to fight back and get on the front pages, lead the newscasts and influence public debate. *$10.95*
165 pages Paperback
ISBN 0-962706-43-4

4444 Medicare and Medicaid Patient and Program Protection Act of 1987
William Hein & Company
2350 North Forest Rd.
Getzville, NY 14068-1296 716-882-2600
800-828-7571
FAX: 716-883-8100
e-mail: mail@wshein.com
www.wshein.com
Bernard D Reams Jr, Editor
Enables the HHS to protect patients and federal health care programs from censured practitioners. The Act broadens the authority of HHS to exclude practitioners from Medicare and Medicaid programs; strengthens the monetary penalities HHS may impose on violators; provides for criminal penalties in certain cases; and requires states to inform HHS regarding sanctions against health care providers. *$195.00*
3 Volumes
ISBN 0-899416-95-0

4445 Mental & Physical Disability Law Reporter
American Bar Association
1050 Connecticut Ave. N.W.
Suite 400
Washington, DC 20036-1019 202-662-1570
800-285-2221
FAX: 202-442-3439
e-mail: cmpdl@abanet.org
www.abanet.org
Robert M Carlson, Chair
James R Silkenat, President
Jack L Rives, Executive Director
G. Nicholas Casey, Treasurer
Contains over 2,000 summanes per year of federal and state court decisions and legislation that affect persons with mental and physical disabilities. Includes bylined articles by experts in the field regarding disability law developments and trends. *$384.00*
350+ pages BiMonthly

4446 Mental Disabilities and the Americans with Disabilities Act
Greenwood Publishing Group
130 Cremona Drive
Santa Barbara, CA 93117 805-968-1911
800-368-6868
FAX: 866-270-3856
e-mail: CustomerService@abc-clio.com
www.greenwood.com
John Gosden, Library Resource Consultants
Lina Gosden, Library Resource Consultants
Steve Pearson, Library Resource Consultants
Lou Pingitore, Library Resource Consultants
A clear, practical compliance guide, written by a psychologist, to help organizations conform to provisions on mental disabilities in the Americans with Disabilities Act. Hardcover. *$91.95*
216 pages Hardcover
ISBN 0-899308-26-5

4447 Mental Disability Law, Evidence and Testimony
ABA Commission on Mental & Physical Disability Law
1050 Connecticut Ave. N.W.
Suite 400
Washington, DC 20036-1019 202-662-1000
800-285-2221
www.abanet.org
Robert M Carlson, Chair
James R Silkenat, President
Jack L Rives, Executive Director
G. Nicholas Casey, Treasurer
Provides a comprehensive analysis of federal and state statues and case law with a disability discrimination focus. *$95.00*
491 pages Paperback
ISBN 1-590318-32-3

4448 Mental Health Law Reporter
Business Publishers
2222 Sedwick Drive
Durham, NC 27713 240-514-0600
800-223-8720
FAX: 800-508-2592
e-mail: custserv@bpinews.com
www.bpinews.com
Leonard A Eiserer, Publisher
Jeremy Bond, Editor MHLR
Bob Grupe, Editor MHLR
Adam Goldstein, President
MHLR brings you the most timely, focused and thorough information on the legal issues that concern mental health practitioners in mental health litigation. Topics include: malpractice litigation, patient-therapist confidentiality, sexual victimization of patients, the insanity defense, social security administrative case law and much more.. *$286.00*
8 pages Monthly

4449 Mental and Physical Disability Law Reporter
American Bar Association
1050 Connecticut Ave. N.W.
Suite 400
Washington, DC 20036-1019 202-662-1000
800-285-2221
e-mail: service@americanbar.org
www.americanbar.org

Wm T Robinson III, President
The only periodical that comprehensively covers civil and criminal mental disability law and disability discrimination law. *$ 324.00*
150+ pages Bimonthly

4450 Mentally Disabled and the Law
William S Hein & Company
2350 North Forest Rd.
Getzville, NY 14068-1296 716-882-2600
800-828-7571
FAX: 716-883-8100
e-mail: mail@wshein.com
www.wshein.com

Samuel Brakel, Author
John Parry, Co-Author
Barbara A Weiner, Co-Author
Chapters retained from 1961 and 1971 editions have been substantially rewritten. Two subjects-sterilization and sexual psychopathy-have been integrated into chapters on family law. Three new chapters on treatment rights, provider-patient relationship and rights of mentally disabled persons in the community. Sixteen new tables supplement the existing revised 41. *$92.00*
845 pages
ISBN 0-910059-05-5

4451 Myths and Facts
US Department of Justice
950 Pennsylvania Ave NW
Washington, DC 20530-9 202-307-0663
800-514-0301
FAX: 202-307-1197
TTY: 800-514-0383
www.ada.gov

Rebecca B. Bond, Chief
Zita Johnson Betts, Deputy Chief
Sally Conway, Deputy Chief
James Bostrom, Deputy Chief
A 3-page publication dispelling some common misconceptions about the ADA's requirements and implementation.

4452 NAD Broadcaster
National Association of the Deaf
8630 Fenton Street
Suite 820
Silver Spring, MD 20910- 3819 301-587-1789
FAX: 301-587-1791
TTY:301-587-1789
e-mail: nad.info@nad.org
www.nad.org

Christopher Wagner, Board Chair
Howard A. Rosenblum, Chief Executive Officer
Marc P. Charmatz, Staff Attorney
Lizzie Sorkin, Director of Communications
National newspaper published 11 times a year by the nation's largest organization safeguarding the accessbility and civil rights of 28 million deaf and hard of hearing Americans in education, employment, health care, and telecommunications. Membership: individual $30 per year. *$7.00*

4453 No Longer Disabled: the Federal Courts & the Politics of Social Security Disability
Greenwood Publishing Group
130 Cremona Drive
Santa Barbara, CA 93117 805-968-1911
800-368-6868
FAX: 866-270-3856
e-mail: CustomerService@abc-clio.com
www.greenwood.com

John Gosden, Library Resource Consultants
Lina Gosden, Library Resource Consultants
Steve Pearson, Library Resource Consultants
Lou Pingitore, Library Resource Consultants
This book is a case study of judicial policy making. It focuses on the role of adjudication in the making and refining of federal policy. *$107.95*
208 pages Hardcover
ISBN 0-313254-24-9

4454 Nolo's Guide to Social Security Disability Getting and Keeping Your Benefits
NOLO
950 Parker St
Berkeley, CA 94710-2524 800-955-4775
FAX: 800-645-0895
www.nolo.com

David Morton, Author
This guide demystifies the program and tells you everything you need to know about qualifying and applying for benefits, maintaining your benefits, and appealing the denial of a claim. *$25.49*
512 pages paperback
ISBN 1-413311-04-4

4455 Opening the Courthouse Door: An ADA Access Guide for State Courts
American Bar Association
1050 Connecticut Ave. N.W.
Suite 400
Washington, DC 20036-1019 202-662-1000
800-285-2221
e-mail: service@americanbar.org
www.americanbar.org

Wm T Robinson III, President
Practical step-by-step guide walks the reader through the courthouse and court process, presenting a menu of straightforawrd access ideas to enhance communications in court, make the facility more accessbile, and nodify rules and procedures. *$12.00*
78 pages

4456 PAL News
Parent Professional Advocacy League
45 Bromfield Street
10th Floor
Boston, MA 02108-4106 866-815-8122
FAX: 617-542-7832
e-mail: info@ppal.net
www.ppal.net

Earl N. Stuck, Chair
Lisa Lambert, Executive Director
Deborah A. Fauntleroy, Associate Director
Anne Metzger, Treasurer
Parent/Professional Advocacy Leage (PPAL) is an organization that promotes a strong voice for families of children and adolescents with mental health needs. PAL advocates for supports, treatment and policies that enable families to live in their communities in an environment of stability and respect.
Quarterly

4457 Power of Attorney for Health Care
Center for Public Representation
P.O.Box 260049
Madison, WI 53726-49 608-251-4008
800-369-0388
FAX: 606-251-1263

132 pages
ISBN 0-93262 -38-0

4458 **Title II & III Regulation Amendment Regarding Detectable Warnings**
U S Department of Justice
950 Pennsylvania Ave NW
Washington, DC 20530-9
202-307-0663
800-514-0301
FAX: 202-307-1197
TTY: 800-514-0383
www.ada.gov

Rebecca B. Bond, Chief
Zita Johnson Betts, Deputy Chief
Sally Conway, Deputy Chief
James Bostrom, Deputy Chief
This document suspends the requirements for detectable warnings at curb ramps, hazardous vehicular areas, and reflecting pools.

4459 **Title II Complaint Form**
US Department of Justice
950 Pennsylvania Ave NW
Washington, DC 20530
202-307-0663
800-514-0301
FAX: 202-307-1197
www.ada.gov

Rebecca B. Bond, Chief
Zita Johnson Betts, Deputy Chiefs
James Bostrom, Deputy Chiefs
Sally Conway, Deputy Chiefs
Standard form for filing a complaint under title II of the ADA or section 504 of the Rehabilitation Act of 1973, which prohibit discrimination on the basis of disability by State and local governments and by recipients of federal financial assistance.

4460 **Title II Highlights**
US Department of Justice
950 Pennsylvania Ave NW
Washington, DC 20530
202-307-0663
800-514-0383
FAX: 202-307-1197
www.ada.gov

Rebecca B. Bond, Chief
Zita Johnson Betts, Deputy Chiefs
James Bostrom, Deputy Chiefs
Sally Conway, Deputy Chiefs
Outline of the key requirements of the ADA for State and local governments. Provides detailed information in bullet format for quick reference.
8 pages

4461 **Title III Technical Assistance Manual and Supplement**
U S Department of Justice
950 Pennsylvania Ave NW
Washington, DC 20530
202-307-0663
800-574-0301
FAX: 202-307-1197
www.ada.gov

Rebecca B. Bond, Chief
Zita Johnson Betts, Deputy Chiefs
James Bostrom, Deputy Chiefs
Sally Conway, Deputy Chiefs
Explains in lay terms what businesses and non-profit agencies must do to ensure access to their goods, services, and facilities.
83 pages

4462 **Toward Independence**
National Council on Disability
81 E. Main Street
Xenia, OH 45385
937-376-3996
FAX: 937-376-2046
e-mail: info@ti-inc.org
www.ti-inc.org

Mary Rose Zink, Chair
Paul Osterfeld, Vice Chair
Mark Schlater, Executive Director
Bob Groskopf, Treasurer
A 1986 report to the U.S. Congress on the federal laws and programs serving people with disabilities, and recommendations for legislation.

4463 **UCP Washington Wire**
United Cerebral Palsy
1825 K Street NW
Suite 600
Washington, DC 20006-1601
202-776-0406
800-872-5827
FAX: 202-776-0414
e-mail: info@ucp.org
www.ucp.org

Stephen Bennett, President/CEO
Publication that provides a comprehensive source of information on federal legislation, agency regulations, court decisions and other issues of interest to the disability community.
weekly

4464 **US Department of Health and Human Services Office for Civil Rights**
200 Independence Ave SW
Room 509F, HHH Building
Washington, DC 20201
202-619-0403
800-368-1019
TTY:800-537-7697
e-mail: ocrmail@hhs.gov
www.hhs.gov

Georgina Verdugo, Director
The Department's civil rights and health privacy law enforcement agency, OCR investigates complaints, enforces rights, and promulgates regulations, develops policy and provides technical assistance and public education to ensure understanding of and compliance with non-discrimination and health information privacy laws.

4465 **US Department of Labor**
200 Constitution Ave NW
Washington, DC 20210
866-487-2365
e-mail: talktosolis@dol.gov
www.dol.gov

Hilda L Solis, Secretary of Labor
Seth D Harris, Deputy Secretary
To foster, promote, and develop the welfare of the wage earners, job seekers, and retirees of the United States; improve working conditions, advance opportunities for profitable employment; and assure work-related benefits and rights.

4466 **US Department of Labor Office of Federal Contract Compliance Programs**
200 Constitution Ave NW
Washington, DC 20210
312-596-7010
866-487-2365
FAX: 312-596-7044
e-mail: OFCCP-MW-PreAward@dol.gov
www.dol.gov

Melissa L Speer, Interim Regional Director
To enforce, for the benefit of job seekers and wage earners, the contractual promise of affirmative action and equal employment opportunity required of those who do business with the Federal government.

4467 **University Legal Services AT Program**
Ste 130
220 i St NE
Washington, DC 20002-4364
202-547-4747
877-221-4638
FAX: 202-547-2083
TTY: 202-547-2657
e-mail: atpdc@uls-dc.org
dcpanda.org

Jane Brown, Executive Director
Designed to empower individuals with disabilities; to promote consumer involvement and advocacy, and provide information, referral and training as they relate to accessing assistive technology services and devices; and to identify and improve access to funding resources..

4468 **William S Hein & Company**
2350 North Forest Rd.
Getzville, NY 14068-1296
716-882-2600
800-828-7571
FAX: 716-883-8100
e-mail: mail@wshein.com
www.wshein.com

Kevin Marmion, President
Offers a catalog of periodicals, publications and reprints, microforms and government publications on medical, handicapped and health law.

Libraries & Research Centers

Alabama

4469 **Alabama Institute for Deaf and Blind Library and Resource Center**
205 East South Street
Talladega, AL 35160
256-761-3207
FAX: 256-761-3352
aidb.org

Dr. John Mascia, President
Dr. Frieda Meacham, Vice President
Mike Hubbard, Director
Jessica W Parker, Assistant Director

Book collection includes discs, cassettes, braille and large print. Also closed-circuit TV and magnifiers. Offers braille production and binding.

4470 **Alabama Radio Reading Service Network(ARRS)**
650 11th St South
Birmingham, AL 35233-1
205-934-2606
800-444-9246
FAX: 205-934-5075
wbhm.org

Audrey Atkins, Marketing Manager
Scott E Hanley, General Manager
Theresa Kidd, Office Manager
Michael Krall, Program Director

Services and readings are broadcast over a subcarrier service of public radio WBHM. This is a statewide service devoted to Alabama's blind and handicapped community.

4471 **Alabama Regional Library for the Blind and Physically Handicapped**
Alabama Public Library Service
6030 Monticello Dr
Montgomery, AL 36130-1
334-213-3900
800-723-8459
FAX: 334-213-3993
e-mail: revans@apls.state.al.us
www.apls.state.al.us

Rebecca Mitchell, Executive Director
Vanessa Carr, Executive Secretary
Carol Burchett, Finance
Christine Bowman, Consultants

Recreational reading in special format for persons unable to use standard print. Reference materials offered include materials on blindness and other handicaps, films, local subjects and authors.

4472 **Houston-Love Memorial Library**
212 W Burdeshaw St
Dothan, AL 36303-4421
334-793-9767
e-mail: houstonlove@houstonlovelibrary.org
houstonlovelibrary.org

Steve Roy, Chairman
Bettye Forbus, Director

Offers magnifiers, summer reading programs and more for the blind and physically handicapped. Scanner, software, jaws for Windows.

4473 **Huntsville Subregional Library for the Blind & Physically Handicapped**
915 Monroe St SW
Huntsville, AL 35801-5007
256-532-5940
FAX: 256-532-5994
e-mail: askus@hpl.lib.al.us
www.hpl.lib.al.us

Regina Cooper, Executive Director

Talking books for people who are blind or disabled offering reference materials on the blind and other disabilities, large-print photocopier, thermaform duplicator and more.

4474 **Public Library Of Anniston-Calhoun County**
108 E 10th St
Anniston, AL 36201
256-237-8501
publiclibrary.cc

4475 **Research for Rett Foundation**
P.O.Box 50347
Mobile, AL 36605-347
251-479-8293
800-422-7388
FAX: 251-479-8293

Jack Tillman, CEO
Anna Luce, Executive Director

National, not-for-profit, voluntary organization dedicated to raising funds for critical ongoing medical research into Rett Syndrome, hosting medical research symposia, and funding grant applications. Committed to expanding public awareness of and encouraging Rett Syndrome research within the National Institute of Child Health and Human Development. Provides a variety of educational mateials including brochures and fact sheets..

4476 **Technology Assistance for Special Consumers**
1856 Keats Drive
Huntsville, AL 35810-3859
256-859-4900
FAX: 256-859-4900
e-mail: tasc@ucphuntsville.org
ucphuntsville.org

Cathy Scholl, President
Theresa Ball, Vice President Campaigns
Jo Layne Hall, Vice President Facilities
Cheryl Smith, Executive Director

Provide individuals with disabilities, their families and/or advocates, and associated professionals access to assistive technology devices and services to increase independence at home, school, and work.

4477 **Tuscaloosa Subregional Library for the Blind & Physically Handicapped**
1801 Jack Warner Parkway
Tuscaloosa, AL 35401-1027
205-345-5820
FAX: 205-752-8300
e-mail: info@tuscaloosa-library.org
www.tuscaloosa-library.org

Dr Marcia Burke, Chairman
Harry Shumaker, Vice Chairman
Dr. Samory Pruitt, Secretary
J. Brad Springer, Treasurer

Provide talking books to patrons who are unable to use standard print because of a visual or physical limitation. Deliver playback equipment to qualified patrons. Provides reference and referral service to this special population also.

Alaska

4478 **Alaska State Library Talking Book Center**
344 W 3rd Ave
Suite 125
Anchorage, AK 99501-2338
907-269-6575
800-776-6566
FAX: 907-269-6580
e-mail: aslanc@alaska.gov
library.state.ak.us/dev/libdev.html

Stephanie Schott, Library Assistant
Beverly Griffin, Library Assistant
Linda Thibodeau, Director
Bob Banghart, Deputy Director

The Alaska State Library Talking Book Center is a cooperative effort between the Library of Congress National Library Service for the Blind and Physically Handicapped and the Alaska State Library to provide print handicapped Alaskans with talking book and Braille service. The Talking Book Center has 55,000 audiobooks that can be checked out to eligible Alaskans whose visual or physical handicap prevents them from reading standard print materials.

Arizona

4479 **Arizona Braille and Talking Book LibraryArizona State Library**
1030 N 32nd St
Phoenix, AZ 85008-5108 602-255-5578
800-255-5578
FAX: 602-286-0444
e-mail: btbl@lib.az.us
www.azlibrary.gov

Linda Montgomery, Director
Audio and braille books and magazines, summer reading program, volunteer-produced audio books, audo described, films and more.

4480 **Books for the Blind of Arizona**
Unit A107
6120 E 5th St
Tucson, AZ 85711-2536 602-792-9153
FAX: 520-886-9839

Betty Evans, Chairperson
Offers large print photocopier, textbooks, recreational, career, vocational, braille books, talking books, cassettes, large print books and more for the visually impaired K-12, college students and adults.

4481 **Children's Center for Neurodevelopmental Studies**
5430 W Glenn Dr
Glendale, AZ 85301-2628 623-915-0345
FAX: 623-937-5425
e-mail: admin@ccnsaz.org
www.thechildrenscenteraz.org

Kent Rideout, Executive Director
Dawna Sterner, Preschool & Education Informatio
Catherine Orsak, Therapy Information
Alicia Bolan, Teaching Staff
The Center is a non-profit school and therapy center for children with autism and other developmental delays specializing in the use of sensory integration.

4482 **Flagstaff City-Coconino County Public Library**
300 W Aspen Ave
Flagstaff, AZ 86001-5304 928-779-7670
TTY:928-214-2417
www.flagstaffpubliclibrary.org

4483 **Fountain Hills Lioness Braille Service**
P.O.Box 18332
Fountain Hills, AZ 85269-8332 480-837-3961

Jean Hauck, Chairperson
Braille and large print books on the subjects of recreation, career and vocations, religion, novels and cookbooks for the visually impaired..

4484 **Prescott Public Library**
215 E Goodwin St
Prescott, AZ 86303-3911 928-777-1500
FAX: 928-771-5829
prescottlibrary.info

Roger Saft, Director
Martha Baden, Public Services Manager
Teresa Vonk, Support Services Manager
Lisa Zierke, Technical Services
Large print, braille and audio books; magnifiers; text to voice scanner; talking book machine application; toy library for children with special needs; special needs product catalogs; home book delivery; descriptive videos; 43 point PC monitor..

4485 **Special Needs Center/Phoenix Public Library**
1221 N Central Ave
Phoenix, AZ 85004-1867 602-262-4636
TTY:602-254-8205
www.phoenixpubliclibrary.org

4486 **World Research Foundation**
P.O. Box 20828
Sedona, AZ 86341-8804 928-284-3300
FAX: 928-284-3530
e-mail: info@wrf.org
wrf.org

Steven A Ross, President
LaVerne Boeckmann, Co-Founder
Large research library of alternative medicine; offers a computer search and printout of specific health issues for a nominal fee.

Arkansas

4487 **Arkansas Regional Library for the Blind and Physically Handicapped**
900 West Capitol Avenue
Suite 100
Little Rock, AR 72201-3108 501-682-2053

www.library.arkansas.gov

J D Hall, Manager of BPH Services
Dwain Gordon, Deputy Director
Danny Koonce, Public Information Specialist
Ruth Hyatt, Manager of Extension Services
Public library books in recorded or braille format. Popular fiction and nonfiction books for all ages, books and players are on free loan, sent to patrons by mail and may be returned postage free. Anyone who cannot see well enough to read regular print with glasses on or who has a disability that makes it difficult to hold a book or turn the pages is eligible.

4488 **Arkansas School for the Blind**
P.O.Box 668
Little Rock, AR 72203-668 501-296-1810
800-362-4451
FAX: 501-296-1831
www.arkansasschoolfortheblind.org

Khayyam Eddings, Chairperson
Jennifer Benedetti, Elementary Principal
Teresa Doan, Special Education Supervisor
William Harrison, Technology Director
Students at the ASB receive a quality education from specially trained instructors of the Visually Impaired in all academic areas. ASB features a comprehensive Music and Art program, as well as extensive extra-curricular activities. ASB is a proud member of the Arkansas Activities Association and The North Central Association of Schools for the Blind.

4489 **Educational Services for the Visually Impaired**
2402 Wildwood Avenue
Suite 112
Sherwood, AR 72120-5085 501-835-5448
FAX: 501-835-6840
e-mail: Angyln.Young@arkansas.gov
www.esvi.org

Angyln Young, State Coordinator
Cindy Lester, Data Management Specialist
Cynthia Kelly, ESVI Office Manager
Offers textbooks, braille books and more to the visually impaired grades K-12 in the Arizona area.

4490 **Library for the Blind and Physically Handicapped SW Region of Arkansas**
P.O.Box 668
2057 North Jackson St
Magnolia, AR 71754-668 870-234-1991
FAX: 870-234-5077
e-mail: library@cocolib.org
www2.youseemore.com/Columbia

Rhonda Rolen, Director
Dana Thornton, Assistant Director
Becky Verschage, Processing Clerk
Lisa Lewis, Bookkeeping
A free library service that serves adults and children who meet the eligiblity requirements, offers free loan of cassette machine and

recorded books, which meet the reading preferences of a highly diverse clientele.

4491 **Northwest Ozarks Regional Library for the Blind and Handicapped**
Fayetteville, AR 72701
479-575-2000
www.uark.edu

California

4492 **Braille Institute Library**
741 N Vermont Ave
Los Angeles, CA 90029-3594
323-663-1111
800-808-2555
FAX: 323-663-0867
e-mail: la@brailleinstitute.org
brailleinstitute.org

Leslie E. Stocker, President
Sally H. Jameson, Vice President of Programs and S
Peter A. Mindnich, Executive Vice President
Reza Rahman, Vice President of Finance/Chief
Braille Institute provides an environment of hope and encouragement for people who are blind and visually impaired through integrated educational, social and recreational programs and services.

4493 **Braille Institute Santa Barbara Center**
2031 De La Vina St
Santa Barbara, CA 93105-3895
805-682-6222
800-272-4553
FAX: 805-687-6141
e-mail: sb@brailleinstitute.org
brailleinstitute.org
Leslie E. Stocker, President
Sally H. Jameson, Vice President of Programs and S
Peter A. Mindnich, Executive Vice President
Reza Rahman, Vice President of Finance/Chief
Offers programs, services and information for persons with visual impairments.

4494 **Braille Institute Sight Center**
741 N Vermont Ave
Los Angeles, CA 90029-3594
323-663-1111
800-808-2555
FAX: 323-663-0867
e-mail: la@brailleinstitute.org
brailleinstitute.org

Sally H. Jameson, Vice President of Programs and S
Leslie E Stocker, President
Peter A. Mindnich, Executive Vice President
Reza Rahman, Vice President of Finance/Chief
Offers help, programs, services and information to the blind and visually impaired children and adults.

4495 **Braille and Talking Book Library: California**
P.O. Box 942837
Sacramento, CA 94237-0001
916-654-0640
800-952-5666
www.library.ca.gov/services/btbl.html
Stacey A. Aldrich, State Librarian
Debbie Newton, Bureau Chief, Administrative Ser
Phyllis Smith, Manager, Human Resources and Bus
Sharleen Finn, Budget Officer, Fiscal Services
Free service for eligible Northern California residents.

4496 **California State Library Braille and Talking Book Library**
P.O. Box 942837
Sacramento, CA 94237-0001
916-654-0640
800-952-5666
www.library.ca.gov/services/btbl.html

Stacey A. Aldrich, State Librarian
Debbie Newton, Bureau Chief, Administrative Ser
Phyllis Smith, Manager, Human Resources and Bus
Sharleen Finn, Budget Officer, Fiscal Services
Provides library services to people in Northern California who are unable to read standard print books because of visual or physical disabilities. Braille and talking books, magazines, machines, catalogs and postage are provided free to qualified appicants. The service is conducted by mail.

4497 **Clearinghouse for Specialized Media and Translations**
1430 N St
Ste 3207
Sacramento, CA 95814-5901
916-319-0800
FAX: 916-323-9732
e-mail: EHughes@cde.ca.gov.
www.cde.ca.gov/re/pn/sm
Jonn Paris-Salb, Manager
Provides materials in accessible formats; aural media, braille, large print, digital talking books and electronic media access technology.

4498 **Dental Amalgam Syndrome (DAMS) Newsletter**
725-9 Tramway Ln NE
Albuquerque, NM 87122-1672
505-291-8239
FAX: 505-294-3339

4499 **Fresno County Free Library Blind and Handicapped Services**
2420 Mariposa Street
Fresno, CA 93721-3640
559-600-7323
800-742-1011
e-mail: wendy.eisenberg@fresnolibrary.org
www.fresnolibrary.org/tblb
Wendy Eisenberg, Manager
Laurel Prysiazny, County Librarian
Magnifiers, home visits, volunteer-produced cassette books, discs and cassettes.

4500 **Glaucoma Research Foundation**
251 Post St
Ste 600
San Francisco, CA 94108-5017
415-986-3162
800-826-6693
FAX: 415-986-3763
e-mail: question@glaucoma.org
glaucoma.org
Tom Brunner, President and CEO
Nancy Graydon, Executive Director of Development
Andrew L. Jackson, Director of Communications
Catalina San Agustin, Director of Operations
Clinical and laboratory studies of glaucoma. We work to prevent vision loss from glaucoma by investing in innovative research, education and support with the ultimate goal of finding a cure..

4501 **Herrick Health Sciences Library**
Alta Bates Medical Center
2001 Dwight Way
Berkeley, CA 94704-2608
510-869-6777
FAX: 510-204-4091
www.altabatessummit.org
Laurie Bagley, Librarian
Carol Hirsch-Butler, Administrator
Carolyn Kemp, Regional Manager of Public Relations
Information on rehabilitation, psychiatry and psychoanalysis.

4502 **Kuzell Institute for Arthritis and Infectious Diseases**
Medical Research Institute Of San Francisco
2200 Webster St
San Francisco, CA 94115-1821
415-923-3262
FAX: 415-441-8548
Lowell S Young, Director
Edward Byrd, Owner
One of seven units comprising the Medical Research Institute of San Francisco that offers basic and applied research in arthritis and related diseases.

4503 **New Beginnings: The Blind Children's Center**
4120 Marathon St
Los Angeles, CA 90029-3584 323-664-2153
800-222-3566
FAX: 323-665-3828
blindchildrenscenter.org

Lena French, Executive Director
Kimberlee Jones, Director of Development
Ross Vergara, Director of Finance
Manuel Ayala, Director of Facilities
The purpose of the Center is to turn initial fears into hope. Helps children and their families become independent by creating a climate of safety and trust. Children learn to develop self confidence and to master a wide range of skills. Services include an infant stimulation program, educational preschool, interdisciplinary assessment services, family services, correspondence program, toll free national hotline and a publication and research service.

4504 **Research & Training Center on Mental Health for Hard of Hearing Persons**
California School of Professional Psychology
Ste 140
6215 Ferris Sq
San Diego, CA 92121-3279 619-282-4443
800-HEA-R619
FAX: 800-642-0266

Raymond J Trybus, Director
Thomas J Goulder, Associate Director
Funded by the National Institute on Disability and Rehabilitation Research, this training center aims to address issues of psychological relevance to persons who are hard of hearing or late deafened (as distinct from prelingually, culturally deaf persons). Also serves as information clearinghouse on this topic.

4505 **Rosalind Russell Medical Research Center for Arthritis**
Suite 600
350 Parnassus Ave
San Francisco, CA 94117 415-476-1141
FAX: 415-476-3526
e-mail: rrac@medicine.ucsf.edu
www.rosalindrussellcenter.ucsf.edu

Ephraim P Engleman, MD, Center Director
David Wofsy, MD, Associate Director
Paula R. Gambs, Chair
Christine Abele, Volunteer
Arthritis research and its probable causes.

4506 **San Francisco Public Library for the Blindand Print Handicapped**
100 Larkin St
San Francisco, CA 94102-4705 415-557-4400
FAX: 415-557-4252
TTY:415-557-4433
e-mail: webmail@sfpl.org
www.sfpl.org

Toni Cordova, Chief of Communications, Program
Toni Bernardi, Special Projects Manager
Laura Lent, Chief of Collections & Technical
Edward Melton, Chief of Branches
Foreign-language books on cassette, children's books on cassettes and more.

4507 **San Jose State University Library**
150 E San Fernando St
San Jose, CA 95112-3580 408-808-2000
FAX: 408-924-1118
e-mail: office@wahoo.sjsu.edu
www.sjlibrary.org

Don W Kassing, President
Jane Light, Library/Executive Director
Jeff Barber, Security Officer
Luann Budd, Administrative Officer
Information on physical disabilities, accessibility and learning disabilities.

Colorado

4508 **AMC Cancer Research Center**
3401 Quebec Street
Suite 3200
Denver, CO 80207 303-233-6501
800-321-1557
FAX: 303-239-3400
e-mail: contactus@amc.org
amc.org

Gary Kortz, Chairman
Steven D. Toltz, Treasurer
Cheryl Kisling, Secretary
Karen Padgett, President and CEO
Provides trained counselors who provide understanding and support for cancer patients; information and referral services; and screening programs.

4509 **Boulder Public Library**
1001 Arapahoe Ave
Boulder, CO 80302-6015 303-441-3100
www.boulderlibrary.org

Melinda Mattling, Manager
Priscilla Hudson, Manager
Offers braille books, cassettes, talking books, large print photocopier, large print books and more for the visually impaired.

4510 **Colorado Talking Book Library**
180 Sheridan Blvd
Denver, CO 80226-8101 303-727-9277
800-685-2136
FAX: 303-727-9281
e-mail: ctbl.info@cde.state.co.us
www.cde.state.co.us/ctbl/index.htm

Debbie Macleod, Executive Director
Provides free library service to Coloradans of all ages who are unable to read standard print due to visual, physical or learning disabilities whether permanent or temporary. Provides audio, braille and large-print books and magazines.

4511 **National Jewish Medical & Research Center**
1400 Jackson St
Denver, CO 80206-2762 303-388-4461
877-225-5654
www.nationaljewish.org

Michael Salem, MD, President and CEO
Richard A. Schierburg, Chair
Robin Chotin, Vice Chair
Robin Chotin, Secretary
The only medical center in the country whose research and patient care resources are dedicated to respiratory and immunologic diseases.

Connecticut

4512 **Connecticut Braille Association**
107 Vanderbilt Ave
West Hartford, CT 6110-1514 860-953-4445
FAX: 860-378-0205

Nick Martino, Owner
Offers textbooks, cassettes, large print books, braille books and more.

4513 **Connecticut Library for the Blind and Physically Handicapped**
231 Capitol Avenue
Hartford, CT 06106-1569
860-757-6500
860-866-4478
FAX: 860-721-2056
e-mail: ctaylor@cslib.org
www.cslib.org

Kendall Wiggin, State Librarian
Ursula Hunt, Administrative Assistant
Shelley Delisle, IT Manager
Jane Beaudoin, Administrative Assistant

Network library of the National Library Service for the Blind and Physically Handicapped, Library of Congress. Lends books and magazines in Braille or recorded formats along with the necessary playback equipment, free, for any Connecticut adult or child who is unable to read regular print due to a visual or physical disability. All materials are mailed to and from library patrons by postage-free mail

4514 **Connecticut State Library**
Connecticut State Government
231 Capitol Ave
Hartford, CT 06106-1569
860-757-6500
866-866-4478
FAX: 860-721-2056
e-mail: isref@cslib.org
www.cslib.org

Kendall Wiggin, State Librarian
Ursula Hunt, Administrative Assistant
Shelley Delisle, IT Manager
Jane Beaudoin, Administrative Assistant

Discs, cassettes, braille, reference materials on blindness and other handicaps, closed-circuit TV and large-print photocopier.

4515 **Connecticut Tech Act Project: Connecticut Department of Social Services**
Bureau of Rehabilitations Services
25 Sigourney St
11th Floor
Hartford, CT 06106-5041
860-424-4881
800-537-2549
FAX: 860-424-4850
TTY: 860-424-4839
e-mail: arlene.lugo@ct.gov
www.cttechact.com

Arlene Lugo, Program Director

Single point of entry, advocacy, information and referral, peer counseling, and access to objective expert advice and consultation for people with disabilities.

4516 **Prevent Blindness Connecticut**
101 Whitney Avenue
New Haven, CT 06510
203-722-4653
800-850-2020
FAX: 203-722-4691
e-mail: info@preventblindnesstristate.org
tristate.preventblindness.org

Kathryn Garre-Ayars, President and CEO
Tahesha Bryan, Administrative Assistant
Naomi Hayner, Connecticut Program Manager
Maria Giarratana, Grants Manager

The mission of Prevent Blindness Connecticut is to save sight and prevent blindness through eye screenings, education, safety activities and research.

4517 **Yale University: Vision Research Center**
310 Cedar St, LH 108
PO Box 208023
New Haven, CT 06520- 8023
203-785-2759
800-395-7949
FAX: 203-785-7303
e-mail: pamela.berkheiser@yale.edu
medicine.yale.edu/pathology

George Shafranov, Chairman
Pam Burkheiser, Manager
Robert J. Alpern, Dean

Vision including studies on growth and development.

Delaware

4518 **Delaware Assistive Technology Initiative (DATI)**
Alfred I. duPont Hospital for Children
461 Wyoming Road
Newark, DE 19716-0269
302-831-0354
800-870-3284
FAX: 302-831-4690
TTY: 302-651-6794
e-mail: dati@asel.udel.edu
www.dati.org

Beth Mineo Mollica, Director
Sonja Rathel, Project Coordinator

The Delaware Assistive Technology Initiative (DATI) connects Delawareans who have disabilities with the tools they need in order to learn, work, play and participate in community life safely and independently. DATI services include: Equipment demonstration centers in eah county; no-cost, short-term equipment loans that let you try before you buy; Equipment Exchange Program; AT workshops and other training sessions; advocacy for improved AT access policies and funding and several more.

4519 **Delaware Library for the Blind and Physically Handicapped**
Government
121 Duke of York Street
Dover, DE 19901-7430
302-739-4748
800-282-8676
FAX: 302-739-6787
e-mail: debph@lib.de.us
libraries.delaware.gov/default.shtml

Dr. Annie E. Norman, Director
Sonja Brown, Administrative Specialist
Beth-Ann Ryan, Deputy Director
Diann Colose, Administrative Librarian

Books on cassette and playback equipment are provided to patrons who are unable to read regular printed books.

4520 **Elwyn Delaware**
111 Elwyn Road
Elwyn, PA 19063-3499
610-891-2000
FAX: 302-654-5815
e-mail: info@elwyn.org
www.elwyn.org

Vicki Haschak, Contact
Kendra Johnson, Contact

Provides work training, job placement and supported employment, and elder care services.

District of Columbia

4521 **District of Columbia Public Library: Services for the Deaf Community**
District of Columbia Public Library
901 G St NW, Room 215
Washington, DC 20001-4531
202-727-0321
FAX: 202-727-0321
TTY:202-559-5368
e-mail: library_deaf_dc@yahoo.com
dclibrary.org

Venetia Demson, Chief Adaptive Services
Janice Roseu, Library for the Deaf Community

Offers reference services through videophone, signers for library programs, sign language classes, information about deafness, print and non-print materials for persons who have hearing disabilities. Book talks on deaf culture and American Sign Language story hours for kids, and Saturday sessions on employment-related skills are offered. Videophones for public use are available at the MLK Library.

4522 **District of Columbia Regional Library for the Blind and Physically Handicapped**
901 G St NW
Washington, DC 20001-4531 202-727-0321
FAX: 202-727-1129
TTY:202-727-2145
e-mail: lbphb_2000@yahoo.com
www.dclibrary.org

Richard Reyes-Gavilan, Executive Director
Jonathan Butler, Director of Business Services
Barbara Kirven, Director of Human Resources
Joi Mecks, Director of Communications

Regional library/RPH is network library in the Library of Congress, National Library Services for the Blind and Physically Handicapped.

4523 **Georgetown University Center for Child and Human Development**
P.O.Box 571485
Washington, DC 20057-1485 202-687-5000
FAX: 202-687-8899
TTY:202-687-5000
e-mail: gucdc@georgetown.edu
gucchd.georgetown.edu

Phyllis R Magrab, Phd, Director
John J DeGioia, President

Established over four decades ago to improve the quality of life for all children and youth, especially those with, or at risk for, special needs and their families. Located in the nation's capital, this center both directly serves vulnerable children and their families, as well as influences local, state, national and international programs and policy.

4524 **National Institute on Disability and Rehabilitation Research**
U S Department of Education
400 Maryland Ave SW
Washington, DC 20202-1 202-401-2000
800-872-5327
FAX: 202-401-0689
TTY: 800-437-0833
e-mail: customerservice@inet.ed.gov
ed.gov

Arne Duncan, Secretary of Education
Jim Shelton, Deputy Secretary
Ted Mitchell, Secretary

A national leader in sponsoring research. Mission is to generate, disseminate and promote new knowledge to improve the options available to disabled persons.

Florida

4525 **Brevard County Talking Books Library**
Brevard County Libraries
2725 Judge Fran Jamieson Way
Viera, FL 32940 321-633-2000
FAX: 321-633-1964
TTY:321-633-1838
e-mail: kbriley@brev.org
www.brevardcounty.us/PublicLibraries

Camille Johnson, Manager
Catherine J Schweinsburg, Library Services Director

Subregional library for the blind and physically handicapped, assistive reading devices collection, reference materials on blindness and other handicaps, descriptive videos, CCTV, phonic ear, reading edge and LOUD-R assistive listening devices available.

4526 **Broward County Talking Book Library**
100 S Andrews Ave
Fort Lauderdale, FL 33301-1830 954-357-7444
FAX: 954-357-5548
www.broward.org

Robert E. Cannon, Director
Carolyn Kayne, Manager

Reference materials on blindness and other handicaps, films, closed-circuit TV, discs, cassettes and a book discussion group is offered.

4527 **Dade County Talking Book Library**
Miami Dade Public Library System
101 West Flagler Street
Miami, FL 33130 305-375-2665
800-451-9544
FAX: 305-757-8401
e-mail: talkingbooks@mdpls.org
www.mdpls.org

Raymond Sanpiago, Executive Director
Lainey Brooks, Development Officer
Sylvia Mora Oria, Assistant Director
Ian D. Rosenior, Operations Administrator

A free Outreach Service of the Miami-Dade Public Library System. A network library, or subregional, of the National Library Service for the Blind and Physically Handicapped, Library of Congress, and of the Florida Bureau of Braille and Talking Books Library Service.

4528 **Florida Division of Blind Services**
Regional Library
325 West Gaines Street
Turlington Building, Suite 1114
Tallahassee, FL 32399-0400 850-245-0300
800-342-1828
FAX: 850-245-0363
e-mail: mike-gunde@dbs.doe.state.fl.us
dbs.myflorida.com

Mike Gunde, Manager
Susan Roberts, Bureau Chief
Robert Doyle, Director
Edward Hudson, Bureau Chief

Discs, cassettes, closed-circuit TV, large-print photocopier, films, children's books on cassettes and more.

4529 **Florida Instructional Materials Center forthe Visually Impaired (FIMC-VI)**
4210 W Bay Villa Ave
Tampa, FL 33611-1206 813-837-7826
800-282-9193
FAX: 813-837-7979
e-mail: FloridaBrailleChallenge@gmail.com
www.fimcvi.org

Mary Stoltz, Database Manager
Jeffrey Fitterman, Technology Specialist
Teresa Gutierrez, Administrative Secretary
Kay Ratzlaff, Coordinator

Operates a clearinghouse depository and production center for braille, large print and digital texts. Provides assistance in assessment of materials and specialized apparatus, organizes and trains volunteers for material production for the visually impaired, and provides professional development for teachers of the visually impaired. Provides electronic texts to NIMAS-eligible students in Florida.

4530 **Hillsborough County Talking Book Library Tampa-Hillsborough County Public Library**
900 N Ashley Dr
Tampa, FL 33602-3704 813-273-3652
FAX: 813-273-3707
TTY:813-273-3610
www.hcplc.org

Joe Stines, Director of Libraries
Marcee Challener, Assitant Director
David Wullschleger, Chief of Operations
Linda Gillon, Manager of Staff & Administrativ

Serves as the reference hub and resource center for all citzens of Hillsborough County and as the flagship library of the Tampa-Hillsborough County Public Library System.

4531 Jacksonville Public Library: Talking Books/Special Needs
303 N Laura St
Jacksonville, FL 32202-3505 904-630-2665
FAX: 904-630-0604
e-mail: jerryr@coj.net
www.jpl.coj.net/lib/talkingbooks.html
Barbara Gubbin, Executive Director
Offers cassettes and digital books, reference materials on blindness and ADA issues, newsline, descriptive videos, and some assistive devices.

4532 Lee County Library System: Talking Books Library
2001 N. Tamiami Trail N.E.
North Fort Myers, FL 33903-4855 239-533-4320
800-854-8195
FAX: 239-485-1146
TTY: 239-995-2665
e-mail: talkingbooks@leegov.com
www.lee-county.com/library
Cynthia N Cobb, Director
Terri Crawford, Deputy Director
Debbie Parrott, Manager
Karen McLeish-Delgado, Librarian
Provides free books and magazines to Lee County residents of all ages who have any disability that prevents them from reading printed material. Books are played on special players provided free by the National Library Service. Circulates low tech assistive aids and devices for temporary loan to Lee County Library card holders. Directs people to assistive technology and disability related resources.

4533 Louis de la Parte Florida Mental Health Institute Research Library
University of South Florida
4202 E. Fowler Ave. LIB122
Tampa, FL 33620 813-974-2729
FAX: 813-974-7242
e-mail: library@fmhi.usf.edu
lib.usf.edu/fmhi
William A. Garrison, Dean
Florence Jandreau, CAP, Senior Assistant to the Dean
Claudia Dold, Assistant University Librarian
Tomaro Taylor, Associate University Librarian / Certified Archivist
Information offered on mental illness, autism and pervasive development disabilities mental health research and archives management.

4534 Orange County Library System: Audio-Visual Department
101 E Central Blvd
Orlando, FL 32801-2429 407-835-7323
FAX: 407-835-7649
TTY:407-835-7641
e-mail: comments@ocls.info
www.ocls.info
Ted Maines, President
Lisa Franchina, Vice President
Bob Tessier, Comptroller
Craig Wilkins, Public Service Administrator
Serves the residents of the Orange County Library District, with headquarters in downtown Orlando.

4535 Pearlman Biomedical Research Institute
Mt Sinai Medical Center
1600 NW 10th Ave
Miami Beach, FL 33140 305-674-2121
FAX: 305-674-2198
e-mail: william-abraham@msmc.com
William Abraham, Director
A 32,000 square feet facility located on the main campus of Mount Sinai. The institute consists of laboratory space, research and administrative offices. The studies conducted within the facility are primarily pre-clinical research.

4536 Pinellas Talking Book Library for the Blind and Physically Handicapped
1330 Cleveland St
Clearwater, FL 33755-5103 727-441-8408
FAX: 727-441-8398
TTY:727-441-3168
e-mail: contactus@pplc.us
www.pplc.us
William Horne, Chair
Cheryl Morales, Executive Director
David Saari, Facilities Manager
Rosa Rodriguez, Deaf Literacy Coordinator at Saf
The Pinellas Public Library Cooperative serves Pinellas County residents in member cities and the unincorporated county. The Cooperative Office provides cooridination of activities and funding as well as marketing services for the the member counties. The Talking Book Library servces Pinellas, Manatee, and Sarasota counties.

4537 Talking Book Service: Mantatee County Central Library
1112 Manatee Avenue West
Bradenton, FL 34206-1000 941-748-4501
FAX: 941-751-7098
www.mymanatee.org
Patricia Schubert, Manager
Offers children's books on disc and cassette and more reference materials for the blind and physically handicapped.

4538 Talking Books Library for the Blind and Physically Handicapped
Palm Beach County Library
3650 Summit Blvd
West Palm Beach, FL 33406-4114 561-233-2600
888-780-4962
FAX: 561-233-2627
e-mail: webmaster@pbclibrary.org
www.pbclibrary.org
John Callahan, Executive Director
Bill Rautenberg, Chair
Harriet Helfman, Vice Chair
John Callahan III, Library Director
Established in 1967, today the County Library system serves Palm Beach County through the Main Library, 2 Regional Libraries, 11 Branch Libraries, a Bookmobile and a library annex. It continues to expand through our involvement with library networks, the Internet, and the World Wide Web.

4539 Talking Books/Homebound Services
Brevard County Library System
2725 Judge Fran Jamieson Way
Viera, FL 32940 321-633-2000
FAX: 321-633-1838
e-mail: kbriley@brev.org
www.brevardcounty.us/PublicLibraries
Kay Briley, Librarian
Camille Johnson, Executive Director
Offers reference materials on blindness and other handicaps. Subregional library for the blind and physically handicapped, assistive reading devices collection, reference materials on blindness and other handicaps; CCTV, phonic ear, reading edge and LOUD-R assistive listening devices available.

4540 University of Miami: Bascom Palmer Eye Institute
Department Of Ophthalmalogy
900 NW 17th St
Miami, FL 33136-1119 305-243-2020
888-845-0002
FAX: 305-326-7000
www.bascompalmer.org
Michael Gittelman, CEO
Teresa Spaulding, Manager
Eduardo C. Alfonso, M.D., Professor and Chairman
Jennifer Cohen, Executive Director
Clinical and basic research into blindness and visual impairments.

4541 University of Miami: Mailman Center for Child Development
1601 NW 12th Ave
Miami, FL 33136-1005 305-243-6395
FAX: 305-326-7594
e-mail: pedsinformation@med.miami.edu
pediatrics.med.miami.edu
William Donelan, Vice President for Medical Admin
William W. O'Neill, M.D., Executive Dean, Chief Medical Of
Pascal J. Goldschmidt, M.D., SVP, Dean, CEO
Steven Falcone, M.D., Executive Dean
Focuses on birth defects and children's illnesses.

4542 West Florida Regional Library
200 W Gregory St
Pensacola, FL 32502-4822 850-436-5060
FAX: 850-436-5039
TTY:850-436-5063
e-mail: hhudson@ci.pensacola.fl.us
wfrl.lib.fl.us
Eugene Fischer, Executive Director
Helen Hudson, Outreach Librarian
Offers children's print/braille books.

Georgia

4543 Athens Talking Book Center-Athens-Clarke County Regional Library
2025 Baxter St
Athens, GA 30606-6331 706-613-3655
800-531-2063
FAX: 706-613-3660
www.clarke.public.lib.ga.us/talkingbooks/inde
Stacey Chandler, Manager
Discs, cassettes, large print books, reference materials on blindness, descriptive videos, films, closed-circuit TV, magnifiers, braille writer, summer reading programs, cassette books and magazines and more.

4544 Augusta Talking Book Center
823 Telfair Street
Augusta, GA 30901-2232 706-821-2600
FAX: 706-724-6762
TTY:706-722-1639
e-mail: priced@ecgrl.org
www.ecgrl.org
Lillie Hamilton, Board Of Trustee
Audrey Bell, Manager
Loran Gray, Board Of Trustee
Brenda Morton, Board Of Trustee
Discs, cassettes, braille writer, films, large print books, summer reading program, magnifiers and reference materials on blindness and other handicaps.

4545 Bainbridge Subregional Library for the Blind & Physically Handicapped
S W Georgia Regional Library
301 S Monroe St
Bainbridge, GA 39819-4029 229-248-2665
800-795-2680
FAX: 229-248-2670
e-mail: lbph@swgrl.org
www.swgrl.org
Susans Wittle, Manager
Kathy Hutchins, Supervisor
The library houses a large collection of recorded materials as well as reference materials. For recorded and Braille materials that are provided by the National Library Service (NLS) but not currently in stock at the Bainbridge Library, the Regional Library in Atlanta can be contacted to Interlibrary Loan the requested materials.

4546 Columbus Subregional Library For The Blind And Physically Handicapped
1120 Bradley Dr
Columbus, GA 31906-2813 706-649-0780
800-652-0782
FAX: 706-649-1914
TTY: 706-649-0974
Dorothy Bowen, Librarian
Braille writer, magnifiers, closed-circuit TV, large-print photocopier, cassette books and magazines, children's books on cassette, home visits and other reference materials on blindness and other handicaps.

4547 Emory Autism Resource Center
Emory University
1551 Shoup Ct
Decatur, GA 30033 404-727-8350
FAX: 404-727-3969
e-mail: tohannon@emory.edu
www.emory.edu/HOUSING/CLAIRMONT/autism.html
James W. Wagner, President
Larry Hagan, IT Manager
Paul B. Pruett, MD, Director of Residency Education
Terri Trotter, Coordinator of Residency Educati
Offers on-line bulletin boards which are relevant to autism.

4548 Emory University Laboratory for Ophthalmic Research
1365b Clifton Rd NE
Atlanta, GA 30322-1013 404-778-4530
FAX: 404-778-4002
e-mail: pbennet@emory.edu
www.eyecenter.emory.edu/education/resi
James W. Wagner, President
Larry Hagan, IT Manager
Paul B. Pruett, MD, Director of Residency Education
Terri Trotter, Coordinator of Residency Educati
Various studies into the aspects of blindness.

4549 Georgia Library for the Blind and Physically Handicapped
Georgia Public Library
1800 Century Place
Suite 150
Atlanta, GA 30345-4304 404-235-7200
800-248-6701
FAX: 404-756-4618
e-mail: dscott@georgialibraries.org
georgialibraries.org
Stella Cone, Director
Deborah Scott, Business Manager
Dr. Lamar Veatch, Librarian
Julie Walker, State Librarian
Discs, cassettes, braille, films, closed-circuit TV, braille writer, large-print photocopier, cassette books and magazines.

4550 Hall County Library: East Hall Branch and Special Needs Library
127 Main St NW
Gainesville, GA 30501-3614 770-532-3311
FAX: 770-532-4305
TTY:770-531-2520
e-mail: info@hallcountylibrary.org
www.hallcountylibrary.org
Adrian Mixson, Manager
Summer reading programs, braille writer, magnifiers, scanners and readers, audio described videos, closed captioned videos, closed-circuit TV, large-print photocopier, cassette books and magazines, large print books, children's books on cassette, home visits and other reference materials on blindness and other handicaps.

4551 **Macon Library for the Blind and Physically Handicapped**
Washington Memorial Library
1180 Washington Ave
Macon, GA 31201-1762
478-744-0800
FAX: 478-742-3161
e-mail: jonest@bibblib.org
www.co.bibb.ga.us/library

Thomas Jones, Director
Leila Brittain, Finance Officer
Hannah Warren, Office Manager
Viveca Jackson, Librarian, West Bibb Branch

Summer reading programs, braille writer, magnifiers, closed-circuit TV, large-print photocopier, cassette books and magazines, children's books on cassette, home visits and other reference materials on blindness and other handicaps.

4552 **National Center on Birth Defects and Developmental Disabilities**
Centers for Disease Control and Prevention
1600 Clifton Rd NE
MS E-87
Atlanta, GA 30333
404-639-3311
800-232-4636
FAX: 404-498-3070
TTY: 888-232-6348
e-mail: cdcinfo@cdc.gov
www.cdc.gov/ncbddd/

Coleen A. Boyle, PhD, MSHyg, Director
Stephanie Dulin, MBA, Deputy Director
Vicki Kipreos, PMP, Management Officer
Lisa Richardson, MD, Director, Division of Blood Diso

Promotes child development, prevents birth defects and developmental disabilities.

4553 **North Georgia Talking Book Center**
LaFayette-Walker Public Library
305 S Duke St
La Fayette, GA 30728-2936
706-638-8312
888-506-0509
888-506-0509
FAX: 706-638-4028
e-mail: cstubblefield@chrl.org
www.chrl.org

Tim York, Manager
June DeLong, Library Assistant
Martha McKeehan, Library Assistant
Kaylee Smith, Library Assistant

We offer books on cassette for the visual and physically disabled induvidual, books in braille, magazines on cassette, zoom text screen magnifier, computer voice program, large-print photocopier, summer reading program, home visits na dother reference materials on blindness and other disabilities.

4554 **Oconee Regional Library**
801 Bellevue Ave
Dublin, GA 31021-4847
478-272-5710
FAX: 478-275-5381
georgialibraries.org

Stella Cone, Director
Deborah Scott, Business Manager
Dr. Lamar Veatch, Librarian
Leard Daughety, Director

Summer reading programs, braille writer, magnifiers, closed-circuit TV, large-print photocopier, cassette books and magazines, children's books on cassette, home visits and other reference materials on blindness and other handicaps.

4555 **Rome Subregional Library for the Blind and Physically Handicapped**
205 Riverside Pkwy
Rome, GA 30161-2922
706-236-4611
888-263-0769
FAX: 706-236-4631
TTY: 706-236-4618
www.floyd.public.lib.ga.us

Diana Mills, Librarian
Delana Hickman, Manager

The regional library system serves Floyd and Polk counties. System headquarters are located in Rome, Georgia, within the Rome/Floyd County Library Branch.

4556 **South Georgia Regional Library-Valdosta Talking Book Center**
300 Woodrow Wilson Dr
Valdosta, GA 31602-2532
229-333-0086
FAX: 229-333-0364
e-mail: commissioner@lowndescounty.com
sgrl.org

Chuck Gibson, Manager

Summer reading programs, Braille writer, magnifiers, closed-circuit TV, large print photocopier, cassette books and magazines, children's books on cassette, home visits and other reference materials on blindness and other handicaps.

4557 **Talking Book Center Brunswick-Glynn County Regional Library**
208 Gloucester St
Brunswick, GA 31520-7007
912-267-1212
FAX: 912-267-9597
e-mail: bransom@trll.org
www.trrl.org/tbc

Betty Ransom, Librarian
Joe Shinnick, Executive Director

The Three Rivers Regional Library system is named for 3 rivers that flow through all 7 counties of the library system. The Three Rivers Regional Library system serves patrons in Brantley, Camden, Charlton, Glynn, Long, McIntosh, and Wayne counties in southeast Georgia.

Hawaii

4558 **Assistive Technology Resource Centers of Hawaii (ATRC)**
200 North Vineyard Boulevard
Suite 430
Honolulu, HI 96817-5362
808-532-7110
800-645-3007
FAX: 808-532-7120
TTY: 808-532-7110
e-mail: atrc-info@atrc.org
www.atrc.org

Barbara Fischlowitz-Leong, Executive Director
Jeff Ah Sam, Technical Assistant
Jodi Asato, Deputy Director
Edna Kaahaaina, Office Manager

Provides information and training on assistive technology devices, services, and funding resources. Conducts presentations and demonstrations in the community to increase AT awareness and promote self-advocacy among people with disabilities.

4559 **Hawaii State Library for the Blind and Physically Handicapped**
874 Dillingham Blvd
Honolulu, HI 96817-4505
808-845-9221
800-559-4096
FAX: 808-733-8449
e-mail: honcclib@hawaii.edu
www2.honolulu.hawaii.edu/library

Fusako Miyashiro, Manager

Supported by the Hawaii State Public Library System and the National Library Service for the Blind and Physically Handicapped, Library of Congress. Staff with knowledge of sign language; Special interest periodicals; Books on deafness and sign language; captioned media; Special Services: Radio Reading Service, Talking Books Reader's Club, educational and cultural programs, machine lending agency. Braille, cassette and large type. Regional and National service, quarterly newsletter.

Idaho

4560 Idaho Assistive Technology Project
University of Idaho
121 West Sweet Ave
Moscow, ID 83843-2268 208-885-3557
800-432-8324
FAX: 208-885-6145
e-mail: idahoat@uidaho.edu
www.idahoat.org

Janice Carson, Project Director
Irene Lunsford, Loan Program Manager
Julie Magelky, Loan Program Coordinator
Dan Dyer, Training Coordinator

A federally funded program managed by the Center on Disbailities and Human Development at the University of Idaho. The goal of the IATP is to increase the availability of assistive technology devices and services for Idahoans with disabilities. The IATP offers free trainings and technical assistance, a low-interest loan program, assistive technology assessments for children and agriculture workers, and free informational materials.

4561 Idaho Commission for Libraries: Talking Book Service
325 W State St
Boise, ID 83702-6055 208-334-2150
800-458-3271
FAX: 208-334-4016
e-mail: talkingbooks@libraries.idaho.gov
www.libraries.idaho.gov/tbs

Ann Joslin, Manager
Irene Lunsford, Library Consultant
David Harrell, IT & Telecommunications Resources Manager
Erica Compton, Project Coordinator

Offers audio and braille books and magazines, equipment, and accessories. All materials are mailed free to users' homes. Service is available free to all Idaho residents with a disability which limits their ability to use print materials.

Illinois

4562 Chicago Public Library Talking Book Center
400 S State St
Chicago, IL 60605-1216 312-747-4300
800-757-4654
FAX: 312-747-4962
e-mail: dtaylor@chipublib.org
www.chipublib.org

Linda Johnson Rice, President
Christopher Valenti, Vice President
Cristina Benitez, Secretary
Joselyn Bell, Director, Finance

Summer reading programs, braille writer, closed-circuit TV, large print photocopier, cassette books and magazines, children's books on cassette, home visits and other reference materials on blindness and other handicaps. Three assistive technology centers designed and equipped for the blind and visually impaired, funded by the National Library Service for the Blind and Handicapped, a division of the Library of Congress. All services FREE!

4563 Department of Ophthalmology and Visual Science
1855 W Taylor St
Chicago, IL 60612-7242 312-996-7000
800-625-2013
FAX: 312-996-7770
TTY: 312-413-0123
e-mail: adriadel@uic.edu
www.uic.edu

Paula Allen-Meares, Chancellor
Lon S. Kaufman, Vice Chancellor for Academic Aff
Mitra Dutta, Vice Chancellor for Research
Barbara Henley, Vice Chancellor for Student Affa

Offers help, support, information and research for persons with vision problems, including Retinitis Pigmentosa.

4564 Guild for the Blind
65 E. Wacker Place
Suite 1010
Chicago, IL 60601-7463 312-236-8569
FAX: 312-236-8128
e-mail: info@guildfortheblind.org
www.second-sense.org

Brett Christenson, President
Laura Rounce, Vice President
Michael P. Wagner, Treasurer
Toria Emas, Secretary

provides worship on vision rehabilitation, training on computers and other adaptive technology, career counseling, and professional development workshops and offers assistive devices for sale.

4565 Horizons for the Blind
125 Erick Street
A103
Crystal Lake, IL 60014-4404 815-444-8800
800-318-2000
FAX: 815-444-8830
TTY: 815-444-8800
e-mail: mail@horizons-blind.org
www.horizons-blind.org

Camille Caffarelli, Executive Director
Jeff T. Thorsen, First Vice President/Treasurer
Keith Myers, Second Vice President
Maryann Bartkowski, Secretary

HORIZONS for the BLIND is a nonprofit organization dedicated to providing products and services to people who are blind or visually impaired. In addition, Horizons is a leading provider of Braille transcription services to the business community; specialing in partnering with companies and nonprofits to provide billing and financial statements, newsletters, and documents in Braille, large print, and audio formats.

4566 Illinois Early Childhood Intervention Clearinghouse
51 Gerty Drive
Champaign, IL 61820-7469 217-333-1386
877-275-3227
FAX: 217-244-7732
e-mail: Illinois-eic@illinois.edu
www.eiclearinghouse.org

Charlton Brandt, Manager
Patricia Traylor, Project Associate

Free lending library of materials related to early childhood and disability. Books, audiovisuals and articles available. Computerized database with more than 31,000 items available to Illinois residents.

4567 Illinois Machine Sub-Lending Agency
607 S Greenbriar Rd
Carterville, IL 62918-1602 618-985-8375
800-455-2665
FAX: 618-985-4211
e-mail: imsastaff@imsa.lib.il.us
www.imsa.lib.il.us

Loretta Broomfield, Director

The Illinois Machine Sublending Agency (IMSA) is a division of the Illinois Network of Talking Book and Braille Libraries. The primary responsibility of IMSA is to maintain Talking Book equipment and accessories and to issue Talking Book equipment and accessories to Illinois residents who are registered for the service. IMSA is also the support center for patrons in need of assistance with the Braille and Audio Reading Download (BARD) service.

4568 Illinois Regional Library for the Blind and Physically Handicapped
1055 W Roosevelt Rd
Chicago, IL 60608-1559 312-746-9210
800-331-2351
FAX: 312-746-9192

Shawn Thomas, Reference Librarian
Barbara Perkins, Acting Director

Summer reading programs, braille writer, magnifiers, closed-circuit TV, large-print photocopier, cassette books and magazines, descriptive videos, children's books on cassette, home visits and other reference materials on blindness and other handicaps.

4569 Mid-Illinois Talking Book Center
600 High Point Ln
East Peoria, IL 61611-9396
309-694-9200
800-426-0709
e-mail: info@mitbc.org
mitbc.org

Rose Chenoweth, Director
Michelle Moran, Assistant
Rebecca Rollings, Assistant
Jane Furrh, Assistant
Providing a free library service to anyone unable to read regular print because of a visual or physical disability. There are books and magazines on tape and playback equipment; and also in Braille. Books and magazines are mailed free to and from library patrons, wherever they reside.

4570 National Eye Research Foundation (NERF)
Ste 207a
910 Skokie Blvd
Northbrook, IL 60062-4033
847-564-4652
800-621-2258
FAX: 847-564-0807
e-mail: info@nerf.org
www.nerf.org

Joel Tenner, Manager
Dedicated to improving eye care for the public and meeting the professional nees of eye care practitioners; sponsors eye research projects on contact lens applications and eye care problems. Special study sections in such fields as orthokertology, primary eyecare, pediatrics, and through continuing education programs. Provides eye care information for the public and professionals. Educational materials including pamphlets. Program activities include education and referrals.

4571 National Lekotek Center
2001 N. Clybourn
Chicago, IL 60614
773-528-5766
800-366-7529
FAX: 773-537-2992
e-mail: lekotek@lekotek.org
www.lekotek.org

Elaine D. Cottey, Chair
Joanna Horsnail, Chair Elect
Eric Gastevich, Treasurer
Carol Neiger, Secretary
Toy library and play-centered programs for children with special needs and their families with branches in 17 states. Sliding fee scale. Lekotek also has a Toy Resource Helpline that provides individualized assistances in the selection of toys and play materials and general resources for families with children with disabilities.

4572 Northwestern University Multipurpose Arthritis & Musculoskeletal Center
420 East Superior Street
Chicago, IL 60611-4296
312-503-8194
FAX: 312-503-1204
e-mail: med-webteam@northwestern.edu
www.feinberg.northwestern.edu

Cynthia Barnard, MBA, Director, Quality Strategies
John Vozenilek, MD, Assistant Professor
Eric G. Neilson, MD, Vice President for Medical Affairs
Sherri L. LaVela, PhD, MPH, MBA, Assistant Professor
Conducts biomedical, educational and health services research into musculoskeletal diseases.

4573 Skokie Accessible Library Services
Skokie Public Library
5215 Oakton St
Skokie, IL 60077-3680
847-673-7774
FAX: 847-673-7797
TTY:847-673-8926
e-mail: tellus@skokielibrary .info
www.skokie.lib.il.us

Carolyn A. Anthony, Director
John J. Graham, President
Diana Hunter, Vice President/President Emerita
Karen Parrilli, Secretary
Library services for people with disabilities, including electronic aids, materials in special formats, programs and special services.

4574 University of Illinois at Chicago: Lions of Illinois Eye Research Institute
University of Illinois at Chicago
1855 West Taylor Street, m/c 648
Room 3.138
Chicago, IL 60612
312-996-6591
FAX: 312-996-7770
e-mail: eyeweb@uic.edu
www.uic.edu

Rolanda Geddis, Manager
Paula Alen Meares, Chancellor
Jerry Bauman, Vice President for Health Affairs
James Schmidt, Director of Athletics
Visual impairments and blindness research, including glaucoma studies.

4575 Voices of Vision Talking Book Center at DuPage Library System
125 Tower Drive
Burr Ridge, IL 60527-2771
630-734-5055
800-426-0709
FAX: 630-208-0399
e-mail: info@illinoistalkingbooks.org
www.illinoistalkingbooks.org

Karen L. Odean, Director
Provides library service to persons who are unable to use standard printed material because of visual or physical disabilities. Part of the Illinois network of Talking Book Libraries. The service is free to those who are eligable. Provides books and magazines on audio-cassettes. Special playback equipment needed to use the books is also loaned. Braille books and magazines are also available. The collection includes popular books, classics and children's literature.

Indiana

4576 Allen County Public Library
900 Library Plaza
Fort Wayne, IN 46802-3699
260-421-1200
FAX: 260-421-1386
TTY:260-421-1302
e-mail: Genealogy@ACPL.Info
www.acpl.lib.in.us

Jeffrey R. Krull, Director
Martin E. Seifert, President
Alan McMahan, Vice President
Paul G. Moss, Secretary
Summer reading programs, braille writer, magnifiers, closed-circuit TV, large-print photocopier, cassette books and magazines, children's books on cassette, home visits and other reference materials on blindness and other handicaps.

4577 Bartholomew County Public Library
536 5th St
Columbus, IN 47201-6225
812-379-1255
FAX: 812-379-1275
e-mail: library@barth.lib.in.us
barth.lib.in.us

Beth Poor, Executive Director
Summer reading programs, braille writer, magnifiers, closed-circuit TV, large-print photocopier, cassette books and magazines,

children's books on cassette, home visits and other reference materials on blindness and other handicaps.

4578 Elkhart Public Library for the Blind and Physicly Handicapped
300 S 2nd St
Elkhart, IN 46516-3109 574-522-2223
800-622-4970
FAX: 574-522-2174
e-mail: webmaster@myepl.org
www.myepl.org/epl

Connie Jo Ozinga, Executive Director
Barbara G. Anderson, President
Janice E. Dean, Vice-President
Krystal Anderson, Secretary

Summer reading programs, braille writer, magnifiers, closed-circuit TV, large-print photocopier, cassette books and magazines, children's books on cassette, home visits and other reference materials on blindness and other handicaps.

4579 Indiana Resource Center for Autism
2853 E 10th St
Bloomington, IN 47408-2696 812-855-6508
800-825-4733
FAX: 812-855-9630
TTY: 812-855-9396
e-mail: iidc@indiana.edu
www.iidc.indiana.edu/irca

Dr Cathy Pratt Ph.D., BCBA, Director
Donna Beasley, Administrative Program Secretary
Pamela Anderson, Outreach/Resource Specialist
Marci Wheeler, M.S.W., Social Work Specialist

The Indiana Resource Center for Autism staff conduct outreach training and consultations, engage in research and develop and disseminate information focused on building the capicity of local communities, organizations, agencies and families to support children and adults across the autism spectrum in typical work, school, home and community settings. Please check our website for a complete list of publications.

4580 Indiana University: Multipurpose Arthritis Center
School Of Medicine, Rheumatology Division
509 E. 3rd Street
Bloomington, IN 47401-3654 812-855-0516
FAX: 812-855-9943
e-mail: dbrandt@iupui.edu
research.iu.edu

Dr. Kenneth Brandt MD, Director
Carmichael Center, Vice President for Research
Steven A Martin, Associate Vice President for Research
Marisa Pratt, Executve Financial & Operations Officer

The mission of the center is to pursue major biomedical research interests relevant to the rheumatic diseases. Current areas of emphasis include; articular cartilage biology, pathogenesis of articular cartilage breakdown in osteoarthritis, causes of pain and disability in QA, the pathogenesis and treatment of various forms of amyloidosis, the pathogenesis of dermatomyositis, and immunologic and biochemical markers of cartilage breakdown and repair.

4581 Lake County Public Library Talking Books Service
1919 W 81st Ave
Merrillville, IN 46410-5488 219-769-3541
FAX: 219-769-0690
e-mail: webmaster@lakeco.lib.in.us
www.lcplin.org

Larry Acheff, Manager

Large-print books, descriptive videos, braille writer, magnifiers, closed-circuit TV, large-print photocopier, cassette books and magazines, children's books on cassette, and other reference materials on blindness and other handicaps.

4582 Special Services Division: Indiana State Library
140 N Senate Ave
Indianapolis, IN 46204-2207 317-232-3675
800-622-4970
FAX: 317-253-3209
TTY: 317-232-7763
e-mail: delivery@statelib.lib.in.us
www.in.gov/isloutage

Roberta Brooker, Manager
Barbara Maxwell, State Librarian
C Ewick, Manager

Circulates a collection of braille, recorded, and large print books and magazines and the special equipment needed to play the recorded materials to anyone in Indiana who cannot read regular print due to a visual or physical disability.

4583 St. Joseph Hospital Rehabilitation Center
700 Broadway
Fort Wayne, IN 46802-1402 260-425-3000
FAX: 260-425-3741
www.stjoehospital.com

Kirk Ray, CEO
Bob Hailes, Vice President

Information offered on rehabilitation.

4584 Talking Books Service Evansville Vanderburgh County Public Library
200 SE Martin Luther King Jr Blvd
Evansville, IN 47713- 1802 812-428-8200
866-645-2536
FAX: 812-428-8397
e-mail: tbs@evpl.org
www.evpl.org

Marcia Learned Au, COO
Connie Davis, Vice President
Marcia Au, Executive Director
Barbara Shanks, Talking Book Manager

The Talking Book Service of the Evansville Vanderburgh Public Library is part of a nationwide network of cooperating libraries headed by the National Library Service & a division of the Library of Congress. This free program provides library services and materials in alternative formats to person who are unable to use standard print material due to a visual or physical handicap.

Iowa

4585 Iowa Department for the Blind Library
State Of Iowa
524 4th Street
Des Moines, IA 50309-2364 515-281-1333
800-362-2587
FAX: 515-281-1263
TTY: 515-281-1355
e-mail: contact@blind.state.ia.us
www.IDBonline.org

Richard Sorey, Director
Mike Hoenig, Chair
Steve Hagemoser, Commision Board Member
Peggy Elliott, Commision Board Member

Summer reading programs, large print, disc, Braille and cassette books and magazines, descriptive videos and reference materials on blindness and other handicaps.

4586 **Iowa Registry for Congenital and Inherited Disorders**
University of Iowa
Department of Epidemiology, Univers
100 BVC, Room W260
Iowa City, IA 52242-5000 319-335-4107
866-274-4237
FAX: 319-335-4030
e-mail: ircid@uiowa.edu
www.public-health.uiowa.edu/ircid/

Paul Romitti, Ph.D, Director
Kim Keppler-Noreuil, M.D, Clinical Director for Birth Defects
Katherine. Mathews, M.D, Clinical Director for Neuromuscular Disorders
James Torner, Ph.D., Chair

The mission of the Iowa Registry for Congenital and Inherited Disorders is; maintain statewide surveillance for collecting information on selected congenital and inherited disorders in Iowa, monitor annual trends in occurrence and mortality of these disorders, provide data for research studies and educational activities for the prevention and treatment of these disorders.

4587 **Library Commission for the Blind**
State Of Iowa
524 4th Street
Des Moines, IA 50309-2364 515-281-1333
800-362-2587
FAX: 515-281-1263
TTY: 515-281-1355
e-mail: contact@blind.state.ia.us
www.blind.state.ia.us

Karen A Keninger, Director
Aldini Jodi, Library Support Staff
Barber Kim, Independent Living Supervisor
Bauer Marcia, Rehabilitation Teacher

Summer reading programs, Braille writer, magnifiers, closed-circuit TV, large print photocopier, cassette books and magazines, children's books on cassette and other reference materials on blindness and other handicaps.

Kansas

4588 **Center for the Improvement of Human Functioning**
3100 N Hillside St
Wichita, KS 67219-3904 316-682-3100
FAX: 316-682-5054
e-mail: information@riordanclinic.org
www.riordanclinic.org

Hugh D Riordan, President
Ron Hunninghake MD, Chief Medical Officer
Brian Riordan, Chief Executive Officer
Danae, Certified Medical Assistant

Medical, research, and educational facility specializing in the treatment of chronic illness.

4589 **Central Kansas Library Systems Headquarters (CSLS)**
1409 Williams St
Great Bend, KS 67530-4020 620-792-4865
800-362-2642
FAX: 620-793-7270
e-mail: cbobbitt@ckls.org
www.ckls.org

Harry Williams, Administrator
Vickie Herl, Adminstrative Manager
Marquita Boehnke, Department Head
Connie Bobbitt, Assistant

Summer reading programs, braille writer, magnifiers, closed-circuit TV, large-print photocopier, cassette books and magazines, children's books on cassette, home visits and other reference materials on blindness and other handicaps. Assistive technology available. Serving 17 counties in Central Kansas.

4590 **Kansas State Library**
Esu Memorial Union
300 SW 10th Avenue
Room 312-N
Topeka, KS 66612-1593 785-296-3296
800-432-3919
FAX: 620-343-7124
e-mail: infodesk@library.ks.gov
kslib.info

Christie Brandau, Manager
Jo Kord, Manager
Budler Jo, State Librarian
Turner Barbara, Administrative Officer

Summer reading programs, braille writer, magnifiers, closed-circuit TV, large-print photocopier, cassette books and magazines, children's books on cassette, home visits and other reference materials on blindness and other handicaps.

4591 **Kansas Talking Books Regional Library**
300 SW 10th Avenue
Room 312-N
Topeka, KS 66612-4401 785-296-3296
800-432-3919
FAX: 620-343-7124
e-mail: talkingbooks@kslb.info
kslib.info

Toni Harrell, Director
Christie Brandau, Manager
Jo Kord, Manager
Budler Jo, State Librarian

Summer reading programs, Braille writer, closed-circuit TV, large-print photocopier, cassette books and magazines, children's books on cassette, home visits and other reference materials on blindness and other handicaps.

4592 **Manhattan Public Library**
629 Poyntz Ave
Manhattan, KS 66502-6131 785-776-4741
800-432-2796
FAX: 785-776-1545
e-mail: refstaff@mhklibrary.org
manhattan.lib.ks.us

Linda Knupp, Director
John Pecoraro, Assistant Director
Brice Hobrock, President
Thomas Giller, Vice President

Summer reading programs, Braille writer, magnifiers, closed-circuit TV, large-print photocopier, cassette books and magazines, children's books on cassette, home visits and other reference materials on blindness and other disabilities.

4593 **Northwest Kansas Library System Talking Books**
2 Washington Square
Norton, KS 67654-1615 785-877-5148
800-432-2858
FAX: 785-877-5697
e-mail: tbook@ruraltel.net
www.nwkls.org

George Seamon, Director
Alice Evans, Business Manager & Acquisitions
David Fischer, Technology Consultant
Marry Boller, Children's and Talking Book Consultant

Offers books on disc and cassette. Library of Congress talking book and program for qualified individuals. Also offers descriptive videos to eligible persons.

4594 **South Central Kansas Library System**
321 North Main Street
South Hutchinson, KS 67505-1145 620-663-3211
800-234-0529
FAX: 620-663-9797
sckls.info

Paul Hawkins, Director
Sharon Barnes, Technology Consultant
Larry Papenfuss, Director of Information Technology
Jill Stern, Continuing Education Specialist

Serving public, school, academic and special libraries in 12 counties since 1968, the South Central Kansas Library System

(SCKLS) is the "go to" resource for innovative services, quality member awareness and assistance.

4595 Topeka & Shawnee County Public Library Talking Books Service
1515 SW 10th Ave
Topeka, KS 66604-1374
785-580-4400
800-432-2925
FAX: 785-580-4496
TTY: 785-580-4544
e-mail: tbooks@tscpl.lib.ks.us
www.tscpl.org

Stephanie Hall, Manager
Gina Millsap, Chief Executive Officer
Robert Banks, Chief Operating Officer
Sheryl Weller, Chief Financial Officer
Talking books is a free service that provides cassette and digital books and equipment to people who are unable to read or use standard print materials because of a visual or physical impairment. There are no fees. To apply for Talking Books you must fill out and submit an application, have it certified by the appropriate authority and return it to the library. You can find an application on our website or have one mailed out to you by contacting our office.

4596 Wichita Public Library/Talking Book Service
Wichita Public Library
223 S Main St
Wichita, KS 67202-3795
316-261-8500
FAX: 316-262-4540
TTY:316-262-3972
e-mail: admin@wichita.lib.ks.us
www.wichita.lib.ks.us

Cynthia Berner-Harris, Executive Director
Eric J. Larson, Member of the Board
Furnish recorded reading material (books and magazines) for visually and physically challenged citizens.

4597 Wichita Public Library/Talking Book Service
223 S Main St
Wichita, KS 67202-3795
316-261-8500
FAX: 316-262-4540
TTY:316-262-3972
e-mail: admin@wichita.lib.ks.us
www.wichita.lib.ks.us

Cynthia Berner-Harris, Executive Director
Eric J. Larson, Member of the Board
Furnish recorded reading material (books and magazines) for visually and physically challenged citizens.

Kentucky

4598 EnTech: Enabling Technologies of Kentuckiana
Spaulding University
851 South 3rd Street
Louisville, KY 40203-2115
502-585-9911
800-896-8941
FAX: 502-585-7103
e-mail: admissions@spalding.edu
www.spalding.edu

Laura Strickland, Manager
Mary Kaye Steinmietz, Outreach Coordinator
Tori Murden McClure, President
Assistive technology resource and demonstration center, serving persons of all ages and disabilities in Kentucky and Southern Indiana. Services include: assistive technology information, demonstration, evaluation, training, technical support and short-term loan of equipment.

4599 Kentucky Talking Book LibraryKentucky Dept. for Libraries and Archives
300 Coffee Tree Road
PO Box 537
Frankfort, KY 40602-0537
502-564-8300
800-372-2968
FAX: 502-564-5773
e-mail: ktbl.mail@ky.gov
www.kdla.ky.gov

Barbara Penegor, Regional Librarian
Lauren Abner, Field Services
Katherine K. Adelberg, E-Rate Coordinator
Jackie Arnold, Local Records Regional Administrator
Provides library service to those who are physically unable to read print. Audio and braille books and magazines are available via mail or download.

4600 Louisville Free Public Library
301 York Street
Louisville, KY 40203-2257
502-574-1611
FAX: 502-574-1666
e-mail: webteam@lfpl.org
lfpl.org

Craig Buthod, Manager
Summer reading programs, braille writer, magnifiers, closed-circuit TV, large-print photocopier, cassette books and magazines, children's books on cassette, home visits and other reference materials on blindness and other handicaps.

Louisiana

4601 Central Louisiana State Hospital Medical and Professional Library
P.O.Box 5031
Pineville, LA 71361-5031
318-484-6200
FAX: 318-484-6501
http://wwwprd.doa.louisiana.gov/laservices/pu

Patrick Kelly, CEO
Carol Gee, Manager
Information offered on psychiatry, psychology and mental health.

4602 Louisiana State Library
701 North 4th St
Baton Rouge, LA 70802-5345
225-342-4913
800-543-4702
FAX: 225-219-4804
e-mail: admin@state.lib.la.us
www.state.lib.la.us

Rebecca Hamilton, Assistant Secretary, State Libra
Diane Brown, Deputy State Librarian
Beverly Dugas, Business Manager
Meg Placke, Associate State Librarian
Summer reading programs, braille writer, magnifiers, closed-circuit TV, large-print photocopier, cassette books and magazines, children's books on cassette. Descriptive videoss and other reference materials on blindness and other handicaps.

4603 Louisiana State University Genetics Section of Pediatrics
533 Bolivar St
New Orleans, LA 70112-1349
504-568-6151
FAX: 504-568-8500
e-mail: postmaster@lsuhsc.edu
www.medschool.lsuhsc.edu

Steve Nelson, MD, Dean
Janis Letourneau, MD, Associate Dean for Faculty & Ins
Cathi Fontenot, MD, Associate Dean for Alumni Affair
Charles Hilton, MD, Associate Dean for Academic Affa
Our goal is to continue building a strong department in which all of the faculty are successful in attracting funding, and committed to establishing productive programs that bring credit to the Department and to the Health Sciences Center as a whole.

4604 State Library of Louisiana: Services for the Blind and Physically Handicapped
701 North 4th St
Baton Rouge, LA 70802-5345 225-342-4913
800-543-4702
FAX: 225-219-4804
e-mail: sbph@state.lib.la.us
www.state.lib.la.us

Rebecca Hamilton, Assistant Secretary, State Libra
Diane Brown, Deputy State Librarian
Beverly Dugas, Business Manager
Meg Placke, Associate State Librarian

Summer reading programs, braille publications, cassette books and magazines, children's books on cassette and other reference materials on blindness and other handicaps. Louisiana Hotlines - quarterly newsletter. Affiliated with National Library Service for the Blind and Physically Handicapped, Washington, DC. Louisiana Voices recording program uses volunteers to record books for the blind.

Maine

4605 Bangor Public Library
145 Harlow St
Bangor, ME 04401-4900 207-947-8336
FAX: 207-945-6694
e-mail: bpill@bpl.lib.me.us
www.bpl.lib.me.us

Barbara Mc Dade, Executive Director
Norman Minsky, President
Franklin E. Bragg II, MD, Vice President
Lee Chick, Treasurer

Summer reading programs, braille writer, magnifiers, closed-circuit TV, large-print photocopier, cassette books and magazines, children's books on cassette, home visits and other reference materials on blindness and other handicaps.

4606 Cary Library
107 Main Street
Houlton, ME 04730-2196 207-532-1302
FAX: 207-532-4350
e-mail: faucher!@carey.lib.me.us
www.cary.lib.me.us

Iva Sussman, Chair
Forrest Barnes, Treasurer
Gary Hagan, Secretary
Linda Faucher, Library Director

Summer reading programs, braille writer, magnifiers, closed-circuit TV, large-print photocopier, cassette books and magazines, children's books on cassette, home visits and other reference materials on blindness and other handicaps.

4607 Lewiston Public Library
200 Lisbon St
Lewiston, ME 04240-7234 207-513-3004
FAX: 207-784-3011
TTY:207-200-1511
e-mail: LPLReference@LewistonMaine.gov
lplonline.org

Rick Speer, Library Director
Marcela Peres, Adult Services Librarian
David Moorhead, Children's Librarian
Beth Martel, Circulation Services Supervisor

Summer reading programs, braille writer, magnifiers, closed-circuit T.V., large-print photocopier, cassette books and magazines, children's books on cassette, home visits and other reference materials on blindness and other handicaps.

4608 Maine State Library
Maine State
64 State House Sta
Augusta, ME 04333-64 207-287-5650
800-762-7106
FAX: 207-287-5624
TTY: 888-577-6690
e-mail: benitad@ursus3.ursus.maine.edu
maine.gov

Chris Boynton, Manager
J Gary Nichols, State Librarian
Melora Norman, Manager

Summer reading programs, cassette books and magazines, children's books on cassette, home visits and other reference materials on blindness and other handicaps.
Newsl./BiAnnual

4609 New England Regional Genetics Group
P.O.Box 920288
Needham, MA 02492-4 781-444-0126
FAX: 781-444-0127
e-mail: mfgnergg@verizon.net
www.nergg.org

Marinell Newtown, President
Jennifer Walsh, Secretary
Merrill Henderson, Treasurer
Mary Frances Garber, MS, CGC, Executive Director

New Englands primary network for collaborative exchange of genetic health information and education.

4610 Portland Public Library
5 Monument Sq
Portland, ME 04101-4072 207-871-1700
FAX: 207-871-1703
e-mail: reference@portland.lib.me.us
portlandlibrary.com

Stephen J. Podgajny, Executive Director
Clare E. Hannan, Head of Finance and Operations
Linda Albert, Head of Human Resources
Linda Putnam, Head of Reference and Informatio

Summer reading programs, magnifiers, closed-circuit T.V., large-print photocopier, cassette books and magazines, children's books on cassette, home visits and other reference materials on blindness and other handicaps.

4611 Waterville Public Library
73 Elm Street
Waterville, ME 04901-6078 207-872-5433
FAX: 207-873-4779
e-mail: wplhelpdesk@waterville.lib.me.us
www.watervillelibrary.org

Sarah Sugden, Executive Director
Marnie Terhune, President
William Grant, Treasurer
Cindy Jacobs, Secretary

Summer reading programs, braille writer, magnifiers, closed-circuit T.V., large-print photocopier, cassette books and magazines, children's books on cassette, home visits and other reference materials on blindness and other handicaps.

Maryland

4612 Johns Hopkins University Dana Center for Preventive Ophthalmology
Wilmer Ophthalmology Institute
600 N Wolfe St
Wilmer Suite 122
Baltimore, MD 21287-9019 410-955-2777
FAX: 410-955-2542
e-mail: boland@jhu.edu
www.hopkinsmedicine.org/wilmer/danacenter

Harry Quigley, Director
Emily W. . Gower, Ph.D, Director
Joanne . Katz, Sc.D, Director/Professor and Associate Chair
Oliver D. Schein, M.D., MPH, MBA, Director

Established in 1979, the Dana Center for Preventive Ophthalmology is dedicated to improving knowlege of risk factors for ocular disease and public health approaches to the prevention of these diseases and their ensuing visual impairment and blindness worldwide.

4613 Johns Hopkins University: Asthma and Allergy Center
5501 Hopkins Bayview Cir
Baltimore, MD 21224-6821 410-550-0545
FAX: 410-550-1733
e-mail: jhuallergy@jhmi.edu
hopkins-arthritis.org

Lawrence Lichtenstein, Director
Studies of allergic diseases and individuals with allergic disease, pulmonary diseases and diseases involving inflammation and immunological processes.

4614 Maryland State Library for the Blind and Physically Handicapped
Maryland State Department of Education
415 Park Avenue
Baltimore, MD 21201-3603 410-230-2424
800-964-9209
FAX: 410-333-2095
TTY: 800-934-2541
e-mail: referenc@lbph.lib.md.us
www.lbph.lib.md.us

Jill Lewis, Manager
Diana Jarvis, Administrative Specialist
LaTarsha Wilson, Secretary
Provide comprehensive library services to the eligible blind and physically handicapped residents of the State of Maryland. The vision is to provide innovative and quality services to meet the needs and expectations of the patrons of Maryland.

4615 Montgomery County Department of Public Libraries/Special Needs Library
6400 Democracy Blvd
Bethesda, MD 20817-1638 240-777-0922
TTY:301-897-2203
http://www6.montgomerycountymd.gov/apps/libra
Susan F Cohen, Assistant Head Librarian
James Montgomery, Owner
Joseph Eagan, Branch Manager
Serves the library information and reading needs of people with disabilities, family members, students and service providers. Some of its services include books, periodicals, and videos on disability issues, adaptive technology, community information; the National Library for the Blind and Physically Handicapped Talking Book program; large print books; and computer room with adaptive technology.

4616 National Epilepsy Library (NEL)
Epilepsy Foundation
8301 Professional Pl
Landover, MD 20785-7223 866-330-2718
800-332-1000
FAX: 877-687-4878
e-mail: ContactUs@cfa.org
www.epilepsyfoundation.org

Marl A Finucane, Executive Vice President
Patty Dukes, Vice President Operations/Human
Mimi Browne, Director, HRSA programs
Chad Hartman, Director of Major Gifts
Contains information about epilepsy and seizure disorders and serves physicians and other health professionals. Provides in-house bibliographic database (ESDI), searches and documents delivery and interlibrary loans. Maintains the Albert and Ellen Grass Archives.

4617 National Federation of the Blind JerniganInstitute
200 East Wells Street
at Jernigan Place
Baltimore, MD 21230 410-659-9314
FAX: 410-685-5653
nfb.org/jernigan-institute
Mark A. Riccobono, Executive Director
Anne Taylor, Director of Access Technology
Natalie Shaheen, Director of Education
Patricia Maurer, Director of Reference, Jacobus t
Cutting-edge research and training is conducted through the NFB Jernigan Institute to address the real problems of blindness, such as model education and rehabilitation methods to empower the blind or improved instruction in Braille.

4618 National Rehabilitation Information Center(NARIC)
8400 Corporate Drive
Suite 500
Landover, MD 20785-2245 301-459-5984
800-346-2742
FAX: 301-459-4263
TTY: 301-459-5984
e-mail: naricinfo@heitechservices.com
www.naric.com

Heidi W Gerding, CEO
Mark X. Odum, Project Director
Jessica H. Chaiken, Media and Information Services Manager
Birgitta Chaiken, Research Associate
NARIC is a federally-funded library and information center that focuses on disability and rehabilitation information.

4619 Red Notebook
Friends of Libraries for Deaf Action
2930 Craiglawn Rd
Silver Spring, MD 20904-1816 301-572-5168
FAX: 301-572-5168
TTY:301-572-5168
e-mail: folda86@aol.com
www.folda.net

Alice L Hagemeyer, MLS, Founder/President
Merrie A. Davidson, Associate
Ricardo Lopez, MS, Associate
Joan Naturale, M.Ed, MLIS, Associate
A binder containing fact sheets, library reprints, announcements and other printed informational materials that are related to both deaf and library issues. It is designed to help build communication among individuals and groups within the deaf community. The focus is on assisting libraries in providing cost-effective and efficient library and information services to these consumers in a unbiased fashion.

4620 Social Security Library
U S Social Security Administration
6401 Security Blvd
Baltimore, MD 21235-6401 800-772-1213
TTY:800-325-0778
www.socialsecurity.gov

Bill Vitek, Manager
Jo B Barnhart, Chief Executive Officer
Information on social security and disability insurance.

4621 Warren Grant Magnuson Clinical Center
National Institue Health
9000 Rockville Pike
Bethesda, MD 20892-1 301-496-2563
800-411-1222
FAX: 301-480-2984
TTY: 866-411-1010
e-mail: prpl@mail.cc.nih.gov
www.cc.nih.gov

John I Gallin, MD, Clinical Center Director
Clare Hastings, PhD, RN, FAA, Chief Nurse Officer
Maureen E. Gormley, MPH, MA, RN, Chief Operating Officer
Maria D. Joyce, MBA, CPA, Chief Financial Officer
Established in 1953 as the research hospital of the National Institutes of Health. Designed so that patient care facilities are close to research laboratories so new findings of basic and clinical scientists can be quickly applied to the treatment of patients. Upon

referral by physicians, patients are admitted to NIH clinical studies.

Massachusetts

4622 **Boston University Arthritis Center**
Boston University
715 Albany St
Boston, MA 02118-2526
617-638-4640
FAX: 617-638-5226
www.bumc.bu.edu
Karen Antman, Dean & Provost, Medical School
Meg Aranow, Director
Barbara A. Cole, Associate VP for Research Admin
Christopher Dorney, Director
The Arthritis Center focuses its educational, research and patient care efforts on the diagnosis and treatment of rheumatic diseases. These include the many forms of arthritis; the auto-immune diseases such as Scleroderma, Systemic Lupus, Erythematosus, Rheumatoid Arthritis; localized pain syndromes such as tendonitis, bursitis, and carpal tunnel syndrome; and metabolic bone disorders such as osteoporosis.

4623 **Boston University Center for Human Genetics**
840 Memorial Drive
Suite 101
Cambridge, MA 02139
617-638-7083
FAX: 617-638-7092
e-mail: amilunsk@bu.edu
www.chginc.org
Aubrey Milunsky, Co-Director
Jeff Milunsky, M.D., F.A.C., Director of Clinical Genetics
Research and molecular diagnosis.

4624 **Boston University Robert Dawson Evans Memorial Dept. of Clinical Research**
75 East Newton St
Boston, MA 02118-2657
617-247-5019
FAX: 617-638-8728
Norman G Levinsky, Director
Jack Ansel, MD
Integral unit of the University Hospital specializing in arthritis and connective tissue studies.

4625 **Braille and Talking Book Library, Perkins School for the Blind**
175 North Beacon Street
Watertown, MA 02472-2751
617-972-3434
800-852-3133
FAX: 617-926-2027
e-mail: Info@Perkins.org
www.perkins.org
Frederic M. Clifford, Chairman
Philip L. Ladd, Vice Chairman
Dave Power, CEO & President
Michael Schnitman, Secretary
The Braille and Talking Book Library loans braille and recorded reading materials and the playback equipment necessary to use them. You are eligible for services if you are unable to read print due to a disability.

4626 **Brigham and Women's Hospital: Asthma and Allergic Disease Research Center**
75 Francis St
Boston, MA 02115-6110
617-732-5500
855-278-8010
FAX: 617-730-2858
e-mail: arc@partners.org
www.brighamandwomens.or
Matthew H Liang, Director
Elizabeth G Nabel, President
Arthur Mombourquette, Vice President of Support Servic
Joel T. Katz, M.D., Director
Integral unit of the hospital focusing research attention on asthma and allergy related disorders.

4627 **Brigham and Women's Hospital: Robert B Brigham Multipurpose Arthritis Center**
Brigham and Women s Hospital
75 Francis St
Boston, MA 02115-6110
617-732-5500
855-278-8010
FAX: 617-432-0979
www.brighamandwomens.org
Matthew H Liang, Director
Elizabeth G Nabel, President
Arthur Mombourquette, Vice President of Support Servic
Joel T. Katz, M.D., Director
Research studies into arthritis and rheumatic diseases.

4628 **Caption Center**
One Guest Street
Boston, MA 02135
617-300-3600
FAX: 617-300-1020
e-mail: access@wgbh.org
www.wgbh.org/caption
Pat McDonald, Director
Lauren Madden, Business Manager
Ian McDonald, Business Manager
Ira Miller, Production Manager
Has been pioneering and delivering accessible media to disabled adults, students and their families, teachers and friends for over 30 years. Each year, the Center captions more than 10,000 hours worth of broadcast and cable programs, feature films, large-format and IMAX films, home videos, music videos, DVDs, teleconferences and CD-Roms.

4629 **Center for Interdisciplinary Research on Immunologic Diseases**
Childrens Hospital Medical Center
300 Longwood Avenue
Boston, MA 02115-5724
617-355-6000
800-355-7944
FAX: 617-355-0443
TTY: 617-730-0152
e-mail: webteam@tch.harvard.edu
www.childrenshospital.org
Sandra L. Fenwick, President and Chief Executive Officer
Kevin Churchwell, MD, Executive Vice President
Dick Argys, Senior Vice President and Chief Administrative Officer
Jean Mixer, Vice President, Strategy
Organizational research unit of the Children's Hospital that focuses on the causes, prevention and treatments of asthma, infections and allergies.

4630 **Harvard University Howe Laboratory of Ophthalmology**
Massachusetts Eye & Ear Infirmary
243 Charles Street
Boston, MA 02114-3002
617-523-7900
FAX: 617-573-4380
TTY:617-573-5498
e-mail: richard.godfrey@schepens.harvard.edu
www.masseyeandear.org/
Wycliffe Grousbeck, Chairman
John Fernandez, President and CEO
Jonathan Uhrig, Treasurer
Lily H. Bentas, Secretary
Development ophthalmology and eye research.

4631 **Laboure College Library**
303 Adams Street
Dorchester Center, MA 02124-5698
617-296-8300
FAX: 617-296-7947
e-mail: admissions@laboure.edu
laboure.edu
Andrew Callo, Manager
Maureen A. Smith, President
Offers information on physical disabilities, independent living, peer counseling and advocacy.

4632 **Massachusetts Rehabilitation Commission**
600 Washington Street
Boston, MA 02111
617-204-3603
800-245-6543
FAX: 617-727-1354
TTY: 800-245-6543
www.mass.gov/mrc

Elmer C Bartels, Commissioner
Deval L. Patrick, Governor
Timothy P. Murray, Lieutenant Governor
John Polanowicz, Secretary
Vacational Rehabilitation and Independent Living for people with disabilities.

4633 **Schepens Eye Research Institute**
20 Staniford Street
Boston, MA 02114-2508
617-912-0100
FAX: 617-912-0118
e-mail: geninfo@vision.eri.harvard.edu
www.theschepens.org

John Fernandez, President and CEO
Debra Rogers, Vice President for Ophthalmology
Alan A Ryan, Director Research Finance
Frances Ng, M.B.A., Director of Human Resources
Prominent center for research on eye, vision, and blinding diseases; dedicated to research that improves the understanding, management, and prevention of eye diseases and visual deficiencies; fosters collaboration among its faculty members; trains young scientists and clinicians from around the world; promotes communication with scientists in allied fields; leader in the worldwide dispersion of basic scientific knowledge of vision.

4634 **Talking Book Library at Worcester Public Library**
3 Salem Sq
Worcester, MA 01608-2015
508-799-1730
800-762-0085
FAX: 508-799-1676
e-mail: talkbook@cwmars.org
www.worcpublib.org/talkingbook

James Izatt, Dept Head
Braille embosser, magnifiers, closed-circuit TV, adapted computers, cassette books and magazines, children's books on cassette, reference materials on blindness and other disabilities.

Michigan

4635 **Artificial Language Laboratory**
Michigan State University
220 Trowbridge Rd
East Lansing, MI 48824-1042
517-353-5940
FAX: 517-353-4766
e-mail: finaid@msu.edu
www.msu.edu

Dr. John B Eulenberg, Phd, Director
Stephen R. Blosser, BSME, Technical Director
Shawn A. Miller, Laboratory Manager
Rebecca Ann Baird, Editor, Communication Outlook
Multidisciplinary research center in the Audiology & Speech Science department, Michigan State University. Its basic research program includes speech analysis and synthesis. Applied research is carried out on computer-based systems for persons who are blind and for persons with cerebral palsy and head injury. The laboratory develops physical, cognitive and linguistic assessment technology.

4636 **Burger School for the Autistic**
31735 Maplewood St.
Garden City, MI 48135-1993
734-793-1830
FAX: 734-762-8533
garden-city.lib.mi.us

James B Lenze, Library Director
Dan Lodge, Adult Librarian
Lindsay Fricke, Youth Librarian
Marti Boyn Tamaroglio, Library Aide
Burger school for students with autism is the largest public school in the United States that specializes in the education of students with autism.

4637 **Chi Medical Library**
Ingham Regional Medical Center
401 West Greenlawn
Lansing, MI 48910-2819
517-975-6000
irmc.org

Judy Barnes, Manager
Consumer health and patient education collection in books, videotapes, pamphlets. Open to the public.

4638 **Glaucoma Laser Trial**
Sinai Hospital of Detroit: Dept. of Opthalmology
31 Center Drive
Bethesda, MI 20892-2510
301-496-5248
e-mail: kcl@nei.nih.gov
www.nei.nih.gov/neitrials

Paul A. Sieving, M.D., Ph.D., Director
The purpose of the trial is to compare the safety and long-term efficacy of argon laser treatment of the trabecular meshwork with standard medical treatment for primary open-angle glaucoma.

4639 **Grand Traverse Area Library for the Blind and Physically Handicapped**
610 Woodmere Ave
Traverse City, MI 49686-3103
231-932-8500
877-931-8558
FAX: 231-932-8578
e-mail: webmaster@tadl.tcnet.org
www.tadl.org

Metta Lansdale, Library Director
Thomas Kachadurian, President
Jason Gillman, Vice President
Jerry Beasley, Secretary
The LBPH was established as a sub-regional library in 1972 and currently provides services for 783 registered individuals in 16 counties, 171 of these registrants are Grand Traverse County residents. Anyone unable to read regular printed materials because of visual or physical limitations may be eligible.

4640 **Kent District Library for the Blind and Physically Handicapped**
814 West River Center Dr. NE
Comstock Park, MI 49321-3420
616-784-2007
877-243-2466
FAX: 616-336-3256
e-mail: WyomingYouthStaff@kdl.org
www.kdl.org

Charles R Myers, Chair
Vickie Hoekstra, Vice Chair
Carol Simpson, Secretary
Lance Werner, Director
Summer reading programs, braille writer, magnifiers, large-print photocopier, cassette books and magazines, children's books on cassette, and other reference materials on blindness and other handicaps.

4641 **Library of Michigan Service for the Blind**
P.O.Box 30007
702 W. Kalamazoo St
Lansing, MI 48909-7507
517-373-5614
877-932-6424
FAX: 517-373-4480
e-mail: sbph@michigan.gov
www.michigan.gov

Sue Chinault, Manager
Braille writer, magnifiers, closed-circuit T.V., large-print photocopier, cassette books and magazines, children's books on cassette, and other reference materials on blindness and other handicaps.

4642 **Macomb Library for the Blind & Physically Handicapped**
40900 Romeo Plank
Clinton Township, MI 48038-1132 586-226-5020
800-203-5274
FAX: 586-286-0634
e-mail: mlbph@cmpl.org
www.cmpl.org

Larry Neal, Library Director
Fred L. Gibson, Jr., President
Peter M. Ruggirello,, Vice Chairman
Barbara S. Brown, Treasurer
Braille writer, closed-circuit T.V., large-print books, cassette books and magazines, children's books on cassette, other reference materials on blindness and other handicaps, descriptive videos and bifokal kits. Assistive technology including JAWS, Zoomtext, OpenBook, and Duxbury.

4643 **Michigan's Assistive Technology Resource**
Physically Impaired Association of Michigan
1023 S Us Highway 27
Saint Johns, MI 48879-2423 989-224-0333
800-274-7426
FAX: 989-224-0330
e-mail: matr@edzone.net
www.cenmi.org/mits

Jeff Diedrich, Manager
Maryann Jones, Coordinator
Barbara Warren, Information Specialist
Provides information services, support materials, technical assistance, and training to local and intermediate school districts in michigan to increase their capacity to address the needs of students with disabilities for assistive technology.

4644 **Mideastern Michigan Library Co-op**
503 S Saginaw St
Suite 711
Flint, MI 48502-1807 810-232-7119
800-641-6639
FAX: 810-232-6639
e-mail: dhooks@mmlc.info
www.mmlc.info

Denise Hooks, Director
Irene Bancroft, Admin. Assistant
Ruth Helwig, Board Member
Robert Cierzniewski, Board Member
Summer reading programs, braille writer, magnifiers, closed-circuit T.V., large-print photocopier, cassette books and magazines, children's books on cassette, home visits and other reference materials on blindness and other handicaps.

4645 **Muskegon Area District Library for the Blind and Physically Handicapped**
4845 Airline Rd
Unit 5
Muskegon, MI 49444-4503 231-737-6248
877-569-4801
FAX: 231-737-6307
TTY: 231-722-4103
e-mail: mclsm@llcoop.org
madl.org

Stephen Dix, Director
Richard Schneider, Assistant Director
Brenda Hall, Business Manager
Michele Wittkopp, Youth Services Coordinator
Braille typewriter, magnifiers, closed-circuit TV, large-print photocopier, cassette books and magazines, children's books on cassette, home visits and other reference materials on blindness and other handicaps, The Reading Edge, and large print books.

4646 **Northland Library Cooperative**
Library Cooperative/ Library for the blind
220 W. Clinton St.
Charlevoix, MI 49720 231-855-2206

e-mail: webmaster@nlc.lib.mi.us
www.nlc.lib.mi.us

Jennifer Dean, Director
Christine Johnston, Executive Director
Roger Mendel, Director
Summer reading programs, Braille writer, magnifiers, closed-circuit TV, large-print photocopier, cassette books and magazines, children's books on cassette and other reference materials on blindness and other handicaps.

4647 **Oakland County Library for the Visually & Physically Impaired**
1200 N Telegraph Rd
Pontiac, MI 48341-1032 248-858-5050
800-774-4542
FAX: 248-858-1153
TTY: 248-452-2247
e-mail: lvpi@.oakgov.com
www.oakgov.com/lvpi

Dave Conklin, Manager
The Oakland County Library for the Visually and Physically Impaired was established in 1974 to provide access to free library service for County residents who are unable to read standard printed material because of a visual impairment or physical limitation.

4648 **St. Clair County Library Special Technologies Alternative Resources (S.T.A.R.)**
210 McMorran Blvd
Port Huron, MI 48060-4014 810-982-3600
800-272-8570
FAX: 810-982-3600
TTY: 810-455-0200
e-mail: lbph@sccl.lib.mi.u
www.sccl.lib.mi.us/LBPH.aspx

Arnold H. Larson, Chairperson
Arlene M. Marcetti, Trustee
Kathleen J. Wheelihan, Trustee
Laurie Crisenbery, Trustee
Offers library services to the blind, deaf and blind, visually disabled, phsyically disabled, and reading disabled.

4649 **University of Michigan: Orthopaedic Research Laboratories**
1500 E. Medical Center Drive
Ann Arbor, MI 48109 734-936-6641
800-211-8181
FAX: 734-647-0003
e-mail: patient-customer-service@umich.edu
www.med.umich.edu

Steve Goldstein, Lab Director
Paul Castillo, C.P.A., Chief Financial Officer
Michael ME Johns, M.D., Interim Executive Vice President for Medical Affairs
Quinta Vreede, Chief Administrative Officer,
Develops and studies the causes and treatments for arthritis including new devices and assistive aids.

4650 **Upper Peninsula Library for the Blind**
1615 Presque Isle Ave
Marquette, MI 49855-2811 906-228-7697
800-562-8985
FAX: 906-228-5627
TTY: 906-228-7697
e-mail: webmaster@uproc.lib.mi.us
www.uplibraries.org

Suzanne Dees, Executive Director
Summer reading programs, braille writer, magnifiers, closed-circuit T.V., large-print photocopier, cassette books and magazines, children's books on cassette, home visits and other reference materials on blindness and other handicaps.

4651 Washtenaw County Library for the Blind & Physically Handicapped
P.O.Box 8645
Ann Arbor, MI 48107-8645 734-222-6860
FAX: 734-222-6803
e-mail: lbpd@ewashtenaw.org
ewashtenaw.org

Mary Udoji, Manager
Michigan Subregional Library, Library of Congress National Library Service network. General library service for persons unable to use standard print materials for various physical reasons. Lends audio books and listening equipment, large type books, descriptive videos. Provides reference information and programs. Kurzweil scanner with components which convert standard print to Braille, large type or audio and closed circuit TV magnifier on site.

4652 Wayne County Regional Library for the Blind
30555 Michigan Ave
Westland, MI 48186-5310 734-727-7300
888-968-2737
FAX: 734-727-7333
TTY: 734-727-7330
e-mail: wcrlbph@wayneregional.lib.mi.us
www.wayneregional.lib.mi.us

Vanessa Morris, Regional Librarian
Sue Steiger, Librarian
Rebecca Farmer, Student Intern
Mariya Webb, Student Intern
Summer reading programs, braille writer, magnifiers, closed-circuit T.V., large-print photocopier, cassette books and magazines, children's books on cassette, and other reference materials on blindness and other handicaps.

4653 Wayne State University: CS Mott Center for Human Genetics and Development
42. W. Warren Avenue
Detroit, MI 48202-1405 313-577-1485
FAX: 313-577-8554
e-mail: rsokol@med.wayne.edu
www.media.wayne.edu

Robert Sokol, Director
Matthew Lockwood, Director of Communications
Tom Reynolds, Associate Director of Public Relations
Mike Brinich, Associate Director of Communicaitons
Human growth and development disorders.

Minnesota

4654 Century College
3300 Century Ave North
White Bear Lake, MN 55110-1252 651-779-3300
800-228-1978
FAX: 651-779-3417
TTY: 651-773-1715
century.edu

Dr. Ron Anderson, President
Steven Ritt, Vice President
Harold M. Johnson, Treasurer
Ralph Olsen, Jr., Secretary
Programs of study - Orthotic Practitioner, Orthotic Technician, Prosethetic Practitioner, Prosthetic Technician. In addition, Century College offers more than 50 other programs in liberal arts, career and occupational programs.

4655 Communication Center/Minnesota State Services for the Blind
Services for the Blind
332 Minnesota Street
Suite 200
Saint Paul, MN 55101-1351 651-642-0500
800-652-9000
FAX: 651-649-5927
e-mail: DEED.CustomerService@state.mn.us
www.mnssb.org

Katie Clark Sieben, Commissioner
Brian Allie, Chief Information Officer
Kim Babine, Director Government Affairs
Richard Strong, Executive Director
Special library service for the blind and physically handicapped providing tape and Braille transcription of textbooks and vocational materials; Minnesota Radio Talking Book providing current newspaper, magazines and best selling books; Dial-in-News, a touch tone phone accessed newspaper service; Library of Congress cassette and phonograph talking book equipment; repair services for special audio reading equipment, with most services free to Minnesota Residents.

4656 Duluth Public Library
520 W Superior St
Duluth, MN 55802-1578 218-730-4200
FAX: 218-723-3822
e-mail: webmail@duluth.lib.mn.us
www.duluth.lib.mn.us

Carla Powers, Library Manager
Renee Zurn, Digital & Outreach Manager
Davis Ouse, Public Services Manager
Dave Lull, Technical Services Manager
Main library computer lab contains one Sorenson Relay and accessibility computer with zoom text JAWS software.

4657 Minnesota Library for the Blind and Physically Handicapped
Department of Education
1500 Highway 36 West
Roseville, MN 55113 651-582-8200
800-722-0550
FAX: 507-333-4832
e-mail: charlene.briner@state.mn.us
education.state.mn.us

Catherine A. Durivage, Manager
Rene Perrance, Librarian
Charlene Briner, Chief of Staff
Dr. Brenda Cassellius, Commissioner
Provides books and magazines in Braille, large print, records, and cassettes to qualified residents of Minnesota who have a visual or physical impairment, including reading disabilities due to an organic cause certified by a medical doctor, that prevents residents from reading standard print or physically handling a book. Equipment for in-house use include magnifiers, braillers, listening equipment, and CCTV. Reference collection for in-house use only on visual impairment topics.

4658 Special U
University of Minnesota
P.O.Box 721-Umhc
Minneapolis, MN 55455 612-625-3846
800-276-8642
FAX: 612-624-0997
e-mail: kdwb-var@umn.edu

Mississippi

4659 Blind and Physically Handicapped Library Services
Mississippi Library Commission
3881 Eastwood Dr
Jackson, MS 39211-6473
601-432-4492
877-594-5733
FAX: 601-432-4478
e-mail: mlcref@mlc.lib.ms.us
www.mlc.lib.ms.us

Shellie Zeigler, BPHLS Director
Christy Williams, Director of Administrative Services Bureau
Gloria Washington, Public Relations Director
Jennifer Walker, Director of Development Services Bureau

BPHLS serves as the MS Regional Library for the Library of Congress, NLS for the Blind and Physically Handicapped. Book collections include audio cassette, CDs, digital books, Braille, large print, children's 18-20 point large print, and standard print reference collection. Descriptive videos, magazines in Braille or on cassette are available, as well as equipment: adaptive workstation, Braille embosser, closed-circuit TV, magnifier, speech input/output, and more. Check for eligibility.

4660 Mississippi Library Commission
3881 Eastwood Dr
Jackson, MS 39211-6473
601-432-4111
800-647-7542
FAX: 601-354-4181
TTY: 601-354-6411
e-mail: mslib@mlc.lib.ms.us
www.mlc.lib.ms.us/index.html

Susan Cassagne, Executive Director
Katherine Buntin, Senior Library Consultant
Tracy Carr, Library Services Bureau Director
David Collins, Grant Program Director

Summer reading programs, braille writer, magnifiers, closed-circuit T.V., large-print photocopier, cassette books and magazines, children's books on cassette, home visits and other reference materials on blindness and other handicaps.

4661 Mississippi Library Commission\Talking Book and Braille Services
3881 Eastwood Dr
Jackson, MS 39211-6473
601-432-4111
800-446-0892
FAX: 601-354-4181
e-mail: mslib@mlc.lib.ms.us
www.mlc.lib.ms.us/index.html

Susan Cassagne, Executive Director
Katherine Buntin, Senior Library Consultant
Tracy Carr, Library Services Bureau Director
David Collins, Grant Program Director

Library service for the print handicapped braille, cassette and disc materials (books & periodicals) for children and adults. Large print RG production (copier & printer), braille embosser and other handicaps.

Missouri

4662 Assemblies of God Center for the Blind
1445 N Boonville Ave
Springfield, MO 65802-1894
417-862-2781
855-642-2011
FAX: 417-863-6614
e-mail: blind@ag.org
myhealthychurch.com

Thomas Trask, Manager
Caryl Weingartner, Administrative Assistant

Offers braille and cassette lending library, braille and cassette Sunday School materials for all ages, braille and cassette periodicals, resource assistance, and resources for blind children and children of blind parents. CHildren's braille books with tactile graphics for purchase or loan. Books in digital media for adaptive reading services.

4663 Church of the Nazarene
Nazarene Publishing House
P.O. Box 843116
Kansas City, MO 64184-3116
816-333-7000
800-877-0700
FAX: 800-849-9827
e-mail: it@nazarene.org
www.nazarene.org

Dr.Eugenio R Duarte, Board of General Superintendents
Dr.Jerry D. Porter, Board of General Superintendents
Dr. David A Busic, Board of General Superintendents
Dr. David W. Graves, Board of General Superintendents

Offers braille and large print books. Also offers a lending library and cassettes for the blind.

4664 Judevine Center for Autism
1333 W Lockwood Avenue
Saint Louis, MO 63132-3252
314-432-6200
800-780-6545
FAX: 888-507-4453
e-mail: judevine@judevine.org
www.judevine.org

Becky Blackwell, President

Evaluations and assessments, parent and professional training programs, consultations, workshops, seminars, family support, clinical therapies, adult programs and support, residential services.

4665 Lutheran Blind Mission
7550 Watson Rd
Saint Louis, MO 63119-4409
314-918-0415
888-215-2455
FAX: 314-963-0738
e-mail: blind.mission@blindmission.org
www.blindmission.org

Sherry Lambing, Manager
Dave Andrus, Executive Director
Nancy Crawford, Manager

Offers Christian books in braille and large print books and cassettes for the blind and visually impaired, on loan, as well as Christian periodicals in braille, large print and cassette tape.

4666 University of Missouri: Columbia Arthritis Center
University of Missouri
1 Hospital Dr
Columbia, MO 65212-1
573-882-4141
FAX: 573-884-3996
e-mail: webeditor@missouri.edu
www.muhealth.org

James Ross, Chief Executive Officer
Mitch Wasden, Chief Operating Officer
Anita Larsen, Chief Nurse Executive
Jeri Doty, Chief Planning Officer

Research into arthritis and rheumatic diseases. One of the most comprehensive health-care networks in Missouri, our 5 hospitals and numerous clinics, all staffed by University Physicians, offer the finest primary, secondary, and tertiary health-care services. We also provide education for future health-care providers and participate in important research.

4667 Wolfner Talking Book & Braille Library
Secretary State Office
600 West Main Street
PO Box 387
Jefferson City, MO 65101-387
573-751-4936
800-392-2614
FAX: 573-526-2985
TTY: 800-347-1379
e-mail: wolfner@sos.mo.gov
www.sos.mo.gov/wolfner/

Richard J Smith, Division Director
Paul Mathews, Reader Advisor, A-CO
Brandon Kempf, Reader Advisor, CP-G & Wi-Z
Virginia Ryan, Reader Advisor, H-L

Wolfner Library provides reading material for Missouri State residents unable to read standard print due to a visual or physical disability. Book formats are recorded books on digital cartridge and cassette, braille and some childrens books in large print. Wolfner

Library also lends out descriptive videos, playback equipment for the cartridges and cassettes are also on loan.

Montana

4668 **MonTECH, Montana's Statewide Assistive Technology Program**
700 SW Higgins Ave
Suite 250
Missoula, MT 59803 406-243-5751
877-243-5511
e-mail: montech@ruralinstitute.umt.edu
montech.ruralinstitute.umt.edu

Kathy Laurin PhD, Project Director
Chris Clasby MSW MATP, Project Coordinator
James Poelstra MA, Info Technology Specialist
Specializing in Assistive Technology and oversee a variety of AT related grants and contracts. The overall goal is to develop a comprehensive, statewide system of assistive technology related assistance. Striving to ensure that all people in Montana with disabilities have equitable access to assistive technology devices and services in order to enhance their independence, productivity, and quality of life.

4669 **Montana State Library-Talking Book Library**
1515 East 6th Ave
P.O. Box 201800
Helena, MT 59620-1800 406-444-2064
800-332-5087
FAX: 406-444-0266
TTY: 406-444-4799
e-mail: mtbl@mt.gov
msl.mt.gov/talking_book_library
Christie Briggs, Regional Librarian/Supervisor
Erin Harris, Director Recording and Volunteer Programs
Carolyn Meier, Library Clerk/Circulation
Martin Landry, Readers' Advisor
The Library offers FREE alternative audio and Braille reading materials for Montana citizens who cannot read standard print materials because of a visual, physical or reading handicap. Over 50,000 titles on 4-track cassette, WebBraille, Web0pac, WebBlud, summer reading programs, braille writer, magnifiers, closed-circuit T.V., large-print photocopier, cassette books and magazines, children's books on cassette, home visits and other reference materials on blindness and other handicaps.

Nebraska

4670 **Nebraska Assistive Technology Partnership Nebraska Department of Education**
Ste C
5143 S 48th St
Lincoln, NE 68516-2261 402-471-0734
888-806-6287
888-806-6287
FAX: 402-471-6052
TTY:402-471-0734
e-mail: atp@atp.state.ne.us
nlc.nebraska.gov/tbbs/

Steve Miller, Manager
Lilly Blase, Program Coordinator
Provides statewide assistive technology and home modification services for Nebraskans of all ages and disabilities.

4671 **Nebraska Library Commission: Talking Book and Braille Service**
Talking Book and Braille Service
Ste 120
1200 N St
Lincoln, NE 68508-2020 402-471-4016
800-307-2665
FAX: 402-471-6244
TTY: 402-471-4083
e-mail: talkingbook@nlc.state.ne.us
nlc.nebraska.gov

David Oertli, Executive Director
Kay Goehring, Reader Services Coordinator
Bill Ainsley, Audio Production Studio Manager
Scott Scholz, Circulation & Audio Prod. Coor.
Summer reading programs, braille writer, magnifiers, closed-circuit T.V., large-print photocopier, audio books and magazines, children's audio books, and in braille and reference materials on blindness and other disabilities.

Nevada

4672 **Las Vegas-Clark County Library District**
7060 W. Windmill Lane
Las Vegas, NV 89113 702-734-7323
FAX: 702-507-6187
e-mail: administration@lvccld.org.
www.lvccld.org
Keiba Crear, Chair
Michael Saunders, Vice Chair
Randy Ence, Secretary
Ydoleena Yturralde, Treasurer
Summer reading programs, braille writer, magnifiers, closed-circuit T.V., large-print photocopier, cassette books and magazines, children's books on cassette, home visits and other reference materials on blindness and other handicaps.

4673 **Nevada State Library and Archives**
100 North Stewart Street
Carson City, NV 89701-4285 775-684-3313
800-922-2880
FAX: 775-684-3330
e-mail: ddeleon@nevadaculture.org
nsla.nevadaculture.org
Michael Fischer, Director
Ann Brinkmeyer, Head of Government Publications
Kathy Edwards, Government Publications Libraria
Sherry Glick, Library Assistant
Summer reading programs, braille writer, magnifiers, closed-circuit T.V., large-print photocopier, cassette books and magazines, children's books on cassette, home visits and other reference materials on blindness and other handicaps.

New Hampshire

4674 **New Hampshire State Library: Talking Book Services**
117 Pleasant St
Concord, NH 03301-3852 603-271-3429
800-491-4200
FAX: 603-271-8370
TTY: 800-735-2964
e-mail: michael.york@dcr.nh.gov
www.nh.gov/nhsl/talking_books
Michael York, State Librarian
Janet Eklund, Administrator of Library Operations
Donna Gilbreth, Supervisor
Marilyn Stevenson, Supervisor
Regional Library for National Library Service for the Blind & Physically Handicapped offers digital and cassette books, magazines on cassette, children's books on digital and on cassette, descriptive videos, playaways, and downloadable digital audio books, and Braille services.

New Jersey

4675 **Children's Specialized Hospital Medical Library - Parent Resource Center**
150 New Providence Rd
Mountainside, NJ 07092-2590
908-518-5806
888-244-5373
FAX: 908-233-4176
e-mail: jbrooks@childrens-specialized.org
www.childrens-specialized.org

Amy B Mansue, President and CEO
Robin A. Walton, Chairwoman
Victoria Wicks, Treasurer
Sueanne D. Korn, Secretary

Contains some 3,000 books, and journals specializing in nursing, pediatrics, child neurology, and rehabilitation. Also provides a Parent Resource Center, a special collection of books, videos and pamphlets designed to meet the information needs of parents and families, as well as the local community.

4676 **Christopher & Dana Reeve Foundation Resource Center**
636 Morris Turnpike
Suite 3A
Short Hills, NJ 07078-2608
973-379-2690
800-539-7309
FAX: 973-912-9433
e-mail: infospecialist@christopherreeve.org
www.christopherreeve.org

John M. Hughes, Chairman
John E. McConnell, Vice Chairman
Peter T. Wilderotter, President and CEO
Robert L. Guyett, Treasurer

A national clearinghouse for information, referral and educational materials on paralysis. Offers a free book 'Paralysis Resource Guide' in English or Spanish. Free lending library.

4677 **Eye Institute of New Jersey**
New Jersey Medical School
Suite 6100
PO Box 1709
Newark, NJ 07101-1709
973-972-2065
FAX: 973-972-2068
e-mail: bhagatne@umdnj.edu
www.umdnj.edu/eyeweb

Jacinta Ogbonna, Administrative director
Department A
Tatiana Forofonova, Program Coordinator

Ophthamology, including research into cornea, retina and neuro-ophthamalogy.

4678 **Mycoclonus Research Foundation**
Apt 17d
200 Old Palisade Rd
Fort Lee, NJ 7024-7060
201-585-0770
FAX: 201-585-0770
e-mail: research@myoclonus.com
http://www.pspinformation.com/index.html

Mark Seiden, VP

Supports clinical and basic research into the cause and treatment of myoclonus; four international workshops facilitated the sharing of information by physicians, scientists, and investigators active in the field, resulted in three publications; supports promising research projects, clinical neurological fellows, with special emphasis on posthypoxic myoclonus and encourages all who are interested in futhering the understanding, treatment, and cure of myoclonus.

4679 **New Jersey Center for Outreach and Services for the Autism Community (COSAC)**
500 Horizon drive
Suite 530
Robbinsville, NJ 8691-2951
609-588-8200
800-4AU-TISM
FAX: 609-588-8858
e-mail: information@autismnj.org
www.autismnj.org

Suzanne Buchanan, Executive Director
Genare A. Valiant, President
Kathleen Moore, Vice President
James Grasselino, Treasurer

Purpose is to assist families, individuals and agencies concerned with the welfare and education of children and adults with autism and other pervasive development disorders.

4680 **New Jersey Library for the Blind and Handicapped**
2300 Stuyvesant Ave
Trenton, NJ 8618-3226
609-530-4000
800-792-8322
FAX: 609-406-7181
TTY: 609-530-4000
e-mail: tbbc@njstatelib.org
njlbh.org

Adam Szczepaniak, Director
Maria Baratta, Assistant Director
Information Technology

Summer reading programs, braille writer, magnifiers, closed-circuit T.V., large-print, cassette, braille books and magazines, children's books on cassette, and other reference materials on blindness and other handicaps. Provides reading material on audio, cassette, large print and braille to eligible NJ residents.

New Mexico

4681 **New Mexico State Library for the Blind and Physically Handicapped**
1209 Camino Carlos Rey
Santa Fe, NM 87507-4400
505-476-9700
1 -0 -6 5
FAX: 505-476-9776
TTY: 800-659-4915
e-mail: lbph@state.nm.us
www.nmstatelibrary.org

David L. Caffey, Chairperson
Norice Lee, Vice Chairperson
Eugene Gant, Public Education Department Appointee
Dean Smith, Professional Member

Summer reading programs, braille writer, magnifiers, closed-circuit T.V., large-print photocopier, cassette books and magazines, children's books on cassette, home visits and other reference materials on blindness and other handicaps.

New York

4682 **Andrew Heiskell Braille and Talking Book Library**
New York Public Library
40 W 20th St
New York, NY 10011-4211
212-206-5400
FAX: 212-206-5418
TTY:212-206-5458
e-mail: ahlbph@nypl.org
www.nypl.org/locations/heiskell

Tony Marx, President and CEO
Mary Lee Kennedy, Chief Library Officer
Anne L. Coriston, Vice President for Public Service
Jeff Roth, Vice President for Finance and Strategy

The library provides talking books and talking book players to the five boroughs of New York City, and braille books to New York City and Long Island. These items may be circulated in person or through the mail without charge to the borrower. Deposit collections may be arranged with agencies that provide service to people with visual impairments. The library also circulates large print books and materials in other formats.

4683 **Center on Human Policy: School of Education**
Syracuse University
805 S Crouse Ave
Syracuse, NY 13244-2280
315-443-3851
800-894-0826
FAX: 315-443-4338
e-mail: thechp@syr.edu
www.thechp.syr.edu

Steven Taylor, Executive Director
Rachael Zubal-Ruggieri, Information Coordinator
The Center on Human Policy is a disability policy organization concerned with ensuring the rights of people with disabilities.

4684 **DREAMMS for Kids**
190 Whispering Oaks Dr
Longs, SC 29568-6973
607-539-3027
FAX: 607-539-9930
e-mail: janet@dreamms.org
www.dreamms.org

Janet Hosmer, Executive Director
DREAMMS is committed to increasing the use of computers, high quality instructional technology, and assistive technologies for students with special needs in schools, homes and the workplace.

4685 **Ehrman Medical Library**
New York University Medical Center
577 First Avenue
Room 117
New York, NY 10016-6402
212-263-5394
FAX: 212-263-6534
e-mail: HSL_admin@nyumc.org
hsl.med.nyu.edu

N. Rambo, Chair/Director
D. Peters, Executive Assistant
N. Romanosky, Department Administrator
J. Williams, Associate Director
Our mission of the Fredrick L. Ehrman Library is to enhance learning, research and patient care and New York University Medical Center by effectively managing knowledge-based resources, providing client-centered information services and education, and extending access through new initiatives in information technology.

4686 **Finger Lakes Developmental Disabilities Service Office**
44 Holland Avenue
Albany, NY 12229-0001
518-474-3625
866-946-9733
FAX: 585-461-8764
e-mail: folwelbe@nysomr.emi.com
www.opwdd.ny.gov/opwdd_contacts/local_

Mike Feeney, Director
Carolyn Bassett, Manager
Andrew M Cuomo, Governor
Information on mental retardation and developmental disabilities.

4687 **Helen Keller International**
Fl 12
352 Park Ave S
New York, NY 10010-1723
212-532-0544
877-535-5374
FAX: 212-532-6014
e-mail: info@hki.org
hki.org

Henry C. Barkhorn III, Chairman
Desmond G. FitzGerald, Vice Chairman
Mary Crawford, Secretary
Nonprofit international organization whose mission is to combat the causes and consequences of blindness and malnutrition.

4688 **Helen Keller National Center for Deaf - Blind Youths And Adults**
141 Middle Neck Rd
Sands Point, NY 11050-1218
516-944-8900
FAX: 516-944-7302
TTY:516-944-8637
e-mail: hkncinfo@hknc.org
www.hknc.org

Joseph McNulty, Executive Director
HKNC is the only national vocational and rehabilitation program providing services exclusively to youth and adults who are deaf-blind.

4689 **Institute for Basic Research in Developmental Disabilities**
1050 Forest Hill Rd
Staten Island, NY 10314-6399
718-494-0600
FAX: 718-698-3803
e-mail: ibr@opwdd.ny.gov
www.opwdd.ny.gov

W. Ted Brown, MD, PhD, Director
Joseph Maturi, MS, Deputy Director
Ann Marie Pannell, Director of Human Resources
Theresa Troiano, Head of Grants Management Office
More than 40 years after IBR opened its doors, its mission has grown from solely conducting research in the developmental disabilities to also providing services and offering educational programs: in 1980, IBR's George A. Jervis Diagnostic and Research Clinic opened, and since 1987, IBR has been providing educational, training and mentoring opportunities, and access to resources for neuroscience research and scholarship to over 125 graduate-level students through the Programs in Developmental Ne

4690 **Institute for Visual Sciences**
221 E 71st St
New York, NY 10021-4139
212-517-0400
FAX: 212-472-0295
www.mmm.edu/

Judson R. Shaver, Ph.D., President
Paul Ciraulo, Executive Vice President for Administration and Finance
Carol L Jackson, Vice President for Student Affairs and Dean of Students
David Podell, Vice President for Academic Affairs & Dean of the Faculty
Ophthalmology with emphasis on the development of care for the eye.

4691 **JGB Cassette Library International**
15 W 65th St
New York, NY 10023-6601
212-769-6200
800-284-4422
FAX: 212-769-6266
e-mail: info@guildhealth.org
www.guildhealth.org

Jerry Bechhofer, President
Summer reading programs, braille writer, magnifiers, closed-circuit T.V., large-print photocopier, cassette books and magazines, children's books on cassette, home visits and other reference materials on blindness and other handicaps.

4692 **Nassau Library System**
900 Jerusalem Ave
Uniondale, NY 11553-3097
516-292-8920
FAX: 516-565-0950
e-mail: outreach@nassaulibrary.org
nassaulibrary.org

Ken Ulric, President
Barbara Behrens, Vice President
Kathy Seyfried, Treasurer
Joe Carroll, Secretary
Information about public library services in Nassau County, including services for people with disabilities and the Senior Connections volunteer project (information and referral for seniors and their families).

4693 National Braille Association
95 Allens Creek Road
95 Allens creek road
Suite 202
Rochester, NY 14618 585-427-8260
FAX: 585-427-0263
e-mail: nbaoffice@nationalbraille.org
www.nationalbraille.org

David Shaffer, Executive Director
Jan Carroll, President
Cindi Laurent, Vice President
Heidi Lehmann, Secretary
Only national organization dedicated to the professional development of individuals who prepare and produce braille materials.

4694 New York State Talking Book & Braille Library
New York State Library and Education
Cultural Education Center
222 Madison Avenue
Albany, NY 12230-1 518-474-5930
800-342-3688
FAX: 518-474-5786
e-mail: tbbl@mail.nysed.gov
nysl.nysed.gov/tbbl

Loretta Ebert, Research library director
Lends audio and braille books and specialized playback equipment to eligible borrowers with print disabilities. Service is completely free. Serves 55 counties of upstate NY (Westchester and above). Also provides service to schools, nursing homes, and other facilities.

4695 Postgraduate Center for Mental Health
124 E 28th St
New York, NY 10016-8402 212-576-4150
FAX: 212-696-1679
www.dvguide.com/newyork/postgrad.html

Marge Slobetz, Assistant Director
Marie Serrano, Manager
Evaluations and psychotherapy by social workers psychologists for children, adolescents, families and couples. Neuropsychological testing and remedation for learning disabilities.

4696 Rehabilitation Research Library
Human Resources Center
Albertson, NY 11507 516-741-2010
FAX: 516-746-3298

Amnon Tishler, Research Librarian
Susan Feifer, Manager
Information on rehabilitation and occupational rehabilitation.

4697 State University of New York Health Sciences Center
450 Clarkson Avenue
Brooklyn, NY 11203-2098 718-270-1000
FAX: 718-778-5397
www.downstate.edu

Meg O'Sullivan, Assistant Vice President
Jennifer Hayes, Staff Assistant
Child psychiatry research programs.

4698 Suffolk Cooperative Library System: Long Island Talking Book Library
Long Island Talking Book Library System
2 Penn Plaza
Suite 1102
New York, NY 10121 212-502-7600
888-545-8331
FAX: 631-286-1647
TTY: 631-286-4546
e-mail: communications@afb.net
www.afb.org

Carl R Augusto, President & CEO
Kelly Bleach, Chief Administrative Officer
Rick Bozeman, Chief Financial Officer
Robin Vogel, Vice President Resource Development
Offers a variety of support services to its 55 member libraries and other patrons including, an extensive talking book program, assistive technology and other services for people with disabilities.

4699 United Spinal Association
75-20 Astoria Blvd
Suite 100
East Elmhurst, NY 11370- 1177 718-803-3782
800-404-2898
FAX: 718-803-0414
e-mail: info@unitedspinal.org
www.unitedspinal.org

Lex Frieden, Chairman of the Board
Denise A. Mc Quade, Vice Chairman of the Board
Michael B. Kinne, Secretary
Paul J. Tobin, President
United Spinal Association's mission is to improve the quality of life of all people living with spinal cord injuries and disorders (SCI/D).

4700 Wallace Memorial Library
Rochester Institute Of Technology
90 Lomb Memorial Dr
Rochester, NY 14623-5603 585-475-2551
FAX: 585-475-7220
TTY:585-475-2760
e-mail: twc@rit.edu
wallacecenter.rit.edu

Lynn Wild, Associate Provost for Faculty Development
Shirley Bower, Director RIT Libraries
Julia Lisuzzo, Director of TWC Administration
Steven Wunrow, Director of RIT Production Services
Information on physical disabilities and deafness.

4701 Xavier Society for the Blind
Two Penn Plaza,
Suite 1102
New York, NY 10121-4595 212-473-7800
800-637-9193
FAX: 212-473-7801
e-mail: info@xaviersocietyfortheblind.org
www.xaviersocietyfortheblind.org

Fr. John Sheehan, SJ, Chairman of the Board / CEO
Fr. Claudio Burgaleta, SJ, Vice-President
Mr. Victor Gainor, Secretary
Ms.Margaret O'Brien, Operations Manager
Provides spiritual and inspirational reading material to visually impaired persons in suitable format: braille, large print and cassette, throughout U.S. and Canada. Services are provided both by way of regular periodical publications sent through the mail and non-returnable; and by means of a lending library where books are returned. All services are provided free.

North Carolina

4702 Genova Diagnostics
63 Zillicoa St
Asheville, NC 28801-1038 828-253-0621
800-522-4762
FAX: 828-252-9303
gdx.net

Ted Hull, President and Chief Executive Officer
Darrly Landis, Vice President and Chief Medical Officer
Ceco Ivanov, Chief Information Officer
Jennifer Gillen, Director of Marketing
Laboratory serves over 8000 primary/specialty physicians and healthcare providers, offering over 125 specialized diagnostic assessments. These innovative tests cover a wide range of physiological areas, including digestive, immune, nutritional, endocrine, and metabolic function. To date, the lab has performed over 2 million individual diagnostic tests.

4703 **North Carolina Library for the Blind and Physically Handicapped**
109 East Jones Street
Raleigh, NC 27635-1
919-807-7450
888-388-2460
FAX: 919-733-6910
TTY: 919-733-1462
e-mail: nclbph@ncdcr.gov
statelibrary.dcr.state.nc.us

Francine Martin, Manager
Carl Ginger Rush, Secretary
James Benton, President
Dennis Thurman, Vice president
Free loan of large print, braille, and cassette tape books and magazines and specialized playback equipment to registered eligible North Carolinians. Call for an application form. Collection contains general fiction and nonfiction titles. Registered borrowers may subscribe to receive descriptive videos for a one time fee.

4704 **Pediatric Rheumatology Clinic**
Duke Medical Center
P.O.Box 3212
Durham, NC 27708-3212
919-684-8111
FAX: 919-684-6616
e-mail: rabin001@mc.duke.edu
www.duke.edu

Rebecca H. Buckley, Medical Director
Michael Duke, Owner
Clinical and laboratory pediatric rheumatoid studies.

4705 **University of North Carolina at Chapel Hill: Neuroscience Research Building**
115 Mason Farm Road
Chapel Hill, NC 27599-7250
919-843-8536
FAX: 919-966-9605
www.med.unc.edu/ophth/

Ricky D. Bass, MBA, MHA, Associate Chair for Administration
Sandy Scarlett, Development Director
Cassandra J. Barnhart, MPH, Manager of Research Administration
An interdepartmental research center on the campus of the UNC-Chapel Hill School of Medicine. Mission is to promote neuroscience research with specific emphasis on developmental, cellular, and disease-related processes.

North Dakota

4706 **North Dakota State Library Talking Book Services**
604 E Boulevard Ave
Bismarck, ND 58505-0800
701-328-4622
800-472-2104
FAX: 701-328-2040
TTY: 800-892-8622
e-mail: statelib@snd.gov
ndsl.lib.state.nd.us

Doris Ott, Manager
Hullen E. Bivins, State Lbirarian
Susan Hammer-Schneider, Head Disability Serves
The Talking Books Program provides patrons with free access to cassette books and magazines. The Talking Books Program is administered by the National Library Service for the Blind and Physically Handicapped.

Ohio

4707 **Case Western Reserve University**
10900 Euclid Ave
Cleveland, OH 44106-4901
216-368-2000
e-mail: president@case.edu
www.case.edu

Barbara R. Snyder, President
Stanton L. Gerson, MD
W.A. Bud Baeslack, Provost and Executive Vice President
Steven M. Altschuler, M, Chief Executive Officer
Programs which encompass the arts and sciences, engineering, health sciences, law, management, and social work.

4708 **Case Western Reserve University Northeast Ohio Multipurpose Arthritis Center**
11100 Euclid Ave
Cleveland, OH 44106-1716
216-844-3969
888-844-8447
www.uhhs.com

Fred Rothstein, Executive Director
Basic and clinical research into the causes, diagnosis and treatment of arthritis.

4709 **Cincinnati Children's Hospital Medical Center**
University Of Cincinnati Uap
3333 Burnet Ave
Cincinnati, OH 45229-3026
513-636-4200
800-344-2462
FAX: 513-636-2837
TTY: 513-636-4900
e-mail: oopes0@chmcc.org
www.cincinnatichildrens.org

James Anderson, CEO
James M Anderson, Chief Executive Officer
David Schonfeld, Executive Director
Richard G Azizkhan, Member of the Board
Dedicated to providing the highest level of pediatric care. As Greater Cincinnati's only pediatric hospital, Cincinnati Children's is committed to bringing the very best medical care to children in our community.

4710 **Cleveland FES Center**
11000 Cedar Ave
Suite 230
Cleveland, OH 44106-3056
216-231-3257
FAX: 216-231-3258
TTY:216-231-3257
e-mail: info@fesc.org
fescenter.case.edu

Robert Kirsch, Executive Director
Peckham P Hunter, Director
Research and development center on functional electrical stimulation. Houses the FES Information Center, a resource center with a library. Publications, newsletters and videotapes for persons with disabilities and others interested in electrical stimulation are offered.

4711 **Cleveland Public Library**
325 Superior Ave E
Cleveland, OH 44114-1271
216-623-2800
FAX: 216-623-2800
e-mail: info@library.cpl.org
cpl.org

Felton Thomas, Executive Director
Thomas D. Corrigan, President
Maritza Rodriguez, Vice President
Alan Seifullah, Secretary
Summer reading programs, braille writer, magnifiers, closed-circuit T.V., large-print photocopier, cassette books and magazines, children's books on cassette, and other reference materials on blindness and other handicaps.

4712 **Ohio Regional Library for the Blind and Physically Handicapped**
National Library Office
800 Vine St
Cincinnati, OH 45202-2009
513-369-6900
800-582-0335
FAX: 513-369-3111
TTY: 516-665-3384
e-mail: info@cincinnatilibrary.org
www.cincinnatilibrary.org

Kimber L. Fender, Director
Ross A Wright, President
Paul G Sittenfeld, Vice President
Elizabeth H LaMachhia, Secretary
Summer reading programs, braille writer, magnifiers, closed-circuit T.V., large-print photocopier, cassette books and magazines,

children's books on cassette, and other reference materials on blindness and other handicaps.

4713 State Library of Ohio: Talking Book Program
National Library Service in Washington
Ste 100
274 E 1st Ave
Columbus, OH 43201-3692
614-644-7061
800-686-1531
FAX: 614-466-3584
e-mail: jbudler@sloma.state.oh.us
library.ohio.gov

Jo Budler, Manager
Jim Buchman, Dir Patron & Catalog Services
Peter Bates, Deputy Director
A machine-lending agency for the visually impaired. Provides free recorded books, and magazines to approximately 26,000 eligible blind, visually impaired, physically handicapped, and reading disabled Ohio residents.

Oklahoma

4714 Oklahoma Library for the Blind & Physically Handicapped
300 NE 18th St
Oklahoma City, OK 73105-3296
405-521-3514
800-523-0288
FAX: 405-521-4582
TTY: 405-521-4672
e-mail: library@drs.state.ok.us
www.library.state.ok.us

Paul Adams, Library Director
Vicky Golightly, Public Information Officer
Braille writer, magnifiers, closed-circuit T.V., large-print photocopier, cassette books and magazines, children's books on cassette, home visits and other reference materials on blindness and other handicaps.

4715 Oklahoma Medical Research Foundation
825 NE 13th St
Oklahoma City, OK 73104-5097
405-271-6673
800-522-0211
FAX: 405-271-7510
e-mail: contact@omrf.org
www.omrf.org

Dr. Stephen Prescott, President
Mike D. 'Chip' Morgan, Executive VP and COO
Adam Cohen, Senior VP and General Counsel
Lisa Day, VP of Business and Government Affairs
Focuses on arthritis and muscoloskeletal disease research.

4716 Tulsa City-County Library System: Outreach Services
Tulsa City: County Library System
400 Civic Centre
Tulsa, OK 74103-3857
918-549-7323
FAX: 918-596-2841
e-mail: os@tulsalibrary.org
www.ohsu.edu

Susan Babbitt, Manager
Linda Saferite, Director
Homebound delivery of library services for the physically disabled.

Oregon

4717 Oregon Health Sciences University, Elks' Children's Eye Clinic
Casey Eye Institute
3181 S.W. Sam Jackson Park Rd.
Portland, OR 97239-3098
503-494-3000
888-222-8311
FAX: 503-494-4286
e-mail: Roystere@ohsu.edu
www.ohsucasey.com

Earl A Palmer, Director
Eleen Reyster, Clinic Manager
James Rosenbaum, Manager
The elks children's eye clinic is the major charitable project of the Oregon State Elks association. The clinic would not be possible without the organization's dedication and commitment to providing eye care for babies and children.

4718 Oregon Talking Book & Braille Services
250 Winter St NE
Salem, OR 97301-3950
503-378-5389
800-452-0292
FAX: 503-585-8059
TTY: 503-378-4334
e-mail: tbabs.info@state.or.us
www.oregon.gov/OSL/TBABS/Pages/index.aspx

Mary Kay Dahlgreen, Interim State Librarian
Robin Speer, Fund Development Officer
Susan Westin, Program Manager
Joel Henderson, Admin Program Coordinator
We serve the blind and physically disabled. Cassette books and magazines, Braille books-magazines, for children and adults. Descriptive videos. Audiocassette machines are provided free of charge. Call us for an application.

4719 Talking Book & Braille Services Oregon State Library
250 Winter St NE
Salem, OR 97301-3950
503-378-5389
800-452-0292
FAX: 503-585-8059
TTY: 503-378-4334
e-mail: tbabs.info@state.or.us
www.oregon.gov/OSL/TBABS/Pages/index.aspx

Mary Kay Dahlgreen, Interim State Librarian
Robin Speer, Fund Development Officer
Susan Westin, Program Manager
Joel Henderson, Admin Program Coordinator
Braille writer, magnifiers, large-print photocopier, cassette books and magazines, children's books on cassette and braille books.

Pennsylvania

4720 Associated Services For The Blind & Visually Impaired
919 Walnut St
Philadelphia, PA 19107-5237
215-627-0600
FAX: 215-922-0692
e-mail: asbinfo@asb.org
asb.org

Patricia C. Johnson, President and CEO
Dolores Ferrara-Godzieba, Director
John Corrigan, Director
Derby Ewing, Director HumanService
A service of Associated Services for the Blind. 26 magazines are available on cassette through this subscription service. A magazine list can be sent, in both large print and on audio cassette.
$18.00

4721 Carnegie Library of Pittsburgh Library for the Blind & Physically Handicapped
4400 Forbes Ave
Pittsburgh, PA 15213-4007 412-622-3114
800-242-0586
FAX: 412-687-2442
e-mail: info@carnegielibrary.org
carnegielibrary.org

Cathy Chaparro, Manager
Sue Murdock, Manager
Jane Dayton, Assistant Director
Jacqueline Flanagan, Executive Director

Loans recorded books/magazines and playback equipment, large print books and described videos to western PA residents unable to use standard printed materials due to a visual, physical, or physically-based reading disability.

4722 Free Library of Philadelphia: Library for the Blind and Physically Handicapped
1901 Vine Street
Philadelphia, PA 19103 215-686-5322
e-mail: reardons@freelibrary.org
www.library.phila.gov

Tobey Gordon Dichter, Chair
Richard A. Greenawalt, First Vice Chair
Miriam Spector, Vice Chair
Siobhan A. Reardon, President and Director

Summer reading programs for children and teens. Closed-circuit T.V.for enlarging print for low vision; computers with screen readers and large print; cassette books and magazines; braille books and magazines; and descriptive videos for the blind and visually impaired. Unique and acclaimed adult education program for all disabilities. State of the art book recording facilities.

4723 Pennsylvania College of Optometry Eye Institute
8360 Old York Rd
Elkins Park, PA 19027-1598 215-780-1400
FAX: 215-780-1336
www.pco.edu

4724 Reading Rehabilitation Hospital
Box 250
Rr 1
Reading, PA 19607 610-796-6297
FAX: 610-796-6353
rehab.fsnhospitals.com/USA/PA/Pottstow

Richard Kruczek, CEO
Doug Mehrkam, Owner

Information on physical disabilities, stroke, head injuries, aging and spinal cord injuries.

Rhode Island

4725 Office Of Library & Information Services for the Blind and Physically Handicapped
1 Capitol Hill
4th Floor
Providence, RI 02908-5803 401-574-9300
FAX: 401-574-9320
e-mail: olis.webmaster@olis.ri.gov
www.olis.ri.gov

Howard Boksenbaum, Chief Library Officer
Chaichin Chen, Library Program Specialist: LORI
Debbie Cullerton, Information Services Technician:
Jeremy Cutler, Information Services Technician

Offers information and services for the visually impaired including reference materials, braille printers, braille writers, large-print books and more.

4726 Talking Books Plus
Library for the Blind & Physically Handicapped
1 Capitol Hill
4th Floor
Providence, RI 02908-5803 401-574-9300
FAX: 401-574-9320
e-mail: olis.webmaster@olis.ri.gov
www.olis.ri.gov

Howard Boksenbaum, Chief Library Officer
Chaichin Chen, Library Program Specialist: LORI
Debbie Cullerton, Information Services Technician:
Jeremy Cutler, Information Services Technician

Offers talking book services for the blind and physically handicapped. Collection includes reference materials, braille printer, braille writer, large-print books, adaptive computer workstations and referrals to appropriate agencies/programs for other services.

South Carolina

4727 Medical University of South Carolina Arthritis Clinical/Research Center
171 Ashley Avenue
Charleston, SC 29425-100 843-792-1414
800-424-MUSC
FAX: 843-792-7121
academicdepartments.musc.edu/musc/

Jennie Ariail, Director
Tom Gasque Smith, Associate Director
Dr. David Cole, President
Mark S Sothmann, Ph.D., Vice President for Academic Affairs and Provost

Offers patient care services and basic and clinical research on various types of arthritis and connective tissue diseases.

4728 South Carolina State Library
1500 Senate Street
P.O.Box 11469
Columbia, SC 29211-1469 803-734-8026
FAX: 803-734-4757
e-mail: reference@statelibrary.sc.gov
statelibrary.sc.gov

Debbie Anderson,, Administrative Coordinator
Flora A. DuBose, Administrative Specialist
Leesa Benggio, Acting Director
Paula James, Director of Finance and Administration

Summer reading programs, braille writer, magnifiers, closed-circuit T.V., large-print photocopier, cassette books and magazines, children's books on cassette, home visits and other reference materials on blindness and other handicaps.

South Dakota

4729 South Dakota State Library
800 Governors Dr
Pierre, SD 57501-2294 605-773-3131
800-423-6665
FAX: 605-773-6962
TTY: 605-773-4950
e-mail: library@state.sd.us
library.sd.gov

Dr. Lesta V. Turchen, President
Monte Loos, Vice President
Sarah Easter, Secretary
Daria Bossman, State Librarian

Summer reading programs, braille writer, magnifiers, closed-circuit T.V., large-print photocopier, cassette books and magazines, children's books on cassette, home visits and other reference materials on blindness and other handicaps.

Tennessee

4730 **Tennessee Library for the Blind and Physically Handicapped**
Tennessee State Library Archives
403 7th Ave N
Nashville, TN 37243-1409
615-741-3915
800-342-3308
FAX: 615-532-8856
e-mail: tlbph.tsla@tn.gov
www.tennessee.gov/tsla/lbph/
Ruth Hemphill, Director
Ed Byrne, Assistant Director
Blake Fontenay, Communications Director
Provides free public library service to residents of Tennessee who are unable to read standard print due to a physical disability. Co-operating library with national network of libraries serving people with print disabilities, operating under the auspices

Texas

4731 **Baylor College of Medicine Birth Defects Center**
One Baylor Plaza
Houston, TX 77030-2348
713-798-4951
FAX: 832-825-3141
www.bcm.edu/obgyn/tcfs
Frank Greenberg, Director
Dr. Paul Klotman, President
One of the few centers in the world that performs fetal surgery. Provides integrated, multidisciplinary care for mothers, carrying babies with genetic or anatomic birth defects requiring therapy before or immediately after birth. This collaboration enable.

4732 **Baylor College of Medicine: Cullen Eye Institute**
Baylor College of Medicine
One Baylor Plaza
Houston, TX 77030-2743
713-798-4951
888-562-3937
FAX: 713-798-1521
http://www.bcm.edu/eye/index.cfm?pmid=0
Dan B. Jones, Professor and Chair
Al Vaughan, Manager
Michael Cassidy, Plant Manager
Dr. Paul Klotman, President
Research activities focus on restoring vision and preventing blindness through a better understanding of the disease.

4733 **Brown-Heatly Library**
4800 N Lamar Blvd
P O Box 149198
Austin, TX 78756-2316
800-252-5204
800-628-5115
e-mail: DARS.Inquiries@dars.state.tx.us
www.dars.state.tx.us
Veronda L. Durden, Commissioner
Glenn Neal, Deputy Commissioner
Daniel Bravo, Chief Operating Officer
Rebecca Trevino, Chief Financial Officer
Houses a collection of books, audio and video tapes and periodicals focusing on rehabilitation, disabilities, employment skills and practices and management for the Texas Rehabilitation Commission. Houses materials on developmental and other disabilities.

4734 **Center for Research on Women with Disabilities**
Baylor College of Medicine
One Baylor Plaza
Houston, TX 77030-3411
713-798-5782
800-443-7693
FAX: 713-798-4688
e-mail: crowd@bcm.tmc.edu
www.bcm.edu/crowd
Kathy Fire, Administrator
Margaret A. Nosek, Executive Director
Martha Mendez, Secretary
Susan Robin Whelen, Investigator
Research organization dedicated to conducting research and promoting, developeing, and disseminating information to expand the life choices of women with disabilities. Conducts research and training activities on issues related to the health, independence

4735 **Christian Education for the Blind**
Suite 702
4200 S Freeway Dr
Fort Worth, TX 76115
817-920-0044
FAX: 817-920-0777
e-mail: bceb@evl.net
Rodger Dyer, Executive Director
Offers braille and large print books and cassettes for the visually impaired.

4736 **Houston Public Library: Access Center**
500 McKinney St
Houston, TX 77002-5000
832-393-1313
FAX: 832-393-1474
TTY:832-393-1539
e-mail: website@hpl.lib.tx.us
houstonlibrary.org
Rhea Brown Lawson, Director
Roosevelt Weeks, Deputy Director
Greg Simpson, Assistant Director
Offers full library services to the visually and hearing impaired in Houston, TX at no charge. Houses unique and critical services for its users including online access to the Internet in a private and secure area.

4737 **Talking Book Program/Texas State Library**
Talking Book Program
1201 Brazos St.
PO Box 12927
Austin, TX 78711-2927
512-463-5458
800-252-9605
FAX: 512-936-0685
e-mail: tbp.services@tsl.state.tx.us
www.texastalkingbooks.org
Ava M Smith, Director
Providing free library service to Texans of all ages who are unable to read standard print material due to visual, physical, or reading disabilities-whether permanent or temporary. The program offers more than 80,000 titles in fiction and nonfiction, plus 80 national magazines for adults and children.

4738 **University of Texas Southwestern Medical Center/Allergy & Immunology**
5323 Harry Hines Blvd
Dallas, TX 75390-7208
214-648-3111
e-mail: philip.schoch@utsouthwestern.edu
www.utsouthwestern.edu
Diane Jeffries, Director
Priscilla Alderman, Executive Assistant
Daniel K Podolsky, President
Mission is to improve the health care in our community, Texas, our nation, and the world through innovation and education. To educate the next generation of leaders in patient care, biomedical science and disease prevention. To conduct high-impact, intern

4739 **University of Texas at Austin Library**
101 E 21st St
Austin, TX 78712-900
512-495-4350
FAX: 512-495-4347
e-mail: webform@lib.utexas.edu
www.lib.utexas.edu

Douglas Dempster, Manager
Sheldon Ekland-Olson, Chief Executive Officer
Dr. Fred Heath, Vice Provost and Director
Provides access to information for all users, including those with disabilities, in accordance with the overall mission of the General Libraries of the University of Texas at Austin.

Utah

4740 **Utah State Library Division: Program for the Blind and Disabled**
250 North 1950 West
Suite A
Salt Lake City, UT 84116- 7901
801-715-6789
800-662-5540
FAX: 801-715-6767
TTY: 801-715-6721
e-mail: blind@utah.gov
www.blindlibrary.utah.gov

Donna Morris, Director
Lisa Nelson, Program Manager
Michael Sweeney, Readers Advisor Librarian
Scott Brooks, Multistate Manager
The Program for the Blind and Disabled provides the kinds of materials found in public libraries in formats accessible to the blind and disabled. Books and magazines are available in braille, in large print, on audio cassettes, and on audio digital books. Services are provided by the Utah State Library Division in cooperation with the Library of Congress, National Library Service for the Blind and Physically Handicapped. Services are provided free of charge to eligible readers.

Vermont

4741 **Vermont Department of Libraries - Special Services Unit**
578 Paine Tpke N
Berlin, VT 05602
802-828-3273
800-479-1711
FAX: 802-828-3109
e-mail: lib.ssu@state.vt.us.
www.libraries.vermont.gov/ssu

Teresa Faust, Special Services Librarian
Sara Blow, Library Assistant
Jennifer Hart, Librarian
Aidan Sammis, Library Assistant
Regional network library pf the National Library Service for the Blind & Physically Handicapped. The SSU makes available reading material in large print and NLS talking book formats, including these special collections: children's print braille books, audio described videos and DVDs.

4742 **Vermont Department of Libraries -Special Services Unit**
578 Paine Tpke N
Berlin, VT 05602-9139
802-828-3273
800-479-1711
FAX: 802-828-3109
e-mail: lib.ssu@state.vt.us
www.libraries.vermont.gov/ssu

Teresa Faust, Special Services Librarian
Sara Blow, Library Assistant
Jennifer Hart, Librarian
Aidan Sammis, Library Assistant

Virginia

4743 **Access Services**
Fairfax County Public Library
12000 Government Center Pkwy
Suite 123
Fairfax, VA 22035-1
703-324-7329
FAX: 703-222-3193
TTY:703-324-8365
e-mail: access@fairfaxcounty.gov
fairfaxcounty.gov

Janice Kuch, Branch Manager
Beena Pandey, Volunteer Coordinator
Ken Plummer, Outreach Manager
Offers talking books, TDD access, assistive devices such as decoders for three-week loans, support groups for people who are visually impaired, adapted computer work station with braille printer and assistive listening devices.

4744 **Alexandria Library Talking Book Service**
5005 Duke St
Alexandria, VA 22304-2903
703-746-1702
FAX: 703-519-5917
TTY:703-519-5911
e-mail: emccaffrey@alexandria.lib.va.us
www.alexandria.lib.va.us

Rose T. Dawson, Director
Renee DiPilato, Deputy Director
Linda Wesson, Communications Officer
Kym Robertson, Talking Book Service
Summer reading programs, braille writer, magnifiers, closed-circuit T.V., large-print photocopier, cassette books and magazines, children's books on cassette, home visits and other reference materials on blindness and other handicaps.

4745 **Arlington County Department of Libraries**
Arlington County Library
1015 N Quincy St
Arlington, VA 22201-4603
703-228-5990
FAX: 703-228-7720
TTY:703-228-6320
e-mail: libraries@arlingtonva.us
arlingtonva.us

Diane Kresh, Director
Margaret Brown, Chief
Anne Gable, Administrative Services/Technology Division Chief
Peter Golkin, Public Information Officer
Summer reading programs, braille writer, magnifiers, closed-circuit T.V., large-print photocopier, cassette books and magazines, children's books on cassette, home visits and other reference materials on blindness and other handicaps.

4746 **Braille Circulating Library for the Blind**
2700 Stuart Ave
Richmond, VA 23220-3305
804-359-3743
FAX: 804-359-4777
bclministries.org

Rev. Brian J Barton, Sr., Executive Director
Offers library materials for the blind and visually impaired on a free-loan basis. Serves the entire USA and 41 foreign countries with cassette tapes, reel to reel tapes, braille books, large print books along with talking book records.

4747 **Central Rappahannock Regional Library**
1201 Caroline St
Fredericksburg, VA 22401-3701
540-372-1144
FAX: 540-899-9867
TTY:540-371-9165
e-mail: webmaster@crrl.org
www.librarypoint.org

Donna Cote, Executive Director
Alison Heartwell, Librarian
Offers reference materials on blindness and other disabilities.

4748 Council for Exceptional Children
2900 Crystal Drive
Suite 1000
Arlington, VA 22202-3557 888-232-7733
FAX: 703-264-9494
e-mail: service@cec.sped.org
www.cec.sped.org

Robin D. Brewer, President
James P. Heiden, President Elect
Christy A. Chambers, Immediate Past President

Members are teachers, college faculty members, administrators, supervisors and others concerned with the education and welfare of visually handicapped and blind children and youth. This is a division of the Council For Exceptional Children.

4749 James Branch Cabell Library
Virginia Commonwealth University
901 Park Avenue
PO Box 842033
Richmond, VA 23284-2033 804-828-1110
866-828-2665
866-828-2665
FAX: 804-828-0151
e-mail: library@vcu.edu
www.library.vcu.edu

John Birch, Media Specialist II
Wesley Chenault, Head
Yuki Hibben, Assistant Head
Ray Bonis, Coordinator

Provides individualized orientations and assistance with library research and equipment.

4750 Newport News Public Library System
2400 Washington Ave
3rd Floor
Newport News, VA 23607- 4301 757-926-8000
FAX: 757-926-1365
e-mail: icieszyn@ci.newport-news.va.us
newportnewsva.com

Thomas P. Herbert, P.E., Chair
Wendy C. Drucker, Vice Chair
Sam Workman, Assistant Director of Development
Matt Johnson, Business Retention Coordinator

Summer reading programs, braille writer, magnifiers, closed-circuit T.V., large-print photocopier, cassette books and magazines, children's books on cassette, home visits and other reference materials on blindness and other handicaps.

4751 Northern Virginia Resource Center for Deafand Hard of Hearing Persons
3951 Pender Dr
Suite 130
Fairfax, VA 22030-6035 703-352-9056
FAX: 703-352-9058
TTY:703-352-9056
e-mail: info@nvrc.org
nvrc.org

William Boyd, Chair
Jim Faughnan, Vice Chair
Steve Williams, Treasurer
Donna Grossman, Secretary

Empowering deaf and hard of hearing individuals and their families through education, advocacy and community involvement.

4752 Roanoke City Public Library System
706 S Jefferson St
Roanoke, VA 24016-5191 540-853-2473
FAX: 540-853-1781
e-mail: main.library@roanokeva.gov
www.roanokegov.com/library

Michael L. Ramsey, President
Barbara Lemon, Vice President

Summer reading programs, braille writer, magnifiers, closed-circuit T.V., large-print photocopier, cassette books and magazines, children's books on cassette, home visits and other reference materials on blindness and other handicaps.

4753 Staunton Public Library Talking Book Center
1 Churchville Ave
Staunton, VA 24401-3229 540-885-6215
800-995-6215
FAX: 540-332-3906
e-mail: talking books@ci.staunton.va.us
www.talkingbookcenter.org

Lisa Eye, Reader Advisor
Lynn Harris, President
Daniel Swift, Treasurer
Betsy Little, Secretary

Offers free library service by circulating recorded books, magazines, and playback equipment to individuals unable to use standard print materials because of visual or physical impairment.

4754 University of Virginia Health System General Clinical Research Group
P.O.Box 800787
Charlottesville, VA 22908-0787 434-924-2394
FAX: 434-924-9960
e-mail: gcrc@virginia.edu
gcrc.med.virginia.edu

Pamela Sprouse, Administrator
Eugene J. Barrett, Program Director
Mary Lee Vance, Associate Director

Provides investigators with the specialized resources necessary to conduct advanced clinical research. The facility includes ten inpatient beds, skilled research nurses, a core assay laboratory, a metabolic kitchen, outpatient facilities, computing and st

4755 Virginia Autism Resource Center
4100 Price Club Blvd
PO Box 842020
Richmond, Virginia, VA 23284-2020 804-674-8888
877-667-7771
877- -
FAX: 804-276-3970
e-mail: info@varc.org
www.varc.org

Carol Schall, Ph.D., Director
Florence McLeod, Administrative Assistant
Dawn Hendricks, Ph.D., Faculty/instructor

VARC promotes and facilitates best practices for those diagnosed within the autism spectrum. Information, resources, and education and training help parents, educators, service providers and medical professionals provide effective support from early childhood through adulthood.

4756 Virginia Beach Public Library Special Services Library
936 Independence Blvd
Virginia Beach, VA 23455-6006 757-385-2680
FAX: 757-464-6741
e-mail: spaddock@vbgov.com
www.vbgov.com/dept/library

Marcy Sims, Library Director
David Palmer, Public Services Manager
Susan Paddock, Library Manager

A public library for people with visual and physical disabilities, braille writer, magnifiers, closed-circuit T.V., large-print photocopier, cassette books and magazines, children's books on cassette, and other reference materials on blindness and other d

4757 Virginia Chapter of the Arthtitis Foundation
2201 W. Broad St
Suite 100
Richmond, VA 23220-3937 800-365-3811
800-456-4687
FAX: 804-359-4900
e-mail: cmogel@arthritis.org
www.arthritis.org/virginia

Gail Norman, Interim President/CEO
Terri Harris, Chief Financial Officer
Nick Turvas, Senior VP of Health/Wellness
Cecil Wallace, Senior VP Policy and Communication

Provides free information, services and counseling to the public. Services include assistance in locating and accessing government and other health care programs for persons with arthritis, referral to doctors specializing in the treatment of arthritis,

4758 **Virginia State Library for the Visually and Physically Handicapped**
395 Azalea Ave
Richmond, VA 23227-3623
804-266-2477
800-552-7015
FAX: 804-266-2478
e-mail: barbara.mccarthy@dbvi.virginia.gov
virginiavoice.org

Paula I. Otto, President
Susan C. Rucker, Secretary/Treasurer
Nicholas B Morgan, Executive Director
Rebecca Emmett, Office Manager

Summer reading programs, braille writer, magnifiers, closed-circuit T.V., large-print photocopier, cassette books and magazines, children's books on cassette, home visits and other reference materials on blindness and other handicaps.

Washington

4759 **Meridian Valley Clinical Laboratory**
801 SW 16th St
Suite 126
Renton, WA 98057-2632
425-271-8689
855-405-8378
FAX: 425-271-8674
e-mail: meridian@meridianvalleylab.com
www.meridianvalleylab.com

Dr. Jonathan Wright, Medical Director

A clinical test facility dedicated to providing the most accurate and informative data for patient diagnosis and therapeutic monitoring. With our current research and up-to-date information and various aspects of clinical nutritional medicine, our methodo

4760 **Ophthalmic Research Laboratory Eye Institute/First Hill Campus**
747 Broadway
Seattle, WA 98122-4307
206-386-6000
800-833-8879
TTY:206-386-2022
www.swedish.org

Bryan Mueller, CEO
Dan Harris, CFO
Heidi Aylsworth, Chief Strategy Officer
Naren Balasubramaniam, Chief Human Resources Officer

Color vision physiology, vision disorders and blindness research.

4761 **Washington Talking Book and Braille Library**
2021 9th Ave
Seattle, WA 98121-2783
206-615-0400
800-542-0866
FAX: 206-615-0437
TTY: 206-615-0418
e-mail: wtbbl@sos.wa.gov
wtbbl.org

Danielle Miller, Director and Regional Librarian
Amy Ravenholt, Assistant Program Manager
Mandy Gonnsen, Youth Services Librarian
David Gonnsen, Volunteer and Outreach Services

Summer reading programs, braille writer, magnifiers, closed-circuit T.V., large-print photocopier, cassette books and magazines, children's books, and other reference materials on blindness and other handicaps, online catalog, reference station with assis

West Virginia

4762 **Cabell County Public Library/Talking Book Department/Subregional Library for the Blind**
455 9th St
Huntington, WV 25701-1417
304-528-5700
FAX: 304-528-5739
e-mail: cabelllibrary@cabell.lib.wv.us
cabell.lib.wv.us

Judy K. Rule, Director
Angela Straight, Assistant Director
Mary Lou Pratt, Adult Services Coordinator
Breana Brown, Youth Service Manager

Summer reading programs, Braille writer, magnifiers, closed-circuit TV, cassette books and magazines, children's books on cassette reference materials on blindness and other handicaps, enlargers and Arkenstone Reader.

4763 **Division of Rehabilitation Services: Staff Library**
107 Capitol St
Charleston, WV 25301-2609
304-356-2060
800-642-8207
FAX: 304-766-4913
e-mail: carolc@mail.drs.state.wv.us
wvdrs.org

Carol Johnson, Manager

Specialized library with information on disabilities and the rehabilitation there of special collections: deaf and hard of hearing, visually impaired/blind, wellness center, literacy and career. The library has assistive devices such as CCTV, scanner and

4764 **Kanawha County Public Library**
123 Capitol St
Charleston, WV 25301-2686
304-343-4646
FAX: 304-348-6530
e-mail: webmaster@kanawha.lib.wv.us
kanawha.lib.wv.us

Cheryl Morgan, President
Jennifer Pauer, First Vice President
Elizabeth O. Lord, Second Vice President
Michael Albert, Board Member

Summer reading programs, large print PC option, magnifiers, large type books, cassette books, and magazines, children's books on cassette, home visits and other reference materials on blindness and other handicaps

4765 **Ohio County Public Library Services for the Blind and Physically Handicapped**
52 16th St
Wheeling, WV 26003-3671
304-232-0244
FAX: 304-232-6848
e-mail: ocplweb@weirton.lib.wv.us
wheeling.weirton.lib.wv.us

Jimmie McCamic, Chairman
Michael Baker, Secretary-Treasurer
Greg Marquart, Trustee
Anthony Werner, Trustee

The Ohio Public Library exists to provide books and related materials that will assist the residents of the community in the pursuit of knowledge, information, education, research, and recreation in order to promote an enlightned citizenry and to enrich t

4766 **Talking Book Department, Parkersburg and Wood County Public Library**
3100 Emerson Ave
Parkersburg, WV 26104-2414
304-420-4587
FAX: 304-420-4589
e-mail: bhdept@park.lib.wv.us

Lindsay Place, Talking Books Dept. Coordinator
Brian Raitz, Director

Free program loaning recorded books and magazines, braille books and magazines to people who are unable to read or use standard print due to a visual or physical impairment.

4767 West Virginia Autism Training Center
Marshall University College Of Educational & Human
Old Main 316
1 John Marshall Drive
Huntington, WV 25755-1 304-696-2332
800-344-5115
FAX: 304-696-2846
www.marshall.edu/atc/

Amanda Plumley, Executive Office Manager
Ginny Painter, Communications Director
Joe Ciccarello, Associate Executive Director
J. T. Schneider, Grants Officer

Provides education, training, and treatment programs for W Virginians who have autism, pervasive devolopmental disorders or Asperger's disease and have formally been registered with the center.

4768 West Virginia Library Commission
1900 Kanawha Blvd E
Charleston, WV 25305-9 304-558-2041
800-642-9021
FAX: 304-558-2044
e-mail: web_one@wvlc.lib.wv.us
www.librarycommission.wv.gov

Karen Goff, Secretary
Deborah McNeal, Personnel Officer
Steve Tyler, Supervisor
Denise Seabolt, Library Administrative Services Director

Summer reading programs, braille writer, magnifiers, closed-circuit T.V., large-print photocopier, cassette books and magazines, children's books on cassette, home visits and other reference materials on blindness and other handicaps.

4769 West Virginia School for the Blind Library
301 E Main St
Romney, WV 26757-1828 304-822-4840
FAX: 304-822-3370
e-mail: cjohn@access.mountain.net
wvde.state.wv.us

Patsy Shank, Administrator
Cynthia Johnson, Librarian

Summer reading programs, braille writer, magnifiers, closed-circuit T.V., large-print photocopier, cassette books and magazines, children's books on cassette, home visits and other reference materials on blindness and other handicaps.

Wisconsin

4770 Brown County Library
Central Library Downtown
515 Pine Street
Green Bay, WI 54301-3743 920-448-4400
FAX: 920-448-4376
TTY:920-448-4400
e-mail: bc_library@co.brown.wi.us
www.co.brown.wi.us/library

Terry Watermelon, President
Kathy Pletcher, Vice President
Carla Buboltz, Secretary
John Hickey, Financial Secretary

Summer reading programs, braille writer, magnifiers, closed-circuit TV, large-print photocopier, cassette books and magazines, children's books on cassette, home visits and other reference materials on blindness and other handicaps.

4771 Eye Institute of the Medical College of Wisconsin and Froedtert Clinic
925 N 87th St
Milwaukee, WI 53226-4812 414-456-2020
FAX: 414-456-6300
e-mail: eyecare@mcw.edu
doctor.mcw.edu

Jane D Kivlin, Director
Richard Schultz, MD, Director

A national leader as a full-service academic opthalmology program. Dedicated to the highest quality patient care, education, and vision research, the faculty and staff strive to provide state-of-the-art clinical and surgical patient care in a compassionat

4772 Trace Research and Development Center
2107 Ecb
Madison, WI 53706 608-262-6966
FAX: 608-262-8848
e-mail: info@trace.wisc.edu
trace.wisc.edu

Kate Vanderheiden, Program Manager

Research focused on how standard information and communication technology products may be designed so that more people with disabilities can use them.

4773 Wisconsin Regional Library for the Blind& Physically Handicapped
813 W Wells St
Milwaukee, WI 53233-1436 414-286-3045
800-242-8822
FAX: 414-286-3102
TTY: 414-286-3548
e-mail: lbph@mpl.org
talkingbooks.dpi.wi.gov

Marsha J Valance, Manager
Meredith Wittmann, Regional Librarian

Circulates recorded materials, playback equipment and braille materials to print-handicapped Wisconsin residents.

Wyoming

4774 Wyoming Services for the Visually Impaired
Wyoming Department of Education
2300 Capitol Ave
Cheyenne, WY 82002-0050 307-777-7690
FAX: 307-777-6234
e-mail: jackie.miller@wyo.gov
edu.wyoming.gov/in-the-classroom/special-prog

Ron Micheli, Chairman
Scotty Ratliff, Vice-Chair
Pete Ratliff, Treasurer
Cindy Hill, Superintendent

Services for the Visually Impaired assists people of all ages who have low vision or are blind. The goal is to provide information, education, and support to individuals with low vision in order that they may lead enjoyable and productive lives with maxim

4775 Wyoming's New Options in Technology(WYNOT) - University of Wyoming
1000 E University Ave
Laramie, WY 82071-2000 307-766-2761
888-989-9463
FAX: 307-766-2763
TTY: 800-908-7011
e-mail: wind.uw@uwyo.edu
wind.uwyo.edu/wynot

William MacLean Jr., Ph.D., Executive Director

Designed to develop and implement a consumer oriented statewide system of technology-related assistance for people with disabilities of all ages.

Media, Print

Children & Young Adults

4776 A Christian Approach to Overcoming Disability: A Doctor's Story
Haworth Press
10 Alice St
Binghamton, NY 13904-1503
607-722-5857
800-429-6784
FAX: 607-722-6362
e-mail: orders@haworthpress.com
www.haworthpress.com
S Harrington-Miller, Advertising
William Cohen, Owner
This is the personal account of a Christian physician who changed her career specialty from obstetrics and gynecology when she was diagnosed with a genetic disease that would cause her to become blind. Dr. Elaine Eng offers faith-based and psychological techniques for coping with disability. *$29.95*
174 pages Hardcover
ISBN 0-789022-57-5

4777 ABCD Newsletter Volume Reprints
Birth Defect Research for Children
976 Lake Baldwin Lane
Suite 104
Orlando, FL 32814
407-895-0802
FAX: 407-895-0824
e-mail: staff@birthdefects.org
www.birthdefects.org
Betty Mekdeci, Executive Director
Offers a variety of reprints from the ABCD newsletter on birth defects
Monthly

4778 AT for Infants and Toddlers with Disabilities
Idaho Assistive Technology Project
121 W. Sweet Avenue
Moscow, ID 83843-2268
208-885-3557
800-432-8324
FAX: 208-885-6145
e-mail: idahoat@uidaho.edu
www.idahoat.org
Janice Carson, Project Director
Sue House, Information Specialist
This handbook is designed as a guide for parents and families in Idaho who have infants and toddlers with developmental delays or disabilities. *$5.00*
68 pages

4779 Assistive Technology for School Age Children
Idaho Assistive Technology Project
121 W. Sweet Avenue
Moscow, ID 83843-2268
208-885-3559
800-432-8324
FAX: 208-885-6145
e-mail: idahoat@uidaho.edu
www.educ.uidaho.edu/idatech
Janice Carson, Project Director
Sue House, Information Specialist
$5.00
84 pages

4780 Birth Defect News
Birth Defect Research for Children
976 Lake Baldwin Lane
Suite 104
Orlando, FL 32814
407-895-0802
FAX: 407-895-0824
e-mail: staff@birthdefects.org
www.birthdefects.org
Betty Mekdeci, Executive Director
Offers updated information on the association activities, events and updates regarding birth defects and environmental exposures.
Monthly

4781 Caring for Children with Chronic Illness
Springer Publishing Company
11 West 42nd Street
15th Floor
New York, NY 10036
212-431-4370
877-687-7476
FAX: 212-941-7842
e-mail: marketing@springerpub.com
www.springerpub.com
James C. Costello, Vice President, Journal Publishing
Diana Osborne, Production Manager
Megan Larkin, Managing Editor, Journals
Theodore C. Nardin, Chief Executive Officer and Publisher
A critical look at the current medical, social, and psychological framework for providing care to children with chronic illnesses. Emphasizing the need to create integrated, interdisciplinary approaches, it discusses issues such as the roles of families, professionals, and institutions in providing health care, the impact of a child's illness on various family structures, financing care, the special problems of chronically ill children as they become adolescents and more. *$36.95*
320 pages Hardcover
ISBN 0-82615 -00-1

4782 Complete IEP Guide: How to Advocate for Your Special Ed Child
Spina Bifida Association of America
4590 Macarthur Blvd NW
Suite 250
Washington, DC 20007- 4226
202-944-3285
800-621-3141
FAX: 202-944-3295
e-mail: sbaa@sbaa.org
www.spinabifidaassociation.org
Sara Struwe, President/ CEO
Glenrae Brown, Staff Accountant
Elizabeth Merck, Development Manager
Lisa Raman, Director, National Resource Center
This all-in-one guide will help you understand special education law, identify your child's needs, prepare for meetings, develop the IEP and resolve disputes. *$28.95*

4783 Coping with Being Physically Challenged
Rosen Publishing Group
29 E 21st St
New York, NY 10010-6209
212-777-3017
FAX: 212-777-0277
e-mail: rosenpub@tribeca.ios.com
www.rosenpublishing.com
Roger Rosen, President
Ratto deals with strong emotions, such as general anger and depression, which affect these young adults and their families. The author shows them how to deal and cope on a day-to-day basis.
$15.95
ISBN 0-82391 -44-9

4784 Delicate Threads
Woodbine House
6510 Bells Mill Rd
Bethesda, MD 20817-1636
301-897-3570
800-843-7323
FAX: 301-897-5838
woodbinehouse.com
Irv Shapell, Owner
How do friendships between children with and without disabilities develop? How do they compare to friendships between typically developing children? What happens to these friendships over time? In Delicate Threads, author Debbie staub helps to answer these questions through careful observations of friendships between seven pairs of children - each including a child with a

moderate to severe disability - who are classmates in an inclusive Pacific Northwest elementary school. *$16.95*

250 pages Paperback

ISBN 0-933149-90-5

4785 Don't Call Me Special: A First Look at Disability

Barron's Educational Series
250 Wireless Blvd
Happaugue, NY 11788
800-645-3476
FAX: 631-494-3723
e-mail: barrons@barronseduc.com
www.barronseduc.com

Pat Thomas, Author

This picture book explores questions and concerns about physical disabilities in a simple and reassuring way. Youger children can find out about individual disabilities, special equipment that is available to help the disabled, and how people of all ages can deal with disabilities and live happy and full lives. *$6.26*

32 pages Paperback

ISBN 0-764121-18-0

4786 Enabling Romance: A Guide to Love, Sex & Relationships for the Disabled

Spina Bifida Association of America
4590 Macarthur Blvd NW
Suite 250
Washington, DC 20007- 4226
202-944-3285
800-621-3141
FAX: 202-944-3295
e-mail: sbaa@sbaa.org
www.sbaa.org

Cindy Brownstein, President/ CEO

An uncensored, illustrated guide to intimacy and sexual expression for persons with physical disabilities. *$15.95*

4787 For Siblings Only

Family Resource Associates
35 Haddon Ave
Shrewsbury, NJ 07702-4007
732-747-5310
FAX: 732-747-1896
e-mail: info@frainc.org
www.frainc.org

Sue Levine, Program Administrator
Nancy Phalanukorn, Executive Director
Rose Lloyd, Financial Operations Manager
Bill Sheeser, President

A newsletter for brothers and sisters, aged 4 through 10, whose sibling has a disablilty. Includes stories, library resources, activities and discussion of feelings. $12/year for families, $20/year for professionals. *$12.00*

12 pages Quarterly

4788 Helping Children Understand Disabilities

Brookline Books
34 University Rd
Brookline, MA 02445-4533
800-666-2665
FAX: 617-734-3952
e-mail: brbooks@yahoo.com
www.brooklinebooks.com

Hardcover

ISBN 0-91479 -09-3

4789 It isn't Fair!: Siblings of Children with Disabilities

Greenwood Publishing Group
130 Cremona Drive
Santa Barbara, CA 93117
805-968-1911
800-368-6868
FAX: 866-270-3856
e-mail: CustomerService@abc-clio.com
www.abc-clio.com

Matt Laddin, Vice President of Marketing
Mike Saltzman, Director-Eastern Territories & National Accounts
James Lingle, International Sales & Marketing

This book presents a wide range of perspectives on the relationship of siblings to children with disabilities. These perspectives are written in the first person by parents, young adult siblings, younger siblings, and professionals.

200 pages $39.95 - $45

ISBN 0-897893-32-8

4790 Kid Kare News

3101 SW Sam Jackson Park Rd
Portland, OR 97239-3009
503-241-5090
FAX: 503-221-3701
e-mail: mthoreson@shrinenet.org
www.shrinershq.org

Craig Patchin, Administrator
Michael D. Aiona, M.D., Chief of Staff
Mark Thoreson, Development Officer
Kay Weber, Public Relations

Bi-annual publication from the Shriners Hospital for Children in Portland, Oregon. Free. Produced by the medical staff.

4791 Kidz Korner

Children's Hopes & Dreams Wish Foundation
280 Us Highway 46
Dover, NJ 7801-2084
706-482-2248
FAX: 706-482-2289
e-mail: chdfdover@juno.com
www.helpingnow.org

Mariann Oswald, Manager

6 pages Monthly

4792 Laugh with Accent, #3

Accent Books & Products
P.O.Box 700
Bloomington, IL 61702-700
309-378-2961
800-787-8444
FAX: 309-378-4420
e-mail: acmtlvng@aol.com

Raymond C Cheever, Publisher
Betty Garee, Editor

These special cartoons prove laughter is the best medicine of all. It's when the laughter stops that we become truly disabled, say readers. *$3.50*

89 pages Paperback

ISBN 0-91570 -16-7

4793 Life Beyond the Classroom: Transition Strategies for Young People

Brookes Publishing
P.O.Box 10624
Baltimore, MD 21285-0624
410-337-9580
800-638-3775
FAX: 410-337-8539
e-mail: custserv@brookespublishing.com
www.brookespublishing.com

Paul H. Brooks, Chairman
Jeffrey D. Brookes, President
Melissa A. Behm, Executive Vice President
George S. Stamathis, Vice President & Publisher

This textbook is an essential guide to planning, designing, and implementing successful transition programs for students with disabilities. *$44.00*

496 pages

ISBN 1-55766 -05-7

4794 Life Planning Workbook

Exceptional Parent Library
P.O.Box 1807
Englewood Cliffs, NJ 7632-1207
201-947-6000
800-535-1910
FAX: 201-947-9376
e-mail: eplibrary@aol.com
www.eplibrary.com

4795 **Little Children, Big Needs**
Exceptional Parent Library
P.O.Box 1807
Englewood Cliffs, NJ 7632-1207 201-947-6000
800-535-1910
FAX: 201-947-9376
e-mail: eplibrary@aol.com
www.eplibrary.com

4796 **Mandy**
William Morrow & Company
1350 Avenue of the Americas
New York, NY 10019-4702 212-974-3100
FAX: 212-261-6595
www.harpercollins.com

32 pages

4797 **Mayor of the West Side**
32 Court Street
21st Floor
Brooklyn, NY 11201 718-488-8900
800-876-1710
FAX: 718-488-8642
e-mail: info@fanlight.com
www.fanlight.com

Ben Achtenberg, Owner
Anthony Sweeney, Marketing Director
What happens when love gets in the way of letting go? As a teenager with multiple disabilities prepares for his Bar Mitzvah, his family and community consider what Mark's life will be like when they are no longer able to protect him. *$199.00*
ISBN 1-572953-95-0

4798 **Me, Too**
JB Lippincott
227
227 S 6th St
Philadelphia, PA 19106-3713 215-463-3393
800-777-2295
FAX: 215-824-7390
Robert Scalia, Owner
Lydia and Lornie were twins. Lydia was a bright twelve year old who vowed to spend her summer vacation teaching her retarded sister, Lornie, how to be normal.
158 pages Hardcover
ISBN 0-39731 -85-X

4799 **Miles Away and Still Caring: A Guide for Long Distance Caregivers**
AARP Fulfillment
601 E St NW
Washington, DC 20049-1 202-434-2277
800-424-3410
FAX: 202-434-3443
e-mail: member@aarp.org
www.aarp.org

A. Barry Rand, CEO
Hop Backus, Executive Vice President
Hollis Bradwell III, Executive Vice President & CIO
Steve Cone, Executive Vice President
This is one of the most helpful and frequently requested publications. Helps people who must coordinate the care of a loved one from a long distance.
18 pages

4800 **My Buddy**
Exceptional Parent Library
P.O.Box 1807
Englewood Cliffs, NJ 7632-1207 201-947-6000
800-535-1910
FAX: 201-947-9376
e-mail: eplibrary@aol.com
www.eplibrary.com

Library Binding
ISBN 0-785799-24-9

4801 **Negotiating the Special Education Maze: A Guide for Parents and Teachers**
Spina Bifida Association of America
4590 Macarthur Blvd NW
Suite 250
Washington, DC 20007- 4226 202-944-3285
800-621-3141
FAX: 202-944-3295
e-mail: sbaa@sbaa.org
www.spinabifidaassociation.org
Cindy Brownstein, President/ CEO
An excellent aid for the development of an effective special education program. *$19.00*

4802 **New Horizons Independent Living Center**
8085 E Manley Dr
Prescott Valley, AZ 86314-6154 928-772-1266
800-406-2377
FAX: 928-772-3808
TTY: 928-772-1266
e-mail: dhenderson@newhorizonsilc.org
www.newhorizonsilc.org
Liz Toone, Executive Director
Vicky McLane, President
Nick Perry, Vice President
Cheryl Rolland, Secretary/Treasurer
The Mission Of New Horizons Independent Living Center is to provide programs and services in Northern Arizona which encourage and empower people with disabilities to self-determine the goals and activities of their lives.

4803 **NoBody's Perfect....Educating Children about Disabilities**
Aquarius Health Care Videos
30 Forest Road
PO Box 249
Millis, MA 02054 508-376-1244
FAX: 508-376-1245
e-mail: lann@aquariusproductions.com
www.aquariusproductions.com
Leslie Kussmann, President/Producer
An upbeat, inclusion-friendly program for kids that profiles three children with disabilties. Viewers discover that accepting differences is an essential part of growing up. We learn how the kids cope and, in the process, are introduced to signing, prosthetics, and assistive technology and Braille. Videocassette, preview option is available. *$ 99.00*

4804 **On Our Own Terms: Children Living with Physical Disabilities**
Gareth Stevens Publishing
1 Readers Digest Rd
Pleasantville, NY 10570-7000 914-242-4100
FAX: 914-242-4187
www.garethstevens.com
Lisa Herrington, Senior Managing Editor
Meet Kicki, a three-year-old with Spina Bifida, battling to walk for the first time. Meet Annelie, nine years old, learning to walk again after a bad car accident. Face the physical challenges with her. *$13.95*
48 pages
ISBN 1-555329-42-X

4805 **Recognizing Children with Special Needs**
Aquarius Health Care Videos
P.O.Box 1159
Sherborn, MA 01770-7159 508-650-6905
FAX: 508-650-4216
e-mail: aqvideos@tiac.net
www.aquariusproductions.com
Video

4806 Reflections on Growing Up Disabled
Council for Exceptional Children
Ste 300
1110 N Glebe Rd
Arlington, VA 22201-5704 703-264-9454
FAX: 703-264-1637
e-mail: service@cec.sped.org
www.cec.sped.org

Robin D. Brewer, President
James P. Heiden, President Elect
Christy A. Chambers, Immediate Past President
Understand how it feels to be a disabled person in school by tuning in to the first-hand accounts of people who have disabilities.
$10.00
112 pages

4807 Rolling Along with Goldilocks and the Three Bears
Spina Bifida Association of America
4590 Macarthur Blvd NW
Suite 250
Washington, DC 20007- 4226 202-944-3285
800-621-3141
FAX: 202-944-3295
e-mail: sbaa@sbaa.org
www.spinabifidaassociation.org

Cindy Brownstein, President/ CEO
The familiar fairytale with a special needs twist. Ages 3-7.
$17.00

4808 Sibling Forum
Family Resource Associates
35 Haddon Ave
Shrewsbury, NJ 07702-4007 732-747-5310
FAX: 732-747-1896
e-mail: info@frainc.org
www.frainc.org

Sue Levine, Program Administrator
Nancy Phalanukorn, Executive Director
Rose Lloyd, Financial Operations Manager
Bill Sheeser, President
A newsletter for brothers and sisters, aged 10 through teen, whose sibling has a disablilty. Includes input from readers, library resources and discussion of feelings. $12/year for families, $20/year for professionals. *$12.00*
8-12 pages Quarterly

4809 Sibshops: Workshops for Siblings of Children with Special Needs
Brookes Publishing
P.O.Box 10624
Baltimore, MD 21285-0624 410-337-9580
800-638-3775
FAX: 410-337-8539
e-mail: custserv@brookespublishing.com
readplaylearn.com

Paul H. Brooks, Chairman
Jeffrey D. Brookes, President
Melissa A. Behm, Executive Vice President
Sibshops is a program that brings together 8-to 13-year-old brothers and sisters of children with special needs. The siblings receive support and information in a recreational setting, so they have fun while they learn. *$32.00*
256 pages Paperback
ISBN 1-55766 -69-3

4810 Special Education Report
Aspen Publishers
7201 McKinney Cir
Frederick, MD 21704-8356 301-698-7100
800-638-8437
FAX: 301-695-7931
e-mail: customer.service@aspenpubl.com
www.aspenpublishers.com

Bob Lemmond, President and CEO
Gustavo Dobles, Vice President & Chief Content Officer
Susan Pikitch, Vice President & CFO
Alan Scott, Vice President & Chief Marketing Officer
Published biweekly, Special Education Report is the independent news service on law, policy and funding of programs for disabled children. *$16.00*
8-12 pages Newsletter

4811 Special Format Books for Children and Youth Ages 3-19
Cultural Education Center
222 Madison Avenue
Albany, NY 12230-1 518-474-5935
800-342-3688
FAX: 518-486-2142
e-mail: tbbl@mail.nysed.gov
www.nysl.nysed.gov/tbbl/index.html

Jane Somers, Director

4812 Special Format Books for Children and Youth: Ages 3-19.Serving New York City/Long Islan
Fifth Avenue at 42nd Street
New York, NY 10018-2788 917-275-6975
FAX: 212-921-2546
e-mail: pleclerc@nypl.org
nypl.org

Tony Marx, President and CEO
Mary Lee Kennedy, Chief Library Officer
Anne L. Coriston, Vice President for Public Service
Jeff Roth, Vice President for Finance and Strategy

4813 The Comprehensive Directory: Programs and Services And Special Needs In The Metro NY Area.
Resources for Children with Special Needs
116 E 16th St
5th Floor
New York, NY 10003-2164 212-677-4650
FAX: 212-254-4070
e-mail: info@resourcesnyc.org
www.resourcesnyc.org

Rachel Howard, Executive Director
Stephen Stern, Director of Finance & Administration
Todd Dorman, Director of Communications & Outreach
Helen Murphy, Director of Program & Fund Development
The second edition of this publication from resources for children with special needs, inc. covers more than 3000 agencies providing all types of services, education, child care, after school, employment, residential, medical and health care, parenting programs and family support. provides 1500 pages of valuable and timely information. *$ 22.00*
308 pages Yearly
ISBN 0-967836-57-3

4814 Transition Matters: from School to Independence: A Guide and Directory of Services
Resources for Children with Special Needs
116 E 16th St
5th Floor
New York, NY 10003-2164 212-677-4650
FAX: 212-254-4070
e-mail: info@resourcesnyc.org
www.resourcesnyc.org

Rachel Howard, Executive Director
Stephen Stern, Director of Finance & Administration
Todd Dorman, Director of Communications & Outreach
Helen Murphy, Director of Program & Fund Development
A guide to the need for transition planning; plus 1000 agencies and organizations that provide post secondary education, vocational services, learning options and family support to children with disabilities transitioning out of high school. *$35.00*
496 pages
ISBN 0-967836-56-5

4815 **Understanding Cub Scouts with Disabilities**
Boy Scouts of America
1325 W Walnut Hill Ln
Irving, TX 75015-2079
972-580-2000
800-323-0732
e-mail: stacy.huff@scouting.org
www.scouting.org
Stacy Huff, Director
Colin Vv. French, Director of Administration
Chris Blum, Major Gifts Director
Drew Glassford, Major Gifts Director
Manual on how to teach and understand boy scouts with handicaps.
10 pages

4816 **Views from Our Shoes**
Spina Bifida Association of America
4590 Macarthur Blvd NW
Suite 250
Washington, DC 20007- 4226
202-944-3285
800-621-3141
FAX: 202-944-3295
e-mail: sbaa@sbaa.org
www.spinabifidaassociation.org
Cindy Brownstein, President/ CEO
Siblings share what it is like to have a brother or sister with a disability. Age 9 and up. *$17.00*
106 pages Paperback

4817 **What About Me? Growing Up with a Developmentally Disabled Sibling**
Perseus Publishing
1094 Flex Drive
Jackson, TN 38301
800-343-4499
FAX: 800-351-5073
e-mail: celeste.winters@perseusbooks.com
www.perseusdistribution.com
316 pages Paperback
ISBN 0-738206-30-X

4818 **What It's Like to be Me**
Friendship Press
P.O.Box 37844
Cincinnati, OH 45222-844
513-948-8733
FAX: 513-761-3722
www.ncccusa.org
Nancy Kennedy, Customer Service
Robert Bray, Manager
This was written and illustrated entirely by children with handicapped conditions. These contributions invite the reader to set aside any pity or prejudices and listen. Black and white, and color drawings and photographs make this book visually appealing, enjoyable for all ages. *$10.95*

Community

4819 **A Commitment to Inclusion: Outreach to Unserved/Underserved Populations**
Independent Living Research Utilization ILRU
1333 Moursund
Houston, TX 77030
713-520-0232
FAX: 713-520-5785
e-mail: ilru@ilru.org
ilru.org
Lex Frieden, Director, ILRU
Richard Petty, Program Director
Darrell Jones, Program Director
Vinh Nguyen, Program Director
Carol Bradley describes Independent Living Resource Center San Francisco's community organizing/outreach approach to serving under-represented consumers. This organization successfully reaches persons with pychiatric disabilities, environmental illness/multiple chemical sensitivities, chronic fatigue immune deficiency syndrome, learning disabilities, institutionalized persons, Chinese, Latinos, deaf/hard of hearing, and lesbian/bisexual populations.
10 pages

4820 **California Community Care News Community Residential Care Association of CA**
Charles W Skoien Jr
P.O.Box 163270
1924 Alhambra Blvd.
Sacramento, CA 95816-9270
916-455-0723
FAX: 916-455-7201
e-mail: information@crcac.com
www.crcac.com
Charles W Skoien Jr, Director/Lobbyist
Denise Johnson, Consultant
Forum for the exchange of ideas, information and opinions among clients, families and service providers. Information regarding services and assisted living programs for the elderly, mentally ill and disabled. *$45.00*
24 pages Monthly

4821 **Community Recreation and People with Disabilities: Strategies for Inclusion**
Brookes Publishing
P.O.Box 10624
Baltimore, MD 21285-0624
410-337-9580
800-638-3775
FAX: 410-337-8539
e-mail: custserv@brookespublishing.com
readplaylearn.com
Paul H. Brooks, Chairman
Jeffrey D. Brookes, President
Melissa A. Behm, Executive Vice President
Offers creative ideas and new techniques for including people with disabilities in community recreation programs. *$39.00*
368 pages Paperback
ISBN 1-55766-59-2

4822 **Crossing the River: Creating a Conceptual Revolution in Community & Disability**
Brookline Books
34 University Rd
Brookline, MA 02445-4533
800-666-2665
FAX: 617-734-3952
e-mail: brbooks@yahoo.com
www.brooklinebooks.com
238 pages Paperback
ISBN 0-91479-82-4

4823 **Disablement in the Community**
Oxford University Press
2001 Evans Rd
Cary, NC 27513-2009
919-677-0977
800-451-7556
FAX: 919-677-1303
e-mail: jnlorders@oupjournals.org
www.oup-usa.org
248 pages Illustrated

4824 **Getting the Most Out of Consultation Services**
Independent Living Research Utilization I LR U
1333 Moursund
Houston, TX 77030
713-520-0232
FAX: 713-520-5785
e-mail: ilru@ilru.org
ilru.org
Lex Frieden, Director, ILRU
Richard Petty, Consultant
A practical, nuts-and-bolts approach to help make working with a consultant a positive, helpful experience for independent living centers.
10 pages

4825 **Home and Community Care for Chronically Ill Children**
Oxford University Press
2001 Evans Rd
Cary, NC 27513-2009 919-677-0977
800-451-7556
FAX: 919-677-1303
e-mail: jnlorders@oupjournals.org
www.oup-usa.org

192 pages

4826 **Housing, Support, and Community**
Brookes Publishing
P.O.Box 10624
Baltimore, MD 21285-0624 410-337-9580
800-638-3775
FAX: 410-337-8539
e-mail: custserv@brookespublishing.com
readplaylearn.com

Paul H. Brooks, Chairman
Jeffrey D. Brookes, President
Melissa A. Behm, Executive Vice President
Choices and strategies for adults with disabilities. *$32.00*
416 pages Paperback
ISBN 1-55766 -90-5

4827 **Inclusive Child Care for Infants and Toddlers: Meeting Individual and Special Needs**
Brookes Publishing
P.O.Box 10624
Baltimore, MD 21285-0624 410-337-9580
800-638-3775
FAX: 410-337-8539
e-mail: custserv@brookespublishing.com
readplaylearn.com

Paul H. Brooks, Chairman
Jeffrey D. Brookes, President
Melissa A. Behm, Executive Vice President
This book gives child care providers the practical guidance they need to serve infants and toddlers with and without disabilities in inclusive settings. It offers information and helpful advice on handling daily care tasks, teaching responsively, meeting individual needs, developing rapport with parents, understanding toddlers' behavior, working with IFSPs, and maintaining high standards of care. *$34.95*
400 pages Paperback
ISBN 1-55766 -96-7

4828 **Independence & Transition to Community Living: The Role of Independent Living Centers**
Independent Living Research Utilization ILRU
1333 Moursund
Houston, TX 77030 713-520-0232
FAX: 713-520-5785
e-mail: ilru@ilru.org
ilru.org

Lex Frieden, Director, ILRU
Richard Petty, Consultant
This publication covers important information on why we all should make assistance to people living in nursing homes a priority. Just as important, this is an excellent summary of all the facts - quality of life, health, and costs - which support deinstitutionalization.
10 pages

4829 **Independent Living Matters**
DisAbility Resources of Southwest Washington
Ste N
5501 NE 109th Ct
Vancouver, WA 98662-6174 360-260-2253
FAX: 360-694-6910
e-mail: ilrswwa@lqwest.net

Jim Baker, Executive Director
Angela Hartford, Editor/Administrative Technician
Scott Anfinson, Independent Living Specialist
To promote the philosophy of independent living by creating opportunities, encouraging choices, advancing equal access and furthering the level of independence for all people with disabilities.
8-10 pages Quarterly

4830 **Keys to Independence**
Coalition for Independence
1281 Eisenhower Rd
Leavenworth, KS 66048 913-250-0287
FAX: 913-250-0167
e-mail: kolson@cfikc.org
www.cfikc.org

Kathy Cooper, Manager

Bi-Monthly

4831 **National Survey Of Americans With Disabilities**
National Organization on Disability
Ste 600
910 16th St NW
Washington, DC 20006-2903 202-872-4710
FAX: 202-293-7999
e-mail: ability@nod.org
www.nod.org

Michael Deland, President
Nancy Starnes, Senior Vice President
John Hershey, Advice/Resource Manager
National cross-disability organization, specializing in employment and emergency preparedness.

4832 **Part Two: A Preview of Independence and Transition to Community Living**
Independent Living Research Utilization ILRU
1333 Moursund
Houston, TX 77030 713-520-0232
FAX: 713-520-5785
e-mail: ilru@ilru.org
ilru.org

Lex Frieden, Director, ILRU
Richard Petty, Consultant
This publication covers important strategies for helping people leave nursing homes. It includes several important recommendations which CIL leaders and staffs will find useful in organizing transition activities.
10 pages

4833 **Resourceful Woman**
Rehabilitation Institute of Chicago
345 E Superior St
Chicago, IL 60611-2654 312-238-2231
FAX: 312-238-1205
TTY:312-908-8523
e-mail: hrcwd@rehabchicago.org
rehabchicago.org

Luciano Dias, Director
Kristi Kirchner, MD, Medical Director
Linda E Miller, Domestic Violence Coordinator
Wayne Lerner, CEO
Annual publication of national, not-for-profit, general health and service center providing accessible medical services for women with disabilities. Conducts research into health issues concerning disabled women and offers educational resources for healthcare professionals and women with disabilities.

4834 **Transitioning Exceptional Children and Youth Into the Community**
Haworth Press
10 Alice St
Binghamton, NY 13904-1503 607-722-5857
800-429-6784
FAX: 607-722-6362
e-mail: orders@haworthpress.com
www.haworthpress.com

William Cohen, Owner
Focusing on the dynamic process of mainstreaming exceptional children and youth into the community, experts examine some of

the exciting technological advances made to accompany the social changes enacted over the years. *$44.95*
202 pages Hardcover
ISBN 0-866567-33-X

4835 Transitions to Adult Life
Books on Special Children
P.O.Box 305
Congers, NY 10920-305 845-638-1236
FAX: 845-638-0847
e-mail: irene@boscbooks.com
385 pages Softcover

Employment

4836 A Guide for People with Disabilities Seeking Employment
US Department of Justice
950 Pennsylvania Ave NW
Washington, DC 20530-9 202-586-5000
800-574-0301
FAX: 202-307-1197
TTY: 800-514-0383
www.ada.gov
James Bostrom, Deputy Chiefs
Zita Johnson Betts, Deputy Chiefs
Sally Conway, Deputy Chiefs
Jana Erickson, Deputy Chiefs
A 2-page pamplet for people with disabilities providing a general explanation of the employment provisions of the ADA and how to file a complaint with the Equal Employment Opportunity Commission.

4837 ADA Questions and Answers
US Department of Justice
950 Pennsylvania Ave NW
Washington, DC 20530-9 202-586-5000
800-574-0301
FAX: 202-307-1197
TTY: 800-514-0383
www.ada.gov
James Bostrom, Deputy Chiefs
Zita Johnson Betts, Deputy Chiefs
Sally Conway, Deputy Chiefs
Jana Erickson, Deputy Chiefs
A 31-page booklet giving an overview of the ADA's requirements affecting employers, businesses, nonprofit service agencies, and state and local governments programs, including public transportation.

4838 ANCOR Wage and Hour Handbook
American Network of Community Options & Resources
1101 King St
Suite 380
Alexandria, VA 22314-2962 703-535-7850
FAX: 703-535-7860
e-mail: ancor@ancor.org
ancor.org
Dave Toeniskoetter, President
Chris Sparks, Vice President
Julie Manworren, Secretary/Treasurer
Bob Bond, Director
This useful publication contains the latest rules and interpretations from the U.S. Department of Labor relative to employment in residential support services for people with disabilities, including copies of enforcement policies and letters of interpretation. It outlines in detail when exemptions from miniimum wage and overtime rules can be applied,a nd when and how employees may be paid on a salary basis. Sample staffing patterns are provided.
121 pages

4839 Ability Magazine
Jobs Information Business Service
8941 Atlanta Ave.
Huntington Beach, CA 92646 949-854-8700
FAX: 949-548-5966
www.abilitymagazine.com

4840 Americans with Disabilities
Federal Consumer Information Center
Department 513j
Pueblo, CO 81009-1 719-295-2675
888-878-3256
FAX: 719-948-9724
e-mail: catalog.pueblo@gsa.gov
www.pueblo.gsa.gov
Alfred Pino, Manager
Judi Mahaney, Public Affairs
Explains how civil rights of persons with disabilities are protected at work and in public places.

4841 Americans with Disabilities Act: Questionsand Answers
Federal Consumer Information Center
Department 513j
Pueblo, CO 81009-1 719-295-2675
888-878-3256
FAX: 719-948-9724
e-mail: catalog.pueblo@gsa.gov
www.pueblo.gsa.gov
Judi Mahaney, Public Affairs
Alfred Pino, Manager
Explains how the Civil Rights of Persons with disabilities are protected at work and in public places. Free.

4842 Career Education for Handicapped Individuals
McGraw-Hill, School Publishing
220 E Danieldale Rd
Desoto, TX 75115-2490 972-224-4772
800-442-9685
FAX: 972-228-1982
mcgraw-hill.com
Joseph Gavigan, President
Based on a life-centered career education program that goes beyond elementary school level to include handicapped people of all ages.
454 pages

4843 Earning a Living
Accent Books & Products
P.O.Box 700
Bloomington, IL 61702-700 309-378-2961
800-787-8444
FAX: 309-378-4420
e-mail: acmtlvng@aol.com
Raymond C Cheever, Publisher
Betty Garee, Editor
Discusses how to prepare a person for a career, what to say in an interview, and gives examples of both home businesses and jobs away from home. Tells how to modify a worksite and how to be successful on the job. *$9.50*
88 pages Paperback
ISBN 0-91570-23-0

4844 Employment in the Mainstream
Mainstream
Ste 830
3 Bethesda Metro Ctr
Bethesda, MD 20814-6301 301-961-9299
800-247-1380
FAX: 301-891-8778
e-mail: info@mainstreaminc.org
www.mainstreaminc.org
David Pichette, Executive Director
Fritz Rumpel, Editor
Charles Moster

Reports on issues, ideas, problems and solutions in employing persons with any kind of physical or mental disability. Quarterly magazine. *$25.00*

32 pages

4845 Encyclopedia of Basic Employment and Daily Living Skills

Phillip Roy, Inc
13064 Indian Rocks Road
PO Box 130
Indian Rocks Beach, FL 33785-3377
727-593-2700
800-255-9085
FAX: 727-595-2685
e-mail: info@philliproy.com
www.philliproy.com

Ruth Bragman PhD, President
Phil Padol, Consultant

Contains developmental skills for special education students. Contains lessons in 6 curriculum areas covering 80 objects with 541 lessons. Also includes objectives, instructional strategies, and assessment tasks. *$495.00*

1200 pages
ISBN 1-568182-25-2

4846 Handbook of Career Planning for Special Needs Students

Sage Publications
2455 Teller Road
Thousand Oaks, CA 91320
805-499-9774
800-818-7243
FAX: 800-583-2665
e-mail: info@sagepub.com
www.sagepub.com

Sara Miller McCune, Founder, Publisher, Chairperson
Blaise R Simqu, President & CEO

The practitioner's guide will show you how to help special needs adolescents and young adults overcome barriers to employment by identifying goals and problems, assessing interests and aptitudes, involving client families and developing communication skills. *$46.00*

358 pages Hardcover
ISBN 0-890797-06-4

4847 Making News

Avacado Press
PO Box 406781
Louisville, KY 40204
888-739-1920
FAX: 502-899-9562
e-mail: contact145@advocadopress.org
www.advocadopress.org

165 pages
ISBN 0-962706-43-4

4848 Making Self-Employment Work for People with Disabilities

Brookes Publishing
P.O.Box 10624
Baltimore, MD 21285-0624
410-337-9580
800-638-3775
FAX: 410-337-8539
e-mail: custserv@brookespublishing.com
readplaylearn.com

Paul H. Brooks, Chairman
Jeffrey D. Brookes, President
Melissa A. Behm, Executive Vice President

Practical support for individuals with significant disabilities in starting and maintaining a small business. Covers building a business plan; pinpointing interests, strengths, and goals; and finding helpful information and support *$35.00*

288 pages
ISBN 1-557666-52-0

4849 Making the Workplace Accessible: Guidelines, Costs and Resources

Spina Bifida Association of America
4590 Macarthur Blvd NW
Suite 250
Washington, DC 20007- 4226
202-944-3285
800-621-3141
FAX: 202-944-3295
e-mail: sbaa@sbaa.org
www.spinabifidaassociation.org

Cindy Brownstein, President/ CEO

A 20 page reference guide on how to provide physical access to persons with disabilities in a cost effective manner. *$9.00*

4850 People with Hearing Loss and the Workplace Guide for Employers/ADA Compliances

Hearing Loss Association of America
7910 Woodmont Ave
Suite 1200
Bethesda, MD 20814-7022
301-657-2248
FAX: 301-913-9413
e-mail: info@hearingloss.org
www.hearingloss.org

Anna Gilmore Hall, Executive Director
Barbara Kelley, Deputy Executive Director and Editor-In-Chief
Lise Hamlin, Director of Public Policy
Nancy Macklin, Director of Events and Marketing

A guide for both people with hearing loss and their employers to learn about accommodations under the law. Includes employment guidelines, resource list of manufacturers and case studies. *$15.00*

40 pages Paperback

4851 Road Ahead: Transition to Adult Life for Persons with Disabilities

Training Resource Network
PO Box 439
St. Augustine, FL 32085-0439
FAX: 904-823-3554
e-mail: info@trninc.com
www.trninc.com

223 pages
ISBN 1-883302-46-3

4852 Supported Employment for Disabled People

Human Sciences Press
233 Spring St
New York, NY 10013-1522
877-283-3229
800-644-4831
FAX: 212-460-1575
e-mail: ainy@aveda.com
www.aveda.edu

288 pages Cloth
ISBN 0-89885 -46-6

4853 WORK

Suite 9
64511 Via Real
Carpinteria, CA 93013
805-566-9000
FAX: 805-566-9070

Kathy Webb, Executive Director

Vocational and residential training and support services for adults with developmental disabilities.

General Disabilities

4854 A Guide to Disability Rights Law
US Department of Justice
950 Pennsylvania Ave NW
Washington, DC 20530-9
202-514-4609
800-574-0301
FAX: 202-514-0293
TTY: 800-514-0383
www.ada.gov

James Bostrom, Deputy Chiefs
Zita Johnson Betts, Deputy Chiefs
Sally Conway, Deputy Chiefs
Jana Erickson, Deputy Chiefs

A 21-page booklet providing a brief description of the ADA, the Telecommunications Act, Fair Housing Act, Air Carrier Access Act, Voting Accessibility for the Elderly and Handicapped Act, National Voter Registration Act, Civil Rights of Institutionalized Persons Act, Individuals with Disabilities in Education Act, Rehabilitation Act, Architectural Barriers Act, and the federal agencies to contact for more information.

4855 A Practical Guide to Art Therapy Groups
Haworth Press
10 Alice St
Binghamton, NY 13904-1503
607-722-5857
800-429-6784
FAX: 607-722-6362
e-mail: orders@haworthpress.com
www.haworthpress.com

S Harrington-Miller, Advertising
William Cohen, Owner

Unique approaches, materials, and device will inspire you to tap into your own well of creativity to design your own treatment plans. It lays out the ingredients and the skills to get the results you want. *$64.95*

115 pages Hardcover
ISBN 0-789001-36-5

4856 A World Awaits You
Mobility International USA
132 E. Broadway
Suite 343
Eugene, OR 97401
541-343-1284
FAX: 541-343-6812
e-mail: info@miusa.org
www.miusa.org

Susan Sygall, Executive Director
Cindy Lewis, Director of Programs
Cerise Roth-Vinson, Chief Operating Officer
Stephanie Gray, Program Manager

Free publication from Mobility International USA.

44 pages Yearly

4857 AAPD News
American Association of People with Disabilities
Ste 503
1629 K St NW
Washington, DC 20006-1634
202-457-0046
800-840-8844
FAX: 202-457-0473
e-mail: aapd@aol.com
www.aapd-dc.org

Anelie Bush, Editor

Quarterly

4858 ADA Guide for Small Businesses
US Department of Justice
950 Pennsylvania Ave NW
Washington, DC 20530-9
202-586-5000
800-574-0301
FAX: 202-307-1197
TTY: 800-514-0383
www.ada.gov

James Bostrom, Deputy Chiefs
Zita Johnson Betts, Deputy Chiefs
Sally Conway, Deputy Chiefs
Jana Erickson, Deputy Chiefs

A 15-page booklet for businesses that provide goods and services to the public. This publication explains basic ADA requirements, illustrates ways to make facilities accessible, and provides information about tax credits and deductions.

4859 ADA Guide for Small Towns
US Department of Justice
950 Pennsylvania Ave NW
Washington, DC 20530-9
202-586-5000
800-574-0301
FAX: 202-307-1197
TTY: 800-514-0383
www.ada.gov

James Bostrom, Deputy Chiefs
Zita Johnson Betts, Deputy Chiefs
Sally Conway, Deputy Chiefs
Jana Erickson, Deputy Chiefs

A 21-page guide that presents an informal overview of some basic ADA requirements and provides cost-effective tips on how small towns can comply with the ADA.

4860 ADA Information Services
US Department of Justice
950 Pennsylvania Ave NW
Washington, DC 20530-9
202-586-5000
800-574-0301
FAX: 202-307-1197
TTY: 800-514-0383
www.ada.gov

James Bostrom, Deputy Chiefs
Zita Johnson Betts, Deputy Chiefs
Sally Conway, Deputy Chiefs
Jana Erickson, Deputy Chiefs

A 2-page list with the telephone numbers and internet addresses of federal agencies and other organizations that provide information and technical assistance to the public about the ADA.

4861 ADA Pipeline
DRTAC: Southeast ADA Center
1419 Mayson Street NE
Atlanta, GA 30324
404-385-0636
800-949-4232
FAX: 404-385-0641
e-mail: sedbtacproject@law.sgr.edu
www.sedbtac.org

Cyndi Smith, B.S., Office Assistant
Mary Morder, Information Technology Support
Sally Z. Weiss, B.A., Director
Rebecca Williams, B.A., M.S., Information Specialist / Technical Assistance

16 pages Quarterly

4862 ADA Questions and Answers
US Department of Justice
950 Pennsylvania Ave NW
Washington, DC 20530-9
202-586-5000
800-574-0301
FAX: 202-307-1197
TTY: 800-514-0383
www.ada.gov

James Bostrom, Deputy Chiefs
Zita Johnson Betts, Deputy Chiefs
Sally Conway, Deputy Chiefs
Jana Erickson, Deputy Chiefs

A 31-page booklet giving an overview of the ADA's requirements affecting employers, businesses, nonprofit service agencies, and state and local governments programs, including public transportation.

4863 ADA Tax Incentive Packet for Business
US Department of Justice
950 Pennsylvania Ave NW
Washington, DC 20530-9 202-586-5000
800-574-0301
FAX: 202-307-1197
TTY: 800-514-0383
www.ada.gov

James Bostrom, Deputy Chiefs
Zita Johnson Betts, Deputy Chiefs
Sally Conway, Deputy Chiefs
Jana Erickson, Deputy Chiefs

A 13-page packet of information to help businesses understand and take advantage of the tax credit and deduction available for complying with the ADA.

4864 ADA and City Governments: Common Problems
US Department of Justice
950 Pennsylvania Ave NW
Washington, DC 20530-9 202-586-5000
800-574-0301
FAX: 202-307-1197
TTY: 800-514-0383
www.ada.gov

James Bostrom, Deputy Chiefs
Zita Johnson Betts, Deputy Chiefs
Sally Conway, Deputy Chiefs
Jana Erickson, Deputy Chiefs

A 9-page document that contains a sampling of common problems shared by city governments of all sizes, provides examples of common deficiencies and explains how these problems affect persons with disabilities.

4865 ADA-TA: A Technical Assistance Update from the Department of Justice
US Department of Justice
950 Pennsylvania Ave NW
Washington, DC 20530-9 202-586-5000
800-574-0301
FAX: 202-307-1197
TTY: 800-514-0383
www.ada.gov

James Bostrom, Deputy Chiefs
Zita Johnson Betts, Deputy Chiefs
Sally Conway, Deputy Chiefs
Jana Erickson, Deputy Chiefs

A serial publication that answers Common Questions about ADA requirements and provides Design Details illustrating particular design requirements. The first edition addresses Readily Achievable Barrier Removal and Van Accessible Packing Spaces.

4866 AEPS Family Report: For Children Ages Birth to Three
Brookes Publishing
P.O.Box 10624
Baltimore, MD 21285-0624 410-337-9580
800-638-3775
FAX: 410-337-8539
e-mail: custserv@brookespublishing.com
www.brookespublishing.com

Paul H. Brooks, Chairman
Jeffrey D. Brookes, President
Melissa A. Behm, Executive Vice President

This is a 64-item questionnaire that asks parents to rank their child's abilities on specific skills. In packages of 10. *$17.00*
20 pages Saddle-stiched
ISBN 1-557660-99-9

4867 ARC's Government Report
Arc of the District of Columbia
817 Varnum St NE
Washington, DC 20017-2144 202-636-2950
FAX: 202-636-2996
e-mail: arcdc@arcdc.net
www.arcdc.net

Mary Lou Meccariello, Executive Director
Ed Cabatic, Director of Finance
Randy Shingler, Chief Operating Officer
Denize Stanton-Williams, Director of Supports & Services

Reports on government activities related to individuals with disabilities with a focus on persons with mental retardation. *$50.00*

4868 ARCA Newsletter
ARCA - Dakota County Technical College
1300 145th St E
Rosemount, MN 55068-2932 651-423-8301
877-937-3282
FAX: 651-423-7028
dctc.edu

Ron Thomas, President

Offers information on support groups, conventions, books, manuscripts and programs for the rehabilitation professional and the disabled.
Monthly

4869 Accent on Living Magazine
Cheever Publishing
P.O.Box 700
Bloomington, IL 61702-700 309-378-2961
800-787-8444
FAX: 309-378-4420

Julie Cheever, Marketing Manager

A magazine published for forty four years, serves physically disabled people, with general interest, travel, and home modification features. *$12.00*
112 pages Quarterly

4870 Access Design Services: CILs as Experts
Independent Living Research Utilization ILRU
1333 Moursund
Houston, TX 77030 713-520-0232
FAX: 713-520-5785
e-mail: ilru@ilru.org
ilru.org

Lex Frieden, Director, ILRU
Richard Petty, Consultant
Rose Shepard, Office Manager

Featuring the Access Design Services of Alpha One in Maine, this month's Readings is another of the winners of the recent competition for innovative CIL programs.
10 pages

4871 Access To Independence Inc.
Access to Independence
3810 Milwaukee Street
Madison, WI 53714 608-242-8484
800-362-9877
FAX: 608-242-0383
TTY: 608-242-8485
e-mail: info@accesstoind.org
www.accesstoind.org

Dee Truhn, Executive Director
Jason Belaungy, Assistant Director
Geri, Finances/HR
Janie, Administrative Assistant

Independent Living Center serving people of any age and all types of disabilities in south-central Wisconsin. Empower people with disabilities, through advocacy, education, and support.
24 pages Semi-Annual

4872 Access for 911 and Telephone Emergency Services
US Department of Justice
950 Pennsylvania Ave NW
Washington, DC 20530-9
202-586-5000
800-574-0301
FAX: 202-307-1197
TTY: 800-514-0383
www.ada.gov

James Bostrom, Deputy Chiefs
Zita Johnson Betts, Deputy Chiefs
Sally Conway, Deputy Chiefs
Jana Erickson, Deputy Chiefs
A 10-page publication explaining the requirements for direct, equal access to 911 for persons who use teletypewritters (TTYs).

4873 Achieving Diversity and Independence
Independent Living Research Utilization ILRU
1333 Moursund
Houston, TX 77030
713-520-0232
FAX: 713-520-5785
e-mail: ilru@ilru.org
ilru.org

Lex Frieden, Director, ILRU
Richard Petty, Consultant
Rose Shepard, Office Manager

10 pages

4874 Activity-Based Intervention: 2nd Edition
Brookes Publishing
P.O.Box 10624
Baltimore, MD 21285-0624
410-337-9580
800-638-3775
FAX: 410-337-8539
e-mail: custserv@brookespublishing.com
readplaylearn.com

Paul H. Brooks, Chairman
Jeffrey D. Brookes, President
Melissa A. Behm, Executive Vice President
This 14 minute video illustrates how activity-based intervention can be used to turn everyday events and natural interactions into opportunities to promote learning in young children who are considered at risk for developmental delays or who have mild to significant disabilities. *$39.00*
ISBN 1-55766-86-3

4875 Ad Lib Drop-In Center: Consumer Management, Ownership and Empowerment
Independent Living Research Utilization ILRU
1333 Moursund
Houston, TX 77030
713-520-0232
FAX: 713-520-5785
e-mail: ilru@ilru.org
ilru.org

Lex Frieden, Director, ILRU
Richard Petty, Consultant
Rose Shepard, Office Manager
Joe describes how Ad Lib ensured consumer control in their Drop-In Center: the DIC came about because of consumer input, and consumers are involved in planning the program; members can choose to become volunteers or paid staff members. All of the staff at the DIC are consumers; and active consumer advisory board helps develop policies and programs and provides input to the Ad Lib board.
10 pages

4876 Adobe News
Santa Barbara Foundation
15 E Carrillo St
Santa Barbara, CA 93101-2706
805-963-1873
805-966-2345
FAX: 805-966-2345

Ron Gallo, CEO

8 pages Bi-Annually

4877 Advocate
Arc Massachusetts
217 South St
Waltham, MA 02453-2710
781-891-6270
FAX: 781-891-6271
e-mail: arcmass@arcmass.org
www.arcmass.org

Leo V. Sarkissian, Executive Director
Judy Zacek, Associate Editor
Beth Rutledge, Production Coordinator/Ad
Brenda Asis, Director of Development
Advocate is The Arc of Massachusetts' quarterly newsletter. This is one of the ways in which we inform and educate people about current topics in the field of developmental disabilities. *$20.00*
8-12 pages Quarterly

4878 After School and More
Resources for Children with Special Needs
116 E 16th St
5th Floor
New York, NY 10003-2164
212-677-4650
FAX: 212-254-4070
e-mail: info@resourcesnyc.org
www.resourcesnyc.org

Rachel Howard, Executive Director
Stephen Stern, Director of Finance & Administration
Todd Dorman, Director of Communications & Outreach
Helen Murphy, Director of Program & Fund Development
More than 450 programs provide a wealth of resources for children in out-of-high school- time program. Information includes contact information, age, disability program capacity, hours, days, transportation, medication administration. *$25.00*
240 pages
ISBN 0-967836-55-7

4879 American Herb Association Newsletter
P.O.Box 353
Nevada City, CA 95959-353
530-265-9552
FAX: 530-274-3140
www.ahaherb.com

4880 Americans with Disabilities Act Checklist for New Lodging Facilities
US Department of Justice
950 Pennsylvania Ave NW
Washington, DC 20530-9
202-586-5000
800-574-0301
FAX: 202-307-1197
TTY: 800-514-0383
www.ada.gov

James Bostrom, Deputy Chiefs
Zita Johnson Betts, Deputy Chiefs
Sally Conway, Deputy Chiefs
Jana Erickson, Deputy Chiefs
This 34-page checklist is a self-help survey that owners, franchisors, and managers of lodging facilities can use to identify ADA mistakes at their facilities.

4881 Americans with Disabilities Act Handbook
Aspen Publishers
76 9th Ave
7th Floor
New York, NY 10011-4962
212-790-2000
FAX: 212-771-0885
e-mail: customerservice@aspenpublishers.com
www.aspenpublishers.com

Henry H Perritt Jr Esq, Author
Bob Lemmond, President and CEO
Gustavo Dobles, Vice President & Chief Content Officer
Susan Pikitch, Vice President & CFO
The Americans With Disabilities Act (ADA) Handbook provides comprehensive coverage of the ADA's employment, commercial facilities, and public accommodations provisions as well as coverage of the transportation, communication, and federal, local, and state government requirements. *$599.00*
1671 pages 2X per year
ISBN 0-735531-48-X

4882 An Interdisciplinary Journal for the Social Study of Health, Illness and Medicine

Sage Publications
2455 Teller Rd
Thousand Oaks, CA 91320-2218
805-499-0721
800-818-7243
FAX: 805-499-0871
hea.sagepub.com

Alan Radley, Editor
Blaise Simqu, Chief Executive Officer

Quarterly

4883 Annual Report Sarkeys Foundation

530 E Main St
Norman, OK 73071-5823
405-364-3703
FAX: 405-364-8191
e-mail: susan@sarkeys.org
sarkeys.org

Kim Henry, Executive Director
Lorri Sutton, Executive Assistant
Susan C. Frantz, Senior Program Officer
Linda English Weeks, Senior Program Officer

Yearly

4884 Applied Kinesiology: Muscle Response in Diagnosis, Therapy and Preventive Medicine

Inner Traditions
P.O.Box 388
Rochester, VT 05767-388
802-767-3174
800-246-8648
FAX: 802-767-3726
e-mail: orders@innertraditions.com
www.InnerTraditions.com

Jessica Arsenault, Sales Associate
Rob Meadows, VP Sales & Marketing
$12.95
144 pages
ISBN 0-892813-28-8

4885 Arc Connection Newsletter

Arc of Tennessee
151 Athens Way
Suite 100
Nashville, TN 37228-1367
615-248-5878
800-835-7077
FAX: 615-248-5879
e-mail: pcooper@thearctn.org
thearctn.org

Carrie Hobbs Guiden, Executive Director
Peggy Cooper, Membership, Chapter and Communications Manager
Nicole Davidson, Business Manager
Lori Israel, Office Manager

The Arc of Tennessee is a nonprofit organization that offers advocacy, information, referral and support to people with intellectual or developmental disabilities and their families. This is their publication. It is free to members. *$10.00*
12 pages Quarterly

4886 Aromatherapy Book: Applications and Inhalations

North Atlantic Books
1435a 4th St
Berkeley, CA 94710
510-559-8277
FAX: 510-559-8279
e-mail: info@northatlanticbooks.com
www.northatlanticbooks.com

Alla Spector, Director of Finance & Office Operations
Doug Reil, Executive Director
Ed Angel, Director of Office Administration
Janet Levin, Senior Director of Sales & Distribution

Considered a bible for those interested in aromatherapy. *$18.95*
ISBN 1-556430-73-6

4887 Aromatherapy for Common Ailments

Simon & Schuster
100 Front St
Delran, NJ 8075-1181
856-461-6500
800-323-7445
FAX: 856-824-2402
www.simonsays.com

David Schaeffer, VP

Explains aromatherapy with emphasis on medicinal uses.
96 pages
ISBN 0-671731-34-3

4888 As I Am

Fanlight Productions
32 Court Street
21st Floor
Brooklyn, NY 11201
718-488-8900
800-876-1710
FAX: 718-488-8642
e-mail: info@fanlight.com
www.fanlight.com

Ben Achtenberg, Owner
Anthony Sweeney, Marketing Director

Three young people with developmental disabilities speak for themselves about their lives, the problems they face and their hopes and expectations for the future. *$99.00*
ISBN 1-572950-58-7

4889 Attitudes Toward Persons with Disabilities

Springer Publishing Company
11 West 42nd Street
15th Floor
New York, NY 10036
212-431-4370
877-687-7476
FAX: 212-941-7842
e-mail: marketing@springerpub.com
www.springerpub.com

James C. Costello, Vice President, Journal Publishing
Diana Osborne, Production Manager
Megan Larkin, Managing Editor, Journals
Theodore C. Nardin, Chief Executive Officer and Publisher

This volume examines what is known of people's complex and multifaceted attitudes toward persons with disabilities. Divided into five areas of concern: theory, origin of attitudes, attitude measurement, attitudes of specific groups and attitude change.
$38.95
352 pages Hardcover
ISBN 0-82616-90-1

4890 Authoritative Guide to Self- Help Resourcein Mental Health

Guilford Press
72 Spring St
New York, NY 10012-4019
212-431-9800
800-365-7006
FAX: 212-966-6708
e-mail: info@guilford.com
www.guilford.com

Linda F Campbell PhD, Author
Thomas P Smith PsyD, Author
Robert Sommer PhD, Author
Bob Matloff, President

Reviews and rates 600+ self-help books, autobiographies, and popular films, and evaluates hundreds of Internet sites. Addresses 28 of the most prevalent clinical disorders and life challenges- from ADHD, Alzheimer's, and anxiety disorders, to marital problems, mood disorders and weight management. Also in cloth at $45.00 (ISBN# 1-57230-506-1) *$25.00*
377 pages Paperback
ISBN 1-572305-80-0

4891 **AwareNews**
Services for Independent Living
26250 Euclid Ave
Suite 801
Euclid, OH 44132
216-731-1529
FAX: 216-731-3083
e-mail: sil@stratos.net
www.sil-oh.org

Molly Foos, Executive Director
Katherine Foley, Director of Advocacy
Lisa Marn, Assistant Director
Laura A. Gold, Director

12 pages Quarterly

4892 **Bach Flower Therapy: Theory and Practice**
Inner Traditions
1 Park St
Rochester, VT 05767
802-767-3174
FAX: 802-767-3726
e-mail: customerservice@InnerTraditions.com
www.innertraditions.com

Ehud Sperling, Owner
Contemporary study of Bach's techniques, intended for practitioners and lay readers alike. Includes lists of symptoms to facilitate diagnosis, ans aims to provide an understanding of psychosomatic elements in relation to physical complaints.
ISBN 0-892812-39-7

4893 **Barrier Free Travel**
Demos Health Publishing
11 West 42nd Street 15th Floor
New York, NY 10036
212-683-0072

barrierfreetravel.net
Candy Harrington, Author
Billed as the definitive guide to accessible travel, this indispensable resource contains detailed information about the logistics of planning accessible travel by plane, train, bus and ship. *$17.49*
200 pages paperback

4894 **Beliefs, Values, and Principles of Self Advocacy**
Brookline Books
34 University Rd
Brookline, MA 02445-4533
800-666-2665
FAX: 617-734-3952
e-mail: brbooks@yahoo.com
www.brooklinebooks.com

48 pages Paperback
ISBN 0-57129 -22-2

4895 **Beliefs: Pathways to Health and Well Being**
Metamorphous Press
P.O.Box 10616
Portland, OR 97296-616
503-228-4972
FAX: 503-223-9117
www.metamodels.com/meta/bks/hea1.htm

David Balding, Publisher
Explores behavioral technologies and belief change strategies that can alter beliefs that support unhealthy habbits such as smoking, overeating, and drug use. Also covers the changing of thinking processes that create phobias and unreasonable fears, retraining the immune system to eliminate allergies and to deal optinally with cancer, AIDS, and other diseases. Includes strategies to transform unhealthy beliefs into lifelong constructs of wellness.

4896 **Bench Marks**
Govennor's Council on Developmental Disabilities
1717 W Jefferson St
Phoenix, AZ 85007-3202
602-542-4049
800-889-5893
FAX: 602-542-5320
e-mail: mward@mail.dc.state.us

Micheal Ward, Executive Director
Susan Madison, Manager

Quarterly

4897 **Bodie, Dolina, Smith & Hobbs, P.C.**
21 W Susquehanna Ave
Suite 110
Towson, MD 21204-5218
410-823-1250
877-739-1013
FAX: 443-901-0802
e-mail: chobbs@bodie-law.com
www.bodie-law.com

Chester Hobbs, Esquire
Thomas G. Bodie, Lawyer
Wallace Dann, Lawyer
Thomas J. Dolina, Lawyer
Law firm; provides estates, trusts and guardianship administration, estate planning, elder law, tax issues, bankruptcy, foreclosures, and real estate issues. *$25.00*
Quarterly

4898 **Body Reflexology: Healing at Your Fingertips**
Parker Publishing Company
Ste 2605
1501 Broadway
New York, NY 10036-5600
212-869-6350

Hy Dubin, President
Features step-by-step instructions of how to send healing flows of energy through the body to relieve back pain, headaches, arthritis, and other afflictions. Illustrated.
343 pages Hardcover
ISBN 0-132997-36-3

4899 **Body Silent: The Different World of the Disabled**
WW Norton & Company
324 State St
Santa Barbara, CA 93101-2362
800-333-6867
FAX: 805-962-5087
www.specialneeds.com/store/

256 pages
ISBN 0-393320-42-1

4900 **Body of Knowledge/Hellerwork**
406 Berry St
Mount Shasta, CA 96067-2548
530-926-2500
e-mail: theheller@aol.com
www.josephheller.com

Joseph Heller, Owner
Information, referral directory, training and certification.

4901 **Bridge Newsletter**
Arizona Bridge to Independent Living
1229 E Washington St
Phoenix, AZ 85034-1101
602-256-2245
800-280-2245
FAX: 602-254-6407
e-mail: azbridge@abil.org
abil.org

Phil Pangrazio, President & CEO
Regina Mitzel, V. P. & Chief Administrative Officer
Amina Kruck, V.P. of Advocacy
Ann Pasco, V.P. of Operations

12 pages Monthly

4902 **Bridging the Gap: A National Directory of Services for Women & Girls with Disabilities**
Educational Equity Concepts
71 Fifth Avenue
New York, NY 10016-5506
212-725-1803
FAX: 212-725-0947
TTY:212-725-1803
e-mail: infomration@edequity.org
www.edequity.org

Ellen Rubin, Coordinator Disability Programs
Merle Froschl, Editor

Contains a resource section of publications and videos geared specifically to women and girls with disabilities. Available in print, on cassette, and also in braille. *$24.95*
ISBN 0-931629-16-0

4903 Bulletin of the Association on the Handicapped
Assoc. on Handicapped Student Service Program
P.O.Box 21192
Columbus, OH 43221-0192 614-365-5216
FAX: 614-365-6718

4904 CDR Reports
Council for Disability Rights
Ste 1540
20 N Wacker Dr
Chicago, IL 60606-2903 312-201-4800
FAX: 312-444-1977
e-mail: cdrights@interaccess.com
www.disabilityrights.org

Jo Holzer, Executive Director/Editor
Bruce Moore, Employment Specialist
$15.00
8 pages Monthly

4905 California Financial Power of Attorney
NOLO
950 Parker St
Berkeley, CA 94710-2524 510-549-1976
800-955-4775
FAX: 510-548-5902
www.nolo.com

Maira Dizgalvis, Trade Customer Service Manager
Susan McConnell, Director Sales
Natasha Kaluza, Sales Assistant
David Rothenberg, CEO
A plain-English book packed with forms and instructions to give a trusted person the legal authority to handle your financial affairs.
Paperback

4906 Caring for America's Heroes
Oklahoma City VA Medical Center
921 NE 13th St
Oklahoma City, OK 73104-5007 405-270-0501
FAX: 405-270-1560
www.oklahoma.va.gov

Steven Gentlin, Director
Kathleen Fogarty, Associate Director
D Robert McCaffree MD, Chief of Staff
Tom Duchene, Plant Manager

4907 Center for Health Research: Eastern Washington University
Showalter 209a
Cheney, WA 99004 509-359-2279
800-221-9369
FAX: 509-359-2778
e-mail: sharon.wilson@mail.ewu.edu
iceberg.ewu.edu

4908 Center for Libraries and Educational Improvement
400 Maryland Ave SW
Washington, DC 20202-1 202-260-2226
800-872-5327
FAX: 202-401-0689
TTY: 800-437-0833
www.ed.gov

4909 Centering Corporation Grief Resources
7230 Maple Street
Omaha, NE 68134 402-553-1200
866-218-0101
FAX: 402-533-0507
e-mail: j1200@aol.com
www.centering.org

Joy Johnson, Founder
Dr. Marvin Johnson, Founder
Janet Roberts, Executive Director
Kelsey Novacek, Director of Marketing
A full catalog of all our available bereavement resources. We are a small, non-profit organization providing help to families in crisis situations.
32 pages BiAnnually

4910 Centers for Disease Control and Prevention
US Department of Health and Human Services
1600 Clifton Rd NE
Atlanta, GA 30329-4018 404-639-3311
800-232-4636
FAX: 404-498-1177
e-mail: inquiry@cdc.gov
www.cdc.gov

Robert Delaney, Plant Manager
Publishes an annually updated list of infectious and communicable diseases transmitted through the handling of food in accordance with Section 103 of Title I.

4911 Child With Special Needs: Encouraging Intellectual and Emotional Growth
Addison-Wesley Publishing Company
Ste 300
75 Arlington St
Boston, MA 02116-3988 617-848-7500
800-238-9682
FAX: 617-944-7273
www.awprofessional.com

Bill Barke, CEO
Covering all kinds of disabilities — including cerebral palsy, autism, retardation, ADD, and language problems — this guide offers parents specific ways of helping all special needs chidren reach their full intellectual and emotional potential. *$32.00*
496 pages
ISBN 0-201407-26-4

4912 Chinese Herbal Medicine
Shambhala Publications
300 Massachusetts Avenue
Boston, MA 02115 617-424-0030
FAX: 617-236-1563
e-mail: editors@shambhala.com
shambhala.com

Richard Reoch, President
Gives an in-depth look into herbal medicine.
176 pages
ISBN 0-877733-98-8

4913 Christian Approach to Overcoming Disability: A Doctor's Story
Haworth Press
10 Alice St
Binghamton, NY 13904-1503 607-722-5857
800-429-6784
FAX: 607-722-6362
e-mail: orders@haworthpress.com
www.haworthpress.com

William Cohen, Owner
$29.95
128 pages
ISBN 0-789022-57-5

4914 Closing the Gap
526 Main Street
P.O.Box 68
Henderson, MN 56044-68
507-248-3294
FAX: 507-248-3810
e-mail: info@closingthegap.com
www.closingthegap.com
Dolores Hagen, Founder
Delores Hagen, Founder
Connie Kneip, Vice President
Megan Turek, Managing Editor
Explores use of microcomputers as personal and educational tools for persons with disabilities.
36+ pages BiMonthly

4915 Comprehensive Directory of Programs and Services
Resources for Children with Special Needs
116 E 16th St
5th Floor
New York, NY 10003-2164
212-387-7091
FAX: 212-254-4070
e-mail: info@resourcesnyc.org
www.resourcesnyc.org
Rachel Howard, Executive Director
Stephen Stern, Director of Finance & Administration
Todd Dorman, Director of Communications & Outreach
Helen Murphy, Director of Program & Fund Development
Published every 24-36 months. *$55.00*
1096 pages
ISBN 0-976836-51-4

4916 Constellations
Minnesota STAR Program
Ste 309
50 Sherburne Ave
Saint Paul, MN 55155-1402
651-296-2771
800-657-3862
FAX: 651-282-6671
e-mail: star.program@state.mn.us
www.admin.state.mn.us/assistivetechnology
Chuck Rassbach, Executive Director
Free quarterly publication from the Minnesota STAR Program.
8 pages Quarterly

4917 Consumer Buyer's Guide for Independent Living
American Occupational Therapy Association (AOTA)
4720 Montgomery Ln
Bethesda, MD 20814-5320
301-652-2682
800-SAY-AOTA
FAX: 301-652-7711
TTY: 800-377-8555
www.aota.org
Florence Clark, President
A buyer's directory of products and publications for the general public listing suppliers' names, addresses and telephone numbers. This directory lists AOTA publications on numerous topics (back pain, Alzheimers, Carpal Tunnel Syndrome, etc.) and suppliers of equipment to assist in activities of daily living for individuals with disabilities.
60 pages Annual

4918 Coping+Plus: Dimensions of Disability
Greenwood Publishing Group
130 Cremona Drive
Santa Barbara, CA 93117
805-968-1911
800-368-6868
FAX: 866-270-3856
e-mail: CustomerService@abc-clio.com
www.abc-clio.com
Matt Laddin, Vice President of Marketing
Mike Saltzman, Director-Eastern Territories & National Accounts
James Lingle, International Sales & Marketing
Everyone can learn new or more effective coping skills and strategies to deal with times of loss, crisis and disability. $55-$59.95
280 pages Hardcover
ISBN 0-275945-44-8

4919 Council News
Northern Nevada Center for Independent Living
999 Pyramid Way
Sparks, NV 89431-4471
775-353-3599
FAX: 775-353-3588
e-mail: nncil@sbcglobal.net
www.nncil.org
Lisa Bonie, Executive Director
Hilda Velasco, Operations Manager
Joni Inglis, Independent Living Advocate
Patti Rodriguez, Life Skills Coordinator
NNCIL was founded in 1982 by a small group of people with disabilities, who believe that each person, regardless of the severity of his or her disability, has the potential to grow, develop and share fully the joys and responsibilities of our society.
12 pages Quarterly

4920 Counseling in Terminal Care & Bereavement
Brookes Publishing
P.O.Box 10624
Baltimore, MD 21285-0624
410-337-9580
800-638-3775
FAX: 410-337-8539
e-mail: custserv@brookespublishing.com
readplaylearn.com
Paul H. Brooks, Chairman
Jeffrey D. Brookes, President
Melissa A. Behm, Executive Vice President
Provides practical suggestions for addressing the needs of patients and family members who are anticipating or currently dealing with grief and bereavement, such as hospice care, hospitals, or at home care. *$34.00*
210 pages Paperback
ISBN 1-85433 -78-7

4921 Creating Wholeness: Self-Healing Workbook Using Dynamic Relaxation, Images and Thoughts
Plenum Publishing Corporation
233 Spring St
7th Floor
New York, NY 10013-1522
212-620-8000
800-644-4831
FAX: 212-460-1575
e-mail: ainy@aveda.com
www.aveda.edu
232 pages
ISBN 0-306441-72-1

4922 DRS Connection
Disabled Resource Services
Ste 101
424 Pine St
Fort Collins, CO 80524-2421
970-482-2700
FAX: 970-407-7072
e-mail: drs@frii.com
Nancy Jackson, Executive Director
4 pages Quaterly

4923 Demand Response Transportation Through a Rural ILC
Independent Living Research Utilization ILRU
1333 Moursund
Houston, TX 77030
713-520-0232
FAX: 713-520-5785
e-mail: ilru@ilru.org
ilru.org
Lex Frieden, Director, ILRU
Richard Petty, Consultant
Rose Shepard, Office Manager
Oklahomans for Independent Living's transportation program was selected as exemplary becuase they marketed it by emphasizing people with disabilities as economic constituency.
10 pages

4924 Developing Organized Coalitions and Strategic Plans
Independent Living Research Utilization ILRU
1333 Moursund
Houston, TX 77030 713-520-0232
FAX: 713-520-5785
e-mail: ilru@ilru.org
ilru.org

Lex Frieden, Director, ILRU
Richard Petty, Consultant
Rose Shepard, Office Manager

10 pages

4925 Dictionary of Congenital Malformations& Disorders
Informa Healthcare
Fl 16
52 Vanderbilt Ave
New York, NY 10017-3846 212-520-2777
FAX: 212-661-5052
e-mail: orders@crcpress.com
www.tandfonline.com

193 pages
ISBN 0-850705-77-1

4926 Dictionary of Developmental Disabilities Terminology
Brookes Publishing
P.O.Box 10624
Baltimore, MD 21285-0624 410-337-9580
800-638-3775
FAX: 410-337-8539
e-mail: custserv@brookesopublishing.com
www.brookespublishing.com

Paul H. Brooks, Chairman
Jeffrey D. Brookes, President
Melissa A. Behm, Executive Vice President
George S. Stamathis, Vice President & Publisher
With more than 3,000 easy-to-understand entries, this dictionary provides thorough explanations of terms associated with developmental disabilities and disorders. *$55.95*
368 pages Hardcover
ISBN 1-557662-45-2

4927 Directory of Members
American Network of Community Options & Resources
1101 King St
Suite 380
Alexandria, VA 22314-2962 703-535-7850
FAX: 703-535-7860
e-mail: ancor@ancor.org
ancor.org

Dave Toeniskoetter, President
Chris Sparks, Vice President
Julie Manworren, Secretary/Treasurer
Wendy Swager, Past president
The Directory lists over 600 agencies that provide residential services and supports in 48 states and the District of Columbia. The listings include the name of the Executive Directors, the name, address, and phone number of the agency, describe the types of services that are provided and how many individuals receive services from that agency. *$25.00*
189 pages

4928 Disability Awareness Guide
Central Iowa Center for Independent Living
655 Walnut St
Suite 131
Des Moines, IA 50309-3930 515-243-1742
FAX: 515-243-5385
e-mail: cicil@raccoon.com
centraliowacil.com

Bob Jeppesen, Executive Director
Frank Strong, Assistant Director Programs
Bob Jepson, Manager
The Disability Awareness Guide contains information about our center; who we are and what we do. It also contains the telephone numbers of local and national agencies and resources available for people with disabilities.

4929 Disability Rights Movement
Children's Press
Sherman Tpke
Danbury, CT 6813 800-621-1115
FAX: 800-374-4329

Elena Rockman, Marketing Manager
Author Deborah Kent illuminates both the history of the National Disability Rights Movement and the inspiring personal stories of individuals with various disabilities. *$18.00*
32 pages Hardcover
ISBN 0-53106-32-3

4930 Disabled People's International Fifth World Assembly as Reported by Two US Participants
Independent Living Research Utilization ILRU
1333 Moursund
Houston, TX 77030 713-520-0232
FAX: 713-520-5785
e-mail: ilru@ilru.org
ilru.org

Lex Frieden, Director, ILRU
Richard Petty, Consultant
Rose Shepard, Office Manager
This report describes the international conference on independent living held in Mexico City in December 1998 as experienced by staff members from two U.S. centers. Kaye Beneke interviewed Luis Chew and Marco Antonio Coronado for this edition of Readings in Independent Living.
10 pages

4931 Disabled We Stand
Brookline Books
34 University Rd
Brookline, MA 02445-4533 800-666-2665
FAX: 617-734-3952
e-mail: brbooks@yahoo.com
www.brooklinebooks.com

Paperback
ISBN 0-25331 -80-0

4932 Disabled, the Media, and the Information Age
Greenwood Publishing Group
130 Cremona Drive
Santa Barbara, CA 93117 805-968-1911
800-368-6868
FAX: 866-270-3856
e-mail: CustomerService@abc-clio.com
www.abc-clio.com

Matt Laddin, Vice President of Marketing
Mike Saltzman, Director-Eastern Territories & National Accounts
James Lingle, International Sales & Marketing
A short and easy-to-read overview of how disabled Americans have been portrayed by the media and how images and the role of the handicapped are changing. *$55.00*
264 pages Hardcover
ISBN 0-313284-72-5

4933 Discovery Newsletter
North Dakota State Library Talking Book Services
Dept 250
604 E Boulevard Ave
Bismarck, ND 58505-605 701-328-2000
800-843-9948
FAX: 701-328-2040
e-mail: sbschneider@nd.gov
ndsl.lib.state.nd.us/DisabilityServices.html

Doris Ott, Manager
The North Dakota State Library Disability Services produces the Doscovery Newsletter containing information on services, books, catalogs and of interest to the patron.
6 pages Bi-Annually

4934 EP Resource Guide
Exceptional Parent Library
P.O.Box 1807
Englewood Cliffs, NJ 7632-1207 201-947-6000
800-535-1910
FAX: 201-947-9376
e-mail: eplibrary@aol.com
www.eplibrary.com

4935 ESCIL Update Newsletter
Eastern Shore Center for Independent Living
9 Sunburst Ctr
Cambridge, MD 21613-2057 410-221-7701
800-705-7944
FAX: 410-221-7714
e-mail: escil@comcast.net
www.escil.org

Shirley Tarbox, Executive Director
Jean Reed, Administrative Assistant
Lisa Morgan, Director IL Services

6 pages Quarterly

4936 Easy Things to Make Things Simple: Do It Yourself Modifications for Disabled Persons
Brookline Books
34 University Rd
Brookline, MA 02445-4533 800-666-2665
FAX: 617-734-3952
e-mail: brbooks@yahoo.com
www.brooklinebooks.com

160 pages Paperback
ISBN 1-571290-24-9

4937 Encyclopedia of Disability
Sage Publications
2455 Teller Rd
Thousand Oaks, CA 91320-2218 805-499-0721
e-mail: info@sagepub.com
www.sagepub.com

Gary L Albrecht, Editor
Blaise Simqu, Chief Executive Officer
A five volume set that covers disabilities A-Z *$850.00*
2500 pages
ISBN 0-761925-65-1

4938 EveryBody's Different: Understanding and Changing Our Reactions to Disabilities
Brookes Publishing
P.O.Box 10624
Baltimore, MD 21285-0624 410-337-9580
800-638-3775
FAX: 410-337-8539
e-mail: custserv@brookespublishing.com
readplaylearn.com

Paul H. Brooks, Chairman
Jeffrey D. Brookes, President
Melissa A. Behm, Executive Vice President
This book discusses the emotions, questions, fears, and stereotypes that people without disabilities sometimes experience when they interact with people who do have disabilities. The author teaches readers to become more at ease with the concept of disability and to communicate more effectively with each other. Features activities and exercises that encourage self-examination, helping people to create more enriching personal relationships and work toward a fully inclusive society.
Paperback
ISBN 1-55766 -59-9

4939 Everybody's Guide to Homeopathic Medicines
Jeremy P Tarcher
375 Hudson St
New York, NY 10014-3658 212-366-2000
e-mail: academic@penguin.com
www.us.penguingroup.com

John Makinson, Chairman and CEO
Coram Williams, CFO
Covers alternative treatments in homeopathic medicines.
375 pages
ISBN 0-874778-43-3

4940 Everyday Social Interaction: A Program for People with Disabilities
Brookes Publishing
P.O.Box 10624
Baltimore, MD 21285-0624 410-337-9580
800-638-3775
FAX: 410-337-8539
e-mail: custserv@brookespublishing.com
readplaylearn.com

Paul H. Brooks, Chairman
Jeffrey D. Brookes, President
Melissa A. Behm, Executive Vice President
This source guides teachers and human services professionals in helping people with disabilities acquire social interaction skills and develop satisfying relationships. Included is a checklist and task analyses that shows how complex skills can be broken down into major components for easy performance monitoring accompanied by tips on social courtesies, rewards, praise, and criticism.
$41.95
342 pages Paperback
ISBN 1-55766 -58-4

4941 Family Challenges: Parenting with a Disability
Aquarius Health Care Videos
P.O.Box 1159
Sherborn, MA 01770-7159 508-650-1616
888-440-2963
FAX: 508-650-4216
e-mail: aqvideos@tiac.net
www.aquariusproductions.com

Lesile Kussmann, Owner
When a parent has a disability, everyone in the family is affected. For children, these experiences may profoundly influence their lives and views of the world. In this sensitive film, you will hear about different roles that all the family members take on at varying times. *$195.00*

4942 Force A Miracle
Writer's Showcase Press

244 pages
ISBN 0-595226-88-4

4943 Forum
Coalition for the Education of Disabled Children
165 W Center St
Marion, OH 43302-3742 740-382-7362
800-374-2806
FAX: 740-382-3428
e-mail: oceed@gte.net
www.oceed.org

Tracie Wilson, Manager
Leeann Derugen, Manager
Forum is a newsletter reporting on legislative and other developments affecting persons with disabilities.
Quarterly

4944 Foundation Fundamentals for Nonprofit Organizations
Foundation Center
Department Ze
79 5th Ave
New York, NY 10003-3034 212-620-4230
800-424-9836
FAX: 212-807-3677
e-mail: order@foundationcenter.org
www.fdncenter.org

Bradford K. Smith, President
Lisa Philip, Vice President for Strategic Philanthropy
Lawrence T. McGill, Vice President for Research
Lisa Brooks, Director of Knowledge Management Systems
This video is designed to give fundraisers a general overview of the foundation funding process and to introduce them to the many resources available through our libraries and cooperating collections. The video gives clear, step-by-step instructions on how to build a fundraising program. *$24.00*
Video

4945 Four-Ingredient Cookbook
Laurel Designs
Apt A
1805 Mar West St
Belvedere Tiburon, CA 94920-1962 FAX: 415-435-1451
e-mail: laureld@ncal.verio.com

Janet Sawyer, Owner
Lynn Montoya, Owner
Simple, easy to follow recipes, each containing four ingredients. Particularly suited to persons with limited physical ability. Includes 400 recipes, appetizers to desserts. *$9.00*

4946 Frequently Asked Questions About Multiple Chemical Sensitivity
Independent Living Research Utilization ILRU
1333 Moursund
Houston, TX 77030 713-520-0232
FAX: 713-520-5785
e-mail: ilru@ilru.org
ilru.org

Lex Frieden, Director, ILRU
Richard Petty, Consultant
Rose Shepard, Office Manager
This FAQ covers important information about multiple chemical sensitivity and environmental illness. The FAQ describes the conditions, recommends strategies for improving access, and lists resources for CILs and other organizations. As the fact sheet states, centers must set an example in assuring that all people can enter their offices.
10 pages

4947 Genetic Disorders Sourcebook
Omnigraphics
155 W. Congress
Suite 200
Detroit, MI 48226-3900 313-961-1340
800-234-1340
FAX: 800-875-1340
e-mail: contact@omnigraphics.com
www.omnigraphics.com

Paul Rogers, Publicity Associate
Georgiann Fratoni, Customer Service Manager
Provides information on hereditary diseases and disorders. *$7800.00*
650 pages
ISBN 0-789892-41-1

4948 Genetic Nutritioneering
McGraw-Hill Company
2460 Kerper Blvd
Dubuque, IA 52001-2224 563-588-1451
800-338-3987
FAX: 614-755-5654
www.mhhe.com/hper/physed

Kurt Strand, VP
Describes how to modify the expression of genetic traits, potentially preventing heart disease, cancer, arthritis, and hormone-related problems. Features how to slow biological aging and reduce the risk of age-related diseases. *$16.95*
288 pages
ISBN 0-879839-21-X

4949 Going to School with Facilitated Communication
Syracuse University, School of Education
230 Huntington Hall
Syracuse, NY 13244-1 315-443-4752
FAX: 315-443-2258
e-mail: jhrusso@syr.edu
www.soe.syr.edu

Shirley Adamczyk, Administrative Assistant
Rachael Gazdick, Executive Director
Isabelle M. Glod, Administrative Assistant
Angela Flanagan, Development Assistant
A video in which students with autism and/or severe disabilities illustrate the use of facilitated communication focusing on basic principles fostering facilitated communication.
Video

4950 Grief: What it is and What You Can Do
Centering Corporation
7230 Maple Street
Omaha, NE 68134 402-553-1200
866-218-0101
FAX: 402-533-0507
e-mail: j1200@aol.com
www.centering.org

Joy Johnson, Founder
Dr. Marvin Johnson, Founder
Janet Roberts, Executive Director
Kelsey Novacek, Director of Marketing
General grief information for all grief issues. *$3.50*
32 pages Paperback

4951 Guidelines on Disability
US Department of Housing & Urban Development
451 7th St SW
Washington, DC 20410-1 202-708-1112
TTY:202-708-1455
portal.hud.gov/hudportal/HUD

Shaun Donovan, Secretary
Helen R. Kanovsky, Acting Deputy Secretary
Jennifer Ho, Senior Advisor to the Secretary
Mike Anderson, Chief Human Capital Officer
Contains information on housing and accessibility for persons with disabilities.

4952 Handbook of Services for the Handicapped
Greenwood Publishing Group
130 Cremona Drive
Santa Barbara, CA 93117 805-968-1911
800-368-6868
FAX: 866-270-3856
e-mail: CustomerService@abc-clio.com
www.abc-clio.com

Matt Laddin, Vice President of Marketing
Mike Saltzman, Director-Eastern Territories & National Accounts
James Lingle, International Sales & Marketing
A handy reference book offering information and services for disabled individuals. $59.95-$65.00.
291 pages Hardcover
ISBN 0-313213-85-2

4953 Healing Herbs
Rodale Press
33 E Minor St
Emmaus, PA 18098-1 610-967-5171
FAX: 610-967-8963
www.rodale.com

Maria Rodale, Chairman/Chief Executive Officer
Scott D. Schulman, President
Heather Rodale, Board Member/Vice President/ Leadership Development
Thomas A. Pogash, EVP/Chief Financial Officer
Covers everything from growing the herbs to home remedies.

4954 Helen Keller National Center for Deaf- Blind Youths And Adults
141 Middle Neck Rd
Sands Point, NY 11050-1218 516-944-8900
FAX: 516-944-7302
e-mail: hkncinfo@hknc.org
www.hknc.org
Joseph McNulty, Executive Director
HKNC is the only national vacational and rehabilitation program providing services exclusively to youth and adults who are deaf-blind.

4955 Hospice Alternative
Harper Collins Publishers/Basic Books
10 E 53rd St
New York, NY 10022-5244 212-207-7000
800-242-7737
FAX: 212-207-7203
Jane Friedman, CEO
An account of the hospice experience. An innovative and humane way of caring for the terminally ill. *$8.95*
256 pages
ISBN 0-46503 -61-0

4956 How to File a Title III Complaint
US Department of Justice
950 Pennsylvania Ave NW
Washington, DC 20530-9 202-307-0663
800-574-0301
FAX: 202-307-1197
TTY: 800-514-0383
www.ada.gov
Rebecca B. Bond, Chief
Zita Johnson Betts, Deputy Chiefs
Sally Conway, Deputy Chiefs
James Bostrom, Deputy Chiefs
This publication details the procedure for filing a complaint under Title III of the ADA.

4957 How to Live Longer with a Disability
Accent Books & Products
PO Box 700
Bloomington, IL 61702-700 309-378-2961
800-787-8444
FAX: 309-378-4420
e-mail: acmtlvng@aol.com
Raymond C Cheever, Publisher
Betty Garee, Editor
Eleven chapters to help you enjoy every aspect of your life, and live easier and happier. Includes sexuality and disability, getting more from the medical community and benefit programs. Co-authored by Robert Mauro, sociologist and Elle Becker, counselor and psychologist, both disabled. *$11.50*
266 pages Paperback
ISBN 0-19570 -38-8

4958 Ideas for Kids on the Go
Accent Books & Products
PO Box 700
Bloomington, IL 61702-700 309-378-2961
800-787-8444
FAX: 309-378-4420
e-mail: acmtlvng@aol.com
Raymond C Cheever, Publisher
Betty Garee, Editor
This guide shows kids with physical disabilities how to go for it! Lists products and where to get them, and includes tips from others for having fun and getting ahead. Ages 1-18. *$6.95*
69 pages Paperback
ISBN 0-91570 -17-5

4959 If I Only Knew What to Say or Do
AARP Fulfillment
601 E St NW
Washington, DC 20049-1 202-434-2277
800-424-3410
FAX: 202-434-3443
TTY: 877-434-7598
e-mail: member@aarp.org
www.aarp.org
Carol Raphael, Chair
Ronald E. Daly, Sr., Board Vice Chair
Jeannine English, President
A. Barry Rand, Chief Executive Officer
Provides a concise discussion of how to help a friend in crisis. Learn what to say and what not to say.

4960 If it Weren't for the Honor: I'd Rather Have Walked
Accent Books & Products
PO Box 700
Bloomington, IL 61702-700 309-378-2961
800-787-8444
FAX: 309-378-4420
e-mail: acmtlvng@aol.com
Raymond C Cheever, Publisher
Betty Garee, Editor
Revealing, often humorous, highly interesting and important reading. This book offers an account told by the author who was on the scene and actually saw and participated in many events that paved the way for progress for all those with disabilities. *$14.50*
262 pages Paperback
ISBN 0-91570 -41-8

4961 Imagery in Healing Shamanism and Modern Medicine
Shambhala Publications
300 Massachusetts Avenue
Horticultural Hall
Boston, MA 02115 617-424-0030
888-424-2329
FAX: 617-236-1563
e-mail: editors@shambhala.com
www.shambhala.com
Richard Reoch, President
Patients use self imagery to fight sickness and pain throughout their lives. *$15.95*
272 pages
ISBN 1-570629-34-x

4962 Independence
Easter Seals
1219 Dunn Ave
Daytona Beach, FL 32114-2405 386-255-4568
877-255-4568
FAX: 386-258-7677
e-mail: info@eseals-vf.org
www.easterseals-volusiaflagler.org
Jeff Blass, Chairman
Austin Brownlee, Chair-Elect
Becky Rutland, Vice Chair
Lynn Sinnott, President/ CEO
4-6 pages Quarterly

4963 Independent Living Centers and Managed Care: Results of an ILRU Study on Involvement
Independent Living Research Utilization ILRU
1333 Moursund
TIRR Memorial Hermann Research Cent
Houston, TX 77030-7031 713-520-0232
FAX: 713-520-5785
e-mail: ilru@ilru.org
www.ilru.org
Lex Frieden, Director, ILRU
Richard Petty, Program Director
Vinh Nguyen, Program Director
Roxy Funchess, Administrative Secretary
This month's Readings presents findings from an ILRU study of roles centers are taking vis-a-vis managed care. Initiated in

spring 1998, we asked Drew Batavia to take the lead in conducting this study for us. We were interested in collecting data on frequency with which centers are contacted by consumers with managed care problems. This is a study that will need to be repeated periodically as our experiences with managed care evolves. Meanwhile, here are the initial findings.
10 pages

4964 Independent Living Challenges the Blues
Independent Living Research Utilization ILRU
1333 Moursund
TIRR Memorial Hermann Research Cent
Houston, TX 77030-7031 713-520-0232
FAX: 713-520-5785
e-mail: ilru@ilru.org
www.ilru.org

Lex Frieden, Director, ILRU
Richard Petty, Program Director
Vinh Nguyen, Program Director
Roxy Funchess, Administrative Secretary
Patricia's article highlights the Georgia SILC's health care advocacy efforts: the Georgia legislature passed a bill enabling Georgia Bleu to convert to for-profit status without a distribution of assets to similar nonprofit corporations; the Georgia SILC joined other health care advocates in filing a class action law suit to challenge the legality of the conversion; the Georgia SILC continues advocacy efforts to involve people with disabilities in developing and monitoring health care policy.
10 pages

4965 Independent Living Office
Department of Housing & Urban Development (HUD)
451 7th St SW
Washington, DC 20410-1 202-863-2800

www.portal.hud.gov

Ted Tozer, President
Rafael Diaz, Chief Information Officer/Chief Information Officer
Mike Anderson, Chief Human Capital Officer
Shaun Donovan, Secretary
This office within HUD is charged with encouraging the construction of housing that is accessible to handicapped persons. The Office of Independent Living encourages modifications of apartments and other dwellings so that handicapped persons can enter without assistance.

4966 Independent Newsletter
Easter Seals Nebraska
12565 West Center Road
Suite 100
Omaha, NE 68144-8144 402-345-2200
800-650-9880
FAX: 402-345-2500
e-mail: kginder@ne.easterseals.com
www.easterseals.com/ne/

James C. Summerfelt, President/Chief Executive Officer
Angela Howell, Vice President
Lily Sughroue, Director of Camp
Terrific fun for campers and a much needed respite for families and care givers from the daily challenges of caring for special needs indviduals
4 pages Quarterly

4967 Information Services for People with Developmental Disabilities
Greenwood Publishing Group
130 Cremona Drive
Santa Barbara, CA 93117 805-968-1911
800-368-6868
FAX: 866-270-3856
e-mail: CustomerService@abc-clio.com
www.abc-clio.com

Matt Laddin, Vice President of Marketing
Mike Saltzman, Director - Eastern Territories
James Lingle, International Sales & Marketing
Overviews the information needs of people with developmental disabilities and tells librarians how to meet them. $65.oo-$75.00.
368 pages Hardcover
ISBN 0-313287-80-5

4968 Innovative Programs: An Example of How CILs Can Put Their Work in Context
Culture
1333 Moursund
TIRR Memorial Hermann Research Cent
Houston, TX 77030-7031 713-520-0232
FAX: 713-520-5785
e-mail: ilru@ilru.org
www.ilru.org

Lex Frieden, Director, ILRU
Richard Petty, Program Director
Vinh Nguyen, Program Director
Roxy Funchess, Administrative Secretary
Another winner in the innovative CIL competition- Steve Brown describes the Talking Books Program of Southeast Alaska Independent Living, discussing their efforts to record the oral history and life experiences of people with disabilities in the larger context of disability culture.
10 pages

4969 Insurance Solutions: Plan Well, Live Better
Demos Medical Publishing
11 West 42nd Street
15th Floor
New York, NY 10036 212-683-0072
800-532-8663
FAX: 212-683-0118
e-mail: support@demosmedical.com
www.demosmedpub.com
Paul Choi, Vice-President of Finance and Operations
Matt Conmy, Sr. Director of Sales
Thomas Hastings, Marketing Manager
Beth Kaufman Barry, Publisher
Learn how to look at various insurance options from a new perspective — including life, disability, health, and long-term care. Concrete information for dealing with potential problems in your coverage, to secure your financial future. *$24.95*
192 pages 2002
ISBN 1-888799-55-2

4970 International Directory of Libraries for the Disabled
KG Saur/Division of RR Bowker
121 Chanlon Rd
New Providence, NJ 7974-1541 908-286-1090
800-521-8110
Michael Cairns, CEO
An essential resource for improving the quality and quantity of materials available to the print-handicapped audience. Featuring talking books, braille books, large print books as well as production centers for these materials. *$46.00*
257 pages
ISBN 3-59821 -81-1

4971 Issues in Independent Living
Independent Living Research Utilization
1333 Moursund
TIRR Memorial Hermann Research Cent
Houston, TX 77030-7031 713-520-0232
FAX: 713-520-5785
e-mail: ilru@ilru.org
www.ilru.org

Laurie Redd, Executive Director
Lex Frieden, Manager
Vinh Nguyen, Program Director
Roxy Funchess, Administrative Secretary
This booklet is a report of the National Study Group on the Implications of Health Care Reform for Americans with Disabilities and Chronic Health Conditions.
30 pages

4972 JAMA: The Journal of the American Medical Association
American Medical Association
PO Box 10946
Chicago, IL 60654-4820
312-670-7827
800-262-2350
FAX: 312-464-5909
e-mail: subscriptions@jamanetwork.com
www.jama.jamanetwork.com

Howard Bauchner, MD, Editor-in-Chief
Articles cover all aspects of medical research and clinical medicine. *$66.00*

4973 JCIL Advocate Times
Jackson Center for Independent Living
409 Linden Ave
Jackson, MI 49203-4065
517-782-6054
FAX: 517-782-3118

Lesia Pikaart, Executive Director
JoAnn Lucas, Associate Director

Quarterly

4974 Jason & Nordic Publishers, Inc.
PO Box 441
Hollidaysburg, PA 16648-441
814-696-2929
FAX: 814-696-4250
e-mail: turtlbks@jasonandnordic.com
www.jasonandnordic.com

Norma Mc Phee, Owner/CEO
Norma Phee
Turtle Books for children with disabilities present heroes who look like them, have problems like theirs, have similar doubts and feelings in non-threatening, fun stories. They are motivational, bridge the gap and promote understanding among peers and siblings. 22 children's books (grades preK-3) plus Sensitivity and Awareness Guide containing lesson plans, activities, background information keyed to the series. Disabilities include: Down syndrome, cerebral palsy, blindness, deafness and more.

4975 Journal of Social Work in Disabilty & Rehabilitation
Haworth Press
10 Alice St
Binghamton, NY 13904-1503
607-722-5857
800-429-6784
FAX: 607-722-6362
e-mail: orders@haworthpress.com
www.haworthpress.com

William Cohen, Owner
John T Oardeck PhD, Editor
S Harrington-Miller, Advertising
Presents and explores issues related to disabilities and social policy, practice, research, and theory. Reflecting the broad scope of social work in disabilty practice, this interdisciplinary journal examines vital issues aspects of the field — from innovative practice methods, legal issues, and literature reviews to program descriptions and cuttinf-edge practice research.
Quarterly

4976 Just Like Everyone Else
World Institute on Disability
3075 Adeline Street
Suite 155
Oakland, CA 94703-1520
510-225-6400
FAX: 510-225-0477
TTY:510-225-0478
e-mail: wid@wid.org
www.wid.org

Paul W. Schroeder, Chair
Linda M. Dardarian, Vice Chair
Mary Brooner, Treasurer
Cassandra Malry, Secretary
The oversize-format publication, intended for general audiences, provides perspective, inspiration and information about the Independent Living Movement and the Americans with Disabilities Act. *$5.00*
16 pages

4977 Keep the Promise: Managed Care and People with Disabilities
American Network of Community Options & Resource
1101 King St
Ste 380
Alexandria, VA 22314-2962
703-535-7850
FAX: 703-535-7860
e-mail: ancor@ancor.org
www.ancor.org

Dave Toeniskoetter, President
Chris Sparks, Vice President
Julie Manworren, Secretary/Treasurer
Renee L. Pietrangelo, PhD, Chief Executive Officer
This publication presents a detailed review of the process and the lessons learned. Details a way for all stake holders to work together for a state or local system.
119 pages $18 - $22

4978 Keeping Our Families Together
Through the Looking Glass
3075 Adeline St.
Ste. 120
Berkeley, CA 94703-2212
510-848-1112
800-644-2666
FAX: 510-848-4445
TTY: 510-848-1005
e-mail: tlg@lookingglass.org
www.lookingglass.org

Maureen Block, J.D., Board President
Thomas Spalding, Board Treasurer
Alice Nemon, D.S.W.,, Board Secretary
Report of the National Task Force on parents with disabilities and their families. Available in braille, large print or cassette. *$2.00*
12 pages

4979 Learn About the ADA in Your Local Library
US Department of Justice
950 Pennsylvania Ave NW
Washington, DC 20530-9
202-307-0663
800-574-0301
FAX: 202-307-1197
TTY: 800-514-0383
www.ada.gov

Rebecca B. Bond, Chief
Zita Johnson Betts, Deputy Chiefs
Sally Conway, Deputy Chiefs
A 10-page annotated list of 95 ADA publications and one videotape that are available in 15,000 public libraries throughout the country.

4980 LifeLines
Disabled & Alone/Life Services for the Handicapped
1440 Broadway
23rd Floor
New York, NY 10018-2326
212-532-6740
800-995-0066
FAX: 212-532-3588
e-mail: info@disabledandalone.org
www.disabledandalone.org

Leslie D. Park, Chairman
Rex L. Davidson, Vice President
William G. Shannon, J.D., Treasurer
Lee Alan Ackerman, B.A., Executive Director
Newsletter providing current and valuable information about lifetime care and planning for persons with disabilities and their families and the organizations serving them. Free upon request.
4-10 pages BiAnnual

4981 Lifelong Leisure Skills and Lifestyles for Persons with Developmental Disabilities
Brookes Publishing
PO Box 10624
Baltimore, MD 21285-0624
410-337-9580
800-638-3775
FAX: 410-337-8539
e-mail: custserv@brookespublishing.com
www.readplaylearn.com

Paul H. Brooks, Chairman
Jeffrey D. Brookes, President
Melissa A. Behm, Executive Vice President

This instructional manual offers ideas and detailed examples that describe how to guide individuals of all ages through popular activities using adaptations that foster skill acquisition and inclusion. Some of the concepts explored are home-school-community collaboration, choice making and the dignity of risk, and leisure skill acquisition for the life span. *$35.00*

352 pages Paperback
ISBN 1-55766-47-2

4982 Livin'
Lehigh Valley Center for Independent Living
435 Allentown Dr
Allentown, PA 18109-9121
610-770-9781
FAX: 610-770-9801
e-mail: info@lvcil.org
www.lvcil.org

Amy Beck, Executive Director
Cara Steidel, Director of Finance
Greg Bott, Director of Development
Jessica DeMaio, Administrative Services Coordinator

4 pages Quarterly

4983 Living in a State of Stuck
Brookline Books
8 Trumbull Rd
Suite B-001
Northampton, MA 01060
413-584-0184
800-666-2665
FAX: 413-584-6184
e-mail: brbooks@yahoo.com
www.brooklinebooks.com

3rd ed., paper
ISBN 1-571290-27-3

4984 Living in the Community
Independent Living Research Utilization ILRU
1333 Moursund
TIRR Memorial Hermann Research Cent
Houston, TX 77030-7031
713-520-0232
FAX: 713-520-5785
e-mail: ilru@ilru.org
www.ilru.org

Lex Frieden, Director, ILRU
Richard Petty, Program Director
Vinh Nguyen, Program Director
Roxy Funchess, Administrative Secretary

James, Lori, and Jamey describe the elements of their successful program to move people out of nursing homes and into the community: providing funding for deposits, first month's rent and other neccessities, including assistive technology; providing training and the other core services before and after consumers leave the nursing home; developing relationships with housing and other service providers.

10 pages

4985 Loud, Proud and Passionate
Mobility International USA
132 E. Broadway, Suite 343
PO Box 10767
Eugene, OR 97401
541-343-1284
FAX: 541-343-6812
e-mail: info@miusa.org
www.miusa.org

Susan Sygall, CEO
Cerise Roth-Vinson, COO
Cindy Lewis, Director of Programs
Stephanie Gray, Program Managers

A resource book for international development and women's organization about including women with disabilities in projects in the community. Informs women sith disabilities about the efforts and successes of their peers worldwide. *$30.00*

4986 Love: Where to Find It, How to Keep It
Accent Books & Products
PO Box 700
Bloomington, IL 61702-700
309-378-2961
800-787-8444
FAX: 309-378-4420
e-mail: acmtlvng@aol.com

Raymond C Cheever, Publisher
Betty Garee, Editor

Offers ideas such as how to meet other single people, avoid the wrong type; communications skills and much more for the disabled person wanting to date. *$6.95*

104 pages Paperback
ISBN 0-91570-31-0

4987 MOOSE: A Very Special Person
Brookline Books
8 Trumbull Rd
Suite B-001
Northampton, MA 01060
413-584-0184
800-666-2665
FAX: 413-584-6184
e-mail: brbooks@yahoo.com
www.brooklinebooks.com

Paperback
ISBN 0-91479-73-5

4988 Mainstream Magazine
2973 Beech St
San Diego, CA 92102-1529
619-232-2727
FAX: 619-234-3155
e-mail: editor@mainstream.mag.com
www.mainstream-mag.com

Cyndi Jones, Executive Director

The authoritative, national voice of people with disabilities, publishes in-depth reports on employment, education, new products and technology, legislation and disability rights advocacy, recreation and travel, disability arts and culture, plus personality profiles and challenging commentary. *$24.00*

Monthly

4989 Making Changes: Family Voices on Living Disabilities
Brookline Books
8 Trumbull Rd
Suite B-001
Northampton, MA 01060
413-584-0184
800-666-2665
FAX: 413-584-6184
e-mail: brbooks@yahoo.com
www.brooklinebooks.com

216 pages Paperback
ISBN 0-91479-93-

4990 Making Informed Medical Decisions: Where to Look and How to Use What You Find
Patient-Centered Guides
1005 Gravenstein Highway North
Sebastopol, CA 95472-3836 707-827-7019
800-889-8969
FAX: 707-824-8268
e-mail: orders@oreilly.com
www.patientcenters.com

Tim O'Reilly, CEO
Making Informed Medical Decisions acts like a friendly reference librarian, explaining: tips for researching for someone else; medical journal articles; statistics and risk; standard treatment options; clinical trial; making an ally of your doctor; and determining your own best course. Authors Oster, Thomas, and Joseff-a patient advocate, medical librarian, and medical doctor-also share examples and stories. *$17.95*
280 pages Paperback
ISBN 1-565924-59-2

4991 Making Wise Decisions for Long-Term Care
AARP Fulfillment
601 E St NW
Washington, DC 20049-1 202-434-2277
800-424-3410
FAX: 202-434-3443
TTY: 877-434-7598
e-mail: member@aarp.org
www.aarp.org

Carol Raphael, Chair
Ronald E. Daly, Sr., Board Vice Chair
Jeannine English, President
A. Barry Rand, Chief Executive Officer
Here's a comprehensive consumer education effort in the area of long-term care.
28 pages

4992 Making a Difference
Georgia Council On Developmental Disabilities
2 Peachtree St N.W.
Suite 26-246
Atlanta, GA 30303-3141 404-657-2126
888-275-4233
FAX: 404-657-2132
TTY: 404-657-2133
e-mail: eejacobson@dhr.state.ga.us
www.gcdd.org

Eric E Jacobson, Executive Director
Pat Nobbie, Deputy Director
Dottie Adams, Family/Individual Support Dir.
Valerie Meadows Suber, Public Information Director
The Georgia Council on Developmental Disabilities collaborates with Georgia's citizens, public and private advocacy organizations and policymakers to positively influence public policies that enhance the quality of life for people with disabilities and their families. GCDD provides this through education and advocacy activities, program implementation, funding and public policy analysis and research.

4993 Making a Difference: A Wise Approach
Easter Seals
233 South Wacker Drive
Suite 2400
Chicago, IL 60606-4703 312-726-0653
800-221-6827
FAX: 312-726-1494
www.easterseals.com

Richard W. Davidson, Chairman
Sandra L. Bouwman, 1st Vice Chairman
Joseph G. Kern, 2nd Vice Chairman
Ralph F. Boyd, Jr., Treasurer
The town of Wise, Virginia, and its leading citizen, Virgil Craft, personify what Making a Difference is all about when a community supports implementing the provisions of the Americans with Disabilities Act. Craft, a person with a disability, has spent his life giving back to the community. The community, in turn, has supported Craft's efforts to improve the environment, education, healthcare and access for disabled persons. A must buy for companies of all sizes, clubs and organizations. *$50.00*

4994 Managing Your Activities
Arthritis Foundation
PO Box 78423
Atlanta, GA 30357-0669 404-237-8771
800-933-7023
FAX: 404-872-0457
e-mail: help@arthritis.org
www.arthritis.org

John H Klippel, CEO/ President

4995 Managing Your Health Care
Arthritis Foundation
PO Box 78423
Atlanta, GA 30357-0669 404-237-8771
800-933-7023
FAX: 404-872-0457
e-mail: help@arthritis.org
www.arthritis.org

John H Klippel, CEO/ President

4996 Medical Aspects of Disability: A Handbook For The Rehabilitation Professional
Springer Publishing Company
11 West 42nd Street
15th Floor
New York, NY 10036 212-431-4370
877-687-7476
FAX: 212-941-7842
e-mail: cs@springerpub.com
www.springerpub.com

Ursula Springer, President
Theodore C. Nardin, CEO/Publisher
Jason Roth, VP/Marketing Director
James C. Costello, Vice President, Journal Publishing
$62.92
744 pages
ISBN 0-826179-71-1

4997 Meeting the Needs of Employees with Disabilities
Resources for Rehabilitation
22 Bonad Road
Ste 19a
Winchester, MA 01890-4330 781-368-9080
FAX: 781-368-9096
e-mail: orders@rfr.org
www.rfr.org

Susan Greenblatt, Editor
Provides information to help people with disabilities retain or obtain employment. Information on government programs and laws, supported employment, training programs, environmental adaptations and the transition from school to work are included. Chapters on mobility impairment, vision impairment and hearing and speech impairments. *$ 47.95*
167 pages Biennial
ISBN 0-92971 -13-5

4998 NCD Bulletin
National Council on Disability
1331 F Street Northwest
Suite 850
Washington, DC 20004- 1138 202-272-2004
FAX: 202-272-2022
e-mail: ncd@ncd.gov
www.ncd.gov

Jeff Rosen, Chairperson
Kamilah Oni Martin-Proctor, Co-Vice Chair
Lynnae Ruttledge, Co-Vice Chair
Rebecca Cokley, Executive Director
Reports on the latest issues and news affecting people with disabilities.
2 pages Monthly

4999 NCDE Survival Strategies for Oversease Living for People with Disabilities
National Clearinghouse on Disability and Exchange
132 E. Broadway, Suite 343
PO Box 10767
Eugene, OR 97401
541-343-1284
FAX: 541-343-6812
e-mail: info@miusa.org
www.miusa.org

Susan Sygall, CEO
Cerise Roth-Vinson, COO
Cindy Lewis, Director of Programs
Stephanie Gray, Program Managers
This book will provide individuals with disablilities information, resources and guidance on pursuing international exchange opportunities. It addresses disability-related aspects of the international exchange process such as choosing a program, applying, preparing for the trip, adjusting to a new country and returning home.

5000 NOD E-Newsletter
National Organization on Disability
77 Water Street
Suite 204
New York, NY 10005
646-505-1191
FAX: 646-505-1184
e-mail: zchizar@a-g.com
www.nod.org

George H W Bush, President
Thomas J. Ridge, Chairman
Charles F. Dey, Vice Chairman
Carol Glazer, President
Monthly E-Newsletter from the National Organization on Disability. Free.
3 pages Monthly

5001 National Hookup
ISC
16 Liberty St
Larkspur, CA 94939-1520
415-924-3549
FAX: 415-927-9556
e-mail: russbo@microweb.com

Russ Bohlke, Manager
Newsletter published by ISC, a national organization of people with physical disabilities. *$6.00*
12-16 pages Quarterly

5002 New Horizons in Sexuality
Accent Books & Products
PO Box 700
Bloomington, IL 61702-700
309-378-2961
800-787-8444
FAX: 309-378-4420
e-mail: acmtlvng@aol.com

Raymond C Cheever, Publisher
Betty Garee, Editor
This manual helps both males and females progress toward a satisfying post-injury relationship. *$7.95*
50 pages Paperback
ISBN 0-91570-42-6

5003 New Voices: Self Advocacy By People with Disabilities
Brookline Books
8 Trumbull Rd
Suite B-001
Northampton, MA 01060
413-584-0184
800-666-2665
FAX: 413-584-6184
e-mail: brbooks@yahoo.com
www.brooklinebooks.com

274 pages Paperback
ISBN 1-57129-04-4

5004 North Star Community Services
3420 University Ave
Waterloo, IA 50701-2050
319-236-0901
888-879-1365
FAX: 319-236-3701
e-mail: jmuller@northstarcs.org
www.northstarcs.org

Mark Witmer, Executive Director
Matt Hinders, Director of Operations & Safety
Bridget Hartmann, Director of Human Resources
Terri Davis, Director of Financial Services
North Star Community Services is a rehabilitative services organization with home office in Waterloo, IA and several branch offices in Northeast, Northern and Central Iowa. North Star helps indiviuals with disabilities live and work in their communities. Services include: adult day services, supported community living services, employment services, and case management/service coordination.

5005 Nothing is Impossible: Reflections on a New Life
Ballantine Books
1745 Broadway
10th Floor
New York, NY 10019
212-782-9000
e-mail: rhkidspublicity@randomhouse.com
www.atrandom.com

Edward Warren, Owner
Reeve offers a uniquely powerful message of hope on topics ranging from the controversial stem cell debate to the mind-body connection he credits with his recent physical improvements. *$6.99*
224 pages
ISBN 0-345470-73-7

5006 Nutritional Desk Reference
Keats Publishing
P.O.Box 876
New Canaan, CT 06840
203-966-8721
800-323-4900

5007 Nutritional Influences on Illness:
Third Line Press
4751 Viviana Dr
Tarzana, CA 91356-5038
818-996-0076
third-line.com

Melvyn R Werbach, Owner
A comprehensive summary of the world's knowledge concerning the relationship between dietary and nutrtional factors and illness. This book does not try to promote any particular school of thought. Instead of the author telling readers his opinion as to what research says, he makes it easy for them to see data for themselves and then form their own opinions.
504 pages
ISBN 0-879835-31-1

5008 Oregon Perspectives
Oregon Council on Developmental Disabilities
540 24th Pl NE
Salem, OR 97301-4517
503-945-9941
800-292-4154
FAX: 503-945-9947
e-mail: ocdd@ocdd.org
www.ocdd.org

Laura Bronson, Office Manager
Beth Kessler, Planning & Communications Coordi
A quarterly publication from the Oregon Council on Developmental Disabilities.

5009 **Organ Transplants: Making the Most of Your Gift of Life**
Patient-Centered Guides
1005 Gravenstein Highway North
Sebastopol, CA 95472-3836
707-827-7000
800-998-9938
FAX: 707-824-8268
e-mail: orders@oreilly.com
www.patientcenters.com

Linda Lamb, Series Editor
Shawnde Paull, Marketing
Tim O'Reilly, CEO

Over 64,000 people in the US are awaiting an organ transplant. Although transplant surgeries are now fairly routine and can give their recipients the gift of new life, the road to getting a transplant can be long and harrowing. Living with immunosuppressive drugs and strong emotional responses can also be more challenging than families imagine. Medical journalist Robert Finn answers the concerns of these families, with the latest facts about transplantation - as well as the stories behind them. *$19.95*
326 pages Paperback
ISBN 1-565926-34-X

5010 **PEAK Parent Center**
611 N Weber St
Suite 200
Colorado Springs, CO 80903-1072
719-531-9400
800-284-0251
FAX: 719-531-9452
e-mail: info@peakparent.org
www.peakparent.org

Barbara Buswell, Executive Director

PEAK Parent Center is a federally-designated Parent Training and Information Center (PTI). As a PTI, PEAK supports and empowers parents, providing them with information and strategies to use when advocating for their children with disabilities. PEAK works one-on-one with families and educators helping them realize new possibilities for children with disabilities by expanding knowledge of special education and offering new strategies for success.

5011 **Parallels in Time**
MN Governor's Council on Development Disabilities
658 Cedar St
Saint Paul, MN 55155-1603
651-296-4018
877-348-0505
FAX: 651-297-7200
e-mail: admin.dd@state.mn.us
www.mncdd.org

Colleen Wieck PhD, Executive Director

Parallels in Time traces present attitudes and the treatment of people with disabilities, and supplements the first weekend seesion of Partners in Policymaking. This CD-ROM includes the History of the Parent Movement and the History of the Independent Living Movement, as well as personal stories of self advocates, leaders in the self advocacy movement.

5012 **Part of the Team**
Easter Seals
Ste 1800
230 W Monroe St
Chicago, IL 60606-4851
312-726-6800
FAX: 312-726-1494

Janet D Jamieson, Communications Manager
James Williams Jr, Chief Executive Officer

Designed for employers of all sizes, rehabilitation organizations and all others concerned with the employment of people with disabilities. It addresses managers' concerns and questions about supervising persons with disabilities and can be used as a discussion/team-building tool for employees with and without disabilities. The video recognizes people with disabilities as strong contenders for almost any job. *$15.00*

5013 **Partnering with Public Health: Funding& Advocacy Opportunities for CILs and SILCs**
Independent Living Research Utilization ILRU
1333 Moursund
Houston, TX 77030-7031
713-520-0232
FAX: 713-520-5785
e-mail: ilru@ilru.org
ilru.org

Lex Frieden, Director, ILRU
Richard Petty, Program Director
Roxy Funchess, Administrative Secretary
George Powers, Legal Specialist

Laura Rauscher discusses how CILs and SCILs can use funding from the Centers for Disease Control and partnerships with public health agencies to provide innovative programs promoting the health of people with disabilities.
10 pages

5014 **Peer Counseling: Roles, Functions, Boundaries**
Independent Living Research Utilization ILRU
1333 Moursund
Houston, TX 77030-7031
713-520-0232
FAX: 713-520-5785
e-mail: ilru@ilru.org
ilru.org

Lex Frieden, Director, ILRU
Richard Petty, Program Director
Roxy Funchess, Administrative Secretary
George Powers, Legal Specialist

In this article, the following points were discussed: describing peer support as counseling suggests safeguards and expectations which cannot be provided by nonprofessionals; the purpose of peer counseling is to promote the independent living philosophy and encourage consumers to embrace it; peer counseling cannot and is not intended to help individuals deal with intense emotional stress, whether it is related to their disability or to something else.
10 pages

5015 **Peer Mentor Volunteers: Empowering People for Change**
Independent Living Research Utilization ILRU
1333 Moursund
Houston, TX 77030-7031
713-520-0232
FAX: 713-520-5785
e-mail: ilru@ilru.org
ilru.org

Lex Frieden, Director, ILRU
Richard Petty, Program Director
Roxy Funchess, Administrative Secretary
George Powers, Legal Specialist

Arizona Bridge to Independent Living (ABIL) in Phoenix, featured in this issue, is another winner in the innovative CIL program competition.
10 pages

5016 **People and Families**
New Jersey Council on Developmental Disabilities
20 West State Street, 6th Floor
P.O.Box 700
Trenton, NJ 08625-0700
609-292-3745
800-792-8858
FAX: 609-292-7114
TTY: 609-777-3238
e-mail: njcdd@njcdd.org
www.njcdd.org

Elaine Buchsbaum, Chairman
Christopher Miller, Vice Chair
Alison M. Lozano, Ph.D, Executive Director
Shirla Rufo Simpson, M.A., DRCC, Deputy Director

A free magazine for people with disabilities, their families and the public about disability topics such as personal assistance, deinstitutionalization, health care and community living. Published by the New Jersey council on Developmental Disabilities, a federally funded advocacy and policy advisory body. The council has 25 members - 15 consumer/product volunteers and 10 professionals.
48 pages Quarterly

5017 **People with Disabilities & Abuse: Implications for Center for Independent Living**
Independent Living Research Utilization ILRU
1333 Moursund
P.O.Box 700
Houston, TX 77030-7031
713-520-0232
FAX: 713-520-5785
e-mail: ilru@ilru.org
ilru.org
Lex Frieden, Director, ILRU
Richard Petty, Program Director
Roxy Funchess, Administrative Secretary
George Powers, Legal Specialist

10 pages

5018 **People with Disabilities Who Challenge the System**
Brookes Publishing
P.O.Box 10624
Baltimore, MD 21285-0624
410-337-9580
800-638-3775
FAX: 410-337-8539
e-mail: custserv@brookespublishing.com
readplaylearn.com
Paul H. Brooks, Chairman
Jeffrey D. Brookes, President
Melissa A. Behm, Executive Vice President
Jeffrey D. Brookes, President
Helpful forms, tables, and case studies plus an emphasis on self-determination point the way to the development of supports so that people who are deaf-blind, have severe to profound physical and cognitive disabilities, or have serious behavior problems can be fully included in the classroom, workplace, and community. *$34.00*
464 pages Paperback
ISBN 1-55766-29-0

5019 **People's Voice**
Independence CIL
300 3rd Ave SW
Suite F
Minot, ND 58701-4346
701-839-4724
800-377-5114
FAX: 701-838-1677
e-mail: independencecil@independencecil.org
independencecil.org
Susan Ogurek, Chair
Heather Wittliff, Vice Chair
Scott Burlingame, Executive Director
Emily Rodacker, Secretary/Treasurer

8 pages Quarterly

5020 **Personal Perspectives on Personal Assistance Services**
World Institute on Disability
3075 Adeline Street
Suite 155
Berkeley, CA 94703
510-225-6400
FAX: 510-225-0477
TTY:510-225-0478
e-mail: wid@wid.org
www.wid.org
Anita Shafer Aaron, Executive Director
Thomas Foley, Deputy Director
Bruce Curtis, International Program Director
Marsha Saxton, Director of Research and Training.
This collection of personal essays explores a wide range of perspectives on Personal Assistance Services. Family issues and PAS concerns for people with various different disabilities, of different ages and as members of minority groups are addressed.
$5.00
80 pages Paperback

5021 **Perspectives**
National Assoc of State Directors of DD Services
113 Oronoco St
Alexandria, VA 22314-2015
703-683-4202
FAX: 703-684-1395
e-mail: dberland@nasddds.org
Nancy Thaler, Executive Director
Nancy Thaler, Executive Director
Provides a concise summary of national policy developments and initiatives affecting persons with devlopmental disabilities and the programs that serve them. From bills pending before Congress, to the growth in Medicaid-funded services, to changes in federal-state Medicaid policies and the shift of responsibility from Washington to the states, keeps readers in tune with the latest national issues shaping publically funded disability services.
$95.00
Monthly

5022 **Place to Live**
Accent Books & Products
P.O.Box 700
Bloomington, IL 61702-700
309-378-2961
800-787-8444
FAX: 309-378-4420
e-mail: acmtlvng@aol.com
Raymond C Cheever, Publisher
Betty Garee, Editor
Raymond C Cheever, Publisher
Many disabled people have found that group housing or accessible apartments are the best alternative to living in a nursing home. These articles tell about some of the alternatives people have found so they can live independently. Just one idea might be the answer for better living for you. *$4.95*
64 pages Paperback
ISBN 0-91570-30-2

5023 **Proceedings**
AHEAD
107 Commerce Center Drive
Suite 204
Huntersville, NC 28078
704-947-7779
FAX: 704-948-7779
e-mail: information@ahead.org
www.ahead.org
Stephan Haml Smith, Director
Bea Awoniyi, President
Michael Johnson, Treasurer
Terra Beethe, Secretary
National conferences, innovative programs, research, evaluation services, auxiliary aids, career information and other vital information.

5024 **Psychological & Social Impact of Disability**
Springer Publishing Company
11 West 42nd Street
15th Floor
New York, NY 10036
212-431-4370
877-687-7476
FAX: 212-941-7842
e-mail: cs@springerpub.com
www.springerpub.com
James C. Costello, Vice President, Journal Publishing
Diana Osborne, Production Manager
Megan Larkin, Managing Editor, Journals
$49.95
488 pages
ISBN 0-826122-13-2

5025 Psychology and Health
Springer Publishing Company
11 West 42nd Street
15th Floor
New York, NY 10036 212-431-4370
877-687-7476
FAX: 212-941-7842
e-mail: cs@springerpub.com
www.springerpub.com
James C. Costello, Vice President, Journal Publishing
Diana Osborne, Production Manager
Megan Larkin, Managing Editor, Journals
Content of this book spans a wide range of clinical conditions, including somatization disorders, chronic pain, migraine, anxiety and cancer. *$29.95*
256 pages

5026 Psychology of Disability
Springer Publishing Company
11 West 42nd Street,
15th Floor
New York, NY 10036-3915 212-431-4370
877-687-7476
FAX: 212-941-7842
e-mail: cs@springerpub.com
www.springerpub.com
James C. Costello, Vice President, Journal Publishing
Diana Osborne, Production Manager
Megan Larkin, Managing Editor, Journals
Theodore C Nardin, Chief Executive Officer
Reactions to the disabled. *$27.95*
288 pages
ISBN 0-82613 -40-1

5027 Quality of Life for Persons with Disabilities
Brookline Books
8 Trumbull Road
Suite B-001
Northampton, MA 01060 413-584-0184
800-666-2665
FAX: 413-584-6184
e-mail: brbooks@yahoo.com
www.brooklinebooks.com
James C. Costello, Vice President, Journal Publishing
Quality of life generally refers to a person's subjective experience of his or her life and focuses attention on how the individual with a disabling condition experiences the world. This book presents a comprehensive and international view of this concept as applied to a broad range of settings in which persons with disabilities live, work and play. *$35.00*
Paperback
ISBN 0-91479 -92-1

5028 REACHing Out Newsletter
REACH of Dallas Resource on Independent Living
8625 King George Drive
Suite 210
Dallas, TX 75235-2286 214-630-4796
FAX: 214-630-6390
TTY:214-630-5995
e-mail: reachdallas@reachcils.org
reachcils.org
Charlotte A. Stewart, Executive Director
Kiowanda Jasso, Information & Referral Specialist
Kevan Johnson, Employment Consultant
Janie Peachee, Administrative Assistant
Quarterly newsletter from REACH of Dallas Resource Center on Independent Living.
16 pages Quarterly

5029 RTC Connection
Research and Training Center
University of Wisconsin Stou
Menomonie, WI 54751 715-232-2236
FAX: 715-232-2251
e-mail: menz@uwstout.edu
www.rtc.uwstout.edu
Julie Larson, Program Assistant
Bi-annual reports on disability and rehabilitation research and policy topics.
Newsletter

5030 Rehabilitation Gazette
Gazette International Networking Institute
4207 Lindell Blvd
Suite 110
Saint Louis, MO 63108-2930 314-534-0475
FAX: 314-534-5070
e-mail: info@post-polio.org
www.post-polio.org
Joan L Headley, Executive Director
William G. Stothers, President/Chairperson
Saul J. Morse, Vice President
Marny K. Eulberg, Secretary
International journal of independent living for people with disabilities. *$12.00*
8 pages Bi-Annually

5031 Relaxation: A Comprehensive Manual for Adults and Children with Special Needs
Research Press
2612 N. Mattis Ave.
P.O.Box 7886
Champaign, IL 61822- 9177 217-352-3273
800-519-2707
FAX: 217-352-1221
e-mail: orders@researchpress.com
www.researchpress.com
Paperback
ISBN 0-878221-86-8

5032 Resources for People with Disabilities and Chronic Conditions
Resources for Rehabilitation
Ste 19a
33 Bedford St
Lexington, MA 02420-4330 781-890-6371
FAX: 781-861-7517
Susan Greenblatt
A comprehensive resource directory that helps people with disabilities and chronic conditions achieve their maximum level of independence. Chapters on spinal cord injuries, low back pain, diabetes, hearing and speech impairments, epilepsy, multiple sclerosis. Describes organizations, products and publications. *$49.95*
215 pages Biennial
ISBN 0-92971 -12-7

5033 Role Portrayal and Stereotyping on Television
Greenwood Publishing Group
130 Cremona Drive
P O Box 1911
Santa Barbara,, CA 93117-4208 203-226-3571
800-368-6868
805-968-1911
FAX: 866-270-3856
e-mail: customerservice@abc-clio.com
www.abc-clio.com
214 pages $55 - $59.95
ISBN 0-313248-55-9

5034 Screening in Chronic Disease
Oxford University Press
2001 Evans Rd
Cary, NC 27513-2009
800-445-9714
877-773-4325
FAX: 919-677-1303
e-mail: custserv.us@oup.com
global.oup.com

Thomas Carty, Senior Vice President

Early detection, or screening, is a common strategy for controlling chronic disease, but little information has been available to help determine which screening procedures are worthwhile, until this textbook. *$42.50*

256 pages

5035 Sexual Adjustment
Accent Books & Products
P.O.Box 700
Bloomington, IL 61702-700
309-378-2961
800-787-8444
FAX: 309-378-4420
e-mail: acmtlvng@aol.com

Raymond C Cheever, Publisher
Betty Garee, Editor

Essential information concerning sexual adjustment for the paraplegic male. *$4.95*

73 pages Paperback
ISBN 0-19570 -00-0

5036 Sexuality and Disabilities: A Guide for Human Service Practitioners
Haworth Press
2&4 Park Square
Abingdon, FL 33487-1503
561-994-0555
FAX: 561-241-7856
e-mail: orders@taylorandfrancis.com
taylorandfrancisgroup.com

159 pages Hardcover
ISBN 1-560243-75-9

5037 Sickened: The Memoir of a Muchausen by Proxy Childhood
Bantam Books
1745 Broadway
10th Floor
New York, NY 10019-4039
212-782-9000
FAX: 212-572-6066
e-mail: crownpublicity@randomhouse.com
www.randomhouse.com

256 pages Hardcover
ISBN 0-553803-07-7

5038 Socialization Games for Persons with Disabilities
Charles C. Thomas
2600 South 1st St
Springfield, IL 62704-4730
217-789-8980
800-258-8980
FAX: 217-789-9130
e-mail: books@ccthomas.com
ccthomas.com

Michael P. Thomas, President

This text will assist those who want to teach severely multiple disabled students by providing information on: general principles of intervention and classroom organization; managing the behavior of students; physically managing students and using adaptive equipment; teaching eating skills; teaching toileting, dressing, and hygiene skills; teaching cognition, communication, and socialization skills; teaching independent living skills; and teaching infants and preschool students. *$38.95*

176 pages Paperback
ISBN 0-398067-46-5

5039 Sometimes You Just Want to Feel Like a Human Being
Brookes Publishing
P.O.Box 10624
Baltimore, MD 21285-0624
410-337-9580
800-638-3775
FAX: 410-337-8539
e-mail: custserv@brookespublishing.com
readplaylearn.com

Paul Brooks, Owner

Case studies of empowering psychotherapy with people with disabilities. This text reveals how counseling can be beneficial to individuals with disabilities of all kinds, including autism, mental retardation, sensory impairment, cerebral palsy, or HIV infection. *$ 26.95*

272 pages Paperback
ISBN 1-55766 -96-0

5040 South Carolina Assistive Technology Program
8301 Farrow Road
University Center for Excellence
Columbia, SC 29203-2920
803-935-5263
800-915-4522
FAX: 803-935-5342
e-mail: carol.page@uscmed.sc.edu
www.sc.edu/scatp/

Carol Page, Ph.D, Program Director
Mary r Alice Bechtle, Program Coordinator
Janet Jendron, Program Coordinator
Lydia Durham, Administrative Assistant

The South Carolina Assistive Technology Program (SCATP) is a federally funded program concerned with getting technology into the hands of people with disabilities so that they might live, work, learn and be a more independent part of the community. We provide an equipment loan and demonstration program, an on-line equipment exchange program, training, technical assistance, publications, an interactive CDROM (SC Curriculum Access through AT), an information listserv and work with various state com

7-8 pages Bi-annually

5041 Space Coast CIL News
Space Coast Center for Independent Living
571 Haverty Court,
Suite W
Rockledge, FL 32955-2566
321-633-6011
FAX: 321-633-6472
TTY:321-784-9008
e-mail: agrau@bellsouth.net
www.sccil.net

Michael Lavoie, President
Howard Fetes, Vice-President

Non-profit organization that provides services which enable people with disabilities to live as independently as possible.

12 pages Quarterly

5042 Special Needs Trust Handbook
Aspen Publishers
7th Fl
76 9th Ave
New York, NY 10011-4962
301-644-3599
800-638-8437
e-mail: customerservice@aspenpublishers.com
www.aspenpublishers.com

Bob Lemmond, President and CEO
Gustavo Dobles, Vice President and Chief Content Officer
Susan Pikitch, Vice President and Chief Financial Officer
Alan Scott, Vice President & Chief Marketing Office

The Special Needs Trusts Handbook is the single-volume, comprehensive resource that provides information on how to handle the complex requirements of drafting and administering trusts for clients who are mentally or physically disabled, or who wish to provide for others with disabilities. *$245.00*

900 pages
ISBN 0-735572-88-7

5043 Special Siblings: Growing Up With Someone with A Disability
Brookes Publishing
P.O.Box 10624
Baltimore, MD 21285-0624 410-337-9580
800-638-3775
FAX: 410-337-8539
e-mail: custserv@brookespublishing.com
readplaylearn.com

Paul Brooks, Owner
The author reveals what she experienced as the sister of a man with cerebral palsy and mental retardation — and shares what others have learned about being and having a special sibling. Weaving a lifetime of memories and reflections with relevant research and interviews with more than 100 other siblings and experts, McHugh explores a spectrum of feelings — from anger and guilt to love and pride — and helps readers understand the issues siblings may encounter. *$21.95*
256 pages Paperback
ISBN 1-557666-07-5

5044 TERI
251 Airport Rd
Oceanside, CA 92058-1321 760-721-1706
teriinc.org

Cheryl Kilmer, CEO & Founder
William E. Mara, Chief Operating Officer
Krysti DeZonia, Ed.D, Director of Education & Research
Joe Michalowski, Chief Financial Officer
A private, nonprofit corporation which has been developing and operating programs for individuals with developmental disabilities since 1980. Offers staff training videos, staff training tools and technique manuals.

5045 To Live with Grace and Dignity
World Institute on Disability
3075 Adeline Street
Suite 155
Berkeley, CA 94703-1520 510-225-6400
FAX: 510-225-0477
TTY:510-225-0478
e-mail: wid@wid.org
www.wid.org

Anita Shafer Aaron, Executive Director
Thomas Foley, Deputy Director
Bruce Curtis, International Program Director
Marsha Saxton, Director of Research and Training.
This unique book combines photographs and essays to allow the reader to enter some of the real day to day relationships that develop between individuals with disabilities and their personal assistants. Looking at and listening to what these relationships are all about is what motivated and inspired this book, says author Lydia Gans. The individuals included in this book represent a wide range of ages, disabilities and cultural backgrounds. *$26.00*
72 pages Paperback

5046 Touch/Ability Connects People with Disabilities & Alternative Health Care Pract.
Independent Living Research Utilization ILRU
1333 Moursund
Houston, TX 77030-7031 713-520-0232
FAX: 713-520-5785
e-mail: ilru@ilru.org
ilru.org

Lex Frieden, Director, ILRU
Richard Petty, Program Director
Roxy Funchess, Administrative Secretary
George Powers, Legal Specialist
The people at DIRECT center for Independence and Touch/Ability in Tuscon, Arizona, have collaborated to develop a wellness program that makes alternative health care choices available to people with disabilities. The Touch/Ability Wellness program was selected as one of last year's winners in the Innovative CILs competition because of this outcome of increased options open to people with disabilities.
10 pages

5047 US Role in International Disability Activities: A History
World Institute on Disability
3075 Adeline Street
Suite 155
Berkeley, CA 94703-1520 510-225-6400
FAX: 510-225-0477
TTY:510-225-0478
e-mail: wid@wid.org
www.wid.org

Anita Shafer Aaron, Executive Director
Thomas Foley, Deputy Director
Bruce Curtis, International Program Director
Marsha Saxton, Director of Research and Training.
This study was undertaken to present an initial introduction to US involvement in the field of international rehabilitation and disability. *$12.00*
169 pages Paperback

5048 Understanding and Accommodating Physical Disabilities: Desk Reference
Greenwood Publishing Group
130 Cremona Drive
P O Box 1911
Santa Barbara,, CA 93117-4208 203-226-3571
800-368-6868
805-968-1911
FAX: 866-270-3856
e-mail: customerservice@abc-clio.com
www.abc-clio.com

200 pages $52.95 - $55
ISBN 0-899308-14-7

5049 Vestibular Disorders Association
Vestibular Disorders Association
5018 NE 15th Ave
PO Box 13305
Portland, OR 97211-305 503-229-7705
800-837-8428
FAX: 503-229-8064
e-mail: info@vestibular.org
www.vestibular.org

Cynthia Ryan MBA, Executive Director
Tony Staser, Development Director
Kerrie Denner, Outreach Coordinator
Karen Ilari, Administrative Support Coordinator
The mission of the Vestibular Disorders Association is to serve people with vestibular disorders by providing access to information, offering a support network, and elevating awareness of the challenges associated with these disorders. *$15.00*
ISBN 0-963261-15-0

5050 Visions & Values
Idaho Council on Developmental Disabilities
650 W. State St., Room 100
P. O. Box 83720
Boise, ID 83720-5840 208-332-1824
800-544-2433
FAX: 208-334-2307
www.state.id.us/icdd

C. L. Butch Otter, Governor
A quarterly publication from the Idaho Council on Developmental Disabilities.

5051 Weiner's Herbal
Quantum Books
355 Middlesex Avenue
Wilmington, MA 01887-1406 978-988-2470
FAX: 617-577-7282
e-mail: orders@quantumbk.com
www.quantumbooks.com

William Szabo, Owner
A-Z index covering all aspects of herbs.
Paperback
ISBN 0-812825-86-1

5052 When the Brain Goes Wrong
Fanlight Productions
32 Court Street,
21st Floor
Brooklyn, NY 11201-1731
718-488-8900
800-876-1710
FAX: 718-488-8642
e-mail: info@fanlight.com
www.fanlight.com

Ben Achtenberg, Owner
Nicole Johnson, Publicity Coordinator
Anthony Sweeney, Marketing Director

An extraordinary and provocative series of seven short films which profile individuals with a range of brian dysfunctions. The seven brief segments focus on schizophrenia, manic depression, epilepsy, head injury, headaches and addiction. In addition to the personal stories, the segments include interviews with physicians who speak briefly about what is known about the disorders and treatment. #131 *$245.00*
ISBN 1-572951-31-1

5053 Women with Physical Disabilities: Achieving & Maintaining Health & Well-Being
Spina Bifida Association of America
1600 Wilson Blvd.
Suite 800
Arlington, VA 22209-4226
202-944-3285
800-621-3141
FAX: 202-944-3295
e-mail: sbaa@sbaa.org
www.spinabifidaassociation.org

Ana Ximenes, Chair
Sara Struwe, President & CEO
Cindy Brownstein, CEO
George Sturm, Treasurer

Introduces the critical concept of womens health in the context of physical disabilities. *$42.00*

5054 Work in the Context of Disability Culture
Independent Living Research Utilization ILRU
1333 Moursund
Houston, TX 77030-7031
713-520-0232
FAX: 713-520-5785
e-mail: ilru@ilru.org
ilru.org

Lex Frieden, Director, ILRU
Richard Petty, Program Director
Roxy Funchess, Administrative Secretary
George Powers, Legal Specialist

Another winner in the innovative CIL competition-Steve Brown describes the Talking Books Program of Southeast Alaska Independent Living, discussing their efforts to record the oral history and life experiences of people with disabilities in the larger context of the disability culture.
10 pages

Parenting: General

5055 AEPS Family Report: For Children Ages Three to Six
Brookes Publishing
P.O.Box 10624
Baltimore, MD 21285-0624
410-337-9580
800-638-3775
FAX: 410-337-8539
e-mail: custserv@brookespublishing.com
readplaylearn.com

Paul Brooks, Owner

This is a 64-item questionnaire that asks parents to rank their child's abilities on specific skills. In packages of 10 paperback. *$23.00*
28 pages Saddle-stiched
ISBN 1-557662-50-9

5056 AT for Parents with Disabilities
Idaho Assistive Technology Project
875 Perimeter Drive
Moscow, ID 83843-2268
208-885-6111
800-432-8324
e-mail: idahoat@uidaho.edu
www.uidaho.edu

Chuck Staben, President
Kathy Aiken, Provost and Executive VP
Keith Ickes, Executive Director for Planning and Budget
Jack Mciver, VP for Research
$5.00
80 pages

5057 Adapted Physical Activity Programs
Human Kinetics
1607 N Market Street
P.O.Box 5076
Champaign, IL 61820- 5076
800-747-4457
FAX: 217-351-1549
e-mail: info@hkusa.com
www.humankinetics.com

Quarterly
ISSN 0736-58 9

5058 All of Us: Talking Together, Sex Educationfor People with Developmental Disabilities
Aquarius Health Care Videos
30 Forest Road
P.O. Box 249
Millis, MA 02054-7159
508-376-1244
FAX: 508-376-1245
e-mail: aqvideos@tiac.net
www.aquariusproductions.com

Lesile Kussmann, President
Joyce Farmer, Assistant Director

For parents, caregivers and young people with developmental disabilities often feel isolated and unsure when approaching sex education with their children. In this video, parents of children with developmental disabilities share their difficulties in talking to their children about the social/sexual arena. Real life conversations between parents and their children demonstrate their discomfort, concerns, thoughts and hopes. *$195.00*
Video

5059 Baby Book for the Developmentally Challenged Child
Exceptional Parent Library
P.O.Box 1807
Englewood Cliffs, NJ 7632-1207
201-947-6000
800-535-1910
FAX: 201-947-9376
e-mail: eplibrary@aol.com
www.eplibrary.com

48 pages Hardcover

5060 Babyface: A Story of Heart and Bones
Spina Bifida Association of America
1600 Wilson Blvd.
Suite 800
Arlington, VA 22209-4226
202-944-3285
800-621-3141
FAX: 202-944-3295
e-mail: sbaa@sbaa.org
www.spinabifidaassociation.org

Ana Ximenes, Chair
Sara Struwe, President & CEO
Cindy Brownstein, CEO
George Sturm, Treasurer

A must read for families that seek insight into coping with a chronic condition. Many useful resources provided. *$32.90*

5061 Backyards and Butterflies
Brookline Books
8 Trumbull Road
Suite B-001
Northampton, MA 01060
413-584-0184
800-666-2665
FAX: 413-584-6184
e-mail: brbooks@yahoo.com
www.brooklinebooks.com

72 pages Paperback
ISBN 1-57129 -11-7

5062 Books on Special Children
BOSC
P.O.Box 305
Congers, NY 10920-305
845-638-1236
FAX: 845-638-0847
e-mail: irene@boscbooks.com
www.boscbooks.com

Irene Slovak, Owner
Distributes books by mail to professionals and parents of handicapped children. The BOSC Directory contains facilities for people with learning disabilities (all disabilities, published annually)
300+ pages Hardcover
ISBN O-G61386-08-8

5063 Brothers, Sisters, and Special Needs
Brookes Publishing
P.O.Box 10624
Baltimore, MD 21285-0624
410-337-9580
800-638-3775
FAX: 410-337-8539
e-mail: custserv@brookespublishing.com
readplaylearn.com

Paul Brooks, Owner
Information and activities for helping young siblings of children with chronic illnesses and developmental disabilities. *$30.00*
224 pages Paperback
ISBN 1-55766 -43-3

5064 Building the Healing Partnership: Parents, Professionals and Children
Brookline Books
8 Trumbull Road
Suite B-001
Northampton, MA 01060
413-584-0184
800-666-2665
FAX: 413-584-6184
e-mail: brbooks@yahoo.com
www.brooklinebooks.com

Paperback
ISBN 0-91479 -63-8

5065 Children with Disabilities
Brookes Publishing
P.O.Box 10624
Baltimore, MD 21285-0624
410-337-9580
800-638-3775
FAX: 410-337-8539
e-mail: custserv@brookespublishing.com
www.brookespublishing.com

Mark L Batshaw MD, Editor
Paul Brooks, Owner
Lauren Rohe, Regional Sales Consultant
Cary Gold, Educational Sales Representative
Extensive coverage of genetics, heredity, pre- and postnatal development, specific disabilities, family roles, and intervention. Features chapters on substance abuse, HIV and AIDS, Down syndrome, fragile X syndrome, behavior management, transitions to adulthood, and health care in the 21st century. Also reveals the causes of many conditions that can lead to developmental disabilities. *$69.95*
912 pages Hardcover
ISBN 1-557665-81-8

5066 Conditional Love: Parents' Attitudes Toward Handicapped Children
Greenwood Publishing Group
130 Cremona Drive
P O Box 1911
Santa Barbara,, CA 93117-4208
203-226-3571
800-368-6868
805-968-1911
FAX: 866-270-3856
e-mail: customerservice@abc-clio.com
www.abc-clio.com

312 pages
ISBN 0-89789 -24-7

5067 Coordinacion De Servicios Centrado En La Familia
Brookline Books
8 Trumbull Road
Suite B-001
Northampton, MA 01060
413-584-0184
800-666-2665
FAX: 413-584-6184
e-mail: brbooks@yahoo.com
www.brooklinebooks.com

34 pages Paperback
ISBN 0-91479 -90-5

5068 Developing Personal Safety Skills in Children with Disabilities
Brookes Publishing
P.O.Box 10624
Baltimore, MD 21285-0624
410-337-9580
800-638-3775
FAX: 410-337-8539
e-mail: custserv@brookespublishing.com
readplaylearn.com

Paul Brooks, Owner
A guide for teachers, parents, and caregivers, this volume explores the issue of personal safety for children with disabilities and offers strategies for empowering and protecting them at home and in school. Recognizing that children with disabilities are vulnerable to abuse, this work explores why children with disabilities need personal safety skills, offers, curriculum ideas and exercises, and advocates the development of self-esteem and assertiveness so that children can protect themselves. *$34.00*
220 pages Paperback
ISBN 1-557661-84-7

5069 Developmental Disabilities in Infancy and Childhood
Brookes Publishing
P.O.Box 10624
Baltimore, MD 21285-0624
410-767-6100
800-638-3775
FAX: 410-767-5850
e-mail: custserv@brookespublishing.com
readplaylearn.com

Paul Brooks, Owner
This two volume set explores advances in assessment and treatment, retains a clinical focus, and incorporates recent developments in research and theory. Can be purchased individually or as a set (Vol. 1: Neurodevelopmental Diagnosis and Treatment Vol. 2: The Spectrum of Developmental Disabilities). *$210.00*
Hardcover
ISBN 1-55766O-CA-P

5070 Dictionary of Developmental Disabilities Terminology
Brookes Publishing
P.O.Box 10624
Baltimore, MD 21285-0624
410-337-9580
800-638-3775
FAX: 410-337-8539
e-mail: custserv@brookespublishing.com
readplaylearn.com

Paul Brooks, Owner
Answers thousands of questions for medical or human services professionals, parents or advocates of children with disabilities, or students preparing for their careers. Provides thorough expla-

nations of the most common terms associated with disabilities. *$ 55.95*
368 pages Hardcover
ISBN 1-557662-45-2

5071 Encyclopedia of Genetic Disorders & Birth Defects
Facts on File
132 W 31st St
17th Floor
New York, NY 10001-3406 800-322-8755
FAX: 800-678-3633
e-mail: custserv@factsonfile.com
www.infobasepublishing.com/
Mark Donnell, President
Layperson-accessible entries on genetic terminology and genetically-influenced conditions. *$71.50*
474 pages
ISBN 0-816038-09-0

5072 Exceptional Parent Magazine
Psy-Ed Corporation
416 Main Street
Johnstown, PA 15901-2032 814-361-3860
877-372-7368
FAX: 814-361-3861
e-mail: cmellott@eparent.com
www.eparent.com
Vanessa B Ira, Contributing Writer / Editor
Joseph M. Valenzano, Jr., President, CEO & Publisher
Rick Rader, MD, Editor-in-Chief
Lois Keegan, Human Resources Manager
Magazine that provides information, support, ideas, encouragement, and outreach for parents and families of children with disabilities and the professionals who work with them. *$39.95*
85 pages Monthly

5073 Face of Inclusion
Special Needs Project
Ste H
324 State St
Santa Barbara, CA 93101-2364 805-962-8087
800-333-6867
FAX: 805-962-5087
e-mail: eplibrary@aol.com
www.eplibrary.com
Hod Gray, Owner
A unique and moving parents' perspective of inclusion for administrators, teachers, and parents of children with disabilities. *$99.00*

5074 Families Magazine
New Jersey Developmental Disabilities Council
20 West State Street, 6th Floor
P.O.Box 700
Trenton, NJ 08625-0700 609-292-3745
800-792-8858
FAX: 609-292-7114
TTY: 609-777-3238
e-mail: njcdd@njcdd.org
www.njddc.org
Elaine Buchsbaum, Chairman
Christopher Miller, Vice Chair
Alison M. Lozano, Ph.D, Executive Director
Shirla Rufo Simpson, M.A., DRCC, Deputy Director
Quarterly magazine for people with disabilities, their families and the public, features family profiles, news, columns and the New Jersey Family support councils newsletter.
Quarterly

5075 Families, Illness & Disability
Through the Looking Glass
3075 Adeline St
Ste. 120
Berkeley, CA 94703-2212 510-848-1112
800-644-2666
FAX: 510-848-4445
TTY: 510-848-1005
e-mail: tlg@lookingglass.org
www.lookingglass.org
Maureen Block, J.D., Co-Founder
Karen Fessel, Ph.D., Executive Director
$35.00
320 pages

5076 Family Interventions Throughout Disability
Springer Publishing Company
11 West 42nd Street,
15th Floor
New York, NY 10036-3915 212-431-4370
877-687-7476
FAX: 212-941-7842
e-mail: cs@springerpub.com
www.springerpub.com
Theodore C Nardin, Chief Executive Officer
James C. Costello, Vice President, Journal Publishing
Diana Osborne, Production Manager
Megan Larkin, Managing Editor, Journals
Family attitudes throughout chronic illness and disability. *$31.95*
320 pages
ISBN 0-82615 -80-4

5077 Family-Centered Service Coordination: A Manual for Parents
Brookline Books
8 Trumbull Road
Suite B-001
Northampton, MA 01060 413-584-0184
800-666-2665
FAX: 413-584-6184
e-mail: brbooks@yahoo.com
www.brooklinebooks.com
34 pages Paperback
ISBN 0-91479 -90-5

5078 Handbook About Care in the Home
AARP Fulfillment
601 E St NW
Washington, DC 20049-1 202-434-2277
888-687-2277
TTY:877-434-7598
e-mail: member@aarp.org
www.aarp.org
24 pages

5079 LifeLines
Disabled & Alone/Life Services for the Handicapped
1440 Broadway,
23rd Floor
New York, NY 10006-2734 212-532-6740
800-995-0066
FAX: 212-532-6740
e-mail: info@disabledandalone.org
www.disabledandalone.org
Leslie D. Park, Chairman
Rex L Davidson, Vice President
Disabled and Alone is a national, nonprofit organization whose sole purpose is to assure the well being of disabled individuals, particularly those whose families have died and have engaged Disabled and Alone to provide advocacy and oversight for the lifetime of their disabled children. This newsletter provides information about 'future planning' for a person with a disability.
8-16 pages Bi-annual

5080 Loving & Letting Go
Centering Corporation
7230 Maple Street
Omaha, NE 68134-5064
402-553-1200
866-218-0101
FAX: 402-533-0507
e-mail: j1200@aol.com
www.centering.org

Joy Johnson, Founder
Dr. Marvin Johnson, co-Founder
For parents who decide to turn away from aggressive medical intervention for their critically ill newborn. *$5.95*
48 pages Paperback

5081 Mobility Training for People with Disabilities
Charles C. Thomas
2600 South 1st St
Springfield, IL 62704-4730
217-789-8980
800-258-8980
FAX: 217-789-9130
e-mail: books@ccthomas.com
www.ccthomas.com

Michael P. Thomas, President

5082 Mother to Be
Through the Looking Glass
3075 Adeline St
Ste. 120
Berkeley, CA 94703-2212
510-848-1112
800-644-2666
FAX: 510-848-4445
TTY: 510-848-1005
e-mail: tlg@lookingglass.org
www.lookingglass.org

Maureen Block, J.D., Co-Founder
Karen Fessel, Ph.D., Executive Director
Guide to pregnancy and birth for women with disabilities. *$34.00*
410 pages

5083 New Language of Toys: Teaching Communication Skills to Children with Special Needs
Spina Bifida Association of America
1600 Wilson Blvd.
Suite 800
Arlington, VA 22209-4226
202-944-3285
800-621-3141
FAX: 202-944-3295
e-mail: sbaa@sbaa.org
www.spinabifidaassociation.org

Ana Ximenes, Chair
Sara Struwe, President & CEO
Cindy Brownstein, CEO
George Sturm, Treasurer
A guide for parents and teachers and a reader-friendly resource guide that provides a wealth of information on how play activities affect a child's language development and where to get the toys and materials to use in these activities. *$19.00*

5084 NewsLine
Federation for Children with Special Needs
45 Bromfield Street
10th Floor
Boston, MA 02108
866-815-8122
FAX: 617-542-7832
e-mail: info@ppal.net
www.ppal.net

Lisa Lambert, Executive Director
Deborah A. Fauntleroy, MSW, Associate Director
Offers information for parents and families on resources, medical updates, activities, fund-raising events and association news for their disabled children.
Quarterly

5085 On the Road to Autonomy: Promoting Self- Competence in Children & Youth with Disabilities
Brookes Publishing
P.O.Box 10624
Baltimore, MD 21285-0624
410-337-9580
800-638-3775
FAX: 410-337-8539
e-mail: custserv@brookespublishing.com
readplaylearn.com

Paul Brooks, Owner
This book provides detailed conceptual, practical, and personal information regarding the promotion of self-esteem, self-determination, and coping skills among children and youth with and without disabilities. *$48.00*
432 pages Paperback
ISBN 1-55766 -35-5

5086 Pain Erasure
M Evans and Company
216 E 49th St
New York, NY 10017-1546
212-979-0880
FAX: 212-486-4544

Mary Evans, Owner
This book explains Bonnie Prudden's method for pain relief using myotherapy, a method hailed by doctors and patients.
ISBN 0-345331-02-8

5087 Parent Centers and Independent Living Centers: Collectively We're Stronger
Independent Living Research Utilization ILRU
1333 Moursund
Houston, TX 77030-7031
713-520-0232
FAX: 713-520-5785
e-mail: ilru@ilru.org
ilru.org

Lex Frieden, Director, ILRU
Richard Petty, Program Director
Roxy Funchess, Administrative Secretary
George Powers, Legal Specialist
This article describes several examples of effective working relationships of PTIs and CILs. The examples highlight how parent and consumer organizations have identified complimentary strengths and formed partnerships to better support children with disabilities and their families. These partnerships can also be a very important way of involving youth in the disability movement so they may become leaders of tomorrow.
10 pages

5088 Parent-Child Interaction and Developmental Disabilities
Greenwood Publishing Group
130 Cremona Drive
P O Box 1911
Santa Barbara,, CA 93117
800-368-6868
805-968-1911
FAX: 866-270-3856
e-mail: customerservice@abc-clio.com
www.abc-clio.com

395 pages Hardcover
ISBN 0-275928-35-7

5089 Parenting
Accent Books & Products
P.O.Box 700
Bloomington, IL 61702-700
309-378-2961
800-787-8444
FAX: 309-378-4420
e-mail: acmtlvng@aol.com

Raymond C Cheever, Publisher
Betty Garee, Editor
Experienced parents (who are disabled) discuss: raising children from infant to teens, balancing career and motherhood, discipline methods and more when both parents are disabled. *$7.95*
83 pages
ISBN 0-91570 -26-4

5090 Parenting with a Disability
Through the Looking Glass
3075 Adeline St
Ste. 120
Berkeley, CA 94703-2212 510-848-1112
800-644-2666
FAX: 510-848-4445
TTY: 510-848-1005
e-mail: tlg@lookingglass.org
www.lookingglass.org

Maureen Block, J.D., Board President
Rusty Hendlin, M.A., LMFT, Director of Medi-Cal Services
Thomas Spalding, Board Treasurer
Alice Nemon, D.S.W., Board Secretary
International newsletter. Available in braille, large print or cassette.
3 per year

5091 Perspectives on a Parent Movement
Brookline Books
8 Trumbull Rd
Suite B-001
Northampton, MA 1060-4533 413-584-0184
800-666-2665
FAX: 413-584-6184
e-mail: brbooks@yahoo.com
www.brooklinebooks.com

Paperback
ISBN 0-91479 -74-3

5092 Sexuality and the Developmentally Handicapped
Edwin Mellen Press
P.O.Box 450
Lewiston, NY 14092-450 716-754-2266
FAX: 716-754-4056
e-mail: jrupnow@mellenpress.com
mellenpress.com

Herbert Richardson, Owner
Presents the knowledge, attitudes, and skills pertinent to responding to the sexual problems of developmentally handicapped persons, their families and communities. Details fully documented cases, issues concerning the law, and resource materials available. *$89.95*
245 pages Hardcover
ISBN 0-88946 -32-5

5093 Shattered Dreams-Lonely Choices: Birth Parents of Babies with Disabilities
Greenwood Publishing Group
130 Cremona Drive
Santa Barbara, CA 93117-4208 203-226-3571
800-368-6868
805-968-1911
FAX: 866-270-3856
e-mail: customerservice@abc-clio.com
www.abc-clio.com

208 pages Hardcover
ISBN 0-897892-86-0

5094 Since Owen, A Parent-to-Parent Guide for Care of the Disabled Child
Special Needs Project
Ste H
324 State St
Santa Barbara, CA 93101-2364 818-718-9900
800-333-6867
FAX: 818-349-2027
e-mail: editor@specialneeds.com
www.specialneeds.com

Hod Gray, Owner
Against the background of his experience as the parent of a severely disabled young man, Callahan writes conscientiously to other parents. *$16.95*
486 pages

5095 Sleep Better! A Guide to Improving Sleep for Children with Special Needs
Brookes Publishing
P.O.Box 10624
Baltimore, MD 21285-624 410-337-9580
800-638-3775
FAX: 410-337-8539
e-mail: custserv@brookespublishing.com
readplaylearn.com

Paul Brooks, Owner
This book offers step-by-step, how to instructions for helping children with disabilities get the rest they need. For problems ranging from bedtime tantrums to night waking, parents and caregivers will find a variety of widely tested and easy-to-implement techniques that have already helped hundreds of children with special needs. *$21.95*
288 pages Paperback
ISBN 1-55766 -15-7

5096 Something's Wrong with My Child!
Charles C. Thomas
2600 S 1st Street
Springfield, IL 62704-4730 217-789-8980
800-258-8980
FAX: 217-789-9130
e-mail: books@ccthomas.com
www.ccthomas.com

Michael P. Thomas, President
This text provides professionals and parents with the opportunity to gain insights into a family that has benefited positively and constructively from the presence of a member with a disability. The author presents a compilation of easy-to-read material that's based on real-life experiences. *$39.95*
234 pages Paperback 1998
ISBN 0-398068-99-8

5097 Sometimes I Get All Scribbly
Exceptional Parent Library
P.O.Box 1807
Englewood Cliffs, NJ 7632-1207 201-947-6000
800-535-1910
FAX: 201-947-9376
e-mail: eplibrary@aol.com
www.eplibrary.com

5098 Son-Rise: The Miracle Continues
2080 South Undermountain Road
Sheffield, MA 01257-9643 413-229-2100
877-766-7473
FAX: 413-229-3202
e-mail: sonrise@option.org
www.son-rise.org

Barry Neil Kaufman, Co-Founder/ Co-Originator/Senior Teacher/Trainer
Samahria Lyte Kaufman, Co-Founder/ Co-Originator/Senior Teacher/Trainer
Bryn Hogan, ATCA Senior Staff
William Hogan, ATCA Senior Staff
Documents Raun Kaufman's astonishing development from a lifeless, autistic, retarded child into a highly verbal, lovable youngster with no traces of his former condition. Details Raun's extraordinary progress from the age of four into young adulthood, also shares moving accounts of five families that successfully used the Son-Rise Program to reach their own special children.
372 pages
ISBN 0-915811-53-7

5099 Special Kids Need Special Parents: A Resource for Parents of Children With Special Needs
Berkley Publishing Group
375 Hudson Street
New York, NY 10014-3657 212-366-2372
FAX: 212-366-2933
e-mail: ecommerce@us.penguingroup.com
www.us.penguingroup.com

319 pages Paperback
ISBN 0-425176-62-2

5100 Special Parent, Special Child
Exceptional Parent Library
P.O.Box 1807
Englewood Cliffs, NJ 7632-1207 201-947-6000
800-535-1910
FAX: 201-947-9376
e-mail: eplibrary@aol.com
www.eplibrary.com

Hardcover

5101 Strategies for Working with Families of Young Children with Disabilities
Brookes Publishing
P.O.Box 10624
Baltimore, MD 21285-624 410-337-9580
800-638-3775
FAX: 410-337-8539
e-mail: custserv@brookespublishing.com
readplaylearn.com

Paul Brooks, Owner
This text offers useful techniques for collaborating with and supporting families whose youngest members either have a disability or are at risk for developing a disability. The authors address specific issues such as cultural diversity, transitions to new programs, and disagreements between families and professionals. *$33.00*
272 pages Paperback
ISBN 1-55766-57-6

5102 That's My Child
Exceptional Parent Library
P.O.Box 1807
Englewood Cliffs, NJ 7632-1207 201-947-6000
800-535-1910
FAX: 201-947-9376
e-mail: eplibrary@aol.com
www.eplibrary.com

5103 They Don't Come with Manuals
Fanlight Productions
32 Court Street, 21st Floor
Brooklyn, NY 11201-1731 718-488-8900
800-876-1710
FAX: 718-488-8642
e-mail: orders@fanlight.com
www.fanlight.com

Ben Achtenberg, Owner
Anthony Sweeney, Marketing Director
Nicole Johnson, Publicity Coordinator
The parents and adoptive parents in this video speak candidly of their day to day experiences caring for children with physical and mental disabilities. *$145.00*

5104 They're Just Kids
Aquarius Health Care Videos
30 Forest Road
P.O. Box 249
Millis, MA 02054-7159 508-376-1244
FAX: 508-376-1245
e-mail: aqvideos@tiac.net
www.aquariusproductions.com

Lesile Kussmann, President
Joyce Farmer, Assistant Director
The importance and value of inclusion, excellent for anyone working with kids with disabilities. The documentary explores the advantages of the inclusion of disabled children in the classroom, cub scouts and other extracurricular activities. *$99.00*
Video

5105 To a Different Drumbeat
Alliance for Parental Involvement in Education
P.O.Box 59
East Chatham, NY 12060-59 518-392-6900
FAX: 518-392-6900

5106 Uncommon Fathers
Woodbine House
6510 Bells Mill Rd
Bethesda, MD 20817-1636 301-897-3570
800-843-7323
e-mail: info@woodbinehouse.com
woodbinehouse.com

Irv Shapell, Owner
Nineteen fathers talk about the life-altering experience of having a child with special needs and offer a welcome, seldom-heard perspective on raising kids with disabilities, including autism, cerebral palsy, and Down syndrome. Uncommon Fathers is the first book for fathers by fathers, but it is also helpful to partners, family, friends, and service providers. *$14.95*
206 pages Paperback
ISBN 0-933149-68-9

5107 We Can Speak for Ourselves: Self Advocacy by Mentally Handicapped People
Brookline Books
8 Trumbull Rd
Suite B-001
Northampton, MA 1060-4533 413-584-0184
800-666-2665
FAX: 413-584-6184
e-mail: brbooks@yahoo.com
www.brooklinebooks.com

246 pages Paperback
ISBN 0-25336 -65-9

5108 You May Be Able to Adopt
Through the Looking Glass
3075 Adeline St
Ste. 120
Berkeley, CA 94703-2212 510-848-1112
800-644-2666
FAX: 510-848-4445
TTY: 510-848-1005
e-mail: tlg@lookingglass.org
www.lookingglass.org

Maureen Block, J.D., Board President
Rusty Hendlin, M.A., LMFT, Director of Medi-Cal Services
Thomas Spalding, Board Treasurer
Alice Nemon, D.S.W., Board Secretary
A guide to the adoption process for prospective mothers with disabilities and their partners. Available in braille, large print or cassette. *$10.00*
112 pages

5109 You Will Dream New Dreams
Kensington Publishing
119 West 40th Street
New York, NY 10018 800-221-2647
www.kensingtonbooks.com

Steven Zacharius, Chairman, President & CEO
A parent's support group in print. The shared narratives come from those with newly diagnosed children, adult disabled children, and everything in between. *$13.00*
278 pages Paperback
ISBN 1-575665-60-3

5110 **Your Child Has a Disability: A Complete Sourcebook of Daily and Medical Care**
Brookes Publishing
P.O.Box 10624
Baltimore, MD 21285-624
410-337-9580
800-638-3775
FAX: 410-337-8539
e-mail: custserv@brookesopublishing.com
readplaylearn.com
Paul Brooks, Owner
Offers expert advice on a wide range of issues-from finding the right doctor and investigating the medical aspects of a child's condition to learning care techniques and fulfilling education requirements. *$24.95*
368 pages Paperback
ISBN 1-557663-74-2

Parenting: Specific Disabilities

5111 **Cancer Clinical Trials: Experimental Treatments and How They Can Help You**
Patient-Centered Guides
1005 Gravenstein Hwy N
Sebastopol, CA 95472-3836
707-827-7019
800-889-8969
FAX: 707-824-8268
e-mail: orders@oreilly.com
www.patientcenters.com
Tim O'Reilly, CEO
Most cancer patients face treatment options that are less than ideal, whether because of a risk of recurrence or side effects. Finally, however, basic research on cell biology is leading to promising new treatments. If you are not evaluating potential experimental treatments alongside the standard treatment protocols, you aren't considering all the facts you need. Cancer Clinical Trials guide you through understanding your options and finding and considering experimental treatments. *$14.95*
222 pages Paperback
ISBN 1-565925-66-1

5112 **Children with Acquired Brain Injury: Education and Supporting Families**
Brookes Publishing
P.O.Box 10624
Baltimore, MD 21285-624
410-337-9580
800-638-3775
FAX: 410-337-8539
e-mail: custserv@brookespublishing.com
www.brookespublishing.com
Ann Glang PhD, Editor
Janet M Williams MSW, Editor
Paul Brooks, Owner
$28.95
288 pages Paperback
ISBN 1-557662-33-9

5113 **Children with Autism**
Woodbine House
6510 Bells Mill Rd
Bethesda, MD 20817-1636
301-897-3570
800-843-7323
e-mail: info@woodbinehouse.com
woodbinehouse.com
Irv Shapell, Owner
Recommended as the first book parents should read, this volume offers information and a complete introduction to autism, while easing the family's fears and concerns as they adjust and cope with their child's disorder. *$17.95*
368 pages Paperback
ISBN 0-933149-16-6

5114 **Final Report: Adapting Through the Looking Glass**
Through the Looking Glass
3075 Adeline St
Ste. 120
Berkeley, CA 94703-2212
510-848-1112
800-644-2666
FAX: 510-848-4445
TTY: 510-848-1005
e-mail: tlg@lookingglass.org
www.lookingglass.org
Maureen Block, J.D., Board President
Rusty Hendlin, M.A., LMFT, Director of Medi-Cal Services
Thomas Spalding, Board Treasurer
Alice Nemon, D.S.W., Board Secretary
Adapting Through the Looking Glass intervention model for deaf parents and their children. Available in braille, large print or cassette. *$2.00*
24 pages

5115 **Final Report: Challenges and Strategies of Disabled Parents: Findings from a Survey**
Through the Looking Glass
3075 Adeline St
Ste. 120
Berkeley, CA 94703-2212
510-848-1112
800-644-2666
FAX: 510-848-4445
TTY: 510-848-1005
e-mail: tlg@lookingglass.org
www.lookingglass.org
Maureen Block, J.D., Board President
Rusty Hendlin, M.A., LMFT, Director of Medi-Cal Services
Thomas Spalding, Board Treasurer
Alice Nemon, D.S.W., Board Secretary
Available in braille, large print or cassette. *$25.00*
24 pages

5116 **Negotiating the Special Education Maze: A Guide for Parents and Teachers**
Spina Bifida Association of America
Ste 250
4590 Macarthur Blvd NW
Washington, DC 20007-4226
202-944-3285
800-621-3141
FAX: 202-944-3295
e-mail: sbaa@sbaa.org
www.sbaa.org
Cindy Brownstein, CEO
Carmen J Head, Director
An excellent aid for the development of an effective special education program. *$19.00*

5117 **Pervasive Developmental Disorders; Findinga Diagnosis and Getting Help**
Patient-Centered Guides
1005 Gravenstein Hwy N
Sebastopol, CA 95472-3836
707-827-7019
800-889-8969
FAX: 707-824-8268
e-mail: orders@oreilly.com
www.patientcenters.com
Tim O'Reilly, CEO
This unique book encompassess both the practical aspects as well as ther personal stories and emotional facets of living with PDD-NOS, the most common pervasive developmental disorder. Parents of an undiagnosed child may suspect many things, from autism to servere allergies. Pervasive Developmental Disorders is for parents (or newly diagnosed adults) who struggle with this neurological condition that profoundly impacts the life of child and family. *$24.95*
580 pages Paperback
ISBN 1-565925-30-0

5118 Raising Kids with Special Needs
Aquarius Health Care Videos
18 North Main Street
P.O. Box 1159
Sherborn, MA 1770- 7159 508-650-1616
FAX: 508-650-1665
e-mail: tm@aquariusproductions.com
www.aquariusproductions.com
Lesile Kussmann, President
Joyce Farmer, Assistant Director
An intimate look into the lives of parents of three kids with very different disabilities. The objective of this video is an understanding of paprenting a child with special nees. This outstanding program looks at safety concerns, issues of anger and grief, the importance of a support network and other important issues. Ultimately, this is a narrative about raising and educating a child with disabilities. Preview option is available. *$89.00*
Video

5119 Your Child in the Hospital: A Practical Guide for Parents
Patient-Centered Guides
1005 Gravenstein Hwy N
Sebastopol, CA 95472-3836 707-827-7019
800-889-8969
FAX: 707-824-8268
e-mail: orders@oreilly.com
www.patientcenters.com
Linda O'Reilly, CEO
This book offers advice from dozens of veteran parents on how to cope with a child's hospitalization, relieving anxious parents so they can help dispel their child's fears and concerns. Parents will find easy-to-read tips on preparing their child, handling procedures without trauma, and preventing insurance snafus. The second edition features a journal to help open communication and give the child a measure of control over the experience. *$11.95*
166 pages Paperback
ISBN 1-565925-73-4

Parenting: School

5120 Allergy and Asthma Network Mothers of Asthmatics
8229 Boone Boulevard
Suite 260
Vienna, VA 22182-4343 800-878-4403
FAX: 703-288-5271
e-mail: mgieminiani@aanma.org
www.breatherville.org
Tonya Winders, President
Marcela Gieminiani, Director of Administration and P
Brenda Silvia-Torma, Project Manager
Michael Amato, Chair
Practical, medical,information for school patients, physicians, caregivers and families. *$7.00*

5121 Carolina Curriculum for Infants and Toddlers with Special Needs
Brookes Publishing
P.O.Box 10624
Baltimore, MD 21285-624 410-337-9580
800-638-3775
FAX: 410-337-8539
e-mail: custserv@brookespublishing.com
readplaylearn.com
Paul Brooks, Owner
This book includes detailed assessment and intervention sequences, daily routine integration strategies, sensorimotor adaptations, and a sample 24-page Assessment Log that shows readers how to chart a child's individual progress. *$41.95*
384 pages Spiral-bound
ISBN 1-557660-74-3

5122 Choosing Outcomes and Accommodations for Children (COACH)
Brookes Publishing
P.O.Box 10624
Baltimore, MD 21285-624 410-337-9580
800-638-3775
FAX: 410-337-8539
e-mail: custserv@brookespublishing.com
readplaylearn.com
Paul Brooks, Owner
A guide to educational planning for students with disabilities, second edition. Focuses on life outcomes such as social relationships and participation in typical home, school, and community activities. *$37.95*
400 pages Spiral bound
ISBN 1-55766 -23-8

5123 Complete IEP Guide: How to Advocate for Your Special Ed Child
Spina Bifida Association of America
Ste 250
4590 Macarthur Blvd NW
Washington, DC 20007-4226 202-944-3285
800-621-3141
FAX: 202-944-3295
e-mail: sbaa@sbaa.org
www.sbaa.org
Cindy Brownstein, CEO
Carmen J Head, Director
This all-in-one guide will help you understand special education law, identify your child's needs, prepare for meetings, develop the IEP and resolve disputes. *$28.95*

5124 Exceptional Student in the Regular Classroom
McGraw-Hill, School Publishing
P.O. Box 182604
Columbus, OH 43272-2490 877-833-5524
FAX: 614-759-3749
e-mail: customer.service@mcgraw-hill.com
mcgraw-hill.com
Louise Raymond, Vice President
Offers good, solid information through a practical understandable presentation unencumbered by specialized jargon. Covers topics associated with special learners.
480 pages

5125 Negotiating the Special Education Maze: A Guide for Parents and Teachers
Spina Bifida Association of America
Ste 250
4590 Macarthur Blvd NW
Washington, DC 20007-4226 202-944-3285
800-621-3141
FAX: 202-944-3295
e-mail: sbaa@sbaa.org
www.sbaa.org
Cindy Brownstein, CEO
Carmen J Head, Director
An excellent aid for the development of an effective special education program. *$19.00*

5126 Parent Teacher Packet
Spina Bifida Association of America
Ste 250
4590 Macarthur Blvd NW
Washington, DC 20007-4226 202-944-3285
800-621-3141
FAX: 202-944-3295
e-mail: sbaa@sbaa.org
www.sbaa.org
Cindy Brownstein, CEO
Carmen J Head, Director
Includes educational material, learning disabilities literature, children's book, social development and the person with spina bifida and one copy of each fact sheet. *$14.00*

5127 **Study Power: Study Skills to Improve Your Learning and Your Grades: A Workbook**
Brookline Books
8 Trumbull Rd
Suite B-001
Northampton, MA 1060-4533
413-584-0184
800-666-2665
FAX: 413-584-6184
e-mail: brbooks@yahoo.com
www.brooklinebooks.com
Paperback
ISBN 1-57129 -46-X

Parenting: Spiritual

5128 **A Miracle to Believe In**
Option Indigo Press
2080 S Undermountain Rd
Sheffield, MA 01257-9643
413-229-8727
800-714-2779
FAX: 413-229-8727
e-mail: happiness@option.org
www.optionindigo.com
379 pages Paperback
ISBN 0-44920 -08-2

5129 **After the Tears**
Centering Corporation
7230 Maple Street
Omaha, NE 68134-5064
402-553-1200
866-218-0101
FAX: 402-533-0507
e-mail: j1200@aol.com
www.centering.org
Joy Johnson, Founder
Dr. Marvin Johnson, co-Founder
Offers talk, articles on raising a child with a disability. This one book combines feelings and emotions of parents on the subject of raising their disabled child. *$11.00*
87 pages Paperback
ISBN 0-15602 -00-6

5130 **Before and After Zachariah**
Special Needs Project
Ste H
324 State St
Santa Barbara, CA 93101-2364
805-962-8087
800-333-6867
FAX: 805-962-5087
www.specialneeds.com
Hod Gray, Owner
This intimate chronicle of one family's life with a severely brain damaged child is recently back in print. *$7.95*
241 pages

5131 **Bethy and the Mouse: A Father Remembers His Children with Disabilities**
Brookline Books
8 Trumbull Rd
Suite B-001
Northampton, MA 1060-4533
413-584-0184
800-666-2665
FAX: 413-584-6184
e-mail: brbooks@yahoo.com
www.brooklinebooks.com
184 pages Paperback
ISBN 0-57129 -35-4

5132 **Disabled God: Toward a Liberatory Theologyof Disability**
Abingdon Press
201 8th Ave S
Nashville, TN 37203-3919
615-749-6000
800-251-3320
FAX: 800-836-7802
www.abingdon.org
Dr. Rex Matthews, Senior Editor
Neil Alexander, President
Draws on themes of the disability rights movement to identify people with disabilities as members of a socially disadvantaged minority group rather than as individuals who need to adjust. Highlights the history of people with disabilities in the church and society. *$13.95*
27 pages Paperback
ISBN 0-68710 -01-2

5133 **Dying and Disabled Children: Dealing with Loss and Grief**
Haworth Press
6000 Broken Sound Parkway, NW
Suite 300,
Boca Raton, FL 33487-1503
561-994-0555
FAX: 561-241-7856
e-mail: orders@taylorandfrancis.com
www.tandf.co.uk
153 pages Hardcover
ISBN 0-866567-59-3

5134 **In Time and with Love: Caring for the Special Needs Infant and Toddler**
Newmarket Press
18 E 48th St
New York, NY 10017-1014
212-832-3575
FAX: 212-832-3629
e-mail: sales@newmarketpress.com
newmarketpress.com
Esther Margolis, President
Heidi Sachner, Associate Publisher/Sales/Mktg
For families and caregivers of preteen and handicapped children in their first three years - more than one hundred tips for adjusting and coping. *$15.95*
208 pages
ISBN 1-557044-45-7

5135 **Journal of Religion, Disability & Health**
Haworth Press
6000 Broken Sound Parkway, NW
Suite 300,
Boca Raton, FL 33487-1503
561-994-0555
FAX: 561-241-7856
e-mail: orders@taylorandfrancis.com
www.tandf.co.uk
Quarterly

5136 **Nobody's Perfect: Living and Growing with Children Who Have Special Needs**
Brookes Publishing
P.O.Box 10624
Baltimore, MD 21285-624
410-337-9580
800-638-3775
FAX: 410-337-8539
e-mail: custserv@brookespublishing.com
readplaylearn.com
Paul Brooks, Owner
This book offers parents who have children with special needs a new and positive perspective on the challenges of family life. This book guides parents through the process of adaptation, describing specific strategies for success in balancing one's own life, developing a parenting partnership, and interacting with children, friends, relatives, professionals, and others. *$21.00*
352 pages Paperback
ISBN 1-55766 -43-X

5137 **Special Education Teacher Packet**
LifeWay Christian Resources Southern Baptist Conv.
One LifeWay Plaza
Nashville, TN 37234-2 615-741-2851
800-458-2772
FAX: 615-532-9412
www.lifeway.com

Ellen Beene, Editor
Wade Stapleton, Manager
Thom S. Rainer, President and CEO
Brad Waggoner, Executive Vice President
Resources to help teachers who lead Sunday School classes for adults and older youth with mental retardation. Includes teaching plans, posters, and one copy of Special Education Bible Study. *$10.00*
Quarterly

5138 **Special Kind of Parenting**
La Leche League International
957 N. Plum Grove Road
Schaumburg, IL 60173-4079 847-519-7730
800-525-3243
FAX: 847-969-0460
e-mail: LLLI@llli.org
www.lalecheleague.org

172 pages Softcover
ISBN 0-912500-27-1

5139 **That All May Worship**
Exceptional Parent Library
2013 H Stree
NW, 5th Floor
Washington, DC 20006-1207 202-457-0046
800-840-8844
FAX: 866-536-4461
e-mail: mailto:eplibrary@aol.com
www.eplibrary.com

Fred Maahs, Chair
Mary P. Davis, Vice Chair
Ralph Boyd, Jr., Treasurer
Merrill Friedman, Secretary
An interfaith handbook to assist congregations in welcoming people with disabilities to promote acceptance and full participation. *$10.00*

5140 **Why Mine?**
Centering Corporation
7230 Maple Street
Omaha, NE 68134-5064 402-553-1200
866-218-0101
FAX: 402-533-0507
e-mail: j1200@aol.com
www.centering.org

Joy Johnson, Founder
Dr. Marvin Johnson, co-Founder
Offers quotes from parents all across the country on their fears, feelings, marriage, the ill child and other children. *$3.25*
32 pages Paperback

5141 **Worst Loss: How Families Heal from the Death of a Child**
Exceptional Parent Library
2013 H Stree NW,
5th Floor
Washington, DC 2006-1207 202-457-0046
800-840-8844
FAX: 866-536-4461
e-mail: mailto:eplibrary@aol.com
www.eplibrary.com

ISBN 0-805032-41-X

Professional

5142 **American Journal of Physical Medicine**
Lippincott, Williams & Wilkins
2001 Market Street
Philadelphia, PA 19103-1551 215-521-8300
800-638-3030
FAX: 301-824-7390
www.lww.com

Walter R. Frontera, MD, PHD, Editor-in-Chief
Larwrence C. Pencak, MA, Executive Editor
Ernest W. Johnson, MD, Emeritus Editor
Emily Babcock, Managing Editors
Journal of the Association of Academic Psychiatrists. Articles covering research and clinical studies and applications of new equipment, procedures and therapeutic advances. *$45.00*

5143 **American Journal of Psychiatry**
American Psychiatric Publishing
Suite 1825
1000 Wilson Blvd
Arlington, VA 22209-3924 703-907-7322
800-368-5777
FAX: 703-907-1091
e-mail: ajp@psych.org
psychiatryonline.org

Nancy Frey, Executive Director
James Scully, Manager
Robert Freedman, M.D., Editor-in-Chief
David A. Lewis, M.D., Deputy Editors
Peer-reviewed articles focus on developments in biological psychiatry as well as on treatment innovations and forensic, ethical, economic, and social topics. *$56.00*
Monthly

5144 **American Journal of Public Health**
American Public Health Association
3141 Fairview Park Drive
Suite 625
Falls Church, VA 22209-2605 571-533-1919
855-863-2762
FAX: 855-883-2762
e-mail: comments@msmail.apha.org
www.apna.org

Nicholas Croce, Jr., MS, Executive Director
Patricia L. Black, PhD, RN, Associate Executive Director
Karla Lewis, Director of Finance & Administration
Lisa Deffenbaugh Nquven, MS, Director of Operations
Association journal containing professional articles and sections such as Notes from the Field and Association News. Single copies are $15.00. $50.00 per year for special consumer membership.
Monthly
ISSN 0090-00 6

5145 **American Rehabilitation**
Rehabilitation Services Administration
9700 West Bryn Mawr Avenue
Suite 200
Rosemont, IL 60018-5701 847-737-6000
800-872-5327
FAX: 847-737-6001
TTY: 800-437-0833
e-mail: info@aapmr.org
www.ed.gov

Kiran Ahuja, Executive Director
Covers medical, social and employment aspects of vocational rehabilitation. *$15.00*
40 pages Quarterly

5146 Art Therapy
American Art Therapy Association
4875 Eisenhower Avenue
Suite 240
Alexandria, VA 22304- 3302
703-548-5860
888-290-0878
FAX: 703-783-8468
e-mail: info@arttherapy.org
www.americanarttherapyassociation.org
Sarah Deaver, PhD, ATR-BC, President
Charlotte Boston, MA, ATR, Secretary
Joseph Jaworek, MA, ATR-BC, Treasurer
Juliet King, MA, ATR-BC, LPC, Director
Publishes articles on the uses of art in the education, enrichment, development and treatment of disabled people. *$10.00*
76+ pages Quarterly
ISSN 0742-16 6

5147 Brown University Long Term Care Advisor
Manisses Communications Group
208 Governor St
Providence, RI 02906-3246
401-831-6020
800-333-7771
FAX: 401-861-6370
e-mail: manisses@manisses.com
www.manisses.com
Fraser Lang, Publisher
Contains practical reports for health care professionals working in long-term care facilities. Published monthly. *$329.00*
8 pages Newsletter
ISSN 1088-92 8

5148 CAREERS & the disABLED Magazine
Equal Opportunity Publications
Suite 425
445 Broadhollow Rd
Melville, NY 11747-3615
631-421-9421
FAX: 631-421-1352
e-mail: info@eop.com
eop.com
John R. Miller, Chairman & Chief Executive Offic
James Schneider, Editorial Director
Laura Lang, Art Director
Tamara Flaum-Dreyfuss, President & Publisher
A career magazine for professional career seekers who have disabilities. Profiles disabled people who have achieved successful careers. Features a career section in Braille, career guide. *$10.00*
64 pages 3X

5149 Clinician's Practical Guide to Attention-Deficit/Hyperactivity Disorder
Brookes Publishing
P.O.Box 10624
Baltimore, MD 21285-624
410-337-9580
800-638-3775
FAX: 410-337-8539
e-mail: custserv@brookespublishing.com
readplaylearn.com
Paul Brooks, Owner
Quick reference volume with comprehensive data on psychoeducational and neuropsychological assessment, related symptoms, drug and counseling therapies and critical issues. *$39.95*
368 pages
ISBN 1-557663-58-0

5150 Counseling Parents of Children with Chronic Illness or Disability
Brookes Publishing
P.O.Box 10624
Baltimore, MD 21285-624
410-337-9580
800-638-3775
FAX: 410-337-8539
e-mail: custserv@brookespublishing.com
readplaylearn.com
Paul Brooks, Owner
$23.00
144 pages Paperback
ISBN 1-85433 -91-8

5151 Cystic Fibrosis: Medical Care
Lippincott, Williams & Wilkins
227
N8904 Lake Park Rd
Menasha, WI 54952-3713
920-739-1901
800-777-2295
FAX: 301-824-7390
e-mail: lakeparkpub@new.rr.com
www.lpub.com
J Lippincott, CEO
A guide to the medical community to the principles and practices of cystic fibrosis care. After chapters on the molecular and cellular bases of CF and its diagnosis, they cover the major organ systems affected by CF and deal with surgery for CF patients, transplantation (lung and liver), hospitalization, and terminal care. Also included are chapters on special populations, exercise, and laboratory testing. *$ 47.95*
365 pages
ISBN 0-781717-98-1

5152 Disability Analysis Handbook
American Board of Disability Analysts
4525 Harding Road
Second Floor
Nashville, TN 37205-1520
615-327-2978
FAX: 615-327-9235
e-mail: americanbd@aol.com
www.americandisability.org
Alexander Horowitz, MD, ABDA, Executive Officer Emeritus
Kenneth Anchor, President
Official newsletter of the American Board of Disability Analysts; features Healthnews Headlines, Meeting Calendar, Application Packet and much more. Free to members; $20 per year for non-members. *$60.00*
396 pages
ISBN 0-787226-70-x

5153 Ethical Conflicts in Management of Home Care
Springer Publishing Company
11 West 42nd Street,
15th Floor
New York, NY 10036-3915
212-431-4370
877-687-7476
FAX: 212-941-7842
e-mail: cs@springerpub.com
www.springerpub.com
Theodore C Nardin, Chief Executive Officer and Publisher
Nancy Hale, Editorial Director
James C. Costello, Vice President, Journal Publishing
Diana Osborne, Production Manager
Offers answers to the questions what is case management and why does it raise ethical issues. *$29.95*
288 pages

5154 Families in Recovery
Brookes Publishing
P.O.Box 10624
Baltimore, MD 21285-624
410-337-9580
800-638-3775
FAX: 410-337-8539
e-mail: custserv@brookespublishing.com
readplaylearn.com
Paul Brooks, Owner
This book teaches professionals how to use each families strengths to promote recovery. The authors demonstrate effective, family-focused intervention techniques developed in their combined 35 years of practice. Motivational techniques and stress reducers for counselors are also provided. *$34.00*
352 pages Paperback
ISBN 1-55766 -64-9

5155 **Journal of Children's Communication Development**
CEC Div for Childrens' Communication Development
267 Wallace Hall
Princeton University
Princeton, NJ 08544-1500 609-258-5894
FAX: 703-312-9193
e-mail: foc@princeton.edu
futureofchildren.org

Alexander Brice, Editor
Contains scholarly articles pertaining to the many aspects of communication disorders in children, encompassing speech, language, hearing and learning disabilities. *$16.00*
2x Year

5156 **NHIF Newsletter**
National Head Injury Foundation
1400 16th Street NW
Suite 430
Washington, DC 20036-1904 202-745-8092
800-444-6443
FAX: 202-478-2534
e-mail: worldwatch@worldwatch.org
worldwatch.org

Robert Engelman, President
Tom Crain, Managing Director
Contains news and articles for families and professionals concerned with head injury. *$25.00*

5157 **National Clearinghouse of Rehabilitation Training Materials**
6524 Old Main Hill
Logan, UT 84322-6524 866-821-5355
FAX: 435-797-7537
e-mail: ncrtm@usu.edu
www.nchrtm.okstate.edu

Michael Millington, Ph.D, Director
Sylvia Sims, Office Assistant
Chenyong Zhu, M.S., Instructional Designer
Jared C. Schultz, Ph.D., Principal Investigator
Newsletter produced quarterly to provide information and opportunities to learn more about related fields.
Quarterly

5158 **Partners in Everyday Communicative Exchanges**
Brookes Publishing
P.O.Box 10624
Baltimore, MD 21285-624 410-337-9580
800-638-3775
FAX: 410-337-8539
e-mail: custserv@brookespublishing.com
readplaylearn.com

Paul Brooks, Owner
A Guide to Promoting Intervention Involving people with Severe Intellectual Disability. This book helps improve communication with people with severe disabilities using practical forms, numerous examples, and illustrative case studies. *$43.00*
192 pages Paperback
ISBN 1-55766-41-X

5159 **Professional Report**
National Rehabilitation Association (NRA)
633 S Washington St
P.O. Box 150235
Alexandria, VA 22315-4109 703-836-0850
888-258-4295
FAX: 703-836-0848
TTY: 703-836-0849
e-mail: info@nationalrehab.org
www.nationalrehab.org

Fredric Schroeder, Executive Director
Sandra Mulliner, Administrative Assistant
Ellen Sokolowski, President
Rosemary Chitwood, Secretary
Association newsletter containing news, programs and information of interest to the Association and its members.

5160 **Provider Magazine**
American Health Care Association
1201 L Street, N.W.
Washington, DC 20005-4024 202-842-4444
800-321-0343
FAX: 202-842-3860
ncal.org

72 pages Monthly
ISSN 0888-03 2

5161 **Public Health Reports**
Oxford Journals
1900 M Street NW
Suite 710
Washington, DC 20036 513-636-0257
FAX: 617-565-4260
e-mail: robert.rinsky@chmcc.org
phr.oupjournals.org

Robert Rinsky PhD, Editor
Scholarly articles on issues that relate to public health and the healthcare system. *$13.00*
BiMonthly

5162 **Public Health/State Capitols**
Wakeman/Walworth
300 N Washington St
Alexandria, VA 22314-2530 703-768-9600
800-876-2545
FAX: 703-768-9690
e-mail: newsletters@statecapitals.com
www.statecapitals.com

Keyes Walworth, Publisher
Christine Ryan, Editor
Digest of state and municipal health care financing and legislation, including disease control, medicaid, AIDS, abortion, substance abuse programs, cancer prevention such as smoking restrictions, mental health and disability programs, regulation of hospitals & nursing homes, food safety, medical policies, health insurance for children, home regulation, managerial care, public health issues, pest control, and water quality. Issued weekly-52 issues/year. *$245.00*
10 pages

5163 **Sexuality and Disability**
Human Sciences Press
233 Spring St
New York, NY 10013-1522 212-460-1500
800-221-9369
FAX: 212-647-1898
www.springer.com

Rudiger Gebauer, President
A journal devoted to the psychological and medical aspects of sexuality in rehabilitation and community settings. The journal features original scholarly articles that address the psychological and medical aspects of sexuality in the field of rehabilitation, case studies, clinical practice reports, and guidelines for clinical practice. Plenum Publishers is now part of Kluner Academic Publishers. Journal fulfillment in the NYC office as before for HSP and Plenum Journals. *$160.00*
64 pages Quarterly
ISSN 0146-10 4

5164 **Sociopolitical Aspects of Disabilities**
Charles C. Thomas
2600 South First Street
P.O. Box 19265
Springfield, IL 62704-4730 217-789-8980
800-258-8980
FAX: 217-789-9130
e-mail: books@ccthomas.com
www.ccthomas.com

Michael P. Thomas, President
Provides understanding of the social and political histories of people with disabilities in the United States. This understanding is pivotal in working with persons with disabilities, to provide

background and perspective on current policies and attitudes. *$41.95*
324 pages Paperback
ISBN 0-398072-40-7

5165 Starting and Sustaining Genetic Support Groups
Johns Hopkins University Press
2715 North Charles Street
Baltimore, MD 21218-4363 410-516-6900
FAX: 410-516-6968
e-mail: webmaster@jhupress.jhu.edu
www.press.jhu.edu

Joan O. Weiss, M.S.W., Author
Guide to the establishment and maintenance of genetic support groups for individuals with genetic disorders and their families. For therapists and group leaders. Discusses practical matters including finding a leader, fund-raising, organizing peer support training programs. *$21.95*
152 pages
ISBN 0-801852-64-1

5166 Substance Abuse and Physical Disability
Haworth Press
6000 Broken Sound Parkway, NW
Suite 300,
Boca Raton, FL 33487-1503 561-994-0555
FAX: 561-241-7856
e-mail: orders@taylorandfrancis.com
www.tandf.co.uk

289 pages Hardcover
ISBN 1-560242-89-2

5167 TeamRehab Report
33900 Harper
Suite 104
Clinton Twp, MI 48035-8987 586-416-9100
800-543-4116
FAX: 586-416-9103
www.team-rehab.com

Meghan Scheidel, Accounts Manager
A magazine for rehab professionals who prescribe, purchase or recommend assistive technology and related services for clients who are permanently disabled. *$24.00*
48 pages Monthly

5168 What Psychotherapists Should Know about Disabilty
Through the Looking Glass
3075 Adeline St
Ste. 120
Berkeley, CA 94703-2212 510-848-1112
800-644-2666
FAX: 510-848-4445
TTY: 510-848-1005
e-mail: tlg@lookingglass.org
www.lookingglass.org

Maureen Block, J.D., Board President
Rusty Hendlin, M.A., LMFT, Director of Medi-Cal Services
Thomas Spalding, Board Treasurer
Alice Nemon, D.S.W., Board Secretary
$24.00
368 pages

5169 Women with Visible & Invisible Disabilitiees: Multiple Intersections, Issues, Therapies
Haworth Press
6000 Broken Sound Parkway, NW
Suite 300,
Boca Raton, FL 33487-1503 561-994-0555
FAX: 561-241-7856
e-mail: orders@taylorandfrancis.com
www.tandf.co.uk

418 pages Hardcover
ISBN 0-789019-36-1

Specific Disabilities

5170 Applying Concepts and Data from the NHIS Child Disability Supplements
HRSA Information Center
P.O.Box 2910
Merrifield, VA 22116-2910 888-275-4772
FAX: 703-821-2098
TTY:877-489-4772
e-mail: ask@hrsa.gov
www.ask.hrsa.gov

Tony Louis, Project Officer
HT Ireys, Author
Assists State public health programs in meeting the accountability mandates of Title V of the Social Security Act.

5171 Dental Care Considerations of Disadvantaged and Special Care Populations
HRSA Information Center
P.O.Box 2910
Merrifield, VA 22116-2910 888-275-4772
FAX: 703-821-2098
TTY:877-489-4772
e-mail: ask@hrsa.gov
www.ask.hrsa.gov

Tony Louis, Project Officer
HT Ireys, Author
These conference proceedings present a list of recommendations for HRSA's Bureau of Health Professions on how to modify Title VII and VIII programs to better meet the dental needs of disadvantaged and special care populations. It include tables and figures.

5172 HIV/AIDS in the Deaf and Hard of Hearing
HRSA Information Center
P.O.Box 2910
Merrifield, VA 22116-2910 888-275-4772
FAX: 703-821-2098
TTY:877-489-4772
e-mail: ask@hrsa.gov
www.ask.hrsa.gov

Tony Louis, Project Officer
HT Ireys, Author
Details the prevalence of HIV disease among deaf and hard of hearing in the United States. It defines deaf and hard the of hearing. It discusses the lack of HIV information among the deaf and hard of hearing population and barriers to care. It includes the HRSA Care ACTION Calendar of Events.

5173 The Patterns of English Spelling
AVKO Educational Research Foundation
Ste W
3084 Willard Rd
Birch Run, MI 48415-9404 810-686-9283
866-285-6612
FAX: 810-686-1101
e-mail: webmaster@avko.org
avko.org

Don McCabe, President
Barry Chute, President
Linda Vice-President, Michael Lane, Treasurer
A 10-volume reference book with all of the words in the English language organized by word family, including CV structures, advanced patters, prefixes, and rimes. Each volume may also be purchased individually. Free as an E-book for Foundation members. *$359.90*
1635 pages

Vocations

5174 Ability
George J DePontis
Unit 18, Gatwick Metro Centre
Balcombe Road
Horley, RH 33137-788
www.ability.com

5175 Case Management in the Vocational
Berkeley Planning Associates
P.O. Box 68
Osceola, IA 50213-5012
641-342-4598
888-342-6019
FAX: 641-342-3411
e-mail: c.oppedal@yourohs.com
www.yourohs.com
Connie Oppedal, MS, CDMS, President
Mark Blankespoor, P.T., M.S, Ergonomic Consultant
Patricia Wright, RN, Medical Case Manager
Ann Short, RN, M.S., Medical Services Consultant
Journal examining the effectiveness of case management services in the context of vocational rehabilitation for persons with psychiatric disabilities.

5176 Demystifying Job Development: Field-Based Approaches to Job Development for the Disabled
Training Resource Network
PO Box 439
St. Augustine, FL 32085
FAX: 904-823-3554
e-mail: info@trninc.com
www.trninc.com

105 pages
ISBN 1-883302-37-4

5177 Economics, Industry and Disability
Paul H Brookes Publishing Company
P.O.Box 10624
Baltimore, MD 21285-624
410-337-9580
800-638-3775
FAX: 410-337-8539
e-mail: custserv@brookespublishing.com
readplaylearn.com
Paul Brooks, Owner
An analysis of the movement toward nonsheltered employment, this book addresses the expanding opportunities, future challenges and economic changes surrounding efforts to ensure the development of positive and constructive employment for persons with disabilities. *$42.00*
Hardcover

5178 Hiring Idahoans with Disabilities
Idaho Assistive Technology Project
500 S 8th Street
Boise, ID 83702-2268
208-342-5884
800-242-4785
FAX: 208-342-1408
e-mail: idahoat@uidaho.edu
www.educ.uidaho.edu/idatech

Angela Lindig, Executive Director
Jennifer Zielinski, Program Coordinator
James Turner, Vice President
Preston Roberts, Treasurer

5179 Life Beyond the Classroom: Transition Strategies for Young People with Disabilities
Paul H Brookes Publishing Company
P.O.Box 10624
Baltimore, MD 21285-624
410-337-9580
800-638-3775
FAX: 410-337-8539
e-mail: custserv@brookespublishing.com
readplaylearn.com

Paul Brooks, Owner
Specialists in a variety of disciplines use creative and practical techniques to ensure careful transition planning, to build young people's confidence and competence in work skills, and to foster support from businesses and community organizations for training and employment programs. *$64.95*
543 pages
ISBN 1-557664-76-5

5180 Mentally Retarded Individuals
Mainstream
Ste 830
660 Third Street
San Francisco, CA 94107-6301
415-281-3100
800-247-1380
FAX: 301-654-6714
e-mail: info@mainstreaminc.org
www.healthline.com
Charles Moster
Philip Dur, Co-Chair
Michael Barber, Vice President
Kevin Brown, General Partner
Mainstreaming mentally retarded individuals into the workplace. *$2.50*
12 pages

5181 OT Practice
American Occupational Therapy Association
Ste 301
4720 Montgomery Ln Ste 200
Bethesda, MD 20814- 3449
301-652-6611
800-729-2682
FAX: 301-652-7711
TTY: 800-377-8555
www.aota.org/publications-news/otp.aspx
Jeanette Bair, Executive Director
Offers information on conferences, books, resources, materials and information and referral services for persons with disabilities.

5182 Options
Anixter Center
2001 N. Clybourn
3rd Floor
Chicago, IL 60614-4062
773-973-7900
FAX: 773-973-5268
TTY:773-973-2180
e-mail: AskAnixter@anixter.org
www.anixter.org

Elaine D. Cottey, Chair
Eric Gastevich, Treasurer
Carol Neiger, Secretary
Jason Adess, Director
Anixter Center's quarterly publication. Free.
Quarterly

5183 Preparation and Employment of Students
Paul H Brookes Publishing Company
P.O.Box 10624
Baltimore, MD 21285-624
410-337-9580
800-638-3775
FAX: 410-337-8539
e-mail: custserv@brookespublishing.com
readplaylearn.com

Paul Brooks, Owner
A practical guide on vocational training and employment issues for persons with severe multiple and physical disabilities. *$ 213.00*
224 pages Paper

5184 Teaching Chemistry to Students with Disabilities
American Chemical Society
1155 16th St NW
Washington, DC 20036-4839
202-872-4570
800-227-5558
FAX: 202-872-4574
TTY: 202-872-6355
e-mail: cwd@acs.org
membership.acs.org

Elizabeth Zubritsky, Manager
James M Landis, CWD Chair
Anne Swanson, Editor
Madeleine Jacobs, Editor

Promotes the full involvement of individuals with physical and learning disabilities in educational and career opportunities in the chemical and allied sciences. CWD members lead the American Chemical Society's efforts to help: individuals with disabilities who seek education or employment in chemical and allied sciences; employers and educators of persons with disabilities; other committees, offices and members of ACS who are interested in the full involvement of persons with disabilities.

148 pages
ISBN 0-841238-16-2

5185 Transition from School to Work
Paul H Brookes Publishing Company
P.O.Box 10624
Baltimore, MD 21285-624
410-337-9580
800-638-3775
FAX: 410-337-8539
e-mail: custserv@brookespublishing.com
readplaylearn.com

Paul Brooks, Owner

A hands-on guide to planning and implementing successful transition programs for adolescents with disabilities. *$25.00*

336 pages Paper

5186 Transition from School to Work for Personswith Disabilities
Longman Publishing Group
9th Fl
8004 Franklin Farms Drive
Henrico, VA 23229-5019
804-662-7000
800-552-5019
FAX: 804-662-9532
TTY: 800-464-9950
e-mail: dars@dars.virginia.gov
www.vadars.org/transitionservices.htm

Joanne Dresner, President

Examines the multidimensional process needed to effectively prepare persons with disabilities for life beyond school and addresses the key issues in the transition process.

251 pages Paper
ISBN 0-801302-28-5

Pamphlets

5187 A Guide for People with Disabilities Seeking Employment
US Department of Justice
950 Pennsylvania Ave NW
Washington, DC 20530-9
202-307-0663
800-574-0301
FAX: 202-307-1197
TTY: 800-514-0383
www.ada.gov

Rebecca B. Bond, Chief
Zita Johnson Betts, Deputy Chiefs
Kathleen P. Wolfe, Special Litigation Counsel
Sheila Foran, Special Legal Counsel

A 2-page pamplet for people with disabilities providing a general explanation of the employment provisions of the ADA and how to file a complaint with the Equal Employment Opportunity Commission.

5188 ADA Business Brief: Restriping Parking Lots
US Department of Justice
950 Pennsylvania Ave NW
Washington, DC 20530-9
202-307-0663
800-574-0301
FAX: 202-307-1197
TTY: 800-514-0383
www.ada.gov

Rebecca B. Bond, Chief
Zita Johnson Betts, Deputy Chiefs
Kathleen P. Wolfe, Special Litigation Counsel
Sheila Foran, Special Legal Counsel

A 2-page illustrated design guide explaining the number of accessible parking spaces that are required and the restriping requirements for accessible parking spaces for cars and vans.

5189 ADA Business Brief: Service Animals
US Department of Justice
950 Pennsylvania Ave NW
Washington, DC 20530-9
202-307-0663
800-574-0301
FAX: 202-307-1197
TTY: 800-514-0383
www.ada.gov

Rebecca B. Bond, Chief
Zita Johnson Betts, Deputy Chiefs
Kathleen P. Wolfe, Special Litigation Counsel
Sheila Foran, Special Legal Counsel

A 1-page publication summarizing the ADA rules on service animals.

5190 Accessible Stadiums
US Department of Justice
950 Pennsylvania Ave NW
Washington, DC 20530-9
202-307-0663
800-574-0301
FAX: 202-307-1197
TTY: 800-514-0383
www.ada.gov

Rebecca B. Bond, Chief
Zita Johnson Betts, Deputy Chiefs
Kathleen P. Wolfe, Special Litigation Counsel
Sheila Foran, Special Legal Counsel

A 4-page publication highlighting features that must be accessible in new stadiums including line of sight for wheelchair seating locations.

5191 Arthritis in Children and La Artritis Infantojuvenil
American Juvenile Arthritis Organization
1330 W. Peachtree Street
Suite 100
Atlanta, GA 30309-669
404-872-7100
800-283-7800
e-mail: help@arthritis.org
arthritis.org

John H Klippel, CEO
Daniel T. McGowan, Chair
Rowland W. Chang, Vice Chairs
Patricia Novak Nelson, Secretary

A medical information booklet about juvenile rheumatoid arthritis. This booklet is written for parents or other adults and includes details about different forms of JRA, medications, therapies and coping issues.

5192 Assistance at Self-Serve Gas Stations
US Department of Justice
950 Pennsylvania Ave NW
Washington, DC 20530-9
202-307-0663
800-574-0301
FAX: 202-307-1197
TTY: 800-514-0383
www.ada.gov

Rebecca B. Bond, Chief
Zita Johnson Betts, Deputy Chiefs
Kathleen P. Wolfe, Special Litigation Counsel
Sheila Foran, Special Legal Counsel

A 1-page document providing guidance on the ADA and refueling assistance for customers with disabilities at self-serve gas stations.

5193 Attention Deficit-Hyperactivity Disorder: Is it a Learning Disability?
Georgetown University, School of Medicine
6001 Executive Boulevard
Rockville, MD 20852-2113 202-298-6775
e-mail: NIMHinfo@mail.nih.gov
www.nimh.nih.gov/health
Joy Drass, President
Offers information on learning disabilities and related disorders.

5194 BVA Bulletin
Blinded Veterans Association
477 H St NW
Washington, DC 20001-2694 202-371-8880
800-669-7079
FAX: 202-371-8258
e-mail: bva@bva.org
bva.org
Mark Cornell, President
Robert Dale Stamper, Vice President
Joe Parker, Secretary
Paul Mimms, Treasurer

Bi-Monthly

5195 Blind and Vision-Impaired Individuals
Mainstream
2 Penn Plaza
Suite 1102
New York, NY 10121-3534 212-502-7600
FAX: 888-545-8331
e-mail: info@mainstreaminc.org
www.afb.org
Carl R. Augusto, President and CEO
Stacy Rollins, Executive Administrative Assistant to the President
Rick Bozeman, Chief Financial Officer
Sonya Shiflet, Chief Human Resources & Planning Officer
Mainstreaming blind individuals into the workplace. *$ 2.50*
12 pages

5196 Cataracts
National Eye Institute
Drive MSC 2510
31 Center Drive
Bethesda, MD 20892-2510 301-496-5248
FAX: 301-402-1065
e-mail: 2020@nei.nih.gov
www.nei.nih.gov
Paul A. Sieving, M.D., Ph.D., Director
A cataract is a clouding of the lens in the eye that affects vision. Most cataracts are related to aging. Cataracts are very common in older people. By age 80, more than half of all Americans either have a cataract or have had cataract surgery.

5197 Common ADA Problems at Newly Constructed Lodging Facilities
US Department of Justice
950 Pennsylvania Ave NW
Washington, DC 20530-9 202-307-0663
800-574-0301
FAX: 202-307-1197
TTY: 800-514-0383
www.ada.gov
Rebecca B. Bond, Chief
Zita Johnson Betts, Deputy Chiefs
Kathleen P. Wolfe, Special Litigation Counsel
Sheila Foran, Special Legal Counsel
This 11-page document lists a sampling of common accessibility problems at newly constructed lodging facilities that have been identified through the Department of Justice's ongoing enforcement efforts.

5198 Commonly Asked Questions About Service Animals in Places of Business
US Department of Justice
950 Pennsylvania Ave NW
Washington, DC 20530-9 202-307-0663
800-574-0301
FAX: 202-307-1197
TTY: 800-514-0383
www.ada.gov
Rebecca B. Bond, Chief
Zita Johnson Betts, Deputy Chiefs
Kathleen P. Wolfe, Special Litigation Counsel
Sheila Foran, Special Legal Counsel
A 3-page publication providing information about service animals and ADA requirements.

5199 Connect Information Service
150 S Progress Ave
P.O. Box 2675
Harrisburg, PA 17109- 2675 717-657-5113
800-692-7288
www.dpw.state.pa.us/forchildren

5200 Easy Access Housing
Easter Seals
PO Box 355
Level 1/274 Taranaki Street
Wellington, 6140-4851 404-499-1064
e-mail: enquiries@atareira.org.nz
www.atareira.org.nz
Leo McIntyre, Manager
Rebecca Etuale, Family/Whanau Coordinator
Zap Haenga, Consumer Services Coordinator
Dominic Howley, Administrator
Booklet with a checklist for finding homes that are already accessible or structurally adaptable to accommodate changes in physical abilities and needs. Includes suggestions for solving common accessibility problems such as narrow doors, high thresholds and round knob fixtures.
12 pages

5201 Facts: Books for Blind and Physically Handicapped Individuals
Nat'l Lib Svc/Blind And Physically Handicapped
1291 Taylor St NW
Washington, DC 20011-2 202-707-5100
FAX: 202-707-0712
TTY:202-707-0744
e-mail: nls@loc.gov
www.loc.gov/nls
Karen Keninger, Director
Administers a national library service that provides braille and recorded books and magazines free on loan to anyone who cannot read standard print because of visual or physical disabilities.
Annual

5202 Heart to Heart
Blind Children's Center
4120 Marathon St
Los Angeles, CA 90029-3584 323-664-2153
FAX: 323-665-3828
e-mail: info@blindchildrenscenter.org
blindchildrenscenter.org
Midge Horton, Executive Director
Lena French, Director of Finance
Parents of blind and partially sighted children talk about their feelings. *$10.00*
12 pages

5203 How to Find More About Your Child's Birth Defect or Disability
Birth Defect Research for Children
BDRC
976 Lake Baldwin Lane, Suite 104,
Orlando, FL 32814-3753 407-895-0802
e-mail: staff@birthdefects.org
www.birthdefects.org
Betty Mekdeci, Executive Director/Manager
An informational fact sheet that encourages parents who have a child with a birth defect or disability to become the expert on the child's disability with some suggestions on how to educate themselves.

5204 Individuals with Arthritis
Mainstream
2200 Lake Boulevard NE
Atlanta, GA 30319-3534 404-633-3777
FAX: 404-633-1870
e-mail: info@mainstreaminc.org
https://www.rheumatology.org
12 pages

5205 Learning to Play
Blind Children's Center
4120 Marathon St
Los Angeles, CA 90029-3584 323-664-2153
FAX: 323-665-3828
e-mail: info@blindchildrenscenter.org
blindchildrenscenter.org
Midge Horton, Executive Director
Lena French, Director of Finance
Discusses how to present play activities to the visually impaired preschool child. *$10.00*
12 pages

5206 Marfan Syndrome Fact Sheet
1275 Mamaroneck Ave
White Plains, NY 10605-5201 914-997-4488
FAX: 914-428-8203
www.marchofdimes.com

5207 Marriage & Disability
Accent Books & Products
P.O.Box 700
Bloomington, IL 61702-700 309-378-2961
800-787-8444
FAX: 309-378-4420
e-mail: acmtlvng@aol.com
Raymond C Cheever, Publisher
Betty Garee, Editor
This guide can help you make the right decision and it can help smooth the way to a happier life. *$7.95*
Paperback
ISBN 0-91570 -34-5

5208 Medical Herbalism
Bergner Communications
P.O. Box 13758
Portland, OR 97213-3512 303-541-9552
e-mail: inquiries@naimh.com
www.medherb.com
Paul Bergner, Editor
Newsletter written by physicians and published six times a year.

5209 Midtown Sweep: Grassroots Advocacy at its Best
Independent Living Research Utilization ILRU
Ste 1000
1333 Moursund
Houston, TX 77030-7031 713-520-0232
FAX: 713-520-5785
e-mail: ilru@ilru.org
ilru.org
Lex Frieden, Director
Laurie Gerke Redd, Administrative Director
Linda CoVan, Grant Coordinator
Maria Del Bosque, Project Associate
Josie, Janetta, and Linda describe the steps their center's advocacy group have taken to ensure enforcement of the ADA: target one neighborhood; survey and collect information on businesses that are inaccessible; send letters offering to work with the businesses to help them become accessible and providing information on tax incentives; file lawsuits against businesses that do not respond; involve the media.
10 pages

5210 Move With Me
Blind Children's Center
4120 Marathon St
Los Angeles, CA 90029-3584 323-664-2153
FAX: 323-665-3828
e-mail: info@blindchildrenscenter.org
blindchildrenscenter.org
Midge Horton, Executive Director
Lena French, Director of Finance
A parent's guide to movement development for visually impaired babies. *$10.00*
12 pages

5211 Newsletter of PA's AT Lending Library
1755 North 13th Street
Student Center, Room 411S
Philadelphia, PA 19122-6005 215-204-1356
FAX: 215-204-6336
TTY:215-204-1805
e-mail: iod@temple.edu
disabilities.temple.edu
Celia Feinstein, Co-Executive Director
Ann Marie White, Deputy Director
Yvette Bolden, Administrative Assistant
Anthony Brown, Project Assistant

5212 Reaching, Crawling, Walking....Let's Get Moving
Blind Children's Center
4120 Marathon St
Los Angeles, CA 90029-3584 323-664-2153
FAX: 323-665-3828
e-mail: info@blindchildrenscenter.org
blindchildrenscenter.org
Midge Horton, Executive Director
Lena French, Director of Finance
Orientation and mobility for preschool children who are visually imapired. *$10.00*
24 pages

5213 Selecting a Program
Blind Children's Center
4120 Marathon St
Los Angeles, CA 90029-3584 323-664-2153
FAX: 323-665-3828
e-mail: info@blindchildrenscenter.org
blindchildrenscenter.org
Midge Horton, Executive Director
Lena French, Director of Finance
A guide for parents of infants and preschoolers with visual impairments. *$10.00*
28 pages

5214 Standing On My Own Two Feet
Blind Children's Center
4120 Marathon St
Los Angeles, CA 90029-3584
323-664-2153
FAX: 323-665-3828
e-mail: info@blindchildrenscenter.org
blindchildrenscenter.org

Midge Horton, Executive Director
Lena French, Director of Finance

A step-by-step guide to designing and constructing simple, individually tailored, adaptive mobility devices for preschool-age children who are visually impaired. *$10.00*
36 pages

5215 Talk to Me
Blind Children's Center
4120 Marathon St
Los Angeles, CA 90029-3584
323-664-2153
FAX: 323-665-3828
e-mail: info@blindchildrenscenter.org
blindchildrenscenter.org

Midge Horton, Executive Director
Lena French, Director of Finance

A language guide for parents of deaf children. *$10.00*
11 pages

5216 Talk to Me II
Blind Children's Center
4120 Marathon St
Los Angeles, CA 90029-3584
323-664-2153
FAX: 323-665-3828
e-mail: info@blindchildrenscenter.org
blindchildrenscenter.org

Midge Horton, Executive Director
Lena French, Director of Finance

A sequel to Talk To Me, available in English and Spanish. *$10.00*
15 pages

5217 Teaching Social Skills to Youngsters with Disabilities
Federation for Children with Special Needs
45 Bromfield Street
10th Floor
Boston, MA 02108
617-542-7860
866-815-8122
FAX: 617-542-7832
e-mail: info@ppal.net
www.ppal.net

Lisa Lambert, Executive Director
Deborah A. Fauntleroy, MSW, Associate Director
Earl N. Stuck, Chair
Anne Metzger, Treasurer

Explains the importance of instruction and training to learn appropriate social behavior.

5218 Understanding
Easter Seals
Ste 1800
230 W Monroe St
Chicago, IL 60606-4851
312-726-6800
FAX: 312-726-1494

Janet D Jamieson, Communications Manager
James Williams Jr, Chief Executive Officer

A brochure series for use in patient, family and public education programs and in career recruitment and counseling.
10 Brochures

5219 Without Sight and Sound
Helen Keller National Center
141 Middle Neck Road
Sands Point, NY 11050-1218
516-944-8900
FAX: 516-944-7302
TTY:516-944-8637
e-mail: hkncinfo@hknc.org
www.hknc.org

Media, Electronic

Audio/Visual

5220 A Place for MeEducational Productions
Educational Productions
9000 SW Gemini Dr
Beaverton, OR 97008-7151
503-644-7000
800-950-4949
FAX: 503-350-7000
e-mail: custserve@edpro.com
www.teachingstrategies.com
Diane Trister Dodge, Founder/President/Lead Author
Arnitra Duckett, VP, Sales & Strategic Marketing
In this video, parents discuss the issues they face in planning for their child's future. This program is designed to stimulate discussion of these issues and help increase awareness of the options available in your local community.

5221 Able to LaughFanlight Productions/Icarus Films
Fanlight Productions
32 Court St.
21st Floor
Brooklyn, NY 11201-4421
718-488-8900
800-876-1710
FAX: 718-488-8642
e-mail: info@fanlight.com
www.fanlight.com
Jonathan Miller, President
Patricio Guzman, Director
Meredith Miller, Sales Manager
Anthony Sweeney, Acquisitions
An exploration of the world of disability as interpreted by six professional comedians who happen to be disabled. It is also about the awkward ways disabled and able-bodied people relate to one another. *$199.00*
ISBN 1-572951-05-2

5222 Acting BlindFanlight Productions/Icarus Films
Fanlight Productions
32 Court St.
21st Floor
Brooklyn, NY 11201-4421
718-488-8900
800-876-1710
FAX: 718-488-8642
e-mail: info@fanlight.com
www.fanlight.com
Jonathan Miller, President
Patricio Guzman, Director
Meredith Miller, Sales Manager
Anthony Sweeney, Acquisitions
Takes audiences behind the scenes as a company of non-professional actors rehearse a play about life without sight. The performers have no problem imagining themselves in these roles: they are blind themselves. *$229.00*

5223 Adaptive Baby Care
Through the Looking Glass
3075 Adeline St
Suite 120
Berkeley, CA 94703-2577
510-848-1112
800-644-2666
FAX: 510-848-4445
TTY: 510-848-1005
e-mail: tlg@lookingglass.org
www.lookingglass.org
Megan Kirshbaum, Executive Director
Paul Preston, Assoc. Dir
This publication is presented as a catalyst for problem-solving regarding the development of adaptive baby care equipment. This newest publication is designed for parents, family members and professionals. It includes: guidelines for problem-solving baby care barriers; photographs and descriptions of prototypes and resources for adaptive baby care equipment; adaptive baby care techniques; adaptive baby care equipment checklist; commercial product safety commission guidelines; and local and natio
$250.00

5224 Adaptive Baby Care Equipment Video and Book Through the Looking Glass
Through the Looking Glass
3075 Adeline St
Suite 120
Berkeley, CA 94703-2577
510-848-1112
800-644-2666
FAX: 510-848-4445
TTY: 510-848-1005
e-mail: tlg@lookingglass.org
www.lookingglass.org
Stephanie Miyashiro, Board President
Thomas Spalding, Board Treasurer
Alice Nemon, D.S.W., Board Secretary
Christina Jopes, Board Members
Includes Adaptive Baby care Equipment: Guide Lines; Prototypes and Resources, plus a twelve minute video. Available in braille, large print or cassette. *$79.00*

5225 All About Attention Deficit Disorders, Revised
Parent Magic
800 Roosevelt Rd
B-309
Glen Ellyn, IL 60137-5839
630-208-0031
800-442-4453
FAX: 630-208-7366
e-mail: ordercenter@parentmagic.com
www.parentmagic.com
Nancy Roe, Administrator/Exec Admin
Thomas Phelan, Owner/President/CEO
A psychologist and expert on ADD outlines the symptoms, diagnosis and treatment of this neurological disorder. Video ($49.95 - 2 parts) and audio cassette ($24.95). Also in DVD format (1 disk-$39.93).

5226 AutismAquarius Health Care Media
Aquarius Health Care Media
30 Forest Rd
PO Box 249
Millis, MA 2054-1511
508-376-1244
FAX: 508-376-1245
e-mail: lann@aquariusproductions.com
www.nmm.net/storage/guide-2011/Aquarius_Hea lt
Lesile Kussmann, Owner/President/Producer
Kathy Newkirk, Director
Jane Hutchinson, Assoc. Director
This video takes you into the lives of autistic people and their families to understand more about autism. What defines autism and how can we help those living with the disability? Children, teens, and adults are also profiled and we begin to see the varying levels of development and new technology to help these people communicate. Preview Available. *$149.00*
Video

5227 Basic Course in American Sign Language(B100) Harris Communications, Inc.
Harris Communications
15155 Technology Dr
Eden Prairie, MN 55344-2273
952-906-1180
800-825-6758
FAX: 952-906-1099
TTY: 800-825-9187
e-mail: info@harriscomm.com
www.harriscomm.com
Robert Harris, Owner/President
Kevin Horsky, Business Director
Randall Moore, Manager
This series of four one-hour tapes is designed to illustrate the various exercises and dialogues in the text. *$39.95*
Video

5228 Beginning ASL Video CourseHarris Communications, Inc.
Harris Communications
15155 Technology Dr
Eden Prairie, MN 55344-2273
952-906-1180
800-825-6758
FAX: 952-906-1099
TTY: 800-825-9187
e-mail: info@harriscomm.com
www.harriscomm.com

Robert Harris, Owner/President
Kevin Horsky, Business Director
Randall Moore, Manager
You'll watch a family teach you to learn American Sign Language during funny and touching family situations. A total of 15 tapes in the course. *$599.40*
Video

5229 BlindnessLandmark Media, Inc.
Landmark Media
3450 Slade Run Dr
Falls Church, VA 22042-3940
703-241-2030
800-342-4336
FAX: 703-536-9540
e-mail: info@landmarkmedia.com
www.landmarkmedia.com

Michael Hartogs, President/Owner
Joan Hartogs, Owner/Vice President
Peter Hartogs, Vice President
Richard Hartogs, Vice President
Landmark Media is an independent family-owned company currently celebrating our 28th anniversary. We have been fortunate to be able to offer the finest quality educational DVDs available. *$250.00*
Video

5230 Braille Documents
Metrolina Association for the Blind
704 Louise Ave
Charlotte, NC 28204-2128
704-887-5118
800-926-5466
FAX: 704-372-3872
e-mail: bschmiel@mabnc.org
www.mabnc.org

Robert Scheffel, President
Richard Hartness, Vice President, Product Design & Development
Barbara Schmiel, Vice President, Accessible Braille Services
Chris Wilkins, Vice President, Information Technology
This production shop creates Braille and large-print documents. We work with our clients to find the most cost effective solutions for their needs. Unlike other modified statement service providers, we accept your existing style of statement or allow you to design your own statement.Documents may be received in electronic data files as encrypted data sent over public networks, data sent to a file transfer protocol drop box, or data sent over a dedicated data line. ABS also accepts paper hardcopi

5231 Bringing Out the Best
PO Box 9177
Dept. 11W
Champaign, IL 61826-9177
217-352-3273
800-519-2707
FAX: 217-352-1221
e-mail: orders@researchpress.com
www.researchpress.com

David Parkinson, Chairman
Russell Pence, President
Gail Salyards, Dir. Of Marketing/President

5232 Business as UsualFanlight Productions/Icarus Films
Fanlight Productions
32 Court St.
21st Floor
Brooklyn, NY 11201-4421
718-488-8900
800-876-1710
FAX: 718-488-8642
e-mail: info@fanlight.com
www.fanlight.com

Jonathan Miller, President
Patricio Guzman, Director
Meredith Miller, Sales Manager
Anthony Sweeney, Acquisitions
An enlightening documentary, brings a unique international perspective to this struggle. This film examines five innovative programs which create opportunities for people with mental and physical disabilities to own and operate their own businesses. *$145.00*

5233 Buying Time: The Media Role in Health CareFanlight Productions/Icarus Films
Fanlight Productions
32 Court St.
21st Floor
Brooklyn, NY 11201-4421
718-488-8900
800-876-1710
FAX: 718-488-8642
e-mail: info@fanlight.com
www.fanlight.com

Jonathan Miller, President
Patricio Guzman, Director
Meredith Miller, Sales Manager
Anthony Sweeney, Acquisitions
This video program is a thoughtful and disturbing examination in the role of the media in determining the allocation of health care resources. This program is a powerful tool on ethics, policy, journalism, sociology, medicine and nursing as well as for professional workshops, and continuing education programs. *$99.00*

5234 Caring for Persons with Developmental Disabilities
PO Box 9177
Dept. 11W
Champaign, IL 61826-9177
217-352-3273
800-519-2707
FAX: 217-352-1221
www.researchpress.com

David Parkinson, Chairman
Russell Pence, President
Gail Salyards, Dir. Of Marketing/President

5235 Clockworks
Learning Corporation of America
6493 Kaiser Dr
Fremont, CA 94555-3610
510-490-7311

Oonchia Chia, Owner
Scotty, who has Down Syndrome, is fascinated by clocks. This film follows him on his adventures of employment in the clock shop.
Film

5236 Close Encounters of the Disabling Kind
Mainstream
6930 Carroll Ave
Suite 204
Takoma Park, MD 20912-4468
301-891-8777
FAX: 301-891-8778
e-mail: info@mainstreaminc.org
www.mainstreaminc.org

Lillie Harrison, Information Programs Clerk
Fritz Rumpel, Editor
A training video that provides a hiring manager with information on how to learn the basics of disability etiquette and, by the end of the video, seems much better prepared and willing to interview

qualified individuals with disabilities. Includes trainer and trainee guides. *$99.95*
Video

5237 **Deaf Children Signers**
Harris Communications
15155 Technology Dr
Eden Prairie, MN 55344-2273
952-906-1180
800-825-6758
FAX: 952-906-1099
TTY: 800-825-9187
e-mail: info@harriscomm.com
www.harriscomm.com
Robert Harris, Owner
Kevin Horsky, Business Director
Randall Moore, Manager
Graduate to voicing for Deaf children ages 5-11. Adding new meaning to the phrase, Out of the mouths (hands?) of babes..., this unique tape lets eleven young children demonstrate their abilities by signing about what is important to them. *$39.95*
Video

5238 **Deaf Culture Series**
Harris Communicatin
15155 Technology Dr
Eden Prairie, MN 55344-2273
952-906-1180
800-825-6758
FAX: 952-906-1099
TTY: 800-825-9187
e-mail: info@harriscomm.com
www.harriscomm.com
Robert Harris, Owner
Kevin Horsky, Business Director
Randall Moore, Manager
Each video in this five-part series features a topic dealing with the unique culture of deaf people. It is an excellent resource for deaf studies programs, Interpreter Preparation programs and Sign Language programs. *$49.95*
Video

5239 **Deaf Mosaic**
Harris Communications
15155 Technology Dr
Eden Prairie, MN 55344-2273
952-906-1180
800-825-6758
FAX: 952-906-1099
TTY: 800-825-9187
e-mail: info@harriscomm.com
www.harriscomm.com
Robert Harris, Owner
Kevin Horsky, Business Director
Randall Moore, Manager
Deaf Mosaic: Deaf President Now documents the most extraordinary week in deaf history, including interviews with student leaders; exclusive footage of the demonstrations; and an interview with Gallaudet president, Dr. I. King Jordan. *$29.95*
Video

5240 **Do You Hear That?**
Alexander Graham Bell Association
3417 Volta Pl NW
Washington, DC 20007-2737
202-337-5220
FAX: 202-337-8314
e-mail: info@agbell.org
www.agbell.org
Todd Houston, Executive Director
This video shows auditory-verbal therapy sessions of a therapist working individually with 11 children who range in age from 7 months to 7 years old and have hearing aids or cochlear implants.
Video

5241 **Doing Things Together**
Britannica Film Company
345 4th St
San Francisco, CA 94107-1206
415-928-8466
FAX: 415-928-5027
Dave Bekowich, Owner
Steve went with his parents to an amusement park. He met another boy named Martin who at first was shocked by Steve's prosthetic hand.
Film

5242 **Emerging Leaders**
Mobility International USA
132 E. Broadway
Suite 343
Eugene, OR 97401-2767
541-343-1284
FAX: 541-343-6812
e-mail: info@miusa.org
www.miusa.org
Susan Sygall, CEO/Founder
Susan Dunn, Exec. Asst./Project Specialist
Cindy Lewis, Director of Programs
Estelle Coreris-Moore, Financial Manager
Pioneering short-term international disability leadership programs in the U.S. and abroad with 2,000 youth, young adults and professionals from over 100 countries. *$49.00*
Video

5243 **Face FirstFanlight Productions/Icarus Films**
Fanlight Productions
32 Court St.
21st Floor
Brooklyn, NY 11201-4421
718-488-8900
800-876-1710
FAX: 718-488-8642
e-mail: info@fanlight.com
www.fanlight.com
Jonathan Miller, President
Patricio Guzman, Director
Meredith Miller, Sales Manager
Anthony Sweeney, Acquisitions
In this documentary, the stories told reflect the reality faced by all those who are seen as different. Despite their difficult experiences, the survival of the profiled individuals affords comic relief &, by adulthood, they possess unusual strengths that shape their careers in pediatrics, disability care, public speaking, and journalism. *$ 195.00*

5244 **Family-Guided Activity-Based Intervention for Toddlers & Infants**
Brookes Publishing
PO Box 10624
Baltimore, MD 21285-0624
410-337-9580
800-638-3775
FAX: 410-337-8539
e-mail: custserv@brookespublishing.com
www.readplaylearn.com
Paul Brooks, Owner
This 20-minute video was created to assist early childhood professionals to incorporate therapeutic intervention into daily living. It includes a discussion and demonstration of how intervention professionals actively may involve caregivers in the planning and implementation of activities aimed at encouraging development of a child's target skills *$37.00*
20 Minutes
ISBN 1-55766-19-3

5245 **Filmakers Library**
124 E 40th St
Suite 901
New York, NY 10016-1798
212-808-4980
FAX: 212-808-4983
e-mail: info@filmakers.com
www.filmakers.com
Sue Oscar, Co-President
Linda Gottesman, Co-President
Andrea Traubner, Dir., Broadcast Sales
Filmakers Library has been a leading source of outstanding films for the education, library, and non-theatrical markets. Now, as an imprint of award-winning online publisher Alexander Street Press, Filmakers Library is able to offer online streaming access to most of our titles, ensuring that our films receive the greatest possible exposure and accessibility through the most flexible de-

livery platforms. We market and promote our films throughout the world by direct mail, print advertising, exhib

5246 Filmakers Library: An Imprint Of AlexanderStreet Press
124 E 40th St
Suite 901
New York, NY 10016-1798 212-808-4980
FAX: 212-808-4983
e-mail: info@filmakers.com
www.filmakers.com

Sue Oscar, Co-President
Linda Gottesman, Co-President
Andrea Traubner, Dir., Broadcast Sales

Filmakers Library has been a leading source of outstanding films for the education, library, and non-theatrical markets. Now, as an imprint of award-winning online publisher Alexander Street Press, Filmakers Library is able to offer online streaming access to most of our titles, ensuring that our films receive the greatest possible exposure and accessibility through the most flexible delivery platforms. We market and promote our films throughout the world by direct mail, print advertising, exhib
$100 - $300

5247 Films & Videos on Aging and Sensory Change
Lighthouse International
111 E 59th St
New York, NY 10022-1202 212-821-9200
800-829-0500
FAX: 212-821-9706
e-mail: info@lighthouse.org

Joanna Mellor, VP Information Services
Tara Cortes, President

An annotated list of over 80 films and videos dealing with age-related sensory change, divided into sections on vision impairment, hearing impairment, and multiple sensory impairments. *$5.00*

5248 Heart to HeartBlind Childrens Center, Inc
Blind Children's Center
4120 Marathon St
Los Angeles, CA 90029-3584 323-664-2153
800-222-3567
FAX: 323-665-3828
e-mail: info@blindchildrenscenter.org
www.blindchildrenscenter.org

Lena French, Executive Director
Fernanda Armenta-Schmitt, PhD, Director of Education & Family Services/Assistant Executive
Muriel Scharf, Director of Development
Ross Vergara, Director of Finance

Parents of blind and partially sighted children talk about their feelings. *$35.00*
Video

5249 Helping HandsFanlight Productions/Icarus Films
Fanlight Productions
32 Court St.
21st Floor
Brooklyn, NY 11201-4421 718-488-8900
800-876-1710
FAX: 718-488-8642
e-mail: info@fanlight.com
www.fanlight.com

Jonathan Miller, President
Patricio Guzman, Director
Meredith Miller, Sales Manager
Anthony Sweeney, Acquisitions

The ADA mandates equal access and opportunity for the 43 million people with disabilities in the United States. These individuals may have limited speech, sight or mobility; a developmental disability; or a medical condition which limits some life activities. Many, however, are ready, willing and very able to join the workforce. This video demonstrates that many modifications or adaptations can be made simply by using ingenuity or common sense — such as keeping the aisles clear, etc. *$145.00*
37 Minutes

5250 Home is in the Heart: Accommodating Peoplewith Disabilities in the Homestay Experience
Mobility International USA
132 E. Broadway
Suite 343
Eugene, OR 97401-2767 541-343-1284
FAX: 541-343-6812
e-mail: info@miusa.org
www.miusa.org

Susan Sygall, CEO/Founder
Susan Dunn, Exec. Asst./Project Specialist
Cindy Lewis, Director of Programs
Estelle Coreris-Moore, Financial Manager

Provides information and ideas for exchange organizations. Discusses how to recruit homestay families, meet accessibility needs and accommodate international participants with disabilities.
$49.00
Video

5251 How Difficult Can This Be ? (Fat City)Rick Lavoie
CACLD
PO Box 210
Barnstable, MA 02630-210 508-362-1052
e-mail: scheduling@ricklavoie.com
www.ricklavoie.com

Rick Lavoie, Film Maker

This unique program allows viewers to experience the same frustration, anxiety and tension that children with learning disabilities face in their daily lives. Teachers, social workers, psychologists, parents and friends who have participated in Richard Lavoie's workshop reflect upon their experience and the way it changed their approach to L.D. children. 1989.

5252 How We PlayFanlight Productions/Icarus Films
Fanlight Productions
32 Court St.
21st Floor
Brooklyn, NY 11201-4421 718-488-8900
800-876-1710
FAX: 718-488-8642
e-mail: info@fanlight.com
www.fanlight.com

Jonathan Miller, President
Patricio Guzman, Director
Meredith Miller, Sales Manager
Anthony Sweeney, Acquisitions

Though most of the people in this new, short documentary are in wheelchairs, and one is blind, they are anything but handicapped. Playing tennis, snorkeling, whitewater canoeing, practicing karate - they are living proof that a disability can be a challenge, not an obstacle. *$99.00*

5253 I'm Not DisabledLandmark Media, Inc.
Landmark Media
3450 Slade Run Dr
Falls Church, VA 22042-3940 703-241-2030
800-342-4336
FAX: 703-536-9540
e-mail: info@landmarkmedia.com
www.landmarkmedia.com

Michael Hartogs, President
Joan Hartogs, Vice President
Peter Hartogs, Vice President
Richard Hartogs, Vice President

Young people talk about their disabilities and the importance of sports in their lives. The afflictions range from blindness and missing limbs to paralysis. Through physical education and therapy they enjoy freedom of movement and participate in sports such as tennis, basketball, kayaking, skiing, and swimming.
$195.00
Video

5254 **Imagery Procedures for People with Special Needs**
Research Press
PO Box 9177
Dept. 11W
Champaign, IL 61826-9177 217-352-3273
800-519-2707
FAX: 217-352-1221
e-mail: rp@researchpress.com
www.researchpress.com
David Parkinson, Chairman
Russell Pence, President
Gail Salyards, Dir. Of Marketing/President
This video was developed at the Groden Center and illustrates imagery based procedures including the use of positive reinforcement, covert modeling, and a self-control triad to assists individuals to self-regulate their behaviors in stressful situations or under conditions that may evoke extreme fear. Recommended for professionals and family members interested in teaching self-control strategies that individuals with autism spectrum disorders can use in community settings. *$195.00*
32 Minutes

5255 **Include Us**
Exceptional Parent Library
PO Box 1807
Englewood Cliffs, NJ 7632-1207 201-947-6000
800-535-1910
FAX: 201-947-9376
e-mail: eplibrary@aol.com
www.eplibrary.com

5256 **Intensive Early Intervention and Beyond**
PO Box 9177
Dept. 11W
Champaign, IL 61826-9177 217-352-3273
800-519-2707
FAX: 217-352-1221
www.researchpress.com
David Parkinson, Chairman
Russell Pence, President
Gail Salyards, Dir. Of Marketing/President

5257 **Invisible Children**
Learning Corporation of America
6493 Kaiser Dr
Fremont, CA 94555-3610 510-490-7311
Oonchia Chia, Owner
Renaldo was blind, Mandy was deaf, and Mark had Cerebral Palsy and used a wheelchair. These child-size puppet characters interacted with non-handicapped puppets.
Film

5258 **Look Who's LaughingAquarius Health Care Media**
Aquarius Health Care Videos
30 Forest Rd
PO Box 249
Millis, MA 2054-1511 508-376-1244
FAX: 508-376-1245
e-mail: aqvideos@tiac.net
www.aquariusproductions.com
Lesile Kussmann, Owner/President/Producer
Kathy Newkirk, Director
Jane Hutchinson, Assoc. Director
This video is packed with laugh-out-loud comedic moments, but is also full of intelligent and inspiring messages. Look Who's Laughing introduces viewers to some of today's funniest comedians - who just happen to be physically disabled. We hear them talk openly and honestly about their limitations as well as their abilities and talents. Helpful for those who work with the disabled and motivational to both the disabled and able-bodied. Preview option available. *$95.00*
Video

5259 **My Body is Not Who I AmAquarius Health Care Media**
Aquarius Health Care Videos
30 Forest Rd
PO Box 249
Millis, MA 2054-1511 508-376-1244
FAX: 508-376-1245
e-mail: aqvideos@tiac.net
www.aquariusproductions.com
Lesile Kussmann, Owner/President/Producer
Kathy Newkirk, Director
Jane Hutchinson, Assoc. Director
This thought-provoking video introduces viewers to people who openly discuss the struggles and triumphs they have experienced living in a body that is physically disabled. They talk honestly about the social stigma of their disability and the problems they face in terms of mobility, health care and family relationships, as well as the challenges of emotional and sexual intimacy. Preview option available. *$195.00*
Video

5260 **My CountryAquarius Health Care Media**
Aquarius Health Care Videos
30 Forest Rd
PO Box 249
Millis, MA 2054-1511 508-376-1244
FAX: 508-376-1245
e-mail: aqvideos@tiac.net
www.aquariusproductions.com
Lesile Kussmann, Owner/President/Producer
Kathy Newkirk, Director
Jane Hutchinson, Assoc. Director
By telling the stories of three people with disabilities and their struggle for equal rights under the law, this film draws a powerful parallel between the efforts of disability rights activists and the civil rights struggle of the 1960s. Great for disability awareness programs, and for discussions of disability rights issues. Should be part of every college curriculum on disabilities. Awarded Best of Show Superfest 98. Preview option available. *$195.00*
Video

5261 **No BarriersAquarius Health Care Media**
Aquarius Health Care Videos
30 Forest Rd
PO Box 249
Millis, MA 2054-1511 508-376-1244
FAX: 508-376-1245
e-mail: aqvideos@tiac.net
www.aquariusproductions.com
Lesile Kussmann, Owner/President/Producer
Kathy Newkirk, Director
Jane Hutchinson, Assoc. Director
Everyone faces the world with different abilities and disabilities. But everyone has at least one goal in common...to break through their own barriers says Mark Wellman. Mark, a paraplegic, knows this well. No Barriers takes us into Mark's world where he defies the odds for most able bodied individuals by climbing Yosemite's Half Dome and El Capitan. This video is more than inspiring and fun to watch...it helps one make that paradigm shift from can't do to can do! Preview option available *$90.00*
Video

5262 **On The SpectrumFanlight Productions/Icarus Films**
Fanlight Productions
32 Court St.
21st Floor
Brooklyn, NY 11201-4421 718-488-8900
800-876-1710
FAX: 718-488-8642
e-mail: info@fanlight.com
www.fanlight.com
Jonathan Miller, President
Patricio Guzman, Director
Meredith Miller, Sales Manager
Anthony Sweeney, Acquisitions
Adults living with Asperger syndrome describe the ways AS has affected their lives, their work and their relationships. They discuss learning to cope with the disorder and the comfort and rein-

forcement of participating with others 'like them' in an Asperger's support group. 53 min. *$199.00*

5263 Open for Business
Disability Rights Education and Defense Fund
3075 Adeline Street
Suite 210
Berkeley, CA 94703-2219
510-644-2555
800-841-8645
FAX: 510-841-8645
e-mail: info@dredf.org
www.dredf.org
Sue Henderson, Executive Director
Jenny . Kern, Esq, President/Chair
Claudia Center, Esq, Treasurer
Vikki Davis, Secretary
Documentary video captures the drama and emotions of the historic civil rights demonstration of people with disabilities in 1977, resulting in the signing of the 504 Regulations, the first Federal Civil Rights Law protecting people with disabilities. Includes contemporary news footage and news interviews with participants and demonstration leaders. *$179.00*

5264 Open to the PublicAquarius Health Care Media
Aquarius Health Care Videos
30 Forest Rd
PO Box 249
Millis, MA 2054-1511
508-376-1244
FAX: 508-376-1245
e-mail: aqvideos@tiac.net
www.aquariusproductions.com
Lesile Kussmann, Owner/President/Producer
Kathy Newkirk, Director
Jane Hutchinson, Assoc. Director
Provides an overview of the Americans with Disabilities Act as it applies to state and local governments. The ADA doesn't provide recommendations for solving common problems, but this film could provide enough information for governments to solve some common problems without turning to high-priced consultants. Preview option available. *$125.00*
Video

5265 Our Own RoadAquarius Health Care Media
Aquarius Health Care Videos
30 Forest Rd
PO Box 249
Millis, MA 2054-1511
508-376-1244
FAX: 508-376-1245
e-mail: aqvideos@tiac.net
www.aquariusproductions.com
Lesile Kussmann, Owner/President/Producer
Kathy Newkirk, Director
Jane Hutchinson, Assoc. Director
This video shows the disabled helping other people who are disabled and portrays the sense of pride they get from helping others. This multicultural program features many different healing techniques, and teaches the importance of helping those who are disabled become independent and productive. *$99.00*

5266 Outsider: The Life and Art of Judith ScottFanlight Productions/Icarus Films
Fanlight Productions
32 Court St.
21st Floor
Brooklyn, NY 11201-4421
718-488-8900
800-876-1710
FAX: 718-488-8642
e-mail: info@fanlight.com
www.fanlight.com
Jonathan Miller, President
Patricio Guzman, Director
Meredith Miller, Sales Manager
Anthony Sweeney, Acquisitions
Judith Scoot has Down Syndrome, is deaf, and does not speak. Yet after 35 years of institutionalization, with the help of a sister who never gave up on her, she emerged to create a series of sculptures that have fascinated and mystified art experts and collectors around the world. 26 minutes. *$199.00*

5267 Passion for Justice
Fanlight Productions
32 Court St.
21st Floor
Brooklyn, NY 11201-4421
718-488-8900
800-876-1710
FAX: 718-488-8642
e-mail: info@fanlight.com
www.fanlight.com
Jonathan Miller, President
Patricio Guzman, Director
Meredith Miller, Sales Manager
Anthony Sweeney, Acquisitions
An unusually penetrating examination of the question of inclusion, this is an engaging portrait of Bob Perske, the author of Unequal Justice, and a crusader for the legal rights of people with developmental disabilities. A Passion for Justice asks challenging questions about society's responsibility to this population, and about ways to protect everyone's rights to equality and justice. *$99.00*
29 Minutes

5268 Phoenix DanceFanlight Productions/Icarus Films
Fanlight Productions
32 Court St.
21st Floor
Brooklyn, NY 11201-4421
718-488-8900
800-876-1710
FAX: 718-488-8642
e-mail: info@fanlight.com
www.fanlight.com
Jonathan Miller, President
Patricio Guzman, Director
Meredith Miller, Sales Manager
Anthony Sweeney, Acquisitions
A heroic journey of transformation and healing, Phoenix Dance challenges our expectations of what it means to be disabled. In March, 2001, renowned dancer Homer Avila discovered that the pain in his hip was cancer. A month later, his right leg and most of his hip were amputated. *$199.00*

5269 Pool Exercise ProgramArthritis Water Exercise / Arthritis Foundation
Arthritis Foundation Distribution Center
PO Box 932915
Atlanta, GA 31193-2915
440-872-7100
800-283-7800
FAX: 404-872-0457
e-mail: aforders@arthritis.org
www.arthritis.org
John Klippel, President/CEO
This video features water exercises that will help you increase and maintain joint flexibility, strengthen and tone muscles, and increase endurance. All exercises are performed in water at chest level. No swimming skills are necessary. *$19.50*

5270 Potty Learning for Children who Experience Delay
Exceptional Parent Library
PO Box 1807
Englewood Cliffs, NJ 7632-1207
201-947-6000
800-535-1910
FAX: 201-947-9376
e-mail: eplibrary@aol.com
www.eplibrary.com

5271 Pushin' ForwardFanlight Productions/Icarus Films
Fanlight Productions
32 Court St.
21st Floor
Brooklyn, NY 11201-4421
718-488-8900
800-876-1710
FAX: 718-488-8642
e-mail: info@fanlight.com
www.fanlight.com
Jonathan Miller, President
Patricio Guzman, Director
Meredith Miller, Sales Manager
Anthony Sweeney, Acquisitions

Growing up poor and Latino, James Lilly was a gang member and drug dealer until, at fifteen, he was shot in the back and paralyzed. Today, he shares his story with inner city kids, and tells them about one thing that helped him move on; wheelchair racing. In Pushin' Forward he takes on the world's longest wheelchair race, from Fairbanks to Anchorage, Alaska, in six days! 39 minutes. *$229.00*

5272 Relaxation Techniques for People with Special Needs
Research Press
PO Box 9177
Dept. 11W
Champaign, IL 61826-9177 217-352-3273
800-519-2707
FAX: 217-352-1221
e-mail: rp@researchpress.com
www.researchpress.com

David Parkinson, Chairman
Russell Pence, President
Gail Salyards, Dir. Of Marketing/President
The developers discuss and demonstrate how to use special relaxation procedures with children and adolescents who have developmental disabilities. They emphasize the need for students to learn relaxation as a means of coping with stress and developing self-control. During the scenes of Dr June Groden conducting relaxation training, viewers will see how to correctly use the training procedures, how to use reinforcement during training and how to use guided imagery. 23 minutes. Includes book. *$195.00*
Video

5273 Right at HomeAquarius Health Care Media
Aquarius Health Care Videos
30 Forest Rd
PO Box 249
Millis, MA 2054 508-376-1244
FAX: 508-376-1245
e-mail: aqvideos@tiac.net
www.aquariusproductions.com

Lesile Kussmann, Owner/President/Producer
Kathy Newkirk, Director
Jane Hutchinson, Assoc. Director
Shows simple solutions for complying with the Fair Hoiusing Act amendments. Emphasizes low-cost, practical solutions, and working with people with disabilities to find the best applicable solution. Ideal for people with disabilities and their families, as well as housing providers, university courses, and disability awareness organizations. Preview option is available. *$99.00*
Video

5274 Seat-A-Robics
PO Box 630064
Little Neck, NY 11363-64 718-631-4007

Daria Alinovi, President
Offers a variety of safe, affordable and medically approved video exercise programs that are listed in our video chapter. In addition the company offers two resources. The first Healthy Eating & Facts For Kids is geared specifically to health professionals and educators that work with disabled children ($39.95). The second is a recreational resource guide that stimulates children to be creative and get involved. It keeps them actively engaged while having fun and getting fit ($29.95).

5275 Shining Bright: Head Start Inclusion
Brookes Publishing
PO Box 10624
Baltimore, MD 21285-624 410-337-9580
800-638-3775
FAX: 410-337-8539
e-mail: custserv@brookespublishing.com
www.readplaylearn.com

Paul Brooks, Owner
This documentary depicts the collaborative efforts of a Head Start and a local education agency to include children with severe disabilities in a Head Start program. This video addresses issues such as support for children with severe health impairments, benefits of participating in Head Start, ability of teachers with a general education background to serve children with severe disabilities, and staff relations. Includes a 28-page saddle-stitched booklet. *$45.00*
23 Minutes
ISBN 1-55766-95-9

5276 Small DifferencesAquarius Health Care Media
Aquarius Health Care Videos
30 Forest Rd
PO Box 249
Millis, MA 2054-1511 508-376-1244
FAX: 508-376-1245
e-mail: aqvideos@tiac.net
www.aquariusproductions.com

Lesile Kussmann, Owner/President/Producer
Kathy Newkirk, Director
Jane Hutchinson, Assoc. Director
What happens when you give children with and without disabilities a camera and ask them to produce a video about disabilities? The result is an uplifting, award-winning disability video that both children and adults can relate to. The kids interviewed adults and children with physical and sensory disabilities. A top-quality production that increases understanding and awareness. Winner, Columbus International Film & Video Festival. Winner, National Education Media Network. Preview option availabe *$110.00*
Video

5277 Someday's ChildEducational Productions
Educational Productions
9000 SW Gemini Dr
Beaverton, OR 97008-7151 503-644-7000
800-950-4949
FAX: 503-350-7000
e-mail: custserv@edpro.com
www.edpro.com

Diane Trister Dodge, Founder/President/Lead Author
Arnitra Duckett, VP, Sales & Strategic Marketing
This video focuses on three families' search for help and information for their children with disabilities.

5278 Sound & FuryAquarius Health Care Media
Aquarius Health Care Videos
30 Forest Rd
PO Box 249
Millis, MA 2054-1511 508-376-1244
FAX: 508-376-1245
e-mail: aqvideos@tiac.net
www.aquariusproductions.com

Lesile Kussmann, Owner/President/Producer
Kathy Newkirk, Director
Jane Hutchinson, Assoc. Director
This film takes viewers inside the seldom seen world of the deaf to witness a painful family struggle over a controversial medical technology called the cochlear implant. Some of the family members celebrate the implant as a long overdue cure for deafness while others fear it will destroy their language and way of life. This documentary explores this seemingly irreconcilable conflict as it illuminates the ongoing struggle for identity among deaf people today. *$195.00*
Video

5279 Special Children/Special Solutions
Option Indigo Press
2080 S Undermountain Rd
Sheffield, MA 1257-9643 413-229-8727
800-714-2779
FAX: 413-229-8727
e-mail: indigo@option.org
www.optionindigo.com

Barry Kaufmans, Owner/Founder/Author
Samahria Kaufmans, Owner/Founder
This four-tape audio series presents concrete, down-to-earth, no-nonsense alternatives which are full of love and acceptance for the special child while being wholly supportive of parents, professionals and helpers who want to reach out. The accepting (nonjudgmental) attitude presented is the basis of all Samahria's work and is the foundation for the nurturing teaching process that

has encouraged and helped parents, children and others to accomplish more than most would have believed. *$55.00*
Audio

5280 Technology for the DisabledLandmark Media, Inc.
Landmark Media
3450 Slade Run Dr
Falls Church, VA 22042-3940
703-241-2030
800-342-4336
FAX: 703-536-9540
e-mail: info@landmarkmedia.com
landmarkmedia.com
Michael Hartogs, President
Joan Hartogs, Vice President
Peter Hartogs, Vice President
Richard Hartogs, Vice President
Physically disabled people cope with the frustrations of a body they cannot control. The computer age has made many disabled more self-reliant; armless feed themselves, the blind read newspapers and the voiceless speak through marvelous technological breakthroughs. *$195.00*
Video

5281 The Boy InsideFanlight Productions/Icarus Films
Fanlight Productions
32 Court St.
21st Floor
Brooklyn, NY 11201-4421
718-488-8900
800-876-1710
FAX: 718-488-8642
e-mail: info@fanlight.com
www.fanlight.com
Jonathan Miller, President
Patricio Guzman, Director
Meredith Miller, Sales Manager
Anthony Sweeney, Acquisitions
Filmmaker Marianne Kaplan tells the personal and often distressing story of her son Adam, a 12-year-old with Asperger Syndrome, during a tumultuous year in the life of their family.

5282 Three R's for Special Education: Rights, Resources, Results
Brookes Publishing
PO Box 10624
Baltimore
MD, 21 0624-624
410-337-9580
800-638-3775
FAX: 410-337-8539
e-mail: custserv@brookespublishing.com
www.readplaylearn.com
Paul Brooks, Owner
This is a guide for parents, and a tool for educators. Through this video parents learn how to work through the steps of the special education system and work toward securing the best education and services for their children. Reviews the laws to protect children with disabilities in easy to understand language. Also provides a list of national organizations that can offer resources, information and advice to parents. *$49.95*
50 Minutes
ISBN 0-96461 -80-7

5283 Tools for StudentsAquarius Health Care Media
Aquarius Health Care Videos
30 Forest Rd
PO Box 249
Millis, MA 2054-1511
508-376-1244
FAX: 508-376-1245
e-mail: aqvideos@tiac.net
www.aquariusproductions.com
Lesile Kussmann, Owner/President/Producer
Kathy Newkirk, Director
Jane Hutchinson, Assoc. Director
Provides a series of 26 fun occupational therapy sensory processing activities. Designed as an in-home, in-workshop, and in-class exercise leader with students. Activities include: Strenghten the muscles necessary for normal activities, provide the muscles necessary to enhance alertness and concentration, increase the ability to use good posture, help social skills and fitting in and increase coordination; concludes with emphasis on team collaboration between the student, teacher, and parents. *$99.00*
Video

5284 Video Guide to Disability AwarenessAquarius Health Care Media
Aquarius Health Care Videos
30 Forest Rd
PO Box 249
Millis, MA 2054-1511
508-376-1244
FAX: 508-376-1245
e-mail: aqvideos@tiac.net
www.aquariusproductions.com
Lesile Kussmann, Owner/President/Producer
Kathy Newkirk, Director
Jane Hutchinson, Assoc. Director
President Clinton opens and concludes this informative video about disability awareness. A series of candid interviews with people who have a wide range of disabilities provide personal insights into the issues surrounding visual, hearing, physical and mental disabilities. Video comes with written reference guide and is also available with open or closed captioning. Preview option available. *$195.00*
Video

5285 Video Intensive Parenting
Systems Unlimited/LIFE Skills
1556 S 1st Ave
Iowa City, IA 52240-6007
319-356-5412
Geoffrey Lauer, Program Director
Bill Gorman, President
Ginny Kirschling, Public Information Specialist
Parents who have children with special needs share their reactions to their child's diagnosis and how they have learned to cope with their feelings. *$69.95*

5286 Vital Signs: Crip Culture Talks BackFanlight Productions/Icarus Films
Fanlight Productions
32 Court St.
21st Floor
Brooklyn, NY 11201-4421
718-488-8900
800-876-1710
FAX: 718-488-8642
e-mail: info@fanlight.com
www.fanlight.com
Jonathan Miller, President
Patricio Guzman, Director
Meredith Miller, Sales Manager
Anthony Sweeney, Acquisitions
This edgy, raw video documentary explores the politics of disability through the performances, debates and late-night conversations of artists at a recent national conference of disabilities and the art's. Vital Signs conveys the intensity, variety and vitality of disability culture today. *$225.00*
Video

5287 What About Me?Educational Productions
Educational Productions
9000 SW Gemini Dr
Beaverton, OR 97008-7151
503-644-7000
800-950-4949
FAX: 503-350-7000
e-mail: custserve@edpro.com
www.teachingstrategies.com
Diane Trister Dodge, Founder/President/Lead Author
Arnitra Duckett, VP, Sales & Strategic Marketing
This video focuses on two siblings of children with disabilities. The siblings (Brian and Julie) share their perspectives, their worries, concerns and victories about living with a sibling with a disability.

5288 When Billy Broke His Head...and OtherFanlight Productions/Icarus Films

Fanlight Productions
32 Court St.
21st Floor
Brooklyn, NY 11201-4421
718-488-8900
800-876-1710
FAX: 718-488-8642
e-mail: info@fanlight.com
www.fanlight.com

Jonathan Miller, President
Patricio Guzman, Director
Meredith Miller, Sales Manager
Anthony Sweeney, Acquisitions

When Billy Golfus, an award-winning journalist, became brain damaged as the result of a motor scooter accident, he joined the ranks of the 43 million Americans with disabilities, this country's largest and most invisible minority. He helped create this video, which blends humor with politics and individual experience with a chorus of voices, to explain what it is really like to live with a disability in America. #136 *$195.00*

ISBN 1-57295 -36-2

5289 When I Grow Up

Britannica Film Company
345 4th St
San Francisco, CA 94107-1206
415-928-8466
FAX: 415-928-5027

Dave Bekowich, Owner

At a costume party each child was to come as what they wanted to be when they grew up. Some of the children had handicaps, and they talked about why their handicaps would not prevent them from fulfilling their desires.

Film

5290 When Parents Can't Fix ItFanlight Productions/Icarus Films

Fanlight Productions
32 Court St.
21st Floor
Brooklyn, NY 11201-4421
718-488-8900
800-876-1710
FAX: 718-488-8642
e-mail: info@fanlight.com
www.fanlight.com

Jonathan Miller, President
Patricio Guzman, Director
Meredith Miller, Sales Manager
Anthony Sweeney, Acquisitions

This documentary looks at the lives of five families who are raising children with disabilities - the problems they face, how they have learned to cope, and the rewards and stresses of adapting to their child's condition. It explores the medical complexities and financial pressures families encounter, the emotional and physical toll on parents and siblings, and the dangers of child abuse in this population. It offers a very realistic look at different family strengths and coping styles.

58 Min. DVD/VHS
ISBN 1-572958-76-6

5291 White Cane and WheelsFanlight Productions/Icarus Films

Fanlight Productions
32 Court St.
21st Floor
Brooklyn, NY 11201-4421
718-488-8900
800-876-1710
FAX: 718-488-8642
e-mail: info@fanlight.com
www.fanlight.com

Jonathan Miller, President
Patricio Guzman, Director
Meredith Miller, Sales Manager
Anthony Sweeney, Acquisitions

Carmen and Steve once dreamed of lives on stage and screen, but their plans were cut short by her blindness and his muscular dystrophy. This program is a funny and touching exploration of a relationship filled with frustration, but held together with patience, stubborness, forgiveness, and love. 26 minutes. *$169.00*

5292 Why My Child

976 Lake Baldwin Lane
Suite 104
Orlando, FL 32814
407-895-0802
800-313-ABDC
e-mail: staff@birthdefects.org
www.birthdefects.org

Web Sites

5293 AbleApparelAffordable Adaptive Clothing and Accessories

2121 Hillside Ave
New Hyde Park, NY 11040-2712
516-873-6552
FAX: 516-248-7308
e-mail: sales@abledata.com
www.ableapparel.com

Mary Ann Tenaglia, Partner
Marie Harmon, Partner
Donna Lo Monica, Partner/Designer

AbleApparel is always designing and creating new products that will make Matty's life and others with disabilities a little easier. Most of the people spoken to regardless of age want to be able to wear clothes that are functional, affordable and, above all, fashionable.

5294 Abledata

8630 Fenton Street
Suite 930
Silver Spring, MD 20910- 3820
301-608-8998
800-227-0216
FAX: 301-608-8958
TTY: 301-608-8912
e-mail: abledata@macrointernational.com
www.abledata.com

Katherine Belknap, Project Director
Steve Lowe, Associate Project Manager/Webmaster
David Johnson, Publications Director
Juanita Hardy, Information Specialist

AbleData provides objective information on assistive technology and rehabilitation equipment available from domestic and international sources to consumers, organizations, professionals, and caregivers within the United States. We serve the nation's disability, rehabilitation, and senior communities.

5295 Access Unlimited

570 Hance Rd
Binghamton, NY 13903-5700
607-669-4822
800-849-2143
FAX: 607-669-4595
www.accessunlimited.com

Thomas Egan, President/Owner
Tom 'TC' Cole, National Sales Manager

Adaptive transportation and mobility equipment for people with disabilities. ccess Unlimited products empower people with disabilities to regain control of their mobility.

5296 Ai Squared

130 Taconic Business Park
Manchester Center, VT 05255-9752
802-362-3612
800-859-0270
FAX: 802-362-1670
e-mail: sales@aisquared.com
www.aisquared.com

David Wu, CEO
Jost Eckhardt, VP of Engineering
Doug Hacker, VP of Business Development
Scott Moore, VP of Marketing

Ai Squared has been a leader in the assistive technology field for over 20 years. Our flagship product, ZoomText, is the world's best magnification and reading software for the vision impaired. We pride ourselves on delivering the highest quality software products and superior technical support.

5297 Alternatives in Education for the Hearing Impaired (AEHI)
9300 Capitol Drive
Wheeling, IL 60090-7207
847-850-5490
FAX: 847-850-5493
e-mail: info@agbms.org
www.agbms.org

Sandra L. Mosetick, Board President Emeritus
Bridget Chevez, Board President
Daniel Konopacki, Treasurer
Debra Trude-Suter, Ph.D., CEO/Executive Director

AEHI is a program of the Alexander Graham Bell Montessori School in Mt. Prospect, IL, that fosters literacy and empowers people with hearing impairments to achieve their full potential through unique educational options. AEHI provides Cued Speech workshops, individualized parental training and support, educational consulting, professional development opportunities, and access to a wide variety of information on Cued Speech and its benefits.

5298 American Academy of Audiology
11480 Commerce Park Drive
Suite 220
Reston, VA 20190- 4748
800-222-2336
FAX: 703-476-5157
e-mail: infoaud@audiology.org
www.audiology.org

Cheryl Kreider Carey, Executive Director
Edward Sullivan, Deputy Executive Director
Deborah Carlson, PhD, President
Shilpi Banerjee, PhD, Board Member

The American Academy of Audiology is the world's largest professional organization of, by, and for audiologists. The active membership of more than 11,000 is dedicated to providing quality hearing care services through professional development, education, research, and increased public awareness of hearing and balance disorders.

5299 American Association of People with Disabilities
2013 H Street, NW
5th Floor
Washington, DC 20006-1675
202-457-0046
800-840-8844
FAX: 866-536-4461
www.aapd.com

Mark Perriello, President/CEO
Henry Claypool, Executive Vice President
Ginny Thornburgh, Director of Interfaith Initiative
TaKeisha Walker, Director of Workplace & Leadership Initiatives

The American Association of People with Disabilities is the nation's largest disability rights organization. We promote equal opportunity, economic power, independent living, and political participation for people with disabilities. Our members, including people with disabilities and our family, friends, and supporters, represent a powerful force for change.

5300 American Botanical Council
6200 Manor Rd
PO Box 144345
Austin, TX 78723-4345
512-926-4900
800-373-7105
FAX: 512-926-2345
e-mail: abc@herbalgram.org
www.abc.herbalgram.org

Mark Blumenthal, Founder/Executive Director
Gayle Engels, Special Projects Director
Matthew Magruder, Art Director
Denise Meikel, Development Director

Provide education using science-based and traditional information to promote responsible use of herbal medicine - serving the public, researchers, educators, healthcare professionals, industry and media.

5301 American College of Rheumatology, Researchand Education Foundation
2200 Lake Boulevard NE
Atlanta, GA 30319-5310
404-633-3777
FAX: 404-633-1870
e-mail: acr@rheumatology.org
www.rheumatology.org

Audrey B. Uknis, MD, President
David I. Daikh, MD, PhD, Foundation President
Jan K. Richardson, PT, PhD, O, ARHP President
E. William St.Clair, MD, Treasurer

The American College of Rheumatology's mission is advancing rheumatology.The organization represents over 8,500 rheumatologists and rheumatology health professionals around the world. The ACR offers its members the support they need to ensure that they are able to continue their innovative work by providing programs of education, research, advocacy, and practice support.

5302 American Liver Foundation
39 Broadway
Suite 2700
New York, NY 10006-3054
212-668-1000
FAX: 212-483-8179
www.liverfoundation.org

Ryan Reczek, National Director, Field Development
Rolf Taylor, National Director, Corporate Relations
Pritha Kuchaculla, National Director, Programs
David Ticker, Chief Financial Officer

Is the only national voluntary health organization dedicated to preventing, treating, and curing hepatitis and other liver and gall bladder diseases through research and education.

5303 American Mobility: Personal Mobility Solutions
60 Island St
Lawrence, MA 1840-1835
978-794-3030
www.americanmobility.com

David Lacroix, President

Source of Pride Scooters, Jazzy Power Chairs, personal mobility vehicles, and lift and recline chairs.

5304 American Speech-Language and Hearing Association
2200 Research Blvd
Rockville, MD 20850-3289
301-296-5700
800-638-8255
FAX: 301-296-8580
TTY: 301-296-5650
e-mail: actioncenter@asha.org
www.asha.org

Wayne A. Foster, PhD, CCC-SLP/A, Chair, Audiology Advisory Council
Patricia A. Prelock, PhD, CCC-SLP, President
Carolyn W. Higdon, EdD, CCC-SLP, Vice President for Finance
Howard Goldstein, PhD, CCC-SL, Vice President for Science and Research

Exhibits by companies specializing in alternative and augmentative communications products, publishers, software and hardware compinies, and hearing aid testing equipment manufacturers.

5305 Americans with Disabilities Act: ADA Home Page
800-514-0301
TTY:800-514-0383
e-mail: webmaster@usdoj.gov
www.ada.gov

5306 Appliance 411
www.appliance411.com

5307 Arc of the United States
1825 K Street, NW
Suite 1200
Washington, DC 20006-5689
202-534-3700
800-433-5255
FAX: 202-534-3731
e-mail: info@thearc.org
www.thearc.org

Gary Bass, Director
Carol Wheeler, Director
Nancy Webster, President
Ronald Brown, Vice President

We are the largest national community-based organization advocating for and serving people with intellectual and developmental disabilities and their families. We encompass all ages and all spectrums from autism, Down syndrome, Fragile X and various other developmental disabilities.

5308 Association for the Cure of Cancer of the Prostate (CaP CURE)-Prostate Cancer Foundation
1250 Fourth St
Suite 360
Santa Monica, CA 90401-1444
310-570-4700
800-757-2873
FAX: 310-570-4701
e-mail: info@pcf.org
www.pcf.org

Mike Milken, Founder/Chairman
Jonathon Simons, MD, President/CEO
Ralph Finerman, Chief Financial Officer/Treasurer/Secretary
Howard R. Soule, PhD, Executive Vice President /Chief Science Officer

CURE is a nonprofit public charity that is dedicated to supporting prostate cancer research and hastening the conversion of research into cures or controls.

5309 Asthma and Allergy Foundation of America
8201 Corporate Drive
Suite 1000
Landover, MD 20785-2266
800-727-8462
e-mail: info@aafa.org
www.aafa.org

Lynn Hanessian, Chair
Michele Abu Carrick, LICSW, Co-Chair, Governance
Judi McAuliffe, RN, Co-Chair, Programs & Services
Calvin Anderson, Chair/Finance/Treasurer

AAFA is dedicated to improving the quality of life for people with asthma and allergic diseases through education, advocacy and research.

5310 Auditory-Verbal InternationalAG Bell
3417 Volta Place, NW
Washington, DC 20007-2737
202-204-4700
FAX: 202-337-8314
e-mail: academy@agbell.org
www.agbell.org

Anita Bernstein, Director
Kathleen Treni, President of the Association
Cheryl Dickson, President

Focus on education, guidance, advocacy, family support and the rigorous application of techniques to promote optimal acquision of spoken language

5311 Cancer Immunology Research Foundation(CIRF) Cancer Research Institute National Headquar
Concern Foundation
One Exchang Plaza, 55 Broadway
Suite 1802
New York, NY 10006-3724
212-688-7515
800-992-2623
FAX: 212-832-9376
e-mail: bbrewer@cancerresearch.org
www.cancerresearch.org

Brian M. Brewer, Director of Marketing and Communications
Lynne Harmer, Director of Grants Administration and Special Events
Alfred R. Massidas, Chief Financial Officer and Director of Human Resources
Alexandra S. Mulvey, Associate Director of Communications

Immunology research will discover why the immune system fails and cancer develops. Herein lies the cure for cancer, AIDS, and other autoimmune diseases.

5312 Cancer Immunotherapy and Gene Therapy
www.skcc.org

5313 Cancer Research Institute
One Exchang Plaza, 55 Broadway
Suite 1802
New York, NY 10006-3724
212-688-7515
800-992-2623
FAX: 212-832-9376
e-mail: bbrewer@cancerresearch.org
www.cancerresearch.org

Brian M. Brewer, Director of Marketing and Communications
Lynne Harmer, Director of Grants Administration and Special Events
Alfred R. Massidas, Chief Financial Officer and Director of Human Resources
Alexandra S. Mulvey, Associate Director of Communications

Immunology research will discover why the immune system fails and cancer develops. Herein lies the cure for cancer, AIDS, and other autoimmune diseases.

5314 Center on the Social & Emotional Foundations for Early Learning (CSEFEL)
Vanderbilt University 110 Magnolia
Box 328 GPC
Nashville, TN 37203
615-322-8150
FAX: 615-343-1570
e-mail: ml.hemmeter@vanderbilt.edu
www.csefel.vanderbilt.edu

Mary-Louise Hemmeter, Principal Investigator
Rob Corso, Project Coordinator
Tweety Yates, Project Coordinator
Glen Dunlap, Key Center Personnel

The center will: focus on promoting the social and emotional developmental of children as a means of preventing challenging behaviors; collaborate with existing T/TA providers for the purpose of ensuring the implementation and sustainability of practices at the local level; provide ongoing identification of training needs and preferred delivery formats of local programs and T/TA providers; disseminate evidence-based practices.

5315 Damon Runyon Cancer Research Foundation
Walter Winchell Foundation
One Exchange Plaza, 55 Broadway
Suite 302
New York, NY 10006-3720
212-455-0500
877-722-6237
e-mail: info@damonrunyon.org
www.damonrunyon.org

Lorraine Egan, President/Chief Executive Officer
Elizabeth Portland, Director of Development
Marialice C. Pagnotta, Director of the Damon Runyon Broadway Tickets Service
Kimberly Kubert, Director of Special Events

The Damon Runyon Cancer Research Foundation funds early career cancer researchers who have the energy, drive and creativity to become leading innovators in their fields. We identify the best young scientists in the nation and support them through four award programs: our Fellowship, Pediatric Cancer Fellowship, Clinical Investigator and Innovation Awards.

5316 DisAbility Information and Resources

e-mail: jlubin@eskimo.com
www.makoa.org

Jim Lubin, Creator/Owner

Offers dozens of links to sites with information, services and products for the disabled.

5317 Disability Net

www.bargione.co.uk/disabled.htm

5318 Disability Rights Activist

www.disrights.org

5319 Disability and Medical Resources Mall

www.icdri.org/Medical/disabilitymall.hmt

5320 DisabilityResources.org
Four Glatter Lane
Dept. IN
Centereach, NY 11720-1032
631-585-0290
FAX: 631-585-0290
e-mail: info@disabilityresources.org
www.disabilityresources.org

Julie Klauber, Co-founder/Managing Editor
Avery Klauber, Co-Founder/Executive Director
Sally Rosenthal, Contributing Editor
Ruth Porfert, Editorial Assistant

Disability Resources, inc. is a nonprofit 501(c)(3) organization established to promote and improve awareness, availability and accessibility of information that can help people with disabilities live, learn, love, work and play independently.

5321 Discover Technology
Houston, TX
713-885-1519
e-mail: dtinc8888@hotmail.com
www.discovertechnology.com

Amantha Cole, Founder

The primary mission of Discover Technology, Inc.is to create and administer computer labs for persons with disabilities, to encourage communication between persons with and without disabilities and to educate the general population about the disabled population.

5322 Dynamic Living
125 Old Iron Ore Road
Bloomfield, CT 06002-1315
860-683-4442
888-940-0605
FAX: 860-243-1910
e-mail: info@dynamic-living.com
www.dynamic-living.com

Andrea Tannenbaum, Owner

Kitchen products, bathroom helpers, and unique daily living products that provide a convienient, comfortable, and safe environment for people with disabilities.

5323 ElderLawAnswers.com
150 Chesnut St
4th Floor, Box #15
Providence, RI 02903
866-267-0947
e-mail: support@elderlawanswers.com
www.elderlawanswers.com

Harry S. Margolis, Founder/President
Ken Coughlin, Editor
Mark Miller, Director of Product and Business Development
Wendy Miki Glaus, Attorney

Provides information about legal issues facing senior citizens and a searchable directory of attorneys.

5324 Exploring Autism: A Look at the Genetics of Autism
Box 3445 DUMC
Durham, NC 27710
FAX: 919-684-0952
e-mail: info@exploringautism.org
www.exploringautism.org

Chantelle Wolpert, Project Director

Dedicated to helping families who are living with the challenges of autism stay informed about the exciting breakthroughs involving the genetics of autism. Report and explain new genetic research findings. Explain genetic principles as they relate to autism, provide the latest research news, and seek your imput.

5325 FHI 360
1825 Connecticut Ave., NW
Suite 800
Washington, DC 20009-5721
202-884-8000
FAX: 202-884-8400
e-mail: CareerCenterSupport@fhi360.org
www.fhi360.org

Willard Cates Jr, MD, MPH, President Emeritus
Albert J. Siemens, PhD, Chief Executive Officer
Patrick C. Fine, MS, Chief Operating Officer
Robert S. Murphy, MBA, Chief Financial Officer

FHI 360 is a nonprofit human development organization dedicated to improving lives in lasting ways by advancing integrated, locally driven solutions.

5326 Foundation Fighting Blindness
7168 Columbia Gateway Dr
Suite 100
Columbia, MD 21046- 3256
410-423-0600
800-683-5555
TTY:800-683-5551
e-mail: info@fightblindness.org
www.blindness.org

Susan Brumley, Sr. National Director
Susan Gloor, Sr. National Director, Events
Michele Mercer, Senior Director, Database Operations
Anastasia Staten, Senior Director, Membership

The urgent mission of the Foundation Fighting Blindness, Inc. is to drive the research that will provide preventions, treatments and ures for people affected by retinitis pigmentosa (RP), macular degeneration, Usher syndrome, and the entire spectrum of retinal degenerative diseases.

5327 Freedom Scientific
11830 31st Court North
St. Petersburg, FL 33716-1805
727-803-8000
800-444-4443
FAX: 727-803-8001
e-mail: info@freedomscientific.com
www.freedomscientific.com

Lee Hamilton, President/CEO/Chairman
Mike Self, Sales Representative
Joseph McDaniel, Sales Representative
Bobby Lakey, Sales Representative

Assistive technology for blind and visually impaired computer users.

5328 Gallaudet University Press
800 Florida Ave, NE
Washington, DC 20002-3695
202-651-5488
FAX: 202-651-5489
e-mail: gupress@gallaudet.edu
www.gupress.gallaudet.edu

5329 Glaucoma Research Foundation
251 Post Street
Suite 600
San Francisco, CA 94108-5017
415-986-3162
800-826-6693
e-mail: question@glaucoma.org
www.glaucoma.org

Andrew Iwach, MD, Board Chair/Executive Director
Thomas r M. Brunne, President/CEO
H. Allen Bouch, Vice Chair
Fred H. Brinkmann, Treasurer

Our mission is to prevent vision loss from glaucoma by investing in innovative research, education, and support with the ultimate goal of finding a cure.

5330 Helen Beebe Speech and Hearing Center

www.helenbeebe.org

5331 Herb Research Foundation
5589 Arapahoe Ave
Suite 205
Boulder, CO 80303-8115 303-449-2265

www.herbs.org

Rob McCaleb, President
John Lowe, Director of Research

Research and public education on the health benefits of medicinal plants. Dedicated to world health through the informed use of herbs.

5332 Hypokalemic Periodic Paralysis Resource Page
155 West 68th St
Suite 1732
New York, NY 10023-5830 407-339-9499

e-mail: lfeld@cfl.rr.com
www.periodicparalysis.org

Jacob Levitt, President/Medical Director
Linda Feld, Vice President

Provides understandable information on HKPP, dynamia linkage to several additional sources of helpful information on the Internet, and offers several online networking opportunities.

5333 Innovation Management Group
179 Niblick Road
Suite 454
Paso Robles, CA 93446-4845 818-701-1579
800-889-0987
FAX: 818-936-0200
e-mail: sales@imgpresents.com
www.imgpresents.com

5334 Interstitial Cystitis Association
1760 Old Meadow Road
Suite 500
McLean, VA 22102-2651 703-442-2070
800-435-7422
FAX: 703-506-3266
e-mail: icamail@ichelp.org
www.ichelp.org

Barbara Gordon, Co-Chair/Executive Director
Eric Zarnikow, MBA, Co-Chair
Marilynn Schreibstein, CFO
F. Neal Thompson, Treasurer

The Interstitial Cystitis Association (ICA) advocates for interstitial cystitis (IC) research dedicated to discovery of a cure and better treatments, raises awareness, and serves as a central hub for the healthcare providers, researchers and millions of patients who suffer with constant urinary urgency and frequency and extreme bladder pain called IC. (IC is also referred to as painful bladder syndrome, bladder pain syndrome, and chronic pelvic pain.)

5335 LD OnLineWETA Public Television
2775 S. Quincy Street
Arlington, VA 22206-2269 703-998-2060
FAX: 703-998-2060
e-mail: ldonline@weta.org
www.ldonline.org

Noel Gunther, Executive Director
Christian Lindstrom, Director
Tina Chovanec, Director
Shalini Anand, Senior Mangager

LD OnLine seeks to help children and adults reach their full potential by providing accurate and up-to-date information and advice about learning disabilities and ADHD.The site features hundreds of helpful articles, multimedia, monthly columns by noted experts, first person essays, children's writing and artwork, a comprehensive resource guide, very active forums, and a Yellow Pages referral directory of professionals, schools, and products.

5336 Lyme Disease Foundation
PO Box 332
Tolland, CT 6084-332 860-870-0070
FAX: 860-870-0080
e-mail: info@lyme.org
www.lyme.org

Karen Forschuer, Chairman
Thomas Forschuer, Executive Director

Provides critical information about tick-borne disease prevention, improves healthcare and funds research for solutions. 500,000 children, adults, and professionals assisted 25 countries.

5337 Mainstream Online Magazine of the Able-Disabled

www.mainstream-mag.com

Cyndi Jones, Publisher
William G. Stothers, Editor

The leading news, advocacy and lifestyle magazine for people with disabilities.

5338 Microsoft Accessibility Technology for Everyone
One Microsoft Way
Redmond, WA 98052-6399 425-882-8080
800-642-7676
FAX: 425-936-7329
TTY: 800-892-5234
www.microsoft.com/enable

William Gates III, Chairman
Steven Ballmer, CEO/Director

Information about accessibility features and options included in Microsoft products.

5339 MossRehab ResourceNet
1200 West Tabor Road
Philadelphia, PA 19141-3099 215-456-9900
800-225-5567
e-mail: NOSPAMkennedyd@einstein.edu
www.mossresourcenet.org

John Whyte, Owner
Ruth Lefton, COO
Anthony Allonardo, Director of Technology

MossRehab, a modern, 147-bed facility, offers comprehensive care to people with a broad range of conditions—including stroke, brain injury, orthopaedic and musculoskeletal disabilities, spinal cord dysfunction, pulmonary disorders, amputations, and other forms of disability.

5340 Multiple Sclerosis National Research Institute
11350 SW Village Parkway
Port St. Lucie, FL 34987-2352 858-597-3872
866-676-7400
FAX: 858-597-3804
e-mail: info@ms-research.org
www.ms-research.org

Robin Offord, Chairman
Richard Houghten, President/CEO
Donald B. Cooper, C.F.O
Karen Douthitt, VP & Corporate Secretary

Multiple Sclerosis National Research Institute is a division of Torrey Pines Institute for Molecular Studies, a not-for-profit basic research center dedicated to the discovery and development of innovative research methods that lead to treatments for major medical conditions, including multiple sclerosis, AIDS, Alzheimer's disease, pain, heart disease, many types of cancer, and more.

5341 National Alliance of the Disabled(NAOTD)

e-mail: turtle@dnaco.net
www.naotd.wheelboat.com

Walton Dutcher, Executive Director/Operations
Fred Temple, Director
Spike Spikberg, Director
Donna Eustice, Director

The National Alliance OF The DisAbled is an online informational and advocacy organization dedicated to working towards gaining equal rights for the disAbled in all areas of life.

5342 National Association for Visually Handicapped Lighthouse International

111 E 59th St
New York, NY 10022-1202
212-821-9497
800-829-0500
FAX: 212-821-9707
TTY: 212-821-9713
e-mail: kcampbell@lighthouse.org
www.lighthouse.org/navh

Karen Campbell, Director of Social Services
Mark Ackermann, President/CEO
Jonathan Wainwright, VP & Secretary

Since 1905, Lighthouse International has led the charge in the fight against vision loss through prevention, treatment and empowerment.

5343 National Brain Tumor FoundationNational Brain Tumor Society

55 Chapel Street
Suite 200
Newton, MA 02458-2599
617-924-9997
800-770-8287
FAX: 617-928-9998
e-mail: info@braintumor.org
www.braintumor.org

Jeffrey Kolodin, Chair
Michael Nathanson, Vice Chair
N. Paul TonThat, Executive Director
Michele Rhee, Director of Program Initiatives

An organization serving people whose lives are affected by brain tumors. The organization is dedicated to promoting a cure for brain tumors, improving the quality of life and giving hope to the brain tumor community by funding meaningful research and providing patient resources, timely information and education.

5344 National Business & Disability Council

201 I.U. Willets Road
Albertson, NY 11507-1516
516-465-1516
e-mail: lfrancis@viscardicenter.org
www.business-disability.com

Michael C. Pascucci, Executive Leadership Team Chairman
Laura Francis, Executive Director
John D. Kemp, President

The NBDC is the leading resource for employers seeking to integrate people with disabilities into the workplace and companies seeking to reach them in the consumer marketplace.

5345 National Organization on Disability

77 Water Street
Suite 204
New York, NY 10005-538
646-505-1191
FAX: 646-505-1184
e-mail: info@nod.org
www.nod.org

Kate Brady, Director of Research and Public Funding
Erika Byrnes, Director of Development
Dwayne D. Beason, Sr, Deputy Director, Wounded Warrior Careers Program
Howard Green, Deputy Director, Corporate Programs

Promotes full and equal participation of America's 54 million men, women, and children with disabilities in all aspects of life. Today, NOD focuses on increasing employment opportunities for the 79 percent of working-age Americans with disabilities who are not employed.

5346 National Rehabilitation Information Center

8400 Corporate Drive
Suite 500
Landover, MD 20785-2266
301-459-5900
800-346-2742
FAX: 301-459-4263
TTY: 301-459-5984
e-mail: naricinfo@heitechservice.com
www.naric.com

Mark X. Odum, Director
Jessica H. Chaiken, Media and Information Services Manager
Natalie J. Collier, Library and Acquisitions Manager
Tamara J. Pyle, Library and Information Services Coordinator

Serves both professionals and the general public intersted in disability and rehabilitation.

5347 National Women's Health Resource Center

157 Broad Street
Suite 200
Red Bank, NJ 07701-2029
877-986-9472
FAX: 732-530-3347
e-mail: info@healthywomen.org
www.healthywomen.org

Eve Dryer, Chair
Kathleen Dyer, Board Member
Erin Graves, Director of Communications and New Media
Elizabeth Battaglino Cahill, Chief Executive Officer

Provides information for women with disabilities, health professionals, researchers, and caretakers.

5348 NeuroControl Corporation

8333 Rockside Rd
Valley View, OH 44125-6134
216-912-0101
800-378-6955
FAX: 216-912-0129
e-mail: skrebs@neurocontrol.com
www.neurocontrol.com

5349 Newsletter of PA's AT Lending Library

Temple University Institute on Disabilities
1755 N 13th Street
Student Center, Room 411S
Philadelphia, PA 19122-6024
215-204-1356
800-204-PIAT
FAX: 215-204-6336
TTY: 215-204-1805
e-mail: iod@temple.edu
www.disabilities.temple.edu/atlend

Celia Feinstein, Co-Executive Director of the Institute on Disabilities
Amy Goldman, Co-Executive Director of the Institute on Disabilities
Ann Marie, Deputy Director
Kristin Ahrens, PA Consumer & Family Training Project Assistant Director

Newsletter from the Assistive Technology Lending Library in Pennsylvania. It is produced quarterly, is free of charge, and is available online only.

4-8 pages Quarterly

5350 Office of Juvenile Justice and Delinquency Prevention

810 Seventh St NW
Washington, DC 20531-3718
202-307-5911
800-851-3420
FAX: 301-519-5600
e-mail: Robert.L.Listenbee@usdoj.gov
www.ojjdp.gov

Kathi Grasso, Director, Concentration of Federal Efforts Program
Robert Listenbee, Jr., Administrator
Melodee Hanes, Principal Deputy Administrator
Nancy Ayers, Deputy Administrator for Operations

The Office of Juvenile Justice and Delinquency Prevention (OJJDP) provides national leadership, coordination, and resources to prevent and respond to juvenile delinquency and victimization. OJJDP supports states and communities in their efforts to develop and implement effective and coordinated prevention and intervention programs and to improve the juvenile justice system so that it protects public safety, holds offenders accountable, and provides treatment and rehabilitative services tailored

5351 Osteogenesis Imperfecta Foundation
804 W. Diamond Ave.
Suite 210
Gaithersburg, MD 20878- 1414
301-947-0083
800-981-2663
FAX: 301-947-0456
e-mail: bonelink@oif.org
www.oif.org

Mary Beth Huber, Director of Program Services
Tom Costanzo, Director of Finance & Administration
Erika r Ruebensaal Carte, Director of Communications & Development
Tracy Smith Hart, Chief Executive Officer
Strives to improve the quality of life for indivduals with this brittle bone disorder through research, education, awareness, and mutual support.

5352 Quantum Technologies
25242 Arctic Ocean Drive
Lake Forest, CA 92630-6217
949-930-3400
FAX: 949-399-4600
e-mail: info@qtww.com
www.qtww.com

Dale Rasmussen, Chairman
Alan Niedzwieck, President/Director
W. Brian Olson, Chief Executive Officer
Bradley J. Timon, Chief Financial Officer
Provides access to information and tools for independence to serve the visually impaired and those with a learning disability.

5353 Regional Resource Centers Program
1 Quality Street
Suite 721
Lexington, KY 40507
859-257-4921
FAX: 859-257-4353
TTY:859-257-2903
e-mail: mike.abell@uky.edu
www.rrcprogram.org

Shauna Crane, RRCP Coordinator
Perry Williams, OSEP, Team Member
Mike Abell, Team Member
Betty Beale, Team Member
The Regional Resource Centers Program provides service to all states as well as the Pacific jurisdictions, the Virgin Islands, and Puerto Rico. The six regional program centers are funded by the federal Office of Special Education Programs (OSEP) to assist state education agencies in the systemic improvement of education programs, practices, and policies that affect children and youth with disabilities.

5354 Research!America
1101 King Street
Suite 520
Alexandria, VA 22314-2960
703-739-2577
800-366-2873
FAX: 703-739-2372
e-mail: info@researchamerica.org
www.researchamerica.org

Hon. John Edward Porter, Chair
Hon. Michael Castle, Vice Chair
Mary Woolley, President/CEO
Barbara Love, Executive Assitant to the President
Builds active public support for more government and private-industry research to find treatments and cures for both physical and mental disorders.

5355 Social Security Online
5 Park Centre Court
Suite 100
Owings Mills, MD 21117-1
800-772-1213
TTY:800-325-0778
www.ssa.gov

Carolyn W. Colvin, Commissioner
James A. Kissko, Chief of Staff
Katherine A. Thornton, Deputy Chief of Staff
Karena L. Kilgore, Executive Secretary,Office of Executive Operations
Official website of the Social Security Administration.

5356 Special Clothes for Children
PO Box 333
E. Harwich, MA 02645-333
508-430-2410
FAX: 508-430-2410
TTY:508-430-2410
e-mail: lou@lnrmusic.com
www.special-clothes.com

A catalog of adaptive clothing for children with disabilities - helping boys and girls with special needs meet the world with pride and confidence since 1987.

5357 V Foundation for Cancer Research
106 Towerview Court
Cary, NC 27513-3595
919-380-9505
800-454-6698
e-mail: info@jimmyv.org
www.jimmyv.org

Sherrie Mazur, Director of Marketing & Communication
Danielle Smith, Director of Corporate and Market Development
Mark Steudel, Associate Director of Development for Prospect Research
Nick Valvano, President Emeritus
Named after basketball coach and broadcaster, Jim Valvano. The V Foundation funds critical stage research conducted by young researchers at NCI approved cancer research facilities.

5358 ValueOptions
240 Corporate Blvd.
Norfolk, VA 23502-4900
757-459-5100
FAX: 501-707-0940
TTY:877-334-0077
www.valueoptions.com

Heyward R. Donigan, President/CEO
Scott Tabakin, Chief Financial Officer
Kyle A. Raffaniello, Executive Vice President and Chief Strategy Officer
Paul Rosenberg, Executive Vice President and General Counsel
Serves over 22 million people in behavioral healthcare through publicaly funded, federal, and commercial contracts.

5359 Wardrobe Wagon: The Special Needs Clothing Store
258B Route 46 E
Fairfield, NJ 7004-2324
973-244-2414
800-992-2737
e-mail: wardrobew@aol.com
www.wardrobewagon.com

E Oppenberg, President
Bonnie Oppenberg
Jerome Oppenberg, Owner
Wearing apparel for individuals with special clothing needs.

5360 We Magazine
130 William St
New York, NY 10038
646-769-2722
FAX: 212-375-6266
TTY:212-375-6235
e-mail: sales@wemedia.com
www.icdri.org/NEWS/WEMedia.htm

5361 We Media
1801 Reston Parkway
Suite 300
Reston, VA 20190-4303
703-880-2659

e-mail: help@wemedia.com
www.wemedia.com

Andrew Nachison, Founder
Dale Peskin, Founder
Online network for people with disabilities.

5362 WebABLE

www.hisoftware.com/press/webable.html

5363 WheelchairNet
6425 Penn Ave
Suite 401 BAKSQ, Department of Reha
Philadelphia, PA 15206
412-624-6279

e-mail: ruffing@pitt.edu
www.wheelchairnet.org

Joseph Ruffing, Communications Specialist
A virtual community of people who care about wheelchairs.

5364 World Association of Persons with Disabilities
2441 N Sterling Ave
302W
Oklahoma, OK 73127-2009
405-672-4440

e-mail: execvp@wapd.org
www.wapd.org

Byron R. Kerford, Founder/Leader
Thomas J. Mecke, Executive Director
Sierra Hebron, Director of Human Resources
Ashley Wardle, Director of Internet Marketing
Dedicated to improving the quality of life for those with disabilities.

Toys & Games

General

5365 Age Appropriate Puzzles
7756 Winding Way
Fair Oaks, CA 95628-5735
916-961-3507
FAX: 916-961-0765
e-mail: miltcher@spcglobal.net

Cheryl Meyers, President

These unique puzzles teach numerous concepts: picture, name, color and shape recognition. Each of the two themes (holidays, and clothing) comes with self-adhesive stickers that name each picture in English, Hmong, Russian, Spanish and Vietnamese. A notch at each puzzle piece makes grasping and lifting the pieces easy to use., They are designed for children from 18 months and up. Special needs children, preschool through high school would also benefit. *$9.95*

5366 All-Turn-It Spinner
AbleNet, Inc.
2625 Patton Road
Roseville, MN 55113-1308
651-294-2200
800-322-0956
FAX: 651-294-2222
e-mail: customerservice@ablenetinc.com
www.ablenetinc.com

Jennifer Thalhuber, President/CEO
Cheryl Volkman, Co-founder
Bill Sproull, Chairman of the Board
William Mills, Board of Directors

The All-Turn-It Spinner is a random spinner that comes with a dice overlay allowing user's to participate in any commercially-available game that require dice. Activate the spinner with its built-in switch or connect an external switch. Overlays are interchangeable with AbleNet designed spinner games or create your own overlay. A great inclusion tool!. *$89.00*

5367 Anthony Brothers Manufacturing
Convert-O-Bike
9 Capper Drive
Dailey Industrial Park,
Pacific, MO 63069-5196
636-257-0533
800-346-6313
FAX: 636-257-5473
www.angelesstore.com

Tim Lynch, Director of Sales
David Curry, General Manager
Michelle Vondera, Customer Service Manager
Sally Perrin, National Account Manager

Manufacture wheeled toys and goods for disabled children.

5368 Automatic Card Shuffler
Maxi Aids
42 Executive Blvd
Farmingdale, NY 11735-4710
631-752-0521
800-522-6294
FAX: 631-752-0689
TTY: 631-752-0738
e-mail: sales@maxiaids.com
www.maxiaids.com

5369 Backgammon Set: Deluxe
Maxi Aids
42 Executive Blvd
Farmingdale, NY 11735-4710
631-752-0521
800-522-6294
FAX: 631-752-0689
TTY: 631-752-0738
e-mail: sales@maxiaids.com
www.maxiaids.com

5370 Board Games: Snakes and Ladders
Maxi Aids
42 Executive Blvd
Farmingdale, NY 11735-4710
631-752-0521
800-522-6294
FAX: 631-752-0689
TTY: 631-752-0738
e-mail: sales@maxiaids.com
www.maxiaids.com

5371 Board Games: Solitaire
Maxi Aids
42 Executive Blvd
Farmingdale, NY 11735-4710
631-752-0521
800-522-6294
FAX: 631-752-0689
TTY: 631-752-0738
e-mail: sales@maxiaids.com
www.maxiaids.com

5372 Braille Playing Cards: Plastic
Maxi Aids
42 Executive Blvd
Farmingdale, NY 11735-4710
631-752-0521
800-522-6294
FAX: 631-752-0689
TTY: 631-752-0738
e-mail: sales@maxiaids.com
www.maxiaids.com

5373 Braille: Bingo Cards, Boards and Call Numbers
Maxi Aids
42 Executive Blvd
Farmingdale, NY 11735-4710
631-752-0521
800-522-6294
FAX: 631-752-0689
TTY: 631-752-0738
e-mail: sales@maxiaids.com
www.maxiaids.com

5374 Braille: Rook Cards
Maxi Aids
42 Executive Blvd
Farmingdale, NY 11735-4710
631-752-0521
800-522-6294
FAX: 631-752-0689
TTY: 631-752-0738
e-mail: sales@maxiaids.com
www.maxiaids.com

5375 Card Holder Deluxe
Maxi Aids
42 Executive Blvd
Farmingdale, NY 11735-4710
631-752-0521
800-522-6294
FAX: 631-752-0689
TTY: 631-752-0738
e-mail: sales@maxiaids.com
www.maxiaids.com

5376 Cards: Musical
Sense-Sations
919 Walnut St
Philadelphia, PA 19107-5237
215-627-0600
FAX: 215-922-0692
e-mail: asbinfo@asb.org
www.asb.org

Richard Forsythe, Director
Patricia Johnson, CEO
Robert Bivenour, IT Manager
Brian Rusk, Public Relations Officer

These cards, for all occasions, play music when they are opened, for the visually impaired and blind persons. *$2.50*

5377 Cards: UNO
Maxi Aids
42 Executive Blvd
Farmingdale, NY 11735-4710
631-752-0521
800-522-6294
FAX: 631-752-0689
TTY: 631-752-0738
e-mail: sales@maxiaids.com
www.maxiaids.com

5378 Checker Set: Deluxe
Maxi Aids
42 Executive Blvd
Farmingdale, NY 11735-4710
631-752-0521
800-522-6294
FAX: 631-752-0689
TTY: 631-752-0738
e-mail: sales@maxiaids.com
www.maxiaids.com

5379 Chess Set: Deluxe
Maxi Aids
42 Executive Blvd
Farmingdale, NY 11735-4710
631-752-0521
800-522-6294
FAX: 631-752-0689
TTY: 631-752-0738
e-mail: sales@maxiaids.com
www.maxiaids.com

5380 Dice: Jumbo Size
New Vision Store
919 Walnut St
Philadelphia, PA 19107-5237
215-629-2990
www.asb.org

Richard Forsythe, Director
Patricia Johnson, CEO
Robert Bivenour, IT Manager
Brian Rusk, Public Relations Officer

The large white and black dice are over-sized and have grooved dots to indicate the numbers, for easy reading for the visually handicapped. *$4.95*

5381 Early Learning 1
MarbleSoft
12301 Central Ave NE
Suite 205
Blaine, MN 55434-4902
763-755-1402
888-755-1402
FAX: 763-862-2920
e-mail: sales@marblesoft.com
www.marblesoft.com

Vicki Larson, Manager

Early learning 2.1 includes four activities that teach prereading skills. Single and dual-switch scanning are built in and special prompts allow blind students to use all levels of difficulty. Includes Matching Colors, Learning Shapes, Counting Numbers and Letter Match. Runs on Windows 98 or later and MAC OS 9 or OSX (classic not required). *$70.00*

5382 Enabling Devices
50 Broadway
Hawthorne, NY 10532-2837
914-747-3070
800-832-8697
FAX: 914-747-3480
e-mail: info@enablingdevices.com
www.enablingdevices.com

Steven Kanor, Owner
Karen O'Connor, Vice President Operations
Elizabeth Bell, Marketing Manager

Enabling Devices is a company dedicated to developing affordable learning and assistive devices to help people of all ages with disabling conditions. Founded by Steven E. Kanor, Ph.D. and orginally known as Toys for Special Children, the company has been creating innovative communicators, adapted toys and switches for the physically challenged for more than 35 years.

5383 Hands-Free Controller
Nintendo
PO Box 957
Redmond, WA 98073-957
800-255-3700
www.nintendo.com

Yoshio Tsuboike, Editor-in-Chief

Nintendo controller for the physically disabled.

5384 Let's Count Braille and Tactile Numbers Poster
Maxi Aids
42 Executive Blvd
Farmingdale, NY 11735-4710
631-752-0521
800-522-6294
FAX: 631-752-0689
TTY: 631-752-0738
e-mail: sales@maxiaids.com
www.maxiaids.com

5385 National Lekotek Center
2001 N. Clybourn Av.
1st Floor
Chicago, IL 60614-3716
773-528-5766
800-366-PLAY
FAX: 773-537-2992
TTY: 773-973-2180
e-mail: lekotek@lekotek.org
www.lekotek.org

Elaine D. Cottey, Chair
Joanna Horsnail, Chair
Eric Gastevich, Treasurer
Carol Neiger, Secretary

Maximizes the development of children with special needs through play. Supports families through nationwide family play centers, toy lending libraries and computer play programs. Publishes six-page newsletter three times per year.

5386 New Language of Toys: Teaching Communication Skills to Children with Special Needs
Spina Bifida Association of America
4590 MacArthur Blvd,NW,
Suite 250
Washington, DC 20007- 4226
202-944-3285
800-621-314
FAX: 202-944-3295
e-mail: sbaa@sbaa.org
www.spinabifidaassociation.org

Lisa Raman, Director-National Resource Center
Mary Nethercutt, National Walk Director
Christopher Vance, Director of Development
Cindy Brownstein, President /CEO

A guide for parents and teachers and a reader-friendly resource guide that provides a wealth of information on how play activities affect a child's language development and where to get the toys and materials to use in these activities. *$19.00*

5387 Puzzle Games: Cooking, Eating, Community and Grooming
PCI
PO Box 34270
San Antonio, TX 78265-4270
210-670-3866
800-594-4263
FAX: 218-210-3771
www.pci.edu.com

Janie Haugen, Program Director
Jeff McLane, President/CEO
Rebecca Phillips, Executive Director

Each game has 63 pieces which are 2 inches in size. The completed full color puzzle is 19 inch x 15 inch. Step 1 - Work the puzzle. Step 2 - Match picture or word cards to the correct space on the puzzle. These puzzles teach basic life skills. *$19.95*

5388 Single Switch Games
MarbleSoft
12301 Central Ave NE
Suite 205
Blaine, MN 55434-4902
763-755-1402
888-755-1402
888-755-1402
FAX: 763-862-2920
e-mail: sales@marblesoft.com
www.marblesoft.com

Vicki Larson, Manager
Mark Larson

Theres alot of educational software for single switch users, but how about something that's just fun? We've taken some games similar to the ones you enjoyed as a kid and made them work just right for single switch users. Includes Single Switch Maze, A Frog's Life, Switching Lanes, Switch Invaders, Slingshot Gallery and Scurry. Runs on Windows 98 or later and MAC OS9 or OSX (classic not required) *$60.00*

5389 Single Switch Latch and Timer
AbleNet
2625 Patton Road
Roseville, MN 55113-1308
651-294-2200
800-322-0956
FAX: 651- 29- 225
e-mail: customerservice@ablenetinc.com
www.ablenetinc.com

Bill Sproull, Chairman of the Board
William Mills, Board of Directors, Chair
Jennifer Thalhuber, President/CEO
Paul Sugden, Vice President of Finance, IT & CFO, Trustee

A Single Switch Latch and Timer allows a user to activate a battery-operated toy or appliance in the latch, timed seconds and timed minutes modes of control. Choose for one user and one device at a time. *$63.00*

5390 Socialization Games for Persons with Disabilities
Charles C. Thomas
2600 S 1st St
Springfield, IL 62704-4730
217-789-8980
800-258-8980
FAX: 217-789-9130
e-mail: books@ccthomas.com
www.ccthomas.com

Michael P. Thomas, President
Nevalyn Nevil, Author
Marna Beatty, Author
David Moxley, Author

This text will assist those who want to teach severely multiple disabled students by providing information on: general principles of intervention and classroom organization; managing the behavior of students; physically managing students and using adaptive equipment; teaching eating skills; teaching toileting, dressing, and hygiene skills; teaching cognition, communication, and socialization skills; teaching independent living skills; and teaching infants and preschool students. *$38.95*
176 pages Paperback
ISBN 0-398067-46-5

5391 Take a Chance
Speech Bin
1965 25th Ave
Vero Beach, FL 32960-3062
772-770-0007
800-477-3324
FAX: 772-770-0006
e-mail: info@speechbin.com
www.store.schoolspecialty.com

Jan J Binney, Senior Editor

Card game for practice of commonly misarticulated speech sounds. *$18.75*
16 pages Book & Cards
ISBN 0-93785 -46-7

5392 Tic Tac Toe
Maxi Aids
42 Executive Blvd
Farmingdale, NY 11735-4710
631-752-0521
800-522-6294
FAX: 631-752-0689
TTY: 631-752-0738
e-mail: sales@maxiaids.com
www.maxiaids.com

5393 Turnabout Game
Maxi Aids
42 Executive Blvd
Farmingdale, NY 11735-4710
631-752-0521
800-522-6294
FAX: 631-752-0689
TTY: 631-752-0738
e-mail: sales@maxiaids.com
www.maxiaids.com

Travel & Transportation

Newsletters & Books

5394 **A Guide for the Wheelchair Traveler**
Access for Disabled Americans
3240 Burnt Mill Drive
Orinda, CA 94563-2317
925-254-1499
FAX: 925-254-6167
e-mail: psmither@aol.com
www.accessfordisabled.com

Neal Smither, President
Patricia Smither, Editor/Secretary
All you need to know when traveling in a wheelchair. *$30.00*
165 pages Paperback
ISBN 1-928616-00-3

5395 **A World Awaits You**
Mobility International USA
132 E. Broadway
Suite 343
Eugene, OR 97401-2767
541-343-1284
FAX: 541-343-6812
e-mail: info@miusa.org
www.miusa.org

Susan Sygall, CEO/Founder
Susan Dunn, Exec. Asst./Project Specialist
Cindy Lewis, Director of Programs
Estelle Coreris-Moore, Financial Manager
A journal of success stories and tips of people with disabilities participating in international exchange programs.
40 pages Yearly

5396 **Access Travel: Airports**
Consumer Information Center
Department 575a
Pueblo, CO 81009-1
719-948-3334
e-mail: catalog.pueblo@gsa.gov

Michael Clark, Public Affairs
Alfred Pino, Manager
Tips and suggestions for easier travel for persons with disabilities and the elderly. Lists designs, facilities, and services at 553 airport terminals worldwide.

5397 **Architectural Barriers Action League**
PO Box 57088
Tucson, AZ 85732-7088
520-628-8118

Martin Floerchinger, Owner
Offers guides to accessible hotels and motels across the country.

5398 **Directory of Travel Agencies for the Disabled**
Twin Peaks Press
PO Box 129
Vancouver, WA 98666-129
206-694-2462
800-637-2256
e-mail: twinpeak@pacifier.com

David Lynch, Director
Directory lists more than 360 travel agents specializing in arrangements for people with disabilities. Handbook provides information about accessibility. *$19.95*
40 pages Paperback
ISBN 0-93326 -04-8

5399 **Elderly Guide to Budget Travel/Europe**
Pilot Books
PO Box 2102
Greenport, NY 11944-893
631-477-1094
FAX: 631-661-4379

5400 **Ideas for Easy Travel**
Accent Books & Products
PO Box 700
Bloomington, IL 61702-700
309-378-2961
800-787-8444
FAX: 309-378-4420
e-mail: acmtlvng@aol.com

Raymond C Cheever, Publisher
Betty Garee, Editor
Ideal for helping the new traveler get started having fun. Points out favorite accessible high-spots as reported by two travel experts (one is disabled), and offers basic ideas to help wherever you go. *$3.25*
55 pages Paperback
ISBN 0-91570 -36-1

5401 **Sports n' Spokes Magazine**
Paralyzed Veterans of America
801 18th St NW
Washington, DC 20006-3517
202-872-1300
800-424-8200
888-888-2201
FAX: 202-785-4432
TTY:800-795-4327
e-mail: info@pva.org
www.pva.org

Homer S. Townsend, Jr., Executive Director
Larry Dodson, National Secretary
Bill Lawson, National President
Al Kovach, Jr, Natonal Senior Vice President
Publication of the PVA, a congressionally chartered veterans service organization, with unique expertise on a wide variety of issues involving the special needs of our members— veterans of the armed forces who have experienced spinal cord injury or dysfunction.

5402 **Survival Strategies for Going Abroad, A Guide for People with Disabilites**
132 E. Broadway
Suite 343
Eugene, OR 97401-2767
541-343-1284
FAX: 541-343-6812
e-mail: info@miusa.org
www.miusa.org

Susan Sygall, Executive Director
Melissa Mitchell, Public Relations
$16.95
225 pages

5403 **Travel Information Service/Moss Rehab Hospital**
Moss Rehabilitation Hospital
1200 W Tabor Rd
Philadelphia, PA 19141-3099
215-456-9900
800-225-5667
e-mail: staff@mossresourcenet.org
www.mossresourcenet.org

John Whyte, Owner
Ruth Lefton, COO
Anthony Allonardo, Director of Technology
Alberto Esquenazi, Plant Manager
Offers information and resources, to telephone callers only, for persons with special traveling/accessibility needs.

5404 **United States Department of the Interior National Park Service**
Superintendent of Documents
1849 C St NW
Washington, DC 20240-1
202-208-3100
FAX: 202-619-7302
e-mail: feedback@ios.doi.gov
www.doi.gov

Mainella, Director
Gale Norton, Chief Executive Officer
Offers an informational packet containing books, guides and tours for the disabled and elderly.

5405 **Wheelin Around**
Wheelers Handicapped Accessible Van Rentals
6614 W Sweetwater Ave
Glendale, AZ 85304-1040 602-776-8830
800-456-1371
FAX: 623-412-9920
e-mail: info@wheelersvanrentals.com
www.wheelersvanrentals.com

Tammy Smith, President
Ron Smith, Corporate Treasurer
Wheelers has been breaking travel barriers through innovative service and products since 1989. Our mission is to have Wheelers rental affiliates available in every city in the United States, Canada and all around the globe. Wheelers' objective is to connect you to the best possible solution for your transportation challenges and continue to find new and innovative ways in making the world a more accessible place.

5406 **Where to Stay USA**
Council On International Educational Exchange
633 3rd Ave
New York, NY 10017-6706 212-822-2600
888-COU-NCIL
FAX: 212-822-2649
Priscilla Tovey, Information Services
A guide to low-cost lodging throughout the United States including information on whether the establishment is accessible. *$ 15.95*
250 pages
ISBN 0-67179 -49-5

Associations & Programs

5407 **Access America**
Northern Cartographic
4050 Williston Rd
South Burlington, VT 5403-6062 802-860-2886
FAX: 802-865-4912
Cynthia Belliveau, President
Offers information on 36 national parks, providing detailed information on accessibility.

5408 **Access Yosemite National Park**
Special Needs Project
324 State Street
Santa Barbara, CA 93101-2364 805-962-8087
800-333-6867
e-mail: books@specialneeds.com
www.specialneeds.com

Hod Gray, Owner
Represents unprecedented combinations of intensive information survey data with high quality cartography. *$7.95*
31 pages

5409 **American Hotel and Lodging Foundation**
1201 New York Ave NW
Suite 600
Washington, DC 20005-3931 202-289-3100
FAX: 202-289-3199
e-mail: membership@ahla.com
www.ahla.com

Barbara DiRocco, Director, Conventions & Events
Katherine Lugar, President/CEO
Pam Inman, IOM, CAE, CMHS, Executive Vice President/COO
Joori Jeon, CPA, CAE, Executive Vice President/CFO, President of AH&LEF
Will disseminate information, develop and conduct a series of seminars for the hotel and motel industry at state-level association conferences, and develop and distribute an ADA Compliance handbook for use by the lodging industry.

5410 **Amtrak**
50 Massachusetts Ave NE
Washington, DC 20002-4214 202-000-1111
800-872-7245
FAX: 202-906-4564
TTY: 800-523-6590
e-mail: access@w0.amtrak.com
www.amtrak.com

Joseph H. Boardman, President/CEO
Eleanor D. Acheson, Vice President, General Counsel and Corporate Secretary
Stephen J. Gardner, Vice President, NEC Infrastructure and Investment Developmen
DJ Stadtler, Vice President, Operations
Amtrak is committed to making travel for passengers with disabilities more accessible. Anyone interested should contact Amtrak's Special Services Desk at 1-800-USA-RAIL at least 24 hours in advance to arrange for special assistance. The type of equipment and accessibility vary from train to train and station to station.

5411 **Easter Seals Project ACTION**
1425 K St NW
Suite 200
Washington, DC 20005-3508 202-347-3066
800-659-6428
FAX: 202-737-7914
TTY: 202-347-7385
e-mail: project_action@easterseals.com
www.projectaction.org
Judy Shanley,Ph. D, Director
Donna Smith, Director of Training
C. Marie Maus, Assistant Director
Mary Leary, Vice President
A national technical assistance program designed to improve access to transportation services for people with disabilities and assist transit providers in implementing the Americans with Disabilities Act. Publishes quarterly newsletter.

5412 **General Motors Mobility Program for Persons with Disabilities**
GM Mobility Program
PO Box 5053
Troy, MI 48007 800-323-9935
TTY:800-833-9935
www.gmmobility.com

Frederick A Henderson, CEO
GM Mobility Program provides up to $1000 reimbursement toward mobility adaptations for drivers or passengers and/or vehicle alerting devices for drivers who are deaf or hard of hearing. Provided on eligible new Chevrolet, Pontiac, Oldsmobile, Buick, Cadillac, and GMC vehicles. Complete GMC financing available. GM Mobility also offers free resource information, including list of area adaptive equipment installers, plus free resource video.

5413 **Kenny Foundation**
21700 Northwestern Hwy
Suite 730
Southfield, MI 48075- 4930 810-552-0202
800-237-3422
e-mail: comnet@uwcs.org
Susan Burstein, Executive Director
Provides education, advocacy & direct services to people with mobility impairments throughout Michigan. Services include Equipment Connection, a database, available online, that connects buyers & sellers of used adaptive equipment; Attitudes is a disability awareness program for 1st & 2nd graders; Information & Referral services; and Accessbility, a program that uses volunteer labor and donated materials to buid ramps for people who can't afford them.

5414 **MedEscort International**
PO Box 8766
Allentown, PA 18105-8766
610-791-3111
800-255-7182
FAX: 610-791-9189
e-mail: serice@medescort.com
www.medescort.com
Craig Poliner, President
MedEscort International was founded over a decade ago with these basic principles and philosophies as its foundation. MedEscort has served the health care community, throughout the world, and has strived to perfect the techniques of moving patients from one place to another. Our medical staff includes registered nurses, respiratory therapists, paramedics, and physicians. MedEscort has developed comprehensive, individual aeromedical services to meet each patient's needs with a personal touch.

5415 **Nantahala Outdoor Center**
13077 Highway 19 W
Bryson City, NC 28713-9165
828-488-2176
888-905-7238
FAX: 828-488-2498
TTY:800-877-8339
e-mail: rafting@noc.com
www.noc.com
Sutton Bacon, CEO
Nantahala Outdoor Center, the leader in outdoor recreation and education for more than 30 years, strongly encourages and supports participants with disabilities. We offer whitewater rafting adventures on six rivers in the Southeast for all skill and thrill levels for groups, also kayak and canoe adaptive instruction. NOC will tailor a whitewater program to your skill and ability level, modify the gear, and pace instruction for you. We also offer a Ropes Challenge Course and team building program

5416 **Paralysis Society of America**
Paralyzed Veterans of America
801 18th St NW
Washington, DC 20006-3517
202-872-1300
800-424-8200
FAX: 202-785-4432
TTY: 800-795-4327
e-mail: info@pva.org
www.pva.org
Homer S. Townsend, Jr., Executive Director
Larry Dodson, National Secretary
Bill Lawson, National President
Al Kovach, Jr, Natonal Senior Vice President
A national organization whose members are people with spinal cord injury or disease, their family members and caregivers, health-care professionals, and others with an interest in the disciplines of spinal cord medicine and paralsis. One year membership includes NewsWheels, a quarterly newsletter.

5417 **Shilo Inns & Resorts**
11707 NE Airport Way
Portland, OR 97220-5995
503-252-7500
800-222-2244
FAX: 503-254-0794
e-mail: franchiseinfo@shiloinns.com
www.shiloinns.com
Mark S. Hemstreet, Founder/Owner
Ivan Mc Affee, VP
Shilo Inns offers affordable excellence with special assist rooms at many of our locations throughout the western United States. These rooms include larger sized bathrooms equipped with assistance railings and wheelchair access. Special assist dogs are welcome free of charge ar most Shilo Inns. Call 1-800-222-2244 for details or make reservations or check out www.shiloinns.com

5418 **Travelers Aid International**
1612 K St. NW
Suite 206
Washington, DC 20006-2849
202-546-0599
FAX: 202-546-9112
e-mail: info@travelersaid.org
www.travelersaid.org
Joan Lowden, Chair
Brian Rogers, Vice Chair
Edward Powers, Vice Chair
Jessica M. Rooney, Treasurer
Provides crisis intervention and casework services, limited financial assistance, protective travel assistance and information and referrals for travelers, transients and newcomers.

5419 **US Airways/America West Airlines**
4000 E Sky Harbor Blvd
Phoenix, AZ 85034-3802
480-693-0800
800-327-7810
FAX: 480-693-3702
TTY: 800-245-2966
www.usairways.org
Douglas Parker, CEO
This airline trains employees to make sure that passengers with disabilities enjoy convenient, safe and comfortable travel.

5420 **US Servas**
1125 16th Street
Suite 201
Arcata, CA 95521-5585
707-825-1714
FAX: 707-825-1762
e-mail: info@usservas.org
www.usservas.org
Judy Sears, Administrator
International network that links travelers with hosts in 130+ countries with the hope of building world peace through understanding and friendship.
Quarterly

5421 **Westin Hotels and Resorts**
270 West 43rd Street
New York, NY 10036
212-201-2700
FAX: 212-201-2701
e-mail: info@westinny.com
www.starwoodhotels.com
Sue A Brush, Senior VP
Westin Hotels & Resortsr indulge our guests in elements of well-being. Our refreshing ambience, innovative programs and thoughtful amenities help provide a stay that leaves you feeling better than when you arrived.

5422 **Wheelers Handicapped Accessible Van Rentals**
6614 W Sweetwater Ave
Glendale, AZ 85304-1040
602-418-5076
800-456-1371
FAX: 623-412-9920
e-mail: info@wheelersvanrentals.com
www.wheelersvanrentals.com
Tammy Smith, President
Rental wheelchairs and scooter accessible vans. Technically advanced engineering features bring a world of independence to the user. Locations throughout the U.S. call 800-456-1371 to make reservations at any of our locations nationwide.

5423 **Wilderness Inquiry**
808 14th Ave SE
Minneapolis, MN 55414-1516
612-676-9400
800-728-0179
FAX: 612-676-9401
TTY: 612-676-9475
e-mail: info@wildernessinquiry.org
www.wildernessinquiry.org
Greg Lais, Executive Director
Lee Friedman, Business and Outreach Director
Megan O'Hara, Youth Outdoor Employment Director
Beth Dooley, Communications Director

Allows people of all ages and abilities to share the adventure of wilderness travel. This nonprofit organization was formed in 1978 and conducts tours to some of the most beautiful and remote parts of the world.

Tours

5424 **Able Trek Tours**
P.O. Box 384
Reedsburg, WI 53959
608-524-3021
800-205-6713
FAX: 608-524-8302
e-mail: info@abletrektours.com
abletrektours.com

5425 **AccessToThePlanet**
Accessible Journeys
35 W Sellers Ave
Ridley Park, PA 19078-2113
610-521-0339
800-846-4537
FAX: 610-521-6959
e-mail: sales@disabilitytravel.com
www.accessiblejourneys.com

Howard Mc Coy, Owner
Kathy Pagliei, Director
Howard J. McCoy, President/CEO

Contains new product announcements, organizing land groups and world travel news.
Monthly

5426 **Accessible Journeys**
35 West Sellers Ave
Ridley Park, PA 19078-2113
610-521-0339
800-846-4537
FAX: 610-521-6959
e-mail: sales@accessiblejourneys.com
www.accessiblejourneys.com

Howard Mc Coy, Owner
Kathy Pagliei, Director
Howard J. McCoy, President/CEO

Accessible Journeys is a vacation planner and tour operator exclusively for wheelchair travelers, their families and friends.

5427 **American The Beautiful; National Parks & Federal Recreation Lands**
National Parks Service
1849 C St NW
Washington, DC 20240-1
202-208-6843
888-275-8747
FAX: 202-219-0910
e-mail: webteam@ios.doi.gov
www.nps.gov

Mary A Bomar, CEO

A free lifetime passport to federally operated parks, monuments, historic sites, recreation areas and wildlife refuges for persons who are blind or permanently disabled.

5428 **Anglo California Travel Service**
4250 Williams Rd
San Jose, CA 95129-3344
408-257-2257
FAX: 408-257-2664
www.acts4travel.com

Audrey Cooper, President

Plans for one and two week accessible tours.

5429 **Cunard Line**
24305 Town Center Drive
Suite 200
Valencia, CA 91355- 2079
305-463-3000
800-528-6273
FAX: 305-463-3010
www.cunard.com

Pamela C Conover, CEO

Cunard Line, one of the world's most recognized brand names with a classic British heritage, operated by Cunard Line Limited, has provided the ultimate in deluxe ocean travel experience for the past 158 years. The fleet consists of famed liner Queen Elizabeth 2 and the Caronia, a classic ship formerly identified as Vistafjord. The Cunard Line brand, the epitome of British essence, focuses on recalling the golden age of sea travel for those who missed the first.

5430 **Dell Rapids Sportsmens Club**
PO Box 126
Dell Rapids, SD 57022-126
605-428-3522
FAX: 605-428-5502
e-mail: billybuckww@sio.midco.net
www.sdshootingsports.org

Wayne Coffaa, President
Pat Weinacht, Vice President
Bill Weber, Secretary/Treasurer
Robin Anderson, Board Member

Offers leage shooting for trap, as well as shooting on individual basis for archery, trap and pistol.

5431 **Diabetic Cruise Desk**
Hartford Holidays
500 Old Country Rd
Suite 110
Garden City, NY 11530-536
516-746-6670
800-828-4813
FAX: 516-746-6690
e-mail: info@hartfordholidays.com
www.hartfordholidays.com

Scott M. Kertes, President
Les Kertes, Chief Executive Officer
Stacey Ganca, Chief Financial Officer
Sally Kertes, Business Development Manager / Senior Travel Counselor

Offers a seven-day cruise to Alaska for people with diabetes. Includes seminars on diabetes, self management, planning, special guidance for exercise classes and individual dietary advice.

5432 **Dialysis at Sea Cruises**
2504 Merchant Ave
Odessa, FL 33556-3468
813-775-4040
800-544-7604
001-813-775
FAX: 727-372-7396
e-mail: info@dialysisatsea.com
www.dialysisatsea.com

Steve Debroux, Owner

Been in the business of providing travel opportunities for persons on hemodialysis and CAPD since 1977. Handle all aspects of their travel and medical requirements. Not Sold Through Travel Agents! Make all reservations and coordinates the total set-up and operation of an onboard ship mobile dialysis clinic. Cruises run from seven days to three weeks and have departures from cities around the world on a variety of cruise lines.

5433 **Directions Unlimited Acccessible Tours**
Empress Travel
720 N. Bedford Rd
Bedford Hills, NY 10507-1508
914-241-1700
800-533-5343
FAX: 914-241-0243

Lois Bonanni, Director
Charles Digiacomo, Manager

Arrange vacations throughout the world for all disabilities including accessible cruises, African safari, rafting and scuba diving, European and Caribbean vacations.

5434 **Dvorak Expeditions**
17921 Us Highway 285
Nathrop, CO 81236-9701
719-539-6851
800-824-3795
FAX: 719-539-3378
e-mail: info@dvorakexpeditions.com
www.dvorakexpeditions.com

Bill Dvorak, Owner
Jaci Dvorak, Co-Owner

This organization does river trips for people who are deaf, visually impaired, physically or mentally disabled. Rafting trips with groups and families and whitewater instruction.

5435 Environmental Traveling Companions
Fort Mason Center, 2 Marina Blvd.
Bldg. C
San Francisco, CA 94123 415-474-7662
FAX: 415-474-3919
e-mail: info@etctrips.org
www.etctrips.org

Diane Poslosky, Executive Director
Maureen O'Hagan, Associate Director
Jessica Heyman, Development Manager
Davido Crow, River Program Manager
Aids travelers regardless of physical or financial limitations to experience the beauty and challenge of the wilderness.

5436 Flying Wheels Travel
143 W. Bridge St.
PO Box 382
Owatonna, MN 55060-382 507-451-5005
877-451-5006
FAX: 507-451-1685
e-mail: barbaraj@flyingwheelstravel.com
www.flyingwheelstravel.com

Barbara Jacobson, Owner
Timothy Holtz
Arranges worldwide custom independent travel and cruises for the physically challenged.

5437 Guide Service of Washington
734 15th St NW
Suite 701
Washington, DC 20005-1023 202-628-2842
FAX: 202-638-2812
e-mail: sales@dctourguides.com
www.dctourguides.com

Neil Amrine, President
A guide service offering tours of Washington DC and vicinity.

5438 Guided Tour for Persons 17 & Over with Developmental and Physical Challenges
7900 Old York Rd
Suite 111-B
Elkins Park, PA 19027-2310 215-782-1370
800-783-5841
FAX: 215-635-2637
e-mail: gtour400@aol.com
www.guidedtour.com

Irv Segal, DCSW, LSW, Owner/Director
Jon Fash, Administration
Lynsey Trohoske, Office/Program Co-ordinator
The Guided Tour is a very special program that offers opportunities for personal growth, recreation and socialization through travel.

5439 Hostelling North America
Hostelling International
8401 Colesville Road
Suite 600
Silver Spring, MD 20910- 6339 301-495-1240
FAX: 240-650-2094
e-mail: netanya.trimboli@hiusa.org
www.hiusa.org

Russ Hedge, CEO
Demetria Trent, Manager
Netanya Trimboli, Communications & PR Manager
Hostels are very inexpensive accommodations for travelers of all ages. They provide dorm-style sleeping rooms with separate quarters for males and females, fully equipped self-service kitchens, dining areas and common rooms for relaxing and socializing. HI-AYH has hostels in major cities, in national and state parks, near beaches and in the mountains. Send for a copy of Hostelling North America, a directory of hostels in U.S. and Canada, which lists hostels that are handicap accessible. *$ 3.00*
400 pages Yearly

5440 New Courier Travel
532 Duane St
Glen Ellyn, IL 60137-4695 630-469-0511
888-777-4453
FAX: 630-469-7390
www.travelcourierinc.com

Fred Mueller, Owner
Offers specialized assistance for independent travel or tours for persons with disabilities including cruises and travel in the USA and abroad. Fee charged for out-of-state clients, long-distance calls and clients who have free air.

5441 New Directions For People With Disabilities, Inc.
5276 Hollister Avenue
Suite 207
Santa Barbara, CA 93111-3068 805-967-2841
888-967-2841
FAX: 805-964-7344
e-mail: hello@newdirectionstravel.org
www.newdirectionstravel.org

Dee Duncan, Executive Director
Jeanne Mohle, Director of Operations
Danna Mead, Program Director
Colette Piacentini, Business Manager
A non-profit organization providing high quality local, national, and international travel vacations and holiday programs for people with mild to moderate developmental disabilities.

5442 Norwegian Cruise Line
7665 Corporate Center Drive
Miami, FL 33126-1201 866-234-0292
800-327-7030
FAX: 305-436-4117
www.ncl.com

Tan Sri Lim Kok Thay, Director
David Chua Ming Huat, Director
Marc J. Rowan, Director
Steve Martinez, Director
Has accessible cabins but urges mobility impaired passengers to travel in the same cabin with a person who is not mobility impaired. Cruise fares vary.

5443 ROW Adventures
202 Sherman Ave
PO Box 579
Coeur D Alene, ID 83816 208-765-0841
800-451-6034
FAX: 208-667-6506
e-mail: info@rowadventures.com
www.rowadventures.com

Brad Moss, Adventure Administration - Director - Marketing & Sales
Betsy Bowen, Adventure Administration - Founder
Morag Prosser, Adventure Administration - International Sales Manager
Candy Bening, Adventure Administration - Domestic Sales Manager
Offers one to six day rafting trips to physically disadvantaged people. Designs custom itineraries, or trips with a special focus for small groups. For those with special dietary needs, they prepare special meals. So come ride the rapids and enjoy life. They also offer canoe trips aboard 34' voyager canoes along the trail of Lewis and Clark on Montana's upper Missouri River. Free brochure upon request.

5444 Sundial Special Vacations
750 Marine Dr.
Suite 100
Astoria, OR 97103 503-325-4536
800-547-9198
FAX: 503-325-4536
e-mail: thomas@sundial-travel.com
www.sundialtour.com

Terry Conner, VP
Provides special vacations for developmentally disabled persons. Provides quality vacations for persons with developmental disabilities. Ratio is 1 for 7 or 1 for 5 depending on tour. Only two people to a room. Exciting destinations. 3 to 4 star properties. Great fun.

5445 **Trips Inc.**
P.O. Box 10885
Eugene, OR 97440
541-686-1013
800-686-1013
e-mail: trips@tripsinc.com
tripsinc.com

5446 **Ventures Travel**
3600 Holly Lane N.
Suite 95
Plymouth, MN 55447-1619
952-852-0107
866-692-7400
FAX: 952-852-0123
e-mail: vt@venturestravel.org
www.venturestravel.org

Nikki Adegun, Director
Lisa Moore, Director
Maggie Venell
A limited liability company is a service of Friendship Ventures-a nonprofit organization that has been enriching the lives of people with mental retardation and related developmental disabilities since 1985. Contact us to learn about our other programs, employment information, volunteer openings or donor opportunities.

5447 **Wheelchair Getaways**
PO Box 1098
Mukilteo, WA 98275-1098
425-353-8213
800-536-5518
FAX: 425-355-6159
e-mail: info@wheelchairgetaways.com
www.wheelchairgetaways.com

Edward Van Artsdalen, Director
Wheelchair Getaways, the largest wheelchair/scooter accessible van rental company in the US, has 50 franchise locations serving major cities and airports throughout the continental US and Hawaii. Rentals by the day, week, month or longer. Delivery/pickup available.

5448 **Wilderness Inquiry**
808 14th Avenue SE
Minneapolis, MN 55414
612-676-9400
FAX: 612-676-9401
e-mail: info@wildernessinquiry.org
wildernessinquiry.org

Vehicle Rentals

5449 **ABC Union, ACE, ANLV, Vegas Western Cab**
5010 S Valley View Blvd
Las Vegas, NV 89118-1705
702-798-3498
FAX: 702-736-8813
www.lvcabs.com

Phyllis Frias, President
Charles Frias, President
Taxi service in Las Vegas that uses vans with wheelchair lifts at regular taxi rates.

5450 **Accessible Vans Of America**
866-224-1750
www.accessiblevans.com

5451 **Avis Rent A Car**
379 Parsippany Road
Parsippany, NJ 07054-5111
973-428-3900
TTY:800-331-2323
e-mail: access@avis.com
www.avis.com

F Robert Salerno, President
Avis Access is a program of Avis Rent A Car that provides a full range of complementary products and services to drivers and passengers with physical disabilities. Renters can simply call the designated Avis Access Reservation line (888-TRY-HARDER) at 24 hours in advance. Products or services include transfer boards, hand controls, swivel seats, and more.

5452 **Consulting & Engineering for the Handicapped (CEH)**
4457 63rd Cir
Pinellas Park, FL 33781-5981
727-522-0364
866-244-1150
FAX: 727-522-9024
e-mail: ceh@liftsandramps.com
www.liftsandramps.com

Al Crisp, Owner
Brenda Crisp, Owner
New vans, used vans, specializing in quad conversions, all types of handicap equipment. Celebrating 33 years in business. Hand controls, lifts & ramps, porch lifts, hand-crank bikes.

5453 **Mobile Care**
6201 Riverdale Rd
Suite 101
Riverdale, MD 20737-2174
301-277-7371
FAX: 301-699-1865
e-mail: jaklimo@aol.com

Maurice Naccache, Manager
Specializing in non-emergency wheelchair service for the elderly and physically challenged.

5454 **National Car Rental System**
600 Terminal Drive
Suite 202
Fort Lauderdale, FL 33315- 3618
954-359-3020
877-222-9058
888-826-6890
FAX: 954-359-8313
www.nationalcar.com

William Decker, Manager
Accommodates special requests subject to availability. Offers hand controls, bench seats, extra mirrors and vans with lifts at many major locations.

5455 **Northwest Limousine Service**
9950 Lawrence Ave
Suite 314
Schiller Park, IL 60176-1216
847-698-0000
800-376-5466
e-mail: chiohare@aol.com
www.oharelimousine.com

Sam Malas, Manager
Offers wheelchair accessible mini vans, sedans, stretch and super stretch limousines for hourly or daily rental.

5456 **Over the Rainbow Disabled Travel Services& Wheelers Accessible Van Rentals**
186 Mehani Cir
Kihei, HI 96753-8072
808-879-5521
800-303-3750
FAX: 808-871-7533

David McKown, VP
Offers the disabled traveler Hawaii airport arrangements and ticketing accessible accommodations, hotels and condos including roll-in showers, Wheelers' Accessible Van Rentals on Maui and Honolulu or cars with hand controls, personal care attendants, medical or recreational equipment rentals and activities such as: helicopter rides, luau's, whalewatching, boating and more. Airfare varies from departure points and time of the year.

5457 **Public Technology**
US Department of Transportation
1301 Pennsylvania Ave NW
Washington, DC 20004
202-626-2400
FAX: 202-626-2498

J Rutter, CEO
One of a series of reports concerned with improving transportation for elderly and disabled persons.
28 pages

5458 Rehabiliation Engineering Center for Personal Licensed Transportation
University Of Virginia School Of Engineering
PO Box 400246
Charlottesville, VA 22904-4246 434-924-3072

Tom Connors, VP
Mitch Rosen, Director

5459 Wheelchair Getaways Wheelchair/Scooter Accessible Van Rentals
4443 Dixie Highway
PO Box 1098
Mukilteo, WA 98275-2864 425-353-8213
800-536-5518
FAX: 425-355-6159
e-mail: info@wheelchairgetaways.com
www.wheelchairgetaways.com

Jennifer Richardson, Owner
Dale Richardson, Owner
Rebecca Heim, Manager
Moon Ko, Owner

Rents wheelchair/scooter accessible vans by the day, week, month or longer and offers delivery to major airports and other convenient locations in more than 200 cities in 42 states and Puerto Rico. Also offers full size and mini vans with automatic lifts and ramps. Some vans are equipped with hand controls, six-way power seats and remote controls for powered door operation and lifts.

5460 WheelersMarauatha Baptist Church
9120 N 95th Avenue
Peoria, AZ 85345-2501 623-937-7866
800-456-1371
FAX: 623-934-3971

Greg Iehl, Religious Leader, Pastor
Gene Noel, Assn't Pastor

Offers delivery to airports in 29 states and Washington, D.C. In about 40 cities, Wheelers works directly with Avis Rent-a-Car. Wheelers offers a variety of van configurations with capacity for up to three wheelchairs, automatic ramps or lifts and nylon tie-downs, hand controls or other modifications.

5461 Wheelers Handicapped Accessible Van Rentals
6614 W Sweetwater Ave
Glendale, AZ 85304-1040 602-418-5076
800-456-1371
FAX: 623-412-9920
e-mail: info@wheelersvanrentals.com
www.wheelersvanrentals.com

Tammy Smith, President
Ron Smith, Corporate Treasurer

Wheelers has been breaking travel barriers through innovative service and products since 1989. Our mission is to have Wheelers rental affiliates available in every city in the United States, Canada and all around the globe. Wheelers' objective is to connect you to the best possible solution for your transportation challenges and continue to find new and innovative ways in making the world a more accessible place.

Veteran Services

National Administrations

5462 **DAV National Service Headquarters**
807 Maine Ave SW
Washington, DC 20024-2410 202-554-3501
FAX: 202-554-3581
e-mail: feedback@davmail.org
www.dav.org

Donald L. Samuels, Chairman
Joseph W. Johnston, Vice-Chairman
Marc Burgess, Secretary
Joseph R. Lenhart, Treasurer

Serves America's disabled veterans and their families. Direct services include legislative advocacy; professional counseling about compensation, pension, educational and job training programs and VA health care; and assistance in applying for those entitlements.

5463 **Department of Medicine and Surgery Veterans Administration**
810 Vermont Ave NW
Washington, DC 20420 202-273-8504
FAX: 202-273-9108
TTY:800-273-8255
www.va.gov

Eric K. Shinseki, Secretary
Stephen W. Warren, Principal Deputy Assistant Secretary
W. Todd Grams, Chief Financial Officer
Glenn D. Haggstrom, Principal Executive Director

Provides hospital and outpatient treatment as well as nursing home care for eligible veterans in Veterans Administration facilities. Services elsewhere provided on a contract basis in the United States and its territories. Provides non-vocational inpatient residential rehabilitation services to eligible legally blinded veterans of the armed forces of the United States.

5464 **Department of Veterans Affairs Regional Office - Vocational Rehab Division**
380 Westminster St
Providence, RI 02903-3246 401-222-2488
800-827-1000
FAX: 401-254-1340
e-mail: dhs.state.ri.us/dhs/dvetsff.htm
www.va.gov

Eric K. Shinseki, Secretary
Stephen W. Warren, Principal Deputy Assistant Secretary
W. Todd Grams, Chief Financial Officer
Glenn D. Haggstrom, Principal Executive Director

Vocational rehabilitation is a program of services administered by the Department of Veterans Affairs for service members and veterans with service-connected physical or mental disabilities. If persons are compensibly disabled and are found in need of rehabilitation services because they have an employment handicap, this program can prepare them for a suitable job; get and keep that job; assist persons to become fully productive and independent.

5465 **Department of Veterans Benefits**
810 Vermont Ave NW
Suite 727
Washington, DC 20420 202-461-6913
800-827-1000
FAX: 202-275-3689
e-mail: vacoOAO@va.gov
www.va.gov

Eric K. Shinseki, Secretary
Stephen W. Warren, Principal Deputy Assistant Secretary
W. Todd Grams, Chief Financial Officer
Glenn D. Haggstrom, Principal Executive Director

Furnishes compensation and pensions for disability and death to veterans and their dependents. Provides vocational rehabilitation services, including counseling, training, assistance and more towards employment, to blinded veterans disabled as a result of service in the armed forces during World War II, Korea and the Vietnam era; also provides rehabilitation services to certain peace-time veterans.

5466 **Disabled American Veterans**
PO Box 14301
Cincinnati, OH 45250-0301 859-441-7300
877-426-2838
877-426-2838
FAX: 859-441-1416
www.dav.org

Donald L. Samuels, Chairman
Joseph W. Johnston, Vice-Chairman
Marc Burgess, Secretary
Joseph R. Lenhart, Treasurer

Advises veterans of their rights and employers of their obligations, under the Rehabilitation Act, the Americans with Disabilities Act, and legislation governing the employment and training of Vietnam era veterans with disabilities.

5467 **Federal Benefits for Veterans and Dependents**
Government Printing Office
810 Vermont Ave NW
Washington, DC 20420 202-273-6763
800-827-1000
FAX: 202-275-3689
www.benefits.va.gov

Eric K. Shinseki, Secretary
Stephen W. Warren, Principal Deputy Assistant Secretary
W. Todd Grams, Chief Financial Officer
Glenn D. Haggstrom, Principal Executive Director

Offers information on benefits for veterans and their families.
93 pages
ISBN 0-16048 -58-

5468 **Hospitalized Veterans Writing Project**
5920 Nall Ave
Room 101
Mission, KS 66202-3456 913-432-1214
FAX: 913-432-1214
e-mail: veteransvoices@sbcglobal.net
www.veteransvoices.org

Margaret (Th Clark, Veterans' Voices Editor in Chief/President HVWP/ VAVS Deputy
Jerry D. Brown, Vice President HVWP
Eileen Wirtz, Recording Secretary HVWP
Tess (John) Raydo, Treasurer HWVP

Individuals and organizations united to encourage VA veterans to write for pleasure and rehabilitation. Maintains speakers' bureau and audio tape version for the blind in Cooperation with Ku Audio. Bestows numerous monetary awards including article; book review; cartoon and drawing; light verse; poetry and short story.
$15.00
64 pages Magazine
ISSN 0504-07 9

5469 **US Department of Veterans Affairs National Headquarters**
1120 Vermont Ave NW
Washington, DC 20420-2 202-273-5400
800-827-1000
e-mail: washingtondc.query@vba.va.gov
www.va.gov

Eric K. Shinseki, Secretary
Stephen W. Warren, Principal Deputy Assistant Secretary
W. Todd Grams, Chief Financial Officer
Glenn D. Haggstrom, Principal Executive Director

Administers the laws providing benefits and other services to veterans, their dependents, and their beneficiaries. Acts as their principal advocate in ensuring that they recieve medical care, benefits, social support, and lasting memorials promoting the health, welfare, and dignity of all veterans in recognition of their service to this nation. As the DVA heads into the 21st century, they will strive to meet the needs of the Nation's veterans today and tomorrow. Publishes a monthly magazine.
80 pages

5470 **US Veteran's Affairs**
810 Vermont Ave NW
Washington, DC 20420-2
202-273-5400
800-827-1000
e-mail: veteransvoices@sbcglobal.net
www.va.gov

Eric K. Shinseki, Secretary
Stephen W. Warren, Principal Deputy Assistant Secretary
W. Todd Grams, Chief Financial Officer
Glenn D. Haggstrom, Principal Executive Director

Provides a wide range of services for those who have been in the military and their dependents, as well as offering information on driver assessment and education programs.

Alabama

5471 **Alabama VA Regional Office**
Veterans Benefits Administration, U S Dept. of V A
345 Perry Hill Rd
Montgomery, AL 36109-4551
800-827-1000
FAX: 334-213-3565
e-mail: montgomery.query@vba.va.gov
www.va.gov

Eric K. Shinseki, Secretary
Stephen W. Warren, Principal Deputy Assistant Secretary
W. Todd Grams, Chief Financial Officer
Glenn D. Haggstrom, Principal Executive Director

The facility represents the Veterans Benefits Administration's first endeavor at designing, constructing, and activating a new building.

5472 **Alabama Veterans Facility**
809 Green Springs Hwy
Homewood, AL 35209-4917
205-916-2700
www.birmingham.va.gov

Robert B Herndon, Manager

Veterans medical clinic offering disabled veterans medical treatments.

5473 **Birmingham VA Medical Center**
Veterans Health Administration U S Dept. of V A
700 South 19th Street
Birmingham, AL 35233-1927
205-933-8101
800-827-1000
e-mail: g.vhacss@forum.va.gov
www.birmingham.va.gov

Thomas Smith, Medical Center Director
Phyllis Smith, MBA, FACHE, Associate Director
Cynthia Cleveland, Assistant Director
Jane Hebb, MSN, RN, Acting Associate Director for Patient/Nursing Services

The medical center serves as a referral center for this population area with 136 operating beds currently. Recent construction provides state-of-the-art facilities and equipment in all clinical programs.

5474 **Central Alabama Veterans Healthcare System**
Veterans Health Administration, US Dept. of VA
215 Perry Hill Rd
Montgomery, AL 36109-3798
334-272-4670
800-214-8387
e-mail: g.vhacss@forum.va.gov
www.centralalabama.va.gov

James R. Talton, PA-C, MBA, M.S, Director
Roderick F. Byrne, Jr., Acting Associate Director
Roselia Adams-Bean, MSN, RN, Interim Associate DirectorPatient Care Services
Cliff Robinson, MD, FAAFP, Chief of Staff

CAVHCS exists to provide excellent services to veterans across the continuum of healthcare. We take pride in providing delivery of timely quality care by staff who demonstrate outstanding customer service, the advancement of health care through research, and the education of tomorrow's health care providers.

5475 **Tuscaloosa VA Medical Center**
Veterans Health Administration, U S Dept. of V A
3701 Loop Rd
Tuscaloosa, AL 35404-5015
205-554-2000
888-269-3405
FAX: 205-554-2845
www.tuscaloosa.va.gov

Maria R. Andrews, MS, FACHE, Director
Paula Stokes, CTRS, CPM, M.E, Associate Director
Patricia A. Mathis, RN, MSN, Associate Director for Patient Care Services
Martin S. Schnier, DO, FACOFP, Chief of Staff

To serve America's Heroes by improving their health and well-being through Veteran and Family Centered Care.

Alaska

5476 **Anchorage Regional Office**
Veterans Benefits Administration, U S Dept. of V A
1201 North Muldoon Rd
Anchorage, AK 99504
800-827-1000
e-mail: anchorage.query@vba.va.gov
www.va.gov

Claude M Kicklighter, Chief Staff
Alex Spector, Executive Director

The Anchorage Regional Office is remotely managed by the Salt Lake City Regional Office.The VBA operation includes a one-stop Veterans Service Center made up of the merged Adjudication and Veterans Service Divisions. There is also a one person Loan Guaranty Division and a Vocational Rehabilitation and Employment Division.

5477 **DAV Department of Alaska**
2925 Debarr Rd
Room 3101
Anchorage, AK 99508-2983
907-257-4803
FAX: 907-258-9828
www.davmembersportal.org

Walter Crary, Treasurer
Robert Boles, Sr. Vice President

Arizona

5478 **Carl T Hayden VA Medical Center**
Veterans Health Administration, U S Dept. of V A
650 E Indian School Rd
Phoenix, AZ 85012-1839
602-277-5551
800-554-7174
FAX: 602-222-6472
e-mail: g.vhacss@forum.va.gov
www.phoenix.va.gov

D Gregg Gordon, President
Marva Greene, Vice President
John Fears, CEO
Linda Herrly MSW, LCSW, Caregiver Support Coordinator

5479 **Northern Arizona VA Health Care System**
Veterans Health Administration, US Dept. of VA
500 Hwy 89N
Prescott, AZ 86313-5001
928-445-4860
800-949-1005
FAX: 928-768-6076
e-mail: g.vhacss@forum.va.gov
www.prescott.va.gov

Deborah Thompson, Manager

5480 **Southern Arizona VA Healthcare System**
Veterans Health Administration, U S Dept. of V A
3601 S 6th Ave
Tucson, AZ 85723 520-792-1450
800-470-8262
FAX: 520-629-1818
e-mail: g.vhacss@forum.va.gov
www.tucson.va.gov

Jonathan H. Gardner, MPA, FACHE, Director
Jennifer S Gutowski, MHA, FACHE, Associate Director
Katie A. Landwehr, MBA, Assistant Director
Fabia Kwiecinski, MD, FACP, Chief of Staff

The Southern Arizona VA Health Care System (SAVAHCS) located in Tucson AZ serves over 170,000 Veterans located in eight counties in Southern Arizona and one county in Western New Mexico.

Arkansas

5481 **Eugene J Towbin Healthcare Center**
Veterans Health Administration, U S Dept. of V A
2200 Fort Roots Dr
North Little Rock, AR 72114-1706 501-257-1000
800-827-1000
FAX: 501-257-1779
e-mail: g.vhacss@forum.va.gov
www.littlerock.va.gov

Michael R. Winn, Director
Toby T. Mathew, MHA/MBA, Deputy Director
Cyril O. Ekeh, MHA, Associate Director
Julie A. Brandt, MSN, RN, CNA-B, Associate Director for Patient Care Service/Nurse Executive

CAVHS is reaching out to veterans through its community-based outpatient clinics in Mountain Home, El Dorado, Hot Springs, Mena, Pine Bluff, Searcy, Conway, Russellville, its Home Health Care Service Center in Hot Springs, and a VA Drop-In Day Treatment Center for homeless veterans in downtown Little Rock.

5482 **Fayetteville VA Medical Center**
Veterans Health Administration, US Dept. of VA
1100 N College Ave
Fayetteville, AR 72703-1944 479-443-4301
800-691-8387
e-mail: g.vhacss@forum.va.gov
www.fayettevillear.va.gov

W. Todd Grams, Chief Financial Officer
Glenn D. Haggstrom, Principal Executive Director
Stephen W. Warren, Principal Deputy Assistant Secretary

Honor America's Veterans by providing exceptional health care that improves their health and well-being.

5483 **John L McClellan Memorial Hospital**
Veterans Health Administration, US Dept. of VA
4300 W 7th St
Little Rock, AR 72205-5446 501-257-1000
800-827-1000
e-mail: g.vhacss@forum.va.gov
www.littlerock.va.gov

Michael R. Winn, Director
Toby T. Mathew, MHA/MBA, Deputy Director
Cyril O. Ekeh, MHA, Associate Director
Julie A. Brandt, MSN, RN, CNA-B, Associate Director for Patient Care Service/Nurse Executive

CAVHS is reaching out to veterans through its community-based outpatient clinics in Mountain Home, El Dorado, Hot Springs, Mena, Pine Bluff, Searcy, Conway, Russellville, its Home Health Care Service Center in Hot Springs, and a VA Drop-In Day Treatment Center for homeless veterans in downtown Little Rock. Throughout its rich 90 year history, CAVHS has been widely recognized for excellence in education, research, and emergency preparedness, and -first and foremost -for a tradition of quality an

5484 **North Little Rock Regional Office**
Veterans Benefits Administration, U S Dept. of V A
2200 Fort Roots Drive
Building 65
N Little Rock, AR 72114-1756 501-370-3820
800-827-1000
FAX: 501-370-3829
e-mail: littlerock.query@vba.va.gov
www.va.gov

Eric K. Shinseki, Secretary
Stephen W. Warren, Principal Deputy Assistant Secretary
W. Todd Grams, Chief Financial Officer
Glenn D. Haggstrom, Principal Executive Director

The Little Rock VA Regional Office offers services to veterans in the State of Arkansas and the city of Texarkana in Bowie County, Texas. Based on 2004 information provided by the Office of Policy, Planning, and Preparedness, the veteran population of Arkansas is 268,000 and the city of Texarkana, Texas, has a veteran population of 3,545. With a staff of approximately 124 employees, the Regional Office determines entitlement to disability compensation and pension, survivors' benefits, vocational

California

5485 **Jerry L Pettis Memorial VA Medical Center**
Veterans Health Administration, U S Dept. of V A
11201 Benton St
Loma Linda, CA 92357-1000 909-825-7084
800-741-8387
e-mail: g.vhacss@forum.va.gov
www.lomalinda.va.gov

Barbara Fallen, RD, MPA, FACHE, Acting Director
Prachi V. Asher, FACHE, Assistant Director
Dwight C. Evans, M.D., Chief of Staff
Shane M. Elliott, MBA, AD for Administration

Since 1977, VA Loma Linda Healthcare System has been improving the health of the men and women who have so proudly served our nation. We consider it our privilege to serve your health care needs in any way we can.

5486 **Long Beach VA Medical Center**
Veterans Health Administration, U S Dept. of V A
5901 E 7th St
Long Beach, CA 90822-5201 562-826-8000
800-827-1000
888-769-8387
e-mail: g.vhacss@forum.va.gov
www.longbeach.va.gov

Isabel Duff, Medical Center Director
John M. Tryboski, MSN, Associate Director
Anthony DeFrancesco, FACHE, Associate Director
Sherrie Schuldheis, Ph.D., RN, Assistant Director, Systems Redesign

5487 **Los Angeles Regional Office**
Veterans Benefits Administration, U S Dept. of V A
11000 Wilshire Blvd
Los Angeles, CA 90024-3602 800-827-1000
e-mail: losangeles.query@vba.va.gov
www.va.gov

Eric K. Shinseki, Secretary
Stephen W. Warren, Principal Deputy Assistant Secretary
W. Todd Grams, Chief Financial Officer
Glenn D. Haggstrom, Principal Executive Director

The Los Angeles Regional Office (RO) provides benefits and services to approximately 706,000 veterans residing in the Southern California counties of Los Angeles, San Bernardino, Riverside, Ventura, Santa Barbara, San Luis Obispo, and Kern. VA benefits expenditures for veterans residing within the jurisdiction of the RO exceed $800 million annually. All Loan Guaranty activities for the six counties are under jurisdiction of the Phoenix Regional Office.

5488 Martinez Outpatient Clinic
Veterans Health Administration, U S Dept. of V A
150 Muir Rd
Martinez, CA 94553-4668 925-372-2000
800-382-8387
e-mail: g.vhacss@forum.va.gov
www.va.gov

John H Simms, Director
Brian E. Schuman, Chief of Police

The Martinez Outpatient Clinic offers a full range of medical, surgical, mental health, and diagnostic outpatient services, including nuclear medicine, ultrasound, CT and MRI. The Center for Rehabilitation and Extended Care is located adjacent to the outpatient clinic.

5489 Oakland VA Regional Office
Veterans Benefits Administration U S Dept. of V A
1301 Clay Street
12th Floor
Oakland, CA 94612-5217 800-827-1000
e-mail: oakland.query@vba.va.gov
www.benefits.va.gov/oakland

Geri Spearman, Director

The jurisdiction includes all Northern California, except for Modoc, Lassen, Alpine and Mono counties, which are assigned to the Reno Regional Office. All Loan Guaranty activities are under the jurisdiction of the Phoenix Regional Office. Seven service organizations are collocated on the eleventh floor of the Federal Office building occupied by the regional office.

5490 Rehabilitation Research and Development Center
Department of Veteran s Affairs
810 Vermont Avenue, NW
Washington, DC 94304-1207 202-443-0575
FAX: 202-495-6153
e-mail: tiffany.asqueri@va.gov
www.rehab.research.va.gov

Patricia A. Dorn, Ph.D., Acting Director, Rehab R&D Service
Ricardo Gonzalez, Administrative Officer
Gloria Winford, Staff Assistant
Sarah Armstrong, Budget Technician

The VA Center of Excellence on Mobility in Palo Alto, CA is dedicated to developing innovative clinical treatments and assistive devices for veterans with physical disabilities to increase their independence and improve their quality of life. The clinical emphasis of the center is to improve mobility, either ambulation or manipulation, in individuals with neurologic impairments or orthopaedic impairments. We do not publish any printed books, journals or periodicals.

5491 Sacramento Medical Center
Veterans Health Administration U S Department of V
10535 Hospital Way
Mather, CA 95655-4200 916-843-7000
800-382-8387
e-mail: g.vhacss@forum.va.gov
www.northerncalifornia.va.gov

David G. Mastalski, Interim Director
Donna Iatarola, RN, MSN, Associate Director
William T. Cahill, MD, Chief of Staff

It is an integrated health care delivery system, offering a comprehensive array of medical, surgical, rehabilitative, mental health and extended care to veterans in Northern California. The health system is comprised of a medical center in Sacramento; a rehabilitation and extended care facility in Martinez, and seven outpatient clinics.

5492 San Diego VA Regional Office
Veterans Benefits Administration, U S Dept. of V A
8810 Rio San Diego Dr
San Diego, CA 92108-1698 858-552-8585
800-827-1000
FAX: 858-552-7436
e-mail: oakland.query@vba.va.gov
www.benefits.va.gov/sandiego

Janet M Peyton, Administrative Officer

The San Diego VA Regional Office provides benefit services for over 600,000 Veterans and their dependents in the Southern California Counties of Imperial, Orange, Riverside and San Diego. Since the Regional Office shares occupancy of the building with a VA Outpatient Clinic and the Employment Development Department of the State of California, it truly offers a one stop Service Center.

5493 VA Central California Health Care System
Veterans Health Administration, U S Dept. of V A
2615 E Clinton Ave
Fresno, CA 93703-2223 559-225-6100
888-826-2838
FAX: 559-268-6911
e-mail: g.vhacss@forum.va.gov
www.fresno.va.gov

Joanne Krumberger, Director
Susan Shyshka, Associate Director
Patricia Richardson Ed.D, RN, N, Nursing Executive
Wessel Meyer MB ChB, FCP (SA), Chief of Staff

VA Central California Health Care System (VACCHCS) has been improving the health of the men and women who have so proudly served our nation. We consider it our privilege to serve your health care needs in any way we can.

5494 VA Greater Los Angeles Healthcare System
Veterans Health Administration U S Deptartment of
11301 Wilshire Blvd
Los Angeles, CA 90073-1003 310-478-3711
800-827-1000
FAX: 310-268-4848
e-mail: g.vhacss@forum.va.gov
www.losangeles.va.gov

Donna M. Beiter, RN, MSN, Director
Christopher Sandles, Assistant Director
Marlene Brewster, RN, MSN, Acting Associate Director, Nursing and Patient Care Services
Carrie J Dekorte, Associate Director for Administration / Operations

The VA Greater Los Angeles Healthcare System is the largest, most complex healthcare system within the Department of Veterans Affairs.GLA consists of three ambulatory care centers, a tertiary care facility and 10 community based outpatient clinics. GLA serves veterans residing throughout five counties: Los Angeles, Ventura, Kern, Santa Barbara, and San Luis Obispo. There are 1.4 million veterans in the GLA service area. GLA is affiliated with both UCLA School of Medicine and USC School of Medici

5495 VA Northern California Healthcare System
Veterans Health Administration, U S Dept. of V A
150 Muir Rd
Martinez, CA 94553-4668 925-372-2000
800-382-8387
e-mail: g.vhacss@forum.va.gov
www.northerncalifornia.va.gov

David G. Mastalski, Interim Director
Donna Iatarola, RN, MSN, Associate Director
William T. Cahill, MD, Chief of Staff

VA Northern California Health Care System (VANCHCS) is an integrated health care delivery system, offering a comprehensive array of medical, surgical, rehabilitative, mental health and extended care to veterans in Northern California. The health system is comprised of a medical center in Sacramento; a rehabilitation and extended care facility in Martinez, and seven outpatient clinics.

5496 VA San Diego Healthcare System
Veterans Health Administration, U S Dept. of V A
3350 La Jolla Village Dr
San Diego, CA 92161 858-552-8585
800-331-8387
e-mail: g.vhacss@forum.va.gov
www.sandiego.va.gov

Jeffrey T. Gering, FACHE, Director
Cynthia Abair, MHA, Associate Director
Robert M. Smith, MD, Chief of Staff/Medical Director
Sandra Solem, PhD, RN, Associate Director, Patient Care Services/Nurse Executive

We provide medical, surgical, mental health, geriatric, spinal cord injury, and advanced rehabilitation services. VASDHS has

296 authorized beds, including skilled nursing beds and operates several regional referral programs including cardiovascular surgery and spinal cord injury. The facility also supports three Vet Centers at the following locations: Chula Vista, San Diego, and San Marcos.

Colorado

5497 **Boulder Vet Center**
4999 Pearl East Circle
Suite 106
Boulder, CO 80301 303-440-7306
877-927-8387
FAX: 303-449-3907
www.va.gov

Gail N Bennett, Office Manager
Michael J Pantaleo, Team Leader
Annette Matlock, Counselor
Collette M Archibald, Counselor
Offers trauma and readjustment from military and civilian life counseling and assistance with disability claims, military benefits and employment are provided.

5498 **Colorado/Wyoming VA Medical Center**
Veterans Benefits Administration U S Dept. of V A
155 Van Gordon St
Suite 395
Lakewood, CO 80225 303-914-2680
800-827-1000
e-mail: denver.query@vba.va.gov
www.denver.va.gov

Forest Farley Jr, Medical Center Director
Thomas E Bowen, Chief of Staff

5499 **Denver VA Medical Center**
Veterans Health Administration, U S Dept. of V A
1055 Clermont St
Suite 6A138
Denver, CO 80220-3808 303-393-2869
888-336-8262
e-mail: judi.guy@va.gov
www.denver.va.gov

Lynnette Roth, Executive Director
Peggy Kearns MS, RD, FACHE, Associate Director
Judith Burke RN, MS, NEA-BC, Associate Director, Patient Care Services
Rebecca Keough MPA, VHA-CM, Assistant Director
Construction of our 1.1m sq foot, $800m replacement facility is well under way! Concrete is being poured, steel is being put in, and we're working hard to open in 2015.

5500 **Grand Junction VA Medical Center**
Veterans Health Administration
2121 North Ave
Grand Junction, CO 81501-6428 970-242-0731
866-206-6415
FAX: 970-244-1300
e-mail: g.vhacss@forum.va.gov
www.grandjunction.va.gov

Patricia A. Hitt, MS, Acting Director
Michael Murphy, Manager
Randal France, M.D., Chief Psychiatry Service/ Int. Chf. of Staff
Angela T Brothers, AD/ Patient Care Svcs
The VAMC operates 53 beds comprised of 23 acute care and 30 Transitional Care Unit beds. The VAMC provides primary and secondary care including acute medical, surgical, and psychiatric inpatient services, as well as a full range of outpatient services.

Connecticut

5501 **Hartford Regional Office**
Veterans Benefits Administration U S Department of
555 Willard Ave
Building 2E
Newington, CT 6111-2631 860-666-6951
800-827-1000
e-mail: hartford.query@vba.va.gov
www.vba.va.gov/ro/hartford

Jeanette A Chirico Post, Network Director
The Hartford Regional Office now provides one-stop service to veterans and their families seeking assistance in compensation, pension, and vocational rehabilitation and employment in an accessible campus environment.

5502 **Hartford Vet Center**
25 Elm St
Suite A
Rocky Hill, CT 06067-2305 860-563-8800
877-927-8387
FAX: 860-563-8805
e-mail: donna.hryb@med.va.gov
www.va.gov

Donna Hryb LCSW, Team Leader
Pedro Ortiz, Counselor
Amy Otzel, Counselor
Laura Hall, Military Sexual Trauma Counselor
A U.S. Department of Veterans Affairs counseling center offering counseling to Vietnam era and combat veterans. Sexual trauma/harassment counseling, medical screening and benefit referral is available to all veterans.

5503 **VA Connecticut Healthcare System: Newington Division**
Veterans Health Administration U S Department. of
555 Willard Ave
Newington, CT 6111-2631 860-666-6951
800-827-1000
FAX: 860-667-6764
e-mail: g.vhacss@forum.va.gov
www.connecticut.va.gov

Janice M. Boss, MS, Director
Margaret Veazey, RN, MSN, Associate Director for Patient Care Services
John Callahan, Associate Director
Al Montoya, Assistant Director
The mission of VA Connecticut Healthcare Systems is to fulfill a nation's commitment to its veterans by providing quality healthcare, promoting health through prevention and maintaining excellence in teaching and research. Provides primary, secondary and tertiary care in medicine, geriatrics, neurology, psychiatry and surgery with an operating capacity of 211 hospital beds.

5504 **VA Connecticut Healthcare System: West Haven**
Veterans Health Administration, U S Dept. of V A
950 Campbell Ave
West Haven, CT 06516-2770 203-932-5711
800-827-1000
FAX: 203-937-3868
e-mail: g.vhacss@forum.va.gov
www.connecticut.va.gov

Janice M. Boss, MS, Director
Margaret Veazey, RN, MSN, Associate Director for Patient Care Services
John Callahan, Associate Director
Al Montoya, Assistant Director
The mission of VA Connecticut Healthcare Systems is to fulfill a nation's commitment to its veterans by providing quality healthcare, promoting health through prevention and maintaining excellence in teaching and research. Provides primary, secondary and tertiary care in medicine, geriatrics, neurology, psychiatry and surgery with an operating capacity of 211 hospital beds.

Delaware

5505 Delaware VA Regional Office
Veterans Benefits Administration U S Dept. of V A
1601 Kirkwood Hwy
Wilmington, DE 19805-4917 302-994-2511
800-461-8262
FAX: 302-633-5516
e-mail: wilmington.query@vba.va.gov
www.wilmington.va.gov

Daniel D. Hendee, FACHE, MHA, Director
Mary Alice Johnson, MS, RN, Associate Director for Patient Care Services
William E. England, Associate Director for Finance and Operations
Enrique Guttin, MD, MMM, CPE,, Chief of Staff

We offer comprehensive services ranging from preventive screenings to long-term care. Wilmington VAMC proudly serves Veterans in multiple locations for convenient access to the services we provide.

5506 Wilmington VA Medical Center
Veterans Health Administration, US Dept. of VA
1601 Kirkwood Hwy
Wilmington, DE 19805-4917 302-994-2511
800-461-8262
FAX: 302-633-5516
e-mail: g.vhacss@forum.va.gov
www.wilmington.va.gov

Daniel D. Hendee, FACHE, MHA, Director
Mary Alice Johnson, MS, RN, Associate Director for Patient Care Services
William E. England, Associate Director for Finance and Operations
Enrique Guttin, MD, MMM, CPE,, Chief of Staff

We offer comprehensive services ranging from preventive screenings to long-term care. Wilmington VAMC proudly serves Veterans in multiple locations for convenient access to the services we provide.

5507 Wilmington Vet Center
2710 Centerville Road
Suite 103
Wilmington, DE 19808- 4917 302-994-1660
877-927-8387
FAX: 302-994-8361
www.va.gov

Joan Spencer, Team Leader
Patricia Elwood, Office Manager
Valerie Feeley, Counselor
Barbara F Blevins, Counselor

Veterans counseling program offering individual counseling services, advocacy services and group counseling. The focus is the counseling of all veterans coping with the aftermath of war, sexual abuse/harassment in the military and all veterans of the Vietnam era. The center also has an active outreach program to seek veterans needing services. Hours of operation are between 8:00 AM - 4:30 PM, Monday - Friday and other times by appointment only. Services are free.

District of Columbia

5508 Disabled American Veterans, National Service & Legislative Headquarters
807 Maine Ave SW
Washington, DC 20024-2410 202-554-3501
FAX: 202-554-3581
www.dav.org

Donald L. Samuels, Chairman
Joseph W. Johnston, Vice-Chairman
Marc Burgess, Secretary
Joseph R. Lenhart, Treasurer

Our mission simply is one of service and advocacy on behalf of the men and women who put their lives on the line to ensure our safety, to protect our freedoms and cherished way of life.

5509 PVA Sports and Recreation Program
Paralyzed Veterans of America
801 18th St NW
Washington, DC 20006-3517 202-872-1300
800-424-8200
888-888-2201
FAX: 202-785-4432
TTY:800-795-4327
e-mail: info@pva.org
www.pva.org

Randy Pleva, President
Homer S. Townsend, Jr., Executive Director
Larry Dodson, National Secretary
Bill Lawson, National President

Today, the work continues to create an America where all veterans and people with disabilities, and their families, have everything they need to live full and productive lives.

5510 VA Medical Center, Washington DC
50 Irving St NW
Washington, DC 20422-1 202-745-8000
800-827-1000
877-328-2621
e-mail: g.vhacss@forum.va.gov
www.washingtondc.va.gov

Brian A. Hawkins, MHA, Medical Center Director
Bryan C. Matthews, MBA, Associate Medical Center Director
Natalie Merckens, Assistant Medical Center Director
Ross D. Fletcher, MD, Chief of Staff

Acute general and specialized services in medicine, surgery, neurology, and psychiatry.

5511 Washington DC VA Medical Center
Veterans Health Administration, U S Dept. of V A
50 Irving St NW
Washington, DC 20422-1 202-745-8000
800-827-1000
877-328-2621
FAX: 202-754-8530
e-mail: g.vhacss@forum.va.gov
www.washingtondc.va.gov

Brian A. Hawkins, MHA, Medical Center Director
Bryan C. Matthews, MBA, Associate Medical Center Director
Natalie Merckens, Assistant Medical Center Director
Ross D. Fletcher, MD, Chief of Staff

Acute general and specialized services in medicine, surgery, neurology, and psychiatry.

Florida

5512 Bay Pines VA Medical Center
Veterans Health Administration, U S Dept. of V A
10000 Bay Pines Blvd
PO Box 5005
Bay Pines, FL 33744 727-398-6661
800-827-1000
888-820-0230
e-mail: g.vhacss@forum.va.gov
www.baypines.va.gov

Suzanne M. Klinker, Medical Center Director
Kristine Brown, MPH, Associate Director
Teresa Kumar, RN, MSN, CPHQ,, Associate Director for Patient / Nursing Services
Keith Neeley, FACHE, Assistant Director

Since 1933, Bay Pines VA Healthcare System has been improving the health of the men and women who have so proudly served our nation. We consider it our privilege to serve your health care needs in any way we can. Our services are available to Veterans living in a ten county catchment area in west central Florida.

5513 **Gainesville Division, North Florida/South Georgia Veterans Healthcare System**
Veterans Health Administration, U S Dept. of V A
1601 SW Archer Rd
Gainesville, FL 32608-1611 352-376-1611
800-324-8387
FAX: 352-379-7445
e-mail: g.vhacss@forum.va.gov
www.northflorida.va.gov/northflorida

Thomas Wisnieski, MPA, FACHE, Director
Nancy Reissener, Deputy Director
Maureen Wilkes, Associate Director
LeAnne Whitlow, RN, MSHSA, MB, Associate Director, Nursing Service

In addition to our medical centers in Gainesville and Lake City, we offer services in three satellite outpatient clinics and several community-based outpatient clinics across North Florida and South Georgia.

5514 **James A Haley VA Medical Center**
Veterans Health Administration, U S Dept. of V A
13000 Bruce B Downs Blvd
Suite T72
Tampa, FL 33612-4745 813-972-2000
800-827-1000
888-811-0107
e-mail: g.vhacss@forum.va.gov
www.tampa.va.gov

Kathleen R. Fogarty, Director
Roy L. Hawkins Jr., Deputy Director
David J. VanMeter, Associate Director
Suzanne Tate, Assistant Director

Comprehensive health care is provided through primary care, tertiary care, and long-term care in areas of medicine, surgery, psychiatry, physical medicine and rehabilitation, spinal cord injury, neurology, oncology, dentistry, geriatrics, and extended care.

5515 **Miami VA Medical Center**
Veterans Health Administration, U S Dept. of V A
1201 NW 16th St
Suite B822
Miami, FL 33125-1693 305-575-7000
800-827-1000
888-276-1785
FAX: 305-575-3266
e-mail: g.vhacss@forum.va.gov
www.miami.va.gov

Paul M. Russo, Director
Mark E. Morgan, Associate Director
Marcia Lysaght, Associate Director, Patient Care Services
P. Gwendolyn Findley, Ph.D., Assistant Director

The Miami VA is an accredited comprehensive medical provider, providing general medical, surgical, inpatient and outpatient mental health services, the Miami VA Healthcare System includes an AIDS/HIV center, a prosthetic treatment center, spinal cord injury rehabilitative center, and Geriatric Research, Education, and Clinical Center (GRECC).

5516 **St. Petersburg Regional Office**
Veterans Benefits Administration, U S Dept. of V A
9500 Bay Pines Blvd
St Petersburg, FL 33708 727-319-7492
800-827-1000
e-mail: stpete.query@vba.va.gov
www.va.gov

Warren McPherson, Executive Director

5517 **West Palm Beach VA Medical Center**
Veterans Health Administration, U S Dept. of V A
7305 N Military Trl
West Palm Beach, FL 33410-7417 561-422-8262
800-972-8262
FAX: 561-882-6707
e-mail: g.vhacss@forum.va.gov
www.westpalmbeach.va.gov

Charleen R. Szabo, FACHE, Medical Center Director
Cristy McKillop, FACHE, MHA, Medical Center Associate Director
Gloria A. Bays, MSN, ARNP, NE-BC, Associate Director for Patient Care Services
Deepak Mandi, MD, Chief of Staff

The medical center is a general medical, psychiatric and surgical facility. It is a teaching hospital, providing a full range of patient care services, with state-of-the-art technology as well as education and limited research. Comprehensive healthcare is provided through primary care and long-term care in the areas of dentistry, extended care, medicine, neurology, oncology, pharmacy, physical medicine, psychiatry, rehabilitation and surgery. The West Palm Beach VA Medical Center operates a Blin

Georgia

5518 **Atlanta Regional Office**
Veterans Benefits Administration, U S Dept. of V A
1700 Clairmont Road
Decatur, GA 30033-1210 404-463-3100
800-827-1000
FAX: 404-929-5819
e-mail: atlanta.query@vba.va.gov
www.va.gov

Chick Krautler, Executive Director

The Atlanta VA Regional Office is responsible for delivering non-medical VA benefits and services to Georgia Veterans and their dependent family members. This is accomplished through the administration of comprehensive and diverse benefit programs established by Congress. Our goal is to deliver these benefits and services in a timely, accurate, and compassionate manner.

5519 **Atlanta VA Medical Center**
Veterans Health Administration, U S Dept. of V A
1670 Clairmont Rd
Decatur, GA 30033-4004 404-321-6111
800-827-1000
FAX: 404-728-7734
e-mail: g.vhacss@forum.va.gov
www.atlanta.va.gov

Leslie B. Wiggins, Director
Tom Grace, MBA/MHA, Associate Director
Sheila Meuse, PhD, Assistant Director
Sandy Leake, MSN, RN, Associate Director for Nursing/Patient Services

The Atlanta VA Medical Center (VAMC), located on 26 acres in Decatur, is one of eight medical centers in the VA Southeast Network. It is a teaching hospital, providing a full range of patient care services complete with state-of-the-art technology, education, and research.

5520 **Augusta VA Medical Center**
Veterans Health Administration, U S Dept. of V A
950 15th Street Downtown/1 Freedom
Augusta, GA 30904-6258 706-733-0188
800-827-1000
FAX: 706-731-7227
e-mail: g.vhacss@forum.va.gov
www.agusta.va.gov

Robert U. Hamilton, MHA, FACHE, Medical Center Director
Richard Rose, Associate Director
Michelle Cox-Henley, MS, RN, Associate Director for Nursing/Patient Services
Luke M. (Mik Stapleton, MD, Chief of Staff

The Charlie Norwood VA Medical Center is a two-division Medical Center that provides tertiary care inmedicine, surgery, neurology, psychiatry, rehabilitation medicine, and spinal cord injury. The Downtown Division is authorized 155 beds (58 medicine, 37 surgery, and 60 spinal cord injury). The Uptown Division, located approximately three miles away, is authorized 315 beds (68 psychiatry, 15 blind rehabilitation and 40 medical rehabilitation. In addition, a 132-bed Restorative/Nursing Home C

5521 **Carl Vinson VA Medical Center**
Veterans Health Administration, U S Dept. of V A
1826 Veterans Blvd
Dublin, GA 31021-3699 478-272-1210
FAX: 478-277-2717
e-mail: dana.doles@med.va.gov
www.dublin.va.gov

John S. Goldman, Director
Gerald M. DeWorth, Associate Director
Sue Preston, RN, Associate Director for Patient and Nursing Services
Nomie Finn, M.D, Chief of Staff

Since 1948, Carl Vinson VA Medical Center has been improving the health of the men and women who have so proudly served our nation. We consider it our privilege to serve your health care needs in any way we can. Services are available to veterans living in the Middle Georgia area.

5522 **Southeastern Paralyzed Veterans of America(PVA)**
4010 Deans Bridge Rd
U.S. Highway 1
Hephzibah, GA 30815-5616 706-796-6301
800-292-9335
FAX: 706-796-0363
e-mail: homercpva@gmail.com
www.southeasternpva.org

Dr. Chuck Turek, National Director
Linda Hutchinson, Advocacy & Legislative Director for North and South Carolina
Homer Cole, Chapter President
Larry Dodson, Chapter Vice President

Works to maximize the quality of life for its members and all people with SCI/D as a leading adovocate for healthcare, SCI/D research and education, veteran's benefits, and rights, accessibility and the removal of architectural barriers, sports programs, and disability rights.

Hawaii

5523 **Hilo Vet Center**
70 Lanihuli St
Suite 102
Hilo, HI 96720-2067 808-969-3833
877-927-8387
FAX: 808-969-2025
www.va.gov

Felipe Sales, Team Leader
Samuelito Labasan, Office Manager
Peter Ehlich, Counselor
Nancy G Waller, Counselor

Veterans medical clinic offering disabled veterans medical treatments, readjustment and PTSD counseling to combat veterans

5524 **Honolulu VBA Regional Office**
Veterans Benefits Administration, U S Dept. of V A
459 Patterson Road, E-Wing
Honolulu, HI 96819-1522 808-566-1412
800-827-1000
FAX: 808-433-0478
e-mail: honolulu.query@vba.va.gov
www.vba.va.gov/ro/honolulu

Claude M Kicklighter, Chief of Staff
Alan Furuno, Manager
Alvin Kalawe, Elderly Program Coordinator
Karin Frazier, Women Veteran's Program Coordinator

The Honolulu Regional Office is responsible for administering VA's benefit programs under the leadership and direction of the Under Secretary for Benefits for the Veterans Benefits Administration. Formerly part of the Honolulu VA Medical & Regional Office Center (VAMROC), the Honolulu Regional Office (RO) was renamed as a stand alone RO on June 2, 2003. The office is co-located with the Spark M. Matsunaga Pacific Islands Health Care System medical center, on the grounds of the Tripler Army Medic

5525 **Pacific Islands Health Care System**
Veterans Health Administration, US Dept. of VA
459 Patterson Rd
Honolulu, HI 96819-1522 808-433-0600
800-214-1306
FAX: 808-433-0390
e-mail: g.vhacss@forum.va.gov
www.hawaii.va.gov

William F. Dubbs, M.D., Acting Director
Brandon K. Yamamoto, Acting Associate Director
Jane Wellman, APRN, Associate Director of Patient Care Services
David M. Bernstein, M.D, Acting Chief of Staff

The VA Pacific Islands Health Care System (VAPIHCS) Honolulu provides a broad range of medical care services, serving an estimated 127,600 veterans throughout Hawaii and the Pacific Islands. The VAPIHCS provides outpatient medical and mental health care through a main Ambulatory Care Clinic on Oahu (Honolulu) and through five Community Based Outpatient Clinics (CBOCs) on the neighboring islands including: Hawaii (Hilo and Kona), Maui, Kauai, and Guam. Traveling clinicians also provide episodi

Idaho

5526 **Boise Regional Office**
Veterans Benefits Administration, U S Dept. of V A
444 W. Fort Street
Boise, ID 83702-4531 800-827-1000
e-mail: boise.query@vba.va.gov
www.va.gov

Jim Vance, Director
Pat Teague, Service Officer
Tom Ressler, Manager

The Boise Regional Office administers monetary benefits to 17,283 veterans in Idaho, Utah, and Oregon. The Regional Office issued monthly disability and death benefit payments of over $15 million in January 2007. VBA's annual compensation and pension benefits for veterans residing within the RO's jurisdiction now exceed $185 million

5527 **Boise VA Medical Center**
Veterans Health Administration, U S Dept. of V A
500 W Fort St
Boise, ID 83702-4531 208-422-1000
800-827-1000
FAX: 208-422-1326
e-mail: g.vhacss@forum.va.gov
www.boise.va.gov

Jennifer T Shalz, Chief of Staff

We truly hope to improve your health and well-being and will make your visit or stay as pleasant as possible. We are committed to veterans and the nation and strive to continually enhance the care we provide. We also train future healthcare professionals, conduct research and support our nation in times of emergency. In all of these activities, our employees will respect and support your rights as a patient.

Illinois

5528 **Edward Hines Jr Hospital**
Veterans Health Administration, U S Dept. of V A
5000 South 5th Avenue
Hines, IL 60141 708-202-8387
800-827-1000
FAX: 708-202-2684
e-mail: g.vhacss@forum.va.gov
www.hines.va.gov

Joan Ricard, FACHE, Hospital Director
Dr. Daniel Zomchek, Associate Director
Carol A. Gouty, RN, MSN, PhD, Associate Director of Patient Care
Karandeep Sraon, Assistant Director

Specialized clinical programs include Blind Rehabilitation, Spinal Cord Injury, Neurosurgery, Radiation Therapy and Cardiovascular Surgery. The hospital also serves as the VISN 12 southern tier hub for pathology, radiology, radiation therapy, human resource management and fiscal services. Hines VAH currently operates 471 beds and six community based outpatient clinics in Elgin, Kankakee, Oak Lawn, Aurora, LaSalle, and Joliet.

5529 **Marion VA Medical Center**
Veterans Health Administration U S Department of V
2401 W Main St
Marion, IL 62959-1188 618-997-5311
800-827-1000
e-mail: kimberly.travelstead@va.gov
www.marion.va.gov
Paul Bockelman, Medical Center Director
Frank Kehus, Associate Director
The VA Medical Center in Marion, Illinois, is a general medical and surgical facility that operates 55 acute care beds and a 60 bed Community Living Center. Ten Outpatient Clinics that provide primary care and behavioral medicine services are located in Harrisburg; Carbondale; Effingham; and Mt. Vernon, IL; Paducah; Hanson; Owensboro; and Mayfield, Kentucky; Vincennes and Evansville, IN.

5530 **North Chicago VA Medical Center**
Veterans Health Administration, U S Dept. of V A
3001 North Green Bay Rd
North Chicago, IL 60064-3048 847-688-1900
800-393-0865
e-mail: g.vhacss@forum.va.gov
www.lovell.fhcc.va.gov
Patrick L. Sullivan, Director
Captain Jos, A. Acosta, MC, US, Commanding Officer/Deputy Director
Captain Jami Kersten, Associate Director
Dr. Sarah Fouse, Associate Director of Patient Services/Nurse Executive
The arrangement incorporates facilities, services and resources from the North Chicago VA Medical Center (VAMC) and the Naval Health Clinic Great Lakes (NHCGL). A combined mission of the health care center means active duty military, their family members, military retirees and veterans are all cared for at the facility.

5531 **VA Illiana Health Care System**
Veterans Health Administration, U S Dept. of V A
1900 E Main St
Danville, IL 61832-5198 217-554-3000
800-320-8387
FAX: 217-554-4552
e-mail: g.vhacss@forum.va.gov
www.danville.va.gov
Emma Metcalf, MSN, RN,, Director
Diana Carranza, Associate Director
Alesia Coe, MSN, RN,, Associate Director for Patient Care Services
Nirmala Rozario, M.D., Ph.D, Chief of Staff
Since 1898, our buildings, facilities, patients, and missions have changed, but remaining constant is VA Illiana Health Care System's endeavor in improving the health of the men and women who have so proudly served our nation. Being the 8th oldest VA facility, we consider it our privilege to serve your health care needs in any way we can.

Indiana

5532 **Indianapolis Regional Office**
Veterans Benefits Administration U S Department of
575 N Pennsylvania St
Indianapolis, IN 46204-1563 317-226-7860
800-827-1000
TTY:800-829-4833
e-mail: indianapolis.query@vba.va.gov
www.benefits.va.gov/indianapolis

5533 **Richard L Roudebush VA Medical Center**
Veterans Health Administration, U S Dept. of V A
1481 W 10th St
Indianapolis, IN 46202-2803 317-554-0000
800-827-1000
FAX: 317-554-0127
e-mail: g.vhacss@forum.va.gov
www.indianapolis.va.gov
Thomas Mattice, Director
Jeff Nechanicky, Associate Director
Kimberly Radant, Associate Director for Patient Care Services
Cathy Lee, Assistant Director
Since 1932, Richard L. Roudebush VA Medical Center has been improving the health of the men and women who have so proudly served our nation. We consider it our privilege to serve your health care needs in any way we can. Services are available to more than 196,000 veterans living in a 45-county area of Indiana and Illinois.

5534 **VA North Indiana Health Care System: Fort Wayne Campus**
Veterans Health Administration, U S Dept. of V A
2121 Lake Ave
Fort Wayne, IN 46805-5100 260-426-5431
800-360-8387
e-mail: g.vhacss@forum.va.gov
www.northernindiana.va.gov
Denise M. Deitzen, Medical Center Director
Audrey L. Frison, MHA, RN, Associate Director
Helen Rhodes MPA, RN, Associate Director for Operations
Ajay Dhawan MD FACHE, Chief of Staff
The Fort Wayne Campus offers primary and secondary medical and surgical services. Primary care clinics are available at both medical center campuses and at Community Based Outpatient Clinics (CBOCs) located in South Bend, Goshen, Peru and Muncie Indiana. Recently completed renovations and construction, and continuous maintenance, ensure an attractive, state-of-the-art healthcare environment.

5535 **VA Northern Indiana Health Care System: Marion Campus**
Veterans Health Administration, U S Dept. of V A
1700 E 38th St
Marion, IN 46953-4568 765-674-3321
800-360-8387
e-mail: g.vhacss@forum.va.gov
www.northernindiana.va.gov
Denise M. Deitzen, Medical Center Director
Audrey L. Frison, MHA, RN, Associate Director
Helen Rhodes MPA, RN, Associate Director for Operations
Ajay Dhawan MD FACHE, Chief of Staff
The Marion Campus offers a full range of mental health, nursing home care, and extended care services. Primary care clinics are available at both medical center campuses and at Community Based Outpatient Clinics (CBOCs) located in South Bend, Goshen, Peru and Muncie Indiana.

Iowa

5536 **Des Moines VA Medical Center**
Veterans Health Administration, U S Dept. of V A
3600 30th St
Des Moines, IA 50310-5753 515-699-5999
800-294-8387
FAX: 515-699-5862
e-mail: g.vhacss@forum.va.gov
www.centraliowa.va.gov
Donald Cooper, Director
Susan Martin, Associate Director for Resources and Operations
Tammy Neff, RN, MBA, MSN, M, Acting Associate Director for Patient Services/Nurse Executi
Fredrick Bahls, MD, Chief of Staff
The VA Central Iowa Health Care System (VACIHCS) operates a Veterans Health Administration (VHA) medical facility in Des Moines, with Community Based Outpatient Clinics (CBOCs) in Mason City, Fort Dodge, Knoxville, Marshalltown and Carroll. The medical center provides acute and specialized medical and

surgical services, residential outpatient treatment programs in substance abuse and post-traumatic stress and a full range of mental health and long-term care services, as well as sub-acute and r

5537 Des Moines VA Regional Office
Veterans Benefits Administration, U S Dept. of V A
210 Walnut Street
Des Moines, IA 50309-2115
515-323-7580
800-827-1000
FAX: 515-323-7580
e-mail: leander@vba.va.gov
www.va.gov

Rich Anderson, Service Director

The Des Moines VA Regional Office provides Compensation, Pension and Vocational Rehabilitation and Counseling services for all military veterans in the State of Iowa. The Des Moines VA Regional Office currently provides approximately $260 million in benefits to the approximately 270,000 veterans in Iowa.

5538 Iowa City VA Medical Center
Veterans Health Administration, U S Dept. of V A
601 Highway 6 West
Iowa City, IA 52240-2202
319-338-0581
800-637-0128
866-687-7382
FAX: 319-339-7171
e-mail: g.vhacss@forum.va.gov
www.iowacity.va.gov

Barry Sharp, Director
Timothy McMurry, Associate Director for Operations
Dawn Oxley, RN, Associate Director Patient Care Services/Nurse Executive
Stanley Parker, MD, Acting Chief of Staff

Tertiary care facility, affiliated teaching hospital, and research center seving an aging veteran populatiaon in eastern Iowa and western Illinois. Satellite clinics are located in Bettendord, Dubuque, and Waterloo, Iowa and in Quincy and Galesburg, Illinois.

5539 Knoxville VA Medical Center
Veterans Health Administration, U S Dept. of V A
1515 W Pleasant St
Knoxville, IA 50138-3399
641-842-3101
800-816-8878
FAX: 641-828-5124
e-mail: g.vhacss@forum.va.gov
www.centraliowa.va.gov

Claudia M Kicklighter

5540 VA Central Iowa Health Care System
3600 30th St
Des Moines, IA 50310-5753
515-699-5999
800-294-8387
FAX: 515-699-5862
www.centraliowa.va.gov

Donald Cooper, Director
Susan Martin, Associate Director for Resources and Operations
Tammy Neff, RN, MBA, MSN, M, Acting Associate Director for Patient Services/Nurse Executi
Fredrick Bahls, MD, Chief of Staff

The VA Central Iowa Health Care System (VACIHCS) operates a Veterans Health Administration (VHA) medical facility in Des Moines, with Community Based Outpatient Clinics (CBOCs) in Mason City, Fort Dodge, Knoxville, Marshalltown and Carroll. The medical center provides acute and specialized medical and surgical services, residential outpatient treatment programs in substance abuse and post-traumatic stress and a full range of mental health and long-term care services, as well as sub-acute and r

Kansas

5541 Colmery-O'Neil VA Medical Center
Veterans Health Administration, U S Dept. of V A
2200 SW Gage Blvd
Topeka, KS 66622
785-350-3111
800-574-8387
e-mail: g.vhacss@forum.va.gov
www.topeka.va.gov

A. Rudy Klopfer, FACHE, Director
John Moon, Associate Director
Nelson L. Dean, RN, BSN, MA, Associate Director for Patient Care Services
Christine M Kleckner, MBA, RD, Assistant Director

Since 1946, the staff of the Colmery-O'Neil VA Medical Center has been serving veterans. Today, we proudly serve our nation's veterans with excellent health care as part of the VA Eastern Kansas Health Care System (VAEKHCS). We consider it our privilege to serve your health care needs in any way we can.

5542 Dwight D Eisenhower VA Medical Center
Veterans Health Administration, U S Dept. of V A
4101 4th Street Trafficway
Leavenworth, KS 66048-5014
913-682-2000
800-952-8387
e-mail: g.vhacss@forum.va.gov
www.leavenworth.va.gov

A. Rudy Klopfer, FACHE, Director
John Moon, Associate Director
Nelson L. Dean, RN, BSN, MA, Associate Director for Patient Care Services
Christine M Kleckner, MBA, RD, Assistant Director

Since 1886, the staff of the Dwight D. Eisenhower VA Medical Center has been serving veterans. Today, we proudly serve our nation's veterans with excellent health care as part of the VA Eastern Kansas Health Care System (VAEKHCS). We consider it our privilege to serve your health care needs in any way we can.

5543 Kansas VA Regional Office
Veterans Benefits Administration, U S Dept. of V A
5500 E Kellogg Dr
Wichita, KS 67218-1607
800-827-1000
e-mail: wichita.query@vba.va.gov
www.benefits.va.gov/wichita

Edgar L Tucker, Medical Center Director

5544 Robert J Dole VA Medical Center
Veterans Health Administration, U S Dept. of V A
5500 E Kellogg Dr
Wichita, KS 67218-1607
316-685-2221
800-827-1000
888-827-6881
FAX: 316-651-3666
e-mail: g.vhacss@forum.va.gov
www.wichita.va.gov

Kevin Inkley, MA, Director
Vicki Bondie, MBA, Associate Director
Carol A. Kaster, MA, RN, Associate Director of Patient Care/Nurse Executive
M. Ganga Hematillake, MD, Chief of Staff

For over 70 years, the Dole VA Medical and Regional office center has been honored to serve Kansas area veterans. The center provides a full range of primary and specialty acute and extended care services to veterans in 59 counties of Kansas. Special emphasis programs include substance abuse, post traumatic stress disorder (PTSD), women's health, spinal cord injury, visual impairment, prosthetic and sensory aids, and homeless services.

Kentucky

5545 Lexington VA Medical Center
Veterans Health Administration, U S Dept. of V A
1101 Veterans Dr
Lexington, KY 40502-2235
859-281-4900
800-352-4000
e-mail: g.vhacss@forum.va.gov
www.lexington.va.gov

Martin J. Traxler, Acting Medical Center Director
Patricia Breeden, MD, Acting Chief of Staff
Laura Faulkner, Acting Associate Medical Center Director
Agnes Therady, RN, NEA-BC, F, Acting Associate Director Patient Care Services

The Lexington Veterans Affairs Medical Center is a fully accredited, two-division, tertiary care medical center with an operating bed complement of 199 hospital beds. Acute medical, neurological, surgical and psychiatric inpatient services are provided at the Cooper Division, located adjacent to the University of Kentucky Medical Center. Other available services include: emergency care, medical-surgical units, acute psychiatry, ICU, progressive care unit, (includes Cardiac Cath Lab) ambulatory s

5546 Louisville VA Medical Center
Veterans Health Administration, U S Dept. of V A
800 Zorn Ave
Louisville, KY 40206-1433
502-287-4000
800-376-8387
e-mail: g.vhacss@forum.va.gov
www.louisville.va.gov

Wayne L. Pfeffer, MHSA, FACHE, Medical Center Director
Douglas V Paxton, Sr, Associate Director / Operations
Pamala Thompson, RN, MSA, MSN, Associate Director for Patient Care Services
Marylee Rothschild, M.D., Chief of Staff

Since 1952, Robley Rex VAMC has been improving the health of the men and women who have so proudly served our nation. We consider it our privilege to serve your health care needs in any way we can. Services are available to more than 166,000 veterans living in a 35-county area of the Kentuckiana area.

5547 Louisville VA Regional Office
Veterans Benefits Administration, U S Dept. of V A
800 Zorn Avenue
Louisville, KY 40206-1433
502-287-4000
800-376-8387
e-mail: louisville.query@vba.va.gov
www.louisville.va.gov

Wayne L. Pfeffer, MHSA, FACHE, Medical Center Director
Douglas V Paxton, Sr, Associate Director / Operations
Pamala Thompson, RN, MSA, MSN, Associate Director for Patient Care Services
Marylee Rothschild, M.D., Chief of Staff

Since 1952, Robley Rex VAMC has been improving the health of the men and women who have so proudly served our nation. We consider it our privilege to serve your health care needs in any way we can. Services are available to more than 166,000 veterans living in a 35-county area of the Kentuckiana area.

Louisiana

5548 Alexandria VA Medical Center
Department of Veterans Affairs
2495 Shreveport Highway
Pineville, LA 71360-9004
318-466-4000
800-375-8387
FAX: 318-483-5029
e-mail: richard.wright2@va.gov
www.alexandria.va.gov

Martin J. Traxler, Medical Center Director
Yolanda Sanders-Jackson, Associate Director
Jose N Rivera, MD, Acting Chief of Staff
Amy Lesniewski, RN MS, Nurse Executive

The VAMC Alexandria is categorized as a primary and secondary care facility. It is a teaching hospital, providing a full range of primary care services with state-of-the-art technology and education. Comprehensive acute and extended health care is provided on a primary and secondary basis in areas of medicine, surgery, psychiatry, physical medicine and rehabilitation, neurology, oncology, dentistry, geriatrics, and extended care. The Medical Center serves a potential veteran population of over 1

5549 New Orleans VA Medical Center
Veterans Health Administration, U S Dept. of V A
1601 Perdido St
New Orleans, LA 70112-1262
504-412-3700
800-935-8387
FAX: 504-589-5210
e-mail: Stacie.Rivera@med.va.gov
www.neworleans.va.gov

John D Church Jr, Medical Director/President
Fernando Rivera, Association Medical Center Direc
Sam Lucero, Special Assistant to Director
Stacie M Rivera, Public Affairs Officer

A teaching hospital, providing a full range of patient care services, with state-of-the-art technology as well as education and research. Comprehensive health care is provided through primary care, tetiary care, and long-term care in areas of medicine, surgery, psychiatry, physical medicine and rehabilitation, neurology, oncology, dentistry, geriatrics, and extended care.

5550 Shreveport VA Medical Center
Veterans Health Administration, U S Dept. of V A
510 E Stoner Ave
Shreveport, LA 71101-4295
318-221-8411
800-827-1000
www.shreveport.va.gov

Shirley M. Bealer, Medical Center Director
Todd M. Moore, Assistant Medical Center Director
Erik J. Glover, Associate Medical Center Director
Ruth Davis, DNS, Associate Director for Patient Care Services

Maine

5551 Maine VA Regional Office
Veterans Benefits Administration, U S Dept. of V A
1 VA Center
Augusta, ME 4330-6719
207-623-8411
877-421-8263
e-mail: togus.query@vba.va.gov
www.va.gov

Dale Demers, Director
Scott Karczewski, Manager

5552 Togus VA Medical Center
Veterans Health Administration, U S Dept. of V A
1 VA Center
Augusta, ME 04330-6795
207-623-8411
877-421-8263
FAX: 207-623-5792
e-mail: g.vhacss@forum.va.gov
www.togus.va.gov

Scott Karczewski, Regional Office Director
Denise Benson, Veterans Sevice Center Manager
Gregg Morin, Assistant Veterans Service Center Manager
Tracy Sinclair, Support Services Chief

Maryland

5553 Baltimore Regional Office
Veterans Benefits Administration, U S Dept. of V A
31 Hopkins Plz
Baltimore, MD 21201-2825
800-827-1000
e-mail: baltimore.query@vba.va.gov
www.va.gov

Jerry L Calhoun

The Baltimore Regional Office serves 484,013 veterans living in the State of Maryland, 2% of the national veteran population. The Regional Office's jurisdiction includes all counties in the State of Maryland. The Baltimore Regional Office has an assigned staffing of 218. We provide services at the VA Medical Center in Baltimore and Transition Assistance throughout the State. We actively participate in a homeless veterans outreach program based at the Maryland Center for the Veterans Educatio

5554 Baltimore VA Medical Center
Veterans Health Administration, U S Dept. of V A
10 N Greene St
Baltimore, MD 21201-1524 410-605-7000
800-463-6295
FAX: 410-605-7901
e-mail: g.vhacss@forum.va.gov
www.maryland.va.gov

Dennis H. Smith, Director
Nancy Quailey-Giannopoulis, Associate Director for Operations
Frederick P. Soetje, Associate Director for Finance
David O. Barrett, Acting Chief of Staff

The Baltimore Medical Center is nationally recognized for its outstanding patient safety and state-of-the-art technology, the VA Maryland Health Care System is proud of its reputation as a leader in veterans' health care, research and education.

5555 Fort Howard VA Medical Center
Veterans Health Administration, U S Dept. of V A
9600 N Point Rd
Fort Howard, MD 21052-3050 410-477-1800
800-351-8387
FAX: 410-477-7177
e-mail: md.veterans@erols.com
www.mdva.state.md.us

Thomas Hutchins, Secretary

5556 Maryland Veterans Centers
10 N Greene St
Baltimore, MD 21201-1524 410-605-7000
800-463-6295
FAX: 410-605-7901
www.maryland.va.gov

J Y Jacks, Manager
Dennis H Smith, Executive Director

Veterans medical clinic offering disabled veterans medical treatments.

5557 Perry Point VA Medical Center
Veterans Health Administration, U S Dept. of V A
Circle Drive
Perry Point, MD 21902 410-642-2411
800-949-1003
FAX: 410-642-1165
e-mail: g.vhacss@forum.va.gov
www.maryland.va.gov

Dennis H. Smith, Director
Nancy Quailey-Giannopoulis, Associate Director for Operations
Frederick P. Soetje, Associate Director for Finance
David O. Barrett, Acting Chief of Staff

It is nationally recognized for its outstanding patient safety and state-of-the-art technology, the VA Maryland Health Care System is proud of its reputation as a leader in veterans' health care, research and education.

5558 VA Maryland Health Care System
10 N Greene St
Baltimore, MD 21201-1524 410-605-7000
800-463-6295
FAX: 410-605-7900
www.maryland.va.gov

Dennis H. Smith, Director
Nancy Quailey-Giannopoulis, Associate Director for Operations
Frederick P. Soetje, Associate Director for Finance
David O. Barrett, Acting Chief of Staff

A dynamic and exciting health care organization that is dedicated to providing quality, compassionate and accessible care and service to Maryland's veterans. As a part of one of the largest health care systems in the United States, the VAMHCS has a reputation as a leader in veterans' health care, reserch and education. Provides comprehensive service to veterans including medical, surgical, rehabilitative, nurological and mental health care on both an inpatient and outpatient basis.

Massachusetts

5559 Boston VA Regional Office
Veterans Benefits Administration, U S Dept. of V A
15 New Sudbury Street
JFK Bldg
Boston, MA 2203-9928 617-232-9500
800-827-1000
e-mail: boston.query@vba.va.gov
www.boston.va.gov

Liza Catucci, Administrative Officer
Michael Lawson, President

5560 Edith Nourse Rogers Memorial Veterans Hospital
Veterans Health Administration U S Deptartment of
200 Springs Rd Bldg #23
Bedford, MA 1730-1114 781-687-2000
800-827-1000
FAX: 781-687-3536
e-mail: g.vhacss@forum.va.gov
www.bedford.va.gov

Michael Mayo-Smith, Manager

5561 Northampton VA Medical Center
Veterans Health Administration, U S Dept. of V A
421 N Main St
Leeds, MA 1062 413-584-4040
800-827-1000
e-mail: g.vhacss@forum.va.gov
www.northhampton.va.gov

Richard Woloss, Manager

5562 VA Boston Healthcare System: Brockton Division
Veterans Health Administration, U S Dept. of V A
940 Belmont St
Brockton, MA 02301-5596 508-583-4500
800-865-3384
FAX: 617-323-7700
e-mail: g.vhacss@forum.va.gov
www.boston.va.gov

Vincent Ng, Acting Director
Susan A. MacKenzie, PhD, Associate Director
Cecilia McVey, BSN, MHA, CAN, Associate Director Nursing & Patient Care Services

VA Boston Healthcare System's consolidated facility consists of the Jamaica Plain campus, located in the heart of Boston's Longwood Medical Community; the West Roxbury campus, located on the Dedham line; and the Brockton campus, located 20 miles south of Boston in the City of Brockton.

5563 VA Boston Healthcare System: Jamaica Plain Campus
Veterans Health Administration, U S Dept. of V A
150 S Huntington Ave
Boston, MA 2130-4817 617-232-9500
800-865-3384
FAX: 617-278-4549
e-mail: g.vhacss@forum.va.gov
www.boston.va.gov

Vincent Ng, Acting Director
Susan A. MacKenzie, PhD, Associate Director
Cecilia McVey, BSN, MHA, CAN, Associate Director Nursing & Patient Care Services

VA Boston Healthcare System's consolidated facility consists of the Jamaica Plain campus, located in the heart of Boston's Longwood Medical Community; the West Roxbury campus, located on the Dedham line; and the Brockton campus, located 20 miles south of Boston in the City of Brockton.

5564 **VA Boston Healthcare System: West Roxbury Division**
Veterans Health Administration, U S Dept. of V A
1400 VFW Pkwy
West Roxbury, MA 2132-4927 617-323-7700
800-865-3384
e-mail: g.vhacss@forum.va.gov
www.boston.va.gov

Susan A Mac Kenzie, Associate Director

VA Boston Healthcare System's consolidated facility consists of the Jamaica Plain campus, located in the heart of Boston's Longwood Medical Community; the West Roxbury campus, located on the Dedham line; and the Brockton campus, located 20 miles south of Boston in the City of Brockton.

Michigan

5565 **Aleda E Lutz VA Medical Center**
Veterans Health Administration, U S Dept. of V A
1500 Weiss St
Saginaw, MI 48602-5251 989-497-2500
800-827-1000
FAX: 989-791-2428
e-mail: g.vhacss@forum.va.gov
www.saginaw.va.gov

Jeff Nechanicky, Acting Medical Center Director
Stephanie Young, Associate Director
Penny Holland, R.N., MSN, Associate Director for Patient Care Svcs
Robert W. Dorr, D.O., JD, CHCQM,, Chief of Staff

Since 1950, the Aleda E. Lutz VA Medical Center has been improving the health of the men and women who have so proudly served our nation. We consider it our privilege to serve your health care needs in any way we can. Services are available to more than 31,000 veterans living in the Central and Northern 35 counties of Michigan's Lower Peninsula.

5566 **Battle Creek VA Medical Center**
Veterans Health Administration, U S Dept. of V A
5500 Armstrong Rd
Battle Creek, MI 49037-7314 269-966-5600
888-214-1247
888-214-1247
FAX: 269-966-5483
e-mail: g.vhacss@forum.va.gov
www.battlecreek.va.gov

Mary Beth Skupien, Director
Edward Dornoff, Associate Director
Kay Bower, Associate Director for Patient Care Services
Dr. Shah, Acting Chief of Staff

Since 1924, the Battle Creek, Michigan VA Medical Center has been improving the health of the men and women who have so proudly served our nation. The Battle Creek VA Medical Center consists of 104 medical and psychiatric beds, 32 residential rehabilitation beds, and 103 nursing home care unit beds. In addition, specialized services offered include a Palliative Care Unit, a Substance Abuse Clinic, a Post Traumatic Stress Disorder Program and a Domiciliary.

5567 **Iron Mountain VA Medical Center**
Veterans Health Administration, U S Dept. of V A
325 East H Street
Iron Mountain, MI 49801-4760 906-774-3300
800-827-1000
FAX: 906-779-3114
e-mail: g.vhacss@forum.va.gov
www.ironmountain.va.gov

James W. Rice, Medical Center Director
William Caron, FACHE, Associate Medical Center Director
Andrea Collins, RN, MSN, Associate Director for Nursing and Patient Care Service
Grace L. Stringfellow, M.D., Chief of Staff

OGJVAMC is a primary and secondary level care facility with 17 acute care beds, 13 in the medical/surgical ward and 4 in the intensive care unit (ICU). The main facility provides limited emergency and acute inpatient care, and collaborates with larger VA Medical Centers in Milwaukee and Madison, WI, to provide higher-level emergency and specialty care services. OGJVAMC also provides rehabilitation and extended care, including palliative and hospice care, in its 40-bed Community Living Center.

5568 **John D Dingell VA Medical Center**
Veterans Health Administration, U S Dept. of V A
4646 John R St
Detroit, MI 48201-1916 313-576-1000
800-827-1000
FAX: 313-576-1112
e-mail: g.vhacss@forum.va.gov
www.detroit.va.gov

Pamela J. Reeves, M.D., Director
Annette Walker, M.S.H.A., B.S., Associate Director
Ann M. Herm, R.N., B.S.N., M., Associate Director, Patient Care Services
Scott A. Gruber, M.D., Ph.D.,, Chief of Staff

Our mission is to provide timely, compassionate and high quality care to those we serve by encouraging teamwork, education, research, innovation, and continuous improvement.

5569 **Michigan VA Regional Office**
Veterans Benefits Administration, U S Dept. of V A
477 Michigan Ave
Patrick V McNamara Federal Building
Detroit, MI 48226-1217 800-827-1000
e-mail: detroit.query@vba.va.gov
www.benefits.va.gov/detroit

David Leonard, Director
Dennis W Paradowski, Assistant Director

The Regional Office Staff are dedicated to providing responsive and timely service to the veterans of Michigan and their families. Their duties include processing and making decisions on claims for disability compensation, and assisting with applications for a wide range of VA benefits.

5570 **VA Ann Arbor Healthcare System**
Veterans Health Administration, U S Dept. of V A
2215 Fuller Rd
Ann Arbor, MI 48105-2303 734-769-7100
800-361-8387
FAX: 734-761-7870
e-mail: g.vhacss@forum.va.gov
www.annarbor.va.gov

Robert P. McDivitt, FACHE, Director
Randall E. Ritter, Associate Director
Stacey Breedveld, R.N., Associate Director Patient Care
Ginny Creasman, Assistant Director

Since 1953, the VA Ann Arbor Healthcare System (VAAAHS) has provided state-of-the-art healthcare services to the men and women who have so proudly served our nation. We consider it our privilege to serve your healthcare needs in any way we can.

5571 **Vet Center Readjustment Counseling Service**
1940 Eastern Ave SE
Grand Rapids, MI 49507-2771 616-285-5795
800-905-4675
FAX: 616-285-5898
www.va.gov

William Busby, Executive Director
Branden K Lyon, Counselor
Lynn Hall, Clinical Coordinator

Providing a broad range of counseling outreach and referral services to eligible veterans in order to help make readjustments to cilvilian life.

Minnesota

5572 Minneapolis VA Medical Center
Veterans Health Administration, U S Dept. of V A
1 Veterans Dr
Minneapolis, MN 55417-2399
612-725-2000
866-414-5058
FAX: 612-725-2049
e-mail: g.vhacss@forum.va.gov
www.minneapolis.va.gov

Judy Johnson-Mekota, Director
Erik J. Stalhandske, Associate Director
Kent Crossley, Chief of Staff
Helen Pearlman, Nurse Executive

Minneapolis VA Health Care System (VAHCS) is a teaching hospital providing a full range of patient care services with state-of-the-art technology, as well as education and research. Comprehensive health care is provided through primary care, tertiary care and long-term care in areas of medicine, surgery, psychiatry, physical medicine and rehabilitation, neurology, oncology, dentistry, geriatrics and extended care.

5573 St. Cloud VA Medical Center
Veterans Health Administration, U S Dept. of V A
4801 Veterans Dr
Saint Cloud, MN 56303-2015
320-252-1670
800-247-1739
FAX: 320-255-6472
e-mail: g.vhacss@forum.va.gov
www.stcloud.va.gov

Barry I. Bahl, Director
Cheryl Thieschafer, Associate Director
Meri Hauge, BSN, MSN Nurse, Executive/Associate Director for Patient Care Services
Susan Markstrom, MD, Chief of Staff

Specialty care services include audiology, cardiology, dentistry, hematology, oncology, optometry, orthopedics, podiatry, pulmonology, urology and rheumatology. A new Ambulatory Surgery (same-day) Center opened in the fall of 2011 and will provide access to additional outpatient surgical procedures. The medical center offers extensive mental health programming, including acute psychiatric care, Residential Rehabilitation Treatment programs and an outpatient mental health clinic. The programs u

5574 St. Paul Regional Office
Veterans Benefits Administration, U S Dept. of V A
1 Federal Dr
Fort Snelling, MN 55111-4080
800-827-1000
e-mail: stpaul.query@vba.va.gov
www.benefits.va.gov/stpaul

Vincent Crawford, Director

5575 Vet Center
405 E Superior St
Ste 160
Duluth, MN 55802-2240
218-722-8654
877-927-8387
FAX: 218-723-8212
www.vetcenter.va.gov

Cynthia Macaulay MEd, Counselor
Rob Evanson, Counselor
Debbie Burt, Office Manager

Counseling, social services and benefits assistance for combat veterans and those sexually traumatized in the military.

Mississippi

5576 Biloxi/Gulfport VA Medical Center
Veterans Health Administration, U S Dept. of V A
400 Veterans Ave
Biloxi, MS 39531-2410
228-523-5000
800-296-8872
FAX: 228-563-2898
e-mail: g.vhacss@forum.va.gov
www.biloxi.va.gov

Anthony L. Dawson, Director
Nancy Weaver, Associate Director
Kenneth Shimon, Chief of Staff
Margaret G Givens, Assciate Director

5577 Jackson Regional Office
Veterans Benefits Administration, U S Dept. of V A
1600 E Woodrow Wilson Ave
Jackson, MS 39216-5100
601-364-7000
800-827-1000
FAX: 601-364-7007
e-mail: jackson.query@vba.va.gov
www.benefits.va.gov/jackson

Neil Anthony Mcphie, Chairman
Barbara Sapin, Vice Chairman

Missouri

5578 Harry S Truman Memorial Veterans' Hospital
Veterans Health Administration, U S Dept. of V A
800 Hospital Dr
Columbia, MO 65201-5275
573-814-6000
800-827-1000
FAX: 573-814-6551
e-mail: g.vhacss@forum.va.gov
www.columbiamo.va.gov

Sallie Houser-Hanfelder, Director
Robert Ritter, Associate Director
Lana Zerrer, Chief of Staff

5579 John J Pershing VA Medical Center
Veterans Health Administration, U S Dept. of V A
1500 N Westwood Blvd
Poplar Bluff, MO 63901-3318
573-686-4151
888-557-8262
FAX: 573-778-4156
e-mail: g.vhacss@forum.va.gov
www.poplarbluff.va.gov

Merk Hedstrom, Medical Center Director
Linda Haga, Research Contact

5580 Kansas City VA Medical Center
Veterans Health Administration, U S Dept. of V A
4801 E Linwood Blvd
Kansas City, MO 64128-2226
816-861-4700
800-827-1000
e-mail: g.vhacss@forum.va.gov
www.kansascity.va.gov

Kenneth Grasing, Research/Development
Ram Sharma, Administrative Officer
Kent Hill, Executive Director

The Kansas City VA Medical Center is a modern, well-equipped teriary care inpatient and outpatient center. As the third largest teaching hospital in the metropolitan area, it maintains educational affiliations with the University of Kansas School of Medicine.

5581 **St. Louis Regional Office**
Veterans Benefits Administration, U S Dept. of V A
400 S 18th St
Saint Louis, MO 63103-2265
800-827-1000
e-mail: stlouis.query@vba.va.gov
www.stlouis.va.gov

5582 **St. Louis VA Medical Center**
Veterans Health Administration, U S Dept. of V A
915 N Grand Blvd
Saint Louis, MO 63106-1621
314-652-4100
800-228-5459
FAX: 314-289-7009
e-mail: g.vhacss@forum.va.gov
www.stlouis.va.gov
Dolores Minor, Administrative Officer

Montana

5583 **Montana VA Regional Office**
3633 Veterans Drive
Fort Harrison, MT 59636-188
406-442-7310
800-827-1000
www.va.gov

5584 **V A Montana Healthcare System**
U S Dept. of V A
3687 Veterans Drive
PO Box 1500
Fort Harrison, MT 59636-1500
406-442-6410
877-468-8387
FAX: 406-447-7916
e-mail: ftharrison.query@vba.va.gov
www.montana.va.gov
Christine Gregory, Director
Vicki Thennis, Interim Associate Director
Trena Bonde, Chief of Staff
Norlynn Nelson, Associate Director for Patient Care
This is a complete, medically reliable dictionary of congenital malformations and disorders. As the authors explain, 'Down syndrome is the only common congenital disorder, the other defects and disorders are rare or very rare, some having been reported fewer than 20 times worlwide.' This dictionary covers them all. Examples: Aagenaes syndrome, Acrocallosal syndrome, and Acrodysostosis

5585 **VA Montana Healthcare System**
Veterans Health Administration, U S Dept. of V A
1892 William St
Fort Harrison, MT 59636
406-447-7945
800-827-1000
FAX: 406-447-7965
e-mail: g.vhacss@forum.va.gov
www.montana.va.gov
Joseph Underkofel, Executive Director
Gregory Johnson, MD

5586 **Vet Center**
Readjusment Counciling Service Western Mountain Re
2795 Enterprise Ave.
Suite 1
Billings, MT 59102-3238
406-657-6071
FAX: 406-657-6603
www.va.gov
Bob Phillips, Manager
Luanne Anderson, Office Manager
Barry Osgard MS, Counselor
Readjustment counseling service for counseling veterans who are having difficulty adjusting from military service especially those diagnosed with PTSD.

Nebraska

5587 **Grand Island VA Medical System**
Veterans Health Administration, U S Dept. of V A
2201 N Broadwell Ave
Grand Island, NE 68803-2153
308-382-3660
866-580-1810
e-mail: g.vhacss@forum.va.gov
www.nebraska.va.gov/visitors/grand_island.asp
John Hilbert, Executive Director
Daniel L Parker, Deputy Director

5588 **Lincoln Regional Office**
Veterans Benefits Administration, U S Dept. of V A
3800 Village Dr.
Lincoln, NE 68501-4103
402-471-4444
800-827-1000
FAX: 402-479-5124
e-mail: lincoln.query@vba.va.gov
www.veteranprograms.com
Bill Gibson, CEO
Daniel Parker, Deputy Director

5589 **Lincoln VA Medical Center**
Veterans Health Administration, U S Dept. of V A
600 S 70th St
Lincoln, NE 68510-2451
402-489-3802
800-827-1000
FAX: 402-486-7860
e-mail: g.vhacss@forum.va.gov
www.nebraska.va.gov/visitors/lincoln.asp
Ryon L Adams, Research/Development Coordinator

5590 **VA Nebraska-Western Iowa Health Care System**
Veterans Health Administration, U S Dept. of V A
4101 Woolworth Ave
Omaha, NE 68105-1850
402-449-0610
800-451-5796
FAX: 402-449-0684
www.nebraska.va.gov
Marci Mylan, Director
Rowen Zetterman, Chief of Staff

Nevada

5591 **Las Vegas Veterans Center**
1919 S. Jones, Suite A
Las Vegas, NV 89146-905
702-251-7873
FAX: 702-388-6664
www.lasvegas.va.gov
Daryl Harding, Resident Counselor LCSW
Matt Watson, Team Leader MSW
Veterans clinical counseling center for veterans and their dependent individual and group counseling, marital and family counseling, alcohol and drug assessment referral or treatment. Community education and consultation, employment counseling.

5592 **Reno Regional Office**
Veterans Benefits Administration U S Deptartment o
1000 Locust St
Reno, NV 89502-2597
775-328-1486
800-827-1000
FAX: 775-328-1447
e-mail: reno.query@vba.va.gov
www.reno.va.gov
Joseph E Dardillo, Administrative Officer

5593 **VA Sierra Nevada Healthcare System**
Veterans Health Administration, U S Dept. of V A
957 Kirman Ave
Reno, NV 89502-2597 775-786-7200
888-838-6256
FAX: 775-328-1816
e-mail: https://iris.custhelp.com
www.reno.va.gov
Kurt W. Schlegelmich, Director
Michael C. Tadych, Associate Director
Rachel Crossley, Associate Director
Steve E. Brilliant, Chief of Staff

5594 **VA Southern Nevada Healthcare System**
Veterans Health Administration, U S Dept. of V A
6900 North Pecos Rd
Las Vegas, NV 89086 702-791-9000
800-827-1000
FAX: 707-636-3027
e-mail: g.vhacss@forum.va.gov
www.lasvegas.va.gov
Isabel M. Duff, Acting Director
Ramu Komanduri, Chief of Staff
Sandra L. Solem, Acting Nurse Executive
John L. Stelsel, Assistant Director

New Hampshire

5595 **Manchester Regional Office**
Veterans Benefits Administration, U S Dept. of V A
275 Chestnut St
Manchester, NH 3101-2411 800-827-1000
e-mail: manchester.query@vba.va.gov
www.va.gov
Jerry Beale, Director

5596 **Manchester VA Medical Center**
Veterans Health Administration, U S Dept. of V A
718 Smyth Rd
Manchester, NH 03104-7007 603-624-4366
800-892-8384
e-mail: g.vhacss@forum.va.gov
www.manchester.va.gov
Susan MacKenzie, Acting Med Center Director
Tammy A. Krueger, Associate Director
Andrew J. Breuder, Chief of Staff
Carol Williams, Associate Director for Patients

5597 **New Hampshire Veterans Centers**
103 Liberty St
Manchester, NH 3104-3118 603-668-7060
800-562-3127
FAX: 603-666-7404
www.va.gov
Caryl Ahern, Manager
Paulette Landry, Office Manager
Veterans clinic offering combat veterans outpatient counseling

New Jersey

5598 **Disabled American Veterans: Ocean County**
P.O.Box 1806
Toms River, NJ 8754-1806 732-929-0907
e-mail: bvenga@thecore.com
community.nj.com/cc/dav24
Mary Bencivenga, Contact

5599 **East Orange Campus of the VA New Jersey Healthcare System**
385 Tremont Ave
East Orange, NJ 07018-1023 973-676-1000
FAX: 973-676-4226
www.newjersey.va.gov
Kenneth Mizrach, Director
Glen Giaquinto, Associate Director
John A. Griffith, Associate Director
Patrick J. Troy, Nurse Executive

5600 **Lyons Campus of the VA New Jersey Healthcare System**
Veterans Health Administration, U S Dept. of V A
151 Knollcroft Rd
Lyons, NJ 7939-5001 908-647-0180
800-827-1000
FAX: 908-647-3452
e-mail: g.vhacss@forum.va.gov
www.newjersey.va.gov
James J Farsetta, Director
Donna Henderson, Coordinator

5601 **Newark Regional Office**
Veterans Benefits Administration, U S Dept. of V A
20 Washington Pl
Newark, NJ 07102-3174 973-645-1441
800-827-1000
e-mail: newark.query@vba.va.gov
www.newjersey.va.gov
Stephen G Abel, Deputy Commissioner for Veterans

New Mexico

5602 **New Mexico State Veterans' Home**
992 South Broadway
Truth or Consequences, NM 87901-927 575-894-4200
800-964-3976
FAX: 575-894-4270
www.nmveteranshome.org/index/shtml
Lori S Montgomery, Administrator
Carol B Wilson, Admission Coordinator
Veterans medical clinic offering disabled veterans medical treatments.

5603 **New Mexico VA Healthcare System**
Veterans Health Administration, US Dept. of VA
1501 San Pedro Dr SE
Albuquerque, NM 87108-5154 505-265-1711
800-465-8262
FAX: 505-256-2855
e-mail: g.vhacss@forum.va.gov
www.albuquerque.va.gov
George Marnell, Executive Director
Pamela Crowell, Acting Associate Director
Peter Woodbridge, Chief of Staff
Jennifer DeWinne, Acting Assistant Director

New York

5604 Albany VA Medical Center: Samuel S Stratton
Veterans Health Administration, U S Dept. of V A
113 Holland Ave
Albany, NY 12208-3410
518-626-5000
800-233-4810
888-838-7890
FAX: 518-626-5500
e-mail: g.vhacss@forum.va.gov
www.albany.va.gov

Donald W Stuart, Associate Director (Interim)
Linda W Weiss, Director
Laurdes Irzarry, Chief of Staff
Deborah Spath, Associate Director for Patient/N

5605 Albany Vet Center
Ste 2
17 Computer Dr W
Albany, NY 12205-1618
518-458-7998
FAX: 518-458-8613

Lloyd Mc Omber, Owner
Melodie Krahula, Team Leader

Provides readjustment counseling for combat veterans and also provides benefits and job counseling for all veterans.

5606 Bath VA Medical Center
Veterans Health Administration U S Deptartment of
76 Veterans Avenue
Bath, NY 14810
607-664-4000
877-845-3247
888-823-9659
FAX: 607-664-4000
e-mail: g.vhacss@forum.va.gov
www.bath.va.gov

Michael Swartz, Medical Center Director
David B. Krueger, Associate Director
Felipe Diaz, Chief of Staff
Shirley A. Pikula, Associate Director for Patient Services

5607 Bronx VA Medical Center
Veterans Health Administration, U S Dept. of V A
130 W Kingsbridge Rd
Bronx, NY 10468-9938
718-584-9000
800-877-6976
FAX: 718-733-1223
e-mail: g.vhacss@forum.va.gov
www.bronx.va.gov

Eric Langhoff, Director
Vincent F Immiti, Associate Director
Kathleen M. Capitulo, Chief of Staff
Kathleen M Capitulo, Associate Director for Patient C

5608 Brooklyn Campus of the VA NY Harbor Healthcare System
Veterans Health Administration, U S Dept. of V A
800 Poly Place
Brooklyn, NY 11209-7104
718-836-6600
800-827-1000
e-mail: g.vhacss@forum.va.gov
www.nyharbor.va.gov

Martina A Parauda, Director
Veronica J Foy, Associate Director, Facilities &
Michael S Simberkoff, Executive Chief of Staff
Elizabeth H Weinshel, Deputy Chief of Staff

5609 Buffalo Regional OfficeDepartment of Veterans Affairs
Veterans Benefits Administration
130 South Elmwood Avenue
Buffalo, NY 14202-2465
716-852-3028
800-827-1000
www.va.gov

5610 Canandiagua VA Medical Center
Veterans Health Administration, U S Dept. of V A
400 Fort Hill Ave
Canandaigua, NY 14424-1159
585-394-2000
800-204-9917
e-mail: g.vhacss@forum.va.gov
www.canandaigua.va.gov

Craig S Howard, Medical Center Director
Margaret Owens, Associate Director
Dr. Robert B Babcock, Chief of Staff
Patricia Hryzak Lind, Associate Director for Patient/N

5611 Castle Point Campus of the VA Hudson Valley Healthcare System
Veterans Health Administration, U S Dept. of V A
Route 9D
Castle Point, NY 12511
845-831-2000
800-827-1000
FAX: 845-838-5193
e-mail: g.vhacss@forum.va.gov
www.hudsonvalley.va.gov

Gerald F Culliton, Director
John M. Gary, Associate Director
Patricia A. Burke, Associate Director
Joanne J. Malina, Chief of Staff

5612 New York City Campus of the VA NY Harbor Healthcare System
Veterans Health Administration, U S Dept. of V A
423 E 23rd St
New York, NY 10010-5011
212-686-7500
800-827-1000
FAX: 718-567-4082
e-mail: g.vhacss@forum.va.gov
www.nyharbor.va.gov

Camille R Varacchi, Administrative Officer

5613 New York Regional Office
Veterans Benefits Administration, U S Dept. of V A
245 W Houston St
New York, NY 10014-4805
212-714-0699
800-827-1000
FAX: 212-807-4042
e-mail: newyork.query@vba.va.gov
www.va.gov

Ronna Brown, President

5614 Northport VA Medical Center
Veterans Health Administration, U S Dept. of V A
79 Middleville Rd
Northport, NY 11768-2296
631-261-4400
800-827-1000
FAX: 631-266-6710
e-mail: g.vhacss@forum.va.gov
www.northport.va.gov

Philip C Moschitta, Medical Center Director
Rosie A Chatman, Associate Director for Patient &
Maria Favale, Associate Director
Edward Mack, Chief of Staff

5615 Syracuse VA Medical Center
Veterans Health Administration, U S Dept. of V A
800 Irving Ave
Syracuse, NY 13210-2716
315-425-4400
800-792-4334
888-838-7890
e-mail: g.vhacss@forum.va.gov
www.syracuse.va.gov

James Cody, VA Medical Center Director
Judy Hayman, Associate Medical Center Director
William H Marx, Chief of Staff
Nancy Schmid, Associate Director for Patient/N

5616 **Torah Alliance of Families of Kids with Disabilities**
T AF KI D
1433 Coney Island Ave
Brooklyn, NY 11230-4119
718-252-2236
FAX: 718-252-2216
e-mail: tafkid@worldnet.att.net
www.tafkid.org

Juby Shapiro, Manager

Serves over 1k families whose children have a variety of disabilities and special needs. Many of these families are large families in the low socioeconomic level. Offers monthly meetings, guest lectures, parent matching, information of new developments in software, technology and techniques, sibling support groups, pen pal lists, audio and video library, alternative medicine and nutrition information and education on legal awareness and rights of disabled citizens.

5617 **VA Hudson Valley Health Care System**
Veterans Health Administration, U S Department of
2094 Albany Post Road
Montrose, NY 10548-1454
914-737-4400
FAX: 845-788-4244
www.hudsonvalley.va.gov

James J Farsette, Network Director
Michael Sabo, Executive Director

5618 **VA Western NY Healthcare System, Batavia**
Veterans Health Administration, U S Dept. of V A
222 Richmond Ave
Batavia, NY 14020-1227
585-297-1000
800-827-1000
FAX: 585-786-1258
e-mail: g.vhacss@forum.va.gov
www.va.gov

William F Feeley, Medical Center Director
Miguel Rainstein, Chief of Staff
Jason C Petti, Associate Medical Center Directo
Royce Calhoun, Assistant Director

5619 **VA Western NY Healthcare System, Buffalo**
Veterans Health Administration, U S Dept. of V A
3495 Bailey Ave
Buffalo, NY 14215-1129
716-834-9200
800-532-8387
www.buffalo.va.gov

Brian Stiller, Medical Center Director
Jason C. Petti, Chief of Staff
Royce Calhoun, Associate Medical Center Directo
Miguel Rainstein, Chief of Staff

North Carolina

5620 **Asheville VA Medical CenterCharles George**
Veterans Health Administration, U S Dept. of V A
1100 Tunnel Rd
Asheville, NC 28805-2043
828-298-7911
800-932-6408
FAX: 828-299-2502
e-mail: g.vhacss@forum.va.gov
www.asheville.va.gov

Cynthia Beyfogle, Executive Director
David A. Pattillo, Assistant Medical Director
James Wells, Chief of Staff
Dennis J. Mehring, Public Affairs Officer

5621 **Charlotte Vet Center**
2114 Ben Craig Drive
Charlotte, NC 28262-2350
704-549-8025
FAX: 704-549-8261
www.va.gov

Loretta Deaton, Team Leader
Cynthia Algra, Office Manager
Billy Moore, Counselor
Melissa L Saunders, Counsilor

Preadjustment Counseling for Combat Veterans with Post Traumatic Stress Disorder (PTSD).

5622 **Durham VA Medical Center**
Veterans Health Administration, U S Dept. of V A
508 Fulton St
Durham, NC 27705-3875
919-286-0411
800-827-1000
888-878-6890
FAX: 919-286-5944
e-mail: leola.jenkins@med.va.gov
www.durham.va.gov

Deanne M Seekins, Director
Rudy A Klopfer, Associate Director
John D Shelburne, Chief of Staff
Kathryn Ward-Presson, Associate Director for Nursing P

Since 1953, Durham Veterans Affairs Medical Cetner has been improving the health of the men and women who have so proudly served our nation. We consider it our privilege to serve your health care needs in any way we can. Services are available to more than 200,000 veterans living in a 26-county area of central and eastern North Carolina.

5623 **Fayetteville VA Medical Center**
Veterans Health Administration, U S Dept. of V A
2300 Ramsey St
Fayetteville, NC 28301-3856
910-488-2120
800-771-6106
FAX: 910-822-7926
e-mail: g.vhacss@forum.va.gov
www.va.gov

Elizabeth Goolsby, Director
James Galkowski, Associate Director, Operations
Jesse Howard III, Acting Chief of Staff
Joyce Alexander-Hines, Associate Director, Patient Care

Since 1940,the Fayetteville VA Medical Center (VAMC) hasimproved the health of the men and women who have so proudly served our nation. We consider it our privilege to serve your health care needs in any way we can. Medical, mental health, women's health careand specialty servicesare available to more than 157,000 veterans living in a 21-county area of North Carolina and South Carolina.

5624 **WG Hefner VA Medical CenterSalisbury**
Vet Health Administration U S Department of VA
1601 Brenner Ave
Salisbury, NC 28144-2515
704-638-9000
800-469-8252
FAX: 704-638-3395
e-mail: g.vhacss@forum.va.gov
www.salisbury.va.gov

Kaye Green, Director
Linette Barker, Associate Medical Center Directo
Subbarao Pemmaraju, Chief of Staff (Interim)
Michele Hilll, Associate Director for Patient C

Since 1953, Hefner VAMC has been improving the health of the men and women who have so proudly served our nation. We consider it our privilege to serve your health care needs in any way we can. Primary and secondary inpatient health care are available to more than 287,000 veterans living in a 24-county area of the Central Piedmont Region of North Carolina. This includes the Charlotte area with over 100,000 veterans, and the Winston-Salem area with 65,000 veterans.

5625 **Winston-Salem Regional Office**
Veterans Benefits Administration, U S Dept. of V A
251 N Main St
Winston-Salem, NC 27155-2 336-768-5560
800-827-1000
FAX: 336-768-7295
TTY: 800-829-4833
e-mail: winsalem.query@vba.va.gov
www.va.gov

Glenn Cobb, Executive VP

North Dakota

5626 **Fargo VA Medical Center**
Veterans Health Administration, U S Dept. of V A
2101 North Elm
Fargo, ND 58102-2417 701-232-3241
800-410-9723
FAX: 701-239-7166
e-mail: g.vhacss@forum.va.gov
www.va.gov

Michael J Murphy, Healthcare Center Director
Dale DeKrey, Associate Director for Operation
J Brian Hancock, Chief of Staff
Julie Bruhn, Associate Director for Patient C

5627 **North Dakota VA Regional OfficeFargo Regional Office**
Veterans Benefits Administration, U S Dept. of V A
2101 Elm St N
Fargo, ND 58102-2417 701-451-4690
800-410-9723
FAX: 701-451-4690
e-mail: fargo.query@vba.va.gov
www.fargo.va.gov

Thomas Santoro, Director Research Department

Ohio

5628 **Chillicothe VA Medical Center**
Veterans Health Administration, U S Dept. of V A
17273 State Route 104
Chillicothe, OH 45601-9718 740-773-1141
800-358-8262
888-838-6446
FAX: 740-772-7023
e-mail: g.vhacss@forum.va.gov
www.chillicothe.va.gov

Wendy J. Hepker, Medical Center Director
Keith Sullivan, Associate Medical Center Directo
Deborah M Meesig, Chief of Staff
Ruth Yerardi, Associate Director for Patient C

The Chillicothe VA Medical Center provides acute and chronic mental health services, primary and secondary medical services, a wide range of nursing home care services, specialty medical services as well as specialized women Veterans health clinics. The facility is an active ambulatory care setting and serves as a chronic mental health referral center for VA Medical Center in southern Ohio and parts of West Virginia and Kentucky

5629 **Cincinnati VA Medical Center**
Veterans Health Administration, U S Dept. of V A
3200 Vine St
Cincinnati, OH 45220-2213 513-861-3100
800-827-1000
888-267-7873
FAX: 513-475-6500
e-mail: g.vhacss@forum.va.gov
www.cincinnati.va.gov

Linda Smith, Director
David Ninneman, Associate Director
Robert Falcone, Chief of Staff
Katheryn Cook, Nurse Executive

5630 **Cleveland Regional Office**
Veterans Benefits Administration, U S Dept. of V A
1240 E 9th St
Cleveland, OH 44199-2068 800-827-1000
FAX: 216-522-8262
e-mail: cleveland.query@vba.va.gov
www.va.gov

P Hunter Peckham, Director
Robert Ruff, Assistant Director
William Bunkley, Minority Veterans Program Coordi

5631 **Dayton VA Medical Center**
Veterans Health Administration U S Department of V
4100 W 3rd St
Dayton, OH 45428-9000 937-268-6511
800-368-8262
888-838-6446
FAX: 937-262-2170
e-mail: g.vhacss@forum.va.gov
www.dayton.va.gov

Glenn Costie, Acting Director
Mark Murdock, Associate Director
James T. Hardy, Chief of Staff
Anna Jones, Associate Director, Patient Care

The Dayton VAMC is a state of the art teaching facility that has been serving Veterans for 146 years, having accepted its first patient in 1867. The Dayton VA Medical Center provides a full range of health care through medical, surgical, mental health (inpatient and outpatient), home and community health programs, geriatric (nursing home), physical medicine and therapy services, neurology, oncology, dentistry, and hospice.

5632 **Louis Stokes VA Medical CenterWade Park Campus**
Veterans Health Administration, U S Dept. of V A
10701 East Blvd
Cleveland, OH 44106-1702 216-791-3800
877-838-8262
888-838-6446
FAX: 440-838-6017
e-mail: g.vhacss@forum.va.gov
www.cleveland.va.gov

Susan M Fuehrer, Medical Center Director
Darwin Goodspeed, Associate Medical Center Director
Murray D. Altose, Chief of Staff
Inette Sarduy, Associate Director Patient

Oklahoma

5633 **Jack C. Montgomery VA Medical Center**
Veterans Benefits Administration, U S Dept. of V A
1011 Honor Heights Dr
Muskogee, OK 74401-1318 918-577-3000
800-827-1000
e-mail: muskogee.query@vba.va.gov
www.muskogee.va.gov

Alef Nancy Graham, Manager

5634 **Jack C. Montomery VA Medical Center**
1011 Honor Heights Dr
Muskogee, OK 74401-1318
918-577-3000
800-827-1000
e-mail: muskogee.query@vba.va.gov
www.muskogee.va.gov

James R. Floyd, Medical Director
Inez Reitz, Acting Associate Director
Thomas D. Schneider, Chief of Staff
Bonnie R Pierce, Associate Director for Patient C

5635 **Oklahoma City VA Medical Center**
Veterans Health Administration, U S Dept. of V A
921 NE 13th St
Oklahoma City, OK 73104-5007
405-456-1000
800-827-1000
FAX: 405-270-1560
www.oklahoma.va.gov

Jimmy A. Murphy, Director
Debra A. Colombe, Associate Director
Mark Huycke, Chief of Staff
Donna DeLise, Associate Director for Patient C

5636 **Oklahoma Veterans Centers Vet Center**
3033 N Walnut Ave
Ste W101
Oklahoma City, OK 73105-2833
405-270-5184
FAX: 405-270-5125

Peter Sharp, Manager
Steve Kenzie, Owner

PTSP counseling for all combat Veterans and victims of sexual trauma/sexual harassment.

Oregon

5637 **Oregon Health Sciences University**
3181 SW Sam Jackson Park Rd
Portland, OR 97239-3098
503-494-8311
ohsu.edu

Joe Robertson, President
James Morgan, Executive Director

Offers services for the totally blind, legally blind, visually impaired, mentally retarded blind and more with health, counseling, educational, recreational, rehabilitation, computer training and professional training services.

5638 **Portland Regional Office**
Veterans Benefits Administration, U S Dept. of V A
100 SW Main St, Floor 2
Portland, OR 97204-2802
503-373-2388
800-827-1000
e-mail: portland.query@vba.va.gov
www.va.gov

5639 **Portland VA Medical Center**
Veterans Health Administration, U S Dept. of V A
3710 SW U.S. Veterans Hospital Rd.
Portland, OR 97239-2964
503-220-8262
800-949-1004
FAX: 503-273-5319
e-mail: g.vhacss@forum.va.gov
www.portland.va.gov

John E Patrick, Director
David Stockwell, Deputy Director of Administratio
Tom Anderson, Chief of Staff
Kathleen M Chapman, Deputy Director for Patient Care

The Portland VA Medical Center (PVAMC) is a 303-bed consolidated facility with two main divisions. The medical center serves as the quaternary referral center for Oregon, Southern Washington, and parts of Idaho for the U.S. Department of Veterans Affairs. The Portland VAMC is located atop Marquam Hill on 28.5 acres overlooking the city of Portland. In addition to comprehensive medical and mental health services, the Portland VAMC supports ongoing research and medical education, including nati

5640 **Roseburg VA Medical Center**
Veterans Health Administration, U S Dept. of V A
913 NW Garden Valley Blvd
Roseburg, OR 97471-6523
541-440-1000
800-549-8387
FAX: 541-440-1225
e-mail: g.vhacss@forum.va.gov
www.roseburg.va.gov

Jim Willis, Director
Mark Traines, MD

5641 **Southern Oregon Rehabilitation Center & Clinics**
Veterans Health Administration, U S Dept. of V A
8495 Crater Lake Hwy
White City, OR 97503
541-826-2111
800-809-8725
FAX: 541-830-3500
e-mail: g.vhacss@forum.va.gov
www.southernoregon.va.gov

George Andries, Executive Director

Pennsylvania

5642 **Butler VA Medical Center**
Veterans Health Administration, U S Dept. of V A
325 New Castle Rd
Butler, PA 16001-2418
724-282-7171
800-362-8262
FAX: 724-282-7640
e-mail: g.vhacss@forum.va.gov
www.butler.va.gov

John Gennaro, Director
Rebecca Hubscher, Associate Director
Sharon Parson, Nurse Executive
Timothy Burke, Chief of Staff

VA Butler Healthcare is located in the heart of Butler County, on the bus line, and convenient to community support services for Western Pennsylvania and Eastern Ohio-area Veterans. We have been attending to Veterans' total care since 1947 and are the health care choice for over 18,000 Veterans - providing comprehensive Veteran care including primary, specialty, and mental health care - as well as health maintenance plans, management of chronic conditions and preventative medicine needs.

5643 **Coatesville VA Medical Center**
Veterans Health Administration, U S Dept. of V A
1400 Blackhorse Hill Rd
Coatesville, PA 19320-2040
610-384-7711
800-290-6172
888-558-3812
e-mail: g.vhacss@forum.va.gov
www.coatesville.va.gov

Gary Devansky, Director
Sheila Chelleppa, Chief of Staff
Nancy Schmid, Associate Director Patient Care
Jonathan Eckman, Associate Director

5644 **Erie VA Medical Center**
Veterans Health Administration, U S Dept. of V A
135 E 38th Street Blvd
Erie, PA 16504-1559
814-868-8661
800-274-8387
888-860-2124
FAX: 814-860-2425
e-mail: g.vhacss@forum.va.gov
www.erie.va.gov

Michael Adelman, Medical Center Director
Melissa Sundin, Associate Medical Center Directo
Dr. Anthony Behm, Chief of Staff
Dorene Sommers, Associate Director for Patient C

5645 **James E Van Zandt VA Medical Center**
Veterans Health Administration, U S Dept. of V A
2907 Pleasant Valley Blvd
Altoona, PA 16602-4377
814-943-8164
800-827-1000
FAX: 814-940-7898
e-mail: g.vhacss@forum.va.gov
www.va.gov
Cecil B Hengeveld, Director
Gerald Williams, Executive Director

5646 **Lebanon VA Medical Center**
Veterans Health Administration, U S Dept. of V A
1700 S Lincoln Ave
Lebanon, PA 17042-7597
717-272-6621
800-409-8771
FAX: 717-228-5907
e-mail: g.vhacss@forum.va.gov
www.lebanon.va.gov
Robert (Bob) Callahan Jr., Director
Robin C. Aube-Warren, Associate Director
Kanan Chatterjee, Chief of Staff
Margaret G Wilson, Associate Director for Patient C

5647 **Pennsylvania Veterans Centers**
Veterans Health Administration, U S Department of
135 E 38th St
Erie, PA 16504
814-868-8661
800-274-8387
FAX: 717-861-8589
www.erie.va.gov
Michael Aldeman, medical Center Director
Melissa Sundin, Associate Director
Anthony Behm, Chief of Staff
Veterans medical clinic offering disabled veterans medical treatments.

5648 **Philadelphia Regional Office and Insurance Center**
Veterans Benefits Administration, U S Dept. of V A
5000 Wissahickon Ave
Philadelphia, PA 19144-4867
215-336-3003
800-827-1000
FAX: 215-336-5542
e-mail: phillyro.query@vba.va.gov
www.va.gov
Sonny Dicrecchio, Executive Director

5649 **Philadelphia VA Medical Center**
Veterans Health Administration, U S Dept. of V A
3900 Woodland Avenue
Philadelphia, PA 19104
215-823-5800
800-949-1001
e-mail: g.vhacss@forum.va.gov
www.philadelphia.va.gov
Joseph M Dalpiaz, Director
Ralph Schapira, Chief of Staff
Margaret O'Shea Caplan, Associate Director for Finance
Patricia O'Kane, Acting Associate Director for Cl

5650 **Pittsburgh Regional Office**
Veterans Benefits Administration U S Deparment of
1000 Liberty Avenue
Pittsburgh, PA 15222
412-688-6100
800-827-1000
FAX: 412-688-6121
e-mail: pittsburgh.query@vba.va.gov
www.pittsburgh.va.gov
Micahel E Moreland

5651 **VA Pittsburgh Healthcare System, University Drive Division**
Veterans Health Administration, U S Dept. of V A
University Dr
Pittsburgh, PA 15240-2400
412-688-6000
866-482-7488
FAX: 412-688-6901
e-mail: g.vhacss@forum.va.gov
www.pittsburgh.va.gov
Timothy Mar Carlos, CEO

5652 **VA Pittsburgh Healthcare System, Highland Drive Division**
Veterans Health Administration, U S Dept. of V A
7180 Highland Dr
Pittsburgh, PA 15206-1206
412-688-6000
800-827-1000
FAX: 412-365-4213
e-mail: g.vhacss@forum.va.gov
www.pittsburgh.va.gov
Kristin Best, Deputy Adjutant General
Roger Sutton, MD

5653 **Wilkes-Barre VA Medical Center**
Veterans Health Administration, U S Dept. of V A
1111 E End Blvd
Wilkes Barre, PA 18711-30
570-824-3521
877-928-2621
FAX: 570-821-7278
e-mail: g.vhacss@forum.va.gov
www.wilkes-barre.va.gov
William H Mills, Director (Interim)
Douglas V Paxton Sr., Associate Director
Mirza Z Ali, Chief of Staff
Linda Stout, Associate Director for Nursing S

Rhode Island

5654 **Providence Regional Office**
Veterans Benefits Administration, U S Dept. of V A
380 Westminster St
Providence, RI 2903-3246
401-462-0324
800-827-1000
FAX: 401-254-2320
e-mail: providence.query@vba.va.gov
www.va.gov
Daniel Evangelista, Acting Associate Director

5655 **Providence VA Medical Center**
Veterans Health Administration, U S Dept. of V A
830 Chalkstone Ave
Providence, RI 02908-4799
401-273-7100
866-363-4486
FAX: 401-457-3360
e-mail: g.vhacss@forum.va.gov
www.providence.va.gov
Vincent W Ng, Medical Center Director
William J Burney, Medical Center Associate Directo
Gregory M Gillette, Medical Center Chief of Staff
Deborah A Clickner, Medical Center Associate Directo
To fulfill President Lincoln's promise To care for him who shall have borne the battle, and for his widow, and his orphan by serving and honoring the men and women who are America's veterans.

South Carolina

5656 Columbia Regional Office
Veterans Benefits Administration, U S Dept. of V A
6437 Garners Ferry Rd
Columbia, SC 29209-2401
803-401-1094
800-827-1000
e-mail: columbia.query@vba.va.gov
www.va.gov

Jimmie Ruff, Executive Director

5657 Ralph H Johnson VA Medical Center
Veterans Health Administration, U S Dept. of V A
109 Bee St
Charleston, SC 29401-5703
843-577-5011
800-827-1000
888-878-6884
FAX: 843-876-5384
e-mail: g.vhacss@forum.va.gov
www.charleston.va.gov

Carolyn L Adams, Director
Scott Isaacks, Associate Director
Florence N Hutchinson, Chief of Staff
Mary C Fraggos, Associate Director for Patient/N

5658 William Jennings Bryan Dorn VA Medical Center
Veterans Health Administration U S Department of V
6439 Garners Ferry Rd
Columbia, SC 29209-1638
803-776-4000
800-293-8262
FAX: 803-695-6739
e-mail: Carolyn.Adams@va.gov
www.columbiasc.va.gov

Carolyn L Adams, Director
Barbara Temeck, Chief of Staff
David L. Omura, Chief of Staff
Ruth Mustard, Director for Patient Care/Nursin

South Dakota

5659 Royal C Johnson Veterans Memorial Medical Center
Veterans Health Administration, U S Dept. of VA
2501 W. 22nd St
Sioux Falls, SD 57105-5046
605-336-3230
800-316-8387
FAX: 605-333-6878
e-mail: g.vhacss@forum.va.gov
www.siouxfalls.va.gov

Patrick J Kelly, Director
Sara Ackert, Associate Director
Victor Waters, Chief of Staff
Barbara Teal, Associate Director, Patient Care

5660 Sioux Falls Regional Office
Veterans Benefits Administration, U S Dept. of V A
2501 W. 22nd St
Sioux Falls, SD 57105-5046
605-336-3230
800-827-1000
FAX: 605-333-5316
e-mail: siouxfalls.query@vba.va.gov
www.siouxfalls.va.gov

Tennessee

5661 Alvin C York VA Medical Center
Veterans Health Administration, U S Dept. of V A
3400 Lebanon Pike
Murfreesboro, TN 37129-1237
615-867-6000
800-876-7093
FAX: 615-867-5768
e-mail: g.vhacss@forum.va.gov
www.tennesseevalley.va.gov

Juan Morales, Medical System Director
Janice Cobb, Associate Director, Nursing Serv
Emma Metcalf, Chief Operating Officer

5662 Memphis VA Medical Center
Veterans Health Administration, U S Dept. of V A
1030 Jefferson Ave
Memphis, TN 38104-2127
901-523-8990
800-636-8262
e-mail: g.vhacss@forum.va.gov
www.memphis.va.gov

Jay Robinson III, Associate Medical Center Directo
Douglas D Southall, Assistant Medical Center Directo
Margarethe Hagemann, Chief of Staff
Marilyn Kerkhoff, Interim Associate Medical Center

5663 Mountain Home VA Medical CenterJames H Quillen VA Medical Center
Veterans Health Administration, US Dept. of VA
Corner of Lamont & Veterans Way
Mountain Home, TN 37684
423-926-1171
877-573-3529
e-mail: g.vhacss@forum.va.gov
www.mountainhome.va.gov

Charlene S Ehret, Medical Center Director
Jimmy H McGlawn, Associate Director
David R Reagan, Chief of Staff
Linda M McConnell, Associate Director, Patient/Nurs

5664 Nasheville Regional Office
Veterans Benefits Administration, U S Dept. of V A
110 9th Ave S
Nashville, TN 37203-3817
800-827-1000
e-mail: nashville.query@vba.va.gov
www.va.gov

Michael R Walsh, Administrative Officer
Donald H Rubin, Research/Development Coordinator

5665 Nashville VA Medical Center
Veterans Health Administration, US Dept. of VA
1310 24th Ave S
Nashville, TN 37212-2637
615-327-4751
800-228-4973
FAX: 615-321-6350
e-mail: g.vhacss@forum.va.gov
www.tennesseevalley.va.gov

Juan Morales, Medical System Director
Michael A Doukas, Chief of Staff
Gary D Trende, Associate Director, Nursing Serv
Gary D Trende, Chief Operating Officer

Texas

5666 Amarillo VA Healthcare System
Veterans Health Administration, U S Dept. of V A
6010 Amarillo Blvd West
Amarillo, TX 79106-1991
806-355-9703
800-687-8262
FAX: 806-354-7869
e-mail: g.vhacss@forum.va.gov
www.amarillo.va.gov

David Welch, Director
Lance Robinson, Associate Director
Grace Stringfelow, Chief of Staff
Louise Anderson, Executive/Chief, Nursing Service

5667 Amarillo Vet Center
Department of Veterans Affairs
3414 Olsen Blvd
Suite E
Amarillo, TX 79109-3072
806-351-1104
FAX: 806-351-1104
www.va.gov

Pedro Garcia Jr., Team Leader
Simon Camarillo, Counsilor
William C Santer, Family Therapist
Cathy L Williams, Office Manager
Provides individual, group and family counseling to veterans who served in combat theaters of World War II and Korea, veterans of the Vietnam Era, and veterans of conflicts zones in Lebanon, Grenada, Panama, the Persian Guld and Somalia.

5668 El Paso VA Healthcare Center
Veterans Health Administration, U S Dept. of V A
5001 N Piedras
El Paso, TX 79930-4210
915-564-6100
800-672-3782
FAX: 915-564-7920
e-mail: g.vhacss@forum.va.gov
www.elpaso.va.gov

John A. Mendoza, Director
Elizabeth Lowery, Associate Director
Homer LeMar, Interim Chief of Staff
Timothy McMurry, Associate Director, Patient Care

5669 Houston Regional Office
Veterans Benefits Administration, U S Dept. of V A
6900 Almeda Rd
Houston, TX 77030-4200
713-791-1414
800-827-1000
e-mail: houston.query@vba.va.gov
www.va.gov

Cecil Aultman, Executive Director
Edgar Tucker, Chief Executive Officer

5670 Michael E. Debakey VA Medical Center
Veterans Health Administration, U S Dept. of V A
2002 Holcombe Blvd
Houston, TX 77030-4211
713-791-1414
800-553-2278
e-mail: g.vhacss@forum.va.gov
www.houston.va.gov

Adam C Walmus, Director
J Kalavar, Chief of Staff
Francisco Vazquez, Associate Director
Thelma Grey-Becknell, Associate Director for Patient C

5671 South Texas Veterans Healthcare System
Veterans Health Administration, U S Dept. of V A
7400 Merton Minter
San Antonio, TX 78229-4404
210-617-5300
877-469-5300
888-686-6350
e-mail: g.vhacss@forum.va.gov
www.southtexas.va.gov

Marie L. Wedon, Director
Wade Vlosich, Associate Director
Joe A. Perez, Assistant Director
Julianne Flynne, Chief of Staff

5672 VA North Texas Health Veterans Affairs Care System: Dallas VA Medical Center
Veterans Health Administration, U S Dept. of V A
4500 S Lancaster Rd
Dallas, TX 75216-7167
214-742-8387
800-849-3597
FAX: 214-857-1171
www.northtexas.va.gov/index.asp

Jeffrey Milligan, Director
Peter Dancy, Associate Director
Clark R. Gregg, Chief of Staff
Alan Bernstein, Assistant Director
Health care system which serves veterans with medical care and rehabilitation services including spinal cord injury center. For VA benefit inquiries contact 1-800-827-1000. This system has locations in Bonham, Dallas, and Fort Worth.

5673 Waco Regional Office
Veterans Benefits Administration, U S Dept. of V A
4800 Memorial Dr
Waco, TX 76711-1
254-752-6581
800-423-1111
TTY:800-829-4833
e-mail: waco.query@vba.va.gov
www.centraltexas.va.gov

William F. Harper, Chief of Staff
Russell E. Lloyd, Associate Director of Resources
Karen Spada, Associate Director for Patients
Andrew Garcia, Assistant Director for Operations
Mission is to honor America's Veterans by providing exceptional health care that improves their health and well being.

5674 West Texas VA Healthcare System
Veterans Health Administration, U S Dept. of V A
300 Veterans Blvd
Big Spring, TX 79720-5566
432-263-7361
800-472-1365
FAX: 915-264-4834
e-mail: g.vhacss@forum.va.gov
www.bigspring.va.gov

Andrew M. Welch, Interim Director
Kenneth Allensworth, Associate Director
Raul Zambrano, Chief of Staff
Charles V. Silveri, Associate Director
The West Texas VA Health Care System (WTVAHCS) proudly serves Veterans in 33 counties across 53,000 square miles of rural geography in West Texas and Eastern New Mexico. The George H. O'Brien, Jr. VA Medical Center is located in Big Spring, Texas and the six Community Based Outpatient Clinics (CBOC's) that comprise the remainder of the health care system are located in Abilene, TX, Stamford, TX, San Angelo, TX, Odessa, TX, Fort Stockton, TX, and Hobbs, NM.

Utah

5675 Utah Division of Veterans Affairs
Utah Division of Veterans Affairs
550 Foothill Blvd
Ste 202
Salt Lake City, UT 84113-1106
801-582-1565
800-894-9497
FAX: 801-326-2369
e-mail: tandrews@utah.gov
www.saltlakecity.va.gov

David J Peifer, Director
Todd Andrews, Assistant to the Director
Karen H. Gribbin, Manager

Our mission is to serve the veteran who served us. The VA Salt Lake City Health Care System is committed to providing our patients with the highest Quality of Care in an environment that is safe. We do this by focusing on Continuous Process Improvement and by supporting a Culture of Safety

5676 VA Salt Lake City Healthcare System
Veterans Health Administration, U S Dept. of V A
500 Foothill Drive
Salt Lake City, UT 84148-1
801-582-1565
800-613-4012
FAX: 801-584-1289
www.saltlakecity.va.gov

Steven W Young, Director
Warren E Hill, Associate Director
Karen H. Gribbin, Chief of Staff
Shella Stovall, Associate Director, Patient Care

Our mission is to serve the veteran who served us. The VA Salt Lake City Health Care System is committed to providing our patients with the highest Quality of Care in an environment that is safe. We do this by focusing on Continuous Process Improvement and by supporting a Culture of Safety

Vermont

5677 Vermont VA Regional Office Center
Veterans Benefits Administration U S Department V
215 N Main St
White River Junction, VT 05009-1
802-295-9363
866-687-8387
FAX: 802-290-6354
e-mail: whiteriver.query@vba.va.gov
www.whiteriver.va.gov

Deborah Amdur, Executive Director
Danielle S. Ocker, Associate Director
Melanie Thompson, Acting Chief of Staff
Laura F. Miraldi, Associate Director for Nursing

The White River Junction VA Medical Center (WRJ VAMC) is responsible for the delivery of health care services to eligible Veterans in Vermont and the 4 contiguous counties of New Hampshire. These services are delivered at the Medical Center's main campus located in White River Junction, Vermont, and at its seven Outpatient Clinics (Bennington, Brattleboro, Colchester, Newport, and Rutland, Vermont; Keene and Littleton, New Hampshire). The White River Junction VA is closely affiliated with the Ge

5678 Vermont Veterans Centers
359 Dorset St
South Burlington, VT 05403-6210
802-862-1806
877-927-8387
FAX: 802-865-3319
www.va.gov

Fred Forehand, Team Leader
William Newkirk, Counsilor
George Troutman, Counsilor
Tamara R Thompson, Family Therapist

Veterans medical clinic offering disabled veterans medical treatments.

Virginia

5679 Hampton VA Medical Center
Veterans Health Administration, U S Dept. of V A
100 Emancipation Dr
Hampton, VA 23667-1
757-722-9961
800-827-1000
FAX: 757-728-3135
e-mail: mike.eisenberg@med.va.gov
www.hampton.va.gov

Deanne M Seekins, Medical Center Director
Benita K Stoddard, Associate Director for Operation
G. Arul, Chief of Staff
Shedale Tindall, Associate Director for Patient C

5680 Hunter Holmes McGuire VA Medical Center
Veterans Health Administration, U S Dept. of V A
1201 Broad Rock Blvd
Richmond, VA 23249-1
804-675-5000
800-784-8381
FAX: 804-675-5236
e-mail: g.vhacss@forum.va.gov
www.richmond.va.gov

Charles E Sepich, Director
David P Budinger, Associate Director
Julie Beales, Interim Chief of Staff
Rita A Duval, Associate Director for Patient C

5681 Roanoke Regional Office
Veterans Benefits Administration, U S Dept. of V A
116 North Jefferson St
Roanoke, VA 24016-1906
540-362-1999
800-827-1000
FAX: 540-563-4838
e-mail: anne.atkins@vdvs.viginia.gov
www.va.gov

Roger Bohm, Executive
Bert Boyd, COO/Executive Director

5682 Salem VA Medical Center
Veterans Health Administration, U S Dept. of V A
1970 Roanoke Blvd
Salem, VA 24153-6478
540-982-2463
800-827-1000
888-982-2463
FAX: 540-983-1096
e-mail: g.vhacss@forum.va.gov
www.salem.va.gov

Miguel H LaPuz, Director
Carol S Bogedain, Associate Director
Maureen McCarthy, Chief of Staff
Pearl Washington, Nurse Executive

5683 Virginia Department of Veterans Services
270 Franklin Rd SW
Roanoke, VA 24011-2204
540-857-7102
FAX: 540-857-6437
e-mail: pmigrand131@worldnet.att.net
dvs.virginia.gov

Colbert Boyd, Manager

Washington

5684 **Jonathan M Wainwright Memorial VA Medical Center**
Veterans Health Administration, U S Dept. of V A
77 Wainwright Dr
Walla Walla, WA 99362-3975
509-525-5200
888-687-8863
FAX: 509-946-3062
www.va.gov

Michael W Parnicky, R and D Coordinator

5685 **Seattle Regional Office**
Veterans Benefits Administration U S Department of
915 2nd Ave
Seattle, WA 98174-1060
206-762-1010
800-827-1000
e-mail: seattle.query@vba.va.gov
www.va.gov

Va Ad Harabanim, Executive Director
Timothy Williams, Chief Executive Officer

5686 **Spokane VA Medical Center**
Veterans Health Administration, U S Dept. of V A
4815 N Assembly St
Spokane, WA 99205-6185
509-434-7000
800-325-7940
FAX: 509-434-7119
e-mail: g.vhacss@forum.va.gov
www.spokane.va.gov

Alan Prentiss, Chief of Staff
Dirk Minatre, Coordinator
Joseph Manley, Executive Director

5687 **VA Puget Sound Health Care System**
Veterans Health Administration, U S Dept. of V A
1660 S Columbian Way
Seattle, WA 98108-1532
206-762-1010
800-329-8387
e-mail: g.vhacss@forum.va.gov
www.pugetsound.va.gov

Michael Fisher, Director
Michael Tadych, Deputy Director
Walt Dannenberg, Assistant Director
William Campbell, Chief of Staff

West Virginia

5688 **Huntington Regional Office**
Veterans Benefits Administration, U S Dept. of V A
640 4th Ave
Huntington, WV 25701-1340
304-525-5131
800-827-1000
FAX: 304-399-9344
e-mail: huntington.query@vba.va.gov
www.va.gov

Mark Bugher, President

5689 **Huntington VA Medical Center**
Veterans Health Administration, U S Dept. of V A
1540 Spring Valley Dr
Huntington, WV 25704-9300
304-429-6741
800-827-8244
FAX: 304-429-6713
www.huntington.va.gov

Edward H Seiler, Director
Suzanne Jene, Associate Director
Jeffery B Breaux, Chief of Staff
Catherine J Locher, Associate Director for Nursing S

5690 **Louis A Johnson VA Medical Center**
Veterans Health Administration, U S Dept. of V A
1 Medical Center Drive
Clarksburg, WV 26301-4155
304-623-3461
800-733-0512
FAX: 304-626-7048
e-mail: g.vhacss@forum.va.gov
www.clarksburg.va.gov

William E Cox, Director
Jeffrey A Beiler II, Associate Director
Glenn R Snider, Chief of Staff
Theresa J White, Nurse Executive

5691 **Martinsburg VA Medical Center**
Veterans Health Administration, U S Dept. of V A
510 Butler Avenue
Martinsburg, WV 25405-9990
304-263-0811
800-817-3807
FAX: 304-262-7433
e-mail: g.vhacss@forum.va.gov
www.martinsburg.va.gov

Ann R Brown, Director
Timothy J Cooke, Associate Medical Center Directo
Jonathan E Fierer, Chief of Staff
Susan George, Nursing Programs and Education

5692 **US Department Veterans Affairs Beckley Vet Center**
200 Veterans Ave
Beckley, WV 25801-4301
304-255-2121
877-902-5142
FAX: 304-254-8711
www.beckley.va.gov

Karin L. McGraw, Director

Vet Center services includes individual and group readjustment counseling, referral for benefits assistance, liason with community agencies, marital and family counseling, substance abuse counseling, job counseling and referral, sexual trauma counseling, and community education.

Wisconsin

5693 **Clement J Zablocki VA Medical Center**
Veterans Health Administration U S Department of V
5000 W National Ave
Milwaukee, WI 53295-1
414-384-2000
888-827-1000
888-469-6614
FAX: 414-382-5319
www.milwaukee.va.gov

Robert H Beller, Director
Michael D Erdmann, Chief of Staff
Judith A Murphy, Associate Director for Patient/N

In an effort to improve access to veterans in Milwaukee County, the VAMC has deployed a mobile clinic that provides primary care four days a week to veterans. The Medical Center also assists the Vet Center located in the City of Milwaukee. In addition, this Medical Center participates in a four-way partnership with the WDVA, the Center for Veterans Issues, Ltd., and the Social Development Commission, to operate Vets Place Central, a 72-bed transitional housing program.

5694 **Tomah VA Medical Center**
Veterans Health Administration, U S Dept. of V A
500 E Veterans St
Tomah, WI 54660-3105
608-372-3971
800-872-8662
FAX: 608-372-1224
e-mail: g.vhacss@forum.va.gov
www.tomah.va.gov

Mario V. DeSanctis, Medical Center Director
David Huffman, Associate Director
David J. Houlihan, Chief of Staff
Judith E. Broad, Associate Director

VAMCTomah has been improving the health of the men and women who have so proudly served our nation. We consider it our privelege to serve your health care needs in any way we can. Services are available to veterans living in a Western/Central area of Wisconsin.

5695 William S Middleton Memorial VA Hospital Center
Veterans Health Administration, U S Dept. of V A
2500 Overlook Ter
Madison, WI 53705-2254 608-256-1901
888-478-8321
888-256-1901
FAX: 608-280-7244
e-mail: g.vhacss@forum.va.gov
www.madison.va.gov

Judy McKee, Director
John Rohrer, Associate Director
Alan J. Bridges, Chief of Staff
Rebecca Kordahl, Associate Director

5696 Wisconsin VA Regional Office
Veterans Benefits Administration, U S Dept. of V A
5000 W National Ave
Milwaukee, WI 53295-1 414-384-2000
800-827-1000
FAX: 414-382-5374
e-mail: milwaukee.query@vba.va.gov
www.milwaukee.va.gov

Philip L Cook, Executive Director
Neil S Mandel, Research/Development Coordinator
Glen Grippen, CEO

In an effort to improve access to veterans in Milwaukee County, the VAMC has deployed a mobile clinic that provides primary care four days a week to veterans. The Medical Center also assists the Vet Center located in the City of Milwaukee. In addition, this Medical Center participates in a four-way partnership with the WDVA, the Center for Veterans Issues, Ltd., and the Social Development Commission, to operate Vets Place Central, a 72-bed transitional housing program.

Wyoming

5697 Casper Vet Center
1030 N. Poplar Suite B
Casper, WY 82601-2665 307-261-5355
FAX: 307-261-5439
www.vetcenter.va.gov

James Whipps, Office Manager

Vet Center offering re-adjustment counseling for combat veterans.

5698 Cheyenne VA Medical Center
Veterans Health Administration, U S Dept. of V A
2360 E Pershing Blvd
Cheyenne, WY 82001-5356 307-778-7370
877-927-8387
888-483-9127
FAX: 307-638-8923
e-mail: g.vhacss@forum.va.gov
www.va.gov

Cynthia McCormack, Medical Center Director
Elizabeth Lowery, Associate Director
Jerry Zang, Chief of Staff
Polly Baird, Associate Director

5699 Sheridan VA Medical Center
Veterans Health Administration, U S Dept. of V A
1898 Fort Rd
Sheridan, WY 82801-8320 307-672-3473
800-827-1000
866-822-6714
FAX: 307-672-1639
e-mail: g.vhacss@forum.va.gov
www.sheridan.va.gov/index.asp

Debra L Hirschman, Director
Michele Beach, Director
Wendell Robison, Chief of Staff
Jane Votaw, Nurse Executive

5700 Wyoming/Colorado VA Regional Office
Veterans Benefits Administration, U S Dept. of V A
155 Van Gordon St
Lakewood, CO 80228-1709 303-894-7474
800-827-1000
FAX: 303-894-7442
e-mail: denver.query@vba.va.gov
www.va.gov

E William Belz, Director

Vocational Programs

Alabama

5701 **Coffee County Training Center**
P.O.Box 311343
Enterprise, AL 36331-1343
334-393-1732
FAX: 334-347-0252

Vickie Florence, Manager
Clients 21 years and up receive training in Independent Living Skills, Self-Care, Language Skills, Learning, Self-Direction and Economic Self-Sufficiency. Transportation is also provided to clients of the center.

5702 **Easter Seal: Opportunity Center**
6300 McClellan Blvd
Anniston, AL 36206
256-820-9960
FAX: 256-820-9592
www.opportunity-center.com

Mike Almaroad, Administrator
Barbara Bradley, Vocational Instructor
Lisa Fincher, Employment Specialist
A nationally accredited non-profit organization providing vocational evaluation/assessment, paid work training, and employment services for people with disabilities in Calhoun, Cleburne, Clay, Talladega, Coosa and Randolph counties.

5703 **Easter Seals: Achievement Center**
Easter Seals of Alabama
510 W Thomason Circle
Opelika, AL 36801-5499
334-745-3501
866-239-2237
FAX: 334-749-5808
e-mail: info@achievement-center.org
www.achievement-center.org

Jason Lazenby, Chairman
Kenneth Burton, Vice-Chairman
Phyllis Horace, Secretary
Lorna Roberts, Treasurer
Provides vocational development and extended employment programs for physically, mentally, and developmentally disabled individuals and to non-disabled persons who are culturally, socially, or economically disadvantaged.

5704 **Employment Service Division: Alabama**
Department of Industrial Relations
649 Monroe St
Montgomery, AL 36131-1
334-242-8990
FAX: 334-242-3960
e-mail: director@dir.alabama.us
www.dir.alabama.gov

Tom Surtees, Director Of Industrial Relations
Robert Brantley, Director Of Employment Services

5705 **Lakeshore Rehabilitation Facility**
3830 Ridgeway Drive
PO Box 59127
Birmingham, AL 35259
331-293-7500
800-441-7609
FAX: 334-293-7371
www.rehab.state.al.us

5706 **Montezuma Day Treatment**
402 Academy Dr
Andalusia, AL 36420
334-222-8411
FAX: 334-427-1832

Michelle Mc Lendon, Administrator
W Underwood, Executive Director
Individuals served in this program must be at least 21 years of age and have a primary diagnosis of mental retardation. Clients receive training in independent living skills, learning, self-direction and economic self-sufficiency. Special Olympic activities are also emphasized.

5707 **Vocational Rehabilitation Service Opelika**
520 W Thomason Circle
Opelika, AL 36801
334-749-1259
800-671-6835
FAX: 334-749-8753
www.rehab.state.al.us

Patricia Floyd, Manager
Available through any of the 21 VRS offices statewide, services can include educational services, vocational assessment, evaluation and counseling, job training, assistive technology, orientation and mobility training and job placement.

5708 **Vocational Rehabilitation Service: Scottsboro**
203 S Market Street
PO Box 296
Scottsboro, AL 35768-0296
256-574-5813
800-418-8823
FAX: 256-574-6033
www.rehab.state.al.us

5709 **Vocational Rehabilitation Service: Dothan**
795 Ross Clark Circle NE
Dothan, AL 36303
334-699-8600
800-275-0132
FAX: 334-792-1783
www.rehab.state.al.us

5710 **Vocational Rehabilitation Service: Gadsden**
1100 George Wallace Drive
Gadsden, AL 35903-6501
256-547-6974
800-671-6839
FAX: 256-543-1784
www.rehab.state.al.us

5711 **Vocational Rehabilitation Service: Homewood**
236 Goodwin Crest Drive
Birmingham, AL 35209
205-290-4400
800-671-6837
FAX: 205-290-0486
www.rehab.state.al.us

Roger McCullough, Manager
Availiable through any of the 21 VRS offices statewide, services can include educational services, vocational assesment, evaluation and counseling, job training, assistive technology, orientation and mobility training, and job placement.

5712 **Vocational Rehabilitation Service: Huntsville**
3000 Johnson Rd SW
Huntsville, AL 35805-5847
256-650-1700
800-671-6840
FAX: 256-650-1795
www.rehab.state.al.us

Eddie C. Williams, Manager
Available through any of the 21 VRS offices statewide, services can include educational services, vocational assesment, evaluation and counseling, job training, assistive technology, orientation and mobility training, and job placement.

5713 **Vocational Rehabilitation Service: Jackson**
1401 Forest Ave
PO Box 1005
Jackson, AL 36545
251-246-5708
800-671-6836
FAX: 251-246-5224
www.rehab.state.al.us

5714 **Vocational Rehabilitation Service: Jasper**
301 N Walston Bridge Road
Suite 116
Jasper, AL 35504
205-221-7840
800-671-6841
FAX: 205-221-1062
www.rehab.state.al.us

5715 Vocational Rehabilitation Service: Mobile
2419 Gordon Smith Drive
Mobile, AL 36617
251-479-8611
800-671-6842
FAX: 251-478-2197
www.rehab.state.al.us
Stephen G. Kayes, Manger
Available through any of the 21 VRS offices statewide, services can include educational services, vocational assesment, evaluation and counseling, job training, assistive technology, orientation and mobility training, and job placement.

5716 Vocational Rehabilitation Service: Muscle Shoals
1450 E Avalon Ave
Muscle Shoals, AL 35661
256-381-1110
800-275-0166
FAX: 256-389-3149
www.rehab.state.al.us

5717 Vocational Rehabilitation Service: Selma
2906 Citizens Pkwy
Selma, AL 36701-3915
334-872-8422
888-761-5995
FAX: 334-877-3796
www.rehab.state.al.us
Richard Weishaupt, Manager
Available through any of the 21 VRS offices statewide, services can include educational services, vocational assesment, evaluation and counseling, job training, assistive technology, orientation and mobility training, and job placement.

5718 Vocational Rehabilitation Service: Talladega
4 Medical Office Park
Talladega, AL 35160
256-362-1300
800-441-7592
FAX: 256-362-6387
www.rehab.state.al.us

5719 Vocational Rehabilitation Service: Troy
1109 Troy Plaza Street
Troy, AL 36081
334-566-2491
800-441-7608
FAX: 334-566-9415
www.rehab.state.al.us

5720 Vocational Rehabilitation Service: Tuscaloosa
1305 James I Harrison Jr Parkway E
Tuscaloosa, AL 35405
205-554-1300
800-331-5562
FAX: 205-554-1369
www.rehab.state.al.us
William Strickland, Manager
Available through any of the 21 VRS offices statewide, services can include educational services, vocational assesment, evaluation and counseling, job training, assistive technology, orientation and mobility training, and job placement.

5721 Vocational Rehabilitation Services: Andalusa
1082 Village Square Drive
Suite 1
Andalusia, AL 36420
334-222-4114
800-671-6833
FAX: 334-427-1216
www.rehab.state.al.us

5722 Vocational Rehabilitation Services: Anniston
1105 Woodstock Ave
Anniston, AL 36207
256-238-9300
800-671-6834
FAX: 256-231-4852
www.rehab.state.al.us

5723 Vocational and Rehabilitation Service: Decatur
621 Cherry St NE
Decatur, AL 35601
256-353-2754
800-671-6838
FAX: 256-351-2476
www.rehab.state.al.us

5724 Vocational and Rehabilitation Services: Montgomery
602 S Lawrence St
Montgomery, AL 36104
334-293-7500
800-441-7578
FAX: 334-293-7372
www.rehab.state.al.us
Jimmy Varando, Manager
Available through any of the 21 VRS offices statewide, services can include educational services, vocational assessment, evaluation and counseling, job training, assistive technology, orientation and mobility training and job placement.

5725 Wiregrass Rehabilitation Center
795 Ross Clark Circle
Dothan, AL 36303
334-792-0022
800-395-7044
FAX: 216-521-9460
e-mail: jls@wrcjobs.com
www.wrcjobs.com
Cliff Mendheim, Chairman
Denise Hattaway, Vice-Chairman
Les Moreland, Chair Elect
Blaine Stewart, Treasurer
Trains individuals to become employable and assists them in finding jobs withing their communities. Also assists individuals who have difficulty maintaining employment, those who are on forms of public assistance such as welfare and those who are employable and underemployed.

5726 Workshops Inc.
4244 3rd Ave S
Birmingham, AL 35222-2008
205-592-9683
888-805-9683
FAX: 205-592-9687
TTY: 205-592-8006
e-mail: email@workshopsinc.org
www.workshopsinc.org
Martha Johnson, President
Martha Ann-Rich, President-Elect
Bart Trench, Treasurer
Kathy Myatt, Secretary
Provides vocational training, sheltered employment and other support services to people with disabilities in central Alabama.

Alaska

5727 Alaska Division of Vocational Rehabilitation
Department of Labor & Workforce Development
801 W 10th Street
Suite A
Juneau, AK 99801
907-465-2814
800-478-2815
FAX: 907-465-2856
TTY: 800-478-2815
e-mail: dol.dvr.info@alaska.gov
www.labor.state.ak.us/dvr
Cheryl Walsh, Director
Assist individuals with disabilities to obtain and maintain employment.

5728 Anchorage Job Training Center
235 E 8th Ave
Anchorage, AK 99501-3615
907-277-0693
FAX: 907-334-2286
www.ci.anchorage.ak.us

5729 **Fair Employment Practice Agency**
Alaska State Commission for Human Rights
Ste 204
800 a St
Anchorage, AK 99501-7500
907-274-4692
800-478-4692
FAX: 907-278-8588
www.gov.state.ak.us/aschr/aschr.htm
Paula Haley, Executive Director

Arizona

5730 **Downtown Neighborhood Learning Center**
1001 W Jefferson St
Phoenix, AZ 85007-2913
602-254-6524
800-869-8521
FAX: 602-256-2524
e-mail: dnlc@swlink.net
www.swlink.net
Scott Ritchey, Manager
Mattie Johnson, Receptionist
Peg Osinski, El Mirage Learning Lab
Adult education agency providing basic skills, GED, ESOL, life skills, computer skills, resume assistance and career testing.

5731 **Fair Employment Practice Agency: Arizona**
Arizona Civil Rights Division
1275 W Washington St
Phoenix, AZ 85007-2926
602-542-5025
800-352-8431
FAX: 602-542-4085
www.azag.gov
Virginia Gonzales, Director
Bruna Pedrini, Manager
Provides legal advice to most state agencies. The office also investigates and prosecutes consumer fraud, white collar crime, organized crime, public corruption, and civil rights.

5732 **JOBS Administration Job Opportunities & Basic Skills**
1717 W Jefferson St
Phoenix, AZ 85007-3202
602-542-9596
FAX: 602-542-5171
Gretchen Evans, Program Administrator
Assist applicants and recipients of temporary assistance to needy families to obtain job training and employment that will lead to economic independence.

5733 **TETRA Services**
Beacon Group SW Inc
2222 N 24th Street
Phoenix, AZ 85008
602-685-9703
FAX: 602-244-2435
e-mail: info@tetraservices.org
www.tetraservices.org

5734 **Vocational and Rehabilitation Agency Rehabilitation Services Administrations**
Division of Employment & Rehabilitation Services
1789 W Jefferson St
Phoenix, AZ 85007-3202
602-604-8835
800-563-1221
800-563-1221
FAX: 602-604-8901
TTY:602-542-6049
e-mail: tazrsa@azdes.gov
azdes.gov/rsa
Michelle Nitschke, Manager
Katharine Levandowsky, Administrator
Moises Gallegos, Manager
This program serves individuals with disabilities seeking jobs and job training.

5735 **Yavapai Regional Medical Center-West**
1003 Willow Creek Rd
Prescott, AZ 86301-1668
928-445-2700
877-843-9762
FAX: 928-445-0994
yrmc.org
Tim Barnett, CEO
Widely recognized for the quality and success of the physical, occupational, and speech therapy programs it offers. Provides a wide range of programs and services that enable our patients to reach their maximum level of function and independence- and enjoy the highest possible quality of life.

Arkansas

5736 **Arkansas Employment Service Agency and Job Training Program**
Arkansas Employment Security Department
Capitol Mall
Ste 2
Little Rock, AR 72201-2981
501-682-2033
FAX: 501-682-2273
www.arkansas.gov/esd
Artee Williams, Manager
Wide range of services including employment services, unemployment insurance, and labor market information.

5737 **Easter Seal Work Center**
3920 Woodland Heights Rd
Little Rock, AR 72212-2406
501-227-3600
FAX: 501-227-7180
e-mail: mail@ar.easterseals.com
www.ar.easterseals.com
Lauren Zilk, Administrator
Mission is to provide exceptional services to ensure that all people with disabilities or special needs have equal opportunities to live,learn work and play in their communities.

5738 **VCT/A Job Retention Skill Training Program**
Arkasas Rehab Services
P.O.Box 1358
Hot Springs, AR 71902-1358
501-624-4411
FAX: 501-624-0019
Barbara Lewis, Administrator
Mae Robinson, Assistant Administrator
A training program designed for use in rehabilitation and educational settings. Using a social skill training strategy, VCT helps participants learn how to solve on-the-job problems and cope with common supervisory demands.

5739 **Vocational and Rehabilitation Agency Division of Services for the Blind**
700 Main St
Little Rock, AR 72201-4608
501-686-9433
800-960-9270
FAX: 501-686-9418
TTY: 501-682-0093
e-mail: jim.hudson@mail.state.ar.us
www.state.ar.us
Lyndel Lybarger, Field Adminstrator
James Hudson, Executive Director

5740 **Vocational and Rehabilitation Agency for Persons Who Are Visually Impaired**
Arkansas Department of Human Services
P.O.Box 3237
Little Rock, AR 72203-3237
501-686-9433
800-960-9270
FAX: 501-686-9418
TTY: 501-324-9271
e-mail: arkblind@edu.gte.net
James C Hudson, Executive Director
Furnishes a wide variety of services to help people with disabilities return to work.

California

5741 ABLE Industries
8127 Avenue 304
Visalia, CA 93291
559-651-8150
888-813-2253
FAX: 559-651-0357
www.ableindustries.org
Wende-Leigh Ayers, Executive Director
Committed to improving the lives of people with disabilities by creating opportunities to maximize their independence.

5742 ARC-Adult Vocational Program
1500 Howard St
San Francisco, CA 94103-2525
415-255-7200
FAX: 415-255-9488
e-mail: info@thearcsanfrancisco.org
www.thearcsanfrancisco.org
Timothy Hornbecker, Executive Director
Job placement programs, remunerative work services and work adjustment training programs.

5743 AbilityFirst
1300 E Green Street
Pasadena, CA 91106
626-396-1010
877-768-4600
FAX: 626-396-1021
e-mail: info@abilityfirst.org
www.abilityfirst.org
Lori E Gangemi, President
Steve S. Schultz, CFO
Keri Castaneda, Chief Program Officer
Syed Kazmi, Controller
Provides programs and services to help children and adults with physical and developmental disabilities reach their full potential throughout their lives. Offers a broad range of employment, recreational and socialization programs and operate 12 accessible residential housing complexes.

5744 Achievement House & NCI Affiliates
496 Linne Road
Paso Robles, CA 93446
805-238-6630
FAX: 805-239-9073
e-mail: conact@nciaffiliates.org
www.achievementhouse.org

5745 Bakersfield ARC
2240 S Union Ave
Bakersfield, CA 93307-4158
661-834-2272
800-834-3160
FAX: 661-834-1694
e-mail: lplank@barc-inc.org
www.barc-inc.org
Jim Baldwin, President/CEO
William Froning, Senior VP/CFO
Dave Kyle, Senior VP/Chief Compliance Officer
Mike Grover, Senior VP/Chief Programmes Officer
A non-profit organization that has been providing essential job training, employment and support services for the developmentally disabled and their families.
1949

5746 California Department of Fair Employment& Housing
2218 Kauden Drive
Suite 100
Elk Grove, CA 95758
916-478-7251
800-884-1684
e-mail: contact.center@dfeh.ca.gov
www.dfeh.ca.gov
Phyllis W Cheng, Director
Annmarie Billotti Esq, Chief Deputy Director
To protect Californians from employment, housing and public accomodation discrimination, and hate violence.

5747 Career Connection Transition Program
Whittier Union High School District
9401 Painter Ave
Whittier, CA 90605-2729
562-698-8121
FAX: 562-693-4414
e-mail: Richard.Rosenberg@wuhsd.k12.ca.us
www.wuhsd.k12.ca.us
Richard L Rosenberg PhD, Vocational Coordinator
Bonnie Bolton, Transition Department Head
Job placement programs, remunerative work services and work adjustment training programs. Transition services.

5748 Career Development Program (CDP)
260 W Grand Ave
Escondido, CA 92025-2604
760-738-0277
FAX: 760-741-9452
Richard Brady MD
Wendy Hope, Supported Employment
Jill Hennessy, Independent Living
Work hardening and disciplinary programs.

5749 Colton-Redlands-Yucaipa Regional Occupational Programs
1214 Indiana Ct
PO Box 8640
Redlands, CA 92374-2896
909-793-3115
FAX: 909-793-6901
www.cryrop.org
Stephanie Houston, Superintendent
Sandra Moritensen, Manager Student Services
Provides quality hands-on training programs in over 40 high demand career fields to assist high school students and adults in acquiring marketable job skills. Works in cooperation with local high schools, adult education colleges, and employers providing a collaborative team of academic and ROP occupational teachers who integrate academic and vocational competencies to provide sequenced paths within career majors. Support services, career guidance and services are provided to disabled people.

5750 Community Outpatient Rehabilitation Center
2823 Fresno Street
Fresno, CA 93721
559-459-6000
FAX: 559-459-1004
e-mail: complaint@jointcommission.org
www.communitymedical.org
Tim A. Joslin, Chief Executive Officer
Thomas Utecht, M.D., Senior Vice President
Craig S. Castro, Senior Vice President
Vicki Anderson, Vice President, Managed Care
Physical, occupational and speech therapy, neuropsychology services available for orthopedic and neurological diagnosis. Lymphedema program.

5751 Desert Haven Enterprises
43437 Copeland Circle
PO Box 2110
Lancaster, CA 93535
661-948-8402
FAX: 661-948-1080
e-mail: kmiller@desrthaven.org
www.deserthaven.org
Jenni Moran, Executive Director
Kathleen Miller, Program Services Director
Lisa Enos, Director Contract Services
Kathy Burcina, Job Developer
A private, nonprofit organization dedicated to developing, enhancing, and promotingthe capabilities of persons with mental retardation and other developmental disabilities.

5752 ESS Work Center
858 Stanton Rd
Burlingame, CA 94010-1404
650-697-2642
FAX: 650-697-2405
Ed Mentzer, Owner
Work adjustment and remunerative work programs.

5753 **Employment Service: California**
Employment Development Department
800 Capitol Mall
P.O. Box 826880
Sacramento, CA 95814- 0001 916-653-0707
www.edd.ca.gov

5754 **Feather River Industries**
1811 Kusel Rd
Oroville, CA 95966-9528 530-534-1112
FAX: 530-534-3137
www.featherriverindustries.com
Randy Guild, Rehabilitation Counselor
Ed Turner, Production Coordinator
Judy Smith, President
Steve Wattenberg, Vice President
Vocational training for persons with developmental disabilities provided through wood products fabrication and assembly tasks. Instructor to trainer rating ranging from 1 to 12, 1 to 8, 1 to 6, and 1 to 4 depending on individual needs and complexity of tasks.

5755 **Fit to Work**
Ste 401
3581 Palmer Dr
Cameron Park, CA 95682-8238 530-676-7485
FAX: 530-676-9114
www.trueyellow.com
Helen Cheng
Provides remunerative work.

5756 **Fresno City College: Disabled Students Programs and Services**
Fresno City College
1101 E University Ave
Fresno, CA 93741-1 559-442-4600
FAX: 559-489-2281
e-mail: janice.emerzian@fresnocitycollege.edu
fresnocitycollege.edu
Dr Janice Emerzian Ed D, District Director
Tony Cantu, President
Ginna Bearden, Director of TRIO Programs
Cris Monahan Bremer, Director of Marketing and Commun
This program offers programs and services to students with physical, learning and/or psychological disabilities beyond those provided by conventional Fresno City College Programs and enables students to successfully pursue their individual educational, vocational and personal goals.

5757 **Heartland Opportunity Center**
323 N E Street
Madera, CA 93638 559-674-8828
FAX: 559-674-8857
e-mail: kanderson@heartlandopportunity.com
www.heartlandopportunity.com
Kristy Anderson, CEO
Maria Alvarado, CFO
Provides employment, job placement, vocational and life skills training to adults with mental, physical and/or emotional disabilities in order to help them reach their personal and vocational goals.

5758 **Hollister Workshop**
Hope Rehabilitation Services
185 Berry Street
Suite 4000
San Francisco, CA 94107-2536 415-243-4200
888-567-7442
415-764-1622
FAX: 831-637-8726
e-mail: salesteam@loopnet.com
www.loopnet.com
Fred Saint, President
Wayne Warthen, CTO & SVP, Information Technology
Curtis Kroeker, President, LoopNet Marketplace Verticals
Leah McMurtry, Vice President, Member Services
Work adjustment and remunerative work programs.

5759 **Job Training Program Liaison: California**
Employment Development Department
800 Capitol Mall
Sacramento, CA 95814-4807 916-654-8210
800-300-5616
FAX: 916-657-5294
edd.ca.gov
Patrick Henning, Manager
Provides information on filing an Unemployment Insurance or Disability Insurance claim, on-line job and resume bank which boasts thousands of job openings.

5760 **King's Rehabilitation Center**
494 E Hanford-Armona Road
Hanford, CA 93232 559-583-5051
FAX: 559-582-1182
www.kingsrehab.com
Robert Knudseon, President
Steve Mendoza, Executive Director
Pat Vestal, VP
Renee Castro, Treasurer
To enhance the lives of adults with disabilities by providing day program services, vocational training and employment opportunities to assist such persons to attain their full potential.

5761 **Morongo Basin Work Activity Center**
74325 Joe Davis Dr
Twentynine Palms, CA 92277 760-366-8474
www.guidestar.org
Sheree Fraser
Job placement programs, remunerative work services and work adjustment training programs.

5762 **Mother Lode Rehabilitation Enterprises**
399 Placerville Dr
Placerville, CA 95667 530-622-4848
FAX: 530-622-0204
www.morerehab.org
Susan Peters, Chair
Henry Jeter, VP Finance
Christa K. Campbell, Secretary
A private, non-profit organization dedicated to supporting persons with disabilities. MORE was established by a group of parents, educators, rehabilitation professionals and concerned citizens and first began serving adults with disabilities in 1973.

5763 **Napa Valley PSI Inc.**
P.O.Box 600
Napa, CA 94559-600 707-255-0177
FAX: 707-255-0802
e-mail: admin@napavalleypsi.org
http://www.napavalleypsi.org
Kimberly Alexander-Yarbor, President
Carol Gonsalves , Vice President
Eleanor Cullum, Secretary
Worthy Brooks, Directors
Work adjustment, work training and educational services for developmentally disabled adults. Emphasis is on manufacture of quality wood products, primarily wooden office furniture.

5764 **Oakland Work Activity Area**
6315 San Leandro St
Oakland, CA 94621-3727 510-639-9350
oaklandlocal.com
Greg Whalley
Dennis Scharssenberg, Manager
Susan Mernit, Editor/Publisher
Abraham Hyatt, Editor
Job placement programs, remunerative work services and work adjustment training programs.

5765 Opportunities for the Handicapped
P.O.Box 322
New York, NY 10040-0322 419-855-2742
www.giveindia.org
Kathy Dodd
Pradeep Jayaraman, President
Harendra Guturu, Secretary
Uttara Diwan, Treasurer
Work adjustment and remunerative work programs.

5766 Orange County ARC
225 W Carl Karcher Way
Anaheim, CA 92801 714-744-5301
FAX: 714-744-5312
e-mail: jhearn2001@yahoo.com
ocarc.net
Joyce Hearn, CEO
Richard Farmer, VP Finance
Michael Galliano, VP Operations
Patrick Faraday, VP Sales
To provide quality care, training and services to our intellectually/developmentally disabled clients.

5767 PRIDE Industries
10030 Foothills Boulevard
Roseville, CA 95747-7102 916-788-2100
800-550-6005
FAX: 800-888-0447
e-mail: info@prideindustries.com
http://www.prideindustries.com
Michael Ziegler, CEO
Tim Yamauchi, Executive Vice President and Chi
John Vaughan, Senior Vice President, Manufactu
Pete Berghuis, Senior Vice President, Integrate
Vocational rehabilitation and employment services creating jobs for people with disabilites; services include career counseling, vocational assessment, work adjustment, work services, job seeking skills, job development, job placement, on-the-job support (coaching), mentoring, independent living skills, transition services and case management.

5768 Parents and Friends, Inc
350 Cypress St
PO Box 656
Fort Bragg, CA 95437 707-964-4940
FAX: 707-964-8536
e-mail: rmoon@parentsandfriends.org
www.parentsandfriends.org
Rick Moon, Executive Director
Serves people with developmental disabilities.

5769 PathPoint
315 W Haley Street
Ste 102
Santa Barbara, CA 93101 805-966-3310
e-mail: info@pathpoint.org
www.pathpoint.org
Barbara Stevenson, Chair
Christopher Jones, Vice Chair/Treasurer
Mary E. Tiffany, Secretary
Jeffery Dodds, Director
To provide comprehensive training and support serviceds that empower people with disabilities of disadvantages to live and work as valued members of the community.

5770 People Services, Inc
4195 Lakeshore Blvd
Lakeport, CA 95453 707-263-3810
FAX: 707-263-0552
e-mail: idumont@nctac.com
www.peopleservices.org
Ilene Dumont, Executive Director
To serve as the local community agency, providing the delivery of quality services for people with disabilities.

5771 Pomona Valley Workshop
4650 Brooks St
Montclair, CA 91763 909-624-3555
FAX: 909-624-5675
e-mail: karen@pvwonline.org
www.pvwonline.org
Karen Jones, Executive Director
Mitch Gariador, Director of Administration
Kitty Dubois, Director of Human Resources
Terri Perkins, Director of Work Services
To assist adults with disabilities reach their potential in vocationsl and socialization skills in order tthat they may achieve their highest level of employment and community integration.

5772 Porterville Sheltered Workshop
194 West Poplar Avenue
Porterville, CA 93257-3449 559-784-1399
FAX: 559-781-5651
e-mail: info@pswrehab.com
http://www.portervilleshelteredworkshop.com/
Steve Tree, Executive Director
Work adjustment and remunerative work programs. Mission is to assist disabled individuals achieve a more independent and productive life.

5773 Project Independence
3505 Cadillac Ave
Suite O-103
Costa Mesa, CA 92626 714-549-3464
877-444-0144
FAX: 714-549-3559
e-mail: info@proindependence.org
www.proindependence.org
Debra Marsteller, Executive Director
Promote civil rights for people with developmental disabilities through services which expand independence and choice.

5774 Sacramento Vocational Services
6950 21st Ave
Sacramento, CA 95820 916-381-1300
FAX: 916-381-9026
e-mail: info@inallianceinc.com
inallianceinc.com

5775 San Francisco Vocational Services
Ste 600
490 Golf Club Road
Pleasant Hill, CA 94523-1553 925-682-6343
FAX: 925-682-6375
e-mail: sfvs@sfvocational.org
rsnc-centers.org
Gina Chenoweth, Executive Director
Jeffrey Faircloth, Manager Case Management
Rita Hays, Chair/President
William Wilson, Vice Chair
Comprehensive vocational rehabilitation center offering vocational evaluation, rehabilitative counseling, business office training, work experience, and job placement.

5776 Shasta County Opportunity Center
1265 Redwood Blvd
Redding, CA 96003-1965 530-225-5781
FAX: 530-225-5751
e-mail: oppcenter_info@co.shasta.ca.us
www.co.shasta.ca.us
Del Lockwood, Manager
Leonard Moty, 2012 Chairman
David A. Kehoe, Board of Supervisor
Glenn Hawes, Board of Supervisor
An employment training program for people with disabilities in Shasta County. These individuals perform paid work in a number of different work environments and at the same time learn the skills necessary to obtain competetive employment in the local community.

5777 **Social Vocational Services**
Ste A104
350 Crenshaw Blvd
Torrance, CA 90503-1725
310-783-0633
FAX: 310-783-0636
e-mail: nto@svsinc.org
socvoc.org
Sabrina Silva, Manager
Dan Strohm, Manager
The leading provider of services for people with developmental disabilities in the state of California

5778 **South Bay Vocational Center**
1526 W 240th St
Harbor City, CA 90710
310-784-2032
FAX: 310-539-6342
e-mail: corey@sbvc1.com
www.sbvc1.com
Corey Sylve, President/CEO
Clare Grey, Vice President/COO
Santiago Lindo, Operations Specialist
Celia Bennett, CFO
A not-for-profit organization that has been providing excellent vocational programs and services for individuals with disabilities.

5779 **Tri-County Independent Living Center**
2822 Harris Street
Eureka, CA 95503
707-445-8404
877-576-5000
FAX: 707-445-9751
e-mail: aa@tilinet.org
http://www.tilinet.org
Chris Jones, Executive Director
Allan Daniel, Information & Referral / Indepen
Mary Bullwinkel, Outreach & Resource Development
Cindy Calderon, Systems Change Advocate
To provide programs, services and information for people with disabilities living in Humboldt, Del Norte and Trinity Counties in northern California in an effort to allow choices for individuals to optimize their independence.

5780 **Unyeway**
Suite E
2330 Main Street
Ramona, CA 92065-2595
760-789-5960
FAX: 760-789-8156
http://www.unyeway.com
Kim Metli, Executive Director
Lisa Oertling, President
Dr. Richard Ferguson, Vice President/Audit Committee C
Pearl Aiello, Director
Job placement programs, remunerative work services and work adjustment training programs.

5781 **V-Bar Enterprises**
720 Gordon Cir
Suisun City, CA 94585
707-864-1334
government-contractors.findthebest.com
Lu Brunet
Job placement programs, remunerative work services and work adjustment training programs.

5782 **Valley Light Industries**
5360 Irwindale Avenue
Irwaindale, CA 91706
626-332-6200
e-mail: info@valleylightindustries.org
valleylightind.org

5783 **Visalia Workshop**
2031 S. Mooney Blvd.
Visalia, CA 93277-6711
559-622-9650
FAX: 866-575-6627
www.buildabear.com
Hortensia Venegas
Work hardening and disciplinary programs.

5784 **Westside Opportunity Workshop**
9503 Jefferson Blvd
Culver City, CA 90232-2917
310-836-4262
FAX: 310-825-0676
e-mail: ayokota@mednet.ucla.edu
http://www.semel.ucla.edu
Peter Whybrow, Director
Fawzy Fawzy, Associate Director
Mark Wheeler, Media Relations
Alan Han, Director of Development
Job placement programs, remunerative work services and work adjustment training programs.

5785 **Work Training Center**
2255 Fair Street
Chico, CA 95928
530-343-7994
FAX: 530-343-4619
e-mail: carlo@ewtc.org
www.wtcinc.org
Carl Ochsner, Executive Director
Brett Barker, Vocational Services Director
Deb Royat, Rehabilitation Services Director
A nonprofit organization providing services to people with disabilities.

Colorado

5786 **Blue Peaks Developmental Services**
703 Fourth Street
Alamosa, CO 81101-2638
719-589-5135
FAX: 719-589-0680
e-mail: info@bluepeaks.org
http://www.bluepeaks.org
John Kreiner, Director
Randall P. Johnson, Human Resources/Staff Developmen
Brooke Hayden, Residential Director
George Garcia, Operations Director
Provides remunerative work.

5787 **Cheyenne Village**
6275 Lehman Drive
Colorado Springs, CO 80918
719-592-0200
FAX: 719-548-9947
TTY:719-592-0224
e-mail: info@cheyennevillage.org
www.cheyennevillage.org
Ann M Turner, Executive Director
B. Jeanne Solze, Business Director
Serves adults with developmental disabilities such as Autism, Down syndrome, Cerebral Palsy, and Mental Retardation in El Paso, Teller and Park Counties.

5788 **Colorado Civil Rights Divsion**
1560 Broadway
Ste 110
Denver, CO 80202
303-894-7855
800-866-7675
FAX: 303-894-7885
www.dora.state.co.us
Barbara J. Kelly, Executive Director
Fred J. Joseph, Banking Division
Steven Chavez, Civil Rights Division
Chris Mykelbust, Division of Financial Services
Embraces the Department's mission of consumer protection and works to protect individuals from discrimination in employment, housing and at places of public accommodation through enforcement and outreach consistent with the Colorado Civil Rights Laws.

5789 Colorado Employment Service
Department of Labor and Employment
Suite 400
1800 Grant Street
Denver, CO 80203-3528
303-860-4200
855-216-7740
FAX: 303-860-4299
e-mail: employeeservices@cu.edu
www.cu.edu/employee-services
Clara Capano, Manager
Job placement programs, remunerative work services and work adjustment training programs.

5790 Developmental Training Services
4600 North Fairfax Drive
Suite 402
Arlington, VA 22203
703-465-9388
FAX: 703-465-9344
www.onlinedts.com
Roger Jensen, CEO
Linda Davis, Administrator
Indira Kaur Ahluwalia,, Founder and President
Viresh Desai, Vice President
Residential and employment programs for adults with developmental disabilities.

5791 Dynamic Dimensions
701 Cypress Street
Sulphur, LA 70663
337-527-7034
FAX: 719-346-6010
https://www.wcch.com
Cheryl Reese, Executive Director
Vocational, evaluation and assessment, training and placement for most disabilities. Group homes and day programs for the developmentally disabled.

5792 Gray Street Workcenter
11177 West 8th Avenue
Lakewood, CO 80215-2821
303-233-3363
FAX: 303-467-2793
http://services.ddrcco.com
Tammy Drumright, Manager
C. David Pemberton, II, President
Neal Berlin, Vice President
Joanne Elliott, M.A., Secretary
Residential and employment programs for adults with developmental disabilities.

5793 Hope Center
3400 Elizabeth St
Denver, CO 80205-4801
303-388-4801
FAX: 303-388-0249
e-mail: gghope@comcast.net
www.hopecenterinc.org
Charlse T. Smith, Chairperson
Sid Davidson, Vice Chairperson
John Hanson, Treasurer
Barbara Batey, Secretary
Provides educational and vocational opportunities for special-needs and at-risk children and adults from 2 1/2 to adulthood.

5794 Imagine: Innovative Resources for Cognitive & Physical Challenges
1400 Dixon St
Lafayette, CO 80026-2790
303-665-7789
FAX: 303-665-2648
e-mail: caroline@imaginecolorado.org
www.imaginecolorado.org
Mark Emery, Executive Director
Judy James-Anderson, Behavioral Health Services Dir
Provides support services to more than 2,600 people of all ages with developmental delays and cognitive disabilities including autism, cerebral palsy and Down syndrome.

5795 Las Animas County Rehabilitation Center
P.O.Box 781
Trinidad, CO 81082-781
719-846-3388
FAX: 719-846-4543
www.scdds.com
Duane Roy, Executive Director
Bernice Whalen, Human Resources Manager
Jeannette Vialobos, SPCC Director
Leslie Lark, Finance Director
Job placement programs, remunerative work services and work adjustment training programs.

5796 NORESCO Workshop
903 E Burlington Ave
Fort Morgan, CO 80701-3637
970-867-5702
fort-morgan.gopickle.com
Ramona Proctor, Executive Director
Nancy Study, Manager
Provides remunerative work.

5797 Regional Assessment and Training Center
1145 Gayley Avenue
Suite 304
Los Angeles, CA 90024-3108
303-866-7253
www.srphtc.ucla.edu
Russell Porter, Executive Director
Work adjustment and renumerative work programs.

5798 Sedgwick County Workshop
7001 W. 21 st St.
North Wichita, KN 67205-1759
316-660-0100
FAX: 316-722-1432
e-mail: sedgwickinfo@k-state.edu
www.sedgwick.ksu.edu
Maria Contreras, Manager
Provides remunerative work.

5799 Vocational and Rehabilitation Agency
Unit B
2 Peachtree Street, NW
Atlanta, GA 30303-3855
404-232-1998
866-489-0001
FAX: 404-232-1800
TTY: 303-866-3980
e-mail: GVRAcustomer-service@gvra.ga.gov
https://gvra.georgia.gov
Diana Huerta, Director
James N. Defoor, Chair
Louise Hill, Vice Chair
Purpose is to assist eligible individuals with disabilities to become productive members of the Colorado workforce and to live independently.

5800 Yuma County Workshop
710 E 2nd Ave
Yuma, CO 80759
970-848-2874
www.yellowpages.com/yuma-co
Robert Stephens
Andrea Anderson, Manager
Provides remunerative work.

Connecticut

5801 Abilities Without Boundaries
615 W Johnson Avenue
Cheshire, CT 06410
203-272-5607
FAX: 203-272-4284
e-mail: cconway@abilitieswithoutboundaries.org
www.abilitieswithoutboundaries.or g

Charlie Conway, Executive Director
Christopher Fanelli, Business Manager
Nancy Knapp, Office Manager
Richard Ambro Jr., Employment Specialist

Formerly known as Cheshire Occupational & Career Opportunities (COCO), provides opportunities in the community through employment and social experiences for people with developmental disabilities.

5802 Allied Community Services
Six Craftsman Road
East Windsor, CT 06088
860-741-3701
FAX: 860-741-6870
TTY:860-741-3701
www.alliedgroup.org

Dean M Wern, President/CEO

Provides individuals with disabilities or other challenges the opportunity to live and enjoy a productive, independent, and fulfilling life

5803 Area Cooperative Educational Services(ACES)
350 State St
North Haven, CT 06473
203-498-6800
e-mail: acesinfo@aces.org
www.aces.org

Craig W Edmondson EdD, Executive Director
Claudette J. Beamon, Human Resources Director
Carolyn McNally, Program Development Director

Exists to improve public education through high quality, cost effective programs and services.

5804 CW Resources
200 Myrtle Street
New Britain, CT 06053
860-229-7700
FAX: 860-229-6847
e-mail: info@cwresources.org
www.cwresources.org

Ronald H Buccilli, President

CW Resources is dedicated to serving the needs of persons with disabilities through the creation of integrated vocational training and employment opportunities for those individuals who are physically, developmentally, emotionally and/or socio-economically challenged.

5805 Central Connecticut Association For Retarted Citizens
950 Slater Rd
New Britain, CT 06053-1658
860-229-6665
FAX: 860-826-6883
e-mail: ccarc@ccarc.com
www.ccarc.com

Anne Ruwet, CEO
Julie Erickson, Senior Vice President
William allyn, Vice President of Residential Services
Anna Cardona, Vice President

Empowerment through Employment

5806 Community Enterprises
441 Pleasant Street
Northampton, MA 01060
413-584-1460
e-mail: info@communityenterprises.com
www.communityenterprises.com

Dick Venne, President/CEO
William Donohue, Chairman
Donald Milner, Vice Chairman
Joanne Carlisle, Clerk

Support self-determination for individuals with disabilities and/or other challenges to actively live, learn, and work in the community.

5807 Connecticut Governor's Committee on Employment of People With Disabilities
200 Folly Brook Boulevard
Wethersfield, CT 06109-1153
860-263-6000
FAX: 860-263-6039
e-mail: dol.webhelp@ct.gov
http://www.ctdol.state.ct.us

Dennis Murphy, Acting Commissioner
Dannel P. Malloy, Governor

Work adjustment and remunerative work programs.

5808 Fotheringhay Farms
84 Waterhole Rd
Colchester, CT 06415-2323
860-267-4463
FAX: 860-267-7628
http://caringcommunityct.org

Wesley Martins, Executive Director

Job placement programs, remunerative work services and work adjustment training programs.

5809 George Hegyi Industrial Training Center
5 Coon Hollow Rd
Derby, CT 06418-1149
203-735-8727
FAX: 203-735-2204
e-mail: bob.wood@snet.net
http://www.varcainc.com

Joan Bucci, Executive Director
Robert Wood, President
Cecelia Staiano-Hayes, Program Manager

Work adjustment and remunerative work programs.

5810 Kennedy Center
2440 Reservoir Ave
Trumbull, CT 06611-4757
203-365-8522
FAX: 203-365-8533
e-mail: info@kennedyctr.org
www.thekennedycenterinc.org

Martin D. Schwartz, President & CEO
Stuart Gordon, Vice President of Finance
Lynn Pellegrino, Vice President of HR
Marie Farina, HR Generalist

Provides vocational rehabilitation, job training and job placement services to 1,000 adults with disabilities including mental retardation, traumatic brain injury, psychiatric disabilities and more. Residential services, well integrated within the community, serve 97 individuals on a daily basis. Children's programs provide support to 85 children age birth to three, in addition to after hours and recreation programs to appromxately 100 school age children. Staff size is presently 450 employees.

5811 Quaezar
285 Riverside Avenue
Suite 300
Westport, CT 06880-4806
203-226-8711
FAX: 203-454-5780
sterlinglp.com

William J Sedarweck, President

Agency for adult mentally retarded/autistic people providing residential care in a group home or apartment setting. Also provides placement in community employment.

5812 Valley Memorial Health Center
435 E Main St
Ansonia, CT 06401-1964
203-736-2601
FAX: 203-736-2641
e-mail: info@bghealth.org
www.bghealth.org

Marilyn Cormack, CEO

Provides innovative, exceptional behavioral health care through quality services and programs that focus on, and respect the consumer.

5813 Vocational and Rehabilitation Agency
2 Peachtree Street, NW
Atlanta, GA 30303-4536
404-232-1998
866-489-0001
FAX: 404-232-1800
TTY: 860-602-4221
e-mail: GVRAcustomer-service@gvra.ga.gov
https://gvra.georgia.gov
Keith Maynard, Deputy Director
Brian Sigman, Executive Director
Alan Sylvestre, Chairman
Mission is to provide quality educational and rehabilitative services to all people who are legally blind or deaf/blind and children who are visually impaired at no cost to our clients or their families.

5814 Vocational and Rehabilitation Agency: State Department of Social Services
Department of Social Services
25 Sigourney St
11th Floor
Hartford, CT 06106-5041
860-424-4844
800-537-2549
FAX: 860-424-4850
TTY: 860-424-4839
e-mail: brs.dss@po.state.ct.us
www.ct.gov/brs
Amy L Porter, Director
Roderick L Bremby, Commissioner
Provides a broad range of services to the elderly, disabled, families, and individuals who need assistance in maintaining or achieving their full potential for self-direction, self-reliance and independent living.

Delaware

5815 Delaware Division of Vocational Rehabilitation
Delaware Department of Labor
4425 N Market Street
Wilmington, DE 19802
302-761-8085
www.delawareworks.com
John McMahon, Secretary of Labor
The state's public program that helps people with physical and mental disabilities obtain or retain employment. Also, and Independent Living Program helps people with disabilities function in the community. DVR's commitment is to help people with disabilities increase independence through employment.

5816 Delaware Fair Employment Practice Agency
Delaware Department of Labor
Ste 6
820 North French Street
Wilmington, DE 19801-3509
302-577-8278
FAX: 302-577-6561
e-mail: delarts@state.de.us
artsdel.org
Karen Gimbutas, VP
Paul Weagraff, Director
Susan Salkin, Deputy Director
Dana Wise, Administrative Specialist
Provides opportunities and resources to eligible individuals with disabilities leading to success in employment and independent living.

5817 Delaware Job Training Program Liaison
Division of Employment & Training
P.O.Box 9828
820 N. French Street
Wilmington, DE 19801- 828
302-577-8977
FAX: 302-577-3996
www.jobaps.com
Harold Stafford, Manager
Work adjustment and remunerative work programs. Also offers career guidance, supported employment, work readiness and job placement.

5818 Service Source
3030 Bowers St
Wilmington, DE 19802
302-762-0300
800-738-1733
FAX: 302-762-8797
www.servicesource.org
Michelle Lee, President/CEO
Rhonda VanLowe, Legal Counsel
Joseph J. Sorota, President
Marilynn Bersoff, BTG
ServiceSource is a leading nonprofit disability resource organization with regional offices and programs located in eight states and the District of Columbia. We serve more than 14,000 individuals with disabilities annually through a range of innovative and valued employment, training, habilitation, housing and other support services. ServiceSource directly employs more than 1,500 individuals on government and commercial affirmative employment contracts.

District of Columbia

5819 District of Columbia Department of Employment Services
4058 Minnesota Avenue NE
Washington, DC 20019
202-724-7000
FAX: 202-673-6993
e-mail: does@dc.gov
does.dc.gov

5820 District of Columbia Dept. of Employment Services: Office of Workforce Development
4058 Minnesota Avenue, NE
Washington, DC 20019
202-671-1633
877-319-7346
FAX: 202-673-6993
TTY: 202-673-6994
e-mail: does@dc.gov
www.does.dc.gov
Diana C Johnson, Public Information Officer
Marianna Lourenco, Specialist/ADA Coordinator
To foster economic development and growth in the District of Columbia by providing workforce training, bringing together job seekers and employers, compensating unemployed and injured workers and promoting safe and healthy workplaces.

5821 District of Columbia Fair Employment Practice Agencies
D C Office of Human Rights
Ste 570n
441 4th Street NW
Washington, DC 20001-2714
202-727-3400
FAX: 202-347-8922
TTY:202-727-3400
e-mail: oag@dc.gov
http://oag.dc.gov
Elizabeth Noel, Executive Director
Irvin B. Nathan, Attorney General
Ariel B. Levinson-Waldman, Senior Counsel to the Attorney G
Victor Bonett, Legislative Director FOIA Office
Investigations and discrimination complaints.

5822 Goodwill of Greater Washington
2200 South Dakota Ave NE
Washington, DC 20018-1622
202-636-4225
888-817-4323
FAX: 202-526-3994
e-mail: info@dcgoodwill.org
dcgoodwill.org
Catherine Meloy, CEO
Brendan Hurley, Vice President Marketing & Commu
Judy Sklar, Regional Director Retail Operati
Colleen Paletta, Vice President Workforce Develop
Offers vocational training, job training, sheltered employment and work experience.

5823 Green Door
1221 Taylor Street, NW
Washington, DC 20011-3063 202-464-9200
FAX: 202-464-5730
e-mail: info@greendoor.org
www.greendoor.org

Judith Johnson, Executive Director
Brenda Randall, Assistant Director
Richard R. Bebout, Ph.D., President and CEO
Linda Wheeler Banton, Chair

Green Door is a community program which prepares people with a severe and persistent mental illness to live and work independently. Since 1976, Green Door has provided comprehensive services to mentally ill people, including housing, job training, job placement, education, homeless outreach, case management, support for people with substance abuse problems, family support,and specialized help for people who have had repeated hospitalizations.

5824 Operation Job Match
National Multiple Sclerosis Society
Suite 750 South
1800 M St NW
Washington, DC 20036-5802 202-887-0136
FAX: 202-296-3425
e-mail: OJM@nmss.org
operationjobmatch.org

Steven Nissen, Manager
Jeanne Angulo, Executive Director

Job readiness program for individuals with adult-onset physical disabilities.

5825 Rehabilitation Services Administration
10th Floor
810 First Street NE
Washington, DC 20002-4227 202-442-8663
FAX: 202-442-8742
e-mail: dds@dc.gov
rsa.dhs.dc.gov

Elizabeth Parker, Administrator
Mark D. Back, FOIA Officer
Laura L. Nuss, Director, Department on Disabili

State Rehabilitation Agency providing services to eligible persons with disabilities.

5826 WAVE Work, Achievement, Value, & Education
Suite 500
525 School St SW
Washington, DC 20024-2762 202-484-0103
800-274-2005
FAX: 202-488-7595
e-mail: wave4kids@aol.com
www.waveinc.org

Dr. Steven W Edwards, President & CEO
Arthur Griffin, Senior Vice President
Dr. Beth P. Reynolds, Executive Director
Dr. Sandy Addis, Associate Director

Job placement programs, remunerative work services and work adjustment training programs for 18 and 21 years of age in many cities across the country including Drop-Out Recovery Programs and Drop-Out Prevention Programs. Programs also available for youth ages 12-18. Youth Professionals Development and Training and key aspects of WAVE services, as well.

Florida

5827 Abilities of Florida: An Affiliate of Service Source
2735 Whitney Road
Clearwater, FL 33760-1610 727-538-7370
FAX: 727-538-7387
e-mail: abilities@ourpeoplework.org
servicesource.org

Janet Samuelson, President & CEO
Mark Hall, Executive Vice President
David Hodge, Executive Vice President & CEO
Bruce Patterson, Executive Vice President & CEO

Provides a full range of employment services including work evaulation, training, job coaching, job placement, advocacy and education. Also provides housing assistance and specialized to adults with cystic fibrosis.

5828 Career Assessment & Planning Services
Goodwill Industries - Suncoast Incorporated
10596 Gandy Blvd
St Petersburg, FL 33702-1422 727-523-1512
888-279-1988
FAX: 727-563-9300
TTY: 727-579-1068
e-mail: gw.marketing@goodwillhisuncoast.com
www.goodwill-suncoast.org

Oscar J. Horton, Chair
Martin W. Gladysz, Sr. Vice Chair
Heather Ceresoli, Vice Chair
Deborah A. Passerini, President

Career assessment and planning services help determine how prepared an individual is for employment, training, or future education. It is a comprehensive assessment that can predict current and future employment and potential adjustment factors for physically, emotionally or developmentally disabled persons who may be unemployed or underemployed.

5829 Choices to Work Program
Goodwill Industries-Suncoast
10596 Gandy Blvd
St Petersburg, FL 33702-1422 727-523-1512
888-279-1988
FAX: 727-563-9300
TTY: 727-579-1068
e-mail: gw.marketing@goodwill-suncoast.com
goodwill-suncoast.org

Oscar J. Horton, Chair
Martin W. Gladysz, Sr. Vice Chair
Heather Ceresoli, Vice Chair
Deborah A. Passerini, President

Assisting individuals currently eligible for Workman's Compensation, this program allows those recovering from injury on the job to prepare to return to independent employment, either through increasing ability and confidence in using adaptive behaviors and/or equipment to return to related employment, or adjusting to a more compatible employment environment.

5830 Florida Division of Vocational Rehabilitation
Bldg A
4070 Esplanade Way
Tallahassee, FL 32399-7016 800-451-4327
800-451-4327
FAX: 850-245-3316
TTY: 866-515-3692
e-mail: ombudsman@vr.fldoe.org
rehabworks.org

Bill Palmer, Manager
Debra Thompson, Florida Rehabilitation Council
Roy Cosgrove, Administrator
Andrea Schwendinger, Government Analyst

Rehabilitation services are important when a physical or mental handicap interferes with your ability to work. Our purpose is to help prepare for, and return to, gainful employment.

5831 Florida Fair Employment Practice Agency
Florida Commission on Human Relations
Suite 100
2009 Apalachee Parkway
Tallahassee, FL 32301- 4830 850-488-7082
800-342-8170
FAX: 850-488-5291
TTY: 800-955-1339
e-mail: fchrinfo@fchr.myflorida.com
http://fchr.state.fl.us

Michelle Wilson, Executive Director
Gilbert Singer, Chairman
Mario Valle, Vice Chairman
Gayle Cannon, Commissioner

The Commission is the state agency charged with enforcing the state's civil rights laws and serves as a resource on human relations for the people of Florida.

5832 **Goodwill Industries-Suncoast Adult Day Training**
10596 Gandy Blvd N
St Petersburg, FL 33702-1422 727-523-1512
888-279-1988
FAX: 727-563-9300
e-mail: gw.marketing@goodwill-suncoast.com
goodwill-suncoast.org

Lee Waits, President

Goodwill's adult day training programs enable people with developmental disabilities to set and achieve personal goals within a work-like setting. Participants work at various jobs throughout Goodwill and engage in a variety of activities that will allow them to become more self-sufficients.

5833 **Goodwill Industries-Suncoast Inc. Adult Day Training**
10596 Gandy Blvd.
St. Petersburg, FL 33702-3305 727-523-1512
888-279-1988
FAX: 727-563-9300
TTY: 727-579-1068
e-mail: gw.marketing@goodwill-suncoast.com
www.goodwill-suncoast.org

Oscar J. Horton, Chair
Martin W. Gladysz, Sr. Vice Chair
Heather Ceresoli, Vice Chair
Deborah A. Passerini, President

Goodwill's adult day training programs enable people with developmental disabilities to set and achieve personal goals within a work-like setting. Participants work at various jobs throughout Goodwill and engage in a variety of activities that will allow them to become more self-sufficients.

5834 **Goodwill Industries-Suncoast Inc. Adult Day Training**
10596 Gandy Blvd.
St. Petersburg, FL 33702-3704 727-523-1512
888-279-1988
FAX: 727-563-9300
TTY: 727-579-1068
e-mail: gw.marketing@goodwill-suncoast.com
www.goodwill-suncoast.org

Oscar J. Horton, Chair
Martin W. Gladysz, Sr. Vice Chair
Heather Ceresoli, Vice Chair
Deborah A. Passerini, President

Goodwill's adult day training programs enable people with developmental disabilities to set and achieve personal goals within a work-like setting. Participants work at various jobs throughout Goodwill and engage in a variety of activities that will allow them to become more self-sufficients.

5835 **Goodwill Industries-Suncoast Non-Residential Supports And Services Program**
10596 Gandy Blvd N
St Petersburg, FL 33702-1422 727-523-1512
888-279-1988
FAX: 727-563-9300
TTY: 727-579-1068
e-mail: gw.marketing@goodwill-suncoast.com
goodwill-suncoast.org

Lee Waits, President
Jean-Marie Moore, Director Of Operations

Goodwill's adult day training programs enable people with developmental disabilities to set and achieve personal goals within a work-like setting. Participants earn paychecks working at various jobs throughout Goodwill and engage in a variety of activities that will allow them to become more self-sufficients.

5836 **Goodwill Industries-Suncoast Supported Living**
10596 Gandy Blvd
St Petersburg, FL 33702-1422 727-523-1512
888-279-1988
FAX: 727-563-9300
TTY: 727-579-1068
e-mail: gw.marketing@goodwill-suncoast.com
goodwill-suncoast.org

Oscar J. Horton, Chair
Martin W. Gladysz, Sr. Vice Chair
Heather Ceresoli, Vice Chair
Deborah A. Passerini, President

Goodwill's supported living program helps people with developmental disabilities expand their skills so they can lead increasingly independentlives. Individuals receive training and assistance with daily living activities while living in the community. Additional support includes assistance with legal issues, adocacy, community resources, banking, safety procedures, self-medication, household management, meal preparation, interpersonal relationships and parenting training.

5837 **Goodwill Industries-Suncoast,Adult Day Training**
10596 Gandy Blvd
St Petersburg, FL 33702-5654 727-523-1512
888-279-1988
FAX: 727-563-9300
TTY: 727-579-1068
e-mail: gw.marketing@goodwill-suncoast.com
goodwill-suncoast.org

Oscar J. Horton, Chair
Martin W. Gladysz, Sr. Vice Chair
Heather Ceresoli, Vice Chair
Deborah A. Passerini, President

Goodwill's adult day training programs enable people with developmental disabilities to set and achieve personal goals within a work-like setting. Participants work at various jobs throughout Goodwill and engage in a variety of activities that will allow them to become more self-sufficients.

5838 **Goodwill Temporary Staffing**
Goodwill Industries- Suncoast
10596 Gandy Blvd
St Petersburg, FL 33702-1422 727-523-1512
888-279-1988
FAX: 727-576-1314
TTY: 727-579-1068
e-mail: gw.marketing@goodwill-suncoast.com
goodwill-suncoast.org

Oscar J. Horton, Chair
Martin W. Gladysz, Sr. Vice Chair
Heather Ceresoli, Vice Chair
Deborah A. Passerini, President

Provides employment links from potential employees, both disabled and non-disabled alike to employers with immediate employment opportunities seeking qualified candidates. Pre-screening on all applicants include: Employment history, personal references, law enforcement background checks and substance screening.

5839 **Impact: Ocala Vocational Services**
Goodwill Industries- Suncoast
10596 Gandy Blvd
St Petersburg, FL 33702-1422 727-523-1512
888-279-1988
FAX: 727-563-9300
TTY: 727-579-1068
e-mail: gw.marketing@goodwill-suncoast.com
goodwill-suncoast.org

Oscar J. Horton, Chair
Martin W. Gladysz, Sr. Vice Chair
Heather Ceresoli, Vice Chair
Deborah A. Passerini, President

Designed to enable individuals with disabilities to work in integrated settings in the community, receiving wages and benefits matching those of non-handicapped workers.

5840 JobWorks NISH Food Service
Goodwill Industries- Suncoast
10596 Gandy Blvd
St Petersburg, FL 33702-1422
727-523-1512
888-279-1988
FAX: 727-563-9300
TTY: 727-579-1068
e-mail: gw.marketing@goodwill-suncoast.com
goodwill-suncoast.org

Oscar J. Horton, Chair
Martin W. Gladysz, Sr. Vice Chair
Heather Ceresoli, Vice Chair
Deborah A. Passerini, President

An enclave style (or group) supported employment program designed to give consumers additional supports that allow and encourage increasingly independent employment opportunities within a food services environment.

5841 JobWorks NISH Postal Service
Goodwill Industries - Suncoast
10596 Gandy Blvd
St Petersburg, FL 33702-1422
727-523-1512
888-279-1988
FAX: 727-563-9300
TTY: 727-579-1068
e-mail: gw.marketing@goodwill-suncoast.com
goodwill-suncoast.org

Oscar J. Horton, Chair
Martin W. Gladysz, Sr. Vice Chair
Heather Ceresoli, Vice Chair
Deborah A. Passerini, President

An enclave style (or group) supported employment program designed to give consumers additional supports that allow and encourage increasingly independent employment opportunities within a mailroom environment.

5842 Lighthouse Central Florida
215 East New Hampshire Street
Orlando, FL 32804-6403
407-898-2483
888-898-2483
FAX: 407-898-0236
e-mail: lvaneepoel@lcf-fl.org
lighthousecentralflorida.com

Lee Nasehi, Executive Director
Lee Van Eepoel, Program Service Director
Donna Esbensen, Vice President, Chief Financial
Kimberly Pawling, Director of Education & Rehabili

Lighthouse Central Florida (LCF) is the only non-profit organization offering comprehensive, professional, vision rehabilitation services to Central Floridians of all ages with low vision or blindness.

5843 MAClown Vocational Rehabilitation Workshop
6390 NE 2nd Ave
Miami, FL 33138-6036
305-759-0212

Sabrina Shelton, Manager

Provides remunerative work.

5844 One-Stop Service
Goodwill Industries- Suncoast
10596 Gandy Blvd.
St Petersburg, FL 33702-1422
727-523-1512
888-279-1988
FAX: 727-563-9300
TTY: 727-579-1068
e-mail: gw.marketing@goodwill-suncoast.com
goodwill-suncoast.org

R. Lee Waits, President and CEO
Deborah A. Passerini, Executive Vice President and Chi
Gary Hebert, Corporate Treasurer and Chief Fi
Lee C. Zeh, Corporate Secretary and Vice Pre

Provides universal job search and placement related services are available to any person entering the service center. Each One-Stop Services Center provides on-site representation from a variety of employment-related service providers. All One-Stops host and/or facilitate local employment fairs and provides access to computerized job-postings.

5845 Palm Beach Habilitation Center
4522 South Congress Avenue
Lake Worth, FL 33461-4797
561-965-8500
FAX: 561-433-8816
e-mail: postman@pbhab.com
pbhab.com

Jeffrey Chapman, Chief Financial Officer
David Lin, Vice President of Programs & Services
Roxanne Jacobs, Director of Developmen
Tina Philips, President/CEO

Providing work evaluation, work adjustment, job placement, employment, residential and retirement services for mentally, emotionally and physically disabled adults.

5846 Primrose Supported Employment Programs
2733 South Ferncreek Ave
Orlando, FL 32806-5538
407-898-7201
FAX: 407-898-2120
www.primrosecenter.org

Mary Vanburen, Executive Director
Leslie North, Chairman
Helen Galloway, Board Director
Faye Scott-Evans, Board Director

Mission is to transform the lives of people with developmental disabilities by providing opportunities to achieve their fullest potential.

5847 Quest
500 E. Colonial Drive
Orlando, FL 32803-4504
407-218-4300
888-807-8378
FAX: 407-218-4301
e-mail: contact@questinc.org
questinc.org

John Gill, President / CEO
Todd Thrasher, Chief Financial Officer
Eb Blakely, Vice President, Behavioral Services
Karenne Levy, Chief Operating Officer

Quest has built communities where people with disabilities have achieved their goals for nearly 50 years. Through a variety of residential and employment options, behavioral therapy, therapeutic day programs, charter schools and even a recreational summer camp, Quest serves more than 1000 individuals each day in the Orlando and Tampa areas.

5848 Quest - Tampa Area
1404 Tech Blvd
Tampa, FL 33619
813-423-7700
888-807-8378
FAX: 813-423-7701
e-mail: contact@questinc.org
www.questinc.org

John Gill, President / CEO
Todd Thrasher, Chief Financial Officer
Eb Blakely, Vice President, Behavioral Services
Karenne Levy, Chief Operating Officer

Quest has built communities where people with disabilities have achieved their goals for nearly 50 years. Through a variety of residential and employment options, behavioral therapy, therapeutic day programs, charter schools and even a recreational summer camp, Quest serves more than 1000 individuals each day in the Orlando and Tampa areas.

5849 SCARC, Inc Evaluation, Training + Emploment Center
213 West McCollum Avenue
Bushnell, FL 33513-5916
352-793-5156
FAX: 352-793-6545
e-mail: marshaperkins@embargmail.com
http://scarcinc.com

Marsha Perkins, Administrator

Training and employment program for adults with disabilities. SCARC offers vocational evaluation, training, work services, transportation, supported independent living and community based training.

5850 Seagull Industries for the Disabled
3879 Byron Drive
West Palm Beach, FL 33404-3311 561-842-5814
FAX: 561-881-3554
e-mail: main@seagull.org
www.seagull.org

Fred Eisinger, Executive Director
Linda Moore, Assistant Executive Director, Se
Joyce Hambrick, Director of Program Services
Ellen Hoffacker, Director of Finance

Dedicated to improving the quality of life of mentally, physically and emotionally challenged adults in Palm Beach County, Florida through advocacy and the provision of a variety of social service, vocational training and residential programs designed to encourage self reliance and independence.

5851 Supported Employment Program
Goodwill Industries - Suncoast
10596 Gandy Blvd.
St Petersburg, FL 33702-1422 727-523-1512
888-279-1988
FAX: 727-563-9300
TTY: 727-579-1068
e-mail: gw.marketing@goodwill-suncoast.com
www.goodwill-suncoast.org

R. Lee Waits, President and CEO
Deborah A. Passerini, Executive Vice President and Chi
Gary Hebert, Corporate Treasurer and Chief Fi
Lee C. Zeh, Corporate Secretary and Vice Pre

Goodwill's supported employment program enables people with developmental disabilities to work in the community, earning wages and benefits marching those of non-disabled workers. Participants receive intensive on-the-job training at job sites that have been carefully chosen for their suitability. A support facilitator provides follow-up job coaching to ensure success. Serving people in Pinellas, Hillsborough and Pasco counties.

5852 The Able Trust
3320 Thomasville Road
Suite 200
Tallahassee, FL 32308 850-224-4493
888-838-2253
888-838-2253
FAX: 850-224-4496
TTY:850-224-4493
e-mail: info@abletrust.org
www.abletrust.org

Susanne Homant, President & CEO
Guenevere Crum, Senior Vice President
Ray Ford, Assistant Director of Communicat
Jessica Taylor, Assistant to the President & CEO

Provides grant funds for employment-related programs for non-profit agencies in Florida. Assists families, individuals and agencies through educational conferences, and youth training programs. Provides businesses free resources for hiring people with disabilities.

5853 Vocational and Rehabilitation Agency Department of Education
Bldg A
4070 Esplanade Way
Tallahassee, FL 32399-7016 850-245-3399
800-451-4327
FAX: 850-245-3316
TTY: 850-488-0867
e-mail: speaker@vr.fldoe.org
rehabworks.org

Bill Palmer, Manager
Aleisa McKinlay, Director

Work adjustment and remunerative work programs.

5854 Vocational and Rehabilitation Agency: Division of Blind Services
401 Platt Street
Daytona Beach, FL 32114-2803 386-254-3856
800-522-5078
FAX: 386-252-3800
e-mail: craig_kiser@dbe.doe.state.fl.us
www.state.fl.us/dbs

Bill Palmer, Manager
Carl Augusto, President and CEO
Kelly Bleach, Chief Administrative Officer
Rick Bozeman, Chief Financial Officer

Mission is to ensure blind and visually impaired Floridians have the tools, support, and opportunity to achieve success.

5855 Work Exploration Center
3000 N West 83rd Street i 40
Gainesville, FL 32606 352-395-5265
FAX: 352-395-5271
admin.sfcc.edu

Karla Wooten, Coordinator

The Work Exploration Center embraces a holistic approach to Comprehensive Vocational Evaluation and Community Employment services, encouraging individual understanding, hope and growth for a productive and fulfilling future.

Georgia

5856 Employment and Training Division, Region B
Goodwill Industries of North Georgia
1123 Progress Rd
Ellijay, GA 30540-5504 706-276-4722
888-514-8112
FAX: 706-276-4732
e-mail: vti@ellijay.com

Linda Rau, Director Programs/Services

Employment training, assessment and job placement for people who have disabilities and/or are disadvantaged. Serving 15 counties in Northern Georgia.

5857 Fair Housing and Equal Employment
Georgia Commission on Equal Opportunity
7 Martin Luther King, Jr. Drive, S.
3rd Floor
Atlanta, GA 30334-9000 404-656-1736
800-473-6736
FAX: 404-656-4399
e-mail: gceo@gceo.state.ga.us
www.gceo.state.ga.us

Teresa Chappell, Fair Housing Division Director
Stephanie Randolph, Intake Coordinator/Housing
Abdul Wali Khadeem, Equal Employment Division Director
Melvin J. Everson, Executive Director/Administrator

To investigate housing and employment discrimination in the state of Georgia.

5858 Griffin Area Resource Center Griffin Community Workshop Division
931 Hamilton Boulevard
Post Office Box 83
Griffin, GA 30224 770-229-4212
FAX: 770-229-4212
e-mail: united_way@bellsouth.net
http://www.gscunitedway.org

Cary Grubbs, Executive Director
Charles Cary Grubbs, Garc Executive Director
Rodney Shurman, President
Dr. Curtis Jones, Vice-President

A CARF (The Rehabilitation Accreditation Commission) accredited Employment and Community Support organization providing daily services to participants with disabilities from 16 years of age and up in a 5 county area.

5859 IBM National Support Center
Special Needs Systems
P.O.Box 2150
Atlanta, GA 30301-2150 404-577-7995
800-426-2133
FAX: 561-982-6059
TTY: 800-284-9482
www.skepticfiles.org/md001/mobility.htm

5860 Kelley Diversified
P.O.Box 967
Athens, GA 30603-967 706-549-4398
FAX: 706-549-4479
ibizprofile.com/biz/kelley-diversified-inc-30
Mary Patton, Executive Director
Sherry Burns, Rehabilitation Services Director
Jenny Taylor, Business Operations Manager
Patricia Horne, Bookkeeper
Work adjustment and remunerative work programs.

5861 New Ventures
306 Fort Dr
Lagrange, GA 30240-5900 706-882-7723
FAX: 706-882-5401
e-mail: customersvc@newventures.org
newventures.org
Dave Miller, CEO
Kelly Anderson, Quality Director
Jeff Chamberlain, Director of Business Services
Mike Wilson, Director of Industrial Marketing
A rehabilitation and work training facility for individuals with barriers to employability. The program utilizes community based industrial work of varying levels of difficulty. A return to work conditioning program for the industrially injured is offered which features: first-day contact, workers compensation rehabilitation team management, and light-duty work conditioning. A training stipend is paid to defray costs associated with training.

Hawaii

5862 Assets School
One Ohana Nui Way
Honolulu, HI 96818-4497 808-423-1356
FAX: 808-422-1920
e-mail: info@assets-school.net
assets-school.net
John F. Morton, Chairman
Kristi L. Maynard, Vice Chairman
Robert W. Wo, Secretary
Russell J. Lau, Treasurer
ASSETS is an independent school for gifted and or dyslexic children that provides an individualized, integrated learning enviroment. ASSETS' enviroment empowers these children to maximize their potential and to find their place as lifelong learners in school and society.

5863 Hawaii Fair Employment Practice Agency
Room 411
830 Punchbowl St
Honolulu, HI 96813-5080 808-586-8636
800-586-8800
FAX: 808-586-8655
TTY: 808-586-8692
e-mail: DLIR.HCRC.INFOR@hawaii.gov
http://hawaii.gov/labor/hcrc
Michael O Yamamoto
William Hoshijo, Executive Director
HCRC enforces state laws prohibiting discrimination in employment.

5864 Hawaii Vocational Rehabilitation Division
1901 Bachelot St.
Honolulu, HI 96817 808-586-9744
FAX: 808-586-9755
TTY:808-586-9744
e-mail: info@hawaiivr.org
hawaiivr.org
Jonathan Chun, Chair
Albert Perez, Administrator
Susan Foard, Assistant Administrator
Katie Keim, Staff Specialist
Mission is our committed staff strive, day-in day-out, to provide timely efficient and effective programs, services and benefits, for the purpose of achieving the outcome of empowering those who are the most vulnerable in our state to expand thier capacity for self sufficiency, self-determination, independence, healthy choices, quality of life and personal dignity.

5865 Lanakila Rehabilitation Center
1809 Bachelot St
Honolulu, HI 96817-2430 808-531-0555
FAX: 808-533-7264
TTY:808-531-0555
e-mail: info@lanakilahawaii.org
www.lanakilahawaii.org
Marian Tsuji, President
Wayne Fujishige, Vice President
Dwayne MASUTANI, Director Budget & Finance
Rachael Young, Director Human Resources
Lanakila is a private nonprofit organization whose mission is to provide services and supports that assist individuals with physical, mental, or age-related challenges to live as independently as possible within our community. A broad range of services are offered which include meal/senior services, community based adult day programming for individuals with disabilities, work training opportunities, and extended/supported employment for individuals with special needs.

5866 Vocational and Rehabilitation Agency
P.O.Box 339
601 Kamokila Boulevard, Room 515
Kapolei, HI 96707-339 808-692-7719
FAX: 808-692-7727
TTY:808-692-7715
e-mail: sfoard@dhs.hawaii.gov
http://www.hawaiivr.org/
Albert Perez, Manager
Work adjustment and remunerative work programs.

5867 Wahiawa Family
302 California Ave
#204
Wahiawa, HI 96786-1883 808-621-7407
wpf-dentalcare.com/
Leslie Chinna
Work adjustment and remunerative work programs.

Idaho

5868 Idaho Employment Service and Job Training Program Liaison
Idaho Department of Employment
317 W Main St
Boise, ID 83735-1 208-332-3578
FAX: 208-327-7470
e-mail: idahocis@labor.idaho.gov
http://labor.idaho.gov
Roger Madsen, Manager
C.L Butch Otter, Governor
Roger B. Madson, Director
Renee Cox, Program Manager
Work adjustment and remunerative work programs.

5869 Idaho Fair Employment Practice Agency
Idaho Human Rights Commission
P.O.Box 83720
450 West State Street
Boise, ID 83720-3 208-334-2873
FAX: 208-334-2664
www2.state.id.us/ihrc/ihrchome.htm

David Rogers, Administrator

Mission is to admininster state and federal anti-discrimination laws in Idaho in a manner that is fair, accurate, and timely; and to work towards ensuring that all people withink the state are treated with dignity and respect in their places of employment, housing, education, and public accomodations.

5870 Idaho Governor's Committee on Employment of People with Disabilities
317 W Main St
Boise, ID 83735-1 208-332-3750
FAX: 208-327-7331
www.dol.gov

5871 Idaho Vocational Rehabilitation Agency
Room 150
650 W. State St.
Boise, ID 83704-8780 208-334-3390
FAX: 208-327-7417
TTY:208-327-7040
e-mail: department.info@vr.idaho.gov
vr.idaho.gov

Darrell Quist, Manager
Janet Thaldorf, Supervisor

Vocational Rehabilitation assists many individuals with disabilities to go to work. With VR assistance, these individuals have overcome numerous obstacles and disability related barriers to achieve employment.

5872 Vocational and Rehabilitation Agency
Idaho Commission for the Blind & Visually Impaired
341 W Washington St
PO Box 83720
Boise, ID 83720-0012 208-334-3220
800-542-8688
FAX: 208-334-2963
e-mail: aroan@icbvi.state.id.us
icbvi.state.id.us

Angela Roan, Manager
Raelene Thomas, Management Assistant
Bruce Christopherson, Rehabilitation Services Chief
Dana Ard, Vocational Rehabilitation Counse

Vocational rehabilitation, independent living training, medical intervention, adaptive technology and devices and employer advocacy.

Illinois

5873 Ada S McKinley Vocational Services
1359 W Washington Blvd
Chicago, IL 60607-4577 312-554-0600
FAX: 312-554-0292
TTY:312-697-9794
e-mail: info@adasmckinley.org
adasmckinley.org

George Jones, Jr., Executive Director
Marion G. Sleet, Chief Operating Officer
Hans J. Schuster, Chief Financial Officer
Kathleen D. Chappell, Chief Development Officer

Mission is to serve those who, because of disabilities or other limiting conditions, need help in finding and pursuing paths leading to healthy, productive, and fulfilling lives.

5874 Anixter Center
2001 N. Clybourn Ave.
3rd Floor
Chicago, IL 60614 773-973-7900
FAX: 773-973-5268
TTY:773-973-2180
e-mail: AskAnixter@anixter.org
anixter.org

Kevin Limbeck, President and CEO
Stacy Brown, Executive Vice President
Lauren K. Hill, Managing Director
Dan Sabol, Vice President and Business Deve

A Chicago-based human services agency that assists people with disabilities to live and work successfully in the community. Anixter Center provides vocational training, employment services, residences, special education, prevention programs, community services and health care. In addition, Anixter Center offers Illinois' only substance abuse treatment programs specifically for people with disabilities including Addiction Recovery of the Deaf.

5875 C-4 Work Center
4740 North Clark St.
Chicago, IL 60640 773-769-0205
e-mail: infoc4@c4chicago.org
www.c4chicago.org

Eileen Durkin, President and CEO
Bruce Seitzer, LCPC, Senior Vice President
John Troy, MBA, CPA, Vice President of Finance
Danielle Byron, MS, Vice President of Information Systems

Aftercare, case finding, information and referrals, vocational training and work activities offered to mentally ill persons.

5876 Clearbrook
1835 W Central Rd
Arlington Heights, IL 60005-2410 847-870-7711
FAX: 847-870-7741
TTY:847-870-2239
e-mail: info@clearbrook.org
www.clearbrook.org

Carl M La Mell, President
Tracy Martin, Admissions Director
Bernie Andersen, Assistant to the President
Rosa Baez-Lopez, Vice President of Human Resource

Offers educational, employment and residential services to the developmentally disabled children and adults.

5877 Cornerstone Services
777 Joyce Rd
Joliet, IL 60436-1876 815-741-7600
FAX: 815-723-1177
e-mail: jhogan@cornerstoneservices.org
cornerstoneservices.org

James A Hogan, CEO
Susan Murphy, Coordinator Public Relations
Ben Stortz, President/Chief Executive Officer
Don Hespell, Vice-President/Chief Operating Officer

Cornerstone Services provides progressive, comprehensive services for people with disabilities, promoting choice, dignity and the opportunity to live and work in the community. Established in 1969, the agency provides developmental, vocational, employment, residential and behavioral health services at various community-based locations. The nonprofit social service agency helps approximately 750 people each day.

5878 Fulton County Rehab Center
500 N Main St
Canton, IL 61520-1844 309-647-6510
FAX: 309-647-7965
www.fultoncountyrehabilitationcenter.com

Rex L. Lewis, Executive Director
John C. Harmon, Public Relations / Marketing
Rhonda S. Dawson, Production Director

Residential rehab center with health care incidental; manufactures wood pallets and skids; job training and vocational rehabilitation services.

5879 Glenkirk
3504 Commercial Ave
Northbrook, IL 60062-1863
847-272-5111
FAX: 847-272-7350
e-mail: info@glenkirk.org
glenkirk.org

Allan G. Spector, CEO

Helps infants, children and adults with developmental disabilities reach higher levels of independence. A non-profit organization serving people in north and northwest Chicago suburbs. Glenkirk's residential, vocational, educational and support programs include services which provide individual evaluation, therapeutic treatment and training.

5880 Illinois Employment Service
Department of Employment Security
Fl 4
401 S State St
Chicago, IL 60605-1293
312-793-4880
800-247-4984
www.state.il.us/agency/

5881 Jewish Vocational Services
216 West Jackson Blvd.
Suite 700
Chicago, IL 60606-4602
312-673-3400
FAX: 312-553-5544
e-mail: jvschgo@jvschicago.org
http://jvschicago.org/

H. Debra Levin, President
Alan S. Crane, Vice President
Marc Jacobs, Vice President
Benn Feltheimer, Secretary

Occupational training and job placement for handicapped persons of all religions.

5882 JoDavies Workshop
P.O.Box 6087
706 West Street
Galena, IL 61036-6087
815-777-2211
FAX: 815-777-3386
e-mail: theworkshopgalena@theworkshopgalena.org
www.jdwi.org

Jean Muchow, Treasurer
Peg Tonne, Chairperson
Dale Gereau, Plant Manager
Lynn Berning, Vice Chairperson

Intake and referral, early intervention for children only, vocational evaluation and work adjustment training services offered.

5883 Kennedy Job Training Center
18350 Crossing Drive
Tinley Park, IL 60487-6122
708-342-5246
FAX:708-594-7156
e-mail: Information@stcolettail.org
http://www.stcolettail.org

Robin Mertes, Placement Manager
Kandy Stamer, QMRP/Intake Coordinator
Bob Loquercio, Board of Director
Wayne A. Kottmeyer, Executive Director

Offers vocational evaluation, vocational training work adjustment training, and job placement services for developmentally disabled and hearing impaired persons.

5884 Knox County Council for Developmental Disabilities
2015 Windish Dr
Galesburg, IL 61401-9774
309-344-2600
FAX: 309-344-1754
e-mail: mcrittenden@kccdd.com
kccdd.com

Mary Crittenden, Executive Director
Pam Green, Director of Operations
Jeff Gomer, Director of Finance
Lynndel Messmore, Director of Rehabilitation

Developmental training, vocational evaluation, work adjustment training, extended training, placement, supported employment.

5885 Kreider Services
500 Anchor Road
Dixon, IL 61021-366
815-288-6691
FAX: 815-288-1636
TTY:815-288-5931
e-mail: info@kreiderservices.org?subject=Kreider%20Se
kreiderservices.org

Dr. Richard Piller, President
Dr. Vernon Brickley, Vice President
Cheryl Ebens, Director
Mike Hickey, Director

Offers day service programs, vocational training programs, job placement, supported employment, respite care, residential and family support for ages birth to three years.

5886 Lambs Farm
14245 W Rockland Rd
Libertyville, IL 60048-9745
847-362-4636
FAX: 847-362-9688
e-mail: info@lambsfarm.org
lambsfarm.org

Dianne Yaconetti, President & CEO
Kathy Buresch, Director, Operations, Marketing
Nikki Bonamarte, Director, Development
Jose Martinez, Director, Quality Assurance

Person-centered, comprehensive program of residential, vocational and social support service for adults with developmental disabilities.

5887 Land of Lincoln Goodwill Industries
1220 Outer Park Drive
Springfield, IL 62704
217-789-0400
FAX: 217-789-0540
e-mail: info@llgi.org
www.llgi.org

Sharon Durbin, CEO and President
Valerie Ausmus, VP of Finance
Deborah Clark, VP of Retail Operations
Kim Wonnell, VP of Human Resources

Empowers people with special needs to become self-sufficient through the power od work.

5888 Orchard Village
7660 Gross Point Road
Skokie, IL 60077-2628
847-967-1800
FAX: 847-967-9543
e-mail: info@orchardvillage.org
www.orchardvillage.org

Joy Decker, President & CEO
Sally Ruecking, Vice President, Development
Allison Stark, Vice President, Programs
Jennifer Burgess, Director, Residential Services

Vocational program and counseling, respite services and community living group homes for the disabled and cognitively impaired. Orchard village also operates a private hope school especially devoted to teaching young adults independent living and skills necessary to flourish in the community.

5889 President's Committee on Employment of Employment of the Disabled
1331 F Street, NW,
Suite 300
Washington, DC 20004-1614
202-376-6200
800-ASK-DORI
FAX: 202-376-6219
TTY: 202-376-6205
e-mail: info@pcepd.gov
www.usccr.gov/pubs/crd/federal/pcepd.htm

Carol Adams, President
John Lancaster, Executive Director

Work adjustment and remunerative work programs.

5890 Sertoma Centre
4343 W 123rd St
Alsip, IL 60803-1807
708-371-9700
FAX: 708-371-9747
e-mail: info@sertomacentre.org
sertomacentre.org
Gus Vanden Brink, Executive Director
Paula Phillips, Assistant Director
A nationally accredited, not-for-profit agency that provides services to students and adults with developmental disabilities and mental illness. MIssion is to provide opportunities that empower individuals with disabilities to achieve success.

5891 Shore Training Center
Shore Community Services
4232 Dempster Street
Skokie, IL 60076
847-982-2030
FAX: 847-982-2039
TTY:847-581-0076
e-mail: info@shoreservices.org
shoreinc.org
Debora K. Braun, Executive Director
Kirsten Luna, Director of Residential Services
Debbie Shulruf, Director of SHORE Lois Lloyd Cen
Lisa Wright, Director, SHORE Joseph Koenig, S
Mission is to improve the quality of life for citizens with developmental disabilities through community based services providing education/training.

5892 Skills Inc.
44 Morris Street
Webster, MA 01570-1233
508-943-0700
FAX: 508-949-6129
e-mail: life-skills@life-skillsinc.org
skills-inc.org
Robert Miller, President
Pamela Guanci, Vice President
Raymond Bembenek, Treasurer
Janice Smith, Secretary
Accredited through the Commission on Accreditation of Rehabilitation Facilities; offers job training partnership act and vocational evaluation services offered.

5893 Thresholds AMISS
12145 Western Ave
Blue Island, IL 60406-1387
708-597-7997
FAX: 708-597-8073
Julia Rupp, Executive Director
Camille Rucks, Team Leader
Services offered include psychosocial, vocational and residential programs for ages 18 or older with a primary diagnosis of mental illness. Facility is wheelchair accessible.

5894 Vocational and Rehabilitation Agency
207 Staehouse
Springfield, IL 62706-1
217-782-0244
800-843-6154
FAX: 217-524-6262
TTY: 888-261-3336
e-mail: ITTF.Web@illinois.gov
www.state.il.us
Pat Quinn, Governor
Provides work adjustment and remunerative skills.

5895 Washington County Vocational Workshop
781 E Holzhauer Dr
Nashville, IL 62263-2055
618-327-4461
FAX: 618-327-4477
www.mapquest.com
Keith Curran, Executive Director
Provides job training and related services and vocational rehabilitation services.

5896 Westside Parents Work Activity Center
3395 Mottman Road SW
Olympia, WA 98512
360-339-7297
blackhillsgym.com/family-activity-center
Theresa McKenzieSullivan, General Manager
Offers developmental training programs providing basic skills in self care for multiply and physically handicapped persons.

Indiana

5897 ADEC Resources for Independence
19670 State Road 120
Bristol, IN 46507-9162
574-848-7451
877-342-8954
FAX: 574-848-5917
e-mail: shivelyp@adecinc.com
adecinc.com
Donna Belusar, President & CEO
Mitch Walorski, CFO
Sally Russell, Vice President
Joe Blocher, Vice President of Human Relation
Serves Elkhart County and surrounding area.

5898 ARC of Allen County
4919 Coldwater Rd
Fort Wayne, IN 46825-5532
260-456-4534
800-234-7811
FAX: 260-745-5200
e-mail: delbrecht@esarc.org
www.easterseals.com
Bill Martin, Chairperson
Larry Graham, Senior Vice Chairperson
Donna K. Elbrecht, President/CEO
Susan Klug, Chief Operating Officer
Primary list of services includes: community living services, production and work training services, residential services, 24 hour medicaid waiver services, employment services, child care center, adult day services, and recreation.

5899 Arc Bridges
2650 W 35th Ave
Gary, IN 46408-1416
219-985-6562
FAX: 219-980-7315
e-mail: mailbox@thearcnwindiana.com
www.thearcnwindiana.com
Brian Davis, Contact
Kris Prohl, Executive Director
Mission is to improve the welfare of people with intellectual and development disabilities and their families.

5900 BI-County Services
425 East Harrison Rd
Bluffton, IN 46714-9013
260-824-1253
FAX: 260-824-1892
e-mail: info@adifferentlight.com
www.bi-countyservices.com
John Whicker, President
Serves Wells and Adam Counties. Infant services, Medicaid waivers, music therapy, ICF, MR, group homes, sheltered employment, pay program and supported employment services available.

5901 Balance Centers of America
3831 Hughes Ave.
Ste 504B
Culver, CA 90232-2630
310-625-5657
americanbalancecenters.com/
Jane Labar, Contact
Offers developmental training programs providing basic skills in self care for physically handicapped persons.

5902 **Bridge Pointe Services & Goodwill of Southern Indiana, Inc**
Goodwill International
1329 Applegate Lane
P.O. Box 2488
Clarksville, IN 47131-2488
812-283-7908
800-660-3355
FAX: 812-283-6248
e-mail: comments@goodwillsi.org
http://www.goodwillsi.org/

Candice C. Barksdale, Chief Executive Director
Joel Henderson, PHR, Vice President of Human Resource
Bonnie Davis, Vice President of Donated Goods
Michelle Dayvault, Vice President of Development an

Career assesment, job readiness and placement, office skills training. Pediatric family support services. Childrens Academy, a developmental preschool.

5903 **Carey Services**
2724 S Carey St
Marion, IN 46953-3515
765-668-8961
FAX: 765-664-6747
www.careyservices.com

Bonnie Smith, Human Resources Manager
James Allbaugh, Chief Executive Officer
Gary Hendricks, Corporate Compliance
David Sprowl, Intake Coordinator

The mission of Carey Services is to create pathways towards self-sufficiency with personal satisfaction.

5904 **Evansville Association for the Blind**
500 North 2nd Avenue
Evansville, IN 47710-2355
812-422-1181
FAX: 812-424-3154
e-mail: eabcdc@evansville.net
http://www.evansvilleblind.org/

Karla Horrell, Executive Director
Daniel Dana, President
Larry Arp, Vice President
Pam Doerter, Vice President

An community rehabilitation facility untilizing individual goals to assist persons with disabilities achieve or maintain potenial

5905 **Four Rivers Resource Services**
P.O.Box 249
Hwy. 59 South
Linton, IN 47441-249
812-847-2231
FAX: 812-847-8836
e-mail: fourrivers@frrs.org
frrs.org

Kenton Barnes, President
Mary Lou Chapman, Vice-President
Ray Hart, Treasurer
Kathy Pennington, Secretary

Employment, community living, connections, follow-along, early intervention, preschool, healthy families, child care resource and referral and child care voucher program, impact, and transpotation services.

5906 **Gateway Services/JCARC**
P.O.Box 216
3500 North Morton Street
Franklin, IN 46131-216
317-738-5500
888-494-8069
FAX: 317-738-5522
www.gatewayarc.com

Karen Luehmann, Executive Director

Utilizes individual goals to assist persons with disabilities achieve or maintain potential.

5907 **Goodwill Industries of Central Indiana**
1635 West Michigan St
Indianapolis, IN 46222-3852
317-524-4313
FAX: 317-524-4336
TTY:317-524-4309
e-mail: goodwill@goodwillindy.org
goodwillindy.org

James M. Mc Clelland, President & CEO
Nicki Washburn, Disability Services Coordinator
Kent A. Kramer, Senior Vice President and Chief Operating Officer
Daniel J. Riley, Senior Vice President, Administration and Chief Financial Of

Goodwill is in the business of helping people find jobs and provides programs and services for people who want to work. Goodwill is a community resource committed to deploying our assets and leveraging our resources with those of others in the community to create more opportunities for people who need assistance to improve their ability to earn a living.

5908 **Indiana Civil Rights Commission**
100 North Senate Avenue
Suite N103
Indianapolis, IN 46204-2208
317-232-2600
800-628-2909
FAX: 317-232-6580
TTY: 800-743-3333
e-mail: info@icrc.in.gov
www.in.gov/icrc

Jamal Smith, Executive Director

Works to develop public policies that ensure equal opportunity in education to all.

5909 **Indiana Employment Services and Job Training Program Liaison**
10 North Senate Avenue
Indianapolis, IN 46204-2201
317-232-6702
FAX: 317-233-5499
www.in.gov/dwd

5910 **Michigan Resources**
4315 East Michigan Blvd
Michigan City, IN 46360-3151
219-874-4288
FAX: 219-874-2689
TTY:219-873-2245
e-mail: michiana@michianaresources.org
michianaresources.org

Nancy J Matela, Board Member
Matt Hollander, Chair
Gretchen Kalk, Treasurer
Andie Wolfinsohn, Secretary

Vocational training center for persons 16 and older with disabilities.

5911 **New Hope Services**
725 Wall Street
Jeffersonville, IN 47130-3616
812-288-8248
800-237-6604
FAX: 812-288-1206
e-mail: info@newhopeservices.org
newhopeservices.org

James A. Bosley, President and CEO
John Broady, Senior Vice President and CFO
Bonnie Long, Senior Vice President, CAO
Jody Kitch, Chief Operating Officer

Mission is to provide hope through services which are responsive to individual needs.

5912 **New Horizons Rehabilitation**
P.O.Box 98
237 Six Pine Ranch Road
Batesville, IN 47006-98
812-934-4528
FAX: 812-934-2522
e-mail: mdausch@nhrinc.org
www.nhrehab.org

Marie Dausch, Executive Director

Serves Ripley, Franklin, Ohio, Switzerland Dearborn, and Decatur. Provides training and services to adults with mental/physical disabilities and infants birth to age 3 with developmental delays or conditions of risk which could result in a developmental delay.

5913 Noble Of Indiana
Noble, Inc.
7701 East 21st Street
Indianapolis, IN 46219-2406
317-375-2700
FAX: 317-375-2719
e-mail: rita.davis@nobleofindiana.org
www.nobleofindiana.org
Julia Huffman, President & CEO
Rita Davis, Director, Community Relations
Julie Brown, Director of Human Resources
Jeanine Coleman, Director of Community Living
Since 1953, Noble of Indiana has been dedicated to its mission: to create opportunities for people with developmental disabilities to live meaningful lives.

5914 Office of State Coordinator of Vocational Education for Students with Disability
Rm 212
10 N Senate Ave
Indianapolis, IN 46204-2201
317-232-1829
800-891-6499
e-mail: tfields@dwd.state.in.us
www.state.in.us/dwd/techd
Scott B. Sanders, Commissioner
Randy Gillespie, Chief Financial Officer
Jeff Gill, General Counsel
Michelle Marshel, Deputy Commissioner of Communica
Manages and impliments innovative employment programs, unemployment insurance systems, and facilitates regional economic growth initiatives for Indiana.

5915 Putnam County Comprehensive Services
630 Tennessee St
Greencastle, IN 46135-2102
765-653-9763
877-653-9763
FAX: 765-653-3646
e-mail: cns_pccs@yahoo.com
www.pccsinc.org
Chuck Schroeder, CEO
Charles Schroeder, Executive Director
Teresa Human, Community Living Services Director
Josi Blunton, Residential Director
A not-for-profit organization serving individuals with disabilities and similar characteristics in Indiana. Their mission is to provide services to individuals with disabilities in order for them to reach their optimum potential in attitudes, habits, and skills through training and integration, making them contributing members of their community, and to promote community awareness and acceptance of people with different abilities.

5916 Southern Indiana Resource Solutions
1579 S Folsomville Rd
Boonville, IN 47601-9465
812-897-4840
FAX: 812-897-0123
e-mail: kelly@sirs.org
www.sirs.org
Kelly Mitchell, CEO/President
Don Critchlow, Chairperson
Larry Oathout, Vice-Chairperson
Jeff Hagedorn, Board Member
Adult services including jobs, community connections, and residential, childrens services, including service coordination and all therapies.

5917 Sycamore Rehabilitation Services
1001 Sycamore Lane
Danville, IN 46122-1474
317-745-4715
888-573-0817
FAX: 317-745-8271
e-mail: info@sycamoreservices.com
sycamoreservices.com
Ralph Dunkin, President
Terry Kessinger, Vice President
Steve Patterson, Treasurer
Peg Murphy, Secretary
Provides individuals training and services for persons with disabilities that enhance independence in all areas of life.

5918 Vocational and Rehabilitation Agency
P.O.Box 7083
2 Peachtree Street, NW
Atlanta, GA 30303- 7083
404-232-1998
800-545-7763
FAX: 404-232-1800
e-mail: GVRAcustomer-service@gvra.ga.gov
gvra.georgia.gov
Mike Hedden, Executive Director
James N. Defoor, Chair
Louise Hill, Vice Chair
Vocational training center for persons with disabilities.

5919 Wabash/Employability Center
201 I.U. Willets Road
S C6395 Earl Ave
Albertson, NY 11507
516-465-1400
FAX: 765-447-6456
e-mail: info@viscardicenter.org
http://www.nbdc.com
Bill Carmichael, Contact
John D. Kemp, Esq., President & CEO
Kenneth J. Kunken, Esq., County Court Deputy Bureau Chief
Constantina Petallides-Markou, Human Resources Manager
Serves Tippecanoe County.

Iowa

5920 ACT Assessment Test Preparation Reference Manual
American College Testing Program
P.O.Box 168
500 ACT Drive
Iowa City, IA 52243-168
319-337-1000
FAX: 319-339-3021
act.org
Jon Whitmore, Chief Executive Officer
Janet E. Godwin, Chief of Staff and Accountability Officer
Jon L. Erickson, President, Education and Career Solutions
Martin L. Scaglione, President, Workforce Development
This reference manual was developed as a resource for high school teachers and counselors in assisting students with test preparation.

5921 Franklin County Work Activity Center
20 5th St NW
Hampton, IA 50441-1908
641-456-2532
FAX: 641-456-4682
www.accessincorportated.org
Harry Jacoby, Executive Director
Jim Koenen, Owner
Nonprofit organization providing residential and vocational services in Franklin and Hardin counties in the state of Iowa. Residential Services include RCF/MR services, Supported Community Living Services and Community Supervised Apartment Living Arrangement Services. Vocational Services include Work Services and Supported Employment Services. Accredited by the Commission on Accreditation of rehabilitation Facilities since 1984, and serves individuals with a wide range of needs.

5922 Innovative Industries
405 E Madison St
Box 41205
Cleveland, OH 44141-2402
330- 46- 260
800-THE-M IR
FAX: 330- 46- 260
e-mail: info@innovativeindustries.com
www.innovativeindustries.com
Duane Nelson, Program Manager

5923 Iowa Civil Rights Commission
400 E 14th Street
Des Moines, IA 50319-201
515-281-4121
800-457-4416
FAX: 515-242-5840
e-mail: don.grove@iowa.gov
www.state.ia.us/government/crc

Ralph Rosenberg, Executive Director
Ron Pothast, Acting Executive Director
Corlis Moody, Executive Director
Beth Townsend, Executive Director

A neutral, fact-finding administrative agency that enforces the 'Iowa Civi Rights Act of 1965,' Iowa's anti-discrimination law. The commission doesn not provide legal representation. The commission's vision is a state free of discrimination.

5924 Iowa Employment Service
1000 East Grand Ave
Suite 140
Des Moines, IA 50309
515-282-5823
FAX: 515-288-2184
e-mail: fering@iowacareerconnection.com
www.iowacareerconnection.com

L.M. (Al) Fering, SPHR, FLMI, President
Miles Morrow, CPC

Specializes in accounting and human resources talent aquisition in the Upper-Midwest.

5925 Iowa Job Training Program Liaison
Iowa Department of Economic Development
200 East Grand Ave
Des Moines, IA 50309-1856
515-725-3000
FAX: 515-725-3010
e-mail: info@iowa.gov
iowalifechanging.com

David Lyons, President
Debi Durham, Director
Kathy Anderson, Director, Communications Team
Jody Benz, Director, Iowa Commission on Vol

To engender and promote economic development policies and practices which stimulate and sustain Iowa's economic growth and climate and that integrate efforts across public and private sectors.

5926 Iowa Valley Community College
3700 S. Center St.
Marshalltown, IA 50158-4783
641-752-7106
866-622-4748
FAX: 641-752-5909
e-mail: mccinfo@iavalley.edu.
http://www.iavalley.edu/

Dr. Chris Wynes, Chancellor
Robin Anctil, Director of Marketing
Dr. Lisa Breja, Institutional Researcher/AQIP Li
Nate Chua, MCC Director of Retention & Lear

Offers two levels of specialized vocational preparatory programming for adults with disabilities. The Career Development Center serves dependent adults. The goal of the program is to maintain or improve skills to enable persons served to enter sheltered or supported employment. The IRP/CBVT programs are non-credit specialized vocational programs for independent adults served by Vocational Rehabilitation and our programs. The goals are for competitive placements in jobs. CARF accredited.

5927 Iowa Vocational Rehabilitation Services
510 East 12th Street
Jessie Parker Building
Des Moines, IA 50319-0240
515-281-4211
FAX: 515-281-7645
TTY:515-281-4211
e-mail: Victoria.Carrington@iowa.gov
www.ivrs.iowa.gov

David Mitchell, Administrator
Matthew Coulter, Chief Financial Officer
Kenda Jochimsen, Bureau Chief
Charlie Levine, Assistant Bureau Chief

The mission is to work for and with individuals who have disabilities to achieve their employment, independence and economic goals.

5928 New Focus
102 W Washington St
Centerville, IA 52544-1550
641-437-1722
FAX: 641-437-1028

Peggy Oden, Executive Director

Provides vocational services for adults with disabilities. Includes work activity, supported employment and supported community living.

5929 Second Time Around
560 Harrison Ave
Suite 501
Boston, MA 02118-1709
641-437-7355
e-mail: press@secondtimearound.net.
www.secondtimearound.net/

Monica Blizeck, Manager
Debbie Steen, Store Supervisor
Deana Edwards, Manager

Work training site for adults with disabilities.

Kansas

5930 Clay Center Adult Training Center
40 Beech Street
Port Chester, NY 10573-2903
914-937-2047
FAX: 914-935-1205
e-mail: mail@clayartcenter.org
www.clayartcenter.org

Michael Spielman, Manager
Robert Rattet, President
Bruce Fern, Vice President
Reena Kashyap, Treasurer

Work training site for adults with disabilities.

5931 Kansas Fair Employment Practice Agency
Suite 568-South
900 SW Jackson St
Topeka, KS 66612-2818
785-296-3206
FAX: 785-296-0589
e-mail: khrc@ink.org
www.state.ks.us/public/khrc

Mostafa Kamal, Manager
William V. Minner, Executive Director
Melvin Neufeld, Chair
Terry Crowder, Vice Chair

5932 Kansas Vocational Rehabilitation Agency
915 SW Harrison
8th Floor West
Topeka, KS 66612-1995
785-368-7471
866-213-9079
FAX: 785-368-7467
TTY: 785-368-7478
e-mail: jac@srkspo.wpo.state.ks.us
www.srskansas.org/rehab

Michael Donnelly, Director

Helps people with disabilities achieve employment and self-sufficiency. Also links employers with qualified and productive individuals to meet thier work force needs.

Kentucky

5933 **Kentucky Committee on Employment of Peoplewith Disabilities**
2nd Floor
275 East Main St
Frankfort, KY 40601-2321
502-564-7456
800-648-6057
FAX: 502-564-7459
e-mail: VivianL.Bettis@ky.gov
www.oet.ky.gov

Greg Higgins, Manager
Tom Bowell, Manager
Shane Smith, Manager
Terri Bradshaw, Communications Director
Provides qualified people for jobs, quality jobs for people, temporary financial support for the unemployed, comprehensive labor market information, and preserve the integrity and viability of the Unemployment Insurance Trust Fund.

5934 **Kentucky Department for Employment Serviceand Job Training Program Liaison**
275 E Main Street 2-W
Frankfort, KY 40621-1
502-564-5331
FAX: 502-564-7452
e-mail: VivianL.Bettis@ky.gov
http://www.oet.ky.gov

Gina Oney, Assistant Director
Linda Prewitt, Acting Division Director/ Assist
Linda Pierce, Compliance Support Branch Manage
Gregory Higgins, Acting Unemployment Insurance Di
Provides qualified people for jobs, quality jobs for people, temporary financial support for the unemployed.

5935 **Kentucky Department for the Blind**
275 East Main Street
Frankfort, KY 40621
502-564-7456
800-321-6668
FAX: 502-564-2951
TTY: 502-564-2929
e-mail: JenniferN.Wright@ky.gov
www.blind.ky.gov

Christopher Smith, Executive Director
Michelle McElmurray, Executive Assistant
Allison Jessee, Director of Consumer Services
Cora McNabb, VR Administrator, Training and H
Provides career services and assistance to adults with severe visual handicaps who want to become productive in the home or work force. Also provides the Client Assistance Program established to provide advice, assistance and information available from rehabilitation programs to persons with handicaps.

5936 **Kentucky Office for the Blind**
275 East Main Street
Frankfort, KY 40621
502-564-7456
800-321-6668
FAX: 502-564-2951
TTY: 502-564-2929
e-mail: JenniferN.Wright@ky.gov
blind.ky.gov
Christopher Smith, Executive Director
Michelle McElmurray, Executive Assistant
Allison Jessee, Director of Consumer Services
Cora McNabb, VR Administrator, Training and H
Our mission is to provide opportunities for employment and independence to individuals with visual impairments.

5937 **Kentucky Vocational Rehabilitation Agency**
275 East Main Street
Frankfort, KY 40621
502-564-4440
800-372-7172
FAX: 502-564-6745
e-mail: WFD.VOCREHAB@ky.gov
http://ovr.ky.gov
Dr. David Beach, Executive Director
Holly Hendricks, Assistant Director of Program Se
Jason Jones, Director of Community Relations
Mindy Yates, Administrative Services Branch M
Assists eligible individuals with disabilities achieve their employment goals.

5938 **Pioneer Vocational/Industrial Services**
150 Corporate Drive
P.O Box 1396
Danville, KY 40422-1396
859-236-8413
800-527-4198
FAX: 859-238-7115
TTY: 859-236-1251
e-mail: pioneer@pioneerservices.org
pioneerservices.org
Mike Pittman, Chief Executive Officer / Executive Director
Danny Rigney, Director of Marketing and Operations
Dot Carman, Office Administration Director / Safety / Compliance Officer
Mike Fayne, Director of Services Assistant
Mission is to provide vocational development and extended employment programs to people who are disabled and or disadvantaged to assist them in obtaining employment and maximizing independent living skills.

5939 **Work Enhancement Center of Western Kentucky**
1906 College Heights Blvd.
Bowling Green, KY 42101-3576
270-745-0111
FAX: 502-767-3600
e-mail: wku@wku.edu
www.wku.edu

Steve Passmore, Director
John O'Shaughnessy, Chief Executive Officer
J. David Porter, Chair
Frederick A. Higdon, Vice Chair
The center has been established in order to service industry in the three state area surrounding Kentucky. This service includes job/skill evaluation, job design consultation, pre-employment employee evaluations and economic evaluation.

Louisiana

5940 **Community Opportunities of East Ascension**
1121 E Ascension Complex Blvd
Gonzales, LA 70737
225-621-2000
FAX: 225-621-2022
http://coea.homestead.com
Mark Thomas, Director
Committed to affording individuals the opportunities that reflect and support choices, dignity, individuality, self-determination, community, coherency and commen sense. Programs incloude Respite, Personal Care Attendant, Support Living, Support Environment, Adult Day Training, and Elderly/Adult Waiver Services.

5941 **Louisiana Employment Service and Job Training Program Liaison**
1001 North 23rd Street
Post Office Box 94094
Baton Rouge, LA 70804-9094
225-342-3111
800-259-5154
FAX: 225-342-7960
e-mail: owd@lwc.la.gov
http://www.laworks.net

Curt Eysink, Executive Directo
Carey Foy, Deputy Executive Director
Jay Augustine, Executive Counsel
Renee Ellender Roberie, Chief Financial Officer

Provides services for job seekers and job training programs.

5942 Louisiana Vocational Rehabilitation Agency
950 N 22nd St
Baton Rouge, LA 70802-6109 225-219-2225
800-737-2958
FAX: 225-219-4993
www.dss.state.la.us/departments/lrs

James Gaston, Manager
Ed Barras, Manager
Mark Martin, Director
Offers individuals with disabilities a wide range of services designed to provide them with skills, resources, attitudes, and expectations needed to compete in the interview process, get the job, keep the job, and develop a lifetime career.

5943 St. James Association for Retarded Citizens
29150 Health Unit St
Vacherie, LA 70090-4221 225-265-2181
FAX: 225-265-7427
e-mail: info@brightscope.com
www.brightscope.com

Judy Bastian, Manager
Bruce Hansen, Chairman
John Sarkisian, Board of Directors
A private sheltered work program for mentally retarded and developmentally disabled adults.

5944 Westbank Sheltered Workshop
606 OPELOUSAS AVE
New Orleans, LA 70114-4344 504-362-1311
www.taxexemptworld.com

Maine

5945 Addison Point Specialized Services
P.O.Box 207
Addison, ME 04606-207 207-483-6500
FAX: 207-483-2817
www.faqs.org

Paula Chartrand, Owner
Provides services to individuals who are deaf/blind, mentally retarded, autistic, behaviorally challenged and/or dual diagnosed. Training services to place these individuals in community employment.

5946 Bangor Veteran Center: Veterans Outreach Center
Veteran's Administration
368 Harlow St
Bangor, ME 04491 207-947-3391
FAX: 207-941-8195
e-mail: Patricia.Albert-Dehetre@va.gov
http://www.maine.va.gov

Joseph A Degrasse, Team Leader
Robert L Daisey LCSW, Clinical Coordinator
Eric K. Shinseki, Secretary
W. Scott Gould, Deputy Secretary
Readjustment counseling services for veterans of Vietnam, Vietnam Era, Persian Gulf, Panama, Grenada, Lebanon, Somalia, WWII and Korean conflicts, as well as Iraq, Afganistan, and military sexual trauma.

5947 Creative Work Systems
619 Brighton Ave
Portland, ME 04102 207-879-1140
FAX: 207-879-1146
e-mail: kraye@creativeworks.com
creativeworksystems.com

Susan Percy, Executive Director
Edward McGeachey, President
Jim Houle, Vice President
Provides residential, day habilitation and supported emploment in Central and Southern Maine.

5948 Maine Department Of Labor
45 Commerce Drive
Augusta, ME 04330 207-623-7900
FAX: 207-287-3042
e-mail: mdol@maine.gov
www.state.me.us/labor

Patrick Fleming, Executive
Jeanne Shorey Paquette, Commissioner
Provides a wide range of services such as employment, labor market information, rehabilitation/disability and others.

5949 Maine Governor's Committee on Employment of the Disabled
45 Commerce Drive
Augusta, ME 04330-7880 207-621-5087
800-794-1110
FAX: 207-624-5302
www.maine.gov

5950 Maine Human Rights Commission
Maine Human Rights Commission
51 State House Station
Augusta, ME 04333-51 207-624-6290
FAX: 207-624-8729
e-mail: Amy.Sneirson@maine.gov
www.maine.gov/mhrc

Amy Sneirson, Executive Director
Barbara Archer Hirsch, Commission Counsel
Victoria Ternig, Chief Investigator
Jill Duson, Compliance Manager
State agency with the responsibility of enforcing Maine's anti-discrimination laws. The commission investigates complaints of unlawful discrimination in employment, housing, education, access to public accommodations, extension of credit and offensive names.

5951 Northeast Occupational Exchange
29 Franklin Street
Bangor, ME 04401-3857 207-942-3685
800-857-0500
FAX: 207-561-4725
TTY: 207-992-2298
www.noemaine.org

Charles O Tingley, Executive Director
A fully licensed, comprehensive mental health and substance abuse treatment and rehabilitation facility.

5952 Vocational and Rehabilitation Agency
Division for the Blind and Visually Impaired
55 State House Station
Augusta, ME 04333-55 207-623-7981
888-457-8883
FAX: 207-624-5980
TTY: 800-794-1110
e-mail: jobbank.careercenter@maine.gov
www.mainecareercenter.com

Jill Busond, Bureau Director
The Maine CareerCenter provides a variety of employment and training services at no charge for Maine workers and businesses. Whether you are looking to improve your job qualifications, explore a different profession, find a new career or hire an employee, the CareerCenter can help.

Maryland

5953 Ardmore Developmental Center
3000 Lottsford Vista Road
Bowie, MD 20721-4001 301-577-2575
FAX: 301-306-9799
e-mail: grow@ArdmoreEnterprises.org
www.ardmoreenterprises.org

Patrick L. Carter, President
Eileen Baker, Vice-President
Marilynn W. Riley, Secretary
Daphne Pallozzi, Chief Executive Officer

Offers supported employment programs and vocational education for persons who are mentally retarded as well as residential services and Emergency Respite Care.

5954 **Job Opportunities for the Blind**
National Federation of the Blind
200 East Wells Street at Jernigan P
Baltimore, MD 21230- 4914 410-659-9315
FAX: 410-685-5653
e-mail: nfb@nfb.org
www.nfb.org

Marc Mauer, President
John Berggren, Executive Director for Operations
John G. Paré Jr., Executive Director for Strategy
Mark Riccobono, Executive Director, NFB Jernigan

This free service allows individuals touch-tone telephone access to the thousands of jobs listed in America's Job Bank, and internet service run by the Department of Labor. Any person registered with either a state rehabilitation agency or a state employment service can search across the country for jobs by either type of work or location.

5955 **Mainstream**
9800 Mt. Pyramid Ct.
Suite 360
Englewood, CO 80112-6301 303-268-1920
FAX: 303-268-1926
e-mail: mainstrm@aol.com
investigativerisk.com

Patricia M Jackson, Executive Director
Charles Moster

Nonprofit organization dedicated to improving competitive employment opportunities for persons with disabilities. Provides specialized services and acts as a bridge that links service providers, employers and persons with disabilties. Provides training, educational publications, and videos on disablityemployment issues. Educationa materials include a magazine, brochures, and audio-visual aids.

5956 **Maryland Employment Services and Job Training Program Liaison**
500 North Calvert Street
#401
Baltimore, MD 21202-2201 410-230-6001
e-mail: det@dllr.state.md.us
http://www.dllr.state.md.us

Maria Simms
Maureen O'Connor, Communications and Media Relatio
Jill Porter, Director of Legislative Services
Kathleen Spencer, Human Resources

Provides job development and placement and services

5957 **Maryland Fair Employment Practice Agency**
9th Fl
6 Saint Paul St
Baltimore, MD 21202-6806 410-767-8600
800-637-6247
FAX: 410-333-1841
TTY: 410-333-1737
e-mail: nbell@mccr.state.md.us
www.mchr.state.md.us

Adrienne Jones, Executive Director
James Neil Bell, Deputy Director
Glendora Hughes, General Counsel
Benny F. Short, Assistant Director

Mission is to ensure equal opportunity to all through the enforcement of Maryland's laws against discrimination in employment, housing, and public accomodations; to provide educational and outreach services related to the provisions of this law: and to promote and improve human relations in Maryland.

5958 **Maryland State Department of Education**
Division of Rehabilitation Services (DI RS)
200 West Baltimore Street
Baltimore, MD 21218-1628 410-767-0100
888-246-0016
FAX: 410-554-9412
TTY: 410-333-6442
http://www.marylandpublicschools.org

Robert Burns, Manager

The Vocational Rehabilitation Program delivers to eligible individuals with physical and/or mental disabilities to enable them to become employed. The Independent Living Program's goal is to assist people in remaining in their homes and communities. The Division operates the Maryland Rehabilitation Center, a comprehensive evaluation and training center that has dormitory space. There are field offices located statewide with counselors to advise and manage the provision of services offered.

5959 **Melwood**
5606 Dower House Road
Upper Marlboro, MD 20772-3432 301-599-8000
FAX: 301-599-0180
e-mail: services@melwood.org
www.melwood.org

Donald A. Donahue, DHEd, MBA, FA, Chair
Richard Mahan, CPA, Vice Chair
George Watkins, CPA, Treasurer
Shelly Gardeniers, Secretary

Melwood is a dynamic nonprofit that creates jobs and opportunities to improve the lives of people with disabilities. Melwood serves more than 1900 people with disabilities in the greater Washington DC area.

5960 **PWI Profile**
Projects W Industry Goodwill Industries of America
16120 W Bernardo Dr
San Diego, CA 92127 858-673-6050
FAX: 858-673-0085
kicthermal.com/process-window-index-pwi

5961 **Project LINK**
Mainstream
Suite 700
3 Bethesda Metro Ctr
Bethesda, MD 20814-6301 301-215-9100
800-247-1380
FAX: 301-891-8778
e-mail: info@cosmoscorp.com
cosmoscorp.com

Charles Moster

Provides job development and placement in services to dislocated workers with disabilities in the Washington, DC and Dallas, TX areas.

5962 **Treatment and Learning Centers (TLC)**
14901 Dufief Mill Road
Suite 100
North Potomac, MD 20878 301-738-6424
FAX: 301-340-6082
TTY:301-424-5203
www.ttlc.org

Dr Patricia Ritter, Executive Director
Suellyn Sherwood, Operations Director
Rhona Schwartz, High School Program Director
Janet Graves-Wright, Outpatient Services Director

A non-profit organization that specializes in educational, therapeutic and vocational services for invididuals with special needs. Programs include speech-language and occupational therapy, psycho-educational testing, tutoring, audiology, employment opportunities and the Katherine Thomas School for students with moderate to severe language and learning disabilities and/or high-functioning autism.
Preschool-12

Massachusetts

5963 **Department Of Workforce Development**
State of Massachusetts
Rm 2112
1 Ashburton Pl
Boston, MA 02108-1518 617-626-7100
800-439-0183
TTY:800-439-2370
e-mail: Dhurley@detma.org
www.massworkforce.org

Suzanne M. Bump, Secretary
Deval L. Patrick, Governor
Timothy P. Murray, Lt. Governor
Serves as the Governor's principal advisory board on workforce development.

5964 **Gateway Arts Center: Studio, Craft Store& Gallery**
Vinsen Corporation
60-62 Harvard St
Brookline, MA 02445-7993 617-734-1577
FAX: 617-734-3199
e-mail: gateway@vinfen.org
www.gatewayarts.org

Rae Edelson, Director
Stephanie Schmidt, Program Director
Mona Thaler, Marketing Director
Stephen De Fronzo, Artistic Director
Award winning, nationally recoginized Arts based rehabilitation service with over 100 talented adults with disabilities.

5965 **Massachusetts Fair Employment Practice Agency**
Rm 601
1 Ashburton Pl
Boston, MA 02108-1524 617-994-6000
FAX: 617-720-6053
TTY:617-994-6196
e-mail: Barbara.Green@massmail.state.ma.us
www.state.ma.us/mcad

Julian T. Tynes, Chairman
Sunila Thomas George, Commissioner
Jamie R. Williamson, Commissioner
Joel Berner, Esq., Chief of Enforcement
The commission works to eliminate discrimination on a variety of bases and areas, and strives to advance the civil rights of the people of commonwealth through law enforcement, outreach and training.

5966 **Massachusetts Governor's Commission on Employment of Disabled Persons**
11th Floor
One Ashburton Place
Boston, MA 02108-2502 617-573-1600
appointments.state.ma.us

Theodore Schipani, Owner
John Polanowicz, Secretary
Kathleen Betts, Assistant Secretary
Claudia Henderson, Chief of Staff
State vocational rehabilitation agency.

5967 **Vocational Rehabilitation Agency**
2 Peachtree Street, NW
Atlanta, GA 30303-1616 404-232-1998
866-489-0001
FAX: 404-232-1800
TTY: 800-764-0200
e-mail: elmer.bartels@mrc.state.ma.us
disabilitycompendium.org

Charles Carr, Commissioner of Rehabilitation
Kasper M. Goshgarian, Deputy Commissioner
Debra Kamen, Assistant Commissioner, Communit
Barbara Kinney, Assistant Commissioner, Disabili
Provides residential, day habilitation and supported employment

5968 **Vocational and Rehabilitation Agency Massachusetts Commission for the Blind**
600 Washington Street
Boston, MA 02111-4718 617-727-5550
800-392-6450
FAX: 617-626-7685
TTY: 800-392-6556
e-mail: Ronald.Gallagher@MassMail.State.MA.US
www.mass.gov/eohhs/gov/departments/mcb/

Charles Carr, Commissioner of Rehabilitation
Kasper M. Goshgarian, Deputy Commissioner
Debra Kamen, Assistant Commissioner, Communit
Barbara Kinney, Assistant Commissioner, Disabili
Provides residentail, habilitation, and supported employment

5969 **Work Inc.**
25 Beach Street
Dorchester, MA 02122-2734 617-691-1500
FAX: 617-691-1595
workinc.org

James Cassetta, CEO
James R. Flanagan, Chairman
Philip Dould, Vice Chairman
David Anderson, Treasurer (CFO)
Mission is all individuals have the ability to grow, the right to make choices and to participate in community life. It is the mission of WORK inc. to join with others in creating the conditions under which all persons with disablities will experience.

Michigan

5970 **Department Of Human Services**
P.O.Box 30037
235 S. Grand Ave.
Lansing, MI 48909-8152 517-887-9400
800-292-4200
FAX: 517-335-5140
TTY: 5173734025
e-mail: kreinerc@state.mi.us
www.michigan.gov.dhs

Maura D. Corrigan, Director
Duane Berger, Chief Deputy Director/Chief Oper
Terrence Beurer, Director, Field Operations
Susan Kangas, Deputy Director, Financial Servi
The DHS is Michigan's public assistance, child and family welfare agency. DHS directs the operations of public assistance and service programs through a network of over 100 county department of human service offices around the state.

5971 **Lamplighter's Work Center**
1320 W State St
Cheboygan, MI 49721-1402 231-627-4319
www.usa.com/frs/lamplighters-work-center.html

Robert Spinella, Executive Director
Offers small business counseling and training to individuals with disabilities

5972 **Michigan Department of Civil Rights**
3054 W Grand Blvd
Ste 3-600
Detroit, MI 48202-6054 313-456-3700
800-482-3604
FAX: 313-456-3791
TTY: 877-878-8464
e-mail: MDCR-INFO@michigan.gov
www.michigan.gov/mdcr

Daniel H. Krichbaum, Director
Investigates and resolves discrimination complaints and works to prevent discrimination through educational programs that promote voluntary compliance with civil rights laws

5973 Michigan Employment Service
201 N. Washington Square
Lansing, MI 48913-3165
517-335-5858
888-605-6722
FAX: 517-241-8217
TTY: 888-605-6722
www.michigan.gov/mdcd
Christine Quinn, Director, Michigan Rehabilitatio
Job development and placement in services to dislocated workers with disabilities

5974 Michigan Rehabilitation Services: Dept ofLabor & Regulatory Affairs
235 S Grand Ave
PO Box 30037
Lansing, MI 48909-7510
517-373-3390
800-605-6722
FAX: 517-335-7277
TTY: 888-605-6722
e-mail: porterj3@michigan.gov
www.michigan.gov/mrs
Jaye N Porter, Director
Laurie Eggers, Administrative Assistant
State vocational rehabilitation agency.

5975 Small Business Development Center
Ann Arbor Center for Independent Living
409 3rd St, SW
Washington, DC 20416-6832
800-827-5722
FAX: 313-971-0826
e-mail: answerdesk@sba.gov
www.sba.gov
Sarah Bard, Director
Phil Zepeda, Manager
Maria Contreras-Sweet, SBA Administrator
Fred Baldassaro, Assistant Administrator
Offers small business counseling and training to individuals with disabilities in the state of Michigan.

Minnesota

5976 Jewish Vocational Service of Jewish Familyand Children's Services
401 N 3rd St
Suite 605
Minneapolis, MN 55401-1388
612-692-8920
FAX: 612-692-8921
e-mail: jfcs@jfcsmpls.org
http://www.jfcsmpls.org
Nancy Rhein, Vice President of Board Development
Howard Zack, President
Sherri Feuer, Vice President of Fund Development
Eileen Kohn, Vice President of Marketing
The mission of JVS is to be a recognized leader in delivering employment, training, and career development services that positively impact individuals of all backgrounds, business and society.

5977 Minnesota Department of Employment and Economic Development - Vocational Rehab Services
332 Minnesota St
1st National Bank Bldg #E-200
Saint Paul, MN 55101-1314
651-259-7114
800-657-3858
FAX: 651-296-3900
TTY: 800657397373
e-mail: DEED.CustomerService@state.mn.us
www.positivelyminnesota.com
Kim Peck, Director
Service for people with disabilities who need skills to prepare for work, or to find and keep a job.

5978 Minnesota Employment Practice Agency
Minnesota Dept. Of Human Rights
Freeman Building
625 Robert Street North
Saint Paul, MN 55155
651-539-1100
800-657-3704
FAX: 651-296-9042
TTY: 651-296-1283
e-mail: Info.MDHR@state.mn.us
humanrights.state.mn.us
Kevin Lindsey, Commissioner
Denise Romero-Zasada, Executive Assistant to the Commi
Ytmar Santiago, Deputy Commisioner
Gregory Torrence, Assistant Commisioner
Mission and vision is to make Minnesota discrimination free.

5979 PWI Forum
Multi Resource Centers
1900 Chicago Ave
Minneapolis, MN 55404-1903
612-752-8138
pwi-forum.perfectworld.com/

5980 Vocational and Rehabilitation Agency
332 Minnesota Street
Suite E200
Saint Paul, MN 55101- 1351
651-259-7114
800-657-3858
FAX: 651-649-5927
TTY: 612-642-0506
e-mail: info@ngwmail.des.state.mn.us
www.mnssb.org
Richard Strong, Executive Director
People seeking work, businesses seeking employees, students, and those looking for a first job or returning to the workforce, will find services to meet their needs.

Mississippi

5981 Allied Enterprises of Tupelo
Ability Works Incorporated
1281 Highway 51
Madison, MS 39110
800-443-1000
FAX: 662-287-1463
mdrs.state.ms.us
Michael Byrd, Manager
Jack Virden, Chairman
Jean Massey, Associate State Superintendentof Education
Carey Wright, Superintendentof Education
Vocational evaluation, work adjustment and job placement of disabled persons in a rehabilitation workshop.

5982 Mississippi Department of Rehabilitation Services
1281 Highway 51
Madison, MS 39110-1698
601-853-5100
800-443-1000
FAX: 601-359-1695
TTY: 800-443-1000
e-mail: bmcmillan@mdrs.state.ms.us
http://www.mdrs.state.ms.us/
Ed LeGrand, Executive Director
Shelia Browning, Deputy Director
Chris Howard, Deputy Director
Richard Sorey, Director
Offers low vision aids and appliances, counseling, social work, educational and professional training, residential services, recreational services, computer training and employment opportunities for the handicapped.

5983 **Mississippi Employment Secutity Commission**
P.O.Box 1699
1235 Echelon Parkway
Jackson, MS 39215-1699 601-321-6000
FAX: 601-961-7405
e-mail: comments@mdes.ms.gov.
www.mdes.ms.gov

Mark Henry, Executive Director
Phil Bryant, Governor
A federally funded state agency. The programs of MDES, under direction of the governor of Mississippi, report to the federal government.

5984 **Worksight**
Mississippi State University
PO Drawer 6189
108 Herbert - South, Room 150
Mississippi State, MS 39762-6189 662-325-2001
800-675-7782
FAX: 662-325-8989
TTY: 662-325-2694
e-mail: nrtc@colled.msstate.edu
www.blind.msstate.edu

Michele Capella McDonnall, Research Professor and Interim D
Jacqui Bybee, Research Associate II
Jessica Thornton, Business Manager
Angela Shelton, Coordinator of Instructional Mat
Discusses news, activities, research projects and training programs of the Center.

Missouri

5985 **Missouri Commission on Human Rights**
421 EastDunklinSt.
P.O. Box 59
Jefferson City, MO 65102-0059 573-751-3215
800-320-2519
FAX: 573-751-4945
e-mail: mchr@labor.mo.gov
http://www.labor.mo.gov

Alisa Warren, Executive Director
Tracey Allan, Intake Officer
Nia Ray, Director
The Missouri Commission on Human Rights enforces the state's anti-discrimination law that prohibits discrimination in housing, employment and places of public accommodations. It prohibits discrimination due to race, color, religion, national origin, ancestry, sex, disability, age and familial status. Complaints must be filed within 180 days of the alleged discrimination. If discrimination is found after investigation, the Commission can hold hearings to enforce the law.

5986 **Missouri Governor's Council on Disability**
P.O. Box 687
1706 East Elm
Jefferson City, MO 65102-1668 573-751-8676
800-877-8249
FAX: 573-526-4109
TTY: 573-751-2600
e-mail: gcd@oa.mo.gov
www.gcd.oa.mo.gov

Douglas E. Nelson, Acting Commissioner
James Trout, Acting Chair and Council Members
Linda Baker, Executive Director Governor's Co
Dawn Evans, Disability Program Specialist
Advocate training, civil rights, community education services, community resource referral, conferences, consumer education, disability awareness program, educational information and resources, information and education services, information and referral, newsletter, policy issues and services, publications, resource directory, seminars, technical assistance, training and seminars.

5987 **Missouri Job Training Program Liaison**
221 Metro Dr
Jefferson City, MO 65109-4412 573-634-2321

Joe Jerkins, Manager
Services for individuals with disabilities who want to become employed.

5988 **Missouri Vocational Rehabilitation Agency**
205 Jefferson St.
Jefferson Cty, MO 65101-6188 573-751-4212
877-222-8963
FAX: 573-751-1441
TTY: 573-751-0881
e-mail: info@vr.dese.mo.gov
www.vr.dese.mo.gov

Jeanne Loyd, Assistant Commissioner
Michelle Scherer, Administrator
A team of decicated individuals working for the continuous improvement of education and services for all citizens.

5989 **WX: Work Capacities**
Suite 103
17331 E 40th Hwy
Independence, MO 64055 816-478-2333
FAX: 816-478-2335

Chris Walters, Manager
Mike Heinz, Manager
Services for individuals with disabilities who want to become employed.

Montana

5990 **Montana Fair Employment Practice Agency**
1805 Prospect Avenue
PO Box 1728
Helena, MT 59624-1728 406-444-2840
800-542-0807
FAX: 406-444-2978
TTY: 406-444-9696
e-mail: erdquestions@mt.gov
www.erd.dli.mt.gov

Marieke Chief, Bureau Chief
Kathleen Hel, Case Manager
Advocate training, civil rights, community education services, community resource referral and conferences

5991 **Montana Governor's Committee on Employment of Disabled People**
PO Box 200801
Helena, MT 59620-127 406-444-4405
800-243-4091
FAX: 406-444-4151
e-mail: Boards@mt.gov
svc.mt.gov/gov/boards/

Nebraska

5992 **Nebraska Employment Services**
Department of Labor
140 S 27th St Ste C
Lincoln, NE 68510-2601 402-474-9675

www.yellowpages.com

5993 **Nebraska Fair Employment Practice Agency**
301 Centennial Mall South, 5th Floo
PO Box 94934
Lincoln, NE 68509-4394
402-471-2024
800-642-6112
FAX: 402-471-4059
www.nol.org/home/neoc

Royce Jeffries, Chairperson
Kristin Yates, Vice-Chairman
Ms.Barbara Albers, Executive Director
he Nebraska Equal Opportunity Commission is a neutral administrative agency created by statute in 1965 to enforce the public policy of the state against discrimination. The principal function of the NEOC is to receive, investigate and pass upon charges of unlawful discrimination occurring anywhere within the State of Nebraska in the areas of Employment, Housing, and Public Accommodations.

5994 **Nebraska Vocational Rehabilitation Agency**
3901 N 27th St, Ste 6
Lincoln, NE 68521-2529
402-471-3231
800-472-3382
FAX: 402-471-0788
e-mail: vr_stateoffice@vocrehab.state.ne.us
vocrehab.state.ne.us

Cheryl Ferree, Manager
Rod Armstrong, Vice President of Strategic Part
Mitch Arnolds, President
Amanda Jedlicka, Executive Director
Services for individuals with disabilities who want to become employed. Services are free to those who qualify.

Nevada

5995 **Nevada Equal Rights CommissionDepartment Of Employment,Training & Rehabilitation**
1820 E Sahara Ave
Ste 314
Las Vegas, NV 89104-6512
702-486-7161
800-326-6868
FAX: 702-486-7054
http://detr.state.nv.us/nerc

5996 **Nevada Governor's Committee on Employment of Persons with Disabilities**
Suite#202
896 W. Nye Lane
Carson City, NV 89703-5062
775-684-8619
FAX: 775-684-8626
www.nevadaddcouncil.org

Sherry Manning, Executive Director
Kari Horn, Projects Manager
Diana Peachay, Executive Assistant
Services for individuals with disabilities who want to become employed.

5997 **Vocational and Rehabilitation Agency**
State of Nevada
Ste 502
1933 N. Carson Street
Carson City, NV 89701-3705
775-684-0400
FAX: 775-684-4186
TTY:775-684-0360
e-mail: mryasmer@nvdetr.org
detr.state.nv.us

Frank Woodbeck, Director
Dennis Perea, Deputy Director
Renee Olson, Administrator for the Employment
William Anderson, Chief Economist for the Research

New Hampshire

5998 **Fit for Work at Exeter Hospital**
5 Alumni Drive
Exeter, NH 03833-2160
603-778-7311
FAX: 603-580-6592
http://www.exeterhospital.com

Kevin Calahan, President
Staffed by a team of allied health professionals, our outpatient rehabilitation program offers functional restoration, work therapy, diagnostic testing and physical therapy.

5999 **New Hampshire Employment Security**
32 S Main St
Concord, NH 03301-4857
603-224-3311
800-852-3400
FAX: 603-228-4010
TTY: 800-735-2964
e-mail: webmaster@nhes.state.nh.us
www.nh.gov/nhes

George Copadis, Commissioner
Darrell Gates, Deputy Commissioner
Zandy L. Dezonie, Administrative Assistant
Operates a free public employment service and provides assisted and self directed employment and career related services and labor market information for employers and the general public.

6000 **New Hampshire Fair Employment Practice Agency**
2 Chenell Dr Unit 2
Concord, NH 03301-8501
603-271-2767
FAX: 603-271-6339
e-mail: humanrights@nhsa.state.nh.us
www.nh.gov/hrc

Joni N. Esperian, Esquire, Executive Director
Roxanne Juliano, Assistant Director
Deborah M Evans, Administrative Secretary
Nancy Rodgers, Secretary
Established for the purpose of eliminating discrimination in employment, public accomodations and the sale or rental of housing or commercial property.

6001 **New Hampshire Job Training Program Liaison**
26 College Drive
Concord, NH 03301-7317
603-230-3500
FAX: 603-271-2725
e-mail: info@ccsnh.edu
www.ccsnh.edu/

Dr. Ross Gittell, Chancellor
Ron Rioux, Vice Chancellor
Michael Marr, Director of Financial Operations
Sara Sawyer, Director of Human Resources
Services for individuals with disabilities who want to become employed.

6002 **Vocational and Rehabilitation Agency**
Department of Education
101 Pleasant Street
Concord, NH 03301-3860
603-271-3494
FAX: 603-271-1953
TTY:603-271-3471
e-mail: Lori.Temple@doe.nh.gov
www.ed.state.nh.us

Paul K Leather, Manager
Virginia Barry, Commissioner
Trisha Allen, Administrative Assistant
Steven Aylward, Rehabilitation Counselor
Offers services for the totally blind, legally blind, visually impaired, mentally retarded blind and more with health, counseling, educational, recreational, rehabilitation, computer training and professional training services.

New Jersey

6003 **ARC of Gloucester County**
1555 Gateway Blvd
West Deptford, NJ 08096-1018 856-629-9061
FAX: 856-848-7753
e-mail: webmaster@thearcgloucester.org
www.thearcgloucester.org

Robert.H Weir, President
Charles Funk, VP
Ethel Lucas, Board Member
Ralph Sundy, Board Member
Non-profit organization serving people with intellectual and related developmental disabilities and their families through education, advocacy and direct services.

6004 **ARC of Mercer County**
180 Ewingville Road
Ewing, NJ 08638-2425 609-406-0181
FAX: 609-406-9258
e-mail: arc@arcmercer.org
www.arcmercer.org

Geoffrey Morris, President
Rick Koreyva, 1st Vice President
Ethel Lucas, Board Member
Ralph Sundy, Board Member
Committed to securing for all people with disabilities mental retardation and developmental disabilities the opportunity to choose and realize their goals.

6005 **ARC of Monmouth**
1158 Wayside Road
Tinton Falls, NJ 7712-3148 732-493-1919
FAX: 732-493-3604
e-mail: info@arcofmonmouth.org
www.arcofmonmouth.org

Joyce Quarles, President
Roger Trendowski, Immediate Past President
Rachel Weiss, First Vice-President
Bill Mirkin, Treasurer
A non-profit organization providing services and supports for individuals who have cognitive and developmental disabilities and for their families.

6006 **Abilities Center of New Jersey**
1208 Delsea Drive
Westville, NJ 08093-2227 856-848-1025
FAX: 856-848-8429
e-mail: info@abilities4work.com
abilities4work.com

Susan Spies Perron, President/CEO
Sharon Kneubuehl, VP
Karen Weitzman, Director of Finance and Adminidt
Bill Urie, Director of Operations
A non-profit organization dedicated to developing employment opportunities for people with disabilities or other disadvantages through education, training and job placement.

6007 **Abilities of Northwest New Jersey**
264 Rt 31 North
Washington, NJ 07882 908-689-1118
e-mail: info@abilitiesnw.com
abilities-nw.com

a.B Wildermuth, CEO
Private not-for-profit community rehabilitation program providing vocational training and employment services since 1974 to the disabled and disadvantaged population.

6008 **Alliance for Disabled in Action New Jersey**
629 Amboy Ave
Edison, NJ 08837-3579 732-738-4388
FAX: 732-738-4416
TTY:732-738-9644
e-mail: ctonks@adacil.org
www.adacil.org

Carole Tonks, Executive Director
Luke Koppisch, Deputy Director
Salma Harris, Office Manager
Iris Hernandez, Bookkeeper
A private not-for-profit center for independence living. A dynamic membership organization run by people with disabilities for people with disabilities.

6009 **Alternatives for Growth: New Jersey**
137 W. Hanover St.
Trenton, NJ 08618 609-393-0008
FAX: 609-393-1189
e-mail: experts@afg-lca.com
www.njfuture.org

Donna Flannery, Contact
Peter Kasabach, Executive Director
Elaine Clisham, Director of Communications and Development
Nicholas Dickerson, Planning and Policy Analyst
Serves all New Jersey.

6010 **Arc of Bergen and Passaic Counties**
223 Moore Street
Hackensack, NJ 7601-7402 201-343-0322
FAX: 201-343-0401
e-mail: arc@arcbp.com
arcbergenpassaic.org

Kathy Walsh, President/CEO
Alice Siegel, Senior VP
Olga Podolsky, Director of Family Support Servi
Anne Gallucci, Vocational Services Director
Serving persons with disabilities and their families in Bergen and Passaic Counties, NJ.

6011 **Career Opportunity Development of New Jersey**
901 Atlantic Avenue
Egg Harbor City, NJ 08215-1810 609-965-6871
FAX: 609-965-3099
njcodi.org

Linda L. Carney, President & CEO
Ellen Loughney, Vice Chairperson
Joe Silipena, Board Chairperson
Joe Cella, Secretary
Serves Bergen and Passaic Counties. Provides services to individuals with varying forms of physical, mental and economic disabilities and disadvantages. Provides services to more than 1,000 unduplicated consumers annually.

6012 **Center for Educational Advancement New Jersey**
11 Minneakoning Road
Flemington, NJ 08822-5726 908-782-1480
FAX: 908-782-5370
e-mail: jkunz@ceaemployment.com
ceaemployment.com

Michael Skoczek, President & CEO
John Reardon, Secretary
Michael Collins, Treasurer
Nancy Vargas, Employee Relations
Serves Somerset and Hunterdon Counties. Skills training in office technology and food service. Job placement and job coaching services are available. Employer Network for Ticket to Work.

6013 Cerebral Palsy Association of Middlesex County
10 Oak Drive
Edison, NJ 08837-2313
732-549-6187
800-852-7897
FAX: 732-549-0629
e-mail: Info@cpamc.org
cpamc.org

Dominic M. Ursino, President
Robert Ferrara, Executive Director
Rob Gross, MBA, Controller
Debra Gilbert, M.S.I.L.R, Director of Human Resources

Dedicated to the provision of comprehensive, superior, multi-faceted programs of service to individuals with developmental and related disabilities

6014 Easter Seal Society of New Jersey Highlands Workshop
Easter Seals
133 Main St
Franklin, NJ 7416-1542
973-827-9066
FAX: 973-827-3828
e-mail: pskipp@nj.easterseals.com
www.nj.easterseals.com

Peggy Skipp, Manager

Enabling indidividuals with special needs or disabilities and their families to learn, live, work and play in their communities with equality, dignity and independence.

6015 Easter Seal of Ocean County
25 Kennedy Blvd.
Suite 600
East Brunswick, NJ 08816
732-257-6662
FAX: 732-257-7373
http://nj.easterseals.com

Brian.J Fitzgerald, President/CEO

Helping people and families with disabilities and special needs live, work, and play in their communities with equality, dignity and independence.

6016 Easter Seals New Jersey
25 Kennedy Blvd
Ste 600
E Brunswick, NJ 08816-2035
732-257-6662
FAX: 732-257-7373
TTY:732-545-1317
www.eastersealsnj.org

Brian Fitzgerald, CEO
Cheryl Young, CFO
Helen Drobnis, VP Corporate Affairs

To enable individuals with disabilities or special needs and their families to live, work and play in their communities with equality, dignity, and independence.

6017 Eden Acres Administrative Services
2 Merwick Road
Princeton, NJ 08540-5711
609-987-0099
FAX: 609-734-0069
www.nj.com/mercer/index.ssf/

Peter H. Bell, President & CEO
Jennifer Bizub, Chief Operating Officer
Carol Markowitz, M.A., M.Ed, Chief Program Officer
Melinda Gorny McAleer, Chief Development Officer

Provides services for the disabilitated.

6018 Edison Sheltered Workshop
328 Plainfield Avenue
Edison, NJ 08817-3117
732-985-8834
FAX: 732-985-2216
e-mail: info@eswnj.org
http://www.eswnj.org

Veronica Valez, Executive Director
Robert.A Ellymer, President
John J. Hogan, First Vice President
Pat Colletto, Treasurer

Serves Middlesex County. Vocational training and job placement services.

6019 First Occupational Center of New Jersey
861 Asbury Avenue
Ocean City, NJ 08226-2809
609-399-6111
800-894-6265
FAX: 973-672-0065
e-mail: ocnj@idt.net
www.ocnj.org

Rocco Meola, CEO
Tanya M. Edghill, VP Of Program Services

A private, nonprofit multi-service community rehabilitation program. Services are offered to all people, such as developmentally disabled, visually impaired, hearing impaired and welfare recipients. Services include vocational evaluation and training, respite care, basic and remedial education and job placement and community support services.

6020 Goodwill Industries of Southern New Jersey
2835 Route 73
Maple Shade, NJ 08052-1620
856-439-0200
FAX: 856-439-0843
e-mail: esmith@goodwillnj.org
goodwillnj.org

Mark B Boyd, President and CEO
Michael Shaw, Chief Operating Officer
Stephen Castro, Chief Financial Officer
Deb Eckenhoff, Vice President of Goodwill Home Medical Equipment

A non profit, community-based organization governed by a volunteer bard of trustees.

6021 Hausmann Industries
130 Union Street
Northvale, NJ 7647-2290
201-767-0255
888-428-7626
FAX: 201-767-1369
e-mail: info@hausmann.com
hausmann.com

David Hausmann, CEO
George Batchelor, Director Sales & Marketing
Michelle Riley, Mail order Sales
Julie Skoda, Sales and Marketing Adminitrator

Wheelchair acessible exam tables, treatment tables and mat platforms.

6022 Jersey Cape Diagnostic Training & Opportunity Center
152 Crest Haven Road
Cape May Court House, NJ 08210-1651
609-465-4117
FAX: 609-465-3899
e-mail: paulann@capeworkshop.com
www.sjworks.org/

George J Plewa, Executive Director
George Plewa, Executive Director

Serves Cape May County. Employment training services. A vocational rehabilitation center that serves individuals with disabilities, the disabled, and the handicapped or others having barriers to work.

6023 New Jersey Commission for the Blind and Visually Impaired
Department of Human Services
153 Halsey St
6th Floor, PO Box 47017
Newark, NJ 07101- 8004
973-648-3333
877-685-8878
FAX: 973-648-3388
e-mail: Vito.DeSantis@cbvi.nj.us
www.state.nj.us/humanservices/cbvi/home/index

Vito J Desantis, Executive Director
Bernice Davis, Executive Assistant
Marcus Stabile Esq., Manager Human Resources
Frank Scheik, Fiscal Operations

The Commission for the Blind and Visually Impaired (CBVI) promotes and provides services in the areas of education, employment, independence and eye health for persons who are blind or visually impaired, their families and the community. It seeks to provide or ensure access to services that will enable consumers to obtain their fullest measure of self-reliance and quality of life and fully integrated into their community.

6024 **New Jersey Employment Service and Job Training Program Services**
Department of Labor
John Fitch Plaza
Trenton, NJ 08625
609-292-1040
wd.dol.state.nj.us/
Roland Machold, Manager
Harold J. Wirths, Commissioner
Aaron R. Fichtner, Ph.D., Deputy Commissioner
Frederick J. Zavaglia, Chief of Staff
Services for individuals with disabilities who want to become employed.

6025 **Occupational Center of Hudson County**
68-70 Tuers Avenue
Jersey City, NJ 07306
201-434-3303
FAX: 201-434-3660
e-mail: info@hudsoncommunity.org
http://www.hudsoncommunity.org
Christine Remler, Executive Director
Services for individuals with disabilities who want to become employed.

6026 **Occupational Center of Union County**
301 Cox St
Roselle, NJ 07203-1797
908-241-7200
FAX: 908-241-2025
e-mail: ocuc@OCUCNJ.com
www.occupationalcenter.org
Michele Ford, VP
The Occupational Center is the only agency in the State of New Jersey which offers a unique combination of individualized training leading to long term employment for people with disabilities in the competitive job market or in our on-site industrial work center. This comprehensive package helps ensure on-the-job success and a productive, dignified life for those with disabilities.

6027 **Occupational Training Center of Burlington County**
2 Manhattan Drive
Burlington, NJ 08016-4408
609-267-6677
otcbc.org
Joseph S Bender, CEO
Mission is to assist individuals with disabilities in reaching their maximum potential.

6028 **Occuptational Training Center of Camden County, New Jersey**
520 Market Street
Suite 306
Camden, NJ 08102-1300
866-226-3362
FAX: 856-767-1378
e-mail: camcofreeholders@gmail.com
www.camdencounty.com
Matt Treihart, President
Serves Camden County.

6029 **Pathways to Independence, Inc.**
60 Kingsland Ave
Kearny, NJ 07032-3305
201-997-6155
FAX: 201-997-7070
e-mail: PTI450@aol.com
www.pathwaysnj.org
Alvin Cox, Executive Director
Tessa Farrell, Program Director
Marie Yakabofski, Financial Director
Lisa M.Johnson, Qualilty Assurance Director
Pre-vocational and vocational programming for people with disabilities. Specializing in Developmental Disabilities, Learning Disabilities and Mental Health issues. Serving over 100 people in Hudson, South Bergen, Passaic and East Essex counties. CARF accredited.

6030 **Somerset Training and Employment Program**
900 Hamilton Street
Somerset, NJ 08873-3206
732-846-8888
FAX: 732-246-7257
www.somersetcap.org/
Laurie Falka, Executive Director
Courtney Throckmorton, Owner
Services for individuals with disabilities who want to become employed.

6031 **St. John of God Community Services Vocational Rehabilitation**
1145 Delsea Dr
Westville, NJ 8093-2252
856-848-4700
FAX: 856-848-3965
e-mail: devctr@stjohnofgod.org
www.stjohnofgod.org
Dr. Jerome Knast, Manager
Serves Gloucester and Camden Counties providing exemplary special education, vocational and habilitative services to residents of southern New Jersey since 1967.

6032 **The ARC of Hunterdon County**
1465 Route 31 South
Suite 23
Annandale, NJ 08801-3127
908-730-7827
FAX: 908-730-7726
e-mail: jeff@archunterdon.org
www.archunterdon.org
Jeffrey Mattison, Executive Director
Colleen Dennis, Deputy Executive Director
Gail Stepka, Executive Assistant
Our mission is to support, training and opportunities to individuals with intellectual & developmental disabilities to achieve the greatest degree of independence and productivity to become contributing, responsible, and proud members of society.

6033 **United Cerebral Palsy Associations of New Jersey**
Suite 1
1005 Whitehead Road Ext
Ewing, NJ 08638-2424
609-882-4182
888-322-1918
FAX: 609-882-4054
TTY: 609-882-0620
cpofnj.org
Warren Kelemen, President
Jim Bartolomei, CPA, Vice President
Elizabeth R. Faircloth, Secretary
Michael Yarrow, Treasurer
Dedicated to changing lives and bringing independence to people with all types of disabilities.

6034 **Vocational and Rehabilitation Agency**
P.O.Box 398
Trenton, NJ 08625
609-659-3045
FAX: 609-292-8347
TTY:609-292-2919
e-mail: tjennings@dol.state.nj.us
http://lwd.dol.state.nj.us
Brian Fitzgibbons, Manager
Frederick J. Zavaglia, Chief of Staff
Harold J. Wirths, Commissioner
Programs and services for people with disabilities.

6035 **West Essex Rehab Center**
83 Walnut St
C
Montclair, NJ 07042-4088
973-744-7733
FAX: 973-744-3744
businessfinder.nj.com
Eugene Sefanelli, Executive Director
Shannon Williams, Contact
Eugene Stefanelli, Executive Director
Services and programs for individuals with disabilities who want to become employed.

New Mexico

6036 Adelante Development Center
3900 Osuna Rd Ne
Albuquerque, NM 87109 505-341-2000
FAX: 505-341-2001
e-mail: info@GoAdelante.org
www.goadelante.org

Mike Kivitz, President
Pamela Sullivan, Board Chair
Mike Lowrimore, Borad Treasurer
Richard Cronin, Physician
Serves Albuquerque and Belen.

6037 Goodwill Industries of New Mexico
5000 San Mateo Blvd NE
Albuquerque, NM 87109-2499 505-881-6401
866-376-0182
FAX: 505-884-3157
goodwillnm.org

Mary Best, President/CEO
Michael P. Keoghan, Chief Operating Officer
Roberta Valesquez, Finance Director
Ricky Sanchez, Facilities Logistics Director
Serves Albuquerque, Santa Fe and Rio Rancho.

6038 New Mexico Employment Services and Job Training Liaison
P.O.Box 1928
Albuquerque, NM 87103-1928 505-898-3599
FAX: 505-827-6812
e-mail: djones2@state.nm.us
http://www.dws.state.nm.us
Reese Suliten, Director
Celina Bussey, Secretary
Provides employment to improve economic progress.

6039 RCI
1111 Menaul Blvd NE
Albuquerque, NM 87107-1614 505-255-5501
FAX: 505-255-9971
e-mail: info@LifeROOTSnm.org
http://www.liferootsnm.org
Kathleen Cates, President/CEO
Gwendolyn Kiwanuka, Director of Adult Services
Trudy Eberhardt, Director of Finance
David Griffis, Director of Contracts
Serves Bernalillo County. Mission is to improve the abilities, interests, and choices of children and adults with physical, developmental or behavioral challenges toward achieving their highest levels of self-sufficiency.

6040 Tohatchi Area of Opportunity & Services
100 Manuelita Drive, P.O.Box 49
Tohatchi, NM 87325 505-733-2027
FAX: 505-733-2161
e-mail: patkeptner@yahoo.com
http://taos-inc.org
Patrick Keptner, CEO
Carol Charles, Administrative Assistant
Judith Woodie, Accounting Clerk
Melinda Golden, Program Manager
Serves McKinley County, San Jose County and the Havanjo Nation.

6041 Vocational Rehabilitation Agency
Ste D
435 Saint Michaels Dr
Santa Fe, NM 87505-7679 505-954-8500
800-224-7005
FAX: 505-954-8562
TTY: 877-954-8583
e-mail: dvris@state.nm.us
www.dvrgetsjobs.com
Gary Beene, Manager
Purpose is to help people with disabilities achieve a suitable employment outcome.

6042 Vocational and Rehabilitation Agency
Bldg 4
2905 Rodeo Park Dr E
Santa Fe, NM 87505-6342 505-827-4479
888-513-7968
e-mail: greg.trapp@state.nm.us
www.state.nm.us/cftb
Greg Trapp, Executive Director
James Salas, Deputy Director
Adelmo Vigil, Deputy Director-IL/OB
Catherine Cross-Maple, Manager
The Commission for the Blind provides vocational rehabilitation and independent living services designed to enable persons who are blind to become more participating and contributing members of society. Blind people lead normal lives, have families, raise children, participate in community activities, and work in a wide range of jobs. They are secretaries, lawyers, teachers, engineers, machinists, scientists, supervisors and business owners.

New York

6043 JOBS VI and SAGE
P ES CO International
21 Paulding St
Pleasantville, NY 10570-3108 914-769-4266
800-431-2016
FAX: 914-769-2970
e-mail: pesco@pesco.org
www.pesco.org
Joseph Kass, President
A computerized matching system matching people to occupations, training, local jobs, local employers and giving job outlooks for the year 2005. Computerized Sage is online computerized testing with the ability for system to read all questions, and job descriptions. Manual Sage is a hands on-computer scored test battery with various adaptation. Braille, large print, bi-lingual and special devices.

6044 Just One Break (JOBS)
6th Floor
570 Seventh Aveune
New York, NY 10018-1653 212-785-7300
FAX: 212-785-4513
TTY:212-785-4515
e-mail: jobs@justonebreak.com
www.justonebreak.com

Orin Lehman, Founder
John D Kemp, President
Angela Burgess, Board of Director
C.Jeffrey Knittel, Board of Director
A not-for-profit organization that is dedicated to supporting and increasing the employment of people with disabilities.

6045 New York State Department of Labor
Building 12
State Office Campus
Albany, NY 12240 518-457-9000
888-469-7365
TTY:800-662-1220
e-mail: nysdol@labor.state.ny.us
www.labor.state.ny.us
James J Mcgowan, Commissioner
Fredda Peritz, Employment Service Division Dire
Thomas Malone, Unemployment Insur Div Dir
The missin of the New York State Department of Labor is to help New York work by preparing individuals for the jobs of today and tomorrow. Provides direct job search and counseling services to job seekers, and can refer people who have disabilities for training opportunities. Provides unemployment insurance for those out of work through no fault of their own.

6046 Rational Effectiveness Training Systems
IRET Corporate Services Division
45 E 65th St
New York, NY 10021-6508
212-535-0822
FAX: 212-249-3582
www.yelp.com

Michael Broder, Owner
Offers advanced training for employee assistance professionals, full service outpatient counseling, consulting services and on-site workshops for the disabled.

6047 Special Education and Vocational Rehabilitation Agency: New York
Room 580 EBA
89 Washington Ave.
Albany, NY 12234
518-474-2925
800-222-5627
e-mail: accesadm@mail.nysed.gov
www.vesid.nysed.gov

Richard Mills, Manager
Mission is to promote educational equity and excellence for students with disabilitites while ensuring that they receive the rights and protection to which they are entitled.

North Carolina

6048 Division Of Workforce Development
NC Department Of Commerce
313 Chapanoke Road
Suite 120
Raleigh, NC 27603
919-814-0400
800-562-6333
FAX: 919-662-4770
http://www.nccommerce.com

Sherry Allen, Accountant
Delores Amogida, Program Assistant V
Barbara Barner, Business & Technology Applicatio
Robbin Broome, Training Manager
Offers vocational assessment and training, adult developmental activities.

6049 Iredell Vocational Workshop
200 Clanton Rd
Charlotte, NC 28217-1446
704-944-5100
www.lifespanservices.org

John Cervantes, Secretary
Davan Cloninger, President & CEO
Robert L. Mendenhall, Vice Chairperson
Jeff Hay, Chairperson
Mission of lifespan is to transform the lives of children and adults with developmental disabilities by providing education, employment, and enrichment programs that promote inclusion, choice, family supports, and other best practices.

6050 North Carolina Division of Services for the Blind
Department of Health and Human Services
2601 Mail Service Center
Raleigh, NC 27699-2601
919-733-9822
800-222-1546
FAX: 919-715-8711
TTY: 919-733-9700
e-mail: VRStatePlan2015@dhhs.nc.gov
www.dhhs.state.nc.us/dsb

Eddie Weaver, Director
Carla Parker, Executive Assistant
Mary Flanagan, Assistant Director
Marvin Gilmore, LAN Administrator
Since 1935, the mission of the North Carolina Division of Services for the Blind has been to enable people who are blind or visually impaired to reach their goals of independence and employment.

6051 Rowan County Vocational Workshop
2728 Old Concord Rd
Salisbury, NC 28146-1338
704-637-9592
FAX: 704-633-6224
salisbury.marketplaceminer.com

Carl Rapsher, Executive Director
Offers vocational assessment and training, adult developmental activities.

6052 Rutherford Vocational Workshop
230 Fairground Rd
Spindale, NC 28160
828-286-4352
FAX: 828-287-3295
rutherfordlifeservices.com

Amanda Freeman, Program Supervisor
Christy Beddinfield, Staff
Larry Brown, Executive Director
John Jarrett, Human Resource Director
Offers vocational assessment and training, adult developmental activities.

6053 Transylvania Vocational Services
11 Mountain Industrial Drive
P.O. Drawer 1115
Brevard, NC 28712-6723
828-884-3195
e-mail: info@tvsinc.org
tvsinc.org

Nancy Stricker, Executive Director
A private non-profit corporation with the mission to provide skills development, career opportunities and related services in a supportive environment for people with barriers to employment.

6054 Vocational and Rehabilitation Agency
2001 Mail Service Center
Raleigh, NC 27699-2001
919-855-4800
800-689-9090
FAX: 919-733-7968
TTY: 919-733-9700
e-mail: dvr.WebInfoRequest@dhhs.nc.gov
http://www.ncdhhs.gov

Albert Delia, Acting Secretary
Beth Melcher, PhD, Chief Deputy Secretary for Healt
Maria. F Spaulding, Deputy Secretary for Long-Term C
Steven Cline, DDS, Assistant Secretary for Health I
Mission statement is to promote employment and independence for people with disabilities through customer partnership and community leadership.

6055 Vocational and Rehabilitation Agency: Department of Health and Human Services
2001 Mail Service Center
Raleigh, NC 27699-2001
919-855-4800
800-689-9090
FAX: 919-733-7968
TTY: 919-733-5924
e-mail: dvr.WebInfoRequest@dhhs.nc.gov
dvr.dhhs.state.nc.us

Albert Delia, Acting Secretary
Beth Melcher, PhD, Chief Deputy Secretary for Healt
Maria. F Spaulding, Deputy Secretary for Long-Term C
Steven Cline, DDS, Assistant Secretary for Health I
Mission statement is to promote employment and independence for people with disabilities through customer partnership and community leadership.

6056 Webster Enterprises Inc.
140 Little Savannah Rd
Sylvia, NC 28779-220
828-586-8981
800-978-2681
FAX: 828-586-8125
e-mail: grobinson@websterenterprises.org
www.websterenterprises.org

Gene Robinson, Executive Director
Wendy Cagle, Vice-Chair
Bob Cochran, Secretary/Treasurer
Tom Stovall, Chair

A community based employment and training program for people with disabilities. A full service program which includes a youth transitional program for life beyond high school, job coaching, vocational assessment and job placement.

6057 Western Regional Vocational Rehabilitation Facility Clifford File, Jr.
P.O.Box 1443
200 Enola Rd.
Morganton, NC 28655 828-433-2423
dvr.dhhs.state.nc.us

Connie Barnette, Facility Director
Elizabeth Watson, Executive Director
Frances Battle, Director of Training
Karen Romito, Program Assistant
Vocational Evaluation, Work Adjustment, Job Placement, On-site Work Services Program. Serves most disability groups including CMI, DD, Deaf and Physically impaired.

North Dakota

6058 North Dakota Department of Labor, Human Rights Division
Dept 406
600 East Boulevard Avenue
Bismarck, ND 58505- 0340 701-328-2660
800-582-8032
800-366-6888
FAX: 701-328-2031
e-mail: humanrights@nd.gov
www.nd.gov

Mark Nelson, Manager
Kathy Kulesa, Human Rights Director
Robin Bosch, Business Manager
Peg Haug, Compliance Investigator
Through a work-sharing agreement with the Equal Employment Opportunity Commission (EEOC), the North Dakota Department of Labor's Human Rights Division enforces the Americans with Disabilities Act (ADA) as related to employment discrimination.

6059 North Dakota Employment Service and Job Training Program Liaison
Job Service North Dakota
1601 E. Century Avenue
PO Box 5507
Bismarck, ND 58506- 5507 701-328-2825
FAX: 701-328-4000
TTY:800-366-6888
www.jobsnd.com/

Leslie Weiss, Manager
Offers vocational assessment and training, adult developmental activities.

6060 North Dakota Vocational Rehabilitation Agency
Suite 1b
Prairie Hills Plaza 1237 W D
Bismarck, ND 58501-1208 701-328-8950
800-756-2745
FAX: 701-328-8969
e-mail: dhsvr@nd.gov
www.nd.gov/dhs/dvr/

Russ Cusack, State Director
Cheryl Wescott, Chief of Field Services
Harley Engelman, Business Relations/Marketing Dir
Robin Throlson, Planning and Evaluation Administ
Offers services for the totally blind, legally blind, visually impaired, mentally retarded blind and more with health, counseling, educational, recreational, rehabilitation, computer training and professional training services.

Ohio

6061 Cornucopia
18120 Sloane Ave
Lakewood, OH 44107-3108 216-521-4600
FAX: 216-521-9460
e-mail: Ronda.mohammad@cornucopia-inc.org
www.cornucopia-inc.org

Wm. Scott Duennes, Executive Director
Anthony Rospert, President
Judy DeFrancesco, 1st Vice President
David Westerfield, Treasurer
Provides work adjustment training for people with and developmental disabilities in a unique community based setting; Nature's Bin, a natural fresh foods market. Consumers learn through participation in retail operations in produce, grocery, bakery, deli, maintenance and customer service areas. Retail revenues help offset the cost of the program. Job search skills training and placement assistance available to program graduates.

6062 Great Oaks Joint Vocational School
3254 E Kemper Rd
Cincinnati, OH 45241-1581 513-771-8881
800-441-6257
FAX: 513-771-4932
http://www.greatoaks.com/

Harold Carr, Medical Director
Deb Graw, Manager
Jim Perdue, Chair
Sue Steele, Vice Chair
Offers vocational assessment and training, adult developmental activities.

6063 Hearth Day Treatment and Vocational Services
8301 Detroit Ave
Cleveland, OH 44102-1805 216-281-2660

Don Cook, Manager
Hearth offers time-limited, paid work adjustment experiences to consumers with mental illness. The goal of Hearth Programs is to prepare the consumer for success in the competitive workforce.

6064 Highland Unlimited Business Enterprises of CRI
1501 Madison Road
Cincinnati, OH 45206-2223 513-354-5200
FAX: 513-354-7115
e-mail: ddutton@cricincy.com
gcbhs.com

Tony Datillo, CEO
Debbie Dutton Lambert, Director Employment Programs
Tony Carter, Chairman of GCB Board
Adrienne Russ, Secretary
Offers vocational assessment and training, adult developmental activities.

6065 Ohio Civil Rights Commission
Rhodes State Office Tower
30 East Broad Street, 5th Floor
Columbus, OH 43215-3414 614-466-5928
TTY:614-753-2391
http://crc.ohio.gov

Leonard Hubert, Chairman
Eddie Harrell, Jr, Commissioner
Rashmi Yajnik, Commissioner
Stephanie Mercado, Commissioner
Primary function is to enforce state laws against discrimination.

6066 **Ohio Commission On Minority Health**
77 S High Street
18th Floor
Columbus, OH 43215-6108 614-466-4000
FAX: 614-752-9049
e-mail: minhealth@mih.ohio.gov
www.mih.ohio.gov

Angela C Dawson, Executive Director
Sheronda Whitner, Executive Assistant
Reina M. Sims, MSA, Program Manager
Venita O'Bannon, Fiscal Specialist
Offers vocational assessment and training, adult developmental activities.

6067 **Vocational and Rehabilitation Agency**
400 East Campus View Boulevard
Columbus, OH 43235-4604 614-438-1210
800-282-4536
FAX: 614-438-1257
TTY: 614-438-1334
e-mail: john.connellyu@rsc.state.oh.us
www.state.oh.us

John M Connelly, Administrator
Rose Reed, Manager
State agency that provides vocational rehabilitation services to help people with disabilities become employed and independent.

Oklahoma

6068 **Oklahoma Department of Rehabilitation Services**
Ste 500
3535 NW 58th St
Oklahoma City, OK 73112-4824 405-424-4932
800-845-8476
FAX: 405-951-3529
e-mail: jharlan@okdrs.gov
www.okrehab.org

Michael O'Brien, Director
Jody Harlan, Public Information Administrator
The Oklahoma Department of Rehabilitation Services (DRS) provides assistance to Oklahomans with disabilities through vocational rehabilitation, employment, independent living, residential and outreach programs, and the determination of medical eligibility for disability benefits.

6069 **Oklahoma Employment Services and Job Training Program Liaison**
2401 North Lincoln Boulevard
Oklahoma City, OK 73105-4409 405-557-7100
FAX: 405-557-5368
TTY:800-722-0353
http://www.ok.gov

Richard McPherson, Executive Director
Teresa Keller, Deputy Director
Mike Evans, Chief Information Technology Officer
Lisa Graven, Reemployment Services/Customer Service Division Director
As the primary agency dedicated to disability services in Oklahoma, we offer a wide range of programs for many individuals each year.

6070 **Oklahoma Governor's Committee on Employment of People with Disabilities**
Ste 90
2401 NW 23rd
Oklahoma City, OK 73107-2423 405-521-3756
800-522-8224
FAX: 405-522-6695
www.odc.ok.gov

Steve Stokes, Executive Director
Doug MacMillan, Director
William Ginn, Disability Program Specialist
Dalene Barton, Office Manager
Mission is to promote the employment of people with disabilities. The vision of the committee is to facilitate partnerships with commitment to full, high quality employment of people with disabilities.

Oregon

6071 **Bend Work Activity Center**
P.O. Box 430 835 E Hwy 126
Redmond, OR 97756 541-548-2611
FAX: 541-548-9573
e-mail: info@ofco.org
www.ofco.org

James Booth, Chairperson
Bill Schertzinger, Vice Chairperson
Cam Chambers, Manager
Seth Johnson, Executive Director
Offers vocational assessment and training, adult developmental activities and programs.

6072 **Oregon Fair Employment Practice Agency**
Oregon Bureau of Labor & Industry
Suite 1045
800 NE Oregon St
Portland, OR 97232-2180 971-673-0761
FAX: 971-673-0762
e-mail: mailb@boli.state.or.us
www.boli.state.or.us/civil

6073 **State of Oregon Office of Vocational Rehabilitation Service**
Ste 500
3165 10th St
Baker City, OR 97814-1480 541-524-1800
800-578-9990
FAX: 541-523-5667
e-mail: wendy.m.wall@state.or.us
www.oregon.gov/dhs/vr

Wendy Wall, Voc Rehab Counselor
Allan McCandless, Voc Rehab Counselor
Offers vocational assessments and training, adult developmental activities, and helps remove disability related barriers to employment.

6074 **Vocational and Rehabilitation Agency**
500 Summer St NE E-87
Salem, OR 97301-1063 503-945-5880
877-277-0513
FAX: 503-947-5010
e-mail: vr.info@state.or.us
www.oregon.gov/dhs/vr/index.shtml

Stephanie Taylor, Administrator
Offers vocational assessments and training, adult developmental activities and programs.

6075 **Vocational and Rehabilitation Agency: Oregon Commission for the Blind**
535 SE 12th Avenue
Portland, OR 97214-2408 971-673-1588
888-202-5463
FAX: 503-234-7468
TTY: 971-673-1577
e-mail: ocb.mail@state.or.us
www.oregon.gov/Blind

Linda Mock, Administrator
Frank Armstrong, Representative
Pat MacDonell, Director
Jodi.C Roth, Chair
A resource for visually impaired Oregonians, as well as their families, friends, and employers. Nationally recognized programs and staff that make a difference in people's lives every day.

Pennsylvania

6076 ACLD/An Association for Children and Adults with Learning Disabilities: Greater Pittsburgh
4900 Girard Rd
Pittsburgh, PA 15227-1440 412-881-2253
e-mail: info@acldonline.org
acldonline.org

Thomas Fogarty, Administrator
Kathleen Donahoe, Director ACLD Tillotson School
Jackie Lulich, Director Business Services

Dedicated to helping children, adolescents, and adults with Specific Learning Disabilities and related disorders succeed in school, employment and life.

6077 Office of Vocational Rehabilitation
7th and Forester St
Harrisburg, PA 17120-1 717-787-4746
FAX: 717-783-5221
www.dli.state.pa.us

Barry Brandt, Rehabilitation Specialist

Information in vocational counseling and the governor's committee on Employment of People with Disabilities. Also serves persons with disabilities that present a substantial handicap to employment and independence. Services are provided when there is a reasonable expectation that employment is possible as a result of those services.

6078 Pennsylvania Employment Services and Job Training
P A Department of Labor and Industry
Room 1700
7th and Forster St
Harrisburg, PA 17120-1 717-787-2500
FAX: 717-772-8284
www.dli.state.pa.us

Edward G Rendell, Manager
Stephen Schmerin, Manager

Administers benefits to unemployed individuals, oversees the administration of worker's compensation benefits to individuals with job related injuries, and provides vocational rehabilitation to individuals with disabilities.

6079 Pennsylvania Governor's Committee on Employment of Disabled Persons
121 N Sixth Street
Harrisburg, PA 17120-1 717-772-6382
FAX: 717-783-5221
www.dli.state.pa.us/landi/cwp

6080 Pennsylvania Human Relations Commission Agency
8th Floor
333 Market St.
Harrisburg, PA 17101-2210 717-787-4410
FAX: 717-772-4340
TTY:717-787-7279
e-mail: phrc@pa.gov
phrc.state.pa.us

JoAnn. L Edwards, Executive Director
Gerald.S Robinson, Chairman
Tom Corbett, Governor
Dr. Raquel O Yiengst, Vice Chairperson

Mission is to administer and enforce the PHRAct and the PFEOA of the Commonwealth of Pennsylvania for the identification and elimination of discrimination and the providing of equal opportunity for all persons.

6081 US Healthworks
25124 Springfield Court
Suite 200
Valencia, CA 91355- 3333 661-678-2600
800-720-2432
FAX: 610-926-6225
www.ushealthworks.com

Beverly Shaeff, Manager
Stephanie Makovsky, Sales Consultant
Daniel D. Crowley, President & Chief Executive Officer
Joseph T. Mallas, Chief Operating Officer

Offers employers comprehensive occupational health services and state-of-the-art physical and occupational therapy. Staff works as a team to produce the best possible patient care while delivering cost savings through workers compensation disability management programs.

6082 Vocational and Rehabilitation Agency
1521 North Sixth Street
Harrisburg, PA 17102-1100 717-787-5244
800-442-6351
FAX: 717-783-5221
TTY: 717-787-4885
e-mail: ovr@dli.state.pa.us
dli.state.pa.us

William Gannon, Manager
Thomas Washic, Manager

Mission is to assist with disabilities, to secure and maintain employment and independence.

6083 Vocational and Rehabilitation Agency: Department of Labor and Industry
909 Green St
Harrisburg, PA 17102-2913 717-236-6211
800-622-2842
FAX: 717-236-3390
TTY: 717-787-6176
e-mail: cboone@state.pa.us

Thomas Carlock, CEO

Mission is to assist people with disabilities, to serve and maintain employment and independence.

Rhode Island

6084 Goodwill Industries of RI
100 Houghton Street
Providence, RI 02904-1013 401-861-2080
FAX: 401-454-0889
TTY:401-331-2830
www.goodwillri.org

Jeffrey D. Machado, President/CEO
Justine Beatini, Transitional Resource Specialist
Shirl Berger, Employee Development & Program
Daniel Burgess, Finance Director

The mission of Goodwill Industries of Rhode Island is to provide training, education and other services which result in employment and expanded opportunities for people with disabilities and other barriers to employment in order to enhance their capacity for independent living, increased quality of life and work.

6085 Groden Center
86 Mount Hope Avenue
Providence, RI 02906-1648 401-274-6310
grodencenter.org

Helen Morcos, Chief Executive Officer
Jane I Carlson, Ph.D., BCBA, Vice President Day & Residential Programs
Cooper Woodard, Ph.D., Vice President Clinical Services
Peggy H. Stocker, Admissions Coordinator

The Groden Center is a school and residential treatment center in Rhode Island enhancing the lives of children and youth with autism, behavioral disorders, and developmental disabilities by providing early autism intervention services, an early childhood education program as well as providing functional and social development instruction to school-age children with learning disabilities.

6086 Newport County Chapter of Retarded Citizens
P.O.Box 4390
906 Aquidneck Avenue
Middletown, RI 02842 401-846-0340
FAX: 401-847-9459
e-mail: danam@mahercenter.org
mahercenter.org

John Maher, Executive Director
Daniel J Oakley, VP
Barbara Burns, Secretary
Walter Jachna, Chairman
Vocational training and job placement services.

6087 Office of Rehabilitation Services
40 Fountain Street
Providence, RI 02903-1898 401-421-7005
FAX: 401-222-3574
TTY:401-421-7016
e-mail: garyw@ors.ri.gov
ors.ri.gov

Ron Racine, Deputy Administrator
Steve Brunero, Acting Deputy Administrator-ORS
John Microulis, Deputy Administrator-Disability
Walter Jachna, Chairman Board of Directors
Their goal is to help individuals with physical and mental disabilities prepare for and obtain appropriate employment.

6088 Vocational and Rehabilitation Agency: Department of Human Services
RI Services for the Blind and Visually Impaired
40 Fountain St
Providence, RI 02903-1830 401-421-7005
FAX: 401-222-3574
TTY:401-421-7016
e-mail: garyw@ors.ri.gov
ors.ri.gov

Ron Racine, Deputy Administrator
Steve Brunero, Acting Deputy Administrator-ORS
John Microulis, Deputy Administrator-Disability
Walter Jachna, Chairman Board of Directors
Their goal is to help individuals with physical and mental disabilities prepare for and obtain appropriate employment.

South Carolina

6089 South Carolina Employment Security Commission South Carolina Center
P.O.Box 567
Columbia, SC 29201 803-777-2400
800-436-8190
e-mail: jobs@sces.org
www.sces.org

Camille Fallow, Disability Program Navigator
Regina Ratterros, Program Coordinator/State Office
Public agency taht offers job search assistance. Unemployment Benefits and WIA program. Also offered is Disability Program Navigator who helps persons with disabilities to find needed resources

6090 South Carolina Governor's Committee on Employment of the Handicapped
1410 Boston Avenue
P.O.Box 15
West Columbia, SC 29171-15 803-896-6500
800-832-7526
FAX: 803-896-1224
TTY: 806-896-6553
http://www.scvrd.net/

Barbara G. Hollis, Executive Director
Derle A. Lowder Sr., Agency Board Chairman
Dr. Roxzanne Breland, Vice Chair
Joseph A. Thomas, Vice Chair
Goal is to help individuals with physical and mental disabilities prepare for and obtain appropriate employment.

6091 South Carolina Vocational Rehabilitation Department
P.O.Box 15
1410 Boston Avenue
West Columbia, SC 29171-15 803-896-6500
800-832-7526
TTY:806-896-6553
e-mail: info@scvrd.state.sc.us
www.scvrd.net

Larry C Bryant, Commissioner
Barbara G Hollis, Executive Director
Dr. Roxzanne Breland, Vice Chair
Derle A Lowder Sr., Agency Board Chairman
The SCVRD's mission is to enable eligible South Carolinians with disabilities to prepare for, achieve and maintain competitive employment.

6092 Vocational and Rehabilitation Agency: Commission for the Blind
Vocational and Rehabilitation Agency
P.O.Box 79
1430 Confederate Avenue
Columbia, SC 29201-79 803-898-8764
800-922-2222
FAX: 803- 89- 879
e-mail: publicinfo@sccb.sc.gov
http://www.sccb.state.sc.us/

Zertie Johnson, Manager
James Kirby, Commissioner
Don Bradley, Director Consumer Affairs
Rhonda Thompson, Director, Prevention
Goal is to help individuals with physical and mental disabilities prepare for and obtain appropriate employment.

South Dakota

6093 South Dakota Governor's Advisory Committeeon Employment of the Disabled
700 Governors Drive
Pierre, SD 57501-2291 605-773-3101
FAX: 605-773-6184
http://dlr.sd.gov

Patrick Keating, Manager
Marcia Hultman, Secretary of Labor and Regulation
Lyle Harter, Director of Administrative Services
Bret Afdahl, Director of the Division of Banking
Goal is to help individuals with physical and mental disabilities prepare for and obtain appropriate employment.

6094 South Dakota State Vocational Rehabilitation
Department of Human Services
3800 E Highway 34 Hillview Plz
Pierre, SD 57501 605-773-3195
FAX: 605-773-5483
e-mail: eric.weiss@state.sd.us
www.state.sd.us

Jeff Pierce, Manager
Bernie Grimme, Assistant Director, DRS
Eric Weiss, Director
South Dakota State Vocational Rehabilitation consists of two agencies; Rehab Services and service to the Blind and Visually Impaired. There mission is the same to provide individualized rehabilitation services that result in optimal employment and independent living outcomes for individuals with disabilities.

6095 **South Dakota Workforce Investment Act Training Programs**
700 Governors Dr
Pierre, SD 57501-2291
605-773-3101
800-952-3216
FAX: 605-773-6184
www.sdjobs.org

Michael Ryan, Administrator
Patrick Keating, Manager
Marcia Hultman, Secretary of Labor and Regulation
Lyle Harter, Director of Administrative Services

Mission is to enhance the South Dakota workforce by providing business with employment-related solutions and helping people with job placement and career transition services

6096 **Vocational and Rehabilitation Agency: Division of Services to the Blind/Visually Impaired**
3800 E Highway 34 Hillview Plz
Pierre, SD 57501
605-773-3195
FAX: 605-773-5483
e-mail: gaye.mattke@state.sd.us
www.state.sd.us

Dawn Backer, Manager, Rehabilitation Center for the Blind
Eric Weiss, Director
Gaye Mattke, Division Director, Service to the Blind and Visually Impaire
Nancy Hoyme, Program Specialist

To provide individualized rehabilitation services that result in optimal employment and independent living outcomes for people with disabilities.

Tennessee

6097 **Division of Rehabilitative Services**
Tennessee Department Human Services
400 Deaderick Street
15th Floor
Nashville, TN 37243-1403
615-313-4700
FAX: 615-741-4165
e-mail: mandy.johnson@tn.gov
www.state.tn.us/humanserv/rehabilitation.htm

Raquel Hatter, Commisioner

6098 **Tennessee Department of Labor: Job Training Program Liaison**
220 French Landing Drive
Nashville, TN 37243-1712
615-741-6642
FAX: 615-741-5078
www.tn.gov

Ruth S Letson, Manager
Burns Phillips, Commissioner
Dustin Swayne, Deputy Commissioner
Stephanie Mitchell, Mitchell

Goal is to help individuals with physical and mental disabilities prepare for and obtain appropriate employment.

6099 **Tennessee Fair Employment Practice Agency**
Human Rights Commission
23rd floor
312 Rosa L Parks Ave
Nashville, TN 37243-1
615-741-5825
800-251-3589
FAX: 615-253-1886
www.state.tn.us/humanrights

Tricia Crawford, Manager
Beverly L. Watts, Executive Director
Sabrina Hooper, Deputy Director
Shalini Rose, General Counsel

An independent state agency charged with preventing and eradicating discrimination in employment, public accomodations, and housing.

Texas

6100 **C-CAD Center of United Cerebral Palsy of Metropolitan Dallas**
8802 Harry Hines Blvd.
Dallas, TX 75235
800-999-1898
e-mail: info@ucpdallas.org
www.ucpdallas.org

Mark Denzin, President/Chief Operating Officer
Frank Pickens, CPA, Chief Financial Officer
April Allen, Chief Program Officer
Shea Needham, Regional Director

Offers a wide range of technology opportunities for persons with all types of disabilities, their families and the professionals who serve them. Services include assesments, traiing, technology access showroom, and workshops for rehabilitation and educational personnel.

6101 **Handbook of Career Planning for Students with Special Needs**
Pro- Ed Publications
8700 Shoal Creek Boulevard
Austin, TX 78757-6897
512-451-3246
800-897-3202
FAX: 512-451-8542
e-mail: general@proedinc.com
www.proedinc.com

Donald D Hammill, Owner
Courtney King, Marketing Coordinator
Thomas F. Harrington, Editor

The practitioner's guide will show you how to help special needs adolescents and young adults overcome barriers to employment by identifying goals and problems, assessing interests and aptitudes, involving client families and developing communication skills. *$42.00*
358 pages

6102 **Texas Employment Services and Job Training Program Liaison**
Texas Workforce Commission
101 E 15th St
Rm 665
Austin, TX 78778-0001
512-463-2236
866-938-4444
TTY:700-735-2989
e-mail: ombudsman@twc.state.tx.us
http://www.twc.state.tx.us

Larry Temple, Executive Director
Lasha Lenzy, Division Director
Reagan Miller, Division Director
Tom McCarty, Division Director

State government agency charged with overseeing and providing workforce development services to employers and job seekers of Texas. Offers career development information, job search resources, training programs, and, as appropriate, unemployment benefits.

6103 **Vocational and Rehabilitation Agency: State Rehabilitation Commission**
Vocational and Rehabilitation Agency
4800 N Lamar Blvd
Austin, TX 78756-3106
512-383-7000
800-628-5115
FAX: 512-424-4730
TTY: 800-628-5115
e-mail: DARS.Inquiries@dars.state.tx.us
www.dars.state.tx.us

Marilyn Hancock, Executive Director
Michelle Crain, Executive Director
Veronda L. Durden, Commissioner
Glenn Neal, Deputy Commissioner

Helps people with disabilities prepare for, find and keep jobs. Work related services are individualized and may include counseling, training, medical treatment, assistive devices, jon placement assistance and other services.

Utah

6104 Utah Employment Services
P.O. Box 45249
2292 South Redwood Road
West Valley, UT 84119-0249
801-978-0378
FAX: 801-978-0374
e-mail: info@utahemploy.com
www.utahemploy.com
Kristen Cox, Executive Director
To help individuals prepare and obtain appropriate employment.

6105 Utah Governor's Committee on Employment ofthe Handicapped
195 North 1950 West?
Salt Lake City, UT 84116-5238
801-538-4200
800-837-6811
FAX: 801-538-4279
e-mail: dspd@utah.gov
dspd.utah.gov
George Kelner, Executive Director
Promotes opportunities and provide support for persons with disabilities to lead self-determined lives.

6106 Utah Veterans Centers
Ste 105
200 South Central Campus Drive
Salt Lake City, UT 84112-1686
801-587-7722
800-246-1197
FAX: 801-377-0227
www.military.com/benefits/veteran-benefits
Dennis Stevens, Executive Director
Brent Price, Manager
Roger Perkins, Director of Veterans Support
Sylvia O'Hara, Executive Assistant
Readjustment counseling services to veterans.

6107 Utah Vocational Rehabilitation Agency
Utah State Office of Rehabilitation
P.O.Box 144200
1501 M Street, NW Seventh Floor
Washington, DC 20005-4200
202-466-6550
800-473-7530
FAX: 202-785-1756
e-mail: duchida@utah.gov
www.ppsv.com/
Donald Uchida, Executive Director
Heidi Kubbe, Executive Assistant
Jennifer Smart, Training Coordinator
Coy Jackson, Program Specialist
Vocational Rehabilitation Services for individuals with disabilities. To assist individuals with disabilities to prepare for and obtain employment and increase their independence.

6108 Vocational and Rehabilitation Agency: Division of Services for the Blind/Visually Imp.
1st Floor
160 E 300 S
Salt Lake City, UT 84111-7902
801-530-4849
877-526-3994
FAX: 801-530-6438
e-mail: wgibson@utah.gov
utah.gov
Willam G Gibson, Executive Director
Cheryl Ritchie, Administrative Secretary
LuWana Martin, Network Specialist
Sharon Pipkin, Office Specialist
Mission is to assist individuals who are blind or visually impaired to obtain employment or increase their independence.

Vermont

6109 State of Vermont Department of Disabilities, Aging and Independent Living
Agency of Human Services
103 South Main Street
Weeks IC
Waterbury, VT 05671-2304
802-241-2210
888-405-5005
FAX: 802-241-2128
e-mail: Info@ahs.state.vt.us
www.ahs.state.vt.us/dbvi
Fred Jones, Director
Stacy Rollins, Executive Administrative Assistant
Carl Augusto, President and CEO
Rick Bozeman, Chief Financial Officer
Mission is to support the efforts of Vermonters who ar blind and visually impaired to achieve or sustain their economic independence, self reliance, and social integration to a level consistent with thier interests, abilities and informed choices.

6110 Vermont Employment Services and Job Training
5 Green Mountain Drive P.O.Box 488
Montpelier, VT 05601- 488
802-828-4000
FAX: 802-828-4022
TTY:802-828-4203
e-mail: tdouse@labor.state.vt.us
www.labor.vermont.gov
Annie Noonan, Commissioner
Deborah Bruce, Human Resource Administrator
Richard Gray, State Director
Tracy Phillips, Director, Unemployment Insurance & Wages
The primary focus is to help support the efforts to make Vermont a more competitive place to do business and create good jobs.

6111 Vermont Governor's Committee on Employmentof People with Disabilities
103 South Main Steet
Weeks 1A
Waterbury, VT 05671-2303
802-241-6757
866-879-6757
FAX: 802-241-3359
e-mail: melita@gcepd.org.
www.vocrehabvermont.org
Diane Dalmasse, Manager
Melita DeBeliss, Staff
Committed to facilitating successful, long-term relationships between employers and people with disabilities in Vermont.

Virginia

6112 Alexandria Community Y Head Start
418 S Washington St
Alexandria, VA 22314-3673
703-549-0111
FAX: 703-549-2097
www.campagnacenter.org/
Tammy.L Mann, Ph.D, President and CEO
Raj Kapur, Chief Financial Officer
Karla Kelley, Senior Director of Out-of-School
Chrystal Starr Brown, Senior Director, Early Childhood
Offers social services, on-the-job-training for parents, play therapy, physical therapy, speech therapy and any other specialized services.

6113 Department Of Rehabilitative Services
8004 Franklin Farms Drive
Henrico, VA 23229-5019
804-662-7000
FAX: 804-662-9532
e-mail: dars@dars.virginia.gov
vadrs.org
Jay Windsor, Contact Pers
Jim Rothrock, Commissioner
Helps people with disabilities get ready for,find, and keep a job.

6114 **Didlake**
8641 Breeden Ave
Manassas, VA 20110-8431
703-361-4195
866-361-4195
FAX: 703-369-7141
www.didlake.com

Rex Parr, CEO
John S Craig, VP Rehabilitation Services
Tammara L. Hoover, Treasurer
Patty Tracy, Secretary
Offers situational assessments, work training, employment and job placement services to people with disabilities.

6115 **Learning Services: Shenandoah**
204 Howe Hall
1460 University Drive
Winchester, VA 22601-5829
540-665-4928
FAX: 540-665-3470
www.su.edu/academic

Peter Patrick, Administrator
Michelle Shenk, Director of Learning Resources and Services
Jeremai Santiago, M.S., Assistant Director & Learning Enrichment Coach
Erin Beaupre, Learning Services Specialist
Postacute rehabilitation program.

6116 **NISH**
8401 Old Courthouse Road
Vienna, VA 22182-3820
571-226-4660
FAX: 703-849-8916
nish.org

E. Robert Chamberlin, President and CEO
Dennis.A Fields, Chief Operating Officer
Elizabeth W. Goodman, Chief Financial Officer
Paul W. Plattner, Vice President of Operations
A nonprofit agency desigated by the Committee for Purchase from People Who Are Blind or Severely Disabled to provide technical assistance to rehabilitation programs interested in obtaining federal contracts under Public Law 92-28, the Javits-Wagner-O'Day Act. NISH's primary objective is to assist community rehabilitation programs in providing jobs for people with severe disabilities.

6117 **Richmond Research Training Center**
P.O.Box 842011
1314 West Main Street
Richmond, VA 23284-2011
804-828-1851
FAX: 804-828-2193
TTY:804-828-2494
e-mail: RRTC@vcu.edu
http://www.worksupport.com

Paul Wehman Ph.D., Professor and Director
Dolores Taylor, Executive Director
John Kregel, Ed.D, Associate Director
Vicki Brooke, M. Ed., Director of Training and Knowledge Translation
Research and training center report on the supported employment of persons with developmental and other disabilities.

6118 **ServiceSource**
Suite 175
6295 Edsall Rd
Alexandria, VA 22312-2670
703-461-6000
800-244-0817
FAX: 703-461-3906
www.ourpeoplework.org

Janet Samuelson, President & CEO
Edie Castner, Assistant Director
Mark Hall, Executive Vice President, Corporate Development
David Hodge, Executive Vice President & Chief Financial Officer
Provides training, job placement and employment services in private sector and government contract employment.

6119 **Sheltered Occupational Center of Virginia**
750 23rd St
Arlington, VA 22202-2452
703-521-4441
FAX: 703-521-3443
socent.org

Perla Ni, CEO
Hayley Gefell, Chief Business Development Offic
Marshall Henson, Chief Operating Officer
Donnell Karimah, Chief Administrative Officer
Assists, empowers and supports people with disabilities to achieve employment, independence and integration in the workplace and community. Our services include: printing, copying, hand work, mail shop, fulfillment and distribution.

6120 **Vocational and Rehabilitation Agency: Department for the Blind/Visually Impaired**
397 Azalea Avenue
Richmond, VA 23227-3623
804-371-3140
800-622-2155
FAX: 804-371-3154
e-mail: Kimberley.Jennings@dbvi.virginia.gov
www.vdbvi.org

Raymond E. Hopkins, Commissioner
James A Taylor, Chief Deputy
Kimberley Jennings, Contact Person
Dr. Rick L. Mitchell, Deputy Commissioner, Services Delivery
DBVI envisions a world in which blind, vision impaired and deafblind people can access all that society has to offer and can, in turn, contribute to the greater community. We believe this is achievable.

Washington

6121 **Career Connections**
P.O.Box 141806
431 East Colfax Ave.
South Bend, IN 46617-1806
574-232-5400
866-404-5867
FAX: 574-245-5822
e-mail: caronn@mindspring.com
www.peoplelinking.com

Susan Warwick, Executive Director
Teresa Antosyn, Program Coordinator
Dan Moody, CFO
Sadie Takila, Production Manager
Offers structured work sites at several locations. Production work at various skill levels, with training as needed.

6122 **Department of Services for the Blind National Business & Disability Council**
Department of Services for the Blind
P.O.Box 40933
4565 7th Avenue SE
Olympia, WA 98504-933
360-725-3830
FAX: 360-407-0679
e-mail: info@dsb.wa.gov
www.dsb.wa.gov

Louana Durand, Executive Director
A state rehabilitation agency that offers assistance to persons who are blind or visually impaired. Also provides various services for employers interested in accomodating or hiring workers with vision loss.

6123 **Division of Developmental Disabilities: Department of Social & Health Services**
P.O.Box 45310
Olympia, WA 98504-5310
360-725-3413
800-737-0617
FAX: 360-407-0955
e-mail: dddcoreception@dshs.wa.gov
www1.dshs.wa.gov/ddd/index.shtml

Robin Arnold-Williams, Secretary
Colleen Cawston, Senior Director
Steve Lowe, Senior Director
Tracy Guerin, Chief of Staff

The Division of Developmental Disabilities offers persons with developmental disabilities quality supports and services that are individual/family driven, stable and flexible, satisfying to the person and their family, and able to meet individual needs.

6124 **SL Start and Associates**
901 N Monroe St.
Suite 200
Spokane, WA 99201-4800
509-328-2740
888-355-7155
FAX: 509-326-9207
e-mail: info@slstart.com
slstart.com

Stephen L Start, Owner
A diversified and innovative human and health services company focused on a wide range of social, employment and long-term services.

6125 **School of Piano Technology for the Blind**
2510 E Evergreen Blvd
Vancouver, WA 98661-4323
360-693-1511
FAX: 360-693-6891
e-mail: info@pianotuningschool.org
pianotuningschool.org

Len Leger, Executive Director
Jeff Lane, Executive Director
Donald L. Mitchell, Director of Instructional Operat
Les Fitzpatrick, Technician/Instructor
Teaches piano tuning and repair to blind and visually impaired menand women, leading to employment and/or self-employment in the piano service industry. Licensed by Washington State and accredited by the Accrediting Commission of Career Schools and Colleges of Technology (ACCSCT). 20-month course.

6126 **Vocational and Rehabilitation Agency: Division of Vocational Rehabilitation**
Department of Social and Health
P.O.Box 45340
Olympia, WA 98504-5340
360-704-3560
800-637-5627
FAX: 360-570-6941
TTY: 360-438-8000
e-mail: krulik@dshs.wa.gov
www1.dshs.wa.gov/dvr

Patrick Raines, Manager
Andres, Director
Mission is to empower individuals with disabilities to achieve a greater quality of life by obtaining and maintaining employment.

West Virginia

6127 **West Virginia Division of Rehabilitation Services**
P.O.Box 50890
107 Capitol Street
Charleston, WV 25301- 2609
304-356-2060
800-642-8207
FAX: 304-766-4905
TTY: 304-766-4809
www.wvdrs.org

Deborah Lovely, Director
Donna Ashworth, Assistant Director
DRS specializes in helping people with disabilities who want to find a job or maintain current employment. Rehabilitation counselors at more than 30 field offices help with applications. Once eligibility is determined, counselors & clients work as a team to develop a plan to meet the individuals employment goal. Services may include work-related counseling/guidance, evaluation/assessment, job development & placement assistance, vocational training, college assistance & assistive technology.

6128 **West Virginia Employment Services and Job Training Programs Liaison**
112 California Ave
Charleston, WV 25305-12
304-558-2660
FAX: 304-558-1343
e-mail: workforcelmi@wv.gov
http://workforcewv.org

Valerie Comer, Director
Allan Galloway, Manager
Workforce West Virginia, a division of the Department of Commerce, effectively coordinates all availiable state and federal resources by orchestrating the efforts of state agencies and local organizations.

6129 **West Virginia Vocational Rehabilitation**
P.O.Box 1004
107 Capitol Street
Charleston, WV 25301- 2609
304-356-2060
800-642-8207
www.wvdrs.org

Earl Wolfe, Director
Offers services for the totally blind, legally blind, visually impaired, mentally retarded blind and more with health, counseling, educational, recreational, rehabilitation, computer training and professional training services.

Wisconsin

6130 **Vocational and Rehabilitation: State of Wisconsin**
201 E Washington Ave
Madison, WI 53702-1
608-266-0050
800-442-3477
FAX: 608-266-3131
TTY: 888-877-5939
e-mail: dvr@dwd.wisconsin.gov
www.dwd.state.wi.us/dvr

Tamara Monsees, Office Manager/Admin. Support
Offers vocational rehabilitation services for the totally blind, legally blind, visually impaired, mentally retarded blind and more with health, counseling, educational, rehabilitation, computer training and professional training services, and displaced worker.

Wyoming

6131 **Division of Vocational Rehabilitation of Wyoming**
Wyoming Department of Workforce Services
1100 Herschler Buiding
Cheyenne, WY 82002-1
307-777-7364

wyomingworkforce.org/how/vr.aspx

Jim Mcintosh, Administrator
Kathy Emmones, Director Workforce Services
Provides only those services which are necessary for eligible individuals to reach the employment goal agreed to in the Individualized Plan for Employment.

6132 **Vocational Rehabilitation, Division of Department of Workforce Services**
Suite 1e
1510 East Pershing Blvd.
Cheyenne, WY 82002-1
307-777-7364
866-804-3678
FAX: 307-777-3759
TTY: 307-777-7386
e-mail: jmcint@state.wy.us
www.wyomingworkforce.org

Jim McIntosh, Administrator
Joan K. Evans, Director
Lisa M. Osvold, Deputy Director
Provides only those services which are necessary for eligible individuals to reach the employment goal agreed to in the individualized plan for employment.

6133 **Wyoming Department of Employment Unemployment Insurance**
P.O.Box 2760
100 West Midwest
Casper, WY 82602-2760
307-235-3264
FAX: 307-235-3277
doe.state.wy.us
Randy Hopper, Manager
A combined state/federally funded agency of the state of Wyoming, headed by a Department Director who is appointed by the Governor.

6134 **Wyoming Governor's Committee on Employment of the Handicapped**
Room 1126
1510 East Pershing Blvd.
Cheyenne, WY 82002-1
307-777-3700
FAX: 307-777-5870
e-mail: workforceservices@state.wy.us
doe.state.wy.us/Inetclaims
Brenda Oswald, Manager
Joan K. Evans, Director
Lisa M. Osvold, Deputy Director
Assists, empowers and supports people with disabilities to achieve employment, independence and intergration in the workplace and community.

Rehabilitation Facilities, Acute

Alabama

6135 HealthSouth Rehabilitation Hospital of North Alabama
3660 Grandview Parkway
Suite 200
Birmingham, AL 35243- 4326
205-967-7116
FAX: 256-428-2608
www.healthsouth.com

Doug Beverley, CEO
Holly Ray, PHR, HR Director
Will Craig, Director of Marketing Operations
Mary Ann Arico, Chief Investor Relations Officer

A comprehensive 50 bed rehabilitation hospital serving the need of patients in the North Alabama area. Guides patients with physically disabling conditions along an individualized treatment pathway so they can reach their highest level of physical, social and emotional well-being. A wide range of medical and theraputic services are delivered by qualified and experienced professionals.

6136 Lakeshore Rehabilitation Hospital
3800 Ridgeway Dr
Birmingham, AL 35209-5599
205-868-2000
FAX: 205-868-2029
www.healthsouthlakeshorerehab.com

Terry Brown, Administrator
Barbie Reedy, Contact

A 100 bed facility whos key services is physical rehabilitation. Also specialized services (inpatient) infection isolation room. In addition, also has outpatient physical rehabilitation and sports medicine. Patient family support services include patient representative, transportation for elderly/handicapped and patient support groups. Imaging services(diagnostic & theraputic) include ct scanner, diagnostic diagnostic radioisotope facility, MRI, and ultrasound.

6137 Mobile Infirmary Medical Center: Rotary Rehabilitation Division
5 Mobile Infirmary Circle
Mobile, AL 36652-3513
251-435-4700
800-826-2085
FAX: 251-435-3403
e-mail: resource@mobileinfirmary.org
www.mobileinfirmary.org

Joe Stough, VP
Kevin O'Connor, CEO
Ben Taylor, Senior Editor
Dan Tobin, Director Healthcare Group

Our vision is to appreciably enhance in a proactive manner the healthcare status and related quality of life of the residents and communities we serve.

6138 More Than Just a Job
Institute On Disability/UCED
60 5th Avenue
Suite 101
New York, NY 10011
212-366-8900
FAX: 603-862-0555
www.forbes.com

6139 Rocky Mountain Resource & Training Institute
3630 Sinton Road
Suite 103
Colorado Springs, CO 80907- 5072
719-444-0268
800-949-4262
FAX: 719-444-0269
TTY: 800-949-4232
www.adainformation.org

Jana Copeland, Principal Investigator
Patrick Going, Senior Advisor

Serves people with disabilities and provides training to the agencies that assist them. Facilitates disabled individuals' transition from school to adult life; provides information and resources concerning assistive technology, devices, and services; promotes and ensures compliance with the federal Americans with Disabilities Act (ADA) and other legislation promoting the rights and inclusion of people with disabilities; promotes supported employment, strategic planning and development.

Arkansas

6140 Central Arkansas Rehab Hospital
2201 Wildwood Ave
Sherwood, AR 72120-5074
501-834-1800
FAX: 501-834-2227
www.stvincentrehabhospital.com

Lee Frazier, MPH, Dr, CEO
Dr. Sean Foley, Medical Director
Debbie Taylor, Director of Marketing Operations
Stacy Sawyer, Director Of Therapy Operations

A nonprofit hospital licensed for 69 acute care beds with all private rooms. Opened in 1999the hospital offers a full range of outpatient diagnostic services, including MRI,CT,PET along with surgical procedures, cardiology, neurology, neurosurgery, othopedic, rehab and a 24 hour emergency department staffed with board certified emergency room physicians. Includes an outpatient surgery center, rehabilitation hospital, senior health program, diabetic program and physician offices.

6141 HealthSouth Rehabilitation Hospital
1401 South J St
Fort Smith, AR 72901-5158
479-785-3300
FAX: 479-785-8599
www.healthsouth.com

Juli Stec, CEO

Provides physical rehabilitation as its key services. Also provides other services such as end-of-life services, pain management and an infection isolation room.

6142 Northwest Arkansas Rehabilitation Hospital
153 E Monte Painter Dr
Fayetteville, AR 72703-4002
479-444-2233
FAX: 479-444-2390
www.healthsouthfayetteville.com

Marty Hurlbut, Medical Director
Denise Wilson, Director Of Clinical Services

A 60-bed acute medical rehabilitation hospital that offers comprehensive inpatient and outpatient rehabilitation services.

6143 Rebsamen Rehabilitation Center
P.O.Box 159
Jacksonville, AR 72078-159
501-985-7000
FAX: 501-985-7384
www.rebsamenmedicalcenter.com

Mack McAlister, Chairperson
Murice Green, Vice Chairman
Tommy Swaim, Secretary

Mission is to provide personal healthcare for your family. Vision is to develop a family of caregivers to become your community hospital. A 113 bed acute care facility operated by a volunteer Board of Directors made up of community leaders. Rebsamen Medical Center is accredited by the Joint Commission on Accredidation of Healthcare Organizations as well as the Arkansas Department of Health. Through JCAHO we voluntary sumbit to evaluations of our compliance with nationwide hospital standards.

Arizona

6144 Barrow Neurological Institute Rehab Center
350 W Thomas Rd
Phoenix, AZ 85013-4409
602-406-3000
FAX: 602-406-4104
www.stjosephs-phx.org

Jackie Aragon, VP Care Management
Linda Hunt, President

Dedicated resources to delivering compassionate, high-quality, affordable health services; serving and advocating for our sisters and brothers who are poor and disenfranchised; and partnering with others in the community to improve the quality of life. Our vision:a growing and diversified health care ministry distinguished by excellent quality and committed to expanding access to those in need.

6145 **HealthSouth Sports Medicine Center**
5111 N Scottsdale Rd
Ste 100
Scottsdale, AZ 85250-7076 480-990-1379
FAX: 480-423-8458
e-mail: chamine@wiley@healthsouth.com
www.healthsouth.com

Troy Meiners, Manager
An out patient facility specialising in sports medicine and treatment of sports injuries.

6146 **Healthsouth Rehab Institute of Tucson**
2650 N Wyatt Dr
Tucson, AZ 85712-6108 520-325-1300
800-333-8628
FAX: 520-327-4045
www.rehabinstituteoftucson.com

Lee Sanford, Plant Manager
Jon Larson, Medical Director
An accredited member of the Joint Commission On Accreditation of Health Care Organizaions (JCAHO) An 80 bed facility specializing in rehabilitation

6147 **Scottsdale Healthcare**
9630 E Shea Blvd
Scottsdale, AZ 85260-6285 480-551-5400
FAX: 480-551-5401
e-mail: preiley@shc.org
www.shc.org

Thomas Sadvary, CEO
Pegg Reiley, Chief Nursing Officer
Kathy Zarubi, Associate VP of Nursing Practice
Lisa Sandoval, Director fo Marketing
A 343 bed full-service hospital providing medical/surgical, critical care, obstetrics, pediatrics, surgery, cardiovascular, and oncology services, as well as the Sleep Disorder Center. All patient rooms are private. Emergency department is a level II Trauma Center. The Radiology Department offers state-of-the-art diagnostic equipment, including MRI, PET/CT scanning, nuclear medicine and ultrasound. Also located are the Piper Surgery Center, Cancer Center, and several medical office plazas.

6148 **St. Joseph Hospital and Medical Center**
350 W Thomas Rd
Phoenix, AZ 85013-4496 602-406-3000
FAX: 602-406-4190
http://hospitals.dignityhealth.org/stjosephs/

Linda Hunt, President
Rehabilitation programs offered by the clinic assists clients with rehabilitation health needs in the comfort of their own home. The home care rehabilitation team of professionals focuses on correcting deficiencies in self-care, mobility skills and communication. Services offered include physical therapy, occupational therapy, speech pathology, rehabilitative nursing and restorative nursing assistants.

California

6149 **Bakersfield Regional Rehabilitation Hospital**
5001 Commerce Dr
Bakersfield, CA 93309-648 661-323-5500
800-288-9829
FAX: 661-633-5254
www.healthsouthbakersfield.com

Chris Yoon, Medical Director
Sandra Hegland, Chief Executive Officer
A specialty hospital that treats an array of physical disabilities. It has 60 beds and offers physical rehabilitation services including support groups and education classes on illnesses such as arthritis, asthma and strokes. No surgery facilities on site.

6150 **Brotman Medical Center: RehabCare Unit**
3828 Delmas Ter
Culver City, CA 90232-6806 310-836-7001
FAX: 310-202-4141
e-mail: info@brotmanmed.com
www.brotmanmedicalcenter.com

Howard Levine, CEO
The mission of Brotman Medical Center is to deliver innovative, quality health care to our patients and their families in an environment of compassion, respect, patient saftey, education, and fiscal responsibility.

6151 **Casa Colinas Centers for Rehabilitation**
255 E Bonita Ave
Pomona, CA 91767-1923 909-596-7733
866-724-4127
FAX: 909-593-0153
TTY: 909-596-3646
e-mail: rehab@casacolina.org
www.casacolina.org

Felice Loverso, CEO/President
Steve Norin, Chairman
Stephen W. Graeber, Vice Chairman
Mary Lou Jensen, Secretary
Casa Colina will provide individuals the opportunity to maximize their medical recovery and rehabilitation potential efficiently in an environment that recognizes their uniqueness, dignity and self esteem. The vision is to strategically reposition themselves at the forefront of the post-acute continuum by becoming the center of excellence in the provision of services to persons who can benefit from rehabilitation care.

6152 **Community Hospital of Los Gatos Rehabilitation Services**
815 Pollard Rd
Los Gatos, CA 95032-1400 408-378-6131
FAX: 408-866-4003
communityhospitallosgatos.com

Ned Borgstrom, CEO
Rehabilitation Services provide individualized treatment programs for inpatient/outpatient care. The team is supervised by a Physiatrist and may include Nurses, Physical Therapists, Occupational Therapists, Speech/Language Therapists, Psychologists, Case Managers, Dietitians, Respiratory Therapists, Recreation Therapists and/or Prosthetists/Orthotists.

6153 **Garfield Medical Center**
525 N Garfield Ave
Monterey Park, CA 91754-1205 626-573-2222
FAX: 626-571-8972
www.garfieldmedicalcenter.com

Philip Cohen, CEO
Provides quality care to all citizens of all ages. We are foreward looking to meet the changing health care needs of Forsyth and the surrounding area. At the same time, we are a stable organization that is financially sound. We involve all of our medical staff through good communication. We support them by trying to meet their professional needs in training, equipment and services. We emphasize good communication with all county citizens who support us financially and through the use of services

6154 **Grossmont Hospital Rehabilition Center**
5555 Grossmont Center
La Mesa, CA 91942 619-740-6000
800-827-4277
FAX: 619-644-4159
www.sharp.com

Michael Murphy, President/CEO
Daniel Gross, EVP
It is our mission to improve the health of those we serve with a commitment to excellence in all that we do. Our goal is to offer quality care and programs that set community standards, exceed patients' expectations and are provided in a caring, convenient, cost-effective and accessible manner.

6155 Health South Tustin Rehabilitation Hospita
14851 Yorba St
Tustin, CA 92780-2925
714-832-9200
FAX: 714-508-4550
www.healthsouth.com
Sandra Yule, CEO

6156 Holy Cross Comprehensive Rehabilitation Center
15031 Rinaldi St
Mission Hills, CA 91345-1207
818-365-8051
888-432-5464
FAX: 818-898-4472
www.providence.org
Larry Bowe, CEO
Derek Berz, COO
Known for providing exceptional treatment through its Cancer Centers, Heart Center, Orthopedics, Neurosciences and Rehabilitation Services, as well as Woman's and Children's Services. As a 254-bed, not-for-profit facility, Providence offers a full continuum of health services, from outpatient to inpatient to home health care. Providence operates one of the only round-the-clock trauma centers in the San Fernando Valley and surrounding communities.

6157 Job Hunting Tips for the So-Called Handicapped
Special Needs Project
324 State St
Ste H
Santa Barbara, CA 93101-2364
805-962-8087
800-333-6867
FAX: 805-962-5087
e-mail: editor@specialneeds.com
www.specialneeds.com
Hod Gray, Owner
This nifty booklet from the guru of job hunting himself is sincere, useful and brief. *$4.95*

6158 Kentfield Rehabilitation Hospital & Outpatient Center
1125 Sir Francis Drake Blvd
Kentfield, CA 94904-1418
415-456-9680
FAX: 415-485-3563
e-mail: info@kentfieldrehab.com
www.kentfieldrehab.com
Deborah Doherty, MD
Provides specialized inpatient and outpatient programs. We provide quality services that are patient centered and family-oriented. Under the medical direction of board-certified hospitalists and other physician specialists, our decicated interdisciplinary teams provide a coordinated, comprehensive treatment approach to a wide range of neurological, orthopedic, pulmonary and complex medical problems.

6159 Laurel Grove Hospital: Rehab Care Unit
20103 Lake Chabot Rd
Castro Valley, CA 94546-4093
510-537-1234
FAX: 510-727-2778
e-mail: nissims@sutterhealth.org
www.edenmedcenter.org
George Bischalaney, CEO & President
Kent Myers, Treasurer
Jeffrey Randall, Secretary
David Davini, CPA Chairman
The mission of Eden Medical Center is carried out by our Board of Directors, employees, physicians and volunteers who are committed to providing our patients and their families with the highest quality medical care and customer service. Creating standards of excellence to ensure quality and value for our patients. Maintaining a financially sound organization through effective clinical and administrative support. Encouraging a culture that supports employees and physicians in development.

6160 Lodi Memorial Hospital West
Lodi Memorial Hospital
975 S Fairmont Ave
Lodi, CA 95240
209-334-3411
800-323-3360
FAX: 209-333-7131
e-mail: lmh@lodihealth.org
www.lodihealth.org
Joseph Harrington, President
Ron Kreutner, Vice President And CFO
Judy Begley RN, MSN, Chief Nursing Officer
Our vision is to provide a system of health-care services which is clinically effective, quality driven and community focused in an environment that supports and encourages excellence. In partnership with our medical staff, we will assume accountability for the health of our community, be responsible for illness and injury prevention and provide care for the ill and injured. We will measure our success on quality outcomes and customer satisfaction.

6161 Long Beach Memorial Medical Center Memorial Rehabilitation Hospital
2801 Atlantic Ave
Long Beach, CA 90806-1701
562-933-2000
FAX: 562-933-9018
www.memorialcare.org
Nissar Syed, Administrator
Barry Arbuckle, President
The hospital offers rehabilitation after catastrophic injury of disabling disease to give patients the opportunity for maximum recovery. The Hospital offers many of the area's finest rehabilitation specialists and most advanced technology, making it one of Southern California's most respected rehabilitation centers.

6162 North Coast Rehabilitation Center
1165 Montgomery Drive
Santa Rosa, CA 95405-4869
707-546-3210
FAX: 707-525-8413
www.santarosamemorial.org
Joyce Cavagnaro, Admissions
Combines state-of-the-art medicine, compassionate care, and the widest array of resources to enhance your health and promote healthy communities. Dedicated to continually introducing new programs and services that help you live life to the fullest.

6163 Northridge Hospital Medical Center
18300 Roscoe Blvd
Northridge, CA 91328
818-885-8500
FAX: 818-885-5435
www.northridgehospital.org
Mike Wall, CEO
dedicating resources to delivering compassionate, high-quality, affordable health services; serving and advocating for our sisters and brothers who are poor and disinfranchised; and partnering with others in the community to improve the quality of life.

6164 PEERS Program
8912 W Olympic Blvd
Beverly Hills, CA 90211-3514
310-553-4833
FAX: 310-553-4833
Paul Berns, Medical Director
Offers a new approach for wheelchair users. PEERS uses a combination of modern physical therapy, the DOUGLAS Reciprocating Gait System and when necessary, functional electrical stimulation to assist selected individuals to walk with recently patented specially made lightweight braces.

6165 PIRS Hotsheet
Placer Independent Resource Services
11768 Atwood Rd
Ste 29
Auburn, CA 95603
530-885-6100
800-833-8453
FAX: 530-885-3032
TTY: 530-885-0326
e-mail: lbrewer@pirs.org
pirs.org
Susan Miller, Executive Director
Harry Powell, President
Paul Opper, Vice President
Dawn Davidson, Secretary
Monthly newletter to customers and other constituents.
6 pages Monthly

6166 Providence Holy Cross Medical Center
Providence Health System
15031 Rinaldi St
Mission Hills, CA 91345-1285
818-365-8051
818-898-4603
FAX: 818-365-4472
www.providence.org
Kerry Carmody, CEO
Physicains and nurses are among the best and are recognized nationally for clinical excellence. We are committed to improving your health and wellness as you journey through life. Our services span beyond the latest advancements in medical procedures, equipment and medication to also include education and wellness services-all provided with compassion and respect. We help our patients understand and use some of the healthiest tools at their disposal, including nutrition & excercise.

6167 Queen of Angels/Hollywood Presbyterian Medical Center
1300 N Vermont Ave
Los Angeles, CA 90027-6005
213-413-3000
FAX: 213-413-3500
e-mail: info@hollywoodpresbyterian.com
www.hollywoodpresbyterian.com
Kathy Wong, Manager
A 434 bed acute-care facility that has been caring for the Hollywood community and surrounding areas since 1924. The hospital is committed to serving local multicultural communities with quality medical and nursing care. With more then 500 physicians representing virtually every speciality. Ready to serve your medical needs and those of your loved ones and strive to distinguish itself as a leading healthcare provider, recognized for providing quality, innovative care in a compassionate manner.

6168 Queen of the Valley Hospital
1000 Trancas St
Napa, CA 94558-2941
707-252-4411
FAX: 707-257-4032
www.thequeen.org
Walt Mickens, President
Vincent Morgese, Vice President
For more then 40 years, Queen of the Valley Hospital has been the premiere medical facility in the Napa Valley. Our long history of providing high quality and caring service is founded on 4 core values:Dignity, Service, Excellence and Justice. These central principals inspire us to reach out to those in need and to help heal the whole person-mind, body and spirit.They are the driving force behind our mission to improve the health and quality of life of people in the community we serve.

6169 Rancho Los Amigos National Rehabilitation Center
7601 E Imperial Hwy
Downey, CA 90242-3496
562-401-7111
877-726-2461
888-RAN-CHO1
FAX: 562-401-6690
TTY:562-401-8450
e-mail: inquiry@rancho.org
www.rancho.org
Jorge Orozco, CEO
Mindy Lipson Aisen, Chief Medical Officer
Michelle Sterling, Interim Chief Nursing Officer
Robin Bayus, CFO
Internationally renowned in the field of medical rehabilitation, consistently ranked in the top Rehabilitation Hospitals in the United States by U.S. News and World Report. It is one of the largest comprehensive rehabilitaion centers in the United States. Licensed for 395 beds, providing service through over 20 centers of excellence.

6170 San Joaquin Valley Rehabilitation Hospital
7173 N Sharon Ave
Fresno, CA 93720-3329
559-436-3600
FAX: 559-436-3606
e-mail: jpage@svjrehab.com
sjvrehab.com
Edward Palacios, CEO
Complete comprehensive rehabilitation services from acute rehab, outpatient and community fitness services.

6171 Santa Clara Valley Medical Center
County of Santa Clara
751 S Bascom Ave
San Jose, CA 95128-2699
408-885-5000
www.scvmed.org
Paul E. Lorenz, CEO
Jeffrey Arnold, Medical Officer
Trudy Johnson, Director of Patient Care Services & Nursing
Carolyn Brown, Director of Quality & Patient Safety
The mission of the medical center is to provide high-quality, cost-effective medical care to all residence of Santa Clara County regardless of their ability to pay. Make availiable a wide range of inpatient, outpatient, emergency services within resource constraints. Maintain an environment within which the needs of our patients are paramount and where patients, their families and all our visitors are treated in a compassionate, supportive, friendly, and dignified manner.

6172 Scripps Memorial Hospital at La Jolla
9888 Genesee Ave
La Jolla, CA 92037-1205
858-626-4123
800-727-4777
FAX: 858-626-6122
www.scripps.org
Sean A Deitch, President/CEO
Gary Fybel, Executive Director/Administrator
One of the county's 6 designated trauma centers, offers a wide range of clinical and surgical services including 24-hour emergency services; intensive care; interventional cardiology and radiology; radiation oncology; cardiothoracic and orthopedic services; neurology; ophthalmology; and mental health and psychology services.

6173 South Coast Medical Center
12 Mason
Ste A
Irvine, CA 92618-2733
714-669-4446
FAX: 714-669-4448
e-mail: info@southcoastmedcenter.com
www.southcoastmedcenter.com
Leigh Erin Connealy, Manager
Bruce Christian, President
A 208 bed acute care hospital. Services include maternity, surgical, subacute care, psychiatric program, eating disorder treatment, chemical dependency treatment, radiology, ICU/CCU, comprehensive rehabilitation services, bariatric surgery and movement disorders program..

6174 **St. Joseph Rehabilitation Center**
St. Joseph Health System
2200 Harrison Ave
Eureka, CA 95501-3215
707-441-4414
FAX: 707-441-4429
www.stjosepheureka.org

6175 **St. Jude Brain Injury Network**
St. Jude Hospital
130 W Bastanchury Rd
Fullerton, CA 92835-1058
714-446-5626
866-785-8332
FAX: 714-446-5979
e-mail: ocrcuser@stjoe.org
www.tbioc.org

Jana Gable, Program Coordinator
David Bogdan, Service Coordinator
Lina Marroquin, Servicer Coordinator
Provides comprehensive planning, program referral, assists with funding possibilities, and interagency coordination of services. Areas of emphasis include day treatment, vocational and housing options, and the requirements are adults who have suffered a brain injury from an external force.

6176 **St. Jude Medical Center**
101 E Valencia Mesa Dr
Fullerton, CA 92835-3809
714-871-3280
800-627-8106
FAX: 714-992-3029
stjudemedicalcenter.org

Robert Fraschetti, President
We are one of Southern California's most respected and technologically advanced hospitals, and our four core values: dignity, excellence, service and justice are the guiding principles for everything we do. St. Jude is synonymous with exceptional care that extends beyond good medicine to a commitment to caring for you - mind, body and spirit.

6177 **St. Mary Medical Center**
1050 Linden Ave
Long Beach, CA 90813-3393
562-491-9000
FAX: 562-491-9053
www.stmarymedicalcenter.org

Chris Desicco, CEO

6178 **Sunnyside Nursing Center**
22617 S Vermont Ave
Torrance, CA 90502-2595
310-320-4130
FAX: 310-212-3232
e-mail: businessdevelopment@sunnysidenursing.com
www.sunnysidenursing.com

Shane Dahl, Administrator
Manny Cordero, Director of Nursing
El Sayad, Medical Director
Skilled nursing care facility; residential care facility; intermediate care facility; specialty hospital.

6179 **UCLA Medical Center: Department of Anesthesiology, Acute Pain Services**
U CLA Medical Center
1245 16th Street Medical Plz
Ste 225
Santa Monica, CA 90404
310-794-1841
FAX: 310-794-1511
e-mail: access@mednet.ucla.edu
www.medcnt.ucla.edu

Michael Ferrante, Clinical Director
A 337-bed acute-care medical center, has been serving the healthcare needs of West Los Angeles and Santa Monica since 1926. Highly regarded for its primary and specialty care, the medical center features many outstanding clinical programs, including its women's and children's services, emergency services, and family medicine programs.

Colorado

6180 **Children's Hospital Rehabilitation Center**
University of Colorado Health Sciences Center
1056 E 19th Ave
Denver, CO 80218-1007
303-861-8888
800-624-6553
e-mail: webmaster@tchden.org
chipteam.org

Lou Blankenship, CEO
Michael J Farrell, Chief Operating Officer
Helen Martinez, Manager
Private not-for-profit pediatric healthcare network, the hospital is 100 percent dedicated to caring for kids of all ages and stages of growth. That dedication is evident in more then 1000 pediatric specialists and more then 2400 employees. It is also our continual dedication that has placed us at the forefront of research in childhood disease with several nationally and internationally recognized medical programs.

6181 **Craig Hospital**
3425 S Clarkson St
Englewood, CO 80113-2899
303-789-8000
FAX: 303-789-8214
e-mail: khosack@craighospital.org
www.craighospital.org

Michael Fordyce, President
Thomas Balazy, Medical Director
Julie Keegan, VP of Finance
Dona Polonsky, VP of Clinical Services
A 93-bed, private, not-for-profit, free-standing, acute care and rehabilitation hospital that provides a comprehensive system of inpatient and outpatient medical care, rehabilitation, neurosurgical rehabilitative care, an equipment company, and long-term follow up services.

6182 **HealthSouth Rehabilitation Hospital of Colorado Springs**
HealthSouth Corporation
325 S Parkside Dr
Colorado Springs, CO 80910-3134
719-630-8000
FAX: 719-520-0387
www.healthsouthcoloradosprings.com

Steve Schaefer, CEO
A 56 bed rehabilitation hospital, its key services are: cardiology department, physical rehabilitation, and orthopedics department. Accredidted to the Joint Commission on Accreditation of Health Care Organizations (JCAHO)

6183 **Mapleton Center**
North Broadway & Balsam
Boulder, CO 80301-9130
303-440-2273
FAX: 303-441-0536
e-mail: pr@bch.org
www.bch.org

David Gehant, President/CEO
Comprehensive inpatient and outpatient rehabilitation services for all age groups. Treatment provided by interdisciplinary teams and staff physicians. CARF accredited in brain injury rehabilitation, pediatric rehabilitation, pain management, work hardening and inpatient rehabilitation.

6184 **Mediplex Rehab: Denver**
Vibra Health Care
8451 Pearl St
Thornton, CO 80229-4804
303-288-3000
FAX: 303-496-1120
e-mail: info@vhdenver.com
www.northvalleyrehab.com

Walter Sackett, CEO
Encompasses the broadest mix of professional talent, the finest technology and a total commitment by our people to deliver the highest quality care today, and well into the future. The services can be divided into 4 main categories: long term Acute Care and rehab. Skilled nursing facility and residential ventilator program. Outpatient services and pain management. Adult and Geriatric inpatient psychiatric services.

Connecticut

6185 Mariner Health Care: Connecticut
23 Liberty Way
Niantic, CT 06357
860-739-4007
FAX: 860-701-2202

District of Columbia

6186 National Rehabilitation Hospital
102 Irving St NW
Washington, DC 20010-2949
202-877-1760
FAX: 202-829-2789
www.nrhrehab.org

Edward Healton, Medical Director
Robert Bunning, Associate Medical Director

A private facility dedicated solely to medical rehabilitation. The hospital offers intensive inpatient programs and full-service outpatient programs.

Florida

6187 Florida Hospital Rehabilitation Center
601 E Rollins St
Orlando, FL 32803-1248
407-303-1527
855-303-3627
FAX: 407-303-7566
e-mail: fh.web@flhosp.org
www.flhosp.org

Rex Alleyne, President

Florida Hospital Orlando uses the latest technology to treat over 32,000 inpatients and 53,600 outpatients annually. This 881-bed, acute-carecommunity hospital also serves as a major tertiary facility for much of the Southeast, the Caribbean and South America

6188 HealthSouth Regional Rehab Center/Florida
20601 Old Cutler Rd
Miami, FL 33189-2441
305-251-3800
FAX: 305-259-0498
www.healthsouth.com

Murray Rolnick, Medical Director
Elizabeth Izquierdo, Chief Executive Officer

HealthSouth Rehabilitation Hospital of Miami is a member of the HealthSouth Corporation, the nation's largest healthcare services provider. The hospital is accredited by the Joint Commission on Accreditation of Healthcare Organizations (JCAHO) and Commission on Accreditaion of Rehabilitation Facilities (CARF). Services offered include dietary services, occupational therapy, and respitory care.

6189 HealthSouth Rehab Hospital: Largo
901 Clearwater Largo Rd N
Largo, FL 33770-4121
727-586-2999
FAX: 727-588-3404
www.healthsouthlargo.com

Elaine Ebaugh, CEO
Linda Russo, Director, Therapies

A specialty hospital devoted to providing comprehensive medical rehabilitation services. The hospital is licensed as a Comprehensive Medical Rehabilitation Hospital by the state of Florida, and accredited by the Joint Commission on Accreditation of Healthcare Organizations (JCAHO). HealthSouth of Largo is the only free standing Rehabilitation Hospital in the Tampa Bay region, and serves patients of all ages. Provides inpatient medical rehabilitation services as well as outpatient programs.

6190 HealthSouth Sports Medicine & Rehabilitation Center
3280 Ponce De Leon Blvd
Coral Gables, FL 33134-7252
305-444-0909
FAX: 305-444-5760
www.healthsouth.com

Jay Greeney, President
Ray Jaffet, Administrator

Provides specialized medical and therapeutic services designated to help physically disabled individuals reach their optimum level of independence and function by providing inpatient and outpatient comprehensive medical rehabilitation services.

6191 HealthSouth Sports Medicine and Rehabilitation Center
2141 South Highway A1A Alt
Jupiter, FL 33477
561-743-8890
FAX: 561-743-8795

Diane Reiley, Manager

Outpatient orthopedic and sports medicine/physical therapy.

6192 HealthSouth Treasure Coast Rehabilitation Hospital
Health South Corporation of Alabama
1600 37th St
Vero Beach, FL 32960-4863
772-778-2100
FAX: 772-567-7041
www.healthsouthtreasurecoast.com

Jimmy Lockhart, Medical Director

HealthSouth Treasure Coast Rehabilitation Hospital is a 90-bed inpatient comprehensive rehabilitation hospital serving Indian River, St. Lucie, Martin and Okeechobee counties. Outpatient services are available at the hospital and at four other clinics. Therapies include physical, occupational, speech and psychology services.

6193 Manatee Springs Care & Rehabilitation Center
5627 9th St E
Bradenton, FL 34203-6105
941-753-8941
FAX: 941-739-4409
e-mail: info@manateespringsrehab.com
www.manateespringsrehab.com

Donna Steiermann, Administrator

Skilled rehabilitation facility specializing in PT, OT, speech therapy, aquatic therapy and an indoor pool. Piped oxygen bed for specialized respiratory care. Compassionate end of life care. Some Medicare, private insurance, and Medicaid.

6194 Perry Health Facility
207 Marshall Dr
Perry, FL 32347-1897
850-584-6334
FAX: 850-838-1801

Rebkah Hatch, Administrator

Full rehabilitation team available, Physiatrist, DOR, Psychiatrist, Psychologist, RD, Geriatric Nursing, PT/OT/ST/RT, Orthotiet/Prosthetist. Provider for PPO's & HMO's as well as medicare, private insurance and medicare/medicaid.

6195 Pinecrest Rehabilitation Hospital and Outpatient Centers
Tenet South Florida
5352 Linton Blvd
Delray Beach, FL 33484-6514
561-498-4440
800-283-8326
FAX: 561-495-3103
www.pinecrestrehab.com

Mark Bryan, CEO

Pinecrest Rehabilitation Hospital is a 90 bed, accredited hospital and is comprised of a Specialty Unit, a Neuro Trauma Unit and Joint Replacement Unit. Additional services at Pincrest include six outpatient rehab centers throughout Palm Beach County. The Outpatient Centers each focus on various specialties such as orthopedic and neurological rehab, pain management, cardiac and pulmonary rehab, occupational medicine, Hearing Institute, dizziness and balance and wellness.

6196 Rehabilitation Institute of Sarasota
3251 Proctor Rd
Sarasota, FL 34231-8538
941-921-8796
FAX: 941-922-6228

Stacy Shepherd, Director Clinical Services

a 75-bed hospital that offers individualized medical and theraputic services tailored to patients and clinics for those affected with stroke, multiple sclerosis, Parkinson's, muscular dystrophy and Lou Gehrig's disease (ALS)

6197 **Sea Pines Rehabilitation Hospital**
101 E Florida Ave
Melbourne, FL 32901-8398 321-984-4600
FAX: 321-727-7440
e-mail: ellen.lyons-olski@healthsouth.com
www.healthsouthseapines.com

Stuart Miller, Medical Director
Donna Bohdal, Director of Therapy Operations
Denise McGrath, Administrator

A 90-bed facility specializing in rehabilitation of brain and spinal injuries.

6198 **Shriners Hospitals for Children: Tampa**
12502 USF Pine Dr
Tampa, FL 33612-9411 813-972-2250
813-281-0300
FAX: 813-975-7125
e-mail: aargiz-lyons@shrinenet.org
www.shrinershq.org/hospitals/tampa

David Ferrell, FACHE
Maureen Maciel, Chief of Staff
Alicia Argis-Lyons, Develpoment Officer

Recognizing that the family plays a vital role in a child's ability to overcome an illness or injury, Shriners Hospitals helps the family provide the support the child needs by involving the family in all aspects of the child's care and recovery. The purpose of all Shriners Hospitals for Children is to provide care to children with orthopedic problems and burn injuries to help them lead fuller, more productive lives.

6199 **South Miami Hospital**
6200 SW 73rd St
South Miami, FL 33143-4679 786-662-4000
FAX: 786-662-5302
www.baptisthealth.net

Brian E. Keely, CEO

The mission is to improve the health and well-being of individuals, and to promote the sanctity and preservation of life, in the communities we serve. We are committed to maintaining the highest standards of clinical and service excellence, rooted in utmost integrity and moral practice.

6200 **St. Anne's Nursing Center**
11855 Quail Roost Dr
Miami, FL 33177-3956 305-252-4000
FAX: 305-969-6752
www.catholichealthservices.org

Tony Farinella, Executive Director
Francisco Cruz, Medical Director
Julia Shillingford, Director of Nursing

Provides spacious, comfortable accommodations with ample recreational areas in a beautifully landscaped setting.

6201 **St. Anthony's Hospital**
1200 7th Ave N
St Petersburg, FL 33705-1388 727-825-1100
www.stanthonys.com

William Ulbricht, President
James McClint, VP
Ron Colaguori, VP Operations
Mary McNally, VP Mission

A not-for-profit, 395-bed hospital established in 1931. St. Anthony's is dedicated to improving the health of the community through community-owned health care that sets the standard for high-quality, compassionate care.

6202 **St. Anthony's Rehabilitation Hospital**
3487 NW 35th Ave
Lauderdale Lakes, FL 33311-1107 954-485-4023
954-739-6233
www.catholichealthservices.org

Linda Motte, Hospital Administrator
Kathy Torbertsonn, Dir. Rehab.

Provides spacious, comfortable accommodations with ample recreational areas in a beautifully landscaped setting.

6203 **St. Catherine's Rehabilitation Hospital and Villa Maria Nursing Center**
1050 NE 125th St
North Miami, FL 33161-5805 305-357-1735
305-891-3361
www.catholichealthservices.org

Virginia Irving, Hospital Administrator
Jim Reiss, Executive Director
Greg Hartley, Director Rehab

St. Catherine's Rehabilitation Hospital is a CARF accredited, 60 bed facility offering inpatient and outpatient rehabilitation and medical clinics; including physical, occupational, and speech therapy, neurology, neurodiagnostics, wound care, and hyperbaric medicine. Villa Maria Nursing center is a JCAHO accredited, 212 bed skilled nursing center providing short term nursing and rehabilitation, as well as long term care.

6204 **St. John's Nursing Center**
3075 NW 35th Ave
Lauderdale Lakes, FL 33311-1107 954-739-6233
FAX: 954-733-9579
www.catholichealthservices.org

Ralph E. Lawson, Chairman
Elizabeth Worley, Vice Chairman
Thomas Marin, Assistant Secretary

Provides spacious, comfortable accommodations with ample recreational areas in a beautifully landscaped setting.

6205 **Successful Job Accommodation Strategies**
LRP Publications
36- Hiatt Dr
Palm Beach Gardens, FL 33418 561-622-6520
800-341-7874
FAX: 561-622-0757
e-mail: webmaster@lrp.com
www.lrp.com

Honora McDowell, Product Group Manager
Kenneth Kahn, Chief Executive Officer

This monthly newsletter provides you with quick tips, new accommodation ideas and innovative workplace solutions. You learn the outcomes of the latest cases involving workplace accommodations. *$ 140.00*
12 pages Monthly

6206 **Tampa General Rehabilitation Center**
1 Tampa General Circle
Tampa, FL 33601-1289 813-844-7000
FAX: 813-844-1477
e-mail: jstone@tgh.org
tgh.org

Ron Hytoff, President/CEO
Devanand Mangar MD, Vice Chief of Staff
Thomas L. Bernasek MD, Chief of Staff

Offers a full range of inpatient and outpatient programs all aimed at helping patients achieve their full potentials. JCAHO and CARF accredited and V.R. designated center. A wide range of inpatient and outpatient programs are available such as Brain and Spinal Cord Injury Programs, Comprehensive Medical Rehabilitation, Pain Management, Cardiac Rehab, Pediatric Therapy Service, Sleep Disorders, Epilepsy, and Wheelchair Seating.Hosts the Florida Alliance for Assistive Services and Technolgy.

6207 University of Miami: Jackson Memorial Rehabilitation Center
University of Miami
1611 NW 12th Ave
Miami, FL 33136-1005
305-585-6970
FAX: 305-585-6092
e-mail: info@jhsmiami.org
www.jhsmiami.org
Michael Butler, Chief Medical Officer
An accredited, non-profit, tertiary care hospital and the major teaching facility for the University of Miami School of Medicine. With more then 1,550 beds, Jackson Memorial is a referral center, a magnet for medical research, and home to the Ryder Trauma Center- the only adult and pediatric level 1 trauma center in Miami-Dade County.

6208 Winter Park Memorial Hospital
Florida Hospital
200 N Lakemont Ave
Winter Park, FL 32792-3273
407-646-7000
FAX: 407-646-7639
e-mail: healthcare@winterparkhospital.com
www.winterparkhospital.com
Ken Bradley, CEO
Offers Acute Rehabilitation.

Georgia

6209 Candler General Hospital: Rehabilitation Unit
5353 Reynolds St
Savannah, GA 31405-6015
912-819-6000
FAX: 912-819-8829
www.sjchs.org/body.cfm?id=383
Paul Hinchey, President/CEO
Special Physical Therapy Services at Candler Outpatient Center: Aquatic therapy, pediatric services, outpaitient neurological rehabilitation program, woman's health therapy, orthotics, and spine specialty

6210 Children's Healthcare of Atlanta at Egleston
1405 Clifton Rd NE
Atlanta, GA 30322-1060
404-785-6000
FAX: 404-315-2158
www.choa.org
Donna Hyland, President/CEO
Ruth Fowler, CFO
Patrick Friars, Chief Children's Physician
Ron Frieson, Chief Public Policy Officer
Rehabilitation Center at Egleston accepts children from birth to age 18 with acute or chronic problems. The length of rehab stay varies for each child according to the determined program of care. The center offers inpatient, outpatient & day rehab programs for comprehensive evaluation & treatment. The program emphasizes the development of the child's abilities & concentrates on helping the family & child compensate for any long-term disabilities. Short term stays require one or two weeks.

6211 Cobb Hospital and Medical Center: Rehab Care Center
3950 Austell Rd
Austell, GA 30106-1121
770-732-5126
e-mail: generalinfo@wellstar.org
www.wellstar.org
David Anderson, Executive VP
Michael Andrews, Chief Cancer Network Officer
Avril Beckford, Chief Pediatrics Officer
To deliver world class healthcare we equip our healthcare facilities and employees with the best technology, resources and education availiable. To deliver world class healthcare we keep seeking ways to improve the way we deliver care knowing each day holds more miracles, more life, more chances, more compassion, and more opportunities.

6212 HealthSouth Central Georgia Rehabilitation Hospital
3351 Northside Dr
Macon, GA 31210-2587
478-201-6500
FAX: 478-471-6536
www.centralgarehab.com

6213 Specialty Hospital
Floyd Healthcare Resources
304 Turner McCall Blvd SW
Rome, GA 30165-5621
706-509-5000
FAX: 706-802-4175
e-mail: contactus@floyd.org
www.floyd.org
Kurt Stuenkel, CEO
Dee Russell, Chief Medical Officer
Our mission is to be responsive to the communities we serve with a comprehensive and technologically advanced heal care system commited to the delivery of care that is characterized by continually improving quality, accessability, affordability and personal dignity.

Hawaii

6214 Shriners Hospital for Children: Honolulu
1310 Punahou St
Honolulu, HI 96826-1099
808-941-4466
888-888-6314
FAX: 808-942-8573
e-mail: jburda@shrinenet.org
www.shrinershospitalsforchildren.org
Kenneth Guidera, Chief Medical Officer
Eugene D'Amore, Vice President
Kathy A. Dean, Vice President Human Resources
Sharon Russell, VP Finance & Accounting
One of 22 hospitals across North America that provide excellent, no-cost medical care to children with orthopedic problems and burn industries.

Idaho

6215 Pocatello Regional Medical Center
777 Hospital Way
Pocatello, ID 83201-2797
208-234-6154
FAX: 208-239-3719
e-mail: robbieo@portmed.org
www.portmed.org
Mark Bukalew, Chairman
John Abreu, VP Finance
Stephen Weeg, Vice-Chairman
David Swindell, Treasurer
Pocatello Regional Medical Center offers 24-hour emergency care, specialized heart services, a dialysis center, a full service rehabilitation unit including transition care, and the Woman's Center For Health including obstetrics.

Illinois

6216 Builders of Skills
515 Busse Hwy
Park Ridge, IL 60068-3154
847-318-0870
FAX: 847-292-0873
e-mail: avenues@avenuesonline.org
www.avenuestoindependence.org
Jacqueline Kinmel, Chair
Peg O'herron, Vice Chair
Eric Johnson, Treasurer
Bob Healy, Secretary
Residential setting for hearing-impaired, developmentally disabled adults who are assisted with daily living skills.

6217 Center for Learning
National-Louis University
2840 Sheridan Rd
Evanston, IL 60201-1730 847-256-5150
FAX: 845-256-1057
e-mail: kadamle@nl.edu

Jerry Dachs, Manager

Psycho-educational evaluations for children, adolescents, and adults. Individualized remedial academic programs, individual counseling

6218 DBTAC-Great Lakes ADA Center
1640 W Roosevelt Road
Room 405
Chicago, IL 60608-1316 312-413-1407
800-949-4232
FAX: 312-413-1856
e-mail: gldbtac@uic.edu
www.adagreatlakes.org

Robin Jones, Project Director
Glenn Fujiura, PhD, Director of Research and Co-Inve
Claudia Diaz, Associate Project Director
Peter Berg, Project Coordinator for Technica

Provides training, technical assistance and consultation on the rights and resposibilities of indiviualsand entities covered by the ADA. Toll free number for technical assistance and materials provided electronically or via mail at no cost.

6219 Institute of Physical Medicine and Rehabilitation
6501 N Sheridan Rd
Peoria, IL 61614-2932 309-692-8110
800-957-4767
FAX: 309-692-8673
e-mail: foundation@ipmr.org
ipmr.org

Lisa Snyder, Medical Director

Comprehensive CARF accredited programs in outpatient medical rehabilitation services. Eight outpatient locations, specialty programs include adult day services, driving evaluations, balance and visual rehabilitation board certified physiatrists.

6220 LaRabida Children's Hospital and Research Center
E 65th At Lake Michigan
Chicago, IL 60649 773-363-6700
FAX: 773-363-9554
e-mail: pr@larabida.org
www.larabida.org

Brenda Wolf, President/CEO

Dedicated to excellence in caring for children with chronic illness, disabilitiesm or who have been abused, allowing them to achieve their fullest potential through expertise and innovation within the health care and academic communities.

6221 Marianjoy Rehabilitation Hospital and Clinics
26W171 Roosevelt Rd
Wheaton, IL 60187-6078 630-909-8000
800-462-2366
FAX: 630-909-8001
e-mail: dlebloch@marianjoy.org
www.marianjoy.org

Maureen Beal, Chairperson
John Oliverio, Vice Chairman
Kathleen Dvorakk, Treasurer
Thomas A. Keiser, Secretary

Goal at Marianjoy Rehabilitation Hospital is to help you and your family return to the lifestyle you enjoyed before your illness or injury. To meet this goal, we provide you with a dedicated team of experienced professionals to assist you every step of the way.

6222 Rush Copley Medical Center-Rehab Neuro Physical Unit
2040 Ogden Ave
Ste 303
Aurora, IL 60504-7222 630-898-3700
866-426-7539
FAX: 630-898-3681
e-mail: clord@rsh.net
www.rushcopley.com

Barry Finn, CEO
Mary Shilkaitis, VP, Patient Care Services

The mission of the medical center and the medical staff is to work together to serve your healthcare needs through excellence in education, technology and a caring touch. Rush-Copley Medical Center will be the leading healthcare provider of the greater Fox Valley area. At Rush-Copley we pride ourselves on providing everyone with extrodinary service.

Indiana

6223 ATTAIN
U S Department of Education/ NI DR R
32 E Washington St
Ste 1400
Indianapolis, IN 46204-3552 317-534-0236
800-528-8246

Gary Hand, Executive Director

The mission of Attain is to create solutions that enable people with functional limitations to live, learn, work and play in the community of their choice. All will have access to assistive devices. We will do this in partnership with people with functional limitations, families and members of the community through training, system change, services and support, research, dissemination and consumer advocacy.

6224 About Special Kids
7172 Graham Rd
Suite 100
Indianapolis, IN 46250-2879 317-257-8683
800-964-4746
FAX: 317-251-7488
e-mail: FamilyNetw@aboutspecialkids.org
www.aboutspecialkids.org

Joe Brubaker, Executive Director
Jane Scott, Director Of Information
Nancy Stone, Project Director

A Parent to Parent organization that works throughout the state of Indiana to answer questions and provide support, information and resources. We are parents and family members of children with special needs and we help other families and professionals understand the various systems that are encountered related to special needs. Our central office is where parents from the entire state can access information, resources and support.

6225 Clark Memorial Hospital: RehabCare Unit
1220 Missouri Ave
Jeffersonville, IN 47130-3743 812-282-6631
FAX: 812-283-2656
e-mail: humanresources@clarkmemorial.org
clarkmemorial.org

Martin Padgett, CEO

The mission of Clark Memorial Hospital is to provide superior health services to the people and communities we serve. The vision of Clark Memorial Hospital is to be the best community healh care provider in the United States. We value each individual and work together to explore new ways to improve the quality of life of all. We persue excellence in all we do. We treat all individuals with the same compassion, dignity, and privacy that we want in ourselves.

6226 Developmental Disabilities Planning Council
402 W Washington St
Indianapolis, IN 46204-2855 317-232-7770
FAX: 317-233-3712
e-mail: gpcpd@gpcpd.org
www.state.in.us/gpcpd

Suellen Jackson-Boner, Executive Director
Christine Dahlberg, Associate Director
Jim Geswein, CFO
Betty Jones, Secretary

The mission of the Indiana Governor's Council is to promote public policy which leads to the independence, productivity and inclusion of people with disabilities in all aspects of society. This mission is accomplished through planning, evaluation, collaboration, education, research and advocacy. The Council is consumer-driven and is charged with determining how the service delivery system in both the public and private sectors can be most responsible to the people with disabilities.

6227 Easter Seals Wayne/Union Counties
P.O.Box 86
Centerville, IN 47330-86 765-855-2482
FAX: 756-855-2482
e-mail: eastersealswu@comcast.net
eastersealswu.tripod.com

Kathy Stephen, Treasurer
Vickey Allen, President
Leslie Mayl Whitney, Secretary

Helps people discover nature and much more at camps equipped to offer physcial, social and emotional support and fun for campers with physical and/or developmental disabilities.

6228 IN-SOURCE
Indiana Resource Center for Families with Special
1703 S Ironwood Dr
South Bend, IN 46613-3414 574-234-7101
800-332-4433
FAX: 574-234-7279
e-mail: insource@insource.org
insource.org

Richard Burden, Executive Director
Scott Carson, Assistant Director
Dory Lawrence, Project Director
Sally Hamburg, Project Director

The mission of IN*SOURCE is to provide parents, families and service providers in Indiana the information and training necessary to assure effective educational programs and appropriate services for children and young adults with disabilities.

6229 Indiana Congress of Parent and Teachers
2525 N Shadeland Ave
Ste D4
Indianapolis, IN 46219-1770 317-357-5881
FAX: 317-357-3751
e-mail: info@indianapta.org
www.indianapta.org

Sharon Wise, President
Theresa Distelrath, VP
Job Wise, Secretary
Julie Klingenberger, Treasurer

The mission of the Indiana PTA is three-fold: to support and speak on behalf of children and youth in the schools, community and before governmental agencies and other organizations that make decisions affecting children; to assist parents in developing the skills they need to raise and protect their children; and, to encorage parent and community involvement in the public schools of this state and nation.

6230 Indiana Protection and Advocacy Services Commission
4701 N Keystone Ave
Ste 222
Indianapolis, IN 46205-1561 317-722-5555
800-838-1131
FAX: 317-722-5564
e-mail: dward@ipas.IN.gov
www.in.gov/ipas

Karen Pedevilla, Education and Training Director

IPAS was created in 1977 by state law to protect and advocate the rights of people with disabilities and its Indiana's federally designated Protection (P&A) system and client assist program. It is an independent state agency, with receives no state funding and is independent from all service providers, as required by federal and state law.

6231 Kokomo Rehabilitation Hospital
829 N Dixon Rd
Kokomo, IN 46901-7709 765-452-6700
FAX: 765-452-7470

Brenda Harry, Admissions Director

a 60 bed facility specializing in rehabilitation services to the people of Indiana.

6232 Memorial Regional Rehabilitation Center
615 N Michigan St
South Bend, IN 46601-1033 574-647-1000
www.qualityoflife.org

6233 Methodist Hospital Rehabilitation Institute
8701 Broadway
Merrillville, IN 46410-7035 219-738-5500
FAX: 219-755-0448
methodisthospitals.org

Ian McFadden, President/CEO
Matthew Doyle, VP & CFO
Wright Alcorn, VP Operations
Michael Davenport, Vp Medical Affairs

Methodist Hospitals, of all the hospitals in Northwest Indiana, attracts the most complex cases across a range of specialties, including stroke, brain tumor, cancer, trauma and high-risk pregnancy. This is the result of our commitment to providing the expertise and technology needed to offer the most advanced clinical care.

6234 NAMI Indiana
P.O.Box 22697
Indianapolis, IN 46222-697 317-925-9399
800-677-6442
FAX: 317-925-9398
e-mail: info@namiindiana.org
www.namiindiana.org

Marilynn Walker, President
Joshua Sprunger, Executive Director
Linda Williams, Program Coooridnator
Leslie Gay, Office Manager

NAMI Indiana is a non-profit grassroots organization dedicated to improving the lives of people afflicted by serious and persistant mental illness. We are dedicated to helping families through a network of support, education, advocacy, and promotion of research. NAMI's goal is to help establish a system of care that provides community based services for persons with serious mental illness, as well as support for them and their families.

6235 Parkview Regional Rehabilitation Center
2200 Randallia Dr
Fort Wayne, IN 46805-4638 260-373-4000
888-480-5151
FAX: 260-373-4288
www.parkview.com

Mike Packnett, President & CEO
Mike Browning, CFO
Rick Henvey, Chief Administrative Officer
Sue Ehinger, President (Parkview & Affiliates)

Provides a full range of inpatient, theraputic services and programs for patients as young as 3 years of age to the very elderly. Our accute care rehabilitation center, is well equipped to care for patients with neurological and orthopedic injuries and diseases.

6236 **Programs for Children with Disabilities: Ages 3 through 5**
Indiana Department of Education
151 W Ohio St
Indianapolis, IN 46204-1905 317-232-0570
877-851-4106
FAX: 317-232-0589
e-mail: specialed@doe.in.gov
www.doe.in.gov/exceptional

Heather Neal, Chief of Staff

The division provides leadership and state-level support for public school gifted and talented (grades K-12) programs and for students with disabilities from ages 3-21. The division ensures that Indiana, in its compliance with the federal Individuals With Disabilities Education Act, through monitoring of special education programs, oversight of community and residential programs, provision of mediation and due process rights, and sound fiscal management.

6237 **Programs for Children with Special Health Care Needs**
Indiana State Department of Health
2 N Meridian St
Indianapolis, IN 46204-3021 317-233-1325
e-mail: wgettelf@isdh.state.in.us
www.in.gov/isdh/

Sean Keefer, Chief of Staff

The Children's Special Health Care Services (CSHCS) program provides financial assistance for needed medical treatment to children with serious and chronic medical conditions to reduce complications and promote maximum quality of life.

6238 **Programs for Infants and Toddlers with Disabilities: Ages Birth through 2**
402 W Washington St
Indianapolis, IN 46204-2773 317-232-1144
800-441-7837
e-mail: firststepsweb@fssa.state.in.us

6239 **Riley Child Development Center**
705 Riley Hospital Drive
Rm 5837
Indianapolis, IN 46202-5128 317-274-7819
FAX: 317-944-9760
e-mail: info@child-dev.com
child-dev.com

Cristy James, Communication Coordinator

Riley Hospital for Children is Indiana's only comprehensive children's hospital, with pediatric specialists in evry field of medicine and surgery. Riley is committed to providing the highest quality health care to children in a compassionate, family-centered environment. Riley is a national leader in cutting edge research and medical education, ensuring health care excellence for children for generations to come. Riley provides medical care to all children, regardless of family's ability to pay.

6240 **St. Anthony Memorial Hospital: Rehab Unit**
301 W Homer St
Michigan City, IN 46360-4358 219-879-8511
FAX: 219-877-1409
www.saintanthonymemorial.org

Joseph Allegreti, Board of Directors
Calvin Bellamy, Board of Directors

Saint Anthony Memorial is an acute care hospital located in Michigan City, primary serving La Porte and Porter Counties in Indiana as well as Berrien County Michigan.

6241 **State Division of Vocational Rehabilitation**
402 W Washington St
P O Box 7083
Indianapolis, IN 46207-7083 317-233-4475
800-545-7763
FAX: 317-232-6478
e-mail: vrcommission@fssa.in.gov
www.state.in.us/fssa

Megan Ornellas, Chief of Staff
Susie Howard, Deputy Chief of Staff

6242 **VSA Indiana**
Harrison Center for the Arts
1505 N Delaware St
Indianapolis, IN 46202-4466 317-974-4123
FAX: 317-974-4124
e-mail: info@vsai.org
www.vsai.org

Gayle Holtman, President
Linda Wisler, Vice President
Ron Lenz, Chairman of the Board
Bruce Westpahl, Vice Chairman

For over 25 years VSA arts of Indiana has led the movement to make the arts accessable to people with disabilitites. VSA arts of Indiana offers a variety of opportunities for people with disabilities of all ages to engage the power of the arts as a means of education, creative self-expression, and personal and professional growth. As a result, VSA promotes change in public perceptions and raises public awareness, and advocates for increased accessability in providing art experiences for all.

Iowa

6243 **Younker Rehabilitation Center of Iowa Methodist Medical Center**
1776 W Lakes Pkwy
Des Moines, IA 50266 515-241-6161
888-584-6311
FAX: 515-241-5137
www.ihs.org

Bill Leaver, President
Kevin Vermeer, EVP
Danny Drake, VP
Kara Dunham, VP Finance

Iowa Health System is the state's first and largest integrated healthcare system. We are physicians, hospitals, civic leaders and local volunteers committed to providing the highest possible quality and the lowest possible cost. We serve over 70 communities in Iowa, Western Illinois, and Eastern Nebraska.

Kansas

6244 **Kansas Rehabilitation Hospital**
1504 SW 8th Ave
Topeka, KS 66606-2714 785-235-6600
FAX: 785-232-8545
www.kansasrehabhospital.com

Mark LeNeave, CEO
Mindy Mitchell, Chief Nursing Officer

A free standing physical rehabilitation hospital located in Topeka Kansas. Designated to provide a barrier-free access to all treatment and patient service areas. This 79-bed facility offers a total rehabilitation environment in a warm, caring setting that encourages patient, family and staff interaction.

6245 **Mid-America Rehabilitation Hospital HealthSouth**
Health South Corporation
5701 W 110th St
Overland Park, KS 66211-2503 913-491-2400
FAX: 913-491-1097
e-mail: tiffany.kiehl@healthsouth.com
www.midamericarehabhospital.com

Kristen De Hart, CEO
Tiffany Kiehl, Director Marketing/Operations
Paul Matlack, Director Therapy Operations
Damon Parker, Chief Nursing Officer

97 bed Acute Rehab hospital offering full continuum from in-patient, day treatment and outpatient services for individuals with physical limitations due to CVA, TBI, SCI, other traumas, joint replacement, etc.

Kentucky

6246 **Cardinal Hill Rehabilitation Hospital**
2050 Versailles Rd
Lexington, KY 40504-1499 859-254-5701
800-233-3260
FAX: 859-231-1365
e-mail: webmaster@cardinalhill.org
www.cardinalhill.org

Kerry Gillihan, CEO
William J. Lester, Medical Director
Russell Travis, Assistant Medical Director

CARF-accredited rehab center provides comprehensive inpatient and outpatient services in two locations to people with physical and cognitive disabilities. We provide diagnosis-specific programs to 100 inpatients, outpatient clinics, outpatient therapies, pain management and therapeutic pool services. The Pediatric Center serves children from birth to age 18 years of age.

6247 **HealthSouth Rehabilitation of Louisville**
1227 Goss Ave
Louisville, KY 40217-1287 270-769-3100
FAX: 502-636-0351
www.healthsouth.com

Tim Nichol, Manager
Regina Durbin, Administrator

HealthSouth Rehabilitation Hospitals lead the way, consistently outperforming peers with a unique, intensive approach to rehabilitative care, partnering with every patient to find a treatment plan that works for them. We offer a wide range of comprehensive rehabilitation programsfor a wide variety of diagnoses. At HealthSouth, we provide access to independent private practice physicians, specializing in physical medicine and rehabilitation, who work in conjunction with HealthSouth's highly qual

6248 **Lakeview Rehabilitation Hospital**
134 Heartland Dr
Elizabethtown, KY 42701-2778 270-769-3100
FAX: 270-769-6870
www.healthsouthlakeview.com

Lori Jarboes, CEO
Chris Koford, Medical Director

HealthSouth Rehabilitation Hospitals lead the way, consistently outperforming peers with a unique, intensive approach to rehabilitative care, partnering with every patient to find a treatment plan that works for them. We offer a wide range of comprehensive rehabilitation programsfor a wide variety of diagnoses. At HealthSouth, we provide access to independent private practice physicians, specializing in physical medicine and rehabilitation, who work in conjunction with HealthSouth's highly qual

6249 **Shriners Hospitals for Children, Lexington**
1900 Richmond Rd
Lexington, KY 40502-1204 859-266-2101
800-444-8314
FAX: 859-268-5636
e-mail: Dwallenius@shrinenet.org
www.shrinershq.org/hospitals/lexington

Warren E. Hopkins, Chairman
Kirk E. Carter, Vice Chairman
Ken R. Dougherty, Treasurer
David E. Hager, Secretary

Shriners Hospitals for Childrenr - Lexington, is a 50-bed pediatric orthopaedic hospital. Our family-centered approach to care is designed to support the whole family during the acute and reconstructive phases of a child's injury. Located in Lexington, Ky., our hospital treats children from all over the country and around the world, and has unique relationships with some of the top hospitals and universities in the world.

Louisiana

6250 **HealthSouth Specialty Hospital Of North Louisiana**
1401 Ezelle St
Ruston, LA 71270-7218 318-251-3126
800-548-9157
FAX: 318-251-1594
e-mail: mark.rice@lifecare-hospitals.com
www.healthsouth.com

Mark Rice, CEO

A 90-bed specialty hospital offering both inpatient and outpatient services. Acute long term care.

6251 **Our Lady of Lourdes Rehabilitation Center**
4801 Ambassador Caffery Pkwy
Lafayette, LA 70508 337-470-2000
FAX: 318-289-2681
e-mail: info@lourdesrmc.com
www.lourdesrmc.com

William Barrow, CEO
Gerald R. Boudreaux, Chairman of the Board
D. Wayne Elmore, Secretary

Our Lady of Lourdes outpatient physical medicine and rehabilitation department is compprised of a multi-disciplinary team of physical therapists, oppcuptational therapists and speech languare pathologists.

6252 **Rehabilitation Center of Lake Charles Memorial Hospital**
1701 Oak Park Boulevard
Lake Charles, LA 70601-8911 337-494-3000
FAX: 337-494-2656
e-mail: webmaster@lcmh.com
www.lcmh.com

Dale Shearer, Director
Larry Graham, President/CEO
Ben F. Thompson, MD, Medical Staff President
Ronald Lewis, Jr., Medical Staff President - Elect

Rehabilitation center offering intensive physical, occupational, speech, neuropsychology, recreational therapies along with rehabilitation nursing.

6253 **Shriners Hospital for Children-Shreveport**
3100 Samford Ave
Shreveport, LA 71103-4239 318-222-5704
FAX: 318-424-7610
e-mail: jburda@shrinenet.org
www.shrinershospitalsforchildren.org

Richard McCall, Chief of Staff
Phillip Gates, Assistant Chief

An interdisciplinary approach is used in patient care programs to ensure comprehensive care for each patient. The staff includes orthopaedists, pediatricians, nurses, therapists, social workers, child life specialists, and more. The Shreveport Hospital is equipped and staffed to provide care for virtually all pediatric orthopaedic problems, with the exception of acute trauma.

6254 **South Louisiana Rehabilitation Hospital**
715 W Worthy Rd
Gonzales, LA 70737-3844 225-647-8277
FAX: 225-647-2446
e-mail: sober@powerhouseprograms.com
www.powerhouseprograms.com

Cody Gautreux, Executive Director
Tonja Randolph, President

Power House Programs is a male only facility for the treatment of Chemical Dependency/Dual Diagnosis, located in Gonzales, Louisiana. Applicants must have participated in a primary treatment program for substance abuse prior to acceptance. Our program is divided into 3 phases and is staffed by Board Certified Social Workers and Board Certified Substance Abuse Counselors. We provide individual, group and family therapy; plus 12 step meetings in a community setting.

6255 **St. Frances Cabrini Hospital: Rehab Unit**
St Frances Cabrini Hospital
3330 Masonic Dr
Alexandria, LA 71301-3899 318-487-1122
FAX: 318-448-6822
www.christusstfrancescabrini.org

Curman Gaines, Chairperson
Dallas Hixson, Vice Chairperson
CHRISTUS St. Frances Cabrini Hospital is a 265-bed facility located in Alexandria, Louisiana. Employing approximately 1,400 Associates and with a staff of neary 320 physicians, CHRISTUS St. Frances Cabrini Hospital offers a comprehensive array of services providing the highest quality patient care in a compassionate setting.

6256 **St. Patrick Hospital: Rehab Unit**
524 Doctor Michael Debakey Dr
Lake Charles, LA 70601-5725 337-491-7577
888-722-9355
FAX: 337-430-4284
www.christusstpatrick.org

Ellen Jones, CEO
Committed to providing care and service of the highest quality for children and adults, and to ensuring that the basic human rights of expression, decision making and personal dignity are preseved. We are also committed to treating our patients with respect, understanding and Christian love. We realize that this committment involves much more then attending to your medical needs.

6257 **Thibodaux Regional Medical Center**
602 N Acadia Rd
PO Box 1118
Thibodaux, LA 70301-4847 985-447-5500
800-822-8442
FAX: 985-449-4600
e-mail: info@thibodaux.com
www.thibodaux.com

Greg Stock, CEO
Jacob Giardina, Chairman
Andrew Hoffman, Chief of Staff
Mission is to provide the highest quality, most cost effective health care services possible to the people of Thibodaux and surrounding areas. The vision is to be the regional medical center of choice for health care services in the southeast Louisiana by recognizing the value of physicians and employees, committing to quality improvement, partnering with other health care providers, and remaining financially viable in a competitive environment.

Maine

6258 **Brewer Rehab and Living Center**
74 Parkway S
Brewer, ME 04412-1628 207-989-7300
800-359-7412
FAX: 207-989-4240
www.brewerrehab.com

Janet Hope, Executive Director
Brewer Rehab and Living Center accomodates 106 residents. We are located in Brewer, Maine. We have a 24-hour nursing staff and experienced dedicated on-site physical therapists, occupational therapists and speech language pathologists. We have a specialized inpatient program for individuals with brain injury resulting from a traumatic injury or neurological event such as a stroke. We also have a specialized care unit for individuals with Alzheimer's disease and other dementias.

6259 **New England Rehabilitation Hospital of Portland**
335 Brighton Ave
Portland, ME 04102-2363 207-662-8000
FAX: 207-879-8168
e-mail: jaye.sewall@healthsouth.com
www.nerhp.org

Elissa Charbonneau, Medical Director
Amy Morse, CEO
Mission is to provide individuals with guidance, education, support, and motivation while helping them achieve maximum independence and function. Our professionals work with the patient and family through a team approach, to establish and implement an individualized rehabilitation plan designed to meet specific patient goals.

Maryland

6260 **Mt. Washington Pediatric Hospital**
1708 W Rogers Ave
Baltimore, MD 21209-4596 410-578-8600
FAX: 410-466-1715
www.mwph.org

Sheldon Stein, President
Richard Katz, VP, Medical Affairs
Provides inpatient, outpatient and day programs for infants and children with rehabilitation and/or complex medical needs. We are dedicated to maximizing the rehabilitation and development of our patients through the delivery of interdisciplinary services and programs and providing every resource availiable to enable our patients to attain the highest quality of life within their families and their communities.

Massachusetts

6261 **New Bedford Rehabilitation Hospital**
4499 Acushnet Ave
New Bedford, MA 02745-4707 508-995-6900
FAX: 508-998-8131
www.newbedfordrehab.com

6262 **New England Rehabilitation Hospital: Massachusetts**
2 Rehabilitation Way
Woburn, MA 01801-6098 781-939-5050
FAX: 781-933-9257
www.newenglandrehab.com

Deniz Ozel, Medical Director
A 168-bed comprehensive inpatient rehabilitation hospital, which includes 2 off-campus satellite units. Offers an array of area outpatient rehabilitation centers. New England Rehabilitation Hospital remains committed to a personal caring approach. The vision is to provide the communities with a complete continuum of acute rehabilitative programs and services.

6263 **Shriners Burns Hospital: Boston**
51 Blossom St
Boston, MA 02114-2623 617-722-3000
800-255-1916
FAX: 617-523-1684
e-mail: sberkowitz@shrinenet.org
www.shrinershospitalsforchildren.org/Hospital

Thomas D'Esmond, Administrator
Matthias Donelan, Chief of Staff
Provides treatment for children to their 18th birthday with acute, fresh burns, plastic reconstructive surgery for patients with healed burns, severe scarring and facial deformity. Some non-burn conditions such as Scalded Skin Syndrome, Cleft Lip, Cleft Palate and purpura fulminians are also treated. Call the Hospital for information. All medical treatment is without cost to the patient, parents, or any third party.

6264 **Shriners Hospital Springfield Unit Springfield Unit for Crippled Children**
516 Carew St
Springfield, MA 01104-2330 413-787-2000
800-237-5055
FAX: 413-787-2009
www.shrinershospitalsforchildren.org

Kenneth Guidera, Chief Medical Officer
Eugene D'Amore, Vice President
Kathy A. Dean, Vice President Human Resources
Sharon Russell, VP Finance & Accounting

Shriners Hospital for Children is fully equipped and staffed to provide care for pediatric orthopaedic conditions and disorders.

Michigan

6265 Covenant Healthcare Rehabilitation Program
1447 N Harrison
Saginaw, MI 48602-4316
989-583-2930
FAX: 989-583-0000
www.covenanthealthcare.com

Spence Maidlow, President
Juli Martin, Program Director

Offers a broad spectrum of programs and services ranging from obstetrics, neonatal and pediatric care, to acute care including cardiology, oncology, surgery and many other services on the leading edge of medicine. All our programs and services exemplify our commitment to providing quality, compassionate care. As a medical facility with more then 700 beds, and a complete range of medical services, Covenant stands ready to meet the healthcare needs of the 15 counties in Michigan we serve.

6266 Farmington Health Care Center
34225 Grand River Ave
Farmington, MI 48335-3440
248-477-7373
FAX: 248-477-2888
www.farmingtonhealthcarecenter.com

Brian Garavaglia, Administrator

Skilled nursing facility specializing in ventilator dependent residents.

6267 Flint Osteopathic Hospital: RehabCare Unit
3921 Beecher Rd
Flint, MI 48532-3602
810-606-5000
FAX: 810-762-2153
TTY:888-633-2368
www.genesys.org

Susan Malone, Program Manager
Joy Finkenbiner, Executive Director

Genesys Health System takes great pride in the fact that we strive to deliver the highest quality health care, in a model healing environment, for the entire continuum of care needed throughout one's life. From birth to the twilight years, and everywhere in between, Genesys is there to get you back to the things you love to do.

6268 Integrated Health Services of Michigan at Clarkston
4800 Clintonville Rd
Clarkston, MI 48346-4297
248-674-0903
FAX: 248-674-3359
e-mail: donna.cook@fundltc.com
www.clarkstonspecialtyhealthcare.com

Carol Doll, Admissions Director
Margaret Canny, Administrator

At Clarkston Specialty Healthcare Center, our mission is to deliver personalized care to the members of our community at a time when our support is most needed. We strive to maximize and enhance the quality of life in a compassionate and professional environment.

6269 St. John Hospital: North Shore
Ascension Health
26755 Ballard St
Harrison Township, MI 48045-2419
586-465-5501
866-501-3627
FAX: 586-466-5352
e-mail: webcenter@stjohn.org
www.stjohnprovidence.org

David Sessions, CEO

A 96-bed specialty hospital that provides comprehensive physical medicine and rehabilitation, along with a wide range of medical and surgical services. St. John North Shores Hospital also provides emergency and urgent care, extensive outpatient rehabilitation services, and most ancillary diagnostic services.

Minnesota

6270 Alinna Health
800 E 28th St
Minneapolis, MN 55407-3798
612-863-4200
866-880-3550
FAX: 612-863-5698
e-mail: sisterkenny@allina.com
www.allinahealth.org/ahs/ski.nsf/

Helen Kettner, Nurse-Liaison

Courage Kenny Rehabilitation Institute provides a continuum of rehabilitation services for people with short- and long-term conditions and disabilities in communities throughout Minnesota and western Wisconsin. Our goal is to improve health outcomes, make it easier for clients and families to get the right services for their needs, and reduce costs by preventing complications.

Missouri

6271 Columbia Regional Hospital: RehabCare Unit
404 N Keene St
Columbia, MO 65201-6698
573-882-2501
FAX: 573-449-7588
www.muhealth.org

James Ross, CEO
Anita Larsen, COO

A medical and physical rehabilitation program serving patients throughout Mid-Missouri with functional deficits due to neurologic, orthopaedic or other medical conditions.

6272 Jewish Hospital of St. Louis: Department of Rehabilitation
1 Barnes Jewish Hospital Plz
Saint Louis, MO 63110-1003
314-747-3000
855-925-0631
FAX: 314-454-5277
www.barnesjewish.org

Richard Liedweg, President
Mark Krieger, VP/CFO
John Lynch, Chief Medical Officer
Craig D. Schnuck, Chairman

We take exceptional care of people by providing world-class healthcare, delivering care in a compassionate, respectful and responsive way. By advancing medical knowledge and continously improving our practices. By educating current and future generations of healthcare professionals.

6273 St. Mary's Regional Rehabilitation Center
201 NW R D Mize Rd
Blue Springs, MO 64014-2513
816-228-5900
FAX: 816-655-5348
www.stmarkyskc.com

Fleury Yelvington, President/CEO
Amy McKay, Executive Director of Nursing

A 143-bed inpatient physical rehabilitation unit offering PT, OT, ST, recreational therapy, psychiatry and all other ancillary services of a full-service hospital. Specialize in orthopedic and neurologic disabilities.

6274 Three Rivers Health Care
2620 N Westwood Blvd
Poplar Bluff, MO 63901-3396
573-785-7721
800-582-9533
FAX: 573-686-5388
e-mail: info@pbrmc.hma-corp.com
www.poplarbluffregional.com

Charles Stewart, Market CEO
Gerald Faircloth, Administrator
Melissa Samuelson, Chief Nursing Officer
Kevin Fowler, CFO

Poplar Bluff Regional Medical Center is a regional medical center with 2 hospital campuses and more then 100 active physicians. The 423-bed facility is the largest medical center in Southeast Missouri and is located in ButlerCounty. With outreach clinics in Bloomfield, Dexter, Malden, Piedmont, and Puxico, Poplar Bluff

Regional Medical Center is committed to serving its 6 county region.

Montana

6275 **St. Vincent Hospital and Health Center**
1233 N 30th St
Billings, MT 59101-165 406-657-7000
FAX: 406-657-8817
www.svhhc.org

Jason Barker, CEO
Steve Loveless, COO
Joan Thullberry, Chief Nursing Officer
Ron Oldfield, VP Finance
Vision is to be recognized for our vitality, best in class performance and providing easy access to compassionate and trust-worthy healthcare. The healthcare we offer is based on community need. We strive to improve the health status of the community, with a special concern for the poor and those who have limited access to healthcare.

Nebraska

6276 **Madonna Rehabilitation Hospital**
5401 South St
Lincoln, NE 68506-2150 402-489-7102
800-676-5448
FAX: 402-483-9406
e-mail: info@madonna.org
www.madonna.org

Marsha Lommel, CEO
Provides a complete range of inpatient and outpatient rehabilitation for patients of all ages and abilities. Through highly specialized programs and services, Madona offers individualized treatment and support to help every patient.

Nevada

6277 **University Medical Center**
1800 W Charleston Blvd
Las Vegas, NV 89102-2386 702-383-2000
FAX: 702-383-2536
e-mail: feedback@umcsn.com
www.umcsn.com

Brian Brannman, CEO
Lawrence Barnard, Chief Operating Officer
Joan Brookhyser, Chief Medical Officer
Stephanie Merril, Chief Financial Officer
University Medical Center is dedicated to providing the highest level of health care possible by maintaining its ongoing commitment to personal, individualized care for each patient.Through the latest treatment techniques, comfortable surroundings and a dedicated staff, that commitment is expressed every day, in every area of the hospital.

New Hampshire

6278 **Head Injury Treatment Program at Dover**
307 Plaza Dr
Dover, NH 03820-2455 603-742-2676
FAX: 603-749-5375
www.doverrehab.com

Sue Mills, Program Rep
Jill Bosa, Administrator
A provider of postacute services in the greater New Hampshire Seacost area. We accomodate 112 residents and are licensed by the state of New Hampshire. We employ nearly 150 licensed nurses, therapists, and other healthcare professionals, who strive to provide quality care. The goal of our patient service model is to bridge the gap between hospitalization and home so that recovery and physical functioning are maximized and hospital re-admission is minimized.

6279 **Lakeview NeuroRehabilitation Center**
244 Highwatch Road
Effingham, NH 03882 603-539-7451
800-473-4221
FAX: 603-539-8815
www.lakeviewsystem.com

Anton Merka, Chairman
Carolyn McDermott, President
Christopher Slover,, Chief Executive Officer
Tina M. Trudel, PhD,, Chief Operating Officer
Residential treatment center serving individuals with neurologic/behavioral disorders. Lakeview serves both children and adults in functionally based program environment. Transistional programs in various group homes also available to clients as they progress in their treatment.

6280 **Northeast Rehabilitation Hospital**
70 Butler St
Salem, NH 03079-3974 603-893-2900
800-825-7292
FAX: 603-893-1638
TTY: 800-439-2370
e-mail: webmaster@northeastrehab.com
www.northeastrehab.com

John Prochilo, CEO
NRHN is an organization characterized by the positive and proactive commitment to the delivery of customer centered care. Our employees exemplify our organizational commitment to providing quality rehabilitation services throughout the continuum. NRHN will be prudent with all resources and will take individual and collective responsibility for fiscal health. NRHN will remain a model by which other rehabilitation and post acute networks seek to emulate.

6281 **St. Joseph Hospital Rehabilitation**
172 Kinsley St
Nashua, NH 03060-3688 603-595-3076
800-210-9000
FAX: 603-595-3635
www.stjosephhospital.com

Judy Grilli, Medical Staff Officer
A comprehensive healthcare system that serves the Greater Nashua area, western New Hampshire and Northern Massachusetts. Our hospital is licensed for 208 beds and includes a Level 2 Trauma Center. In addition to the hospital, St. Joseph Healthcare system also includes a satellite emergency center in Milford, 5 family medical centers, a large network of primary care and specialty physician practices.

New Jersey

6282 **Betty Bacharach Rehabilitation Hospital**
61 W Jimmie Leeds Rd
Pomona, NJ 08240-9102 609-652-7000
FAX: 609-652-7487
e-mail: chrism@bacharach.org
www.bacharach.org

Philip J. Perskie, Esq., Chairman
Roy Goldberg, Vice Chairman
Craig Anmuth, Medical Director
Ross Berlin, Medical Director
Therapists, nurses and other specialists, led by physiatrists - doctors specially trained in the medical practice of physical medicine and rehabilitation.

6283 **Children's Specialized Hospital**
150 New Providence Rd
Mountainside, NJ 07092-2590
908-259-3330
888-344-5373
FAX: 908-233-4176
e-mail: jbrooks@childrens-specialized.org
www.childrens-specialized.org

Robin A. Walton, Chairwoman
Margaret M. Pego, First Vice Chairwoman
Steven M. Rosenberg, Esq, Second Vice Chairman
Victoria Wicks, Treasurer

New Jersey's largest comprehensive pediatric rehabilitation hospital, treats children and adolescents from birth through 21 years of age. Programs include spinal dysfunction, brain injury, respiratory, burn, Day Hospital, early intervention, preschool, and cognitive rehabilitation. Locations in Fairwood, Roselle Park, Newark, Toms River and Hamilton

6284 **HealthSouth Rehabilitation Hospital**
14 Hospital Dr
Toms River, NJ 08755-6402
732-244-3100
FAX: 732-244-7790
www.rehabnj.com/tomsriver/

Patty Ostaszewski, CEO
Joseph Stillo, Medical Director

A comprehensive 131-bed medical rehabilitation hospital dedicated to treating individuals with a variety of physical disabilities resulting from injury and illness. We serve all of New Jersey, Manhattan, and Philiadelphia. Accredited by the Joint Commission on Accredidation of Healthcare Organizations (JCAHO). The mission of the hospital is to get people back to work, to play, to living.

6285 **JFK Johnson Rehab Institute**
65 James St
Edison, NJ 08820-3947
732-321-7070
FAX: 732-321-0994
e-mail: jfkjri@solarishs.org
www.njrehab.org

Krishna Urs, Physician
David Brown, Physician

JRI has developed programs in such specialties as stroke rehabilitation, orthopedic programs, fitness, cardiac rehabilitation, women's health, pediatrics and brain injury rehabilitation. We also offer the most sophisticated diagnostic services available.

6286 **Kessler Institute for Rehabilitation, Welkind Facility**
201 Pleasant Hill Rd
Chester, NJ 07930-2141
973-252-6300
FAX: 973-252-6343
e-mail: jkment@kessler-rehab.com
kessler-rehab.com

Sue Kida, CEO
Sam Bayoumy, Director of Rehabilitation
Bruce Pomeranz, MD, Medical Director
Norma Glennon, Associate Director of Outpatient Rehabilitation

Set in the rolling hills of Morris County, this 72 bed facility provides specialized services to brain injury patients, including our unique Cognitive Redmediation Program, as well as a full range of stroke, amputee and orthopedic services. Kessler's team of dedicated rehabilitation professionals, including physicians, nurses and therapists, work with each patient to build physical strength, optimize movement, maximize independence, increase cognitive skills and address any other issues.

6287 **Mediplex Rehab: Camden**
1 Cooper Plz
Camden, NJ 08103-1461
856-342-2300
FAX: 856-342-7979
www.cooperhealth.org/content/locationsCamden

John P. Sheridan, Jr. President/CEO
Adrienne Kirby, Phd, President/CEO
Raymond L. Baraldi, Interim Chief Medical Officer
Celeste Johnson, Administrator

Cooper University Hospital is the leading provider of comprehensive health services, medical education and clinical research in Southern New Jersey and the Delaware Valley. With over 550 physicians in over 75 specialties, Cooper is uniquely equipped to provide an almost unlimited number of medical services. The hospital is committed to excellence in medical education, patient care, and research. Offers training programs to medical students, residents, and nurses in a variety of specialties.

New Mexico

6288 **HealthSouth Rehabilitation Center: New Mexico**
7000 Jefferson St NE
Albuquerque, NM 87109-4357
505-344-9478
800-293-7226
FAX: 505-345-6722
www.healthsouthnewmexico.com

Sylvia Kelly, CEO
Rocky BigCrane, Director of Plant Operations
Lisa Brower, Director of Therapy Operations
Angela Eaton-Walker, M.D, Medical Director

Our hospital offers highly specialized inpatient rehabilitation services. From hip fractures to joint replacements and stroke to Parkinson's disease - our hospital has the experts, technology and experience to meet your rehabilitation needs.

6289 **St. Joseph Rehabilitation Hospital and Outpatient Center**
Ardence
505 Elm St NE
Albuquerque, NM 87102-2500
505-727-4700
FAX: 505-727-4793
www.sjhs.org

Janelle Raborn, Administrator/CEO
Sherrie Peterson, Director

A member of the four hospital, St. Joseph healthcare system, this facility provides inpatient and outpatient care for those requiring physical medicine and rehabilitation. Specialty programs include brain injury, stroke, spinal cord, orthopedics, occupational and physical therapies, clinical psychology, speech/language pathology, hand clinic and functional capacity evaluations. The only facility in New Mexico accredited in four areas by the commission on accreditation of rehab facilities.

New York

6290 **Burke Rehabilitation Hospital**
785 Mamaroneck Ave
White Plains, NY 10605-2523
914-597-2500
888-99 -URKE
FAX: 914-946-0866
e-mail: web@burke.org
www.burke.org

John Ryan, Executive Director
Mary Beth Walsh, M.D., Executive Medical Director/CEO
Brett Langley, Physician

We provide inpatient and outpatient care for a broad range of neurological, musculoskeletal, cardiac, and pulmonary disabilities caused by disease or injury. Burke treats patients who have suffered a stroke, spinal cord injury, brain injury, amputation, joint replacement, complicated fracture, arthritis, cardiac and pulmonary disease, and neurological disorders. Patients are most frequently transferred to Burke from acute care hospitals once their condition is stable and they are able to partici

6291 **Occupational Therapy Strategies and Adaptations for Independent Daily Living**
Haworth Press
10 Alice St
Binghamton, NY 13904-1503
607-722-5857
800-429-6784
FAX: 607-722-6362
e-mail: orders@haworthpress.com
www.tandf.co.uk

186 pages Softcover
ISBN 0-866563-50-4

6292 Rusk Institute of Rehabilitation Medicine
301 East 17th Street
Second Avenue (in the Hospital for
New York, NY 10016-4901 212-263-6034
FAX: 212-263-8510
e-mail: DevelopmentOffice@nyumc.org
www.med.nyu.edu/rusk

Steven Flanagan, Chairman

Operates under the auspices of the Dept. Of Rehabilitation Medicine of New York University School of Medicine, one of the nations foremost medical schools. The relationship between Rusk and other clinical and research units within the medical center contributes to an environment which provides the optimal rehabilitation setting for patients. Rusk provides patients with access to treatment across a continuum of care depending on their individual medical needs.

6293 Silvercrest Center for Nursing & Rehabilitation
144-45 87th Ave
Briarwood, NY 11435-3109 718-480-4000
800-645-9806
FAX: 718-658-2367
e-mail: admissions@silvercrest.org
www.silvercrest.org

Andrea Gibbon, Clinical Care Coordinator
Penny Blakely, Unit Manager

The Silvercrest Center for Nursing and Rehabilitation has earned a wide-spread reputatiopn for combing the best in clinical care with the best in nursing care and for making available to its communities the broadest menu of services to ease a patients' path to recovery from hospital to home. The Center is for the treatment of medically complex patients beginning their recovery, for the rehabilitation of patients who need restorative therapy before going home and much more.

6294 Vocational Rehabilitation and Employment
Books on Special Children
PO Box 305
Congers, NY 10920-305 845-638-1236
FAX: 845-638-0847
www.vba.va.gov/bln/vre/

372 pages Hardcover

North Carolina

6295 Horizon Rehabilitation Center
Trans Health Incorporated
3100 Erwin Rd
Durham, NC 27705-4505 919-383-1546
800-541-7750
FAX: 919-383-0862

6296 Integrated Health Services of Durham
Duke University Medical Center
3100 Erwin Rd
Durham, NC 27705-4505 919-383-1546
FAX: 919-383-0862

Aaron Lony, Administrator

6297 Learning Services Corporation
Corporate Office
10 Speen St
Ste 4
Framingham, MA 01701-4661 508-626-3671
888-419-9955
FAX: 866-491-7396
www.learningservices.com

Susan Snow, Director of Admissions
Deb. Braunling-McMorrow, Ph, President and CEO

A licensed postacute rehabilitation program for adults who have an acquired brain injury. Individuals who are enrolled in the program participate in active, intensive rehabilitation carried out by a team of neuropsychology, speech/language therapy, physical therapy, occupational therapy, vocational services, family services and life skills training. Services include residential rehabilitation, home based treatment, day treatment, subacute rehabilitation and supported living.

Ohio

6298 Columbus Rehab & Subacute
44 S Souder Ave
Columbus, OH 43222-1539 614-228-5900
FAX: 614-228-3989
e-mail: columbusrehab@extendicare.com
www.columbusrehabskillednursing.com

Kelly Fligor, Administrator

Columbus Rehabilitation and Subacute Institute is a leading provider of long-term skilled nursing care and short-term rehabilitation solutions. Our 120 bed facility offers a full continuum of services and care focused around each individual in today's ever-changing healthcare environment.

6299 Great Lakes Regional Rehabilitation Center
3700 Kolbe Rd
Lorain, OH 44053-1611 440-960-3470
FAX: 440-960-4636

Julie Jones, Manager

Provides excellent, innovative and comprehensive rehabilitation programs to people in our community. Committed to a better quality of life for all individuals, the Rehabilitation Center has grown to become a regional resource for individuals needing all types of rehabilitation services.

6300 HCR Health Care Services
1 Seagate
Toledo, OH 43604-1541 419-321-5470
800-736-4427
FAX: 419-252-5543
www.harborfund.net

6301 Heather Hill Rehabilitation Hospital
Heather Hill
12340 Bass Lake Rd
Chardon, OH 44024-8327 440-285-4040
800-423-2972
FAX: 440-285-0946
e-mail: info@heatherhill.org

Ed Davis, Operations
Donald Goddard, Chief Medical Officer

Individualized treatment programs for adults and adolescents can participate in and benefit from three-plus hours a day of active therapy.

6302 Parma Community General Hospital Acute Rehabilitation Center
7007 Powers Blvd
Parma, OH 44129-5437 440-743-3000
FAX: 440-843-4387
www.parmahospital.org

David Nedrich, Chairman
Thomas P. O'Donnell, First Vice Chairman
Nancy E. Hatgas, Second Assistant Treasurer
Alex I. Koler, First Assistant Treasurer

Parma Hospital offers acute and subacute inpatient care including specialty centers for heart, cancer, robotic surgery, orthopedics, pain management, acute rehabilitation and bariatric care.

6303 Rehabilitation Institute of Ohio at Miami Valley Hospital
1 Wyoming St
Dayton, OH 45409-2793 937-208-8000
TTY:937-208-2006
www.miamivalleyhospital.com

Vanessa Sandarusi, Executive Director
Anita Marie Greer, Program Manager, Acute Therapy Services
Jessica Hallum, Nurse Manager of the Inpatient Rehabilitation Unit
Phillip Boarman, Clinical Coordinator for Acute Care Occupational Therapy and

The Miami Valley Hospital Rehabilitation Institute of Ohio (RIO) is one of the largest and most comprehensive rehabilitation services providers in the United States. RIO offers a full spectrum of specialized rehabilitation programs delivered by the region's most experienced rehabilitation experts.

6304 Shriners Burn Institute: Cincinnati Unit
Shriners Hospitals for Children Cincinnati
3229 Burnet Ave
Cincinnati, OH 45229-3095
513-872-6000
800-875-8580
FAX: 513-872-6999
e-mail: vmosley@shrinenet.org
www.shrinershospitalsforchildren.org

Richard Kagan, Chief of Staff
Petra Warner, Assistant Chief of Staff
Tony Lewgood, Interim Administrator
Vanessa Mosley, Development Officer

All the attention and resources are focused on just one kind of patient-the burn-injured child. Shriners combine excellent clinical skill, compassionate care, and innovative research, providing comprehensive pediatric burn care and reconstructive rehabilitation to achieve the best possible outcome for a child that has suffered a burn injury. There is never a charge to the patient or family for any of the medical care or services provided by the Shriners Hospitals throughout North America.

6305 St. Francis Health Care Centre
401 N Broadway St
Green Springs, OH 44836-9653
419-639-2626
800-248-2552
FAX: 419-639-6225
e-mail: hr@sfhcc.org
www.sfhcc.org

Kim Eicher, CEO
Jane Holmer, Admissions Coordinator

Provides compassionate care for the elderly and physically challenged. We are a healthcare ministry under the sponsorship of the Franciscan Sisters of Our Lady of Perpetual Help. As a Catholic facility, we respectfully offer those we serve, care hope and dignity in a joyful and compassionate manner.

6306 St. Rita's Medical Center Rehabilitation Services
730 W Market St
Lima, OH 45801-4602
419-227-3361
800-232-7762
FAX: 419-226-9750
www.ehealthconnection.com

James Reber, CEO

The St. Rita's Inpatient Acute Care Rehabilitation service provides individualized service to you or your family member 7 days a week, wherever you might stay in the hospital. Acute rehabilitation care includes physical, occupational, and speech therapy services. Our goal is to make you as independent as possible before your discarge to home or, when necessary to extended services in other parts of the hospital.

6307 University of Cincinnati Hospital
Health Alliance
234 Goodman St
Cincinnati, OH 45219-2316
513-584-1000
FAX: 513-584-7712
www.universityhospital.uchealth.com

James Kingsbury, President/CEO

University Hospital has an international reputation, bringing thousands of people, from the region and around the world to Cincinnati to receive care from world renowned physicians in state-of-the-art medical facilities.

6308 Upper Valley Medical/Rehab Services
3130 N County Road
25-A
Troy, OH 45373-1309
937-440-4000
FAX: 937-440-7337
e-mail: info@uvmc.com
www.uvmc.com

Rafay Atiq, Director Rehab Services

A not-for-profit health care system serving the health care needs of Miami County and the surrounding area. The health care system features a state-of-the-art acute care hospital which opened in 1998. Comprehensive inpatient and outpatient services are provided with a full compliment of diagnostic and treatment services and behavioral health care programs.

Oklahoma

6309 Hilcrest Medical Center: Kaiser Rehab Center
1125 S Trenton Ave
Tulsa, OK 74120-5498
918-579-7100
FAX: 918-579-7110
www.hillcrest.com/kaiser

Perri Craven, Medical Director

Kaiser Rehabilitation Center offers a wide range of services to help people regain functionality and independence after a debilitating injury or illness. Our approach to rehabilitation is a team approach, bringing the expertise of physicians, therapists, nurses and other health professionals together with patient family to achieve the best possible outcome. Each patient is given an individualized treatment plan that stimulates and challenges them to achieve their maximum potential.

6310 Jane Phillips Medical Center
Jane Phillips Medical Center
3500 E Frank Phillips Blvd
Bartlesville, OK 74006-2464
918-333-7200
FAX: 918-331-1360
e-mail: webmaster@jpmc.org
www.jpmc.org

David Stire, CEO
Mike Moore, CFO

Jane Phillips Health System is sponsored by St. John Health System. This partnership helps our patients by ensuing access to the most sophisticated levels of care availiable in this area. It offers a wide range of services, including general medicine, surgery, cardiopulmonary care, maternal and infant care, cancer treatment, geriatric care, orthopedics, and physical medicine.

6311 Jim Thorpe Rehabilitation Center at Southwest Medical Center
Southwest Medical Center
4100 S. Douglas Ave.
Oklahoma City, OK 73109
405-644-5445
800-677-1238
FAX: 405-644-5384
www.integris-health.com

Al Moorad, Medical Director

Provides inpatient rehabilitation for people with head injuries, spinal cord injuries, orthopedic conditions, pain management, neurological diseases, strokes and a variety of diagnoses that stop individuals from being able to take care of themselves independently. Services available include medical direction, physical therapy, social work, occupational therapy, speech therapy, recreational therapy, and aftercare follow-up.

6312 Mercy Memorial Health Center-Rehab Center
1011 14th Ave NW
Ardmore, OK 73401-1828
580-223-5400
800-572-1182
FAX: 580-220-6463
www.mercy.net

Jan Shores, Manager
Lynn Britton Britton, President/CEO
Randy Combs, Executive Vice President Strategic Growth
Michael McCurry, Executive Vice President/Chief Operating Officer

A full service tertiary hospital with 176 licensed beds, 913 co-workers and 100 physicians. Four primary care clinics

6313 St. Anthony Hospital: Rehabilitation Unit
St. Anthony Hospital
1000 N Lee Ave
Oklahoma City, OK 73102-1036
405-272-7000
800-851-0888
FAX: 405-272-7075
e-mail: st_anthony@ssmhc.com
www.saintsok.com

S Beaver, President

18 spacious private rooms, each with bathroom, and furnishings designed with patient safety in mind. Horticulture room where patients can work with plants and flowers as part of their rehabilitation. And a residential-style training apartment with fully equipped kitchen, bathroom, and bedroom to make the patient feel more at home.

6314 Valir Health
700 NW 7th St
Oklahoma City, OK 73102-1212
405-609-3600
888-898-2080
FAX: 405-605-8638
e-mail: info@valir.com
www.valir.com

Dirk O'Hara, Principal
Tonya Purvine, Corporate Compliance Officer

Inpatient Rehab Facility including all therapy services serving people who have been injured and had an illness resulting in a decreased level of independence.

Oregon

6315 Shriners Hospitals for Children: Portland
3101 SW Sam Jackson Park Rd
Portland, OR 97239-3095
503-241-5090
800-237-5055
FAX: 503-221-3701
e-mail: mthoreson@shrinenet.org
www.shrinershospitalsforchildren.org

Michael Aiona, Chief of Staff
Craig Patchin, Administrator
Mark Thoreson, Development Officer
Joslyn Davidson, M.D, Anesthesiology

Pediatric orthopedic and plastic surgery; inpatient and outpatient services. No charge for any services provided at the Hospital. Diagnosis, rehabilitation, surgery, sports and recreation for ages 0-18 for people with physical disabilities involving bones, muscles or joints or in need of plastic surgery for burn scars or cleft lip/palate.

Pennsylvania

6316 Allied Services John Heinz Institute of Rehabilitation Medicine
150 Mundy St
MAC III Building, 1st Floor
Wilkes Barre, PA 18702-6830
570-826-3900
FAX: 570-830-2027
e-mail: tpugh@allied-services.org
www.allied-services.org

Gerald Franceski, Chairman
Thomas Speicher, Vice-Chairman
William Conaboy, CEO
Gregory Basting, VP Medical Affairs

John Heinz Rehab is one of the foremost providers of rehabilitation in the country. Under the supervision of board-certified psychiatrists, a team of highly qualified professionals provides a broad range of specialized services and therapies for inpatients, with specialized programs in the areas of brain injury, injured worker recovery and pediatrics. John Heinz Rehab is the only CARF accredited program in northeastern Pennsylvania for treatment of brain injury rehabilitation.

6317 Allied Services Rehabilitation Hospital
475 Morgan Hwy
Scranton, PA 18508-2656
570-348-1359
FAX: 570-341-4548
www.allied-services.org

Gerald Franceski, Chairman
Thomas Speicher, Vice-Chairman
William Conaboy, CEO
Gregory Basting, VP Medical Affairs

We are committed to the people of our commuinity, to help them overcome challenges and reach their greatest potential by providing quality care, people-oriented services and comfort. Our approach is a hands-on, people-oriented style which places the physical and emotional needs of those in our care at the center of all we do. Whether in our rehabilitation hospitals, our skilled nursing facilities, or mental health/mental retardation program, we strive to help people reach their potential.

6318 Brighten Place
131 North Main St
Chalfont, PA 18914-245
215-997-7746
FAX: 215-997-2517
e-mail: brightenplace@enter.net
www.brightenplace.org

William Koffros, CEO

A residential brain injury program with the mission to encourage growth and foster independence on an individual level for each resident. We are CARF accredited and provide additional services which include a day program and respite care.

6319 Chestnut Hill Rehabilitation Hospital
8601 Stenton Ave
Wyndmoor, PA 19038-8312
215-233-6200
FAX: 215-233-6879
www.extendedcare.com

Cammi Lubking, Administrator

Chestnut Hill Rehab Hospital is dedicated to meeting patients' physical, emotional, social, and vocational goals. Through innovative programs, sophisticated equipment, and support by specially trained staff members committed to the progress of every patient, Chestnut Hill achieves results.

6320 Doylestown Hospital Rehabilitation Center
595 W State St
Doylestown, PA 18901-2597
215-345-2200
FAX: 215-345-2512
www.dh.org

James Brexler, President and Chief Executive Officer
Eleanor Wilson, RN, MSN, MHA, Vice President, Patient Services/Chief Operating Officer
Dan Upton, Vice President, Chief Financial Officer
Scott S. Levy, MD, Vice President, Chief Medical Officer

The mission of Doylestown Hospital is to provide a responsive healing environment for patients and their families, and to improve the quality of life for all members of our community. We combine the creative energies of Medical Staff, Board, Associates and Volunteers to make Doylestown Hospital a place where each patient and family feels healed and whole, even when disease cannot be cured.

6321 Health Care Solutions
500 Abbott Dr
Ste B
Broomall, PA 19008-4301
610-544-6023
800-451-1671
FAX: 610-544-6035
www.lincare.com

John Byrnes, CEO
Shawn Schabel, President/COO

Develops unique containment programs, offers equipment set-up, patient instruction, patient assessment and equipment usage. Offers clinical services that include oxygen systems, ventilators, aerosol therapy, suction equipment, T.E.N.S. programs, compression pumps, custom orthotics, enteral feeding.

6322 HealthSouth Harmarville Rehabilitation Hospital
P.O.Box 11460
320 Guys Run Road
Pittsburgh, PA 15238-460
412-828-1300
877-937-7342
FAX: 412-828-7705
www.healthsouthharmarville.com

Ken Anthony, Chief Executive Officer
Thomas Franz, M.D., Medical Director
Catherine M. Birk, M.D., Staff Physiatrist
Brian Cicuto, D.O., Staff Physiatrist

A 202-bed facility providing inpatient and outpatient physical medicine and rehabilitation to adults and adolescents in Pennsylvania, West Virginia, Ohio and Maryland.

6323 HealthSouth Nittany Valley Rehabilitation Hospital
Health South of Nittany Valley
550 W College Ave
Pleasant Gap, PA 16823-7401
814-359-3421
800-842-6026
FAX: 814-359-5898
www.nittanyvalleyrehab.com

Richard Allatt, Medical Director
Susan Hartman, CEO
Sara Godwin, CNO
Ann Foster, Therapy Operations Director

Comprehensive inpatient and outpatient facilities. Treatment for symptoms relating to: stroke, head injury, pulmonary disease, orthopedic conditions, neurological disorders, cardiac illnesses and spinal cord injuries. Healthsouth Nittany Valley Rehabilitation Hospital is a part of Healthsouth's national network of more than 2,000 facilities in 50 states.

6324 HealthSouth Rehab Hospital Of Erie
143 E 2nd St
Erie, PA 16507-1501
814-878-1200
800-234-4574
FAX: 814-878-1399
www.healthsoutherie.com

Douglas Grisier, Medical Director
Shelly Mayes, Director of Therapy Operations

An acute inpatient rehabilitation hospital that was founded in 1986. HealthSouth Erie is one of the only rehabilitation hospitals in the country to hold a triple-certification by the Joint Commission in the areas of Brain Injury, Stroke and Parkinson's disease Rehabilitation.

6325 HealthSouth Rehabilitation Hospital of Altoona
2005 Valley View Blvd
Altoona, PA 16602-4548
814-944-3535
800-873-4220
FAX: 814-944-6160
www.healthsouthaltoona.com

Scott Filler, Chief Executive Officer
Paul Sutton, Director Of Clinical Services
Rakesh (Rock Patel, D.O., Medical Director
Mary Gen Boyles, Director of Nursing Services

Inpatient and outpatient physical rehabilitation programs and services.

6326 Healthsouth Rehabilitation Hospital of Greater Pittsburgh
2380 McGinley Rd
Monroeville, PA 15146-4400
412-856-2400
FAX: 412-856-9320
www.lifecare-hospitals.com

Mary Lee Dadey, Administrator

Rehabilitation and long-term acute care hospital that treats brain injury, stroke, multiple sclerosis, Parkinson's disease, back and spinal cord injuries, cancer, pulmonary disease, cardiac disease, traumatic and work injuries.

6327 Healthsouth Rehabilitation Hospital of Mechanicsburg
175 Lancaster Blvd
Mechanicsburg, PA 17055-3562
717-691-3700
800-933-3831
FAX: 717-697-6524
e-mail: annette.bates@healthsouth.com
www.healthsouthpa.com

Mark Freeburn, CEO
Annette Bates, Director of Marketing Operations
Jeff Brandenburg, MPT, Director of Therapy Operations
Michael F. Lupinacci, M.D, Medical Director

HealthSouth provides comprehensive rehabilitation and recovery services to patients with stroke, brain injury, hip fracture, medically complex, pulmonary, wound, spinal cord injury, amputation, and other neuro-muscular, and orthopedic impairments. Our primary goal is to provide individualized treatment programs to people requiring physical rehabilitation and medical recovery in order to help patients get back to work, to play, to living.

6328 Healthsouth Rehabilitation Hospital of York
1850 Normandie Dr
York, PA 17408-1552
717-767-6941
FAX: 717-767-8776
www.healthsouthyork.com

Sally Arthur, Director of Human Resources
Bruce Sicilia, Medical Director
Elaine Charest, Director of Therapy Operations
Daniel C. DeFalcis, M.D., Associate Medical Director

A 120-bed rehabilitation hospital dedicated to providing advanced, comprehensive services to patients who have suffered head injury, spinal cord injury, stroke, burns, amputation, chronic pain and other neurological and musculoskeletal disorders. HRH of York provides outpatient services in seven locations. Healthsouth is located in York, Pennsylvania, approximately 50 miles north of Baltimore and 25 miles south of Harrisburg.

6329 Magee Rehabilitation Hospital
1513 Race St
Philadelphia, PA 19102-1177
215-587-3000
800-966-2433
FAX: 215-568-3736
e-mail: hskoczen@mageerehab.org
www.mageerehab.org

Jack Carroll, CEO

A not-for-profit health organization which is the home to the nation's first brain injury rehabilitation program to be accredited by the Commission on the Accreditation of Rehabilitation Facilities (CARF) and is one of 14 federally designated Regional Spinal Cord Injury Centers. Our staff and management are committed to restoring the highest level of independence possible to individuals with disabilities.

6330 Moss Rehabilitation Hospital
1200 W Tabor Rd
Philadelphia, PA 19141-3099
215-456-9800
FAX: 215-456-9381
www.mossrehab.com

Alberto Esquenazi, Plant Manager
Alberto Esquenazi, MD, Director
Carmen Angles, MD, Director
Cynthia Farrell, DO, Director

The Philadelphia region's major resource for medical rehabilitation since 1959. This 152 bed facility offers comprehensive care to people with broad ranges of conditions, diagnostic laboratories and a multidisciplinary team of rehabilitation professionals.

6331 Shriners Hospitals for Children, Philadelphia
Shrinners Hospitals for Children
3551 N Broad St
Philadelphia, PA 19140-4131
215-430-4000
800-281-4051
FAX: 215-430-4126
www.shrinershq.org

Alan W. Madsen, Chairman of the Board
John A. Cinotto, 1st Vice President
Dale W. Stauss, 2nd Vice President
Ernest Perilli, Administrator

At Shriners Hospitals for Childrenr - Philadelphia, we provide state-of-the-art medical care for children with spinal cord injuries, as well as a host of orthopaedic and neuromusculoskeletal disorders and diseases

6332 Shriners Hospitals for Children, Erie
1645 W 8th St
Erie, PA 16505-5007
814-875-8700
FAX: 814-875-8756
www.shrinershq.org

John Lubahn, Chief of Staff
Charles Walczak, Administrator

The Shriners Hospitals for Children, Erie, is a 30-bed pediatric orthopaedic hospital providing comprehensive orthopaedic care to children at no charge. The hospital is one of 22 Shriners Hospitals throughout North America. The Erie Hospital accepts and treats children with routine and complex orthopaedic and neuromuscular problems, utilizing the latest treatments and technology available in pediatric orthopaedics, resulting in early ambulation and reduced length of stay.

6333 Shriners Hospitals, Philadelphia Unit, for Crippled Children
3551 N Broad St
Philadelphia, PA 19140-4105 215-430-4000
FAX: 215-430-4079
www.shrinershq.org/hospitals/philadelphia

Randal Betz, Chief of Staff
Ernest Perilli, Administrator
Provides comprehensive medical, surgical and rehabilitative care for children with orthopaedic conditions and spinal cord injuries. All services are provided at no charge. The hospital is one of 22 located throughout North America. In addition to treating children with routine and complex orthopaedic problems, the Philadelphia hospital provides a comprehensive and individualized rehabilitation program for children and adolescents who have sustained a traumatic injury to their spine.

South Carolina

6334 Colleton Regional Hospital: RehabCare Unit
501 Robertson Blvd
Walterboro, SC 29488-5714 843-782-2000
FAX: 843-549-7562
www.colletonmedical.com

Mitchell Mongel, CEO
Colleton Medical Center's 8-bed physical and mental rehabilitation department is the oldest in the Lowcountry and has been serving the community for nearly 20 years. Strives to provide patient-centered care in a family atmosphere. The team includes nurses, physical therapists, occupational therapists, speech therapists, and nutritionists. The typical patient requires rehabilitation following a stroke, spinal injury, close head injury, and orthopedic rehabilitation.

6335 HealthSouth Rehab Hospital: South Carolina
2935 Colonial Dr
Columbia, SC 29203-6811 803-254-7777
FAX: 803-414-1414
www.healthsouthcolumbia.com

W. Anthony Jackson, CEO
Lydia Carpenter, Director of Therapy Operations
Devin Troyer, M.D., Medical Director
Luanne Burton, Director of Human Resources
Offers a wide range of specialized medical and therapeutic services designed to help physically disabled individuals reach their optimum level of function and independence.

6336 Shriners Hospitals for Children, Greenville
950 W Faris Rd
Greenville, SC 29605-4255 864-271-3444
866-459-0013
FAX: 864-271-4471
e-mail: tmcreynolds@shrinenet.org
www.shrinershq.org/hospitals/greenville

Randall Romberger, Administrator
Peter Stasikelis, Chief of Staff
Tracy McReynolds,, Development Officer
A 50-bed pediatric orthopaedic hospital providing comprehensive orthopaedic care to children at no charge to their families. The hospital is one of 22 Shriners Hospitals throughout North America. The hospital accepts and treats children with routine and complex orthopaedic problems, utilizing the latest tretments and technology availiable in pediatric orthopaedics, resulting in early ambulatory and reduced length of stay.

Tennessee

6337 Health South Cane Creek Rehabilitation Center
Health South Corporation
180 Mount Pelia Rd
Martin, TN 38237-3812 731-587-4231
FAX: 731-588-1454
e-mail: dayle.unger@healthsouth.com
www.healthsouthcanecreek.com

Eric Garrard, CEO
William Eason, Medical Director
Lindsey Box-Rotger, BSN, RN, C, Director of Quality and Risk Management
Cindy Cooper, RN, Director of Case Management
Offers a wide variety of programs and services for patients in need of acute rehabilitation. Programs and services are availiable through inpatient and outpaitent. Thereapy services availiable are physical, occupational, speech, and respiratory.

6338 HealthSouth Chattanooga Rehabilitation Hospital
2412 McCallie Ave
Chattanooga, TN 37404-3398 423-697-9129
800-763-5189
FAX: 423-697-9124
www.healthsouthchattanooga.com

Scott Rowe, CEO
Amjad Munir, Medical Director
Karen Jonakin, Director Clinical Services
Offers orthopaedic rehabilitation, stroke rehabilitation, amputee rehabilitation, brain injury program, pain management, ventilator weaning, carpal tunnel screening, low intensity program, oncology program, aquatic therapy, day treatment, burn program and outpatient services.

6339 HealthSouth Rehabilitation Cntr/Tennessee
1282 Union Ave
Memphis, TN 38104-3414 901-722-2000
FAX: 901-729-5171
healthsouthmemphis.com

Tracy Willis, CEO
Toni Wackerfuss, Director of Therapy Operation
An 80-bed acute medical rehabilitation hospital that offers comprehensive inpatient and outpatient rehabilitation services.

6340 James H And Cecile C Quillen Rehabilitation Hospital
2511 Wesley St
Johnson City, TN 37601-1723 423-952-1700
800-235-1994
FAX: 423-283-0906
www.msha.com

Tammy Bishop, Manager
A 60-bed, freestanding comprehensive medical rehabilitation hospital. Full range of outpatient and day treatment, 14-bed traumatic brain injury unit, in ground therapeutic pool, transitional living apartment, outdoor ambulation course. All inpatient and outpatient programs utilize an interdisciplinary team approach designed to improve a patient's physical and cognitive functioning.

6341 Nashville Rehabilitation Hospital
610 Gallatin Ave
Nashville, TN 37206-3225 615-650-2600
800-227-3108
FAX: 615-650-2562
www.nrhcares.com

Alan Miller, CEO
Marc Miller, President
A free-standing physical rehabilitation facility offering services to patients on an inpatient and outpatient basis. Programs include CVA, orthopedic, neuromuscular, traumatic brain injury, spinal cord injury, general rehabilitation and Bridges - geriatric psychiatric unit. Intra-disciplinary team approach is utilized to assist patients in obtaining their maximum fuctional level.

6342 Patricia Neal Rehab Center : Ft. Sanders Regional Medical Center
Covenant Health
1901 W Clinch Ave
Knoxville, TN 37916-2307 865-541-1111
800-728-6325
FAX: 865-541-2247
www.patneal.org

J.E. Henry, Co-Chair
David Kugley, Co-Chair
Mary Dillon, M.D., Medical Director, Patricia Neal Rehabilitation Center
Sharon E. Glass, M.D., Stroke Program Director, Patricia Neal Rehabilitation Center

A CARF accredited 73-bed facility, it offers a comprehensive team approach to care. Physical, occupational, recreational, behavioral medicine and speech language therapists work with physiatrists to develop individual plans of care designed to return patients to a normal lifestyle as quickly as possible. In addition, rehabilitation nurses collaborate with specialists to teach self-care techniques and provide education to help patients reach optimal functionality.

6343 Rehabilitation Center Baptist Hospital
137 E Blount Ave
Suite 6-B
Knoxville, TN 37920-1643 865-632-5520

6344 Rehabilitation Center at McFarland Hospital
University Medical Center
500 Park Ave
Lebanon, TN 37087-3721 615-449-0500
FAX: 615-453-7405
www.universitymedicalcenter.com

Saad Ehtisham, CEO
Matt Caldwell, Chief Executive Officer
Michael Cherry, Chief Financial Officer
Greg Carda, Chief Operating Officer

An Acute Inpatient Rehab, located on the hospital's second floor. The center has 26 patient rooms, three therapy treatment rooms, a patient dining area, and an 'activities of daily living' area which includes a kitchen/laundry area and a patient apartment, for those individuals who will be returning home.

6345 St. Mary's Medical Center: RehabCare Center
900 E Oak Hill Ave
Knoxville, TN 37917-4505 865-545-7962
FAX: 865-545-8133
www.tennova.com

Jeffrey Ashin, President

Committed to providing individualized and flexable treatment programs designed for individuals who have been disabled by an injury or illness. The primary mission of the RehabCare Center is to help patients achieve basic skills that may allow independent living and working.

6346 Sumner Regional Medical Center
555 Hartsville Pike
Gallatin, TN 37066-2400 615-328-8888
FAX: 615-328-3903
www.mysumnermedical.com

Susan Peach, BSN, MBA, CEO
Kevin Rinks, Chief Financial Officer
Michael S. Herman, Chief Operating Officer
Anne Melton, RN, MSN, Chief Nursing Officer

SRMC operates as a 155-bed healthcare facility and provides quality Gallatin hospital and medical care services in numerous areas, including cancer treatment, cardiac care, same- day surgery, orthopaedics, diagnostics, women's health and rehabilitation services. As the community grows, SRMC strives to continually improve its services and programs to meet the changing needs of its service area.

Texas

6347 Bayshore Medical Center: Rehab
4000 Spencer Hwy
Pasadena, TX 77504-1202 713-359-2000
FAX: 713-359-1283
www.bayshoremedical.com

Dr. Charles Bessire, Board
Jeanna Barnard, FACHE,, CEO
Alice Hopkins Adams, Board
Wilfred J. Broussard, Board

A 345-bed facility, providing the award-winning care for which we have been nationally recoginzed. Members are here to care for the physical and emotional well-being of those who arrive at Bayshore Medical Center often frightned, in pain and perhaps even alone. We offer patients solace and security through constant communication and compassionate listening in the midst of their medical emergencies and surgical or diagnostic procedures. Kindness, empathy & quality are triats that patients trust.

6348 Cecil R Bomhr Rehabilitation Center of Nacogdoches Memorial Hospital
1204 N Mound St
Nacogdoches, TX 75961-4027 936-564-4611
FAX: 936-564-4616
e-mail: info@nacmem.org
www.nacmem.org

Jerry Whitaker, Chairperson
Larry Walker, M.D., Vice-Chairperson
Lisa King, Secretary
Walter Scott, Board Member

The goal of Nacogdoches Memorial Hospital's rehabilitation services is to assist patients in attaining their highest potential activity level for independent daily living, thereby reducing the number of necessary hospitalizations. Keeping folks healthy and in their homes lowers healthcare costs for all of us.

6349 Covenant Health Systems Owens White Outpatient Rehab Center
9812 Slide Rd
Lubbock, TX 79424-1116 806-725-5627
FAX: 806-723-6009
www.covenanthealth.org

Walt Cathey, Manager

A comprehensive rehabilitation program designed to help patients attain their maximum level of independence following a debilitating stroke, illness or injury. Our fully accredited program features outpatient physical, occupational and speech language therapies, as well as certified athletic trainers and a certified strength and conditioning specialist.

6350 Gonzales Warm Springs Rehabilitation Hospital
200 Memorial Dr
Luling, TX 78648-3213 830-875-8400
FAX: 830-875-5029
www.warmsprings.org

Anthony Misitano, President/CEO
Vonnie Cromwell, Operations Manager

Statewide not-for-profit system of inpatient and outpatient rehabilitation speciality centers. Throughout the communities we serve, the Warm Springs Rehabilitation System offers hope and acts as a catalyst for achieving an optimal quality of life by providing comprehensive physical and/or cogenitive care. Investing resources in educational and recreational programs. Supporting research efforts.

6351 Harris Methodist Fort Worth Hospital Mabee Rehabilitation Center
1301 Pennsylvania Ave
Fort Worth, TX 76104-2122 817-250-2760
866-847-7342
FAX: 814-250-6846
www.texashealth.org

Lillie Biggins, B.S.N., M.S.N, CEO/President
Elaine Nelson, R.N., M.S.N., Chief Nursing Officer
Joseph Prosser, M.D., M.B.A., Chief Medical Officer

Professionals at the Harris Methodist Fort Worth Hospital's Mabee Rehabilitation Center work closely with each patient to develop a specialzed treatment plan for personal achievement. The center offers highly trained clinical staff members and spacious facilities An incredibly wide range of treatment programs and educational services are provided for both inpatient and outpatient needs.

6352 **HealthSouth Plano Rehabilitation Hospital**
6701 Oakmont Blvd.
Fort Worth, TX 76132-7526 817-370-4700
FAX: 972-423-4293
www.healthsouth.com

Jon F. Hanson, Chairman
John W. Chidsey, Board of director
Donald L. Correll, Board of director
Yvonne M. Curl, Board of director

A 62-bed medical reahabilitation facility serving inpatient and out patient needs in the Northern Dallas area. The team coordinate all aspects of the patient's rehabilitation to maximize results. The overall effort is directed by board-certified physical medicine and rehabilitation physicians who specialize in medical rehabilitation. Whatever the cause of the disability, our services can benefit patients who have functional limitations in such areas as mobility, communication and self care.

6353 **HealthSouth Rehab Hospital Of Arlington**
3200 Matlock Rd
Arlington, TX 76015-2911 817-468-4000
FAX: 817-468-3055
www.healthsouth.com

Jon F. Hanson, Chairman
John W. Chidsey, Board of director
Donald L. Correll, Board of director
Yvonne M. Curl, Board of director

A modern 65-bed hospital dedicated to providng inpatient programs in a general rehabilitation setting for persons recovering for a disabling injury or illness. As part of our continuum of care, we also offer outpatient therapy, a day program, and individual therapy services. Our goal is to help our patients resume a productive and more meaningful life through appropriate rehabilitative care and restorative nursing in a wellness-oriented environment that promotes healing and functional recovery.

6354 **HealthSouth Rehab Hospital Of Austin**
1215 Red River St
Austin, TX 78701-1921 512-474-5700
FAX: 512-479-3765
www.healthsouthaustin.com

Duke Saldiver, CEO
Corey Helm Swartz, Director of Therapy Operations
Maria Arizmendez, M.D., Medical Director
Debbie Belcher, Human Resource Director

A comprehensive 83 bed medical rehabilitation hospital serving the needs of patients in the Central Texas area. The mission is to promote recovery for persons with disabling conditions by providing individualized treatment so they can reach the highest level of physical, social and emotional well-being.

6355 **HealthSouth Rehabilitation Center of Humble Texas**
19002 McKay Blvd
Humble, TX 77338 281-446-6148
FAX: 281-446-5616
www.healthsouthhumble.com

Angie Simmons, CEO
Mikael Simpson, Director of Therapy Operations
Emile Mathurin, Jr., M.D., Medical Director
Christy Dixon, Human Resources Director

Offers comprehensive rehabilitation services for patients with diverse diagnoses. Rehabilitation can be defined as multidisciplinary therapy designed to increase patient's overall functioning to a level that meets or exceeds where the patient was prior to illness or injury or to maximize current level of ability. The benefits of these services to patients and their families is invaluable.

6356 **HealthSouth Rehabilitation Hospital**
6701 Oakmont Blvd
Fort Worth, TX 76132-2957 817-370-4700
FAX: 817-370-4977
www.healthsouthcityview.com

Deborah Hopps, CEO
Mark Bussell, Medical Director
Mark Bussell, M.D., Medical Director
Kenneth Akwar, PharmD, Director of Pharmacy

A 62-bed acute medical rehabilitation hospital that offers comprehensive inpatient and outpatient rehabilitation services.

6357 **HealthSouth Rehabilitation Hospital of Beaumont**
3340 Plaza 10 Dr
Beaumont, TX 77707-2551 409-835-0835
FAX: 409-835-0898
www.healthsouthbeaumont.com

Sam Coco, Director of Therapy Operations
HJ Gaspard, CEO
Linda Smith, M.D., Medical Director
Sam Coco, PT, Director of Therapy Operations

A state of the art freestanding 61-bed comprehensive physical rehabilitation hospital. The hospital is specifically designed to meet the needs of individuals and their families who have experienced a disabling injury or illness or are recovering from a surgery. An experienced team of physicians, nurses, therapists, treat conditions and other disorders.

6358 **HealthSouth Rehabilitation Institute Of San Antonio (RIOSA)**
9119 Cinnamon Hill
San Antonio, TX 78240-5401 210-691-0737
FAX: 210-558-1297
www.hsriosa.com

Scott Butcher, CEO
Richard Senelick, Medical Director
Christine Chesnut, OTR, MPH, Director of Therapy Operations
Linda Hart, LVN, Director of Marketing

HealthSouth Rehabilitation Institute of San Antonio is the largest free-standing physical rehabilitation hospital in San Antonio and is proud to enter our 11th year of delivering quality, comprehensive medical rehabilitation in a pristine environment. HealthSouth annually serves over 1,500 inpatients and more then 20,000 outpatient visits from throughout San Antonio and Mexico. 108-bed hospital has more then 300 personell on staff providing extensive experience.

6359 **Hillcrest Baptist Medical Center: Rehab Care Unit**
100 Hillcrest Medical Blvd
Waco, TX 76712-3239 254-202-2000
FAX: 254-202-8975
e-mail: marketing@hillcrest.net
www.hillcrest.net

Fred Walters, President
Jon Ellis, Secretary

A fully accredited 393-bed acute care facility in Waco including a Level II Trauma Center, Hillcrest Family Health Center, a network of family medicine clinics; and many key services. Hillcrest is a ministry of Texas Baptists and is one of 7 health care institutions affiliated with the Baptist General Convention of Texas.

6360 **Institute for Rehabilitation & Research**
1333 Moursund St
Houston, TX 77030-3405 713-942-6159
800-447-3422
FAX: 713-942-5289
e-mail: tirr.referrals@memorialhermann.org
www.memorialhermann.org

Jeffrey Berliner, Physician
Michelle Pu, Physician

A national center for information, training, research, and technical assistance in independent living. The goal is to extend the body of knowledge in independent living and to improve the utilization of results of research programs and demonstration projects in this field. It has developed a variety of strategies for collecting, synthesizing, and disseminating information related to the field of independent living.

6361 Midland Memorial Hospital & Medical Center
400 Rosalind Redfern Grover Parkway
Midland, TX 79701-9980 432-685-1111
800-833-2916
e-mail: russell.meyers@midland-memorial.com
www.midland-memorial.com

J.T. Lent Jr., President
Russell Meyers, CEO
Greg Wright, Board of Directors
Pete Hulder, Board of Directors

The Occupational and Physical Therapy Center is a specialzed outpatient clinic. The clinic provides a wide variety of rehabilitation services designed to adequately assist you in returning back to your normal duties. Our highly trained professionals are here to help you with all your rehabilitation needs.

6362 Navarro Regional Hospital: RehabCare Unit
Navarro Hospital
3201 W State Highway 22
Corsicana, TX 75110-2469 903-654-6800
FAX: 903-654-6955
www.navarrohospital.com

Xavier Villarreal, CEO
Glenda Teri, Chief Nursing Officer

The rehab unit is located on the 4th floor and is designed for individuals who require intense rehab for an injury or disease process where the goal would be to return home. Our team is committed to helping individuals return to the highest level of functioning. Our team consists of physicians, nurses, physical therapist, occupational therapist, speech therapist, social workers, dieticians and other professionals as needed.

6363 Rebound: Northeast Methodist Hospital
12412 Judson Rd
Live Oak, TX 78233-3255 210-757-7000
FAX: 210-757-5072
www.nemh.sahealth.com

Joe Hernandez, Manager

Methodist Healthcare provides quality, comprehensive rehabilitation services for children and adults. Working as a team, rehabilitation professionals help patients define and achieve individual goals in restoring function and productivity.

6364 Rio Vista Rehabilitation Hospital
1740 Curie Dr
El Paso, TX 79902-2900 915-544-8336
800-999-8392
FAX: 915-544-4838

Gene Miller, Administrator

6365 San Antonio Warm Springs Rehabilitation Hospital
5101 Medical Dr
San Antonio, TX 78229-4801 210-595-2380
FAX: 210-614-0649
www.warmsprings.org

Kurt Meyer, SVP Operations
Rick Marek, VP Post Acute Medical

A statewide not-for-profit system of inpatient and outpatient rehabilitation specialty centers. Warm Springs Rehabilitation System offers hope and acts as a catalyst for achieving an optimal quality of life by providing comprehensive physical and/or cognitive rehabilitative care. Invensting resources in educational and recreational programs. Supporting research efforts.

6366 Shannon Medical Center: RehabCare Unit
120 E Harris Ave
San Angelo, TX 76903-5904 325-653-6741
FAX: 325-657-5706
www.shannonhealth.com

Bryan Horner, CEO
Irv Zeitler, VP Medical Affairs
Shane Plymell, Chief financial officer
Gary Gibian, Executive director

Committed to improving the health of our community, using the latest technologies available in the spirit of caring and integrity. Strives to create an environment committed to the values of accountability, service, pride, integrity, respect and excellence. We foster growth toward the highest quality care and customer service and strive for excellent financial performance. We hire and develop the best people to accomplish these tasks.

6367 Shriners Burn Institute: Galveston Unit
815 Market St
Galveston, TX 77550-2725 409-770-6600
FAX: 409-770-6919
www.totalburncare.com

David Herndon, Chief Of Staff
David Ferrell, F.A.C.H.E., Administrator

Providing expert, orthopaedic and burn care to children under 18 regardless of ability to pay.

6368 Shriners Hospitals for Children, Houston
6977 Main St
Houston, TX 77030-3701 713-797-1616
800-853-1240
FAX: 713-797-1029
www.shrinershq.org

David Ferrell, Administrator
Douglas Barnes, Chief of Staff
Melanie Lux, M.D.,, Director
Gloria Gogola, M.D., Doctor

Shriners Hospitals provides at no charge quality pediatric orthopedic serivces to children ages newborn to 18 years old. These services include both outpatient and inpatient needs. Specialties include cerebrel palsy, spina bifida, scoliosis, hand, hip and feet problems. An application is required and may be completed by phone.

6369 South Arlington Medical Center: Rehab Care Unit
3301 Matlock Rd
Arlington, TX 76015-2908 817-472-4849
FAX: 817-472-4946
e-mail: mca@hcahealthcare.com
www.medicalcenterarlington.com

Patrice Oliver, Manaager

Above all else, we are committed to the care and improvement of human life. In recognition of this committment, we strive to deliver high-quality, cost-effective healthcare in the communities we serve.

6370 South Texas Rehabilitation Hospital
Ernest Health
425 E Alton Gloor Blvd
Brownsville, TX 78526-3361 956-554-6000
FAX: 956-350-6150
e-mail: askus@earnesthealth.com
www.strh.ernesthealth.com

Christopher Wilson, Medical Director
Jessie Eason, CEO
Mary Valdez, Director of Marketing

STRH was designed for the provision of specialized rehabilitative care, in the only freestanding acute rehabilitation hospital serving Brownsville and the Rio Grande Valley. The hospital provides rehabilitative services for patients with functional deficits as a result of debilitating illnesses or injuries.

6371 St. David's Rehabilitation Center
St. David s Medical Center
621 Radam Lane
Suite 200
Austin, TX 78745-4237 512-447-1083
FAX: 512-447-1338
www.stdavids.com

Anisa Godinez, Medical Director
Everett Heinze, MD Neurology, Medical Director
Tom Hill, MD, Medical Director
Albert Horn, MD, Medical Director

Mission is to provide exceptional care to every patient every day with a spirit of warmth, friendliness and personal pride. Values are integrity, compassion, accountability, respect and excellence.

6372 Texas NeuroRehab Center
1106 W Dittmar Rd
Austin, TX 78745-6328 512-444-4835
800-252-5151
FAX: 512-462-6749
www.texasneurorehab.com

Alison Crawford Sinsky, Inpatient and Outpatient Manager
Ed Varando, Occupational Therapy Manager

Internationally recognized provider in brain injury/neurobehavioral treatment for children, adolescents, and adults with complex medical, physical and/or behavioral issues. Medical rehabilitation, neurobehavioral, and neuropsychiatric programs combine traditional therapies with education, vocational, substance abuse, and sensory integration services.

6373 Texas Specialty Hospital at Dallas
7955 Harry Hines Blvd
Dallas, TX 75235-3305 214-637-0000

Robin Burns, CEO

66 beds offering active/acute rehabilitation, brain injury day treatment, cognitive rehabilitation, complex care, extended rehabilitation and short term evaluation.

6374 Touchstone Neurorecovery Center
Nexus Health Systems
9297 Wahrenberger Rd
Conroe, TX 77304-2441 936-788-7770
800-414-4824
FAX: 936-788-7785
e-mail: tncinfo@nhsltd.com
www.touchstoneneuro.com

John W. Cassidy, MD, Executive Medical Director
Jude Theriot, MD, Medical Director
Ron Tintner, MD, Associate Clinical Director
Nelson Valena, MD, Director of Physical Medicine and Rehabilitation

Touchstone provides treatment and rehabilitation in a residential environment on a tranquil, wooded 26-acre site just north of Houston in Conroe, TX. Touchstone offers customized treatment programs designed to help individuals with known or suspected brain injury or neurological deficits progress to their highest functional level possible. Touchstone offers both on-campus and off-campus housing in home-like settings for residents based on their needs.

6375 Valley Regional Medical Center: RehabCare Unit
100A E Alton Gloor Blvd
Brownsville, TX 78526-3328 956-350-7000
FAX: 956-350-7111
www.valleyregionalmedicalcenter.com

Billy Bradford Jr.,, Chair
Francisco Javier Del Castillo, M, Vice Chair
Subramaniam Anandasivam, MD, Board
Christopher Olson, MD, Board

Our mission is to treat our community as family by providing quality compassionate care.

Utah

6376 HealthSouth Rehab Hospital Of Utah
8074 S 1300 E
Sandy, UT 84094-743 801-561-3400
801-565-6666
FAX: 801-565-6576
www.healthsouthutah.com

Phil Eaton, CEO
William McNutt, Director of Therapy Operations
Mark Rada, M.D., Interim Medical Director
Richard Ashby, Western Regional Director of Plant Operations/Safety Officer

A full spectrum of services, including inpatient, outpatient, day hospital and home health. Holistic patient care, education and community assimilation are the hallmarks of our programs, and evidence of our leadership in the field of rehabilitation. Working together as a team, we are able to tailor the needs of our patients and provide the highest quality services. We believe that education and involvement of family and friends, will assist them in maintaining independence after discharge.

6377 LDS Hospital Rehabilitation Center
8th Ave & C Street
Salt Lake City, UT 84143-0001 801-408-1100
800-527-1118
FAX: 801-408-5610
e-mail: contactus@intermountainmail.org
www.intermountainhealthcare.org

Lizz Daley, Administrator
Jim Sheets, Administrator

Located within a Trauma I Center, this facility provides comprehensive inpatient and outpatient rehabilitation to people with physical disabilities. CARF/JCAHO accredited. Low cost family housing is available and Medicaid/Medicare is accepted.

6378 Primary Children's Medical Center
100 Mario Capecchi Dr
Salt Lake City, UT 84113-1100 801-662-1000
FAX: 801-588-2318
www.intermountainhealthcare.org

Scott Parker, President
Kevin Jones, Manager
Ore-Ofe O. Adesina, MD, Ophthalmology
Zeinab A. Afify, MD, Pediatric Hematology Oncology

Primary Children's Medical Center is the pediatric center serving 5 states in the Intermountain West Utah, Idaho, Wyoming, Nevada and Montana. The 289-bed facility is equipped and staffed to treat children with complex illness and injury. PCMC is owned by Intermountain Healthcare, a non-profit health care system. In addition, it is affiliated with the Dept. of Pediatrics, University of Utah, integrating pediatric programs. The hospital is designed to meet the needs of children & their families.

6379 Shriners Hospitals for Children: Intermountain
Fairfax Road at Virginia St
Salt Lake City, UT 84103 801-536-3500
800-313-3745
FAX: 801-536-3782
www.shrinershq.org

Kevin Martin, Administrator
Jacques D'Astous, Chief of Staff

One of nineteen hospitals in North America specializing in pediatric orthopedics (plus four hospitals providing pediatric burn treatment). This hospital serves the Intermountain region. All services provided in the hospital are at no cost to family, insurance company, nor state/federal agency regardless of ability to pay.

6380 Stewart Rehabilitation Center: McKay Dee Hospital
4401 Harrison Blvd
Ogden, UT 84403-3195 801-387-2080
FAX: 801-387-7720
e-mail: contactus@intermountainmail.org
www.intermountainhealthcare.org

Corey Anden, Nurse Coordinator
Judy Grover, Manager

With 10 affiliated clinics, McKay-Dee serves northern Utah, and portions of southeast Idaho and western Wyoming. A part of Intermountain Healthcare's system of 21 hospitals, McKay-Dee Hospital Center offers nationally ranked programs such as the Heart & Vascular Institute, the Newborn ICU and a new Cancer Treatment Center.

6381 University Healthcare-Rehabilitation Center
50 N Medical Dr
Salt Lake City, UT 84132-1 801-587-3422
801-58 -EHAB
FAX: 801-581-2111
www.healthcare.utah.edu/rehab/

David Entwistle, Administrator
Trish Jensen, Program Coordinator

Provides quality, comprehensive, rehabilitation services to persons with complex rehabilitation needs, including spinal cord injuries, head trauma, stroke, and other disabling conditions. Rehabilitation Services has been serving physicians, their patients, and the community since 1965. Rehabilitation Services has been an established leader in comprehensive inpatient, outpatient and home/community rehabilitation programs. Accredited by CARF and JCAHO.

Vermont

6382 Vermont Achievement Center
88 Park St
Rutland, VT 05701-4715
802-775-2395
FAX: 802-773-9656
e-mail: kmcshane@vac-rutland.com
www.vac-rutland.com

Kiki Mc Shane, CEO
Rebecca Wisell, Administrator
Vermont Achievement Center is recognized as a catalyst in building a community where all people are capable of change. Individuals flourish because they are nutured, valued and treated with respect. Education is empowering. The family is the primary influence in a person's life. Children belong in a family. Families are enhanced by support of the community. Children and family services are flexible and responsive to changing needs.

Virginia

6383 Inova Mount Vernon Hospital Rehabilitation Program
Inova Rehabilitation Center
2501 Parkers Ln
Alexandria, VA 22306-3209
703-664-7000
800-554-7342
FAX: 703-664-7423
www.inova.com

Barbara Doyle, CEO
Inova Mount Vernon Hospital is a 237-bed hospital offering patients convenience and state-of-the-art care in a community environment. Our hospital sits on 26 acres of beautifully landscaped open space, where patients can find moments of serenity in our specially designed gardens..

6384 Kluge Children's Rehabilitation Center
University of Virginia
2270 Ivy Rd
Charlottesville, VA 22903-4977
434-924-5161
800-627-8596
FAX: 434-924-5559
www.healthsystem.virginia.edu

Janet Allaire, Administrator
Richard Stevenson, Research Director
The Kluge Childrens's Rehabilitation Center (KCRC) is a place dedicated to serving children with special needs. Children between the ages of birth and 21 come to the KCRC from all over Virginia, the United States, and even overseas for many reasons. Some need specific therapy or rehabilitation after injuries, accidents, or surgery. Others have chronic illness such as diabetes, and cystic fibrosis. Many families come to find out why their child is experiencing behavior problems.

Washington

6385 Good Samaritan Healthcare Physical Medicine and Rehabilitation
Good Samaritan Hospital
407 14th Ave SE
Puyallup, WA 98372-3770
253-697-4000
FAX: 253-697-5157
e-mail: info@goodsamhealth.org
www.multicare.org

Glenn Kassman, President
Vince Schmitz, CFO
Good Samaritan is part of the Multi-Care Health System, a non-for-profit medical system serving the growing populations of Pierce and King Counties in the greater Puget Sound region of Washington. Our medical staff includes 1,600 of the regions most respected primary care physicians and specialists.

6386 Northwest Hospital Center for Medical Rehabilitation
1550 N 115th St
Seattle, WA 98133-9733
206-364-0500
FAX: 206-364-0500
TTY:877-694-4677
www.nwhospital.org

Peter Evans, Chairman
Scott L. Hardman, Vice Chairman
James K. Anderson, Board
C W Schneider, CEO
Provides complete medical and surgical services in both inpatient and outpatient settings. Services across multiple specialties include: 24hr emergency services, critical care, cardiac care, stroke program, cancer care, childbirth center, rehabilitation center, diagnostic imaging and education and wellness services. Mission is to raise the long-term health status of our community by providing personalized, quality care with compassion dignity, and respect.

6387 Providence Medical Center
500 17th Ave
Seattle, WA 98122-5711
206-000-1111
FAX: 206-320-3387
www.providence.org

6388 Providence Rehabilitation Services
Providence Rehabilitation Services
1321 Colby Ave
Everett, WA 98201-1665
425-261-3825
FAX: 425-261-3823
www.providence.org

Jim Phillips, Manager
Leslie Baumgarten, Manager
Continuum of care available: Acute Care, Inpatient Rehabilitation Unit, Transitional Care, Outpatient therapies, and In-home services.

6389 Shriners Hospitals for Children: Spokane
Shriners Hospitals
911 W 5th Ave
Spokane, WA 99204-2901
509-455-7844
FAX: 509-744-1223
www.shrinershq.org/hospitals/spokane

Kristin Monasmith, Public Relations Director
Craig Patchin, Administrator
Paul M. Caskey, M.D., Chief of Staff
Provides pediatric orthopedic services plus burn scar revision to children birth to 18. All services at no charge to the family.

West Virginia

6390 HealthSouth Mountain View Regional Rehab Hospital
1160 Van Voorhis Rd
Morgantown, WV 26505-3437
304-598-1100
800-388-2451
FAX: 304-598-1103
e-mail: healthsouthmountainview.com
www.healthsouthmountainview.com/

Vicki Demers, Chief Executive Officer
Govind Patel, M.D., Medical Director
Robbin Butler, OTR/L, Director of Therapy Operations
Ginger Dearth, RN, Director of Marketing Operations
A 96-bed inpatient accute rehabilitation hospital. Outpatient services, physical, occupational and speech therapy, and interior therapy pool. Programs include neuro/stroke, brain injury, spinal cord injury and pediatric.

6391 HealthSouth Western Hills Regional Rehab Hospital
3 Western Hills Dr
Parkersburg, WV 26105-8122 304-420-1392
FAX: 304-420-1374
www.healthsouthwesternhills.com

Kalapala Rao, Medical Director
Candace Ross, Director of Human Resources
Greg Holland, Director of Marketing Operations
Michelle Lowers, MS, LSW, Director of Care Management

A 40-bed medical rehabilitation hospital serving inpatient and outpatient needs in the western West Virginia area. Our hospital is accredited by the Joint Commission on Accreditation of Healthcare Organizations (JCAHO) Our mission is to guide patients whtih physically disabling conditions along an individualized treatment pathway so they can reach the highest level of physical, social and emotional well-being. We strive to provide the highest quality care for you and your family.

Wisconsin

6392 Extendicare Health Services, Inc.
3540 South 43rd Street
Milwaukee, WI 53220-2903 414-541-1000
800-395-5000
FAX: 414-541-1942
www.extendicare.com

Timothy Lukenda, CEO
Douglas Harris, SVP
David Pearce, Vice President, General Counsel

Sunrise Care Center is a leading provider of long-term skilled nursing care and short-term rehabilitation solutions. Our 99 bed facility offers a full continuum of services and care focused around each individual in today's ever-changing healthcare environment. Our facility is Medicare and Medicaid certified.

6393 St. Catherine's Hospital
9555 76th St
Pleasant Prairie, WI 53158 262-577-8000
FAX: 262-653-5795
www.uhsi.org

Vicki Lewis, Manager

Committed to living out the healing ministries of the Judeo-Christian faiths by providing exceptional and compassionate healthcare service that promotes the dignity and well-being of the people we serve.

6394 St. Joseph Hospital
611 Saint Joseph Ave
Marshfield, WI 54449-1898 715-387-1713
FAX: 715-389-3939
e-mail: sjhweb@stjosephs-marshfield.org
www.ministryhealth.org

Michael Schmidt, CEO
Catherine Olson, Director

A values-driven healthcare delivery network of aligned hospitals, clinics, long-term care facilities, home care agencies, dialysis centers and many other programs and services in Wisconsin and Minnesota.

Wyoming

6395 Spalding Rehabilitation Hospital at Memorial Hospital of Laramie
2301 House Ave
Suite 300
Cheyenne, WY 82001-3748 307-635-4141
800-374-7687
FAX: 307-638-2656
www.imgwy.com

Mitchell Schwarzbach, Executive Director
Tanya Boerkircher, Wyoming Endoscopy Center Manager
Andrea Bailey, Charge Entry Supervisor
Michelle Flanagan, Front Office Supervisor

We are a professional corporation of physicians trained in various medical specialties and subspecialties including Internal Medicine, Gastroenterology and Chest Diseases.It is our mission to provide the highest quality, cost-effective primary and subspecialty medical care, and education to the people of southern Wyoming, western Nebraska, and northern Colorado.

Rehabilitation Facilities, Post-Acute

Alabama

6396 **Alabama Department of Rehabilitation Services**
602 S Lawrence St
Montgomery, AL 36104-4787
334-293-7500
800-441-7607
FAX: 334-293-7383
rehab.state.al.us

Cary F. Boswell, Commissioner

State agency which provides services and assistance to Alabama's children and adults with disabilities.

6397 **Alabama Goodwill Industries**
2350 Green Springs Highway S
Birmingham, AL 35205-6834
205-323-6331
FAX: 205-324-9059
e-mail: caroline.goodwill@yahoo.com
www.alabamagoodwill.org/

Don Smith, President/CEO
Rayford L. Coleman, Chairman
Paul Beasley, Vice Chairman
Herbert L. Boring, Treasurer

The mission of Goodwill is to provide rehabilitation services, training, employment, and opportunities for personal growth to the disabled/disadvantaged.

6398 **Briarcliff Nursing Home & Rehab Facility**
3201 North Ware Road
McAllen, TX 78501
956-631-5542
FAX: 956-631-5777
http://www.briarcliffnursingcenter.com

6399 **Butler Adult Training Center**
19815 Bay Branch Rd
Andalusia, AL 36420-3615
334-222-2525
FAX: 334-382-9518
http://www.scamhc.org

Diane Baugher, CPA, MBA, Executive Director

Clients 21 years of age and older who are mentally retarded. School age clients are also served at the center and must also be mentally retarded. Clients receive training in Independent Living Skills, Self-Care, Language Skills, Learning, Self Direction and Economic Self-Sufficiency. The clients also participate in Special Olympics activities.

6400 **Cheaha Mental Health**
P.O.Box 1248
351W 3rd Street
Sylacauga, AL 35150-1248
256-245-1340
FAX: 256-245-1343
crmhc.org/

Cynthia L. Atkinson, Executive Director
Dr. Shakil Khan, Medical Director
Kathleen Robinson, Human Resources Coordinator
Karen McKinney, Clinical Director of Mental Health Services

Offers mental health rehabilitation, respite care, residential facilities and more for the mentally disabled. Serves Talladega, Coosa, Clay and Randolph counties.

6401 **Children's Rehabilitation Service**
602 S. Lawrence St.
Montgomery, AL 36104
334-293-7500
800-441-7607
FAX: 334-293-7383
www.rehab.state.al.us/home/services/crs/main

Steve Shivers, Manager

Statewide organization of skilled professionals providng quality medical, rehabilitative, coordination and support services for children with special health care needs and their families.

6402 **Chilton-Shelby Mental Health Center/ The Mitchell Center**
151 Hamilton Lane
Calera, AL 35040
205-668-4308
FAX: 205-668-0894
chiltonshelby.org

Melodie D. Crawford, Chief Executive Officer
Vicki M. Potts, BS, CPA, Chief Financial Officer
Kathryn T. Crouthers, LCSW, Chief Operations Officer
Dena Foster, MS, Intellectual Disabilities Division Director

Offers mental health rehabilitation services and more for the recovery of mentally disabled adults. Serves Chilton and Shelby counties.

6403 **EL Darden Rehabilitation Center**
1001 E Broad Street
Suite C
Gadsden, AL 35903-2400
256-547-5751
FAX: 256-547-5761
e-mail: darden@dardenrehab.org
dardenrehab.org

Brent McCoy, Executive Director
Derek Coburn, Operations Manager
Sam Bishop, Information Systems and Workshop
Lisa Wilson, Executive Assistant

Work adjustment and job placement programs. Serves the counties of Etawah, Marshall, Dekalb, Clair and Cherokee.

6404 **Easter Seals Central Alabama**
2125 East South Boulevard
Montgomery, AL 36116-2409
334-288-0240
FAX: 334-288-7171
e-mail: info@eastersealsca.org
www.eastersealsca.or

Debbie Lynn, Executive Director
Ed Collier, Programs Manager
Sharis LeMay, CNA Instructor
Frankie Thomas, Senior Employment Program

A private, nonprofit organization offering services audiology, physical, occupational, lymphedemia and speech therapy, psychological counseling, vocational evaluation and assessment, person, social and work adjustment training, GED preparation, computer service training, job placement and follow-up, and special learning disabilities service and supported employment service.

6405 **Easter Seals West Alabama**
1110 Dr Edward Hillard Drive
Tuscaloosa, AL 35401-7446
205-759-1211
800-726-1216
FAX: 205-349-1162
e-mail: eswa@eastersealswestal.org
eastersealswestal.org

Ronny Johnston, Administrator
Dusty Beam, Administrative Assistant
Gwen Stewart, Events and Public Relations
Jennifer Goode Davis, Director of Community Relations

Leading organization in helping children and adults with disabilities to live with equality, dignity and independence. Rehabilitation services are provided in two divisions: outpatient rehabilitation division (physical therapy, occupational therapy, speech therapy, hearing evaluation, sell and service hearind aids) and vocational division (vocational evaulation and vocational development). Services are rendered regardless of age, race, sex, color, creed, national origin, veteran's status.

6406 **Geer Adult Training Center**
P.O.Box 419
83 South Canaan Road
Canaan, CT 06018-419
860-824-7067
FAX: 205-367-8032
geercares.org/content/about-geer

Yvonne Williams, Program Coordinator

6407 **Goodwill Easter Seals of the Gulf Coast**
5960 East Shirley Lane
Montgomery, AL 36617-2319 334-395-4489
800-411-0068
FAX: 251-476-4303
e-mail: info@al.easterseals.com
alabama.easterseals.com

Frank Harkins, President
Stephanie Constantine, VP Marketing
Richard W. Davidson, Chairman
Ralph F. Boyd, Jr., Treasurer
Vocational, medical, pre-school education, day care, recreation and other support services.

6408 **Indian Rivers**
2209 9th Street
Tuscaloosa, AL 35401 205-391-3131
FAX: 205-391-3135
http://www.irmhc.org

6409 **MARC Enterprises**
2424 Gordon Smith Drive
Mobile, AL 36617-2397 251-479-7409
FAX: 251-473-7649
e-mail: jzoghby@mobilearc.org
mobilearc.org

Jeff Zoghby, Executive Director
Amy Odom, Public Relations and Development Director
Serving the mentally retarded of Mobile County both locally and through its state and national affiliations. Their united efforts through this voluntary association assure the availability of services and provide the opportunity for achievement.

6410 **North Central Alabama Mental Retardation Authority**
1602 Church Street SE
PO Box 2091
Decatur, AL 35602-597 256-350-1458
FAX: 256-350-1485
www.cddnca.org

Earl Brightwell, Executive Director
NCA, MRA, Inc. functions as an entrance to the service delivery system for the Alabama Department of Mental Health and Mental Retardation and is responsible for planning, development, implementation of programs, sanction, monitoring, referral, and case management for persons with mental retardation/developmental disabilities in Morgan, Lawrence and Limestone Counties.

6411 **Northwest Alabama Easter Seals Children's Clinic Rehabilitation Center**
1450 Avalon Avenue
Muscle Shoals, AL 35660-3110 256-391-1110
FAX: 256-314-5105
e-mail: info@al.easterseals.com
www.alabama.easter-seals.org

Danny Prince, Administrator
John Ives, Chairman
Tommy Hester, Treasurer
Susie White, Secretary
Easter Seals has been helping individuals with disabilities and special needs, and their families live better lives for more then 80 years. From child development centers to physical rehabilitation and job training for people with disabilities, Easter Seals offers a variety of services to help people with disabilities address lif's challenges and achieve personal goals.

6412 **Southeastern Blind Rehabilitation Center**
Department of Veterans Affairs Medical Center
700 South 19th Street
Birmingham, AL 35233-1927 205-558-4706
FAX: 205-933-4484
e-mail: george.sands@med.va.gov
www1.va.gov/blindrehab

George Sands, Director
Kelly Bleach, Chief Administrative Officer
Eric K. Shinseki, Secretary
Carl Augusto, President and CEO
The Center is a 32-bed inpatient blind rehabilitation program which serves the southeastern region. The majority of client services are for basic adjustment and management to sight loss. Basic services include: low vision, orientation and mobility, manual skills, ADL and communications. Training on electronic mobility aids and adapted computers is also available on a restricted basis. The program maintains graduate education affiliations and an active applied research program.

6413 **Tennessee Valley Rehabilitation**
P.O.Box 1926
Decatur, AL 35602-1926 256-350-2041
866-350-2041
FAX: 256-350-2806
www.tvrcdecatur.com

Kathy Cagle, Executive Director
Bill Grissim, Vice President
Mission is to help persons with disabilities gain and maintain employment in the competitive market. The mission is accomplished by providing quality services for individuals. Being attuned to the needs of each individual served. Respecting the rights of individuals served. Promoting the welfare and dignity of each individual served at all times. Not showing partiality to individuals based on race, color, national origin, gender and religion.

6414 **The ARC of Jefferson County**
215 21st Ave S
Birmingham, AL 35205-6801 205-323-6383
FAX: 205-323-0085
www.arcofjeff.org

William Hoehle, Executive Director
Phiip Richards, President
The ARC has four primary components. The HOPE Program provides early intervention therapy services to developmentally delayed infants and toddlers up to the age of three years. The ARC also provides services to adults ages 21 and over with intellectual disabilities. Adult services provides education, pre-vocational screening, and socialization skills training. Employment services provides vocational training, a sheltered workshop, off-site job skills training, job coach services and more.

6415 **UAB Eye Care**
University Of Alabama At Birmingham
1530 3rd Avenue South
Birmingham, AL 35294-0010 205-975-2020
FAX: 205-934-6755
www.main.uab.edu/eyecare

RW Nowakowski, Dean
Dr. Marsha Snow, Chief, Low Vision Patient Care
Brittney Bolen, Optometric Technician
Joseph Fleming, D.D., Chief Of Staff
Complete eye services, including low vision services and materials.

6416 **Vaughn-Blumberg Services**
2715 Flynn Road P.O.Box 8646
Dothan, AL 36304-646 334-793-3102
FAX: 334-793-7740
http://vaughnblumbergservices.com

Ed Dorsey, Executive Director
Linda Cunningham, Director of Human Resources
Billy McCarthy, Director of Finance
Karen Amos, Director of Nursing
Child early intervention services for the mentally handicapped adult including diagnosis and evaluation and physical, speech, and occupational therapies. They also offer counseling, day training,employment assistance and residental homes.

6417 West Central Alabama Easter Seals Rehabilitation Center
2906 Citizens Parkway
P. O. Box 750
Selma, AL 36701-0750
334-872-8421
800-801-4776
FAX: 334-872-3907
e-mail: wcarcdw@tomnet.com
www.al.easter-seals.org

David White, Administrator
Wayne Middlebrooks, Chairman
Glenn King, Treasurer
Shirley Holmes, Vice-Chairman

Vocational evaluation, job development, employment development, job coaching, counseling, medical services, audiology, pre-school development programs.

Alaska

6418 Alaska Center for the Blind and Visually Impaired
3903 Taft Drive
Anchorage, AK 99517-3069
907-248-7770
800-770-7517
FAX: 907-248-7517
e-mail: info@alaskabvi.org
www.alaskabvi.org

CB Brady, President
Dennis P. Cimmings, Vice President
Christina Dobbins, Treasurer
Karla Jutzi, Executive Director

Services to help the adult residential or community-based student become independent and self-sufficient by offering independent travel, Braille reading and writing, use of assiative technology such as talking computers, manual skills and personal, as well as home management. There is a special program for those 55 years of age and older who are experiencing a vision loss and another program for rural Alaska Native youth who are visually impaired.

6419 Alaska Veterans Facility
Ste 115
1201 North Muldoon Road
Anchorage, AK 99504-5914
907-257-4700
888-353-7574
FAX: 907-561-7183
www.alaska.va.gov/

Bob Erwin, Manager
Robert Nelson, Counselor
Susan M. Yeager, Director
Greg Puckett, Associate Director

Veterans medical clinic offering disabled veterans medical treatments.

Arizona

6420 Arizona Center for the Blind and Visually Impaired
3100 E Roosevelt St
Phoenix, AZ 85008-5036
602-273-7411
FAX: 602-273-7410
e-mail: jlamay@acbvi.org
acbvi.org

James La May, CEO
Frank Vance, Director
Christine Boisen, Chair
Alexia Matek, Secretary

A private, nonprofit organization that provides comprehensive rehabilitation services and more for the blind and visually handicapped. The staff includes 20 instructional and adminstrative professionals.

6421 Arizona Industries for the Blind
Suite 130
515 N 51st Avenue
Phoenix, AZ 85043-2711
602-771-9100
FAX: 602-353-5701
e-mail: DanielMartinez@azdes.gov
www.azdes.gov/aib

Richard Monaco, General Manager
Daniel Martinez, Community Services Liaison

Offers rehabilitation services, vocational/pre-vocational evaluation and training, work adjustment, job development and employment and training opportunties for individuals who are blind.

6422 Banner Good Samaritan Medical Center
1111 E McDowell Road
Phoenix, AZ 85006-2666
602-839-2000
FAX: 602-239-5868
www.bannerhealth.com

Steve Narang, MD, Chief Executive Officer
Lorraine Hudspeth, Controller
Letty Cerpa, Senior Accountant
Larry Mann, IT Manager

Nearly 1,700 physicians representing more than 50 specialties work with Banner Good Samaritan staff to care for more then 36,000 inpatients a year. Houses more then 650 licensed patient care beds. A teaching hospital that trains more then 220 physicians annually and a premier medical center in Arizona and the Southwest. Provides a comprehensive foundation of major programs and an equally impressive offering of highly specialized programs not availiable in most hospitals.

6423 Beacon Foundation for the Mentally Retarded
308 W. Glenn St.
Tucson, AZ 85703
520-622-4874
FAX: 520-620-6620
e-mail: sking@beacongroup.org
http://beacongroup.org

Steven R King, President
Chuck Tiller, Vice President Rehabilitation Se
Greg Natvig, Vice President of Business Opera
Michelle Kroeger, CFO

Committed to effectively assisting adults with disabilities to maximize their personal, social, vocational and educational skills in order to attain a successful and meaningful independence within the Tucson community.

6424 Carondelet Brain Injury Programs and Services (Bridges Now)
2202 N. Forbes Blvd.
Tucson, AZ 85745-2602
520-872-7324
FAX: 520-873-3743
e-mail: comments@carondelet.org
carondelet.org

Daisy M Jenkins, Executive VP, Chief HR/Administr
James K Beckmann, President/Chief Executive Officer
Alan Strauss, Executive VP, Finance and Chief Financial Officer
Christen Castellano, MBA, Executive VP and Chief Strategy Officer

Comprehensive outpatient rehabilitation program. PT, OT, ST, Psychology and Rehab Counseling Services.

6425 Desert Life Rehabilitation & Care Center
1919 W Medical St
Tucson, AZ 85704-1133
520-369-9620
FAX: 520-867-6612
www.desertlifercc.com

Amad Nazifi, Executive Director

Accomodates 240 residents. Provides skilled and intermediate nursing with occupational, physical, speech and respiratory therapy services. Offers special programs including an Alzheimer's Unit and a Young Adult program

6426 Freestone Rehabilitation Center
10617 E Oasis Drive
Mesa, AZ 85208
480-986-1531
FAX: 480-986-1538
e-mail: Marccenter.com
www.manta.com

Randy Gray, Executive Director
Cherie Vance, Manager

6427 HealthSouth Valley Of The Sun Rehabilitation Hospital
13460 N 67th Ave
Glendale, AZ 85304-1000
623-878-8800
FAX: 623-878-5254
healthsouth.com

Beth Bacher, Manager

A 60-bed free-standing hospital that offers acute physical rehabilitation, outpatient therapy services and day hospital treatment. Works in cooperation with local, regional and national managed care organizations and other sources to maximise patient recovery while conserving financial resources.

6428 Institute for Human Development
Northern Arizona University
912 Riordan Rd. P.O.Box 5630
Flagstaff, AZ 86011-5630
928-523-4791
FAX: 928-523-9127
TTY:928-523-1695
e-mail: ihd@nau.edu
www.nau.edu/ihd

Levi Esguerra, Director
Lisa Andrew, Advisory Commitee
Lynn Black, Advisory Commitee
Maria Bravo, Advisory Commitee

The Institute values and supports the independence, productivity and inclusion of Arizona's citizens with disabilities. Based on the values and beliefs, the Institute conducts training, research and services that further these goals.

6429 John C Lincoln Hospital North Mountain
250 E Dunlap Ave
Phoenix, AZ 85020-2871
602-943-2381
FAX: 602-944-8062
e-mail: webmaster@jcl.com
www.jcl.com/content/northmountain/default.htm

Rhonda Forsyth, President
Bruce Pearson, FACHE, Senior Vice President
Maggi Griffin, RN, MS, Vice President & Chief Executive Officer
Jessica Rivas, RN, MSN, Vice President and Chief Nursing Officer

Mission is to assist each person entrusted to our care to enjoy the fullest gift of health possible, and work with others to build a community where a helping hand is available for our most vulnerable members.

6430 La Frontera Center
504 W 29th St
Tucson, AZ 85713-3394
520-884-9920
FAX: 520-792-0654
www.lafronteraaz.org

Kevin Heath, Board Chair
Frank Valenzuela, Vice Chair
Celestino Fernandez, Treasurer
Susan Agrillo, Recording Secretary

A nonprofit community-based behavioral health agency that has been helping southern Arizona children, adults, and families since 1968.

6431 Manor Care Nursing and Rehab Center: Tucson
3705 N Swan Rd
Tucson, AZ 85718-6939
520-299-7088
FAX: 520-529-0038
www.hcr-manorcare.com

Clifton J. Porter II, Vice President - Government Rela
Martin Allen, Vice President

A leading provider of short-term post-acute medical care and rehabilitation and long-term skilled nursing care. High quality medical care is provided through registered (RN) and licensed practical (LPN) nurses and certified nursing assistants (CNA) in concert with physical, occupational and speech rehabilitation therapists. Our more then 275 skilled nursing centers are Medicare-and Medicaid-certified.

6432 Nova Care
Second Floor
680 American Avenue
King of Prussia, PA 19406-2607
800-331-8840
FAX: 602-256-7292
novacare.com

Scott Lusted, General Manager
Brian Beal, Market Manager

NovaCare Rehabilitation's highly respected clinical team provides preventative and rehabilitative services that maximize functionality and promote well-being. NovaCare Rehabilitation also provides physical therapy and athletic training services to more then 20 professional sports teams and 300 universities, colleges, and highschools thoughout the nation.

6433 Perry Rehabilitation Center
3146 E Windsor Avenue
Phoenix, AZ 85008-1199
602-956-0400
FAX: 602-957-7610
e-mail: perrycenter@qwest.net
www.azafh.com

Diana Casillas, Human Resources Director
Jim Musick, President

Provides services for people with disabilities, cognitive disabilities including residential services, day treatment, job training and job placement.

6434 Phoenix Veterans Center
Ste 100
1544 W. Grant St.
Phoenix, AZ 85004-1554
602-358-8494
FAX: 602-379-4130
www.azcremationcenter.com/?

Ken Benckwitz, Manager

Veterans medical clinic offering disabled veterans medical treatments.

6435 Progress Valley: Phoenix
10505 North 69th Street
Suite 1100
Paradise Valley, AZ 85253-6106
480-922-9427
FAX: 602-274-5473
e-mail: mailto:recovery@progressvalley.org
alcoholism.about.com

Susanne Lambert, Executive Director
Jennifer White, Director of Programs
Cathie Scott, Sober Housing Manager
Kristine Peltier, Finance Director

Residential aftercare for alcoholism and chemical dependency. Certified chemical dependency counselors provide individual treatment.

6436 Rehabilitation Services Administration
Suite 102
3425 East Van Buren
Phoenix, AZ 85008-3202
602-771-9100
800-563-1221
FAX: 602-250-8584
TTY: 855-475-8194
e-mail: azrsa@azdes.gov
azdes.gov/rsa

Katharine Levandowsky, Administrator

Provides a variety of specialized services to assist in removing barriers to employment and/or independent living for individuals with physical or mental disabilities. RSA offers 3 major service programs and several specialized programs/services.

6437 **Southern Arizona Association For The Visually Impaired**
3767 East Grant Rd
Tucson, AZ 85716-2935 520-795-1331
FAX: 520-795-1336
e-mail: reception@saavi.us
www.saavi.us

Michael Gordon, Executive Director
Amy Murillo, Associate Director
Carol Lopez, Finance Director
Lenetta Lefko, Tucson Services Manager
Offers health services, counseling, social work, home and personal management, computer training, low vision aids and more for the visually handicapped 18 years or older.

6438 **Toyei Industries**
Hc 58 Box 55
Ganado, AZ 86505-55 928-736-2417
888-45T-OYEI
FAX: 928-736-2495
www.yelp.com/biz/toyei-industries-inc-ganado-

Anthony Lincoln, CEO
Serves the needs of developmentally disabled and the severely mentally impaired adult citizens of the Navajo Nation and other Indian Nations. Staff of 60+ serves the needs of all the Navajo adults. Services include day treatment programs, and residential and group home services.

6439 **Yuma Center for the Visually Impaired**
328 W. Spears Street
Yuma, AZ 85365-6580 928-247-8890
FAX: 928-344-1863
https://www.azdes.gov

Calvin Roberts, Executive Director
Kathy Lucero, Store Manager
Dana Clayton, Human Resources Specialist
Lorraine Hudspeth, Controller
A private nonprofit agency offering services for totally blind and legally blind children and adults in the Arizona area.

Arkansas

6440 **Arkansas Lighthouse for the Blind**
P.O.Box 192666
6818 Murray St.
Little Rock, AR 72209- 2666 501-562-2222
FAX: 501-568-5275
e-mail: info@arkansaslighthouse.org
arkansaslighthouse.org

Bill Johnson, Chief Executive Officer
Danny Novielli, COO
John McAtee, Chief Financial Officer
Ronnie Cates, Director of Communications & Procurement
Manufacturer of textiles, apparel and paper products and employs blind and legally blind individuals.

6441 **Beverly Enterprises Network**
1 Thousand Beverly
Fort Smith, AR 72901-2629 479-201-2000
800-666-9996
FAX: 479-452-5131
www.yelp.com/biz/beverly-enterprises-inc-fort

Randy Churchey, CEO
Offers a progressive approach to subacute care. The goal of this organization is to assist injured and disabled individuals regain the level of independence to which they have been accustomed. Provides support and training programs, patient and family services and specialty programs for patients.

6442 **Easter Seals: Arkansas**
3920 Woodland Heights Rd
Little Rock, AR 72212-2495 501-227-3600
877-533-3700
FAX: 501-227-4021
TTY: 501-227-3686
e-mail: lrogers@ar.easterseals.com
www.eastersealsar.com

Sharon Moone-Jochums, President/ CEO
Linda Rogers, VP Programs
Michael E. Stock, Treasurer
Cindy Nash, Secretary
Their mission is to provide exceptional services to ensure that all people with disabilities or special needs have equal opportunities to live, learn, work and play in their communitites.

6443 **HealthSouth Rehabilitation Hospital Of Fort Smith**
1401 South J. Street
Fort Smith, AR 72901-5158 479-785-3300
FAX: 479-785-8599
healthsouth.com

Ryan Cassedy, CEO
Cygnet Schroeder, M.D., Medical Director
Donna Beallis, D.O., Director of Medical Management
Brandi Denham, Director of Human Resources
A free-standing 80-bed comprehensive physical medicine and rehabilitation hospital offering inpatient and outpatient services. Provides specialized medical and therapy services, designed to assist physically challenged persons to reach their highest level of independent function.

6444 **Lions World Services for the Blind**
2811 Fair Park Blvd
Little Rock, AR 72204-5044 501-664-7100
800-248-0734
FAX: 501-664-2743
e-mail: training@lwsb.org
www.wsblind.org/

Larry Dickerson, President/ CEO
Tony Woodell, President & Chief Executive Officer
Bill Smith, Director of Development
Melanie Jones, Marketing & Communications Director
Offers services in the areas of health education, recreation, rehabilitation, counseling, employment, computer training and more for all legally blind residents of the U.S. The staff includes 56 full time employees.

6445 **Little Rock Vet Center #0713**
Department of Veterans Affairs of Washington DC
Suite A
201 W Broadway St
North Little Rock, AR 72114- 5505 501-324-6395
877-927-8387
FAX: 501-324-6928
www.hud.gov/offices/cpd/about/hudvet/state/ar

Elizabeth N Ruggiero, Team Leader
Ida L Fogle, Counselor
Van A Hall, Counselor
Darryl A Lasker, Office Manager
Vet Center provides PTSD counseling to veterans of a combat zone. No medical care provided.

6446 **Timber Ridge Ranch NeuroRestorative Services**
4500 W Commerce Dr
North Little Rock, AR 72116 501-758-8799
800-743-6802
FAX: 501-758-8778
e-mail: neuroinfo@thementornetwork.com
www.neurorestorative.com

Bill Duffy, Chief Operating Officer
Michael E. Hofmeister, MS, MBA, Vice President of Operations
Sean Byrne, MBA, Chief Financial Officer
Roger P. Carrillo, M.Ed, Vice President of Business Development
Comprehensive, individualized services from a transdisciplinary team of licensed professionals assist clients along a course to greater independence. A separate team is dedicated to the needs of children, adolescents, and their families. A clinical team may include professionals from the disciplines of: behavior analysis,

neuropsychology, physiatry, psychology, speech-language pathology, occupational therapy, physical therapy, social work, couseling, education, nursing, and case management.

California

6447 **ARC Fresno-Kelso Activity Center**
4567 N Marty Ave
Fresno, CA 93722-7810
559-226-6268
FAX: 559-226-6269
e-mail: arcfresno@arcfresno.org
arcfresno.org

Lori Ramirez, Executive Director
Catherine Wooliever, Director of Human Resources
Jamie Marrash, Director of Program Services
Pamela Wirth, Director of Finance
The Arc Fresno is a private, non-profit 501(c)(3) organization who was founded in 1953. They provide services and supports for over 550 individuals with developmental disabilities throughout Fresno County. They currently offer eight (8) programs, and do so with the help of 145 employees.

6448 **ARC Of San-Diego-South Bay**
1280 Nolan Avenue
Chula Vista, CA 91911-3738
619-427-7524
FAX: 619-427-4657
e-mail: info@arc-sd.com
www.arc-sd.com/locations

Becky Thaller, Director
Steve Hojsan, Arc Enterprises Director
Michael Bruce, Workshop Manager
David W. Schneider, President & CEO
Provides remunerative work.

6449 **ARC Of Southeast Los Angeles-Southeast Industries**
9501 Washburn Rd
Downey, CA 90242-2913
562-803-1556
FAX: 562-803-4080
e-mail: sales@arcselac.org
www.arcselac.org/

6450 **ARC: VC Community Connections West**
5103 Walker Street
Ventura, CA 93003-7358
805-650-8611
FAX: 805-644-7308
www.arcvc.org

Robert Hogan, President
Gene West, First Vice President
Eve Liebman, Recording Secretary
Kathy Raffaelli, Treasurer
Caring and experienced staff is dedicated to serving participants with a variety of physical, mental and social disabilities who require a higher level of support and supervision. Using a person-centered planning approach, Arc Ventura County promotes self-directed services for all clients and families served. Adult development centers serve individuals with physical and mental disabilities, as well as people with challenging behaviors, who require assistance with basic skills such as self care.

6451 **ARC: VC Ventura**
5103 Walker Street
Ventura, CA 93003-7358
806-650-8611
FAX: 806-644-7308
www.arcvc.org

Robert Hogan, President
Gene West, First Vice President
Eve Liebman, Recording Secretary
Kathy Raffaelli, Treasurer
Arc Ventura County is a private, nonprofit organization that provides educational, vocational and residential services for people with developmental disabilities. Informed decisions, positive changes, and integration in the community are fundamental principals in all programs. As evidence of our programming excellence, Arc Ventura County has been accredited by CARF (The Rehabilitation Accreditation Commission.

6452 **AbilityFirst**
1300 E Green Street
Pasadena, CA 91106-2606
626-396-1010
877-768-4600
FAX: 626-396-1021
e-mail: info@abilityfirst.org
www.abilityfirst.org

Lori E. Gangemi, President
Steve S. Schultz, Chief Financial Officer
Keri Castaneda, Chief Program Officer
Syed Kazmi, Controller
AbilityFirst serves children and adults with special needs through 24 locations in Southern California.

6453 **Accentcare**
17855 North Dallas Pkwy
Dallas, TX 75287-2468
972-201-3800
800-834-3059
e-mail: info@accentcare.com
accentcare.com

Mark Pacala, Chairman of the Board and CEO (i
Vincent E. Cook, EVP and Chief Financial Officer
Melvin Warriner, SVP and Chief Culture Officer
Mel Deutsch, General Counsel
Postacute rehabilitation program: home care aides follow through with rehabilitation instructions given by physical, occupational and speech therapists. Other home care services are available, serving special needs for Alzheimer's, blind, brain injury, MS, ostomies, parkinsonism, spinal injury and stroke.

6454 **Anaheim Veterans Center**
859, South Harbor Blvd
Anaheim, CA 92805-4680
714-776-0161
800-225-8387
FAX: 714-776-8904
e-mail: anaheimvetcenter@yahoo.com
www.longbeach.va.gov/visitors/vet_center.asp

6455 **Association for Retarded Citizens: Alameda County**
1101 Walpert St
Hayward, CA 94541-3721
510-582-8151
FAX: 510-639-4684
www.sbn.com

Ram Sirck, Director
Offers the Right Track program in which selected workers are grouped together on a contract basis to maximize work productivity. Provides a full benefit package, as well as a permanent supervisor. A worker is matched to a job of at least 20 hours per week and then trained by the staff of The Right Track.

6456 **Azure Acres Recovery Center**
5777 Madison Avenue
Suite 1210
Sacramento, CA 95841-9034
877-977-3755
877-762-3735
FAX: 707-823-8972
e-mail: info@azureacres.com
azureacres.com

Joe Tinervin, MSW, Executive Director
Michael Roeske, Psy.D., Clinical Director
Christie Splitstone, MA, Counselor/Case Manager
James Canter, CATC, Counselor/Case Manager
Offers rehabilitation services and residential care for the person with an alcohol or drug abuse related problems.

6457 **Back in the Saddle**
2 BITS Trail
P.O. Box 3336
Chelmsford, MA 01824-0936
800-865-2478
877-756-5068
FAX: 800-866-3235
e-mail: help@BackInTheSaddle.com
www.thesaddle.com

Richard Smith PhD, Owner
Erika Reed, Co-Director
A long term community residential facility for head injured adults. House parents live on-site; and oversee a variety of programs which are individually designed and might include classes

in community college, placement in a workshop or on a workstation, volunteer positions and home skills assignments. Recreational outing range from horseback riding to weekend camping. Apartment programs available as set-up. Price: $2800-$3000 per month.

6458 **Ballard Rehabilitation Hospital**
1760 W 16th St
San Bernardino, CA 92411-1150
909-473-1200
800-761-1226
FAX: 909-473-1276
www.ballardrehab.com

Edward C. Palacios, RN,MPH, Administrator
Mary Hunt, Chief Operating Officer
Patty Meinhardt, Director Marketing/Admissions

Ballard Rehab Hospital is a free standing specialty hospital and provides the complete continuum of acute rehabilitation and outpatient rehabilitation, dedicated to providing rehab care to adults and children. The following inpatient and outpatient programs are available: CNA (Stroke) Rehab; Spinal Cord Injury Rehab; Brain Injury Rehab; Pain Management Rehab; Bariatric program, pulmonary program, injured Worker Programs; and Post Amputation Rehab.

6459 **Bayview Nursing and Rehabilitation**
516 Willow Street
Alameda, CA 94501-6132
510-521-5600
FAX: 510-865-6441
TTY:800-735-2922
e-mail: kleger.org@comcast.net.
http://www.bayviewnursing.com/

Richard S Espinoza, Administrator

Offers a full range of medical services to meet the individual needs of our residents, including short-term rehabilitative services and long termed skilled care. Working with the resident's physician, our staff-including medical specialists, nurses, nutritionists, dietitians, and social workers-establishes a comprehensive treatment plan intended to restore you or your loved one to the highest practicable potential.

6460 **Belden Center**
606 Humboldt St
Santa Rosa, CA 95404-4219
707-579-2735
FAX: 707-579-4145

Casey Harding, Owner
Pamela Fadden, Owner

Postacute rehabilitation program.

6461 **Blind Babies Foundation**
Suite 300
1814 Franklin St
Oakland, CA 94612-3487
510-446-2229
FAX: 510-446-2262
e-mail: bbfinfo@blindbabies.org
blindbabies.org

Dottie Bridge, President
Aben Hill, 1st Vice President
Clare Friedman, PhD, 2nd Vice President
Beverly Libaire, Treasurer

Mission: when an infant or pre school child is identified as blind or visually impaired, provides family-centered services to support the child's optimal development and access to the world.

6462 **Brotman Medical Center: RehabCare Unit**
Brotman Medical Center
3828 Delmas Terrace
Culver City, CA 90232-2713
310-836-7000
800-677-1238
FAX: 310-202-4105
e-mail: info@brotmanmed.com
phvc.com

Jennifer Cortez, Program Manager
Kevin O'Connor, CEO
Scott Leonard, CTO
Ben Taylor, Senior Editor

Culver City is centrally located within the city of Los Angeles. These are two programs offering inpatient rehabilitation. The acute rehab program is designed for patients who need physical rehabilitation due to injury or medical disability. This program requires patients to participate in 3 hours therapy per day. The sub-acute program is designed especially for patients who need rehab but cannot tolerate the intensity of the acute rehab program..

6463 **Build Rehabilitation Industries**
12432 Foothill Blvd
Sylmar, CA 91342
818-898-0020
FAX: 818-898-1949
buildindustries.com

6464 **California Elwyn**
18325 Mt. Baldy Circle
Fountain Valley, CA 92708-6115
714-557-6313
FAX: 714-963-2961
e-mail: info@elwyn.org
elwyn.org

Sandra S. Cornelius, President of Elwyn
Daniel M. Reardon, Senior Vice President and Chief Operating Officer
Stan H. Retif, Vice President for Development a
Richard T. Smith, Vice President for Information Technology

Provides opportunities for people challenged by physical and mental disabilities who are 18 or older. California Elwyn develops an Individual Rehabilitation Plan for all consumers. Contract work, shrinkwrap, janitorial are just some of the types of jobs done. Supported Employment Services are available and over 100 consumers currently are employed. Funded by the State Department of Rehabilitation and Vocational Rehabilitation.

6465 **California Eye Institute**
1360 E Herndon Ave
Fresno, CA 93720-3326
559-449-5000
www.samc.com

Nancy Hollingsworth, President and CEO
Michael W. Martinez, EVP/Chief Operating and Financial Officer
Stephen Soldo, Chief Medical Officer
Christine Sarrico, Chief Financial Officer

A private, nonprofit agency offering services such as health, educational, recreational, rehabilitation and employment counseling to the totally blind, legally blind and visually impaired. The staff includes two full time workers.

6466 **Camp Recovery Center**
3192 Glen Canyon Rd
Scotts Valley, CA 95066-4916
877-557-6237
FAX: 831-438-2789
camprecovery.com

Michael Johnson, Ph.D, Executive Director
Tim Sinnott, Clinical Director
Zoe R., Case Manager
Jeff Geiger, Clinical Tech Director

A free-standing social model recovery center for chemical dependency located on 25 wooded acres in the Santa Cruz Mountains. The services include: medical detoxification, complete medical evaluation, psychiatric evaluation and counseling, psychological testing, individual counseling and more. Helps the recovery from chemical dependency in a easier, warm and caring environment.

6467 **Campobello Chemical Dependency Recovery Center**
2448 Guerneville Road
Suite 400
Santa Rosa, CA 95402- 4030
707-546-1547
800-805-1833
FAX: 707-579-1603
campobello.org

6468 **Casa Colina Centers for Rehabilitation**
P.O.Box 6001
255 East Bonita Avenue
Pomona, CA 91767- 6001 909-596-7733
866-724-4127
FAX: 909-593-0153
TTY: 909-596-3646
casacolina.org

Steve Norin, Chairman
Felice L Loverso, President
Chandrahas Agarwal, Medical Director
Elmer B. Pineda, M.D., Chief Of Medical Staff
Casa Colina, has pioneered effective programs to create opportunity for health, productivity and self-esteem for persons with disability since 1936. Through medical rehabilitation, transitional living, residential, community, and prevention and wellness programs. Casa Colina serves more than 7,000 persons annually. Casa Colina, a non-profit organization, offers a unique spectrum of opportunities, achievement and results to patients and their families.

6469 **Casa Colina Padua Village**
P.O.Box 6001
255 East Bonita Avenue
Pomona, CA 91767- 6001 909-596-7733
866-724-4127
FAX: 909-593-0153
TTY: 909-596-3646
casacolina.org

Steve Norin, Chairman
Chandrahas Agarwal, Medical Director
Felice L Loverso, President
Elmer B. Pineda, M.D., Chief Of Medical Staff
Long term residential services for adults with developmental disability. Residences include Malmquist House, Woodbend House, and Hillsdale House, all located in Claremont, California.

6470 **Casa Colina Residential Services: Rancho Pino Verde**
Casa Colina Center for Rehabilitation
P.O.Box 6001
255 East Bonita Avenue
Pomona, CA 91767- 7517 909-596-7733
866-724-4127
FAX: 909-593-0153
TTY: 909-596-3646
www.casacolina.org

Steve Norin, Chairman
Randy Blackman, Vice Chairman
Felice L. Loverso, President
Elmer B. Pineda, M.D., Chief Of Medical Staff
Long term residential services in rural environment for adults with brain injury.

6471 **Casa Colina Transitional Living Center**
255 East Bonita Avenue
P.O.Box 6001
Pomona, CA 91767- 1923 909-596-7733
866-724-4127
FAX: 909-593-0153
TTY: 909-596-3646
casacolina.org

Steve Norin, Chairman
Felice L Loverso, President
Chandrahas Agarwal, Medical Director
Elmer B. Pineda, M.D., Chief Of Medical Staff
Postacute rehabilitation program.

6472 **Casa Colina Transitional Living Center: Pomona**
P.O.Box 6001
255 East Bonita Avenue
Pomona, CA 91767- 6001 909-596-7733
866-724-4127
FAX: 909-593-0153
TTY: 909-596-3646
casacolina.org

Steve Norin, Chairman
Felice L Loverso, President
Chandrahas Agarwal, Medical Director
Elmer B. Pineda, M.D., Chief Of Medical Staff
Post acute short term residential program for persons with brain injury. In a home-like setting, therapy promotes successful re-entry to home and community living.

6473 **Cedars of Marin**
PO Box 947
Ross, CA 94957-947 415-454-5310
FAX: 415-454-0573
e-mail: lauren@thecedarsofmarin.org
thecedarsofmarin.org

Jefferson Rice, Board Chair
James Brentano, Board Vice President
Andrew Hinkelman, Board Treasurer
Chuck Greene, Executive Director
The Cedars of Marin has provided residential and day programs for adults with developmental disabilities for over 91 years. Our award-winning programs help our clients to live creative, productive, joyous lives.

6474 **Center for Neuro Skills**
5215 Ashe Rd.
Bakersfield, CA 93313-2988 661-872-3408
800-922-4994
FAX: 661-872-5150
e-mail: skatomski@neuroskills.com
neuroskills.com

Mark J Ashley, President/CEO and Co-Founder
A comprehensive, post-acute, community based head-injury rehabilitation program serving over 100 clients per year. Since 1980, CNS has effectively treated the entire spectrum of head-injured clients, including those with severe behavioral disorders, cognitive/perceptual impairments, speech/language problems, physical disabilities and post-concussion syndrome.

6475 **Center for the Partially Sighted**
Suite 150
6101 W. Centinela Ave.
Culver City, CA 90230 310-988-1970
FAX: 310-988-1980
e-mail: info@low-vision.org
low-vision.org

La Donna S. Ringering, Ph.D, President/CEO
Pam Thompson, Director of Psychological Servic
Phyllis Amaral, Clinical Director
Laura Valencia, Psychosocial Services Coordinato
Services for partially sighted and legally blind people include low vision evaluations, the design and prescription of low vision devices and adaptive technology, as well as counseling and rehabilitation training (independent living skills and orientation/mobility training). Special programs include children's program, diabetes and vision loss program, Technology demonstrations. Store carries low vision aids. Catalog available.

6476 **Central Coast Neurobehavioral Center OPTIONS**
P.O.Box 877
800 Quintana Road Suite 2C
Morro Bay, CA 93442-877 805-772-6066
FAX: 805-772-6067
e-mail: info@optionsccnbc.org
www.optionsccnbc.org

Michael Mamot, CEO
Ole von Frausing-Borch, COO
Serves adults with developmental disabilities, traumatic head injuries, or other neurological impairments. OPTIONS operates two transitional living centers, eight licensed residential facilities, two licensed community integration day programs and a li-

censed short term stabilization center. Services offered include: supported and independent living services, group and individual vocational services, neuropsychological assessment, occupational therapy, cognitive therapy, speech therapy and more.

6477 Cerebral Palsy: North County Center
#209
8525 Gibbs Drive
San Diego, CA 92123-1758 858-571-7803
FAX: 858-571-0919
e-mail: info@ucpsd.org
www.ucpsd.org

David Carucci, Executive Director
Mary Krieger, Associate Executive Director
Bruce Neufeld, Chief Financial Officer
Sophia Williams, Director of Human Resources

The mission of UCP San Diego County is to advance the independence, productivity and full citizenship of people affected by cerebral palsy and other disabilities. By making solid steps, UCP can build a better community for all in the process.

6478 Children's Hospital Central California Rehabilitation Center
9300 Valley Childrens Place
Madera, CA 93636-8762 559-353-3000
www.valleychildrens.org

Todd Suntrapak, President & Chief Executive Officer
David Christensen, MD, SVP Medical Affairs & Chief Medical Officer
Beverly Hayden-Pugh, Vice President & Chief Nursing Officer
Kirk Larson, Vice President & Chief Informati

A 297-bed pediatric medical center on a 50-acre campus. We now have more then 500 doctors practicing in over 40 pediatric subspecialties with clinics and services throughout the state.

6479 Children's Hospital Los Angeles Rehabilitation Program
4650 W Sunset Blvd
Los Angeles, CA 90027-6062 323-361-4155
888-631-2452
FAX: 323-361-8101
e-mail: webmaster@chla.usc.edu
www.childrenshospitalla.org

Richard D. Cordova, President & CEO
Rodney B. Hanners, Senior Vice President and Chief
Henri R. Ford, M.D.
Lawrence L. Foust, J.D.,, Secretary

Designated as a Level I Pediatric Trauma Canter by the Los Angeles County EMS Agency, the hospital treats more then 1,500 pediatric trauma patients per year. Performs more then 13,900 pediatric surgeries a year, including more complex surgical procedures then any other hospital in Southern California

6480 Children's Therapy Center
Ste 120
770 Paseo Camarillo
Camarillo, CA 93010-6092 805-383-1501
FAX: 805-383-1504
e-mail: ctcinc@islc.net

Beth Maulhardt, Owner

Provides individual occupational therapy, speech/language therapy, family/child consulting, education services and physical therapy consultation for children. Evaluations and treatment are on an individual basis and special emphasis is placed on a multidisciplinary approach with information sharing, and often team treatment.

6481 Clausen House
88 Vernon Street
Oakland, CA 94610-4217 510-839-0050
e-mail: info@clausenhouse.org
clausenhouse.org

Deborah Levy, Interim Executive Director
Michael A. Scott, Director of Development
Stan Nicholson, Director of Human Resources
Jaynette Underhill, Director of Program Services

Residential, supported employment, independent and supported living, adult education, and social recreation activities. Serving the developmentally disabled since 1967.

6482 Community Gatepath
1764 Marco Polo Way
Burlingame, CA 94010-4503 650-259-8544
e-mail: helpmychild@gatepath.com
communitygatepath.com

Sheryl Young, Chief Executive Officer
John Marvuqlio, Chief Financial Officer
Gabrielle Karampelas, Vice President of Strategic Initiatives & Collaborations
Anne Jarchow, Director of Internal Communications and Culture

Popular center and Peninsula Care merged into a new organization named Community Gatepath. Driving forces behind the merger were to be able to provide expanded and/or better services to indidviduals throughout San Mateo County, using the best practices of both organizations.

6483 Community Hospital and Rehabilitation Center of Los Gatos-Saratoga
815 Pollard Rd
Los Gatos, CA 95032-1438 408-378-6131
FAX: 408-866-4003
communityhospitallosgatos.com

Gary Honts, CEO

Offers rehabilitation services, inpatient and outpatient care, physical therapy, occupational therapy and more for the physically challenged adult. We have a commitment to health care excellence. It is in this commitment that we have dedicated ourselves to provide personal and professional service to our patients. Our goal is to work closely with staff, physicians and the community to attain shared goals and positive changes, now and in the future..

6484 Contra Costa ARC
1340 Arnold Drive
Suite 127
Martinez, CA 94553-4189 925-370-1818
FAX: 925-370-2048
e-mail: feedback@arcofcc.org
www.ContraCostaARC.com

Barbara Maizie, Executive Director
Diana Jorgensen, Program Coordinator
Andrey George, Administrative Coordinator

A private nonprofit membership-based organization dedicated to enhancing the quality of life of individuals with mental retardation and other developmental disabilities.

6485 Corona Regional Medical Center- Rehabiltation Center
800 S. Main St.
Corona, CA 92882-3117 951-737-4343
FAX: 951-736-7276
www.coronaregional.com

Diane Mc Donald, Manager
Mark Uffer, Chief Executive Officer
Doreen Dann, Chief Nursing Officer
Douglas Crouse, Chairman of the Board

Offers inpatient and outpatient rehabilitation services. The Center consists of an acute rehab unit, a subacute rehab unit containing modules for long-term ventilator care, respiratory rehab, coma intervention and orthopedics. In addition to inpatient therapies, the Center's outpatient programs include sports and industrial medicine.

6486 Critical Air Medicine
Montgomery Field
8775 Aero Drive
Suite 235
San Diego, CA 92123-1705 858-300-0224
800-247-8326
FAX: 858-300-0228
e-mail: criticalair.ops@criticalair.com
www.aircharterguide.com

Frank Craven, Publisher of the Air Charter Guide

Offers emergency medical care by air medical transport carriers. These carriers are fully equipped with medical equipment and supplies for cardiovascular emergencies, respiratory supplies, orthopedic supplies and medications..

6487 Crutcher's Serenity House
P.O.Box D
50 Hillcrest Drive
Deer Park, CA 94576-504 707-963-3192
FAX: 707-963-2309
e-mail: crutcherssh@earthlink.net
www.crutcherssh.com
Robert Crutcher, Owner/CEO
Lu Crutcher, Executive Director
A privately owned and operated facility that introduces to residents a new lifestyle free of all chemicals, and a new awareness of their total being. The length of the program is four weeks and is within five minutes of an acute care hospital. The Center is licensed for 19 beds, male and female located in a home-like setting with an emphasis on maintaining a family atmosphere.

6488 Daniel Freeman Rehabilitation Centers
333 N Prairie Ave
PO Box 28990
Santa Ana, CA 92799-4501 714-230-3150
FAX: 714-850-0153
e-mail: advertising@acupuncturetoday.com
www.acupuncturetoday.com
H Arndt, Associate Administrator
Gabrielle Lindsley, Business Development Manager
Evelyn Petersen, Human Resources / Payroll Manager
Andrea Weeks, Accountant
Comprehensive rehabilitation services which address needs and issues of the physically diabled and their families. We offer accute input rehabilitation, outpatient and short term skilled nursing rehabilitaion. Specialty areas include: brain injury, stroke, spinal chord injury, chronic pain, arthritis..

6489 Delano Regional Medical Center
1401 Garces Highway
Delano, CA 93215-3690 661-725-4800
e-mail: info@drmc.com
drmc.com
Bahram Ghaffari, President
Jeremy Klemm, HealthStream Regional Director
Robert A. Frist, HealthStream CEO
Delano Regional Medical Center (DRMC) is proud to be known throughout California & beyond as an innovative regional hospital, deeply rooted in the local communities and committed to providing an exceptional patient experience. A non-profit acute-care facility serving a region of 10 rural central Californiatowns. With over 100 physicians on our active medical staff and additional courtesy or consulting physicians, patients are assured of receiving high-quality care in multiple specialties.

6490 Desert Regional Medical Center
1150 N Indian Canyon Dr
Palm Springs, CA 92262 760-323-6511
800-491-4990
www.desertmedctr.com
Carolyn Caldwell, Chief Executive Officer
Tracey Cowles, Physician Relations Manager
Jeanne Stanton, RN, Chair
Lee Bledsoe, Physician Relations Manager
Our dedicated physicians and caregivers provide a broad array of quality programs and services, including comprehensive cancer care, women's health services, heart care, surgical weight loss reduction and orthopedics.

6491 Devereux California
P.O.Box 6784
Santa Barbara, CA 93160-6784 805-968-2525
FAX: 805-968-3247
e-mail: johnso3@devereux.org
www.devereux.org
Amy Evans, M.F.T., Executive Director
Commodore Dixon, Marketing & Admissions Manager
Janis Johnson, Manager of External Affairs
Alan Purucker, Clinical Case Manager
Serves adults age 18 through life span, who have intellectual and developmental disabilities, emotional disturbances, neurological impairments, brain injuries, schizophrenia, autism, and dual diagnosis. Devereux California currently provides a continuum of services, including on-campus residential, day programs, behavior management, and supported living services in the community.

6492 Division of Physical Medicine and Rehabilitation
San Joaquin General Hospital
500 W Hospital Rd
French Camp, CA 95231-9693 209-468-6000
FAX: 209-468-6501
e-mail: pmradministration@sjgh.hs.co.san-joaquin.ca.u
www.sjphysicalmedicine.com

6493 Dr. Karen H Chao Developmental Optometry Karen H. Chao. O.D.
Suite A
121 S Del Mar Ave
San Gabriel, CA 91776-1345 626-287-0401
FAX: 626-287-1457
e-mail: drkhchao@yahoo.com
www.healthgrades.com
Karen Chao, Owner
Karen Chao OD, Owner
Roger C. Holstein, Chief Executive Officer
Jeff Surges, President
Developmental optometrist specializing in the testing and treatment of vision problems and the enhancement of visual performance. Performs visual perceptual testing and training for children and adults. Undetected vision problems interfere with the ability to achieve and are highly correlated with learning difficulties and developmental problems. Provides the opportunity to overcome vision and visual-perceptual dysfunctions..

6494 Early Childhood Services
Desert Area Resources and Training
201 E Ridgecrest Blvd
Ridgecrest, CA 93555-3919 760-375-9787
FAX: 760-375-1288
e-mail: dart@dartontarget.org
www.dartontarget.org/
Peter V. Berns, Chief Executive Officer
Cris Bridges, Chief of Client Services
Bob Beecroft, Chief Operations Officer
Jeannie Luke, Human Resources Director/Risk Ma
Provides early intervention services to children who have disabilities or are experiencing delays in development. Provides developmental activities to promote the attainment of developmental milestones so that each child may reach his/her maximum potential. The program also provides therapeutic and educational intervention and offers support and guidance to families.

6495 East Los Angeles Doctors Hospital
4060 Whittier Boulevard
Los Angeles, CA 90023-2526 323-268-5514
www.elalax.com
Hector Hernandez, Chief Executive Officer
Kamlesh Dhawan, Chief Of Staff
Michael Austerlitz, Vice-Chief Of Staff
Horacio Fleischman, Secretary Treasurer
Postacute rehabilitation program.

6496 Easter Seals Disability Svcs: Bay Area
Suite 250
391 Taylor Boulevard
Pleasant Hill, CA 94523- 4851
925-849-8999
800-221-6827
FAX: 312-726-1494
e-mail: info@easterseals.com
www.bayarea.easterseals.com

6497 Easter Seals Superior California
Sacramento Center & Regional Offices
2617 A & B Alta Arden Expy.
Sacramento, CA 95825-1306
916-679-3113
888-877-3257
FAX: 916-485-2653
www.superiorca.easterseals.com
Harry Johns, President and CEO
Kathie Wright, Program Director
Terry Colborn, VP Programs/Government Affairs
Joanne Budge, Chief Financial Officer
Provides outpatient rehabilitation services including day training programs for adults with disabilities and traumatic brain injuries, warm water therapy, non-public agency services to children including pediatric OT and PT services, work training/employment services, medical equipment loans, early intervention services for infants and toddlers. Serving the counties of Alpine, Calaveras, El Dorado, Sacramento, San Joaquin, Sutter, Tuolumne, Yolo, Yuba, Amador, Stanislaus, Nevada and Placer, CA.

6498 Exceed: A Division of Valley Resource Center
P.O.Box 1773
1285 N. Santa Fe
Hemet, CA 92543-1773
951-766-8659
800-423-1227
FAX: 951-929-9758
e-mail: vrctwohip@aol.com
www.exceed-solutions.org
Pattie Robert, Business Development Specialist
Mary Morse, Marketing Director
Kathy Cooke, Manager
Our vision is an environment where each client is valued as an individual and is provided the opportunity to reach his/her maximum potential. Our mission is to provide service and advocacy, which creates choices and opportunities, for adults with disabilities to reach their maximum potential.

6499 Eye Medical Center of Fresno
Eye Medical Center
1360 E. Herndon Avenue
Suite 301 & 210
Fresno, CA 93720-1498
559-486-5000
emcfresno.com

6500 Fontana Rehabilitation Workshop
Industrial Support Systems
8333 Almeria Ave
Fontana, CA 92335-3283
909-428-3883
800-755-4755
FAX: 909-428-3835
e-mail: ceo@industrialsupport.org
www.industrial-support.org
Silvia Anderson, Executive Director
U. Jones, CFO
C.Steven Bowen Plant, Operations manager
Bonnie Edwards, Operations Manager
The Fontana Rehabilitation Workshop, Inc., through its business divisions is committed to maintaining a stable environment wherein people with disabilities are provided with those services and supports that enable them to overcome barriers to employment and empower them to maximize their employment potential.

6501 Foothill Vocational Opportunities
789 North Fair Oaks Avenue
Pasadena, CA 91103-3045
626-449-0218
FAX: 626-449-0218
e-mail: info@foothillvoc.org
foothillvoc.org

6502 Fred Finch Youth Center
3800 Coolidge Ave
Oakland, CA 94602-3399
510-482-2244
FAX: 510-488-1960
e-mail: receptionist@fredfinch.org
fredfinch.org
Vonza Thompson, President/CEO
Kathie Jacobson, COO
Ed Hsu, CFO
Sue Guy, Chief Human Resource Officer
Seeks to provide a continuum of high quality programs for the care and treatment of children, youth, young adults and their families, whose changing needs can best be met by a variety of mental health and social services. The goal is for clients to be professionally served in the least restricitive environment appropriate to their needs so that they may function at their highest potential.

6503 Gateway Center of Monterey County
850 Congress Ave
Pacific Grove, CA 93950-4898
831-372-8002
FAX: 831-372-2411
e-mail: info@gatewaycenter.org
gatewaycenter.org
Stephanie Lyon, Executive Director
Mike Price, Chief Financial Officer
Desiree Boller, Accounting Assistant
Heidy Welch, Human Resources
Our mission is to be a caring and stimulating environment for the Developmentally Disabled where all people can achieve their individual goals safely and with dignity. Our goal is to continue our programs and to find new and innovative ways of assisting the developmentally disabled to live in our community in surroundings compatable with their ability to live and work at the highest level possible.

6504 Gateway Industries: Castroville
7055 Veterans Blvd
Unit A
Burr Ridge, IL 60527
630-321-1333
888-473-3744
FAX: 630-321-1321
e-mail: growth@redshft.com
www.redshift.com

6505 Gilroy Workshop
7471 Monterey Street
Gilroy, CA 95020-3629
408-430-2810
FAX: 408-842-6770
e-mail: info@leadershipgilroy.org
www.leadershipgilroy.org/
Kristi Alarid, Manager
Sally French, Manager
Denise Martin, Executive Director
Andrea Gamble, Administrative Director
Work adjustment and remunerative work programs..

6506 Glendale Adventist Medical Center
1509 Wilson Ter
Glendale, CA 91206-4098
818-409-8000
FAX: 818-546-5609
www.glendaleadventist.com/services/rehab
Kevin Roberts, President/CEO
Warren Tetz, Sr. Vice President and COO
Kelly Turner, Sr. Vice President and CFO
Judy Blair, Sr. Vice President and CNO
Rehabilitative team is made up of physician specialists, as well as professional and certified staff nurses, thereapists and others who meet regularly to ensure tht each patients progress is carefully planned and closely monitored.

6507 Glendale Memorial Hospital and Health Center Rehabilitation Unit
Glendale Memorial Hospital and Health Center
1420 South Central Ave
Glendale, CA 91204-2508
818-502-1900
FAX: 818-409-7688
www.glendalememorialhospital.org

Catherine M. Pelley, President
Offers rehabilitation services, occupational therapy, physical therapy, residential services and more for the disabled.

6508 Goleta Valley Cottage Hospital
Cottage Health System
351 S Patterson Ave
Santa Barbara, CA 93111-2496
805-967-3411
FAX: 805-681-6437
e-mail: cverkiak@cottagehealthsystem.org
www.sbch.org

Ronald C. Wreft, President & CEO
Rosemary Bray, Clinical Manager
Diana Gray Miller, Administrator
Betty Jane Petrich, Manager
A 122-bed acute care hospital was founded in 1966 to serve the growing community of Goleta Valley. Today, we admit more then 2,000 patients a year, see more then 17,000 emergency visits, and welcome nearly 400 newborns to our designated 'Baby Friendly' Birth Center each year. We are also recognized for our Level IV trauma designation. We take great pride in fulfilling our goal of providing each patient with comfortable, personalized care.

6509 HealthSouth Tustin Rehabilitation Hospital
Health South Corporation
14851 Yorba St
Tustin, CA 92780-2925
714-832-9200
www.tustinrehab.com/

Diana Hanyak, Chief Executive Officer
Rodric Bell, Medical Director
Lindsey Barrett, Director of Case Management
Maryam Jouharzadeh, Pharm.D., Director, Pharmacy
HealthSouth Tustin Rehabilitation Hospital is part of the HealthSouth Corporation, the nation's largest provider of rehabilitative healthcare services, we are the only facility of its kind in Orange County. Fully accredited by the Joint Commission on Accreditation of Healthcare Organizations (JACHO) we provide inpatient and outpatient care designed to meed individual needs of patients and their families.

6510 Hi-Desert Medical Center
6601 White Feather Road
Joshua Tree, CA 92252-760
760-366-3711
hdmc.org

Lionel Chadwick, Chief Executive Officer
Tom Duda, Chief Financial Officer
Judy Austin, Chief Operating Officer & Chief
Barbara Staresinic, Director, Human Resources
Postacute rehabilitation program.

6511 Home of the Guiding Hands
Suite 200
1825 Gillespie Way
El Cajon, CA 92020-0501
619-938-2850
FAX: 619-938-3055
e-mail: info@guidinghands.org
guidinghands.org

Mary Miller, President
Debby McNeil, Vice President
Michael Harris, Treasurer
Mark Klaus, Executive Director
The mission of Home og the Guiding Hands is to provide quality services, training and advocacy for people with developmental disabilities, their families, and others who will benefit.

6512 Hospital of the Good Samaritan Acute Rehabilitation Unit
1225 Wilshire Blvd
Los Angeles, CA 90017-1901
213-977-2121
800-366-8338
FAX: 213-482-2770
e-mail: info@goodsam.org
goodsam.org

Andrew B Leeka, President and CEO
Charles T. Munger, Chairman
Physicians, researchers and staff are united by a common mission: to foster growth into one of the most comprehensive medical centers in the West. Services offered include: cardiology and cardiovascular services, neurosciences, movement disorders and Parkinsons disorder, wound care center and transfusion-medicine and surgery center.

6513 Innovative Rehabilitation Services
Hacienda La Puente Unified School District
15959 E. Gale Ave
City Of Industry, CA 91745
626-933-1000
FAX: 626-934-2900
e-mail: info@hlpusd.k12.ca.us
www.hlpusd.k12.ca.us

Matthew Smith, Site Administrator
George Stransky, Counselor
Crystal Ontiveros, Counselor
Provides innovative student-centered learning opportunities and support services to a diverse population that enable individuals to achieve thier goals as lifelong learners, productive workers and effective communicators.

6514 Janus of Santa Cruz
Suite 150
200 7th Ave
Santa Cruz, CA 95062-4669
831-462-1060
866-526-8772
janussc.org

Rod Libbey, Executive Director
Bill Morris, Medical Director
Margie Storms, Clinical Director
Chris Storms, Intake Manager
A private not-for-profit corporation, licensed by the state of California. The Janus Clinic has a 3 year accreditation by the Council on Accreditation for Health Care Facilities.

6515 John Muir Medical Center Rehabilitation Services, Therapy Center
1601 Ygnacio Valley Rd
Walnut Creek, CA 94598-3122
925-939-3000
FAX: 925-308-8944
www.johnmuirhealth.com

Calvin Knight, President and CEO
Helen Doughty, Librarian
A 324-bed acute care facility that is designated as the only trauma center for Contra Costa County and portions of Solano County. Recognized as one of the region's premier healthcare providers, areas of specialty include high-and low-risk obstetrics, orthopedics, neurosciences, cardiac care and cancer care. The campus is accredited by the Joint Commission on Accreditation of Healthcare Organizations (JCAHO), a national surveyor of quality patient care.

6516 Kindred Hospital-La Mirada
14900 E. Imperial Hwy
La Mirada, CA 90638-2172
562-944-1900
FAX: 562-906-3455
TTY:800-735-2922
www.kindredlamirada.com

April Myers, Administrator
Adam Darvish, Executive Director
Committed to the delivery of high quality care in a cost-effective manner to enable us to become 'a model of excellence' in Long-Term Acute Care. Committed to treat our patients and families with dignity and respect, in the same manner we would want to be treated.

6517 King's View Work Experience Center- Atwater
559 East Bardsley Avenue
P. O. Box 688
Tulare, CA 93275-0688
559-688-7531
FAX: 559-688-3509
e-mail: info@kingsview.org
www.kingsview.org

Leon Hoover, Chief Executive Officer
Vida Jalali, Chief Financial Officer Interim
Sue Essman, Director of Human Resources
Jeff Gorski, Director of Business Development

The primary mission of the Kings View Work Experience Center (KVWEC) is to serve people who have developmental disabilities. We believe in the dignity and worth of each person and in their right to rehabilitation, education and community integration. It is Kings View's aim to provide quality services to people who need assistance in the development of social, vocational and independent living skills.

6518 LaPalma Intercommunity Hospital
7901 Walker St
La Palma, CA 90623-1764
714-670-7400
e-mail: LPIHInfo@primehealthcare.com
www.lapalmaintercommunityhospital.com

Virg Narbutas, Regional CEO
Sami Shoukair, Chief Medical Officer
Linda Gonzaba, Medical Staff Office Director
Hilda Manzo-Luna, Chief Nursing Officer

Lapalma Intercommunity Hospital endeavors to provide comprehensive, quality healthcare in a convenient, compassionate and cost effective manner. Lapalma is consistenty at the forefront of evolving national healthcare reform. Our organization provides an innovative and integrated healthcare delivery system. We remain ever cognizant of our patient's needs and desires for high quality affordable healthcare.

6519 Learning Services of Northern California
131 Langley Drive
Suite B
Lawrenceville, GA 30046-9315
408-848-4379
888-419-9955
FAX: 866-491-7396
www.learningservices.com

Dr. Debra Braunling-McMorrow, President and CEO
Jeanne Mack, Chief Financial Officer and Vice President of Operations
Michael Weaver, Chief Development Officer
Susan Snow, Director of Admissions

Located on 10 acres of ranchland in rural Santa Clara Valley, our Gilroy Program offers treatment, structure, and support in a spacious, campus-based living environment. Sharing living residences are complimented by a treatment and recreation facility for individuals who require intensive support.

6520 Learning Services: Morgan Hill
131 Langley Drive
Suite B
Lawrenceville, GA 30046-9315
408-848-4379
888-419-9955
FAX: 866-491-7396
www.learningservices.com

Dr. Debra Braunling-McMorrow, President and CEO
Jeanne Mack, Chief Financial Officer and Vice President of Operations
Michael Weaver, Chief Development Officer
Susan Snow, Director of Admissions

Located in the quaint rural town within walking distance from the old main street of Morgan Hill. Our Morgan Hill program offers the convenience and amenities of small-town living within the supportive community of Morgan Hill.

6521 Learning Services: Supported Living Programs
131 Langley Drive
Suite B
Lawrenceville, GA 30046-9315
408-848-4379
888-419-9955
FAX: 866-491-7396
www.learningservices.com

Dr. Debra Braunling-McMorrow, President and CEO
Jeanne Mack, Chief Financial Officer and Vice President of Operations
Michael Weaver, Chief Development Officer
Susan Snow, Director of Admissions

We offer a variety of diverse and stimulating environments for people with different needs, capabilities and personal goals. Within comfortable, homelike, age-appropriate settings we provide the structure and support necessary to ensure the richest possible quality of life. Program offered in both Northern and Southern facilities of California

6522 Leon S Peters Rehabilitation Center
2823 Fresno St
Fresno, CA 93721-1324
559-459-6000
www.communitymedical.org

Florence Dunn, Chairwoman
John McGregor, Esquire, Secretary
Tim A. Joslin, President, Chief Executive Officer
Patrick Rafferty, Executive Vice President, Chief Operating Officer

Community's flagship hospital that offers world class specialized critical care with the area's only stroke unit with 24-hour vascular neurology and neurosurgery coverage and a team of specially trained stroke nurses. The world's first G4 CyberKnife. The table Mountain Rancheraia Level 1 Trauma Center. The Leon S. Peters burn center. The region's only perinatology program for high rish pregnancies and deliveries. The Da-Vinci robotic surgical system, and 3 helicopeter landing pads.

6523 Lion's Blind Center of Diablo Valley, Inc. Lions Center For The Visually Impaired
175 Alvarado Ave
Pittsburg, CA 94565-4862
925-432-3013
800-750-3937
FAX: 925-432-7014
e-mail: edward.329@comcast.net
www.seniorvision.org

Edward Schroth, Executive Director
Barbara Cronin, President
Charles Dunham, First Vice President
Phillis Neitling, Secretary

A private, nonprofit agency offering services such as health, educational, recreational, rehabilitation, employment and counseling to the totally blind, legally blind and visually impaired. The staff includes two full time workers..

6524 Lion's Blind Center of Oakland
2115 Broadway
Oakland, CA 94612-2698
510-450-1580
FAX: 510-654-3603
e-mail: info@lbcenter.org
lbcenter.org

Michelle Taylor Lagunas, Executive Director/ CEO
Christina Easiley, Administrative Manager
Scott Blanks, Director of Rehabilitation Servi
Danette Davis, Orientation & Mobility Instructor

A private nonprofit organization offering services for the totally blind, legally blind, deaf-blind and multihandicapped blind. Services include: professional training, rehabilitation, education, counseling, social work, self help and more. The staff includes 12 full time and 1 part time worker.

6525 **Living Skills Center for the Visually Impaired**
2430 Road 20
#B112
San Pablo, CA 94806-5005
510-234-4984
FAX: 510-234-4986
e-mail: info@hcblind.org
www.hcblind.org

Patricia Williams, Executive Director
Patricia Maffei, Program Director
Ronald Hideshima, Adaptive Technology Instructor
Lee Staub, Orientation and Mobility Instruc
A private, nonprofit agency offering services such as independent living skills training, recreational, employment and accessible technology training to the totally blind, legally blind and visually impaired. The staff includes six full time teachers.

6526 **Loma Linda University Orthopedic and Rehabilitation Institute**
25333 Barton Rd
Loma Linda, CA 92354-3123
909-558-1000
FAX: 909-558-0308
www.llu.edu

Richard H. Hart, MD, DrPH, President & Chief Executive Officer
Ronald L. Carter, PhD, Senior Vice President, Educational Affairs
Cari Dominguez, DHS, Senior Vice President, Human Resources
Mark L. Hubbard, Senior Vice President, Risk Management
Offers a full range of clinical programs for both inpatients and outpatient. The specific diagnosis leading to patient admission includes stroke, spinal cord injury, traumatic or anoxic brain damage, amputation, post neurosurgery, chronic neurological disease, Guillain-Barre syndrome, arthritis, multiple trauma or other complex orthopedic problems. The facilities and professional services are comprehensive and ensure that the best care is provided to pediatric and adult patients..

6527 **Manor Care Health Services- Citrus Heights**
7807 Uplands Way
Citrus Heights, CA 95610-7500
916-967-2929
FAX: 916-965-8439
hcr-manorcare.com

Steven M. Cavanaugh, Chief Financial Officer
Paul A. Ormond, Chairman, President and Chief Ex
The nations leader in skilled nursing and rehabilitation care. Our facility has been serving the Sacramento area for more then 12 years. We are known for our beautiful decor, outstanding rehabilitation staff and loving nursing care. We offer short term rehabilitation, long term skilled nursing care, respite care and post hospital surgical care.

6528 **Manor Care Health Services- Palm Desert**
74-350 Country Club Dr
Palm Desert, CA 92260-1608
760-341-0261
FAX: 760-779-1563
hcr-manorcare.com

Steven M. Cavanaugh, Chief Financial Officer
Paul A. Ormond, Chairman, President and Chief Ex
Centrally located in the Coachella Valley, specializing in skilled nursing whith an emphasis on rehabilitation, post surgery recovery, hospice, alzheimer's care and long term care. In addition, we offer 2 unique service options for the discriminating consumer. Our Arcadia unit offers a specialized Alzheimer's care program in a dedicated secure wing. ManorCare offers rehabilitation services including physical, occupational and speech therapies for those recovering from illness injury or surgery.

6529 **Manor Care Health Services-Fountain Valley**
11680 Warner Ave
Fountain Valley, CA 92708-2513
714-241-9800
FAX: 714-966-1654
hcr-manorcare.com

Steven M. Cavanaugh, Chief Financial Officer
Paul A. Ormond, Chairman, President and Chief Ex
Provides 24-hour skilled nursing, rehabilitative therapies and specialized Alzheimer's care. Our in-house therapists provide physical, occupational and speech therapies in our rehabilitation area. Our team is goal oriented and focuses on producing positive outcomes for those recovering from illness, injury or surgery. Our respite care program provides a full range of services for a few days, a week or even a season.

6530 **Manor Care Health Services-Hemet**
1717 W Stetson Ave
Hemet, CA 92545-6882
951-925-9171
FAX: 951-925-8186
hcr-manorcare.com

Steven M. Cavanaugh, Chief Financial Officer
Paul A. Ormond, Chairman, President and Chief Ex
Provides skilled nursing, Rehabilitation services, and specialized Alzheimer's care. In addition we offer short term respite stays for family caregivers that simply need a break from the stress of daily care. Our Arcadia unit staff is specially trained in the care of residents with Alzheimer's disease. The secured unit is designed to provide a soothing and homelike environment while enhancing each resident's remaining abilities.

6531 **Manor Care Health Services-Sunnyvale**
1150 Tilton Dr
Sunnyvale, CA 94087-2440
408-735-7200
FAX: 408-736-8629
hcr-manorcare.com

Steven M. Cavanaugh, Chief Financial Officer
Paul A. Ormond, Chairman, President and Chief Ex
Our in-house therapists provide physical, occupational and speech therapies in our rehabilitation area. Our team is goal oriented and focuses on producing positive outcomes for those recovering from illness, injury or surgery. Our skilled nursing staff works with our therapy department and dietary department to provide positive wound care programs for patients requiring skin management care.

6532 **Manor Care Health Services-Walnut Creek**
1226 Rossmoor Pkwy
Walnut Creek, CA 94595-2538
925-975-5000
FAX: 925-937-1132
hcr-manorcare.com

Steven M. Cavanaugh, Chief Financial Officer
Paul A. Ormond, Chairman, President and Chief Ex
Provides luxurious long term care and rehabilitation services. In house therapists provide, physical, occupational and speech therapies in our rehabilitation area. Our team is goal oriented and focuses on producing positive outcomes for those recovering from illness, injury or surgery. Our years of combined management experience add value to our resident's quality of life.

6533 **Maynord's Chemical Dependency Recovery Centers**
19325 Cherokee Road
Tuolumne, CA 95379-1657
209-928-3737
800-228-8208
FAX: 209-928-1152
maynords.com

James Berry, Director
Maynord's Recovery Centers has always been dedicated to the recovery of good people whose lives are being destroyed by alcohol and drugs. Since 1978, Maynord's residential program has helped thousands of people put their lives back together after addiction has taken its toll. Today, Maynord's offers a treatment system over much of the San Joaquin Valley and the San Francisco Bay Area.

6534 **Maynord's Ranch for Men**
19325 Cherokee Road
Tuolumne, CA 95379-1657
209-928-3737
800-228-8208
FAX: 209-928-1152
maynords.com

James Berry, Director
Provides treatment for chemical dependency problems to men. The treatment addresses their recovery through a comprehensive plan created for their individual needs. Also offers a program for women called the Meadows.

6535 **Meadowbrook Manor**
431 West Remington Boulevard
Bolingbrook, IL 60440
630-759-1112
FAX: 630-759-6925
e-mail: jmolen@meadowbrookmanor.com
www.meadowbrookmanor.com

6536 **Meadowview Manor**
41 Crestview Terrace
Bridgeport, WV 26330
304-842-7101
FAX: 304-842-7104
e-mail: info@meadowviewmanor.com
www.meadowviewmanor.com

6537 **Memorial Hospital of Gardenia**
1145 West Redondo Beach Blvd
Gardena, CA 90247-3528
310-532-4200
800-782-2288
www.avantihospitals.com/memorial-hospital-of-
Edward Mirzabegian, Corporate Chief Executive Officer
Postacute rehabilitation program..

6538 **Mercy Medical Group**
Mercy Hospital
3000 Q Street
Sacramento, CA 95816
916-733-3333
www.mymercymedicalgroup.org

6539 **Napa County Mental Health Department**
2344 Old Sonoma Road
Bldg. D
Napa, CA 94559-3708
707-259-8151
800-648-8650
www.countyofnapa.org/MentalHealth/

6540 **Napa Valley Support Systems**
1700 Second Street Suite 212
Napa, CA 94559-1344
707-253-7490
FAX: 707-253-0115
napavalleysupportservices.org
Beth Kahiga, Executive Director
Heather Jump, Administrative Manager
Katy Vanzant, Program Director
Emmy Lesko, Program Supervisor
Work hardening and disciplinary programs.

6541 **North Valley Services**
1040 Washington
Red Bluff, CA 96080-4509
530-527-0407
FAX: 530-527-7091
www.northvalleyservices.org
Joe Brown, President
Larry Donnelley, Vice President
Lynn DeFreece, CEO
Delbert Brownfield, COO
Provides vocational rehabilitation services, such as job counseling, job training, and work experience, to unemployed and underemployed persons, persons with disabilities.

6542 **Northridge Hospital Medical Center Rehabiltation Medicine**
18300 Roscoe Blvd
Northridge, CA 91328-4167
818-885-8500
FAX: 818-701-7367
www.northridgehospital.org/index.htm
Mike L. Wall, President
Thomas L. Hedge, Medical Director
Joel S. Rosen, Associate Medical Director
Alex L. Lin, Managing Director
A full service, comprehensive rehabilitation program suited to treat patients of all ages who have suffered catastrophic or debilitating injury or illness. The goal of the program is to deliver exceptional patient care to maximise each individual's skills and independence.

6543 **Northridge Hospital Medical Center: Centerfor Rehabilitation Medicine**
18300 Roscoe Blvd
Northridge, CA 91328-4167
818-885-8500
FAX: 818-701-7367
www.northridgehospital.com
Mike L. Wall, President
Thomas L. Hedge, Medical Director
Joel S. Rosen, Associate Medical Director
Alex L. Lin, Managing Director
Committed to serving the health needs of our communities with particular attention to the needs of the poor, the disadvantaged, and vulneralbe, and the comfort of the suffering and dying. Catholic Healthcare West has a commitment to quality-quality healthcare services and the promotion of optimal quality of life for all of life.

6544 **Old Adobe Developmental Services**
1301A Rand Street
Suite A
Petaluma, CA 94954-5697
707-763-9807
FAX: 707-763-7708
e-mail: webmaster@oadsinc.org
www.oadsinc.org
Elizabeth Clary, Executive Director
Marie Padgett, Controller
The mission of Old Adobe to provide opportunities for individuals with developmental challenges to reach thier fullest potentials. Our job at OADS is to find ways for these individuals to find full expression in all parts of their lives. We have a partnership with the Adult Education Department of the Petaluma School District in providing services to persons with developmental challenges. We are funded by the Dept. of Rehabilitation and the Dept. Of Developmental services.

6545 **Old Adobe Developmental Services-Rohnert Park Services (Behavioral)**
5401 Snyder Ln.
Rohnert Park, CA 94928-3124
707-584-5859
FAX: 707-664-8057
www.oadsinc.org
Elizabeth Clary, Executive Director
Helen Gunderson, Administrative Assistant
The program services are designed to assist individuals who demonstrate basic work skills, to develop social skills and work habits necessary to succeed in supported or competitive employment. Most often individual program services involve working with the client to replace those behavioral excesses that have been a barrier to vocational placement.

6546 **PRIDE Industries**
10030 Foothills Blvd
Roseville, CA 95747-7102
916-788-2100
800-550-6005
FAX: 800-888-0447
e-mail: info@prideindustries.com
prideindustries.com
Michael Ziegler, President & CEO
Bob Selvester, Vice Chair
Mike Snegg, Treasurer
Tim Yamauchi, Executive Vice President and Chi
To provide opportunities through employment, training, evaluation and placement maximizing community access, independence and quality of life for people with barriers to employment.

6547 **Pacific Hospital Of Long Beach-Neuro Care Unit**
2776 Pacific Ave
Long Beach, CA 90806-2613
562-997-2000
e-mail: webmaster@phlb.org
www.phlb.org
Michael D. Drobot, CEO
Clark Todd, President
Teri Plemmons, Administrative Assistant
Our mission is to heal with compassion and to perform with distinction. Our vision: to improve the hospital's orthopedic and Spine Center of Excellence. Achieve exceptional financial performance to enhance hospital services. Improve the vertically in-

tegrated ancillary, outpatient and inpatient surgery system. Develop a professionally challenging work environment that reflects an agile, peak performance culture.

6548 Paradise Vally Hospital-South Bay Rehabilitation Center
2400 East 4th St
National City, CA 91950-2026 619-470-4321
paradisevalleyhospital.net
Prem Reddy, Chairman
Neerav Jadeja, Administrator
Luis Leon, President
Gemma Rama-Banaag, Chief Nursing Officer
South Bay Rehabilitation Center, offers a complete range of treatment for patients with physical disabilities. Our specialized inpatient and outpatient programs are designed to meet each person's individual needs or injuries, with the goal of restoring as much independence as possible and significantly improving their lives.

6549 Parents and Friends
350 South Main Street
Fort Bragg, CA 95437-5408 707-964-4940
e-mail: moon@parentsandfriends.org
parentsandfriends.org
Rick Moon, Executive Director
Jessica Dickey, Administrative Assistant
Kristy Tanguay, Manager
Kathy Connell, Bookkeeper
Parents and Friends provides opportunities for persons with developmental challenges and similar needs to participate fully in our community.

6550 People Services
4195 Lakeshore Blvd
Lakeport, CA 95453-6411 707-263-3810
e-mail: idumont@nctac.com
peopleservices.org
Ilene Dumont, Executive Director
Martin Diesman, Director
Vicki Cole, Director
Kathy Ryan, Director
Providing an array of services for adults with developmental disabilities and other people with disabilities. Services include supported employment, work services, supported living, personal, social and community training, transportation, specialized individual services and much more.

6551 Petaluma Recycling Center
Old Adobe Developmental Services
315 2nd St
Petaluma, CA 94952-4230 707-763-4761
FAX: 707-763-4921
e-mail: davide@oadsinc.org
www.oadsinc.org/petarecycle
Elizabeth Clary, Executive Director
Began in 1974; has been one of the major employers of persons with developmental challenges for 26 years; is the primary recycling facility in the growing city of 52,000; accepts over 20 different kinds of recyclables; employs 20-25 persons a day.

6552 Pomerado Rehabilitation Outpatient Service
15615 Pomerado Rd
Poway, CA 92064-2405 858-485-6511
FAX: 858-613-4248
Bob Blake, Director Rehab Services
Jonathan Pee, Manager
A 107-bed acute care hospital. In addition to a round-the-clock Emergency Department, Pomerado offers the area's finest outpaitent surgery center and general medical/surgical services. Pomerado Hospital also is home to a world-class Birth Center and a Level II NICU. Fully JCAHO-accrediddted, Pomerado is well-known for offering only private rooms, each with a scenic view of the North Countryside, which enhances the healing atmosphere..

6553 Pride Industries: Grass Valley
12451 Loma Rica Dr
Grass Valley, CA 95945-9059 530-477-1832
800-550-6005
FAX: 530-477-8038
e-mail: info@prideindustries.com
www.prideindustries.com
Bob Olsen, Chairman
Bob Selvester, Vice Chairman
Walt Payne, President/CEO
Mike Snegg, Treasurer
Work adjustment and remunerative work programs. We offer an adult day program as well.

6554 Rancho Adult Day Care Center
Rancho Los Amigos Medical Center
7601 Imperial Hwy
Downey, CA 90242-3456 562-401-7111
FAX: 562-401-7991
TTY:562-401-8450
e-mail: radscenter@aol.com
www,rancho.org/ser_adultday
Valerie Orange, CEO
Margaret L Campbell, Research Director
Provides personal care, social services and a therapeutic program to older adults in order to improve their quality of life. Offers a Clinical Gerontology Service, an Alzheimer's Disease Diagnostic and Treatment Center and a Geriatric Assessment and Rehabilitation Unit..

6555 Regional Center for Rehabilitation
2288 Auburn Blvd
Sacramento, CA 95821-1618 916-421-4167
FAX: 916-925-1586

6556 Rehabilitation Institute of Santa Barbara
2415 De La Vina St
Santa Barbara, CA 93105-3819 805-569-8999
FAX: 805-687-3707
risb.org
Ralph Pollock, President
Scott Silic MBA, Vice President Of Operations
Cheryl Ellis MD, MHA, VP Medical Services
A regional rehabilitation system with an acute care hospital at the center, the Institute provides specialized inpatient and outpatient programs for brain injury, spinal cord injury, stroke, work-related injury, chronic pain, orthopedic problems and more. Offers a 46-bed acute-care rehabilitation hospital, a free-standing outpatient center, the brain injury continuum, chronic pain program..

6557 Rehabilitation Institute of Southern California
1800 E La Veta Ave
Orange, CA 92866-2902 714-633-7400
FAX: 714-633-4586
e-mail: adults@rio-rehab.com
riorehab.org
Praim S. Singh, Executive Director
Carol Reese, Executive Assistant
Grace Lee, Administrative Assistant
Dana Patton, Personnel Officer
Outpatient rehabilitation serving physically and disabled children and adults. Child development programs, adult day care for disabled seniors, child care for disabled and non-disabled children, outpatient therapy, aquatics, adult day healthcare, independent living, vocational services, social services, and housing.

6558 Rubicon Programs
2500 Bissell Avenue
Richmond, CA 94804-1815 510-235-1516
FAX: 510-235-2025
e-mail: rubicon@rubiconpgms.org
www.rubiconprograms.org
Rob Hope, Chief Program Officer
Jane Fischberg, President and Executive Director
Roger Contreras, CFO
Kelly Dunn, General Counsel and Director of Legal Services
Rubicon Programs Inc. helps people and communities build assets to achieve greater independence. Since 1973, Rubicon has

built and operated affordable housing and provided employment, job training, mental health, and other supportive services to individuals who have disabilities, are homeless, or are otherwise economically disadvantaged.

6559 San Bernardino Valley Lighthouse for the Blind
762 North Sierra Way
San Bernardino, CA 92410-4438 909-884-3121
FAX: 909-884-2964
e-mail: lighthouse4blind@aol.com
www.afb.org

Robert Mc Bay, Executive Director
Sandra Wood, Administrative Assistant

Provides training in independent living skills - cooking, mobility and orientation, sewing, Braille and typing. Also, we have classes in macrame, ceramics and basket weaving. Weekly support group and Bible study..

6560 Santa Clara Valley Blind Center, Inc.
101 N Bascom Ave
San Jose, CA 95128-1805 408-295-4016
FAX: 408-295-1398
e-mail: info@visionbeyondsight.org
visionbeyondsight.org

Arnold Chew, President
John Glass, Vice President
Arlene Holmes, Secretary
Sue Szucs, Treasurer

SCVBC's mission is to increase the confidence, independence, and quality of life of the blind and visually impaired through educational, recreational, and rehabilitative programs.

6561 Scripps Memorial Hospital: Pain Center
4275 Campus Point Ct.
San Diego, CA 92121-1205 858-626-4123
800-727-4777
e-mail: clinicalresearch@scrippshealth.com
www.scripps.org

Chris Van Gorder, President and CEO
Richard K Rothberger, Vice President, Chief Financial Officer
Robin B Brown, Chief Executive
Richard R Sheridan, Corporate Senior Vice President

Offers both inpatient and outpatient programs including: physical activity management, individual pain management, group therapy, medication adjustment, pain control classes, occupational therapy, biofeedback training, family counseling, vocational and leisure counseling and recreational therapy.

6562 Sharp Coronado Hospital
250 Prospect Place
Coronado, CA 92118-1999 619-522-3600
e-mail: erica.carlson@sharp.com
sharp.com

Marcia Hall, CEO
Mark Tamsen, Chairman
Tom Smisek, Vice Chairman
Dan Gensler, Secretary

Providing medical and surgical care, intensive care, sub-acute and long-term care, rehabilitation therapies and emergency services in a peaceful setting is part of our live+heal+grow philosophy. We are one of the county's few community-owned hospitals and are proud of our history of providing convenient, award-winning heath care to Coronado and San Diego.

6563 Shriners Hospitals For Children-Northern California
2425 Stockton Blvd.
Sacramento, CA 95817 916-453-2000
e-mail: patientreferrals@shrinenet.org
www.shrinershospitalsforchildren.org

John McCabe, Executive Vice President
Dale W Stauss, Chairman
Jerry G Gantt, 1st Vice President
Chris L Smith, 2nd Vice President

The only hospital in the Shriners system that houses facilities for treatment of all 3 Shriner specialties -spinal cord injuries, orthopaedic, and burns. The hospital features 80 patient beds, 9 parent apartments, 5 state-of-the-art operating rooms, a high-tech Motion Analysis lab, and an entire floor devoted to research.

6564 Shriners Hospitals for Children: Los Angeles
3160 Geneva Street
Los Angeles, CA 90020-1199 213-388-3151
e-mail: patientreferrals@shrinenet.org
www.shrinershospitalsforchildren.org

John McCabe, Executive Vice President
Dale W Stauss, Chairman
Jerry G Gantt, 1st Vice President
Chris L Smith, 2nd Vice President

Shriners Hospitals for Children: Los Angeles, treats children under age 18 with burn scars, orthopedic conditions, cleft lip and palate and limb deficiencies at no cost to the patient or their families.

6565 Society for the Blind
1238 S Street
Sacramento, CA 95811-3256 916-452-8271
FAX: 916-492-2483
e-mail: info@societyfortheblind.org
societyfortheblind.org

William Carter, President
Bryce McAnally, Vice President
Shari Roeseler, Executive Director
Liz Culp, Director of Resource Development

A private, local nonprofit organization providing blind and visually impaired people with the training supplies and support they need to live independent, productive and fulfilled lives with limited vision. Services include the Low Vision Clinic, Braille classes, computer training, support groups, living skills instruction, mobility training and the Products for Independence Store.

6566 Solutions at Santa Barbara: Transitional Living Center
1135 N Patterson Ave
Santa Barbara, CA 93111-1113 805-683-1995
FAX: 805-683-4793
e-mail: sol1135@aol.com
solutionsatsantabarbara.com

Sue Hannigan, Director

Postacute rehabilitation program. Short-term transitional living program for individuals with traumatic brain injury, stroke, aneurysm and other neurological disorders.

6567 St. John's Pleasant Valley Hospital Neuro Care Unit
2309 Antonio Ave
Camarillo, CA 93010-1414 805-389-5800
shw.org

Jerry Conway, President
Maureen M. Malone, Administrator
Raye Burkhardt, Vice President and Chief Nursing

Houses 82 acute-care beds, a 99-bed extended care unit, and the only hyperbaric medicine unit in Ventura County. Employ's 1,800 people and count 250 active medical staff.

6568 St. John's Regional Medica Center- Industrial Therapy Center
1600 North Rose Ave
Oxnard, CA 93030-3723 805-988-2500
www.stjohnshealth.org

Gudrun Moll, Vice President and Chief Nursing
Laurie Harting, President & CEO
Kim Wilson, Vice President
Chris Champlin, Senior Vice President

A non-profit health care facility offering multi-disciplinary programs for pain management and work hardening, as well as physical and occupational therapy.

6569 **Sub-Acute Saratoga Hospital**
13425 Sousa Lane
Saratoga, CA 95070-4663 408-378-8875
FAX: 408-378-7419
subacutesaratoga.com

Jack Stephens, President & CEO
Paul Quintana, Medical Director
Gary Vernon, NHA Administrator
Lindsay Zarcone, Marketing Manager
Dedicated to the fulfillment of human needs, desires, and wishes in illness and in health. The cohesiveness of caring in a family community of staff, patients, and their loved ones. The celebration of each unique life through their therapeutic journey, while preserving their individual spirit. The achievement of advanced medical expertise, knowledge, and skill given with the human touch of caring toward the ultimate goal: enhancing the healing process from acute illness to the joy of going home.

6570 **Synergos Neurological Center: Hayward**
27200 Calaroga Avenue
Hayward, CA 94545-4383 510-264-4000
FAX: 510-264-4007
strosehospital.org

Richard C. Hardwig, Chair
Alan McIntosh, Vice Chair
Lex Reddy, President and CEO
Roger Krissman, Chief Financial Officer
Postacute rehabilitation program.

6571 **Synergos Neurological Center: Mission Hills**
27200 Calaroga Avenue
Hayward, CA 94545-4383 510-264-4000
FAX: 510-264-4007
www.strosehospital.org

Richard C. Hardwig, Chair
Alan McIntosh, Vice Chair
Lex Reddy, President and CEO
Roger Krissman, Chief Financial Officer
For over 30 years, St. Rose Hospital Rehabilitation Services Department has helped thousands of patients recover from illness and injury through the help of our specially trained therapists. These therapists have been trained in specific rehabilitative areas such as physical, occupational, and speech therapies.

6572 **Temple Community Hospital**
235 N Hoover St
Los Angeles, CA 90004-3672 213-382-7252
FAX: 213-382-1874
e-mail: info@templecommunityhospital.com
templecommunityhospital.com

6573 **The ARC Of San Diego-ARROW Center**
3030 Market Street
San Diego, CA 92102-3297 619-685-1175
FAX: 619-234-3759
arc-sd.com

Dwight Stratton, Chair
Jerry Wechsler, 1st Vice Chairman
David W. Schneider, President & CEO
Anthony J. DeSalis, Executive Vice President & COO
The ARC of San Diego will be the premier provider of services to persons with disabilities. Arc-SD will be an advocate for diversity of opportunities, enhancing individual life choices as a member of the communuity. Our values: Everyone will be be treated equally, without prejudice and with respect. Will provide Quality Services and Supports with a well trained and caring staff. State of the art equipment and methods. A willingness to innovate and collaborate.

6574 **The ARC Of San Diego-East County Training Center**
1374 E Lexington Ave
El Cajon, CA 92019-2312 619-444-9417
FAX: 619-234-3759
arc-sd.com

Dwight Stratton, Chair
Jerry Wechsler, 1st Vice Chairman
David W. Schneider, President & CEO
Anthony J. DeSalis, Executive Vice President & COO
Work adjustment and remunerative work programs.

6575 **The ARC Of San Diego-Rex Industries**
9575 Aero Dr
San Diego, CA 92123-1803 858-571-4369
800-748-5575
FAX: 858-715-3788
arc-sd.com

Dwight Stratton, Chair
Jerry Wechsler, 1st Vice Chairman
David W. Schneider, President & CEO
Anthony J. DeSalis, Executive Vice President & COO
Offers many different programs including: North County Parent/Infant Program which is an educational program for children, birth to three years who are showing delays in development or who are at risk for developmental delays. The Adult Development Center is a program for adults, eighteen and over, with a developmental disability in the severe to profound range. The program focuses on self-help, communication, daily living and pre-vocational skills. Other programs are available..

6576 **Tunnell Center for Rehab**
680 South Fourth Street
Louisville, CA 40202-4807 502-596-7300
FAX: 800-545-0749
e-mail: web_administrator@kindred.com
kindredhealthcare.com

Mary R., Activities Assistant
Kristen W., Health and Rehabilitation Center
The Tunnell Center for Rehabilitation and Healthcare accomodates 178 residents. We are dedicated to short-term complex medical and rehabilitative care. Using a holistic care management approach we work with residents who have suffered debilitating injury or illness, and who need comprehensive nursing and rehabilitation services to achieve their highest practicable level of functional ability and independence.

6577 **Ukiah Valley Association for Habilitation**
Ukiah, CA 95482-689 707-468-8824
FAX: 707-468-9149
TTY:800-735-2929
www.uvah.org

Pamela Jensen, Executive Director
Kris Vipond, Business Manager
Sharrae Elston, Director
Suzanne Warner, Employment Training Specialist
Work adjustment and suppoted employment and social and community services.

6578 **Valley Center for the Blind**
2491 W Shaw Avenue
Suite 124
Fresno, CA 93711-3331 559-222-4088
FAX: 559-222-4844
e-mail: info@valleycenterblind.org
www.valleycenterblind.org

Bud Breslin, Executive Director
Millie Marshall, Marriage Family Therapist
Saramarie Katich, Office Mngr/Program Director
Connie Parrick, Secretary
A private, nonprofit organization that offers educational, health, recreational and professional training services to the totally blind, legally blind or severely visually impaired.

6579 **Villa Esperanza Services**
2060 East Villa Street
Pasadena, CA 91107 626-449-2919
FAX: 626-449-2850
e-mail: info@villaesperanzaservices.org
www.villaesperanzaservices.org

Candice Rogers, Chairman
Richard Hubinger, President
Vicky Castillo, CFO
Kelly White, Chief Executive Officer
Serving disabled infants to seniors in a school, adult day program, adult work program and residences and adult day health care program and care management program.

6580 **Village Square Nursing And Rehabilitation Center**
Kindred Healthcare, Inc.
1586 West San Marcos Blvd
San Marcos, CA 92078-4019 760-471-2986
www.villagesquarerehab.com

6581 **Vista Center for the Blind & Visually Impaired**
2470 El Camino Real,
Suite 107
Palo Alto, CA 94306-1715 650-858-0202
800-660-2009
FAX: 650-858-0214
e-mail: info@vistacenter.org
www.vistacenter.org
Pam Brandin, Executive Director
Nacole Barth-Ellis, Co-Director of Development
Terry Kurfess, Co-Director of Development
Meg Faville, Administrative Services Manager
Private nonprofit agency that serves the visually impaired in the San Mateo, Santa Clara, San Benito and Santa Cruz Counties with offices in Palo Alto and Santa Cruz. Offers Low Vision Evaluations, mobility training, daily living skills training, social services, counseling, support groups, computer training, other rehabilitation services, and a store.

6582 **Winways at Orange County**
7732 E Santiago Canyon Rd
Orange, CA 92869-1829 714-771-5276
FAX: 714-771-1452
winwaysrehab.com
Pamela Kauss, Director
The program offers clients highly personalized, comprehensive programs to meet the needs of individuals with traumatic brain injury, stroke, tumors, aneurysm, post concussive syndrome or other neurological disorders. Winways also has a special program that provides services to Spanish speaking clients, called Contigo Adelante with materials in Spanish, and Spanish speaking interpreters to assist in the therapy process.

Colorado

6583 **Capron Rehabilitation Center**
Penrose Hospital/ St. Francis Healthcare System
2222 N Nevada Ave
Colorado Springs, CO 80907-6819 719-776-5000
penrosestfrancis.org
Margaret Sabin, President & CEO
Nate Olson, Chief Executive Officer
Jameson Smith, Senior VP & Chief Admnistrative Officer
Gil Porat, Chief Medical Officer
Southern Colorado's most complete inpatient and outpatient rehabilitation center.

6584 **Cerebral Palsy of Colorado**
801 Yosemite Street
Denver, CO 80230 303-691-9339
FAX: 303-691-0846
abilityconnectioncolorado.org
Judith I Ham, CEO
James Reuter, Chairman of the Board
Penfield Tate, Vice Chairman
Kathy Higgins, Treasurer
Provides services for children birth-5 years, employment services for adults, information and referral, donation pickup and cell phone/ink cartridge recycling services.

6585 **Cherry Hills Health Care Center**
Kindred
3575 S Washington St
Englewood, CO 80110-3807 303-789-2265
www.cherryhillshc.com

6586 **Community Hospital Back and Conditioning Clinic**
1060 Orchard Ave
Grand Junction, CO 81501-2997 970-243-3400
800-621-0926
FAX: 970-856-6510
Amy Hibberd, Executive Director
David Scherman, Manager
Post-accute rehabilitation program .

6587 **Laradon Hall Society for Exceptional Children and Adults**
5100 Lincoln St
Denver, CO 80216-2056 303-296-2400
866-381-2163
FAX: 303-296-4012
laradon.org
William Mitchell, Chair
Suzanne Bradeen, Vice Chair
Jason Adams, Treasurer
Nancy Hodges, Secretary
Laradon provides educational, vocational and residential services to children and adults with developmental disabilities and other special needs. Laradon was founded in 1948. It is among the largest and most comprehensive service providers in Colorado.

6588 **Learning Services: Bear Creek**
7201 W Hampden Ave
Lakewood, CO 80227-5305 303-989-6660
888-419-9955
FAX: 866-491-7396
e-mail: lengland@learningservices.com
learningservices.com
Susan Snow, Director of Admissions
Dr. Debra Braunling-McMorrow, President and CEO
Jeanne Mack, Chief Financial Officer
Michael Weaver, Chief Development Officer
Supported living program for persons with acquired brain injury.

6589 **MOSAIC In Colorado SpringsMOSAIC**
888 W. Garden of the Gods Road
Ste 100
Colorado Springs, CO 80907-6251 719-380-0451
FAX: 719-380-7055
e-mail: mosaic_cosprings@mosaicinfo.org
www.mosaicincoloradosprings.org
Tom Maltais, Executive Director
Mosaic in Colorado Springs provides a variety of services to assist adults and families in achieving positive goals. Services to persons with intellectual disabilities include community living options, vocational training and supported employment, spiritual growth and personal development options, and day programs habilitation and community participation.

6590 **Manor Care Nursing and Rehabilitation Center: Boulder**
Manor Care Ohio
2800 Palo Pkwy
Boulder, CO 80301-1540 303-440-9100
FAX: 303-440-9251
www.hcr-manorcare.com
Steven M. Cavanaugh, Chief Financial Officer
Paul A. Ormond, Chairman, President and Chief Ex
150 bed center offers a full spectrum of nursing care and rehabilitation. This includes our Arcadia Special Care Unit for Alzheimer's patients. Specialized unit for post acute skilled nursing care. Physical and massage therapies. And a 48 bed upscale Heritage unit offering additional amenities and furnishings.

6591 **Manor Care Nursing: Denver**
290 S Monaco Pkwy
Denver, CO 80224-1105 303-355-2525
FAX: 303-333-6960
www.hcr-manorcare.com
Steven M. Cavanaugh, Chief Financial Officer
Paul A. Ormond, Chairman, President and Chief Ex
Our center has delveloped a reputation for its luxurious environment, comprehensive rehabilitation service and focus on quality care. A wide range of individual and group activities and many gracious amenities create the finest combination of elegance and

professional skilled nursing care. Arcadia, our special care unit for persons with Alzheimer's disease and related memory impairments, promotes independence and preserves dignity within a safe and secure environment.

6592 **Mediplex of Colorado**
8451 Pearl St
Thornton, CO 80229-4804
303-288-3000
FAX: 303-286-5136
e-mail: info@vhdenver.com
www.northvalleyrehab.com
Jan Eyer, Chief Executive Officer
Our programs and services help each patient along the road to recovery toward our ultimate aim; the greatest possible restoration of the individual's self-esteem, ability to set goals, and self-sufficiency. Also offer specialized acute inpatient rehabilitative services, including special programs in Trauma Rehabilitation.

6593 **Platte River Industries**
490 Bryant St
Denver, CO 80204-4808
303-825-0041
FAX: 303-825-0564
e-mail: pri01_lil@attglobal.net
Bob Smith, Executive Director
Postacute rehabilitation facility and program..

6594 **Pueblo Diversified Industries**
2828 Granada Blvd
Pueblo, CO 81005-3198
800-466-8393
FAX: 719-564-3407
e-mail: info@pdipueblo.org
www.pdipueblo.net
Karen K Lillie, President & CEO
Robin Forbes, Director Human Services
Tom Drolshagen, Chief Operating Officer
Tom Denslow, Manager, Human Resources
A place where people can turn limitations into opportunities. People can experience the independence, pride and self worth of securing and maintaining a job.

6595 **SHALOM Denver**
2498 W 2nd Ave
Denver, CO 80223-1007
303-623-0251
FAX: 303-620-9584
e-mail: akover@jewishfamilyservice.org
shalomdenver.com
Arnie Kover, Disability and Employment Servic
Sara Leeper, Coordinator of Client Services
Vicky Brittain, Mailing Business Manager
Bari Belinsky, Work Services Manager
SHALOM Denver provides employment, training, and job placement opportunities to people with disabilities, resettled immigrants, and people moving from welfare to work.

6596 **SPIN Early Childhood Care & Education Cntr**
1333 Elm Ave
Canon City, CO 81212-4431
719-275-0550
www.starpointco.com/spin
Diane Trujillo, Manager
SPIN center is a fully inclusive non-discriminating community early childhood program, offering a variety of schedule choices for families. The philosophy of the SPIN program is to promote each child's growth and development. Special attention is given to cognitive, physical, speech language and social-emotional growth. Staff is specifically trained to facilitate and prepare environments that promote exploration, key experiences, creativity and self-expression..

6597 **Schaefer Enterprises**
500 26th Street
P.O. Box 200009
Greeley, CO 80631-8427
970-353-0662
FAX: 970-353-2779
e-mail: schaefenterprises@comcast.net
www.schaeferenterprises.com
Valorie Randall, Executive Director
Alex Witt, Executive Assistant
Veronica Griego, Production Director
Schaefer Enterprises, Inc., located in Greely, Colorado, is a vaulable community resource that has been fulfilling the outsourcing needs of businesses in Weld County and outlying areas since 1952.

6598 **Spalding Rehab Hospital West Unit**
150 Spring St
Morrison, CO 80465
303-697-4334
FAX: 303-697-0570

Connecticut

6599 **ACES/ACCESS Inclusion Program**
350 State Street
North Haven, CT 06473-3218
203-498-6800
FAX: 203-234-1369
e-mail: acesinfo@aces.org
www.aces.org
Thomas M Danehy, Executive Director
Erika Forte, Assistant Executive Director
Evelyn Rossetti, Manager
Provides a person centered planning approach for integrated employment, volunteer community based opportunities for adults who have developmental disabilities..

6600 **Apria Healthcare**
26220 Enterprise Court
Lake Forest, CA 92630-1015
800-277-4288
e-mail: contact_us@apria.com
www.apria.com
Lisa M. Getson, Executive Vice President, Govern
Nichola Denney, Executive Vice President, Revenue Management
Dan Stark, Chief Executive Officer
Debra L Morris, Chief Financial Officer
Provides a broad range of high quality and cost effective specialty infusion therapies and related services to patients in their homes throughout the Northeastern United States. Offer home infusion antibiotic therapy, quality pharmacy services, skilled nursing services and related support services.

6601 **Arc Of Meriden-Wallingford, Inc.**
200 Research Parkway
Meriden, CT 06450
203-237-9975
FAX: 203-639-0946
e-mail: info@mwsinc.net
www.arcmw.org
Pamela Fields, Executive Director
Joseph Palfini, Board President
Becky Blazejowski, Financial Director
Maritza Dell, Director of Program Services
A membership agency that provides comprehensive, full-service, community-based opportunities for people with disabilities. Guided by over 120 community members and an active Board of Directors, the Arc always has its focus on improving the lives of people with disabilities. The Arc of Meriden-Wallingford offers advocacy and assistance to our members along with advocating for the rights and choices of people with disabilities in our community.

6602 Arc of the Farmington Valley
225 Commerce Drive
Canton, CT 06019-2478
860-693-6662
FAX: 860-693-8662
e-mail: rcipolla@favarh.org
favarh.org

George Kral, President
Ernest E Mack, Vice President
Larry Pollock, Treasurer
Robin Dinicola, Secretary

Serving over 300 mentally retarded adults through a comprehensive program of residential and support services. These include three group homes, three apartments, competitive and supported employment options, a day program for mentally retarded seniors, community experience day services for severe and profoundly disabled adults, recreation and leisure services, advocacy, transportation, case management, in-home respite and other support services.

6603 Connecticut Subacute Corporation
19 Tuttle Pl
Middletown, CT 06457-1881
860-347-6300
FAX: 860-347-2446
www.cpl-usa.com

Evan K Lyle, Managed Care Director
Cheri Kauset, Corporate Rep.

Specializes in subacute medical and rehabilitation programming. The strength of our system is in its' ability to service a broad range of clinical and psychosocial needs which enable each individual to attain his/her optimal potential. Programming includes neurological and orthopedic rehabilitation, post-surgical and wound care management, intravenous therapy, pulmonary rehabilitation including ventilator services, and long term care..

6604 Datahr Rehabilitation Institute
4 Berkshire Blvd
Bethel, CT 06801-1001
203-775-4700
888-8DA-TAHR
FAX: 203-775-4688
abilitybeyonddisability.com

Thomas Fanning, CEO

Providers of comprehensive rehabilitation services with a history of nearly 5 decades of service. This institute is recognized as a leading resource in meeting the needs of those disabled by illness, injury or developmental disorders in Connecticut and New York. A team of rehabilitation and health care professionals offering career development, residential services, supported employment, volunteer services, occupational therapy, day activities and more.

6605 Eastern Blind Rehabilitation Center
810 Vermont Avenue
Washington, DC 20420
202-461-7600
800-273-8255
www1.va.gov/blindrehab

Eric K. Shinseki, Secretary of Veterans Affairs
W. Scott Gould, Deputy Secretary of Veterans Aff
Jose D Riojas, Chief of Staff
Richard J Griffin, Acting Inspector General

Provides residential rehabilitation services to eligible legally blind veterans in the Northeast and Middle Atlantic portions of the country. Referral applications by Veterans Administration Medical Centers and Outpatient Clinics in the geographical area served by the Blind Rehabilitation Center.

6606 FAVRAH Senior Adult Enrichment Program
23 W Avon Rd
Avon, CT 06001
860-674-8839
FAX: 860-676-0275

Nancy Ralston, Manager

Provides remunerative work. Post acute rehabilitation programs and facility.

6607 Gaylord Hospital
Gaylord Farm Road
P.O.Box 400
Wallingford, CT 06492-7048
203-284-2800
866-429-5673
FAX: 203-284-2894
TTY: 203-284-2700
e-mail: lcrispino@gaylord.org
www.gaylord.org

James Cullen, President

Works to restore ability and build courage. Offers rehabilitation care with one goal in mind: to help patients return to their homes, communities and jobs.

6608 Hockanum Greenhouse
Hockanum Industry
290 Middle Tpke
Storrs Mansfield, CT 06268-2908
860-429-6697
FAX: 860-429-7496
hockanumindustries.org

Christopher Campbell, Manager
Beth Chaty, Director
Betsy Treiber, Director

A non profit agency that strives to provide gainful employment, training, support and retirement services for developmentally disabled individuals through the dignity of work, community interaction and structured activities.

6609 Kuhn Employment Oppurtunities
1630 North Colony Road
P.O.Box 941
Meriden, CT 06450
203-235-2583
860-347-5843
www.kuhngroup.org

Paul O'Sullivan, Chairperson
Mark DuPuis, Vice Chairperson
John J. Ausanka III, Treasurer
James Anderson, Secretary

Kuhn is committed to developing quality skill enhancement programs which provide meaningful employment for persons with disabilities so that they will become independentm gain self-esteem, and be accepted by the community. Our vision is that all individuals have the ability to fully participate in the community through work. Kuhn believes that all participants have a right to integrated community employment.

6610 Norwalk Hospital Section Of Physical Medicine And Rehabilitation
34 Maple Street
Norwalk, CT 06856
203-852-2000
FAX: 800-789-4584
e-mail: marketing@norwalkhealth.org
www.norwalkhosp.org

Diane M. Allison, Chair
Edward A. Kangas, Vice Chair
Andrew J. Whittingham, Treasurer
Barbara Butler, Secretary

A 25 bed inpatient Rehabilitation Unit. This CARF and JCAHO accredidted rehab unit is located on the 8th floor of Norwalk Hospital. The focus of the rehab unit is to restore lost function and assist patients in returning to the community. Who have recently experienced a life changing medical event. The progam is tailored to meet individual therapy needs and address activities of daily living. Family and caregiver participation in the program is welcomed and encouraged.

6611 Rehabilitation Associates, Inc.
1931 Black Rock Tpke
Fairfield, CT 06825-3506
203-384-8681
FAX: 203-384-0956
e-mail: info@rehabassocinc.com
www.rehabilitationassociatesinc.com

Carol Landsman, Director

A comprehensive outpatient rehabilitation facility offering physical therapy, occupational therapy, speech-language pathology, clinical social work services and nutritional services to all age groups. Facility locations in Fairfield, Stratford, Milford, Shelton and Westport.

6612 Reliance House
40 Broadway
Norwich, CT 06360-5702
860-887-6536
FAX: 860-885-1970
reliancehouse.org

Jack Malone, President
Jackie Falman, Vice President
Sam Bliven, Secretary
Raul Walker, Treasurer

A residential vocational and recreational support network. An active and productive clubhouse where people with mental illness can gain skills, strength and self-esteem.

6613 Yale New Haven Health System-Bridgeport Hospital
789 Howard Avenue
New Haven, CT 06519
203-384-3000
www.yalenewhavenhealth.org

Marna P. Borgstrom, President and CEO
Richard D'Aquila, Executive Vice President
Peter N. Herbert, MD, Senior VP, Medical Affairs
Kevin Myatt, Senior VP of Human Resources

Medical services are provided by physicians who are specialists in physical medicine and rehabilitation. The physical therapy department provides a variety of services and utilizes sophisticated modalities to restore and reinforce physical abilities.

Delaware

6614 Alfred I DuPont Hospital for Children
Division of Rehabilitation
1600 Rockland Road,
PO Box 269
Wilmington, DE 19803-269
302-651-4000
888-533-3543
FAX: 302-651-4055
e-mail: infodupont@nemours.org
www.nemours.org

William G. Mackenzie, MD, Chair
David J. Bailey, President and Chief Executive Officer
Robert D. Bridges, Executive Vice President, Enterprise Services/Chief Financia
Roy Proujansky, Executive Vice President, Health Operations and Chief Operat

The hospital is a division of Nemours, which operates one of the nations largest subspecialty group practices devoted to pediatric patient care, teaching, and research. A 180-bed hospital that offers all the specialties of pediatric medicine, surgery, and dentistry in a spacious, comfortable, and family focused facility.

6615 Community Systems Inc.
2 Penns Way
Suite 301
New Castle, DE 19720
302-325-1500
FAX: 302-325-1505
e-mail: info@csi-del.org
communitysystems.org

David Paige, Executive Director
Amy Yento, Chair

A 4 state family of non-profit, tax exempt corporations whose mission is helping persons with disabilities to find happiness in their own homes, in their personal relationships, and as contributing members of their community.

6616 DDDS/Georgetown Center
5 Academy St
Georgetown, DE 19947-1915
302-856-5366
FAX: 302-856-5305
dhss.delaware.gov/dhss

6617 Delaware Association for the Blind
2915 Newport Gap Pike
Landis Lodge Building
Wilmington, DE 19808
302-998-5913
888-777-3925
FAX: 302-691-5810
e-mail: contact@dabdel.org
dabdel.org

Janet L. Berry, Executive Director
Ken Rolph, President
Jennifer Smith, Secretary
Robert Mosch, Treasurer

A private, nonprofit organization that offers adjustment to blindness counseling, recreation activities, summer camps and financial assistance for the legally blind. The staff includes five full time, nine part time and twelve seasonal. Operates a store selling items for the blind.

6618 Delaware Veterans Center
810 Vermont Avenue
Washington, DC 20420
302-994-2511
800-273-8255
FAX: 302-633-5591
www1.va.gov/directory/guide

Slaon D Gibson, Acting Secretary of Veterans Affairs
Jose D Riojas, Chief of Staff
Richard J Griffin, Acting Inspector General

A 60-bed hospital and 60-bed NHCU, both accredited by the Joint Commission on Accreditation of Healthcare Organizations with a VBA Regional Office and 2 Vet Centers (one on campus) offering veterans the unique opportunity to obtain heathcare, benefits services, and Readjustment Counseling at one location. The center provides a wide spectrum of primary and tertiary acute and extended care inpatient and outpatient activities an an academic setting..

6619 Easter Seals Delaware & Maryland's Eastern Shore
233 South Wacker Drive
Suite 2400
Chicago, IL 60606
302-324-4444
800-221-6827
FAX: 302-324-4441
TTY: 302-324-4442
easterseals.com

Richard W. Davidson, Chairman
Sandy Tuttle, President
Ralph F. Boyd, Treasurer
Eileen Howard Boone, Secretary

Provides exceptional services to ensure that all people with disabilities or special needs and their families have equal opportunities to live, learn, work and play in their communities.

6620 Edgemoor Day Program
500 Duncan Rd
Wilmington, DE 19809-2369
302-762-9077
FAX: 302-762-1652
www.dhss.delaware.gov/dhss/main/maps/other/ed

Scott Borino, Executive Director
Carol Koyste, Manager, Finance & Administratio
Brandon Furrowh, Director, Recreation & Youth Pro
Avani Patel, Administrative Assistant

Our mission is providing affordable and accessible services which help improve the quality of life for community members of all ages through a broad range of educational, recreational, self-enrichment, and family support services. ECC is a not-for-profit, community-based, multi-service agency located just north of Wilmington. We provide a broad range of educational, recreational, self-enrichment, and family support services.

6621 Elwyn Delaware
321 E 11th St
Wilmington, DE 19801-3422 302-658-8860
FAX: 302-654-5815
e-mail: info@elwyn.org
www.elwyn.org

Sandra S. Cornelius, President of Elwyn
Daniel M. Reardon, Senior Vice President and Chief
H. Scott Campbell, Vice President
Richard T. Smith, Vice President for Information T

A non-profit human services organization recognized nationally and internationally as experts in the education and care of individuals with special challenges and disadvantages. Today Elwyn is a leading provider of services for people with special needs of all ages.

6622 First State Senior Center
291a N Rehoboth Blvd
Milford, DE 19963-1303 302-422-1510
dhss.delaware.gov/dhss/main/maps/other/dddssr

6623 Woodside Day Program
941 Walnut Shade Rd
Dover, DE 19901-7765 302-739-4494
FAX: 302-697-4490

Connie Grace, Supervisor
Joyce Oliver, Manager
.

District of Columbia

6624 Barbara Chambers Children's Center
1470 Irving St NW
Washington, DC 20010-2804 202-387-6755
FAX: 202-319-9066
e-mail: bcchildrencenter@erols.com
barbarachambers.org

Barbara Chambers, Founder

Mission is to provide comprehensive, quality child care services to the community at large, by offering a variety of opportunities for childrens's intellectual, emotional, social and physical development in a clean, safe, and nurturing environment. Our philosophy is to provide a supportive environment in which children can be children..allowing each child to learn at his/her pace and most of all allowing the child to learn through his/her daily play.

6625 District of Columbia General Hospital Physical Medicine & Rehab Services
Room 1358
19th and Mass Ave
Washington, DC 20003 202-727-6055
FAX: 202-675-7819

Dr. Maribel Bieberach, Chairperson PM&R
Dr. Raman Kapur, Staff Physiatrist

Offers comprehensive physical medicine and rehabilitation services including in and outpatient consultations and electrodiagnostic testing; in and outpatient physical and occupational therapy; inpatient recreational therapy, and a multidisciplinary prosthetic clinic which meets once a month..

6626 George Washington University Medical Center
George Washington University Medical Center
2150 Pennsylvania Ave NW
Washington, DC 20037-3201 202-741-3000
FAX: 202-741-3183
www.gwdocs.com

6627 HSC Pediatric Center, The
1731 Bunker Hill Rd NE
Washington, DC 20017-3026 202-832-4400
800-226-4444
FAX: 202-467-0978
e-mail: efowler@cscn.org
www.hscpediatriccenter.org

Debbie Zients, CEO
Dr Murry M Pollack, VP, Medical Affairs
Eva Fowler, Media Contact

Provides the highest quality rehabilitative and transitional care for infants, children, adolescents, and young adults with special health care needs and their families in a supportive environment that respects their needs, strengths, vslues and priorities..

6628 Howard University Child Development Center
1911 5th St NW
Washington, DC 20001-2314 202-797-8134
FAX: 202-986-6580

Connie Siler, Manager

Offers children with developmental problems diagnosis, treatment, evaluation and follow along visits..

6629 Psychiatric Institute of Washington
4228 Wisconsin Ave NW
Washington, DC 20016-2138 202-885-5600
800-369-2273
FAX: 202-885-5614
e-mail: ceo@piw-dc.com
psychinstitute.com

Ken Courage, Chairman
Carol Desjuns, Chief Operations Officer
Howard Hoffman, Executive Medical Director
Aarti Subramanian, VP/Chief Financial Off

Psychiatric intensive care, crisis intervention, adult day treatment, drug treatment and other services to children and adults who have psychiatric and chemical dependency problems.

6630 Spina Bifida Program of DC Children's Hospital
Department of Physical Medicine and Rehabilitation
111 Michigan Ave NW
Washington, DC 20010-2916 202-476-5000
FAX: 202-476-2270
childrensnational.org

Kurt Newman, President and Chief Executive Of
Elizabeth Flury, Chief Strategy Officer
Kathleen E. Chavanu Gorman, Chief Operating Officer
Mary Anne Hilliard, Chief Risk Counsel

Offers neurosurgery, orthopedics,physical medicine, social work, urology and nursing. Mission is to improve health outcomes for children regionally, nationally, and internationally. Be a leader in creating innovative solutions to pediatric healthcare problems. Excel in Care, Advocacy, Research, and Education to meet the unique needs of children, adolescents and their families.

Florida

6631 Bayfront Rehabilitation Center
Bayfront Medical Center
701 6th St S
St Petersburg, FL 33701-4814 727-823-1234
www.bayfrontstpete.com

Kathryn Gillette, President and CEO
Eric Smith, Chief Financial Officer
Lavah Lowe, Chief Operating Officer
Karen Long, Chief Nursing Executive

Bayfront Medical Center has an Inpatient Rehabilitation Hospital and two outpatient rehabilitation clinics that each provide progressive, comprehensive, individualized treatment. Specialized care in Physiatry (physical medicine), rehab nursing, occupational therapy, speech language pathology, recreational therapy, patient/family services and psychology is tailored to each patient from admission to community and/or school reintegration.

6632 Brain Injury Rehabilitation Center Dr. P. Phillips Hospital
Brain Injury Rehabilitation Center Dr. P. Phillips
9400 Turkey Lake Rd
Orlando, FL 32819-8001 407-351-8580
www.orlandohealth.com/drpphillipshospital/ind
Shannon Elswick, President
Linda Chapin, Chairman
Mark Swanson, Chief Quality Officer
John Hillenmeyer, CEO Emeritus, Orlando Health
Dedicated to restoring brain injured patients with rehabilitation potential to their highest level of functioning. This is accomplished through an interdisciplinary team demonstrating personal responsibility to the patient, their family and each other.

6633 Brooks Memorial Hospital Rehabilitation Center
3599 University Blvd. South
Jacksonville, FL 32207-6215 904-858-7600
FAX: 904-858-7619
e-mail: louise.spierre@brookshealth.org
www.brookshealth.org
Douglas Baer, Chief Executive Officer/ Preside
Holly Morris, Director, Brooks Rehabilitation
Louise Spierre, Medical Director
Floris Singletary, Research Manager, Clinical Resea
An entire care facility featuring five day inpatient evaluation, pre-operative evaluation programs, five week pain management program, referral criteria and treatment goals, therapy services, psychological services and more to the physically challenged.

6634 Center for Pain Control and Rehabilitation
Ste 607
2780 Cleveland Ave
Fort Myers, FL 33901-5858 239-337-4332
Mary Bonnette, Owner
.

6635 Comprehensive Rehabilitation Center at Lee Memorial Hospital
2776 Cleveland Ave
Fort Myers, FL 33901-5864 239-343-2000
leememorial.org
James R. Nathan, Chief Executive Officer System P
Larry Antonucci, Chief Operating Officer
Jon Cecil, Chief Human Resources Officer
Mike German, Chief Financial Officer
Lee Memorial hospital has achieved national recognition as one of the top 100 hospitals for stroke, orthopedics, and Intensive Care Unit (ICU) It is a 367 bed hospital that provides 24-hour emergency and trauma care, inpatient rehabilitation, orthopedics, neuroscience, trauma, cancer, diabetes, digestive, general surgery, urology, endocrinology, gastroenterology, opthamology, and many others.

6636 Comprehensive Rehabilitation Center of Naples Community Hospital
350 7th Street North
Naples, FL 34102 239-436-5000
FAX: 239-436-5250
www.nchmd.org
Allen S. Weiss, CEO
Mariann MacDonald, Chairman
Thomas Gazdic, Chairman/Treasurer
John Lewis, Secretary
Offers rehabilitation services, inpatient and outpatient care at 5 locations in the county and more for the benefit of the disabled.

6637 Conklin Center for the Blind
405 White St
Daytona Beach, FL 32114-2999 386-258-3441
FAX: 386-258-1155
e-mail: info@conklincenter.org
www.conklincenter.org
Robert T Kelly, Executive Director
The Conklin Center's mission is to empower children and adults who are blind and have one or more additional disabilities to develop their potential to be able to obtain competitive employment, live independently and fully participate in community life.

6638 Davis Center for Rehabilitation Baptist Hospital of Miami
8900 N Kendall Dr
Miami, FL 33176-2118 786-596-1960
e-mail: corporatepr@baptisthealth.net
www.baptisthealth.net/bhs
Brian E. Keeley, President and Chief Executive Of
Calvin Babcock, Chairman
A full-service, nonprofit community hospital providing a full range of inpatient and outpatient rehabilitation services. The overall commitment to excellence has extended to this specialized field. Access to medical expertise and services ensures that the best in medical resources are available should an unforeseen medical problem arise.

6639 Division of Blind Services
325 West Gaines Street
Suite 1114
Turlington Building, FL 32399-0400 850-245-0300
800-342-1828
FAX: 850-245-0386
e-mail: ana.saint-ford@dbs.fldoe.org
dbs.myflorida.com
Aleisa McKinlay, Interim Director
Phyllis Vaughn, Bureau Chief, Administrative Services
William Findley, Bureau Chief, Business Enterprise Program
Edward Hudson, Bureau Chief of the Rehabilitation Center for the Blind and
Serves the totally blind, legally blind, visually impaired, deaf-blind, learning disabled, mentally retarded and other multiply handicapped by offering health, counseling, educational, recreational and computer training services.

6640 Easter Seals Broward County
1475 N.W. 14th Ave.
Miami, FL 33125 305-325-0470
FAX: 305-325-0578
www.easterseals.com/southflorida
Loreen Chant, President and Chief Executive Officer
ESBC provides direct services to children and adults with physical, neurological and communications disabilities and their families.

6641 Easter Seals South Florida
1475 NW 14th Avenue
Miami, FL 33125-1616 305-325-0470
FAX: 305-325-0578
e-mail: info@southflorida.easterseals.com
www.southflorida.easterseals.com
Luanne Welch, President
The mission of Easter Seals South Florida is to provide exceptional services to ensure that all children and adults with disabilities or special needs and their families have equal opportunities to live, learn, work and play in their communities.

6642 Easter Seals Southwest Flordia
Sarasota, FL 34243-2001 941-355-7637
themeadowscup.com

6643 Easter Seals: Volusia and Flagler Counties, FL
Easter Seals National
233 South Wacker Drive
Suite 2400
Chicago, IL 60606-2405 800-221-6827
easterseals.com
Richard W. Davidson, Chairman
Ralph F. Boyd, Jr., Treasurer
Eileen Howard Boone, Secretary
James E. Williams, Jr., Assistant Secretary
Provides early intervention services: inclusive pre-school, aquatherapy and sensory processing therapy, OT, PT, ST and

parenting programs, audiology services, equipment loan program, assistive technology information and referral. Residential summer camp and respite.

6644 Florida CORF
Columbia Medical Center: Peninsula
www.memorial-health.com
John Feore, Executive VP
Sandra Trovato, Executive Director
Offers Medicare authorized therapy programs for seniors, disabled and others who need rehabilitation. CORF can provide coordinated and extended services in the home after a hospital stay, or when physical status changes. Patients who are treated at CORF, include amputations, arthritis, chronic/acute pain, depression/anxiety, nerve injury, sports injury, stroke and swallowing problems.

6645 Florida Community College at Jacksonville/ Services for Students with Disabilities
501 State St W
Jacksonville, FL 32202-4086 904-646-2300
877-578-6801
e-mail: equityofficer@fscj.edu
fscj.edu
Steven R. Wallace, President
James E. McCollum, Chairman
Patti Williams, Project Coordinator
Shirley Hendley, Administrative Assistant II
Florida Community College provides educational support services through the Auxiliary Aids Program within the Office of Services for Students With Disabilities.

6646 Florida Institute Of Rehabilitation Education (FIRE)
3071 Highland Oaks Terrace
Tallahassee, FL 32301-4876 850-942-3658
888-827-6033
FAX: 850-942-4518
e-mail: info@lighthousebigbend.org
www.firesight.org
Barbara Ross, Executive Director
Evelyn Worley, Assistant Director
Wayne Warner, Vocational Program Director
Toni King, Independent Living Specialist
Provides independent living and vocational rehabilitation services to Florida residents who are legally blind. Services include instruction in orientation and mobility, accessible technology, daily living skills and employability skills. Information, referral and counseling services are also offered. All services are provided without charge.

6647 Florida Institute for Neurologic Rehabilitation, Inc
1962 Vandolah Road
P O Box 1348
Wauchula, FL 33873-1348 863-773-2857
800-697-5390
FAX: 863-773-0867
finr.net
John Richards, Administrator
Stephanie Ortiz, RN, Director of Nursing
Kevin E. O'Keefe, Program Director
Dana Lucas, Director of Nursing
A residential rehabilitation facility providing a therapeutic environment in which children, adolescents and adults who have survived head-injury can develop the independence and skills necessary to re-enter the community.

6648 Fort Lauderdale Veterans Medical Center
713 NE 3rd Ave
Fort Lauderdale, FL 33304-2619 954-356-7926
FAX: 954-356-7609
www.va.gov/directory/guide/
Robert White, Executive Director
Sloan D Gibson, Acting Secretary
Jose D Riojas, Chief of Staff
Richard J Griffin, Acting Inspector General
Veterans medical clinic offering disabled veterans medical treatments.

6649 Halifax Hospital Medical Center Eye Clinic Professional Center
308 Farmington Avenue
Farmington, CT 06032 860-658-4388
888-444-3598
e-mail: webmaster@evariant.com
www.evariant.com
Bill Moschella, CEO
Rob Grant, Executive Vice President
Michael Clark, Chief Operating Officer
James Orsillo, Chief Financial Officer
Offers services for the totally blind, legally blind, visually impaired, mentally retarded blind and more with health, counseling, educational, recreational, rehabilitation, computer training and professional training services.

6650 HealthQuest Subacute and Rehabilitation Programs
Regenta Park
8700 a C Skinner Pkwy
Jacksonville, FL 32256-836 FAX: 904-641-7896

6651 HealthSouth Emeral Coast Sports & Rehabilitation Center
1847 Florida Avenue
Panama City, FL 32405-3730 850-784-4878
FAX: 850-769-7566
www.healthsouthpanamacity.com
Tony Bennett, CEO
Michelle Miller, Manager
Outpatient sports medicine and rehabilitation center providing physical therapy, occupational therapy, industrial rehab, work hardening/work simulation, worksite and ergonomic analysis, FCE's, work assessment and pre-employment goals of returning the clients back to work, and returning to all recreational, sports and functional activities safely..

6652 HealthSouth Rehabilitation Hospital of Tallahassee
Healthsouth Corporation
1675 Riggins Rd
Tallahassee, FL 32308-5315 850-656-4800
www.healthsouthtallahassee.com
Heath Phillips, Chief Executive Officer
Robert Robert Rowland, Medical Director
Tom Abbruscato, Controller
Deborah Baird, Director of Quality and Risk Man
North Florida's sole acute rehabilitation hospital between Jacksonville \, Panama City, and Gainesville. With 250 employees providing a full continuum of care form its 70 bed facility, the hospital is accredited by JCAHO, CARF and state designated and certified by Vocational Rehabilitation for traumatic brain injury, as well as a wide variety of other diagnoses. With the addition of our outpatients, the facility has served the greater community by touching the lives of over 50,000 patients.

6653 HealthSouth Rehabilitation Hospital Of Miami
20601 Old Cutler Rd
Miami, FL 33189-2441 305-251-3800
www.healthsouthmiami.com
Elizabeth Izquierdo, Chief Executive Officer
Angelo Appio, Director of Marketing Operations
Reyna M. Hernandez, Chief Financial Officer
Paige Keil, Director of Quality and Risk Man
A comprehensive source of medical rehabilitation services for Pinellas County, Florida area residents, their families and their physicians. Offers the people of Florida all the clinical, technical and professional resources of the nation's leading provider of comprehensive rehabilitation care.

6654 HealthSouth Rehabilitation Hospital of Sarasota
Health South Corporation in Burmingham Alabama
6400 Edgelake Drive
Sarasota, FL 34240-8813 941-921-8600
866-330-5822
www.healthsouthsarasota.com

Marcus Braz, Chief Executive Officer
Alexander DeJesus, Medical Director
Nancy Arnold, Director of Marketing Operations
Brenda Benner, Director of Human Resources

HealthSouth Rehabilitation Hospital of Sarasota is a 96-bed inpatient rehabilitation hospital that offers comprehensive inpatient rehabilitation services designed to return patients to leading active and independent lives.

6655 HealthSouth Sea Pines Rehabilitation Hospital
Sea Pines Rehabilitation Hospital
101 E Florida Ave
Melbourne, FL 32901-8398 321-984-4600
FAX: 321-952-6532
www.healthsouthseapines.com

Stuart Miller, Medical Director
Denise McGrath, Chief Executive Officer
Donna Anderson, Director of Human Resources
Jerry Bishop, Director of Quality and Risk Man

Designed to return patients to leading active, independent lives, HealthSouth Sea Pines Rehabilitation Hospital is a 90-bed rehabilitation hospital that provides a higher level of comprehensive rehabilitation services.

6656 Holy Cross Hospital
Catholic Southwest
4725 North Federal Hwy
Fort Lauderdale, FL 33308-4668 954-771-8000
www.holy-cross.com

Patrick Taylor, President & Chief Executive Offi
Luisa Gutman, Senior Vice President & Chief Op
Linda Wilford, Senior Vice President & Chief Fi
Kenneth Homer, Chief Medical Officer & Medical

Holy Cross Hospital in Fort Lauderdale is a full-service, non-profit Catholic hospital, sponsored by the Sisters of Mercy. Holy Cross is a US News & World Report 'Best Hospital' and HealthGrades Distinguished Hospital for Clinical Excellence, 2004 and 2005

6657 Lee Memorial Hospital
2776 Cleveland Ave
Fort Myers, FL 33901-5855 239-343-2000
www.leememorial.org

Sanford Cohen, Chairman
Chris Hansen, Vice Chairman
David Collins, Treasurer
Diane Champion, Secretary

Offers a complete inpatient program of intensive rehabilitation designed to restore a patient to a more independent level of functioning. The comprehensive care includes medical rehabilitation and training for spinal cord injury, brain injury, stroke and neurological disorders.

6658 Lighthouse for the Blind of Palm Beach
1710 Tiffany Drive East
West Palm Beach, FL 33407-3224 561-586-5600
FAX: 561-84- 80
lighthousepalmbeaches.org

Marvin A. Tanck, President and CEO
Dont, Mickens, Chair
John R. Banister, Vice Chairman
David B. Cano, MD

A private, non-profit rehabilitation and education agency in its 55th year of service. Offers programs to assist persons who areblind or visually impaired, an on-site Industrial Center, a technology training center, an Aids and appliances Store, special equipment grant programs, outreach services for children and adults, Early Intervention and Preschool Services, and a variety of support groups. These programs provide services and education for blind children and their parents.

6659 Lighthouse for the Visually Impaired and Blind
8610 Galen Wilson Blvd
Port Richey, FL 34668-5974 727-815-0303
866-962-5254
FAX: 727-815-0203
e-mail: lighthouse@lvib.org
www.lvib.org

Sylvia Stinson-Perez, Executive Director
Dr. John Mann, President
Melissa M. Suess, Orientation and Mobility Instruc
Peter James, Business Development Specialist

The Lighthouse offers services for visually impaired or blind adults and children ages 0-5 years old. Counseling, educational services, recreational services, rehabilitation, computer training and support groups.

6660 MacDonald Training Center
5420 W Cypress Street
Tampa, FL 33607-1706 813-870-1300
866-948-6184
FAX: 813-872-6010
TTY: 813-873-7631
e-mail: jfreyvogel@macdonaldcenter.org
macdonaldcenter.org

Jim Freyvogel, President/CEO
Judith DeStasio, CFO
Debi Hamilton, Director of Services
Joe Donato, COO

A private, non-profit, community-based human services organization serving adults with disabilities (since 1953). Persons are provided the opportunity to achieve their highest potential through the Center's various programs that include day training, employment, community living and various support services.

6661 Medicenter of Tampa
4411 North Habana Avenue
Tampa, FL 33614-7211 813-872-2771
FAX: 813-871-2831
rehabilitationandhealthcarecenteroftampa.com

Dan Davis, President
Mariluz G, Social Services Director
Brenda Pace, Secretary
Hilda B, Medicaid Coordinator

Postacute rehabilitation program. A 174 bed non-profit facility with postacute reahbilitation programs..

6662 Miami Heart Institute Adams Building
4300 Alton Rd
Miami Beach, FL 33140-2997 305-674-2121
www.msmc.com

Steven D. Sonenreich, President/CEO

The mission is to provide high quality health care to our diverse community enhanced through teaching, research, charity care and financial responsibility.

6663 Miami Lighthouse for the Blind
601 SW 8th Ave
Miami, FL 33130-3200 305-856-2288
FAX: 305-285-6967
e-mail: info@miamilighthouse.com
miamilighthouse.org

Virginia A. Jacko, President & Chief Executive Officer
Sharon Caughill, Special Projects Manager
Jeannie Reinoso, Executive Assistant
Arnie Paniagua, Chief Financial Officer

Offers services for the legally blind and severely visually impaired (including those who are developmentally delayed) of all ages in the areas of counseling and educational, recreational, rehabilitation, computer and vocational training services.

6664 Mount Sinai Medical Center Rehabilitation Unit
4300 Alton Rd
Miami Beach, FL 33140-2997 305-674-2121
www.msmc.com

Steven D. Sonenreich, President/CEO

A comprehensive inpatient and outpatient rehabilitation programs have been helping patients recover for more then 20 years. Fully customized treatment plans based on the needs of each patient is 1 reason why our services are among the best in South Florida. Our team approach takes into account the medical, physical, psychological, social, spiritual, cultural and economic needs of patients and their families.

6665 Neurobehavioral Medicine Center
Ste 1
4821 Us Highway 19
New Port Richey, FL 34652-4259 727-849-2005
FAX: 727-849-2087
Otsenre Matos, Medical Director
Gerard Taylor PhD, Counseling/Stress Management
Donna Taylor RN, Manager
Joyce Park Matos ARNP, Clinical Specialist
A multidisciplinary outpatient program for the evaluation and treatment of chronic pain. Consultation services for hospitalized patients are also provided upon request. Comprehensive treatment of individuals with closed traumatic brain injuries..

6666 North Broward Rehab Unit
North Broward Medical Center
201 E Sample Rd
Deerfield Beach, FL 33064-3596 954-941-8300
www.browardhealth.org
Douglas Ford, Chiefs of Staff
Pauline Grant, Chief Executive Officer
CARF accredited, 30-bed inpatient rehabilitation unit treating adults with brain injuries, spinal cord injuries, stroke, orthopedic and neurologic injuries.

6667 Northwest Medical Center
Health Care Corporation of America
2801 North State Road 7
Margate, FL 33063-5727 954-974-0400
866-256-7720
northwestmed.com
Mark Rader, CEO
Above all else, we are committed to the care and improvement of human life. In recognition of this commitment, we strive to deliver high quality, cost effective healthcare in the communities we serve. We recognize and affirm the unique and intrinsic work of each individual. We treat all those we serve with compassion and kindness. We act with absolute honesty, integrity, and fairness in the way we conduct our business and the way we live our lives.

6668 Pain Institute of Tampa
4178 N Armenia Ave
Tampa, FL 33607-6429 813-875-5913
www.barsahealth.com
John E Barsa, Founder & MD
Offers a comprehensive and multidisciplinary approach to pain controll and management. Most services are provided on-site but other services may require you to be referred elswhere. We will monitor and coordinate your care in a manner to provide optimal recovery potential.

6669 Pain Treatment Center, Baptist Hospital of Miami
8900 N Kendall Dr
Miami, FL 33176-2118 786-596-1960
e-mail: corporatepr@baptisthealth.net
www.baptisthealth.net
Calvin Babcock, Chairman
Brian E. Keeley, President and Chief Executive Of
Since 1960, Baptist Hospital of Miami has been one of the most respected medical centers in South Florida. The hospitals full range of medical and technological services is the natural choice for a growing number of people throughout the world.

6670 Pine Castle
4911 Spring Park Rd
Jacksonville, FL 32207-7496 904-733-2650
FAX: 904-733-2681
e-mail: info@pinecastle.org
pinecastle.org
Jonathan May, Executive Director
Randall Duncan, Associate Executive Director
Leigh Griffin, Director of Finance
Cliff Evans, Director of Development
Provides remunerative work, training, community employment and community living options for adults with developmental disabilities.

6671 Polk County Association for Handicapped Citizens
1038 Sunshine Dr E
Lakeland, FL 33801-6338 863-858-2252
FAX: 863-665-2330
e-mail: sbaloghweb@pcahc.org
www.pcahc.org
Kecia Howell, Owner
Anthony J. Senzamici Jr., 1st Vice Chairman
Carol N. Asbill, 2nd Vice Chairman
A private non-profit organization that provides an adult day training program to people with developmental disabilities and is under the direction of a volunteer board of directors. The primary goal for our services is to provide people with knowledge and practical experience to be independent adults so they can become contributing members of their community..

6672 Quest
500 E Colonial Drive
P O Box 531125
Orlando, FL 32853- 4504 407-218-4300
888-807-8378
FAX: 407-218-4301
questinc.org
David Canora, Chair
James Gallagher, Vice-Chair
Suzanne Bennett, Treasurer
Ruth Bresnick, Secretary
Quest has built communities where people with disabilities have achieved their goals for nearly 50 years. Through a variety of residential and employment options, behavioral therapy, therapeutic day programs, charter schools and even a recreational summer camp, Quest serves more than 1000 individuals each day in the Orlando and Tampa areas.

6673 Quest - Tampa Area
1404 Tech Blvd
Tampa, FL 33619 813-423-7700
888-807-8378
FAX: 813-423-7701
e-mail: contact@questinc.org
www.questinc.org
David Canora, Chair
James Gallagher, Vice-Chair
Suzanne Bennett, Treasurer
Ruth Bresnick, Secretary
Quest has built communities where people with disabilities have achieved their goals for nearly 50 years. Through a variety of residential and employment options, behavioral therapy, therapeutic day programs, charter schools and even a recreational summer

6674 Rehabilitation Center for Children and Adults
300 Royal Palm Way
Palm Beach, FL 33480-4305 561-655-7266
FAX: 561-655-3269
e-mail: info@rcca.org
rcca.org
John C. Whelton, Chairman
Jacob L. Lochner, Co-Chairman
Christopher Adams, MD
A private, nonprofit organization whose purpose is to improve physical function, independence and communication of people with physical disabilities. Any child or adult with a physical or speech disability is eligible for services.

6675 Renaissance Center
3599 University Blvd
Suite 604
Jacksonville, FL 32216- 9249
904-399-0905
FAX: 904-743-5109
www.obiplasticsurgery.com/index.php

Lewis Obi, MD

6676 Rosomoff Comprehensive Pain Center, The
5200 NE 2nd Avenue
Miami, FL 33137-2706
305-532-7246
FAX: 305-534-3974
e-mail: painrelief@rosomoffpaincenter.com
www.rosomoffpaincenter.com

Elsayed Abdel-Moty, Director
Hubert Rossomoff, Owner

A state-of-the-art Center of Excellence offering inpatient, outpatient, outpatient rehabilitation services and seniors programs. The Center became an internationally renowned model for the evalutation and treatment of all persons seeking pain relief.

6677 Sarasota Memorial Hospital/Comprehensive Rehabilitation Unit
1700 S Tamiami Trail
Sarasota, FL 34239-3509
941-917-9000
FAX: 941-917-2211
www.smh.com

Marguerite G Malone, Chair
Gregory Carter, First Vice Chair
Alex Miller, Second Vice Chair
Joseph J. DeVirgilio, Jt. Treasurer

The goal of the 34-bed Comprehensive Rehabilitation Unit (CRU) is to increase patient functional independence, adjust to illness or disability and successfully return to the community. The unit is dedicated to patients who have experienced conditions such

6678 Strive Physical Therapy Centers
2620 SE Maricamp RD
Ocala, FL 34471-4517
352-732-8868
FAX: 352-732-8890
www.striverehab.com

R W Shutes, Owner
Johanna Solbato, Administrator
R.W. Shutes, President and CEO

Certified as an Outpatient Rehabilitation Agency, providing a comprehensive approach to patient evaluation and treatment. Our objective is to return our patients back to a productive life as quickly as possible and safely as possible.

6679 Sunbridge Care and Rehabilitation
101 East State Street,
Kennett Square, FL 19348-6105
610-444-6350
FAX: 610-925-4000
e-mail: info@genesishcc.com
www.genesishcc.com

Dan Hirschfeld, President
George V Hager, Chief Executive Officer
Robert A Reitz, Executive Vice President & Chief Operating Officer
Michael Sherman, Senior VP

A comprehensive medical rehabilitation facility that is committed to helping individuals with disabilities improve their quality of life. This is a 120-bed facility offering a full range of acute and sub-acute inpatient programs as well as community-based

6680 Tampa Bay Academy
12012 Boyette Rd
Riverview, FL 33569-5631
813-677-6700
800-678-3838
FAX: 813-671-3145
e-mail: tlamb@tampahope.org
www.tampahope.org

Renee Scott, Chair
Amy McClure, Vice-Chair
Titania Lamb, Executive Director

A psychiatric residential treatment center and partial hospitalization program for ages 7 to 17.

6681 Tampa General Rehabilitation Center
1 Tampa General Circle
P.O.Box 1289
Tampa, FL 33606-3571
813-844-7700
866-844-1411
FAX: 813-844-1477
e-mail: jstone@tgh.org
tgh.org

James R. Burkhart, President & CEO
Bruce Zwiebel, Chief Of Staff
Deana L. Nelson, Chief Operating Officer
Steve Short, Cheif Financial Officer

Offers a full range of programs all aimed at helping patients achieve their full potentials. It is one of three centers in the state that provides Driver Training and Evaluation Programs for persons with disabilities, and also an Assisted Reproduction Pro

6682 Tampa Lighthouse for the Blind
1106 West Platt Street
Tampa, FL 33606-2142
813-251-2407
FAX: 813-254-4305
e-mail: tlh@templelighthouse.org
tampalighthouse.org

Sheryl Brown, Executive Director

Offers services for the totally blind, legally blind, visually impaired, mentally retarded blind and more with health, counseling, educational, recreational, rehabilitation, computer training and professional training services.

6683 Upper Pinellas Association for Retarded Citizens
1501 N Belcher Rd
Suite 249
Clearwater, FL 33765-1300
727-799-3330
FAX: 727-799-4632
e-mail: info@uparc.com
www.uparc.com

Karen Crown, Executive Director

Offers services to more than 500 persons with mental retardation and other developmental disabilities. Services include two early intervention pre-schools, physical, speech and occupational therapies, homebound education and family support for children, b

6684 Visually Impaired Persons of Southwest Florida
35 W Mariana Ave
North Fort Myers, FL 33903-5515
239-997-7797
FAX: 239-997-8462
e-mail: mmcgrael@vipcenter.org
vipcenter.org

Doug Fowler, Executive Director
Margaret Ruhe Lincoln, Director of operations

Provides training in independent living skills, orientation and mobility, counseling, computer and other communication skills, family support groups, peer counseling, socialization and a low vision clinic. Second location in Charlotte County. Phone: 941-6

6685 West Florida Hospital: The Rehabilitation Institute
8383 North Davis Hwy
Pensacola, FL 32514-6039
850-494-4000
800-342-1123
FAX: 850-494-4881
www.westfloridahospital.com

Roman S Bautista, President/CEO
Carol Saxton, Senior VP Patient Care Services

A 58-bed comprehensive rehabilitation facility offering inpatient and outpatient services. JCAHO and CARF accredited and a State designed head and spinal cord injury center. CARF accredited programs include: comprehensive inpatient rehab, spinal cord inju

6686 **West Gables Health Care Center**
2525 SW 75th Ave
Miami, FL 33155-2800
305-262-6800
FAX: 888-453-1928
www.westgablesrehabhospital.com

Jose Vargas, Medical Director
Walter Concepcion, Chief Executive Officer
Cesar Sepulveda, Materials Manager
Zely Santos, Admissions Director
Services provide by West Gables Health Center: activities services are provided onsite to residents. Clinical laboratory services are provided, dental, dietary, housekeeping, mental health services, nursing services, occupational therapy, pharmacy, physic

6687 **Willough at Naples**
9001 Tamiami Trail East
Naples, FL 34113-3397
239-775-4500
800-722-0100
FAX: 239-793-0534
e-mail: info@thewilloughatnaples.com
thewilloughatnaples.com

James O'Shea, President
A licensed psychiatric hospital in Southwest Florida which provides quality management and treatment for eating disorders and chemical dependency in adults.

Georgia

6688 **Annandale Village**
3500 Annandale Ln
Suwanee, GA 30024-2150
770-945-8381
FAX: 770-945-8693
e-mail: administration@annandale.org
annandale.org

Adam Pomeranz, Chief Executive Officer
Melissa Burton, Chief Financial Officer
Keith Fenton, Chief Development & Marketing Officer
Nancy Trujillo, Chief Operating Officer
Private nonprofit residential facility for adults with developmental disabilities. Located on 124 acres just north of Atlanta. Annandale provides full program and 24 hour residential services, pay program services, respite care and skilled nursing services.

6689 **Atlanta Institute of Medicine and Rehabilitation**
Ste E
2911 Piedmont Rd NE
Atlanta, GA 30305-2782
404-365-0160
FAX: 404-365-0751
e-mail: contact@atlantaimr.com
www.atlantaimr.com

Lawrence E Eppelbaum, Founder
Galina Vayner, MD
One of the most famous medical centers in the state of Georgia. The Institute employs more then 40 highly qualified medical professionals and fully equipped with the latest medical equipment. It has gathered recognition and respect from the people of Atla

6690 **Bobby Dodd Institute (BDI)**
2120 Marietta Blvd NW
Atlanta, GA 30318-2122
678-365-0071
FAX: 678-365-0098
TTY:678-365-0099
e-mail: wmcmillan@bdi-atl.org
bobbydodd.org

Rodney Hall, Chair
Christopher Rosselli, Vice Chair
Wayne McMillan, President & CEO
John Ralls, Treasurer
BDI annually serves approximately 400 clients in Atlanta, GA. BDI works primarily with people with developmental disabilities such as autism, down syndrome or mental retardation, but includes clients with physical or acquired disabilities. Client age va

6691 **Cave Spring Rehabilitation Center**
Georgia Department of Labor
7 Georgia Ave
P.O.Box 303
Cave Spring, GA 30124-2718
706-777-2341
FAX: 706-777-2366
e-mail: russell.fleming@dol.state.ga.us
gvra.georgia.gov/cave-spring-center-cont acts-

Russell Fleming, Director
Karen Hulsey, Administrative Operations Coordinator
Renee Lambert, Rehabilitation Assistant
Renaultha Houston, Residential Program Supervisor

6692 **Center for Assistive Technology and Environmental Access**
490 10th St
Atlanta, GA 30332-0156
404-894-4960
800-726-9119
FAX: 404-894-9320
e-mail: catea@coa.gatech.edu
www.catea.org

Carrie Bruce, Research Scientist
Charlie Drummond, Administrative Assistant
Summer Ienuso, Wen Developer
Trin Intra, Financial Administrator
The Center for Assistive Technology and Environmental Access (CATEA) promotes maximum function, activity and access of persons with disabilities through the use of technology. The foci of the Center includes the development, evaluation and utilization of

6693 **Center for the Visually Impaired**
739 West Peachtree St NW
Atlanta, GA 30308-1137
404-875-9011
FAX: 404-607-0062
e-mail: info@cviatlanta.org
cviga.org

Susan Hoy, Chair
Fontaine M. Huey, President
Doreen Zaksheske, Vice President of Finance & Operations
Anisio Correia, Vice President for Programs
Offers services to people of all ages who are blind or visually impaired with training in orientation and mobility, computer technology, activities of daily living, communication skills and employment readiness. Aso offers two children's programs, a comm

6694 **Devereux Georgia Treatment Network**
1291 Stanley Road
Kennesaw, GA 30152-8688
770-427-0147
800-342-3357
FAX: 770-427-4030
e-mail: cfrost@devereux.org
www.devereuxga.org

Helena T. Devereux, Founder
Robert Q. Kreider, President & CEO
Serves ages 10 to 17, males and females with a capacity for up to 187. Serves moderate to severe emotional, behavioral and/or learning disabilities. A specialized psychiatric hospital/intensive residential treatment program for below average to superior i

6695 **Easter Seals East Georgia**
1500 Wrightsboro Road
Augusta, GA 30904-2441
706-667-9695
866-667-9695
FAX: 706-667-8831
e-mail: sthomas@esega.org
www.easterseals.com/eastgeorgia

Sheila H. Thomas, CEO
Patrick Clayton, Chairman
Easter Seals East Georgia assists people with disabilities and other special needs to maximize opportunities for employment, independence and full inclusion into society.

6696 **Georgia Industries for the Blind**
700 Faceville Highway
Bainbridge, GA 39819-218 229-248-2666
FAX: 229-248-2669
gvra.georgia.gov/gib/about-us
James Hughes, Executive Director
Offers services for the totally blind, legally blind, visually impaired, mentally retarded blind and more with health, counseling, educational, recreational, rehabilitation, computer training and professional training services.

6697 **Hillhaven Rehabilitation**
26 Tower Rd NE
Marietta, GA 30060-6947 770-422-8913
800-526-5782
FAX: 770-425-2085
Leslie Ann Marie Parrish, Case Manager
Valerie Hamilton, Administrator
Routine skilled and subacute medical and rehabilitation care including physical therapy, occupational therapy, speech pathology and therapeutic recreation. Programs include stroke and head injury rehab; orthopedic rehab; complex IV therapy; woundcare; can.

6698 **In-Home Medical Care**
Care Master Medical Services
240 Odell Rd
P.O.Box 278
Griffin, GA 30223-4787 770-227-1264
800-542-8889
FAX: 770-412-0014
e-mail: caremaster@accesunited.com
caremastermedical.com
Nancy Frederick, VP
Eddie Grogan, Chief Executive Officer
Offers the devoted attention of a professional nurse, the use of I.V. therapies, pain management and provision of medical equipment and supplies right where the patient wants to be.

6699 **Learning Services: Harris House Program**
131 Langley Drive
Suite B
Lawrenceville, GA 30046-4446 404-298-0144
888-419-9955
FAX: 866-491-7396
learningservices.com
Dr. Debra Braunling-McMorrow, President and CEO
Susan Snow, Director of Admissions
Michael Weaver, Chief Development Officer
Jeanne Mack, Chief Financial Officer
Situated in the small, historic district of Stone Mountain, just outside of Atlanta, this 6 bed program is designed to encourage independence while providing appropriate support for each individuals needs. Community-based productive activities are customi

6700 **Pain Control & Rehabilitation Institute of Georgia**
Ste 120
2784 N Decatur Rd
Decatur, GA 30033-5993 404-297-1400
FAX: 404-297-1427
Shulim Spektor, CEO
Anna Britman, Office Manager
Provides pain management for chronic and acute pain resulted from injuries, diseases of muscles and nerve, Reflex Sympathetic Dystrophy, perform disabilities and impairment ratings.

6701 **Savannah Association for the Blind**
214 Drayton Street
Savannah, GA 31401-4021 912-236-4473
FAX: 912-234-9286
www.sabinc.org
Gregory Hodges, President
Robert Falligant, Vice-president
Gary Sadowski, Treasurer
Lula Baker, Secretary
Offers services for the totally blind, legally blind, visually impaired, mentally retarded blind and more with health, counseling, educational, recreational, rehabilitation, computer training and professional training services.

6702 **Shepherd Center for Treatment of Spinal Injuries**
2020 Peachtree Rd NW
Atlanta, GA 30309-1465 404-352-2020
FAX: 404-350-7479
e-mail: admissions@shepherd.org
www.shepherd.org
Gary R. Ulicny, President & CEO
David F. Apple, Jr., M.D., Medical Director
Angela Beninga, D.O., Staff Physiatrist
ChiChi Berhane, M.D., MBA, Director, Reconstructive Surgery
Dedicated exclusively to the care of patients with spinal cord injuries and other paralyzing spinal disorders. It serves predominately residents of Georgia and neighboring states as one of the only 14 hospitals designated by the U.S. Department of Educati

6703 **Transitional Hospitals Corporation**
Ste 1000
7000 Central Pkwy NE
Atlanta, GA 30328-4592 770-821-5328
800-683-6868
FAX: 770-913-0015
e-mail: staff@csins.com
csins.com
Dean Kozee, Owner
Carolyn Norton, Special Projects Consultant/Broker
Amaury Rentas, Event Insurance/Broker
A national network of intensive care hospitals providing care for patients who suffer from a chronic illness and/or catastrophic accident. The mission is founded on providing quality health care to patients who require highly skilled nursing care and acce.

6704 **Walton Rehabilitation Health System**
1355 Independence Dr
Augusta, GA 30901-1037 706-823-8584
866-492-5866
FAX: 706-724-5752
e-mail: vickig@waltonfoundation.net
www.waltonfoundation.net
Robert Taylor, Chair
Dennis Skelley, President/CEO
David Dugan, Treasurer
Brent Smith, Secretary
A 58-bed comprehensive physical rehabilitation hospital offering inpatient and outpatient services. Services offered include: stroke recovery, orthopedic injury, pediatrics, head injury, pain management for chronic pain syndrome, TMJ/Craniofacial pain and

Hawaii

6705 **Rehabilitation Hospital of the Pacific**
226 N Kuakini St
Honolulu, HI 96817-2498 808-531-3511
FAX: 808-566-3411
e-mail: rehabfoundation@rehabhospital.org
www.rehabhospital.org
John Komeiji, Chair
Glenn O. Sexton, Vice Chair
E. Lynne Madden, Secretary/Treasurer
Timothy J. Roe, President & Chief Executive Officer
The only acute care medical rehabilitation organization serving both Hawaii and the Pacific. For over 52 years, the hospital and its 7 outpatient clinics on Oahu, and Maui and Hawaii have been dedicated to providing comprehensive, cost effective rehabilit

Idaho

6706 Ashton Memorial Nursing Home and Chemical Dependency Center
700 N 2nd
Ashton, ID 83420 208-652-7461
FAX: 208-652-7595
e-mail: ashmem@frtel.com
ashtonmemorial.com
Sheila Kellogg, Administrator

6707 Easter Seals-Goodwill Northern Rocky Mountains
Easter Seals National
1465 S Vinnell Way
Boise, ID 83709-1659 208-378-9924
800-374-1910
FAX: 208-378-9965
www.easterseals.org
Richard W. Davidson, Chairman
Ralph F. Boyd, Jr., Treasurer
Eileen Howard Boone, Secretary
James E. Williams, Jr., Assistant Secretary
Provides services for children and adults with disabilities and other special needs, and support to their families

6708 Idaho Elks Rehabilitation Hospital
600 N Robbins Rd
Boise, ID 83702 208-489-4444
FAX: 208-344-8883
e-mail: info@elksrehab.org
www.elksrehab.org
Joseph P. Caroselli, CEO
Doug Lewis, Chief Financial Officer
Mellisa Honsinger, Chief Operating Officer
A nonprofit hospital serving Idaho and the Pacific Northwest. All inpatient and outpatient programs and services are supervised by the hospital's full-time medical directors whose specialty is physical rehabilitative medicine. Services include: occupation

6709 Portneuf Medical Center Rehabilitation
777 Hospital Way
Pocatello, ID 83201-4004 208-239-1000
e-mail: charlesa@portmed.org
www.portmed.org
Mark Buckalew, Chairman
Michael Nosacka, MD
Dan Ordyna, CEO
John Abreu, Vice President
Provides compassionate, quality health care services needed by the people of eastern Idaho in collaboration with other providers and community resources.

Illinois

6710 Advocate Christ Hospital and Medical Center
4440 W 95th St
Oak Lawn, IL 60453-2600 708-684-8000
FAX: 708-684-4440
advocatehealth.com
Jim Skogsbergh, CEO
Bill Santulli, COO
Kate K, Director
A 665-bed, not-for-profit teaching, research and referral medical center in Oak Lawn, Illinois. It also is home to the Advocate Hope Childrens's Hospital, one of the most comprehensive providers of pediatric care in the state. The medical center is a lead

6711 Advocate Christ Medical Center & Advocate Hope Children's Hospital
4440 W 95th St
Oak Lawn, IL 60453-2600 708-684-8000
FAX: 708-684-4440
advocatehealth.com
Kenneth Lukhard, CEO
Darcie Brazel, Market Chief Nurse Executive
Jan McCrea, Rehab Services Director
William Adair MD, Medical Director/Rehab Services
The largest fully integrated not-for-profit health care delivery system in metropolitan Chicago and is recognized as one of the top 10 systems in the country. The mission of Advocate Health Care is to serve the health needs of individuals, families and co

6712 Advocate Illinois Masonic Medical Center
836 W Wellington Ave
Chicago, IL 60657-5147 773-975-1600
www.advocatehealth.com/immc
Jim Skogsbergh, CEO
Ajay V. Maker, MD
Consultation, education, family counseling, parent training in behavior modification techniques offered to developmentally disabled adults.

6713 Alexian Brothers Medical Center
800 Biesterfield Rd
Elk Grove Village, IL 60007-3396 847-437-5500
e-mail: AlexianBrothersMedicalCenter @alexian.net
www.alexian.org
Mark Frey, President/CEO
Tracy Rogers, Senior Vice President and Chief Operating Officer
Paul Belter, Senior Vice President and Chief Financial Officer
Patricia Cassidy, Senior Vice President and Chief Strategy Officer
A threefold mission: Works toward maximizing physical function, enhance independent social skills and optimize communication skills consistent with an individual's ability. The Center helps those disabled by accident or illness achieve a new personal best

6714 Back in the Saddle Hippotherapy Program
Corcoran Physical Therapy
4200 W Peterson Ave
Chicago, IL 60646-6074 312-286-2266
847-604-4145
FAX: 847-673-8895
e-mail: info@hippotherapychicago.com
Julie Naughton, Program Coordinator
Maureen Corcoran, Physical Therapist
Tom Corcoran, Owner
A direct medical treatment used by licensed physical therapists who have a strong treatment background in posture and movement, neuromotor function and sensory processing. The benefits of Hippotherapy are available to individuals with just about any disab

6715 Barbara Olson Center of Hope
3206 N Central Ave
Rockford, IL 61101-1797 815-964-9275
FAX: 815-964-9607
e-mail: info@b-olsoncenterofhope.org
b-olsoncenterofhope.org
Carm Herman, Executive Director
Pam Sondell, Director of Programs and Services
Pam Carey, Director of Human Resources
Mike Marvell, Director of Business Development
We provide vocational employment, educational and social opportunities for adults with developmental disabilities.

6716 Bartolucci Center, The- ILC Enterprises
6415 Stanley Ave
Berwyn, IL 60402-3130
708-745-5277
FAX: 708-698-5090
www.pillarscommunity.org

Zada Clarke, Chairman
Ann Schreiner, President & CEO
Jennifer Hogberg, Vice Chair
Sheila Eswaran, Secretary
A nonprofit tax exempt private social service agency serving suburban Chicago offering day treatment and vocational counseling to individuals who encountered a pattern of job loss due to emotional problems.

6717 Baxter Healthcare Corporation
1 Baxter Pkwy
Deerfield, IL 60015-4625
224-948-2000
800-422-9837
224-948-1812
FAX: 800-568-5020
baxter.com

Phillip L. Batchelor, Corporate Vice President - Quality and Regulatory Affairs
Jean-Luc Butel, Corporate Vice President - President, International
Robert M. Davis, Corporate Vice President - President, Medical Products
Robert Parkinson Jr, Chairman of the Board and Chief Executive Officer
Baxter International Inc. is a global healthcare company that, through its subsidiaries assists healthcare professionals and their patients with treatment of complex medical conditions including hemophelia, immune disorders, kidney disease, cancer, trauma and other conditions. Baxter applies its expertise in medical devices, pharmaceuticals, and biotechnology to make a meaningful difference in patient's lives.

6718 Beacon Therapeutic Diagnostic and Treatment Center
10650 S Longwood Dr
Chicago, IL 60643-2617
773-881-1005
FAX: 773-881-1164
www.beacon-therapeutic.org

Susan Reyha-Guerrero, President & CEO
Cheryl Thompson, Deputy CEO
Paul Morley, Chief Operating Officer
Offers community day treatment, education, diagnostic services, family counseling, learning disabled, speech and hearing and psychiatric services.

6719 Blind Service Association
17 N State St
Ste 1050
Chicago, IL 60602-3510
312-236-0808
blindserviceassociation.org

Ann Lousin, President
Linda Schwartz, Executive Vice President
Arthur M. Shapiro, Secretary
John Powen, Treasurer
Offers services for the totally blind, legally blind and visually impaired with reading and recording low vision network, social services, referrals and support groups.

6720 Brandecker Rehabilitation Center
1939 West 13th Street
Suite 300
Chicago, IL 60643-6316
312-491-4110
FAX: 312-733-0247
www.easterseals.com/chicago

Richard W. Davidson, Chairman
Ralph F. Boyd, Jr., Treasurer
Eileen Howard Boone, Secretary
James E. Williams, Jr., Assistant Secretary
We offer early intervention services for infants and toddlers with developmental delays and disabilities. Our outpatient Medical Rehabilitation Program offers direct therapy services for children from age birth-16.

6721 Brentwood Subacute Healthcare Center
T HI Brentwood
5400 W 87th St
Burbank, IL 60459-2913
866-300-3257
www.savaseniorcare.com

Audrey Protrowski, Director Business Development
Jill Sattersield, Administrator
John Walton, CEO
Seeks to help patients and their families through what can be a very emotional decision-making process. We provide guidance and consultation on everything from how to properly choose the facility to providing resources that help you cope with the nature of the decision itself.

6722 Caremark Healthcare Services
2211 Sanders Rd
Northbrook, IL 60062-6128
847-559-4700
800-423-1411
FAX: 847-559-3905
e-mail: phu@caremark.com
www.caremark.com

Larry J. Merlo, President & CEO
Mark Cosby, Executive Vice President
An 80-service-center network providing services anywhere in the U.S. Offers 24 hour access to nursing and pharmacy services, case management resource centers, HIV/AIDS services, women's health services, transplant care services, nutrition support services

6723 Centegra Northern Illinois Medical Center
4209 West Shamrock Lane
Suite B
McHenry, IL 60050-8499
815-759-8017
877-236-8347
FAX: 815-759-8062
www.centegra.org

Michael S. Eesley, CEO
Jason Sciarro, President
David L. Tomlinson, Executive Vice President
Kumar Nathan, MD
Providing rehabilitation services in Lake and McHenry Counties, the Rehabilitation Unit is a complete living environment for up to 15 patients after a debilitating illness of trauma. Various locations offering a multitude of services: PT, OT, speech, HT,

6724 Center for Comprehensive Services
Mentor Network
P.O.Box 2825
Carbondale, IL 62902-2825
618-457-4008
800-582-4227
FAX: 618-457-5372
e-mail: dayna.foreman@thementornetwork.com
mentorabi.com

Bill Duffy, Chief Operating Officer
Michael E. Hofmeister, Vice President
Sean Byrne, Chief Financial Officer
Post-acute rehabilitation services for adults and adolescents with acquired brain injuries. Residential, day-treatment and out-patient services tailored to individual needs.

6725 Center for Rehabilitation at Rush Presbyterian: Johnston R Bowman Health Center
1653 W Congress Parkway
Chicago, IL 60612-3833
312-942-5000
FAX: 312-942-3601
TTY:312-942-2207
e-mail: teri_sommerfeld@rush.edu
www.rush.edu

Larry J. Goodman, CEO
A 613-bed hospital serving adults and children, the John R. Bowman Health Center and Rush University is home to one of the first medical colleges in the Midwest and one of the nation's top-ranked nursing colleges, as well as graduate programs in allied he

6726 Center for Spine, Sports & Occupational Rehabilitation
345 E Superior St
Chicago, IL 60611-2654
312-238-7767
800-354-7342
FAX: 312-238-7709
e-mail: webmaster@ric.org
www.rehabchicago.org

Joanne C. Smith, President & CEO
Edward B. Case, Executive Vice President
M. Jude Reyes, Chair

Offers evaluation and treatment of patients with acute and subacute musculoskeletal and sports injuries. RIC offers different levels of care, including inpatient, day rehabilitation, and outpatients services, according to the special needs of each patient

6727 Children's Home and Aid Society of Illinois
125 South Wacker Drive
14th Floor
Chicago, IL 60606-4448
312-424-0200
e-mail: contact@chasi.org
www.childrenshomeandaid.org

Beverley Sibblies, Chairman
Chris Leahy, Vice-Chairman
Mark Tresnowski, Secretary
David Gookin, Treasurer

Private state-wide. Multi-service, racially integrated staff and client populations. Provides educational, placement and community services for children-at-risk and their families. Advocacy, consultation and follow-up services provided according to our ph

6728 Clinton County Rehabilitation Center
1665 North Fourth Street
P O Box 157
Breese, IL 62230- 1791
618-526-8800
FAX: 618-526-2021
e-mail: info@commlink.org
commlink.org

Wesley A. Gozia, President
Judge Joseph L. Heimann, Vice President
John L. Lengerman, Treasurer
Jerry Albers, Secretary

Provides Adult Day Programs (developmental training, work training, job readiness and job placements); Residentail Programs (CILA Intermittent Care, CILA 24 hour care); Infant Programs (early interventions, early head start); Community Services (specializ

6729 Continucare, A Service of the Rehab Institute of Chicago
West Suburban Hospital Medical Center
3 Erie Ct
Oak Park, IL 60302-2519
708-383-6200
800-354-7342
FAX: 312-908-1369
www.westsuburbanmedicalcenter.research.org

Heidi Asbury MD

We respond to the needs of the whole person: body, mind and spirit. We foster a climate of care, hospitality and a spirit of community. We develop systems and structures that attend to the needs of those at risk of discrimination because of age, gender, lifestyle, ethnic background, religious beliefs or socioeconomic status.

6730 Delta Center
1400 Commercial Ave
Cairo, IL 62914-1978
618-734-2665
800-471-7213
FAX: 618-734-1999
e-mail: delta1@midwest.net
deltacenter.org

Lisa Tolbert, Executive Director
Lisa Tholbert, Assistant Executive Director

The Delta Center is a non-profit mental health center, substance abuse counseling facility, and also provides various community services to Alexander and Pulaski County, Illinois. The purpose and mission is to promote, encourage, foster and engage exclusi

6731 Division of Rehabilitation-Education Services, University of Illinois
Beckwith Hall
201 E. John Street
Champaign, IL 61820- 6901
217-333-4603
FAX: 217-333-0248
e-mail: disability@uiuc.edu
www.disability.ui.uc.edu

Ann Fredricksen, Disability Specialist
Jon Gunderson, Coordinator
Pat Malik, Director
Dennis Cable, Accountant

Offers services for the totally blind, legally blind, visually impaired, mentally retarded blind and more with health, counseling, educational, recreational, rehabilitation, computer training and professional training services.

6732 Easter Seals
Easter Seals Joliet Region
233 South Wacker Drive
Suite 2400
Chicago, IL 60606-5272
312-726-6200
800-221-6827
FAX: 312-726-1494
www.easterseals.com

Richard W. Davidson, Chairman
Sandra L. Bouwman, 1st Vice Chairman
Joseph G. Kern, 2nd Vice Chairman
Ralph F. Boyd, Treasurer

Services for children and adults with disabilities and their families. Pediatric outpatient medical rehabilitation, inclusive childcare, fostercare, residential homes, clinics.

6733 Easter Seals DuPage And The Fox Valley Region
830 S Addison Ave
Villa Park, IL 60181-2877
630-620-4433
FAX: 630-620-1148
e-mail: info@eastersealsdfvr.org
www.eastersealsdfvr.org

Theresa Forthofer, President & CEO
Erik Johnson, Vice President of Development
Roger Hendrick, Vice President of Operations
Kathy Schrock, Vice President of Clinical Services

The mission of Easter Seals DuPage & the Fox Valley Region is to enable infants, children & adults with disabilities to achieve maximum independence and to provide support to the families who love and care for them. Key services include: physical, occupational, speech-language, nutrition and assistive technology therapies and audiology services for all ages.

6734 Easter Seals Gilchrist-Marchman Rehab Center
1939 West 13th Street
Suite 300
Chicago, IL 60608-1226
312-491-4110
FAX: 312-733-0247
e-mail: Mcancel@eastersealschicago.org
www.easterseals.com/chicago

David A. Pearre, Chairman
Jeff Buchanan, Vice Chairman
Mark O'Toole, Secretary
John G. Anos, Treasurer

Provides comprehensive services for individuals with disabilities or other special needs and their families to improve quality of life and maximize independence.

6735 Easter Seals Jayne Shover Center
799 S McLean Blvd
Elgin, IL 60123-6704
847-742-3264
FAX: 847-742-9436
e-mail: il-ja.easter-seals.org
dfvr.easterseals.com

Dr. Haydee Muse, Chair
Kelly N. Taira, Vice Chairman
Karen Janousek, Secretary
Roger McDougal, Treasurer

A free-standing, comprehensive outpatient rehabilitation center serving children and adults with physical and developmental disabilities.

6736 El Valor Corporation
Early Intervention Program
1850 W 21st St
Chicago, IL 60608-2799
312-666-4511
FAX: 312-666-6677
e-mail: info@elvalor.net
www.elvalor.org

Paul Gaughan, Chairman
Philip K. Fuentes, Vice Chairman
Rey B. Gonzalez, President & CEO
Michael J. Cabrera, Secretary
Mission is to challenge people with disabilities. It is a center for people with disabilities and their families and serves Chicago and surrounding areas, providing services in English and Spanish to individuals whose lives would be drastically impoverish

6737 Elgin Training Center
Association For Individual Development Elgin Area
1135 Bowes Road
Elgin, IL 60123-1321
847-931-6200
FAX: 847-888-6079
www.the-association.org

Chuck Miles, Chairmen
Patrick Flaherty, Vice Chairmen
Walter Dwyer, Treasurer
Lynn O'Shea, Executive Director
Day training services to develop work habits and attitudes while providing training in small product assembly, sorting, packaging, collating, & material handling. Instruction also offered in job related knowledge & in personal, social and independent living skills. There is also an on-site specialized Autism Program. Additionally, residential programs (group homes & apartments) are also available for people with developmental disabilities.

6738 Family Counseling Center
PO Box 759
Golconda, IL 62938
618-683-2461
FAX: 618-683-2066
e-mail: fccgolconda@shawneelink.com
fccinconline.org

Larry Mizell, Executive Director
Connie Duncan, Director
Nora Beth Hacker, Financial Director
Provides counseling, developmental training, evaluations, assisted living services, referrals, psychosocial rehabilitation, and a variety of work services.

6739 Family Matters
A RC Community Support Systems
1901 S. 4th St
Ste 209
Effingham, IL 62401-4123
217-347-5428
866-436-7842
FAX: 217-347-5119
e-mail: deinhorn@arc-css.org
www.fmptic.org

Debbie Einhorn, Executive Director
Debbie Einhorn, Director Family Support
Nancy Mader, Project Coordinator
Barbara Utz, Vice President
Parent Training and Information Center and family support programs for families of children who have disabilities from the ages of birth through 21. Services include: Parent support and training, school advocacy, home visits, information and referral, pa

6740 Five Star Industries
1308 Wells Street Road
P O Box 60
Du Quoin, IL 62832-60
618-542-5421
FAX: 618-542-5556
e-mail: fivestarinc@5starind.com
5starind.com

Susan Engelhardt, Executive Director
Incorporated as a private, non-profit corporation under the laws of the State of Illinois, is an equal opportunity employer and provides equal opportunity in compliance with the Civil Rights Act of 1964 and all other appropriate laws, rules and regulation

6741 HSI Austin Center For Development
1819 S Kedzie Ave
Chicago, IL 60623-2623
773-854-1676
FAX: 773-854-8300

6742 Hyde Park-Woodlawn
950 E 61st St
Chicago, IL 60637-2623
773-324-0280
FAX: 773-324-0285
e-mail: jvshp@jvschicago.org

Clarissa Williams, Manager

6743 Illinois Center for Autism
548 South Ruby Lane
Fairview Heights, IL 62208-2614
618-398-7500
FAX: 618-394-9869
e-mail: info@illinoiscenterforautism.org
illinoiscenterforautism.org

Hardy Ware, Chairperson
Thomas E. Berry, Vice Chairperson
Gary Guthrie, Secretary
Joy Rick, Treasurer
A community-based mental health/educational treatment center dedicated to serving autistic clients.

6744 Julius and Betty Levinson Center
1825 K Street NW
Suite 600
Washington, DC 60304-1557
202-776-0406
800-872-5827
FAX: 708-383-9025
e-mail: info@ucp.net.org
www.ucp.org

Woody Connette, Chair
Ian Ridlon, Vice Chair
Mark Boles, Treasurer
Pamela Talkin, Secretary
Houses one of its three adult developmental training programs for substantially physically disabled men and women.

6745 Lake County Health Department
18 N. County Street
Waukegan, IL 60085
847-377-2000
FAX: 847-336-1517
www.lakecountyil.gov

Aaron Lawlor, Chairman
Stevenson Mountsier, Vice Chairman
Barry Burton, Administrator
Includes counseling, crisis intervention, emergency management, psychotherapy and chemotherapy management for individuals and families.

6746 Little Friends, Inc.
140 N Wright Street
Naperville, IL 60540-4799
630-355-6533
FAX: 630-355-3176
e-mail: info@lilfriends.com
www.littlefriendsinc.com

Dan Casey, Chairman
Matt Johanson, Vice Chairman
Michele Calbi, Treasurer
Kathy West, Secretary
Little Friends has been serving children and adults with autism and other developmental disabilities for over 40 years. Based in Naperville, Little Friends operates three schools, vocational training programs, community-based residential services and the

6747 MAP Training Center
7th and Mc Kinley St
Karnak, IL 62956
618-634-9401
FAX: 618-634-9090

Larry Earnhart, President
Cindy Earnhart, Community Liaison
Training, employment, residential and support services, targeted for adults with developmental disabilities.

6748 Macon Resources
2121 Hubbard Ave.
P O Box 2760
Decatur, IL 62524-2760
217-875-1910
FAX: 217-875-8899
TTY:217-875-8898
e-mail: jpatterson@maconresources.org
maconresources.org

Tom Hill, President
Michael Breheny, Vice President
Barb Nadler, Secretary
Chris Funk, Treasurer

The purpose is to provide a comprehensive array of habilitative/rehabilitative training programs and support services to assist individuals and/or family units of an individual with a developmental disability, mental illness, or other handicapping conditi

6749 Mary Bryant Home for the Blind
2960 Stanton
Springfield, IL 62703-4385
217-529-1611
888-529-1611
FAX: 217-529-6975
e-mail: mbha@marybryanthome.org
marybryanthome.org

Jerry Curry, Executive Director
Robert E. Maxey, President
Allan J. Rupel, Vice President
Gary Rapaport, Secretary

Supportive living facility for blind or visually impaired adults over the age of 22. A supportive living facility remodeled to foster the move to increased independence for residents. The new apartment style housing combined with personal care and other a

6750 Northern Illinois Special Recreation Association (NISRA)
285 Memorial Drive
Crystal Lake, IL 60014-3650
815-459-0737
FAX: 815-459-0388
e-mail: info@nisra.org
www.nisra.org

Brian Shahinian, Executive Director
Carol Amoroso, Manager of Finance and Personnel
Kerri Ruddy, Manager of Office Services
Sarah Holcombe, Manager of Communications & Marketing

Leisure and recreation services to those with disabilities who are unable to participate successfully in park district and city recreation programs.

6751 Oak Forest Hospital of Cook County
15900 Cicero Ave
Oak Forest, IL 60452
708-687-7200
FAX: 708-687-7979
TTY:708-687-4794
http://www.cchil.org

Robert Weinstein, Department Chair
Suja Mathew, Associate Chair

A 654 bed health care center devoted to the diagnosis, rehabilitation and long-term care of adults suffering from chronic illnesses, diseases and physical impairments.

6752 PARC
1913 W. Townline Road
P.O.Box 3418
Peoria, IL 61615-3418
309-691-3800
FAX: 309-689-3613
e-mail: rricketts@arcpeoria.org
parcway.org

Pat Kawczynski, Chair
Heyl Royster, Vice Chair
Terry Waters, Treasurer
Alexis Duhon, Secretary

Serves all ages that are diagnosed with mental retardation and other developmental and physical disabilities. Programs include early intervention, family support, respite care, vocational training, supported employment, adult day programs and residential

6753 Peoria Area Blind People's Center
2905 W Garden St
Peoria, IL 61605-1316
309-637-3693
FAX: 309-637-3693
e-mail: info@cicbvi.org
cicbvi.org

Carol Warren, President
Cora Quinn, Vice President
Prasad Parupalli, Treasurer

Offers services for the totally blind, legally blind, visually impaired, mentally retarded blind and more with health, counseling, educational, recreational, rehabilitation, computer training and professional training services.

6754 Pioneer Center of McHenry County
4001 W Dayton St
McHenry, IL 60050-8379
815-344-1230
FAX: 815-344-3815
TTY:815-344-6243
e-mail: GetHelp@pioneercenter.org
www.pioneercenter.org

Michael T. Moushey, Chairman
Pam Allen, Secretary
Mark LeFevre, Treasurer
Rebecca Heisler, Board

Pioneer Center is the largest social service agency in McHenry County delivering direct services to more than 2,500 individuals annually. The organization also provides education and outreach to schools and community organizations reaching over 10,000 additional individuals. Pioneer Center delivers community-based services in the areas of:McHenery County PADS, Youth Service Bureau, Autism Services, Developmental Disabilities, Mental Illness, Traumatic Brain Injury and VOICE Sexual Assault.

6755 Prosthetics and Orthotics Center in Blue Island
2310 York St
Blue Island, IL 60406-2411
708-597-2611
800-354-7342
FAX: 800-908-1932
www.rehabchicago.org/about/blue_island.php

6756 RB King Counseling Center
2300 N Edward St
Decatur, IL 62526-4163
217-877-8121
FAX: 217-875-0966

Gordon Cross MD

Offers outpatient, individual, group, divorce and meditation, family and re-adjustment counseling.

6757 REHAB Products and Services
3715 N Vermilion St
Danville, IL 61832-1130
217-446-1146
FAX: 217-446-1191
e-mail: rehab@soltec.net
workse.org

Frank L. Brunacci, President/CEO
Crystal Meece, Vice President Production
Todd Seabaugh, VP Programs
Scott Rudy, VP Operations

janitorial, lawn care, distribution services.

6758 RIC Northshore
Rehabilitation Institute of Chicago
345 E Superior St
Chicago, IL 60611-2654
312-238-1000
800-354-7342
e-mail: webmaster@ric.org
www.rehabchicago.org

Joanne C. Smith, President/CEO
Edward B. Case, Vice President

Provides rehabilitation for sports-related injuries, musculoskeletal conditions, neurological conditions, stroke, arthritis, amputation, burns, and general deconditioning.

6759 RIC Prosthetics and Orthotics Center
Rehabilitation Institute of Chicago
345 E. Superior Street
Suite 101
Chicago, IL 60611-4615 312-238-1000
800-345-7342
FAX: 708-957-8353
e-mail: webmaster@rehabchicago.org
ric.org

Martin Buckner, CPO, Inpatient Coordinator
Nicole T. Soltys, CP, Clinical Coordinator
Robert D. Lipschutz, CP, Director of Prosthetic and Orthotic Education
Walter Afable, CP, Clinical Operations Manager
Offers almost all the prosthetics and orthotics services provided at RIC's main hospital in downtown Chicago, including consultations, fittings and training.

6760 RIC Windermere House
5548 S Hyde Park Blvd
Chicago, IL 60637-1909 773-256-5050
800-354-7342
FAX: 773-256-5060
www.rehabchicago.org

Meghan Scalise, Manager
Evaluation, therapeutic services and patient education are offered in the areas of arthritis, multiple sclerosis, musculoskeletal conditions, orthopedics, stroke, spinal cord injury, brain injury and sports medicine.

6761 Ray Graham Association for People with Disabilities
901 Warrenville Road
Suite 500
Lisle, IL 60532-1038 630-620-2222
FAX: 630-628-2350
TTY:630-628-2352
e-mail: cathyfickerterill@yahoo.com
ray-graham.org

Michael Komoll, Chairperson
Neville Bilimoria, Vice Chairperson
Kim zoeller, President & CEO
Jeff Park, Secretary/Treasurer
Provides developmental services at 15 sites to infants, children and adults with disabilities. Services range from 1 hr/wk respite to full-time residential.

6762 Reach Rehabilitation Program: Americana Healthcare
9401 S Kostner Ave
Oak Lawn, IL 60453-2697 708-423-1505
FAX: 708-423-3822

Jean M Roche, Owner
Postacute rehabilitation program.

6763 Rehabilitation Achievement Center
345 E Superior St
Chicago, IL 60611-4805 312-238-1000
800-354-7342
www.ric.org

M. Jude Reyes, Chair
Mike P. Krasny, Vice Chair
Joanne C. Smith, President & CEO
Ed Case, Treasurer
Rehabilitation Institute of Chicago (RIC) has aquired the assets of the Rehabilitation Achievement Center (RAC).

6764 Rehabilitation Institute of Chicago: Alexian Brothers Medical Center
800 Biesterfield Rd
Elk Grove Village, IL 60007-3361 847-437-5500
866-253-9426
FAX: 847-631-5663
TTY: 847-956-5116
www.alexianbrothershealth.org

Mark Frey, President and Chief Executive Officer
Tracy Rogers, Senior Vice President and Chief Operating Officer
Paul Belter, Senior Vice President and Chief Financial Officer
Janice Jastrowski, Manager
A 32-bed rehabilitation unit under the medical direction and supervision of the Rehabilitation Institute of Chicago.

6765 Riverside Medical Center
Mental Health Unit
350 N Wall St
Kankakee, IL 60901-2991 815-933-1671
FAX: 815-935-8160
e-mail: rhuber@rsh.net
riversidehealthcare.org

Phillip Kambic, CEO
Bill W. Douglas, Vice President
Offers recreation, parenting therapy, emergency services, psychological testing and inpatient treatment programs. Riverside is nationally recognized for its specialty programs in heart care, obstetrics, trauma, oncology, rehabilitation, geriatrics, occupa

6766 Robert Young Mental Health Center Division of Trinity Regional Haelth System
Trinity Health Foundation
2701 17th St
Rock Island, IL 61201-5351 309-779-2800
800-322-1431
FAX: 309-779-2027
www.unitypoint.org

Rick Seidler, President & CEO
Jim Hayes, CFO
Tamara Byram, VP, Legal/Compliance
Matt Behrens, Regional VP, UnityPoint Clinic
Services include comprehensive inpatient rehabilitation, chronic pain management programs, outpatient medical rehabilitation, work hardening programs, vocational evaluation, alcohol and other drug dependency rehabilitation programs, Burn Center, and menta

6767 Sampson-Katz Center
216 West Jackson Blvd
Suite 700
Chicago, IL 60606-2104 312-673-3400
FAX: 312-553-5544
TTY:773-761-6672
e-mail: jvsskc@jvschicago.org
www.jvschicago.org

Andrew M. Glick, Chair
John L. Daniels, Vice Chair
H. Debra Levin, President
Benn Feltheimer, Secretary

6768 Shelby County Community Services
160 North Main Street
Memphis, TN 38103-650 901-222-2300
FAX: 912-222-2090
www.shelbycountytn.gov

Dottie Jones, Director
Primary focus is substance abuse treatment.

6769 Streator Unlimited
305 N Sterling St
P O Box 706
Streator, IL 61364-2369 815-673-5574
FAX: 815-673-1714
e-mail: contact@streatorunlimited.org
www.streatorunlimited.org

Jeffrey Dean, Executive Director
Lynn Fukar, Director of Day Services
Julie Caestens, Director Residential Services
Vocational and personal skills training, residential services, client and family support, supported and computerized employment. Serves adults with intellectual disabilities with the goal of enabling them to reach their fullest potential, live as independ

6770 **Swedish Covenant Hospital Rehabilitation Services**
5145 N California Ave
Chicago, IL 60625-3661
773-878-8200
FAX: 773-561-0490
e-mail: ask_us@schosp.org
www.schosp.org
Mark Newton, President & CEO
Provides acute rehabilitation services, subacute care and outpatient services for many types of disabling injuries and conditions, including amputation, arthritis, brain injury, general deconditioning, multiple sclerosis, musculoskeletal injuries, stroke,

6771 **TCRC Sight Center**
21310 Route 9
Tremont, IL 61568-2558
309-347-7148
FAX: 309-925-4241
e-mail: info@tcrcorg.com
www.tcrcorg.com
Jamie Durdel, President & CEO
Molly Anderson, Vice President
Offers services for persons who are totally blind, legally blind, partially sighted or visually impaired along with other disabilities. Have support group, rehabilitation classes, orientation and mobility services, counseling services, low vision clinic,

6772 **Tazewell County Resource Center**
Box 12
Rr 1
Tremont, IL 61568
309-347-7148
FAX: 309-925-4241
e-mail: info@tcrcorg.com
http://www.tcrcorg.com
Jamie Durdel, President & CEO
Molly Anderson, Vice President
A private, nonprofit agency providing programs for the special needs of infants, adults, children and their families residing in Tazewell County. Services offered include: birth-three infant/parent program, adult day care services, family support, residen

6773 **Thresholds Bridge Deaf North Program**
Thresholds Psychiatric Rehabilitation Centers
4101 N. Ravenswood Ave
Chicago, IL 60613
773-572-5500
FAX: 773-989-1075
e-mail: thresholds@thresholds.org
www.thresholds.org
Jana Barbe, President
Marianne Doan, Vice President
Harold E. D'Orazio, Treasurer
Kathy Graham, Secretary
A private, nonprofit psychosocial rehabilitation center that serves the deaf mental health consumers at the highest risk of hospitalization, those with serious and persistent mental illness. The program provides residential case management services focuse

6774 **Thresholds South Suburbs**
4101 N. Ravenswood Ave
Chicago, IL 60613
773-572-5500
FAX: 708-597-8053
e-mail: thresholds@thresholds.org
www.thresholds.org
Jana Barbe, President
Marianne Doan, Vice President
Harold E. D'Orazio, Treasurer
Kathy Graham, Secretary
Services offered include psychosocial, vocational and residential programs for ages 18 or older with a primary diagnosis of mental illness. Facility is wheelchair accessible.

6775 **Trumbull Park**
10530 S Oglesby Ave
Chicago, IL 60617-6140
773-375-7022
FAX: 773-375-5528
Gregory Terry, Director
Diana Moore, Site Supervisor
Ada McKinley, Manager
Offers consultation, education, general counseling, recreation, self-help and social services for children and adults.

6776 **University of Illinois Medical Center**
1740 West Taylor Street
Chicago, IL 60612-7232
312-355-4000
866-600-2273
FAX: 312-996-7770
hospital.uillinois.edu
Rajiv Pai, Chief
Marilyn Plomann, Manager
Offers services for the totally blind, legally blind, visually impaired, mentally retarded blind and more with health, counseling, educational, recreational, rehabilitation, computer training and professional training services.

6777 **VanMatre Rehabilitation Center**
950 S Mulford Rd
Rockford, IL 61108-4274
815-381-8500
866-754-3347
FAX: 815-484-9953
e-mail: webcontentcoordinator@rhsnet.org
www.vanmatrerehab.com
Gary E. Kaatz, President and Chief Executive Officer
Scott Craig, Medical Director
A CARF-accredited comprehensive rehabilitation center based within the Rockford Memorial Hospital providing inpatient and outpatient services for physically and cognitively challenged persons with debilitating illness and injuries.

6778 **Warren Achievement Center**
1220 E 2nd Ave
Monmouth, IL 61546-2404
309-734-3131
FAX: 309-734-7114
e-mail: info@warrenachievement.com
warrenachievement.com
Rick Barnhill, President
Jim Kesse, Vice President
Sherry Waite, Chief Operations Officer
Linda Baker, Chief Financial Officer
For developmentally disabled children and adults. Parent-infant education programs are for parents of infants with disabilities or developmental delays; Children's Group Homes which serve children on a fulltime basis and can serve additional children on a

Indiana

6779 **Ball Memorial Hospital**
2401 W University Ave
Muncie, IN 47303-3499
765-747-3111
FAX: 765-747-3313
iuhealth.org/ball-memorial
Mike Haley, CEO
Offers rehabilitation services, occupational therapy, physical therapy and more for the physically challenged child or adult.

6780 **Community Health Network**
1500 N Ritter Ave
Indianapolis, IN 46219-3027
317-355-4275
800-775-7775
FAX: 317-351-7723
www.ecommunity.com
Keith Thompson, Manager
Anita Harden, President
A leading not-for-profit health system offering convenient access to expert physicians, advanced treatments and leading edge technology, all focused on getting patients well and back to their lives. With caring compassion, Community's 5 hospitals and 70 + sites of care continually strive to improve the health and well being of those individuals in central Indiana who entrust care to us.

6781 **Crossroads Industrial Services**
8302 E 33rd Street
Indianapolis, IN 46226
317-897-7320
FAX: 317-897-9763
e-mail: info@crossroadsindustrialservices.com
www.crossroadsindustrialservices.c om
Anne Shupe, Finance Executive
Curtiss Quirin, CEO
Assisting customers with short-term, seasonal, and long-term outsourcing needs. Many consider Crossroads an extension of their company

6782 **Department of Veterans Affairs Vet Center #418**
302 W. Washington St
Room E120
Indianapolis, IN 46204- 2738
317-232-3910
800-490-4520
FAX: 317-232-7721
e-mail: vcen418@evansville.net
www.in.gov/veteran/sso/fac
Charles T. Applegate, Director
Provides readjustment counseling to combat veterans. Onsite assistance for employment problems, vocational rehabilitation and sexual trauma counsel.

6783 **Frasier Rehabilitation Center Division of Clark Memorial Hospital**
2201 Greentree N
Clarksville, IN 47129-8957
812-218-6590
FAX: 812-218-6597
http://www.jhsmh.org/Frazier-Rehab-Institute-
Catherine Lucas Spalding, Administrator
Designed to help patients in their adjustment to a physically limiting condition, both psychologically and physically, by helping to maximize each patient's abilities so he or she can function as independently as possible. The program treats patients whos

6784 **HealthSouth Deaconess Rehabilitation Hospital**
4100 Covert Ave
Evansville, IN 47714-5559
812-476-9983
800-677-3422
FAX: 812-476-4270
www.healthsouthdeaconess.com
Barbara Butler, Chief Executive Officer
Ashok . Dhingra, M.D, Medical Director
Brett Hirt, Director, Therapy Operations
Doron Finn, M.D., Wound Care Program Director
AHealthSouth Deaconess Rehabilitation Hospital is a joint venture partner with Deaconess Health System. Our hospital is an 80-bed inpatient rehabilitation hospital that offers comprehensive inpatient and outpatient rehabilitation services designed to return patients to leading active and independent lives. - See more a t : http://www.healthsouthdeaconess.com/en/our-hospital#sthash.RCsNTk1u.dpuf

6785 **Healthwin Specialized Care**
20531 Darden Rd
South Bend, IN 46637-2999
574-272-0100
FAX: 574-277-3233
e-mail: info@healthwin.org
healthwin.org
Connie McCahill, President
Lauren Davis, Vice President
John Cergnul, Treasurer
Stephen J. Gazdick, Chief Financial Officer
No other facility in the area has a homelike environment like ours. Its simply part of our culture. Rehabilitation therapy that includes physical, occupational, speech, respiratory and a full time in-house therapist. Other services include a wound special

6786 **Memorial Regional Rehabilitation Center**
615 N Michigan St
South Bend, IN 46601-1033
574-647-1000
877-282-0964
www.qualityoflife.org/rehab
Johan Kuitse, MSA, PT, Outpatient Clinical Manager
Anne Clifford, DPT, Physical Therapists
Shanti Shrestha Dalson, DPT, Physical Therapists
Brandi DeMont, DPT, Physical Therapists
20-bed CARF accredited inpatient rehabilitation, outpatient orthopedic clinic and work performance program, head injury clinic. Outpatient neuro rehab and a driver education and training program are provided.

6787 **Saint Joseph Regional Medical Center- South Bend**
5215 Holy Cross Parkway
Mishawaka, IN 46545-2814
574-335-5000
FAX: 574-237-7312
e-mail: thefoundation@sjrmc.com
sjmed.com
Albert Gutierrez, President & CEO
Steven Gable, Vice President
Janice Dunn, CFO
Christopher Karam, Chief Operating Officer
Continuum of rehabilitation services offered. Included are: acute rehabilitation, a 26 bed CARF accredited comprehensive inpatient unit, a CARF certified inpatient brain injury program, a CARF outpatient day treatment brain injury program, comprehensive o

Iowa

6788 **Crossroads of Western Iowa**
1 Crossroads Pl
Missouri Valley, IA 51555-6069
712-642-4114
FAX: 712-642-4115
e-mail: info@cwiowa.org
explorecrossroads.com
Brent Dillinger, CEO
Pat Kocour, President
Steven Van Riper, Vice President
Darci Tierney, Secretary
CWI provides services in Missouri Valley, Onawa and Council Bluffs, Iowa. An array of services for people with mental illness, mental retardation and brain injury are provided in each location.

6789 **Des Moines Division-VA Central Iowa Health Care System**
3600 30th St
Des Moines, IA 50310-5753
515-699-5999
800-294-8387
FAX: 515-699-5862
www.centraliowa.va.gov
Judith Johnson-Mekota, Director
Fredrick Bahls, Chief Of Staff
Susan A. Martin, Associate Director
Alton C. Alexander, Associate Director
VA Cental Iowa Health Care System is the result of the 1997 merger of the Des Moines and Knoxville, Iowa, VA Medical Centers. This integrated healthcare system brings 2 previously separate organizational structures, located 40 miles apart, into one cohesi

6790 **Easter Seals Iowa**
Easter Seals National
401 N.E. 66th Avenue
Des Moines, IA 50313-4002
515-289-1933
FAX: 515-289-1281
TTY:515-289-4069
e-mail: infi@easterseals ia.org
ia.easterseals.com
Steve Niebuhr, Chair
Rochelle Burnett, Vice Chair
Sherri Nielsen, President & CEO
David Lester, Treasurer
Easter Seals is a leading nonprofit provider of services to Iowans with disabilities. Services include vocational and employment

training, camping recreation and respite services, craft training and sales, home and farm adaptations, transportation, schola

6791 Genesis Regional Rehabilitation Center
Genesis Health System
1227 E.Rusholme Street
Davenport, IA 52803-3396
563-421-1000
FAX: 563-421-3499
genesishealth.com
Doug Cropper, President & CEO
Kenneth Croken, Vice President
Joseph Lohmuller, Chief Medical Officer
Karen Bolton, Vice President
Serves persons of all ages experiencing a disability, whether acquired at birth or following a serious interdisciplinary service. Rehabilitation programs include acute rehabilitation; adult rehabilitation, pediatric rehabilitation, outpatient orthopaedics

6792 Homelink
Van G Miller & Associates
1101 W S Marnan Drive
Waterloo, IA 50701-2817
319-235-7173
866-575-8483
FAX: 319-235-7822
e-mail: homelinkprivacyofficer@vgm.com
www.vgmhomelink.com
Dave Kazynski, President
Rick Hibben, Coordinator
A national network of home medical equipment, respiratory therapy, rehabilitation and infusion therapy service providers with over 2,500 locations serving all fifty states.

6793 Iowa Central Industries
127 Avenue M
Fort Dodge, IA 50501-5797
515-576-2126
FAX: 515-576-2251
e-mail: bloglines@merchantcircle.com
www.bloglines.com/company/3495669/post
Tom Eckman, Executive Director
Services include evaluation and training in pre-vocational and vocational skills, personal behavior management, cognitive skills, communication skills, self-care skills and social skills. Services arranged include: independent living training, medical ser

6794 Life Skills Laundry Division
1510 Industrial Rd SW
Le Mars, IA 51031-3009
712-546-4785
FAX: 712-546-4985
Don Nore, Executive Director

6795 MIW
909 S 14th Ave
Marshalltown, IA 50158-3610
641-752-3697
FAX: 641-752-1614
Rich Byers, President/CEO
Vocational services for adults with disabilities. Includes organizational employment services, supported employment, job placement.

6796 Mercy Dubuque Physical Rehabilitation Unit
250 Mercy Drive
Dubuque, IA 52001-7320
563-589-8000
FAX: 563-589-8162
www.mercydubuque.com
Russel M. Knight, CEO
Provides services which open the door to improved communication, offering the opportunity to enrich the quality of life. Mercy offers many other branches of services including, rehabilitation services for children and a pulmonary rehabilitation program.

6797 Mercy Medical Center-Pain Services
1111 6th Ave
Des Moines, IA 50314-2611
515-247-3121
FAX: 515-248-8867
e-mail: webmaster@mercydesmoines.org
www.mercydesmoines.org/services/painservice s
Dana L. Simon, MD
Dave Vellinga, President & CEO
Laurie Conner, Vice President
An outpatient program dedicated to helping people with chronic pain live more productive, satisfying lives. The program is not designed for conditions that are surgically curable, but rather approaches the problem using a comprehensive, holistic treatment.

6798 Nishna Productions-Shenandoah Work Center
902 Day Street
Shenandoah, IA 51601-70
712-246-1242
FAX: 712-246-1243
e-mail: nci@nishna.org
nishna.org
Mary Rolf, President
Sherri Clark, Executive Director
Melissa Mueller, Program Manager
Barb Hammer, Team Leader
Shelter, workshop and job training for the disabled. Some of the services we provide are Work Activity, Adult Day Activity Program, Personal & Social Adjustment, Residential Services, Home & Community Based Services & Employment Resources.

6799 Northstar Community Services
3420 University Avenue
Waterloo, IA 50701-2050
319-236-0901
888-879-1365
FAX: 319-236-3701
e-mail: info@northdstarcs.org
www.northstarcs.org
Mark Witmar, Executive Director
Jeff Conrey, President
Kathy Folkerts, Vice President
Mary Wankowicz, Director of operations
Provides adult day services, employment services and supported community living so people with disabilities can live and work in the community.

6800 Options of Linn County
935 2nd street
SW
Cedar Rapids, IA 52404-3100
319-892-5000
FAX: 319-892-5849
e-mail: optons@linncounty.org
linncounty.org
Joel D. Miller, Auditor
Sharon Gonzalez, Treasurer
Options of Linn County works with community businesses in providing employment services to adults with disabilities. Options is a publicly operated service provider within the Linn County Community Services department.

6801 RISE
106 Rainbow Dr
Elkader, IA 52043-9075
563-245-1868
FAX: 563-245-2859
Ed Josten, Manager

6802 Ragtime Industries
116 N 2nd St
Albia, IA 52531-1624
641-932-7813
FAX: 641-932-7814
e-mail: ragtime@cknet.net
www.ragtimeind.com
Lisa Glenn, Executive Director
A work-oriented rehabilitation organization which provides training for mentally and physically disabled adults in Monroe County. A variety of programs which help to develop each person's individual potential are offered.

6803 **Sunshine Services**
1106 East 9th St
Spencer, IA 51301-225
712-262-7805
FAX: 712-262-8369
e-mail: info@sunshine-services.org
www.sunshine-services.org
Ann Vandehar, Executive Director

6804 **Tenco Industries**
710 Gateway Dr
Ottumwa, IA 52501-2204
641-682-8114
FAX: 641-684-4223
e-mail: clogan@tenco.org
www.tenco.org
Ben Wright, Executive Director
Dixie Merritt, Vocational Director
Brenda Miller, Marketing and Development DirectoR
Joanie Lundy, Human Resources Director
To advocate and provide opportunities for people with disabilities, or conditions that limit their abilities, to develop and maintain the skills necessary for personal dignity and independence in all areas of life. Provide a wide array of services to individuals with disabilities. By looking at each person as individuals, we are able to work with them to maximize their skills. Residentials services, including HCBS and CSALA are also provided in all communities.

Kansas

6805 **Arrowhead West**
1100 E Wyatt Earp Blvd
Dodge City, KS 67801-5337
620-227-8803
FAX: 620-227-8812
e-mail: web@arrowheadwest.org
www.arrowheadwest.org
Kelly Mason, Chairperson
Michael Stein, Vice Chairperson
Lori Pendergast, President
Anita Allard, Treasurer
Services and programs offered include: developmental and therapy services for children birth to age 3; adult center-based work services and community integrated employment options; adult life skills and retirement programs; and adult residential services.

6806 **Big Lakes Developmental Center**
1416 Hayes Dr
Manhattan, KS 66502-5066
785-776-9201
FAX: 785-776-9830
e-mail: biglakes@biglakes.org
biglakes.org
Lori Feldkamp, President
Shawn Funk, Community Education Director
A private nonprofit Community Developmental Disability Organization (CDDO) serving individuals with developmental disabilities in Riley, Geary, Clay and Pottawatome counties in Kansas. Big lakes is supported by county mill levy and federal and state fundi

6807 **Developmental Services of Northwest Kansas**
2703 Hall St
Suite 10
Hays, KS 67601-1964
785-625-5678
800-637-2229
FAX: 785-625-8204
e-mail: comments@notes1.dsnwk.org
dsnwk.org
Jerry Michaud, President
Ruth Lang, Administrative Assistant
A private nonprofit organization serving both children and adults with disabilities. Offers services to children ages birth to three years, youth and adults through a network of community-based and outreach programs and inter-agency agreements with other

6808 **ENVISION**
2301 S Water St
Wichita, KS 67213-4819
316-267-2244
FAX: 316-267-4312
e-mail: Info@envisionus.com
www.envisionus.com
Sam Williams, Chair
Jon Rosell, PhD, Vice-Chair
Michael Monteferrante, President and CEO
Greg Unruh, Vice President, CFO
Provides jobs, job training and vision rehabilitation services to people who are blind or low vision. A private not-for-profit agency uniquely combining employment opportunitites with rehabilitation services and public education.

6809 **Heartspring**
8700 E 29th St N
Wichita, KS 67226-2169
316-634-8700
800-835-1043
FAX: 316-634-0555
e-mail: kgrover@heartspring.org
www.heartspring.org
Gary W. Singleton, President and CEO
Paul Faber, Executive Vice President, Operations
Katie Grover, Director Of Marketing
David Dorf, CPA, Chief Financial Officer
Heartspring provides outpatient therapies, evaluations and consultations for children with special needs through Heartspring Pediatric Services. The Heartspring School is a residential and day school for children ages 5-21 with multiple disabilities. Children with autism and their families receive resources through the Heartspring CARE program. The Heartspring Hearing Center provides services to individuals of all ages.

6810 **Indian Creek Nursing Center**
6515 W 103rd St
Overland Park, KS 66212-1798
913-633-7000
FAX: 913-642-3982
www.savaseniorcare.com
Randy Sutterfield, Administrator
Postacute rehabilitation program. A 120-bed nursing home facility.

6811 **Johnson County Developmental Supports**
111 South Cherry Street
Olathe, KS 66061-1223
913-715-5000
FAX: 913-715-0800
e-mail: info@jocogov.org
www.jocogov.org
Ed Eilert, Chairman
Michael Lally, Vice Chair
Scott Tschudy, Treasurer
Jessica Dain, Secretary
JCDS is the community Developmental Disability Organization for Johnson County, Kansas. Provides supports in the form of direct services to people on a daily basis. Through a person-centered process and within availiable resources services are shaped to f

6812 **Ketch Industries**
1006 E Waterman St
Wichita, KS 67211-1525
316-383-8700
800-766-3777
FAX: 316-383-8715
e-mail: webmaster@ketch.org
ketch.org
Fred Badders, Chairman
Carla Bienhoff, Chairman
Loren Anthony, Secretary
Dan Crug, Treasurer
The mission of Ketch is to promote independence for persons with disabilities through innovative learning experiences that support individuals choices for working, living and playing in their community.

6813 **Lakemary Center**
100 Lakemary Dr
Paola, KS 66071-1855
913-557-4000
FAX: 913-557-4910
lakemaryctr.org

William Craig, President
Paul Sokoloff, Chair
Gayle Richardson, Vice Chair
Lydia Marien, Secretary

A private, not-for-profit day and residential training facility which provides for the assessment, education, training, therapy and social development of children and adults, moderate and severe mental retardation. The Center is based 28 miles southwest o

6814 **Northview Developmental Services**
700 E 14th St
Newton, KS 67117-5702
316-283-5170
FAX: 316-283-5196
e-mail: nds@northviewdsi.com
http://northviewdev.mennonite.net/

Mary Holloway, CEO

The mission is to provide quality supportive and coordinating services to persons with developmental disabilities, assisting them to grow as they integrate into the community. Further, our mission is to improve the quality of their lives by providing acce

Kentucky

6815 **Cardinal Hill Rehabilitation Hospital**
Cadinal Hill Medical Center
2050 Versailles Rd
Lexington, KY 40504-1499
859-254-5701
800-233-3260
FAX: 859-231-1365
www.cardinalhill.org

Gary R. Payne, CEO

Provides occupational health services, therapy services and urgent medical treatment of injured workers.

6816 **Frazier Rehab Institute**
220 Abraham Flexner Way
Louisville, KY 40202-1887
502-582-7400
FAX: 502-582-7477
www.frazierrehab.org

Jamie Ochsner, Manager
Steve Ahr, VP Frazier Rehab/Neurscience

Frazier Rehab Institute is a regional healthcare system dedicated entirely to rehabilitation. Through an expansive network of inpatient and outpatient facilites in Kentucky and southern Indiana, Frazier offers a wide array of services based on one common

6817 **HealthSouth Northern Kentucky Rehabilitation Hospital**
201 Medical Village Dr
Edgewood, KY 41017-3407
859-341-2044
800-860-6004
FAX: 859-341-2813
www.healthsouthkentucky.com

Richard Evans, CEO
Mary Pfeffer, Director Therapy Operations
Neal Moser, M.D., Medical Director
Mary Beth Bauer, RD, CSG, LD, Director of Quality and Risk Management

Offers all types of inpatient and outpatient rehabilitation services such as occupational therapy, physical therapy, speech therapy. Respiratory therpay, Psychology, Aquatics, Case Managemenet/Social Work and Nutritional Services.

6818 **King's Daughter's Medical Center's Rehab Unit/Work Hardening Program**
2201 Lexington Ave
Ashland, KY 41101-2843
606-408-4000
888-377-5362
FAX: 606-327-7542
e-mail: info@kdmc.net
www.kdmc.com

Kristie Whitlatch, President & CEO
Matt Ebaugh, VP / Chief Strategy and Information Officer
Philip Fioret, M.D., VP / Chief Medical Officer
Howard Harrison, Vice President, Facilities

Offers a 27-bed, inpatient rehabilitation services unit treating physical disabilities related to accident or illness. The program provides an interdisciplinary inpatient program designed to restore the individual to the highest level of independence. It

6819 **LifeSkills Industries**
380 Suwannee Trail St
Bowling Green, KY 42103-6499
270-901-5000
800-223-8913
FAX: 270-782-0058
e-mail: sbell@lifeskills.com
lifeskills.com

Alice Simpson, CEO

LifeSkills will be the reliable advocate, dependable safety net and provider of choice, for high quality, accessable services and supports for the citizens of south-central Kentucky whos lives are affected by mental illness, developmental disablilities or

6820 **Low Vision Services of Kentucky**
120 N. Eagle Creek Drive
Suite 500
Lexington, KY 40509- 1827
859-263-3900
800-627-2020
FAX: 859-977-1136
e-mail: jvanarsdall@retinaky.com
www.lowvisionky.com

Regina Callihan-May, O.D.
Jeanne Van Arsdall, Co-ordinator
Maryanne Inman, Practice Administrator
William J. Wood, MD, Physician

Offers educational, recreational and rehabilitational services and devices for the visually impaired, legally blind, totally blind.

6821 **Muhlenberg County Opportunity Center**
PO Box 511
Greenville, KY 42345-1416
270-754-5590
FAX: 270-338-5977
muhlon.com

Chuck Hammonds, Manager
Charles Hamonds, Director

Post-acute rehabilitation facility with programs including a workshop with hand packaging of manufactured goods.

6822 **New Vision Enterprises**
1900 Brownsboro Rd
Louisville, KY 40206-2102
502-893-0211
800-405-9135
FAX: 502-893-3885

Larry Sherman, Plant Manager

Offers employment training and services for the blind and legally blind.

6823 **Park DuValle Community Health Center, Inc.**
3015 Wilson Ave
Louisville, KY 40211-1969
502-774-4401
FAX: 502-775-6195
e-mail: rjones@pdchc.org
www.pdchc.org

Richard K Jones, President
John Howard MD, Medical Director
Dave Gerwig, CFO
Ann Hagan, Administrator

Offers services for the totally blind, legally blind, visually impaired, mentally retarded blind and more with health, counseling, educational, recreational, rehabilitation, computer training and professional training services.

Louisiana

6824 Alliance House
427 S Foster Drive
Baton Rouge, LA 70806-2723 225-987-0013
FAX: 225-346-0857

6825 Assumption Activity Center
4201 Highway 1
Napoleonville, LA 70390-8628 985-369-2907
FAX: 985-369-2657
e-mail: arcoa.catbl.net

Warren Gonzales, Manager
A community work center providing prevocational training and extended employment for adults with disabilities. Services include: social services, work activities, specialized training and supported employment.

6826 Bancroft Rehabilitation Living Centers
425 Kings Highway East
P.O. Box 20
Haddonfield, NJ 08033-0018 504-482-3075
800-774-5516
FAX: 504-483-2135
e-mail: lynn.tomaio@bancroft.org
www.bancroft.org

Dr. Robert Voogt, Owner
Toni Pergolin, President & CEO
Cynthia Boyer, Executive Director
Thomas J. Burke, MBA, Chief Financial Officer
Mission is to nurture abilities and independence of people with neurological challenges by providing a broad spectrum of advanced therapeutic and educational programs and by fostering the development of best practices in the field through research and pro

6827 Caddo-Bossier Association for Retarded Citizens
4103 Lakeshore Dr
Shreveport, LA 71109-1998 318-636-0258
FAX: 318-221-4262
Janet Parker, Director
A community operated workshop for male and female mentally retarded individuals. It provides work evaluation and transitional and extended employment.

6828 Deaf Action Center Of Greater New Orleans
Catholic Charities
1000 Howard Ave
Suite 200
New Orleans, LA 70113-1903 504-523-3755
866-891-2210
FAX: 504-523-2789
TTY: 504-615-4944
e-mail: ccano@ccano.org
www.ccano.org

Tommie A. Vassel, Chairman
Sr.Marjorie Hebert, MSC, President & CEO
This community service and resource center serves deaf, deaf-blind, hard of hearing and speech-impaired persons in the greater New Orleans area regardless of age, religion, race or secondary disability. DAC provides interpreting services, equipment distri

6829 Donaldsville Association for Retarded Citizens
1030 Clay St
Donaldsonville, LA 70346-3518 225-473-4516
FAX: 225-473-4517
e-mail: daarc@eatel.net

Marlene Domingue, Executive Director
A private, nonprofit sheltered work program working with the mentally retarded and developmentally disabled adults.

6830 East Jefferson General Hospital Rehab Center
4200 Houma Blvd
Metairie, LA 70006-2996 504-454-4000
www.ejgh.org

Newell D. Normand, Chairman
Ashton J. Ryan, Jr., Vice Chairman
Mark J, Peters, President & CEO
Judy Brown, CPA, MHA, FACHE, Executive Vice President / Chief Operating Officer
Provides the highest quality, compassionate healthcare to the people we serve. East Jefferson General Hospital will be the region's healthcare leader providing the highest quality care through innovation and collaboration with our team members, medical st

6831 Family Service Society
2515 Canal Street
Suite 201
New Orleans, LA 70119-6489 504-822-0800
FAX: 504-822-0831
e-mail: family@fsgno.org
www.fsgno.org

L. Blake Jones, Chair
Jackie Sullivan, 1st Vice Chair
Kathleen Vogt, 2nd Vice Chair
Ronald P McClain JD, President & CEO
Offers services for the totally blind, legally blind, visually impaired, mentally retarded blind and more with health, counseling, educational, recreational, rehabilitation, computer training and professional training services.

6832 Foundation Industries
9995 Highway 64
Zachary, LA 70791 225-654-6288
FAX: 225-654-3988

Jim Lambert-Oswald, President
Jim Oswald, General Manager
A private, nonprofit sheltered workshop providing extended employment and work activities for the mentally retarded and developmentally disabled clients. Objectives are to build work skills through supervision, develop social interaction and manifest basi.

6833 Handi-Works Productions
2700 Lee St
Alexandria, LA 71301-4358 318-442-3377
FAX: 318-473-0858

6834 HealthSouth Rehabilitation Hospital Of Baton Rouge
3660 Grandview Parkway
Suite 200
Birmingham, AL 35243- 2251 225-927-0567
800-765-4772
FAX: 225-928-0317
healthsouth.com

Jacque Shadle, CEO
Derrick Landreneau, Director of Nursing services
Dedicated to one field of medicine - physical rehabilitation medicine - and are committed to one goal, helping patients achieve the highest level of functioning possible after a debilitating injury or illness.

6835 Iberville Association for Retarded Citizens
24615 J.Gerald Berret Blvd
Plaquemine, LA 70764-201 225-687-4062
FAX: 225-687-3272
e-mail: arci@eatel.net
Paul Rhorer, Executive Director
A private sheltered work program operating out of one facility and providing transitional, extended employment and work activities for mentally and developmentally ill adults.

6836 Lighthouse for the Blind in New Orleans
123 State St
New Orleans, LA 70118-5793
504-899-4501
888-792-0163
FAX: 504-895-4162
lighthouselouisiana.org

Curtis Eustis, Chair
Paul Masinter, Chair Elect
Tabatha George, Secretary
Peyton Bush, Treasurer

Offers services for the totally blind, legally blind, visually impaired, mentally retarded blind and more with health, counseling, educational, recreational, rehabilitation, computer training and professional training services.

6837 Louisiana Center for the Blind
101 South Trenton Street
Ruston, LA 71270-4431
318-251-2891
800-234-4166
FAX: 318-251-0109
e-mail: pallen@lcb-ruston.com
www.louisianacenter.org

Pam Allen, Executive Director
Neita Ghrigsby, Office Manager
Janette Woodard, Residential Manager
Jack Mendez, Director of Technology

A new kind of orientation and training center for blind persons. The center is privately operated and provides quality instruction in the skills of blindness. Offers employment assistance, computer literacy training, summer training and employment project

6838 Louisiana State University Eye Center
Lousiana State University
433 Bolivar Street
New Orleans, LA 70112-2272
504-568-4808
FAX: 504-412-1315
www.lsuhsc.edu

Jayne S. Weiss, Director
Kelli McMichael, Manager

The LSU Eye Center is part of the LSU Medical Center complex in downtown New Orleans. It is in the LSU-Lions Building at 2020 Gravier Street between South Bolivar and South Prieur streets.

6839 New Orleans Speech and Hearing Center
1636 Toledano St
New Orleans, LA 70115-4598
504-897-2606
FAX: 504-891-6048
noshc.org

Mary Beth Green, President
Jessica Vinturella, Treasurer
Kindall James, Secretary

This non-residential facility serves male and female clients for purposes of evaluating speech and hearing problems and providing speech therapy, hearing aids and other assistive technology for speech and hearing.

6840 Port City Enterprises
836 North Seventh Street
Port Allen, LA 70767-113
225-344-1142
877-344-1142
FAX: 225-344-1192
www.portcityenterprises.org

William Kleinpeter, President
Mark Graffeo, Vice President
L.J. Treuil Jr, Secretary
Philip Bourgoyne, Treasurer

Offers supported employment, sheltered work and supervised programs for the mentally retarded, ages 22 and over.

6841 Rehabilitation Center at Thibodeaux Regional
Rehab Care
602 N Acadia Rd
Thibodaux, LA 70301-4847
985-493-4731
800-822-8442
FAX: 985-449-4600
e-mail: infoA@thibodaux.com
www.thibodaux.com/rehabilitation.html

Jan Torres, Program Manager
Rose Pipes, Clinical Coordinator

Designed to help patients in their adjustment to a physically limiting condition, both physically and psychologically, by helping to maximize each patients abilities so he or she can function as independently as possible.

6842 St. Patrick RehabCare Unit
RehabCare
524 Doctor Michael Debakey Dr
Lake Charles, LA 70601-5725
337-491-7590
888-722-9355
FAX: 337-491-7157
www.stpatrichospital.org/serv_rehab_main.htm

Larry A Hauskins, Manager
Ruth Thornton, Admissions

A comprehensive physical and cognitive rehabilitation program designed to help individuals who have experienced a disabling injury or illness.

6843 Touro Rehabilitation CenterLCMC (Louisiana Children's Medical Center)
1401 Foucher St
New Orleans, LA 70115-3515
504-897-8565
FAX: 504-897-8393
e-mail: GeneralRehabilitationProgram@touro.com
www.touro.com/rehab

Jeanette Ray, VP of Rehab and Post Acute Srv
Janet Clark, Director of Inpatient Rehabilitation Programs
Marylee Pontillas, Director of Outpatient Rehab Srv
Lynn Drake, Patient Care Manager

Located in New Orleans' Garden District, Touro Rehabilitation is a comprehensive rehabilitation facility dedicated to the restoration of function and independence for individuals with disabilities. The scope of rehabilitation services is broad, with 3 CARF accreditations for Brain Injury, Spinal Cord Injury and General Rehabilitation. TRC opened in 1984 and offers 69 rehab beds. TRC is part of Touro Infirmary which has a proud 150 year history as a nonprofit teaching hospital.

6844 Training, Resource & Assistive-Technology
2000 Lakeshore Drive
New Orleans, LA 70148-1
504-280-6000
888-514-4275
FAX: 504-280-5707
e-mail: ggaglian@uno.edu
www.uno.edu

Ken Zangla, Director
Naomi Moore, Assistant Director
Connie Lanier, Coordinator
Peter J. Fos, President

Provides quality services to persons with disabilities, rehabilitation professionals, educators and employers. Built a solid reputation for its innovative training programs and community outreach efforts. The Center is recognized as a valuable resource st

Maine

6845 Charlotte White Center
572 Bangor Rd
Dover Foxcroft, ME 04426-3373 207-564-2426
888-440-4158
FAX: 207-564-2404
e-mail: info@charlottewhite.org
charlottewhitecenter.com

Richard M. Brown, CEO
Charles G. Clemons, COO
Dale Shaw, CFO
Mary Louis McEwen, President

A nonprofit agency, devoted to assisting adults and children with mental retardation, mental health, physical handicaps, and elder age related issues. With headquarters in Dover-Foxcroft Maine, the agency provides multiple levels of social services, inclu

6846 Iris Network for the Blind
189 Park Avenue
Portland, ME 04102-2909 207-774-6273
FAX: 207-774-0679
e-mail: ashah@theiris.org
theiris.org

Leonard Cole, Chairman
Katharine Ray, 1st Vice Chairman
Bruce Roullard, 2nd Vice Chairman
James E. Phipps MBA/JD, Executive Director

A statewide resource and catalyst for people who are visually impaired or blind so they can attain their determined level of independence and integration into the community.

6847 Roger Randall Center
45 School St
Houlton, ME 04730-2010 207-532-4068
FAX: 207-532-7334
e-mail: rlangworthy@cla-maine.org
www.cla-maine.org

Rob Moran, Executive Director
Tom Moakler, President
Vicki Moody, Vice President
Peter Crovo, Treasurer

The Roger Randall Cneter is one of five Day Habilitation Programs adminsitered by Community Living Association, a private, non-profit agency. These programs may provide a supportive environment that allows the individual to achieve their maximum growth po

6848 Sebasticook Farms-Great Bay Foundation
P.O.Box 65
Saint Albans, ME 04971 207-487-4399
FAX: 207-938-5670
e-mail: tad@tdstelme.net
www.greatbayfoundation.org

Tom Davis, Executive Director
Pam Erskin, Program Coordinator

Provides residential, educational and vocational services to adults who are developmentally disabled in order to maximize independent living and to provide assistance in obtaining an earned income.

6849 Social Learning Center
10 Shelton McMurphey Blvd
Eugene, OR 97401-3363 541-485-2711
877-208-6134
FAX: 541-485-7087
www.oslc.org

Sam Vuchinich, Ph.D, Chair
Gordon Naga Hall, Ph.D., Vice President
Susan Miller, J.D., Secretary/Treasurer
Sally Guyer, Staff Representative

Post accute rehabilitation program.

Maryland

6850 Blind Industries and Services of Maryland
3345 Washington Blvd
Baltimore, MD 21227-1602 410-737-2600
888-322-4567
FAX: 410-737-2665
e-mail: info@bism.org
bism.org

Donald J. Morris, Chairperson
Walter A. Brown, Vice Chairperson
Fredrick J. Puente, President
James R. Berens, Treasurer

Offers a comprehensive residential rehabilitation training program for people who are blind. Areas of instruction: braille, cane travel, independent living, computer, adjustment and blindness seminars.

6851 Center for Neuro-Rehabilitation
2340238 N Cary St
Annapolis, MD 21223 410-263-1704
410-462-4711
e-mail: cnrnhq@erols.com

Jeanne Fryer
Laurent Pierre-Philippe

Provide community-based inpatient and outpatient acute rehabilitation, vocational services and long-term care. Specializing in treating complex neurological conditions including spinal cord injuries, multiple sclerosis, strokes, and other brain injuries resulting from trauma, anoxia, tumors, genetic malformations and other related conditions. Locations in Annapolis, Bethesda, Frederick, Towson, MD and Fairfax, Va. CNR is licensed, a Medicare provider and CARF accredited.

6852 Child Find/Early Childhood Disabilities Unit Montgomery County Public Schools
Ste A4
10731 Saint Margarets Way
Kensington, MD 20895- 2831 301-929-2224
FAX: 301-929-2223

Julie Bader, Supervisor

Offers free developmental screening for children ages 3 years until eligible for kindergarten, evaluation and placement services.

6853 Greater Baltimore Medical Center
6701 N Charles St
Baltimore, MD 21204-6881 443-849-2000
800-597-9142
FAX: 443-849-2631
www.gbmc.org

John B. Chessare MD, President & CEO
Harold J. Tucker MD, Chief Of Staff
Eric L. Melchoir, Vice President & CFO
Keith Poisson, Executive VP & COO

Offers services for the visually impaired and blind with low vision exams. Rehabilitation teaching and orientation and mobility in the home or workplace. Also offers a bimonthly newsletter for $12/yr for Hoover patients and monthly share group.

6854 James Lawrence Kernan Hospital
2200 Kernan Drive
Baltimore, MD 21207-6697 410-285-6566
888-453-7626
FAX: 410-448-6854
www.umrehabortho.org

Michael Jablonover MD,MBA, President & CEO
John P. Straumanis MD, FAAP, Vice President
W. Walter x Augustin, III, CPA, Vice President of Financial Services
Cheryl D. Lee, RN, MSN, CRRN, Vice President, Patient Care Services

Kernan reigns as Maryland's origional orthopaedic hospital with a staff which consists of a support team of orthopaedic physician assistants and dedicated nurses in the Post Anesthesia Care Unit and on the Medical/Surgical Unit, guaranteeing the highest q

6855 Levindale Hebrew Geriatric Center
2401 W. Belvedere Ave.
Baltimore, MD 21215-5267 410-601-9000
FAX: 410-601-2700
www.lifebridgehealth.org

Jason A. Blavatt, Chair
David Uhlfelder, Vice Chair
Edward L. Morris, Treasurer
Sharon Caplan, Secretary

a 292-licensed bed facility, which includes 172-comprehensive care beds, 20 subacute beds, and a 26-bed dementia care unit. Levindale's 120-bed specialty hospital consists of 20 gerospychiatric beds, 80 complex medical beds, some with ventilator capacity

6856 Meridan Medical Center For Subacute Care
770 York Rd
Towson, MD 21204 410-821-5500
FAX: 410-821-6735

Yvette Caldwell, Administrator

Patients receive around-the-clock professional nursing care; physical and occupational, speech and respiratory therapists also assist patients. Each patient's individualized plan of care is reviewed and updated as patient needs change. Careful discharge p.

6857 Rehabilitation Opportunities
5100 Philadelphia Way
Lanham, MD 20706-4412 301-731-4242
FAX: 301-731-4191
roiworks.org

Tom Purcell, President
Bruce Shapiro, Vice President
David Fierst, Secretary
Henry Neloms, Treasurer

Organization offering day programs, evaluation, work adjustments and sheltered workshops for persons who are mentally retarded or developmentally disabled.

6858 Rosewood Center
410-951-5000
888-300-7071
FAX: 410-581-6157
www.dhmh.state.md.us/dda/rosewood

Leslie Smith, Program Director
James Anzalone, Director

Rosewood Center is a State residential Center that supports adults with mental retardation from the central Maryland region. Rosewood will provide comprehensive supports to Maryland citizens with developmental disabilities and their families in a setting .

6859 TLC: Treatment and Learning Centers
2092 Gaither Road
Suite 100
Rockville, MD 20850-3316 301-424-5200
FAX: 301-424-8063
e-mail: dpaton@ttlc.org
www.ttlc.org

Patricia Ritter Ph.D., CCC-SLP, Executive Director
Cathleen Burgess Ms Ed, CCC-SLP, Director
Bill McDonald, President
Michael Cogan, Vice President

Provides audiological evaluations, testing and hearing aids, physical and occupational therapy and evaluation; speech-language evaluation and therapy, psycho-educational testing and tutoring services for learning disabled students, head injury services an

6860 Workforce and Technology Center
Division of Rehabilitation Services
2301 Argonne Drive
Baltimore, MD 21218-1628 410-554-9442
888-554-0334
FAX: 410-554-9112
www.dors.state.md.us

Dan Frye, Chairperson
Josie Thomas, Vice Chairperson

Is one of nine state operated comprehensive rehabilitation facilities in the country providing a wide range of services to individuals with disabilities. The Maryland Division of Rehabilitation Services operates the Workforce and Technology Program. Avail

Massachusetts

6861 Baroco Corporation
136 West Street
Northampton, MA 01060-2711 413-534-9978
FAX: 413-585-9019
www.baroco.com

Rick Barnard, President/Owner
Suzanne Darby, Executive Administrator
Julia McLaughlin, Executive Administrator
Janet Lawlor, Executive Administrator

Provides training and therapeutic support for its recipients with developmental disabilities in order to aid them in securing and maintaining placement in a less-restrictive setting.

6862 Berkshire Meadows
160 Gould Street
Suite 300
Needham, MA 02494-2300 781-559-4900
FAX: 413-528-0293
e-mail: lkelly@jri.org
berkshiremeadows.org

Andy Pond, President
Gregory Canfield, Vice President
Deborah Reuman, CFO
Stephen H. Webster, Executive Advisor

Private, non profit school for children, adolescents, young adults who are severely, developmentally disabled. Approved special education learning center, work site program and foster care. Physical therapy, speech and language development, behavioral pro *$8200.00*

6863 Blueberry Hill Healthcare
75 Brimbal Ave
Beverly, MA 01915-6009 978-927-2020
FAX: 978-922-5213
e-mail: admissions@BlueberryHillRehab.com
www.blueberryhillrehab.com

Ralph Epstein, Medical Director

Accomodates 146 residents. We are centrally located close to Route 128 and Route 1A in Beverly Massachusetts. We offer short-term rehab care, long term care and Alzheimer's Special Care Programs. Our interdisciplinary team designs individual care plans fo

6864 Boston University Hospital Vision Rehabilitation Services
One Boston Medical Center Place
Boston, MA 02118-2371 617-638-8000
FAX: 617-638-7769
www.bmc.org/rehab.htm

Simona Manasian, Medical Director
Karen Mattie, Director
Jenn Blake, Clinical Outpatient Supervisor
Kara Schworm, Clinical In-patient Supervisor

Offers services for the totally blind, legally blind, visually impaired, mentally retarded blind and more with health, counseling, educational, recreational, rehabilitation, computer training and professional training services.

6865 Burbank Rehabilitation Center
275 Nichols Rd
Fitchburg, MA 01420-1919 978-343-5000
888-840-3627
FAX: 978-343-5342
www.umassmemorialhealthcare.org

David Bennett, Chair
Eric Dickson, President & CEO

The largest community hospital and regional referral center in the area. Offers the most extensive high quality, cost-effective healthcare services in the region. The hospital provides outstanding hospital-based services such as case management of high ri

6866 CPB/WGBH National Center for Access Media
W GB H Educational Foundation
One Guest Street
Boston, MA 02135
617-300-3400
FAX: 617-300-1035
TTY:617-300-2489
e-mail: ncam@wgbh.org
www.wgbh.org/ncam

Larry Goldberg, Director
Marcia Brooks, Project Director
Geoff Freed, Director of Technology
Richard Caloggero, Technology Specialist
Dedicated to the issues of media and information technology for people with disabilities in their homes, schools, workplaces, and communities. NCAM's mission is to expand access to present and future media for people with disabilities; explore how existin

6867 Carroll Center for the Blind
770 Centre St
Newton, MA 02458-2597
617-969-6200
800-852-3131
FAX: 617-969-6204
e-mail: joe.abely@carroll.org
www.carroll.org

Joseph Abely, President
Arthur O'Neill, Vice President
Brian Charlson, Director of Computer Training Services
Robert McGillivray, Director of Low Vision Services
Offers services for the totally blind, legally blind, visually impaired, mentally retarded blind and more with health, counseling, educational, in dependent living, tronell skills, computer traing, recreational, rehabilitation, computer training and professional training services.

6868 Center for Psychiatric Rehabilitation
Boston University
940 Commonwealth Ave
West
Boston, MA 02215-1203
617-353-3549
FAX: 617-353-7700
e-mail: psyrehab@bu.edu
cpr.bu.edu

Kim T. Mueser, Executive Director
Deborah Dolan, Director of operations
Larry Kohn, Director of Development
E. Sally Rogers, Director of Research
The mission of the Center is to increase knowledge, to train treatment personnel, to develop effective rehabilitation programs and to assist in organizing both personnel and programs into efficient and coordinated service delivery systems for people with

6869 Clark House Nursing Center At Foxhill Village
Kindred Healthcare
30 Longwood Dr
Westwood, MA 02090-1132
781-326-5652
800-359-7412
FAX: 781-326-4034
www.clarkhousefhv.com

Chris Wasel, Administrator
Clark House At Fox Hill Village accomodates 70 residents. We are part of the Fox Hill Village Assisted Living and Retirement Center campus. Clark House Nursing center has been named a recipient of a 2005 step II quality Award from the American Health Care

6870 College Internship Program at the Berkshire Center
18 Park St
Lee, MA 01238-1702
413-243-2576
FAX: 413-243-3351
e-mail: admissions@berkshirecenter.org
berkshirecenter.org

Lucy Gosselin, Program Director
Laina Hubbard, Admissions Coordinator
Charles D. Houff, Head Therapist
A highly individualized postsecondary program for learning disabled young adults 18-30. Provides job placement services and follow-ups; college support; money management and social skills. Residential students share an apartment and have their own room. T

6871 Eagle Pond Rehabilitation and Living Center
1 Love Lane
P.O.Box 208
South Dennis, MA 02660-3445
508-385-6034
FAX: 508-385-7064
www.eaglepond.com

Paul Marchwat, Executive Director
Ellen Reil, Marketing Director
Eagle Pond accomodates 142 residents. Medicare and Medicaid certified as well as being accredited by the Joint Comission (formerly (JCAHO) which enables us to contract with many insurance companies.

6872 FOR Community Services
75 Litwin Ln
Chicopee, MA 01020-4817
413-592-6142
FAX: 413-598-0478
e-mail: ggolash1@aol.com

Gina Golash, Executive Director
Providing a world of meaning for individuals with developmental disabilities throughout Western Massachusetts since 1967.

6873 Fairlawn Rehabilitation Hospital
189 May Street
Worcester, MA 01602-4399
508-791-6351
FAX: 508-831-1277
www.fairlawnrehab.org

Dave Richer, CEO
Peter Bagley MD, Medical Director
Matthew Akulonis, Director Of Support Operations
Judy Chuli, Chief Nursing Officer
Offers comprehensive rehabilitation on both an inpatient and outpatient basis. Specialty programs include: head injury, spinal cord injury, young/senior stroke, oncology, geriatrics and orthopedics.

6874 Greenery Extended Care Center: Worcester
59 Acton Street
Worcester, MA 01604-4899
508-791-3147
800-633-0887
FAX: 508-753-6267
e-mail: worcester@wingatehealthcare.com
wingatehealthcare.com

Scott Schuster, Founder & President
Brian Callahan, CFO
Michael Benjamin, Vice President
Trent Guthrie, Senior Director
173 beds offering complex care, extended rehabilitation and neurobehavioral intervention. Offering life care homes and Nursing home services. Specialties include life events and physical care, long term and home health care, and nursing homes and nursing

6875 Greenery Rehabilitation & Skilled Nursing Center
P.O.Box 1330
Middleboro, MA 02346-4330
508-947-9295
FAX: 508-947-7974

6876 Harrington House Nursing And Rehabilitation Center
160 Main Street
Walpole, MA 02081-4037
508-660-3080
FAX: 508-660-1634
www.harringtonrehab.com

Joseph Haron, Medical Director
Accomodates 90 residents. Our state-of-the-art center offers post-accute services including rehabilitation and medical management. Our center also provides a long term care program including hospice services.

6877 HealthSouth Rehabilitation Hospital Of Western Massachusetts
222 State Street
Ludlow, MA 01056-3478 413-308-3300
FAX: 413-547-2738
www.healthsouthrehab.org

Victoria Healy, CEO
Adnan Dahdul, M.D., Medical Director
Deborah Cabanas, Chief Nursing Officer
AnnMaria Elder, M.D., Medical Staff President

A 53-bed acute Rehabilitation Hospital. The facility has been operating for 14 years and has provided rehabilitative care to patients and families in the greater Springfield area with an outstanding reputation for attention to detail and compassion. Becau

6878 Holiday Inn Boxborough Woods
242 Adams Pl
Boxborough, MA 01719-1735 978-263-8701
800-465-4329
FAX: 978-263-0518
e-mail: box_sales@fine-hotels.com
www.ihg.com/holidayinn

Kevin Murray, Manager
Marcel Girard, Manager
Nancy Ellen Hurley, Chief Marketing Officer

Located on 35 acres of wooded countryside just off I-495 at exit #28. Minutes from the Mass Turnpike, Route 2, 290 and 9. Conference center located on main level with 30,000 square feet of meeting space. Guest rooms feature two-line telephones, voice mail

$129 - $159

6879 Lifeworks Employment Services
1400 Providence Highway
Suite 2300
Norwood, MA 02062- 4551 781-769-3298
FAX: 781-551-0045
e-mail: able@lifeworksma.org
www.lifeworksma.org

Dan Burke,, President & CEO
Chris Page, Vice President
Brenda Calder, CFO
Mary Hagen, Controller

Providing homes, jobs, education and supportive living for people with developmental disabilities.

6880 Massachusetts Eye and Ear Infirmary & Vision Rehabilitation Center
243 Charles Street
Boston, MA 02114-3002 617-523-7900
FAX: 617-573-4178
TTY:617-523-5498
www.masseyeandear.org

Wycliffe Grousbeck, Chairman
John Fernandaz, President & CEO
Lily H. Bentas, Secretary
Jonathan Uhrig, Treasurer

Visual rehabilitation encompasses a low vision rehabilitation evaluation, occupational therapy evaluation (with home visit if necessary), and social service evaluation.

6881 New England Center for Children
260 Tremont Street
Boston, MA 02116-2108 617-636-4600
FAX: 617-636-4866
e-mail: cwelch@necc.org
necc.org

Lisel Macenka, Chair
James C. Burling, Vice Chair
L.Vincent Strully, President
Michael F. Downey, Treasurer

A comprehensive year-round program for students with autism and PDD who require a highly specialized educational and behavior management program. Students are from all over the country and receive intensive, positive, behavioral counseling and social skil

6882 New England Eye Center, Tufts Medical Center
Vision Rehabilitation Service
260 Tremont Street
Boston, MA 02116-1533 617-636-4600
800-231-3316
FAX: 617-636-4866
e-mail: eli@vision.eri.harvard.edu
www.neec.com

Harry P. Selker, Principal Investigator
Anastassios Pittas, Program Director
Tamsin A. Knox, Associate Director
June S. Wasser, Executive Director

Offers services for the legally blind, visually impaired, mentally retarded blind and more with health, counseling, educational, recreational, rehabilitation, computer training and professional training services.

6883 New Medico Rehabilitation and Skilled Nursing Center at Lewis Bay
89 Lewis Bay Rd
Hyannis, MA 02601-5207 508-775-7601
FAX: 508-790-4239

Edmund Steinle, Executive Director

Post acute rehabilitation services.

6884 Protestant Guild Learning Center
411 Waverley Oaks Rd
Suite 104
Waltham, MA 02452-8449 781-893-6000
FAX: 781-893-1171
e-mail: admin@theguildschool.org
www.theguildschool.org

Eric H. Rosenberger, President
Thomas P. Corcoran, Vice President & Treasurer
Thomas Belski, Chief Executive Officer
Sandra L. Skinner, Clerk

Offers services for the diagnostically disabled children and adolescents with ages 6-22 years with health, counseling, educational, recreational, rehabilitation, computer training and professional training services.

6885 Shaughnessy-Kaplan Rehabilitation Hospital
1 Dove Ave
Salem, MA 01970 978-745-9000
FAX: 978-740-4730
e-mail: skrhinfo@partners.org
spauldingrehab.org

Anthony Sciola, CEO
Maureen Banks, RN, MS, MBA, CN, President
Mary Beth DiFilippo, Vice President
Charles Pu, MD, Chief Medical Officer

A 160-bed private, non-profit hospital. We have been providing care for residents of greater North Shore communities since 1975. Shaughnessy has 120 long-term care hospital beds and a 40-bed transitional care unit sometimes referred to as a skilled nursin

6886 Son-Rise Program
2080 South Undermountain Road
Sheffield, MA 01257-9643 413-229-2100
877-766-7473
FAX: 413-229-3202
e-mail: correspondence@option.org
www.autismtreatmentcenter.org

Barry Neil Kaufman, Co Founder
Samahria Lyte Kaufman, Co Founder

THe Son-Rise Program is a powerful, effective and totally unique treatment for children and adults challengedby Autism, Autuism Spectrum Disorders, Pervasive Developmental Disorder (PDD), Asperger's Syndrome and other developmental difficulties.

6887 **Southern Worcester County Rehabilitation Inc. D/B/A Life-Skills, Inc.**
44 Morris St
Webster, MA 01570-1812 508-943-0700
FAX: 508-949-6129
e-mail: life-skills@lifeskillsinc.org
www.life-skillsinc.org
J Thomas Amick, Executive Director
Kristin Nelson, Board President
Barbara Butrym, Board Vice President
Janice Smith, Board Secretary
Life-Skills, Inc. assists mentally and developmentally challenged adults with meeting their individual needs, and empowering them to take full advantage of meaningful opportunities in their communities. We provide residential, employment, transportation, behavior, and theraputic day habilitation services to 350 adults in MA. We operate thrift & consignment stores, a small cafe, an ice cream shop, mini golf & arcade center, vending and greenhouse businesses, bank courier service, and others.

6888 **Vinfen Corporation**
950 Cambridge Street
Cambridge, MA 02141-1001 617-441-1800
877-284-6336
FAX: 617-441-1858
TTY: 617-225-2000
e-mail: info@vinfen.org
www.vinfen.org
Philip A. Mason, Ph.D., Chairperson
Bruce L. Bird, Ph.D., CEO/ President
Elizabeth K. Glaser, Chief Operations Officer
Glen Mattera, Chief Financial Officer
A private, nonprofit company, Vinfen Corporation is the largest human services provider in Massachusetts. Vinfen offers clinical, educational, residential and support services to individuals of all ages with mental illness and or mental retardation, who also may have another disability (e.g. substance abuse, homelessness, AIDS). The company also trains professionals in the mental health field and helps consumers to learn to live in community-based settings at the highest levels.

6889 **Visiting Nurse Association of North Shore**
5 Federal St
Danvers, MA 01923-3687 508-751-6926
800-728-1862
FAX: 978-777-0308
www.vnacarenetwork.org
Mary Ann O'Connor, CEO/ President
Stephanie Jackman-Havey, Chief Operating Officer/Chief Financial Officer
David Rose, Vice President of Human Resources
Jane Woodbury, Vice President of Fund Development
Home health services including nurses, physical, occupational and speech therapy, home health aides and more. Special programs include nutrition counseling, IV care, pediatric therapy, HIV/AIDS services and wound management. Provides services 7 days a week, 365 days a year and we accept Medicare, Medicaid and most HMO's and health insurers.

6890 **Weldon Center for Rehabilitation**
233 Carew St
Springfield, MA 01104-2377 413-748-6800
FAX: 413-748-6806
mercycares.com
Barbara Haswell, Manager
One of the most vital, necessary health resources in the region by helping thousands of people toward restored health and independence. A comprehensive, integrated, non-profit facility offering inpatient, outpatient, day rehabilitation and pediatric services on one site.

6891 **Youville Hospital & Rehab Center**
1575 Cambridge St
Cambridge, MA 02138-4398 617-876-4344
FAX: 617-547-5501
www.youville.org

Michigan

6892 **Botsford Center For Rehabilitation & Health Improvement-Redford**
28050 Grand River Ave.
Farmington Hills, MI 48336-5919 248-471-8000
877-442-7900
FAX: 313-387-3838
e-mail: info@botsfordsystem.org
www.botsford.org
John Darin, Manager
A 20 bed inpatient physical rehabilitation unit, servicing individuals who have experienced a stroke, amputation, orthopedic fracture, or other neurological impairment.

6893 **Chelsea Community Hospital Rehabilitation Unit**
775 South Main Street
Chelsea, MI 48118-1383 734-593-6000
800-231-2211
FAX: 734-475-4191
www.stjoeschelsea.org
Nancy K. Graebner, CEO/ President
Kathy Brubaker, RN, Vice President and Chief Nursing Officer
Randall Forsch, MD, Chief Medical Officer
Barbara Fielder, VP Finance
A private, non-profit, acute care facility that combines the best of small town values with national standards of healthcare excellance. The hospital has a 19-bed acute care inpatient rehabilitation unit with comprehensive outpatient programs, including a coordinated brain injury program.

6894 **Clare Branch**
790 Industrial Dr
Clare, MI 48617-9224 989-386-7707
888-773-7664
FAX: 989-386-2199
e-mail: mail@mmionline.com
www.mmionline.org
Cris Zeigler, Executive Director
MMI will strive to be the premier provider of person-centered services to people with barriers to employment. We will connect individuals with community resources that provide mutual benefit to them and to the community. MMI will be known for excellence in service provision, ethical business practices, a quality work environment, and for providing services that enhance the dignity and value of the people we serve.

6895 **Clarkston Spec Healthcare Center**
4800 Clintonville Rd
Clarkston, MI 48346-4297 800-454-5909
fundltc.com
Margaret Canny, Administrator
120 beds offering active/acute rehabilitation, complex care, day treatment, extended rehabilitation, neurobehavioral intervention and short-term evaluation.

6896 **DMC Health Care Center-Novi**
42005 W 12 Mile Rd
Novi, MI 48377-3113 248-305-7575
FAX: 425-201-1450
e-mail: novi@patch.com
novi.patch.com
Bud Rosenthal, CEO
Leigh Zareli Lewis, COO
Andreas Turanski, CTO
Melanie Pereira, VP of Finance
The Detroit Medical Center's record of service has provided medical excellence throughout the history of the Metropolitan Detroit area. From the founding of the Children's Hospital in 1886, to the creation of the first mechanical heart at Harpers Hospital 50 years ago, to our compassion for the underdeserved, our legacy of caring is unmatched.

6897 Eight CAP, Inc. Head Start
904 Oak Drive
Greenville, MI 48838-9277
616-754-9315
FAX: 616-754-9310
e-mail: laurelm@8cap.org
www.8cap.org

Ralph Loeschner, Executive Director
Nancy Secor, Contact
Post accute rehabilitation programs.

6898 Greater Detroit Agency for the Blind and Visually Impaired
16625 Grand River Ave
Detroit, MI 48227-1419
313-272-3900
FAX: 313-272-6893
e-mail: Information@gdabvi.org
gdabvi.org

Frederick J Simpson, Board Chairman
Charles L. Cone, Vice Chairman
Leonard W Robinson, Board Secretary
John W. Rhinesmith, CPA, Board Treasurer
Offers services for seniors 60 and over who are legally blind. Also provides eye health information, counseling, education and rehabilitation services.

6899 Hope Network Rehabilitation Services
Hope Network
1490 East Beltline Ave SE
Grand Rapids, MI 49506-4336
616-940-0040
800-695-7273
FAX: 616-940-8151
e-mail: jbaker@hopenetwork.org
hopenetwork.org

Margaret Kroese, Vice President/Executive Directo
An office of Hope Network, one of the largest, private, nonprofit organizations of its kind in Michigan. The purpose is to assist people with brain injuries and/or physical disabilities in achieving an optimal level of self-determination, dignity, and independence as they develop and attain goals to overcome environmental barriers and mobilize adaptive skills.

6900 Lakeland Center
26900 Franklin Rd
Southfield, MI 48033-5312
248-350-8070
FAX: 248-350-8078
e-mail: peggys@thelakelandcenter.net
thelakelandcenter.net

Irving Shapiro, CEO
Santhosh Madhavan, Director Physical Medicine
Gary Yashinsky, Associate Medical Director
Subacute rehabilitation program directed toward those with severe neurologic diagnoses, ie: TBI, cerebral aneurysm, anoxic encephalopathy, CVA and cerebral hemorrhage, orthopedic injuries, and spinal cord injury. Subacute rehabilitation is provided for those who recover slowly and require individualized treatment plans. Residential program available as well.

6901 Mary Free Bed Rehabilitation Hospital
235 Wealthy St SE
Grand Rapids, MI 49503-5247
616-493-9657
800-528-8989
FAX: 616-454-3939
e-mail: info@maryfreebed.com
maryfreebed.com

Kent Riddle, CEO
John Butzer, MD, Medical Director
Randy DeNeff, Vice President of Finance
Founded more than 100 years ago, Mary Free Bed Rehabilitation Hospital is and 80-bed, not-for-profit, acute rehabilitation center. Its mission is to restore hope and freedom through rehabilitation to people with disabilities. Mary Free Bed offers comprehensive inpatient and outpatient rehabilitationfor children and adults using an interdisciplinary approach. Also available are numerous specialty programs designed to increase the quality of life and independence of people with disabilities.

6902 Michigan Career And Technical Institute
11611 Pine Lake Rd
Plainwell, MI 49080-9225
269-664-4461
877-901-7360
FAX: 269-664-5850

Dennis Hart, Executive Director
A residential vocational training center for adults with physical, mental or emotional disabilities.

6903 Michigan Commission for the Blind Training Center
1541 Oakland Dr
Kalamazoo, MI 49008
269-337-3848
800-292-4200
FAX: 269-337-3872
e-mail: mossc@michigan.gov
www.mcb1.org

Christine Boone, Director
Bruce Schultz, Assistant Director
Residential facility that provides instruction to legally blind adults in braille, computer operation and assistive technology, handwriting, cane travel, cooking, personal management, industrial arts and also crafts. During training students will develop career plans which may include work experience, internships, volunteer opprtunities and even part-time paid employment.

6904 Mid-Michigan Industries
2426 Parkway Dr
Mt Pleasant, MI 48858-4723
989-773-6918
888-773-7664
888-773-7664
FAX: 989-773-1317
e-mail: mail@mmionline.com
mmionline.com

Alan Schilling, President
Andrea Christopher, Director Admissions
Linda Wagner, Branch Director
Sheri Alexander, Director of Community Employment
Providing jobs and training for persons with barriers to employment. Services include vocational evaluation, job placement, supported employment, work services, prevocational training and case management

6905 New Medico Community Re-Entry Service
216 St Marys Lake Rd
Battle Creek, MI 49017-9710
FAX: 269-962-2241
James Rekshan, Executive Director

6906 Sanilac County Community Mental Health
171 Dawson St
Sandusky, MI 48471-1062
810-648-0330
888-225-4447
888-225-4447
FAX: 810-648-0319
e-mail: deanr@sanilacmentalhealth.org
sanilacmentalhealth.org

Roger Dean, Executive Director
Post-acute rehabilitation facility and programs.

6907 Special Tree Rehabilitation System
600 Stephenson Highway
Troy, MI 48083-1110
248-616-0950
800-648-6885
FAX: 248-616-0957
e-mail: info@specialtree.com
www.specialtree.com

Joseph Richart, CEO
Special Tree exists to provide hope, encouragement, and expertise for people who have experienced life-altering changes. Our team approach to rehabilitation, custom designed for each person's needs and goals, offers these individuals the best opportunity for healing and recovery.

6908 **Thumb Industries**
1263 Sand Beach Rd
Bad Axe, MI 48413-8817 989-269-9229
FAX: 989-269-2587
e-mail: thumbindustries@hotmail.com
www.thumbindustries.com
Rhonda Wisenbaugh, Executive Director
Provides job training and employment for disabled persons. Vocational rehabilitation agency, manufactures household furnishings, direct mail advertising service.

6909 **Visually Impaired Center**
1422 W Court St
Flint, MI 48503-5008 810-767-4014
FAX: 810-767-0020
e-mail: info@vicflint.org
www.vicflint.org
a pages

6910 **Welcome Homes Retirement Community for the Visually Impaired**
1953 Monroe Ave NW
Grand Rapids, MI 49505-6242 616-447-7837
888-939-9292
888-939-9292
FAX: 616-447-9891
e-mail: info@welcomehomes.org
Beth Lucksted, Manager
Offers services for the totally blind, legally blind, visually impaired, mentally retarded blind and more with health, counseling, educational, recreational, rehabilitation, computer training and professional training services.

6911 **William H Honor Rehabilitation Center Henry Ford Wyanclotte Hospital**
Henry Ford Health System
2333 Biddle Ave
Wyandotte, MI 48192-4668 734-246-6000
FAX: 734-246-6926
www.henryfordwyandotte.com
Denise Dailing, Administration Leader/rehabilita
James Sexton, Chief Executive Officer
Henry Ford, Owner
Henry Ford Wyandotte Hospital offers an array of educational programs, health screenings, and support groups. The hospital is CARF accredited and has a CARF certified stroke specialty unit.

Minnesota

6912 **Industries: Cambridge**
601 Cleveland St S
Cambridge, MN 55008-1752 763-689-5434
FAX: 763-552-1281
e-mail: jspicer@industriesinc.org
www.industriesinc.org
Daryl Peterson, Board Chair
Bruce Montgomery, Vice Chair
Marilyn Bachman, Secretary
Kevin Troupe, Treasurer
Nonprofit organization that does vocational assessment and training for people with disabilities.

6913 **Industries: Mora**
500 Walnut St S
Mora, MN 55051-1936 320-679-2354
FAX: 320-679-2355
e-mail: jspicer@industriesinc.org
www.industriesinc.org
Daryl Peterson, Board Chair
Bruce Montgomery, Vice Chair
Marilyn Bachman, Secretary
Kevin Troupe, Treasurer
Nonprofit organization that does vocational assessment and training for people with disabilities.

6914 **Shriners Hospitals for Children: Twin Cities**
2025 E River Pkwy
Minneapolis, MN 55414-3696 612-596-6100
888-293-2832
888-293-2832
FAX: 612-339-5954
e-mail: dengle@shrinenet.org
www.shrinershospitalsforchildren.org
Charles C. Lobeck, Administrator
Cary Mielke, M.D, Interim Chief of Staff
Don Engel, Development Officer
Shriners Hospital for Children-Twin Cities offers quality orthopedic medical care regardless of the patients' ability to pay. Shriners Hospitals provide inpatient and outpatient services, surgery, casts, braces, artificial limbs, x-rays and physical and occupational therapy to any child under the age of 18 who may benefit from treatment.

6915 **Vision Loss Resources**
1936 Lyndale Ave S
Minneapolis, MN 55403-3101 612-871-2222
FAX: 612-872-0189
TTY:612-382-8422
e-mail: info@vlrw.org
www.visionlossresources.org
Barry Shear, Chair
Lisa David, Vice Chair
Mary McDougall, Secretary
Jackie Peichel, Treasurer
Offers services for the totally blind, legally blind, visually impaired, and more with health, counseling, educational, recreational, rehabilitation, computer training and professional training services.

Mississippi

6916 **Addie McBryde Rehabilitation Center for the Blind**
PO Box 5314
Jackson, MS 39296-5314 601-364-2700
800-443-1000
FAX: 601-364-2677
www.mdrs.ms.gov/VocationalRehabBlind/Pages/Ad
H. S. McMillan, Executive Director
Shelia Browning, Deputy Director Non-Vocational P
Offers services for the totally blind, legally blind, visually impaired, mentally retarded blind and more with health, counseling, educational, recreational, rehabilitation, computer training services and orientation and mobility.

6917 **Mississippi Methodist Rehabilitation Center**
1350 E Woodrow Wilson Ave
Jackson, MS 39216-5198 601-981-2611
800-223-6672
FAX: 601-364-3571
www.methodistonline.org
Mark A. Adams, President/ CEO
Matthew L. Holleman, III, Chair
Mike P. Sturdivant Jr, Vice Chairman
David L. McMillin, Secretary
Rebuild lives that have been broken by disabilities and impairments from serious illness or severe injury. The challenge is to help patients regain abilities, restore function and movement, and renew emotionally. It features personal rehabilitation treatment plans administered by specialized teams of health care professionals through a variety of outpatient programs, treatments and other services.

Missouri

6918 Alpine North Nursing and Rehabilitation Center
4700 NW Cliff View Dr
Kansas City, MO 64150-1237 816-741-5105
FAX: 816-746-1301

Mike Stacks, Executive Director
Bob Richard, Administrator
Postacute rehabilitation program.

6919 Christian Hospital Northeast
11133 Dunn Rd
Saint Louis, MO 63136-6119 314-653-5000
877-747-9355
FAX: 314-653-4130
christianhospital.org

Ron McMullen, President
Bryan Hartwick, Vice President Human Resources
Sebastian Rueckert, MD, Vice President and Chief Medical Officer
Jennifer Cordia, Vice President and Chief Nurse Executive
A non-profit organization, a 493 bed acute care facility on 28 acres. Christian Hospital has more then 600 physicians on staff and a diverse workforce of more then 2,5000 health-care professionals who are dedicated to providing the absolute best care with the latest technology and medical advances.

6920 Integrated Health Services of St. Louis at Gravois
10954 Kennerly Rd
Saint Louis, MO 63128-2018 314-843-4242
FAX: 314-843-4031
Lisa Niehaus, Administrator
Subacute, skilled and intermediate care; ventilator/tracheostomy management program; wound management program and complex rehabilitation program.

6921 Metropolitan Employment & Rehabilitation Service
M ER S Goodwill
1727 Locust St
Saint Louis, MO 63103-1703 314-241-3464
FAX: 314-241-9348
e-mail: info@mersgoodwill.org
www.mersgoodwill.org
Lewis C. Chartock, Ph.D., President/ CEO
Dawayne Barnett, CFO
Mark Arens, Executive Vice President, Chief of Program Services
Mark Kahrs, Executive Vice President, Retail Services
Vocational rehabilitation, primarily with the disabled, skills training and placement services.

6922 Missouri Easter Seal Society: Southeast Region
233 South Wacker Drive
Suite 2400
Chicago, IL 60606 312-726-6200
800-221-6827
FAX: 312-726-1494
easterseals.com

Richard W. Davidson, Chairman
Sandra L. Bouwman, 1st Vice Chairman
Ralph F. Boyd, Jr., Treasurer
Eileen Howard Boone, Secretary
The mission of the Easter Seal Society is to work with individuals, their families and the community to enhance the independence and quality of life for persons with disabilities.

6923 Poplar Bluff RehabCare Program
Lucy Lee Hospital
2620 N Westwood Blvd
Poplar Bluff, MO 63901-3396 573-785-7721
FAX: 573-686-5987

Jim Martin, Program Manager
Chris Murray, Care Coordinator
Darlene Hill, Care Admissions Coordinator
Provides physical medicine and rehabilitation to individuals with a physically limiting condition. The program is designed to help individuals function as independently as possible by maximizing their strength and abilities.

6924 Shriners Hospitals for Children St. Louis
2001 S Lindbergh Blvd
Saint Louis, MO 63131-3597 314-432-3600
800-850-2960
FAX: 314-432-2930
www.shrinershq.org/hospitals/st.louis
John McCabe, Executive Vice President
Kenneth Guidera, M.D., Chief Medical Officer
Eugene R. D'Amore, Vice President, Hospital Operations
Kathy A. Dean, Vice President, Human Resources
Medical care is provided free of charge for children 18 and under with orthopaedic conditions.

6925 St. Louis Society for the Blind and Visually Impaired
8770 Manchester Rd
Saint Louis, MO 63144-2724 314-960-9000
FAX: 314-968-9003
e-mail: socscrv@slsbvi.org
www.slsbvi.org

David Ekin, President
Chris Pickel, Chair
Ann Shapiro, Vice Chair
Sherine Apte, Secretary
Offers vision rehabilitation services for the totally blind, legally blind, visually impaired, including counseling, educational, recreational, rehabilitation, computer training and professional training services. Low vision aids and appliance available through low vision clinic by appointment.

6926 Truman Medical Center Low Vision Rehabilitation Program
Eye Foundation of Kansas City
2300 Holmes St.
Kansas City, MO 64108 816-404-1780
FAX: 816-404-1786
www.umkc-efkc.org

Nelson R. Sabates, M.D., Chairman
Monika Malecha, MD, Residency Program Director
Abraham Poulose, MD, Director of Clinics
Our program is designed to maximize daily tasks for a person with low vision. We are able to evaluate a person's home and provide recommendations as needed.

6927 Truman Neurological Center
12404 E. US 40 Highway
Independence, MO 64055-1354 816-373-5060
FAX: 816-373-5787
e-mail: info@tnccommunity.com
tnccommunity.com

James Landrum, Executive Director
Ann Johnson, Finance Director
Terri Boyce, Office Assistant
Mary Beth Johnson, Compliance Director
A licensed habilitation center established for the purpose of assisting persons with developmental disabilities and/or mental retardation. The minimum age is 18. Residential care is provided in four group homes in the community licensed by the DMH and CARF accredited.

Montana

6928 Benefis Healthcare
1101 26th St S
Great Falls, MT 59405-5104 406-455-5000
FAX: 406-455-2110
e-mail: benefis@benefis.org
www.benefis.org

John Goodnow, CEO
Laura Goldhahn-Konen, President
Forrest Ehlinger, Chief Financial & Treasury Officer
Paul Dolan, MD, Chief Medical Information Officer
Benefis Healthcare is a not-for-profit community asses governed by a 15-member local board of directors. Benefis is locally owned and controlled. Benefis is a Level II trauma center- one of only 4 in the state and 107 in the country.

6929 Disability Services Division of Montana
Department of Public Health
Helena, MT 59604 406-444-7734
FAX: 406-444-3465
e-mail: dphhs@mt.gov
www.dphhs.state.mt.us/dsd

Keith Messmer, Manager
Sandi Gory, Administrative Assistant
Janice Frisch, Chief Management Operations
Responsible for coordinating, developing and implementing comprehensive programs to assist Montanans with disabilities with activities of daily living, community base services and coordinated programs of habilitation, rehabilitation and independent living.

Nebraska

6930 Las Vegas Healthcare And Rehabilitation Center
680 South Fourth Street
Louisville, KY 40202 502-596-7300
TTY:800-545-0749
e-mail: web_administrator@kindredhealthcare.com
kindredhealthcare.com

Paul J. Diaz, President/ CEO
Accomodates 79 residents. Serving the community for approximately 40 years. Located in close proximity to local hospitals and surrounded by medical complexes, out center offers both short-term rehabilitation and long term.care.

6931 Sierra Pain Institute
265 Golden Ln
Reno, NV 89502-1205 775-323-7092
FAX: 775-323-5259

Lyle Smith, Owner
The program consists of a medically supervised outpatient program managed by an interdisciplinary team with input from specialties of Pain Medicine, Physical Therapy and Occupational Science. The format insures that each patient receives the full range of behavioral techniques in a well-integrated, individually tailored therapeutic regimen.

New Hampshire

6932 Crotched Mountain Adult Brain Injury Center
Crotched Mountain Foundation
1 Verney Dr
Greenfield, NH 03047-5000 603-547-3311
800-966-2672
FAX: 603-547-3232
e-mail: admissions@crotchedmountain.org
www.crotchedmountain.org

Donald Shumway, President, CEO
Michael Terrian, Vice President of Administration & Facilities
Tom Zubricki, Chief Financial Officer
Kathleen C. Brittan, Vice President of Development
Adult Brain Injury Center provides sub-acute rehabilitative services and individualized care to survivors of acquired (including traumatic) brain injury. Ambulatory and non-ambulatory adults are served. Ages range from 18-59, the staff to client ratio is 3:1 and services are provided by experienced interdisciplinary clinical and therapeutic teams. Crotched Mountain is a licensed Special Hospital providing 24 hour medical coverage and skilled nursing. Clients reside in semi-private rooms w/superv

6933 Department of Physical Medicine and Rehabilitation
Exeter Hospital
5 Alumni Dr
Exeter, NH 03833-2128 603-778-7311
FAX: 603-580-6592
www.exeterhospital.com

Kevin Calahan, President
Offers patient treatment, committed to enhancing the lives of individuals with short and long term physically disabling conditions.

6934 Farnum Rehabilitation Center
580 Court St
Keene, NH 03431-1718 603-354-6630
FAX: 603-355-2078

Susan Loughrey, Program Director
Judy Bell, Manager
Offers rehabilitation services, occupational therapy, physical therapy and more for the physically challenged individual.

6935 Hackett Hill Nursing Center and Integrated Care
191 Hackett Hill Rd
Manchester, NH 03102-8993 603-668-8161
FAX: 603-622-2584

Daniele Peckham, Administrator
Brett Lennerton, Administrator
A 68-bed certified nursing home.Postacute rehabilitation program.

6936 New Hampshire Rehabilitation and Sports Medicine
Catholic Medical Center
Ste 201
769 S Main St
Manchester, NH 03102-5166 603-647-1899
800-437-9666
FAX: 603-668-5348

Stuart Draper, Owner
Victor Carbone, Manager
A specialized facility for comprehensive rehabilitation for individuals who have been injured or have a disability.

6937 New Medico, Highwatch Rehabilitation Center
Highwatch Rd
Center Ossipee, NH 03814 FAX: 603-539-8888
William Burke, Executive Director
Post-acute rehabilitation service.

6938 Northern New Hampshire Mental Health and Developmental Services
87 Washington St
Conway, NH 03818-6044 603-447-3347
FAX: 603-447-8893
www.northernhs.org

Dennis Mackay, CEO
Provides mental health and developmental services to northern New Hampshire, including early intervention, elderly services, residential program, outpatient services, employee assistance programs, inpatient services, etc.

6939 The Mental Health Center: Riverside Courtyard
3 Twelfth St
Berlin, NH 03570-3860 603-752-7404
FAX: 603-752-5194

Eileen Theriault, Manager
A center to help people that have mental disabilities.

New Jersey

6940 All Garden State Physical Therapy
44 Ridge Road
North Arlington, NJ 07031 201-998-6300
FAX: 201-998-6344
gardenstatept.com

6941 **Bancroft**
425 Kings Highway East
PO Box 20
Haddonfield, NJ 08033- 1284
856-429-0010
800-774-5516
FAX: 856-429-1613
TTY: 856-428-2697
e-mail: inquiry@bancroft.org
www.bancroft.org

Cynthia Boyer, PhD, Executive Director, Brain Injury Services
Toni Pergolin, President and Chief Executive
Clair Rohrer, Med, Executive Director, Programs for Adults
Dennis . Morgan, M.Ed, Executive Director of Bancroft Special Education Programs

Private, not-for-profit organization serving people with disabilities since 1883. Based in Haddonfield, New Jersey, help more than 1000 children and adults with autism, developmental disabilities, brain injuries, and other neurological impairments. Operates more than 140 sites throughout the U.S. and abroad.

6942 **Daughters of Miriam Center/The Gallen Institute**
155 Hazel St
Clifton, NJ 07011-3423
973-772-3700
FAX: 973-253-5389
e-mail: administration@daughtersofmiriamcenter.org
www.daughtersofmiriamcenter.o rg

Fred Feinstein, Executive Director

Dedicated to providing the highest quality care, the Center has far exceeded a stereotypical nursing home by offering a continuum of care environment, making us a leader in Jewish eldercare.

6943 **Devereux Center in New Jersey**
444 Devereux Drive
Villanova, PA 19085
856-599-6400
800-345-1292
FAX: 856-423-8916
www.devereux.org

Robert Q. Kreider, President
Carol Poirier, Admissions Assistant

Serves emotionally disturbed females, ages 5-21, who have affective disorders, bi-polar disorders, adjustment reactions, behavioral disorders, specific developmental disorders, identity disorders, attention deficit disorders, schizoid disorders, anxiety disorders, enuresis, runaway behavior, substance abuse, in remission and personality disturbances. The center offers 95-100 full-time staff including, teachers, administrators, counselors, therapists, recreation staff and support services.

6944 **Ladacain Network**
Schroth School & Technical Education Center
1701 Kneeley Blvd
Wanamassa, NJ 07712-7622
732-493-5900
FAX: 732-493-5980
ladacin.org

Patricia Carlesimo, Executive Director

Provides an array of services and programs specifically for children and adults with developmental and physical disabilities. Services include approved Department of Education school programs; adult education and training; vocational training, personal care assistance services, in-home and Saturday respite; child care programs, housing opportunities, and more.

6945 **Lourdes Regional Rehabilitation Center**
Our Lady of Lourdes Medical Center
1600 Haddon Ave
Camden, NJ 08103-3101
856-757-3864
856-757-3500
FAX: 856-968-2511
e-mail: info@lourdesnet.org
www.lourdesnet.org

Alexander J. Hatala, President
Kimberly D. Barnes, Vice President, Planning and Development
Michael Hammond, Chief Financial Officer
Maureen Hetu, Chief Information Officer

The only comprehensive rehabilitation facility located within an acute care hospital in Southern New Jersey. Patients benefit from the proximity to the full range of state of the art medical and surgical services should the need arise.

6946 **Mt. Carmel Guild**
1160 Raymond Blvd
Newark, NJ 07102-4168
973-596-4100
FAX: 973-639-6583

Anita Holland, Manager

Offers services for the totally blind, legally blind, visually impaired, mentally retarded blind and more with health, counseling, educational, recreational, rehabilitation, computer training and professional training services.

6947 **Pediatric Rehabilitation Department, JFK Medical Center**
65 James St
Edison, NJ 08818-3947
732-321-7362
732-321-7000
FAX: 732-548-7751
www.jfkmc.org

Michael A. Kleiman, DMD, Chair
Douglas A. Nordstrom, Vice Chair
John L. Kolaya, PE, Secretary
Leonard Sendelsky, Treasurer

Comprehensive interdisciplinary, family focused outpatient pediatric rehabilitation services including evaluation and individual and group treatment programs for children birth-21.

6948 **REACH Rehabilitation Program: Leader Nursing and Rehabilitation Center**
550 Jessup Rd
West Deptford, NJ 08066-1921
856-848-9551

Karen Fattore, Case Manager
Anthony Stenson, Administrator

Postacute rehabilitation program.

6949 **REACH Rehabilitation and Catastrophic Long-Term Care**
1180 Us Highway 22
Mountainside, NJ 07092-2810
908-654-0020
FAX: 908-654-8661

Allen Swanson, Manager
Archie Ordana, Manager

Postacute rehabilitation program.

6950 **Rehabilitation Specialists**
18-01 Pollitt Drive
Ste 1A
Fair Lawn, NJ 07410-2815
201-478-4200
800-441-7488
FAX: 201-478-4201
e-mail: program@rehab-specialists.com
www.rehab-specialists.com

Virgilio Caraballo, President/CEO
Dustin Gordon, Director of Neuropsychological and Clinical Services
Dr. Brian Greenwald, Medical Director
Cindy Dittfield, Director of Marketing & Public Relations

Rehabilitation Specialists, founded in 1983, is a quality, cost effective community re-entry center treating individuals with acquired brain injury. A non clinical environment based in the community is utilized that offers professional services enabling participants to learn skills they need to return to a productive life. Both our Day and Residential programming emphases focus on Functional Life Skills, Work Skills and Learning Skills. Each participant's program is tailored to meet their needs.

6951 **Somerset Valley Rehabilitation and Nursing Center**
Care-One
11300 Cornell Park Drive
Suite 360
Cincinnati, OH 45242
513-469-7222
FAX: 513-469-7230
e-mail: info@healthbridge.org
healthbridge.org

Trudi Matthews, Director of Policy and Public Re

Subacute rehabilitation program, long term care, respite care.

6952 **Summit Ridge Center**
101 East State Street
Kennett Square, PA 19348
973-736-2000
FAX: 973-736-2764
genesishcc.com

New Mexico

6953 **SJR Rehabilitation Hospital**
525 S Schwartz Ave
Farmington, NM 87401-5955
505-609-2625
FAX: 505-327-6562
e-mail: eniemand@sjrmc.net
www.sjrrh.com

Ena M Niemand, Executive Director
Sue Clay, Program Director
Jill Morgan, Nursing Director
Uses a team of professionals to provide a comprehensive rehabilitation program. Accomplishing the best possible physical and cognitive improvement is the aim of the following treatment members: nurses, physical therapists, physicians, speech and occupational therapists, therapeutic recreation specialist. Providing inpatient and out patient services.

6954 **Southwest Communication Resource**
P.O.Box 788
Bernalillo, NM 87004-788
505-867-3396
FAX: 505-867-3398
e-mail: info@abrazosnm.org
swcr.org

New York

6955 **Aspire of Western New York**
2356 N Forest Rd
Getzville, NY 14068-1224
716-838-0047
FAX: 716-894-8257
e-mail: info@aspirewny.org
aspirewny.org

Thomas A. Sy, Executive Director
Janet Hansen, Chief Operating Officer
Mary Anne Coombe, V.P. of Service Coordination & Fiscal Management Services
Helen Trowbridge Hanes, Vice President of Community Living
Provides comprehensive services to individuals with disabilities from infancy through adulthood. Also serves people with all types of developmental disabilities as well as providing clinical services to persons with other types of disabilities such as: spinal cord injury, head trauma and others. Aspire employs 1500 people.

6956 **Bronx Continuing Treatment Day Program**
1527 Southern Blvd
Bronx, NY 10460-5619
718-893-1414
FAX: 718-893-0707

Mary Jane Purcell, Manager
Post-acute rehabilitation program.

6957 **Brooklyn Bureau of Community Service**
285 Schermerhorn St
Brooklyn, NY 11217-1098
718-310-5600
FAX: 718-855-1517
e-mail: info@WeAreBCS.org
www.wearebcs.org

Marla Simpson, Executive Director
Anthony B. Edwards, MBA, CCF, MFM, CFO
Janelle Farris, Chief Operating Officer
Sonya Shields, Chief Officer for External Relations and Advancement
Offers independent living skills, counseling, work readiness, vocational trianing, job placement and job follow-up services to individuals with disabilities (to include individuals with psychiatric, physical, and developmental disabilities). Special programs to move disabled welfare recipients from welfare to work. Publishes a bi-annual newsletter.

6958 **Buffalo Hearing and Speech Center**
50 E North St
Buffalo, NY 14203-1002
716-885-8318
FAX: 716-885-4229
askbhsc.org

Frank J. Polino, Chairman
Dennis J. Szefel, First Vice Chairman
Kenneth J. Wilson, Treasurer
Gerald Chiari, Esq., Secretary
Assists individuals with speech, language and/or hearing impairments to achieve maximum communication potential.

6959 **Cora Hoffman Center Day Program**
2324 Forest Ave
Staten Island, NY 10303-1506
718-447-8205
FAX: 718-815-2182

Kevin Kenney, Manager
Post-acute rehabilitation program specializing in Cerebral Palsy. Part of the Cerebral Palsey Association of New York State.

6960 **Elmhurst Hospital Center**
7901 Broadway
Elmhurst, NY 11373-1368
718-334-4000
www.nyc.gov/html/hhc/ehc/html/home/home.shtml

Chris D Constantino, Executive Director
Hospital is comprised of 525 beds and is a Level I Trauma Center, and Emergency Heart Care Stattion and a 911 recieving hospital. It is the premiere health care organization for key areas such as Surgery, Cardiology, Women's health, Pediatrics, Rehabilitation Medicine, Renal and Mental Health Services.

6961 **Federation Employment And Guidance Service(F-E-G-S)**
315 Hudson St
New York, NY 10013-1086
212-366-8400
FAX: 212-366-8441
e-mail: info@fegs.org
www.fegs.org

Gail Magaliff, CEO
Ira Machowsky, Executive Vice President
Thomas M. Higgins, CFO
Kristin M. Woodlock, Chief Operating Officer
The largest and most diversified private, not-for-profit health related and human service organization in the United States. With operations in over 258 facilities, residences, and off-site locations, F-E-G-S has served more then 2 million people since its inception.

6962 **Flushing Hospital**
4500 Parsons Blvd
Flushing, NY 11355-2205
718-670-5000
FAX: 718-670-3082
flushinghospital.org

Robert V. Levine, Executive Vice President and COO
Bruce J. Flanz, President/ CEO
Mounir Doss, Executive Vice President/CFO
Offers services for the totally blind, legally blind, visually impaired, mentally retarded blind and more with health, counseling, educational, recreational, rehabilitation, computer training and professional training services.

6963 **Gateway Community Industries Inc.,**
1 Amy Kay Pkwy
Kingston, NY 12401-6444
845-331-1261
800-454-9395
FAX: 845-331-4920
e-mail: info@gatewayindustries.org
gatewayindustries.org

Francoise C. Gunefsky, President/ CEO
Eva Graham, CFO
Ralph Smith, Chief Information Officer
Mary Ann Hildebrandt, Chief Quality and Compliance Officer
Gateway Community Industries, Inc., founded in 1957, is one of the leading independent not-for-profit vocational rehabilitation and training centers for people with mental and/or physical disabilities. The agency provides comprehensive services in vocational evaluation, job training, job placement, vocational work

center employment, supported employment, psychiatric rehabilitation, continuing day treatment, and residential habilitation/rehabilitation.

6964 Henkind Eye Institute Division of Montefiore Hospital
111 East 210th Street
Bronx, NY 10467-2404 718-920-4321
www.montefiore.org
Philip O. Ozuah, MD, PhD, Executive Vice President/ COO
Steven M. Safyer, MD, President/ CEO
Joel A. Perlman, Executive Vice President, Chief Financial Officer
Alfredo Cabrera, Senior Vice President & Chief Human Resources Officer
Offers services for the totally blind, legally blind, visually impaired, mentally retarded blind and more with health, counseling, educational, recreational, rehabilitation, computer training and professional training services. Low vision services offered.

6965 Industries for the Blind of New York State
194 Washington Ave
Ste 300
Albany, NY 12210-6314 518-456-8671
800-421-9010
FAX: 518-456-3587
e-mail: customercare@nyspsp.org
www.abilityone.com
Richard Healey, CEO
Offers services for the totally blind, legally blind, visually impaired, mentally retarded blind and more with health, counseling, educational, recreational, rehabilitation, computer training and professional training services.

6966 Inpatient Pain Rehabilitation Program
550 First Avenue
New York, NY 10016 212-263-7300
FAX: 212-598-6468
www.med.nyu.edu
William Pinter Phd, Administrative Director
The Inpatient Rehabilitation Program, established in 1983 specializes in the treatment of chronic pain. Our inpatient program is one of the oldest and well established pain programs in the country. It is the only interdisciplinary inpatient pain program in the tri-state area and one of only 20 pain programs in the entire US to have CARF accreditation. Upon completion of an extensive evaluation, patients are admitted for an 18-day inpatient stay.

6967 Koicheff Health Care Center
2324 Forest Ave
Staten Island, NY 10303-1506 718-447-0200
FAX: 718-981-1431
Paul Castello, Clinic Director
Post-accute rehabilitation programs.

6968 New York-Presbyterian Hospital
622 W 168th St
New York, NY 10032-3796 212-305-4600
FAX: 212-305-1017
www.nyp.org
Steven J. Corwin, MD, CEO
Robert E. Kelly, MD, President
New York Presbyterian Hospital is internationally recognized for its outstanding comprehensive services. Its medical, surgical, and emergency care services provide each patient with the highest possible level of care. In addition, as part of the Hospital's commitment to the total well-being of each patient, it offers a range of specialized services, as well as special healthcare programs for neighboring communities.

6969 Norman Marcus Pain Institute
30 E 40th St
Ste 1100
New York, NY 10016 212-532-7999
FAX: 212-532-5957
e-mail: support@nmpi.com
backpainusa.com
Norman J Marcus, Medical Director
We focus on muscles as the cause of most common pains, i.e. back, neck, shoulders, and headaches. We make specific muscle diagnoses and have specific treatments that in many cases will eliminate the need for surgery or relieve the pain. Patients diagnosed with herniated disc, spinal stenosis, rotator cuff tear, impingement syndrome, sciatica, fibromyalgia and headache will generally find relief.

6970 Pain Alleviation Center
Comprehensive Pain Management Associates
125 S Service Rd
Jericho, NY 11753-1038 516-997-7246
FAX: 516-997-7281
www.paincenter.com
Alex Weingarten, Director
Phillip Fyman, Director
Marisa French, Manager
One of the first pain clinics to gain national accreditation from the Commission on Accreditation of Rehabilitation Facilities. This is due largely to a patient-centered program based on the latest research.

6971 Pathfinder Village
3 Chenango Rd
Edmeston, NY 13335-2314 607-965-8377
FAX: 607-965-8655
e-mail: info@pathfindervillage.org
www.pathfindervillage.org
Paul Landers, CEO
Caprice S. Eckert, Chief Financial Officer
Kelly A. Meyers, Director of Admissions
Paula B. Schaeffer, Director of Enrichment Programs
Pathfinder Village is a warm, friendly community in the rolling hills of Central New York. Here children and adults with Down Syndrome gain independence, build lasting friendships, become partners in the world and take in all that life has to offer.

6972 Pilot Industries: Ellenville
845-331-4300
48 Canal St
Ellenville, NY 12428-1327 845-647-7711
FAX: 845-647-7711
Peter Pierri, Executive Director
Betty Marks, Plant Manager
Post-accute rehabilitation services.

6973 Skills Unlimited
405 Locust Ave
Oakdale, NY 11769-1695 631-567-3320
FAX: 631-567-3285
e-mail: info@skillsunlimited.org
skillsunlimited.org
Richard Kassnove, Executive Director
Our basic goals is to offer persons with disabilities the opportunity to explore and develop their full vocational potential. Our programs are unique in that by offering comprehensive services, individuals are able to deal with many different issues that could potentially affect their vocational success. Any individual that has an impairment that interferes with their ability to work is entitles to the services that we offer.

North Carolina

6974 Center for Vision Rehabilitation
Academy Eye Associates
3115 Academy Rd
Durham, NC 27707-2652 919-493-7456
800-942-1499
FAX: 919-493-1718
e-mail: henry.greene@academyeye.com
academyeye.com
Henry A Greene, Owner
Vision rehabilitation and low-vision care for the visually impaired, post-stroke, head trauma and for neuro-oncology vision complications.

6975 Diversified Opportunities
1010 Herring Ave E
Wilson, NC 27893-3311 252-291-0378
FAX: 252-291-1402
www.diversifiedopportunitiesinc.com
Cindy Dixon, Executive Director
Carlton Goff, Business Manager
Ericka Simmons, QP Program Manager
Ken Jones, Chairman
Vocational rehabilitation agency, better outcomes, lower cost, guaranteed performance standards.

6976 Forsyth Medical Center
3333 Silas Creek Pkwy
Winston Salem, NC 27103-3090 336-718-5000
FAX: 336-718-9250
www.novanthealth.org
Jeffrey T. Lindsay, President
Denise Mihal, Chief Operating Officer
Stephen J. Motew, MD, Senior Vice President
Bruce D. Walley, MD, Senior Vice President
Provides care that is state-of-the-art and second to none, both because of advanced treatments availiable through our clinical research and technology to the academic excellence-and caring nature-of our doctors and nurses.

6977 Industries of the Blind
914-920 W Lee St
Greensboro, NC 27403-2803 336-274-1591
800-909-7086
FAX: 336-544-3739
e-mail: customerservice@iob-gso.com
industriesoftheblind.com
David Thompson, Chairperson
Scott Thornhill, 1st Vice Chairperson
Ashley S. James, Jr., 2nd Vice Chairperson
Chi Anyansi-Archibong, Secretary
Offers services for the totally blind, legally blind, visually impaired, mentally retarded blind and more with health, counseling, educational, recreational, rehabilitation, computer training and professional training services.

6978 Johnston County Industries
1100 East Preston Street
Selma, NC 27576-3162 919-743-8700
FAX: 919-965-8023
jcindustries.com
John Shallcross, Jr., President
Durwood Woodall, Vice President
Lina Sanders-Johnson, Secretary/Treasurer
JCI is an entrepreneurial not-for-profit corporation dedicated to empowering people with disabilities or disadvantages to succeed through training and employment

6979 Learning Services: Carolina
707 Morehead Ave
Durham, NC 27707-1319 919-688-4444
888-419-9955
FAX: 919-419-9966
learningservices.com
Debra Braunling-McMorrow, President and CEO
Jeanne Mack, Chief Financial Officer and Vice President of Operations
Michael Weaver, Chief Development Officer
Terri Dorman, V.P. of Customer Service and Care Management
Located in an historic neighborhood in the heart of Durham, this campus-style setting offers easy access to resources at 3 outstanding facilities: Duke University, The University of North Carolina at Chapel Hill, and Research Triangle Park. This program provides a range of services and activities that draw upon the many resources availiable in the community.

6980 LifeSpan
200 Clanton Road
Charlotte, NC 28217 704-944-5100
lifespanservices.org
Davan Cloninger, President & CEO
Ralph Adams, Treasurer & CFO
Christopher White, Vice President of Operations & Business Development
Lori Avery, Senior Development Director
Provide vocational and enrichment program for adults with developmental disabilities.

6981 Lions Club Industries for the Blind
4500 Emperor Blvd.
Durham, NC 27703 919-596-8277
800-526-1562
FAX: 919-598-1179
e-mail: inquire@buylci.com
Bill Hudson, President
Offers services for the totally blind, legally blind, visually impaired, mentally retarded blind and more with health, counseling, educational, recreational, rehabilitation, computer training and professional training services.

6982 Lions Services Inc.
5 Penn Plaza
New York, NY 10001 21 -62 -210
e-mail: lsisale@aol.com
Jimmy R Cranford, President
Jimmy Cranford, President
Offers services for the totally blind, legally blind, visually impaired, mentally retarded blind and more with health, counseling, educational, recreational, rehabilitation, computer training and professional training services.

6983 Regional Rehabilitation Center Pitt County Memorial Hospital
2100 Stantonsburg Rd
Greenville, NC 27834-2818 252-847-4448
FAX: 252-816-7552
e-mail: mdixon@pcmh.com
www.uhseast.com/rehab
Martha M Dixon, VP General Services
An accredited, comprehensive rehabilitation center-part of a statewide network- and we're the largest such facility in eastern North Carolina. Our service area covers 29 counties, and we offer a complete array of rehabilitation services for patients of all ages. Because the Regional Rehabilitation Center is associated with both Pitt County Memorial Hospital And the Brody School of Medicine at East Carolina University, patients have access to a full range of state of the art medical services.

6984 Rehab Home Care
2660 Yonkers Rd
Raleigh, NC 27604-3384 800-447-8692
FAX: 919-831-2211
Alan Silver, CEO
Janis Hansen, Chief Operating Officer
A Medicare/Medicaid certified, state-licensed home health agency with emphasis on rehabilitation.

6985 Thoms Rehabilitation Hospital
Thoms Rehabilitation Hospital
68 Sweeten Creek Rd
Asheville, NC 28803-2318 828-277-4800
FAX: 828-277-4812
TTY:800-735-2962
www.carepartners.org
Tracy Buchanan, President & CEO
Gary Bowers, COO
Freestanding physical rehabilitation hospital, founded 1938 - 100 beds, including 90 acute and 10 transitional - JCAHO accredited.

6986 **Winston-Salem Industries for the Blind**
7730 N Point Blvd
Winston Salem, NC 27106-3310
336-759-0551
800-242-7726
FAX: 336-759-0990
e-mail: info@wsifb.com
www.wsifb.com

Mike Faircloth, Chairman
Karen Carey, Vice Chairman, Secretary
W. Robert Newell, Treasurer
David Horton, Executive Director

Offers services for the totally blind, legally blind, visually impaired, mentally retarded blind and more with health, counseling, educational, recreational, rehabilitation, computer training and professional training services.

Ohio

6987 **Bellefaire Jewish Children's Bureau**
22001 Fairmount Blvd
Cleveland, OH 44118-4819
216-932-2800
800-879-2522
FAX: 216-932-6704
e-mail: info@bellefairejcb.org
www.bellefairejcb.org

Adam Jacobs, CEO
Adam G. Jacobs PhD, Executive Vice President

Residential treatment for ages 12 to 17 1/2 at time of admission offering individualized psychotherapy, special education, and group living for severaly emotionally disturbed children and adolescents. Also offers a variety of other programs including specialized and therapeutic foster care, partial hospitilization, outpatient counseling, home-based intensive counseling and adoption services.

6988 **Christ Hospital Rehabilitation Unit**
2139 Auburn Ave
Cincinnati, OH 45219-2906
513-585-2737
FAX: 513-585-4353
www.thechristhospital.com

Mike Keating, President and CEO
Chris Bergman, Vice President and Chief Financial Officer
Berc Gawne, MD, Vice President and Chief Medical Officer
Peter Greis, Vice President and Chief Information Officer

Patients of this 555-bed, not-for-profit acute care facility receive personalized health care provided by trained specialists using the most sophisticated medical technology available, including state-of-the-art intensive care units, surgical facilities, cardiac catheterization labs, three new electrophysiology labs, and the tristates first positron emission tomography (PET) scanning capabilities.

6989 **Cleveland Society for the Blind**
Cleveland Sight Center
P.O.Box 1988
1909 East 101st Street
Cleveland, OH 44106-8696
216-791-8118
FAX: 216-696-2582
e-mail: jcarey@clevelandsightcenter.org
www.clevelandsightcenter.org

William L. Spring, Chair
Thomas J. Gibbons, Vice Chair
Gary W. Poth, Treasurer
Sheryl King Benford, Secretary

Social, rehabilitation, education and support services for blind and visually impaired children and adults, early intervention program for children birth to age 6, low vision clinic, aid and appliance shop, Braille and taping transcription, training for rehabilitation, orientation, mobility and computer access, employment services and job placement, recreation program, resident camping, talking books, radio reading services, food service training and snack bar employment. Free screening.

6990 **Columbus Speech and Hearing Center**
510 E North Broadway St
Columbus, OH 43214-4114
614-263-5151
FAX: 614-263-5365
columbusspeech.org

Dawn Gleason, Au.D., President/ CEO
Karen Deeter, Director of Operations

Serves persons who have speech-language and hearing challenges. Provides vocational rehabilitation services for individuals who are deaf, hard-of-hearing or deaf-blind.

6991 **CommuniCare of Clifton Nursing and Rehabilitation Center**
Communi Care Health Services
4700 Ashwood Drive
Cincinnati, OH 45241
513-489-7100
FAX: 513-281-2559
communicarehealth.com

Stephen L. Rosedale, Founder/ CEO

A long term care facility which specializes in rehabilitation. Offers a full range of rehabilitative services including physical therapy, occupational therapy and speech therapy.

6992 **Doctors Hospital**
5100 W Broad St
Columbus, OH 43228-1672
614-544-1000
800-837-7555
FAX: 614-544-1844
www.ohiohealth.com/homedoctors

David Blom, President/ CEO
Michael Bernstein, Senior Vice President and Chief

We believe our first responsibility is to the patients we serve. We respect the physical, emotional and spiritual needs of our patients and find that compassion is essential to fostering healing and wholeness.

6993 **Dodd Hall at the Ohio State University Hospitals**
410 W 10th Ave
Columbus, OH 43210-1240
614-293-3300
800-293-5123
e-mail: OSUCareConnection@osumc.edu
www.medicalcenter.osu.edu

Steven G. Gabbe, MD, Senior Vice President / CEO
Larry Anstine, CEO
Gail Marsh, Chief Strategy Officer
Phyllis Teater, Chief Information Officer

Dodd Hall is a full service medical rehabilitation hospital offering comprehensive inpatient and outpatient rehabilitation.

6994 **Easter Seal Society of Mahoning**
National Easter Seals Chicago
299 Edwards Street
Youngstown, OH 44502-1599
330-743-1168
800-221-6827
FAX: 330-743-1616
www.easterseals.com/mtc

6995 **Four Oaks Center**
245 N. Valley Road
Xenia, OH 45385-2605
937-562-6500
FAX: 937-562-6520
www.greenedd.org

Todd McManus, President
Jill A. LaRock, Director
Dr. Vijay Gupta, Vice President
Melinda Mays, Recording Secretary

Starts children on the road to discovery by providing a learning environment rich in opportunities and encouragement. The program was designed to give children with delays or disabilities, or those at-risk the extra help needed to develop fully. Any child under the age of six who exhibits developmental delays, handicapping conditions, or is considered at risk may qualify to participate.

6996 Genesis Healthcare System
Rehabilitation Services
800 Forest Ave
Zanesville, OH 43701-2881
740-454-5000
800-322-4762
FAX: 740-455-7527
e-mail: llynn@genesishcs.org
www.genesishcs.org

Matt Perry, President/ CEO
Paul Masterson, CFO
Richard Helsper, COO

A CARF and JACHO accredited 19-bed rehabilitation facility located within Genesis Healthcare System, a 732 bed, non-profit hospital system, located in Zanesville, Ohio. Freestanding outpatient services, including work hardening, pain management, vocational services, audiology, lymphedema, vestibular rehab, off-the-road driving evals, aquatic therpay, womens health and sports enhancement.

6997 George A Martin Center
3603 Washington Ave
Cincinnati, OH 45229-2009
513-221-1017
FAX: 513-221-3817

Karen Doggett, Executive Director

Offers services for the totally blind, legally blind, visually impaired, mentally retarded blind and more with health, counseling, educational, recreational, rehabilitation, computer training and professional training services.

6998 Grady Memorial Hospital
561 W Central Ave
Delaware, OH 43015-1489
740-615-1000
800-487-1115
FAX: 740-368-5114
ohiohealth.com

Bruce Hagen, Regional Executive and President

As a progressive healthcare leader, Grady Memorial Hospital is committed to excellence while providing the Deleware community with comprehensive quality service delivered with compassionate, personal care. Our membership in Ohio's largest healthcare system, Ohio Health, enables us to improve access to a broader range of healthcare services, enhance development of new programs and services, and provide a complete continuum of care for patients in the deleware area.

6999 Hamilton Adult Center
3400 Symmes Rd
Hamilton, OH 45015-1359
513-867-5970
FAX: 513-874-2977

Donald Musnuff, Executive Director

7000 Holzer Clinic
100 Jackson Pike
Gallipolis, OH 45631-1560
740-446-5000
FAX: 740-446-5532
e-mail: info@holzer.org
www.holzer.org

T. Wayne Munro, MD, CEO
Brent A. Saunders, Chair
Christopher Meyer, Chief Medical Officer
John Cunningham, Chief Administrative Officer

Serves medical needs of patients in an 8 county area, including counties in Ohio and West Virginia.

7001 Holzer Clinic Sycamore
Holzer Medical Center
4th Avenue & Sycamore St
Gallipolis, OH 45631-1560
740-446-5244
FAX: 740-446-5448
e-mail: info@holzer.org
www.holzer.org

T. Wayne Munro, MD, CEO
Brent A. Saunders, Chair
Christopher Meyer, Chief Medical Officer
John Cunningham, Chief Administrative Officer

Offers an individualized quality comprehensive rehabilitation program for people with disabilities by an interdisciplinary team including physical therapy, occupational, speech, nursing and social services to restore the patient to the highest degree of rehab outcomes attainable.

7002 IKRON Institute for Rehabilitative and Psychological Services
2347 Vine St
Cincinnati, OH 45213-1745
513-621-1117
FAX: 513-621-2350
e-mail: ikron@ikron.org
ikron.org

Randy Strunk, MA, LPCC-S, Executive Director
Ken Carbonell, BBA, Fiscal Director
Melissa Harmeling, MA, PCC-S, Program Director
Jake Striker, President

An accredited mental health facility and a certified rehabilitation center. Through a variety of creative treatment and rehabilitation services, IKRON assists adults with mental health and/or substance abuse problems to attain greater independence, to lead lives of sobriety, to obtain competitive work and live more satisfying lives. IKRON places a strong emphasis on respect and support for persons with problems of adjustment. Special contracts to persons desiring job placement.

7003 Integrated Health Services at Waterford Commons
955 Garden Lake Pkwy
Toledo, OH 43614-2777
419-382-2200
FAX: 419-381-8508

Nicole Giesige, Executive Director

A subacute and rehabilitation program specializing in ventilator weaning and management, I.V. therapeutics and pain management, wound management and subacute rehabilitation.

7004 Lester H Higgins Adult Center
3041 Cleveland Ave SW
Canton, OH 44707-3625
330-484-4814
FAX: 330-484-9416
http://www.theworkshopsinc.com/

Margalie Belazaire, Manager
Ed Allar, Manager

Post-accute rehabilitation service

7005 Live Oaks Career Development Campus
5936 Buckwheat Rd
Milford, OH 45150
513-575-1906
FAX: 513-575-0805

Harold Carr MD, Superintendent
Robin White, President/CEO
Jim Dixon, Principal

Post-accute rehabilitation facility and services.

7006 Metro Health: St. Luke's Medical Center Pain Management Program
2500 Metrohealth Dr
Cleveland, OH 44109-1900
216-778-7800
www.metrohealth.org

Mark Moran, President

CARF accredited comprehensive multidisciplinary pain management program.

7007 MetroHealth Medical Center
2500 Metrohealth Dr
Cleveland, OH 44109-1900
216-778-7800
www.metrohealth.org

Mark Moran, President

Located on the near west side of Cleveland, is a leader in trauma, emergency, and critical care; women's and childrens's services, including high risk obstetrical care and neonatal intensive care; comprehensive medical and surgical subspecialties.

7008 Middletown Regional Hospital: Inpatient Rehabilitation Unit
105 McKnight Dr
Middletown, OH 45044-4838
513-422-1401
800-338-4057
FAX: 513-422-1520
www.middletownhospital.org

C N Reddy, Owner
Douglas McNeill, Chief Executive Officer
Our mission is to serve and help people, improving the status of their health and the quality of thier lives. Our vision is to be the premier integrated delivery system in Southwest Ohio. Our Values are quality, respect, service and teamwork

7009 Newark Healthcare Center
680 South Fourth Street
Louisville, KY 40202
502-596-7300
TTY:800-545-0749
e-mail: web_administrator@kindred.com
kindredhealthcare.com

Paul J. Diaz, President/ CEO
Accomodates 300 residents. We are located in the heart of Newark, Ohio. Newark Healthcare is a 2004 recipient of the American Health Care Association's Quality Award.

7010 Parma Community General Hospital Acute Rehabilitation Center
7007 Powers Blvd
Parma, OH 44129-5495
440-743-3000
FAX: 440-843-4387
www.parmahospital.org

David Nedrich, Chairman
Thomas P. O'Donnell, First Vice Chairman
Alex I. Koler, First Assistant Treasurer
Sharon Martin, Assistant Secretary
The mission of this CARF accredited unit is to provide the most comprehensive, cost-effective, acute rehabilitation program possible in order for every patient and family to adjust to his/her disability and to achieve the maximum potential of independent functioning when returning to community living.

7011 Peter A Towne Physical Therapy Center
Ste 10
447 Nilles Rd
Fairfield, OH 45014-2626
513-829-7726
FAX: 513-829-7726
www.townept.com/fairfield

Debbie Wilkerson, Office Manager
Outpatient, private practice physical and occupational therapy. Three other offices in Hamilton, Monroe and West Chester.

7012 Philomatheon Society of the Blind
2701 Tuscarawas St W
Canton, OH 44708-4638
330-453-9157
www.philomatheon.com

David Miller, President
Denise Dessecker, Vice President
Angela Randall, Secretary
Paul Williams, Treasurer
Offers services for the totally blind, legally blind, visually impaired, mentally retarded blind and more with health, counseling, educational, recreational, rehabilitation, computer training and professional training services.

7013 Providence Hospital Work
2270 Banning Rd
Cincinnati, OH 45239-6621
513-591-5600
FAX: 513-591-5604

Kay Brogle, Executive Director
Post-acute rehabilitation services.

7014 Six County, Inc.
2845 Bell St
Zanesville, OH 43701-1794
740-454-9766
800-344-5818
FAX: 740-588-6452
e-mail: info@sixcounty.org
www.sixcounty.org

John A Creek, President
Tim Llewellyn, Senior VP/Community Intervention
Robert Santos, Ex Vp & Coo
Mary Denoble, Vp Qip
Six County, Inc., is a private, not-for-profit corporation under contract with the Mental Health and Recovery Services Board. Six County, Inc., provides comprehensive community mental health services to people of all ages in each of the six Southeastern Ohio counties served: Coshocton, Guernsey, Morgan, Muskingum, Noble, and Perry. SCI's counseling centers provide a full range of services including outpatient counseling; diagnostic assessment, referrals, and psychological testing.

7015 Society for Rehabilitation
9290 Lake Shore Blvd
Mentor, OH 44060-1664
440-352-8993
800-344-3159
FAX: 440-352-6632
e-mail: info@societyhelps.org
www.societyhelps.org

Richard Kessler, Executive Director
Vision is to provide individuals with comprehensive services to improve their quality of life. Our mission is to meet the needs of individuals and their families by delivering a wide range of affordable accessible and personalized services, providing treatment by a team of highly qualified, caring professionals. Collaborating with other agencies to meet community needs.

7016 Southeast Ohio Sight Center
425 E. Alvarado Street
Suite E
Fallbrook, CA 92028
800-677-4180
www.charityadvantage.com

7017 St. Francis Rehabilitation Hospital
401 N Broadway St
Green Springs, OH 44836-9638
419-639-2626
800-248-2552
FAX: 419-639-6225
www.sfhcc.org

Kim Eicher, CEO
Dan Schwanke, Chief Executive Officer
Program offers specialized treatment for patients who have suffered a head injury, spinal cord injury, or stroke, or who have an orthopedic injury. The Head Injury Program provides a continuum of care from coma stimulation through transitional living. Their physicians, nurses, counselors and therapists are dedicated to helping our patients develop the motivation, strength and skills needed to overcome or adapt to their disability.

7018 TAC Enterprises
2160 Old Selma Rd
Springfield, OH 45505-4600
937-525-7400
FAX: 937-525-7401
e-mail: info@tacind.com
www.tacind.com

Clifford Meyer, CEO
TAC Enterprises provides employment opportunities for individuals to develop marketable skills by completing contract work in partnership with other industries. Work and self-help skills, social adjustment, and a variety of daily living experiences are offered to the workers by our specialized staff.

Oklahoma

7019 **Dean A McGee Eye Institute**
608 Stanton L Young Blvd
Oklahoma City, OK 73104-5065
405-271-6060
800-787-9012
FAX: 405-271-4442
www.mei.org

Gregory L. Skuta, M.D., President/CEO
Matthew D. Brown, Executive Vice President
Lana G. Ivy, Vice President of Development
Kimberly A. Howard, Chief Financial Officer and Vice President of Finance

Offers services for the totally blind, legally blind, visually impaired, mentally retarded blind and more with health, counseling, educational, recreational, rehabilitation, computer training and professional training services.

7020 **Jane Phillips Medical Center**
Rehab Care
3500 E Frank Phillips Blvd
Bartlesville, OK 74006-2464
918-333-7200
FAX: 918-333-7801
e-mail: webmaster@jpmc.org
jpmc.org

David Stire, President/ COO
Mike Moore, Chief Financial Officer/Vice President Fiscal Services
Susan Herron, RN, Vice President Nursing Services
Paul W. McQuillen, MD, Chief Medical Officer

Comprehensive inpatient rehabilitation services are provided to patients with orthopedic, neurologic, and other medical conditions of recent onset or regression, who have experienced a loss of function in activities of daily living, mobility, cognition and communication.

7021 **McAlester Regional Health Center RehabCare Unit**
1 E Clark Bass Blvd
McAlester, OK 74501-4255
918-426-1800
FAX: 918-421-6832
e-mail: nbrinlee@mrhcok.com
www.mrhcok.com

David Keith, President/ CEO
Cara Bland, Chairman
Evans McBride, Vice-Chairman

A 19-bed inpatient physical rehabilitation unit serving the Southeast Oklahoma area. Offers physical therapy, occupational therapy, social work, speech and psychological services in an interdisciplinary framework.

7022 **Oklahoma League for the Blind**
501 N Douglas Ave
Oklahoma City, OK 73106-5085
405-232-4644
888-522-4644
FAX: 405-236-5438
e-mail: info@newviewoklahoma.org
www.newviewoklahoma.org

Lauren White, President/ CEO
Carol Campbell, Executive Assistant
John Wilson, Chief Financial Officer
Randy Hearn, Chief Operations Officer

Offers services for the blind and visually impaired, counseling, educational, recreational, rehabilitation, computer training and professional training services.

7023 **Valley View Regional Hospital-RehabCare Unit**
430 N Monte Vista St
Ada, OK 74820-4657
580-332-2323
FAX: 580-421-1395
e-mail: valleyview@wrh.com
www.valleyviewregional.org

W. Kent Rogers, President/ CEO

Comprehensive physical medicine and rehabilitation services designed to help patients in their adjustment to a physically limiting condition.

Oregon

7024 **Garten Services**
PO Box 13970
Salem, OR 97309
503-581-1984
FAX: 503-581-4497
e-mail: garten@garten.org
garten.org

Tim Rocak, CEO
Pamela Best, CFO
Steve Babcock, Mail Services Manager
Stacie Braun, Custodial Services Manager

Garten's mission is to support people with disabilities in their effort to contribute to the community through employment, career, and retirement opportunities. Our actions increase society's awareness of human potential. Garten's vision is to be recognized as an organization positively demonstrating to the community that people with disabilities can be contributing and valued employees of a thriving business.

7025 **Legacy Emanuel Rehabilitation Center**
2801 N. Gantenbein
Portland, OR 97227-1542
503-413-2200
FAX: 503-413-1501
www.legacyhealth.org

Gary Guidetta, Executive Director
Gail Weisgerber, Manager

A non-profit tax-exempt corporation that includes 5 full-service hospitals and a children's hospital. The Legacy system provides an integrated network of healthcare services, including acute and critical care, inpatient and outpatient treatment, community health education and a variety of specialty services.

7026 **Oakcrest Care Center**
2933 Center St NE
Salem, OR 97301-4527
503-585-5850
FAX: 503-585-8781

7027 **Oakhill-Senior Program**
1190 Oakhill Ave SE
Salem, OR 97302-3496
503-364-9086
FAX: 503-365-2879

Jan Dillon, Senior Services Manager

Garten Senior Services provides an adult day service program to seniors with and without developmental disabilities. The program will provide community opportunities, college classes and a wide variety of leisure activities in group and individual settings.

7028 **Pacific Spine and Pain Center**
1801 Highway 99 N
Ashland, OR 97520-9152
541-488-2255
866-482-5515
FAX: 541-482-2433

Janel R Guyette, Manager

7029 **Vision Northwest**
9225 SW Hall Blvd
Portland, OR 97223-6794
503-684-8389
800-448-2232
FAX: 503-684-9359
e-mail: marthaz@visionnw.com
visionnw.com

Evelyn Maizels, Executive Director

Offers services for the totally blind, legally blind, visually impaired, mentally retarded blind and more with health, counseling, educational, recreational, rehabilitation, computer training and professional training services.

7030 **Willamette Valley Rehabilitation Center**
1853 W Airway Rd
Lebanon, OR 97355-1233
541-258-8121
FAX: 541-451-1762
wvrc.org

Martin Baughman, Executive Director

Provides the best professional vocational services to those adults in the community who, by virtue of their physical or mental limitations, are negatively impacted by their ability to attain or maintain employment.

Pennsylvania

7031 Alpine Nursing and Rehabilitation Center of Hershey
Pennstate
405 Martin Ter
State College, PA 16803-3426
814-865-1710
FAX: 814-863-9423
e-mail: geron@psu.edu
geron.psu.edu

Melissa A Hardy, Director
Anna Shuey, Administrative Assistant
Postacute rehabilitation program.

7032 Alpine Ridge and Brandywood
444 Devereux Drive
Victoria, TX 19085-2666
361-575-8271
800-345-1292
FAX: 361-575-6520
devereux.org

Robert Q. Kreider, President and CEO
Margaret McGill, SVP, Chief Operations Officer
Robert C. Dunne, SVP & Chief Financial Officer, Treasurer
Marilyn B. Benoit, M.D., SVP, Chief Clinical Officer, Chief Medical Officer

7033 Amity Lodge
Devereux Foundation
444 Devereux Drive
Victoria, TX 19085-2666
361-575-8271
800-345-1292
FAX: 361-575-6520
devereux.org

Robert Q. Kreider, President and CEO
Margaret McGill, SVP, Chief Operations Officer
Robert C. Dunne, SVP & Chief Financial Officer, Treasurer
Marilyn B. Benoit, M.D., SVP, Chief Clinical Officer, Chief Medical Officer
Offers residents a continuum of services ranging from minimal care and supervision to total physical and medical care.

7034 Beechwood Rehabilitation Services A Community Integrated Brain Injury Program
469 E Maple Ave
Langhorne, PA 19047-1600
215-750-4299
800-782-3299
FAX: 215-750-4327
e-mail: dcerra-tyl@wood.org
beechwoodrehab.com

Thomas Felicetti, President
Services include residential, day treatment and community based support services. Individuals with brain injury are served. The facility is Care Accredited.

7035 Beneto Center
Devereux Foundation
444 Devereux Drive
Victoria, TX 19085-2666
361-575-8271
800-345-1292
FAX: 361-575-6520
devereux.org

Robert Q. Kreider, President and CEO
Margaret McGill, SVP, Chief Operations Officer
Robert C. Dunne, SVP & Chief Financial Officer, Treasurer
Marilyn B. Benoit, M.D., SVP, Chief Clinical Officer, Chief Medical Officer
Offers a continuum of services for residents requiring services ranging from minimal care and supervision to total physical and medical care.

7036 Blind & Vision Rehabilitation Services Of Pittsburgh
1800 West St
Homestead, PA 15120-2578
412-368-4400
800-706-5050
FAX: 412-368-4090
www.bvrspittsburgh.org

Erika M. Arbogast, President
Brian Glass, Director of Information Services and Facilities
Leslie Montgomery, Director of Development and Public Relations
Barbara Peterson, Director of Client Services
Offers services for the totally blind, legally blind, visually impaired, mentally retarded blind and more with health, counseling, educational, recreational, rehabilitation, computer training and professional training services.

7037 Bradford Regional Medical Center
116 Interstate Pkwy
Bradford, PA 16701-1036
814-368-4143
FAX: 814-368-4130
www.brmc.com

Marek Dzionara, Owner
Andrew Lehman, Executive Director
Timothy J. Finan, President and CEO
Offers rehabilitation services to individuals with an alcohol or drug related problem.

7038 Bryn Mawr Rehabilitation Hospital
414 Paoli Pike
Malvern, PA 19355-3311
610-251-5400
888-734-2241
888-734-2241
FAX: 610-647-3648
www.mainlinehealth.org

Donna M. Phillips, President
We are dedicated to serving individuals and their families whose lives can be enhanced through physical or cognitive rehabilitation. We continually strive for excellence by providing care and services which are valued by those we serve and by contributing to the community through education, research and prevention of disability.

7039 Daman Villa
Devereux Foundation
444 Devereux Drive
Victoria, TX 19085-2666
361-575-8271
800-345-1292
FAX: 361-575-6520
devereux.org

Robert Q. Kreider, President and CEO
Margaret McGill, SVP, Chief Operations Officer
Robert C. Dunne, SVP & Chief Financial Officer, Treasurer
Marilyn B. Benoit, M.D., SVP, Chief Clinical Officer, Chief Medical Officer
Offers residents a continuum of services ranging from minimal care and supervision to total physical and medical care.

7040 Devereux
444 Devereux Dr
Villanova, PA 19085-1932
610-520-3000
800-345-1292
FAX: 610-542-3100
e-mail: knash@devereux.org
www.devereux.org

Samuel G. Coppersmith, Esq., Chairman
Francis Genuardi, Vice Chairman & Chairman Emeritus
hristopher D Butler, Vice Chairman
Robert Q Kreider, President/CEO
Devereux is a leading nonprofit behavioral health organization that supports many of the most underserved and vulnerable members of our communities.

7041 Devereux Pennsylvania
230 Highland Avenue
Devon, PA 19333
610-788-6565
800-345-1292
FAX: 610-430-0567
www.devereux.org
Carol Oliver, M.S., State Director
Melanie Beidler, M.S., Executive Director, Children's Intellectual/Developmental D
Judy Lau, M.S., Executive Director, Adult Services
Mary Seeley LPN, Executive Director, Devereux Poconos
Devereux Pennsylvania has been an innovative leader in helping children and adults with intellectual, behavioral and emotional challenges accomplish their dreams by discovering their strengths and realizing personal fulfillment.

7042 Devereux's Kanner
444 Devereux Drive
Victoria, TX 19085-2666
361-575-8271
800-345-1292
FAX: 361-575-6520
devereux.org
Robert Q. Kreider, President and CEO
Margaret McGill, SVP, Chief Operations Officer
Robert C. Dunne, SVP & Chief Financial Officer, Treasurer
Marilyn B. Benoit, M.D., SVP, Chief Clinical Officer, Chief Medical Officer

7043 Fox Subacute Center
2644 Bristol Rd
Warrington, PA 18976-1404
800-782-2288
e-mail: WebAdmin@rehabcare.com
subacute.com
James Foulke, CEO
Vic Costenko, COO
Walter Dunsmore, CFO
Fox subacute recognizes the great need for alternative programs for today's medically compromised patients. Fox has developed Models of Care and offers subacute programs fore the management of ventilator-dependent patients. We recognize that the best road to recovery for these patients is an environment with special care in an alternative setting. We believe that setting should be outside the hospital, in facilities where the focus is on the management of individual patients.

7044 Fox Subacute at Clara Burke
251 Stenton Ave
Plymouth Meeting, PA 19462-1220
610-828-2272
800-424-7201
FAX: 610-828-7939
e-mail: admissions@foxsubacute.com
www.foxsubacute.com
Terri Herd, Director of Marketing
Amy Swartley, RN,, Director of Admissions
Kathy Palladino, Director of Human Resources
Erik I. Soiferman, DO, FACOI, Chief Medical Officer
Fox Subacute at Clara Burke in Plymouth Meeting, PA offers attentive, nurturing management of ventilator dependent, medically compromised patients in the PA, NJ, DE, Tri-State area. This sixty-bed facility, with its picturesque setting on 16 acres in historic Plymouth Meeting, is ideal for the specialized services and programs offered by Fox. With a team of highly motivated professionals, we offer the discharge alternative to prolonged lengths of stay in more costly acute care settings.

7045 Good Samaritan Health System
4th & Walnut Sts
P.O.Box 1281
Lebanon, PA 17042-1281
717-270-7500
www.gshleb.org
Robin Weiler, Manager
Frederick Davis, VP Clinical Services
Offers services for the totally blind, legally blind, visually impaired, mentally retarded blind and more with health, counseling, educational, recreational, rehabilitation, computer training and professional training services.

7046 Good Samaritan Hospital-Health System Center
Good Samaritan Hospital
4th & Walnut Sts
P.O.Box 1281
Lebanon, PA 17042-1281
717-270-7500
www.gshleb.org
June Nafziger-Eberl, Manager
Stuart Hartman, Medical Director
Comprehensive inpatient rehab unit for adults regarding general physical rehabilitation. Specific programs include orthopedic, neurological, stroke, amputee, etc.

7047 Kanner Center
Devereax Foundation
444 Devereux Drive
Victoria, TX 19085-2666
361-575-8271
800-345-1292
FAX: 361-575-6520
devereux.org
Robert Q. Kreider, President and CEO
Margaret McGill, SVP, Chief Operations Officer
Robert C. Dunne, SVP & Chief Financial Officer, Treasurer
Marilyn B. Benoit, M.D., SVP, Chief Clinical Officer, Chief Medical Officer
A private nonprofit nationwide network of treatment services for individuals of all ages with emotional and/or developmental disabilities.

7048 Pediatric Center at Plymouth Meeting Integrated Health Services
491 Allendale Rd
King of Prussia, PA 19406-1426
610-265-9290
800-220-7337
Fran Currick, Manager
Subacute programs such as intensive respiratory care, stressing ventilator dependent children, pre and post transplant care, total parenteral nutrition, IV therapy, intensive/behavioral oral feeding programs. Provides extensive discharge planning including teaching or review for all the above programs with an emphasis on development and accessing community resources.

7049 Penn State Milton S. Hershey Medical Center College Of Medicine
500 University Dr
Hershey, PA 17033-2360
717-531-8521
800-243-1455
FAX: 717-531-4558
www.pennstatehershey.org
Harold L Paz, CEO
Alan L. Brechbill, Executive Director
Wayne Zolko, Associate Vice President for Finance and Business
Andrew S. Resnick, Chief Quality Officer
a non-sectarian, not-for-profit community hospital whose purpose is to provide high quality acute, rehabilitative and preventive health services for the entire community, regardless of creed, race, nationality, or ability to pay.

7050 Pennsylvania Pain Rehabilitation Center
Ste 2
252 W Swamp Rd
Doylestown, PA 18901-2465
215-230-9707
FAX: 215-348-5106
Kenneth Lefkowitz, Manager
Post acute rehabilitation facility and programs.

7051 The Rehabilitation & Nursing Center at Greater Pittsburgh
890 Weatherwood Ln
Greensburg, PA 15601-5777
724-837-8076
FAX: 724-837-7456
www.healthbridgemanagement.com
Nancy Flenner, Administrator
Marsha Echard, Admissions Coordinator
Craig Stepien, Admissions Director

Subacute care, ventilator and pulmonary managment, comprehensive rehabilitation.

Rhode Island

7052 In-Sight
43 Jefferson Blvd
Warwick, RI 02888-6400
401-941-3322
FAX: 401-941-3356
e-mail: cbutler@in-sight.org
in-sight.org

Chris Butler, Executive Director
Lucille Gaboriault, Director of Community Resources
Paul Hopkins, Director of First Impressions
Richard Andrade, Director of Vision Rehabilitation

Offers services for the totally blind, legally blind, visually impaired, mentally retarded blind and more with health, counseling, educational, recreational, rehabilitation, computer training and professional training services.

7053 Vanderbilt Rehabilitation Center
Newport Hospital
167 Point Street
Providence, RI 02903
401-444-3500
www.lifespan.org

Timothy J. Babineau, President/CEO
Kenneth E. Arnold, SVP, General Counsel
Carole M. Cotter, SVP, Chief Information Officer
Cathy Duquette, EVP, Nursing Affairs

The Vanderbilt Rehabilitation Center at Newport Hospital has been providing comprehensive rehabilitation sercices for more than 40 years and is known throughout the region for its unique programs and high-quality, patient focused care.

South Carolina

7054 Association for the Blind
One Carriage Lane
Building A
Charleston, SC 29407
843-723-6915
FAX: 843-577-4312
www.abvisc.org

J. Douglas Hazelton, President
Capers A. Grimball, Vice President
Lea B. Kerrison, Secretary
Mary Morrison, Executive Director

Offers services for people who are blind, or are visually impaired with health, counseling, educational, recreational, rehabilitation, computer training and professional training services.

7055 Hitchcock Rehabilitation Center
690 Medical Park Dr
Aiken, SC 29801-6348
803-648-8344
800-207-6924
FAX: 803-648-1631
e-mail: mail@hitchcockhealthcare.org
www.hitchcockhealthcare.org

Karen Bowlen, Administrator
Dan Hillman, Case Manager
Carrie Morgan, Finance Director

Comprehensive outpatient rehabilitation for adults, children, geriatrics, pediatric therapy, special needs preschool, sports medicine, home health and hospice.

7056 The Mentor Network
3600 Forest Drive
Suite 100
Columbia, SC 29204-1891
803-799-9025
800-297-8043
FAX: 803-931-8959
thementornetwork.com

Edward Murphy, Executive Chairman
Bruce Nardella, President and CEO
Denis Holler, Chief Financial Officer
Jeffrey Cohen, Chief Information Officer

Mentor provides a full network of individually tailored services for people with development disabilities and their families. Individuals may be served in their homes, shared living home, or in a host home.

Tennessee

7057 Humana Hospital: Morristown RehabCare
726 McFarland St
Morristown, TN 37814-3989
423-522-6000
www.lakewayregionalhospital.com

James Perry, Program Director

Designed to help patients in their adjustment to a physically limiting condition by helping to maximize each patient's abilities so he or she can function as independently as possible.

7058 Opportunity East Rehabilitation Services for the Blind
758 W Morris Blvd
Morristown, TN 37813-2136
423-586-3922
800-278-6274
FAX: 423-586-1479
e-mail: bandit75@charter.net
volblind.org

Fred Overbay, CEO
Vic Mende, Director Rehabilitation Services

Offers services for the totally blind, legally blind, visually impaired, mentally retarded blind and more with health, counseling, educational, recreational, rehabilitation, computer training and professional training services.

7059 Patrick Rehab Wellness Center
Lincoln County Health System
106 Medical Center Blvd
Fayetteville, TN 37334-2684
931-433-0273
FAX: 931-433-0378
www.ichealthsystem.com

Gloria Meadows, Administrator
Jim Stewart, Principal

Provides rehabilitation services of physical, occupational, and speech therapy. Also, wellness memberships are available to the public.

7060 PharmaThera
1785 Nonconnah Blvd
Memphis, TN 38132-2104
901-348-8100
800-767-6714
FAX: 901-348-8270

7061 Siskin Hospital For Physical Rehabilitation
1 Siskin Plz
Chattanooga, TN 37403-1306
423-634-1200
e-mail: info@siskinrehab.org
siskinrehab.org

Bob Main, CEO
Robert P. Main, President

Dedicated exclusively to physical rehabilitation and offers specialized treatment programs in brain injury, amputation, stroke, spinal cord injury, orthopedics, and major multiple trauma. The hospital also provides treatment for neurological disorders and loss of muscle strength and controll following illness or surgery.

7062 **St. Mary's RehabCare Center**
900 E Oak Hill Ave
Knoxville, TN 37917-4556
865-545-7962
FAX: 865-545-8133

Debbie Keeton, Director
Beth Greco, Executive Director
Provides comprehensive rehabilitation services for patients experiencing CVA, head trauma, orthopedic conditions, spinal cord injury or neurological impairment.

Texas

7063 **Baylor Institute for Rehabilitation**
3500 Gaston Avenue
Dallas, TX 75246-2017
214-820-9300
800-4BA-YLOR
FAX: 214-841-2679
www.baylorhealth.com

Joel T. Allison, Chief Executive Officer
Gary Brock, President and Chief Operating Officer
LaVone Arthur, Vice President of Business Development
Wm. Stephen Boyd, Chief Legal Officer
A 92-bed specialty hospital offering comprehensive rehabilitation services for persons with spinal cord injury, traumatic brain injury, stroke, amputation, and other orthopedic and neurological disorders.

7064 **CORE Health Care**
E&J Health Care
400 Highway 290
Bldg B, Suite. 205,
Dripping Springs, TX 78620
512-894-0801
866-683-1007
FAX: 512-858-4627
e-mail: info@corehealth.com
www.corehealth.com

Eric Makowski, CEO
Kristi Jones, Marketing/Admissions Director
Erika Mountz, MBA, OTR/L, Director of Rehabilitation
Annie Freeman, MBA, PHR, Director of Huma Resources
Post acute and transitional rehabilitation, long-term care, community re-entry, for brain injury and complex psychiatric disorders.

7065 **Center for Neuro Skills**
1320 W Walnut Hill Ln
Irving, TX 75038-3007
972-580-8500
800-544-5448
FAX: 972-255-3162
e-mail: srobinson@neuroskills.com
neuroskills.com

John Schultz, Administrator
Mark J. Ashley, President
Centre for Neuro Skills (CNS) seeks to provide medical rehabilitation programs, lifecare programs, advocacy, and research for people with brain injury in order to achieve a maximum quality of life.

7066 **Dallas Services**
4242 Office Pkwy
Dallas, TX 75204-3629
214-828-9900
FAX: 214-828-9901
www.dallasservices.org

Thomas . Turnage, Ph.D, Executive Director
Clark Thomas, Ph.D., Chair
Melissa Malonson, Vice-Chair
Cynthia O'Brien Robinson, Secretary
Offers four programs:1) an early education for children(6weeks-6yrs)with and without special needs.2)low vision clinic-provides low cost eye examsand glasses to low-income families as well as assistance to individuals who vision problems which cannot be corrected with glasses/surgery.3)mesquite day school- an early head start program for infants and toddlers of low-income families.4)special needs advocacy and inclusion program that offers families of special need children guidance and education.

7067 **Devereux Texas Treatment Network Adult Community**
444 Devereux Drive
Victoria, TX 19085-2666
361-575-8271
800-345-1292
FAX: 361-575-6520
devereux.org

Robert Q. Kreider, President and CEO
Margaret McGill, SVP, Chief Operations Officer
Robert C. Dunne, SVP & Chief Financial Officer, Treasurer
Marilyn B. Benoit, M.D., SVP, Chief Clinical Officer, Chief Medical Officer
Provides a permanent home for individuals with chronic psychiatric and/or developmental disabilities who require long term or lifelong care, support or a transitional home for individuals who progress to a less structured setting. Located on a beautiful 400+ acre campus in sunny south Texas, the primary focus is to offer, in keeping with the philosophies of least restrictive alternatives and normalization, active treatment which will facilitate growth.

7068 **El Paso Lighthouse for the Blind**
200 Washington St
El Paso, TX 79905-3897
915-532-4495
FAX: 915-532-6338
www.lighthouse-elpaso.com

Craig Hays, President
Lea Cochran, Vice President
Lola Dawkins, Secretary
Rusty Hooten, Chief Financial Officer
Enables people of all ages to embody blindness and vision impairment through training, rehabilitation, employment opportunity, advocacy and research. Provides access to opportunities and quality of life so that the blind and visually impaired can reach their fullest potential for self-sufficiency and independence.

7069 **Harris Methodist Fort Worth/Mabee Rehabilitation Center**
612 E. Lamar Boulevard
Arlington, TX 76011-2122
877-847-9355
FAX: 817-882-2753
www.texashealth.org

Louise Baldwin, President
Peggyo Ehrlich, Rehab Manager
Karen Mallett, Executive Director
Douglas D. Hawthorne, Chief Executive Officer
A hospital based inpatient rehab program and outpatient day programs in chronic pain management, work hardening and brain injury transitional services.

7070 **HealthSouth Hospital Of Houston**
3660 Grandview Parkway
Suite 200
Birmingham, AL 35243
205-967-7116

e-mail: feedback@healthsouth.com
healthsouth.com

Jerome Lengel, Executive Officer
Dewitt Hilton, Owner
Offers an individualized approach to the process of rehabilitation for severely injured or disabled individuals. The process begins with a pre-admissions assessment of each referred patient. The Center combines state-of-the-art technology and equipment with multi-disciplinary therapy and education in a cheerful, secure environment.

7071 **Heights Hospital Rehab Unit**
1917 Ashland St
Houston, TX 77008-3994
713-861-6161
FAX: 713-802-8660
www.selectmedical.com

Theresa Davis, CEO
Robert A. Ortenzio, Executive Chairman and Co-Founder
Rocco A. Ortenzio, Vice Chairman and Co-Founder
David S. Chernow, President and Chief Executive Officer
This program is designed to assist patients with physical disabilities achieve their maximum functional abilities.

7072 **Hillcrest Baptist Medical Center**
100 Hillcrest Medical Blvd
Waco, TX 76712 254-202-2000
FAX: 254-202-5105
www.sw.org

Anne Hott Kimberly, Program Director
Ann Gammel, Nurse Manager
Debbie Meurer, Manager
Designed to assist patients in adjustment to a physically limiting condition, utilizing interdisciplinary strategies to maximize each patient's ability and capability.

7073 **Institute for Rehabilitation & Research**
1333 Moursund St
Houston, TX 77030-3405 713-799-5000
800-447-3422
FAX: 713-797-5289
tirr.memorialhermann.org

Carl Josehart, CEO
Jean Herzog, President
Gerard E. Francisco, M.D., Chief Medical Officer
Mary Ann Euliarte, CNO/COO
A national center for information, training, research, and technical assistance in independent living. The goal is to extend the body of knowledge in independent living and to improve the utilization of results of research programs and demonstration projects in this field. It has developed a variety of strategies for collecting, synthesizing, and disseminating information related to the field of independent living.

7074 **Integrated Health Services of Amarillo**
6141 Amarillo Blvd. West
Amarillo, TX 79106 806-356-0488
FAX: 806-356-8074
e-mail: cheryl.studer@medcenter.org
www.medcenter.org

Mary Bearden, Chairman
Jay L. Barrett, President
Marvin Franz, Executive Director & CEO
Provides acute, post acute, residential and outpatient health care services. IHS of Amarillo is a 153-bed facility with 120 beds licensed by The Texas Department of Health and Human Services, and is accredited by JCAHO. We serve urban and rural populations of over 500,000, drawing from a 5-state region.

7075 **Lighthouse of Houston**
3602 W Dallas St
Houston, TX 77019-1704 713-527-9561
FAX: 713-284-8451
e-mail: custserv@houstonlighthouse.org
houstonlighthouse.org

Gibson DuTerroil, President
Shelagh Moran, VP/COO
Chelean Zander, VP Community Programs
Serves the blind, visually impaired, deaf-blind and multihandicapped blind. Provides workshops, vocational training and placement, low vision clinic, orientation and mobility, housing, Braille, volunteer services, senior center, visual aid sales, counseling and support, diabetic education and day health activity services and day summer camp, Summer Transition for Youth.

7076 **Mainland Center Hospital RehabCare Unit**
6801 Emmett F Lowry Expy
Texas City, TX 77591-2500 409-938-5000
FAX: 409-938-5501
www.mainlandmedical.com

Michael Ehrat, CEO
The RehabCare program is designed and staffed to assist functionally impaired patients improve to their maximum potential. The opportunities for improvement and adjustments are provided in a pleasant, supportive inpatient environment by therapists from the occupational, physical, recreational and speech therapy disciplines.

7077 **North Texas Rehabilitation Center**
1005 Midwestern Pkwy
Wichita Falls, TX 76302-2211 940-322-0771
FAX: 940-766-4943
ntrehab.org

Mike Castles, President/ CEO
Provides outpatient rehabilitation services to maximize independence or promote development to children and adults with disabilities. Programs include: physical, occupational, speech therapy, closed head injury, infant/child development, support groups, aquatics and wellness program and a child achievement program.

7078 **South Texas Lighthouse for the Blind**
PO BOX 9697
Corpus Christi, TX 78469-3321 361-883-6553
888-255-8011
FAX: 361-883-1041
e-mail: Customer.service@stlb.net
www.stlb.net

Regis Barber, President
Nicky Ooi, Chief Operations Officer
Alana Manrow, Public Affairs Director
Their mission is to Employ, Educate and Empower their neighbors who are blind and visually impaired. They offer job opportunities in manufacturing, retail and administration, as well as orientation and mobility and adaptive technology training.

7079 **Texas Specialty Hospital at Dallas**
7955 Harry Hines Blvd
Dallas, TX 75235-3305 214-637-0000
FAX: 214-637-6512
e-mail: Mary.Alexander@fundltc.com
www.texasspecialtydallas.com

Mary Alexander, CEO
Cathy Campbell, Chief Executive Officer
66 beds offering active/acute rehabilitation, brain injury day treatment, cognitive rehabilitation, complex care, extended rehabilitation and short term evaluation.

7080 **Transitional Learning Center at Gavelston and Lubbock**
1528 Post Office St
Galveston, TX 77550 409-762-6661
FAX: 409-763-3930
www.tlcrehab.org

Brent Masel, MD, President and Medical Director
Gary Seale, Ph.D., VP Clinical Programs
Jim Lovelace, MBA, VP of Operations
Shelley Kessler, CPA, Chief Financial Officer
Specializes solely in post-acute brain injury. A nationally known pioneer in the field and a not for profit with a three fold mission: treatment, research and education. Offers 6 hours of therapy a day from licensed/certified staff, on site physician and nursing services and long-term living for brian injured adults at Tideway on Gavelston Island. Accredited by CARF.
1982

7081 **Treemont Nursing And Rehabilitation Center**
5550 Harvest Hill Rd
Dallas, TX 75230-1684 972-661-1862
FAX: 972-788-1543
e-mail: moreinfo@treemonthealthcare.com
treemonthealthcare.com

Bob Barker, Administrator
Postacute rehabilitation program.

7082 **West Texas Lighthouse for the Blind**
2001 Austin St
San Angelo, TX 76903-8796 325-653-4231
FAX: 325-657-9367
e-mail: customerservice@lighthousefortheblind.org
www.lighthousefortheblind.org

David Wells, Executive Director
Stephen Horton, Operations Manager
Fonda V. Galindo, Finance & Human Resources Manager
Vickie Sanders, Sales & Marketing Manager

Offers services for the totally blind, legally blind, visually impaired, mentally retarded blind and more with health, counseling, educational, recreational, rehabilitation, computer training and professional training services.

Utah

7083 Quincy Rehabilitation Institute of Holy Cross Hospital
1050 E South Temple
Salt Lake City, UT 84102-1507 801-350-8140
FAX: 801-350-4791

Dave Jenson, President
Postacute rehabilitation program.

7084 Wasatch Vision Clinic
849 E 400 S
Salt Lake City, UT 84102-2928 801-328-2020
FAX: 801-363-2201
e-mail: email@wasatchvision.com
eyeappointment.com

Craig Cutler, Owner
Camron Bateman OD, Doctor
Postacute rehabilitation program.

Vermont

7085 Rutland Mental Health Services
78 S Main St
Rutland, VT 05701-4594 802-775-2381
FAX: 802-775-4020
rmhsccn.org

Dan Quinn, President/ CEO
Scott Dikeman, Vice Chairman
Ron Holm, Secretary
Tom Pour, Treasurer
A private, non-profit comprehensive community mental health center. It provides services to individuals and families for mental health and substance abuse related problems and also to persons who are mentally retarded.

Virginia

7086 Bay Pine-Virginia Beach
680 South Fourth Street
Louisville, KY 40202 502-596-7300
TTY:800-545-0749
e-mail: web_administrator@kindred.com
kindredhealthcare.com

Paul J. Diaz, President/ CEO
Postacute rehabilitation program.

7087 Carilion Rehabilitation: New River Valley
2013 S Jefferson Street
Roanoke, VA 24014 540-981-7377
FAX: 540-981-8233
www.carilionclinic.org

Nancy Howell Agee, President/ CEO
James A. Hartley, Chair
Briggs W. Andrews, Corporate Secretary
G. Robert Vaughan, Jr., Treasurer, SVP
CARF-accredited pain management program, work hardening program and comprehensive outpatient therapy clinic, massage therapy, outpatient programs and more. Program emphasis is on interdisiplinary behavioral rehab based pain management and functional restoration in conjunction with medical treatment. Work hardening is a transdisciplinary work simulation program taylored to the individual. Comprehensive outpatient program is multi-disciplinary with emphasis on manual treatment.

7088 Faith Mission Home
3540 Mission Home Ln
Free Union, VA 22940-1505 434-985-2294
FAX: 434-985-7633
www.beachyam.org

Paul Beiler, Manager
Reuben Yoder, Director
A Christian residential center that serves 60 mentally retarded children, including individuals with Down Syndrome, Cerebral palsy and other similar conditions. Children may be admitted from the time they are ambulatory until they reach 15 years of age. He or she may stay as long as it is in the child's best interests. The training program stresses the following areas: self-care, social, academic, vocational, crafts, speech and physical development.

7089 ManorCare Health Services-Arlington
333 N. Summit St.
Toledo, OH 43604 800-366-1232
e-mail: CareLine@hcr-manorcare.com
hcr-manorcare.com

Marcia K Jarrell, Administrator
Ric Birch, Marketing Director
ManorCare-Arlington offers residents a full Continuum of Care in a caring environment. ManorCare's wide range of services includes subacute medical and rehabilitation programs for short term patients transitioning from hospital to home and Skilled Nursing Care.

7090 Pines Residential Treatment Center
825 Crawford Pkwy
Portsmouth, VA 23704-2301 757-393-0061
FAX: 757-393-1029

Lenard J Lexier, Medical Director
Judy Kemp, Admissions Director
A 310-bed residential treatment center in Portsmouth Virginia, providing a therapeutic environment for severely emotionally disturbed children and youth. Five unique programs meet behavioral, educational and emotional needs of males and females, five to twenty-two years of age. Multi-disciplinary teams devise individual service plans to enhance strengths and reverse self-defeating behavior. A highly effective positive reinforcement program with a proven track record.

7091 Resurrection Children's Center
2280 N Beauregard St
Alexandria, VA 22311-2200 703-998-0888
FAX: 703-820-2912
e-mail: office@welcometoresurrection.org
www.welcometoresurrection.org

Jane McCabe, Parish Administrator
Deena Jaworski, Director of Music
Offers children ages 2-5 with varying disabilities academic education, parent education, opportunities including classes, workshops, support groups and individual counseling.

7092 Roanoke Memorial Hospital
Carilion Health System
2013 S Jefferson Street
Roanoke, VA 24014 540-981-7377
FAX: 540-981-8233
www.carilionclinic.org

Nancy Howell Agee, President/ CEO
James A. Hartley, Chair
Briggs W. Andrews, Corporate Secretary
G. Robert Vaughan, Jr., Treasurer, SVP
Carilion Health System exists to improve the health of the communities it serves. The vision is to assure accessible, affordable, high quality healthcare that meets the needs of the community. Motivate and educate individuals to improve their health. Champion community initiatives to reduce health risk

7093 Southside Virginia Training Center
P.O.Box 4030
Petersburg, VA 23803-30 804-524-7000
FAX: 804-524-7228
www.svtc.dbhds.virginia.gov
Bob Kaufman, Director, Administrative Service

Offers residential, vocational, occupational, physical, and speech therapies.

7094 Woodrow Wilson Rehabilitation Center
P.O.Box 1500
Fishersville, VA 22939-1500 540-332-7000
800-345-9972
FAX: 540-332-7132
e-mail: colemawl@wwrc.state.va.lls
www.wwrc.net

Rick Sizemore, Executive Director
Amy Blalock, Admissions and Marketing Director
Comprehensive residential rehabilitation center offering complete medical and vocational rehabilitation services including: vocation evaluation, vocational training, transition from school to work, occupational therapy, physical therapy, speech, language and audiology, assistive technology, rehabilitation engineering, counseling/case management, behavioral health services, nursing and physician services, etc.

Washington

7095 Arden Rehabilitation And Healthcare Center
680 South Fourth Street
Louisville, KY 40202 502-596-7300
TTY:800-545-0749
e-mail: web_administrator@kindred.com
kindredhealthcare.com

Paul J. Diaz, President/ CEO
Arden can accomodate 90 residents- post-acute/rehabilitation patients as well as long term residents. Medicare certified, the center also takes most managed healthcare insurance plans, as well as VA, respite and hospice patients.

7096 Bellingham Care Center
680 South Fourth Street
Louisville, KY 40202 502-596-7300
TTY:800-545-0749
e-mail: web_administrator@kindred.com
kindredhealthcare.com

Paul J. Diaz, President/ CEO
Postacute rehabilitation program.

7097 Division of Vocational Rehabilitation Department of Social and Health Services
P.O.Box 45130
Olympia, WA 98504-5130 360-704-3560
800-737-0617
FAX: 360-570-6941
e-mail: krulik@dshs.wa.gov
www1.dshs.wa.gov/dvr

Patrick Raines, Manager
Lynnea Ruttledge, Manager
Information on computers, supported employment, marketing rehabilitation facilities and transition.

7098 First Hill Care Center
1334 Terry Ave
Seattle, WA 98101 206-682-2661
FAX: 206-624-0188
www.khseattlefirsthill.com

7099 Harborview Medical Center, Low Vision Aid Clinic
Harborview Medical Center
325 9th Ave
Seattle, WA 98104-2499 206-744-3300
TTY:206-744-3246
e-mail: comment@u.washington.edu
www.uwmedicine.org

Eileen Whalen, Executive director
J. Richard Goss, M.D.,, Medical director
Darcy Jaffe, Chief nursing officer and senior associate for patient care
Elise Chayet, Associate administrator, clinical support services and plan
Harborview Medical Center is the only designated Level 1 adult and pediatric trauma and burn center in the state of Washington and serves as the regional trauma and burn referral center for Alaska, Montana and Idaho. UW Medicine physicians and staff based at Harborview provide highly specialized services for vascular, orthopedics, neurosciences, ophthalmology, behavioral health, HIV/AIDS and complex critical care.

7100 Integrated Health Services of Seattle
820 NW 95th St
Seattle, WA 98117-2207 206-783-7649
FAX: 206-781-1448

Jerry Harvey, Administrator
Marlette Basada, Director Nursing
Flavia Lagrange, Director Admissions
Postacute rehabilitation program. IHS provides 24 hour subacute and long-term care. We can handle vent/trach/hemo andritoneal dialysis and provide a full scope of rehabilitation services.

7101 Lakeside Milam Recovery Centers (LMRC)
3315 S. 23rd Street
Ste 102
Tacoma, WA 98405 253-272-2242
800-231-4303
FAX: 253-272-0171
e-mail: help@lakesidemilam.com
www.lakesidemilam.com

Michael Kinder, Administrator
LMRC was established in 1983 with a single mission, to help victims and families recover from the pain of drug/alcohol addiction. Enlightned by the work of Dr. James Milam in the 1960's and 70's, the founders of LMRC created a treatment system based on a bedrock set of principals.

7102 Lakewood Health Care Center
11411 Bridgeport Way SW
Lakewood, WA 98499-3047 253-581-9002
800-359-7412
FAX: 253-581-7016
www.lakewoodhc.com

Gwynn Rucker, Executive Director
Patty Wood, Administrator
Linda Doll, Social Services
Dr. Mian, Medical Director
Accomodates 80 residents. We offer 24 hour skilled nursing services, long-term care and rehab services which include Physical, Occupational and Speech Therapy.

7103 Manor Care Health Services-Tacoma
5601 S Orchard St
Tacoma, WA 98409-1371 253-474-8421
FAX: 253-471-8857
www.hcr-manorcare.com

Tina Irwin, Administrator
124-bed skilled nursing and rehabilitation center provides services for those seeking long term Skilled Nursing Care, short term subacute care, hospice services, Alzheimer's and respite care. Our Acadia Wing, a specialized Alzheimer's care unit, provides specialized programming and trained staff that truly makes us the leader in Alzheimers Services.

7104 ManorCare Health Services-Lynnwood
3701 188th St SW
Lynnwood, WA 98037-7626 425-775-9222
FAX: 425-712-3685
www.hcr-manorcare.com

Liza Loyet, Administrator
Our in-house therapists provide physical, occupational and speech therapies in our state-of-the-art therapy gym. Our team is goal oriented and focuses on producing positive outcomes for those recovering from illness, injury or surgery.

7105 ManorCare Health Services-Spokane
6025 N Assembly St
Spokane, WA 99205-7674 509-326-8282
FAX: 509-326-4790
www.hcrmanorcare.com

Cheri Kubu, Administrator
Sandra Hayes, Administrator
Provides skilled nursing and respite stays for those needing a break from care giving. We specialize in Rehabilitation Services provided by our in-house occupational, physical and speech therapists.

7106 Northwest Continuum Care Center
Kindred Health Care
128 Old Beacon Hill Dr
Longview, WA 98632-5859 360-423-4060
FAX: 360-636-0958
www.nwcontinuum.com

Steve M. Ross, Executive Director
Tami Wilson, Director of Nursing
Mary R., Activities Assistant
Kristen W., Health and Rehabilitation Center
Accomodates 69 residents. Employs the Angel Care Program designed to address any special needs that may arise during a resident's stay in our facility. The program focuses extra attention on residents and, in some cases, family members. The goal is to meet the special needs of the people we provide care to every day.

7107 Park Manor Convalescent Center
1710 Plaza Way
Walla Walla, WA 99362-4362 509-529-4218
FAX: 509-522-1729
e-mail: egines@ensigngroup.net
www.parkmanorcare.com

Jed Gines, Administrator
Krista Maiuri, Directr Of Nursing
Sonya Taylor, Director of Rehabilitation
Mike Henckel, Admissions & Marketing Director
Residents of Park Manor enjoy a range of activities, developed to meet their needs, inculding excercise programs, social and recreational activities, arts and crafts, shopping trips and other excursions. We also offer religious services.

7108 Queen Anne Health Care
Queen Anne Health Care
2717 Dexter Ave N
Seattle, WA 98109-1914 206-284-7012
FAX: 206-283-3936
www.queenannehealthcare.com

Heather Eacker, Executive Director
Mary R., Activities Assistant
Kristen W., Health and Rehabilitation Center
Becky D., Activity Director
Our goal is to provide quality, compassionate care. Our cozy building accomodates 120 residents. We offer semi private rooms with space to add items from home for a special personalized touch

7109 Rainier Vista Care Center
920 12th Ave SE
Puyallup, WA 98372-4920 253-841-3422
FAX: 253-848-3937
www.rainiervistacc.com

Linda Larson, Administrator
Nancy L. Erckenbrack, Executive Director
Kristen W., Health and Rehabilitation Center
Becky D., Activity Director
Accomodates 120 residents. We are certified for Medicare and Medicaid and we offer a continuum of healthcare services from short-term or outpatient rehabilitation to long-term care. We offer semi-private and private rooms as well as rehabilitation and hospice suites. Rainier Vista Care Center is a recipient of the American Health Care Association Quality Award.

7110 Rehabilitation Enterprises of Washington
430 E Lauridsen Blvd
Port Angeles, WA 98362-7978 360-452-9789
FAX: 360-452-9700

Brett White, President
REW is the professional trade association representing community rehabilitation programs before government and other publics. These organizations provide a wide array of employment and training services for people with disabilities. The goal is to assist member organizations to provide the highest quality rehabilitative and employment services to their customers.

7111 Seattle Medical and Rehabilitation Center
Evergreen Healthcare
12040 NE 128th St
Kirkland, WA 98034-3013 425-899-3000
877-601-2271
TTY:425-899-2007
e-mail: comment@evergreenhealthcare.org
evergreenhealthcare.org

Al DeYoung, Chair
Robert H. Malte, Chief Executive Officer
Neil Johnson, RN, MSA, Senior Vice President & Chief Operating Officer
Nancee Hofmeister, Vice President, Chief Nursing Officer
103 beds offering subacute rehabilitation, complex care, subacute treatment and short-term evaluation. Pulmonary unit offering long and short term care for ventilator dependent patients.

7112 Slingerland Institute for Literacy
Educators Publishing Service
12729 Northup Way
Suite 1
Bellevue, WA 98005 425-453-1190
FAX: 425-635-7762
e-mail: mail@slingerland.org
www.slingerland.org

Bonnie Meyer, Executive Director
Elyce Newton, Program Support
A nonprofit public corporation founded in 1977 to carry on the work of Beth H. Slingerland in providing classroom teachers with the techniques, knowledge and understanding necessary for identifying and teaching children with Specific Language Disability. The main objective is to educate teachers in successful methods of identifying, diagnosing and instructing children and adults with SLD and to promote literacy through reading, writing and oral expression.

7113 Timberland Opportunities Association
400 W Curtis St
Aberdeen, WA 98520-7698 360-533-5823
FAX: 360-533-5848
e-mail: jimeddy@techline.com
www.users.olynet.com/timberlandopp

Jim Eddy, Executive Director
Provides training and employment for disabled people.

7114 Vancouver Health and Rehabilitation Center
400 E 33rd St
Vancouver, WA 98663-2238 360-696-2561
FAX: 360-696-9275
www.vancouverhealthcare.com

Jody Wigen, Human Resources
Joe Joy, Executive Director
Kristen W., Health and Rehabilitation Center
Becky D., Activity Director
Postacute rehabilitation program.

Wisconsin

7115 **Colonial Manor Medical And Rehabilitation Center**
1010 E Wausau Ave
Wausau, WI 54403-3101 715-842-2028
FAX: 715-848-0510
www.colonialmanormrc.com

Ericca Ylitalo, Administrator
Shelley Solberg, Executive Director
Colonial Manor Medical and Rehabilitation Center is part of the Kindred Community and is located in Wausau, Wisconsin. The corporate headquarters are based in Louisville Kentucky. Our facility accomodates 150 residents.

7116 **Waushers Industries**
210 E Chicago Rd
Wautoma, WI 54982-6932 920-787-4696
FAX: 920-787-4698

Richard King, Human Resources
Provides various programming for individuals with disabilities in waushara county.

7117 **Woodstock Health and Rehabilitation Center**
3415 Sheridan Rd
Kenosha, WI 53140-1924 262-657-6175
FAX: 262-657-5756
www.woodstockhealth.com

Debra Lamb, Administrator
Darlene Einerson, Executive Director
Kristen W., Health and Rehabilitation Center
Becky D., Activity Director
Offers a full range of medical services to meet the individual needs of our residents, including short term rehabilitative services and long-tern skilled care.

Rehabilitation Facilities, Sub-Acute

Alabama

7118 **Rehabilitation & Healthcare Center Of Birmingham**
2728 10th Ave S
Birmingham, AL 35205-1202
205-933-7010
FAX: 205-933-8720
Jimmie Thompson, Administrator
Rehabilitation and Healthcare Center of Birmingham is conveniently located on Birmingham's beautiful and historic Southside. We accomodate 114 residents and we are Medicare and Medicaid certified. Saint Vincent's Hospital, University of Alabama in Birmingham Hospital, and Baptist Medical Center Montclair are either within walking distance or just minutes away. We have caring professionals who strive to meet the needs of our residents.

Alaska

7119 **Fairbanks Memorial Hospital/Denali Center**
1650 Cowles St
Fairbanks, AK 99701-5998
907-452-8181
FAX: 907-458-5324
www.bannerhealth.com/locations/alaska
Mike Powers, CEO
Offers the following rehabilitation services: Physical Therapy, Occupational Therapy, Speech Therapy, Sub-Acute Rehab.

Arizona

7120 **Desert Life Rehabilitation & Care Center**
Kindred Healthcare
1919 W Medical St
Tucson, AZ 85704-1133
520-297-8311
FAX: 520-544-0930
www.desertlifercc.com
Amad Nazifi, Executive Director
Jane Olmstead, Director of Nursing
Accomodates 240 residents. We provide skilled and intermediate nursing with occupational, physical, speech and respiratory therapy services. We offer special programs including an Alzheimer's Unit and a Young Adult Program, and are located in beautiful Southern Arizona where there is plenty of sunshine, mountains and desert views. Desert Life is a 2005 recipient of the American Health Care Association Quality Award.

7121 **Hacienda Rehabilitation and Care Center**
660 S Coronado Dr
Sierra Vista, AZ 85635-3386
520-459-4900
FAX: 520-458-4082
www.haciendarcc.com
Monica Vandivort, Medical Director
Kristen W., Health and Rehabilitation Center Executive Director
Becky D., Activity Director
Mary R., Activities Assistant
Accomodates 100 residents. We are located in Sierra Vista, near Kartchner Caverns, Fort Huachuca, Coronado National Forest and historic Tombstone. Serving the medical needs of the community since 1983, we strive to provide care with quality, compassion and integrity.

7122 **Kachina Point Health Care & Rehabilitation Center**
505 Jacks Canyon Rd
Sedona, AZ 86351-7856
928-284-1000
FAX: 928-284-0626
www.kindredkachinapoint.com
Michael Amadei, Medical Director
Accomodates 120 residents. We have met the healthcare needs of the community since 1984. Kachina Point is a 2004 recipient of the American Health Care Association's Quality Award.

7123 **Mayo Clinic Scottsdale**
13400 E Shea Blvd
Scottsdale, AZ 85259-5499
480-301-8000
800-446-2279
FAX: 480-301-9310
www.mayoclinic.org/arizona
Neena S. Abraham, Gastroenterology/ Hepatology
Roberta H. Adams, Hematology/Oncology
Charles H. Adler, Parkinson's Disease and Movement Disorders Center
Neera Agarwal, Hospital Internal Medicine
Mayo clinic is a not-for-profit medical practice dedicated to the diagnosis and treatment of virtually every type of complex illness. Mayo clinic staff members work together to meet your needs. You will see as many doctors, specialists, and other health care professionals as needed to provide comprehensive diagnosis, understandable answers and effective treatment.

7124 **Sonoran Rehabilitation and Care Center**
Kindred
4202 N 20th Ave
Phoenix, AZ 85015-5101
602-264-3824
FAX: 602-279-6234
Jeffrey Barrett, Executive Director
Offers the following rehabilitation services: Respiratory Therapy, Physical Therapy, Speech Therapy, Occupational Therapy, Restorative Therapy, Sub-Acute Rehabilitation, Wound Care.

7125 **Valley Health Care and Rehabilitation Center**
Kindred Health Care Center
5545 E Lee St
Tucson, AZ 85712-4205
520-296-2306
FAX: 520-296-4072
www.valleyhcr.com
Dale Pelton, Executive Director
Sandra Lewis, Administrator
Offers the following rehabilitation services: Physical Therapy, Occupational Therapy, Speech Therapy, Sub-Acute Rehab.

California

7126 **Alamitos-Belmont Rehab Hospital**
3901 E 4th St
Long Beach, CA 90814-1699
562-434-8421
FAX: 562-433-6732
www.alamitosbelmont.com
John L. Sorensen, Chairman of the Board of Directors.
Jonathan Sloey, Administrator
Offers the following rehabilitation services: Speech Therapy, Occupational Therapy, Physical Therapy, Sub-Acute Rehab.

7127 **Bay View Nursing and Rehabilitation Center**
Kindred Health Care
516 Willow St
Alameda, CA 94501-6132
510-521-5600
FAX: 510-865-9035
www.kindredhealthcare.com
Richard S Espinoza, Administrator
Say Silva, Assistant Executive Director
Accomodates 180 residents. Bay View is a 2004 recipient of the American Health Care Association's Quality Award. We provide short-term rehabilitative care, traditional long-term skilled care and Alzheimer's/dementia special care. Our combination of clinical skill and comprehensive rehabilitation services enables us to care for a variety of complex medical conditions.

7128 **Foothill Nursing and Rehab Center**
401 W Ada Ave
Glendora, CA 91741-4241
626-335-9810
FAX: 626-963-0720
www.foothillnursing.com
Arnie Shafer, Executive Director
Marianne Schultz, Administrator
Offers the following rehabilitation services: Physical Therapy, Occupational Therapy, Speech Therapy, In and Out Patient Rehab.

7129 Long Beach Memorial Medical Center Memorial Rehabilitation Hospital
2801 Atlantic Ave
Ground Floor
Long Beach, CA 90806-1701 562-933-9001
FAX: 562-933-9019
www.memorialcare.org/long_beach
Barry Arbuckle, President/CEO
The goal of the MemorialCare Rehabilitation Institute is to help persons with disabilities regain independence and rebuild their lives in an environment where loved ones are involved in the rehabilitation process. We are dedicated to the pursuit of our mission, vision and values.

7130 Mercy Medical Center Mt. Shasta
914 Pine St
Mount Shasta, CA 96067-2143 530-926-6111
FAX: 530-926-0517
www.mercymtshasta.org
Greg Lippert, Senior Director of Support and Information Services
Scott Foster, Director of Hospital Finance
Sister Anne Chester, Director of Mission Integration
Joyce Zwanziger, Director Marketing, Community Relations & Volunteer Services
Mercy Medical Center is committed to furthering the healing ministry of Jesus, and to provide high-quality, affordable healthcare to the communities we serve.

7131 Northridge Hospital Medical Center
18300 Roscoe Blvd
Northridge, CA 91328-4167 818-885-8500
www.northridgehospital.org
Michael Wall, CEO
Offers the following rehabilitation services: Physical Therapy, Occupational Therapy, Speech Therapy, Sub-Acute Rehab. As a member of the Catholic Heathcare West Northridge Hospital Medical Center is committed to serving the health needs of our communities with particular attention to the needs of the poor, the disadvantaged and vulnerable, and the comfort of the suffering and dying.

7132 Riverside Community Hospital
4445 Magnolia Ave
Riverside, CA 92501 951-788-3000
FAX: 630-792-5636
e-mail: complaint@jointcommission.org
www.riversidecommunityhospital.com
Jaime Wesolowski, President/CEO
Patrick Brilliant, CEO
At Riverside Community Hospital, we are able to provide the healthcare services that you and your family will need through the many stages of your life. Services like Emergency/Trauma, Labor and Delivery, Cardiac Care, Orthopedics and Transplant are among our many Centers of Excellence.

7133 Saint Jude Medical Center
101 E Valencia Mesa Dr
Fullerton, CA 92835-3809 714-871-3280
800-870-7537
FAX: 714-992-3029
www.stjudemedicalcenter.org
April De Cou, Wellness Educator
Jane Wang, Wellness Programs Supervisor
Offers the following rehabilitation services: Out-patient Rehab, Sub-Acute Rehab, Occupational Therapy, Physical Therapy, Speech and Audiology Therapy, Pain Management Program.

7134 South Coast Medical Center
12 Mason
Suite A
Irvine, CA 92618-2733 714-669-4446
FAX: 714-669-4448
e-mail: info@southcoastmedcenter.com
www.mission4health.com
Leigh Erin Connealy, Manager
Bruce Christian, President
Offers the following services: physical therapy, occupational therapy, speech therapy, cardica rehabilitation, incontinence program, sub-acute rehabilitation.

7135 Valley Garden Health Care and Rehabilitation Center
1517 Knickerbocker Dr
Stockton, CA 95210-3119 209-957-4539
FAX: 209-957-5831
www.valleygardenshealth.com
Dr. Alexande Chan, Medical Director
Accomodates 120 residents. Our center provides short-term nursing and rehabilitative care as well as traditional long-term skilled care. Our combination of clinical skill and comprehensive rehabilitation services enables us to care for a variety of complex medical conditions. Rehabilitative therapies are provided as needed by physical, occupational and speech therapists.

Colorado

7136 Boulder Community Hospital Mapleton Center
1100 Balsam
PO Box 9019
Boulder, CO 80301-9019 303-440-2273
e-mail: info@bch.org
www.bch.org
Lou DellaCava, Chairman
Ric Porreca, Vice Chairman
Jean Dubofsky, Secretary
R. David Hoover, Treasurer
159-bed acute care hospital and 24-hour emergency department.

7137 Fairacres Manor
1700 18th Ave
Greeley, CO 80631-5152 970-353-3370
FAX: 970-353-9347
www.fairacresmanor.com
Kathy Gardner, Admissions/Marketing Director
Marla Trujillo, Director of Nursing
Ben Gonzales, Admissions/Marketing Assistant Director
Kathleen Mekelburg, Administrator
Offers the following rehabilitation services: Physical Therapy, Occupational Therapy, Speech Therapy, Restorative Therapy, Skilled Nursing, and Sub-Acute Rehabilitation.

7138 Rowan Community
4601 E Asbury Cir
Denver, CO 80222-4722 303-757-1228
FAX: 303-759-3390
e-mail: tgleisner@pinonmgt.com
pinonmgt.com
Tammy Gleisner, Director/Admissions/Marketing Director
Jeff Jerebker, President/CEO
Bruce Odenthal, VP Operations
John D. Brammeier, CPA, FHFMA,, Chief Financial Officer
Rowan is a 70-bed community, small enough to support personal relationships between residents and caregivers. Our residents vary in age, reflecting the diversity of a much larger community. Rowan's focus is on a psycho-social model of care with a dynamic activities and social service program. Our staff is specially trained in behavior management and many are certified Eden AlternativeT associates and certifid Elder Care Specialists.

Connecticut

7139 Hamilton Rehabilitation and Healthcare Center
89 Viets St
New London, CT 6320-3355 860-447-1471
FAX: 860-439-0107
Steve Roizen, Executive Director
Offers the following rehabilitation services: Sub-Acute, Occupational Therapy, Speech Therapy, Physical Therapy.

7140 **Hospital For Special Care (HSC)**
2150 Corbin Ave
New Britain, CT 06053-2298 860-223-2761
FAX: 860-827-4849
e-mail: info@hfsc.org
www.hfsc.org

John J. Votto, President/CEO
Paul J. Scalise, M.D., F.C.C.P, Senior Vice President
Thomas J. Soltis, M.D., M.P.H., Chief of Geriatrics
HSC is a private, not-for-profit 200-bed rehabilitation long-term acute and chronic care hospital, widely-known and respected for its expertise in physical rehabilitation, respiratory care, and medically-complex pediatrics. Special programs for spinal cord injuries, pulmonary rehabilitation, acquired brain injuries, stroke, ventilator management and geriatrics, make HSC an important regional resource for patients with special healthcare needs.

7141 **Masonic Healthcare Center**
MasoniCare Corporation
22 Masonic Ave
PO Box 70
Wallingford, CT 06492-3048 203-679-5900
877-424-3537
FAX: 203-679-6459
e-mail: info@masonicare.org
www.masonicare.org

Stephen B. McPherson, President
Arthur Santilli, President
The states leading provider of healthcare and retirement living communities for seniors. We are not-for-profit and have more then 100 years of experience behind us. We're recognized for the quality, compassionate care and steadfast support we provide to our residents and patients.

7142 **Stamford Hospital**
30 Shelburne Rd
Stamford, CT 06904-3628 203-276-1000
FAX: 203-325-7905
e-mail: info@stamhealth.org
www.stamfordhospital.org

Brian Grissler, President/CEO
Kathleen Silard, EVP/Chief Operating Officer
Kevin Gage, Senior Vice President, Finance/Chief Financial Officer
Sharon Kiely, MD, Senior Vice President, Medical Affairs/Chief Medical Officer
A not-for-profit, community teaching hospital that has been serving Stamford and surrounding communities for more then 100 years. We have 305 inpatient beds in medicine, surgery, obstetrics/gynecology, psychiatry, and medical and surgical critical care units and maintain an educational partnership with Columbia University College of Physicians and Surgeons for its teaching program in the internal medicine, family practice, obstetrics/gynecology and surgery

7143 **Windsor Rehabilitation and Healthcare Center**
581 Poquonock Ave
Windsor, CT 06095-2202 860-688-7211
FAX: 860-688-6715
www.windsorrehab.com

Jeffrey Robbins, Medical Director
Accomodates 116 residents. We offer private and semi-private rooms with access to private telephones and cable television. Our goal is to be a comprehensive, leading care center viewed by our community as an excellent resource for patients, families, and professionals.

Delaware

7144 **Arbors at New Castle**
32 Buena Vista Dr
New Castle, DE 19720-4660 302-328-2580
FAX: 302-326-4132
e-mail: newcastle@extendicare.com
www.extendicareus.com/newcastle

Annette Moore, Administrator
A subacute and rehabilitation center offering skilled medical services, infusion therapies, cardiac recovery services, renal disease services, cancer services and digestive disease services. Skilled rehabilitation services include physical therapy, occupational therapy and speech therapy. Also provides case management and discharge planning, general nursing and restorative care and respite care.

Florida

7145 **Avon Oaks Skilled Care Nursing Facility**
37800 French Creek Rd
Avon, OH 44011-1763 440-934-5204
800-589-5204
e-mail: jreidy@avonoaks.net
www.avonoaks.net

Natalie McIntyre, Human Resources Director
Stephanie Auvil, RN, BC, Director of Nursing
Joan Reidy, Administrator
Richard J. Reidy, Technologies & Information Manager
Oaks at Avon provides a full range of skilled nursing services including infusion therapy, enteral therapy, wound care, tracheotomy care, and portable diagnostics.

7146 **Boca Raton Rehabilitation Center**
755 Meadows Rd
Boca Raton, FL 33486-2384 561-391-5200
FAX: 561-391-0685

Stanley Mucinic, Administrator
Tracey Dougherty, Administrator
Offers the following rehabilitation services: Occupational Therapy, Speech Therapy, Physical Therapy, Sub-Acute Rehabilitation

7147 **Cape Coral Hospital**
636 Del Prado Blvd
Cape Coral, FL 33990 239-424-2000
FAX: 239-574-1935
www.leememorial.org

Richard Akin, Chairman
Sanford Cohen, MD, Vice Chairman
Marilyn Stout, Treasurer
Diane Champion, Secretary
A 291-bed acute care facility, Cape Coral Hospital features all private rooms. The hospital currently is undergoing a complete renovation, expansion and modernization of the Weigner-Taeni Center for Emergency Services, which will make the emergency department the largest in Lee County.

7148 **Evergreen Woods Health and Rehabilitation Center**
7045 Evergreen Woods Trl
Spring Hill, FL 34608-1306 352-596-8371
FAX: 352-596-8032

Janet Hanciles, Administrator
Offers the following rehabilitation services: Sub-Acute rehabilitation, Occupational therapy, Speech pathology therapy, Physical therapy.

7149 **Healthcare and Rehabilitation Center of Sanford**
950 Mellonville Avenue
Sanford, FL 32771-2237 407-322-8566
FAX: 407-322-0121
www.healthcareandrehabofsanford.com

Dr. S. Joshi, Medical Director
Kate Hilgar, Administrator
Vicky Smith, Director Admissions
We provide post-acute services, rehabilitative services, skilled nursing, short and long term care through Physical, Occupational, and Speech Therapists; Registered and Licensed Practical Nurses; and Certified Nursing Assistants. This is complemented by Social Services, Activities, Nutritional Services, Housekeeping and Laundry Services. With over 224 years of combined experience, our staff of professionals is here to meet the needs of each and every patient and resident.

7150 **Highland Pines Rehabilitation Center**
1111 S Highland Ave
Clearwater, FL 33756-4432 727-446-0581
FAX: 727-442-9425
Paula Anthony, Administrator
Offers the following rehabilitation services: Sub-Acute rehabilitation, Occupational Therapy, Speech Therapy, Physical Therapy.

7151 **Jupiter Medical Center-Pavilion**
1210 S Old Dixie Hwy
Jupiter, FL 33458-7205 561-747-2234
FAX: 561-744-4467
e-mail: JCouris@jupitermed.com
www.jupitermed.com
John D. Couris, President/Chief Executive Officer
Dale Hocking, Vice President, Finance/Chief Financial Officer
Mike Fehr, Vice President, Information Services/Chief Information Offic
Steven Seeley, Vice President, Chief Operating Officer/Chief Nursing Office
Offers the following rehabilitation services: Sub-Acute Rehabilitation, Occupational Therapy, Speech Therapy, Physical Therapy.

7152 **North Broward Medical Center**
201 E Sample Rd
Deerfield Beach, FL 33064-4441 954-941-8300
FAX: 954-941-4233
www.browardhealth.org
Pauline Grant, CEO
Douglas Ford, Chief of Staff
Offers the following rehabilitation services: Sub-Acute rehabilitation, Physical Therapy, Occupational Therapy, Speech Therapy, Respiratory Therapy.

7153 **Pompano Rehabilitation and Nursing Center**
Senior Health Care Management
51 W Sample Rd
Pompano Beach, FL 33064-3542 954-942-5530
FAX: 954-942-0941
Jeff Nusbusn, Administrator
Offers the following rehabilitation services: Sub-Acute Rehabilitation, Physical Therapy, Occupational Therapy, Speech Therapy

7154 **Rehabilitation Center of Palm Beach**
300 Royal Palm Way
Palm Beach, FL 33480-4385 561-655-7266
FAX: 561-655-3269
e-mail: info@rcca.org
www.rcca.org
Ellen O'Bannon, Manager
Pamela Henderson, Executive Director
Our mission is to improve the physical function, communication & independence of people with disabilities.

7155 **Rehabilitation and Healthcare Center of Tampa**
4411 N Habana Ave
Tampa, FL 33614-7211 813-872-2771
FAX: 813-871-2831
www.rehabilitationandhealthcarecenteroftampa.
Dr. Gustavo Barrazuetta, Medical Director
We provide post-acute services, rehabilitative services, skilled nursing, short and long term care through Physical, Occupational, and Speech Therapists; Registered and Licensed Practical Nurses; and Certified Nursing Assistants. This is complemented by Social Services, Activities, Nutritional Services, Housekeeping and Laundry Services. With over 60 years of combined experience, our staff of professionals is here to meet the needs of each and every patient and resident.

7156 **Shands Rehab Hospital**
4101 NW 89th Blvd
Gainesville, FL 32606-3813 352-265-8938
FAX: 352-265-5420
www.ufhealth.org/shands-rehab-hospital
Tim Goldfarb,M.S., Chief Executive Officer
David S. Guzick, M.D., Ph.D., Senior Vice President
Ed . Jimenez, M.B.A, Senior Vice President/Chief Operating Officer
James Roberts, J.D., Senior Vice President/General Counsel
UF Health Shands Rehab Hospital is a 40-bed acute rehab hospital for patients who have suffered strokes, traumatic brain and spinal cord injuries, amputations, burns or major joint replacements.

7157 **St. Anthony's Hospital**
1200 7th Ave N
St Petersburg, FL 33705-1388 727-825-1100
www.stanthonys.com
William Ulbricht, President
Ron Colaguori, VP Operations
James McClintic, M.D., Vice President, Medical Affairs
Sr. Mary McNally, OSF, Vice President, Mission
We offer outstanding diagnostic and treatment options of all types of cancer. Our Susan Sheppard McGillicuddy Breast Center is unmatched in the community in diagnostic services and helping patients navigate their treatment options should they find a cancer diagnosis.

7158 **Winkler Court**
3250 Winkler Avenue Ext
Fort Myers, FL 33916-9414 239-939-4993
FAX: 239-939-1743
www.winklercourt.com
Michael Collier, Medical Director
Michael Stens, Medical Director
We provide post-acute services, rehabilitative services, skilled nursing, short and long term care through Physical, Occupational, and Speech Therapists; Registered and Licensed Practical Nurses; and Certified Nursing Assistants. This is complemented by Social Services, Activities, Nutritional Services, Housekeeping and Laundry Services. With over 100 years of combined experience, our staff of professionals is here to meet the needs of each and every patient and resident.

7159 **Winter Park Memorial Hospital**
Florida Hospital
200 N Lakemont Ave
Winter Park, FL 32792-3273 407-646-7000
FAX: 407-646-7639
e-mail: healthcare@winterparkhospital.com
www.winterparkhospital.com
Ken Bradley, CEO
Nestled among the oak-shaded, brick-paved streets of one of the most picturesque hometowns in the country, Winter Park Memorial Hospital has continuously served the residents of Winter Park and its surrounding communities for more than 50 years.

Georgia

7160 **Athena Rehab of Clayton**
2055 Rex Rd
Lake City, GA 30260-3944 404-361-5144
FAX: 404-363-6366
Reginald Washington, Administrator
Offers the following rehabilitation services: Sub-Acute rehabilitation, Occupational therapy, Speech therapy, Physical therapy, Restorative care.

7161 **Lafayette Nursing and Rehabilitation Center**
110 Brandywine Blvd
Fayetteville, GA 30214-1500 770-461-2928
FAX: 770-461-8507
www.lafayetterehab.com
Wendy Goza, Medical Director

Lafayette Nursing and Rehab Center accomodates 179 residents. We are Medicare certified and our center also features a 25-bed postacute rehab unit and a 24-bed dementia unit. We have RN's LPN's and CNA's 24 hours a day. We also have physician services availiable seven days a week.

7162 Savannah Rehabilitation and Nursing Center
815 E 63rd St
Savannah, GA 31405-4499 912-352-8615
FAX: 912-355-4642
www.savannahrehab.com

Sandra Casper, Executive Director
At our facility, we provide quality care with modern rehabilitation and restorative nursing techniques. We aim to provide an atmosphere which encourages family involvement in the care-planning process, with the right mix of activities addressing the social, spiritual and intellectual needs of our residents.

7163 Specialty Hospital
PO Box 1566
Rome, GA 30162-1566 706-509-4100
FAX: 706-509-4159
www.thespecialtyhospital.com

7164 Walton Rehabilitation Health System
523 13th St.
Augusta, GA 30901-1037 706-823-8505
866-492-5866
FAX: 706-724-5752
e-mail: postmaster@wrh.org
www.wrh.org

Dennis Skelley, President/CEO
Has Centers of Excellence in Stroke Brain Injury, Complex Orthopedics, Spinal Cord Injury and Pain Management. 58-bed nonprofit facility.

7165 Warner Robins Rehabilitation and Nursing Center
1601 Elberta Rd
Warner Robins, GA 31093-1393 478-922-2241
FAX: 478-328-1984
www.warnerrobinsrehabilitation.com

Laura Fergason, Administrator
Offers the following rehabilitation services: Sub-Acute rehabilitation, Physical Therapy, Occupational Therapy, Speech Therapy.

Hawaii

7166 Aloha Nursing and Rehab Center
45-545 Kamehameha Hwy
Kaneohe, HI 96744-1943 808-247-2220
FAX: 808-235-3676
e-mail: info@alohanursing.com
alohanursing.com

Charles Harris, Executive Director
Amy Lee, Administrator
Our unique nursing care facility is nestled in the picturesque town of Kaneohe, Oahu, amid the towering Koolau Mountains and the panoramic vistas of Kaneohe Bay. In this tranquil setting, our 141-bed facility offers both long and short term care to residents who meet intermediate or skilled level of care criteria.

Idaho

7167 Boise Health And Rehabilitation Center
1001 S Hilton St
Boise, ID 83705-1925 208-345-4464
FAX: 208-345-2998
www.kindredboise.com

Jason Ludwig, Medical Director
Aaron Moorhouse, Medical Director
Debbie Mills, Executive Director
Offers the following rehabilitation services: Sub-acute rehabilitation, occupational therapy, speech therapy, physical therapy.

7168 Eastern Idaho Regional Medical Center
3100 Channing Way
Idaho Falls, ID 83404-7533 208-529-6111
FAX: 208-529-7021
www.eirmc.com

Cindy Smith-Putnam, Executive Director of Business Development, Marketing & Comm
Lou Fatkin, Executive Director of Risk Management, Physician Relations,
Matt Campbell, Director of Human Resources
Jared Rickabaugh, Director of Quality Management
The largest medical facility in the region, Eastern Idaho Regional Medical Center (EIRMC) is a modern, JCAHO-accredidted, full-service hospital. EIRMC serves as the region's healthcare hub, offering specialty services including open-heart surgery, leading-edge cancer treatment, trauma, neurosurgery, intensive care for adults and infants, and a helicopeter service.

7169 Kindred Transitional Care and Rehabilitation
3315 8th St
Lewiston, ID 83501-4966 208-743-9543
FAX: 208-746-8662
www.lewistonrehab.com

Debbie Freeze, Administrator
Lewiston Rehabilitation and Care Center has years of experience providing diversified healthcare services. We have our own staff of physical, occupational and speech therapists. Our therapy gym and rehab kitchen are a lovely atmosphere in which to work toward your therapy goals. We are an Eden Alternative Certified facility.

7170 Mountain Valley Care and Rehabilitation Center
601 West Cameron Avenue
PO Box 689
Kellogg, ID 83837- 2004 208-784-1283
FAX: 208-784-0151
www.mountainvalleycare.com

Maryruth Butler, Executive Director
Mountain Valley Care and Rehabilitation Center accomodates 68 residents. We are conveniently located in the heart of Kellogg Idaho. We strive to offer quality care and superior customer service in a home-like environment. Upon admission, you or your loved one is looked after by an assigned staff member. We call this our 'Angel Care' program. Our rehabilitation program focuses on meething the individual needs of the resident so you or your loved one can see how they are going to progress.

7171 River's Edge Rehabilitation and Healthcare
Kindred Healthcare
714 N Butte Ave
Emmett, ID 83617-2799 208-365-4425
FAX: 208-365-6989
e-mail: GDecker@ensigngroup.net
www.riversedgerehab.com

Janis Shields, Executive Director
Steve Balle, MPT, Director of Rehabilitation
Margaret Williams RN, BSN, Director of Nursing
Patty Alsup, Business Office Manager
Emmett Rehab & healthcare accomodates 95 residents. We are located in Emmett, Idaho, a rural community located an easy 30 minute drive from Boise. Emmett Rehab &'healthcare has served the area for more then 40 years by providing healthcare for residents of Gem County.

Illinois

7172 Chevy Chase Nursing and Rehabilitation Center
3400 S Indiana Ave
Chicago, IL 60616-3841 312-842-5000
FAX: 312-842-3790

Tony Prather, Administrator
Our approach to care is multidisciplinary; our medical staff members work together as a team in a proactive fashion, challenging residents each and every day, in order to motivate them to rehabilitate and achieve their ultimate potential.

7173 Glenview Terrace Nursing Center
1511 Greenwood Rd
Glenview, IL 60026-1513
847-729-9090
FAX: 847-729-9135
www.glenviewterrace.com
Ian Crook, Administrator
We're best known as the industry leader in post-hospital rehabilitation, including orthopedic rehabilitation and stroke recovery. Our highly effective rehabilitation services feature one-on-one physical, occupational, speech and respiratory therapies up to seven days a week.

7174 Halsted Terrace Nursing Center
10935 S Halsted St
Chicago, IL 60628-3189
773-928-2000
FAX: 773-928-9154
Ted O'Brien, Administrator
Offers the following rehabilitation services: Sub-acute rehabilitation, physical therapy, occupational therapy, speech therapy, cardiac rehabilitation.

7175 Harmony Nursing and Rehabilitation Center
3919 W Foster Ave
Chicago, IL 60625-6056
773-588-9500
FAX: 773-588-9533
www.harmonychicago.com
John Sianghio, Administrator
Offers a friendly healthcare experience. You'll find compassionate experts who provide short-term rehabilitation and therapy, wound care, Alzheimer's and memory loss care, long-term nursing care and more.

7176 Imperial
1366 W Fullerton Ave
Chicago, IL 60614-2199
773-248-9300
FAX: 773-935-0036
www.imperialpavilion.com
David Hartman, Administrator
Mary Bangayan, M.D., Pulmonary Care Programme
Sanjay Gill, M.D., Cardiac Management Program
We offer a comprehensive approach to post acute care. One that takes into consideration our guests' unique needs, and utilizes a progressive healthcare model to provide them with a personalized rehabilitation program designed to offer them the fullest possible recovery.

7177 Jackson Square Nursing and Rehabilitation Center
5130 W Jackson Blvd
Chicago, IL 60644-4332
773-921-8000
FAX: 773-287-9302
www.jacksonsquarecare.com
Rick Walworth, Administrator
At Jackson Square, there is one primary goal: to help guests regain maximum independence and functioning so that they can safely, comfortably, and happily get their life back. Our physicians, therapists, and nurses use their experience, compassion, and skill-combined with the latest and best technology-to provide comprehensive rehabilitation for a wide range of physical disabilities and medical conditions.

7178 Renaissance at 87th Street
2940 W 87th St
Chicago, IL 60652-3832
773-434-8787
FAX: 773-434-8717
www.renaissanceat87.com
Juli Foy, Administrator
At Renaissance at 87th, there is one primary goal: to help guests regain maximum independence and functioning so that they can safely, comfortably, and happily get their life back. Our physicians, therapists, and nurses use their experience, compassion, and skill-combined with the latest and best technology-to provide comprehensive rehabilitation for a wide range of physical disabilities and medical conditions.

7179 Renaissance at Hillside
4600 N. Frontage Rd.
Hillside, IL 60162-1761
708-544-9933
FAX: 708-544-9966
www.ariapostacute.com
John Stare, Administrator
Utilizing a progressive healthcare model that takes into account each patient's individual needs, Aria Post Acute Care designs a personalized rehabilitation program offering guests the best chance at the fullest possible recovery.

7180 Renaissance at Midway
4437 S Cicero Ave
Chicago, IL 60632-4333
773-884-0484
FAX: 773-884-0485
www.renaissanceatmidway.com
Jeff Baker, Executive Director
At Renaissance at Midway, there is one primary goal: to help guests regain maximum independence and functioning so that they can safely, comfortably, and happily get their life back. Our physicians, therapists, and nurses use their experience, compassion, and skill-combined with the latest and best technology-to provide comprehensive rehabilitation for a wide range of physical disabilities and medical conditions.

7181 Renaissance at South Shore
2425 E 71st St
Chicago, IL 60649-2612
773-721-5000
FAX: 773-721-6850
www.rensouthshore.com
Dave Schechter, Administrator
The Renaissance at South Shore is a 248 bed skilled nursing facility with multiple services that include short-term rehabilitation, specialized dementia care and long-term care and hospice care. Our highly trained nursing professionals provide loving care in a home-like atmosphere.

7182 Schwab Rehabilitation Hospital
Mt. Sinai
1401 S California Ave
Chicago, IL 60608-1858
773-522-2010
e-mail: schwabinquiries@sini.org
www.schwabrehab.org
Suzan Rayner, Medical Director
Lisa Thornton, Medical Staff President
Alan Channing, President/ Chief Executive Officer
Anita Halvorsen, Vice President of Schwab Rehabilitation Hospital
Schwab Rehabilitation Hospital is a freestanding, not-for-profit, 102-bed rehabilitation hospital located on Chicago's west side. It offers a therapeutic environment of comprehensive inpatient and outpatient rehabilitation, both for adults and children.

Indiana

7183 Angel River Health and Rehabilitation
5233 Rosebud Ln
Newburgh, IN 47630-9283
812-473-4761
FAX: 812-473-5190
e-mail: HSDED0204@kindredhealthcare.com
www.angelriverhc.com
Kay Congleton, Executive Director
Our wide array of services enables our patients and residents to receive the medical care they need, the restorative therapy they require, and the support they and their families deserve. We serve many types of patient and resident needs - from short-term rehabilitation to traditional long-term care. Our resident council meets regularly to ensure that our residents' needs are being met to their satisfaction.

7184 Chalet Village Health and Rehabilitation Center
Magnolia Health Systems
1065 Parkway St
Berne, IN 46711-2366
260-589-2127
FAX: 260-589-3521
e-mail: mwolfe@chalet-village.net
www.chalet-village.net

Vicki Shepherd, Administrator

We provide dedicated, community-centered healthcare which was founded in Indiana, operates in Indiana, for people who live in Indiana.

7185 Columbus Health and Rehabilitation Center
2100 Midway St
Columbus, IN 47201-3722
812-372-8447
FAX: 812-375-5117
www.columbushrc.com

Sherry Harrison, Executive Director
William Lustig, Medical Director

Accomodates 235 residents. We offer a continuum of healthcare services. Our center also provides a Special Care Alzheimer's Unit. We are licensed by the Stat of Indiana and are Medicare and Medicaid approved provider. We are proud to offer a friendly home-like atmosphere while providing comprehensive healthcare services. These services include short-term medical and rehabilitation treatment, which is designed to address the individual needs of our residents and patients.

7186 Harrison Health and Rehabilitation Centre
150 Beechmont Drive
Corydon, IN 47112-1717
812-738-0550
FAX: 812-738-6273
e-mail: HSDED0131@kindredhealthcare.com
www.harrisonrehab.com

Sheila Bieker, Executive Director
Bruce Burton, Medical Director

We serve many types of patient and resident needs - from short-term rehabilitation to traditional long-term care. Working with your physician, our staff - including medical specialists, nurses, nutritionists, therapists, dietitians and social workers - establishes a comprehensive treatment plan intended to restore you or your loved one to the fullest practicable potential.

7187 Indian Creek Health and Rehabilitation Center
240 Beechmont Dr
Corydon, IN 47112-1718
812-738-8127
877-380-7211
FAX: 812-738-2917
e-mail: HSDED0288@kindredhealthcare.com
www.indiancreekhrc.com

Bonnie Fallin, Executive Director
Bruce Burton, Medical Director

140 bed facility offering the following rehabilitation services: Sub-Acute rehabilitation, Physical therapy, Occupational Therapy, Speech Therapy, pain management, Wound rehabilitation. Short and long term skilled nursing care certified for Medicare, Medicaid, Private Pay and Private Insurance. Hospice and respite care rated #1 in clinical care in southern Indiana district for 2002.

7188 Meadowvale Health and Rehabilitation Center
Kindred Health Care
1529 Lancaster St
Bluffton, IN 46714-1507
260-824-4320
800-743-3333
FAX: 260-824-4689
e-mail: HSDED0269@kindredhealthcare.com
www.meadowvalerehab.com

Todd Beaulieu, Executive Director
Yadagiri Jonna, Medical Director

Working with your physician, our staff - including medical specialists, nurses, nutritionists, therapists, dietitians and social workers - establishes a comprehensive treatment plan intended to restore you or your loved one to the fullest practicable potential.

7189 Muncie Health Care and Rehabilitation
680 South Fourth Street
Louisville, KY 40202
502-596-7300
800-545-0749
e-mail: web_administrator@kindred.com
www.kindredhealthcare.com

Dee Harrold, Executive Director
Dr. Jeffery Hiltz, Medical Director

Offers the following rehabilitation services: Sub-Acute rehabilitation, physical therapy, occupational therapy, speech therapy.

7190 Rehabilitation Hospital of Indiana
4141 Shore Dr
Indianapolis, IN 46254-2607
317-329-2000
FAX: 317-329-2104
www.rhin.com

Ian Worden, MHA, MBA, CPA, RHI Board Chair
James G. Terwilliger, MPH, Vice Chair/Secretary
Kyle Netter, MBA, PT, Executive Director of Corporate and Affiliate Relations
Larissa Swan, MS, OTR, Executive Director of Therapies

We approach every patient understanding that every diagnosis, every illness, and every injury are different. It's the collective effort of trained and compassionate team members who value the quality of life of every patient and their caregivers. It's the right kind of treatment- inpatient, outpatient, and follow-up services- provided under the same roof. It's one step closer to home. It's a continuum of care

7191 Sellersburg Health and Rehabilitation Centre
7823 Old State Road 60
Sellersburg, IN 47172-1858
812-246-4272
FAX: 812-246-8160
www.sellersburgrehab.com

Dave Powell, Administrator
Chris Hansen, Executive Director

Sellersburg is a modern healthcare center conveniently located on the edge of the community. Our center accomodates 110 residents and includes a rehabilitative program with a goal of returning residents home as quickly as possible. Sellersburg is a 2006 recipient of the American Health Care Association Quality Award.

7192 Westpark Rehabilitation Center
1316 N Tibbs Ave
Indianapolis, IN 46222-3024
317-634-8330
FAX: 317-263-9442
www.westparkhealthcare.com

Dave Mc Carroll, Owner

Offers the following rehabilitation services: Sub-acute rehabilitation, occupational therapy, physical therapy, speech therapy, respiratory therapy.

7193 Westview Nursing and Rehabilitation Center
1510 Clinic Dr
Bedford, IN 47421-3530
812-279-4494
FAX: 812-275-8313
www.ascseniorcare.com/westview-nursing—rehab

Sholin Montgomery, Executive Director
Mike Spencer, Executive Director

Offers the following rehabilitation services: Sub-acute rehabilitation, physical therapy, occupational therapy, speech therapy.

7194 Windsor Estates Health and Rehab Center
429 W Lincoln Rd
Kokomo, IN 46902-3508
765-453-5600
FAX: 765-455-0110
e-mail: HSDED0294@kindredhealthcare.com
www.kindredkokomo.com

Brenda Alfrey, Administrator
Monica Martin, Executive Director

Our wide array of services enables our patients and residents to receive the medical care they need, the restorative therapy they require, and the support they and their families deserve. We serve many types of patient and resident needs - from short-term rehabilitation to traditional long-term care.

Iowa

7195 Madison County Rehab Services
Madison County Hospital
300 W Hutchings St
Winterset, IA 50273-2109
515-462-2373
FAX: 515-462-4492

Marcia Harris, CEO
Panndee Stebbins, Director
Offers the following rehabilitation services: Sub-acute rehabilitation, occupational therapy, physical therapy, speech therapy, home health rehab, wellness programs.

7196 Mercy Subacute Care
603 E 12th St
Des Moines, IA 50309-5515
515-247-4400
FAX: 515-643-0945

Bonnie Mc Coy, Manager
Pam Nelson, Intake Coordinator
Offers the following rehabilitation services: Sub-acute rehabilitation, physical therapy, speech therapy, occupational therapy.

Kentucky

7197 Danville Centre for Health and Rehabilitation
642 N 3rd St
Danville, KY 40422-1125
859-236-3972
FAX: 859-236-0703
e-mail: HSDED0782@kindredhealthcare.com
www.danvillecentre.com

Debbie Gibson, Executive Director
We offer short-term rehabilitative care as well as long-term care. Our emphasis is on service excellence - providing quality care in a home-like environment to allow for independence and to enable our patients and residents to receive the medical care they need, the restorative therapy they require, and the support they and their families deserve.

7198 Fountain Circle Health & Rehabilitation
Kindred Healthcare
200 Glenway Rd
Winchester, KY 40391
859-744-1800
FAX: 859-744-0285
www.fountaincircle.com

William Whited, Executive Director
Kathryn Jones, Medical Director
Offers the following rehabilitation services: Sub-acute rehabilitation, speech therapy, physical therapy, occupational therapy.

7199 Lexington Center for Health and Rehabilitation
353 Waller Ave
Lexington, KY 40504-2974
859-252-3558
FAX: 859-233-0192

Karole Ward, Administrator
Offers the following rehabilitation services: Sub-acute rehabilitation, speech therapy, occupational therapy, physical therapy.

7200 Paducah Centre For Health and Rehabilitation
Wellsouth Health Systems
501 N 3rd St
Paducah, KY 42001-0749
270-444-9661
FAX: 270-443-9407
www.genesishcc.com/Paducah?

Jean Glisson, RN, Director of Nursing
Elizabeth Kay Chilton, Admissions Director
Tracy Summers, Rehab/Specialty Program Director
Cathy Ortega, Administrator
Paducah Center is an 86-bed skilled and long-term care facility with a 28-bed Alzheimer's secure unit. This unit has a private courtyard and structured activities throughout the day, and is the only true Alzheimer's secure unit in the area.

7201 Pathways Brain Injury Program
4200 Browns Ln
Louisville, KY 40220-1523
502-459-8900
FAX: 502-459-5026
www.hcr-manorcare.com

Pam Pearson, Manager
Offers the following rehabilitation services: Sub-acute rehabilitation, speech therapy, occupational therapy, physical therapy, recreational therapy.

Louisiana

7202 Guest House of Slidell Sub-Acute and Rehab Center
1051 Robert Blvd
Slidell, LA 70458-2011
985-643-5630
800-303-9872
FAX: 985-649-6065

Brandy Wheat, Administrator
116 bed healthcare center offering the following subacute services within the skilled nursing setting: physical, occupational, and speech therapies, infusion therapy, respiratory care, wound care, neurological rehabilitation, cardiac reconditioning, pain management, post surgical recovery, orthopedic rehabilitation.

7203 Irving Place Rehabilitation and Nursing Center
1736 Irving Pl
Shreveport, LA 71101-4606
318-631-9121
FAX: 318-222-2095

Webster Johnson, Administrator
Offers the following rehabilitation services: sub-acute rehabilitation, speech therapy, occupational therapy, physical therapy

Maine

7204 Augusta Rehabilitation Center
188 Eastern Ave
Augusta, ME 04330-5928
207-622-3121
800-457-1220
FAX: 207-623-7666
e-mail: HSDED0544@kindredhealthcare.com
www.augustarehabcenter.com

Malcolm Dean, Executive Director
Cathleen O'Connor
From intensive short term rehabilitation therapy to longer-term restorative care, our Nursing and Rehabilitation Centers provide a full range of nursing care and social services to treat and support each of our patients and residents. Our clinical capabilities allow us to accept patients with greater medical complexity than a traditional nursing home. This is increasingly important as many patients require transitional care before they are ready to return home.

7205 Brentwood Rehabilitation and Nursing Center
370 Portland St
Yarmouth, ME 04096-8101
207-846-9021
800-457-1220
FAX: 207-846-1497
e-mail: HSDED0555@kindredhealthcare.com
www.brentwoodrnc.com

Malcolm Dean, Executive Director
Daniel M. Pierce, Medical Director
Brentwood accomodates 82 residents. We are located at 370 Portland Street in Yarmouth, Maine. We strive to meet the healthcare needs of the greater Yarmouth community, including Portland and Brunswick, which are located within 10 miles of the center. In addition to Brentwood's rehabilitation and skilled nursing services, we also offer Alzheimer's specialty care in a comfortable setting.

7206 **Den-Mar Rehabilitation and Nursing Center**
44 South St
Rockport, MA 01966-1800
978-546-6311
800-439-2370
FAX: 978-546-9185
e-mail: HSDED0542@kindredhealthcare.com
www.denmarrnc.com
Christine Marek, Executive Director
Den-Mar nursing and Rehab center accomodates 80 residents. We provide skilled nursing and rehabilitation services as well as long term care. We are certified for Medicare and Medicaid as well as many insurance carriers. We offer semi-private and private rooms, with many common areas for socializing.

7207 **Eastside Rehabilitation and Living Center**
516 Mount Hope Ave
Bangor, ME 04401-4215
207-947-6131
800-457-1220
FAX: 207-942-0884
e-mail: HSDED0545@kindredhealthcare.com
www.eastsiderehab.com
Ryan Kelley, Executive Director
From intensive short term rehabilitation therapy to longer-term restorative care, our Nursing and Rehabilitation Centers provide a full range of nursing care and social services to treat and support each of our patients and residents. Our clinical capabilities allow us to accept patients with greater medical complexity than a traditional nursing home. This is increasingly important as many patients require transitional care before they are ready to return home.

7208 **Kennebunk Nursing & Rehabilitation Center**
158 Ross Rd
Kennebunk, ME 04043-6532
207-985-7141
800-457-1220
FAX: 207-985-0961
e-mail: HSDED0549@kindredhealthcare.com
www.kennebunknursing.com
Stephen Alaimo, Executive Director
We treat a variety of conditions and provide an array of services including, but not limited to:Respiratory conditions such as pneumonia and post-acute COPD episodes Cardiac conditions and post surgical care (grafts, valves, stints) Wound Stroke Orthopedic Neurological illnesses Diabetes

7209 **Norway Rehabilitation and Living Center**
29 Marion Ave
Norway, ME 04268-5601
207-743-7075
800-457-1220
FAX: 207-743-9269
e-mail: info@norwayresidentialcare.com
www.norwayresidentialcare.com
Carolyn Farley, Administrator
Norway Rehabilitation and Living Center has been a fixture in the Norway community since 1976. We are a 70-bed facility offering short-term rehabilitation, skilled nursing services, long term care and residential care services. Utilizing an interdisciplinary team led by a physician and consisting of qualified health care specialists, we develop individualized plans of care for each patient that are designed to restore maximum health and optimize functional abilities and independence

7210 **Shore Village Rehabilitation & Nursing Center**
201 Camden St
\, ME 04841-2534
207-596-6423
800-457-1220
FAX: 207-596-7235
Phyllis Nickerson, Administrator
Shore Village accomodates 60 residents and is located in the mid-coast region of the state of Maine. We have a cozy size and a primary goal for the staff is to ensure a home-like atmosphere for all the residents. Shore Village provides skilled nursing and rehabilitation, respite care, and long term care. The facility is dually certified for Medicare and Medicaid and accepts many commercial insurance plans.

Maryland

7211 **Greater Baltimore Medical Center**
6701 N Charles St
Baltimore, MD 21204-6881
443-849-2000
FAX: 443-849-3024
TTY:800-735-2258
www.gbmc.org
John B. Chessare, M.D., President/Chief Executive Officer
Eric L. Melchior, Executive Vice President/Chief Financial Officer
Keith Poisson, Executive Vice President/Chief Operating Officer
John W. Ellis, Senior Vice President/Corporate Strategy & Business Developm
The 281-bed medical center (acute and sub-acute care) is located on a beautiful suburban campus and handles more than 26,700 inpatient cases and approximately 60,000 emergency room visits annually.

Massachusetts

7212 **Bolton Manor Nursing Home**
400 Bolton St
Marlborough, MA 01752-3912
508-481-6123
800-439-2370
FAX: 508-481-6130
www.boltonmanor.com
Michele Ricard, Medical Director
Thomas Sullivan, Executive Director
Bolton Manor accomodates 157 residents. We are located in Marlboro, Massachusetts. We provide medical management and long-term care through comprehensive skilled and post-acute nursing services. We also provide physical, occupational, and speech therapy services from an onsite dedicated staff of therapists. The facility is Joint Commission (formerly JCAHO) accredited and has an excellent survey history with the State Department of Public Health.

7213 **Brigham Manor Nursing and Rehabilitation Center**
77 High St
Newburyport, MA 01950-3071
978-462-4221
800-439-2370
FAX: 978-463-3297
www.brighammanor.com
Stephen Cynewski, Executive Director
Brigham Manor accomodates 64 residents. We are a Medicare-certified facility offering private, semi-private and multi-bed suites. Our bright, formal dining room, with French doors that open to a shaded courtyard, provides a warm atmosphere for entertaining family and friends. Each resident's personal tastes and medical needs are considered in the planning of our weekly menus.

7214 **Country Gardens Skilled Nursing and Rehabilitation Center**
2045 Grand Army Hwy
Swansea, MA 02777-3932
508-379-9700
800-439-2370
FAX: 508-379-0723
e-mail: HSDED0534@kindredhealthcare.com
www.cntrygrdns.com
Sandy Sarza, Executive Director
Country Gardens Skilled Nursing and Rehabilitation Center accomodates 86 residents. We are located in a beautiful rural setting conveniently located about 15 minutes east of Providence and 10 minutes west of Fall River. We have provided healthcare service to the greater Swansea area for over 34 years.

7215 **Country Manor Rehabilitation and Nursing Center**
180 Low St
Newburyport, MA 01950-3519
978-465-5361
800-439-2370
FAX: 978-463-9366
www.countryrehab.com
Stephen Doyle, Executive Director
Country Rehabilitation and Nursing Center accomodates 123 residents. We are located in the quaint seaport town of Newburyport,

Massachusetts. We provide medical management and long-term care through comprehensive skilled and intermediate nursing services. We also provide physical, occupational, and speech therapy services from an onsite dedicated staff of therapists. The center offers an Alzheimer's special care unit with staff trained in dimentia care and dementia specific programs.

7216 Franklin Skilled Nursing and Rehabilitation Center
130 Chestnut St
Franklin, MA 02038-3903 508-528-4600
800-439-2370
FAX: 508-528-7976
e-mail: HSDED0584@kindredhealthcare.com
www.franklinskilled.com

Paula Topijan, Executive Director
We treat a variety of conditions and provide an array of services including, but not limited to :Respiratory conditions such as pneumonia and post-acute COPD episodes,Cardiac conditions and post surgical care (grafts, valves, stints),Wound,Stroke,Orthopedic,Neurological illnesses,Diabetes

7217 Great Barrington Rehabilitation and Nursing Center
148 Maple Ave
Great Barrington, MA 01230-1906 413-528-3320
800-439-2370
FAX: 413-528-2302
e-mail: HSDED0585@kindredhealthcare.com
www.greatbarringtonrnc.com

William Kittler, Executive Director
Andrew Potler, Medical Director
Great Barrington Rehabilitation and Nursing Center accomodates 106 residents. As part of a national network of long-term healthcare centers, we have the expertise and resources to provide care appropriate to the individual needs of each and every one of our residents. We provide personal care with minimal daily living assistance to the most skilled treatment for medically complex patients.

7218 Ledgewood Rehabilitation and Skilled Nursing Center
87 Herrick St
Beverly, MA 01915-2773 978-921-1392
800-439-2370
FAX: 978-927-8627
www.ledgewoodrehab.com

Frank Silvia, Executive Director
Ledgewood Rehabilitation and Skilled Nursing Center is a unique provider of healthcare services. We are part of a continuum of services that includes acute care services at Beverly Hospital, subacute care at Ledgewood, and care after discharge through Northeast Homecare. We believe this partnership offers the highest quality post-acute services north of Boston.

7219 Leo P La Chance Center for Rehabilitation and Nursing
59 Eastwood Cir
Gardner, MA 01440-3901 978-632-8776
FAX: 978-632-5048
e-mail: souellet@legendcenter.com
www.lachancecenter.com

Mark Alinger, Administrator
Leo P. LaChance, Founder
A privately owned facility, combines the best of medical technology with the ultimate in healing, compassionate rehabilitation and nursing care. Our goal is to help each client reach that ultimate goal of living life to the fullest.

7220 Oakwood Rehabilitation and Nursing Center
11 Pontiac Ave
Webster, MA 01570-1629 508-943-3889
800-439-2370
FAX: 508-949-6125
e-mail: HSDED0517@kindredhealthcare.com
www.oakwoodrehab.com

Thomas Sullivan, Executive Director
Oakwood Rehabilitation and Nursing Center accomodates 81 residents. We offer 24-hour skilled nursing, inpatient rehabilitation, respite care, and hospice services. Our center has been successfully serving the greater Webster, Massachusetts, community for 35 years. We have a dedicated and caring staff and our common goal is to promote recovery and enhance quality of live whether your needs are short or long term.

7221 Walden Rehabilitation and Nursing Center
785 Main St
Concord, MA 01742-3310 978-369-6889
800-439-2370
FAX: 978-369-8392
e-mail: HSDED0588@kindredhealthcare.com
www.waldenrehab.com

Ladan Azarm, Executive Director
Walden Rehabilitation and Nursing Center accomodates 123 residents. We are located in the quaint town of Concord, Massachusetts, across the street from Emerson Hospital and a short drive from the town center. Walden provides medical management and long-term care through comprehensive skilled and intermediate nursing services. We also provide physical, occupational, and speech therapy services from an onsite dedicated staff of therapists.

Michigan

7222 Boulder Park Terrace
14676 W Upright St
Charlevoix, MI 49720-1201 231-547-1005
FAX: 231-547-1039
www.mclaren.org/northernmichigan/northernmich

Reezie DeVet, President/CEO
Mary-Anne Ponti, COO
A partnership formed with Charlevoix Area Hospital, Boulder Park Terrace is a long-term care facility and Sub-acute Rehabilitation Center located in Chalrevoix near the shores of Lake Michigan. The Sub-acute Rehabilitation Center was created as a transition between an acute care hospital and home. Patients enter into the program to increase their strength, endurance and over-all functioning before returning home.

Minnesota

7223 Park Health And Rehabilitation Center
4415 W 36 1/2 St
St Louis Park, MN 55416-4890 952-927-9717
FAX: 952-927-7687
e-mail: park@extendicare.com
www.extendicare.com

Jennifer Kuhn, Administrator
Park Health & Rehabilitation Center is a leading provider of long-term skilled nursing care and short-term rehabilitation solutions. Our 93 bed facility offers a full continuum of services and care focused around each individual in today's ever-changing healthcare environment.

Missouri

7224 Barnes-Jewish Hospital Washington University Medical Center
1 Barnes Jewish Hospital Plz
Saint Louis, MO 63110-1003 314-747-3000
866-867-3627
FAX: 314-362-8877
www.barnesjewish.org

Richard Liekweg, President
John Beatty, Vice President of Human Resources
John Lynch, MD, Chief Medical Officer
David Jaques, MD, Vice President for Surgical Services
Barnes-Jewish Hospital at Washington University Medical Center is the largest hospital in Missouri and the largest private employer in the St. Louis region. An affiliated teaching hospital of Washington University School of Medicine, Barnes-Jewish Hospital has a 1,700 member medical staff with many who are recognized in the 'Best Doctors in America.

Montana

7225 **Parkview Acres Care and Rehabilitation Center**
200 N Oregon St
Dillon, MT 59725-3624
406-683-5105
866-253-4090
FAX: 406-683-6388
e-mail: HSDED0433@kindredhealthcare.com
www.parkviewacres.com
Claire Miller, Executive Director
We are Medicare and Medicaid certified skilled nursing facility which accomodates 108 residents serving scenic Dillon and surrounding Montana communities.

Nebraska

7226 **Homestead Healthcare and Rehabilitation Center**
4735 S 54th St
Lincoln, NE 68516-1335
402-488-0977
800-833-0920
FAX: 402-488-4507
www.homesteadrehab.com
Matt Romshek, Executive Director
Gay Bate, RN, Director of Nursing
James Murray, Administrator
James Murray,LPN, Clinical Liaison/Admissions
Homestead Healthcare and Rehabilitation Center is one of the area's oldest providers of skilled nursing and rehabilitation services. We are a 163-bed skilled nursing and rehabilitation center nestled in a lovely, quiet established neighborhood in South Lincoln.

7227 **Madonna Rehabilitation Hospital**
5401 South St
Lincoln, NE 68506-2150
402-413-3000
800-676-5448
FAX: 402-486-5448
e-mail: info@madonna.org
www.madonna.org
Marsha Lommel, CEO
Tom Stalder, VP Medical Affairs
Madonna provides intensive rehabilitation and expertise for a wide variety of conditions, such as: orthopedic injuries, work injuries, arthritis, amputation, neuromuscular diseases, cardiac conditions, pulmonary disease and conditions including those dependent upon a ventilator, cancer, lymphedema, osteoporosis, wounds, renal disorders, burns, fibromyalgia, multiple scelerosis, parkinson's disease and degenerative diseases.

7228 **Mary Lanning Memorial Hospital**
715 N Saint Joseph Ave
Hastings, NE 68901-4497
402-463-4521
866-460-5884
e-mail: tanderson@mlmh.org
www.mlmh.org
Beth Schlichtman, Compensation/Benefit Services - Director
Lisa Brandt, Public Relations & Marketing Services - Director
Carrie Edwards, Home Care Services - Director
Chris Page, Ancillary Services - Director
Mary Lanning Healthcare is in its 95th year of providing quality healthcare for residents of the central Nebraska area. We continue to grow and expand, working to provide patient-centered care in a positive environment, while implementing some of the newest technologies available.

Nevada

7229 **Las Vegas Healthcare and Rehabilitation Center**
2832 S Maryland Pkwy
Las Vegas, NV 89109-1502
702-735-5848
800-326-6888
FAX: 702-735-6218
www.lasvegaskindred.com
Randall Fuller, Executive Director
Las Vegas Healthcare accomodates 79 residents. We have been serving the community for approximately 40 years. Located in close proximity to local hospitals and surrounded by medical complexes, our center offers both short-term rehabilitation and long-term care.

New Hampshire

7230 **Dover Rehabilitation and Living Center**
307 Plaza Dr
Dover, NH 03820-2455
603-742-2676
800-735-2964
FAX: 603-749-5375
www.doverrehab.com
Daniel Estee, Executive Director
Dover Rehab is a provider of postacute services in the greater New Hampshire Seacost area. We accomodate 112 residents and are licensed by the state of New Hampshire. We employ nearly 150 licensed nurses, therapists and other healthcare professionals, who strive to provide quality care. The goal of our patient service model is to bridge the gap between hospitalization and home so that recovery and physical functioning are maximized and hospital readmission is minimized.

7231 **Northeast Rehabilitation Clinic**
70 Butler St
Salem, NH 03079-3925
603-893-2900
800-825-7292
FAX: 603-893-1638
TTY: 800-439-2370
e-mail: webmaster@northeastrehab.com
www.northeastrehab.com
John Prochilo, CEO/Administrator
Subacute rehabilitation at NRH was designed for people who have experienced an acutely disabling orthopedic, medical, or neurologic condition but who either do not require or are unable to participate in a full acute inpatient program. Impairment groups pertinent to this level of care include brain injury, spinal cord injury (traumatic/non-traumatic), stroke, orthopedic injury, amputation, and neurologic disorder.

New Jersey

7232 **Atlantic Coast Rehabilitation & Healthcare Center**
485 River Ave
Lakewood, NJ 08701-4720
732-364-7100
FAX: 732-364-2442
e-mail: abby@atlanticcoastrehab.com
www.atlanticcoastrehab.com
Simon Shain, Administrator
Sharon Sckbower, Director of Nursing
Atlantic Coast is family owned and operated. It's a warm, friendly place where caregivers and patients know each other by first name. But it's also an innovative and energetic place, where the most advanced therapies and cutting edge techniques are offered. It's a comprehensive health care center that provides three distinct areas of care:Rehabilitative Therapy & Sub Acute Care, Long Term Care ,Alzheimer's/Memory Impaired Care.

7233 **Crestwood Nursing & Rehabilitation Center**
101 Whippany Rd
Whippany, NJ 7981-1407
973-887-0311
FAX: 973-887-8355
Carol Shepard, Administrator

Sub-acute rehabilitation facility.

7234 Lakeview Subacute Care Center
130 Terhune Dr
Wayne, NJ 7470-7104
973-839-4500
87 -UBA-UTE
FAX: 973-839-2729
e-mail: rgrossojr@lakeviewsubacute.com
www.lakeviewsubacute.com

Richard Grosso, Jr, Director
Sue Ahlers, Director of Admission
Kerry Iamurri, Director of Rehab
Nicole Iacolina, Director Social Services

Our comprehensive medical, nursing and rehabilitation services cater to a diverse patient population. In addition to long-term care, we offer exceptional inpatient subacute programs. We're proud to report that our average length of stay for subacute patients is a brief 14 days.

7235 Merwick Rehabilitation and Sub-Acute Care
79 Bayard Ln
Princeton, NJ 8540-3045
609-497-3000
FAX: 609-497-3024

Ryan Wismer, Administrator

76-bed skilled nursing and residential center as well as a separate 17-bed comprehensive rehabilitation center. Offers rehabilitation, physiatry, occupational therapy, respite care, speech/hearing therapy, sub-acute care.

7236 Seacrest Village Nursing Center
1001 Center St
Little Egg Harbor Twp, NJ 8087-1364
609-296-9292
FAX: 609-296-0508
e-mail: info@seacrestvillagenj.com
seacrestvillagenj.com

Brian T Holloway, Administrator

Seacrest Village Nursing and Rehabilitation Center has specialized in quality rehabilitation, transitional and restorative care for more then a decade and is a perfect alternative for bridging the gap between hospital and home.

7237 St. Lawrence Rehabilitation Center
2381 Lawrenceville Rd
Lawrenceville, NJ 08648-2098
609-896-9500
FAX: 609-895-0242
e-mail: epiechota@slrc.org
www.slrc.org

Kevin McGuigan, MD, Medical Director
Robyn F. Agri, MD, Doctor
Dr. Madhu Jain, Doctor
Charles Terry MD, Doctor

St. Lawrence Rehabilitation Center, a non-profit facility sponsored by the Roman Catholic Diocese of Trenton, is committed to maximizing the quality of human life by providing comprehensive physical rehabilitation and related programs to meet the healthcare needs of our communities.

7238 Summit Ridge Center Genesis Eldercare
20 Summit St
West Orange, NJ 07052-1501
973-736-2000
800-699-1520
FAX: 973-736-2764
e-mail: info@genesishcc.com
www.genesishcc.com

Michele Cartagena, Director of Admissions
Elizabeth (L Orlando, Rehabilitation Program Director
Tsega Asefaha, LNHA, BS, MHA, Administrator
Elizabeth Martin, Customer Relations Manager

Summit Ridge Center provides skilled nursing, medical and rehabilitative care for patients requiring post-hospital, short stay rehabilitation and for longer term residents. Our Clinical Care Teams are focused on implementing your personalized care program to facilitate your recovery and improve your well-being.

New York

7239 Beth Abraham Health Services
612 Allerton Ave
Bronx, NY 10467-7495
718-519-4037
888-238-4223
FAX: 718-547-1366
e-mail: info@bethabe.org
www.bethabrahamhealthservices.org

Maria Provenzano, Program Director
Yolanda Lester, Director of Admissions
Rosalie Bernard, Director of Nursing Services
Vincent Bonadies, Director of Therapeutic Recreation

Offers the following rehabilitation services: Sub-Acute rehabilitation, brain injury rehabilitation, pain management, post-operative recovery. Home visits and a network of community-based programs help patients and their families with a successful transition home.

7240 Central Island Healthcare
825 Old Country Rd
Plainview, NY 11803-4913
516-433-0600
FAX: 516-868-7251
www.centralislandhealthcare.net

Michael Ostreicher, Administrator

Serving the community for over 33 years, Central Island Healthcare is Long Island's largest and most active sub-acute care provider. We offer comprehensive programs focused on restoring our patients to their maximum potential and returning home. Central Island's 202-bed facility provides top notch professionals and the latest in rehabilitation and therapeutic equipment in a beautiful and comfortable setting.

7241 Clove Lakes Health Care and Rehabilitation Center
25 Fanning St
Staten Island, NY 10314-5307
718-289-7900
FAX: 718-761-8701
e-mail: info@clovelakes.com
www.clovelakes.com

Helene Demisay, CEO

Clove Lakes seeks to rehabilitate those who have sustained injury or illness to the highest level of independence possible and support those with disabling conditions to live meaningful and productive lives.

7242 Dr. William O Benenson Rehabilitation Pavilion
36-17 Parsons Blvd
Flushing, NY 11354-5931
718-961-4300
FAX: 718-939-5032
www.flushingmanors.com

Esther Benenson, Executive Director
Liza Marie Dowd, Director of Nursing
Erika Rossi, Director of Social Services
Diane Marron, Director of Admissions

The Dr. William O Benson Reahbilitation Pavilion is a subacute short-term rehabilitation center committed to the excellence of elevated health care for our patients. Through the use of the most comprehensive and specialized services available, our staff of dedicated professionals are devoted to putting patients back to the road to full recovery 24 hours a day.

7243 Flushing Manor Nursing and Rehab
35-15 Parsons Blvd
Flushing, NY 11354-4297
718-961-3500
FAX: 718-461-1784
www.flushingmanors.com

Esther Benenson, Executive Director
Dr. Ion Oltean, Medical Director
Myung Chung, Director of Nursing
Bridgett Brown, Director of Admissions

At the Flusing Manor Nursing and Rehabilitation, we stress the importance of family involvement because it is the true source of strength and stability in ones life...a tie that brings us all together as a team, enhancing the quality of life of the patients in our care.

7244 Glengariff Health Care Center
141 Dosoris Ln
Glen Cove, NY 11542
516-676-1100
FAX: 516-759-0216
e-mail: info@glengariffcare.com
www.glenhaven.org
Jean Campo, Director Admissions
Michael Miness, President
Licensed skilled nursing and subacute medical and rehabilitation facility.

7245 Haym Salomon Home for The Aged
2340 Cropsey Ave
Brooklyn, NY 11214-5706
718-266-4063
FAX: 718-372-4781
Chain Lipschitz, Administrator
Religious nonmedical health care institution.

7246 Kings Harbor Multicare Center
2000 E Gun Hill Rd
Bronx, NY 10469-6016
718-320-0400
FAX: 718-671-5022
e-mail: info@kingsharbor.com
www.kingsharbor.com
Morris Tenenbaum, Owner
Octavio Marin, Vice President
Kings Harbor Multicare Center provides long-term and short-term skilled nursing care for more then 700 residents. Kings Harbor is located in the Pelham Gardens neighborhood of Northeast Bronx, easily accessible to major highways and near public transportation. A 3 building campus facility with surrounding gardens ensures that residents with similar capabilities are grouped together.

7247 Northwoods of Cortland
28 Kellogg Rd
Cortland, NY 13045-3155
607-753-9631
FAX: 607-756-2968
www.northwoodshealth.net
Lawrence Mennig, Administrator
Subacute rehabilitation facility.

7248 Port Jefferson Health Care Facility
141 Dosoris Lane
Glen Cove, NY 11542
631-676-1100
FAX: 631-759-0216
e-mail: info@glenhaven.org
www.glengariffcare.com
Ellen Harte, Administrator
Subacute medical and rehabilitative care and long term residential skilled nursing care.

7249 Rehab Institute at Florence Nightingale Health Center
1760 3rd Ave
New York, NY 10029-6810
212-410-8760
800-786-8968
FAX: 212-410-8792
e-mail: info@rehabinstitute.org

7250 Schnurmacher Center for Rehabilitation and Nursing
Beth Abraham of Family Health Services
12 Tibbits Ave
White Plains, NY 10606-2438
914-287-7200
888-238-4223
FAX: 914-428-1824
e-mail: info@schnurmacher.org
www.schnurmacher.org
Linda Murray, Executive Director
Thomas Camisa, Medical Director
Iryn Obaldo Fontanosa, Director of Rehabilitation
Filomena Cristo, Director of Therapeutic Recreation
The environment at Schnurmacher is tailored to the needs of patients who require medical and nursing services but who do not need the complexity of services associated with an acute-care hospital. And Schnurmacher Subacute Medical patients are out of bed more quickly and as often as possible, which helps them maintain functional status while recovery progresses.

7251 South Shore Healthcare
275 W Merrick Rd
Freeport, NY 11520-3346
516-623-4000
FAX: 516-223-4599
www.northshorelij.com
Winnie Mack, RN, BSN, MPA, Regional Executive Director
Gene Tangney, Senior Vice President/ Regional Executive Director
Michael J. Dowling, President/ CEO
David L. Battinelli, MD, Senior Vice President/Chief Medical Officer
North Shore-LIJ Health System includes 16 award-winning hospitals and nearly 400 physician practice locations throughout New York, including Long Island, Manhattan, Queens and Staten Island. Proudly serving an area of seven million people, North Shore-LIJ delivers world-class services designed for every step of your health and wellness journey.

7252 St. Camillus Health and Rehabilitation Center
813 Fay Rd
Syracuse, NY 13219-3009
315-488-2951
FAX: 315-488-3255
e-mail: info@st-camillus.org
www.st-camillus.org
Aileen Balitz, President
Patrick VanBeveren, PT, DPT, M, Supervisor of Physical Therapy
Nancy, Pirro, RN, Case Manager
Kathy Walsh,PT, DPT, NCS, Designer/Facilitator
Since our founding in 1969, St. Camillus' mission has been to provide high-quality services and facilities emphasizing the rehabilitation of individuals to their maximum potential. The importance of the human spirit drives all we do. We are dedicated to caring for life and helping individuals achieve their highest possible level of independence.

North Carolina

7253 Chapel Hill Rehabilitation and Healthcare Center
1602 E Franklin St
Chapel Hill, NC 27514-2892
919-967-1418
800-735-8262
FAX: 919-918-3811
www.chapelhillhc.com
Turner Prichett, Executive Director
Chapel Hill Rehabilitation and Healthcare Center accomodates 120 residents. We are located in downtown Chapel Hill on Franklin Street and we provide roud the clock nursing care 365 days a year. Intensive rehabilitation services are administered by our licensed speech, occupational and physical therapists. Our staff is trained to care for medically complex patients such as those requiring intensive wound care, dialysis, and artificial nutrition.

7254 Cypress Pointe Rehabilitation and Healthcare Center
2006 S 16th St
Wilmington, NC 28401-6613
910-763-6271
800-735-8262
FAX: 910-251-9803
e-mail: HSDED0188@kindredhealthcare.com
www.cypresspointehc.com
Sara Deiter, Executive Director
Dr. Jose Gonzalez, Medical Director
Cypress Pointe offers comprehensive physical, occupational, speech and respiratory therapy services. Following a physician's referral, patients are evaluated to determine their needs. Recommendations are then made for the appropriate interventions and rehabilitation. If therapy is required, a personalized care plan is developed.

7255 Pettigrew Rehabilitation and Healthcare Center
1551 W Pettigrew St
Durham, NC 27705-4821
919-286-0751
800-735-8262
FAX: 919-286-5992
e-mail: HSDED0116@kindredhealthcare.com
www.pettigrewhc.com
La'Ticia Beatty, Executive Director

Pettigrew Rehabilitation and Healthcare Center accomodates 107 residents. Our healthcare center is certified by Medicare and Medicaid. We have experienced staff members who care for our residents. We strive to improve the quality of life our residents experience as a result of the services they receive from our nursing and therapy departments.

7256 **Raleigh Rehabilitation and Healthcare Center**
616 Wade Ave
Raleigh, NC 27605-1237 919-828-6251
800-735-8262
FAX: 919-828-3294
e-mail: HSDED0143@kindredhealthcare.com
www.raleighrehabhc.com
Steven Jones, Executive Director
Raleigh Rehabilitation and Healthcare Center accomodates 172 residents. We provide short-term rehabilitation-including, physical, occupational, and speech therapies-as well as long-term nursing services. We specialize in neurological disorders, complex diabetes treatment, amputation recovery and pain management. We welcome short stays (respite care). Transportation services are availiable for physician appointments and dialysis treatments.

7257 **Rehabilitation and Healthcare Center of Monroe**
1212 E Sunset Dr
Monroe, NC 28112-4318 704-283-8548
800-735-8262
FAX: 704-283-4664
e-mail: HSDED0707@kindredhealthcare.com
www.monroehc.com
Judy Olson, Executive Director
We accomodate 159 residents and are certified for Medicare and Medicaid. We specialize in short-term rehabilitation as well as long-term care. Our therapists, wound nurse and dietician work closely to administer wound care. We hav 2 dialysis centers within a 10-block radius and gladly accpet their patients. We have an on-staff medical director as well as a psychiatrist.

7258 **Winston-Salem Rehabilitation and Healthcare Center**
1900 W 1st St
Winston Salem, NC 27104-4220 336-724-2821
800-735-8262
FAX: 336-725-8314
Tom Bauer, Administrator
We accommodate 230 residents and we have approximately 250 employees. Our staffing ratio averages 1 licensed nurse for every 20 residents and 1 Certified Nursing Assistant for every 10 residents. We offer a wide range of services including but not limited to respiratory care, tracheotomy care and gastric tube feeding and we also feature an in house licensed therapy program.

Ohio

7259 **Arbors East Subacute and Rehabilitation Center**
5500 E Broad St
Columbus, OH 43213-1476 614-575-9003
FAX: 614-575-9101
e-mail: arborseast@extendicare.com
www.arborseastskillednursing.com

7260 **Arbors at Canton Subacute And Rehabilitation Center**
2714 13th St NW
Canton, OH 44708-3121 330-456-2842
FAX: 330-456-5343
www.laurelsofcanton.com
Amy McDermand, Director of Marketing
Beth Jones, PT, DPT, Rehabilitation Services Director
Cindy Shingler, RN,, Director of Nursing
Jennifer Fess, Administrator
We provide individualized, quality care to guests staying short-term for rehabilitation services or long-term for extended care services. The highest level of independence for our guests is the creed of The Laurels of Canton.

7261 **Arbors at Dayton**
320 Albany St
Dayton, OH 45408-1402 937-496-6200
FAX: 937-496-1990
e-mail: dayton@extendicare.com
www.extendicareus.com/dayton
Dave Maxwell, Administrator
Carlisa Pedalino, Administrator
Arbors at Dayton is a leading provider of long-term skilled nursing care and short-term rehabilitation solutions. Our 106 bed facility offers a full continuum of services and care focused around each individual in today's ever-changing healthcare environment.

7262 **Arbors at Marietta**
400 N 7th St
Marietta, OH 45750-2024 740-373-3597
FAX: 740-376-0004
e-mail: marietta@extendicare.com
www.extendicareus.com/marietta
Joan Florence, Director of Nursing
Kenneth Leopold, Medical Director
Arbors at Marietta is a leading provider of long-term skilled nursing care and short-term rehabilitation solutions. Our 150 bed facility offers a full continuum of services and care focused around each individual in today's ever-changing healthcare environment.

7263 **Arbors at Milford**
5900 Meadow Creek Dr
Milford, OH 45150-5641 513-248-1655
FAX: 513-248-7340
e-mail: milford@extendicare.com
www.extendicareus.com/milford
Bruce Yarwood, President/CEO
Mark Ostendorf, Administrator
Arbors at Milford is a leading provider of long-term skilled nursing care and short-term rehabilitation solutions. Our 139 bed facility offers a full continuum of services and care focused around each individual in today's ever-changing healthcare environment.

7264 **Arbors at Sylvania**
7120 Port Sylvania Dr
Toledo, OH 43617-1158 419-841-2200
FAX: 419-841-2822
e-mail: sylvania@extendicare.com
www.extendicareus.com/sylvania
Sheril Flowers, Administrator
Graig Hopple, Medical Director
Arbors at Sylvania is a leading provider of long-term skilled nursing care and short-term rehabilitation solutions. Our 79 bed facility offers a full continuum of services and care focused around each individual in today's ever-changing healthcare environment.

7265 **Arbors at Toledo Subacute and Rehab Centre**
2920 Cherry St
Toledo, OH 43608-1716 419-242-7458
FAX: 419-242-6514
www.extendicare.com
Jill Schlievert, Administrator
Subacute rehabilitation services and facility.

7266 **Bridgepark Center for Rehabilitation and Nursing Services**
145 Olive St
Akron, OH 44310-3236 330-762-0901
800-750-0750
FAX: 330-762-0905
www.bridgeparkrehab.net
Joseph Burick, Medical Director
A skilled nursing and rehabilitation center located in Akron, Ohio, across the street from St. Thomas Hospital with a beautiful view of the Akron skyline. Access to Interstate 77 and State Route 8 is just minutes away. Our entire staff is committed to providing caring, customer-focused skilled nursing and rehabilitation. For

your convenience, we accept Medicare, Medicaid and most managed care and private insurance.

7267 **Broadview Multi-Care Center**
5520 Broadview Rd
Parma, OH 44134-1605 216-749-4010
FAX: 216-749-0141
e-mail: info@broadviewmulticare.com
www.broadviewmulticare.com

Harold Shachter, Owner
Mike Flank, VP
Broadview Multi-Care Center is a family run business with more than 40 years of experience providing quality care to the community. We are committed to meeting your needs and providing you with a warm, home-like environment. Our family is on-site and our doors are always open for your suggestions or to drop in and say hello. We always try to take and honor requests, whether it's a favorite food, an exciting activity or a particular room.

7268 **Caprice Care Center**
9184 Market St
North Lima, OH 44452-9558 330-965-9200
FAX: 330-726-6097
e-mail: capriceadm@chcccompanies.com
www.chcccompanies.com/CapriceMain.html

Lori Crowl, Owner
Becky Berger, Director of Nursin
Stacey Howell, Administrator
Valerie Conzett, Admission Liaison
A 106-bed skilled nursing, subacute and rehabilitation facility. Our goal is to provide comfortable living to all who are in our care. Caprice Health Care Center is a contemporary Medicare and Medicaid approved facility specializing in short-term rehabilitation services. The inpatient/outpatient rehab department includes physical, occupational, speech therapies, indoor aquatic therapy pool, as well as complimentary van transportation for outpatient services.

7269 **Cleveland Clinic**
9500 Euclid Ave
Cleveland, OH 44195-2 216-444-2200
800-801-2273
FAX: 216-444-7021
my.clevelandclinic.org/default.aspx

Gene Altus, Executive Director
Delos M. Cosgrove, MD, Chief Executive Officer, Preside
Joseph F. Hahn, MD, Chief of Staff, Vice Chairman of
David Bronson, MD, Chief Executive Officer, Clevela
A not-for-profit, multispecialty academic medical center that integrates clinical and hospital care with research and education. Cleveland clinic was founded in 1921 by 4 renowned physicians with a vision of providing outstanding patient care based upon the principals of cooperation, compassion and innovation. Today, Cleveland Clinic is one of the largest and most respected hospitals in the country.

7270 **Columbus Rehabilitation And Subacute Institute**
111 West Michigan Street
Milwaukee, WI 53203-2903 800-395-5000
e-mail: kschaewe@extendicare.com
www.extendicareus.com

Kelly Fligor, Administrator
Jillian Fountain, Secretary
Subacute rehabilitation programs and facility.

7271 **LakeMed Nursing and Rehabilitation Center**
70 Normandy Dr
Painesville, OH 44077-1616 440-357-1311
800-750-0750
FAX: 440-352-9977
www.lakemednursing.com

Connie Eyman, Administrator
Vesta Jones, Executive Director
Our goal is to provide you with quality care and we are known for our successful short-term rehab and care of the clinically complex. We also offer respite services to give caregivers a rest, and hospice services through our local hospice care provider. Our interdisciplinary team works together as they strive to deliver quality care and responsive service to our residents.

7272 **Oregon Nursing And Rehabilitation Center**
904 Isaac Streets Dr
Oregon, OH 43616-3204 419-691-2483
FAX: 419-697-5401
www.extendicareus.com/oregon

Mark Rogers, Administrator
Subacute rehabilitation facility and services.

7273 **Sunset View Castle Nursing Homes Castle Nursing Homes**
434 N Washington St
Millersburg, OH 44654-1188 330-674-0015
FAX: 330-763-2238
e-mail: info@castlenursinghomes.com
www.castlenursinghomes.com

Becky Snyder, Admissions Coordinator
Kathy Edwards, Admissions And Marketing
310 licensed, certified beds. Subacute rehabilitation facility and programs.

Oregon

7274 **Care Center East Health & Specialty Care Center**
Expendicare
11325 NE Weidler St
Portland, OR 97220-1950 503-253-1181
FAX: 503-253-1871
www.extendicareus.com

Glydon Kimbrough, Administrator
Subacute rehabilitation facility and programs

7275 **Medford Rehabilitation and Healthcare Center**
Kindred Healthcare
625 Stevens St
Medford, OR 97504-6719 541-779-3551
800-735-1232
FAX: 541-779-3658
www.medfordrehab.com

Grant Gloor, Administrator
Dane Reeves, Executive Director
Kristen W., Health and Rehabilitation Center
Becky D., Activity Director
We strive to provide quality, compassionate care. Our cozy building accomodates 110 residents. Our smaller size creates an inviting and homelike environment. We offer semi-private rooms with space to add items from home for a special personalized touch.

Pennsylvania

7276 **Dresher Hill Health and Rehabilitation Center**
1390 Camp Hill Rd
Dresher, PA 19034-2805 215-643-0600
FAX: 215-641-0628
www.dresherhillskillednursing.com

Earl Kimble, Administrator
Subacute rehabilitation facility and programs: physical/speech.

7277 **Good Shepherd Rehabilitation**
850 S 5th St
Allentown, PA 18103-3295 610-776-3586
888-447-3422
FAX: 610-776-8336
e-mail: info@goodshepherdrehab.org
goodshepherdrehab.org

John Kristel, MBA, MPT, President & CEO
Mike Bonner, MBA, Vice President, Neurosciences
Ronald J. Petula, CPA, Senior Vice President, Finance and Chief Financial Officer
Joseph Shadid, Administrator, Good Shepherd Home-Bethlehem
A world class rehabilitation network, Good Shepherd provides comprehensive inpatient and outpatient services throughout Pennsylvania's Lehigh Valley. Founded in 1908, Good Shepherd

has steadily expanded over last 95 years. Good Shepherd is one of the most comprehensive rehabilitation institutes in the world.

7278 **Statesman Health and Rehabilitation Center**
2629 Trenton Rd
Levittown, PA 19056-1428 215-943-7777
FAX: 215-943-1240
www.statesmanskillednursing.com
Jamie Tanner, Administrator
Subacute rehabilitation facility and programs.

7279 **UPMC Braddock**
200 Lothrop St.
Pittsburgh, PA 15213-2582 412-647-8762
800-533-8762
FAX: 412-636-5398
e-mail: hospitalbill@upmc.edu
upmc.com
Mark Sevco, Administrator
Rodney Jones, Vice President
With a team of more then 43,000 employees, UPMC serves the health needs of more then 4 million people each year, improving lives in western Pennsylvania-and beyond-through redefined models of health care delivery and superb clinical outcomes.

7280 **UPMC McKeesport**
Presby
1500 5th Ave
McKeesport, PA 15132-2422 412-664-2000
FAX: 412-664-2309
e-mail: fisherpj@upmc.edu
upmc.com
Ronald H Ott, CEO
Offers 56 beds for patients who need skilled nursing care. Offers ongoing rehabilitation and educational programs to patients with cardiac, neurologic, and orthopaedic diagnosis.

7281 **UPMC Passavant**
9100 Babcock Blvd
Pittsburgh, PA 15237-5842 412-367-6700
800-533-8762
e-mail: gloordc@ph.upmc.edu
upmc.com
William Kristan, Dir Inpatient Physical Therapy
Teresa Petrick, Chief Executive Officer
Patients who have had an acute illness, injury, or exacerbation of a disease and no longer need the intensity of services in the acute care setting, but still require some complex medical care or supervision and rehabilitation services, may be appropriate to be transferred into the Subacute Unit.

Rhode Island

7282 **Kindred Heights Nursing & Rehabilitation Center**
Kindred Healthcare
680 South Fourth Street
Louisville, KY 40202 502-596-7300
800-545-0749
e-mail: web_administrator@kindred.com
www.kindredheights.com
Sandra Sarza, Manager
Jean Aubin, Director
Kindred Heights Nursing and Rehabilitation Center accomodates 58 residents and serves the needs of elders in the greater East Bay and Providence area. We are conveniently located on Wampanoag Trail in East Providence. Kindred Heights provides skilled nursing, short-term rehab and long-term care in a family environment, but we are large enough to manage the complex nursing and rehab care needs our residents may have.

7283 **Oak Hill Nursing and Rehabilitation Center**
Kindered Health Care
544 Pleasant St
Pawtucket, RI 02860-5776 401-725-8888
800-745-6575
FAX: 401-723-5720
www.oakhillrehab.com
Scott M. Sandborn, Executive Director
Heidi Capela, Director Nursing
Amybeth Almeida, Director Admissions
Aman Nanda, Medical Director
Accomodates 143 residents. Throughout our 40 year history, Oak Hill has developed a reputation as one of the finest healthcare centers in Rhode Island. Our center consists of 3 separate units. A 34-bed post-acute unit provides care to the medically complex and those in need of extensive rehabilitative services. A 20-bed Alzheimer's Special Care Unit provides a unique style of care utilizing habilitative therapy in comfortable, home-like surroundings.

7284 **Southern New England Rehab Center**
200 High Service Avenue
North Providence, RI 02904 401-456-3801
888-456-4501
FAX: 401-456-3784
www.snerc.com
Vivian Hagstrom, Manager
The Center's skilled staff of over 100 professionals provides a full range of coordinated rehabilitative care. Our clinical expertise and compassion make a big difference as we develop first-rate plans of care for the unique needs of each patient. Our medical staff is comprised of physicians board-certified in rehabilitation medicine and internal medicine.

South Carolina

7285 **Tuomey Healthcare System**
129 N Washington St
Sumter, SC 29150-4949 803-774-9000
FAX: 803-774-8737
www.tuomey.com
R Jay Cox, CEO
Here to anticipte the needs of the communities we serve, responding with proactive healthcare initiatives, providing expert rehabilitative services and delivering life-saving acute care.

Tennessee

7286 **Camden Healthcare and Rehabilitation Center**
680 South Fourth Street
Louisville, KY 40202 502-596-7300
800-545-0749
e-mail: web_administrator@kindred.com
kindredhealthcare.com
Mark Walker, Administrator
Subacute rehabilitation products and services, nursing and life care homes.

7287 **Centennial Medical Center Tri Star Health System**
2300 Patterson St
Nashville, TN 37203-1538 615-342-1000
800-242-5662
FAX: 615-342-1045
e-mail: Laurel.Haskamp@HCAHealthcare.com
tristarcentennial.com
Thomas L Herron, President/Chief Executive Office
Above all else we are committed to the care and improvement of human life by caring for those we serve with integrity, compassion, a positive attitude, respect and exceptional quality.

7288 Cordova Rehabilitation and Nursing Center
955 N Germantown Pkwy
Cordova, TN 38018-6215 901-754-1393
800-848-0299
FAX: 901-754-3332
e-mail: cdadmi@gracehc.com
www.gracehccordova.com

John Palmer, Administrator
Renee Tutor, Executive Director
Our professional staff can help you make an informed decision. Upon admission, our interdisciplinary team develops a comprehensive care plan to meet not only physical and rehabilitative goals, but also social and emotional needs. We understand the importance of family and resident involvement and encourage participation in the development of a personalized plan of care.

7289 Erlanger Medical Center Baronness Campus
975 E 3rd St
Chattanooga, TN 37403-2147 423-778-7000
FAX: 423-778-7615
e-mail: guestrelations@erlanger.org
www.erlanger.org

Kevin M. Spiegel, FACHE, President and CEO
James Creel, MD, Chief Medical Officer
Gregg T. Gentry, Chief Administrative Officer
Robert M. Brooks, FACHE, Executive Vice President and Chief Operating Officer
Our mission is to improve the health of the people we touch. Our vision is to be recognized locally, regionally, and and nationally, as a premiere healthcare system.

7290 Huntington Health and Rehabilitation Center
635 High St
Huntingdon, TN 38344-1703 731-986-8943
FAX: 731-986-3188
e-mail: w.summers@huntingdonhealth.com
huntingdonhealth.com

Heidi Hawkins, Administrator
Windi Summers, Admissions Director
Subacute rehabilitation facility and programs.

7291 Madison Healthcare and Rehabilitation Center
431 Larkin Springs Rd
Madison, TN 37115-5005 615-865-8520
800-848-0299
FAX: 615-868-4455
www.madisonrehab.com

Phyllis Cherry, Executive Director
At our facility, we provide quality care with modern rehabilitation and restorative nursing techniques. We aim to provide an atmosphere which encourages family involvement in the care-planning process, with the right mix of activities addressing the social, spiritual and intellectual needs of our residents.

7292 Mariner Health of Nashville
3939 Hillsboro Cir
Nashville, TN 37215-2708 615-297-2100
FAX: 615-297-2197

David Reeves, Administrator
Amy Artrip, Director of Nursing
Religious nonmedical health care institution. 150-bed subacute rehabilitation facility

7293 Pine Meadows Healthcare and Rehabilitation Center
700 Nuckolls Rd
Bolivar, TN 38008-1531 731-658-4707
FAX: 731-658-4769
e-mail: s.mckeen@pinemeadowshc.com
www.pinemeadowshc.com

Larry Shrader, Administrator
Sharon McKeen, Admissions Director
Our goal is to take care of your loved ones. Our professional team works with skilled hands, is directed by creative minds and is guided by compassionate hearts. Upon your admission, our interdisciplinary team develops a comprehensive care plan designed with a goal of meeting not only physical and rehabilitative objectives, but also social and emotional needs. We understand the importance of family and resident involvement and encourage participation in the development of a plan of care.

7294 Primacy Healthcare and Rehabilitation Center
Kindred Health Care
6025 Primacy Pkwy
Memphis, TN 38119-5763 901-767-1040
800-848-0299
FAX: 901-685-7362
www.primacyrehab.com

Donnie Dubert, Executive Director
Dr. Mark Hammond, Medical Director
Kristen W., Health and Rehabilitation Center
Becky D., Activity Director
Upon a resident's admission, our interdisciplinary team develops a comprehensive care plan with a goal of meeting not only physical and rehabilitative objectives but also social and emotional needs. We understand the importance of family and resident involvement and encourage participation in the development of a personalized plan of care.

7295 Ripley Healthcare and Rehabilitation Center
118 Halliburton St
Ripley, TN 38063-2011 731-635-5180
FAX: 731-635-0663
e-mail: j.hodge@ripleyhc.com
www.ripleyhc.com

Johnny Rea, Executive Director
Brandon Whiteside, Executive Director
Jan Hodge, Admissions Directo
Jennifer Pitts, Administrator
Upon admission, our interdisciplinary team develops a comprehensive care plan to meet not only physical and rehabilitative goals, but also social and emotional needs. We understand the importance of family and resident involvement and encourage participation in the development of a personalized care plan. Our goal is to take care of your loved ones.

7296 Shelby Pines Rehabilitation and Healthcare Center
3909 Covington Pike
Memphis, TN 38135-2281 901-377-1011
FAX: 901-377-0032

Rene Tutor, Executive Director
Subacute rehabiltation facility and programs.

7297 Siskin Hospital for Physical Rehabilitation
1 Siskin Plz
Chattanooga, TN 37403-1306 423-634-1200
FAX: 423-634-4538
TTY:423-634-1201
e-mail: info@siskinrehab.org
siskinrehab.org

Robert Main, CEO
Lindsay Wyatt, Media Coordinator, Marketing Co
Dedicated exclusively to physical rehabilitation and offers specialized treatment programs in brain injury, amputation, stroke, spinal cord injury, orthopeadics, and major multiple trauma.

Texas

7298 North Hills Hospital
4401 Booth Calloway Rd
North Richland Hills, TX 76180-7399 817-255-1000
FAX: 817-255-1991
northhillshospital.com

Randy Moresi, CEO
North Hills Hospital's services include a wide range of cardiovascular services, surgical services, emergency services, radiology, a rehabilitation unit, a senior health center, therapy services, and women's services.

7299 Valley Regional Medical Center
100 E Alton Gloor Blvd
Brownsville, TX 78526-3328
956-350-7000
FAX: 956-350-7111
valleyregionalmedicalcenter.com

Susan Andrews, CEO
Francisco Javier Del Castillo, MD
Subramaniam Anandasivam, MD
Christopher Olson, MD

Above all else, we are committed to the care and improvement of human life. In recognition of this committment, we strive to deliver high quality, cost effective healthcare in the communities we serve. In persuit of our mission, we recognize and affirm the unique and intrinsic worth of each individual. We treat all those we serve with compassion and kindness. We act with absolute honesty and integrity and fairness in the way we conduct our business and the way we live our lives.

Utah

7300 Crosslands Rehabilitation and Healthcare Center
680 South Fourth Street
Louisville, KY 40202
502-596-7300
800-545-0749
e-mail: web_administrator@kindred.com
www.kindredhealthcare.com

John Williams, Executive Director
Lyle Black, Manager

Crossroads Rehabilitation and Healthcare accomodates 120 residents. We are fully Medicare and Medicaid certified. We are proud of our reputation for providing quality, compassionate care. Services availiable include in-house physical, occupational and speech therapies, as well as 24-hour licensed nursing staff coverage. We offer therapeutic recreation, in-house social services and registered dietician services, among many other professional services.

7301 Federal Heights Rehabilitation and Nursing Center
Kindred Health Care
680 South Fourth Street
Louisville, KY 40202
502-596-7300
800-545-0749
e-mail: web_administrator@kindred.com
www.kindredhealthcare.com

Pete Zeigler, Executive Director
Dr. Charles Canfield, Medical Director

Federal Heights accomodates 120 residents. We are located near three major hospitals in the Salt Lake Valley. We specialize in providing nursing services for complex medical and rehabilitation conditions. Our discharge planning works jointly with the family and resident in determining the future needs and goals upon discharge.

7302 St. George Care and Rehabilitation Center
Kindred Health Care Publications
1032 E 100 S
Saint George, UT 84770-3005
435-628-0488
800-346-4128
FAX: 435-628-7362
www.stgeorgecare.com

John Larson, Plant Manager
Erin Hammon, Director of Nursing
Derrick Glum, Executive Director

St. George Care and Rehabilitation accomodates 95 residents. We offer a 4,000 square foot rehabilitation gym with an indoor therapy pool for inpatient and outpatient services. Therapy is provided to meet specific needs seven days a week. There is a dietitian on staff for individualized nutritional needs. We offer an Alzheimer's unit with specialized staff. We provide compassionate health services including physicians, nurses, physical therapists, and occupational therapist and licensed aides.

7303 St. Mark's Hospital
1200 E 3900 S
Salt Lake City, UT 84124-1390
801-268-7111
FAX: 801-270-3489
www.stmarkshospital.com

Steve B. Bateman, CEO

Above all else we are committed to the care and improvement of human life. In recognition of this commitment, we strive to deliver high quality, cost effective healthcare in the communities we serve. We define quality as 'caring people with the commitment to a continuous process of improvement in the services provided, that will better enable the hospital to meet or exceed our customer's needs and expectations.

7304 Wasatch Valley Rehabilitation
Kindred Healthcare
680 South Fourth Street
Louisville, KY 40202
502-596-7300
800-545-0749
e-mail: web_administrator@kindred.com
www.kindredhealthcare.com

Alex Stevenson, Executive Director
Ric Toomer, Executive Director

Wasatch Valley accomodates 110 residents. We are licensed for Medicare and Medicaid and we are conveniently located in the heart of Salt Lake City with easy access from I-15 and I-215. We are known by the area hospitals as a specialist in wound care and for the care we provide to those with complex medical conditions.

Virginia

7305 Nansemond Pointe Rehabilitation and Healthcare Center
200 Constance Rd
Suffolk, VA 23434-4960
757-539-8744
800-828-1140
FAX: 757-539-6128
www.nansemondhc.com

Mel Epelle, Executive Director
Mary R, Activities Assistant
Kristen W., Health and Rehabilitation Center
Becky D., Activity Director

Nansemond Pointe Rehabilitation and Healthcare Center accomodates 160 residents in private and semi-private rooms. We have been serving the needs of Suffolk, Virginia and the surrounding areas for over 38 years. We offer an entire continuum of care from assisted living apartments to skilled nursing to long-term care. Our licensed therapists, working with our dedicated nursing staff, share a common goal- to help our residents improve their level of recovery and independence.

7306 Rehabilitation and Research Center Virginia Commonwealth University
1250 East Marshall Street
Richmond, VA 23298
804-828-9000
FAX: 804-828-5074
www.vcuhealth.org

Michael Rao, Ph.D., VCU President & VCUHS President,
Sheldon M. Retchin, M.D., VP Health Sciences & CEO, VCUHS
John Duval, Chief Executive Officer MCV Hosp
Dominic J. Puleo, Executive VP Finance and CFO, VC

The Rehabilitation and Research Center is a collaborative effort between the Department of Physical Medicine and Rehabilitation and the Medical College of Virginia Hospitals. The goals of the Rehabilitation and Research Center at the Medical College of Virginia Hospitals (MCVH) are to provide highly-skilled, interdisciplinary, inpatient rehabilitative care to adults with complex needs; to be an advocate and educator for patients and people with disabilities.

7307 Warren Memorial Hospital
1000 N Shenandoah Ave
Front Royal, VA 22630-3598
540-636-0300
800-994-6610
FAX: 540-636-0258
e-mail: complaint@jointcommission.org
www.valleyhealthlink.com
Mark H. Merrill, President & Chief Executive Officer
Tonya Smith, Vice President of Operations
Pete Gallagher, Senior Vice President & CFO
Joan Roscoe, Vice President of Information Sy
A nonprofit organization of health care providers, Valley Health offers a full spectrum of services in acute care, rehabilitation and extended care facilities, and outpatient and community settings to help the people of the region manage their health and enjoy a high quality of life. Valley Health has the resources to diagnose, treat and help patients manage virtually any medical problem that may be encountered.

7308 Winchester Rehabilitation Center
333 W Cork St
Suite 230
Winchester, VA 22601-3870
540-536-5114
800-994-6610
FAX: 540-536-1122
e-mail: complaint@jointcommission.org
www.valleyhealthlink.com
Mark H. Merrill, President & Chief Executive Officer
Tonya Smith, Vice President of Operations
Pete Gallagher, Senior Vice President & CFO
Joan Roscoe, Vice President of Information Sy
Offers the following rehabilitation services: Sub-Acute inpatient rehabilitation, Speech therapy, Physical therapy, Occupational therapy, Disability evaluations. 30-bed inpatient center.

Washington

7309 Aldercrest Health and Rehabilitation Center
21400 72nd Ave W
Edmonds, WA 98026-7702
425-775-1961
FAX: 425-771-0116
e-mail: aldercrest@extendicare.com
www.aldercrestskillednursing.com
Rick Milsow, Administrator
Aldercrest Health & Rehabilitation Center is a leading provider of long-term skilled nursing care and short-term rehabilitation solutions. Our 124 bed facility offers a full continuum of services and care focused around each individual in today's ever-changing healthcare environment.

7310 Arden Rehabilitation and Healthcare Center
16357 Aurora Ave N
Seattle, WA 98133-5651
206-542-3103
800-833-6384
FAX: 206-542-7192
www.ardenrehab.com
Matthew Preston, Administrator
Ann Zell, Executive Director
Kristen W., Health and Rehabilitation Center
Becky D., Activity Director
Arden Rehabilitation has been an integral part of the Shoreline community since 1953. It is a one-level building set on mature grounds with several beautiful courtyards for the residents to enjoy. Arden can accomodate 90 residents-post acute/rehabilitation patients as well as long-term residents. Medicare certified, the center also takes most managed healthcare insurance plans, as well as VA, respite and hospice patients.

7311 Bellingham Health Care and Rehabilitation Services
1200 Birchwood Ave
Bellingham, WA 98225-1302
360-734-9295
800-833-6384
FAX: 360-671-4368
www.avamererehabofbellingham.com
Melissa Nelson, Executive Director
Dr. Richard McClenahan, Medical Director
Kristen W., Health and Rehabilitation Center
Becky D., Activity Director
At Bellingham Health Care and Rehab, we strive to provide quality, compassionate care. Our cozy building accomodates 84 residents. Our smaller size creates an inviting and homelike environment for your loved one. We offer semi-private rooms with space to add items from home for a special personalized touch. Provides meals served restaurant style in our dinning room overlooking our beautiful grounds.

7312 Bremerton Convalescent and Rehabilitation Center
2701 Clare Ave
Bremerton, WA 98310-3313
360-377-3951
FAX: 360-377-5443
bremertonskillednursing.com
Stephanie Bonanzino, Administrator
Subacute rehabilitation facility and programs.

7313 Edmonds Rehabilitation & Healthcare Centerer
Kindred Healthcare
21008 76th Ave W
Edmonds, WA 98026-7104
425-778-0107
800-833-6384
FAX: 425-776-9532
www.edmondsrehab.com
Jane Davis, Executive Director
At Edmonds Rehabilitation and Healthcare, we strive to provide quality, compassionate care. Our center accomodates 91 residents. Our smaller size creates an inviting and homelike environment. We offer semi-private rooms with space to add items from home for a special personalized touch. Edmonds Rehabilitation and Healthcare provides delicious meals served restaurant style in our dinning room.

7314 Heritage Health and Rehabilitation Center
Kindred Health Care
3605 Y St
Vancouver, WA 98663-2647
360-693-5839
800-833-6384
FAX: 360-693-3991
www.heritagerehab.com
Michael Moses, Executive Director
Su Patchett, Director of Nursing
Heritage Health & Rehabilitation Center is the smallest free-standing healthcare center in southwest Washington with accomodations of 49, enabling more personal care and a more home-like environment. Heritage has licensed nursing staff, restorative aides, and certified nurses assistants, trained and experienced in providing Alzheimer's care, end of life/hospice care, psychiatric care, rehabilitative care, and respite care.

7315 North Auburn Rehabilitation And Health Center
111 West Michigan Street
Milwaukee, WI 53203-2903
800-395-5000
e-mail: kschaewe@extendicare.com
extendicare.com
Allyson Jenkins, Administrator
Subacute rehabilitation facility and programs.

7316 Northwoods Lodge
2321 NW Schold Pl
Silverdale, WA 98383-9504
360-698-3930
FAX: 360-692-2169
e-mail: mhalverson@encorecommunities.com
www.encorecommunities.com
Leslie Krueger, Owner
Debbie Griffin, Director of Rehab Services
Silverdale Campus, Executive Director

Provides you with a full-range of services from weekly housekeeping and laudry services, to grounds keeping and maintenance. Our monthy fee inculdes utilities and hot, delicious, nutritious meals served table side every day. We offer transportation services, full-time activities directors, and numerous amenities to add to your comfort and enjoyment.

7317 **Pacific Specialty & Rehabilitation Center r**
1015 N Garrison Rd
Vancouver, WA 98664-1313 360-694-7501
FAX: 360-694-8148
www.pacificskillednursing.com
Rebecca Pruett, Administrator
Subacute rehabilitation facility and programs.

7318 **Puget Sound Healthcare Center**
4001 Capitol Mall Dr SW
Olympia, WA 98502-8657 360-754-9792
FAX: 360-754-2455
www.pugetsoundskillednursing.com
Sheila Oberg, Administrator
Our goal is to provide excellence in patient care, veteran's benefits and customer satisfaction. We have reformed our department internally and are striving for high quality, prompt and seamless service to veterans. Our department employees continue to offer their dedication and commitment to help veterans get the services they have earned.

7319 **Vancouver Health & Rhabilitation Center**
400 E 33rd St
Vancouver, WA 98663-2238 360-696-2561
800-833-6384
FAX: 360-696-9275
www.vancouverhealthcare.com
Jody Wigen, Human Resources
Joe Joy, Executive Director
Kristen W., Health and Rehabilitation Center
Becky D., Activity Director
At Vancouver Health and Rehab Center we strive to provide quality, compassionate care. Our cozy building accomodates 98 residents. Our smaller size creates an inviting and homelike environment. We offer semi-private rooms with space to add items from home for a special personalized touch. Provides delicious meals served restaurant style in our dining room.

West Virginia

7320 **War Memorial Hospital**
1 Healthy Way
Berkeley Springs, WV 25411-1743 304-258-1234
FAX: 304-258-5618
e-mail: complaint@jointcommission.org
www.valleyhealthlink.com
Mark H. Merrill, President & Chief Executive Officer
Tonya Smith, Vice President of Operations
Pete Gallagher, Senior Vice President & Chief Financial Officer
Joan Roscoe, Vice President of Information Systems
Offers physical therapy, occupational therapy, speech therapy, social services, and patient/family education for individuals who have experienced a recent physical disability due to disease, dysfunction, or general debilitation. Helps patients to maximize their abilities through activities of daily living, mobility, self-medication, and self-care and restore their ability to return to their previous lifestyle.

Wisconsin

7321 **Cedar Spring Health and Rehabilitation Center**
N27w5707 Lincoln Blvd
Cedarburg, WI 53012-2852 262-376-7676
FAX: 262-376-7808
www.cedarspringsskillednursing.com
Mary Wirth, Executive Director
Subacute rehabilitation facility and programs.

7322 **Clearview-Brain Injury Center**
198 Home Rd
Juneau, WI 53039-1401 920-386-3400
877-386-3400
FAX: 920-386-3800
e-mail: lbertagnoli@co.dodge.wi.us
co.dodge.wi.us/clearview
Jane E. Hooper, Administrator
Jacqueline Kuhl, Household Coordinator
Laura Bertagnoli
Kathy Lorenz, AFH Manager
A 30-bed, state certified, subacute neuro-rehabilitation program in Juneau, WI. We are located just 45 minutes northeast of Madison WI and 10 minutes east of Beaver Dam, WI. We are the first and longest standing of only 2 community re-entry programs in the state of Wisconsin providing subacute neuro-rehabilitation to teens and adults who have experienced a brain injury.

7323 **Colonial Manor Medical and Rehabilitation Center**
1010 E Wausau Ave
Wausau, WI 54403-3101 715-842-2028
800-947-6644
FAX: 715-848-0510
www.colonialmanormrc.com
Ericca Ylitalo, Administrator
Shelley Solberg, Executive Director
Kristen W., Health and Rehabilitation Center
Becky D., Activity Director
Colonial Manor Medical and Rehabilitation Center is part of the Kindred Community and is located in Wausau, Wisconsin. The corporate headquarters are based in Louisville Kentucky. Our facility accomodates 150 residents.

7324 **Eastview Medical and Rehabilitation Center**
729 Park St
Antigo, WI 54409-2745 715-623-2356
800-947-6644
FAX: 715-623-6345
www.eastviewmedrehab.com
Wanda Hose, Administrator
Wanda Hose, Executive Director
Kristen W., Health and Rehabilitation Center
Becky D., Activity Director
Eastview Medical Center and Rehabilitation Center accomodates 165 residents. We are Medicare and Medicaid certified, as well as being Joint Commission accredited. Our 'TEAM' approach means specially trained staff work around the clock to assist in meeting rehabilitative goals established by our team of professionals. We encourage family involvement in our rehabilitative process. The support of loved ones is a major key to a speedy recovery.

7325 **Hospitality Nursing Rehabilitation Center**
8633 32nd Ave
Kenosha, WI 53142-5187 262-694-8300
FAX: 262-694-3622
www.hospitalityskillednursing.com
Marla Benson, Administrator
LaRae Nelson, President
Lisa Behling, Secretary
Scott Miller, Treasurer
Subacute rehabilitation facility and programs.

7326 **Kennedy Park Medical Rehabilitation Center**
Kindred Healthcare
6001 Alderson St
Schofield, WI 54476-3614 715-359-4257
800-947-6644
FAX: 715-355-4867
e-mail: info@kennedyparkrehab.com
www.kennedyparkrehab.com
Judy Kowalski, Manager
Jim Torgerson, Executive Director
Kristen W., Health and Rehabilitation Center
Becky D., Activity Director
Kennedy Park Medical & Rehabilitation Center accomodates 154 residents. We are located in Schofield, WI. At Kennedy Park, we specialize in dementia care, with our Reflections and Passages

Units. Short-term rehabilitation and sub-acute care are provided in a setting conducive to meeting the individual needs of our residents and patients. We also provide general nursing care for persons with long-term care needs.

7327 Middleton Village Nursing & Rehabilitation
Kindred
6201 Elmwood Ave
Middleton, WI 53562-3319 608-831-8300
800-947-6644
FAX: 608-831-4253
www.middletonvillage.com

Nicholas Stamatas, Manager
Ashley Ostrowski, Executive Director
Kristen W., Health and Rehabilitation Center
Becky D., Activity Director

Middleton Village accomodates 97 residents. We specialize in post-surgical and post-acute rehabilitation and long-term care services.

7328 Mount Carmel Health & Rehabilitation Center
5700 W Layton Ave
Milwaukee, WI 53220-4099 414-281-7200
FAX: 414-281-4620
www.milwaukeemtcarmel.com

Mike Berry, Administrator
Darrin Hull, Executive Director
Kristen W., Health and Rehabilitation Center
Becky D., Activity Director

Subacute rehabilitation facility and programs.

7329 Mount Carmel Medical and Rehabilitation Center
680 South Fourth Street
Louisville, KY 40202 502-596-7300
800-545-0749
e-mail: web_administrator@kindred.com
kindredhealthcare.com

Randy Nitschke, Administrator
Jeanne Piccioni, Executive Director

Mount Carmel Medical and Rehabilitation Center accomodates 155 residents. We are located in Burlington Wisconsin. Mount Carmel Medical and Rehabilitation center is a recipient of the American Health Care Association Quality Award.

7330 North Ridge Medical and Rehabilitation Center
1445 N 7th St
Manitowoc, WI 54220-2011 920-682-0314
800-947-6644
FAX: 920-682-0553
e-mail: HSDED0769@kindredhealthcare.com
www.nrmrc.com

Jane Conway, Interim ED
Mary Ann Hamer, Executive Director

North Ridge Medical and Rehabiliation Center accomodates 110 residents. We have been serving the Manitowoc, Wisconsin area for over 25 years. Our goal is to provide services in a warm, homey environment. Many of our staff in all departments have a long history with North Ridge and have worked here for more then 20 years. We also take pride in the fact that we have all in-house staff. Our therapy team is availiable to provide physical, occupational and speech therapy 7 days a week.

7331 Oshkosh Medical and Rehabilitation Center
1580 Bowen St
Oshkosh, WI 54901 920-233-4011
FAX: 920-233-5177
www.northpointmedicalandrehab.com

Tom Wagner, President

Subacute rehabilitation facility and programs.

7332 San Luis Medical and Rehabilitation Center
680 South Fourth Street
Louisville, KY 40202 502-596-7300
800-545-0749
e-mail: web_administrator@kindred.com
www.kindredhealthcare.com

Heather Dreier, Administrator
Tim Dietzen, Executive Director
Dr. John T. Warren, Medical Director
Kristen W., Health and Rehabilitation Center

San Luis Medical and Rehabilitation Center accomodates 126 residents. We are located in Green bay, WI. At San Luis, we strive to meet the needs of our residents and we specialize in dementia care, with our Reflections Unit. Our goal is to provide short-term rehabilitation and sub-acute care in a setting conducive to assisting the needs of our residents.

7333 Strawberry Lane Nursing & Rehabilitation Center
130 Strawberry Lane
Wisconsin Rapids, WI 54494-2156 715-424-1600
FAX: 715-424-4817
e-mail: cglodoski@strawberrylanenursing.com
www.strawberrylanenursing.com

Cyndi Glodoski, Admissions Director
Carrie Russert, Administrator

Skilled nursing facility that provides both long term and short term care. Offer Alzheimer's and Dementia care units, as well as Hospice Care. Medicare and Medicaid certified.

Wyoming

7334 Mountain Towers Healthcare & Rehabilitation Center
3128 Boxelder Dr
Cheyenne, WY 82001-5808 307-634-7901
800-877-9975
FAX: 307-634-7910
www.mttowersrehab.com

Dan Stackis, Administrator
Toni Wyenn, Director of Nursing
Daniel G. Stackis, Executive Director
Dr. Kent Britton, Medical Director

Mountain Towers Healthcare and Rehabilitation Center accomodates 170 residents, including a 16-bed acute secure unit. We offer a full range of nursing and medical care to meet individual needs. We have a full staff to meet the needs of our residents.

7335 South Central Wyoming Healthcare and Rehabilitation
Kindred Healthcare
542 16th St
Rawlins, WY 82301-5241 307-324-2759
800-877-9975
FAX: 307-324-7579
www.kindredrawlins.com

Chris Tanner, Executive Director
Anthony Janusz, Administrator
Kristen W., Health and Rehabilitation Center
Becky D., Activity Director

South Central Wyoming Healthcare and Rehabilitation accomodates 52 residents. We are located in Rawlings, in south central Wyoming. We are Medicare and Medicaid certified by the State of Wyoming. We strive to provide quality personal services, long-term care or short-term rehabilitation to our residents in a comfortable home-like environment.

7336 Wind River Healthcare and Rehabilitation Center
Kindred Health Care
1002 Forest Dr
Riverton, WY 82501-2918 307-856-9471
800-877-9975
FAX: 307-856-1665
www.windriverhealthcare.com

Jo Ann Aldrich, Executive Director
Amelia Asay, Business Office Manager
Kristen W., Health and Rehabilitation Center
Becky D., Activity Director

Offers a full range of medical services to meet the individual needs of our residents, including short-term rehabilitative services and long-term skilled care. Working with the residents physician, our staff-including medical specialists, nurses, nutritionists, dietitians and social workers-establishes a comprehensive treatment plan intended to restore you or your loved one to the highest practicable potential.

Aging

Associations

7337 Aging Services of California
1315 I St
Suite 100
Sacramento, CA 95814-2915
916-392-5111
FAX: 916-428-4250
e-mail: info@aging.org
www.aging.org

Kay Kallander, Chair
Todd Murch, Chair Elect
Robert Edmondson, Vice Chair
Roberta Jacobsen, Vice Chair
The California Association of Homes and Services for the Aging (CAHSA) is the primary statewide association for not-for-profit organizations providing health care, housing and community services to older adults.

7338 Aging Services of Michigan
201 North Washington Square
Suite 920
Lansing, MI 48933
517-323-3687
FAX: 517-323-4569
e-mail: info@leadingagemi.org
www.agingmi.org

David Herbel, President/CEO
Deanna Ludlow Mitchell, Senior Vice President for Perfor
Debra Danai, Director of Finance
Stephanie Shooks Winslow, Vice President for Government St
Aging Services of Michigan represents and promotes the common interests of its members through leadership, advocacy, education and other services in order to enhance members' ability to serve their constituencies.

7339 Aging Services of South Carolina
2711 Middleburg Dr
Suite 309-A
Columbia, SC 29204-2413
803-988-0005
FAX: 803-988-1017
e-mail: information@leadingagesc.org
www.scanpha.org

Vickie Moody, President/CEO
Beth Bouknight, Education Coordinator
Aging Services of South Carolina represents not-for-profit organizations dedicated to providing high-quality health care, housing and services to the seniors of South Carolina.

7340 Aging Services of Washington
1495 Wilmington Driv
Ste 340
Dupont, WA 98327-8773
253-964-8870
FAX: 253-964-8876
e-mail: info@leadingagewa.org
www.agingwa.org

Bonnie Blachly, Director of Clinical Services
Paul Montgomery, Director of Financial Services
Pat Sylvia, Director of Member Development
Julie Martin, Director of Senior Living & Community Services
Washington Association of Housing and Services for the Aging (WASHA) is the state association serving primarily not-for-profit organizations dedicated to providing quality housing, health, community and related services to older persons.

7341 Aging in America
1000 Pelham Pkwy South
Bronx, NY 10461-1198
718-824-4004
877-244-6469
FAX: 718-824-4242
e-mail: admissiondept@aiamsh.org
www.aginginamerica.org

William T Smith, President/CEO
Research and services organization for professionals in gerontology. Objectives are: to produce, implement and share effective and affordable programs and services that improve the quality of life for the elderly community; to better prepare professionals and students interested in or currently involved with, aging and the aged. Conducts research projects, educational and training seminars, and in-service curricula for long-term and acute care facilities.

7342 American Association of Homes and Servicesfor the Aging
2519 Connecticut Ave NW
Washington, DC 20008-1520
202-783-2242
FAX: 202-783-2255
e-mail: info@LeadingAge.org
www.leadingage.org

William L Minnix Jr, President/CEO
Katrinka Smith Sloan, Chief Operating Officer and Seni
Robyn I. Stone, Senior Vice President of Researc
Cheryl Phillips, Senior Vice President, Policy and Advocacy
The American Association of Homes and Services for the Aging (AAHS) represents not-for-profit organizations dedicated to providing high-quality health care, housing and services to the nation's elderly. AAHSA organizations serve more than one million older persons af all income levels, creeds and races.

7343 American Association of Retired Persons
601 E St NW
Washington, DC 20049-2
800-687-2277
TTY:877-434-7589
e-mail: member@aarp.org
www.aarp.org

A Barry Rand, President/CEO
Hop Backus, Executive Vice President, State
Steve Cone, Executive Vice President of Integrated Value and Strategy
Lorraine Cort,s-V zquez, Executive Vice President, Multicultural Markets and Engageme
A nonprofit membership organization of persons 50 and older dedicated to addressing their needs and interests.

7344 Arizona Association of Homes and Housing for the Aging
3877 N 7th St
Ste 240
Phoenix, AZ 85014
602-230-0026
FAX: 602-230-0563
e-mail: azaha@azaha.org
www.azaha.org

Genny Rose, Executive Director
Jon Scott Williams, Chair
The Arizona Association of Homes and Houses for the Aging is a not-for-profit trade association representing more than 100 facilities dedicated to providing quality health care, housing and services to over 12,000 elderly Arizona citizens. AzAHA is the only association in Arizona representing the full continuum of long term care, housing and services including: retirement communities, HUD subsidized senior housing, assisted living and nursing facilities.

7345 Association of Ohio Philanthropic Homes, Housing and Services for the Aging
855 S Wall St
Columbus, OH 43206-1921
614-444-2882
FAX: 614-444-2974
e-mail: info@aopha.org
aopha.org

John Alfano, CEO
Founded in 1937, AOPHA, the advocate of not-for-profit services for older Ohioans, is a statewide nonprofit trade association representing over 335 not-for-profit senior housing apartments, home and community-based service providers, assisted living facilities, nursing homes and continuing care retirement communities (CCRCs).

7346 **Children of Aging Parents**
PO Box 167
Richboro, PA 18954-167 215-945-6900
800-227-7294
FAX: 215-945-8720
e-mail: info@caps4caregivers.org
www.caps4caregivers.org

Karen Rosenberg, Director

A national clearinghouse for caregivers of the elderly. It provides information and referral, educational programs and materials and caregiver support groups. CAPS also produces a quarterly newsletter which is available through the organization. Individuals: $25.00. Organizational/Professional: $100.00.

7347 **Colorado Association of Homes and Services for the Aging**
303 E. 17th Ave.
Suite 502
Denver, CO 80203-1160 303-837-8834
FAX: 303-837-8836
e-mail: Jennifer@LeadingAgeColorado.org
www.cahsa.org

Laura Landwirth, Executive Director
Michael Meehan, Secretary
Dan Stenersen, Treasurer
Jennifer Stone, Member Services Manager

The American Association of Homes and Services for the Aging (AAHS) represents nonprofit organizations dedicated to providing high quality health care, housing and services to the nation's elderly. AAHSA organizations serve more than one million older persons af all income levels, creeds and races.

7348 **Connecticut Association of Not-for-Profit Providers for the Aging**
1340 Worthington Rdg
Berlin, CT 06037-3208 860-828-2903
FAX: 860-828-8694
e-mail: leadingagect@leadingagect.org
www.leadingagect.org

Andrea Bellofiore, Director of Member Programs & Services
Beth Ricker, Finance Manager & Membership Director
Mag Morelli, President
Nurka Carrero, Office Manager

LeadingAge Connecticut is a membership organization representing over 130 not-for-profit mission driven provider organizations serving elderly and disabled individuals across the continuum of care, including nursing homes, residential care homes, housing for the elderly, continuing care retirement communities, adult day centers, home care agencies and assisted living.

7349 **Georgia Association of Homes and Services for the Aging**
1440 Dutch Valley PL NE
Suite 120
Atlanta, GA 30324-5367 404-872-9191
FAX: 404-872-1737
e-mail: selahi@leadingagega.org
www.centerforpositiveaging.org

Susan Watkins, Dir. of Member Services
Walter Coffey, President/C.E.O.
Jacque Thornton, Sr. Vice President

The Georgia Association of Homes and Services for the Aging (GAHSA) is an affiliated partner of the American Association of Homes and Services of the Aging (AASHA), which represents over 5,600 nonprofit facilities, over one million older adults in the United States and maintains an impressive staff of 80 professionals at its headquarters in Washington, D.C.

7350 **Gulf States Association of Homes and Services for the Aging**
PO Box 1748
Marrero, LA 70073-1748 504-442-0483
FAX: 504-689-3982
e-mail: kcontrenchis@gulfstatesahsa.org
www.gulfstatesahsa.org

Cindy Ladnier, Chair
Dennis Adams, Vice-Chair
Scott Crabtree, Secretary/Treasurer
Karen Contrenchis, President

Along term care system which offers accessable, affordable, high-quality and innovative healthcare, housing and comminuty services. Provides value to the the senior population and their families through personal and professional commitment, in a compassionate manner, supported by benevolence and integrity. Socially resposible and accountable for promoting excellence in long-term care and support services.

7351 **Indiana Association of Homes and Services for the Aging**
PO Box 68829
Indianapolis, IN 46268-0829 317-733-2380
FAX: 317-733-2385
e-mail: jimleich@LeadingAgeIndiana.org
www.iahsa.com

Emilie Perkins, CMP, Director of Training
Rebecca (Bec Carter, Director of Association Management
Jim Leich, President
Susan Darwent, Vice President of Operations

LeadingAge Indiana is an association representing not-for-profit services and facilities for the elderly. Members are non-profit organizations, providing high quality health care, services and housing for over 25,000 seniors throughout Indiana. Our members are sponsored by or affiliated with religious, fraternal, governmental, and community organizations.

7352 **Iowa Association of Homes and Services forthe Aging**
4200 University Ave.
Suite 305
West Des Moines, IA 50266-6723 515-440-4630
888-440-4630
FAX: 515-440-4631
e-mail: info@leadingageiowa.org
www.leadingageiowa.org

Bill Nutty, Director of Government Relations
Kathy Strang, Director of Professional Develop
Bill Nutty, Government Relations/Member Services Director
Shannon Strickler, President/CEO

LeadingAge Iowa is the state association serving not-for-profit and missiondriven organizations dedicated to providing quality housing, health, community, and related services to our state's seniors. LeadingAge Iowa represents and promotes the common interests of its members through advocacy, education and collaboration to enhance their ability to provide quality care and service within their community.

7353 **Kentucky Association of Homes and Services for the Aging**
2501 Nelson Miller Pkwy
Suite 200
Louisville, KY 40223- 2221 502-992-4380
FAX: 502-992-4390
e-mail: info@leadingageky.org
www.kahsa.com

Timothy Veno, President

LeadingAge Kentucky (formerly Kentucky Association of Homes and Services for the Aging (KAHSA) was founded in 1977. The association represents not-for-profit community, church, proprietary and government sponsored health care facilities, retirement communities, assisted living, housing and service programs for the elderly and the disabled.

7354 **Life Services Network of Illinois**
1001 Warrenville Rd
Suite 150
Lisle, IL 60532 630-325-6170
FAX: 630-325-0749
e-mail: info@lsni.org
www.lsni.org

Kathy Burke, Director of Business Development
Suzanne Schemm, Director of Finance and Administration
Cathy Nelson RN, MS, LNHA, Director of Clinical Services
Karen Messer, Interim President

With over 500 partners in Illinois, Life Services Network is one of the largest and most respected associations of its type in the country. Founded in the early part of the 20th century by an ecumenical group of long term care providers, LSN has represented the complete continuum of services for older adults for over 75 years.

7355 LifeSpan Network: Maryland
10280 Old Columbia Road
Suite 220
Columbia, MD 21046- 2382 410-381-1176
FAX: 410-381-0240
e-mail: ifirth@lifespan-network.org
www.lifespan-network.org

Kathy Bernetti, Director of Finance
Charlotte Eliopoulos, PULL Grant Program Director
Lisa Fichman, Director of Membership Services and Marketing
Isabella Firth, President

Senior care provider association representing more than 300 senior care provider organizations in Maryland and the District of Columbia. Lifespan members include non-profit and proprietary independent living, assisted living, continuing care retirement communities, nursing facilities, subsidized senior housing and community and hospital based services. Also provide education, advocacy and products and services, as well as networking for our members.

7356 Massachusetts Aging Services Association
246 Walnut Street
Suite 203
Newton, MA 02460-3328 617-244-2999
FAX: 617-244-2995
e-mail: office@LeadingAgeMA.org
www.massaging.org

Sue Pouliot, Director of Education and Events
Don Powell, Director of Member Services
Elissa Sherman, President
Lisa Miano, Officer Manager

LeadingAge Massachusetts, formerly MassAging, is the only organization representing the full continuum of mission-driven, not-for-profit providers of health care, housing, and services for older persons in Massachusetts. Members of LeadingAge Massachusetts provide housing and services to more than 25,000 older persons in the Commonwealth each year.

7357 Missouri Association of Homes for the Aging
3412 Knipp Dr
Suite 102
Jefferson City, MO 65109 573-635-6244
FAX: 573-635-6618
e-mail: diana@moaha.org
www.moaha.org

Denise Clemonds, CEO
Diana Love
Patricia Hubbs
Patricia Hubbs

LeadingAge Missouri's work is dedicated to assisting its members to be the leaders in Missouri in the delivery of innovative, quality long-term health care, housing, and services for older adults. LeadingAge Missouri assists its members in providing quality services for the elderly

7358 National Association of Area Agencies on Aging
1730 Rhode Island Ave NW
Suite 1200
Washington, DC 20036-3109 202-872-0888
FAX: 202-872-0057
e-mail: smarkwood@n4a.org
www.n4a.org

Tom Endres, Director
Joanetta Bolden, Associate Director, Communications
Amy E. Gotwals, Senior Director, Public Policy and Advocacy
Virginia Dize, Program Manager/Assistant Director

The National Association of Area Agencies on Aging (n4a) is the leading voice on aging issues for Area Agencies on Aging and a champion for Title VI Native American aging programs. Through advocacy, training and technical assistance, we support the national network of 629 AAAs and 246 Title VI programs.

7359 National Association of Counties
25 Massachusetts Ave NW
Suite 500
Washington, DC 20001- 1430 202-393-6226
888-407-6226
888-407-6226
FAX: 202-393-2630
e-mail: nacomeetings@naco.org
naco.org

Maeghan Gilmore, Program Director, County Solutions & Innovation
Karon Harden, Director of Professional Development, Education and Training
Emilia Istrate, Director of Research
Kim Struble, Director of Conferences & Meetings

NACO represents elected officials and aging administrators who are interested in providing quality programs to their older constituents. NACO members work with Congress, the Administration on Aging, and other federal agencies to ensure that the nationa maintains an effective and efficient safety net of services for the elderly and their families.

7360 National Association of Nutrition and Aging Services Programs
1612 K St NW
Suite 400
Washington, DC 20006-2829 202-682-6899
FAX: 202-223-2099
e-mail: pcarlson@nanasp.com
www.nanasp.org

Robert Blancato, Executive Director
Shannon Donahue, Associate
Pamela (Pam) Carlson, Membership & Education
Scott Carlson, Finance & Operations

A national membership organization for persons across the country working to provide older adults healthful food and nutrition through community-based services.

7361 National Association of State Units on Aging
1201 15th St NW
Suite 350
Washington, DC 20005-2842 202-898-2578
FAX: 202-898-2583
e-mail: info@nasuad.org
www.nasuad.org

Martha Roherty, Executive Director
Lindsey Copeland, Director of Policy and Legislative Affairs
Rachel Shiffrin Feldman, Director of Communications and Corporate Relations
John Michael Hall, Senior Director of Medicaid Policy and Planning

NASUAD represents the nation's 56 state and territorial agencies on aging and disabilities and supports visionary state leadership, the advancement of state systems innovation and the articulation of national policies that support home and community based services for older adults and individuals with disabilities.

7362 National Council on Aging
1901 L St NW
4th Fl
Washington, DC 20036-3540 202-479-1200
FAX: 202-479-0735
TTY:202-479-6674
e-mail: membership@ncoa.org
www.ncoa.org

James P Firman, EdD, President/CEO
Jay Robertson, Senior Vice President
Richard Birkel, PhD, MPA, Acting Senior Vice President, Ce
Nora Dowd Eisenhower, JD, Acting Senior Vice President, Ec

We are a national voice for older Americans and the community organizations that serve them. We bring together nonprofit organizations, businesses, and government to develop creative solutions that improve the lives of all older adults.

7363 National Hispanic Council on Aging
734 15th St NW
Suite 1050
Washington, DC 20005-1038 202-347-9733
FAX: 202-347-9735
e-mail: nhcoa@nhcoa.org
www.nhcoa.org

Yanira Cruz, DrPH, President/CEO
Eric Rodriguez, Director
B rbara Robles, PhD, Director
Jorge Lambrinos, Director

To achieve its mission, NHCOA has developed a Hispanic Aging Network of community-based organizations across the continental U.S., the District of Columbia, and Puerto Rico that reaches millions of Latinos each year. NHCOA also works to ensure the Hispanic community is better understood and fairly represented in U.S. policies.

7364 National Indian Council on Aging
10501 Montgomery Blvd NE
Suite 210
Albuquerque, NM 87111-3851 505-292-2001
FAX: 505-292-1922
e-mail: info@nicoa.org
www.nicoa.org

Randella Bluehoose, Executive Director
Dorinda Fox, SCSEP Director
Jonnie Gilbert, Finance Director
Darrell Begay, Arizona Central Employment Speci

A non-profit organization, was founded by members of the National Tribal Chairmen's Association that called for a national organization to advocate for improved, comprehensive health and social services to American Indian and Alaska Native Elders.

7365 National Senior Citizens Law Center
1444 Eye Street NW
Suite 1100
Washington, DC 20005-6547 202-289-6976
FAX: 202-289-7224
e-mail: nsclc@nsclc.org
www.nsclc.org

Robert K. Johnson, Esq.,, Chair
Barrett S. Litt, Esq.,, Vice Chair
Paul Nathanson, Executive Director
Kevin Prindiville, Deputy Director

The National Senior Citizens Law Center is a non-profit organization whose principal mission is to protect the rights of low-income older adults. Through advocacy, litigation, and the education and counseling of local advocates, we seek to ensure the health and economic security of those with limited income and resources, and to preserve their access to the courts.

7366 Nebraska Association of Homes and Services for the Aging
900 North 90th Street
Suite 940
Omaha, NE 68114 402-990-2346
e-mail: kaminskij@leadingagene.org
www.leadingagene.org

Julie Kaminski, Executive Director
Cheryl Wichman, Education Coordinator

LeadingAgeNebraska is the only State Association representing the full continuum of mission-driven, non-profit providers of health care, housing, and services for older adults in Nebraska. Members of LeadingAgeNebraska provide housing and services to more than 5,000 Nebraska seniors each year

7367 New Jersey Association of Homes and Services for the Aging
13 Roszel Rd
Suite C-200
Princeton, NJ 08540-6211 609-452-1161
FAX: 609-452-2907
e-mail: mkent@leadingagenj.org
www.leadingagenj.org

Amy S. Greenbaum, Director of Professional Develop
Michele M. Kent, President, CEO
Judy Collett-Miller, Executive Vice President
Darlene Arden, Executive Assistant

LeadingAge New Jersey represents not-for-profit nursing homes, assisted living residences, residential health care centers, independent senior housing, and continuing care retirement communities throughout the entire state of New Jersey. LeadingAge New Jersey serves over 140 member communities, many of which are supported through religious, fraternal and governmental sponsorship.

7368 New York Association of Homes and Services for the Aging
13 British American Blvd
Suite 2
Latham, NY 12110-1431 518-867-8383
FAX: 518-867-8384
e-mail: info@leadingageny.org
www.nyahsa.org

Ellen Quinn, SPHR, Director of Human Resources
Patrick Cucinelli, Sr. Director of Public Policy
Elliott Frost, Director of ProCare
Ami Schnauber, Director of Government Relations

Founded in 1961, LeadingAge New York, formerly the New York Association of Homes & Services for the Aging (NYAHSA), represents not-for-profit, mission-driven and public continuing care providers, including nursing homes, senior housing, adult care facilities, continuing care retirement communities, assisted living and community service providers. Leading Age New York's more than 600 members employ 150,000 professionals serving more than 500,000 New Yorkers annually.

7369 North Carolina Association of Non-Profit Homes for the Aging
100 Carolina Meadows
Chapel Hill, NC 27517 919-571-8333
FAX: 919-571-1297
e-mail: info@leadingagenc.org
www.leadingagenc.org

Tom Akins, President/CEO
Leslie Roseboro, Vice President
Anne Moffat, Chair
Kevin McLeod, Chair Elect

LeadingAge North Carolina is the state association of not-for-profit providers dedicated to providing quality care, housing, health, community and related services to the elderly. As the only Association in North Carolina exclusively representing not-for-profit long term care facilities, a primary goal is to support members in maintaining their 501(c)(3) status and promoting the not-for-profit philosophy of quality long term care and services for the elderly.

7370 Northern New England Association of Homes and Services for the Aging
PO Box 339
New Gretna, NJ 08224-0339 603-391-9881
FAX: 603-391-9881
e-mail: rgoedtel@leadingagemenh.org
www.leadingagemenh.org

Peter Warecki, Chair
Rebecca Smith, Vice Chair
Maureen Carland, Secretary
Lee Karker, Treasurer

The mission of LeadingAge Maine & New Hampshire is to promote the interests of its not-for-profit members in Maine and New Hampshire, which provide healthy, affordable and ethical long-term care to our older citizens through education, advocacy, representation and collaboration.

7371 Oklahoma Association of Homes and Services for the Aging
PO Box 1383
El Reno, OK 73036-1383 405-640-8040
e-mail: inquiry@LeadingAgeOK.org
www.leadingageok.org

Mary Brinkley, Executive Director
Jessica Pfau, President
Lindsay Fick, Secretary
Jim O'Brien, Treasurer

LeadingAge Oklahoma represents an association of members who are forward-thinking in shaping the future of the long-term care profession. Our members lead in innovative practices that transform how we care for our aging population, cutting-edge initiatives to develop services that meet the needs and preferences of older adults and advocacy efforts to advance the interests of the aging consumer.

7372 Oregon Alliance of Senior and Health Services
7340 SW Hunziker St
Suite 104
Tigard, OR 97223-2303 503-684-3788
FAX: 503-624-0870
e-mail: info@leadingageoregon.org
www.oashs.org
Ruth Gulyas, Executive Director
Margaret Cervenka, Deputy Director
Karen Nichols, Manager of Membership Services a
Denise Wetzel, Administrative Coordinator and B
Established in 1979, LeadingAge Oregon is the state association of not-for-profit, mission-directed organizations dedicated to providing quality housing, health, community and related services to the elderly and disabled. LeadingAge Oregon members set the standards for the field through service excellence and mission-driven objectives.

7373 Pennsylvania Association of Nonprofit Senior Services
1100 Bent Creek Blvd
Mechanicsburg, PA 17050-1872 717-763-5724
800-545-2270
FAX: 717-763-1057
e-mail: info@leadingagepa.org
www.panpha.org
Ronald L Barth, President/CEO
Holly Rosini, Senior Vice President/Chief Operating Officer
Beth Greenberg, VP, Strategic Knowledge and Research
Heidi Geist, Communications Manager
LeadingAge PA's mission is to promote the interests of our members by enhancing their ability to provide quality services efficiently and effectively; and by representing our members through cooperative action.

7374 Quality Healthcare Foundation of Wyoming
6909 Foxglove Drive
Cheyenne, WY 82009 307-287-4594
800-773-2273
FAX: 307-638-8472
e-mail: steve@qhcf.org
www.qhcf.org
Steve Bahmer, Executive Director
Eric Boley, President
Sandy Ward, Vice President
Jill Hult, Secretary/Treasurer
The American Association of Homes and Services for the Aging (AAHS) represents not-for-profit organizations dedicated to providing high-quality health care, housing and services to the nation's elderly. AAHSA organizations serve more than one million older persons af all income levels, creeds and races.

7375 Rhode Island Association of Facilities and Services for the Aging
225 Chapman St
2nd Floor
Providence, RI 02905-4533 401-490-7612
866-883-1631
FAX: 401-490-7614
TTY: 401-383-6578
e-mail: info@leadingageri.org
www.leadingageri.org
James P Nyberg, Director
Matt Trimble, President
Sandra Cullen, Vice-President
Wendy Fargnoli, Treasurer
LeadingAge RI is committed to Expanding the World of Possibilities for Aging. As such, LeadingAge RI will continue its focus on advancing excellence in the field by fostering innovation, collaboration, and ethical leadership; advocating for sound public policy; providing education, collaboration, and professional development; valuing older people and their right to make choices; and promoting a continuum of services.

7376 Tennessee Association of Homes and Services for the Aging
5201 Virginia Way
Suite 325
Brentwood, TN 37027-4634 615-256-8240
FAX: 615-242-4803
e-mail: webmaster@tha.com
www.tha.com
Patrick Turri, Senior Director Analysis/Information Technoloy
Joe Burchfield, Senior Director Operations and Member Services
Patrice Mayo, Vice President, Operations Director
Mary Ellen Mooney, Clinical Director
TNAHSA is an association of faclities and professionals providing quality housing, health, community and related services for the elderly. TNAHSA represents and promotes the common interest of its members through leadership, advocacy, education, communication and other services in order to enhance members' ability to serve their constituencies.

7377 Texas Association of Homes and Services for the Aging
2205 Hancock Dr
Austin, TX 78756-2508 512-467-2242
FAX: 512-467-2275
e-mail: info@leadingagetexas.org
www.tahsa.org
Crystal Laza, CAE, Director of Member Services and Operations
Alyse Migliaro, Director of Public Policy
Claire Director of Education, Morris, CASP
George Linial, CAE, CASP, President/CEO
LeadingAge Texas (formerly the Texas Association of Homes and Services for the Aging - TAHSA) was established in 1959 as a Texas not-for-profit corporation. Its purpose is to provide leadership, advocacy, and education for not-for-profit retirement housing and nursing home communities that serve the needs of Texas retirees.

7378 Wisconsin Association of Homes and Services for the Aging
204 S Hamilton St
Madison, WI 53703-3212 608-255-7060
FAX: 608-255-7064
e-mail: info@LeadingAgeWI.org
www.wahsa.org
John Sauer, President/CEO
Pam Walker, Executive Secretary
Janice Mashak, Vice President of Member Services & Innovation
Brian Schoeneck, Vice President of Financial & Regulatory Services
LeadingAge Wisconsin is committed to advancing the fields of long-term care, assisted living and retirement living. We strive to develop a continuum of elderly care and services that meets the holistic needs of seniors and individuals with a disability in order to encourage maximum independence and enhance quality of life. We serve as a resource for our members, assisting them in problem resolution and providing services and programs to meet their needs.

Print: Books

7379 Activities in Action
Routledge
270 Madison Ave
Fl 4 #4
New York, NY 10016-0601 212-695-6599
800-634-7064
FAX: 212-563-2269
e-mail: www.routledgementalhealth.com/contact/
www.routledgementalhealth.com
Jeffrey Lim, Director
Francis Chua, Manager
Tamaryn Anderson, Marketing Manager
An invaluable resource which serves as a catalyst for professional and personal growth and provides a national forum on geriatric and activity issues. *$30.00*
116 pages Hardcover
ISBN 1-560241-32-4

7380 **Activities with Developmentally Disabled Elderly and Older Adults**
Routledge
270 Madison Ave
Fl 4 #4
New York, NY 10016-601 212-695-6599
800-637-7064
FAX: 212-563-2269
e-mail: www.routledgementalhealth.com/contact/
www.routledgementalhealth.com

Jeffrey Lim, Director
Francis Chua, Manager
Tamaryn Anderson, Marketing Manager

Learn how to effectively plan and deliver activities for a growing number of older people with developmental disabilities. It aims to stimulate interest and continued support for recreation program development and implementation among developmental disability and aging service systems. *$42.00*
164 pages Hardcover
ISBN 1-560241-74-4

7381 **Aging and Developmental Disability: Current Research, Programming, and Practice**
Routledge
270 Madison Ave
Fl 4 #4
New York, NY 10016-601 212-695-6599
800-634-7064
FAX: 212-563-2269
e-mail: www.routledgementalhealth.com/contact/
www.routledgementalhealth.com

Joy Hammel, Author
Susan Nochajski, Co-Author

Explores research findings and their implications for practice in relation to normative and disability-related aging experiences and issues. It discusses the effectiveness of specific intervention targeted toward aging adults with developmental disabilities such as Down's Syndrome, cerebral palsy, autism, and epilepsy, and offers suggestions for practice and future research in this area. *$48.00*
112 pages Hardcover
ISBN 0-789010-39-1

7382 **Aging and Family Therapy: Practitioner Perspectives on Golden Pond**
Routledge
270 Madison Ave
Fl 4 #4
New York, NY 10016-601 212-695-6599
800-634-7064
FAX: 212-563-2269
e-mail: www.routledgementalhealth.com/contact/
www.routledgementalhealth.com

George Hughston, Author
Victor Christopherson, Co-Author
Marilyn Bojean, Co-Author

Here are creative strategies for use in therapy with older adults and their families. This significant new book provides practitioners with information, insight, reference tools, and other sources that will contribute to more effective intervention with the elderly and their families. *$48.00*
260 pages Hardcover
ISBN 0-866567-78-7

7383 **Aging in Stride**
IlluminAge Communications Partners
2200 1st Ave South
Suite 400
Seattle, WA 98134-1408 206-269-6363
888-620-8816
FAX: 206-269-6350
e-mail: www.cobaltgroup.com/contact/
www.cobaltgroup.com

Dennis Kenny, Owner
Elizabeth N Oettinger, Co-Author
Dennis E Kenny JD, Co-Author

Guide to aging, the special needs of older adults, and the demands of providing care and support. Experts explain potential conflicts, planning opportunities and strategies for success. Six guides. *$24.95*
Paperback

7384 **Aging in the Designed Environment**
Routledge
270 Madison Ave
Fl 4 #4
New York, NY 10016-601 212-216-7800
800-634-7064
FAX: 212-563-2269
www.routledgementalhealth.com

Margaret Christenson, Author
Ellen D Taira, Co-Author

The key sourcebook for physical and occupational therapists developing and implementing environmental designs for the aging. *$30.00*
146 pages Hardcover
ISBN 1-560240-31-0

7385 **Aging with a Disability**
Special Needs Project
1405 Anderson Lane
Santa Barbara, CA 93111-2946 805-962-8087
800-333-6867
FAX: 805-962-5087
www.specialneeds.com

Hod Gray, Owner
Laura Mosqueda, Co-Author

Aging with a Disability provides clinicians with a complete guide to the care and treatment of persons aging with a disability. Divided into five parts, this book first addresses the perspective of the person with a disability and his or her family. *$ 24.95*
328 pages Paperback

7386 **Assistive Technology and Older Adults**
121 West Sweet Ave
Moscow, ID 83843 208-885-6097
800-432-8324
FAX: 208-885-6145
e-mail: such@uidaho.edu
www.educ.uidaho.edu/idatech

Ron Seiler, Project Director

The Idaho Assistive Technology Project (IATP) is a federally funded program administered by the Center on Disabilities and Human Development at the University of Idaho. IATPO's goal is to increase the availability of assistive technology devices and services for older persons and Idahoians with disabilities.

7387 **Caring for Those You Love: A Guide to Compassionate Care for the Aged**
Horizon Publishers & Distributors
191 N 650 E
Bountiful, UT 84010-3628 801-295-9451
866-818-6277
FAX: 801-298-1305
www.duanescrowther.com

Duane S. Crowther, Author/President
Jean Crowther, Vice President/Sec
David Crowther, Vice President

This book is a practical guide to coping with special problems of the aged and infirm, and examines the many challenges of caring for the elderly on a personal and family level. *$12.98*
108 pages
ISBN 0-882902-70-9

7388 **Chronically Disabled Elderly in Society**
Greenwood Publishing Group
88 Post Rd W
Westport, CT 06880-4208 203-226-3571
800-225-5800
FAX: 877-231-6980
e-mail: customer-service@greenwood.com
www.greenwood.com

Merna J Alpert, Author
Lisa Scott, President
Herman Bruggink, CEO

This timely work increases awareness of and knowledge about problems of societal living among the chronically disabled elderly, with implications for policy makers, educational institutions, advocacy groups, families and individuals. *$76.95*
160 pages Hardcover
ISBN 0-313291-09-8

7389 Coping and Caring: Living with Alzheimer's Disease
AARP Fulfillment
601 E St NW
Washington, DC 20049 800-687-2277
TTY:877-434-7589
e-mail: member@aarp.org
www.aarp.org

Charles Leroux, Author
Steve Cone, Executive Vice President of Inte
Lorraine Cortes-Vazquez, Executive Vice President, Multic
Addresses the questions: What is Alzheimer's? How does the disease progress? How long does it last? How can families cope?
24 pages

7390 Elder Abuse and Mistreatment
Routledge
270 Madison Ave
Fl 4 #4
New York, NY 10016-601 212-695-6599
800-634-7064
FAX: 212-563-2269
e-mail: www.routledgementalhealth.com/contact/
www.routledgementalhealth.com

Joanna Mellor, Author
Patricia Brownell, Co-Author
Elder Abuse and Mistreatment is a comprehensive overview of current policy issues, new practice models, and up-to-date research on elder abuse and neglect. Experts in the field provide insight into elder abuse with newly examined populations to create an understanding of how to design service plans for victims of abuse and family mistreatment. The book addresses all forms of abuse and neglect, examining the value issues and ethical dilemmas that social workers face in providing service to elderl *$120.00*
284 pages Paperback
ISBN 0-789030-22-1

7391 Explore Your Options
Kansas Department on Aging
503 S Kansas Ave
New England Building
Topeka, KS 66603- 3404 785-296-4986
800-432-3535
FAX: 785-296-0256
TTY: 785-291-3167
e-mail: wwwmail@kdads.ks.gov
www.agingKansas.org

Maria Russo, President
This book will help you through the maze of services available to Kansas seniors. It is designed to help you take an active role in making decisions that affect your health care and living situation.

7392 Falling in Old Age
Springer Publishing Company
11 W 42nd St
Fl 15 #15
New York, NY 10036-8002 212-431-4370
877-687-7476
FAX: 212-941-7842
e-mail: cs@springerpub.com
www.springerjournals.com

Ursula Springer, President
Ted Nardin, CEO
Edie Lambiase, CFO
Presented are practical techniques for the prevention of falls and for determining and correcting the causes. *$60.00*
412 pages Hardcover
ISBN 0-826152-91-6

7393 Family Intervention Guide to Mental Illness
New Harbinger Publications
5674 Shattuck Ave
Oakland, CA 94609-1662 510-652-0215
800-748-6273
FAX: 800-652-1613
e-mail: customerservice@newharbinger.com
www.newharbinger.com

Matthew McKay, Owner
Kim T Mueser, Co-Author
Kirk Johnson, CFO
Bodie Morey, Co-Author
The Family Intervention Guide to Mental Illness outlines the nine fundamental steps to recognizing, managing, and recovering from mental illness. It provides both diagnostic information and details about therapy options and useful medications. With the right advice, determined effort, and a lot of love, you can make a difference. *$17.95*
240 pages
ISBN 1-572245-06-8

7394 Handbook of Assistive Devices for the Handicapped Elderly
Routledge
270 Madison Ave
Fl 4 #4
New York, NY 10016-601 212-695-6599
800-634-7064
FAX: 212-563-2269
www.routledgementalhealth.com

Joseph A Breuer, Author
Jeffrey Lin, Director
Francis Chua, Manager
Tamaryn Anderson, Marketing Manager
Concise yet comprehensive reference of assistive devices for handicapped elders. *$42.00*
77 pages Hardcover
ISBN 0-866561-52-5

7395 Handbook on Ethnicity, Aging and Mental Health
Greenwood Publishing Group
88 Post Rd W
Westport, CT 6880-4208 203-226-3571
800-225-5800
FAX: 877-231-6980
e-mail: customer-service@greenwood.com
www.greenwood.com

Deborah K Padgett, Author
Lisa Scott, President
Herman Bruggink, CEO
State-of-the-art reference by leading experts and first book-length appraisal of research, practices and policies concerning mental health needs of the ethnic elderly in America. *$141.95*
376 pages Hardcover
ISBN 0-313282-04-8

7396 Health Care of the Aged: Needs, Policies, and Services
Routledge
270 Madison Ave
Fl 4 #4
New York, NY 10016-601 212-695-6599
800-634-7064
FAX: 212-563-2269
www.routledgementalhealth.com

Abraham Monk, Author
Jeffrey Lim, Director
Francis Chua, Manager
Tamaryn Anderson, Marketing Manager
Focusing on the need for developing new service delivery models for the aged, this book examines fiscal, political, and social criteria influencing this challenge of the 1990's. The aged are caught in the sweeping changes currently occurring in the financing, organizing and delivery of human health care services. *$36.00*
800 pages Hardcover
ISBN 1-560240-65-5

7397 **Health Promotion and Disease Prevention in Clinical Practice**
Lippincott, Williams & Wilkins
2001 Market Street
Two Commerce Square
Philadelphia, PA 19103-3603 215-521-8300
800-638-3030
FAX: 215-521-8902
e-mail: customerservice@lww.com.
www.lww.com

Steven H Woolf MD, Co-Author
Steven Jonas MD, Co-Author
Evonne Kaplan-Liss, Co-Author
Rick Perry, CEO
Incorporating the latest guidelines from major organizations, including the U.S. Preventive Services Task Force, this book offers the clinician a complete overview of how to help patients adopt healthy behaviors and to deliver recommended screening tests and immunizations. *$52.95*
218 pages Softcover
ISBN 0-781775-99-1

7398 **Life Planning for Adults with Developmental Disabilities**
New Harbinger Publications
5674 Shattuck Ave
Oakland, CA 94609-1662 510-652-0215
800-748-6273
FAX: 800-652-1613
e-mail: customerservice@newharbinger.com
www.newharbinger.com

Matthew McKay, Publisher
Kirk Johnson, CFO
Judith Greenbaum PhD, Author
The book begins by assessing the quality of life of the adult with a disability. It offers a wealth of suggestions for making that person's life even better. The book then focuses on long-term planning for the individual with a disability and helps answer the question, Who will take care of my child after I'm gone? *$19.95*
208 pages
ISBN 1-572244-51-1

7399 **Long-Term Care: How to Plan and Pay for It**
NOLO
950 Parker St
Berkeley, CA 94710-2524 510-549-1976
800-728-3555
FAX: 800-645-0895
www.nolo.com

Joseph L Matthews, Author
Ralph Warner, Chariman/CEO
Ann Heron, COO
Bob Dubow, CFO
This book helps you choose a nursing home, or find a viable alternative. Covers how to get the most out of Medicare and other benefit programs.
384 pages Paperback
ISBN 1-413305-21-0

7400 **Mentally Impaired Elderly: Strategies and Interventions to Maintain Function**
Routledge
270 Madison Ave
Fl 4 #4
New York, NY 10016-601 212-695-6599
800-634-7064
FAX: 212-653-2269
www.routledgementalhealth.com

Ellen D Taira, Author
Jeffrey Lim, Director
Francis Chua, Manager
Tamaryn Anderson, Marketing Manager
Provides effective support and sensitive care for the most vulnerable segment of the elderly population, those with mental impairment. *$34.00*
171 pages Hardcover
ISBN 1-560241-68-3

7401 **Mirrored Lives: Aging Children and Elderly Parents**
Praeger Publishers
88 Post Rd W
Westport, CT 06880-4208 203-226-3571
800-225-5800
FAX: 877-231-6980
e-mail: customer-service@greenwood.com
www.greenwood.com

Tom Koch, Author
Lisa Scott, President
Herman Bruggink, CEO
Discusses geriatric decline connected to nonterminal illness in old age. Koch takes a sensitive but thorough look at the declining years of his father. *$117.95*
240 pages Hardcover
ISBN 0-275936-71-6

7402 **Physical & Mental Issues in Aging Sourcebook**
Omnigraphics
155 W Congree St
Suite 200 #200
Detroit, MI 48226-3261 313-961-1340
800-234-1340
FAX: 313-961-1383
e-mail: info@omnigraphics.com
www.omnigraphics.com

Jennifer Swanson, Editor
Frederic Ruffner, Chairman
Kay Gill, Vice President
Laurie Harris, Manager
Basic information about maintaining health through the post-reproductive years. Includes stats, recommendations for lifestyle modifications, a glossary and resrouce information *$84.00*
660 pages Hard cover
ISBN 0-780802-33-9

7403 **Prescriptions for Independence: Working with Older People Who are Visually Impaired**
American Foundation for the Blind/AFB Press
11 Penn Plz
Suite 300
New York, NY 10001-2006 212-502-7600
800-232-3044
FAX: 212-502-7777
e-mail: afborder@abdintl.com
www.afb.org

Carl Augusto, President
Gerda Groff, Co-Author
Richard Obnen, Chairman of the Board
Alan Lindroth, Principal
Easy-to-read manual on how older visually impaired persons can pursue their interests and activities in community residences, senior centers, long-term care facilities and other community settings. Paperback.
99 pages Paperback
ISBN 0-891282-44-0

7404 **Sharing the Burden**
Brookings Institution
1775 Massachusetts Ave NW
Washington, DC 20036-2188 202-797-6000
FAX: 202-797-6004
www.brookings.edu

Joshua N Weiner, Author
Laurel Hixon Illston, Co-Author
Raymond J Hanley, Co-Author
Strobe Talbott, President
The authors examine the cost of public and private initiatives and who would pay for them. Their answers emerge from a large computer simulation model that the authors developed. *$42.95*
342 pages Cloth
ISBN 0-815793-78-2

7405 **Social Security, Medicare, and Government Pensions**
NOLO
950 Parker St
Berkeley, CA 94710-2524
510-549-1976
800-728-3555
FAX: 800-645-0895
www.nolo.com

Joseph L Matthews, Author
Dorothy Matthews Berman, Co-Author
Ralph Warner, Chairman/CEO
Ann Heron, COO
Social Security, Medicare, SSI and more explained in this all-in-one resource that gets you the most out of your retirement benefits. *$24.95*
480 pages Paperback
ISBN 1-413307-53-5

7406 **Successful Models of Community Long Term Care Services for the Elderly**
Routledge
270 Madison Ave
Fl 4 #4
New York, NY 10016-601
212-695-6599
800-637-7064
FAX: 212-563-2269
www.routledgementalhealth.com

Eloise Killeffer, Author
Ruth Bennett, Co-Author
Jeffrey Lim, Director
Francis Chua, Manager
Experienced practitioners provide examples of successful community-based long term care service programs for the elderly. *$ 72.00*
174 pages Hardcover
ISBN 0-866569-87-3

7407 **Therapeutic Activities with Persons Disabled by Alzheimer's Disease**
Sage Publications
804 Anacapa Stree
Sanat Barbara, CA 93101-2212
805-899-8620

e-mail: info@sagepub.com
www.sagepub.com

Sara Miller McCune, Founder, Publisher, Chairperson
Blaise Simqu, CEO
Tracey Ozmina, COO
Stephen Barr, Managing Director
A program of functional skills for activities of daily living. Hardcover. *$86.00*
432 pages
ISBN 0-834211-62-9

7408 **Visually Impaired Seniors as Senior Companions: A Reference Guide**
American Foundation for the Blind/AFB Press
11 Penn Plz
Suite 300
New York, NY 10001-2006
212-502-7600
800-232-3044
FAX: 212-502-7777
e-mail: afborders@abdintl.com
www.afb.org

Carl Augusto, President
Alan Lindroth, Principal
Richard Obnen, Chairman of the Board
Michael Gilliam, Vice Chairman
This useful guide describes the Senior Companion Program that is intended to broaden opportunities for older persons with disabilities. Appendix includes training materials, evaluation forms, recruitment and public relations information. *$15.00*
108 pages Paperback
ISBN 0-891282-38-6

7409 **Work, Health and Income Among the Elderly**
Brookings Institution
1775 Massachusetts Ave NW
Washington, DC 20036-2188
202-797-6000
FAX: 202-797-6004
www.brookings.edu

Gary Burtless, Author
Strobe Talbott, President
Steven Bennett, Vice President/COO
Stewart Uretsky, Vice President/CFO
Employment, health and financial information for the elderly. *$26.95*
276 pages Cloth
ISBN 0-815711-76-6

Print: Journals

7410 **Gerontology: Abstracts in Social Gerontology**
National Council on the Aging
1901 L St NW
4th Floor
Washington, DC 20036-3506
202-479-1200
FAX: 202-479-0735
TTY:202-479-6674
e-mail: info@ncoa.org
www.ncoa.org

James Firman, President/CEO
Jay Greenberg, ScD, Senior Vice President, Social Enterprise
Richard Birkel, PhD, MPA, Senior Vice President, Center for Healthy Aging and Director
Nora Dowd Eisenhower, JD, Senior Vice President, Economic Security and Director
Detailed abstracts are provided for recent major journal articles, books, reports and other materials on many facets of aging, including: adult education, demography, family relations, institutional care and work attitudes. Item No. AB100; Journals $114.00; Member Discount: $94.00.
Quarterly

7411 **Physical & Occupational Therapy in Geriatrics**
Taylor & Francis Group, LLC
325 Chestnut Street
Suite 800 #800
Philadelphia, PA 19106-2608
215-625-8900
800-354-1420
FAX: 215-625-2940
e-mail: haworthpress@taylorandfrancis.com
www.tandf.co.uk

Ellen Dunleavey Taira, Editor
Barbara Pucher, CFO
Focuses on current practices and emerging issues in the care of the older client, including long-term care in institutional and community settings, crisis intervention, and innovative programming; the entire range of problems experienced by the elderly; and the current skills needed for working with older clients. *$99.00*
Quarterly

Print: Magazines

7412 **AARP Magazine**
American Association of Retired Persons
601 E St NW
Washington, DC 20049-3
202-434-7700
888-687-2277
FAX: 202-434-7710
TTY: 877-434-7598
e-mail: member@aarp.org
www.aarp.org

A Barry Rand, President/CEO
Hop Backus, Executive Vice President, State
Steve Cone, Executive Vice President of Integrated Value
Lorraine Cort,s-V zquez, Executive Vice President, Multicultural Markets

A nonprofit membership organization of persons 50 and older dedicated to addressing their needs and interests.

Print: Newsletters

7413 **Aging & Vision News**
Lighthouse International
111 E 59th St
New York, NY 10022-1202
212-821-9216
800-829-0500
FAX: 212-821-9707
e-mail: info@lighthouse.org
www.lightfair.com

Laurie A Silbersweig, Editorial Director
Intended for professionals engaged in research, education or service delivery in the field of vision and aging.
6-12 pages Newsletter

7414 **Aging News Alert**
C D Publications
8204 Fenton St
Silver Spring, MD 20910-4502
301-588-6380
800-666-6380
FAX: 301-588-6385
e-mail: subscription@cdpublications.com
www.cdpublications.com/seniors/ana

Michael Gerecht, President
Ash Gerecht, Co-Owner
Reports on successful senior programs, funding opportunities, and federal actions that effect the elderly. Available in 6, 12 or 24 month subscriptions online and online/print combinations.
$192.00
8 pages Monthly

7415 **Aging and Vision News**
Lighthouse International
111 E 59th St
New York, NY 10022-1202
212-821-9384
800-829-0500
FAX: 212-821-9707
TTY: 212-821-9713
e-mail: info@lighthouse.org
www.lighthouse.org

Robert Rosenberg, Editor
Mark G. Ackermann, President/ Chief Executive Officer
Maura J. Sweeney, Senior Vice President/Chief Operating Officer
John Vlachos, Senior Vice President/Chief Financial Officer

Newsletter

7416 **Enabling News**
Access II Independent Living Centers
101 Industrial Parkway
Gallatin, MO 64640-1280
660-663-2423
888-663-2423
FAX: 660-663-2517
TTY: 660-663-2663
e-mail: access@accessii.org
www.accessii.org

Debra Hawman, Executive Director
Gary Matticks, Owner
Debra Hawman, Executive Director
It is a newsletter published by Access II.
8 pages Quarterly

7417 **Part B News**
DecisionHealth
9737 Washingtonian Blvd
Two Washingtonian Center, Suite. 20
Gaithersburg, MD 20878-7364
301-287-2682
855-225-5341
FAX: 301-287-2535
e-mail: customer@decisionhealth.com
www.decisionhealth.com

Scott Kraft, Editor
Scott Kraft, Director, Content Management
Steve Greenberg, President
Tonya Nevin, Vice President, New Business Development
Each week Part B News brings you comprehensive Medicare Part B regulatory coverage, plain-English interpretive guidance, Fee Schedule updates, claims filing strategies, coding, documentation and payment best practices, and the latest on Congressional health care deliberations and how they affect your practice.
$519.00
Yearly

7418 **Social Security Bulletin**
US Social Security Administration
2100 M Street NW
Suite 829 #829
Washington, DC 20037- 0002
202-358-6066
800-772-1213
FAX: 202-282-7219
TTY: 800-325-0778
www.ssa.gov/policy

Karyn Tucker, Managing Editor
Richard Balkus, Assoc. Comm. Office Of Dis
Carolyn W. Colvin, Commissioner
James A. Kissko, Chief of Staff
Reports on results of research and analysis pertinent to the Social Security and SSI programs. *$16.00*
Monthly

Non Print: Newsletters

7419 **AGRAM**
Assoc of Ohio Philanthropic Homes, Housing/Service
855 S Wall St
Columbus, OH 43206-1921
614-444-2882
FAX: 614-444-2974
e-mail: info@aopha.org
www.aopha.org

John Alfano, CEO
Tim White, Executive Director
P Alfano, President/CEO

Weekly

7420 **Aging News Alert**
C D Publications
8204 Fenton Street
Silver Spring, MD 20910-4502
301-588-6380
800-666-6380
FAX: 301-588-6385
e-mail: subscription@cdpublications.com
www.cdpublications.com

Ash Gerecht, Co-Owner
Sharon Livermore, Businesss Manager
Reports on successful senior programs, funding opportunities, and federal actions that effect the elderly. Available in 6, 12 or 24 month subscriptions online and online/print combinations.
$192.00
8 pages Monthly

7421 CAHSA Connecting
Colorado Assoc of Homes and Services for the Aging
1888 Sherman St
Suite 610
Denver, CO 80203-1160 303-837-8834
FAX: 303-837-8836
e-mail: info@cahsa.org
www.leadingagecolorado.org

Laura Landwirth, Executive Director
Elisabeth Borden, Director
Maureen Hewitt, President
Vennita Jenkins, Secretary
CAHSA Connecting is published monthly by the Colorado Association of Homes and Services for the Aging (CAHSA)

7422 CANPFA-Line
CT Assoc of Not-for-Profit Providers of the Aging
1340 Wilmington Rdg
Berlin, CT 6037 860-828-2903
FAX: 860-828-8694
e-mail: leadingagect@leadingagect.org
www.leadingagect.org

Mag Morelli, President
Nurka Carrero, Office Manager
Andrea Bellofiore, Director of Member Programs & Se
Beth Ricker, Finance Manager & Membership Dir
LeadingAge Connecticut promotes and advocates for a vision of the world in which every community offers an integrated and coordinated continuum of high quality, affordable health care, housing and community based services.
Bi-Monthly

7423 Capitol Focus
Colorado Assoc of Homes and Services for the Aging
1888 Sherman St
Suite 610
Denver, CO 80203-1160 303-837-8834
FAX: 303-837-8836
e-mail: info@cahsa.org
www.leadingagecolorado.org

Laura Landwirth, Executive Director
Elisabeth Borden, Director
Maureen Hewitt, President
Vennita Jenkins, Secretary
Capitol Focus is a weekly activities summary of the Colorado Legislature for CAHSA members, provided by staff of the Colorado Association of Homes and Services for the Aging.

7424 Capsule
Children of Aging Parents
P.O.Box 167
Richboro, PA 18954-167 215-945-6900
800-227-7294
FAX: 215-945-8720
e-mail: info@caps4caregivers.org
www.caps4caregivers.org

Karen Rosenberg, Director
An informative newsletter for caregivers.
Quarterly

7425 Communique
Iowa Association of Homes & Services for the Aging

Bi-weekly

7426 Elder Visions Newsletter
National Indian Council on Aging
10501 Montgomery Blvd NE
Suite 210
Albuquerque, NM 87111-3832 505-292-2001
FAX: 505-292-1922
e-mail: randella@nicoa.org
www.nicoa.org

Traci Mc Clellan, Executive Director
James Delacruz, Chairman Of The Board
Phyllis Antone, Director
Provides information on issues affecting American Indian and Alaska Native Elders.
Quarterly

7427 Innovations
National Council on Aging
1901 L Street NW
4th Floor
Washington, DC 20036-3506 202-479-1200
FAX: 202-479-0735
TTY:202-479-6674
e-mail: info@ncoa.org
www.ncoa.org

Austin Han, Manager
James Firman, President/CEO
Donna Whitt, SVP/CFO
Nancy Whitelaw, SVP/Director
Explores significant developments in the field of aging, keeping individuals informed on a broad range of topics.
Quarterly

7428 NASUA News
National Association of State Units on Aging
1201 15th Street NW
Suite 350
Washington, DC 20005-2842 202-898-2578
FAX: 202-898-2583
e-mail: info@nasua.org
www.nasuad.org

Martha Roherty, Executive Director
Peggie Rice, Director of Policy and Legislative Affairs
Eric Risteen, Chief Operating Officer
Kimberly Fletcher, Conference and Outreach Coordinator
It is the newsletter of the National Association of State Units on Aging
Monthly

7429 NCOA Week
National Council on Aging
1901 L Street NW
4th Floor
Washington, DC 20036-3540 202-479-1200
FAX: 202-479-0735
TTY:202-479-6674
e-mail: info@ncoa.org
www.ncoa.org

James P Firman, President/CEO
Donna Whitt, SVP/CFO
Nancy Whitelaw, SVP/Director
A concise e-newsletters focused on the issues you care about, including policies that affect funding, grants and awards you can apply for, and best practices you can adapt for your center.
Weekly

7430 NNEAHSA
Northn New England Assoc of Homes & Svcs for Aging
PO Box 1428
Standish, ME 04084-1428 207-773-4822
FAX: 207-773-0101
e-mail: sderingis@nneahsa.org
www.agingservicesmenh.org

Sheila Deringis, Editor
Providing healthy, affordable and ethical long-term care to older citizens throughout Maine, New Hampshire and Vermont.

7431 NSCLC Washington Weekly
National Senior Citizens Law Center
1444 Eye St NW
Suite 1100
Washington, DC 20005-6547 202-289-6976
FAX: 202-289-7224
e-mail: nscls@nsclc.org
www.nsclc.org

Paul Nathanson, Executive Director
Edward King, Executive Director
Edward Spurgeon, Executive Director

Provides the latest case information, administration and congressional developments of importance for the elderly.

7432 Quality First
American Assoc of Homes and Services for the Aging
2519 Connecticut Ave NW
Washington, DC 20008-1520
202-783-2242
FAX: 202-783-2255
www.leadingage.org

William L Minnix Jr, President

Features helpful tips for marketing services and earning the public's trust through the web site.

Quarterly

7433 Senior Focus
National Council on Aging
1901 L Street
4th Floor
Washington, DC 20036-3540
202-479-1200
FAX: 202-479-0735
TTY:202-479-6674
e-mail: info@ncoa.org
www.ncoa.org

Austin Han, Manager
James Firman, President/CEO
Donna Whit, SVP/CFO
Nancy Whitelaw, SVP/Director

Contains health, financial, lifestyle tips written for seniors

Quarterly

Support Groups

7434 Area Agency on Aging of Southwest Arkansas
600 Columbia Road 11 East
PO Box 1863
Magnolia, AR 71753
870-234-7410
800-272-2127
FAX: 870-234-6804
e-mail: inref@magnolia-net.com
www.agewithdignity.com

Janet Morrison, Executive Director

The Area Agency on Aging of Southwest Arkansas, Inc. is a non-profit organization serving adults age 60 or older, family care-givers, agencies and organizations working with seniors. It is part of a national network of more than 650 Area Agencies on Aging throughout the United States.

7435 Area Agency on Aging: Region One
1366 E Thomas Rd
Suite 108
Phoenix, AZ 85014-5739
602-264-2255
888-783-7500
FAX: 602-230-9132
www.aaaphx.org

Mary Lynn Kasunic, President
Jeannine Berg, Vice Chairman
Bobbie Garland, Vice Chairman
Richard Peitzmeier, Vice Chairman

We have a vast variety of programs and services to enhance the quality of life for residents of Maricopa County, Arizona. If you would like more information about services mentioned within the website please call.

7436 High Country Council of Governments Area Agency on Aging
468 New Market Blvd
Boone, NC 28607-1820
828-265-5434
FAX: 828-265-5439
e-mail: breece@regiond.org
www.regiond.org

Robert L. Johnson, Chairman
Gary D. Blevins, Vice Chair
Brenda Lyerly, Secretary
Danny McIntosh, Treasurer

High Country Council of Governments is the multi-county planning and development agency for the seven northwestern North Carolina counties of Alleghany, Ashe, Avery, Mitchell, Watauga, Wilkes, and Yancey. The High Country region is a voluntary association of towns and counties located in the northern mountains of North Carolina.

7437 Institute on Aging
3575 Geary Blvd
San Francisco, CA 94118-3212
415-750-4111
877-750-4111
FAX: 415-750-5337
e-mail: info@ioaging.org
www.ioaging.org

J. Thomas Briody, MHSc, President
Dustin Harper, Vice President, Community Living Services
Cindy Kauffman, MS, COO
Roxana Tsougarakis, MBA, Chief Financial Officer

Support Services for Elders (SSE) provides care coordination, household management, personal support, bookkeeping, and other assistance to help protect your financial affairs.

7438 Land-of-Sky Regional Council Area Agency on Aging
339 New Leicester Hwy
Suite 140
Asheville, NC 28806-2087
828-251-6622
FAX: 828-251-6353
e-mail: info@landofsky.org
www.landofsky.org

LeeAnne Tucker, Aging & Volunteer Services Director
Terry Albrecht, Program Director
Joan Tuttle, Director
Joe Mc Kinney, Manager

Is the designated regional organization to meet the needs of persons over 60 in Buncombe, Henderson, Madison, and Transylvania counties, by the North Carolina Division of Aging and Adult Services.

7439 Lumber River Council of Governments Area Agency on Aging
30 Cj Walker Rd
COMtech Park
Pembroke, NC 28372-7340
910-618-5533
FAX: 910-521-7556
e-mail: lrcog@mail.lrcog.dst.nc.us
www.lumberrivercog.org

Michelle Gaitley, Nutrition Program Director
Renee Cooper, Nutrition Program Assistant
Kristen Elk Maynor, Aging Program Coordinator
Margaret Lennon, Division Administrator

The Family Caregiver Support Program was created to assist family members, neighbors, and friends who help care for a person over the age of 60, or minor grandchildren being reared by a grandparent over 60.

7440 Mid-Carolina Area Agency on Aging
130 Gillespie Street
3rd Floor, Post Office Drawer 1510
Fayetteville, NC 28301-1510
910-323-4191
FAX: 910-323-9330
e-mail: gdye@mccog.org
www.mccog.org

James Caldwell, COG Executive Director
Glenda Dye, Aging Director
Lynda Barnett, Aging Care Manager
Carla Smith, Aging Program Specialist

The Mid-Carolina Area Agency on Aging is designated for planning, administration, and advocacy of services for persons aged 60 and older and their spouses who need assistance in order to remain as independent as possible.

7441 Piedmont Triad Council of Governments Area Agency on Aging
2216 W Meadowview Rd
Suite 201
Greensboro, NC 27407-3480 336-294-4950
FAX: 336-632-0457
e-mail: acalhoun@ptcog.org
www.ptcog.org

Blair Barton-Percival, Director
Adrienne Calhoun, Assistant Director
Bob Cleveland, Aging Program Planner
Joe Dzugan, Aging Systems Coordinator
Responsible for planning, developing, implementing, and coordinating aging services for seven counties in the Piedmont Triad (Alamance, Caswell, Davidson, Guilford, Montgomery, Randolph, and Rockingham) and their 185,00 residents age 60 and older.

7442 Southwestern Commission Area Agency on Aging
125 Bonnie Ln
Sylva, NC 28779-8552 828-586-1962
FAX: 828-586-1968
e-mail: mary@regiona.org
www.regiona.org

Ryan Sherby, Executive Director
Beth Cook, Workforce Development Director
Janne Mathews, Aging Program Coordinator
Sarajane Melton, Area Agency on Aging Administrator
The Area Agency on Aging (AAA) works on behalf of older adults and their caregivers in the seven southwestern counties of North Carolina. The Southwestern Commission Area Agency on Aging was established in 1980 as mandated by the 1977 Amendments of the Older Americans Act in order for a Planning and Service Area (PSA) to receive funds from the Act.

7443 Tompkins County Office for the Aging
214 W. Martin Luther King Jr./State
Ithaca, NY 14850-4299 607-274-5482
FAX: 607-274-5495
e-mail: lholmes@tompkins-co.org
www.tompkins-co.org

Lisa Holmes, Director
Lisa Lunas, Aging Services Planner
Katrina Schickel, Aging Services Specialist
David Stoyell, Aging Services Specialist
We provide objective and unbiased information regarding the array of services available for older adults and their caregivers. Established in 1975, our mission is to assist the senior population of Tompkins County to remain independent in their homes as long as is possible and appropriate, and with a decent quality of life and human dignity.

7444 Triangle J Council of Governments Area Agency on Aging
PO Box 12276
Research Triangle Park, NC 27709-2276 919-549-0551
FAX: 919-549-9390
e-mail: ejones@tjcog.org
www.tjaaa.org

Joan Pellettier, Director
Mary Warren, Assistant Director
Ashley Price, Program Associate
Jennifer Link, Regional Ombudsman for Long-Term Care
We serve to facilitate and support the development of programs to address the needs of older adults and to support investment in their talents and interests.

7445 University of California Memory and Aging Center
675 Nelson Rising Lane
Suite 190
San Francisco, CA 94143-1207 415-353-2057
FAX: 415-476-5591
e-mail: webmaster@memory.ucsf.edu
www.memory.ucsf.edu

Bruce L Miller, Director
Mary Koestler, Project Administrator
Carrie Cheung, Clinic Coordinator
Ken Edwards, Administrative Assistant
Provides support for patients and families affected by neurodegenerative diseases. In addition to our established support groups, we continue to develop new support groups.

7446 Upper Coastal Plain Council of Governments Area Agency on Aging
PO Box 9
Wilson, NC 27894-9 252-234-5952
FAX: 252-234-5971
e-mail: helen.page@ucpcog.org
www.ucpcog.org

Greg Godard, Executive Director
Jody Riddle, AAA Program Director
Helen Page, Aging Programs Specialist
Abigail W. Harper, Regional Ombudsman
The Upper Coastal Plain Area Agency On Aging is one of 16 Area Agencies on Aging across the state of NC, serving Region L. Counties include Edgecombe, Halifax, Nash, Northampton, and Wilson. The mission of the Area Agency on Aging is to empower senior adults, family caregivers, and individuals with disabilities residing in Edgecombe, Halifax, Nash, Northampton, and Wilson Counties to live independent, meaningful, healthy, and dignified lives.

Blind & Deaf

Associations

7447 **American Association of the Deaf-Blind**
8630 Fenton Street
PO Box 2831, Suite 121
Kensington, MD 20891-3803
301-495-4403
FAX: 301-495-4404
TTY:301-495-4402
e-mail: aadb-info@aadb.org
www.aadb.org

Jamie Pope, Executive Director
Elizabeth Spiers, Information Services Director
Jill Gaus, President

The American Association of the Deaf-Blind (AADB) is a non-profit 501(c)(3) national consumer organization of, by, and for deaf-blind Americans and their supporters. Deaf-Blind includes all types and degrees of dual vision and hearing loss. Our mission is to ensure that all deaf-blind persons achieve their maximum potential through increased independence, productivity, and integration into the community.
Membership dues

7448 **American Society for Deaf Children**
800 Florida Ave NE
Washington, DC 20002-3695
202-644-9204
800-942-2732
FAX: 410-795-0965
e-mail: asdc@deafchildren.org
www.deafchildren.org

Jodee Crace, President

We believe deaf or hard-of-hearing children are entitled to full communication access in their home, school, and community. We also believe that language development, respect for the Deaf, and access to deaf and hard-of-hearing role models are important to assure optimal intellectual, social, and emotional development.

7449 **Arena Stage**
11101 Sixth St
Washington, DC 20024
202-554-9066
FAX: 202-488-4056
TTY:202-484-0247
e-mail: arena@arenastage.org
www.arenastage.org

David E. Shiffrin, Chair
Zelda Fichandler, Founding Director
Molly Smith, Artistic Director
Chad Bauman, Associate Executive Director

A pioneer in providing access to theater for people with disabilities and the birthplace of Audio Description. Offers infrared assistive listening devices (both loop and headset), program books in Braille, large print and wheelchair accessible seating with adjacent companion seating. Audio cassette format available upon request. Sign Interpretation and Audio Description are offered at selected performances. Cafe menus and shop lists in Braille. Wheelchair-accessible with lifts and ramps.

7450 **Association of Late-Deafened Adults**
8038 Macintosh Ln
Suite 2
Rockford, IL 61107-5300
815-332-1515
866-402-2532
TTY:815-332-1515
e-mail: info@alda.org
www.alda.org

Linda Drattell, President
Matt Ferrara, Region I Director
Marsha Kopp, Region II Directo
Dave Litman, Region III Director

Supports the empowerment of late-deafened people.

7451 **Canadian Deafblind Association (CDBA) National Office**
421 - 1860 Appleby Line
Suite 421
Burlington, ON L7L-7H7
866-229-5832
FAX: 905-319-2027
e-mail: info@cdbanational.com
www.cdbanational.com

Carolyn Monaco, President
Suzanne McConnell, VP Administration
Ericka Dixon-Williams, VP Special Projects
Brad Ramey, Ontario Chapter Representative

The mission of the Canadian Deafblind Association's National organization is to promote and enhance the well-being of people who are deafblind through: advocacy, the development and dissemination of information, and the provision of support to our chapters, members, and community partners.

7452 **Foundation Fighting Blindness**
716B Columbia Gateway Drive
Suite 100
Columbia, MD 21046
410-423-0600
800-683-5555
FAX: 410-363-2393
TTY: 800-683-5551
e-mail: info@fightblindeness.org
www.fightblindness.org

Gordon Gund, Chairman
Edward H. Gollob, President
Joel P. Davis, Senior Vice President
Haynes Lea, Vice President/Treasurer

the urgent mission is to drive the research that will provide preventions, treatments, and cures for people affected by retinitis pigmentosa, macular degeneration, Usher syndrome and the entire spectrum of retinal degenerative diseases.

7453 **Hearing Loss Association of America**
7910 Woodmont Ave
Suite 1200
Bethesda, MD 20814-7022
301-657-2248
FAX: 301-913-9413
TTY:301-657-2248
www.hearingloss.org

Brenda Battat, Executive Director
Barbara Kelley, Dep Exec Dir, Editor-In-Chief
Nancy Macklin, Director of Events & Marketing
Lise Hamlin, Director of Public Policy

The mission of the Hearing Loss Association of America is to open the world of communication to people with hearing loss through information, education, advocacy and support.

7454 **Helen Keller National Center for Deaf- Blind Youths And Adults**
141 Middle Neck Rd
Sands Point, NY 11050-1218
516-944-8900
FAX: 516-944-7302
TTY:516-944-8637
e-mail: hkncinfo@hknc.org
www.hknc.org

Joseph McNulty, Executive Director

Enables each person who is deaf/blind to live and work in his or her community of choice.

7455 **Idaho Commission for the Blind and Visually Impaired**
341 W. Washington St.
PO Box 83720
Boise, ID 83720-0012
208-334-3220
800-542-8688
FAX: 208-334-2963
e-mail: ajones@icbvi.idaho.gov
www.icbvi.state.id.us

Angela Jones, Administrator
Raelene Thomas, Management Assistant
Bruce Christopherson, Rehabilitation Services Chief
Dana Ard, Vocational Rehabilitation Counse

Empowers persons who are blind or visually impaired by providing vocational rehabilitation training, skills training and educational opportunities to achieve self fulfillment through quality employment and independent living; to serve as a resource to families and employers and to expand public awareness regarding the potential of all persons who are blind or visually impaired.

7456 **International Hearing Society**
16880 Middlebelt Rd
Ste 4
Livonia, MI 48154-3374
734-522-7200
FAX: 734-522-0200
e-mail: bdemicoli@ihsinfo.org
www.ihsinfo.org

Kathleen Mennillo MBA, Executive Director
Donna Kinnelly, Member Services Coordinator
Sandra den Boer, Communications Specialist
Marlene Deuby, Continuing Education Specialist

IHS members are engaged in the practice of testing human hearing and selecting, fitting and dispensing hearing instruments.

7457 **Lilac Services for the Blind**
1212 N Howard St
Spokane, WA 99201-2410
509-328-9116
800-422-7893
FAX: 509-328-8965
e-mail: info@lilacblind.org
www.lilacblind.org

Cheryl Martin, Executive Director
Mathew Plank, Marketing Director
Peggy Swanson, Office Manager
Debbie Bowcutt, Rehabilitation Teacher & Low Vis

Lilac Services for the Blind provides independent living instruction, adaptive aids, counseling, low-vision evaluations, support groups, Braille transcription services, and much more for 14 counties in the inland Northwest.

7458 **National Consortium on Deaf-Blindness**
345 Monmouth Ave N
Monmouth, OR 97361-1329
800-438-9376
FAX: 503-838-8150
TTY:800-854-7013
e-mail: info@nationaldb.org
www.nationaldb.org

D. Jay Gense, Director
Kathy McNulty, Associate Director
Joe Mcnulty, Co-Principal Investigator
Amy Parker, ED. D, Associate Director

Promotes academic achievement and results for children and youth who are deaf-blind, through technical assistanve, model demonstration, and information dissemination activities that are supported by evidence-based practices. Information about deaf-blindness is available free of charge through the Consortium's information services branch, DB-Link.

7459 **National Family Association for Deaf-Blind**
141 Middle Neck Rd
Sands Point, NY 11050-1218
516-944-8900
800-255-0411
FAX: 516-883-9060
TTY: 516-944-8637
e-mail: NFADB@aol.com
www.nfadb.org

Susan Green, President
Janette Peracchio, Vice President
Cynthia Jackson-Glenn, Treasurer
Paddi Davies, Secretary

The National Family Association for Deaf-Blind (NFADB) is a non-profit, volunteer-based family association. Our philosophy is that individuals who are deaf-blind are valued members of society and are entitled to the same opportunities and choices as other members of the community. We are the largest national network of families focusing on issues surrounding deaf blindness.

7460 **National Federation of the Blind**
200 East Wells Street
at Jernigan Place
Baltimore, MD 21230-4998
410-659-9314
FAX: 410-685-5653
e-mail: nfb@nfb.org
nfb.org

John Berggren, Executive Director for Operation
John G. Paré Jr., Executive Director for Strategic Initiatives
Mark Riccobono, Executive Director, NFB Jernigan Institute
Joanne Wilson, Executive Director for Affiliate Action

The National Federation of the Blind (NFB) is the largest organization of the blind in the world. The Federation's purpose is to help blind people achieve self-confidence, self-respect, and self-determination. Their goal is the complete integration of the blind into society on a basis of equality.

7461 **National Information Center for Children and Youth with Disabilities (NICHCY)**
1825 Connecticut Ave NW
Ste 700
Washington, DC 20009
202-884-8200
800-695-0285
FAX: 202-884-8441
TTY: 202-884-8200
e-mail: nichcy@aed.org
www.nichcy.org

Suzanne Ripley, Manager

NICHCY is the center that provides information to the nation ondisabilities in children and youth; programs and services for infants, children, and youth with disabilities; IDEA, the nation's special education law; and research-based information on effective practices for children with disabilities.

7462 **National Information Clearinghouse on Children who are Deaf-Blind**
National Consortium on Deaf-Blindness
345 Monmouth Ave N
Monmouth, OR 97361-1329
503-838-8391
800-438-9376
877-877-1593
FAX: 503-838-8150
TTY:800-854-7013
e-mail: dblink@tr.wou.edu
www.tr.wou.edu

Dr. Ella Taylor, Director
Nancy Ganson, Assistant to the Director
Mike Stewart, Grants Management Office
Cindi Mafit, Grants Management Office

Collects, organizes, and disseminates information related to children and youth of ages 0 to 21 who are deaf-blind and connects consumers of deaf-blind information to the appropriate resources. Publishes a number of topical papers and publishes Deaf-Blind Perspective.

7463 **Ultratec**
450 Science Dr
Madison, WI 53711-1166
608-238-5400
800-482-2424
FAX: 608-238-3008
TTY: 800-482-2424
www.ultratec.com

Jackie Morgan, Marketing Director

Ultratec works to make telephone access more convenient and reliable for people with hearing loss.

Camps

7464 Florida Lions Camp
Lions of Multiple District 35
2819 Tiger Lake Road
Lake Wales, FL 33898-9582
863-696-1948
FAX: 863-696-2398
e-mail: bjcage@hotmail.com
www.lionscampfl.org

Barbara Cage, Executive Director
Liz Cage, Program Director
Carissa Moen, Bookkeeping/Registrar

One-week sessions June-August for youths and adults with visual impairments and other challenging disabilities. Coed, ages 5 and up. A variety of traditional summer camp activities which include: swimming, canoeing, fishing, hiking, camping out and cooking over a fire, games, arts & crafts, singing & dancing, hay-wagon rides, challenge course and much more. Activities are adapted to the age and ability of each camper to ensure maximum participation, safety and fun.

7465 Florida School for the Deaf and Blind
207 San Marco Ave
St Augustine, FL 32084-2799
904-827-2200
800-344-3732
FAX: 904-827-2325
e-mail: info@fsdb.k12.fl.us
www.fsdb.k12.fl.us

Dr. Jeanne Glidden Prickett, EdD, Shelter Administrator
Debbie Schuler, Administrator of Instructional S
Cindy Day, Executive Director of Parent Ser
Terri Wiseman, Administrator of Business Servic

Statewide public boarding school for eligible students who are deaf/hard-of-hearing or blind/visually impaired. FSDB serves children who are pre-k through high school.

Print: Books

7466 Communicating with People Who Have Trouble Hearing & Seeing: A Primer
National Association for Visually Handicapped
22 W 21st St
Fl 6
New York, NY 10010-6943
212-255-2804
FAX: 212-727-2931
www.lighthouse.org

Roger O Goldman, Chairman Of The Board

Line drawings that depict problems for those with both deficiencies. $2.00

7467 Helen and Teacher: The Story of Helen & Anne Sullivan Macy
American Foundation for the Blind/AFB Press
11 Penn Plz
Suite 300
New York, NY 10001-2006
212-502-7600
800-232-5463
FAX: 212-502-7777
e-mail: afbinf@afb.net
www.afb.org

Carl Augusto, President
Richard Obnen, Chairman Of The Board
Michael Gilliam, Vice Chairman
Alan Lindroth, Principal

A pictorial biography emphasizing Hellen Keller's accomplishments in public life over a period of more than 60 years. Traces Anne Sullivan's early years and her meeting with Helen Keller, and goes on to recount the joint events of their lives. A definitive biography. $29.95.

Paperback
ISBN 0-891282-89-0

7468 Independence Without Sight and Sound: Suggestions for Practitioners
American Foundation for the Blind/AFB Press
11 Penn Plz
Suite 300
New York, NY 10001-2006
212-502-7600
800-232-8463
FAX: 212-502-7777
e-mail: afbinfo@afb.net
www.afb.org

Carl Augusto, President
Richard Obnen, Chairman Of The Board
Michael Gilliam, Vice Chairman
Alan Lindroth, Principal

This practical guidebook covers the essential aspects of communicating and working with deaf-blind persons. Includes useful information on how to talk with deaf-blind people, and adapt orientation and mobility techniques for deaf-blind travelers. *$39.95*

193 pages Paperback
ISBN 0-891282-46-7

7469 Reclaiming Independence: Staying in the Drivers Seat When You Are no Longer Drive.
American Printing House for the Blind
1839 Frankfort Ave
Louisville, KY 40206-3148
502-895-2405
800-223-1839
FAX: 502-899-2274
e-mail: info@aph.org
www.aph.org

Tuck Tinsley, President
Joseph Paradis, Chairman
Kathleen Huebner, Vice Chairman
Jane Thompson, Executive Director

Useful for both individuals and professionals, this video/resource guide will help you successfuly use rehabilitation and transportation resources. *$60.00*

7470 Verbal View of the Web & Net
American Printing House for the Blind
1839 Frankfort Ave
Louisville, KY 40206-3148
502-895-2405
800-223-1839
FAX: 502-899-2274
e-mail: info@aph.org
www.aph.org

Tuck Tinsley, President
Joseph Paradis, Chairman
Kathleen Huebner, Vice Chairman
Jane Thompson, Executive Director

One of a series of Verbal View titles, Verbal View of the Net & Web explains how to access information on the internet and teaches accessability features of Internet Explorer. *$50.00*

Print: Magazines

7471 Braille Montior
National Federation of the Blind Senior Division
200 E Wells St
Baltimore, MD 21230-4914
410-659-9314
FAX: 410-685-5653
e-mail: nfbpublications@nfb.org
www.nfb.org

Barbara Pierce, Editor

The Braille Monitor is the leading publication of the National Federation of the Blind. It covers the events and activities of the NFB and addresses the many issues and concerns of the blind.

11 times a year

7472 **Deaf-Blind American**
American Association of the Deaf-Blind (AADB)
8630 Fenton Street
PO Box 2831, Suite 121
Kensington, MD 20891-3803
301-495-4403
FAX: 301-495-4404
TTY:301-495-4402
e-mail: aadb-info@aadb.org
www.aadb.org

Jamie Pope, Executive Director
Elizabeth Spiers, Information Services Director
Timothy Jackson, President
We are a consumer membership organization of, by and for people who have dual vision and hearing loss. Services we provide include an information clearinghouse on deaf blindness, a quarterly magazine (The Deaf Blind American), a newsletter, AADB news, a task force to improve interpreting for deaf-blind people, a listen for members, a partnership with the American Red Cross, and national conferences. *$5.00*
Quarterly

7473 **Hearing Loss Magazine**
HearingLoss Association of America
7910 Woodmont Ave
Ste 1200
Bethesda, MD 20814-7022
301-657-2248
FAX: 301-913-9413
www.hearingloss.org

Brenda Battat, Executive Director
Barbara Kelley, Editor-in-Chief/Deputy Executive Director of HLAA
Lisa Hamlin, Director Of Public Policy
Cindy Dyer, Graphic Design
Readers look to Hearing Loss Magazine to provide them with the latest information on products, services, research, and technology in the hearing health care field. They also look for personal stories of hard of hearing people to find encouragement, and give them the feeling that they're not alone in living with a hearing loss. They look for practical and useful information. Hearing Loss Magazine readers view the magazine as a lifeline to help them help themselves and live well with hearing loss.
Bi-Monthly

7474 **Hearing Professional Magazine**
International Hearing Society
Ste 4
16880 Middlebelt Rd
Livonia, MI 48154-3374
734-522-7200
FAX: 734-522-0200
e-mail: knacarato@ihsinfo.org
www.ihsinfo.org

Scott Beall, Treasurer Director
Alan Lowell, President
Kathleen Mennillo, Executive Director
The Hearing Professional magazine is the official publication of the International Hearing Society. This quarterly publication includes industry news, membership highlights and best practices, hearing healthcare legislation, and other information and tools for hearing healthcare professionals.

Print: Newsletters

7475 **Deaf-Blind Perspective**
National Consortium on Deaf-Blindness
345 Monmouth Ave
Monmouth, OR 97361
503-838-8391
800-438-9376
FAX: 503-838-8150
TTY: 800-854-7013
e-mail: dbp@wou.edu
www.tr.wou.edu/dblink

John Reiman PhD, Director
Peggy Malloy, Managing Editor
A free publication with articles, essays, and announcements about topics related to people who are deaf-blind. The primary focus is on the education of children and youth with deaf-blindness. Published two times a year (Spring and Fall) by the national consortium on Deaf-blindness at the Teaching Research Institute at Western Oregon University.

7476 **InFocus**
7168 Columbia Gateway Dri
Suite 100
Columbia, MD 21046
410-423-0600
800-683-5555
FAX: 410-363-2393
TTY: 800-683-5551
e-mail: info@fightblindeness.org
www.blindness.org

Gordon Gund, Chairman
Edward H. Gollob, President
David Brint, VP
Haynes Lea, VP &Treasurer
Presents articles on coping, research updates, and Foundation news.
3x/year

7477 **News from Advocates for Deaf-Blind**
National Family Association for Deaf-Blind
141 Middle Neck Rd
Sands Point, NY 11050-1218
516-944-8900
800-225-0411
FAX: 516-883-9060
TTY: 516-944-8637
e-mail: NFADB@gmail.com
www.NFADB.org

Clara Berg, President
Edgenie Bellah, Affiliate Coordinator
Paddi Davies, Treasurer
Patti McGowan, Secretary
A membership organization which provide resources, education, advocacy, referrals and support for families with children who are deaf-blind; professionals in the field; and individuals who are deaf-blind.
20 pages TriAnnual

Non Print: Newsletters

7478 **AADB E-News**
American Association of the Deaf-Blind
8630 Fenton Street
Suite 121
Silver Spring, MD 20910- 3803
301-495-4403
FAX: 301-495-4404
e-mail: aadb-info@aadb.org
www.aadb.org

Jill Gaus, President
Lynn Jansen, VP
Debby Lieberman, Secretary
Mike Reese, Vice Treasurer
Contains information about the latest events occurring within AADB and in the deaf-blind community.

7479 **ALDA Newsletter**
ALDA
8038 Macintosh Ln
Suite 2
Rockford, IL 61107-5336
815-332-1515
866-402-2532
FAX: 877-907-1738
TTY: 815-332-1515
e-mail: info@alda.org
www.alda.org

Mary Lou Mistretta, President
Dave Litman, President Elect
Brenda Estes, Past President
Articles, stories and poems by and about late-deafened adults.

7480 Beam
1850 W Roosevelt Rd
Chicago, IL 60608-1298
312-666-1331
FAX: 312-243-8539
TTY:312-666-8874
www.chicagolighthouse.org

James Kesteloot, President
Terrence Longo, Assistant Director
Quarterly newsletter of the organization offering progressive programs for the blind, visually impaired, deaf-blind and multi-disabled children and adults, including vocational programs, computer and office skills training, job placement, independent living skills, orientation and mobility training, counseling and a low vision clinic.

7481 Endeavor
American Society for Deaf Children
800 Florida Ave NE
Washington, PA 20002-3695
717-703-0073
800-942-2732
FAX: 717-909-5599
TTY: 202-664-9204
e-mail: asdc@deafchildren.org
www.deafchildren.org

Robert B Wells, Editor
Tami Hossler, Editor
ASDC's qurterly publication featuring committee reports, stories, and fun.
Quarterly

7482 HKNC Newsletter
Helen Keller National Center
141 Middle Neck Rd
Sands Point, NY 11050-1218
516-944-8900
FAX: 516-944-7302
TTY:516-944-8637
e-mail: hkncinfo@hknc.org
www.hknc.org

Joseph McNulty, Executive Director
Highlights recent activities at the national center.

7483 NAT-CENT
Helen Keller National Center
141 Middle Neck Rd
Sands Point, NY 11050-1218
516-944-8900
FAX: 516-944-7302
TTY:516-944-8637
e-mail: hkncinfo@hknc.org
www.hknc.org

Joseph McNulty, Executive Director
Contains articles on legislation, services, aids and devices, human interest and issues related to deaf-blindness.

Non Print: Software

7484 Braille + Mobile Manager
American Printing House for the Blind
1839 Frankfort Ave
Louisville, KY 40206-0085
502-895-2405
800-223-1839
FAX: 502-899-2284
e-mail: info@aph.org
aph.org

Tuck Tinsley, President
Joseph Paradis, Chairman
Kathleen Huebner, Vice Chairman
Jane Thompson, Executive Director
Use it like a hand-held PDA or like a laptop. *$1395.00*

7485 MaximEyes
American Printing House for the Blind
1839 Frankfort Ave
Louisville, KY 40206-0085
502-895-2405
800-223-1839
FAX: 502-899-2284
e-mail: info@aph.org
aph.org

Tuck Tinsley, President
Joseph Paradis, Chairman
Kathleen Huebner, Vice Chairman
Jane Thompson, Executive Director
MaximEyes is a plug-in for Internet Explorer that adds a toolbar that allows you to controll the size of website text and images. *$59.95*

Non Print: Video

7486 Getting in Touch
2612 N Mattis Ave
PO Box 7886
Champaign, IL 61826-1053
217-352-3273
800-519-2707
FAX: 217-352-1221
e-mail: orders@researchpress.com
www.researchpress.com

Russell Pence, President
David Parkinson, Chairman
Cynthia Martin, Principal
Ann Parkinson, Principal

7487 Journey
Landmark Media
3450 Slade Run Dr
Falls Church, VA 22042-3940
703-241-2030
800-342-4336
FAX: 703-536-9540
e-mail: info@landmarkmedia.com
landmarkmedia.com

Michael Hartogs, President
Richard Hartogs, VP Acquisitions
Peter Hartogs, VP New Business & Development
Eric Miller, Sales Representative
A moving portrayal of the extraordinary journey to Japan of 74-year-old Billie Sinclair, who is deaf, blind and mute. He funds his travels by weaving and selling baskets. In Japan he rides a roller coaster, tries judo and visits a deaf and blind acupuncturist. He demonstrates how it is possible to communicate by touch alone. *$195.00*
Video

Support Groups

7488 Aurora pf Central New York
518 James Street
Suite 100
Syracuse, NY 13203-2282
315-422-7263
FAX: 315-422-4792
TTY:315-422-9746
e-mail: auroracny@auroracny.org
auroraofcny.org

John Scala, President
John McCormick, President
Ryan Emery, Treasurer
Leslie Rapson, Secretary
Professional counseling services to assist individuals and their families deal with the trauma of hearing or vision loss.

Cognitive

Associations

7489 **ARC**
1825 K St NW
Suite 1200
Washington, DC 20006
202-534-3700
800-433-5255
FAX: 202-534-3731
e-mail: info@thearc.org
www.thearc.org

Nancy Webster, President
Ronald Brown, VP
Elise McMillan, Secretary
M. J. Bartelmay, Treasurer

The ARC promotes and protects the rights of people with intellectual and developmental disabilities and actively supports their inclusion and participation in the community throughout their lifetimes.

7490 **Autism Research Institute**
4182 Adams Ave
San Diego, CA 92116-2536
619-281-7165
866-366-3361
FAX: 619-563-6840
e-mail: matt@autism.com
www.autismresearchinstitute.com

Steve Edelson Ph.D., Executive Director
Jane Johnson, Managing Director
Valerie Paradiz, Director
Anthony Morgali, Producer

Conducts research on the causes, diagnosis, and treatment of autism and publishes a quarterly newsletter that reviews worldwide research. Literature on causes and treatment available. Refers patients and families to health care professionals and clinics. Request publication list and sample newsletter, Autism Research Review International.

7491 **Autism Services Center**
929 4th Ave
PO Box 507
Huntington, WV 25701-1408
304-525-8014
FAX: 304-525-8026
www.autismservicescenter.org

Mike Grady, CEO
Jimmie Beirne, COO
Nathel Lewis, ASC Training Coordinator

Service agency for individuals with autism and developmental disabilities, and their families. Assists families and agencies attempting to meet the needs of individuals with autism and other developmental disabilities. Makes available technical assistance in designing treatment programs and more. The hotline provides informational packets to callers and assists via telephone when possible.

7492 **Autism Treatment Center of America**
2080 S Undermountain Rd
Sheffield, MA 01257-9643
413-229-2100
877-766-7473
FAX: 413-229-3202
e-mail: correspondence@option.org
www.son-rise.org

Barry Kausman, Co-Founder/ Co-Originator/ Senio
Samahria Lyte Kaufman, Co-Founder/ Co-Originator/ Senio
Bryn Hogan, ATCA Senior Staff
William Hogan, ATCA Senior Staff

Since 1983, the Autism Treatment Center of America has provided innovative training programs for parents and professionals caring for children challenged by Autism, Autism Spectrum Disorders, Pervasive Developmental Disorders (PDD) and other development difficulties. The Son-Rise Program teaches a specific yet comprehensive system of treatment and education designed to help families and caregivers enable their children to dramatically improve in all areas of learning.

7493 **Beck Institute for Cognitive Therapy and Research**
1 Belmont Ave
Suite 700
Bala Cynwyd, PA 19004-1610
610-664-3020
FAX: 610-709-5336
e-mail: info@beckinstitute.org
www.beckinstitute.org

Aaron T Beck, President Emeritus
Judith S Beck PhD, President
Deborah Beck Busis, LSW, Diet Program Coordinator
Norman Cotterell, PhD, Senior Therapist and Clinical Co

Serves as a critically important training ground for cognitive therapists/cognitive behavior therapists.

7494 **Best Buddies**
1243 Islington Ave
Suite 907
Toronto, ON M8X-1Y9
416-531-0003
888-779-0061
FAX: 416-531-0325
e-mail: info@bestbuddies.ca
www.bestbuddies.ca

Steven Pinnock, Executive Director
Emily Bolyea-Kyere, Director of Program and Special
Amy Lynn Taylor, Program Manager
Gemma ', Program Manager

Our program gives people with intellectual disabilities the chance to have experiences which most people take for granted.

7495 **Brain Injury Association of America**
1608 Spring Hill Rd
Suite 110
Vienna, VA 22182
703-761-0750
FAX: 703-761-0755
e-mail: sconnors@biausa.org
www.biausa.org

Susan H Connors, President/CEO
Mary S. Ritter, Executive VP/COO
Marianna Abashian, Director of Professional Service
Gregory Ayotte, Director of Consumer Services

Creates a better future through brain injury prevention, research, education and advocacy.

7496 **Brain Injury Association of New York State**
10 Colvin Ave
Albany, NY 12206-1242
518-459-7911
800-228-8201
FAX: 518-482-5285
e-mail: President@bianys.org
bianys.org

Judith Avner, Executive Director
Marie Cavallo, Ph.D., President
Debbie Berenda, Director of Finance & Administra
Renee Bullis, Family Services Program Assistan

(BIANYS) is a statewide non-profit membership organization that advocates on behalf of individuals with brain injury and their families, and promotes prevention. Established in 1982, BIANYS provides education, advocac, and community support services that lead to improved outcomes for children and adults with brain injuries and their families. BIANYS also offers chapters and support groups throughout the state, prevention programs, mentoring programs, speakers bureau and publications library.

7497 **Brain Injury Association of Texas**
316 W 12th Street
Suite 405
Austin, TX 78701-1845
512-326-1212
800-392-0040
FAX: 512-478-3370
e-mail: info@texasbia.com
www.texasbia.org

Judith Abner, Director
Penny Phillips, President
Donna Kuhlmann, Chairman
Kelly Ramsay, CFO

A online quarterly e-newsletter, as well as news and updates on the Brain Injury Association of Texas.

7498 **Center Academy At Pinellas Park**
6710 86th Ave North
Pinellas Park, FL 33782-4502
727-541-5716
FAX: 727-544-8186
e-mail: infopp@centeracademy.com
www.centeracademy.com

Mack R. Hicks, Founder & CEO
Andrew P. Hicks, CEO & Clinical Director
Eric V. Larson, President & Chief Operating Officer
Steven Hicks, VP Operations

Since 1968, Center Academy has been specifically designed for the learning disabled child and other children with difficulties in concentration, social skills, impulsivity, distractibility and study strategies. Programs offered include: academic day school and 5 week remedial summer program. 11 locations throughout Florida.

7499 **Dynamic Learning Center**
PO Box 112
Ben Lomond, CA 95005
831-336-3457
FAX: 503-738-9546
e-mail: teresanlp@aol.com
www.nlpu.com

Robert B Dilts, President
Teresa Epstein, Coordinator

The vision of NLP (neuro-lingusitic programming)University is to create a context in which professionals of different backgrounds can develop fundamental and advanced NLP skills for applications relevant to their profession. The mission of NLP University is to provide the organizational structure through which the necessary guidance, training, culture, and community support can be brought to the people who are interested in exploring the global potential of Systemic NLP.

7500 **Focus Alternative Learning Center**
126 Dowd Avenue
PO Box 452
Canton, CT 06019-452
860-693-8809
FAX: 860-693-0141
e-mail: info@focuscenterforautism.org
focusalternative.org

Marcia Bok, President
Claudia Godburn, Secretary
Rita Barredo, Treasurer

A private non profit, licensed clinical and learning center specialized in the treatment of creatively wired and socially challenged kids. We treat kids on the autism spectrum who suffer from high anxiety, experience processing difficulties and learning problems.

7501 **Life Development Institute**
18001 N 79th Ave
Suite E71
Glendale, AZ 85308-8396
866-736-7811
FAX: 623-773-2788
e-mail: info@life-development-inst,org
www.life-development-inst.org

Robert Crawford, CEO
Veronica Lieb (Crawford), President
Justin Coller, Manager of Marketing
Shirley Schroeder, CFO

Serves older adolescents and adults with learning disabilities, ADD and related disorders. The purpose of the training is to enable program participants to pursue responsible independent living, enhance academic/workplace literacy skills and facilitate placement in educational/employment opportunities, commensurate with individual capabilities. Includes a stand alone, regionally accredited 2-year college.

7502 **NLP Comprehensive**
PO.Box 348
Indian Hills, CO 80454-648
303-987-2224
800-233-1657
FAX: 303-987-2228
e-mail: learn@nlpco.com
www.nlpco.com

Tom Dotz, President
Sharon DeBault, Director of Community Relations
Jamie Reaser, PhD, Director of Professional Relatio
Christian Miller, Publishing Manager

An online e-newsletter on Neuro-linguistic programming.

7503 **National Alliance on Mental Illness(NAMI)**
3803 N Fairfax Dr
Ste 100
Arlington, VA 22203-3080
703-524-7600
800-950-6264
FAX: 703-524-9094
www.nami.org

Suzanne Vogel-Scibilia, President
Keris J,,n Myrick, Ph.Dc., First Vice President
Henry Acosta, M.A., M.S.W.,, Second Vice President
Ralph E. Nelson, Jr., M.D., Treasurer

Our mission is to provide you with the technical assistance, tools and referrals to resources you need to build organizational capacity and achieve the goals of the NAMI Standards of Excellence.

7504 **National Association for Down Syndrome**
PO Box 206
Wilmette, IL 60091-206
630-325-9112
FAX: 847-723-3138
e-mail: info@nads.org
www.nads.org

Jackie Rotondi, President
Mary Lou Miller, 1st VP
Deanne Medina, 2nd VP
Beata McCann, Treasurer

Works for a strong network of support systems within their own organization and with medical, educational and school service professionals who work with children and adults with Down Syndrome. NADS serves the Chicago Metropolitan area.

7505 **National Association of Cognitive-Behavioral Therapists**
PO Box 2195
Weirton, WV 26062-1395
304-723-3982
800-853-1135
FAX: 304-723-3982
e-mail: nacbt@nacbt.org?subject=General%20Message%20t
www.nacbt.org

Aldo R Pucci, President
Paul A. Hauck, Ph.D., Director
Michael R. Edelstein, Ph.D., Director
Bill Borcherdt, ACSW, BCD, Director

Dedicated exclusively to supporting, promoting, teaching, and developing cognitive-behavioral therapy.

7506 **National Down Syndrome Congress**
30 Mansell Court
Suite 108
Roswell, GA 30076
770-604-9500
800-232-6372
FAX: 770-604-9898
e-mail: info@ndsccenter.org
ndsccenter.org

Jim Faber, President
Marilyn Tolbert, 1st VP
Carole J. Guess, 2nd VP
Lori McKee, Treasurer

Provides information, advocacy and support concerning all aspects of life for individuals with Down syndrome. A world with equal rights and opportunitites for people with Down syndrome. It is the purpose of the NDSC to create a national climate in which all people will recognize and embrace the value and dignity of people with Down syndrome. That purpose is enhanced by the commitment of the NDSC to promote the accessability to a full range of opportunities that meet the needs of the individual.

7507 National Down Syndrome Society
666 Broadway
8th Floor
New York, NY 10012-2317 212-460-9330
800-221-4602
FAX: 212-979-2873
e-mail: info@ndss.org
ndss.org

Jon Colman, President
Patricia Baker, Program Manager
Madeline Alemar, Development Associate
Chris Burke, Goodwill Ambassador/Administrati

Not-for-profit organization increases public awareness about Down syndrome and works to discover its underlying causes through research, education and advocacy. Distributes timely and informative materials, encourages and supports the activities of local parent support groups, sponsors sonferences and scientific symposia and undertakes major advocacy efforts—all to increase awareness and acceptance of people with Down syndrome.

7508 National Institute on Deafness and Other Communication Disorder
Federal Government
31 Center Dr
MSC 2320
Bethesda, MD 20892-2320 301-496-7243
800-241-1044
FAX: 301-402-0018
e-mail: nidcdinfo@nidcd.nih.gov
www.nidcd.nih.gov

James F Battey Jr. Dr., Director
Timothy J. Wheeles, Executive Officer and Chief
Chris Clements, Program Advisor
Chad Wysong, Deputy Executive Officer

The National Institute on Deafness and Other Communication Disorders (NIDCD) one of the National Institude of Health, supports and conducts research and research training on the normal and disordered processes of hearing, balance smell, taste, voice, speech and language.

7509 Oak Leyden Developmental Services
411 Chicago Ave
Oak Park, IL 60302 708-524-1050
FAX: 708-524-2469
e-mail: batkinson@oak-leyden.org
www.oak-leyden.org

Bob Atkinson, President/CEO
Ken Cheatham, Division Chief of Facilities, Ma
Nancy Thomas, Director of Human Resources
Mary Taylor, Vice President of Finance

The mission of Oak-Leyden Developmental Services is to help people with developmental disabilities meet life's challenges and reach their highest potential. Our mission is to achieved through the following programs: Early Intervention Program, Vocational Evaluation, Developmental Training Program, Supported Employment Program, Community Integrated Living Arrangements and Multi-disciplinary Clinic.

7510 St. John Valley Associates
160 Main St
PO Box 419
Madawaska, ME 04756-1219 207-728-3336
800-339-9502
FAX: 207-728-3825
www.sjvalley-times.com

Megan Gendreau, Executive Director

A nonprofit association with the mission of empowering adult citizens with mental retardation to dignify themselves. Three broad-based programs and services (Independence Plus, Job Involvements, People Now) are designed to allow each individual to upgrade learning skills, assert rights, increase independence and accept new responsibilities. *$75.00*

7511 TEACCH
University of North Carolina at Chapel Hill
100 Renee Lynne Ct
Carrboro, NC 27510 919-966-2174
FAX: 919-966-4127
e-mail: teacch@unc.edu
www.teacch.com

Dr. Laura Klinger, Director
Rebecca Mabe, Assistant Director of Business
Walter Kelly, Business Officer
Mark Klinger, Director of Research

Focus on the person with autism and the development of a program around this person's skills, interests and needs.

Camps

7512 Adventure Learning Center at Eagle Village
4507 170th Ave
Hersey, MI 49639-8785 231-832-2234
800-748-0061
FAX: 231-832-1468
e-mail: alcinfo@eaglevillage.org
www.eaglevillage.org

Cathey Prudhomme, President/CEO
Jim McCain, Director of Support Services/CFO
Craig Weidner, Director of Advancement

Offers a variety of fun camp experiences with a low staff-to-camper ratio and exciting, challenging activities. This program accepts youth, ages 5-17, who are high risk or special needs - behavioral problems, emotionally unstable or Attention Deficit. The camping experience includes canoeing, hiking, swimming and high adventure activities. Half-week, one-week, and two-week sessions June-August. Coed.

7513 CNS Camp New Connections
Mclean Hospital Child/Adolescent Program
115 Mill St
Mailstop115
Belmont, MA 02478-1064 617-855-2000
800-333-0338
FAX: 617-855-2833
e-mail: mcleaninfo@mclean.harvard.edu
www.mcleanhospital.org

Roya Ostovar PhD, Center Director
Scott L. Rauch, MD., President and Psychiatrist in Ch
Joseph Gold MD, Clinical Director
Cynthia Kaplan, CAP Administrative Director

Four-week summer day camp for children ages 7-17 who have pervasive developmental disorders, Asperger's Syndrome, autism spectrum disorders and non-verbal learning disabilities. The camp is designed to help children develop social skills through fun activities including: communication games, swimming, field trips, drama, and arts and crafts. *$4500.00*

7514 Camp Baker
Greater Richmond ARC
7600 Beach Rd
Chesterfield, VA 23838-6513 804-748-4789
FAX: 804-796-6880
e-mail: campbaker@RichmondARC.org
richmondarc.org

Robert L. Sommerville, Chair - Officer
Thomas G. Haskins, Vice Chair - Officer
Chriss Mumford, Secretary Officer
Marshall W. Butler Jr., President

An organization created by families, for families that has grown to provide a continuum of programs and services for individuals with developmental disablities acroos the lifespan, helping each person achieve his or her potential and improving the quality of life for everyone in the community.

7515 Camp Betsey Cox
140 Betsey Cox Lane
Pittsford, VT 05763-9456 802-483-6611
e-mail: info@campbetseycox.com
www.campbetseycox.com

Lorrie Byrom, Camp Director
Devri Byrom, Winter Office Director
Mike Byrom, Camp Director

Camp Betsey Cox is a summer camp with an educational mindset. Betsey Cox is a perfect setting to give children the chance to completely make their own choices in the course of the day. For many campers, this is the beggining of learning how to make intelligent and informed choices in life.

7516 Camp Buckskin
4124 Quebec Ave N
Suite 300, PO Box 389
Ely, MN 55731- 389 763-208-4805
FAX: 218-365-2880
e-mail: info@campbuckskin.com
www.campbuckskin.com

Thomas R Bauer CCD, Camp Director
Mary Bauer, Co-Director
Jared Griffin, Program Director

Camp is located in Ely, Minnesota. Buckskin assists LD, AD/HD, Asperger's, and adopted individuals to realize and develop the potentials and abilities which they possess. Teaches a combination of traditional camp, academic activities and social skills so the campers experience success in many areas. Ages 6-18.

7517 Camp Horizons
127 Babcock Hill Rd
PO Box 323
South Windham, CT 06266- 323 860-456-1032
FAX: 860-456-4721
e-mail: scott.lambeck@camphorizons.org
www.camphorizons.org

Adam Milne, Chairman
L. Sanford Rice, Treasurer
Kathleen McNAboe, VP
Deirdhre Delaney, Board Secretary

Bordering Lake Probus, the facilities at the camp are equipped to accomodate a wide range of activities and programs for campers with developmental disabilities, or other challenging emotional and social needs. There is a 5:1 camper-counselor ratio with a schedule of three programs in the morning and four in the afternoon.

7518 Camp Huntington
56 Bruceville St
PO Box 37
High Falls, NY 12440-37 845-687-7840
855-707-2267
FAX: 845-213-4313
e-mail: mbednarz@camphuntington.com
www.camphuntington.com

Michael Bednarz, Executive Director
Amber Allan-Latham, Camp Director
Stacy Kane Greenzeig, Visiting Prgm Supervisor Spec Ed

A co-ed residential summer camp specifically designed to focus on Adaptive and Therapeutic Recreation. Campers include those with learning and developmental disabilities, ADD/HD, Autism Spectrum Disorders, Asperger's, PDD, and other special needs. Three programs are offered that focus on: recreation and social skills; independence; and participation.

7519 Camp Nissokone
YMCA Camping Services
1401 Broadway
Suite A
Detroit, MI 48226-8929 313-267-5300

e-mail: office@ycampingservices.org
www.ymcadetroit.org

Doug Grimm, Vice President Camping Services
David Marks, Director

A six week summer resident camp program for boys and girls whose learning and behavior styles have made successful participation in the traditional camp program difficult. All camp activities have a special emphasis on building self-esteem and peer relationships. Strong in waterfront, nature, campcrafts and a special arts program.

7520 Camp Northwood
132 State Route 365
Remsen, NY 13438-5700 315-831-3621
FAX: 315-831-5867
e-mail: northwoodprograms@hotmail.com
www.nwood.com

Gordon Felt, Camp Director
Donna Felt, International Counselor

Summer sessions for children with ADD. Coed, ages 8-18.

7521 Camp Nuhop
404 Hillcrest Dr
Ashland, OH 44805-4152 419-289-2227
FAX: 419-289-2227
nuhop.org

Trevor Dunlap, Executive Director, CEO
Jim Machin, Director of Facilities and Maint
Terri Ru Lon, Office Manager
Terri Pringle, Director of Dining Services

A summer residential program for any youngster from 6 to 18 with a learning disability, behavior disorder or Attention Deficit Disorder. 84 campers and 41 staff members live on site in groups of to seven campers to every three counselors. Activities focus on positive self-concept and behaviors and teaches children to learn how to find their strengths, abilities and talents from a positive, yet realistic viewpoint.

7522 Camp Ramapo
Route 52 Salisbury Turnpike
P.O.Box 266
Rt. 52 / Salisbury Turnpike
Rhinebeck, NY 12572-266 845-876-8403
FAX: 845-876-8414
e-mail: office@ramapoforchildren.org
ramapoforchildren.org

Mike Kunin, Executive Director
Rachel Flynn, PhD, Senior Program Officer
Bruce Kuziola, Chief Financial and Administrative Officer
Adam Weiss, Chief Executive Officer

Ramapo's specific focus is adventure-based, experiential learning programs that promote positive character values in children and teens with special needs.

7523 Camp Royall
Autism Society of North Carolina
505 Oberlin Road
Suite 230
Raleigh, NC 27605-1345 919-743-0204
800-442-2762
e-mail: info@autismsociety-nc.org
www.autismsociety-nc.org

Sharon Jeffries-Jones, Chair
Elizabeth Phillippi, Vice Chair
Darryl R. Marsch, Secretary
John Delaloye, Treasurer

The best source in North Carolina for connecting people who live with autism (and those who care about them) with resources, support, advocacy and informantion tailored to thier unique needs.

7524 Camp Ruggles
PO Box 353
Chepachet, RI 02814 401-567-8914

e-mail: info@ricamps.org
www.ricamps.org

Peter Swain, President
Jim Field, Camp Director
Mr. Robert Tyler, Treasurer
Ms. Nan Levine, Director

Camp Ruggles is located in Glocester, RI, and is a summer day camp for emotionally handicapped children. The Camp offers a 6 week co-ed summer session for 60 children ages 6-12.

7525 Camp Sisol
Jewish Community Center of Greater Rochester/JCC
1200 Edgewood Ave
Rochester, NY 14618-5408 585-461-2000
FAX: 585-461-0805
e-mail: membership2@jccrochester.org
www.jccrochester.org
Leslie Berkowitz, Executive Director
Dan Irving, Children's Programs/Camp Sisol D
Bill Blodgett, Facilities Director
Anna Gossin, Librarian
Camp is located in Honeoye Falls, New York. Summer sessions for children with autism. Coed, ages 5-16.

7526 Camp World Light
Florida Baptist Convention
1230 Hendricks Ave
Jacksonville, FL 32207-8619 904-396-2351
800-226-8584
FAX: 904-396-6470
www.campworldlight.com
Anne Wilson, Camp Director
Delicia Garland, Ministry Assistant to Director
Camp is located in Marianna, Florida. One-week sessions June-July for girls with ADD. Ages 3-12. Activities include arts/crafts, challenge/rope courses, clowning, community service, dance, drama, drawing/painting, leadership development, performing arts and sailing.

7527 Camp-A-Lot And Leisure Express (PALS Program)
Arc of San Diego
3030 Market Street
San Diego, CA 92102 619-685-1175
FAX: 619-234-3759
e-mail: pals@arc-sd.com
www.arc-sd.com
Lin Taylor, Camp Director
David W Schneider, President/CEO
Anthony J Desalis, Esq, Executive Vice President
Rich Coppa, Vice President Of Infrastructure
Offers one-week sessions for children and adults with attention deficit disorder, autism, mobility limitation and developmental disabilities.

7528 Carroll School Summer Programs
25 Baker Bridge Rd
Lincoln, MA 01773-3199 781-259-8342
FAX: 781-259-8842
e-mail: admissions@carrollschool.org
carrollschool.org
Steve Wilkins, Head of School
Brad Watts, Treasurer
Sam Foster, Chair
Eileen Archambault, Technology Specialist
Academic and recreational programs designed to improve learning skills and build self-confidence. The school is a tutorial program for students not achieving their potential due to poor skills in reading, writing and math. The summer camp complements the summer school offering outdoor activities in a supportive, non-competitive environment.

7529 Casowasco Camp, Conference and Retreat Center
158 Casowasco Dr
Moravia, NY 13118-3498 315-364-8756
FAX: 315-364-7636
e-mail: info@casowasco.org
www.casowasco.org
Mike Huber, Executive Director
Shelly Sherboneau, CRM Coordinating Registrar
Kevin Dunn, Casowasco Assistant Director
Roger Marshall, Property Manager
Camp is located in Moravia, New York. Summer sessions for children with ADD. Coed, ages 6-18 and families.

7530 Center Academy at Pinellas Park
6710 86th Ave North
Pinellas Park, FL 33782-4502 727-541-5716
FAX: 727-544-8186
e-mail: infopp@centeracademy.com
www.centeracademy.com
Patricia Lambert, Principal
Mack R Hicks PhD, Founder/Chairman of the Board
Andrew P Hicks PhD, CEO/Clinical Director
Lisa Hartmann, Director Education
Specifically designed for the learning disabled child and other children with difficulties in concentration, strategy, social skills, impulsivity, distractibility and study strategies. Programs offered include: attention training, visual-motor remediation, socialization skills training, relaxation training, horseback riding and more. The day camp meets weekdays from 9-3 for 3,4 or 5 week sessions.

7531 Council for Extended Care of Mentally Retarded Citizens
11140 So. Towne Square
Ste. 101
Saint Louis, MO 63123 314-845-3900
FAX: 314-845-3901
e-mail: info@sunnyhillinc.org
cecstl.org
Derrick Good, Chairman of the Board
Wes Burns, Vice Chairman
Vicky James, President/CEO
Sean King, Secretary
Services are provided to adults and children with developmental disabilities. Supported living arrangements are located in St. Louis city, St. Louis county and St. Charles County. Group home and camp services are located in Dittmer, MO. Travel program also available.

7532 Dallas Academy
950 Tiffany Way
Dallas, TX 75218-2743 214-324-1481
FAX: 214-327-8537
e-mail: mail@dallas-academy.com
www.dallas-academy.com
Troy Sturrock, Chair
Terrence S. Welch, Vice Chair
Dallas Cothrum, Secretary
Redonna Higgins, Treasurer
7-week summer session for students who are having difficulty in regular school classes.

7533 Eagle Hill School: Summer Program
242 Old Petersham Road
P.O. Box 116
Hardwick, MA 01037- 0116 413-477-6000
FAX: 413-477-6837
e-mail: admission@ehs1.org
www.ehs1.org
Peter J. Mc Donald, Headmaster
Marilyn Waller, President
Alden Bianchi, Vice President
Arthur Langhaus, Treasurer
For children ages 9-19 with specific learning (dis)abilities and/or Attention Deficit Disorder, this summer program is designed to remediate academic and social deficits while maintaining progress achieved during the school year. Electives and sports activities are combined with the academic courses to address the needs of the whole person in a camp-like atmosphere.

7534 Easter Seals Oklahoma
701 NE 13th St
Oklahoma City, OK 73104-5003 405-239-2525
FAX: 405-239-2278
e-mail: sbusch@eastersealsoklahoma.org
www.eastersealsoklahoma.org
Paula K. Porter, President, CEO
Vida Wasinger, Director of Operations
Debora Baden, Activity Coordinator
Samantha Pascoe, Director, Child Development Center
Adult day health center, and child development center.

7535 Englishton Park Academic Remediation
Englishton Park Presbyterian
P.O.Box 228
Lexington, IN 47138-228 812-889-2046
e-mail: ThomasLisaBarnett@etczone.com
www.englishtonpark.org

Lisa Barnett, Director
Thomas Barnett, Co-Director
Camp is located in Lexington, Indiana. Two-week sessions for children with ADD. Boys and girls, ages 7-12.

7536 Florida Sheriffs Caruth Camp
Florida Sheriffs Youth Ranches
2486 Cecil Webb Place
Boys Ranch, FL 32060 386-842-5501
800-765-3797
FAX: 386-842-2429
e-mail: fsyr@youthranches.org
www.youthranches.org

Roger Bouchard, President
Bill Frye, Executive Vice President
Janet Bass, Vice President of Operations
Maria Knapp, Vice President of Donor Relation
Camp is located in Inglis, Florida. One-week sessions for children with ADD. Coed, ages 10-15.

7537 Gow School Summer Programs
2491 Emery Road
P.O. Box 85
South Wales, NY 14139-0085 716-652-3450
FAX: 716-652-3457
e-mail: webmaster@gow.org
www.gow.org

Gayle Hutton, Director of Development
Robert Garcia, Director of Admissions
Eric Bray, Summer Program Director
Rosemary Shields, CPA, Director of Finance
Co-ed summer programs for students ages 8-16 with dyslexia or similar learning disabilities offer a balanced blend of morning academics, afternoon/evening traditional camp activities and weekend overnights. The primary purpose of these programs is to provide a positive experience while balancing these three elements. Committed to the creation of a positive and enjoyable experience for each participant by defining and merging the goals of the camp and the school, with those of camper students.

7538 Hill School of Fort Worth
4817 Odessa Ave
Fort Worth, TX 76133-1640 817-923-9482
FAX: 817-923-4894
e-mail: hillschool@hillschool.org
www.hillschool.org

Roxann Breyer, Principal
Audrey Boda-Davis, Executive Director
Janet Smith, Account & Records Manager
Kathy Edwards, Principal, Grapevine campus
Provides an alternative learning environment for students having average or above-average intelligence with learning differences. Hill school is an established leader in North Texas with a 25 year history of effectively serving LD children. Beginning in 1961 as a tutorial service, Hill became a formal school in 1973. Our mission is to help those who learn differently develop skills and strategies to succeed. We do this by developing academic/study skills, and self-discipline.

7539 Indian Acres Camp for Boys
1712 Main St
Fryeburg, ME 04037-4327 207-935-2300
FAX: 954-349-7812
e-mail: geoff@indianacres.com
www.indianacres.com

Michael Burness, Assistant Director
Mary Beth 'Bert' Wiig, Head Counselor, Camp Forest Acre
Lisa Newman, Director
Geoff Newman, Director
Camp is located in Fryeburg, Florida. Four and seven-week sessions June-August for boys with ADD ages 7-16.

7540 Lab School of Washington
4759 Reservoir Rd NW
Washington, DC 20007-1921 200-965-6600
e-mail: labschool@webmail.org
www.labschool.org

Katherine Schantz, Head of School
Diana Meltzer, Associate Head of School
Laurelle Sheedy McCready, Associate Head of School for Fin
Bob Lane, Director of Admissions
The Lab School six week summer session includes individualized reading, spelling, writing, study skills and math programs. A multisensory approach addresses the needs of bright learning disabled children. Related services such as speech/language therapy and occupational therapy are integrated into the curriculum. Elementary/Intermediate; Junior High/High School.

7541 Lions Den Outdoor Learning Center
600 Kiwanis Dr
Eureka, MO 63025-2212 636-938-5245
FAX: 636-938-5289
e-mail: info@wymancenter.org
www.wymancenter.org

David Hilliard, President
Theresa Mayberry, Executive VP
Kristine Ramsey, Sr. VP
Tony Etzkorn, VP
Varied programs for mentally retarded children, ages 6 and up, includes daily living, socialization and language skills. Sports, tent camping, crafts, and nature study are also offered. Sliding scale tuition for 2 weeks.

7542 Maplebrook School
5142 Route 22
Amenia, NY 12501-5357 845-373-9511
FAX: 845-373-7029
e-mail: admin@maplebrookschool.org
www.maplebrookschool.org

Paul Scherer, Administrator
Donna Konkolics, Head Of School
A coeductional boarding school which offers a six week camp for children with learning differences and ADD.

7543 Marvelwood Summer
Marvelwood School
476 Skiff Mountain Road
PO Box 3001
Kent, CT 06757-3001 860-927-0047
FAX: 860-927-0021
e-mail: summerschool@marvelwood.org
www.marvelwood.org

Alfred C Brooks, President
Arthur F Goodearl, Jr, Head Of School
The emphasis in this summer program is on diagnosis and remediation of individual reading, spelling, writing, mathematics and study problems. Offered to ages 12-16.

7544 New Horisons Summer Day Camp
YMCA
13821 Newport Avenue
Suite 200
Tustin, CA 92780-7803 714-549-9622
FAX: 714-838-5976
www.ymcaoc.org

Jeff Black, Vice Chair
Tom Reyes, Director
Christian Buell, Director
John Rochford, Director
One-week sessions for children with ADD and speech/communication impairment. Coed, ages 5-14.

7545 New Jersey YMHA/YWHA Camps Milford
21 Plymouth St
Fairfield, NJ 07004-1686
973-575-3333
800-776-5657
FAX: 973-575-4188
e-mail: info@njycamps.org
www.njycamps.org

Leonard Robinson, President
Bruce Nussman, President
Camp is located in Milford, Pennsylvania. Summer sessions for children with ADD. Coed, ages 6-17 and families.

7546 Oakland School & Camp
Boyd Tavern
Keswick, VA 22947
434-293-9059
FAX: 434-296-8930
e-mail: information@oaklandschool.net
www.oaklandschool.net

Carol Williams, School Director
Jamie Cato, Admissions Director
A highly individualized program stresses improving reading ability. Subjects taught are reading, English composition, math and word analysis. Recreational activities include horseback riding, sports, swimming, tennis, crafts, archery and camping. For girls and boys, ages 8-14.

7547 Outside In School Of Experiential Education, Inc.
P.O.Box 639
Greensburg, PA 15601-639
724-837-1518
FAX: 724-837-0801
e-mail: administration@outsideinschool.com
myoutsidein.org
Michael C. Henkel, Executive Director
Camp is located in Bolivar, Pennsylvania. Sessions for children with ADD and substance abuse problems. Boys 11-18 and girls 13-18.

7548 Phelps School Summer School
583 Sugartown Rd
Malvern, PA 19355-2800
610-644-1754
FAX: 610-644-6679
e-mail: admis@thephelpsschool.org
www.thephelpsschool.org

Christopher Chirieleison, Principal
Daniel E. Knopp, Head of School
Amy Anderson, Director of College Counseling
Janessa Davis, Director of Student Services
Open for grades 7-11 to make up academic deficiencies or complete studies in English, math and reading. Sports include riding, tennis and swimming. A program is also available to a limited number of international students in English as a Second Language.

7549 Quest Camp
2355 San Ramon Valley Blvd.
Suite 208
San Ramon, CA 94583-1763
925-743-2900
800-313-9733
FAX: 925-820-9761
e-mail: questcamps@mac.com
www.questcamps.com

Robert Field, Founder/Executive Director
Debra Forrester-Field, M.A., Administrative Director
Adam Berman, Psy.D., Director
Aprilyn Artz, MA, Director
Camp is located in Alamo, California. Day camp offering three to eight-week sessions including psychological treatment for children with ADD and other mild to moderate psychological disorders. Coed, ages 6-15.

7550 Raven Rock Lutheran Camp
17912 Harbaugh Valley Road
P.O.Box 136
Sabillasville, MD 21780-136
410-303-2108
800-321-5824
e-mail: ravenrock@innernet.net
Brenda Minnich, Executive Director
Christ-centered program for youth and mentally retarded adults.

7551 Rimland Services for Autistic Citizens
1265 Hartrey Ave
Evanston, IL 60202-1056
847-328-4090
877-395-6937
FAX: 847-328-8364
e-mail: pwatson@rimland.org
www.rimland.org

Pamela Watson, CEO
Dave Work, Assoc Executive Director Program
Brendy Sims, Chief Operating Officer
Terrance Wimberly, Associate Executive Director of
An accessible camp facility that can be utilized by groups for day use or overnight camping experiences. Six winterized cabins, a meeting facility, indoor pool, full food service, and an excellent staff are available. Educational programs can be arranged or you can utilize the facility to manage your own programs.

7552 Rolling Hills Country Day Camp
P.O.Box 172
Marlboro, NJ 07746
732-308-0405
FAX: 732-780-4726
e-mail: info@rollinghillsdaycamp.com
www.rollinghillsdaycamp.com

Billy Breitner, Director
Summer sessions for children with ADD. Coed, ages 3-12.

7553 SOAR Summer Adventures
NC Base Camp
226 SOAR Lane
P.O.Box 388
Balsam, NC 28707-0388
828-456-3435
FAX: 828-456-3449
e-mail: admissions@soarnc.org
www.soarnc.org

John Willson, Executive Director
Catey Terry, CFO
Laura Pate, Director of Operations
Joe Geier, Director of the Academy at SOAR
A nonprofit adventure program working with disadvantaged youth diagnosed with learning disabilities in an outdoor, challenge based environment. Focuses on esteem building and social skills development through rock climbing, backpacking, whitewater rafting, mountaineering, sailing, snorkeling, and much more. Offers two week, one month, and semester programs available. SOAR programs utilize North Carolina, Florida, Colorado, American Southwest, Alaska, and Jamaica as program areas.

7554 Sherman Lake YMCA Outdoor Center
6225 N 39th St
Augusta, MI 49012-9722
269-731-3000
FAX: 269-731-3020
e-mail: shermanlakeymca@ymcasl.org
www.shermanlakeymca.org

Luke Austenfeld, Executive Director
Jean Henderson, Business Manager
Lorrie Syverson, Director of Camping, Education &
Mark VanDaff, Facility Manager
Summer camping sessions for campers with ADD and spina bifida. Coed, ages 6-15 and families, seniors.

7555 Squirrel Hollow Summer Camp
The Bedford School
5665 Milam Rd
Fairburn, GA 30213-2851
770-774-8001
FAX: 770-774-8005
e-mail: bbox@thebedfordschool.org
www.thebedfordschool.org

Betsy Box, Executive Director
Jeff James, Headmaster/Athletic Director./MS
Allisom DaY, Asst. Headmaster/MS Admin./ MS
Susan Blake, Art/After-School Care Coordinato
A remedial summer program for children with academic needs held on the campus of The Bedford School in Fairburn, Georgia. It is a five week day camp held from June 19 to July 21 and serves ages 6-16. For mor information contact Betsy Box at (770) 774-8001.

7556 Summit Camp
322 Route 46 West
Suite 210
Parsippany, NJ 07054
973-732-3230
800-323-9908
FAX: 973-732-3226
e-mail: info@summitcamp.com
www.summitcamp.com

Mayer Stiskin, Owner
Eugene Bell, Senior Director
Debs Hugill, Head Counselor/Program Director
Maryann Santora, Clinical Social Worker & Admissi

Camp is located in Honesdale, Pennsylvania. Summer sessions for children with ADD. Coed, ages 8-17.

7557 Sunnyhill Adventure Center
Council for Extended Care
6555 Sunlit Way
Dittmer, MO 63023-3306
636-274-9044
314-781-4950
FAX: 636-285-1305
e-mail: dropin4fun@aol.com
sunnyhilladventures.org

Victoria James, President/CEO
Kathleen Branson, Director of Finance
Donald Mitchell, Director of ISLA
Rob Darroch, Director of Sunnyhill Adventures

Camp is located in Dittmer, Missouri. Summer sessions for campers with developmental disabilities and autism. Coed, ages 8-99. Sunnyhill Adventures is program that offers campers fun, exciting, educational experiences in a beautiful outdoor setting. Our residential summer camp combines traditional camping activities plus specially selected and adapted events to meet the needs of each camper group.

7558 Talisman Summer Camp
64 Gap Creek Rd
Zirconia, NC 28790-8791
828-697-6249
855-588-8254
e-mail: info@talismancamps.com
www.talismancamps.com

Linda Tatsapaugh, Operations Director & Owner
Robiyn Mims, Admissions Director
Doug Smathers, Summer Camps Director
Cory Greene, Program Manager

Camp is located in Black Mountain, North Carolina. Offers a program of hiking, rafting, climbing, and caving for learning disabled ADD/ADHD and autistic young people. Coed, ages 9-18.

7559 Timbertop Nature Adventure Camp
YMCA Camp Glacier Hollow
1000 Division St
Stevens Point, WI 54481-2724
715-342-2980
FAX: 715-342-2987
e-mail: pmatthai@spymca.org
www.glacierhollow.com

Dave Morgan, Executive Director
Pete Matthai, Camp Director
Tiffany Praeger, Summer Camp Program Director

For children who can benefit from an individualized program of learning in a non-competitive outdoor setting under the skilled leadership of people who understand the environment and the unique potential of these children.

7560 Triangle Y Ranch YMCA
YMCA of Southern Arizona
PO Box 1111
Tucson, AZ 85702
520-623-5511
FAX: 520-624-1518
e-mail: camp@tucsonymca.org
www.tucsonymca.org

Dane Woll, President and CEO
Kerry Dufour, V.P. Chief Development Officer
Cathy Scheirman, Chief Financial Officer
Amanda Thomas, Director of Communications and Special Projects

Summer camp programs for children and young adults ages 6-17. Camp offers horseback riding, sports, story telling, arts & crafts, swimming, archery and nature programs.

7561 Wendell Johnson Speech And Hearing Clinic
University Of Iowa
250 Hawkins Dr
Iowa City, IA 52242-1025
319-335-3500
FAX: 319-335-8851
e-mail: dorothy-albright@uiowa.edu
www.uiowa.edu

Dorothy Albright, Department Administration
Lauren Eldridge, Undergraduate Academic Programs
Mary Jo Yotty, Graduate Programs
Lauren Eldridge, Clinic Appointments

The clinic offers assessment and remediation for communication disorders in adults and children. The clinic also offers a Intensive Summer Residential Clinic for school age children needing intervention services because of speech, language, hearing and/or reading problems.

Print: Books

7562 A Miracle to Believe In
Option Indigo Press
2080 S Undermountain Rd
Sheffield, MA 01257-9643
413-229-8727
800-714-2779
FAX: 413-229-8727
e-mail: indigo@bcn.net
www.optionindigo.com

Barry Neil Kaufman, Author

A group of people from all walks of life come together and are transformed as they reach out, under the direction of the Kaufmans, to help a little boy the medical world had given up as hopeless. This heartwarming journey of loving a child back to life will not only inspire you, the reader, but presents a compelling new way to deal with life's traumas and difficulties.
379 pages
ISBN 0-449201-08-2

7563 ADD: Helping Your Child
Warner Books
1271 Avenue of the Americas
New York, NY 10020-1300
212-522-7200
FAX: 212-522-7989

Barbara Smalley, Author
Bruce Paonessa, Vice President
Elizabeth Nunuz, Manager

The definitive guide to helping children with AD/HD *$ 12.95*
224 pages Paperback
ISBN 0-446670-13-8

7564 ADHD Book of Lists: A Practical Guide for Helping Children and Teens with ADDs
Jossey-Bass
111 River St
Hoboken, NJ 7030-5773
201-748-6000
FAX: 201-748-6008
e-mail: info@wiley.com
www.wiley.com

Sandra F Rief, Author

Information about Attention Deficit/Hyperactivity Disorder including strategies, supports, and interventions that have been found to be the most effective. For teachers, parents, and counselors. *$29.95*
320 pages
ISBN 0-787965-91-X

7565 ADHD in the Schools: Assessment and Intervention Strategies
Guilford Press
72 Spring St
New York, NY 10012-4019
212-431-9800
800-365-7006
FAX: 212-966-6708
e-mail: info@guilford.com
www.guilford.com

George J DuPaul, Author
Gary Stoner, Co-Author
This landmark volume emphasizes the need for a team effort among parents, community-based professionals, and educators. Provides practical information for educators that is based on empirical findings. Chapters focus on: how to identify and assess students who might have ADHD; the relationship between ADHD and learning disabilities; how to develop and implement classroom-based programs; communication strategies to assist physicians; and the need for community-based treatments. $ 36.00
269 pages Hardcover
ISBN 0-898622-45-X

7566 ADHD with Comorbid Disorders: Clinical Assessment and Management
Guilford Press
72 Spring St
New York, NY 10012-4019
212-431-9800
800-365-7006
FAX: 212-966-6708
e-mail: info@guilford.com
www.guilford.com

Steven R Pliszka, MD, Author
Caryn Leigh Carlson, Co-Author
James M Swanson, Co-Author
$44.00
Cloth
ISBN 1-572304-78-2

7567 AT for Individuals with Cognitive Impairment
Idaho Assistive Technology Project
121 West Sweet Ave
Moscow, ID 83843-2268
208-885-3557
800-432-8324
FAX: 208-885-6145
e-mail: idahoat@uidaho.edu
www.idahoat.org

Ron Seiler, Project Director

7568 Adolescents with Down Syndrome: Toward a More Fulfilling Life
Brookes Publishing
P.O.Box 10624
Baltimore, MD 21285-624
410-337-9580
800-638-3775
FAX: 410-337-8539
e-mail: custserv@brookespublishing.com
www.brookespublishing.com

Maria Sustrova, Author
Lauren Smith, Western Region Sales Representat
Jeannine Blimline, Central Region Sales Representat
Kevin Warg, Northeastern Region Sales Repres
Written for health care professionals, psychologists, other developmental disabilities practitioners, educators, and parents, it covers biomedical concerns; behavioral, psychological, and psychiatric challenges; and education, employment, recreation, community, and legal concerns. *$35.95*
416 pages Paperback
ISBN 1-55766-81-9

7569 Adult ADD: The Complete Handbook: Everything You Need to Know About How to Cope with ADD
Prima Publishing
P.O.Box 1260
Rocklin, CA 95677-1260
916-787-7000
800-632-8676
FAX: 916-787-7001

David B Sudderth, Author
In simple and friendly terms, the authors offer help to those leading frustrating lives. They provide coping mechanisms, both psychological and an up-to-date guide to the latest technology *$14.95*
272 pages
ISBN 0-761507-96-5

7570 All About Attention Deficit Disorders, Revised
Parent Magic
800 Roosevelt Rd
Glen Ellyn, IL 60137-5839
630-208-0031
800-442-4453
FAX: 630-208-7366
e-mail: custcare@parentmagic.com
www.parentmagic.com

Thomas Phelan, Owner
A psychologist and expert on ADD outlines the symptoms, diagnosis and treatment of this neurological disorder. *$12.95*
248 pages Paperback
ISBN 1-889140-11-2

7571 Attention Deficit Disorder
Sage Publications
2455 Teller Road
Thousand Oaks, CA 91320
800-818-7243
FAX: 800-583-2665
e-mail: info@sagepub.com
www.sagepub.com

Sara Miller McCune, Founder, Publisher, Chairperson
Blaise R Simqu, President & CEO
A book providing helpful suggestions for both home and classroom management of students with attention deficit disorder.

7572 Attention Deficit Disorder and Learning Disabilities
Books on Special Children
P.O.Box 305
Congers, NY 10920-305
845-638-1236
FAX: 845-638-0847
e-mail: irene@boscbooks.com

Barbara Ingersoll, Author
Introduces ADD and learning disabilities. This is an easy reading book. Gives definitions and discusses some effective and controverial medication, dietary, biofeedback, cognitive therapy, and many more issues. *$15.95*
246 pages Softcover
ISBN 0-385469-31-4

7573 Attention Deficit Disorder in Adults Workbook
Taylor Publishing Company
7211 Circle S. Road
Austin, TX 78745-5007
214-637-2800
800-225-3687
FAX: 214-819-8220
e-mail: Rings@balfour.com
www.balfour.com

Don Percenti, CEO
Workbook for adults with ADD. *$17.99*
192 pages Paperback
ISBN 0-878338-50-0

7574 Attention Deficit Disorder: A Different Perception
Underwood Books
PO Box 1919
Nevada City, CA 95959-1919
800-788-3123
e-mail: rebecca@underwoodbooks.com
www.underwoodbooks.com

Thorn Hartmann, Author

Supports theory linking ADD to the genetic makeup of men and women who hunted for their food in prehestoric times. Also links second hand smoke to disruptive behavior. *$9.95*

180 pages Paperback

ISBN 0-887331-56-4

7575 Attention Deficit Disorders: Assessment & Teaching

Brooks/Cole Publishing Company
10650 Toebben Drive
Independence, KY 41051 859-525-2230
FAX: 859-282-5700
www.brookscole.com

Janet W Lerner, Author

A handy resource that offers teachers, school psychologists, councelors, social workers, administrators, and parents practical advice for working with children who have attention deficit disorders. *$18.95*

258 pages Paperback

ISBN 0-534250-44-0

7576 Attention-Deficit Hyperactivity Disorder: Symptoms and Suggestons for Treatment

Slosson Educational Publications Inc.
538 Buffalo Rd
East Aurora, NY 14052-280 716-652-0930
888-756-7766
FAX: 800-655-3840
e-mail: slosson@slosson.com
www.slosson.com

Thomas W Phelan, Author
Steven Slosson, President
John Slosson, Vice President
David Slossan, Vice President

An exhaustive review of current research and decades of experience as practicing school-based professionals, as well as being a parent of an ADHD child, have culminated in this brief, to-the-point, and yet informed ADHD package which has recieved tremendous reviews. Well-grounded answers and suggestions which would facillitate behavior, learning, social-emotional functioning, and other factors in preschool and adolesence are discussed. Answers most commonly asked questions about ADHD/ADD. *$60.00*

61 pages

7577 Attention-Deficit/Hyperactivity Disorder, What Every Parent Wants to Know

Brookes Publishing
P.O.Box 10624
Baltimore, MD 21285-0624 410-337-9580
800-638-3775
FAX: 410-337-8539
e-mail: custserv@brookespublishing.com
www.brookespublishing.com

Lauren Rohe, Regional Sales Consultant
Jeff Stickler, Educational Sales Representative
Sam Schissler, Educational Sales Representative
Dant Washington, Account Sales Manager

New easy-to-understand, non-technical edition helps teachers and parents get accessible answers to their ADHD. *$21.95*

304 pages Paperback

ISBN 1-557663-98-X

7578 Augmenting Basic Communciation in Natural Contexts

Brookes Publishing
P.O.Box 10624
Baltimore, MD 21285-0624 410-337-9580
800-638-3775
FAX: 410-337-8539
e-mail: custserv@brookespublishing.com
www.brookespublishing.com

Lauren Rohe, Regional Sales Consultant
Jeff Stickler, Educational Sales Representative
Sam Schissler, Educational Sales Representative
Dant Washington, Account Sales Manager

Here you will find the techniques needed to establish a basic communication system for people of all ages with cognitive disabilities or motor sensory impairments. *$41.95*

304 pages Paperback

ISBN 1-55766-43-6

7579 Autism 24/7: A Family Guide to Learning at Home & in the Community

Autism Society of North Carolina Bookstore
505 Oberlin Rd
Suite 230
Raleigh, NC 27605-1345 919-743-0204
800-442-2762
FAX: 919-743-0208
e-mail: info@autismsociety-nc.org
www.autismsociety-nc.org

David Lax, Manager
Martina Ballen, Chair
Beverly Moore, Vice Chair
Elizabeth Phillippi, Secretary

Parents are encouraged to focus on skill sets and behaviors that most negatively affect family functioning, and replacing these behaviors with acceptable alternatives. *$19.95*

7580 Autism Handbook: Understanding & Treating Autism & Prevention Development

Oxford University Press
2001 Evans Rd
Cary, NC 27513-2010 919-677-0977
800-445-9714
FAX: 919-677-1303
e-mail: custserv.us@oup.com
www.oup-usa.org

Thomas Carty, Senior Vice President
Simon Li, Regional Director
Adam Glazer, Director
Thomas McCarty, Manager/VP Operations

$25.00

320 pages

ISBN 0-195076-67-2

7581 Autism and Learning

Taylor & Francis
7625 Empire Dr
Florence, KY 41042-2919 212-695-6599
800-634-7064
FAX: 212-563-2269
e-mail: orders@taylorandfrancis.com
www.taylorandfrancis.com

Rita Jordan, Author
Stuart Powell, Co-Author

This book is about how a cognitive perception on the way in which individuals with autism think and learn may be applied to particular curriculum areas.

160 pages Paperback

ISBN 1-853464-21-X

7582 Autism in Adolescents and Adults

Springer Publishing
11 W 42nd St
Floor 15
New York, NY 10036-8002 212-431-4370
FAX: 212-460-1575
e-mail: service-ny@springer.com
www.springerjournals.com

Eric Schopler, Editor

$63.00

456 pages

ISBN 0-306410-57-5

7583 Autism...Nature, Diagnosis and Treatment
Autism Society of North Carolina Bookstore
505 Oberlin Rd
Suite 230
Raleigh, NC 27605-1345
919-743-0204
800-442-2762
FAX: 919-743-0208
e-mail: jchampion@autismsociety-nc.com
www.autismbookstore.com

David Lax, Manager

Covers perspectives, issues, neurobiological issues and new directions in diagnosis and treatment. *$49.00*

7584 Autism: Explaining the Enigma
Wiley Publishers
111 River St
Suite 2000
Hoboken, NJ 7030-5773
201-748-6000
FAX: 201-748-6088
e-mail: info@wiley.com
www.wiley.com

Uta Firth, Author

Explains the nature of autism. *$27.95*

7585 Autism: From Tragedy to Triumph
Branden Books
Po Box 812094
Wellesley, MA 02482
617-734-2045
FAX: 781-790-1056
www.brandenbooks.com

Carol Johnson, Author
Julia Crowder, Co-Author

A new book that deals with the Lovaas method and includes a foreward by Dr. Ivar Lovaas. The book is broken down into two parts — the long road to diagnosis and then treatment. *$12.95*

7586 Autism: Identification, Education and Treatment
Routledge
7625 Empire Dr
Florence, KY 41042-2919
212-695-6599
800-634-7064
FAX: 212-563-2269
e-mail: orders@taylorandfrancis.com
www.routledge.com

Dianne Zager, Editor
Jeffrey Lin, Director
Francis Chua, Manager
Tamaryn Anderson, Marketing Manager

Chapters include medical treatments, early intervention and communication development in autism. *$36.00*
ISBN 0-805820-44-7

7587 Autism: The Facts
Oxford University Press
2001 Evans Rd
Cary, NC 27513-2010
919-677-0977
800-445-9714
FAX: 919-677-1303
e-mail: custserv.us@oup.com
www.oup-usa.org

Simon Cohen, Author
Patrick Bolton, Co-Author
$22.50
128 pages
ISBN 0-192623-27-3

7588 Autistic Adults at Bittersweet Farms
Routledge
7625 Empire Dr
Florence, KY 41042-2919
212-695-6599
800-634-7064
FAX: 212-563-2269
e-mail: orders@taylorandfrancis.com
www.routledge.com

Norman Giddan PhD, Author
Jane Giddan MA, Co-Author
Jefferey Lin, Director
Francis Chua, Manager

A touching view of an inspirational residential care program for autistic adolescents and adults. Also available in softcover. *$94.95*
Hardcover
ISBN 1-560240-42-3

7589 Be Quiet, Marina!
Star Bright Books
13 Landsdowne St
Cambridge, MA 02139
617-354-1300
FAX: 617-354-1399
e-mail: orders@starbrightbooks.com
www.starbrightbooks.com

Kirsten Debear, Author

A noisy little girl with cerebral palsy and a quiet little girl with Down Syndrome learn to play together and eventually become best friends. *$16.95*
40 pages Hardcover
ISBN 1-887734-79-1

7590 Breakthroughs: How to Reach Students with Autism
Aquarius Health Care Media
30 Forest Road
PO Box 249
Millis, MA 02054
508-376-1244
FAX: 508-376-1245
e-mail: aqvideos@tiac.net
www.aquariusproductions.com

Leslie Krussman, President/Producer
Joseph Wellington, Distribution Coordinator
Anne Baker, Billing & Accounting
Jane Hutchinson, Associate Director William Patte

A hands-on, how-to program for reaching students with autism, featuring Karen Sewell, Autism Society of America's teacher of the year. Here Sewell demonstrates the successful techniques she's developed over a 20-year career. A separate 250 page manual ($59) is also available which covers math, reading, fine motor, self help, social adaptive, vocational and self help skills as well as providing numerous plan reproducibles and an exhaustive listing of equipment and materials resources. Video. *$99.00*

7591 Bus Girl: Selected Poems
Brookline Books
8 Trumbull Rd
Suite B-001
Northampton, MA 01060
617-734-6772
800-666-2665
FAX: 617-734-3952
e-mail: brbooks@yahoo.com
www.brooklinebooks.com

Gretchen Josephson, Author
Lula O Lubchenco, Editor

Poems written over several decades by a young woman with Down Syndrome. *$14.95*
144 pages Paperback
ISBN 1-57129-41-9

7592 Change Your Brain, Change Your Life: The Breakthrough Program for Conquering Depression
Three Rivers Press
3rd Floor
175 Broadway
New York, NY 10019 212-782-9000
FAX: 212-940-7860
www.randomhouse.com
Daniel G Amen MD, Author
Clinical neuroscientist and psychiatrist Amen uses nuclear brain imaging to diagnose and treat behavioral problems. He explains how the brain works, what happens when things go wrong, and how to optimize brain function. Five sections of the brain are discussed, and case studies clearly illustrate possible problems.
$15.00
352 pages
ISBN 0-812929-98-5

7593 Child and Adolescent Therapy: Cognitive-Behavioral Procedures, Third Edition
Guilford Press
72 Spring Street
New York, NY 10012-4019 212-431-9800
800-365-7006
FAX: 212-966-6708
e-mail: info@guilford.com
www.guilford.com
Chris Jennison, Publisher Emeritus, Education
Seymour Weingarten, Editor-in-Chief
Jody Falco, Managing Editor: Periodicals
Natalie Graham, Editor: School Psychology, Liter
Incorporating significant developments in treatment procedures, theory and clinical research, new chapters in this second edition examine the current status of empirically supported interventions and developmental issues specific to work with adolescents.
$45.00
432 pages Cloth
ISBN 1-572305-56-8

7594 Children with Mental Retardation
Woodbine House
6510 Bells Mill Rd
Bethesda, MD 20817-1636 301-897-3570
800-843-7323
FAX: 301-897-5838
e-mail: info@woodbinehouse.com
www.woodbinehouse.com
Irv Shapell, Owner
A book for parents of children with mild to moderate mental retardation, whether or not they have a diagnosed syndrome or condition. It provides a complete and compassionate introduction to their child's medical, therapeutic, and educational needs, and discusses the emotional impact on the family. New parents can rely on Children with Mental Retardation to provide that solid foundation and confidence they need to help their child reach his or her highest potential. *$14.95*
437 pages Paperback
ISBN 0-933149-39-5

7595 Cognitive Behavioral Therapy for Adult Asperger Syndrome
Autism Society of North Carolina Bookstore
505 Oberlin Rd
Ste 230
Raleigh, NC 27605-1345 919-743-0204
800-442-2762
FAX: 919-743-0208
e-mail: jchampion@autismsociety-nc.org
www.autismbookstore.com
David Lax, Manager
Text is prepared with case studies and examples from the author's own experiences working as a cognitive-behavioral therapist specializing in adults and adolescents with dual diagnosis, autism spectrum disorders, mood disorders, and anxiety disorders.

7596 Communication Development in Children with Down Syndrome
Brookes Publishing
P.O.Box 10624
Baltimore, MD 21285-0624 410-337-9580
800-638-3775
FAX: 410-337-8539
e-mail: custserv@brookespublishing.com
www.brookespublishing.com
Lauren Rohe, Regional Sales Consultant
Jeff Stickler, Educational Sales Representative
Sam Schissler, Educational Sales Representative
Dant Washington, Account Sales Manager
This book offers an extensive, detailed explanation of communication development in children with Down syndrome relative to their advancing cognitive skills. It introduces a critical framework for assessing and treating hearing, speech, and language problems and provides explicit intervention methods and tested clinical protocols.
Paperback
ISBN 1-55766-50-5

7597 Comprehensive Guide to ADD in Adults: Research, Diagnosis & Treatment
ADD Warehouse
300 NW 70th Ave
Suite 102
Plantation, FL 33317-2360 954-792-8100
800-233-9273
FAX: 954-792-8545
e-mail: websales@addwarehouse.com
www.addwarehouse.com
Harvey C Parker, Owner
The first to provide broad coverage of the burgeoning field. Written for professionals who diagnose and treat adults with ADD, it provides information from psychologists and physicians on the most current research and treatment issues. *$50.95*
426 pages
ISBN 0-876307-60-8

7598 Concentration Cockpit: Explaining Attention Deficits
Educators Publishing Service
P.O.Box 9031
Cambridge, MA 02139-9031 617-367-2700
800-225-5750
FAX: 617-547-0412
e-mail: CustomerService.EPS@schoolspecialty.com
eps.schoolspecialty.com
Rick Holden, President
Melvin D Levine, Author
This eight-page pamphlet explains the administration of The Concentration Cockpit, a newly revised poster that helps children with attention deficits gain insight into their problems and monitor their progress in grappling with these problems. *$64.50*
ISBN 0-838820-59-X

7599 Coping with ADD/ADHD
Rosen Publishing Group
29 E 21st St
New York, NY 10010-6209 212-420-1600
800-237-9932
FAX: 888-436-4643
e-mail: rosenpub@tribeca.ios.com
www.rosenpublishing.com
Jaydene Morrison, Author
At least 3.5 million American youngsters suffer from attention deficit disorder. This book defines the syndrome and provides specific information about treatment and counseling. *$16.95*
ISBN 0-823920-70-4

7600 Count Us In
Exceptional Parent Library
P.O.Box 1807
Englewood Cliffs, NJ 7632-1207 201-947-6000
800-535-1910
FAX: 201-947-9376
e-mail: eplibrary@aol.com
www.eplibrary.com

Jason Kingsley, Author
Mitchell Levitz, Co-Author
Offers information on growing up with Downs Syndrome. *$9.95*

7601 Culture and the Restructuring of Community Mental Health
Greenwood Publishing Group
130 Cremona Drive
Santa Barbara, CA 93117 805-968-1911
800-368-6868
FAX: 866-270-3856
e-mail: CustomerService@abc-clio.com
www.greenwood.com

William A Vega, Author
John W Murphy, Co-Author
Michael Millman, Editor, American History
Hilary Clagget, Editor, Business, Economics & Finance
Examines treatment, organizational planning and research issues and offers a critique of the theoretical and programmatic aspects of providing mental health services to traditionally underserved populations. $45.00-$52.95. *$95.00*
168 pages Hardcover
ISBN 0-313268-87-8

7602 Difficult Child
Bantam Books
1745 Broadway, 10th Floor
New York, NY 10019 212-782-9000
FAX: 212-302-7985
e-mail: BBDPublicity@randomhouse.com
www.randomhouse.com/bantamdell

Stanley Turecki, Author
Leslie Tonner, Co-Author
The classic and definitive work on parenting hard-to-raise children with new sections on ADHD and the latest medications for childhood disorders. *$15.95*
302 pages Paperback
ISBN 0-553380-36-2

7603 Disability Culture Perspective on Early Intervention
Through the Looking Glass
3075 Adeline Street
Suite 120
Berkeley, CA 94703-2212 510-848-1112
800-644-2666
FAX: 510-848-4445
TTY: 510-848-1005
e-mail: TLG@lookingglass.org
www.lookingglass.org

Megan Kirshbaum PhD, Author
For parents with physical or cognitive disabilities and their families. Available in braille, large print or cassette. *$2.00*
12 pages

7604 Down Syndrome
Aquarius Health Care Media
30 Forest Road
PO Box 249
Millis, MA 02054-1066 508-376-1244
888-440-2963
FAX: 508-376-1245
e-mail: aqvideos@tiac.net
www.aquariusproductions.com

Lesile Kussmann, Owner
This is an excellent video for families who have just had a baby with Down Syndrome as well as professionals in the field of genetics and nursing. Through honest and open discussion, parents of children with Down Syndrome express the feelings and concerns they had during the early years of their child's life. Preview option available. *$150.00*
Video

7605 Driven to Distraction
Simon & Schuster/Touchstone Publishing
1230 Avenue of the Americas
Fl 11
New York, NY 10020- 1513 212-698-7000
FAX: 212-698-7009
www.simonsays.com

Edward M Hallowell, MD, Author
John J Ratey, MD, Co-Author
A practical book discussing adult as well as child attention deficit disorder (ADD). Non-technical, realistic and optimistic, it is an informative how-to manual for parents and consumers. *$23.00*

7606 Dyslexia over the Lifespan
Educators Publishing Service
PO Box 9031
Cambridge, MA 02139-9031 617-367-2700
800-225-5750
FAX: 617-547-0412
e-mail: eps@schoolspecialty.com
www.epsbooks.com

Margaret B Rawston, Author
Discusses the educational and career development of 56 dyslexic boys from a private school that was one of the first to have a program to detect and treat developmental language disabilities. *$ 18.00*
224 pages
ISBN 0-838816-70-3

7607 Embracing the Monster: Overcoming the Challenges of Hidden Disabilities
Paul H Brookes Publishing Company
PO Box 10624
Baltimore, MD 21285-624 410-337-9580
800-638-3775
FAX: 410-337-8539
e-mail: custserv@brokespublishing.com
www.brookespublishing.com

Veronica Crawford M.A., Author
Larry B Silver, MD, Foreword/Commentary
The author shares her experience of living with LD, ADHD and bipolar disorder to give readers an awareness of the challenges of living with hidden disabilities and what can be done to help *$24.95*
272 pages paperback
ISBN 1-557665-22-2

7608 Encounters with Autistic States
Jason Aronson
400 Keystone Industrial Park
Dunmore, PA 18512-1507 800-782-0015
FAX: 201-840-7242

Theodore Mitrani, Author
This book explores and explands the work of the late Frances Tustin, which was devoted to the psychoanalytic understanding of the bewildering elemental world of the autistic child. *$50.00*
448 pages Hardcover
ISBN 0-765700-62-

7609 Equal Treatment for People With Mental Retardation: Having and Raising Children
Harvard University Press
79 Garden St
Cambridge, MA 02138-1423 617-495-1000
800-405-1619
FAX: 617-495-5898
www.hup.harvard.edu

William Sisler, President
Valerie A Sanchez, Co-Author
Martha A Field, co-Author

A Harvard law professor and civil liberties practitioner provide a comprehensive examination of the reproductive and parental rights of mentally retarded citizens. *$19.95*
464 pages Paperback
ISBN 0-674006-97-6

7610 Families of Adults With Autism: Stories & Advice For the Next Generation
Autism Society of North Carolina Bookstore
505 Oberlin Road
Suite 230
Raleigh, NC 27605-1345
919-743-0204
800-442-2762
FAX: 919-743-0208
e-mail: books@autismsociety-nc.org
www.autismbookstore.com
Tracey Sheriff, Chief Executive Officer
Paul Wendler, Chief Financial Officer
David Laxton, Director of Communications
Kristy White, Director of Development
This book's unique point of view is that of a parent who's been there and done that and is now willing to tell the reader what it was like. *$19.95*

7611 Family Therapy for ADHD: Treating Children, Adolescents and Adults
Guilford Press
72 Spring St
New York, NY 10012-4019
800-365-7006
www.guilford.com
Craig A Everett, Author
Sandra Volgy Everett, Co-Author
Presents an innovative approach to assesing and treating ADHD in the family context. *$29.00*
Paperback
ISBN 1-572304-38-3

7612 Fighting for Darla: Challenges for Family Care & Professional Responsibility
Teachers College Press
1234 Amsterdam Ave
New York, NY 10027-6602
212-678-3929
FAX: 212-678-4149
e-mail: tcpress@tc.columbia.edu
Mary Lynch, Manager
Susan M Klein, Co-Author
Samuel Guskin, Co-Author
Samuel Guskin, Co-Author
Follows the story of Darla, a pregnant adolescent with autism. *$18.95*
161 pages
ISBN 0-807733-56-3

7613 Fragile Success
Brookes Publishing
PO Box 10624
Baltimore, MD 21285-624
410-337-9580
800-638-3775
FAX: 410-337-8539
www.brookespublishing.com
Virginia Walker Sperry, Author
A book about the lives of autistic children, whom the author has followed from their early years at the Elizabeth Ives School in New Haven, CT, through to adulthood. *$27.50*
ISBN 1-557664-58-7

7614 Getting Our Heads Together
Thoms Rehabilitation Hospital
68 Sweeten Creek Rd
Asheville, NC 28803-2318
828-274-2400
FAX: 828-274-9452
Kathi Petersen, Director Planning/Communication
Edgardo Diez MD, Medical Director Brain Injury
Kathy Price, Director Admissions
Chat Norvell, CEO
A handbook for families of head injured patients - available in Spanish as well as English. *$4.00*
40 pages Paperback

7615 Getting a Grip on ADD: A Kid's Guide to Understanding & Coping with ADD
Educational Media Corporation
1443 Old York Rd
Warminster, PA 18794
763-781-0088
800-448-9041
FAX: 215-956-9041
e-mail: emedia@educationalmedia.com
www.educationalmedia.com
Kim Frank Ed.S., Author
Susan Smith-Rex Ed.D., Co-Author
Free catalog of resources.
64 pages Yearly

7616 Getting the Best for Your Child with Autism
Autism Society of North Carolina Bookstore
505 Oberlin Road
Suite 230
Raleigh, NC 27605-1345
919-743-0204
800-442-2762
FAX: 919-743-0208
e-mail: books@autismsociety-nc.org
www.autismbookstore.com
Tracey Sheriff, Chief Executive Officer
Paul Wendler, Chief Financial Officer
David Laxton, Director of Communications
Kristy White, Director of Development
This treatment guide helps parents navigate the complex and overwhelming world of Autism. *$16.95*

7617 Group Activity for Adults with Brain Injury
Sage Publications
2455 Teller Road
Thousand Oaks, CA 91320
805-499-0721
800-818-7243
FAX: 805-499-0871
e-mail: info@sagepub.com
www.sagepub.com
Sara Miller McCune, Founder, Publisher, Executive Chairman
Blaise R Simqu, President & CEO
Tracey A. Ozmina, Executive Vice President & Chief Operating Officer
Chris Hickok, Senior Vice President & Chief Financial Officer
This manual addresses attention, memory, reasoning, and language skills in group settings. *$53.00*

7618 Guide to Successful Employment for Individuals with Autism
Brookes Publishing
P.O.Box 10624
Baltimore, MD 21285-0624
410-337-9580
800-638-3775
FAX: 410-337-8539
e-mail: custserv@brookespublishing.com
www.brookespublishing.com
Marcia Daltow Smith, Author
Ronald G Belcher, Co-Author
Patricia D Juhrs, Co-Author
Lauren Smith, Western Region Sales Representat
Describing all aspects of job placement, this book details strategies for assessing workers, networking for job opportunities, and tailoring job supports to each individual. Also illustrates how to help individuals with autism become productive workers, and with detailed descriptions of specific jobs help provide ideas for employment. *$ 32.95*
336 pages Paperback
ISBN 1-55766-71-5

7619 Handbook of Autism and Pervasive Developmental Disorders

Autism Society of North Carolina Bookstore
505 Oberlin Road
Suite 230
Raleigh, NC 27605-1345
919-743-0204
800-442-2762
FAX: 919-743-0208
e-mail: books@autismsociety-nc.org
www.autismbookstore.com

David Laxton, Director of Communications
Paul Wendler, Chief Financial Officer
Tracey Sheriff, Chief Executive Officer
Kristy White, Director of Development

A list of contributors address such topics as characteristics of autistic syndromes and interventions. *$125.00*

7620 Helping People with Autism Manage Their Behavior

Indiana Resource Center For Autism
2853 E 10th St
Bloomington, IN 47408-2696
812-855-6508
FAX: 812-855-9630
e-mail: prattc@indiana.edu
www.iidc.indiana.edu

David Mank, Executive Director
Scott Bellini, Assistant Director

Covers the broad topic of helping people with autism manage their behavior. *$7.00*

7621 Helping Your Child with Attention-Deficit Hyperactivity Disorder

Learning Disabilities Association of America
4156 Library Road
Pittsburgh, PA 15234-1349
412-341-1515
FAX: 412-344-0224
e-mail: info@ldaamerica.org
www.ldaamerica.org

Nancie Payne, President
Ed Schlitt, First Vice President
Nanette Schweitzer, Second Vice President
Beth McGraw, Secretary

LDA is the largest non-profit volunteer organization advocating for individuals with learning disabilities

7622 Helping Your Hyperactive: Attention Deficit Child

Crown Publishing Company (Random House)
1745 Broadway
New York, NY 10019-4305
212-782-9000
800-632-8676
FAX: 212-572-6066
e-mail: websupportlife@primapub.com
crownpublishing.com

John Taylor, Author
$19.95
ISBN 1-559584-23-8

7623 Hidden Child: The Linwood Method for Reaching the Autistic Child

Woodbine House
6510 Bells Mill Road
Bethesda, MD 20817-1636
301-897-3570
800-843-7323
FAX: 301-897-5838
e-mail: info@woodbinehouse.com
www.woodbinehouse.com

Irv Shapell, Owner
Sabine Oishi, Co-Author

Chronicle of the Linwood Children's Center's successful treatment program for autistic children. *$17.95*
286 pages Paperback
ISBN 0-933149-06-9

7624 How To Reach and Teach Children and Teens with Dyslexia

Jossey-Bass
111 River St
Hoboken, NJ 7030-5773
201-748-6000
FAX: 201-748-6008
e-mail: info@wiley.com
www.wiley.com

Cynthia M Stowe, Author

This practical resource gives educators at all levels essential information, techniques, and tolls for understanding dyslexia and adapting teaching methods in all subject areas to meet the learning style, social, and emotional needs of students who have dyslexia. *$ 22.95*
340 pages
ISBN 0-130320-18-8

7625 How to Own and Operate an Attention Deficit Disorder

Learning Disabilities Association of America
4156 Library Road
Pittsburgh, PA 15234-1349
412-341-1515
FAX: 412-344-0224
e-mail: info@ldaamerica.org
www.ldaamerica.org

Nancie Payne, President
Ed Schlitt, First Vice President
Nanette Schweitzer, Second Vice President
Beth McGraw, Secretary

Clear, informative and sensitive introduction to ADHD. Packed with practical things to do at home and school, from a professional and mother of a son with ADHD. *$8.95*
43 pages

7626 Hyperactive Child, Adolescent, and Adult: ADD Through the Lifespan

Oxford University Press
198 Madison Ave
New York, NY 10016-4308
212-726-6000
www.us.oup.com/us

Paul H Wender, Author

Comprehensive general review. Update on previous research by the author, offering a basic text. Published by Connecticut Association for Children & Adults with Learning Disabilities (CACLD). *$8.75*
162 pages
ISBN 0-195113-49-7

7627 Hyperactivity, Attention Deficits, and School Failure: Better Ways

Learning Disabilities Association of America
4156 Library Road
Pittsburgh, PA 15234-1349
412-341-1515
FAX: 412-344-0224
e-mail: info@ldaamerica.org
www.ldaamerica.org

Nancie Payne, President
Ed Schlitt, First Vice President
Nanette Schweitzer, Second Vice President
Beth McGraw, Secretary

LDA is the largest non-profit volunteer organization advocating for individuals with learning disabilities

7628 In Search of Wings: A Journey Back from Traumatic Brain Injury

Lash & Associates Publishing/Training
100 Boardwalk Drive, Suite 150
Youngsville, NC 27596
919-556-0300
FAX: 919-556-0900
e-mail: orders@lapublishing.com
www.lapublishing.com

Marilyn Lash, President
Bob Cluett, CEO
Bill Herrin, Director of Graphics & Design
Nick Vidal, Director of IT

The true story of one woman coping with traumatic brain injury after a car accident that affected her cognitive skills and memory
$14.95
233 pages
ISBN 1-882332-00-8

7629 **In Their Own Way**
Alliance for Parental Involvement in Education
375 Hudson Street
New York, NY 10014 212-366-2000
FAX: 212-366-2933
e-mail: ecommerce@us.penguingroup.com
http://us.penguingroup.com

Thomas Armstrong, Author
John Makinson, Chairman and Chief Executive
Coram Williams, CFO
David Shanks, CEO
For the parents whose children are not thriving in school, Armstrong offers insight into individual learning styles. *$11.95*

7630 **Increasing and Decreasing Behaviors of Persons with Severe Retardation and Autism**
Research Press
PO Box 9177
Champaign, IL 61826-9177 217-352-3273
800-519-2707
FAX: 217-352-1221
e-mail: rp@researchpress.com
www.researchpress.com

Dennis Wiziecki, Marketing
Richard M Fox, Author
These well-organized manuals are written for teachers, aides and persons responsible for designing or evaluating behavioral programs. Offers specific guidelines for arranging and managing the learning environment as well as standards for evaluating and maintaining success. In Volume Two of this series, chapters address more restrictive procedures including physical restraing, punishment, time-out and overcorrection. Set of two volumes.
$39.50
230 pages Paperback
ISBN 0-878222-63-4

7631 **Jumpin' Johnny Get Back to Work, A Child's Guide to ADHD/Hyperactivity**
Ste 15-5
25 Van Zant St
Norwalk, CT 6855-1729 203-838-5010
FAX: 203-866-6108
e-mail: CACLD@optonline.net
www.CACLD.org

Beryl Kaufman, Executive Director
Written primarily for elementary age youngsters with ADHD to help them understand their disability. Also valuable as an educational tool for parents, siblings, friends and classmates. Includes two pages on medication. *$12.50*
24 pages

7632 **Keys to Parenting a Child with Attention Deficit Disorder**
Barron's Educational Series
250 Wireless Blvd
Hauppauge, NY 11788-3924 631-434-3311
800-645-3476
FAX: 631-434-3723
e-mail: barrons@barronseduc.com
barronseduc.com

Manuel H Barron, CEO
Francine McNamara MSW CSW, Co/Author
This book shows how to work with the child's school, effectively manage the child's behavior and act as the child's advocate. *$6.95*
160 pages Paperback
ISBN 0-812014-59-6

7633 **Keys to Parenting a Child with Downs Syndrome**
Barron's Educational Series
250 Wireless Blvd
Hauppauge, NY 11788-3924 631-434-3311
800-645-3476
FAX: 631-434-3723
e-mail: barrons@barronseduc.com
barronseduc.com

Manuel H Barron, CEO
Lucy Guarino
Down Syndrome poses many challenges for children and their families. This book prepares parents and guardians to raise a child with Down Syndrome by discussing adjustment, advocacy, health and behavior, education and planning for greater independence. *$5.95*
160 pages Paperback
ISBN 0-812014-58-8

7634 **Keys to Parenting the Child with Autism**
Barron's Educational Series
250 Wireless Blvd
Hauppauge, NY 11788-3924 631-434-3311
800-645-3476
FAX: 631-434-3723
e-mail: barrons@barronseduc.com
barronseduc.com

Manuel H Barron, CEO
Parents of children with autism will find a solid balance between home and practical information in this book. It explains what autism is and how it is diagnosed, then advises parents on how to adjust to their child and give the best care. *$6.95*
208 pages Paperback
ISBN 0-812016-79-3

7635 **LD Child and the ADHD Child: Ways Parents & Professionals Can Help**
1406 Plaza Dr
Winston Salem, NC 27103-1470 336-768-1374
800-222-9796
FAX: 336-768-9194
e-mail: southern@blairpub.com
www.blairpub.com

Carolyn Sakowski, President
Susan H Stevens, Author
Book about learning disabilities available to parents. Stevens cuts through the jargon and complex theories which usually characterize books on the subject to present effective and practical techniques that parents can employ to help their child succeed at home and at school. New edition adds information about ADHD children. *$12.95*
201 pages Paperback
ISBN 0-895871-42-4

7636 **Labeling the Mentally Retarded**
University of California Press
2120 Berkeley Way
Berkeley, CA 94704-1012 510-642-4247
FAX: 510-643-7127
www.ucpress.edu

Lynne Whity, Executive Director
Jane R Mercer, Author
Clinical and social system perspectives on mental retardation.
$12.95
333 pages Paper

7637 **Let Community Employment be the Goal for Individuals with Autism**
Indiana Resource Center For Autism
2853 E 10th St
Bloomington, IN 47408-2601 812-855-9396
800-825-4733
FAX: 812-855-9630
e-mail: prattc@indiana.edu
www.iidc.indiana.edu

David Mank, Executive Director
Scott Bellini, Assistant Director

A guide designed for people who are responsible for preparing individuals with autism to enter the work force. *$7.00*

7638 Making the Writing Process Work
Brookline Books
8 Trumbull Rd
Suite B-001
Northampton, MA 01060
617-734-6772
800-666-2665
FAX: 617-734-3952
e-mail: brbooks@yahoo.com
www.brooklinebooks.com

Karen R Harris, Author
Steve Grahm, Co-Author
Making the Writing Process Work: Strategies for Composition and Self-Regulation is geared toward students who have difficulty organizing their thoughts and developing their writing. The specific strategies teach students how to approach, organize, and produce a final written product. *$24.95*
240 pages Paperback
ISBN 1-57129-10-9

7639 Management of Autistic Behavior
Sage Publications
2455 Teller Road
Thousand Oaks, CA 91320
805-499-0721
800-818-7243
FAX: 800-583-2665
e-mail: info@sagepub.com
www.sagepub.com

Sara Miller McCune, Founder, Publisher, Executive Chairman
Blaise R Simqu, President & CEO
Tracey A. Ozmina, Executive Vice President & Chief Operating Officer
Stephen Barr, Managing Director/SAGE London
This excellent reference is a comprehensive and practical book that tells what works best with specific problems. *$41.00*
450 pages

7640 Management of Children and Adolescents with AD-HD
Learning Disabilities Association of America
4156 Library Road
Pittsburgh, PA 15234-1349
412-341-1515
FAX: 412-344-0224
e-mail: info@ldaamerica.org
www.ldaamerica.org

Nancie Payne, President
Ed Schlitt, First Vice President
Nanette Schweitzer, Second Vice President
Beth McGraw, Secretary
LDA is the largest non-profit volunteer organization advocating for individuals with learning disabilities

7641 Managing Attention Deficit Hyperactivity in Children: A Guide for Practitioners
John Wiley & Sons Inc
111 River St
Hoboken, NJ 07030-5774
201-748-6000
800-825-7550
FAX: 201-748-6088
e-mail: info@wiley.com
www.wiley.com

Warren J Baker, President
Michael Goldstein, Co-Author
Matthe S Kissner, CEO
Offers information about human personality, structure and dynamics, assessment and adjustment. *$27.50*
214 pages Hardcover
ISBN 0-471121-58-9

7642 Mental Retardation
McGraw-Hill, School Publishing
PO Box 182605
Columbus, OH 43218
800-338-3987
FAX: 609-308-4480
e-mail: customer.service@mheducation.com
mcgraw-hill.com

David Levin, President and CEO
Patrick Milano, Chief Administrative Officer & CFO
Stephen Laster, Chief Digital Officer
David Stafford, SVP & General Counsel
Combines significant findings from the most current research, focusing on a unique relationship between the special educator and the learner with mental retardation.
656 pages Casebound

7643 Mental Retardation: A Life-Cycle Approach
Pearson Publishing
200 Old Tappan Rd
Old Tappan, NJ 07675-7033
201-785-2721
800-922-0579
FAX: 201-797-2993
www.pearsonhighered.com

Clifford J Drew, Author
Michael L Hardman, Co/Author
This text considers the needs of the retarded individual at every stage of life.
512 pages

7644 Neurobiology of Autism
Johns Hopkins University Press
2715 N Charles St
Baltimore, MD 21218-4363
410-516-6900
FAX: 410-516-6968
www.press.jhu.edu

William Brody, President
Thomas L Kemper, Co-Author
Margaret L Bauman, M.D., Co-Author
Thomas L Kemper, M.D., Co-Author
This book discusses recent advances in scientific research that point to a neurobiological basis for autism and examines the clinical implications of this research. *$28.00*
272 pages
ISBN 0-801880-47-5

7645 Out of the Fog: Treatment Options and Coping Strategies for ADD
Hyperion
1500 Broadway
3rd Floor
New York, NY 10036
212-563-6500
800-331-3761
FAX: 212-456-0176
www.hyperionbooks.com

Robert Miller, President
Suzanne Levert, Co-Author
Discusses the recent recognition of attention deficit disorder as a problem that is not outgrown in adolescence, and cogently summarizes the stumbling blocks this affliction creates in the pursuit of a career or attainment of a healthy family life *$14.95*
300 pages
ISBN 0-786880-87-2

7646 Overcoming Dyslexia
Vintage-Random House
3rd Fl
1745 Broadway
New York, NY 10019-4305
212-782-9000
FAX: 212-302-7985
www.randomhouse.com/vintage

Markus Dohle, CEO
Sally Shawitz, M.D., Author
Yale neuroscientist Shaywitz demystifies the roots of dyslexia (a neurologically based reading difficulty affecting one in five chil-

dren) and offers parents and educators hope that children with reading problems can be helped. *$15.00*
432 pages
ISBN 0-679781-59-5

7647 Parent Survival Manual
Springer Publishing Company
11 W 42nd St
15th Floor
New York, NY 10036
212-431-4370
877-687-7476
FAX: 212-941-7842
e-mail: cs@springerpub.com
www.springerpub.com
Ursula Springer, President
Ted Nardin, CEO
Edie Lambiase, CFO
A guide to crises resolution in autism and related developmental disorders. *$39.95*

7648 Parent's Guide to Down Syndrome: Toward a Brighter Future
Brookes Publishing
PO Box 10624
Baltimore, MD 21285-0624
410-337-9580
800-638-3775
FAX: 410-337-8539
e-mail: custserv@brookespublishing.com
www.brookespublishing.com
Siegfried Pueschel MD PhD, Author
Highlights developmental stages and shows the advances that improve a child's quality of life. Includes discussions on easing the transition from home to school and choosing integration and curricular priorities, as well as guidelines for confronting adolescent and adult issues such as social and sexual needs and independent living and vocational options. *$21.95*
352 pages
ISBN 1-557664-52-8

7649 Parenting Attention Deficit Disordered Teens
CACLD
25 Van Zant Street
Norwalk, CT 06855-1729
203-838-5010
FAX: 203-866-6108
e-mail: CACLD@optonline.net
cacld.org
Beryl Kaufman, Executive Director
Detailed outline of the various problems of adolescents with ADHD. Published by Connecticut Association for Children & Adults with Learning Disabilities (CACLD). *$3.25*
14 pages

7650 Parents Helping Parents: A Directory of Support Groups for ADD
Novartis Pharmaceuticals Division
59 State Route 10
East Hanover, NJ 7936-1005
862-778-7500
800-742-2422
Paulo Costa, CEO

7651 Please Don't Say Hello
Human Sciences Press
233 Spring St
New York, NY 10013-1522
212-229-2859
800-221-9369
FAX: 212-463-0742
http://isbndb.com
Charles Stenken, Author
Jaroslav Chobot, Author
Zirul Evany, Author
Bill Feldmaier, Author
Paul and his family moved into a new neighborhood. Paul's brother was autistic. The children thought that Eddie was retarded until they learned that there were skills that he could do better than they could. *$10.95*
47 pages Paperback
ISBN 0-89885 -99-8

7652 Preventable Brain Damage
Springer Publishing Company
11 W 42nd St
15th Floor
New York, NY 10036
212-431-4370
877-687-7476
FAX: 212-941-7842
e-mail: cs@springerpub.com
www.springerpub.com
Donald L Templer, Author
Lawrence C Hartlage, Co-Author
Ursula Springer, President
Ted Nardin, CEO
Offers information on brain injuries from motor vehicle accidents, contact sports and injuries of children. *$35.95*
256 pages

7653 Reading, Writing and Speech Problems in Children
International Dyslexia Association
40 York Rd
4th Floor
Baltimore, MD 21204
410-296-0203
800-509-4980
FAX: 410-321-5069
e-mail: info@idamd.org
www.interdys.org
Samuel Orton, Author
Steve Peregay, Executive Director
Kristin Penczek, Director Of Conferences
Kristi Bauman, Director Of Development
A tribute to the man who more than any other aroused the attention of the scientific community and who provided the sound educational principles on which much teaching of dyslexics today is based. *$27.00*
ISBN 0-89079 -79-1

7654 Reality of Dyslexia
Brookline Books
8 Trumbull Rd
Suite B-001
Northampton, MA 01060
617-734-6772
800-666-2665
FAX: 617-734-3952
e-mail: brbooks@yahoo.com
www.brooklinebooks.com
John Osmond, Author
An informative and sensitive study of living with dyslexia which affects one in 25. He introduces the reader to the subject by sharing the difficulties of his dyslexic son. He then uses the personal accounts of other children and adult dyslexics, even entire dyslexic families, to illuminate the problems they encounter. *$14.95*
150 pages Paperback
ISBN 1-57129 -17-6

7655 Relationship Development Intervention with Young Children
Jessica Kingsley Publishers
400 Market St
Suite 400
Philadelphia, PA 19106
215-922-1161
FAX: 215-992-1417
e-mail: orders@jkp.com
www.jkp.com
Steven E Gustein, Author
Rachelle Sheely, Co-Author
Social and emotional development activities for Asperger Syndrome, Autism, PDD and NLD. Comprehensive set of activities emphasizes foundation skills for younger children between the ages of two and eight. Covers skills such as social referencing, regulating behvior, conversational reciprocity, and synchronized

actions. For use in therapeutic settings as well as schools and parents. *$22.95*
256 pages
ISBN 1-843107-14-7

7656 **Retarded Isn't Stupid, Mom!**
Brookes Publishing
4501 Forbes Blvd
Suite 200
Lanham, MD 20706
301-459-3366
800-638-3775
FAX: 301-429-5748
e-mail: custserv@brookespublishing.com
www.pbrookescom/store/books/kaufman-3785
Sandra Z Kaufman, Author
Sandra Kaufman reveals the feelings of denial, guilt, frustration and eventual acceptance that resulted in a determination to help her daughter, Nicole, live an independent life. This edition, revised on the 10th anniversary of the book's original publication, adds a progress report that updates readers on Nicole's adult years and reflects on the revolutionary changes in society's attitudes toward people with disabilities since Nicole's birth. *$22.95*
272 pages Paperback
ISBN 1-557663-78-5

7657 **Rethinking Attention Deficit Disorder**
Brookline Books
8 Trumbull Rd
Suite B-001
Northampton, MA 01060-4533
617-734-6772
800-666-2665
FAX: 617-734-3952
e-mail: brbooks@yahoo.com
www.brooklinebooks.com
Miriam Cherkes-Julkowski, Author
In contrast to the common focus on behavioral symptoms of attention disorders, this book emphasizes internal factors that make attention regulation difficult. In-depth discussions of social, emotional, and academic consequences and appropriate interventions are provided. *$27.95*
250 pages Paperback
ISBN 1-571290-30-7

7658 **Riddle of Autism: A Psychological Analysis**
Jason Aronson
4501 Forbes Blvd
Suite 200
Lanham, MD 20706-4346
301-459-3366
800-782-0015
FAX: 301-429-5746
www.rowmanlittlefield.com
Jason Aronson, Author
James Lyons, President/CEO
Stanley Plotnick, Chairman
Dr. Victor examines the myths that cloud an understanding of this disorder and describes the meanings of its specific behavioral symptoms. *$30.00*
356 pages Paperback
ISBN 1-568215-73-8

7659 **SCATBI: Scales Of Cognitive Ability for Traumatic Brain Injury**
Sage Publications
2455 Teller Road
Thousand Oaks, CA 91320
805-499-0721
800-818-7243
FAX: 805-499-0871
e-mail: happiness@option.org
www.sagepub.com
Sara Miller McCune, Founder, Publisher, Executive Chairman
Blaise R Simqu, President & CEO
Tracey A. Ozmina, Executive Vice President & Chief Operating Officer
Stephen Barr, Managing Director/SAGE London
Assesses cognitive and linguistic abilities of adolescent and adult parents with head injuries. *$287.00*

7660 **Schools for Children with Autism Spectrum Disorders**
Resources for Children with Special Needs Inc
116 E 16th St
Fl 5
New York, NY 10003-2164
212-677-4650
FAX: 212-254-4070
e-mail: info@resourcesnyc.org
www.resourcesnyc.org
Rachel Howard, Executive Director
Edie Novicki, Director Of Finance
Published every 24-36 months. *$20.00*
160 pages
ISBN 0-967836-53-0

7661 **Sex Education: Issues for the Person with Autism**
Indiana Resource Center For Autism
2853 E 10th St
Bloomington, IN 47408-2696
812-855-6508
800-825-4733
FAX: 812-855-9630
e-mail: iidc@indiana.edu
www.iidc.indiana.edu
David Mank, Executive Director
Scott Bellini, Assistant Director
Discusses issues of sexuality and provides methods of instruction for people with autism. *$4.00*

7662 **Son-Rise: The Miracle Continues**
2080 South Undermountain Road
Sheffield, MA 01257
413-229-2100
800-562-7171
e-mail: happiness@option.org
www.autismtreatmentcenter.org
Samahria Lyt Kaufman, Co-Founder and Co-Director
Dane Griffith, Director of Administrative Services
Bears Kaufman, Co-Founder and Co-Director
Raun Kaufman, Director of Global Education
Part One is the astonishing record of Raun Kaufman's development from an autistic and retarded child into a loving, brilliant youngster who shows no traces of his former condition. Part Two follows Raun's development after the age of four, teaching the limitless possibilities of the Son-Rise Program. Part Three shares moving accounts of five other ordinary families who became extraordinary when they used the Son-Rise Program to reach their own unreachable children. *$12.95*
343 pages
ISBN 0-915811-53-7

7663 **Soon Will Come the Light**
Future Horizons Inc
721 W Abram St
Arlington, TX 76013-6995
817-277-0727
800-479-0727
FAX: 817-277-2270
www.fhautism.com
Wayne Gilpin, Owner
Jennifer Gilpin, Vice President
Annette Vick, Manager
Offers new perspectives on the perplexing disability of autism. *$19.95*

7664 **Successful Job Search Strategies for the Disabled: Understanding the ADA**
Wiley Publishing
605 3rd Ave
New York, NY 10158-180
212-850-6000
FAX: 212-850-6088
www.wiley.com
Jeffrey G Allen, Author
Following a concise overview of the Americans with Disabilities Act (ADA), covers such topics as job identification, self-assessment, job leads, resumes, disability disclosure, interviewing, and accommodating specific disabilities. Includes dozen of relevant and instructive situation analyses, case examples, and answers to commonly asked questions. *$165.00*
229 pages

7665 Taking Charge of ADHD Complete Authoritative Guide for Parents
Guilford Press
72 Spring St
New York, NY 10012-4019
212-431-9800
800-365-7006
FAX: 212-966-6708
e-mail: info@guilford.com
www.guilford.com

Russell A Barkley, Author
Revised and updated to incorporate the most current information on ADHD and its treatment. Provides parents with the knowledge, guidance and confidence they need to ensure that their child receives the best care possible. Also in cloth at $40.00 (ISBN# 1-57230-600-9 *$18.95*
331 pages Paperback
ISBN 1-572305-60-1

7666 Teaching Children with Autism: Strategies for Initiating Positive Interactions
Brookes Publishing
P.O.Box 10624
Baltimore, MD 21285-624
410-337-9580
800-638-3775
FAX: 410-337-8539
e-mail: custserv@brookespublishing.com
www.brookespublishing.com

Robert L Kroegel, Author
Lynn Kern Kroegel, Co-Author
Lauren Smith, Western Region Sales Representative
Jeannine Blimline, Central Region Sales Representative
Stategies for initiating positive interactions and improving learning opportunities. This guide begins with an overview of characteristics and long-term strategies and proceeds through discussions that detail specific techniques for normalizing environments, reducing disruptive behavior, improving language and social skills, and enhancing generalization. *$32.95*
256 pages Paperback
ISBN 1-55766 -80-4

7667 Teaching and Mainstreaming Autistic Children
Love Publishing Company
9101 E Kenyon Ave
Suite 2200
Denver, CO 80237-1854
303-221-7333
FAX: 303-221-7444
e-mail: lpc@lovepublishing.com
www.lovepublishing.com

Stan Love, Owner
Peter Knoblock, Author
Dr. Knoblock advocates a highly organized, structured environment for autistic children, with teachers and parents working together. His premise is that the learning and social needs of autistic children must be analyzed and a daily program designed with interventions that respond to this functional analysis of their behavior. *$24.95*
ISBN 0-89108 -11-9

7668 Techniques for Aphasia Rehab: (TARGET) Generating Effective Treatment
Speech Bin
1965 25th Ave
Vero Beach, FL 32960-3062
772-770-0007
800-477-3324
FAX: 772-770-0006
store.schoolspecialty.com

Mary Jo Santo Pietro, Co-Author
Robert Goldfarb, Co-Author
TARGET is the kind of resource aphasia clinicians beg for. A practical resource that answers not only the what and how questions of treatment, but also the why. It describes dozens of treatment methods and gives you practical exercises and activities to implement each technique. It shows you how to treat all components of the disability, language disorder, overall impairment, communication problems, and the needs of the person with aphasia. *$45.00*
384 pages
ISBN 0-93785 -50-5

7669 Teenagers with ADD
Woodbine House
6510 Bells Mill Rd
Bethesda, MD 20817-1636
301-897-3570
800-843-7323
FAX: 301-897-5838
e-mail: info@woodbinehouse.com
www.woodbinehouse.com

Irv Shapell, Owner
Chris A Ziegler Dendy, M.S., Author
This best selling guide to understanding and coping with teenagers with attention deficit disorder (ADD) provides complete coverage of the special issues and challenges faced by these teens. Based on current diagnostic criteria and the latest literature and research in the field, the book discusses diagnosis, medical treatment, family and school life, intervention, advocacy, legal rights, and options after high school. Parents find strategies for dealing with their teen's difficult behaviors. *$18.95*
370 pages Paperback
ISBN 0-933149-69-7

7670 Traumatic Brain Injury: Cognitive & Communication Disorders
Federal Government
31 Center Drive Msc2320
Bethesda, MD 20892-1
800-241-1044
FAX: 301-402-0018
e-mail: nidcdinfo@nidcd.nih.gov
http://www.nidcd.nih.gov

Dr. James F. Battey, M.D., Ph.D., Director
Timothy J. Wheeles, Executive Officer and Chief
Chad Wysong, Deputy Executive Officer
Chris Clements, Program Advisor
Explains what is traumatic brain injury, who suffer from head trauma, what are the cognitive and communication problems that result from traumatic brain injury, how cognitive and communication probles assessed and how they are treated, and what research is being done for the cognitive and communication prblems caused by traumatic brain injury.

7671 Understanding Down Syndrome: An Introduction for Parents
Brookline Books
8 Trumbull Rd
Suite B-001
Northampton, MA 01060-4533
617-734-6772
800-666-2665
FAX: 617-734-3952
e-mail: brbooks@yahoo.com
www.brooklinebooks.com

Cliff Cunningham, Author
Using positive and readable language, this book helps parents understand Down Syndrome. Medical details are explained in lay terms, and advice is given on working with professionals, obtaining services, and treatment techniques that help the child. Cunningham alerts families to potential problems, the prospects for the child in schooling and the passage to adulthood. Revised 1996. *$14.95*
Softcover
ISBN 1-57129 -09-5

7672 Valley News Dispatch
New York Families For Autistic Children
95-16 Pitkin Avenue
Ozone Park, NY 11417-2834
718-641-3441
FAX: 718-641-2228
e-mail: help@nyfac.org
www.nyfac.org

Cheryl L. Marsh, Chairperson
Robert Burt, Treasurer
Education, recreation and support services for families and children with developmental disabilities.

7673 **Verbal Behavior Approach: How to Teach Children with Autism & Related Disorders**
Autism Society of North Carolina Bookstore
505 Oberlin Road
Suite 230
Raleigh, NC 27605-1345 919-743-0204
800-442-2762
FAX: 919-743-0208
e-mail: books@autismsociety-nc.org
www.autismbookstore.com

David Laxton, Director of Communications
Paul Wendler, Chief Financial Officer
Tracey Sheriff, Chief Executive Officer
Kristy White, Director of Development
Provides full descriptions of how to teach the verbal operants that make up expressive languate which include: manding, tacting, echoing and intraverbal skills. *$19.95*

7674 **Without Reason: A Family Copes with two Generations of Autism**
Books on Special Children
721 W Abram St
Arlington, TX 76013-6995 817-277-0727
800-489-0727
FAX: 817-277-2270
www.futurehorizons-autism.com

Wayne Tilton, President
The author discovers his son has autism. He delves into problems of the autistic person and explains reasons for their actions. *$20.95*
292 pages Hardcover

7675 **Women with Attention Deficit Disorder: Embracing Disorganization at Home and Work**
Underwood-Miller
708 Westover Dr
Lancaster, PA 17601-1242
288 pages
ISBN 1-887424-05-9

7676 **You Mean I'm Not Lazy, Stupid or Crazy?!: A Self-Help Book for Adults with ADD**
Simon & Schuster
1230 Avenue Of The Americas
11th Floor
New York, NY 10020-1513 212-698-7000
FAX: 212-698-7099
www.simonsays.com

Kate Kelly, Author
Peggy Ramundo, Co-Author
Practical advice on controlling adult ADD, a straightforward guide explains how to get along in groups, become organized, improve memory, and pursue professional help. *$15.00*
464 pages
ISBN 0-684815-31-1

7677 **You and Your ADD Child**
Nelson Publications
1 Gateway Plz
Port Chester, NY 10573-4674 914-481-5490
FAX: 914-937-8950

Paul Warren MD, Author
Jody Capehart M.Ed., Co-Author
$12.99
252 pages Paperback
ISBN 0-785278-95-8

Print: Journals

7678 **American Journal on Mental Retardation**
American Association on Mental Retardation
501 3rd Street NW
Suite 200
Washington, DC 20001 202-387-1968
800-424-3688
FAX: 202-387-2193
e-mail: aamr@access.digex.net
www.aamr.org

Leonard Abbeduto, Editor
Articles cover biological, behavioral, and educational research: theory papers; and reviews of research literature on specific aspects of mental retardation. *$142.00*
112 pages BiMonthly

7679 **Annals of Dyslexia**
International Dyslexia Association
40 York Road
4th Floor
Baltimore, MD 21204 410-296-0232
800-ABC-D123
FAX: 410-321-5069
www.interdys.org

Hal Malchow, President
Ben Shifrin, Vice President
Elsa C. Hagen, Vice President
Suzanne Carreker, Secretary
IDA is a clearinghouse of scientific data and practice-based information related to dyslexia. Provides community-based referrals and information fact sheets in response to thousands of emails, calls & letters. Our annual conference attracts thousands of outstanding researchers, clinicians, parents, teachers, psychologists, educational therapists and people with dyslexia. *$15.00*
Paper

7680 **Journal of Cognitive Rehabilitation**
Neuroscience Publishers
6555 Carrollton Ave
Indianapolis, IN 46220-1664 317-257-9672
FAX: 317-257-9674
e-mail: nsc@neuroscience.cnter.com
neuroscience.cnter.com

Odie L Bracy, Executive Director
Publication for therapists, family and patient, designed to provide information relevant to the rehabilitation of impairment resulting from brain injury. *$50.00*
36-48 pages Quarterly

Print: Magazines

7681 **AWARE**
National Fibromyalgia Association
1000 Bristol Street North
Suite 17-247
Irvine, CA 92660 714-921-0150
FAX: 714-921-6920
www.fmaware.org

Lynne Matallana, President/Founder
Mark Dobrilovic, Board of Director
John Fry, PhD, Board of Director
Michael Seffinger, DO, FAAFP, Board of Director
Magazine published three times a year with membership only.

7682 **Attention**
Children & Adults with ADHD
8181 Professional Place
Suite 150
Landover, MD 20785- 2264 301-306-7070
800-233-4050
FAX: 301-306-7090
e-mail: webmaster@chadd.org
www.chadd.org

Bryan Goodman, Director

A bi-monthly publication from CHADD. Free with membership.
Bi-monthly

Print: Newsletters

7683 ADHD Report
Guilford Press
72 Spring St
New York, NY 10012-4019
212-431-9800
800-365-7006
FAX: 212-966-6708
e-mail: info@guilford.com
www.guilford.com

Russell A Barkley PhD, Editor
Presents the most up-to-date information on the evaluation, diagnosis and management of ADHD in children, adolescents and adults. This important newsletter is an invaluable resource for all professionals interested in ADHD. *$49.95*
16 pages BiMonthly
ISSN 1065-8025

7684 Arc Connection Newsletter
Arc of Tennessee
151 Athens Way
Suite 100
Nashville, TN 37228
615-248-5878
800-835-7077
FAX: 615-248-5879
e-mail: info@thearctn.org
thearctn.org

John Lewis, President
John H. Shouse, VP,Planning & Rules committee Chair
Donna Lankford, Secretary
Ann Curl, Treasurer,Budget/Finance Committee Chair
Quarterly publication from the ARC of Tennessee. *$ 10.00*
12 pages Quarterly

7685 Autism Research Review International
Autism Research Institute
4182 Adams Ave
San Diego, CA 92116-2599
619-281-7165
FAX: 619-563-6840
e-mail: br@autismresearchinstitute.com
autism.com

Steve Edelson, Executive Director
The Autism Research Institute has pubished this quarterly newsletter, Autism Research Review International (ARRI), since 1987. The ARRI has received worldwide praise for it's thoroughness and objectivity in reporting the current developments in biomedical and educational research. The latest findings are gleaned from a computer search of the 25,000 scientific and medical articles published every week. *$18.00*
8 pages Quarterly

7686 Chadder
Children & Adults with Attention Deficit Disorder
4601 Presidents Drive
Suite 300
Lanham, MD 20706
301-306-7070
FAX: 301-306-7090
www.chadd.org

Michael MacKay, President
Ruth Hughes, CEO
Susan Buningh, Executive Editor
Christine hoch, Director of Development
Quarterly newsletter
Quarterly

7687 Down Syndrome News
National Down Syndrome Congress
30 Mansell Court
Suite 108
Roswell, GA 30076
770-604-9500
800-232-6372
FAX: 770-604-9898
e-mail: info@ndsccenter.org
www.ndsccenter.org

Jim Faber, President
Marilyn Tolbert, 1st VP
Carole J. Guess, 2nd Vice President
Lori Mckee, Treasurer
Must become a member to receive the newsletter.

7688 Farmington Valley ARC
225 Commerce Dr
Canton, CT 06019-1099
860-693-6662
FAX: 860-693-8662
favarh.org

Diane Brown, President
Stephen Morris, Executive Director
The official newsletter containing information, new ideas, progress and more on the Farmington Valley Association for Retarded and Handicapped Citizens.

7689 Imagine!
Imagine!
1400 Dixon St
Lafayette, CO 80026-2790
303-665-7789
FAX: 303-665-2648
e-mail: gstebick@imaginecolorado.org
imaginecolorado.org

John Taylor, President
Mark Emery, Executive Director
John Nevins, CFO
Susan LaHoda, Foundation Executive Director
For people of all ages with cognitive, developmental, physical & health related needs, so they may live lives of independence & quality in their homes and communities.
12-16 pages quarterly

7690 Pure Facts
Feingold Association of the US
11849 Suncatcher Dr
Fishers, IN 46037
631-369-9340
800-321-3287
FAX: 631-369-2988
e-mail: help@feingold.org
www.feingold.org

Debbie Lehner, Manager
Relationship between foods, food additives and behavior/learning problems, including Attention Deficit Disorder (ADD) and hyperactivity. *$38.00*
10+ pages Monthly

Non Print: Newsletters

7691 Arc Light
Arc of Arizona
5610 S Central Ave
Phoenix, AZ 85040-3090
602-268-6101
800-252-9054
FAX: 602-268-7483
e-mail: thearcaz@gmail.com
www.arcofarizona.org

Cindy Waymire, Editor
For people with intellectual and developmental disabilities.
Quarterly

7692 BIATX Newsletter
Brain Injury Association of Texas
316 W 12th Street
Suite 405
Austin, TX 78701-1845
512-326-1212
800-392-0040
FAX: 512-478-3370
e-mail: info@texasbia.com
www.texasbia.org

Judith Abner, Director
Penny Phillips, President
Donna Kuhlmann, Chairman
Kelly Ramsay, CFO
A online quarterly e-newsletter, as well as news and updates on the Brain Injury Association of Texas.

7693 BIAWV Newsletter
Brain Injury Association of America
PO Box 574
Institute, WV 25112-0574
304-766-4892
800-356-6443
FAX: 304-766-4940
e-mail: biawv@aol.com
biawestvirginia.org

Peggy Brown, Director
Mike Davis, President

7694 Best Buddies Times
Best Buddies Times
907-1243 Islington Ave
Toronto, ON
416-531-0003
888-779-0061
FAX: 416-531-0325
e-mail: info@bestbuddies.ca
www.bestbuddies.ca

Steven Pinnock, Director
Emily Bolyea-Kyere, Regional Program Manager
Bi-annual newsletter.

7695 Cognitive Therapy Today
Beck Institute for Cognitive Therapy & Research
One Belmont Avenue
Ste 700
Bala Cynwyd, PA 19004-1610
610-664-3020
FAX: 610-709-5336
e-mail: info@beckinstitute.org
www.beckinstitute.org
Judith S Beck, Director
Aaron T Beck, President
Cognitive Therapy TodayT features articles on a wide range of topics in CBT by leading clinicians from around the world. Articles have addressed evaluating psychotherapies; CBT and special populations, such as soldiers, the elderly, or diagnoses such as schizophrenia; conceptualizing emotions; cross-cultural issues and many other issues of interest to clinicians. You will also find information on workshops, speaking engagements by Beck Institute faculty and more.

7696 Focus Times Newsletter
Focus Alternative Learning Center
126 Dowd Avenue
PO Box 452
Canton, CT 06019-0452
860-693-8809
FAX: 860-693-0141
e-mail: info@focuscenterforautism.org
www.focus-alternative.org

Marcia Bok, President
Claudia Godburn, Secretary
Rita Barredo, Treasurer
Monthly online newsletter on autism.

7697 NAMI Advocate
National Alliance on Mental Illness
3803 N Fairfax Dr
Suite 100
Arlington, VA 22203-3080
703-524-7600
800-950-6264
FAX: 703-524-9094
www.nami.org
Suzanne Vogel-Scibilia, President
Our mission is to provide you with the technical assistance, tools and referrals to resources you need to build organizational capacity and achieve the goals of the NAMI Standards of Excellence.

7698 NLP News
NLP Comprehensive
PO.Box 348
Indian Hills, CO 80454-648
303-987-2224
800-233-1657
FAX: 303-987-2228
e-mail: learn@nlpco.com
www.nlpco.com

Christian Miller, Editor
Tom Dotz, President
Tom Hoobyar, Director Of Planning
Sharon DeBault, Director Of Community Relations
An online e-newsletter on Neuro-linguistic programming.

7699 REACH
TEACCH
100 Renee Lynn Ct
Carrboro, NC 27510
919-966-2174
FAX: 919-966-4127
e-mail: teacch@unc.edu
www.teacch.com
Dr. Laura Klinger, Director
Walter Kelly, Business Officer
Rebecca Mabe, Assistant Director of Business
Mark Klinger, Director of Research
Free online newsletter.

7700 Weekly Wisdom
Autism Treatment Center of America
2080 S Undermountain Rd
Sheffield, MA 01257-9643
413-229-2100
877-766-7473
FAX: 413-229-3202
www.son-rise.org
Barry Kausman, Owner
Weekly Wisdom is available through a free email subscription.

Non Print: Software

7701 Cogrehab
Life Science Associates
1 Fenimore Rd
Bayport, NY 11705-2115
631-472-2111
FAX: 631-472-8146
e-mail: lifesciassoc@pipeline.com
www.lifesciassoc.home.pipeline.com
Joann Mandriota, President
Divided into six groups for diagnosis and treatment of attention, memory and perceptual disorders to be used by and under the guidance of a professional. $95.-$1,950

Non Print: Video

7702 ADD, Stepping Out of the Dark
Child Development Media
5632 Van Nuys Blvd
Suite 286
Van Nuys, CA 91401-4602
818-989-7221
800-405-8942
FAX: 818-989-7826
e-mail: info@childdevelopmentmedia.com
www.childdevelopmentmedia.com
Margie Wagner, Owner
A powerful, effective video, ideal for health professionals, educators and parents providing a visual montage designed to promote an understanding and awareness of attention deficit disorder. Based on actual accounts of those who have ADD, including a neurologist, an office worker, and parents of children with ADD. The DVD allows the viewer to feel the frustration and lack of attention that ADD brings to many. *$52.95*
Video

7703 ADHD in Adults
Guilford Press
72 Spring St
New York, NY 10012-4019
212-431-9800
800-365-7006
FAX: 212-966-6708
e-mail: info@guilford.com
www.guilford.com
Russell A Barkley, Editor
This program integrates information on ADHD with the actual experiences of four adults who suffer from the disorder. Representing a range of professions, from a lawyer to a mother working at home, each candidly discusses the impact of ADHD on his or her daily life. These interviews are augmented by comments from family members and other clinicians who treat adults with ADHD. *$99.00*
DVD 1906
ISBN 0-898629-86-1

7704 ADHD: What Can We Do?
Guilford Press
72 Spring St
New York, NY 10012-4019
212-431-9800
800-365-7006
FAX: 212-966-6708
e-mail: info@guilford.com
www.gulford.com
Russell A Barkley, Editor
A video program that introduces teachers and parents to a variety of the most effective technologies for managing ADHD in the classroom, at home, and on family outings. *$99.00*
DVD 1906
ISBN 0-898629-72-1

7705 ADHD: What Do We Know?
Guilford Press
72 Spring St
New York, NY 10012-4019
212-431-9800
800-365-7006
FAX: 212-966-6708
e-mail: info@guilford.com
www.guilford.com
Bob Matloff, President
Russell A Barkley, Editor
An introduction for teachers and special education practitioners, school psychologists and parents of ADHD children. Topics outlined in this video include the causes and prevalence of ADHD, ways children with ADHD behave, other conditions that may accompany ADHD and long-term prospects for children with ADHD. *$99.00*
DVD 1906
ISBN 0-898629-71-3

7706 Around the Clock: Parenting the Delayed AD HD Child
Guilford Press
72 Spring St
New York, NY 10012-4019
212-431-9800
800-365-7006
FAX: 212-966-6708
e-mail: info@guilford.com
Joan F Goodman, Editor
Susan Hoban, Editor
This videotape provides both professionals and parents a helpful look at how the difficulties facing parents of ADHD children can be handled. Video. *$150.00*
VHS 1994
ISBN 0-898629-68-3

7707 Attention Deficit Disorder: Adults
Aquarius Health Care Media
30 Forest Road
Millis, MA 02054
508-376-1244
888-440-2963
FAX: 508-376-1245
e-mail: aqvideos@tiac.net
www.aquariusproductions.com
Lesile Kussmann, President/Owner
Joseph Wellington, Distribution Coordinator
Anne Baker, Billing & Accounting
Adults with ADD talk about how the disorder that went undiagnosed for so many years has affected their choice of spouses and work, and what they have found to help them. Biofeedback, which is growing as a treatment, is explained and demonstrated by its founder, Dr. Joel Lubar. Medical treatments like antidepressants and stimulants are also discussed, along with behavioral changes that can help the person with ADD and his or her spouse and family. *$149.00*
Video

7708 Attention Deficit Disorder: Children
Aquarius Health Care Media
30 Forest Rd
PO Box 249
Millisrn, MA 02054-7159
508-376-1244
888-440-2963
FAX: 508-376-1245
e-mail: aqvideos@tiac.net
www.aquariusproductions.com
Lesile Kussmann, President/Owner
Everyone has been impulsive or easily distracted for different periods of time, so these symptoms that are hallmarks of Attention Deficit Disorder (ADD) have also led to criticism that too many people are being diagnosed with this biochemical brain disorder. This program examines who is being diagnosed, and what treatments are working. An innovative private school specializing in alternative education is profiled, and tips on structuring the school and home environment are included. *$149.00*
Video

7709 Autism: A World Apart
Fanlight Productions C/O Icarus Films
32 Court Street
Brooklyn, NY 11201-1731
718-488-8900
800-876-1710
FAX: 718-488-8642
e-mail: info@fanlight.com
www.fanlight.com
Ben Achtenberg, Owner
Nicole Johnson, Publicity Coordinator
Anthony Sweeney, Marketing Director
In this documentary, three families show us what the textbooks and studies cannot: what it's like to live with autism day after day; to raise and love children who may be withdrawn and violent and unable to make personal connections with their families. 29 minutes. *$195.00*
VHS/DVD 1988
ISBN 1-572950-39-0

7710 **Autism: the Unfolding Mystery**
Aquarius Health Care Media
30 Forest Road
PO Box 249
Millis, MA 02054
508-376-1244
FAX: 508-376-1245
e-mail: lkussmann@aquariusproductions.com
www.aquariusproductions.com

Lesile Kussmann, Owner

Explore what it means to be autistic, how you can recognize the signs of autism in your child, and hear about new treatments and programs to help children learn to deal with the disorder. *$145.00*
DVD 1905

7711 **Biology Concepts Through Discovery**
Educational Activities Software
5600 W 83rd Street
Suite 300, 8200 Tower
Bloomington, MN 55437
800-447-5286
FAX: 239-225-9299
e-mail: info@edmentum.com
http://www.ea-software.com

Vin Riera, President/CEO
Rob Rueckel, CFO
Dave Adams, Chief Academic Officer
Paul Johansen, Chief Technology Officer

These videos, available in English and Spanish versions, encourage learning by presenting interactive problem solving in an effective VISUAL/AUDITORY style. *$89.00*
Video

7712 **Concentration Video**
Learning disAbilities Resources
6 E Eagle Road
Havertown, PA 19083
610-446-6126
800-869-8336
FAX: 610-525-8337
e-mail: rcooper-ldr@comcast.net

Video

7713 **Educating Inattentive Children**
ADD Warehouse
300 Northwest 70th Avenue
Suite 102
Plantation, FL 33317-2360
954-792-8100
800-233-9273
FAX: 954-792-8545
e-mail: websales@addwarehouse.com
www.addwarehouse.com

Harvey C Parker, Owner

Ideal for in-service to regular and special educators concerning the problems inattentive, elementarty and secondary students experience. *$49.00*
Video

7714 **Getting Started with Facilitated Communication**
Facilitated Communication Institute, Syracuse Univ
230 Huntington Hal
Syracuse, NY 13244-1
315-443-4752
FAX: 315-443-2258
http://thefci.syr.edu

Annegret Schubert, Director

Describes in detail how to help individuals with autism and/or severe communication difficulties to get started with facilitated communication.
Video

7715 **Getting Together: A Head Start/School District Collaboration**
Brookes Publishing
P.O.Box 10624
Baltimore, MD 21285-624
410-337-9580
800-638-3775
FAX: 410-337-8539
e-mail: custserv@brookespublishing.com
www.brookespublishing.com

David P Lindeman, Producer
Lauren Smith, Western Region Sales Representative
Jeannine Blimline, Central Region Sales Representative

This video describes how to include children with disabilities in the Head Start classrooms. Addresses such issues as leadership, staff support, and policy development. Comes with a 24-page saddle-stitched booklet. *$34.95*
Video
ISBN 1-55766-97-5

7716 **How to Cope with ADHD: Diagnosis, Treatment & Myths**
Aquarius Health Care Media
30 Forest Road
PO Box 249
Millis, MA 02054
508-376-1244
FAX: 508-376-1245
e-mail: lkussmann@aquariusproductions.com
www.aquariusproductions.com

Lesile Kussmann, President/Owner

Learn how ADHD is diagnosed, clear up some of the myths, explain the treatmens that are availiable, and give you tips on how you can help your child at home. *$145.00*
DVD 1905

7717 **I Just Want My Little Boy Back**
Autism Treatment Center Of America
2080 South Undermountain Road
Sheffield, MA 01257
413-229-2100
800-714-2779
e-mail: happiness@option.org
www.option.org

Samahria Lyt Kaufman, Co-Founder and Co-Director
Dane Griffith, Director of Administrative Services
Bears Kaufman, Co-Founder and Co-Director
Raun Kaufman, Director of Global Education

A great video for parents and professionals caring for children with special needs. Join one British family and their autistic son before, during and after their journey to America to attend The Son-Rise Program at The Autism Treatment Center of America. This informative, inspirational and deeply moving story not only captures the joy, tears, challenges and triumps of this amazing little boy and his family, but also serves as a powerful introduction to the attitude and principles of the program. *$25.00*

7718 **It's Just Attention Disorder**
Western Psychological Services
625 Alaska Avenue
Torrance, CA 90503-5124
424-201-8800
800-648-8857
FAX: 424-201-6950
e-mail: customerservice@wpspublish.com
wpspublish.com

Gregg Gillmar, VP

This ground-breaking videotape takes the critical first steps in treating attention-deficit disorder: it enlists the inattentive or hyperactive child as an active participant in his or her treatment. *$99.50*
Video

7719 **Understanding ADHD**
Aquarius Health Care Videos
30 Forest Road
PO Box
Millis, MA 02054
508-376-1244
FAX: 508-376-1245
e-mail: aqvideos@tiac.net
www.aquariusproductions.com

Leslie Kussmann, President/Owner

A look at some of the controversies surrounding Attention Deficit Hyperactivity Disorder. This video shows how the disorder is diagnosed and presents strategies for living with a child with the disorder. Diverse and candid opinions from teachers, social workers, a behavior specialist, a pediatrician and a parent with ADHD twins. Recommended for child development students, social workers, and caregivers. Preview option available. *$120.00*
Video

7720 **Understanding Attention Deficit Disorder**
CACLD
25 Van Zant Street
Norwalk, CT 6855-1713 203-838-5010
FAX: 203-866-6108
e-mail: CACLD@optonline.net
www.CACLD.org

Beryl Kaufman, Executive Director
Helen Bosch, President
A video in an interview format for parents and professionals providing the history, symptoms, methods of diagnosis and three approaches used to ease the effects of attention deficit disorder. Published by Connecticut Association for Children & Adults with Learning Disabilities (CACLD). *$20.00*
45 Minutes VHS

7721 **Understanding Autism**
Fanlight Productions C/O Icarus Films
32 Court Street
Brooklyn, NY 11201 718-488-8900
800-876-1710
FAX: 718-488-8642
e-mail: info@fanlight.com
www.fanlight.com

Ben Achtenberg, Owner
Susan Newman, Editor
Parents of children with autism discuss the nature and symptoms of this lifelong disability and outline a treatment program based on behavior modification principles. 19 minutes *$199.00*
VHS/DVD 1993
ISBN 1-572951-00-1

7722 **We're Not Stupid**
Media Projects Inc
5215 Homer St
Dallas, TX 75206-6623 214-826-3863
FAX: 214-826-3919
e-mail: mail@mediaprojects.org
www.mediaprojects.org
Fonya Naomi Mondell, Producer
We're Not Stupid is an insightful and very personal video that gives a voice to people who are struggling with learning disabilities. It was made by filmmaker Fonya Naomi Mondell, who is also living with learning differences. The filmmaker camptures the personal stories of young people from all walks of life who discuss what it's like to live with Attention Deficit Disorder and Dyslexia. Their comments are open, honest and direct, and their determination to manage their condition shines through. *$125.00*
Video

7723 **Why Won't My Child Pay Attention?**
ADD Warehouse
300 Northwest 70th Avenue
Suite 102
Plantation, FL 33317-2360 954-792-8100
800-233-9273
FAX: 954-792-8545
www.addwarehouse.com

Sam Goldstein, Ph.D, Author
Michael Goldstein, M.D., Co-Author
Practical and reassuring videotape, noted child psychologist tells parents about two of the most common and complex problems of childhood: inattention and hyperactivity. *$49.50*
224 pages Hardcover 1992
ISBN 0-471530-77-8

Support Groups

7724 **Autism Society of America**
4340 East-West Highway
Suite 350
Bethesda, MD 20814 301-657-0881
800-328-8476
FAX: 301-657-0869
e-mail: info@autism-society.org
www.autism-society.org
Scott Badesch, President/CEO
Jennifer Repella, VP Programs
John Dabrowski, CFO
Doreen Allen, Marketing Manager
ASA is the largest and oldest grassroots organization within the autism community, with more than 200 chapters and over 20,000 members and supporters nationwide. ASA is the leading source of education, information and referral about autism and has been the leader in advocacy and legislative initiatives for more than three decades.

7725 **National Autism Hotline**
Autism Services Center
929 4th Ave
PO Box 507
Huntington, WV 25701-1408 304-525-8014
FAX: 304-525-8026
www.autismservicescenter.org

Mike Grady, CEO
Jimmie Beirne, COO
Nathel Lewis, ASC Training Coordinator
Service agency for individuals with autism and developmental disabilities, and their families. Assists families and agencies attempting to meet the needs of individuals with autism and other developmental disabilities. Makes available technical assistance in designing treatment programs and more. The hotline provides informational packets to callers and assists via telephone when possible.

7726 **National Health Information Center**
Office Of Disease Prevention And Health Promotion
P.O.Box 1133
Washington, DC 20013-1133 301-565-4167
800-336-4797
301-468-7394
FAX: 301-984-4256
e-mail: info@nhic.org
www.health.gov/nhic
Jessica Rowden, Sec Dept. Health Human Services
William Corr, J.D., Deputy Secretary
National health information center provides information referral and support. NHIC links consumers and health professionals to organizations that are best able to provide reliable health information.

Dexterity

Associations

7727 **American Amputee Foundation, Inc.**
PO Box 94227
North Little Rock, AR 72190 501-835-9290
FAX: 501-835-9292
e-mail: info@americanamputee.org
www.americanamputee.org
Catherine J Walden LSW MPA CLCP, Executive Director
Serves primarily as a national information clearinghouse and referral center assisting mainly amputees and their families. AAF researches and gathers information including studies, product information, services, self-help publications and review articles written within the field. AAF has helped with claims, justification letters to payers, testimony and life care planning. Free information packet for phone or letter inquiries.

7728 **American Board for Certification in Orthotics & Prosthetics And Pedorthics, Inc.**
330 John Carlyle Street
Suite 210
Alexandria, VA 22314- 5760 703-836-7114
FAX: 703-836-0838
e-mail: info@abcop.org
www.abcop.org
Timothy E. Miller, CPO
Curt A. Bertram, President Elect
James H. Wynne, CPO
Donald D. Virostek, CPO/Past President
The American Board for Certification in Orthotics and Prosthetics (ABC) is the national certifying and accrediting body for the orthotic and prosthetic professions. The public requires and deserves assurance that the persons providing orthotic and prosthetic services and care are qualified to provide the appropriate services, and it was on this basis that the ABC was established as a credentialing organization.

7729 **American Stroke Association**
American Heart Association
7272 Greenville Ave
Dallas, TX 75231-4596 800-242-8721
888-478-7653
FAX: 214-706-5231
e-mail: strokeconnection@heart.org
www.strokeassociation.org/STROKEORG/
Ralph L Sacco MS, President
Fifty-five state affiliates monitoring local chapters offering educational materials, seminars, conferences and transportation for members nationwide. Maintains a listing of over 1,000 stroke support groups across the nation for referral to stroke survivors, their families, caregivers and interested professionals.

7730 **Epilepsy Foundation**
8301 Professional Place
Landover, MD 20785-2353 301-459-3700
800-332-1000
FAX: 301-577-2684
e-mail: ContactUs@efa.org
www.epilepsyfoundation.org
Phil Gattone, President/CEO
Lee Gaston, Vice President Finance
Patty Dukes, VP Operations
Angela Ostrom, VP of Public Policy
The Epilepsy Foundation is the national voluntary agency solely dedicated to the welfare of the 3 million people with epilepsy in the U.S. and their families. The organization works to ensure that people with seizures are able to participate in all life experiences; and to prevent, control and cure epilepsy through research, education, advocacy and services.

7731 **National Amputation Foundation**
40 Church St
Malverne, NY 11565-1735 516-887-3600
516-887-3600
FAX: 516-887-3667
e-mail: amps76@aol.com
www.nationalamputation.org
Paul Bernacchio, President
William Sturges, 1st Vice President
Al Pennacchia, 2nd Vice President
Doanld A. Sioss, Executive Secretary
Information & resources for amputees. Scholarship programs for college students with major limb amputation. Free donated durable medical equipment open to anyone in need locally-as items need to be picked up.
Quarterly

7732 **National Commission on Orthotic and Prosthetic Education**
330 John Carlyle Street
Suite 200
Alexandria, VA 22314- 5760 703-836-7114
FAX: 703-836-0838
e-mail: info@ncope.org
www.ncope.org
Robin C Seabrook, Executive Director
Jonathan D. Day, CPO
Dominique Mungo, Residency Program Manager
Joan M. Dallas, Accreditation Assistant
The mission of NCOPE is to be recognized authority for the development and accreditation of O&P education and residency standards leading to competent patient care in the changing healthcare environment. NCOPE develops, applies, and assures standards for orthotic and prosthetic education through accreditation and approval to promote exemplary patient care.

7733 **National Institute of Neurological Disorde Disorders & Stroke**
PO Box 5801
Bethesda, MD 20824-5801 301-496-5751
800-352-9424
FAX: 301-402-2186
www.ninds.nih.gov
Samahria Lyt Landis, Executive Director
Walter J Koroshetz MD, Deputy Director
Caroline Lewis, Executive Officer
Alfred W. Gordon, Ph.D., Associate Director for Special P
The mission of the National Institute of Neurological Disorders and Stroke is to reduce the burden of neurological disease.

7734 **National Stroke Association**
9707 E Easter Ln
Suite B
Centennial, CO 80112-3754 303-649-9299
800-787-6537
FAX: 303-649-1328
e-mail: info@stroke.org
www.stroke.org
James Baranski, CEO
Sharon Jaunchowski, Executive VP
Teran Nash, Customer Relations
Carol Griffin, Development Manager
The only national health organization solely committed to stroke prevention, treatment, rehabilitation and community reintegration. Provides packaged training programs, on-site assistance, physician, patient and family education materials to acute and rehab hospitals. Develops workshops; operates the Stroke Information & Referral Center and produces professional publications such as Stroke: Clinical Updates and the Journal of Stroke and Cerebrovascular Diseases.

7735 **World Chiropractic Alliance**
2950 N Dobson Rd
Suite 3
Chandler, AZ 85224-1819
480-786-9235
800-347-1011
FAX: 480-732-9313
e-mail: comments@worldchiropracticalliance.org
www.worldchiropracticalliance.org

Terry A Rondberg, Founder/CEO
Richard Barwell, President

Dedicated to protecting and strengthening chiropractic around the world. Serving as a watchdog and advocacy organization, we place our emphasis on education and political action.

Print: Books

7736 **Carpal Tunnel Syndrome**
Arthritis Foundation
1330 W Peachtree St
Suite 100
Atlanta, GA 30309
404-872-7100
800-283-7800
FAX: 404-872-0457
e-mail: help@arthritis.org
www.arthritis.org

John H Klippel, President/CEO
Daniel T. McGowan, Chairman Of The Board
Rowland W. Chang, Vice Chair
Patricia Nov Nelson, Vice Chair

The Arthritis Foundation is committed to raising awareness and reducing the unacceptable impact of arthritis, a disease which must be taken as seriously as other chronic diseases because of its devastatng consequences.

7737 **Don't Feel Sorry for Paul**
Harper Collins Publishing
76 Ninth Ave
New York, NY 10011
800-843-2665
www.barnesandnoble.com

Bernard Wolf, Author
Ann Ledden, Vice President
Lorna Metzler, Manager

Paul is seven but was born with deformities of both hands and feet. Paul must wear a prosthesis on both feet so that he can walk. He has a third prosthesis for his right hand. The third prosthesis has a pair of hoks Paul uses as fingers.
94 pages Hardcover
ISBN 0-39731 -88-0

7738 **Functional Restoration of Adults and Children with Upper Extremity Amputation**
Demos Medical Publishing
11 West 42nd Street
15th Floor
New York, NY 10036-8804
212-683-0072
800-532-8663
FAX: 212-683-0118
e-mail: orderdep@demospub.com
www.demosmedpub.com

Robert Meier III, Author
Diane Atkins, OTR, Co-Author

Provides a comprehensive reference to the surgery, prosthetic fitting, and rehabilitation of individuals sustaining an arm amputation. Covers the recent advancements in prosthetics and rehabilitation. *$165.00*
384 pages
ISBN 1-888799-73-0

Print: Magazines

7739 **ABC Mark of Merit Newsletter**
Amer Board for Cert in Otthotics & Prosthetics
330 John Carlyle St
Suite 210
Alexandria, VA 22314-5760
703-836-7114
FAX: 703-836-0838
e-mail: info@abcop.org
www.abcop.org

Timothy E. Miller, CPO
Curt A. Bertram, President Elect
James H. Wynne, CPO
Donald D. Virostek, CPO/Past President

An online bi-monthly newsletter.

7740 **Active Living Magazine**
American Amputee Foundation
PO Box 94227
North Little Rock, AR 72190
501-835-9290
FAX: 501-835-9292
e-mail: info@americanamputee.org
www.americanamputee.org

Catherine J Walden, Executive Director

A print magazine published four times a year.

7741 **Stroke Connection Magazine**
American Heart Association
7272 Greenville Ave
Dallas, TX 75231-5129
214-373-6300
888-478-7653
FAX: 214-706-5231
www.strokeassociation.org/STROKEORG/

John Caswell, Editor
Debra Lockwood, Chairman
Nancy Brown, CEO
Ralph Sacco, President/Director

Free magazine for stroke survivors and their family caregivers.

Print: Newsletters

7742 **NINDS Notes**
Ntn'l Institute of Neurological Disorders & Stroke
P.O.Box 5801
Bethesda, MD 20284
301-496-5751
800-352-9424
FAX: 202-944-3295
e-mail: sbaa@sbaa.org
www.ninds.nih.org

Caroline Lewis, Executive Officer
Story C. Landis, Director
Denise Dorsey, Chief Administrative Officer
Maryann Sofranko, Deputy Executive Officer

A print newsletter published three times a year.

Non Print: Newsletters

7743 **Advocacy Pulse**
American Stroke Association
7272 Greenville Ave
Dallas, TX 75231-5129
214-373-6300
888-478-7653
FAX: 214-706-5231
www.strokeassociation.org/STROKEORG/

Ralph Sacco, President/Director
Debra Lockwood, Chairman
Nancy Brown, CEO

7744 **Noteworthy Newsletter**
Ntn'l Comm on Orthotic & Prosthetic Education
330 John Carlyle Street
Suite 200
Alexandria, VA 22314- 5760
703-836-7114
FAX: 703-836-0838
e-mail: info@ncope.org
www.ncope.org

Robin C Seabrook, Executive Director
Jonathan D. Day, CPO
Dominique Mungo, Residency Program Manager
Joan M. Dallas, Accreditation Assistant

The mission of NCOPE is to be recognized authority for the development and accreditation of O&P education and residency standards leading to competent patient care in the changing healthcare environment. NCOPE develops, applies, and assures standards for orthotic and prosthetic education through accreditation and approval to promote exemplary patient care.

7745 **Stroke Smart Magazine**
National Stroke Association
9707 E Easter Ln
Suite B
Centennial, CO 80112-3754
303-649-9299
800-787-6537
FAX: 303-649-1328
e-mail: info@stroke.org
www.stroke.org

James Baranski, CEO
Sharon Jaunchowski, Executive VP
Teran Nash, Customer Relations
Carol Griffin, Development Manager

The only national health organization solely committed to stroke prevention, treatment, rehabilitation and community reintegration. Provides packaged training programs, on-site assistance, physician, patient and family education materials to acute and rehab hospitals. Develops workshops; operates the Stroke Information & Referral Center and produces professional publications such as Stroke: Clinical Updates and the Journal of Stroke and Cerebrovascular Diseases.

Hearing

Associations

7746 **Academy of Rehabilitative Audiology**
PO Box 2323
Albany, NY 12220-0323
952-920-0484
FAX: 952-920-6098
e-mail: ARA@audrehab.org
www.audrehab.org

Kathleen Cienkowski, President
Jan Moore, Ph.D, Treasurer
Kristin Vasil-Dilaj, Secretary
Sheila Pratt, Ph.D., JARA Editor

Provides professional education, research and interest in programs for hearing handicapped persons. The primary purpose of the ARAÝis to promote excellence in hearing care through the provision of comprehensive rehabilitative and habilitative services.

7747 **Alexander Graham Bell Association for the Deaf and Hard of Hearing**
3417 Volta Pl NW
Washington, DC 20007-2737
202-337-5220
FAX: 202-337-8314
TTY:202-337-5221
e-mail: info@agbell.org
agbell.org

Lyn Robertson, President
Steven W. Noyce, Secretary/Treasurer
Cheryl L. Dickson, Immediate Past President
Anita Bernstein, Director

The Alexander Graham Bell Association for the Deaf and Hard of Hearing (AG Bell) is the world's oldest and largest membership organization promoting the use of spoken language by children and adults who are hearing impaired. Members include parents of children with hearing loss, adults who are deaf or hard of hearing, educators, audiologists, speech-language pathologists, physicians and other professionals in fields related to hearing loss and deafness.

7748 **American Association of People with Disabilities**
2013 H Street, NW, 5th Floor
5th Floor, Suite 950
Washington, DC 20006
202-457-0046
800-840-8844
FAX: 866-536-4461
www.aapd.com

Mark Perriello, President/CEO
Henry Claypool, Executive VP
TaKeisha Walker, Director of Workplace & Leadership Initiatives
Adam Abosedra, Program Manager

Dedicated to ensuring economic self-sufficiency and political empowerment for more than 50 million Americans with disabilities.

7749 **American Society for Deaf Children**
800 Florida Ave NE
Suite 2047
Washington, DC 20002-3695
800-942-2732
866-895-4206
FAX: 410-795-0965
e-mail: ascd@deafchildren.org
www.deafchildren.org

Beth S Benedict PhD, President

Supports and educates families of deaf and hard of hearing children and advocates for high quality programs and services.

7750 **American Speech-Language-Hearing Association**
2200 Research Blvd
Rockville, MD 20850-3289
301-296-5700
800-638-8255
FAX: 301-296-8255
e-mail: actioncenter@asha.org
www.asha.org

Patricia A. Prelock, PhD, President
Elizabeth S. McCrea, President-Elect
Shelly S. Chabon, Immediate Past President
Perry F. Flynn, Chair

Provides information for both the general public and physicians in an easy-to-access manner, on speech, hearing and language disorders. Exhibits by companies specializing in alternative and augmentative communications products, publishers, software and hardware companies, and hearing aid testing equipment manufacturers.

7751 **American Tinnitus Association**
522 S W Fifth Ave
Suite 825
Portland, OR 97207-0005
503-248-9985
800-634-8978
FAX: 503-248-0024
e-mail: tinnitus@ata.org
www.ata.org

Michael Manusevec, Executive Director
Katie Fuller, Director of Support
Jennifer Born, Director of Public Affairs
Cara James, Development Director

The American Tinnitus Association (ATA) is the national champion of tinnitus awareness, prevention, and treatment. Under its guiding principles—Education, Advocacy, Research and Support—the ATA offers prevention programs in schools, urges governmental and private organizations to support hearing conservation, funds the nation's brightest researchers, and facilitates self-help groups around the country.

7752 **Association of Late-Deafened Adults**
8038 Macintosh Ln
Suite 2
Rockford, IL 61107-5336
815-332-1515
866-402-2532
FAX: 877-907-1738
TTY: 815-332-1515
e-mail: info@alda.org
www.alda.org

Mary Lou Mistretta, President
Dave Litman, President Elect
Brenda Estes, Past President

Articles, stories and poems by and about late-deafened adults.

7753 **Better Hearing Institute**
1444 I St NW
Suite 700
Washington, DC 20005-6542
202-449-1100
800-327-9355
FAX: 202-216-9646
e-mail: mail@betterhearing.org
www.betterhearing.org

Sergei Kochkin, Executive Director
Norm Crosby, Chairman
Shari Lewis, Chairman

The BHI is a not-for-profit corporation that educates the public about the neglected problem of hearing loss and what can be done about it. Founded in 1973 we are working to erase the stigma and end the embarassment that prevents millions of people from seeking help for hearing loss and show the negative consequences of untreated hearing loss for millions of Americans. And to promote treatment and demonstrate that this is a national problem that can be solved.

7754 **Center for Hearing and Communication**
50 Broadway
Fl 6
New York, NY 10004-3810
917-305-7700
FAX: 917-305-7888
TTY:917-305-7999
e-mail: info@chchearing.org
www.chchearing.org

Laurie Hanin PhD CCC-A, Executive Director
Ellen Lafargue, Director of Audiology
Susan E. Adams, Coordinator
Anita Stein, Assistant Director

The Center for Hearing and Communication provides hearing health services to people of all ages who have a hearing loss. With offices in New York City and Florida, CHC meets all of your hearing and communication needs through professional services that offer the highest level of clinical expertise and technical know-how available in the hearing healthcare field. Visit us for a wide array of services including free hearing screenings; complete hearing evaluations; pediatric services; hearing a

7755 **Communication Service for the Deaf**
3520 Gateway Lane
Sioux Falls, SD 57106
866-642-6410
FAX: 605-362-2806
TTY:866-273-3323
e-mail: inquiry@c-s-d.org
www.c-s-d.org

Dr. Benjamin Soukup, Founder, Chairman & CEO
Christopher Soukup, President
Brad Hermes, CFO
Ann Marie Mickleson, VP, CSD Interpreting

CSD's mission is to create greater opportunities for Deaf and hard of hearing individuals to reach their full potential. Through global leadership and the development of innovative technologies, CSD provides tools conducive to a positive and fully integrated life.

7756 **Conference of Educational Administrators of Schools and Programs for the Deaf**
PO Box 1778
St Augustine, FL 32085-1778
904-810-5200
866-697-8805
FAX: 904-810-5525
e-mail: nationaloffice@ceasd.org
www.ceasd.org

Joseph Finnegan, Executive Director
Ronald Stern, President
Nancy Hlibok Amann, Secretary
Peter L. Bailey, Treasurer

CEASD provides an opportunity for professional educators to work together for the improvement of schools and educational programs for individuals who are deaf or hard of hearing. The organization brings together a rich composite of resources and reaches out to both enhance educational programs and influence educational policy makers.

7757 **Council of American Instructors of the Deaf (CAID)**
PO Box 377
Bedford, TX 76095-0377
817-354-8414
FAX: 817-354-8414
e-mail: caid@swbell.net
www.caid.org

Keith Mousley, President
Helen Lovato, Office Manager

The CAID continues to follow the tradition begun in 1850 and recognizes the value of bringing fellow teaching professionals together to share experiences and ideas for the purpose of improving learning opportunities for deaf and hard of hearing children, adolescents and young adults.

7758 **Deaf REACH**
3521 12th St NE
Washington, DC 20017-2545
202-832-6681
FAX: 202-832-8454
e-mail: info@deaf-reach.org
deaf-reach.org

Sarah E. Brown, Executive Director
Annette Reichman, President
Jonathan Tomar, Vice-President
Myrene Sargent, Director of Administration

The psychosocial rehabilitation approach, ulitzed by all Deaf-REACH programs, provides the solid foundation to member's success. Participants are activly involved in establishing the format and level of highly individualized service delivery that they receive. The concept, which has achieved national acclaim, involves teaching members necessary life skills, thus minimizing the need for assistance from a service professional. This is part of what distinguishes the approach at Deaf-REACH.

7759 **Deafness Research Foundation**
363 Seventh Avenue,
10th Floor
New York, NY 10001-3904
212-257-6140
866-454-3924
FAX: 212-257-6139
TTY: 888-435-6104
e-mail: info@hearinghealthfoundation.org
www.drf.org

Shari Eberts, Chairman
Mark Angelo, President
Robert Boucai, Principal
Judy R. Dubno, Dept. of Otolaryngology-Head and Neck Surgery

Founded in 1958, the Deafness Research Foundation is the leading source of private funding for basic and clinical research in the hearing science. The DRF is committed to making lifelong hearing health a national priority by funding research and implementing education projects in both the government and private sectors.

7760 **Dogs for the Deaf**
10175 Wheeler Rd
Central Point, OR 97502-9360
541-826-9220
800-990-3647
FAX: 541-826-6696
TTY: 541-826-9220
e-mail: info@dogsforthedeaf.org
dogsforthedeaf.org

Robin Dickson, CEO
Vaughan Maurice, General Manager
Janine Bol, Finance Director
John Drach, Training Dept. Manager

Rescues dogs from shelters and professionally trains them for people with special needs such as: deafness, autism for children, seniors, stroke victims, cerebral palsy, etc.

7761 **Ear Foundation**
1817 Patterson St
Nashville, TN 37203-2110
615-329-7849
800-545-4327
FAX: 615-329-7935
e-mail: info@earfoundation.org
www.earfoundation.org

Suzanne Wyatt, Executive Director

National, nonprofit organization committed to integrating the hearing and balance impaired into the mainstream of society through public awareness and medical education. Also administers The Meniere's Network, a national network of patient support groups providing people with the opportunity to share experiences and coping strategies.

7762 **Georgiana Institute**
736 Harmony Street
New Orleans, LA 70115
203-994-8215

e-mail: georgianainstitute@snet.net
www.georgianainstitute.org

Annabel Stehli, President

The information source for Auditory Integration Training (AIT)/Digital Auditory Aerobics (DAA).

7763 **HEAR Center**
301 E Del Mar Blvd
Pasadena, CA 91101-2714
626-796-2016
FAX: 626-796-2320
e-mail: info@hearcenter.org
hearcenter.org

Ellen Simon, Executive Director
Deborah Lorino, Office Manager
Berenice Castro, Accounting Supervisor
Maline Medina, Accounts Receivable/Billing Cle

Auditory and verbal program designed to help hearing impaired children, infants and adults lead normal and productive lives. Seeks to develop auditory techniques to aid people who have communication problems due to deafness. Offers diagnostic evaluations for speech and hearing. Individual auditory, verbal training and speech-language therapy.

7764 **Hearing Education and Awareness for Rockers**
1405 Lyon St
San Francisco, CA 94115-2914
415-409-3277
FAX: 415-409-5683
e-mail: info@hearnet.com
www.hearnet.com

Kathy Peck, Executive Director
Joseph Monatano, Chief of Audiology
Flash Gordon, Primary Care Physician
John Doyle, Secretary of the Board

H.E.A.R.'s mission is the prevention of hearing loss and tinnitus among musicians and music fans (especially teens) through education awareness and grassroots outreach advocacy.

7765 **Hearing Loss Association of America**
7910 Woodmont Ave
Suite 1200
Bethesda, MD 20814-7022
301-657-2248
FAX: 301-913-9413
TTY:301-657-2248
hearingloss.org

Brenda Battat, Executive Director
Barbara Kelley, Dep Exec Dir, Editor-In-Chief
Nancy Macklin, Director of Events & Marketing
Lisa Hamlin, Director of Public Policy

The mission of the Hearing Loss Association of America is to open the world of communication to people with hearing loss through information, education, advocacy and support.

7766 **Hearing, Speech and Deafness Center (HSDC)**
1625 19th Ave
Seattle, WA 98122-2848
206-323-5770
888-222-5036
FAX: 206-328-6871
TTY: 206-388-1275
e-mail: hsdc@hsdc.org
www.hsdc.org

Ken Block, Chairman
Norman Guadango, Managing Director
Robert Leining, Treasurer
Mike Redmond, President

Our mission is to enrich lives of all adults and children who experience hearing loss, speech and language impairments or who are deaf, by providing professional services and by promoting community awareness and accessibility.

7767 **House Ear Institute**
2100 W 3rd St
Los Angeles, CA 90057-1944
213-483-4431
800-388-8612
FAX: 213-484-8789
TTY: 213-484-2642
e-mail: info@hei.org
www.hei.org

James Boswell, CEO
John.W House, M.D, President
Daniel. M Graham, Executive Vice President Develop
Neil Segil, Ph.D, Executive Vice President

Offers pediatric hearing tests, otologic and audiologic evaluation and treatment, rehabilitation, hearing aid dispensing, and cochlear implant services. Outreach programs focus on families with hearing impaired children.

7768 **International Catholic Deaf Association**
7202 Buchanan St
Landover Hills, MD 20784-2236
301-429-0697
FAX: 301-429-0698
e-mail: homeoffice@icda-us.org
icda-us.org

Jean Cox, President
Kate Slosar, Vice President
T.K Hill, Secretary
Jimmy Kelly, Treasurer

An organization of Catholic deaf people and hearing people in the church working with the deaf in the united states of America.

7769 **International Hearing Dog**
5901 E 89th Ave
Henderson, CO 80640-8315
303-287-3277
FAX: 303-287-3425
e-mail: info@hearingdog.org
www.pawsforsilence.org

Valerie Foss-Brugger, President
Robert Cooley, Field Representative
Andrea Paul, Vetinary Technician
Larry Norby, Accounting/HR

Trains and places Hearing dogs with deaf or hard-of-hearing persons, with or without multiple disabilities, nationwide, free of charge to the recipient.

7770 **International Hearing Society**
1688 Middlebelt Rd
Suite 4
Livonia, MI 48154-3374
734-522-7200
800-521-5247
FAX: 734-522-0200
e-mail: chelms@ihsinfo.org
ihsinfo.org

Kathleen Mennillo, Executive Director
Joy Wilkins, Director of Education
Fran Vincent, Marketing Manager
Alissa Parady, Manager of Government Affairs

The IHS is the professional association that represents Hearing Instrument Specialists worldwide. IHS members are engaged in the practice of testing human hearing and selecting, fitting and dispensing hearing instruments. Founded in 1951, the Society continues to recognize the need for promoting and maintaining the highest possible standards for its members in the best interestof the hearing impaired it serves.

7771 **League for the Hard of Hearing**
50 Broadway
6th Fl
New York, NY 10004-3810
917-305-7700
TTY:917-305-7999
www.lhh.org

Laurie Hanin, Executive Director
Ellen Pfeffer Lafargue, Au.D, Director
Dorene Watkins, Coordinator
Anita Stein-Meyers, Au.D, C, Assistant Director

The Center for Hearing and Communication is a leading hearing center offering state-of-the-art hearing testing, hearing aid fitting, speech therapy and full range of services for people of all ages with hearing loss. Visit our offices in New York City and Florida for services that meet all of your hearing and communication needs.

7772 **Lexington School for the Deaf: Center for the Deaf**
30th Avenue and 75th St
Jackson Heights, NY 11370
718-350-3300
FAX: 718-899-9846
TTY:718-350-3056
e-mail: generalinfo@lexnyc.org
www.lexnyc.org

Regina Carroll PhD, CEO/Executive Director
Philip W. Bravin, President
Gregory Hlibok, Vice President
Seth Bravin, Treasurer
Offers a comprehensive range of services to deaf, hard of hearing and speech impaired persons from infancy to elderly through its affiliate agencies: The Center for Mental Health Services; The Lexington Hearing and Speech Center, Lexington Vocational Services, and the Lexington School for the Deaf. The Lexington Center also provides services through its research division which houses the only federally funded Rehabilitation Engineering Center.

7773 **Michigan Association for Deaf and Hard of Hearing**
5236 Dumond Court
Suite C
Lansing, MI 48917-6001
517-487-0066
800-968-7327
FAX: 517-487-0202
e-mail: info@madhh.org
www.madhh.org

Nancy Asher, Executive Director
Pat Walton, Office Manager
MADHH is a statewide collaboration agency dedicated to improving the lives of people who are deaf or hard of hearing through leadership in education, advocacy and services.

7774 **National Association of Hearing Officials**
PO Box 4999
Midlothian, VA 23112-17
www.naho.org

Bonny M Fetch CALJ, President
The mission of the National Association of Hearing Officials is to improve the administrative hearing process and thereby benefit hearing officials, their employing agencies, and the individuals they serve through promoting professionalism and by providing trainінf, continuing education, a national forum for discussion of issues, and leadership concerning administrative harings.

7775 **National Association of Special Education Teachers**
1250 Connecticut Ave NW
Suite 200
Washington, DC 20036- 2643
202-296-7739
800-754-4421
FAX: 800-754-4421
e-mail: contactus@naset.org
www.naset.org

Dr Roger Pierangelo, Executive Director
Dr. George Giuliani, Executive Director
The mission of NASET is to render all possible support and assistanve to professionals who teach children with special needs.

7776 **National Association of the Deaf**
8630 Fenton Street
Suite 820
Silver Spring, MD 20910- 3819
301-587-1788
FAX: 301-587-1791
TTY:301-587-1789
e-mail: nadinfo@nad.org
www.nad.org

Howard A. Rosenblum, CEO
Shane H. Feldman, COO
Marc P. Charmatz, Staff Attorney
Lizzie Sorkin, Director of Communications
Nation's largest organization safeguarding the accessability and civil rights of 28 million deaf and hard of hearing Americans in education, employment, health care, and telecommunications. Focuses on grassroots advocacy and empowerment, captioned media deafness-related information and publications, legal assistance, and policy development.

7777 **National Black Association for Speech Language and Hearing**
700 McKnight Park Drive
Pittsburgh, PA 15237-1116
412-366-1177
FAX: 412-366-8804
e-mail: nbaslh@nbaslh.org
www.nbaslh.org

Arnell Brady, Exec Board Chair
Carolyn Mayo, PhD, Secretary
Linda McCabe Smith, PhD, Treasurer
Rachel M. Williams, PhD, Convention Chair
The mission of the National Black Association of Speech-Language and Hearing is to maintain a viable mechanism through which the needs of black professionals, students and individuals with communication disorders can be met.

7778 **National Black Deaf Advocates**
PO Box 32
Frankfort, KY 40602
585-475-2411
800-421-1220
FAX: 585-475-6500
e-mail: president@nbda.org
www.nbda.org

Benro Ogunyipe, President
Cory Parker, VP
Sharon.D White, Secretary
Betty Henderson, Treasurer
The Mission of the National Black Deaf Advocate is to promote the leadership development, economic and educational opportunities, social equality, and to safeguard the general health and welfare of Black deaf and hard of hearing people.

7779 **National Catholic Office of the Deaf**
7202 Buchanan St
Landover Hills, MD 20784-2299
301-577-1684
FAX: 301-577-1684
TTY:301-577-4184
e-mail: info@ncod.org
www.ncod.org

Consuelo Martinez Wild, Executive Director
Helps coordinate efforts of deaf or hard of hearing people who are involved in the ministry, acts as a resource center, assists bishops and pastors become available to the deaf and hard of hearing.

7780 **National Cued Speech Association**
1300 Pennsylvania Avenue, NW
Suite 190-713
Washington, DC 20004
301-915-8009
800-459-3529
e-mail: info@cuedspeech.org
www.cuedspeech.org

Amy Ruberl, Executive Director
Marah Baltzell, Executive Assistant
Shannon Howell, President
Champions effective communication, language development and literacy through the use of cued speech.

7781 **National Deaf Women's Bowling Association**
9244 E Mansfield Ave
Denver, CO 80237-1915
303-771-9018
e-mail: ndwbast@gmail.com
www.ndwba.com

Gayle Willingham, President
Ali Martinez, VP
Holds world Deaf Bowling Torunament annually in July. Also holds Las Vegas Scratch Classic annually in October.

7782 **National Hearing Conservation Association**
3030 W 81st Ave
Westminster, CO 80031 303-224-9022
FAX: 303-458-0002
e-mail: nhcaoffice@hearingconservation.org
www.hearingconservation.org

Jennifer Tufts, President
Beth Cooper, President Elect
Nancy Wojcik, Secretary/Treasurer
Cory Portnuff, Director of Communications

The mission of the NHCA is to prevent hearing loss due to noise and other environmental factors in all sectors of society.

7783 **National Student Speech Language Hearing Association**
2200 Research Blvd
Suite 450
Rockville, MD 20850-3289 301-296-5650
800-498-2071
FAX: 301-296-8580
TTY: 301-296-5650
e-mail: nsslha@asha.org
www.nsslha.org

Patricia A. Prelock, PhD, President
Elizabeth S. McCrea, President-Elect
Shelly S. Chabon, Immediate Past President
Donna Fisher Smiley, Vice President for Audiology Practice

The American Speech-Language-Hearing Association is committed to ensuring that all people with speech, language, and hearing disorders receive services to help them communicate effectively.

7784 **Registry of Interpreters for the Deaf**
333 Commerce St
Alexandria, VA 22314-2801 703-838-0030
FAX: 703-838-0454
TTY:7038380459
e-mail: ridinfo@rid.org
rid.org

Brenda Walke Prudhomme, President
Kelly L. Flores, VP
Dawn Whitcher, Secretary
Chris Grooms, Treasurer

The Registry of Interpreters for the Deaf, Inc. (RID), a national membership organization, plays a leading role in advocating for excellence in the delivery of interpretation and transliteration services between people who use sign language and people who use spoken language. In collaboration with the Deaf community, RID supports our members and encourages the growth of the profession through the establishment of a national standard for qualified sign language interpreters and transliterators, o

7785 **Spring Dell Center**
6040 Radio Station Rd
La Plata, MD 20646-3368 301-934-4561
FAX: 301-870-2439
e-mail: info@springdellcenter.org?subject=I'd like In
www.springdellcenter.org

Patsy Finch, President
Badgley CPA, Treasurer
Jean Hubbard, Secretary
Donna Rretzlaff, Executive Director

Since 1967, Spring Dell center has been, bridging the gap to enhance the lives of developmentally disabled people. Spring Dell's goal is to empower people in every aspect of their lives through the implementation of two programs, employment/vocational services and residential services including transportation. Spring Dell offers transportation door-to-door for persons with developmental disabilities, including day care programs, supportive environment, residential and any other transportation.

7786 **Starkey Hearing Foundation**
6700 Washington Ave S
Eden Prairie, MN 55344-3405 866-354-3254
FAX: 952-828-6900
e-mail: hearingfoundation@starkey.com
www.starkeyhearingfoundation.org

Peter Lecy, President
Brady Forseth, Executive Director
Steven Sawalich, Executive Director
Dr.Paul Nash, Vice President

Continues to provide over 50,000 hearing aids per year to people in the U.S. and all over the world.

7787 **Telecommunications for the Deaf and Hard of Hearing**
8630 Fenton St
Suite 121
Silver Spring, MD 20910-3803 301-563-9122
FAX: 301-589-3797
TTY:301-589-3006
e-mail: info@tdi-online.org
tdiforaccess.org

Claude L Stout, Executive Director
James House, Director of Public Relations
John Skjeveland, Business Manager

Promoting equal access to telecommunications and media for people who are deaf, late-deafened, hard of hearing or deaf-blind through consumer education and involvement; technical assistance and consulting; applications of exisiting and emerging technologies; networking and collaboration; uniformity of standards; and national policy development and advocacy.

7788 **The Davis Center**
19 State Route 10 E
Suite 25
Succasunna, NJ 07876 862-251-4637
FAX: 862-251-4642
e-mail: npdunn@thedaviscenter.com
www.thedaviscenter.com

Dorinne S Davis MA CCC-A FAAA, Director
Elizabeth Meade, Head Sound Therapist
Nancy Puckett-Dunn, Office Manager
Laura Darby, Part Time Sound Therapist

The Davis Center's Sound Therapy Programs make positive changes for children and adults with autism, ADD/ADHD, auditory processing issues, Dyslexia, learning disabilities, and other learning and wellness challenges. Our programs address issues such as phonics, spelling, writing, reading comprehension, hearing only parts of words, following directions, discriminating between sounds, sound sensitivity, behavioral responses, focus, attention, and more.

7789 **Vestibular Disorders Association**
5018 NE 15th Ave
Portland, OR 97213-305 503-229-7705
800-837-8428
FAX: 503-229-8064
e-mail: veda@vestibular.org
www.vestibular.org

Sue Hickey, President
Cynthia Ryan, MBA, Executive Director
Kerrie Denner, Outreach Coordinator
Karen Ilari, Administrative Support Coordinator

The mission of the Vestibular Disorders Association is to serve people with vestibular disorders by providing access to information, offering a support network, and elevating awareness of the challenges associated with these disorders.

Camps

7790 ASD Summer Camp
Alabama School for the Deaf
205 E South St
PO Box 698
Talladega, AL 35106 256-761-3260
FAX: 256-761-3278
e-mail: Pshaw@aidb.state.al.us
www.aidb.org
Pam Shaw, Camp Director
Carl Ponder, PhD, Principal
The Alabama School for the Deaf Summer Enrichment Camp is designed especially for deaf and hard of hearing children ages 6-15. Recreation activities include swimming, skating, outdoor games, horseback riding, field trips, arts and craft. Tuition is free.

7791 Aspen Camp School for the Deafearing
PO Box 1494
Aspen, CO 81612-1494 970-923-2511
FAX: 970-923-0643
e-mail: info@aspencamp.org
www.aspencamp.org
Lesa Thompson, Camp Director
DJ Monahan, Program Coordinator
Katie Murch, Outreach Coordinator
Chelsea Bridges, Advocacy Coordinator
Aspen Camp's mission is to enrich the lives of Deaf and Hard of Hearing individuals by providing experiential educational and recreational activities which increase self-esteem, confidence, and individual skills.

7792 Aspen Camp of the Deaf & Hard of Hearing
PO Box 1494
Aspen, CO 81612 970-923-2511
FAX: 970-923-0643
e-mail: info@aspencamp.org
www.aspencamp.org
Lesa Thompson, Camp Director
Aspen Camp's mission is to enrich the lives of Deaf and Hard of Hearing individuals by providing experiential educational and recreational activities which increase self-esteem, confidence, and individual skills.

7793 CHAMP Camp
1116 East Market St
Suite B-210
Indianapolis, IN 46202- 5629 317-679-1860
FAX: 317-245-2291
e-mail: admin@champcamp.org
www.champcamp.org
Dave Carter, Co-Camp Director/Founder
Jamie Mitchell, Co-Camp Director
Nancy McCurdy, Camp Consultant/Founder
Kristina Watkins, Program Coordinator
We are an ACA accredited camp.

7794 Camp Alexander Mack
Indiana Deaf Camps Foundation
P.O.Box 158
Milford, IN 46542 574-658-4831
www.campmack.org
Galen Jay, Interim Executive Director
Lauren Carrick, Director of Development/Facility Manager
Amber Barrett, Food Service
Norma Miller, Ordained Minister
Our program is intentionally designed to provide campers with life changing experiences that lead to a formation of personal faith within a safe faith community.

7795 Camp Bishopswood
Diocese of Maine Episcopal
143 State St
Portland, ME 04101 207-772-1953
800-244-6062
FAX: 207-773-0095
e-mail: mike@bishopswood.org
www.bishopswood.org
Laurie Kazilionis, President
Robert Johnston, VP
Jeff Mansir, Treasurer
Pam Waite, Secretary
Camp is located in Hope, Maine. One to seven-week sessions for hearing impaired children June-August. Coed, ages 7-16.

7796 Camp Capella
8 Pearl Point Road
Dedham, ME 04429 207-843-5104
e-mail: dana@campcabella.org
www.campcapella.org
Dana Mosher, Religious Leader
Provides an opportunity for children with disabilities to engage in various recreational and social experiences.

7797 Camp Chris Williams
Lions 11 B-2 and MADHH
5236 Dumond Court
Suite C
Lansing, MI 48917-6001 586-778-4188
FAX: 586-285-1842
TTY:586-285-1842
e-mail: info@madhh.org
www.madhh.org
Nancy Asher, Executive Director
An exciting summer camp experience for deaf and hard of hearing youth and their siblings ages 8-14.

7798 Camp Comeca & Retreat Center
United Methodist Church
75670 Road 417
Conzad, NE 69130 308-784-2808
e-mail: comeca@cozadtel.net
www.campcomeca.com
John, Asst. Director
Camp is located in Cozad, Nebraska. Summer sessions for campers with diabetes and hearing impairment. Coed, ages 6-19, families, seniors, single adults.

7799 Camp Emanuel
P.O. Box 752343
Dayton, OH 45475 937-477-5504
e-mail: crawford@campenamuel.org
www.campemanuel.org
Stephanie Ackner, President
Brian Demarke, Vice President
Nan Crawford, Executive Director
Mary Foreman, Secretary
Camp for hearing impaired and normal hearing youth.

7800 Camp Grizzly
NorCal Services For Deaf & Hard Of Hearing, Inc.
4708 Roseville Road
Suite 112
North Highlands, CA 95660-5172 916-349-7500
FAX: 916-349-7580
e-mail: info@nocalcenter.org
www.norcalcenter.org
Cheryl Bella, Chair
Sheri Farinah, CEO
Yim Orsi, Secretary
Andrew Metz, Treasurer
This camp is designed the deaf and hard of hearing youth or hearing youth with deaf or hard of hearing parent. The camp helps

with social interaction, building self esteem, leadership skills while enriching the lives of the deaf and hard of hearing.

7801 Camp Isola Bella On Twin Lakes,Salisbury, Ct.
American School for the Deaf
139 N Main St
West Hartford, CT 06107-1264
860-570-2300
FAX: 860-570-2301
TTY:860-570-2222
e-mail: Steve.Borsotti@asd-1817.org
www.asd-1817.org

Alyssa Pecorino, Director
Edward Peltier, Executive Director
Steve Borsotti, Reunion Chairperson
Jenilee Terry, Camp Registrar

Hearing-impaired children, ages 6-19, blend educational instruction in communications with recreational activities. Qualified deaf and hearing staff members with experience in education, child care and counseling are employed at the camp.

7802 Camp Joy
3325 Swamp Creek Rd
Schwenksville, PA 19473-1518
610-754-6878
FAX: 610-754-7880
e-mail: campjoy@fast.net
www.campjoy.com

Angus Murray, Camp Director

A special needs camp for kids and adults (ages 4-80+) with developmental disabilities such as: mental retardation, autism, brain injury, neurological disorder, visual and/or hearing impairments, Angelman and Down syndromes, and other developmental disabilities.

7803 Camp Juliena
Georgia Council for the Hearing Impaired
4151 Memorial Drive
Suite 103-B
Decatur, GA 30032
404-292-5312
800-541-0710
FAX: 404-299-3642
e-mail: campjuliena@gmail.com
www.gachi.org

Pat Ford, President
Jeanette Lorch, VP
Jimmy Peterson, Executive Director
Faithlyn Peart, Office Manager

A weeklong residential summer camp for youths and teens who are deaf or hard of hearing. Through challenging, team-oriented activities, campers form lasting friendships and acquire valuable leadership, social and communication skills.

7804 Camp Mark Seven
Mark Seven Deaf Foundation
144 Mohawk Hotel Rd
Old Forge, NY 13420
315-357-6089
FAX: 315-357-6403
e-mail: cm7campdirector@gmail.com
www.campmark7.org

Dave Staehle, Camp Director
Chris McQuaid, Office Manager
Kelly Lange, Foundation director
Jenn Legg, KODA Programs Director

Adirondack Mountain camp for hard-of-hearing, deaf and hearing people. Coed, ages 1-99, families, seniors and single adults.

7805 Camp Pacifica, Inc.
California Lions Camp
45895 California Hwy. 49
Ahwahnee, CA 93601
559-683-4660
FAX: 209-543-9418
e-mail: webmaster@camppacifica.org
www.camppacifica.org/

Ann Tognetti, President
Bob Ransom, Treasurer
Russ Custer, VP
Jill Loving, Secretary

Camp Pacifica is a camp for special needs children ages 7-15 years old. The camp offers outdoor recreational activities, along with promoting greater independence and self confidence among the children, and provides opportunities for social interaction, and further development of social skills.

7806 Camp Shocco for the Deaf
AL Baptist State Board of Missions
P.O. Box 6569
Talladega, AL 35161-886
256-761-1100
800-264-1225
FAX: 256-761-1270
e-mail: campshocco@albcdeaf.org
www.campshocco.org

Chad Fleming, Director
Matthew Dixon, Co-Director
Linnea Elliott, Assistant Director

Camp Shocco gives each child and teenager attending camp the opportunity to have an unforgettable one week of fun, games, and spiritual growth. Each camper also learns essence of teamwork, while developing their own unique abilities and talents that can often be overlooked.

7807 Camp Taloali
Lions Club of Oregon and Washington
15934 N Santiam Hwy
PO Box 32
Stayton, OR 97383-9619
971-239-8153
FAX: 503-769-6415
e-mail: camptaloali@comcast.net
www.taloali.org

George Scheler, Chair
Sylvia Hall, Vice Chair
Rolland Hart, Executive Director
Dave Taylor, Secretary

Camp Taholi is a magic world of challenge and excitement where campers learn new skills, goals, care, for the earth and share new experience with both old and new friends.

7808 Camp Tekoa UMC
Western NC Conference/United Methodist Church
211 Thomas Rd.
Hendersonville, NC 28739
828-692-6516
FAX: 828-696-3699
e-mail: director@camptekoa.org
www.camptekoa.org

James Johnson, Executive Director
John Isley, Asst. Director
Melisa Coates, Administrative Assistant
Karen Rohrer, Business Manager

Camping for children with asthma/respiratory ailments, hearing impairment and developmental disabilities. Coed, ages 6-17.

7809 Deaf Kid's Kamp
Sproul Ranch, Inc.
42263 50th Street West
Suite 610
Quartz Hill, CA 93536
661-675-3323
877-399-5449
e-mail: deafkidskamp@earthlink.net
www.deafkidskamp.com

Buffy Sproul, Executive Director

Our purpose is to meet the needs of deaf children outside of the classroom setting. These needs, as we have defined them, would include but are not limited to: social contact with peers; contact with the culture of the Deaf Community; educational and recreational programs not available in most school settings.

7810 Easter Seals Oklahoma
701 NorthEast 13th Street
Oklahoma City, OK 73104
405-239-2525
FAX: 405-239-2278
e-mail: sbusch@eastersealsoklahoma.org
www.eastersealsoklahoma.org

Rodney Burgamy, Chairman
David Adams, Board Member
Kristen Sorocco, Secretary
Jeb Reid, Treasurer

Adult day health center, and child development center.

7811 **Father Drumgoole Connelly Summer Camp**
MIV: Mount Loretto
6581 Hylan Blvd
Staten Island, NY 10309-3830 718-317-2600
FAX: 718-317-2830
www.mountloretto.org

Stephen Rynn, Executive Director
Maryann Virga, Executive Assistant
Loretta Polanish, Executive Secretary
Ed Gani, Facilities Manager
Summer sessions for children with epilepsy, hearing impairment and developmental disabilities. Coed, ages 5-13.

7812 **Lions Camp Crescendo, Inc.**
1480 Pine Tavern Road
P.O. Box 607
Lebanon Junction, KY 40150 502-833-3554
888-879-8884
FAX: 502-833-4427
e-mail: bjflannery@lions-campcrescendo.org
www.lions-campcrescendo.org

Major Wheat, Chairperson
Barbara Walker, Vice Chairperson
Billie J. Flannery, Administrator
Melinda Gilbert, Secretary
The enhancement of the quality of life for youth, especially those with disabilities, through the delivery of a traditional camp experience by caring individuals and to enable others to use our camping and retreat facilities to serve the larger communities humanitarian needs.

7813 **Lions Camp Kirby**
1735 Narrows Hill Rd
Upper Black Eddy, PA 18972-9712 610-982-5731
e-mail: info@lionscampkirby.org
www.lionscampkirby.org

Bob Hunsberger, President
Alice Breon, Camp Director
Offers 4-week camps for deaf and hearing impaired children and their siblings in eastern Pennsylvania.

7814 **Lions Camp Merrick**
Lions Clubs of District 22-C
P.O. Box 56
Nanjemoy, MD 20662 301-870-5858
FAX: 301-246-9108
e-mail: info@LionsCampMerrick.org
lionscampmerrick.org

Wayne Magoon, President
Ray Shumaker, Vice President
Julie Andrew, Board Member
Frank Culhane, Treasurer
This recreational camp for special needs children offers a complete waterfront program including swimming, canoeing and fishing for ages 6-16. Designed for children who are deaf and hard of hearing, children of deaf parents, and children with diabetes. Also helps children to learn to deal with their special conditions.

7815 **Lions Wilderness Camp for Deaf Children, Inc.**
Lions Clubs of California and Nevada
P.O.Box 195
Knightsen, CA 94548 877-896-1598
888-613-1557
e-mail: campdirector@lionswildcamp.org
www.lionswildcamp.org

Richard A. Wilmot, President
Rachel Mix, Camp Program Director
Robin L. Nichol, Camp Manager
Dana Johnson, Secretary
A camp experience where a deaf child age 7 to 15 can learn outdoor skills and enjoy the wonder and beauty of nature to the fullest extent.

7816 **Meadowood Springs Speech and Hearing Camp**
Oregon State Elks Association
P.O. Box 1025
Pendleton, OR 97801 541-276-2752
FAX: 541-276-7227
e-mail: info@meadowoodsprings.org
www.meadowoodsprings.org

Michael Ashton, Executive Director
Kathy Hosek, Administrative Assistant
Patti Hall, Camp Staff Manager
On 143 acres in the Blue Mountains of Eastern Oregon, this camp is designed to help young people who have diagnosed clinical disorders of speech, hearing or language. A full range of activities in recreational and clinical areas is available.

7817 **Ramah in the Poconos**
2618 Upper Woods Road
Suite 734
Lakewood, PA 18439-3725 570-798-2504
FAX: 570-798-2049
e-mail: info@ramahpoconos.org
www.ramahpoconos.org

Todd Zeff, Executive Director
Rabbi Joel Seltzer, Director
Bruce Lipton, Director of Finance & Operations
Deborah Jo Essrog, Development Director
Camp is located in Lake Como, Pennsylvania. Summer sessions for children and adults with hearing impairment. Coed, ages 10-16, families and seniors.

7818 **Sandcastle Day Camp**
Children's Beach House
1800 Bay Ave
Lewes, DE 19958 302-645-9184
FAX: 302-645-9467
e-mail: cterranova@cbhinc.org
www.cbhinc.org

Martha P. Tschantz, President
Maryann Helms, Vice President
Linda M. Fischer, Secretary
Charles H. Sterner, Treasurer
Camp is located in Lewes, Delaware. Four-week sessions June-August for Delaware children with hearing impairment or speech/communication impairment. Coed, ages 6-12.

7819 **Sertoma Camp Endeavor**
Sertoma Camp Endeavor
P.O.Box 910
Dundee, FL 33838-0910 863-439-1300
FAX: 863-439-1300
e-mail: info@sertomacampendeavor.com
www.sertomacampendeavor.org

Jeff Nunemaker, Executive Director
The intergration of deaf, hard of hearing and hearing youngsters is a unique characteristic of our camping program. Both hearing, deaf and hard of hearing children have the opportunity to learn about themselves and each other in an informal and empowering setting.

7820 **Texas Lions Camp**
Lions Club of Texas
P.O.Box 290247
Kerrville, TX 78029 830-896-8500
FAX: 830-896-3666
e-mail: smabry@lionscamp.com
www.lionscamp.com

Stephen Mabry, Executive Director
The primary purpose of the League shall be to provide, without charge, a camp for physically disabled, hearing/vision impaired and diabetic children from the State of Texas, regardless of race, religion, or national origin. Our goal is to create an atmosphere wherein campers will learn the can do philosophy and be allowed to achieve maximum personal growth and self-esteem. The camp welcomes boys and girls ages 7-16.

7821 YMCA Camp Fitch
The YMCA's Camp Fitch on Lake Erie
12600 Abels Rd
North Springfield, PA 16430-1014
814-922-3219
FAX: 814-922-7000
e-mail: info@campfitchymca.org
www.campfitch.com

Brian Rupe, Executive Director
Greg Donahue, Assistant Camp Director
Dann Olin, Operations Director
Barb Olin, Senior Program Director
Camp is located in North Springfield, Pennsylvania. Camping sessions for children and adults with diabetes, hearing impairment, developmental disabilities, mobility limitation and speech/communication impairment. Ages 8-16, families and seniors.

7822 YWCA Camp Westwind
YWCA of Greater Portland
1111 SW 10th Ave
Portland, OR 97205
503-294-7400
FAX: 503-721-1751
e-mail: connect@ywcapdx.org
http://www.ywcapdx.org

Susan Staoltenberg, Executive Director
Tracy Madsen, Development Director
Patricia Martin, Program Manager
Rebecca Alexander, Foundation & Corporate Relations Program Manager
Promotes the understanding of racism and all forms of discrimination and fosters value, respect, and enjoyment of each person's unique contribution.

7823 Youth Leadership Camp
National Association of the Deaf
8630 Fenton Street
Suite 820
Silver Spring, MD 20910
301-587-1788
FAX: 301-587-1791
e-mail: info@nad.org
www.nad.org

Christopher Wagnor, President
Melissa S. Draganac-Hawk, VP
Howard A. Rosenblum, CEO
Joshua Beckman, Secretary
Sponsored by the National Association of the Deaf, this camp emphasizes leadership training for deaf teenagers and young adults. In addition to many recreational activities and sports, there are academic offerings and camp projects.

Print: Books

7824 A Basic Course in American Sign Language
TJ Publishers
2544 Tarpley Rd
Suite 108
Carrollton, TX 75006-2288
972-416-0800
800-999-1168
FAX: 972-416-0944
e-mail: customerservice@tjpublishers.com
www.tjpublishers.com

Tom Humphries, Author
Carol Padden, Co-Author
Terrence J O'Rouke, Co-Author
Tanner Beach, Director
The first three DVDs in this series are designed to illustrate and demonstrate each of the exercises and dialogues presented in A Basic Course in American Sign Language. Four Deaf teachers and three hearing students provide a variety of models for the exercises. *$35.95*
288 pages Spiral Bound
ISBN 0-932666-42-6

7825 A Basic Course in Manual Communication
Gallaudet University Bookstore
800 Florida Ave NE
Washington, DC 20002-3600
202-651-5855
866-204-0504
FAX: 773-660-2235
TTY: 202-651-5855
e-mail: gupress@gallaudet.edu
www.clerccenter.gallaudet.edu

Terrence J O'Rourke, Author
T. Alan Hurwitz, President
Paul Kelly, Vice President Adm and Finance
Teach your students manual communication - that living, changing, growing language of signs.
161 pages Softcover

7826 A Basic Vocabulary: American Sign Languagefor Parents and Children
TJ Publishers
2544 Tarpley Rd
Suite 108
Carrollton, TX 75006-2288
972-416-0800
800-999-1168
FAX: 972-416-0944
e-mail: customerservice@tjpublishers.com
www.tjpublishers.com

Terrence J O'Rouke, Author
Tanner Beach, Director
Carefully selected words and signs include those that children use every day. Alphabetically organized vocabulary incorporates developmental lists helpful to both deaf and hearing children and over 1000 clear sign language illustrations. *$9.95*
240 pages Softcover
ISBN 0-932666-00-0

7827 A Handbook for Writing Effective Psychoeducational Reports
Sage Publications
2455 Teller Road
Thousand Oaks, CA 91320
800-818-7243
FAX: 800-583-2665
e-mail: info@sagepub.com
www.sagepub.com

Sara Miller McCune, Founder, Publisher, Chairperson
Blaise R -imqu, President & CEO
Tracey A. Ozmina, Executive Vice President & Chief Operating Officer
Stephen Barr, Managing Director
This book includes a comprehensive presentation of issues and procedures related to the assessment of hearing-impaired students. *$27.00*
134 pages Paperback
ISBN 1-416401-40-7

7828 A Loss for Words
HarperCollins Publishers
10 E 53rd St
New York, NY 10022-5244
212-207-7901
800-242-7737
FAX: 212-702-2586
e-mail: spsales@harpercollins.com
www.harpercollins.com

Lou Ann Walker, Author
From the time she was a toddler, Lou Ann Walker was the ears and voice for her deaf parents. Their family life was warm and loving, but outside the home, they faced a world that misunderstood and often rejected them. *$13.00*
224 pages Paperback 1987
ISBN 0-060914-25-4

7829 Access for All: Integrating Deaf, Hard of Hearing and Hearing Preschoolers

Gallaudet University Bookstore
800 Florida Avenue NorthEast
Washington, DC 20002-3600
202-651-5530
FAX: 202-651-5489
e-mail: gupress@gallaudet.edu
http://www.gallaudet.edu

Stephanie Cawthon, Ph.D., Book Review Editor
Peter V. Paul, Ph.D., Editor, Literary Issues
Ye Wang, Ph.D., Senior Associate Editor
Feifei Ye, Ph.D., Associate Editor for Research Methodology

This exciting new 90 minute videotape and manual describes a model program for integrating deaf and hard of hearing children in early education.

169 pages Book & Video

7830 Advanced Sign Language Vocabulary: A Resource Text for Educators

Charles C. Thomas
2600 South 1st Street
Springfield, IL 62704
217-789-8980
800-258-8980
FAX: 217-789-9130
e-mail: books@ccthomas.com
www.ccthomas.com

Michael P. Thomas, President
Elizabeth E Wolf, Co-Author

A resource text for educators, interpreters, parents and sign language instructors. *$53.95*

202 pages Spiral Paper
ISBN 0-398057-22-0

7831 American Sign Language Handshape Dictionary

Gallaudet University Press
800 Florida Ave NE
Washington, DC 20002-3600
773-568-1550
800-621-2736
FAX: 773-660-2235
TTY: 888-630-9347
e-mail: gupress@gallaudet.edu
www.gupress.gallaudet.edu

Richard A Tennant, Author
Marianne Gluszak Brown, Co-Author
Valerie Nelson-Metlay, Illustrator
T. Alan Hurwitz, President

The new DVD shows how each sign is formed from beginning to end. Users can watch a sign at various speeds to learn precisely how to master it themselves. Together, the new edition of The American Sign Language Handshape Dictionary and its accompanying DVD presents students, sign language teachers, and deaf and hearing people alike with the perfect combination for enhancing communication skills in both ASL and English. *$45.00*

408 pages Hardcover
ISBN 1-563680-43-2

7832 American Sign Language Phrase Book

TJ Publishers
2544 Tarpley Rd
Suite 108
Carrollton, TX 75006-2288
972-416-0800
800-999-1168
FAX: 972-416-0944
e-mail: customerservice@tjpublishers.com
www.tjpublishers.com

Lou Fant, Author
Terrence O'Rourke, Principal
Tanner Beach, Director

The author provides interesting, realistic and meaningful situations. Sign language is learned through novel remarks cleverly organized around everyday topics. *$18.95*

362 pages Softcover
ISBN 0-809235-00-5

7833 American Sign Language: A Look at Its History, Structure & Community

TJ Publishers
2544 Tarpley Rd
Suite 108
Carrollton, TX 75006-2288
972-416-0800
800-999-1168
FAX: 972-416-0944
e-mail: customerservice@tjpublishers.com
www.tjpublishers.com

Charlotte Baker-Shenk, Author
Carol Padden, Co-Author
Terrence O'Rourke, Principal
Tanner Beach, Director

Answers basic questions about American Sign Language. What is it? What is its history? Who uses it? What is the Deaf community? Why is ASL important? What are the building blocks of ASL? What is the relationship between ASL and body language? What are examples of ASL -grammar? *$4.95*

22 pages Softcover
ISBN 0-93266 -01-9

7834 At Home Among Strangers

Gallaudet University Press
800 Florida Ave NE
Washington, DC 20002-3600
773-568-1550
800-621-2736
FAX: 773-660-2235
TTY: 888-630-9347
e-mail: gupress@gallaudet.edu
www.gupress.gallaudet.edu

Jerome D Schein, Author
T. Alan Hurwitz, President
Paul Kelly, Vice President Adm And Finance

At Home Among Strangers presents an engrossing portrait of the Deaf community as a complex, nationwide social network that offers unique kinship to deaf people across the country. *$36.95*

264 pages Paperback
ISBN 1-563681-41-2

7835 BPPV: What You Need to Know

Vestibular Disorders Association
5018 NE 15th Ave
Portland, OR 97211-5331
503-229-7705
800-837-8428
FAX: 503-229-8064
e-mail: veda@vestibular.org
www.vestibular.org

P J Haybach, Author
Lisa Haven, Executive Director
Jerry Underwood, Managing Director
Vincente Honrubia, Director

The aim of this book is to present basic information about benign paroxysmal positional vertigo (BPPV) including what it is, causes, how it is diagnosed, various treatments currently in use, and strategies for coping with the symptoms associated with BPPV. *$29.95*

207 pages Hardcover
ISBN 0-963261-14-2

7836 Ben's Story: A Deaf Child's Right to Sign

Gallaudet University Bookstore
800 Florida Avenue NorthEast
Washington, DC 20002-3600
202-651-5530
FAX: 202-651-5489
e-mail: gupress@gallaudet.edu
http://www.gallaudet.edu

Stephanie Cawthon, Ph.D., Book Review Editor
Peter V. Paul, Ph.D., Editor, Literary Issues
Ye Wang, Ph.D., Senior Associate Editor
Feifei Ye, Ph.D., Associate Editor for Research Methodology

This is a mother's story of how she responded to the diagnosis of her son's deafness and how she struggled to have her son educated using sign language.

267 pages Softcover
ISBN 0-930323-47-5

7837 Book of Name Signs: Naming in American Sign Language
DawnSign Press
6130 Nancy Ridge Dr
San Diego, CA 92121-3223
858-625-0600
800-549-5350
FAX: 858-625-2336
e-mail: info@dawnsign.com
www.dawnsign.com
Joe Dannis, President
Sam Supalla, Author

To explain how a name sign is chosen in the Deaf community, professor and researcher Sam Supalla wrote this valuable resource book. Revealing fascinating insights about the origins of ASL name signs, Supalla shows how they serve the same function as given names used in the hearing community. He also details how the history of the name sign system dates back to the early years of deaf education in America. Included for reference is a list of more than 500 name signs available for selection. *$12.95*

120 pages Paperback 1992
ISBN 0-915035-30-4

7838 Chelsea: The Story of a Signal Dog
Gallaudet University Bookstore
800 Florida Ave NE
Washington, DC 20002-3600
202-651-5855
866-204-0504
FAX: 773-660-2235
TTY: 202-651-5855
e-mail: gupress@gallaudet.edu
www.clerccenter.gallaudet.edu
Paul Ogden, Author
T. Alan Hurwitz, President
Paul Kelly, Vice President Adm. And Finance

This is a story of a young deaf couple and their Belgian sheepdog, who acts as their ears. It explains how these dogs are trained and paired with their new owners.

169 pages

7839 Children of a Lesser God
Gallaudet University Bookstore
800 Florida Ave NE
Washington, DC 20002-3600
202-651-5855
866-204-0504
FAX: 773-660-2235
TTY: 202-651-5855
e-mail: gupress@gallaudet.edu
www.clerccenter.gallaudet.edu
Mark Medoff, Author
T. Alan Hurwitz, President
Paul Kelly, Vice President Adm. And Finance

The movie that won the hearts of thousands. This is a story of a deaf woman who refuses to succumb to the hearing people's image of what a deaf person should be.

91 pages Softcover
ISBN 0-822202-03-4

7840 Choices in Deafness: A Parent's Guide to Communication Options
Woodbine House
6510 Bells Mill Rd
Bethesda, MD 20817-1636
301-897-3570
800-843-7323
FAX: 301-897-5838
e-mail: info@woodbinehouse.com
www.woodbinehouse.com
Irv Shapell, Owner
Sue Schwartz, PhD., Editor

A useful aid in choosing the appropriate communication option for a child with a hearing loss. Experts present the following communication options: Auditory-Verbal Approach, Bilingual-Bicultural Approach, Cued Speech, Oral Approach, and Total Communication. This new edition explains medical causes of hearing loss, the diagnostic process, audiological assessment, and cochlear implants. Children and parents also offer their personal experiences. *$24.95*

400 pages Paperback
ISBN 1-890627-73-7

7841 Cochlear Implants for Kids
Alexander Graham Bell Association
3417 Volta Pl NW
Washington, DC 20007-2737
202-337-5220
FAX: 202-337-8314
e-mail: info@agbell.org
www.listeningandspokenlanguage.org
Warren Estabrooks MEd, Editor
Alexander T. Graham, Executive Director
Susan Boswell, Director of Communications and Marketing
Judy Harrison, Director of Programs

Designed to educate readers about cochlear implants, including surgery, the importance of rehabilitation and the significance of parents' and professionals' roles. *$12.49*

404 pages Paperback
ISBN 0-882002-08-2

7842 Cognition, Education and Deafness: Directions for Research and Instruction
Gallaudet University Press
800 Florida Ave NE
Washington, DC 20002-3600
773-568-1550
800-621-2736
FAX: 773-660-2235
TTY: 888-630-9347
e-mail: gupress@gallaudet.edu
www.gupress.galladuet.edu
David S Martin, Editor
T. Alan Hurwitz, President
Paul Kelly, Vice President Adm. And Finance

This groundbreaking book integrates the work of 54 contributors to the 1984 symposium on cognition, education, and deafness. It focuses on cognition and deaf students' growth and development, problem-solving strategies, thinking processes, language development, reading methodology, measurement of potential, and intervention programs. *$50.00*

248 pages Paperback
ISBN 1-563681-49-8

7843 College and University Programs for Deaf and Hard of Hearing Students
Gallaudet & NTID
800 Florida Avenue NE
Gallaudet University
Washington, DC 20002
202-651-5000
800-451-8834
FAX: 202-651-5508
www.lulu.com
S. Benaissa, & L. Dunning, Co-Authors
J. DeCaro, M. Karchmer, Co-Authors
J Hochgesang, Co-Author
T. Alan Hurwitz, President

Compiled by Gallaudet University and the National Technical Institute for the Deaf, this publication is a guide to accessibility for deaf and hard of hearing students in American colleges and universities. Available through LuLu Publishing. *$11.50*

240 pages Paperback
ISBN 9-998242-81-9

7844 Come Sign with Us
Gallaudet University Press
800 Florida Ave NE
Washington, DC 20002-3600
773-568-1550
800-621-2736
FAX: 773-660-2235
TTY: 888-630-9347
e-mail: gupress@gallaudet.edu
www.gupress.gallaudet.edu
Jan C Hafer, Author
Robert M Wilson, Co-Author
T. Alan Hurwitz, President
Paul Kelly, Vice President Adm. And Finance

This fun guide for parents and educators on teaching hearing children how to sign has been thoroughly revised with completely new activities that provide contexts for practice. *$39.95*

160 pages Paperback
ISBN 1-563680-51-3

7845 Comprehensive Reference Manual for Signers and Interpreters

Charles C. Thomas
2600 S 1st St
Springfield, IL 62704-4730
217-789-8980
800-258-8980
FAX: 217-789-9130
e-mail: books@ccthomas.com
www.ccthomas.com

Michael P. Thomas, President
Cheryl M. Hoffman, Author

A classic in sign language literature since its introduction over two decades ago, this updated and expanded sixth edition of Comprehensive Reference Manual for Signers and Interpreters contains almost seven thousand entries, including vocabulary and idioms, with cross-references and sign descriptions. It is intended primarily for interpreters, but it can also be used effectively by signers who have at least a working knowledge of sign language. *$59.95*

404 pages Spiral Paper 1909
ISBN 0-398078-58-4

7846 Comprehensive Signed English Dictionary

Gallaudet University Press
800 Florida Ave NE
Washington, DC 20002-3600
773-568-1550
800-621-2736
FAX: 773-660-2235
TTY: 888-630-9347
e-mail: gupress@gallaudet.edu
www.gupress.gallaudet.edu

Harry Bornstein, Editor
Karen L. Saulnier, Editor
Lillian B. Hamilton, Editor
T. Paul Hurwitz, President

The Comprehensive Signed English Dictionary is the premier volume of the Signed English series. This complete dictionary more than 3,100 signs, including signs reflecting lively, contemporary vocabulary. *$45.00*

464 pages Casebound
ISBN 0-913580-81-3

7847 Conversational Sign Language II: An Intermediate Advanced Manual

Gallaudet University Press
800 Florida Ave NE
Washington, DC 20002-3600
773-568-1550
800-621-2736
FAX: 773-660-2235
TTY: 888-630-9347
e-mail: gupress@gallaudet.edu
www.gupress.gallaudet.edu

William J Madsen, Author
T. Alan Hurwitz, President
Paul Kelly, Vice President Adm. And Finance

This book presents English words and their American Sign Language (ASL) equivalents in 63 lessons. Part one covers 750 words and their signs. Part two deals with the interpretation of 220 English idioms (which have over 300 usages in ASL). Part three presents over 300 ASL idioms and colloquialisms prevalent in informal conversations. *$17.95*

236 pages Paperback
ISBN 0-913580-00-7

7848 Deaf Empowerment: Emergence, Struggle and Rhetoric

Gallaudet University Press
800 Florida Ave NE
Washington, DC 20002-3600
773-568-1550
800-621-2736
FAX: 773-660-2235
TTY: 888-630-9347
e-mail: gupress@gallaudet.edu
www.gupress.gallaudet.edu

Katherine A Jankowski, Author
T. Alan Hurwitz, President
Paul Kelly, Vice President Adm. And Finance

Employing the methodology successfully used to explore other social movements in America, this meticulous study examines the rhetorical foundation that motivated Deaf people to work for social change during the past two centuries. *$49.95*

192 pages Hardcover
ISBN 1-563680-61-0

7849 Deaf History Unveiled: Interpretations from the New Scholarship

Gallaudet University Press
800 Florida Ave NE
Washington, DC 20002-3600
773-568-1550
800-621-2736
FAX: 773-660-2235
TTY: 888-630-9347
e-mail: gupress@gallaudet.edu
www.gallaudet.edu

John Vickrey Van Cleve, Editor
T. Alan Hurwitz, President
Paul Kelly, Vice President Adm. And Finance

Deaf History Unveiled features 16 essays, including work by Harlan Lane, Renate Fischer, Margret Winzer, William McCagg, and other noted historians in this field. Readers will discover the new themes driving Deaf history, including a telling comparison of the similar experiences of Deaf people and African Americans, both minorities with identifying characteristics that cannot be hidden to thwart bias. *$ 36.95*

316 pages Paperback
ISBN 1-563680-87-4

7850 Deaf Like Me

Gallaudet University Press
800 Florida Ave NE
Washington, DC 20002-3600
773-568-1550
800-621-2736
FAX: 773-660-2235
TTY: 888-630-9347
e-mail: gupress@gallaudet.edu
www.gupress.gallaudet.edu

Thomas S Spradley, Author
James P Spradley, Co-Author
T. Alan Hurwitz, President
Paul Kelly, Vice President Adm. And Finance

Deaf Like Me is the moving account of parents coming to terms with their baby girl's profound deafness. The love, hope, and anxieties of all hearing parents of deaf children are expressed here with power and simplicity. *$16.95*

292 pages Paperback
ISBN 0-930323-11-4

7851 Deaf Parents and Their Hearing Children

Through the Looking Glass
3075 Adeline Street
Suite 120
Berkeley, CA 94703
510-848-1112
800-644-2666
FAX: 510-848-4445
e-mail: tlg@lookingglass.org
www.lookingglass.org

Maureen Block, J.D., President
Thomas Spalding, Treasurer
Alice Nemon, Secretary
Mega Kirshbaum, Author

The focus of this review article is on families with Deaf parents and hearing children. We provide a brief description of the Deaf community, their language, and culture; describe communication patterns and parenting issues in Deaf-parented families, examine the role of the hearing child in a Deaf family and how that experience affects their functioning in the hearing world; and discuss important considerations and resources for families, educators, and health care and service providers. *$2.00*

8 pages

7852 Deaf in America: Voices from a Culture
TJ Publishers
2544 Tarpley Rd
Suite 108
Carrollton, TX 75006-2288
972-416-0800
800-999-1168
FAX: 972-416-0944
e-mail: customerservice@tjpublishers.com
www.tjpublishers.com

Carol Padden, Author
Tom Humphries, Co-Author
Terrence O'Rourke, Principal
Tanner Beach, Director
Now available in paperback, this book opens deaf culture to outsiders, inviting readers to imagine and understand a world of silence. This book shares the joy and satisfaction many people have with their lives and shows that deafness may not be the handicap most hearing people think. *$15.95*
134 pages Softcover
ISBN 0-674194-24-1

7853 EASE Program: Emergency Access Self Evaluation
Telecommunications for the Deaf (TDI)
8630 Fenton St
Suite 604
Silver Spring, MD 20910-3822
301-589-3786
FAX: 301-589-3797
e-mail: info@tdi-online.org
tdi-online.org

Claude L Stout, Executive Director
Gloria Carter, Executive Secretary
James House, Public Relations Director
Robert McConnell, Advertising Manager
A complete training, testing, maintenance and self evaluation program that helps emergency service providers prepare for emergency calls from TTY users and to comply with the American with Disabilities Act. *$35.00*
48 pages

7854 Encyclopedia of Deafness and Hearing Disorders
Powell's Books
1005 W Burnside St
Portland, OR 97209-3114
503-228-4651
800-873-7323
e-mail: help@powells.com
www.powells.com

Carol Turkington, Author
Michael Powell, Owner
Presents the most current information on deafness and hearing disorders in an authoritative A-to-Z compendium. *$7.50*
294 pages Hardcover
ISBN 0-816056-15-3

7855 Expressive and Receptive Fingerspelling for Hearing Adults
Gallaudet University Bookstore
800 Florida Ave NE
Washington, DC 20002-3600
202-651-5855
866-204-0504
FAX: 773-660-2235
TTY: 202-651-5855
e-mail: gupress@gallaudet.edu
www.clerccenter.gallaudet.edu
LaVera M Guillory, Author
T. Alan Hurwitz, President
Paul Kelly, Vice President Adm. And Finance
Here is a new and meaningful way for adults to increase their comfort with fingerspelling. The system is based on the principles of phonetics rather than letters of the English alphabet.
42 pages Softcover
ISBN 0-875110-55-X

7856 Eye-Centered: A Study of Spirituality of Deaf People
National Catholic Office for the Deaf
7202 Buchanan St
Hyattsville, MD 20784-2236
301-577-1684
FAX: 301-577-1684
e-mail: info@ncod.org
www.ncod.org

Bill Key, Author
Arvilla Rank, Executive Director
Deacon Patrick Graybill, Vice President
Gregory Schott, Member at Large
The findings of the five-year De Sales Project conducted by The National Catholic Office for the Deaf. *$16.70*
167 pages

7857 For Hearing People Only
Harris Communications
15155 Technology Dr
Eden Prairie, MN 55344-2273
952-388-2152
800-825-6758
FAX: 952-906-1099
TTY: 800-825-9187
e-mail: info@harriscomm.com
www.harriscomm.com

Robert Harris, Owner
Linda Levitan, Co-Author
Matthew S. Moore, Co-Author
Harlan Lane, Foreword
For Hearing People Only answers some of the most common questions hearing people ask about Deaf culture and how Deaf people communicate and live. *$35.95*
724 pages Paperback
ISBN 0-963401-63-7

7858 From Gesture to Language in Hearing and Deaf Children
Gallaudet University Press
800 Florida Ave NE
Washington, DC 20002-3600
773-568-1550
800-621-2736
FAX: 773-660-2235
TTY: 888-630-9347
e-mail: gupress@gallaudet.edu
www.gupress.gallaudet.edu

Virginia Volterra, Editor
Carol J. Erting, Editor
In 21 essays on communicative gesturing in the first two years of life, this vital collection demonstrates the importance of gesture in a child's transition to a linguistic system. *$45.95*
358 pages Paperback
ISBN 1-563680-78-5

7859 From Mime to Sign Package
TJ Publishers
2544 Tarpley Rd
Suite 108
Carrollton, TX 75006-2288
972-416-0800
800-999-1168
FAX: 972-416-0944
e-mail: customerservice@tjpublishers.com
www.tjpublishers.com
Gilbert C Eastman, Author
Terrence O'Rourke, Principal
Tanner Beach, Director
More than 1,000 photographs illustrate how natural gestures, mime and facial expressions used every day can become the basis for learning sign language. *$27.95*
183 pages Softcover
ISBN 0-932666-34-5

7860 **GA and SK Etiquette**
Telecommunications for the Deaf
8630 Fenton Street
Suite 604
Silver Spring, MD 20910- 3822
301-589-3786
FAX: 301-589-3797
e-mail: info@tdi-online.org
www.tdi-online.org

Claude L Stout, Executive Director
Keith Cagle, Co-Author
Roy Miller, President
Gloria Carter, Administrator
Promoting equal access to telecommunications and media for people who are deaf, late-deafened, hard-of-hearing or deaf-blind through consumer education and involvement; technical assistance and consulting; applications of exisiting and emerging technologies; networking and collaboration; uniformity of standards; and national policy development and advocacy. *$11.95*
54 pages Paperback
ISBN 0-961462-17-5

7861 **Gallaudet Survival Guide to Signing**
Gallaudet University Press
800 Florida Ave NE
Washington, DC 20002-3600
773-568-1550
800-621-2736
FAX: 773-660-2235
TTY: 888-630-9347
e-mail: gupress@gallaudet.edu
www.gallaudet.edu

Jon Mitchiner, Manager
Leonard G. Lane, Author
Jan Skrobisz, Illustrator
T. Alan Hurwitz, President
Features 500 of the most frequently used signs with clear illustrations and descriptions for each one. *$9.95*
218 pages Paperback
ISBN 0-930323-67-X

7862 **Goldilocks and the Three Bears: Told in Signed English**
Gallaudet University Press
800 Florida Ave NE
Washington, DC 20002-3600
773-568-1550
800-621-2736
FAX: 773-660-2235
TTY: 888-630-9347
e-mail: gupress@gallaudet.edu
www.gupress.gallaudet.edu
Harry Bornstein, Author
Karen L Saulnier, Co-Author
T. Alan Hurwitz, President
Paul Kelly, Vice President Adm. And Finance
Goldilocks and the Three Bears offers children ages 3 - 8 all of the fun their parents had when they first read about the little girl with the golden curls who turned the Bears' house upside down. *$ 21.95*
48 pages Hardcover
ISBN 1-563680-57-2

7863 **Hearing Impaired Children and Youth with Developmental Disabilities**
Gallaudet University Bookstore
800 Florida Ave NE
Washington, DC 20002-3600
202-651-5855
866-204-0504
FAX: 773-660-2235
TTY: 202-651-5855
e-mail: gupress@gallaudet.edu
www.clerccenter.gallaudet.edu
Evelyn Cherow, Editor
T. Alan Hurwitz, President
Paul Kelly, Vice President Adm. And Finance
The insights of 24 experts help clarify relationships between hearing impairment and developmental difficulties and propose interdisciplinary cooperation as an approach to the problems created. *$29.95*
394 pages Hardcover
ISBN 0-913580-97-X

7864 **Hollywood Speaks: Deafness and the Film Entertainment Industry**
University of Illinois Press
1325 S Oak St
MC-566
Champaign, IL 61820-6903
217-333-0950
FAX: 217-244-8082
e-mail: uipress@uillinois.edu
www.press.uillinois.edu

Willis G. Regier, Director
John S. Schuchman, Author
Kathy O'Neill, Assistant To The Director
Laurie Matheson, Editor-in-Chief
How deafness has been treated in movies and how it provides yet another window onto social history in addition to a fresh angle from which to view Hollywood. *$27.00*
200 pages Paperback 1999
ISBN 0-252068-50-8

7865 **I Have a Sister, My Sister is Deaf**
HarperCollins Publishers
10 E 53rd St
New York, NY 10022-5244
212-207-7901
800-242-7737
FAX: 212-702-2586
e-mail: spsales@harpercollins.com
www.harpercollins.com
Jeanne Whitehouse Peterson, Author
Deborah Kogan Ray, Illustrator
Ann Ledden, Vice President
Lorna Metzler, Manager
An emphatic, affirmative look at the relationship between siblings, as a young deaf child is affectionately described by her older sister. This Coretta Scott King Honor Award winner helps young children develop an understanding that deaf children share the same interests as hearing children. *$6.99*
32 pages Paperback 1984
ISBN 0-064430-59-6

7866 **Independence Without Sight or Sound**
AFB Press
2 Penn Plaza
Suite 1102
New York, NY 10121-2006
212-502-7600
800-232-5463
FAX: 888-545-8331
e-mail: afbweb@afb.net
www.afb.org

Richard Obnen, Chairman Of The Board
Carl Augusto, President and CEO
Rick Bozeman, Chief Financial Officer
Kelly Bleach, Chief Administrative Officer
This practical guidebook covers the essential aspects of communicating and working with deaf-blind persons. Full of valuable information on subjects such as how to talk with deaf-blind people, adapt orientation and mobility techniques for deaf-blind travelers, and interact with deaf-blind individuals socially, this useful manual also contains a substantial resource section detailing sources of information and adapted equipment. *$39.95*
193 pages Paperback
ISBN 0-891282-46-4

7867 **Innovative Practices for Teaching Sign Language Interpreters**
Gallaudet University Press
800 Florida Ave NE
Washington, DC 20002-3600
773-568-1550
800-621-2736
FAX: 773-660-2235
TTY: 888-630-9347
e-mail: gupress@gallaudet.edu
www.gupress.gallaudet.edu

Cynthia B Roy, Editor
Researchers now understand interpreting as an active process between two languages and cultures, with social interaction, sociolinguistics, and discourse analysis as more appropriate theoretical frameworks. Roy's penetrating new book acts upon these new insights by presenting six dynamic teaching practices to help interpreters achieve the highest level of skill. *$45.95*
200 pages Hardcover
ISBN 1-563680-88-2

7868 **Intermediate Conversational Sign Language**
Gallaudet University Press
800 Florida Ave NE
Washington, DC 20002-3600
773-568-1550
800-621-2736
FAX: 773-660-2235
TTY: 888-630-9347
e-mail: gupress@gallaudet.edu
www.gupress.gallaudet.edu

Willard J Madsen, Author
This fully illustrated text offers a unique approach to using American Sign Language (ASL) and English in a bilingual setting. Each of the 25 lessons involve sign language conversation using colloquialisms that are prevalent in informal conversations. *$31.50*
400 pages Softcover
ISBN 0-913580-79-1

7869 **Interpretation: A Sociolinguistic Model**
Sign Media
4020 Blackburn Ln
Burtonsville, MD 20866-1167
301-421-0268
800-475-4756
FAX: 301-421-0270
e-mail: info@signmedia.com
www.signmedia.com

Verden Ness, President
Dennis Cokely, Author
This text presents a sociolinguistically sensitive model of the interpretation process. The model applies to interpretation in any two languages although this one focuses on ASL and English. *$22.95*
199 pages
ISBN 0-932130-10-0

7870 **Interpreting: An Introduction**
Registry of Interpreters for the Deaf
333 Commerce St
Alexandria, VA 22314-2801
703-838-0030
FAX: 703-838-0454
TTY:703-838-0459
e-mail: ridinfo@rid.org
www.rid.org

Nancy J Frishberg, Author
Shane Feldman, Executive Director
Don Roose, Director
Emil Ladner, Director
This text is written by a practicing interpreter and includes information on history, terminology, research, competence, setting and a comprehensive bibliography. *$24.95*
249 pages Softcover
ISBN 0-916883-07-8

7871 **Joy of Signing**
Gospel Publishing House
1445 N Boonville Ave
Springfield, MO 65802-1894
417-862-8000
800-641-4310
FAX: 417-862-5881
e-mail: CustSrvOrders@ag.org
www.gospelpublishing.com

Lottie L Riekehof, Author
This manual on signing includes illustrations, information on sign origins, practice sentences, and step-by-step descriptions of hand positions and movements. *$23.99*
352 pages Hardcover
ISBN 0-882435-20-5

7872 **Joy of Signing Puzzle Book**
Harris Communications
15155 Technology Dr
Eden Prairie, MN 55344-2273
952-388-2152
800-825-6758
FAX: 952-906-1099
TTY: 800-825-9187
e-mail: info@harriscomm.com
www.harriscomm.com

Robert Harris, Owner
Lottie L Riekehof, Co-Author
Whether you are learning sign language to communicate with a family member, co-worker, student or friend, this puzzle book makes the learning fun and interesting. *$4.50*
57 pages Softcover
ISBN 0-882436-76-7

7873 **Kid-Friendly Parenting with Deaf and Hard of Hearing Children**
Gallaudet University Press
800 Florida Ave NE
Washington, DC 20002-3600
773-568-1550
800-621-2736
FAX: 773-660-2235
TTY: 888-630-9347
e-mail: gupress@gallaudet.edu
www.gupress.gallaudet.edu

Daria Medwid, Author
Denise Chapman Weston, Co-Author
At each chapter's beginning, experts (some deaf, some hearing), including I. King Jordan, Jack Gannon, Merv Garretson, and others, offer their insights on the subject discussed. Designed for parents with various styles, Kid-Friendly Parenting is a complete, step-by-step guide and reference to raising a deaf or hard of hearing child. *$35.95*
320 pages Paperback
ISBN 1-563680-31-9

7874 **Laurent Clerc: The Story of His Early Years**
Gallaudet University Press
800 Florida Ave NE
Washington, DC 20002-3600
773-568-1550
800-621-2736
FAX: 773-660-2235
TTY: 888-630-9347
e-mail: gupress@gallaudet.edu
www.gupress.gallaudet.edu

Cathryn Carroll, Author
T. Alan Hurwitz, President
Paul Kelly, Vice President Adm. And Finance
In his own voice, Clerc vividly relates the experiences that led to his later progressive teaching methods. Especially influential was his long stay at the Royal National Institute for the Deaf in Paris, where he encountered sharply distinct personalities - the saintly, inspiring deaf teacher Massieu, the vicious Dr. Itard and his heartless experiments on deaf boys, and the Father of the Deaf, Abbe Sicard, who could hardly sign. *$13.95*
208 pages Paperback
ISBN 0-930323-23-8

7875 Linguistics of American Sign Language: An Introduction
Gallaudet University Press
800 Florida Ave NE
Washington, DC 20002-3600
773-568-1550
800-621-2736
FAX: 773-660-2235
TTY: 888-630-9347
e-mail: gupress@gallaudet.edu
www.gupress.gallaudet.edu

Clayton Valli, Author
Ceil Lucas, Co-Author
Kristin J Mulrooney, Co-Author
Miako Villanueva, President
Completely reorganized to reflect the growing intricacy of the study of ASL linguistics, the 5th edition presents 26 units in seven parts. Part One: Introduction presents a revision of Defining Language and an entirely new unit, Defining Linguistics. Part Two: Phonology has been completely updated with new terminology and examples. *$75.00*
560 pages Hardcover
ISBN 1-563682-83-4

7876 Literacy & Your Deaf Child: What Every Parent Should Know
Gallaudet University Press
800 Florida Ave NE
Washington, DC 20002-3600
773-568-1550
800-621-2736
FAX: 773-660-2235
TTY: 888-630-9347
e-mail: gupress@gallaudet.edu
www.gupress.gallaudet.edu
David A Stewart, Author
Bryan R Clarke, Co-Author
T. Alan Hurwitz, President
Paul Kelly, Vice President Adm. And Finance
Literacy and Your Deaf Child begins by introducing some common concepts, among them the importance of parental involvement in a deaf child's education. It outlines how children acquire language and describes the auditory and visual links to literacy.
$24.95
240 pages Paperback
ISBN 1-563681-36-6

7877 Mother Father Deaf: Living Between Sound and Silence
Harvard University Press
79 Garden St
Cambridge, MA 02138-1423
617-495-2600
800-405-1619
FAX: 617- 49- 589
e-mail: contact_hup@harvard.edu
www.hup.harvard.edu
William Sisler, President
Paul Preston, Author
The book explores the intimate intersection of families like his own - families which embody the conflicts and resolutions of two often opposing world views, the Deaf and the Hearing. Although I have normal hearing, both of my parents are profoundly deaf.
$19.50
278 pages Paperback
ISBN 0-674587-48-0

7878 My First Book of Sign
Gallaudet University Press
800 Florida Ave NE
Washington, DC 20002-3600
773-568-1550
800-621-2736
FAX: 773-660-2235
TTY: 888-630-9347
e-mail: gupress@gallaudet.edu
www.gupress.gallaudet.edu

Pamela J Baker, Author
Patricia Bellan Gillen, Illustrator
T. Alan Hurwitz, President
Paul Kelly, Vice President Adm. And Finance
Full-color book gives alphabetically grouped signs for 150 words most frequently used by young children. *$22.95*
80 pages Hardcover
ISBN 0-930323-20-3

7879 My Signing Book of Numbers
Gallaudet University Press
800 Florida Ave NE
Washington, DC 20002-3600
773-568-1550
800-621-2736
FAX: 773-660-2235
TTY: 888-630-9347
e-mail: gupress@gallaudet.edu
www.gupress.gallaudet.edu
Patricia Bellan Gillen, Author
This full-color book helps children learn their numbers in sign language. Each two-page spread of this delightfully illustrated book has the appropriate number of things or creatures for the numbers 0 through 20. *$22.95*
56 pages Hardcover
ISBN 0-930323-37-8

7880 Nursery Rhymes from Mother Goose
Gallaudet University Press
800 Florida Ave NE
Washington, DC 20002-3600
773-568-1550
800-621-2736
FAX: 773-660-2235
TTY: 888-630-9347
e-mail: gupress@gallaudet.edu
www.gupress.gallaudet.edu

Harry Bornstein, Author
Karen L Saulnier, Co-Author
Patricia Peters, Illustrator
Linda Tom, Illustrator
Young readers, both hearing and deaf, will learn the special charm of rhyme while also discovering new vocabulary and new ways to experience English through signing. As they learn and memorize their favorite verses, children will also strengthen their language skills in a fun, entertaining way. *$21.95*
64 pages Hardcover
ISBN 0-930323-99-8

7881 Outsiders in a Hearing World: A Sociology of Deafness
Sage Publications
2455 Teller Rd
Thousand Oaks, CA 91320-2218
805-499-9774
800-818-7243
FAX: 805-499-0871
www.sagepub.com
Paul C Higgins, Author
An introduction to the social world of deaf people. The author gives a sociologists view of what it's like to be deaf. *$72.95*
208 pages Hardcover 1980
ISBN 0-803914-22-3

7882 Perigee Visual Dictionary of Signing
Harris Communications
15155 Technology Dr
Eden Prairie, MN 55344-2273
952-388-2152
800-825-6758
FAX: 952-906-1099
TTY: 800-825-9187
e-mail: info@harriscomm.com
www.harriscomm.com

Robert Harris, Owner
Mickey Flodin, Co-Author
Rod R Butterworth, Co-Author
An A-to-Z guide to American Sign Language vocabulary. *$15.26*
450 pages Softcover
ISBN 0-399519-52-1

7883 Phone of Our Own: The Deaf Insurrection Against Ma Bell
Gallaudet University Press
800 Florida Ave NE
Washington, DC 20002-3600
773-568-1550
800-621-2736
FAX: 773-660-2235
TTY: 888-630-9347
e-mail: gupress@gallaudet.edu
www.gupress.gallaudet.edu
Harry G Lang, Author
T. Alan Hurwitz, President
Paul Kelly, Vice President Adm. And Finance
A recount of the history of the teletypewriter, from the three deaf engineers who developed the acoustic coupler that made mass communication on TTY's feasible, through the deaf community's twenty-year struggle against the government and AT&T to have TTY's produced and distributed. *$36.50*
256 pages Hardcover
ISBN 1-563680-90-4

7884 Place of Their Own: Creating the Deaf Community in America
Gallaudet University Press
800 Florida Ave NE
Washington, DC 20002-3600
773-568-1550
800-621-2736
FAX: 773-660-2235
TTY: 888-630-9347
e-mail: gupress@gallaudet.edu
www.gallaudet.edu
John V Van Cleve, Author
Barry A Crouch, Co-Author
T. Alan Hurwitz, President
Paul Kelly, Vice President Adm. And Finance
Traces development of American deaf society to show how deaf people developed a common language and sense of community. Views deafness as the distinguishing characteristic of a distinct culture. *$22.95*
224 pages Paperback
ISBN 0-930323-49-1

7885 PreReading Strategies
Gallaudet University Bookstore
800 Florida Ave NE
Washington, DC 20002-3600
202-651-5855
866-204-0504
FAX: 773-660-2235
TTY: 202-651-5855
e-mail: gupress@gallaudet.edu
www.clerccenter.gallaudet.edu
David R Schleper, Author
T. Alan Hurwitz, President
Paul Kelly, Vice President Adm. And Finance
Here is a wealth of good advice for preparing students to understand what they read, building comprehension and enjoyment. *$ 14.95*
65 pages

7886 Quad City Deaf & Hard of Hearing Youth Group: Tomorrow's Leaders for our Community
Independent Living Research Utilization ILRU
2323 S Shepherd Dr
Houston, TX 77019-7019
713-520-9058
FAX: 713-520-5785
e-mail: ilru@ilru.org
Lex Frieden, Director
Rose Sheperd, Manager
IICIL staff see this program as a way to develop young leaders for themovement. Emphasis is given to providing oppportunities for members of the youth group to develop skills in planning and organizing activities.

7887 Religious Signing: A Comprehensive Guide for All Faiths
TJ Publishers
P.O. Box 702701
Dallas, TX 75370
972-416-0800
800-999-1168
FAX: 972-416-0944
TTY: 301-585-4440
e-mail: TJPubinc@aol.com
www.tjpublishers.com
Elaine Costello, Author
Terrence O'Rourke, Principal
Tanner Beach, Director
Contains over 500 religious signs for all denominations and their meanings illustrated by clear upper torso illustrations that show movements of hand, body and face. Includes a section on signing favorite verses, prayers and blessings. *$18.95*
219 pages Softcover
ISBN 0-553342-44-4

7888 Seeing Voices
Vintage and Anchor Books
1745 Broadway
3rd Floor
New York, NY 10019
212-782-9000
FAX: 212-572-6066
e-mail: vintageanchor@randomhouse.com
www.randomhouse.com
Oliver Sacks, Author
Madeline McIntosh, President/Sales/Operations
Markus Dohle, Chairman/CEO
Andrew Weber, SVP Operations And Technology
Well known for his exploration of how people respond to neurological impairments, Dr Sacks explores the world of the deaf and discovers how deaf people respond to their loss of hearing and how they develop language. A highly readable introduction to deaf people, deaf culture and American Sign Language. *$13.95*
240 pages Softcover 2000
ISBN 0-375704-07-8

7889 Sign Language Interpreting and Interpreter Education
Oxford University Press
2001 Evans Rd
Cary, NC 27513-2009
919-677-0977
800-445-9714
FAX: 919-677-1303
e-mail: custserv.us@oup.com
www.oup.com
Marc Marschark, Editor
Rico Peterson, Editor
Elizabeth A Winston, Editor
Patricia Sapere, Contributing Editor
Provides a coherent picture of the field as a whole, including evaluation of the extent to which current practices are supported by validating research. The first comprehensive source, suitable as both a reference book and a textbook for interpreter training programs and a variety of courses on bilingual education, psycholinguistics and translation, and cross-linguistic studies. *$65.00*
328 pages Hardcover
ISBN 0-195176-94-4

7890 Signing for Reading Success
Gallaudet University Press
800 Florida Ave NE
Washington, DC 20002-3600
773-568-1550
800-621-2736
FAX: 773-660-2235
TTY: 888-630-9347
e-mail: gupress@gallaudet.edu
www.gupress.gallaudet.edu
Jan C Hafer, Author
Robert M Wilson, Co-Author
T. Alan Hurwitz, President
Paul Kelly, Vice President Adm. And Finance
This booklet provides summaries of four research students on the usefulness of signing for reading achievement. *$7.95*
24 pages Paperback
ISBN 0-930323-18-1

7891 Signing: How to Speak with Your Hands
TJ Publishers
2427 Bond Street
Suite 108
University Park, IL 60466- 2288
972-416-0800
800-999-1168
FAX: 972-416-0944
e-mail: customerservice@tjpublishers.com
www.tjpublishers.com

Elaine Costello, Author
Terrence O'Rourke, Principal
Tanner Beach, Director

Presents 1,200 basic signs with clear illustrations in logical topical groupings. Linguistic principles are described at the beginning of each chapter, giving insight into the rules which govern American Sign Language. *$19.95*

248 pages Softcover
ISBN 0-553375-39-3

7892 Signs Across America
Gallaudet University Press
800 Florida Ave NE
Washington, DC 20002-3600
773-568-1550
800-621-2736
FAX: 773-660-2235
TTY: 888-630-9347
e-mail: gupress@gallaudet.edu
www.gupress.gallaudet.edu

Edgar H Shroyer, Author
Susan P Shroyer, Co-Author
T. Alan Hurwitz, President
Paul Kelly, Vice President Adm. And Finance

A look at regional variations in ASL. Signs for selected words collected from 25 different states. More than 1,200 signs illustrated in the text. *$28.95*

304 pages Paperback
ISBN 0-913580-96-1

7893 Signs for Me: Basic Sign Vocabulary for Children, Parents & Teachers
TJ Publishers
2427 Bond Street
Suite 108
University Park, IL 60466- 2288
972-416-0800
800-999-1168
FAX: 972-416-0944
e-mail: customerservice@tjpublishers.com
www.tjpublishers.com

Ben Bahan, Author
Joe Dannis, Co-Author
Terrence O'Rourke, Principal
Tanner Beach, Director

Sign language vocabulary for preschool and elementary school children introduces household items, animals, family members, actions, emotions, safety concerns and other concepts. *$14.95*

112 pages Softcover
ISBN 0-915035-27-8

7894 Signs for Sexuality: A Resource Manual
Planned Parenthood of Western Washington
2001 E Madison St
Seattle, WA 98122-2959
206-328-7715
FAX: 206-328-6810
www.plannedparenthood.org

Marlyn Minken, Author
Laurie Rosen-Ritt, Co-Author
Cecile Richards, President

An important book for those who want to listen to and talk with other people about feelings, loving and caring. *$40.00*

122 pages Softcover

7895 Signs of the Times
Gallaudet University Press
800 Florida Ave NE
Washington, DC 20002-3600
773-568-1550
800-621-2736
FAX: 773-660-2235
TTY: 888-630-9347
e-mail: gupress@gallaudet.edu
www.gupress.gallaudet.edu

Edgar H Shroyer, Author
Susan P Shroyer, Illustrator
T. Alan Hurwitz, President
Paul Kelly, Vice President Adm. And Finance

An excellent beginner's contact signing book that fills the gap between sign language dictionaries and American Sign Language text. Designed for use as a classroom text. *$34.95*

448 pages Softcover
ISBN 0-913580-76-7

7896 Sing Praise Hymnal for the Deaf
LifeWay Christian Resources
1 Lifeway Plz
MSN 146
Nashville, TN 37234-1001
615-251-2000
800-458-2772
FAX: 615-251-3899
www.lifeway.com

Thom Rainer, President/CEO
Jerry Rhyne, CFO/ VP Finance And Buisness
Tim Vineyard, VP Technology And CIO

Designed to be used by interpreters to the deaf, sign-language students, and deaf members of the congregation, this special combinded hymnal edition offers 234 of the most popular hymns. *$12.95*

Hardcover 2000
ISBN 0-767314-09-3

7897 TDI National Directory & Resource Guide: Blue Book
Telecommunications for the Deaf
8630 Fenton Street
Suite 604
Silver Spring, MD 20910- 3822
301-589-3786
FAX: 301-589-3797
e-mail: info@tdi-online.org
www.tdi-online.org

Claude L Stout, Executive Director

Promoting Equal Access to Telecommunications and Media for People who are Deaf, Late-Deafened, Hard-of-Hearing or Deaf-Blind. *$ 20.00*

600 pages Annual

7898 The Mask of Benevolence: Disabling the Dea Community
DawnSign Press
6130 Nancy Ridge Dr
San Diego, CA 92121-3223
858-625-0600
800-549-5350
FAX: 858-625-2336
e-mail: info@dawnsign.com
www.dawnsign.com

Joe Dannis, President
Harlan Lane, Author

Dr. Harlan Lane does not view deafness as a handicap but rather a different state from hearing. Deaf people are a societal minority and should be treasured, not eradicated. *$12.95*

360 pages Paperback 1992
ISBN 1-581210-09-5

7899 The Signed English Starter
Gallaudet University Press
800 Florida Ave NE
Washington, DC 20002-3600
773-568-1550
800-621-2736
FAX: 773-660-2235
TTY: 888-630-9347
e-mail: gupress@gallaudet.edu
www.gupress.gallaudet.edu
Harry Bornstein, Author
Karen L Saulnier, Co-Author
T. Alan Hurwitz, President
Paul Kelly, Vice President Adm. And Finance
A first course in Signed English for adults and children, the book is fully illustrated (several figures per page), and it is organized in a way that leads to rewarding learning quite rapidly. The authors of this new and exciting text believe firmly that Signed English must be made as easy as possible if it is going to be as useful (and used) as it can and should be. The book explains the rationale for the Signed English system and the conventions used to teach it.
$18.50
232 pages Paperback
ISBN 0-913580-82-1

7900 The Signing Family: What Every Parent Shounow About Sign Communication
Gallaudet University Press
800 Florida Ave NE
Washington, DC 20002-3600
773-568-1550
800-621-2736
FAX: 773-660-2235
TTY: 888-630-9347
e-mail: gupress@gallaudet.edu
www.gupress.gallaudet.edu
David A Stewart, Author
Barbara Luetke-Stahlman, Co-Author
T. Alan Hurwitz, President
Paul Kelly, Vice President Adm. And Finance
This reader-friendly book shows parents how to create a set of goals around the communication needs of their deaf child. Describes in even-handed terms the major signing options available, from American Sign Language to Signed English. *$29.95*
192 pages Paperback
ISBN 1-563680-69-6

7901 The Silent Garden
Gallaudet University Press
800 Florida Ave NE
Washington, DC 20002-3600
773-568-1550
800-621-2736
FAX: 773-660-2235
TTY: 888-630-9347
e-mail: gupress@gallaudet.edu
www.gupress.gallaudet.edu
Paul W Ogden, Author
T. Alan Hurwitz, President
Paul Kelly, Vice President Adm. And Finance
The author explain the broad range of hearing loss types, from minor to profound. Parents also are advised about what type of school their child should attend and what kinds of professional help will be best for the entire family. The book describes all forms of communication, including choices in signing from American Sign Language to the various manual systems based upon English. Technological alternatives are presented also, including when and when not to consider cochler implants. *$34.95*
304 pages
ISBN 1-563680-58-0

7902 The Week the World Heard Gallaudet
Gallaudet University Press
800 Florida Ave NE
Washington, DC 20002-3600
202-651-5000
800-621-2736
FAX: 202-651-5508
e-mail: gupress@gallaudet.edu
www.gupress.gallaudet.edu
Jack R Gannon, Author
T. Alan Hurwitz, President
Paul Kelly, Vice President Adm. And Finance
This day-to-day description of the events surrounding the Deaf President Now movement at Gallaudet University includes full color and black and white photographs and interviews with people involved in the events of that week. *$49.95*
176 pages Hardcover
ISBN 0-930323-54-8

7903 Theoretical Issues in Sign Language Research
University of Chicago Press
1427 E 60th St
Chicago, IL 60637-2902
773-702-7700
FAX: 773-702-9756
e-mail: sales@press.uchicago.edu
www.press.uchicago.edu
Donald A Collins, President
Susan D Fischer, Author
Patricia Siple, Co-Author
These volumes are an outgrowth of a conference held at the University of Rochester in 1986, dealing with the four traditional core areas of phonology, morphology, syntax and semantics.
$29.95
348 pages Paperback 1990
ISBN 0-226251-52-7

7904 We CAN Hear and Speak
Alexander Graham Bell Association
3417 Volta Pl NW
Washington, DC 20007-2737
202-337-5220
FAX: 202-337-8314
e-mail: info@agbell.org
www.agbell.org
Carol Flexer PhD, Author
Catherine Richards MA, Co-Author
K Houston PhD, Executive Director
John Wyant, Owner
Written by parents for families of children who are deaf or hard of hearing, this work describes auditory-verbal terminology and approaches and contains personal narratives written by parents and their children who are deaf or hard of hearing. *$6.98*
184 pages Softcover

7905 What is Auditory Processing?
Abilitations - Speech Bin
P.O.Box 922668
Norcross, GA 30010-2668
770-449-5700
800-850-8602
FAX: 770-510-7290
e-mail: info@speechbin.com
www.speechbin.com
Susan Bell, Author
What is Auditory Processing? It is and information-packed 16-page booklet created to explain auditory processing and it's disorders and offers practical suggestions for coping with this problem. It describes the listening process and tells how to help children with auditory processing problems. It shows what families and teachers can do to help children who have trouble remembering and understanding what they hear and offers easy-to-use activities and practical suggestions. *$ 22.69*
16 pages Softcover

7906 You and Your Deaf Child: A Self-Help Guidefor Parents of Deaf and Hard of Hearing Children
Gallaudet University Press
800 Florida Ave NE
Washington, DC 20002-3600
773-568-1550
800-621-2736
FAX: 773-660-2235
TTY: 888-630-9347
e-mail: gupress@gallaudet.edu
www.gupress.gallaudet.edu

John W Adams, Author
T. Alan Hurwitz, President
Paul Kelly, Vice President Adm. And Finance
Eleven chapters focus on such topics as feelings about hearing loss, the importance of communication in the family, and effective behavior management. Many chapters contain practice activities and questions to help parents retain skills taught in the chapter and check their grasp of the material. Four appendices provide references, general resources, and guidelines for evaluating educational programs. *$29.95*
224 pages Paperback
ISBN 1-563680-60-2

Print: Journals

7907 American Journal of Audiology
American Speech-Language-Hearing Association
2200 Research Blvd
Rockville, MD 20850-3289
240-632-2081
800-638-8255
FAX: 301-296-8580
e-mail: actioncenter@asha.org
www.asha.org

Gary Dunham, Editor-in-Chief
Bridget Murray Law, Managing Editor
Carol Polovoy, Assistant Managing Editor
Kellie Rowden-Racette, Print and Online Writer/Editor
Articles concern screening, assesment, and treatment techniques; prevention; professional issues; supervision; administration. Includes clinical forums, clinical reviews, letters to the editor, or research reports that emphasize clinical practice.
2 x year

7908 Hearing Professional
International Hearing Society
16880 Middlebelt Rd
Ste 4
Livonia, MI 48154-3374
734-522-7200
800-521-5247
FAX: 734-522-0200
e-mail: akovach@ihsinfo.org
www.ihsinfo.org

Kathleen Mennillo, MBA, Executive Director
Kara Nacarato, Editor & Mgr Of Strgc. Alliances
Scott Beall, Treasurer Director
Alan Lowell, President
Provides authoritative technical and business information that will help hearing aid specialists serve the hearing impaired.
bi-monthly

7909 JADARA
ADARA National Office
12461 Stottlemeyer Rd
Myersville, MD 21773-9620
301-293-8969
FAX: 301-293-9698
e-mail: adaraorg@comcast.net
www.adara.org

Gary Dunham, Editor-in-Chief
Bridget Murray Law, Managing Editor
Carol Polovoy, Assistant Managing Editor
Kellie Rowden-Racette, Print and Online Writer/Editor
A professional journal sharing new procedures, thoughts, and research with application to the working professional.

7910 Journal of Speech, Language and Hearing Research
American Speech-Language-Hearing Association
2200 Research Blvd
Rockville, MD 20850-3289
301-296-5700
800-638-8255
FAX: 301-296-8580
e-mail: actioncenter@asha.org
www.asha.org

Gary Dunham, Editor-in-Chief
Bridget Murray Law, Managing Editor
Carol Polovoy, Assistant Managing Editor
Kellie Rowden-Racette, Print and Online Writer/Editor
Pertains broadly to studies of the processess and disorders of hearing, language, and speech diagnosis and treatment of such disorders.

7911 Journal of the Academy of Rehabilitative Audiology
Academy of Rehabilitative Audiology
PO Box 2323
Albany, NY 12220-0323
952-920-0484
FAX: 952-920-6098
e-mail: ara@audrehab.org
www.audrehab.org

Linda Thibodeau, President
Laura A. Wilber, Parlamentarian
Kristin V. Dilaj, Secretary
Sherri Smith, Treasurer
A peer-reviewed journal published annually. *$25.00*

7912 Sign Language Studies
Gallaudet University Press
800 Florida Ave NE
Washington, DC 20002-3695
202-651-5488
800-621-2736
FAX: 202-651-5508
e-mail: gupress@gallaudet.edu
www.gupress.gallaudet.edu

Ceil Lucas, Editor
T. Alan Hurwitz, President
Paul Kelly, Vice President Adm. And Finance
Presents a unique forum for revolutionary papers on signed languages and other related disciplines, including linguistics, anthropology, semiotics, and deaf studies, history, and literature. *$ 55.00*
Quarterly

7913 The Literature Journal
Gallaudet University
800 Florida Ave NE
Washington, DC 20002-3695
202-651-5488
800-621-2736
FAX: 202-651-5508
e-mail: Oluyinka.Fakunle@gallaudet.edu
www.clerccenter.gallaudet.edu

Charles C Welsh-Charrier, Author
T. Alan Hurwitz, President
Paul Kelly, Vice President Adm. And Finance
This book includes extensive examples of student and teacher entries taken from actual journals of deaf high school students. *$12.95*
44 pages Spiral Bound

7914 Volta Review
Alexander Graham Bell Association
3417 Volta Pl NW
Washington, DC 20007-2778
202-337-5220
FAX: 202-337-8314
e-mail: mfelzien@agbell.org
www.agbell.org

Jackson Roush, PhD, Editor
K Houston, PhD, Executive Director
John Wyant, Owner
Professionally refereed journal that publishes articles and research on education, rehabilitation and communicative development of people who have hearing impairments. Also includes

subscription to Volta Voices, up-to-date magazine, bimonthly.
$60.00
Quarterly

Print: Magazines

7915 Endeavor Magazine
American Society for Deaf Children
800 Florida Avenue NorthEast
#2047
Washington, Dc 20002-3695
717-703-0073
866-942-2732
800-942-ASDC
FAX: 410-795-0965
e-mail: asdc@deafchildren.org
www.deafchildren.org

Beth Benedict, President
Avonne Rutowski, VP
Timothy Frelich, Treasurer
Tami Hossler, Executive Secretary

7916 Hearing Health Magazine
Deafness Research Foundation
363 Seventh Avenue
10th Floor
New York, NY 10001-3904
212-257-6140
866-454-3924
FAX: 212-257-6139
e-mail: info@drf.org
www.drf.org

Andrea Boidman, Executive Director
Andrea Delbanco, Senior Editor
Yishane Lee, Editor
Julie Grant, Art Director

Serves as a source of quality information and provides the tools and resources to help people seek treatment for and manage hearing loss. Each issue features relevant and timely information on the latest research, articles written by leading authorities in the field, news about the latest technology, and human interest stories about those living with hearing loss.

7917 Hearing Loss Magazine
Hearing Loss Association of America
7910 Woodmont Ave
Ste 1200
Bethesda, MD 20814-7022
301-657-2248
FAX: 301-913-9413
e-mail: info@hearingloss.org
www.hearingloss.org

Barbara Kelley, Editor-In-Chief/Deputy Ex. Dir.
Cindy Dyer, Graphic Design

Provides the latest information on products, services, research, and technology in the hearing health care field. *$35.00*
40 pages BiMonthly

7918 Tinnitus Today
American Tinnitus Association
PO Box 5
Portland, OR 97207-5
503-493-2550
800-634-8978
FAX: 503-248-0024
e-mail: tinnitus@ata.org
www.ata.org

Nina Rogozen, Editor
Michael Malusevic, Executive Director

The magazine contains up-to-date medical and research news, feature articles on urgent tinnitus issues, questions and answers, self-help suggestions and letters to the editor from others with tinnitus. *$35.00*
28 pages 3 x year

7919 Volta Voices
Alexander Graham Bell Association
3417 Volta Pl NW
Washington, DC 20007-2737
202-337-5220
FAX: 202-337-8314
e-mail: mfelzien@agbell.org
www.agbell.org

Melody Felzien, Editor
K Houston, Executive Director
John Wyant, Owner

Covers a variety of topics, including hearing aids and cochlear implants, early intervention and education, professional guidance, legislative updates and perspectives from individuals from across the United States and around the world. *$60.00*
Bi-Monthly

Print: Newsletters

7920 AAPD Newsletter
American Association of People with Disabilities
1629 K Street NW
Suite 950
Washington, DC 20006-1634
202-457-0046
800-840-8844
www.aapd.com

Mark Perriello, President/CEO
Helena Berger, COO
Robin Shaffert, Senior Director

Provides latest information on a variety of national disability policies and issues.

7921 American Annals of the Deaf
Gallaudet University Press
800 Florida Ave NE
Washington, DC 20002-3600
202-651-5000
800-621-2736
FAX: 202-651-5508
e-mail: paul.3@osu.edu
www.gupress.gallaudet.edu

Peter V. Paul, Editor, Literary Issues
T. Alan Hurwitz, President
Paul Kelly, Vice President Adm. And Finance

Quarterly publication from the Conference of Educational Administrators Serving the Deaf. *$55.00*
Quarterly

7922 CommuniquŠ
Michigan Assoc for the Deaf and Hard of Hearing

Quarterly

7923 Connect - Commmunity News
Hearing, Speech & Deafness Center (HSDC)
1625 19th Ave
Artz Communication Center
Seattle, WA 98122-2848
206-323-5770
888-222-5036
FAX: 206-328-6871
TTY:206-388-1275
e-mail: admin@hsdc.org
www.hsdc.org

David Delmar, Editor

Connect is the quarterly eNews of the Hearing, Speech & Deafness Center.
8 pages Annual

7924 Deaf Catholic
International Catholic Deaf Association
7202 Buchanan St
Landover Hills, MD 20784-2236
301-429-0697
FAX: 301-429-0698
e-mail: homeoffice@icda-us.org
www.icda-us.org

Jean Cox, President
Kate Slosar, Vice President
TK Hill, Treasurer
Aline Shaw, Secretary
Newsletter reporting the news of the Archdiocese, Deaf Apostolate and each of the Catholic Deaf Organizations. *$20.00*
16 pages Quarterly

7925 Hearing, Speech & Deafness Center (HSDC)
1625 19th Ave
Artz Communication Center
Seattle, WA 98122-2848
206-323-5770
888-222-5036
FAX: 206-328-6871
TTY:206-388-1275
e-mail: admin@hsdc.org
www.hsdc.org

David Webster, Director of Finance
Cherylyn McRae, Director of Development
Roger Mauldin, Interim CEO
Gordon Braun, CFO
Newsletter with information on Center services, activities, news, helpful articles.
10 pages Quarterly

7926 League Letter
Center for Hearing and Communication
50 Broadway
6th Floor
New York, NY 10004-3810
917-305-7700
FAX: 917-305-7888
TTY:917-305-7999
e-mail: info@chchearing.org
www.lhh.org

Laurie Hanin, Executive Director
Ellen Lafargue, Au.D., CCC, Director, Hearing Technology
Lois Kam Heymann, M.A., CCC, Director, Communication
Linda Kessler, M.A., CCC-SLP, Assistant Director, Communication

Quarterly

7927 NAHO News
National Association of Hearing Officials
PO Box 4999
Midlothian, VA 23112-17
701-328-3260
e-mail: jwezelman.wezelmanlaw@midconectwork.com
www.naho.org

Joy Wezelman, Editor
Janice Deshais, Editor
National Association of Hearing Officials newsletter.

7928 Newsletter Bulletin
John Tracy Clinic
806 W Adams Blvd
Los Angeles, CA 90007-2505
213-748-5481
800-522-4582
FAX: 213-749-1651
e-mail: ealaniz@jtc.org
www.jtc.org

Gaston Kent, President Director
Blythe Maling, Vice President Of Development
A newsletter for our friends and families.
8 pages Bi-annually

7929 On the Level
Vestibular Disorders Association
5018 NE 15th Ave
Portland, OR 97211-5331
503-229-7705
800-837-8428
FAX: 503-229-8064
e-mail: veda@vestibular.org
www.vestibular.org

Lisa Haven PhD, Executive Director
Jerry Underwood, Director
Vincente Honrubia, Director
Contents of each issue include information about local support groups, a calendar of conferences and training opportunities for health professionals, a list of donors, and special items indexed below. *$5.00*
12 pages Quarterly

7930 Paws for Silence
International Hearing Dog
5901 E 89th Ave
Henderson, CO 80640-8315
303-287-3277
FAX: 303-287-3425
e-mail: info@hearingdog.org
www.ihdi.org

Valerie Foss-Brugger, Executive Director
Robert Cooley, Field Representative/Placement Counselor
Andrea Paul, Veterinary Technician/Hd Trainer
Cindy Horn, Kennel Technician & Assistant Trainer
Paws for Silence is our quarterly newsletter. In this publication you will find up-to-date information on what's going on at IHDI, future plans and in-depth stories.
4-8 pages Quarterly

7931 Soundings Newsletter
American Hearing Research Foundation
8 South Michigan Avenue
Suite 1205
Chicago, IL 60603- 4539
312-726-9670
FAX: 312-726-9695
e-mail: ahrf@american-hearing.org
www.american-hearing.org

Sharon Parmet, Executive Director
Promote, conduct and furnish financial assistance for medical research into the cause, prevention and cure of deafness, impaired hearing and balance disorders; encourage the collaboration of clinical and laboratory research; encourage and improve teaching in the medical aspects of hearing problems; and disseminate the most reliable scientific knowledge to physicians, hearing professionals and the public.
Quarterly

7932 Spring Dell Center Newsletter
Spring Dell Center
6040 Radio Station Rd
La Plata, MD 20646-3368
301-934-4561
FAX: 301-870-2439
e-mail: donnaretzlaf@springdellcenter.org
www.springdellcenter.org

Donna Retzlaff, Executive Director
Jody Loper, President
Brett Hamorsky, Vice President
Jeff Hubbard, Treasurer

Quarterly

7933 The ASHA Leader
American Speech-Language-Hearing Association
2200 Research Blvd
Rockville, MD 20850-3289
301-215-6710
800-638-8255
FAX: 301-296-8580
e-mail: leader@asha.org
www.asha.org

Gary Dunham, Editor-in-Chief
Bridget Murray Law, Managing Editor
Carol Polovoy, Assistant Managing Editor
Kellie Rowden-Racette, Print and Online Writer/Editor

Association publication containing news, notices of events and activities and information for members on issues facing the profession of audiology and speech-language pathology. *$80.00*
35 pages 2 x month

Non Print: Newsletters

7934 **Canine Listener**
Dogs for the Deaf
10175 Wheeler Rd
Central Point, OR 97502 541-826-9220
800-990-3647
800-990-3647
FAX: 541-826-6696
TTY:541-826-9220
e-mail: info@dogsforthedeaf.org
dogsforthedeaf.org

Marvin Rhodes, Chair
Susan Bahr, Vice Chair
Kelly Gonzales, Development Director
Janine Bol, Finance Director
Provides information on Hearing Dogs, placements, dog training, and other news about happenings at Dogs for the Deaf.
Quarterly

7935 **Cochlear Implants In Children: Ethics and Choices**
Gallaudet University Press
800 Florida Ave NE
Washington, DC 20002-3600 202-651-5000
800-621-2736
FAX: 202-651-5508
e-mail: gupress@gallaudet.edu
www.gupress.gallaudet.edu

John B Christiansen, Author
Irene W Leigh, Co-Author
T. Alan Hurwitz, President
Paul Kelly, Vice President Adm. And Finance
Designed to educate readers about cochlear implants, including surgery, the importance of rehabilitation and the significance of parents' and professionals' roles. *$55.00*
340 pages Casebound
ISBN 1-563681-16-1

7936 **Communique**
Michigan Association for Deaf Hard of Hearing
5236 Dumond Court
Suite C
Lansing, MI 48917-6001 517-487-0066
800-968-7327
FAX: 517-487-2586
e-mail: info@madhh.org
www.madhh.org

Nancy Asher, Executive Director
Pat Walton, Office Manager
Provides leadership through advocacy and education. The association conducts leadership training for youth, information and referral services, interpreter referral, legislative advocacy, and a variety of other services.
4-8 pages Bi-annually

7937 **Listner**
HEAR Center
301 E Del Mar Blvd
Pasadena, CA 91101-2714 626-796-2016
FAX: 626-796-2320
e-mail: info@hearcenter.org
www.hearcenter.org

Ellen Simon, Executive Director
Berenice Castro, Accounting Supervisro
Debbie Lorino, Office Manager
Chronicals current events, spotlights pediatric and adult clients as well as community outreach events.
Semi-Quarterly

7938 **NAD E-Zine**
National Association of the Deaf
8630 Fenton Street
Suite 820
Silver Spring, MD 20910- 3819 301-587-1788
FAX: 301-587-1791
TTY:301-587-1789
e-mail: nadinfo@nad.org
www.nad.org

Bobbie Beth Scoggins, President
Christopher Wagner, Vice President
Includes up-to-the-minute information about the NAD, including Board news, advocacy, outreach and community activities, as well as NAD Conference and other information.

7939 **Pinnacle Newsletter**
Academy of Rehabilitative Audiology
PO Box 26532
Minneapolis, MN 55426-532 952-920-0484
FAX: 952-920-6098
e-mail: sherri.smith@va.gov
www.audrehab.org

John Greer Clark, Editor
Diana Derry, Co-Editor
Sherri Smith, Ph.D.,, Content Editor
Academy of Rehabilitative Audiology newsletter.

7940 **So the World May Hear**
Starkey Hearing Foundation
6700 Washington Ave S
Eden Prairie, MN 55344-3405 952-941-6401
866-354-3254
FAX: 952-828-6900
e-mail: info@StarkeyFoundation.org
www.sotheworldmayhear.org

Brady Forseth, Executive Director
Steven Sawalich, Senior Executive Director
Ann Spilker, Director of Operations
Frederic Rondeau, International Director
Our mission, So the World May Hear, is about bringing understanding between people through caring and sharing. We believe caring develops trust and by sharing we find our humanity.
Quarterly

7941 **Vision Magazine**
National Catholic Office of the Deaf
7202 Buchanan St
Hyattsville, MD 20784-2236 301-577-1684
FAX: 301-577-1684
e-mail: info@ncod.org
www.ncod.org

Arvilla Rank, Editor/Executive Director
Published as a pastoral service for the deaf and hard of hearing. Provides information to members and others working in ministry.
$15.00
Quarterly

Non Print: Video

7942 **Christmas Stories**
Video Learning Library
15838 N 62nd St
Scottsdale, AZ 85254-1988 480-596-9970
800-383-8811
FAX: 480-596-9973
e-mail: info@videolearning.com
www.videolearning.com

Jim Spencer, Owner
Told by popular deaf story-tellers, the stories included are A Christmas Carol, Night Before Christmas, Story of the First Christmas Tree, Birth of Christ, The Great Walled City, and Little Match Girl. *$29.95*
Video/80 Mins 1986
ISBN 1-882257-02-2

7943 **Fantastic Series Videotape Set**
Gallaudet University Press
800 Florida Ave NE
Washington, DC 20002-3695 202-651-5488
800-621-2736
FAX: 202-651-5489
e-mail: gupress@gallaudet.edu
www.gupress.gallaudet.edu

Rita Corey, Director
T. Alan Hurwitz, President
Paul Kelly, Vice President Adm. And Finance
These videotapes offer a blend of entertainment and information to both deaf and hearing children ages 6-10. A total of eight tapes in the series. *$254.00*
Video 8 VHS
ISBN 1-563680-12-2

7944 **Fantastic: Colonial Times, Chocolate, and Cars**
Gallaudet University Press
800 Florida Ave NE
Washington, DC 20002-3695 202-651-5488
800-621-2736
FAX: 202-651-5489
e-mail: gupress@gallaudet.edu
www.gupress.gallaudet.edu

Rita Corey, Director
T. Alan Hurwitz, President
Paul Kelly, Vice President Adm. And Finance
Young viewers visit Colonial Williamsburg in Virginia to see various crafts. Other parts show chocolate being made, and films of old cars. *$39.95*
Video
ISBN 1-563680-06-8

7945 **Fantastic: Dogs at Work and Play**
Gallaudet University Press
800 Florida Ave NE
Washington, DC 20002-3695 202-651-5488
800-621-2736
FAX: 202-651-5489
e-mail: gupress@gallaudet.edu
www.gupress.gallaudet.edu

Rita Corey, Director
T. Alan Hurwitz, President
Paul Kelly, Vice President Adm. And Finance
See how dogs are trained, including Fantastic's own hearing-ear dog, police dogs, plus puppies, and dogs in space? *$39.95*
Video
ISBN 1-563680-03-3

7946 **Fantastic: Exciting People, Places and Things!**
Gallaudet University Press
800 Florida Ave NE
Washington, DC 20002-3695 202-651-5488
800-621-2736
FAX: 202-651-5489
e-mail: gupress@gallaudet.edu
www.gupress.gallaudet.edu

Rita Corey, Director
T. Alan Hurwitz, President
Paul Kelly, Vice President Adm. And Finance
Welcomes young viewers for a trip to a crayon factory, a jump rope tournament, and mime by actor Bernard Bragg. *$39.95*
Video
ISBN 1-563680-01-7

7947 **Fantastic: From Post Offices to Dairy Goats**
Gallaudet University Press
800 Florida Ave NE
Washington, DC 20002-3695 202-651-5488
800-621-2736
FAX: 202-651-5489
e-mail: gupress@gallaudet.edu
www.gupress.gallaudet.edu

Rita Corey, Director
T. Alan Hurwitz, President
Paul Kelly, Vice President Adm. And Finance
In this video children follow the route of a letter from the mailbox through the post office to its final destination. Also, they visit dairy goats and other animals. *$39.95*
Video
ISBN 1-563680-05-X

7948 **Fantastic: Imagination, Actors, and 'Deaf Way'**
Gallaudet University Press
800 Florida Ave NE
Washington, DC 20002-3695 202-651-5488
800-621-2736
202-651-5508
FAX: 202-651-5489
e-mail: gupress@gallaudet.edu
www.gupress.gallaudet.edu

Rita Corey, Director
T. Alan Hurwitz, President
Paul Kelly, Vice President Adm. And Finance
Deaf clowns, mimes, and actors display the wonders of imagination, along with performances at the international cultural celebration 'Deaf Way.' *$39.95*
Video
ISBN 1-563680-04-1

7949 **Fantastic: Roller Coasters, Maps, and Ice Cream!**
Gallaudet University Press
800 Florida Ave NE
Washington, DC 20002-3695 202-651-5488
800-621-2736
FAX: 202-651-5489
e-mail: gupress@gallaudet.edu
www.gupress.gallaudet.edu

Rita Corey, Director
T. Alan Hurwitz, President
Paul Kelly, Vice President Adm. And Finance
In this program Mike Montangino leads the way on rides at Kings Dominion, and also to see how maps are drawn, and how ice cream is made. *$39.95*
Video
ISBN 1-563680-07-6

7950 **Fantastic: Skiing, Factories, and Race Hores**
Gallaudet University Press
800 Florida Ave NE
Washington, DC 20002-3695 202-651-5488
800-621-2736
FAX: 202-651-5489
e-mail: gupress@gallaudet.edu
www.gupress.gallaudet.edu

Rita Corey, Director
T. Alan Hurwitz, President
Paul Kelly, Vice President Adm. And Finance
Snow Skiing starts this program, which continues in a factory where 'who-knows-what' is made. Also, young viewers learn about horse care, and also about the making of Oreos. *$39.95*
Video
ISBN 1-563680-08-4

7951 **Fantastic: Wonderful Worlds of Sports and Travel**
Gallaudet University Press
800 Florida Ave NE
Washington, DC 20002-3695 202-651-5488
800-621-2736
FAX: 202-651-5489
e-mail: gupress@gallaudet.edu
www.gupress.gallaudet.edu

Rita Corey, Director
T. Alan Hurwitz, President
Paul Kelly, Vice President Adm. And Finance
In this program, young viewers ride on a train, watch deaf athletes compete, and see actor Bernard Bragg perform 'The Lion and the Mouse.' *$39.95*
Video
ISBN 1-563680-02-5

7952 Fingerspelling: Expressive and Receptive Fluency
DawnSign Press
6130 Nancy Ridge Dr
San Diego, CA 92121-3223
858-625-0600
800-549-5350
FAX: 858-625-2336
e-mail: info@dawnsign.com
www.dawnsign.com

Joe Dannis, President
Joyce Linden Groode, Fingerspelling Teacher
Improve your fingerspelling with this new video guide. A 24-page instructional booklet is included with fingerspelling practice suggestions. *$29.95*
120 Minutes
ISBN 1-581210-46-9

7953 Getting Better
Vestibular Disorders Association
5018 NE 15th Ave
Portland, OR 97211-5331
503-229-7705
800-837-8428
FAX: 503-229-8064
e-mail: veda@vestibular.org
www.vestibular.org

Cynthia Ryan MBA, Executive Director
Tony Staser,, Development Director
Vicente Honrubia, Director
Joel A. Goebel, MD, FACS, Director, Vestibular & Oculomotor Laboratory
Interviews with physicians, physical therapists, psychologists, social workers, and patients on Managing Symptoms, Diagnosis & Treatment, and Cognitive/Psychological Impacts. *$24.95*
Video

7954 Helping the Family Understand
Vestibular Disorders Association
5018 NE 15th Ave
Portland, OR 97211-5331
503-229-7705
800-837-8428
FAX: 503-229-8064
e-mail: veda@vestibular.org
www.vestibular.org

Cynthia Ryan MBA, Executive Director
Tony Staser,, Development Director
Vicente Honrubia, Director
Joel A. Goebel, MD, FACS, Director, Vestibular & Oculomotor Laboratory
Interviews with physicians, physical therapists, psychologists, social workers, and patients on Managing Symptoms, Diagnosis & Treatment and Cognitive/Psychological Impacts. *$24.95*
Video

7955 Managing Your Symptoms
Vestibular Disorders Association
5018 NE 15th Ave
Portland, OR 97211-5331
503-229-7705
800-837-8428
FAX: 503-229-8064
e-mail: veda@vestibular.org
www.vestibular.org

Cynthia Ryan MBA, Executive Director
Tony Staser,, Development Director
Vicente Honrubia, Director
Joel A. Goebel, MD, FACS, Director, Vestibular & Oculomotor Laboratory
Interviews with physicians, physical therapists, psychologists, social workers, and patients. on Managing Symptoms, Diagnosis & Treatment, and Cognitive/Psychological Impacts. *$24.95*
Video

Sports

7956 American Hearing Impaired Hockey Association
4214 W. 77th Place
Chicago, IL 60652-1618
978-922-0955
FAX: 312-829-2098
e-mail: kkmm2won@aol.com
www.ahiha.org

Stan Mikita, President
Cheryl Hager, General Manager
Helen Tovey, Registrar, USA Hockey Reg.
The American Hearing Impaired Hockey Association provides deaf and hard of hearing hockey players the opportunity to learn about and improve their hockey skills through our program. We offer these hockey players the opportunity to be coached by a coaching staff with college, national and international experience.

7957 USA Deaf Sports Federation
102 N Krohn Pl
PO Box 910338
Lexington, KY 40591-0338
605-367-5760
FAX: 605-782-8441
TTY:605-367-5761
e-mail: homeoffice@usadeafsports.org
www.usdeafsports.org

Jack C Lamberton, President
Mark Apodaca, VP Of Financial Affairs
William J Bowman, VP Of International Affairs
Jeffrey L. Salit?, Vice-President of NSO Affairs
The USA Deaf Sports Federation's purpose was to foster and regulate uniform rules of competition and provide social outlets for deaf members and their friends; serve as a parent organization for regional sports organizations; conduct annual athletic competitions; and assist in the participation of U.S. teams in international competition.

Support Groups

7958 Dial-a-Hearing Screening Test
Occupational Hearing Services Inc.
300 S Chester Rd
Suite 301
Swarthmore, PA 19081-1800
610-544-7700
800-622-3277
FAX: 610-543-2802
e-mail: DAHST@aol.com

George Biddle, President/Owner
James Biddle, Vice President
Phyllis Biddle, Treasurer
A national telephone resource providing information about hearing impairments and deafness. Dial-A-Hearing Screening Test: national test number for free telephone hearing test: 1-800-222-EARS, MON-FRI: 9:00 AM to 5:00 PM Eastern time.

Mobility

Associations

7959 American Association of Spinal Cord Injury Psychologists & Social Workers
75-20 Astoria Boulevard
Jackson Heights, NY 11370-1138 718-803-3782
FAX: 718-803-0414
e-mail: info@unitedspinal.org
www.unitedspinal.org/donations/online-
Lex Frieden, Chairman of the Board
Paul Tobin, President and Chief Executive Officer
Michael B. Kinne, Secretary
Janeen Earwood, Treasurer
Organized and operated for scientific and educational purposes to advance and improve the psychosocial care of persons with spinal cord impairment, develop and promote education and research related to the psychosocial care of persons with spinal cord injury, recognize psychologists and social workers whose careers are devoted to the problems of spinal cord impairment.

7960 American Back Society
2648 International Blvd
Ste 502
Oakland, CA 94601-1537 510-536-9929
FAX: 510-536-1812
e-mail: info@americanbacksoc.org
www.americanbacksoc.org
James W Simmons M.D. F.A.C.S., President
Ronald G Donelson M.D. M.S, Vice President
Carol McFarland, Secretary
Thomas E Dreisinger PhD, Treasurer
The American Back Society is a non-profit organization dedicated to providing an interdisciplinary educational forum for healthcare professionals committed to relieving pain and diminishing impairment in patients suffering from neck and back conditions through proper diagnosis and treatment.

7961 American Stroke Association
7272 Greenville Ave
Dallas, TX 75231-4596 800-242-8721
888-478-7653
FAX: 214-706-5231
e-mail: strokeconnection@heart.org
www.strokeassociation.org
Ralph Sacco, President/Director
Donna Arnett, Ph.D., President
Debra Lockwood, Chairman
Nancy Brown, CEO
Fifty-five state affiliates monitoring local chapters offering educational materials, seminars, conferences and transportation for members nationwide. Maintains a listing of over 1,000 stroke support groups across the nation for referral to stroke survivors, their families, caregivers and interested professionals.

7962 Amytrophic Lateral Sclerosis Association
27001 Agoura Rd
Ste 250
Calabasas Hills, CA 91301-5104 818-880-9007
800-782-4747
FAX: 818-880-9006
e-mail: alsinfo@alsa-national.org
www.alsa.org
Janes H Gilbert, President/CEO
Michelle Powers Keegan, Chief Development Officer
Daniel M. Reznikov, CFO
Lance Slaughter, Chief Chapter Relations Officer
The ALS association is the only national not-for-profit health organization dedicated soley to lead the fight against ALS. The Association covers all the bases-research, patient and community services, public education, and advocacy-in providing help and hope to those facing the disease. The mission is to lead the fight to cure and treat ALS through global cutting edge research, and to empower people with Lou Gehrig's disease to live fuller lives & provide them with compassion care and support.

7963 Arthritis Foundation
PO Box 932915
Atlanta, GA 31193-2915 404-872-7100
800-283-7800
FAX: 404-872-0457
e-mail: aforders@arthritis.org
www.arthritis.org
Daniel T. McGowan, Chair
Rowland W. (Bing) Chang, Vice Chairs
Patricia Novak Nelson, Vice Chairs
Michael V. Ortman, Treasurer
Offers information and referrals regarding educational materials and programs, fund-raising, support groups, seminars and conferences offered by 55 local chapters across the United States.

7964 Association for Neurologically Impaired Brain Injured Children
61-35 220th St
Oakland Gardens, NY 11364 718-423-9550
FAX: 718-423-9838
e-mail: mail@anibic.org
www.anibic.org
Gerard Smith, Executive Director
John F DeBiase, Associate Executive Director
Rachel Plakstis, MSC Director
Gail Baquero, Residential Director
ANIBIc is a voluntary, multi-service organization that is dedicated to serving individuals with severe learning disabilities, neurological impairments and other developmental disabilities. Services include: residential, vocational, family support services, recreation (children and adults), respite (adult), in home support services, counseling and tramatic brain injury services (adults).

7965 Christopher & Dana Reeve Paralysis Resource Center
636 Morris Turnpike
Suite 3A
Short Hills, NJ 07078-2608 973-379-2690
800-225-0292
FAX: 973-912-9433
e-mail: information@christopherreeve.org
www.christopherreeve.org
John M. Hughes, Chairman
Arnold H. Snider, Vice Chairman
Henry G. Stifel, III, Vice Chairman
Joel M. Faden, Chairman, Executive Committee
Our goal is to provide you with the information you need to live a healthy life, make informed decisions, and better understand paralysis, spinal cord injury and other conditions.

7966 Epilepsy Foundation
8301 Professional Pl
Landover, MD 20785-2353 800-332-1000
866-330-2718
FAX: 301-459-1569
e-mail: ContactUs@efa.org
www.epilepsyfoundation.org
Diane Rubinstein, Senior Director Finance/Controller
Ken Lowenberg, Senior Director Marketing and Communications
Chad Hartman, Senior Director of Development
Adina Frazier, Director of Special Events
The organization works to ensure that people with seizures are able to participate in all life experiences; to improve how people with epilepsy are perceived, accepted and valued in society; and to promote research for a cure. In addition to programs conducted at the national level, epilepsy clients throughout the United States are served by 48 Epilepsy Foundation affiliates around the country.

7967 **Friends of Disabled Adults and Children**
4900 Lewis Rd
Stone Mountain, GA 30083-1104 770-491-9014
866-977-1204
e-mail: chrisbrand@fodac.org
www.fodac.org

Chris Brand, President

FODAC's mission is to provide durable medical equipment (DME) such as wheelchairs and hospital beds at little or no cost to the disabled and their families. We seek to enhance the quality of life for people of all ages who have any type of illness or physical disability. Since 1986, FODAC has collected and distributed more than 29,000 wheelchairs!

7968 **Head Injury Rehabilitation And Referral Service, Inc. (HIRRS)**
11 Taft Court
Suite 100
Rockville, MD 20850-4162 301-309-2228
FAX: 301-309-2278
e-mail: tbi@headinjuryrehab.org
www.headinjuryrehab.org

Maggie Hunter, Director of Admissions and Quality Assurance
Robert Cousland, Director of Rehabilitation
Debbie Jones, Director of Individual Support
Janet McCloskey, Director of Community Living Services

Head Injury Rehabilitation and Referral Services, Inc. (HIRRS) is a private not-for-profit agency that provides comprehensive brain injury support including long-term living, daily programs, vocational supports and services to individuals that live in the community. The agency is located in Rockville, MD, but serves the DC Metropolitan area.

7969 **Mobility International USA**
132 E. Broadway
Suite 343
Eugene, OR 97401-2767 541-343-1284
FAX: 541-343-6812
e-mail: info@miusa.org
www.miusa.org

Susan Sygall, Executive Director
Alison Ecker, Project Assistant
Cerise Roth Vinson, Chief Operating Officer
Cindy Lewis, Director of Programs

A US based national nonprofit organization dedicated to empowering people with disabilities around the world through leadership development, training and international exchange to ensure inclusion of people with disabilities in international exchange and development programs. The National Clearinghouse on Disability & Exchange, a joint project managed by MIUSA provides free information and referrals.

7970 **Multiple Sclerosis Association of America**
706 Haddonfield Rd
Cherry Hill, NJ 08002-2652 856-488-4500
800-532-7667
FAX: 856-488-8257
e-mail: northeast@mymsaa.org
www.msassociation.org

Robert Manley, Chair
Sue Rehmu, Vice Chair
William Saunders, Treasurer
Monica Derbes Gibson, Secretary

MSAA is a national non-profit organization dedicated to enriching the quality of life for evryone affected by multiple sclerosis.

7971 **National Coalition for Assistive and Rehab Technology**
54 Towhee Court
East Amhurst, NY 14051 716-839-9728
FAX: 716-839-9624
e-mail: info@ncart.us
www.ncart.us

Don Clayback, Executive Director
Gary Gilberi, President
Doug Westerdahl, Treasurer
Bob Gouy, Executive Committee Member

The coalition's mission is to ensure proper and appropriate access to complex rehab and assistive technologies.

7972 **National Council on Independent Living**
1710 Rhode Island Ave NW
5th Floor
Washington, DC 20036-3007 202-207-0334
877-525-3400
FAX: 202-207-0341
TTY: 202-207-0340
e-mail: ncil@ncil.org
www.ncil.org

Kelly Buckland, Executive Director
Tim Fuchs, Operations Director
Dan Kessler, President
Lou Ann Kibbee, Vice President

NCIL advances independent living and the rights of people with disabilities through consumer-driven advocacy.

7973 **National Fibromyalgia Association**
2121 S Towne Centre Place
Ste 300
Anaheim, CA 92806-6124 714-921-0150
FAX: 714-921-6920
e-mail: fmaware.org
www.fmaware.org

Lynne Matallana, President
Mark Dobrilovic, Board of Director
John Fry, PhD, Board of Directors
Michael Seffinger, DO, FAAFP, Board of Directors

National Fibromyalgia Association's mission is to develop and execute programs dedicated to improving the quality of life for people with fibromyalgia.

7974 **National Mobility Equipment Dealers Association**
3327 W Bearss Ave
Tampa, FL 33618-2100 813-264-2697
866-948-8341
FAX: 813-962-8970
e-mail: info@nmeda.org
www.nmeda.org

Sam Cook,, President
Mark DiRosa,, Vice President
Richard May,, Secretary
Bill Koeblitz, Treasurer

NMEDA is a non-profit trade association of mobility equipment dealers, driver rehabilitation specialists, and other professionals dedicated to broadening the opportunities for people with disabilities to drive or be transported in vehicles modified with mobility equipment. All members work together to improve transportation options of people with disabilities.

7975 **Paralyzed Veterans of America**
801 18th St NW
Washington, DC 20006-3517 202-872-1300
800-424-8200
888-888-2201
FAX: 202-785-4432
TTY:800-795-4327
e-mail: info@pva.org
www.pva.org

Homer S. Townsend, Jr., Executive Director
Larry Dodson, National Secretary
Bill Lawson, National President
Al Kovach, Jr, Natonal Senior Vice President

A congressionally chartered veterans service organization, has developed a unique expertise on a wide variety of issues involving the special needs of our members— veterans of the armed forces who have experienced spinal cord injury or dysfunction.

7976 **Post-Polio Health International**
4207 Lindell Blvd
Ste 110
Saint Louis, MO 63108-2930 314-534-0475
FAX: 314-534-5070
e-mail: info@post-polio.org
www.post-polio.org

Joan L Headley, Executive Director
Gayla Hoffman, Editor
Sheryl R. Rudy, Editor
Judith Raymond Fischer, MSLS, Editor

Educates, advocates and networks the survivors of polio and the health professionals who treat them. Funds a research grant, publishes Post Polio Health (Quarterly, 12 page newsletter).

7977 Society for Progressive Supranuclear Palsy
30 E. Padonia Road,
Suite 201
Timonium, MD 21093
800-457-4777
FAX: 410-785-7009
e-mail: info@curepsp.org
www.psp.org

Janet Edmunson, Med, Chair
Dan Johnson, Vice-Chair
George S. Jankiewicz, CPA, CFP,, Treasurer
John T. Burhoe, Secretary
Members of the Board of Directors of CurePSP accept the major responsibility of implementing the mission of the Foundation for PSP | CBD and Related Brain Diseases. Board members are actively involved in continually defining and redefining the mission and participating in strategic planning to review purposes, programs, priorities, funding needs, and levels of achievement.

7978 Vermont Back Research Center
1 S Prospect St
Burlington, VT 05405
802-656-3131
FAX: 802-660-9243
e-mail: learn@uvm.edu
www.uvm.edu

7979 World Chiropractic Alliance
2683 Via De La Valle
Suite G 629
Del Mar, CA 92014
480-786-9235
866-789-8073
FAX: 480-732-9313
e-mail: comments@worldchiropracticalliance.org
www.worldchiropracticalliance.org

Linda Bevel, Manager
Terry A Rondberg DC, Founder/CEO
The World Chiropractic Alliance was founded in 1989 as a non-profit organization dedicated to protecting and strengthening chiropractic around the world. Since its inception, the WCA has played an important role in the global chiropractic community. In 1998, it was granted status as a Non-Governmental Organization (NGO) associated with the United Nations Department of Public Information.

Camps

7980 Autism Day Camp
Hillcroft Services: Isanogel
114 E. Streeter Avenue
Muncie, IN 47304
765-288-1073
FAX: 765-288-3101
TTY:765-288-1073
e-mail: demcintosh@bsu.edu
www.hillcroft.org

Ted Baker, Chair
Brenda Llyod, Vice Chair
Bruce Baldwin, Director
Julie Bering, Secretary/ Treasurer
The camp is designed to improve the academic, social skills, and behaviors of children with autism spectrum disorders. The day camp is an 8-week intensive experience for children classified with autism spectrum disorders.

7981 Camp Esperanza
Southern California Chapter
West 6th Street
Suite 1250
Los Angeles, CA 90017
323-954-5760
800-954-2873
FAX: 213-954-5790
e-mail: jziegler@arthritis.org
www.arthritis.org

Jennifer Ziegler, Camp Director
Lindsey Gonzales, Regional Director, Human Resources
Manuel Loya, Chief Executive Officer
Teri Lim, Chief Marketing Officer
A one-week camp in August that allows children with arthritis to participate in such activities as horseback riding, swimming, etc. in a fun-filled environment.

7982 Camp Oakhurst
New York Service for the Handicapped
111 Monmouth Rd
Oakhurst, NJ 7755-1514
732-531-0215
FAX: 732-531-0292
e-mail: info@nysh.org
www.nysh.org

Robert Pacenza, Executive Director:
Charles Sutherland, Camp Director
Camp Oakhurst, established in 1906, is operated by New York Service for the Handicapped (NYSH), an independent non-profit social service agency with offices in New York City and Oakhurst, New Jersey.

7983 Easter Seals Camp Stand by Me
Easter Seal Society of Washington
17809 S. Vaughn Road KPN
PO Box 289
Vaughn, WA 98394-313
253-884-2722
FAX: 253-590-0594
e-mail: camp@wa.easterseals.com
www.wa.easterseals.com

Cathy Bisaillon, President/Camp Director
Jennifer Ting, Board Chair
Dr. Tim Johnson, Vice Chair
Charissa Manglona, Secretary
Camp Stand By Me provides a safe, barrier-free environment for children and adults to experience all aspects of camp without limitations.

7984 Summer Wheelchair Sports Camp
University of Illinois
1207 S Oak St
Champaign, IL 61820-6901
217-333-4606
FAX: 217-244-0014
TTY:217-244-9738
e-mail: sportscamp@illinois.edu
www.disability.illinois.edu

Brian Walsh, Camp Director
Kim Collins, Asst. Dir., Academic Disability Support Services
Pat Malik, Asst. Dir., Non-Academic Disability Support Services
Angella Anderson, Disability Specialist, Accessible Media
Rigorous camps designed for individuals with lower extremity physical disabilities. Camp attendees will spend an average of 8-9 hours a day, focusing on development and refinement of fitness, techniques and strategies. Strength training, nutrition and mental training sessions will also be included in all camps. The camp staff is comprised of athletic staff and faculty front, the Division of Rehabilitation Education Services and local wheelchair athletes with coaching experience.

7985 Twin Lakes Camp
1451 E Twin Lakes Rd
Hillsboro, IN 47949-8004
765-798-4000
e-mail: outdoors@twinlakescamp.com
www.twinlakescamp.com

Jon Beight, Executive Director
Duane Bush, Guest Service
Dan Daily, Program Director
Donna Beight, Secretary

Provides a summer camp program for special needs children and young adults. Campers suffer from a wide range of maladies including crippling accidents, Spina Bifida, epilepsy, Cerebral Palsy, Muscular Dystrophy, Quadriplegia, Paraplegia, and other disabling diseases. Campers range in age from 8 to 27.

7986 **YMCA Camp Fitch**
Youngstown YMCA
17 N Champion St
P.O. Box 1287
Youngstown, OH 44501 330-744-8411
FAX: 330-744-8415
e-mail: info@campfitchymca.com
www.youngstownymca.org

Thomas Fleming, Chair/ CVO
James B. Greene, 1st Vice chiar
Thomas Gacse, 2nd Vice chiar
Donald Harrison, 3rd Vice chiar

Camp is located in North Springfield, Pennsylvania. Camping sessions for children and adults with diabetes, hearing impairment, developmental disabilities, mobility limitation and speech/communication impairment. Ages 8-16, families and seniors.

Print: Books

7987 **Adapted Physical Education and Sport**
Human Kinetics, Inc.
1607 N Market Street
Champaign, IL 61820-2220 217-351-5076
800-747-4457
FAX: 217-351-1549
e-mail: info@hkusa.com
www.naspem.org

Joseph P Winnick EdD, Author
Scott Kimberly, Owner
Rainer Martens, President/Treasurer
Jill Wikgren, COO

Designed as a resource for both present and future physical education leaders, this book is an exceptional book for teaching exceptional children. It emphasizes the physical education of young people with disabilities. *$68.00*
592 pages Hardcover
ISBN 0-736052-16-X

7988 **Arthritis Bible**
Inner Traditions - Bear & Company
PO Box 388
Rochester, VT 05767-0388 802-767-3174
800-246-8648
FAX: 802-767-3726
e-mail: customerservice@innertraditions.com
www.innertraditions.com

Craig Weatherby, Author
Leonid Gordin MD, Co-Author

A comprehensive guide to the alternative therapies and conventional treatments for Arthritic diseases including Osteoarthritis, Rheumatoid Arthritis, Gout, Fibromyalgia and more. *$16.95*
272 pages Paperback 1999
ISBN 0-892818-25-5

7989 **Arthritis Helpbook: A Tested Self Management Program for Coping with Arthritis**
Da Capo Press
44 Farnsworth Street,
Boston, MA 02210 617-252-5200
FAX: 617-252-5265
www.dacapopress.com

Kate Lorig, Author
James Fries, Co-Author

The Arthritis Helpbook is the world's leading guide to coping with joint pain, and has been used by more than 600,000 readers over its twenty years in print. It succeeds because of its tested advice, its hundreds of useful hints, and its emphasis on self-management-helping people with arthritis and fibromyalgia to achieve their own health goals. *$18.95*
Paperback
ISBN 0-738210-38-2

7990 **Arthritis Sourcebook**
McGraw-Hill Professional
7500 Chavenelle Rd
Dubuque, IA 52002-9655 563-584-6000
877-833-5524
FAX: 614-759-3749
e-mail: pbg.ecommerce_custserv@mcgraw-hill.com
www.mhprofessional.com

Earl J Brewer Jr MD, Author
Kathy Cochran Angel, Co-Author

A comprehensive guide to the latest information on treatments, medications, and alternative therapies for arthritis. *$ 16.95*
272 pages Paperback
ISBN 0-737303-81-6

7991 **Arthritis, What Exercises Work: Breakthrough Relief for the Rest of Your Life**
MacMillan - St. Martin's Press
175 5th Ave
New York, NY 10010-7703 646-307-5151
FAX: 212-420-9314
e-mail: press.inquiries@macmillanusa.com
www.us.macmillan.com

Dava Sorbel, Author
Arthur C Klein, Co-Author

What is the most powerful arthritis treatment ever developed to help restore you to a healthy, pain-free, and vigorous life—for the rest of your life? It's exercise. Here are the right exercised for your kind of arthritis, pain-level, age, occupation, and hobbies. *$14.99*
200 pages Paperback 1995
ISBN 0-312130-25-2

7992 **Arthritis: A Take Care of Yourself Health Guide**
Da Capo Press
44 Farnsworth Street,
Boston, MA 02210 617-252-5200
FAX: 617-252-5265
www.dacapopress.com

James F Fries, Author
Donald M Vickery, Co-Author

In this updated book the author draws on new research to recommend exercises and new pain medications for both arthritis and fibromyalgia. *$18.95*
Paperback 1909
ISBN 0-738202-25-8

7993 **Disability and Sport**
Human Kinetics, Inc.
1607 N Market Street
Champaign, IL 61820-2220 217-351-5076
800-747-4457
FAX: 217-351-1549
e-mail: info@hkusa.com
www.naspem.org

Karen P DePauw, Author
Susan J Gavron, Co-Author
Scott Kimberley, Owner
Rainer Martens, President/Treasurer

Provides a comprehensive and practical look at the past, present, and future of disability sport. Topics covered are inclusive of youth through adult participation with in-depth coverage of the essential issues involving athletes with disabilities. This new edition has updated references and new chapter-opening outlines that assist with individual study and class discussions. *$48.00*
408 pages Hardcover
ISBN 0-736046-38-0

7994 Fitness Programming for Physical Disabilities
Human Kinetics, Inc.
1607 N Market Street
Champaign, IL 61820-2220
217-351-5076
800-747-4457
FAX: 217-351-1549
e-mail: info@hkusa.com
www.naspem.org

Patricia D Miller, Editor
Scott Kimberley, Owner
Rainer Martens, President/Treasurer
Jill Wikgren, COO

A book offering information for developing and conducting exercise programs for groups that included people with physical disabilities. A dozen authorities in exercise science and adapted exercise programming explain how to effectively and safely modify existing programs for individuals with physical disabilities. *$42.00*
232 pages Paperback
ISBN 0-873224-34-5

7995 Freedom from Arthritis Through Nutrition
Tree of Life Publications
PO Box 126
Joshua Tree, CA 92252-0126
760-366-2937
FAX: 760-366-2937
e-mail: office@booxr.us
www.treelifebooks.com

Philip J Welsh DDS ND, Author
Bianca Leonardo ND, Co-Author

Reveals the results of 60 years of research on arthritis by noted nutritionist, Dr. Philip J. Welsh, D.D.S. N.D. Here you will find simple, natural, inexpensive, tested ways of coping with the various forms of arthritis, using only nutrition and other natural methods. There are no drugs or gadgets in this program. *$24.95*
255 pages Softcover

7996 Functional Electrical Stimulation for Ambulation by Paraplegics
Krieger Publishing Company
1725 Krieger Drive
PO Box 9542
Malabar, FL 32950
321-724-9542
800-724-0025
FAX: 321-951-3671
e-mail: info@krieger-publishing.com
www.krieger-publishing.com

Daniel Graupe, Author
Kate H Kohn, Co-Author

FES is employed to enable spinal cord injury patients who are complete paraplegics to stand and ambulate without bracing. The text covers 12 years of amulation experience. *$49.50*
210 pages Paperback 1994
ISBN 0-894648-45-4

7997 Guide to Managing Your Arthritis
Arthritis Foundation
1330 W. Peachtree St
Suite 100
Atlanta, GA 30309
404-872-7100
800-283-7800
FAX: 404-237-8153
e-mail: AFOrders@pbd.com
www.arthritis.org

Mary Anne Dunkin, Author
John Klippel, President/CEO
Cecile Perich, Chairman
William Brackney, Vice Chair

Expert reviewers answer questions about basic arthritis facts, treatments, research, surgery and more. Also, specific information about six common conditions: rheumatoid arthritis, osteoarthritis, osteoporosis, fibromyalgia, lupus and gout. *$9.95*
193 pages Paperback
ISBN 0-912423-28-5

7998 How to Deal with Back Pain and Rheumatoid Joint Pain: A Preventive and Self Treatment Manua
Global Health Solutions
2146 Kings Garden Way
Falls Church, VA 22043-2593
703-848-2333
800-759-3999
FAX: 703-848-0028
e-mail: information@watercure.com
www.watercure.com

Fereydoon Batmanghelidj, Author
Xiaopo Batmanjhelidj, President
Kristin Swan, Administrator

The physiology of pain production and its direct relationship to chronic regional dehydration of some joint spaces is explained: Special movements that would create vacuum in the disc spaces and draw water and the displaced discs into the vertebral joints are demonstrated. *$14.95*
100 pages Paperback
ISBN 0-962994-20-0

7999 Inclusive Games
Human Kinetics
1607 N Market Street
PO Box 5076
Champaign, IL 61825- 5076
217-351-5076
800-747-4457
FAX: 217-351-1549
e-mail: info@hkusa.com
www.humankinetics.com

Susan L Kasser, Author
Scott Kimberley, Owner
Rainer Martens, President/Treasurer
Jill Wikgren, COO

Features more than 50 games, helpful illustrations, and hundreds of game variations. The book shows how to adapt games so that children of every ability level can practice, play and improve their movement skills together. The game finder makes it easy to locate an appropriate game according to its name, approximate grade level, difficulty within the grade level, skills required/developed, and number of players. *$17.95*
120 pages Paperback
ISBN 0-873226-39-9

8000 Inside The Halo and Beyond: The Anatomy of a Recovery
WW Norton & Company
500 5th Ave
New York, NY 10110-2
212-354-5500
FAX: 212-869-0856
www.wwnorton.com

Maxine Kumin, Author
W Drake McFeely, Chairman/President
Stephen King, VP Finance/CFO
Robert Weil, VP/Executive Editor

A skilled horsewoman and lifelong athlete, poet Kumin was 73 when a riding accident left her with two broken vertebrae in her neck. Kumin survived in the face of overwhelming odds that she would be paralyzed for the rest of her life. Miraculously, however, she was walking again within weeks of the accident; now, though one hand and an arm remain partially immobilized, her life has largely resumed its normal course. Here is the journal of her first nine months of recovery. *$ 13.95*
192 pages Softcover
ISBN 0-393049-00-0

8001 Life on Wheels: For the Active Wheelchair User
Patient-Centered Guides
1005 Gravenstein Hwy North
Sebastopol, CA 95472-2811
707-827-7000
800-998-9938
FAX: 707-829-0104
e-mail: order@oreilly.com
www.oreilly.com

Gary Karp, Author

For 1.5 million Americans, life includes a wheelchair for mobility. Life on Wheels is for people who want to take charge of their life experience. Author Gary Karp describes medical issues (paralysis, circulation, rehab, cure research); day-to-day living (exercise, skin, bowel and bladder, sexuality, home access,

maintaining a wheelchair); and social issues (self-image, adjustment, friends, family, cultural attitudes, activism). *$24.95*
565 pages Paperback 1999
ISBN 1-565922-53-0

8002 Paralysis Resource Guide
Christopher and Dana Reeve Paralysis Resource Ctr
636 Morris Turnpike
Suite 3A
Short Hills, NJ 07078
973-467-8270
800-539-7309
FAX: 973-912-9433
e-mail: information@christopherreeve.org
www.paralysis.org

John M. Hughes, Chairman
John E. McConnell, Vice Chair
Matthew Reeve, Vice Chair
Peter T. Wilderotter, President

A comprehensive information tool for people affected by paralysis and for those who care for them. English or Spanish.
336 pages

8003 Primer on the Rheumatic Diseases
Arthritis Foundation
1330 W. Peachtree St
Suite 100
Atlanta, GA 30309-2111
404-872-7100
800-933-7023
FAX: 404-237-8153
e-mail: AFOrders@pbd.com
www.arthritis.org

Rob Shaw, President
Patience White M.D., Editor
John H. Klippel, Editor

The leading professional book about arthritis and related diseases, the Primer is published by Springer and the Arthritis Foundation. *$79.95*
724 pages Softcover
ISBN 0-387356-64-8

8004 Sport Science Review: Adapted Physical Activity
Human Kinetics
1607 N Market Street
Champaign, IL 61820-2220
217-351-5076
800-747-4457
FAX: 217-351-1549
e-mail: info@hkusa.com
www.naspem.org

Rainer Martens, President/Treasurer
Scott Kimberley, Owner
Jill Wikgren, COO

This issue of Sport Science Review examines the newly emerging academic discipline of adapted physical activity. Researchers from diverse academic backgrounds and parts of the world review the issues and controversies surrounding inclusion in physical education and sport. *$15.00*
96 pages Paperback
ISBN -073602-07-9

8005 Still Me
Random House
1745 Broadway
3rd Floor
New York, NY 10019-4305
212-782-9000
FAX: 212-572-6066
e-mail: vintageanchor@randomhouse.com
www.randomhouse.com

Christopher Reeve, Author
Markus Dohle, Chairman/CEO
Madeline McIntosh, President
Andrew Weber, SVP Operations

The man who was Superman begins with his debilitating riding accident, then weaves back and forth between past and present, creating a thorough biography of Reeve's life. *$7.99*
336 pages Paperback 1999
ISBN 0-345432-41-4

8006 When Your Student Has Arthritis
Arthritis Foundation
2970 Peachtree Rd NW
PO Box 932915, Ste 200
Atlanta, GA 31193-2915
404-237-8771
800-933-7023
FAX: 404-237-8153
e-mail: aforders@arthritis.org
www.afstore.org

Rob Shaw, President

An overview of arthritis, including juvenile rhuematoid arthritis and treatment. Also includes a school activities checklist for students, education rights, and how teachers can help.
28 pages

8007 Yoga for Fibromyalgia: Move, Breathe, and Relax to Improve Your Quality of Life
Mobility Limited
PO Box 838
Morro Bay, CA 93443-0838
805-772-3560
800-366-6038
FAX: 805-772-4717
e-mail: shsh@mobilityltd.com
www.mobilityltd.com

Shoosh Lettick Crotzer, Director

The first book devoted exclusively to managing the symptoms of fibromyalgia; the comprehensive program of 26 illustrated poses, breathing techniques, and guided visualization and relaxation sessions can be practiced regardless of age or experience. The Living with Fibromyalgia section discusses lifestyle concerns. *$14.95*
128 pages 1908

Print: Magazines

8008 Arthritis Today
Arthritis Foundation
1330 W. Peachtree St.
Suite 100
Atlanta, GA 30309
404-872-7100
800-933-7023
FAX: 404-237-8153
e-mail: info.ga@arthritis.org
www.arthritis.org

Dan McGowan, Chairman
Rowland W. Chang, Vice Chair
Ann M. Palmer, President and CEO
Patricia N. Nelson, Secretary

Magazine for patients, physicians, public authorities and others with an interest in the field of arthritis. (Price noted paid for yearly subscription) *$12.95*
Bi-Monthly

8009 Fibromyalgia AWARE Magazine
National Fibromyalgia Association
2121 S Towne Centre Pl
suite 30
Orange, CA 92865-6124
714-921-0150
FAX: 714-921-6920
e-mail: paird@fmaware.org
fmaware.org

Lynne Matallana, Editor In Chief
Malina Anderson, CFO
Eroll Landy, Treasurer

Addresses the needs and concerns of people affected by fibromyalgia and overlapping conditions. *$35.00*
3 times a year

8010 **New Mobility**
Leonard Media Group
75-20 Astoria Blvd.
East Elmhurst, NY 11370-2068
215-675-9133
888-850-0344
FAX: 215-675-9376
e-mail: jeff@leonardmedia.com
www.newmobility.com

Amy Blackmore, Vice President Sales
Jean Dobbs, Editorial Director
Tim Gilmer, Editor
Josie Byzek, Managing Editor
The full-service, full-color lifestyle magazine for the disability community. The award-winning magazine is contemporary, witty and candid. Produced by professional journalists and visual artists, the magazine's voice is uncompromising and unsentimental, yet practical, knowing and friendly. The magazine covers issues that matter to readers: medical news, and cure research; jobs, benefits and civil rights; sports, recreation and travel; product news, technology and innovation. *$27.95*
Monthly

8011 **PALAESTRA: Forum of Sport, Physical Education and Recreation for Those with Disabilities**
Challenge Publications Limited
1807 N. Federal Drive
Urbana, IL 61801
217-359-5940
800-327-5557
FAX: 217-359-5975
e-mail: challpub@macomb.com
www.palaestra.com

David P Beaver EdD, Fonding Editor
Martin.E Block, Editor-in-Chief
Julian U. Stein, Associate Editor
Kathleen Stanton, Asst. Editors
The most comprehensive resource on sport, physical education and recreation for individuals with disabilities, their parents and professionals in the field of adapted physical activity. Published in cooperation with US Paralympics and AAHPERD's Adapted Physical Activity Council. Informative yet entertaining and delivers valuable insights for consumers, families and professionals in the field. Published quarterly.

8012 **PN/Paraplegia News**
PVA Publications
2111 E Highland Ave
Suite 180
Phoenix, AZ 85016-4702
602-224-0500
888-888-2201
FAX: 602-224-0507
e-mail: info@pnnews.com
www.pn-magazine.com

Richard Hoover, Editor
Ann Santos, Assistant Editor
Packed with timely information on spinal-cord-injury research, new products, legislation that impacts people with disabilities, accessible travel, computer options, car/van adaptations, news for veterans, housing, employment, health care and all issues affecting wheelers and caregivers around the world.

8013 **Spirit Magazine**
Special Olympics International
1133 19th St NW
Washington, DC 20036-3604
202-628-3630
FAX: 202-824-0200
e-mail: info@specialolympics.org
www.specialolympics.org

Kathy Smallwood, Editor
Timothy P Shriver PhD, Chariman/CEO
J Brady Lum, President/COO
This magazine reflects the power of Special Olympics to build bridges between people with and without intellectual disabilities and spark personal insight, compassion and gratitude for life.
Quarterly

8014 **Strides Magazine**
North American Riding for the Handicapped Assoc
7475 Dakin Street
Suite 600
Denver, CO 80221-6920
303-452-1212
800-369-7433
FAX: 303-252-4610
e-mail: narha@narha.org
www.narha.org

Carol Nickell, CEO
Sheila Dietrich, Executive Director
William Scebbi, CEO
This engaging magazine is a non-technical, yet accurate journal that focuses on the work of NARHA. Rider profiles, how-to articles, editorials and instructional columns seek to educate a general readership of the diverse aspects of equine facilitated therapy and activities. Each seasonal issue carries a theme.
Quarterly

8015 **Stroke Connection Magazine**
American Stroke Association
7272 Greenville Ave
Dallas, TX 75231-5129
214-373-6300
888-478-7653
FAX: 214-706-1191
www.strokeassociation.org

Ralph Sacco, President/Director
Nancy Brown, CEO
Debra Lockwood, Chairman
From in-depth information on conditions such as aphasia, central pain, high blood pressure and depression, to tips for daily living from healthcare professionals and other stroke survivors. Stroke Connection keeps you abreast of how to cope, how to reduce your risk of stroke and how to make the most of each day.
6 issues

Print: Newsletters

8016 **Arthritis Foundation Great West Region**
Arthritis Foundation
115 N.E. 100th St
Suite 350
Seattle, WA 98125
206-547-2707
888-391-9389
FAX: 206-547-2805
e-mail: tzuehl@arthritis.org
www.arthritis.org

Scott Weaver, CEO
Kelsey Birnbaum, Vice President, Development
Deborah Genge, Vice President, Development
Duane Hille, Development Coordinator
Offers regional updates, information on activities and events, resources and medical research for members.
Newsletter

8017 **Arthritis Update**
Arthritis Foundation
1330 W. Peachtree St.
Suite 100
Atlanta, GA 30309
404-872-7100
e-mail: info.uny@arthritis.org
www.arthritis.org

Dan McGowan, Chairman
Rowland W. Chang, Vice Chair
Ann M. Palmer, President and CEO
Patricia N. Nelson, Secretary
Offers chapter updates, information on activities and events, resources and medical research for members.
Newsletter

8018 **Focus**
Arthritis Foundation
1330 W. Peachtree St.
Suite 100
Atlanta, GA 30309
404-872-7100
e-mail: info.coh@arthritis.org
www.arthritis.org

Dan McGowan, Chairman
Rowland W. Chang, Vice Chair
Ann M. Palmer, President and CEO
Patricia N. Nelson, Secretary
Offers chapter updates, information on activities and events, resources and medical research for members.
Newsletter

8019 **Joint Efforts**
Arthritis Foundation
1330 W. Peachtree St.
Suite 100
Atlanta, GA 30309
404-872-7100
800-464-6240
FAX: 415-356-1240
e-mail: info.nca@arthritis.org
www.arthritis.org

Dan McGowan, Chairman
Rowland W. Chang, Vice Chair
Ann M. Palmer, President and CEO
Patricia N. Nelson, Secretary
Offers chapter updates, information on activities and events, resources and medical research for members.
Newsletter

8020 **Post-Polio Newsletter**
Post-Polio Health International
4207 Lindell Blvd
Ste 110
Saint Louis, MO 63108-2930
314-534-0475
FAX: 314-534-5070
e-mail: info@post-polio.org
www.post-polio.org

Joan Headley, Executive Director
Gayla Hoffman, Editor
Contains current information about the late effects of polio, updates about post-polio related and neuromuscular respiratory research, as well as articles that offer practical and useful advice by experienced survivors and health care professionals. Available with membership.
12 pages Quarterly

8021 **SCILIFE**
National Spinal Cord Injury Association
75-20 Astoria Blvd
East Elmhurst, NY 11370
718-803-3782
800-404-2898
FAX: 718-803-0414
e-mail: info@spinalcord.org
www.unitedspinal.org

David C. Cooper, Chairman
Patrick W. Maher, Vice Chairman
Joseph Gaskins, President and CEO
Denise A. McQuade, Secretary
Filled with issue-driven articles, and news of interest to the SCI community and the larger disability community.
Bi-monthly

Non Print: Newsletters

8022 **A World Awaits You**
Mobility International USA
132 E Broadway
Suite 343
Eugene, OR 97401-3155
541-343-1284
FAX: 541-343-6812
e-mail: clearinghouse@miusa.org
www.miusa.org

Susan Sygall, Executive Director
Includes interviews with people with disabilities who have participated in a wide range of international exchange programs.

8023 **ABS Newsletter**
American Back Society
2648 International Blvd
Suite 502
Oakland, CA 94601-1547
510-536-9929
FAX: 510-536-1812
e-mail: info@americanbacksoc.org
www.americanbacksoc.org

Scott Haldeman, President
Aubrey Swartz MD, Executive Director
Keeps subscribers current with timely topics on the diagnosis and treatment of a wide spectrum of painful and disabling conditions of the spine.

8024 **CurePSP Magazine**
Society for Progressive Supranuclear Palsy
2648 International Blvd
Suite 502
Hunt Valley, MD 21031-1002
410-785-7004
800-457-4777
FAX: 410-785-7009
e-mail: info@curepsp.org
www.psp.org

Richard Gordon Dyne DMin, President
Janet Edmunson, Chair
Dan Johnson, Vice Chair
Informs readers of findings in the area of PSP.

8025 **EpilepsyUSA Magazine**
Epilepsy Foundation of America
8301 Professional Pl
Landover, MD 20785-2237
301-459-3700
FAX: 301-577-2684
www.epilepsyfoundation.org

Brien J Smith Md, Chair
Mark E Nini, Senior Vice Chair
Richard P Denness, President/CEO
Alexandra K Finucane Esq, Executive Vice President
The Epilepsy Foundation's award-winning magazine, epilepsyUSA, is published online four times a year. The magazine is one of the only publications of its kind devoted entirely to news and up-to-the-minute information about epilepsy.

8026 **Exchange**
ALS Association
27001 Agoura Rd
Suite 250
Agoura Hills, CA 91301-5105
818-340-0182
800-782-4747
FAX: 818-880-9006
e-mail: webmaster@alsa.org
www.alsa.org

Gary A Leo, CEO
Morton Charlestein, Chairman
Andrew Soffel, Chairman
Julie Sharpe, Executive Director
Covers a broad range of subjects including stories about the lives of ALS patients, special events, research and public policy in the ALS community.
4-6 times/year

8027 Fibromyalgia Online
National Fibromyalgia Association
2121 S Towne Centre Pl
suite 300
Ornage, CA 92865-6124 714-921-0150
FAX: 714-921-6920
www.fmaware.org

Lynne Matallana, President/Editor In Chief
Malina Anderson, CFO
Eroll Landy, Treasurer
An educational resource for patients and healthcare professionals that brings the latest news on fibrmyalgia and overlapping conditions.
Monthly

8028 MIUSA's Global Impact Newsletter
Mobility International USA
132 E. Broadway
Suite 343
Eugene, OR 97401-2767 541-343-1284
FAX: 541-343-6812
e-mail: info@miusa.org
www.miusa.org

Susan Sygall, Executive Director
Cindy Lewis, Director
Olivia Hardin, Information Services Coordinator
Each issue features photos, alumni updates, highlights from recent activities, and new publications.
semi-annually

8029 Motivator
Multiple Sclerosis Association of America
706 Haddonfield Rd
Cherry Hill, NJ 8002-2652 856-488-4500
800-532-7667
FAX: 856-661-9797
e-mail: jmasino@mymsaa.org
www.msassociation.org

Andrea L GriesS, Editor
Susan W Courtney, Sr Writer & Creative Director
Amanda Bednar, Contributing Writer
MSAA's 48-plus page magazine highlights and explains many vital issues of importance to our readers affected by MS. These include cover and feature stories about a variety of topics such as depression, assistive technology, the role of pets and service animals, parents with MS, and clinical trials, to name a few.
48 pages Quarterly

8030 New York Arthritis Reporter
New York Chapter of the Arthritis Foundation
122 East 42nd Street
New York, NY 10168-1898 212-984-8700
FAX: 212-878-5960
e-mail: info.ny@arthritis.org
www.arthritis.org

Phyllis Geraghty, Editor
Ross Alfieri, President
Daniel T. McGowan, Chair
Provides public access to current arthritis information and resources on important health issues.
Quarterly

8031 SCI Psychosocial Process
American Assoc of Spinal Cord Injury Psych/Soc Wor
75-20 Astoria Blvd
East Elmhurst, NY 11370 718-803-3782
800-404-2898
FAX: 718-803-0414
e-mail: info@unitedspinal.org
www.unitedspinal.org

David C. Cooper, Chairman
Patrick W. Maher, Vice Chairman
Joseph Gaskins, President and CEO
Denise A. McQuade, Secretary
The purpose of this e journal is disseminating information of value to psychologists, social workers and other psychological caring for spinal cord injured persons.
2 time a year

Non Print: Video

8032 A Wheelchair for Petronilia
Fanlight Productions C/O Icarus Films
32 Court St.
21st Floor
Brooklyn, NY 11201-1731 718-488-8900
800-876-1710
FAX: 718-488-8642
e-mail: info@fanlight.com
www.fanlight.com

Bob Gliner, Director
Jonathan Miller, President
Meredith Miller, Sales Manager
Anthony Sweeney, Acquisitions
Profiles a program, organized and run by Guatemalans with disabilities, which trains them to manufacture and repair cheap, sturdy wheelchairs designed for conditions in developing countries. 28 Minutes.
VHS/DVD
ISBN 1-572953-98-5

8033 Beyond the Barriers
Aquarius Health Care Videos
30 Forest Road
PO Box 249
Millis, MA 02054 508-376-1244
888-440-2963
FAX: 508-376-1245
www.aquariusproductions.com

Mark Wellman, Director
Leslie Kussmann, President/Producer
For too many years, paraplegics, amputees, quadraplegics and the blind have felt trapped by their disabilities. No more! Mark Wellman and other disabled adventurers, rock climb the desert towers of Utah, sail in British Columbia, body-board the big waves of Pipeline and Waimea Bay, scuba dive with sea lions in Mexico and hand glide the California coast. This film delivers the simple message: Don't give up, and never give in. If you can't ever lose, then you can't ever win. Preview option.
Video/47 Mins

8034 Breathing Lessons: The Life and Work of Mark O'Brien
Fanlight Productions C/O Icarus Films
32 Court St.
21st Floor
Brooklyn, NY 11201-1731 718-488-8900
800-876-1710
FAX: 718-488-8642
e-mail: info@fanlight.com
www.fanlight.com

Jessica Yu, Director
Jonathan Miller, President
Meredith Miller, Sales Manager
Anthony Sweeney, Acquisitions
Breathing Lessons breaks down barriers to understanding by presenting an honest and intimate portrait of a complex, intelligent, beautiful and interesting person, who happens to be disabled.
$225.00
Video/35 Mins 1996
ISBN 1-572958-41-3

8035 Complete Armchair Fitness
CC-M Productions
7755 16th St NW
Washington, DC 20012-1460 202-882-7432
800-453-6280
FAX: 202-882-7432
e-mail: info@armchairfitness.com
www.armchairfitness.com

Robert Mason, Manager

Armchair Fitness video series. 4 DVDs: Armchair Fitness Aerobic, Armchair Fitness Gentle, Armchair Fitness Strength and Armchair Fitness Yoga. *$120.00*
Video

8036 How Come You Walk Funny?
Fanlight Productions C/O Icarus Films
32 Court St.
21st Floor
Brooklyn, NY 11201-1731
718-488-8900
800-876-1710
FAX: 718-488-8642
e-mail: info@fanlight.com
www.fanlight.com

Tina Hahn, Director
Jonathan Miller, President
Meredith Miller, Sales Manager
Anthony Sweeney, Acquisitions
Profiles a unique experiment in reverse integration: a school where non disabled kids attend a kindergarten designed for children with physical disabilities. The kids and families tackle their differences and discover common ground through finding a way that all can play. *$ 179.00*
Video/47 Mins 2004
ISBN 1-572958-84-7

8037 Key Changes: A Portrait of Lisa Thorson
Fanlight Productions C/O Icarus Films
32 Court St.
21st Floor
Brooklyn, NY 11201-1731
718-488-8900
800-876-1710
FAX: 718-488-8642
e-mail: info@fanlight.com
www.fanlight.com

Cindy Marshall, Director
Jonathan Miller, President
Meredith Miller, Sales Manager
Anthony Sweeney, Acquisitions
A documentary profiling Lisa Thorson, a gifted vocalist who uses a wheelchair. Ms. Thorson defines herself as a performer first, a person with a disability second, and this thoughtful portrait respects that distinction. Her work as a jazz singer is at the heart of the film, reflecting her philosophy that the biggest contribution that she can make to the struggle for the rights of people with disabilities is doing her art the best way she can. *$149.00*
Video/28 Mins 1993
ISBN 1-572959-30-4

8038 Wheelchair Bowling
American Wheelchair Bowling Association
PO Box 69
Clover, VA 24534-69
434-454-2269
FAX: 434-454-6276
e-mail: garyryan210@gmail.com
www.awba.org

Dick Schaaf, Author
Dave Roberts, Executive Secretary Treasurer
In addition to providing historical background, it includes principles of the game from keeping score through ball drilling for the wheelchair bowler. Through profiles of wheelchair bowlers, the text covers ball delivery, spare making techniques and special equipment that can be used. *$9.95*
96 pages

8039 Yoga for Arthritis
Mobility Limited
601 Morro Bay Blvd
Suite E
Morro Bay, CA 93442-2000
805-772-3560
800-366-6038
FAX: 805-772-4717
e-mail: shsh@mobilityltd.com
www.mobilityltd.com

Shoosh Crotzer, Owner/Executive Director
A yoga-based program with five separate segments, which includes breathing and relaxation techniques, stretching and strengthening routines, and aerobic exercises. This 52-minute program can also be performed seated. Available on DVD or VHS; DVD includes Spanish version. *$19.95*
Video

8040 Yoga for MS and Related Conditions
Mobility Limited
601 Morro Bay Blvd
Suite E
Morro Bay, CA 93442-2000
805-772-3560
800-366-6038
FAX: 805-772-4717
e-mail: shsh@mobilityltd.com
www.mobilityltd.com

Shoosh Crotzer, Owner/Executive Director
A yoga-based program. Shows assisted versions of each exercise for those who require it; is available with an optional Instructional Guidebook with illustrations, alternative positions, and hints. This 48-minute program can also be performed seated. Available on DVD or VHS; DVD includes Spanish version. *$19.95*
Video

Sports

8041 Access to Sailing
423 E Shoreline Village Drive
Long Beach, CA 90802
562-901-9999

e-mail: info@accesstosailing.org
www.accesstosailing.org

Duncan Milne, Founder/Executive Director
Cliff Larson, Director
Gaile Oslapas, Assistant Director
Provides therapeutic rehabilitation to disabled and disadvantaged children and adults, through interactive sailing outings.

8042 Achilles Track Club
42 West 38th Street
Suite 400
New York, NY 10018-6241
212-354-0300
FAX: 212-354-3978
e-mail: info@achillestrackclub.org
www.achillestrackclub.org

Richard Traum PhD, President/Founder
Mary Bryant, Vice President
Kathleen Bateman, Director
Organization whose goal is to guide disabled athletes into the able-bodied community.

8043 Adaptive Sports Center
PO Box 1639
Crested Butte, CO 81224-1639
970-349-2296
866-349-2296
FAX: 970-349-2077
e-mail: info@adaptivesports.org
www.adaptivesports.org

Christopher Hensley, Executive Director
Chris Read, CTRS Program Director
Ella Fahrlander, Development Director
Erin English, Marketing/Communications Dir.
Year round adaptive, adventure recreation program located at the base of Crested Butte Mountain Resort, Crested Butte ,CO. The Adaptive Sports Centers provides adaptive downhill and cross country ski lessons, ski rentals and snowboarding lessons in the winter. Offers a variety of wilderness based programs in the summer including multi-day trips into the back country, extensive cycling programs, canoeing, and white water rafting.

8044 American Wheelchair Bowling Association
PO Box 69
Clover, VA 24534-69
434-454-2269
FAX: 434-454-6276
e-mail: garyryan210@gmail.com
www.awba.org

Joseph L. Fox, Chairman
Wayne Webber, Vice Chairperson
Paul Kenney, Treasurer
Gary Rayan, Secretary
A non-profit organization, composed of wheelchair bowlers, dedicated to encouraging, developing, and regulating wheelchair bowling and wheelchair bowling leagues.

8045 Basketball School
Alabama Institute for Deaf and Blind
205 South St E
Talladega, AL 35160-2411
256-761-3335
FAX: 256-761-3505
www.aib-aidb.com

Terry Graham, President
John Mascia, Executive Director
Cindy Baker, Director
We offer Class 1A champion football, basketball, volleyball, track and field, soccer and cheerleading. Our students have competed in the international Deaf-Olympics and our teams have won state and national championships in every major sport. We compete against public schools around Alabama and schools for the deaf from across the nation.

8046 Bold Tracks
Big Earth Publishing
3005 Center Green Drive
Suite 225
Boulder, CO 80301
800-258-5830
FAX: 303-443-9687
e-mail: books@bigearthpublishing.com
www.bigearthpublishing.com

Hal O'Leary, Author
Janet Heisz, Sales Manager
This guide is essential for instructor and student alike. It covers skiing for the visually and hearing impaired as well as the physically and developmentally disabled. *$24.95*
156 pages Paperback
ISBN 1-555661-14-4

8047 Chesapeake Region Accessible Boating
PO Box 6564
Annapolis, MD 21401-564
410-626-0273
FAX: 410-626-6070
e-mail: info@crabsailing.org
www.crab-sailing.org

Daniel Jarzynski, President
Lance Hinrichs, Vice President
Ernie Shineman, Treasurer
Loren Barnett, Secretary
Provides opportunities for the disabled and their friends to sail the Chesapeake Bay. Day sails, lessons, organized races. Call for charter information. Sail for free on the fourth Sunday of each month, May through October.

8048 Disabled Sports Program Center
Disabled Sports USA Far West
PO Box 9780
Truckee, CA 96162-7780
530-581-4161
FAX: 530-581-3127
e-mail: dsusa@disabledsports.net
www.dsusafw.org

Doug Pringle, President
Marilyn Cummings,, Office Manager
Haakon Lang-Ree, Manager
Founded in 1967, Disabled Sports USA Far West is dedicated to innovative programs that provide an environment with positive therapeutic and psychological outcomes. Individuals are empowered to reach their full potential. Our programs allow individuals of all abilities to discover their own strengths and interests.

8049 Disabled Sports USA
451 Hungerford Dr
Suite 100
Rockville, MD 20850-5102
301-217-0960
FAX: 301-217-0968
e-mail: information@dusa.org
www.disabledsportsusa.org

Kirk Bauer, Executive Director
Kathy Chandler, Executive Director
Kathy Celo, Operations
Kathy Laffey, Special Projects Manager
Provides year-round sports and recreation opportunities for people with physical disabilities, veterans and non-veterans alike, such as sanctioned regional and national events in alpine and Nordic skiing, cycling, shooting swimming, table tennis, track and field, volleyball, and weightlifiting. The organization handles physical disabilities which restrict mobility, including amputations paraplegia, quadriplegia, cerebral palsy, head injury, mulitple sclerosis, muscular dystrophy, and more.

8050 Disabled Watersports Program
Mission Bay Aquatic Center
1001 Santa Clara Pl
San Diego, CA 92109
858-488-1000
FAX: 858-488-9625
e-mail: mbac@sdsu.edu
www.missionbayaquaticcenter.com

Kevin Starw, Director
Kevin Waldick, Asst. director
Eric Fehrs, Maintenance Director
Amanda Burgess, Office Supervisor
Devoted to providing accessible water sports and recreational opportunities for individuals with disabilities. Specially designed equipment makes water skiing, wake boarding, keelboat sailing, windsurfing, rowing, surfing, and kayaking possible for people with varying levels of mobility and ability.

8051 Galvin Health and Fitness Center
Rehabilitation Institute of Chicago
345 East Suuperior St.
Chicago, IL 60611
312-238-1000
800-354-7342
800-354-REHA
FAX: 312-238-5017
e-mail: sports@ric.org
http://www.ric.org

Jude Reyes, Chair
Mike P. Kransy, Vice Chair
Thomas Reynolds III, Vice Chair
Joanne C. Smith, President & CEO
The RIC Sports and Fitness Program offers people with physical disabilities an on-site fitness center, specialized exercise classes and services, and adult and junior competitive and recreational sports opportunities, including the recreational/social Caring for Kids program for youth ages 7-17. Most programs are provided free of charge or for a nominal fee.

8052 Guide to Wheelchair Sports and Recreation
Paralyzed Veterans of America
801 18th St NW
Washington, DC 20006-3517
202-872-1300
800-424-8200
888-888-2201
FAX: 202-785-4432
TTY:800-795-4327
e-mail: info@pva.org
www.pva.org

Homer S. Townsend, Jr., Executive Director
Larry Dodson, National Secretary
Bill Lawson, National President
Al Kovach, Jr, Natonal Senior Vice President
This guide is published to introduce and increase awareness of people with disabilities to the many sports and recreational opportunities available. It lists descriptions of adaptive sports and recreation, activity and equipment directories, and additional resources for people with disabilities.
28 pages Booklet

8053 Handicapped Scuba Association International
Handicapped Scuba Association
1104 El Prado
San Clemente, CA 92672-4637 949-498-4540
FAX: 949-498-6128
e-mail: hsa@hsascuba.com
www.hsascuba.com
Jim Gatacre, President
Patricia Derk, Vice President
A nonprofit volunteer organization dedicated to improving the physical and social well being of those with special needs through the exhilarating sport of scuba diving. An educational program for able bodied scuba instructors to learn to teach and certify people with special needs. Accessible travel opportunities.

8054 Lakeshore Foundation
4000 Ridgeway Dr
Birmingham, AL 35209-5563 205-313-7400
FAX: 205-313-7475
e-mail: information@lakeshore.org
www.lakeshore.org
Amy Rauworth, Director of Policy and Public Affairs
Ann O'Nihill, Director of Aquatics
Carol Kutik, Director of Fitness & Health Promotion
Damian Veazey, Associate Director of Communications
Promotes independence for persons with physically disabling conditions and provides opportunities to pursue active, healthy lifestyles.

8055 National Disability Sports Alliance
25 W Independence Way
Kingston, RI 02881-1124 401-792-7130
FAX: 401-792-7132
e-mail: info@ndsaonline.org
http://nationaldisabilitysportsalliance.webs.
Jerry McCole, Executive Director
Serves to present disabled athletes with the opportunity to perform in many different sports. Participants range from the beginning athlete to the elite, international caliber athlete.

8056 National Skeet Shooting Association
5931 Roft Rd
San Antonio, TX 78253-9261 210-688-3371
800-877-5338
FAX: 210-688-3014
e-mail: nsca@nssa-nsca.com
www.mynssa.com
Michael Hampton, Jr., Executive Director
Royce Graff, NSSA Director
Amber Schwarz, NSC Assistant Director
Linda Mayes, NSSA Director
Offers information on sporting clay targets for the disabled hunter.

8057 National Sports Center for the Disabled
33 Parsenn Road
PO Box 1290
Winter Park, CO 80482-1290 303-316-1518
FAX: 970-726-4112
e-mail: info@nscd.org
www.nscd.org
Diane Eustace, Marketing Director
Beth Fox, Operations Director,
Erica Mays, Human Resources Director
Ellen White, Finance Director/CFO
Our mission is to provide quality outdoor sports and therapeutic recreation programs that positively impact the lives of people with physical, cognitive, emotional, or behavioral challenges.
6-8 pages Quarterly

8058 National Wheelchair Poolplayers Association
9757 90 Flemons Drive
Somerville, AL 89178-7511 256-778-0449
FAX: 714-486-2048
www.nwpainc.org
Jeffrey Dolezal, President
Bob Calderon, Secretary
Ken Force, Editor
Works together with other groups, organizations, and tournaments to update rules to include wheelchair players.

8059 North American Riding for the Handicapped Association
7475 Dakin Street
Suite 600
Denver, CO 80221-6920 303-452-1212
800-369-7433
FAX: 303-252-4610
e-mail: narha@narha.org
www.pathintl.org
Sheila Dietrich, Executive Director
Carolyn Malcheski,, Director of Finance and Human Resources
Kaye Marks, Director of Marketing and Communications
Kay Green, Chief Executive Officer
Professional Association of Therapeutic Horsemanship International (PATH Intl.), a federally-registered 501(c3) nonprofit, was formed in 1969 as the North American Riding for the Handicapped Association to promote equine-assisted activities and therapies (EAAT) for individuals with special needs. *$35.00*
42 pages Quarterly

8060 Special Olympics
1133 19th St NW
Washington, DC 20036-3604 202-393-1251
FAX: 202-715-1146
e-mail: info@specialolympics.org
www.specialolympics.org
Timothy P Shriver PhD, Chariman/CEO
J Brady Lum, President/COO
Stephen M Carter, Lead Director/CEO/Vice Chair
A year-round worldwide program that promotes physical fitness, sports training and athletic competition for children and adults with intellectual disabilities.

8061 Special Olympics International
1133 19th St NW
Washington, DC 20036-3604 202-393-1251
FAX: 202-715-1146
e-mail: info@specialolympics.org
www.specialolympics.org
Timothy P Shriver PhD, Chariman/CEO
J Brady Lum, President/COO
Stephen M Carter, Lead Director/CEO/Vice Chair
Provides year-round training and athletic competition in a variety of well-coached, Olympic-type sparts for persons with mental retardation. Offers opportunities to develop physical fitness, prepare for entry into school and community sports programs. Athletes express courage, experience joy and participate in gifts, skills and friendship with their families and other Special Olympics athletes. Local information can be provided by regional offices.

8062 United Foundation for Disabled Archers
20 NE 9th Ave. Glenwood,
PO Box 251
Glenwood, MN 56334- 251 320-634-3660
e-mail: info@uffdaclub.com
www.uffdaclub.com
Daniel James Hendricks, President
Russ Kalk, Vice President
Debbie Kalk, Treasurer
It is the mission of the United Foundation for Disabled Archers to promote and provide a means to practice all forms of archery for any physically challenged person.

8063 **Wheelchair Sports, USA**
PO Box 5266
Kendall Park, NJ 08824-5266 732-266-2634
FAX: 732-355-6500
e-mail: office@wsusa.org
www.wsusa.org

Kelly Behlmann, Owner
Gregg Baumgraten, Chairperson
Denise Hutchins, Vice-Chairperson
Jessica Galli, Secretary
Initiates, stimulates and promotes the growth and development of wheelchair sports.

Support Groups

8064 **Information Hotline**
Arthritis Foundation, Southeast Region Inc
1330 W. Peachtree St.
Suite 100
Atlanta, GA 30309 404-872-7100
800-933-7023
FAX: 404-237-8153
e-mail: info.ga@arthritis.org
www.arthritis.org

Dan McGowan, Chairman
Rowland W. Chang, Vice Chair
Ann M. Palmer, President and CEO
Patricia N. Nelson, Secretary
The mission of the Arthritis Foundation is to improve lives through leadership in the prevention, control and cure of arthritis and related diseases.

8065 **Kids on the Block Programs**
9385 Gerwig Lane
Suite C
Maryland, MD 21157-2893 410-290-9095
800-368-5437
FAX: 410-290-9358
e-mail: kob@kotb.com
www.kotb.com

Aric Darroe, President
Jane Thuman, Vice President
Christina Grogan, Marketing Manager
Features life-size puppets in educational programs that enlighten children and adults on the issues of disability awareness, medical and educational differences, and social concerns.

Specific Disorders

Associations

8066 Academy of Dentistry for Persons with Disabilities
330 North Wabash Avenue,
Suite 2000
Chicago, IL 60611- 4245
312-527-6764
FAX: 312-673-6663
e-mail: scda@scdonline.org
www.scdonline.org

Kristin Dee, Executive Director
Kenneth M. Fedor, DDS, MS, President
Jason Grinter, DDS, President-Elect
Nancy J Dougherty, FADPD, DABS, Vice President

Special Care Dentistry (SCD) is headquartered in Chicago and has a wide ranging membership that includes: dentists, dental hygienists; dental assistants; non-dental health care providers; health program administrators; and others who share our mission. There is also a participating membership category for hospitals, agencies that serve people with special needs and other advocacy and heath care organizations.

8067 Academy of Spinal Cord Injury Professionals
801 18th Street NW
Washington, DC 20006
202-416-7704
FAX: 212-416-7641
www.ascipro.org

Maurice L Jordan, Acting Executive Director
Brenda Finkel, Administrative Assistant

The premier, interdisciplinary organization dedicated to advancing the care of people with spinal cord injury/dysfunction.

8068 Acid Maltase Deficiency Association (AMDA)
PO Box 700248
San Antonio, TX 78270-248
210-494-6144
FAX: 210-490-7161
e-mail: TiffanyLHouse@aol.com
www.amda-pompe.org

Tiffany House, President

The Acid Maltase Deficiency Association was established in 1995 to assist in funding research and to promote public awareness of Pompe disease. Pompe disease is one of a family of 49 rare genetic disorders known as Lysosomal Storage Diseases or LSDs. Pompe disease is also known as Acid Maltase Deficiency or Glycogen Storage Disease type II. It affects an estimated 5,000 to 10,000 people in the developed world.

8069 American Academy of Allergy, Asthma and Immunology
555 E Wells St
Ste 1100
Milwaukee, WI 53202-3823
414-272-6071
FAX: 414-272-6070
e-mail: info@aaaai.org
www.aaaai.org

Dr Mark Ballow FAAAAI, President

The American Academy of Allergy, Asthma & Immunology (AAAAI) is a professional organization with more than 6,700 members in the United States, Canada and 72 other countries. This membership includes allergist / immunologists, other medical specialists, allied health and related healthcare professionals-all with a special interest in the research and treatment of allergic and immunologic diseases.

8070 American Academy of Child and Adolescent Psychiatry
3615 Wisconsin Ave NW
Washington, DC 20016-3007
202-966-7300
FAX: 202-966-2891
e-mail: communications@aacap.org
www.aacap.org

Elizabeth Hughes, Asst. Director of Education & Recertification
Alan Ezagui, Deputy Director of Development
Kristin Kroeger Ptakowski, Director & Sr. Deputy Executive Director
Michael Linskey, Assistant Director, Federal Government Affairs

A 501 (C)(3) nonprofit membership organization composed of over 6,500 child and adolescent psychiatrists. Members actively research, evaluate, diagnose and treat psychiatric disorders and pride themselves on giving direction to and responding quickly to new developments in addressing the health care needs of children and their families.
53 pages

8071 American Academy of Osteopathy
3500 Depauw Blvd,
Ste 1080
Indianapolis, IN 46268-1174
317-879-1881
FAX: 317-879-0563
e-mail: dcole@academyofosteopathy.org
www.academyofosteopathy.org

Diana Finley, Executive Director
Michael Seffinger, President

The mission of the American Academy of Osteopathy is to teach, advocate, and research the science, art and philosophy of osteopathic medicine, emphasizing the integration of osteopathic principles, practice and manipulative treatment in patient care.

8072 American Academy of Otolaryngology: Head and Neck Surgery
1650 Diagonal Rd
Alexandria, VA 22314-2857
703-836-4444
TTY:703-519-1585
www.entnet.org

David Nielson, EVP/CEO
Rodney P Lusk, President
John W. House, Secretary/Treasurer
Michael G. Stewart, MD, MPH, Director - Academic

The American Academy of Otolaryngology-Head and Neck Surgery (AAO-HNS) is the world's largest organization representing specialists who treat the ear, nose, throat, and related structures of the head and neck.

8073 American Academy of Physical Medicine and Rehabilitation
9700 W Bryn Mawr Ave
Ste 200
Rosemont, IL 60018-5701
847-737-6000
FAX: 847-737-6001
e-mail: info@aapmr.org
www.aapmr.org

Thomas Stautzenbach, Executive Director
M Elizabeth Sandel, President
Sherry Milligan, Website Content Editor
Beth Binkley, Communications Coordinator

This national medical specialty society represents more than 6,500 physical medicine and rehabilitation physicians, whose patients include people with physical disabilities and chronic, disabling illnesses. The academy's mission is to maximize quality of life, minimize the incidence and prevalence of impairments and disability, promote societal health and enhance the understanding and development of the specialty. The organization offers information, referrals, and patient materials.

8074 American Association For Respiratory Care
9425 N. Macarthur Blvd.
Suite 100
Irving, TX 75063-4706
972-243-2272
FAX: 972-484-2720
e-mail: info@aarc.org
www.aarc.org

Sam Giordano, CEO
Tom Kallstrom, COO

AARC's mission is to advance the science, technology, ethics and art of respiratory care through research and education for its members and to teach the general public about pulmonary health and disease prevention.

8075 American Association of Cardiovascular and Pulmonary Rehabilitation
330 N. Wabash Avenue
Suite 2200
Chicago, IL 60611
312-321-5146
FAX: 312-673-6924
e-mail: aacvpr@aacvpr.org
www.aacvpr.org

Megan Cohen, Executive Director
Abigail Lynn, Operations Manager
Erica Naranjo, Administrative Associate
Jessica Eustice, Development Manager

The mission of American Association of Cardiovascular and Pulmonary Rehabilitation is to reduce morbidity, mortality, and disability from cardiovascular and pulmonary diseases through education, prevention, rehabilitation, research, and aggressive disease management.

8076 American Brain Tumor Association
8550 W. Bryn Mawr
Ste 550
Chicaog, IL 60631-4106
773-577-8750
800-886-2282
FAX: 773-577-8738
e-mail: info@abta.org
www.abta.org

Elizabeth Wilson, Executive Director
Deneen Hesser, MSHSA, RN, OCN, Chief Mission Officer
Kerri Mink, Chief Operating Officer
Garett Auriemma, Director, Marketing and Communications

A non-profit organization founded in 1973 dedicated to the elimination of brain tumors through research and patient education services. Exists to eliminate brain tumors through research and to meet the needs of brain tumor patients and their families.

8077 American Diabetes Association
1701 N Beauregard St
Alexandria, VA 22311-1733
703-549-1500
800-342-2383
FAX: 703-836-7439
e-mail: askada@diabetes.org
www.diabetes.org

Larry Hausner, CEO
Debbie Johnson, CPA, Chief Financial Officer
Greg Elfers, Chief Field Development Officer
M. Vaneeda Bennett, Chief Revenue Officer

Provides diabetes research, information and advocacy. The mission of the Association is to prevent and cure diabetes and to improve the lives of all people affected by diabetes.

8078 American Group Psychotherapy Association
25 East 21st Street
6th Floor
New York, NY 10010-6207
212-477-2677
877-668-2472
FAX: 212-979-6627
e-mail: info@agpa.org
www.agpa.org

Marsha Block, CEO
Kathleen H. Ulman, Ph.D, President
Anne McEneaney, Ph.D, Secretary

AGPA serves as the national voice specific to the interests of group psychotherapy. Its 4,100 members and 31 affiliate societies provide a wealth of professional, educational and social support for group psychotherapists in the United States and around the world.

8079 American Head and Neck Society
11300 W Olympic Blvd
Ste 600
Los Angeles, CA 90064-1663
310-437-0559
FAX: 310-437-0585
e-mail: admin@ahnns.info
www.headandneckcancer.org

Mark Wax, MD, President
Doug Girod, VP
Dennis.H Kraus, Secretary
Ehab Hanna, Treasurer

AHNS is a professional organization, formed in 1998 to promote research and education in head and neck oncology. The website includes clinical practice guidelines, details of events, grants, and patient information. To promote and advance the knowledge of prevention, diagnosis, treatment, and rehabilitation of neoplasms and other diseases of the head and neck.

8080 American Lung Association
1301 Pennsylvania Ave. NW
Ste 800
Washington, DC 20004
202-785-3355
800-586-4872
FAX: 202-452-1085
e-mail: info@lungusa.org
www.lungusa.org

Harold P. Wimmer, President/CEO
Don . Awerkamp, Ph.D., J.D, Board Member
Timothy D. Byrum, MSN, CRNP, Board Member
Michael V. Carstens, Board Member

The American Lung Association is the leading organization working to save lives by improving lung health and preventing lung disease through Education, Advocacy and Research. With the generous support of the public, we are Fighting for Air. When you join the American Lung Association in the fight for healthy lungs and healthy air, you help save lives today and keep America healthy tomorrow.

8081 American Psychiatric Association
Psychiatric Services
1000 Wislon Blvd
Ste 1825
Arlington, VA 22209-3901
703-907-7300
888-35 -7924
FAX: 703-907-1085
e-mail: apa@psych.org
www.psych.org

Dilip Jeste, MD, President
Margaret Cawley Dewar

The American Psychiatric Association is a medical specialty society recognized worldwide. Its over 35,000 U.S. and international member physicians work together to ensure humane care and effective treatment for all persons with mental disorder, including mental retardation and substance-related disorders. It is the voice and conscience of modern psychiatry. Its vision is a society that has avaliable, accessible quality psychiatric diagnosis and treatment.

8082 American SIDS Institute
528 Raven Way
Naples, FL 34110
239-431-5425
FAX: 239-431-5536
e-mail: prevent@sids.org
www.sids.org

Marc Peterzell, JD, Chairman
Betty McEntire, PhD, Executive Director/CEO
Randy Barfield, MD, Board Member
Kristen Marr, Board Member

American SIDS Institute is a national nonprofit health care organization that is dedicated to the prevention of sudden infant death and the promotion of infant health through an aggressive, comprehensive nationwide program of: research, clinical services, education and family support.

8083 American Social Health Association
PO Box 13827
Research Triangle Park, NC 27709-3827
919-361-8400
FAX: 919-361-8425
e-mail: info@ashastd.org
www.ashastd.org

Lynn Barclay, President/CEO
Deborah Arrindell, VP Health Policy
H. Hunter Handsfield, MD, Secretary
Leandro Antonio Mena, M.D., MP, Treasurer

The American Sexual Health Association is a trusted source of reliable information on sexual health and sexually transmitted diseases/infections.

8084 **American Society of Pediatric Hematology/Oncology**
4700 W Lake Ave
Glenview, IL 60025-1468
847-375-4716
FAX: 847-375-6483
e-mail: info@aspho.org
www.aspho.org

Cynthia Porter, Executive Director
Steve Biddle, Director of Education
Jackie Holcomb, Education Manager
Carrie Gremer, Senior Membership Development Senior Manager

ASPHO is multidisciplinary organization dedicated to promoting optimal care of children and adolescents with blood disorders and cancer by advancing research, education, treatment and professional practice.

8085 **American Thoracic Society**
25 Broadway
18th Floor
New York, NY 10004-2755
212-315-8600
FAX: 212-315-6498
e-mail: atsinfo@thoracic.org
www.thoracic.org

Steve Crane, Executive Director
Nicola Black, Associate Director, Governance Activities & External Relatio
Kevin Wilson, MD, Senior Director, Documents & Medical Affairs
Miriam Rodriguez, Senior Director, Assembly Programs and Program Review Subcom

A non-profit, international, professional and scientific society for respiratory, critical care and sleep medicine. The ATS is committed to the prevention and treatment of respiratory disease through research, education, patient care and advocacy. The long-range goal of ATS is to decrease morbidity and mortality from respiratory, critical care and sleep disorders and life threatening acute illnesses in people of all ages.

8086 **Aplastic Anemia and MDS International Foundation**
100 Park Ave
Suite 108
Rockville, MD 20850
301-279-7202
800-747-2820
FAX: 301-279-7205
e-mail: help@aamds.org
www.aamds.org

John Huber, Executive Director
Stephanie Chisolm, Senior Director of Programs and Services
Benita Marcus, Senior Director of Information/Management
Pamela Spears, Senior Director of Resource Development and Marketing

This organization, formerly known as Aplastic Anemia Foundation of America was founded in 1983. It provides a resource directory for patient assistance, produces educational material and supports research into AA and MDS.

8087 **Behavior Therapy and Research Society**
Temple University Medical School
3420 N Broad St
Philadelphia, PA 19140-5104
215-707-3133
800-331-2839
FAX: 215-707-4086
www.medschool.temple.edu

John Daly, Dean
Judith Russo, Manager
Larry R. Kaiser, MD, FACS, Senior Executive Vice President

This organization promotes behavior therapy by conducting and facilitating research in behavioral interventions and providing information through consultations, conferences and publications, about the use of these methods.

8088 **Canadian Cancer Society**
55 St. Clair Avenue West
Suite 300
Toronto, ON M4V-2Y7
416-961-7223
FAX: 416-961-4189
e-mail: webmaster@ontario.cancer.ca
www.cancer.ca

Shirley Auyeung, Director of Finance
Sian Bevan, Director, Research
Gillian Bromfield, Director
Heather Chappell, National Director

A national community based organization of volunteers whose mission is the eradication of cancer and the enhancement of the quality of life of people living with cancer.

8089 **Canadian Diabetes Association**
1400-522 University Avenue
Toronto,, ON M5G-2R5
416-363-3373
800-226-8464
FAX: 416-408-7015
e-mail: info@diabetes.ca
www.diabetes.ca

Suzanne Deuel,, Chair & Secretary
Heath Applebaum, Director of Communications
Aileen Leo, Executive Director, Government Relations and Public Policy
Doug Macnamara, President and CEO

The mission of the Canadian Diabetes Association is to promote the health of Canadians through diabetes research, education, service and advocacy.

8090 **Canadian Lung Association**
1750 Courtwood Crescent
Ottawa,, ON K2C-2B5
613-569-6411
888-566-5864
FAX: 613-569-8860
e-mail: info@lung.ca
www.lung.ca

Janis Hass, Director of Marketing and Communications
Anne Van Dam, Director, Research & Knowledge Translation
Connie C"t,, Senior Director
Mary-Pat Shaw, Acting President and CEO

The Canadian Lung Association has been dedicated to its mission of promoting and improving lung health for all Canadians. A non-profit and volunteer-based health charity, The Lung Associatin depends on donations from the public to support lung health research, education, prevention and advocacy.

8091 **Candlelighters Childhood Cancer Foundation of Canada**
21 St Clair Ave E
Ste 801
Toronto,, ON M4T-1L9
416-489-6440
800-363-1062
FAX: 416-489-9812
e-mail: info@childhoodcancer.ca
www.childhoodcancer.ca

Melody Khodaverdian, Director of Development
Megan Davidson, President/CEO
Zoey Friedman, Manager of National Programs & Services
Jessica MacInnis, Manager of Marketing & Communications

A national, volunteer governed, charitable organization dedicated to improving the qualtiy of life for children with cancer and their families. We will achieve our mission through undertaking and supporting national initiatives resulting in the increased survival and wellbeing of our children, and ultimately a cure for all childhood cancers.

8092 Cerebral Palsy Associations of New York State Annual Conference
90 State Street
Suite 929
Albany, NY 12207-1709 518-436-0178
e-mail: AffiliateServices@cpofnys.org
www.cpofnys.org
Susan Constantino, President & CEO
Michael Alvaro, Executive Vice President
Thomas Mandelkow, Executive Vice President, CAO/CFO
Joseph M. Pancari, Executive Vice President/COO
Offers 50 sessions and features many outstanding presenters in areas such as assitive technology, education, health care, clinical services, public relations and development, and finance and management.
October

8093 Child Neurology Service
Inova Fairfax Hospital For Children
8110 Gatehouse Rd
Falls Church, VA 22042 703-776-2515
855-MY -NOVA
FAX: 703-776-4010
e-mail: tony.raker@inova.org
www.inova.org
Mark Stauder, President/COO
Knox Singleton, CEO
Richard Magenheimer, Chief Financial Officer
Loring Flint, Executive Vice President and Chief Medical Office
Inova is a not-for-profit healthcare system based in Northern Virginia that serves more than two million people each year from throughout the Washington, DC, metro area and beyond.

8094 Children's Hemiplegia & Stroke Association
4101 W Green Oaks Blvd
Suite 305, #149
Arlington, TX 76016 817-478-0861
e-mail: info437@chasa.org
www.chasa.org
Nancy Atwood, Executive Director and Founder
Jana Smoot White, President
Julie Ring, Vice President
Jackie Haley, Treasurer
Offering support and information to families of infants, children and young adults who have hemiplegia or hemiplegic cerebral palsy.

8095 Diabetes Exercise & Sports Association
310 W Liberty St
Ste 604
Louisville, KY 40202-3017 502-581-0207
800-898-4322
FAX: 502-581-0206
e-mail: desa@diabetes-exercise.org
www.mentalhealthamerica.net
Doug Dressman, Executive Director
Exists to enhance the quality of life for people with diabetes through exercise and physical fitness.

8096 Division for Physical and Health Disabilities
1110 N Glebe Rd
Ste 300
Arlington, VA 22201-5704 866-232-7733
FAX: 703-264-9494
TTY:866-915-5000
www.cec.sped.org
Bruce Ramirez, Executive Director
Twanna Clark, Senior Executive Assistant
Sharon Rodriguez, Senior Executive Assistant
Advocates for quality education for individuals with physical disabilities, multiple disabilities, and special health care needs served in schools, hospitals, or home settings. DPHD's members include classroom teachers, administrators, related service personnel, hospital/homebound teachers, and parents.

8097 Emphysema Foundation for our Right to Service
PO Box 20241
Kansas City,, MO 64119-241 816-452-9300
FAX: 816-413-0176
e-mail: efforts-request@home.ease.lsoft.com
www.emphysema.net
Linda Watson, President
Becky Collison, Treasurer
EFFORTS is a nonprofit organization that takes an active role in promoting research for more effective treatment and perhaps a cure for emphysema and related lung diseases. It also works to further education about the disease and provides a support mailing list for members.

8098 Environmental Health Center: Dallas
8345 Walnut Hill Lane
Ste 220
Dallas, TX 75231-4205 214-368-4132
FAX: 214-691-8432
e-mail: contact@ehcd.com
www.ehcd.com
William J Rea, Director
Chris Rea, Business Manager
Yaqin Pan, M.D., Research Physician
Bertie Griffiths, Ph.D., Microbiologist/Immunologist
Clinic providing patient care in the areas of Immunotherapy, Nutrition, Physical Therapy, Chemical Depuration, Energy Balancing, Electromagnetic Sensitivity Testing, Psychological Support Services, Family Practice Medicine and Internal Medicine.

8099 Epilepsy Foundation
8301 Professional Pl
Landover, MD 20785-2353 301-459-3700
800-332-1000
86- 33- 271
FAX: 301-459-1569
e-mail: ContactUs@efa.org
www.epilepsyfoundation.org
Phil Gattone, President/CEO
Brien Smith
The Epilepsy Foundation of Americar is the national voluntary health agency dedicated solely to the welfare of the almost 3 million people with epilepsy in the U.S. and their families. The organization works to ensure that people with seizures are able to participate in all life experiences; to improve how people with epilepsy are perceived, accepted and valued in society; and to promote research for a cure.

8100 Eunice Kennedy Shriver National Institute of Child Health and Human Development (NICHD)
National Institutes of Health (NIH)
PO Box 3006
Rockville, MD 20847-3006 301-496-5097
800-370-2943
FAX: 866-760-5947
TTY: 888-320-6942
e-mail: nichdinformationresourcecenter@mail.nih.gov
www.nichd.nih.gov
Alan Guttmacher, Acting Director
Dexter Collins, Deputy Executive Office
The NICHD, part of the federal National Institutes of Health, conducts and supports research topics related to the health of children, adults, families, and populations, including growth and development; parenting; learning and reading; and mental retardation, autism, and developmental disabilities, and provides information on these topics.

8101 **Families of Spinal Muscular Atrophy**
925 Busse Rd
PO Box 196
Elk Grove Village, IL 60007
847-367-7620
800-886-1762
FAX: 847-367-7623
e-mail: info@fsma.org
www.fsma.org

Jill Jarecki, Research Director
Kenneth Hubby, President
Karen O'Brien, Membership
Colleen McCarthy O'Toole, Family Support Director

Families of Spinal Muscular Atrophy is the largest international organization dedicated solely to: eradicating spinal muscular atrophy (SMA) by promoting and supporting research, helping families cope with SMA through informational programs and support, and educating the public and professional community about SMA.

8102 **Health Education AIDS Liason (HEAL)**
PO Box 1103
New York, NY 10113-1103
212-580-3471
FAX: 212-873-0891
e-mail: revdocnyc@aol.com
www.healaids.com

Michael Ellner, President
Tom DiFerdinando, Executive Director
Barnett.J Weiss, Board Member
Robert Giraldo, Board Member

Nonprofit, community-based educational organization providing information, hope, and support to people who are HIV positive or living with AIDS. The men and women at HEAL are health professionals, people living with life threatening diseases, and concerned volunteers.

8103 **Herpes Resource Center**
American Social Health Association
PO Box 13827
Research Triangle Park, NC 27709-3827
919-361-8400
800-227-8922
FAX: 919-361-8425
e-mail: customerservice@ashastd.org
www.ashastd.org

Tom Beall, Chair
J. Dennis Fortenberry, M.D., M.S, Vice Chair
H. Hunter Handsfield, MD, Secretary
Leandro Antonio Mena, M.D., MP, Treasurer

The Herpes Resource Center (HRC) focuses on increasing education, public awareness, and support to anyone concerned about herpes. Since its formation in 1979, the HRC has helped over five million people. The work of the HRC is funded primarily through individual gifts, subscriptions and product sales, with additional support in the form of corporate contributions. Today, people continue to depend on ASHA and the HRC for educational information about herpes.

8104 **International Academy of Biological Dentistry and Medicine**
19122 Camellia Bend Circle
Ste 101
Spring, TX 77379
281-651-1745
FAX: 281-440-1258
e-mail: drdawn@drdawn.net
www.iabdm.org

Dr. Dawn Ewing, Executive Director
Dr. Blanche Grube, President
Dr. Joan Sefcik, Vice President
Dr. Nick Meyer, 2nd Vice President/Dean of Education

Promotes non-toxic diagnostic and therapeutic approaches in dentistry; hosts seminars on biological diagnosis and therapy.

8105 **International Academy of Oral Medicine and Toxicology**
8297 Champions Gate Blvd
Ste 193
Champions Gate, FL 33896-8387
863-420-6373
FAX: 863-419-8136
e-mail: info@iaomt.org
www.iaomt.org

Maths Berlin, Advisor
Boyd Haley, PhD, FIAOMT, Chairman
Kym Smith, Executive Director

Nonprofit organization dedicated to funding solid peer-reviewed scientific research in the area of toxic substances used in dentistry as well as providing continuing education and carefully reviewed procedures, protocols, and methodologies to reduce the risk for patients and professionals.

8106 **International Association for Cancer Victors: Northern California Chapter**
POB 745
Lakeport, CA 95453
408-834-5300
FAX: 408-264-9659
e-mail: contact@cancervictors.net
www.cancervictors.net

Cecile Pollack Hoffman, Founder

The Cancer Victors and Friends, also known as The International Association of Cancer Victors and Friends, or IACVF, is dedicated to disseminating information about alternative and complimentary methods for treating cancer and other diseases, which encompasses hundreds of clinics and practitioners. Multiple avenues for information include this website, printed information including chapter newsletters and a journal, personal contact with members, monthly chapter meetings with guest speakers, a p

8107 **International Association of Hygienic Physicians-IAHP**
4620 Euclid Blvd
Youngstown, OH 44512-1633
330-788-0526
FAX: 330-788-0093
e-mail: anhs@anhs.org
www.iahp.net

Alec Burton, Co-Founder
Mark A Huberman, Secretary/Treasurer

The International Association of Hygienic Physicians (IAHP) is a professional association for licensed, primary care physicians (Medical Doctors, Osteopaths, Chiropractors, and Naturopaths) who specialize in Therapeutic Fasting Supervision as an integral part of Hygienic Care. Founded in 1978, the IAHP offers an Internship program for Certification in Fasting Supervision. The Association has adopted Standards of Practice and Principles of Ethics for providing Hygienic Care. They further have ado

8108 **International Medical and Dental Hypnotherapy Association**
8852 SR 3001
Rr 2
Laceyville, PA 18623-9417
570-869-1021
800-553-6886
FAX: 570-869-1249
www.imdha.com

Linda Otto, Executive Director
Robert Otto, President/CEO
Christie Boecker, Membership Services Coordinator
Joann Wright, Administrative Assistant

To provide and encourage education programs to further, the knowledge, understanding, and application of hypnosis in complementary healthcare; to encourage research and scientific publication in the field of hypnosis; to promote the further recognition and acceptance of hypnosis as an important tool in healthcare and focus for scientific research.

8109 International Myeloma Foundation
12650 Riverside Dr
Ste 206
North Hollywood, CA 91607- 3421 818-487-7455
800-452-2873
FAX: 818-487-7454
e-mail: theimf@myeloma.org
www.myeloma.org

David Girard, Executive Director
Susie Novis, President
Diane Moran, Senior Vice President, Strategic Planning
Jennifer Scarne, Chief Financial Officer

For 20 years, the IMF has been on a mission, a mission to improve the lives of myeloma patients. With over 196,000 members in 113 countries worldwide, the IMF is the oldest and largest organization dedicated to finding a cure for myeloma.

8110 International Ozone Association
PO Box 28873
Scottsdale, AZ 85255 480-529-3787
FAX: 480-522-3080
e-mail: infO3zone@io3a.org
www.io3a.org

8111 International Rett Syndrome Foundation
4600 Devitt Dr
Cincinnati, OH 45246-1104 513-847-3020
800-818-7388
FAX: 513-874-2520
e-mail: admin@rettsyndrome.org
www.rettsyndrome.org

Stephen E Bajardi, Executive Director
Eva Dillon, Director of Individual Giving
Paige Nues, Director of Family Support
Steven Kaminsky, Ph.D., Chief Science Officer

The core mission of the IRSF is to fund research for treatments and a cure for Rett syndrome while enhancing the overall quality of life for those living with Rett syndrome by providing information, programs, and services.

8112 Leukemia and Lymphoma Society
1311 Mamaroneck Ave
Suite 310
White Plains, NY 10605- 5228 914-949-5213
800-955-4572
FAX: 914-949-6691
e-mail: supportservices@lls.org
www.lls.org

John Walter, CEO
Louis DeGennaro, Chief Mission Officer
George Omiros, CFRE, CAE, Executive Vice President, Chief Campaign & Field Development
Lisa Stockmon, Executive Vice President and Chief Marketing Officer

The Leukemia and Lymphoma Society is the world's largest voluntary health organization dedicated to funding blood cancer research, education and patient services. Thier mission: cure leukemia, lymphoma, Hodgkin's disease and myeloma, and improve the quality of life of patients and their families. Since its founding in 1949, the Society has invested more then $483 million for research specifically targeting blood cancers.

8113 Little People of America
250 El Camino Real
Ste 201
Tustin, CA 92780 714-368-3689
888-572-2001
FAX: 714-368-3367
e-mail: info@lpaonline.org
www.lpaonline.org

Joanna Campbell, Executive Director
Gary Arnold, President
Bill Bradford, Senior Vice President
Jason Rasa, Vice President of Finance

Little People of America, Inc., is a national non-profit organization that provides support and information to people of short stature and their families. Short stature is generally caused by one of the more than 200 medical conditions known as dwarfism. LPA welcomes all 200+ forms of dwarfism.

8114 Lymphoma Foundation Canada
7111 Syntex Drive,
Suite 351
Mississauga,, ON L5N-8C3 905-822-5135
866-659-5556
FAX: 905-814-9152
e-mail: info@lymphoma.ca
www.lpaonline.org

Paul Weingarten, Chair
Mike Joyce, Vice-Chair
John Sutherland, Treasurer
Nick Iozzo, Secretary

We provide information on new treatments and research, as well as support patient education workshops and seminars to help people understand and manage their cancer. We support lymphoma-specific research through the creation of fellowships, as well as provide community-based resources to help people learn about and cope with their cancer.

8115 Medic Alert Foundation International
2323 Colorado Ave
Turlock, CA 95382-2018 209-668-3333
888-633-4298
e-mail: customer_service@medicalert.org
www.medicalert.org

Calvin Bland, Chair
Barton G. Tretheway, CAE, Vice Chair
Colin Rorrie, Jr., PhD, CAE, Treasurer
Margaret Gradison, MD, HHS-CL, Secretary

We protect the health and well-being of more than 4 million members worldwide through our trusted emergency support network. We educate emergency responders and medical personnel - our partners in everyday emergency situations. And we communicate your health information, your wishes, and your directives to ensure you receive the best care possible.

8116 Mental Health America
2000 N Beauregard St
6th Fl
Alexandria, VA 22311 703-684-7722
800-969-6642
FAX: 703-684-5968
www.mentalhealthamerica.net

Julio Abreu,, Senior Director of Public Policy and Advocacy
Erica Ahmed,, Director of Public Education
Trish Enright, Director of Community Outreach & Partnerships
Patrick Hendry, Senior Director of Consumer Advocacy

Nonprofit organization addressing all issues related to mental health and mental illness. With more than 340 affiliates nationwide, NMHA works to improve the mental health of all Americans, especially the 54 million individuals with mental disorders, through advocacy, education, research and service.

8117 Multiple Sclerosis Association of America
706 Haddonfield Rd
Cherry Hill, NJ 8002-2652 856-488-4500
800-532-7667
FAX: 856-661-9797
e-mail: msaa@mymsaa.org
www.msassociation.org

Cindy Richman, Senior Director of Patient & Healthcare Relations
Carla Foote, Director of Administrative Services
Susan Courtney, Senior Writer & Creative Director.
Kimberly Goodrich, CFRE, Senior Director of Development

A national non-profit organization dedicated to enriching the quality of life for everyone affected by multiple sclerosis. MSAA provides ongoing support and direct services to these individuals with MS and the people close to them. MSAA also serves to promote greater understanding of the needs and challenges of those who face physical obstacles.

8118 Multiple Sclerosis Center of Oregon
Oregon Health & Sciences University
3181 SW Sam Jackson Park Rd
Department of Neurology, L226
Portland, OR 97239-3098
503-494-5759
FAX: 503-494-3480
www.ohsu.edu

Dennis Bourdette, M.D., F.A.A, Chair
Michelle H. Cameron, M.D., P.T., Neurologist and a Physical therapist
Joseph Robertson Jr MBA, President
Steven D Stadum JD, Executive VP

OHSU's fundamental purpose is to improve the well-being of people in Oregon and beyond. As part of its multifaceted public mission, OHSU strives for excellence in education, research, clinical practice, scholarship and community service. Through its dynamic interdisciplinary environment, OHSU stimulates the spirit of inquiry, initiative and cooperation among students, faculty and staff.

8119 Multiple Sclerosis Foundation
6350 N Andrews Ave
Fort Lauderdale, FL 33309-2130
954-776-6805
800-225-6495
FAX: 954-938-8708
e-mail: admin@msfocus.org
www.msfocus.org

Jules Kuperberg, Executive Director
Alan Segaloff, Co- Executive Director
Dr. William Mundy, Director Emeritus
William Sheehan, Director

Contemporary national, nonprofit organization that provides free support services and public education for persons with Multiple Sclerosis, newsletters, toll-free phone support, information, referrals, home care, assitive technology, and support groups.

8120 Myositis Association
1737 King Street
Suite 600
Alexandria, VA 22314
703-299-4850
800-821-7356
FAX: 703-535-6752
e-mail: tma@myositis.org
www.myositis.org

Bob Goldberg, Executive Director
Theresa Reynolds Curry, Communications Manager
Aisha Morrow, Operations Manager
Charlia Sanchez, Member Services Coordinator

The Myositis Association is dedicated to finding a cure for inflammatory and other related myopathies, while serving those affected by these diseases. The aim of TMA's programs and services is to provide information, support, advocacy and research for those concerned about myositis. Support groups offer members the chance to share their feelings and discuss their concerns with people in similar situations. These groups encourage an atmosphere of communication and compassion.

8121 National AIDS Fund
1424 K Street, N.W.,
Suite 200
Washington, DC 20005-1511
202-408-4848
888-234-2437
FAX: 202-408-1818
e-mail: info@aidsfund.org
www.aidsfund.org

Victor Barnes, Interim President & CEO
Rob Banaszak, Communications Director
Vignetta Charles, Ph.D., Senior Vice President
Alanna Adams, Program Associate

The National AIDS Fund was founded in 1988 to reduce the incidence and impact of HIV/AIDS by promoting leadership and generating resources for effective community responses to the epidemic. Through its unique expanding network of Community Partnerships, NAF supports over 400 grassroots organizations annually which in turn provide HIV prevention, care and support services to underserved individuals and populations most impacted by HIV/AIDS including communities of color, youth and women.

8122 National Association for Children of Alcoholics
10920 Connecticut Avenue
Suite 100
Kensington, MD 20895-3007
301-468-0985
888-554-2627
FAX: 301-468-0987
e-mail: nacoa@nacoa.org
www.nacoa.org

Sis Wenger, President/CEO
Steve Hornberger, Program Director

National non-profit membership and affiliate organization working on behalf of children of alcohol and drug dependent parents. NACoA has publications available for the individual as well as the professional in the field.

8123 National Association for Continence
PO Box 1019
Charleston, SC 29402-1019
843-377-0900
800-252-3337
FAX: 843-377-0905
e-mail: memberservices@nafc.org
www.nafc.org

Katherine F Jeter EdD, Founder
Nancy Muller, Executive Director
Meghan Hansen, Membership and Fund Development

NAFC's mission is to educate the public about the causes, diagnosis, categories, treatment options and management alternatives for incontinence, voiding disfunction and related pelvic floor disorders. To network with other organizations and agencies to elevate the visibility and priority given to these areas; and to advocate on behalf of consumers who suffer from such symptoms as a result of disease or other illness.

8124 National Association for Home Care & Hospice
228 7th St SE
Washington, DC 20003-4306
202-547-7424
FAX: 202-547-3540
e-mail: webmaster@nahc.org
www.nahc.org

Andrea Devoti, Chair
Lucy Andrews, Vice Chair
Mary Haynor, Secretary
Walter W. Borginis, Treasurer

This is a non-profit trade association representing various home care, hospice and health aid organizations. Website contains a section with information on how to choose a home care provider and a zip code driven locator for home care and hospice. Publishes monthly newsletter.

8125 National Association for Medical Direction of Respiratory Care
8618 Westwood Center Dr
Ste 210
Vienna, VA 22182-2222
703-752-4359
FAX: 703-752-4360
e-mail: execoffice@namdrc.org
www.namdrc.org

Phillip Porte, Executive Director
Vickie Parshall, Member Services Director
Karen Lui, RN, Associate Executive Director
Peter C. Gay, MD, Board Member

Established over three decades ago, the National Association for Medical Direction of Respiratory Care (NAMDRC) is a national organization of physicians whose mission is to educate its members and address regulatory, legislative and payment issues that relate to the delivery of healthcare to patients with respiratory disorders.

8126 National Association for Proton Therapy
1301 Highland Dr
Silver Spring, MD 20910-1623
301-587-6100
FAX: 301-565-0747
e-mail: lenarzt@proton-therapy.org
www.proton-therapy.org

Leonard Arzt, Executive Director

The National Association for Proton Therapy (NAPT) is registered as an independent, non-profit, public benefit corporation providing education and awareness for the public, professional and governmental communities. Founded in 1990, it promotes the therapeutic benefits of proton therapy for cancer treatment in the U.S. and abroad.

8127 National Association for the Dually Diagnosed
132 Fair St
Kingston, NY 12401-4802
845-331-4336
800-331-5362
FAX: 845-331-4569
e-mail: info@thenadd.org
www.thenadd.org

Robert Fletcher, CEO
Edward Seliger, Project Coordinator
Judie Johnston, Administrative Assistant
Cassie Lattin, Office Assistant

Promotes awareness of, and services for individuals who have co-occuring intellectual disability and mental illness. NADD provides training and consultation services.

8128 National Association of Anorexia Nervosa and Associated Disorders
750 E Diehl Road
Suite127
Highland Park, IL 60563
630-577-1333
FAX: 847-433-4632
e-mail: anadhelp@anad.org
www.anad.org

Laura Discipio, Executive Director

A non-profit corporation that seeks to alleviate the problems of eating disorders, especially anorexia nervosa and bulimia nervosa.

8129 National Association of Chronic Disease Directors
2872 Woodcock Blvd
Suite 220
Atlanta, GA 30341-4096
770-458-7400
FAX: 770-458-7401
e-mail: jrobitscher@chronicdisease.org
www.chronicdisease.org

John Robitscher, Executive Director
Sue Grinnell, President
Jill Myers Geadelmann, BS, RN, President-Elect
David M. Vigil, MBA, Treasurer

A national public health association, founded in 1988 to link the chronic disease program directors of each state and US territory to provide a national forum for chronic disease prevention and control efforts. Since its founding, NACDD has made impressive strides in mobilizing national efforts to reduce chronic diseases and the associated risk factors.

8130 National Association of Cognitive Behavioral Therapists
203 Three Springs Drive
Suite 4, PO Box 2195
Weirton, WV 26062-1395
304-723-3982
800-853-1135
FAX: 304-723-3982
e-mail: nacbt@nacbt.org
www.nacbt.org

Aldo R Pucci, President

An organization dedicated solely to the teaching and practice of cognitive-behavioral psychotherapy. The mission of the NACBT is two fold: to promote and support the teaching and practice of cognitive-behavioral psychotherapy and to support those professionals and students seeking to practice it; and to set standards for credentialing that enable the general public to be confident that they will receive quality CBT from our certified members.

8131 National Association of Epilepsy Centers
600 Maryland Avenue, SW,
Suite 835W
Washington, DC 20024-1227
202-484-1100
888-525-6232
FAX: 202-484-1244
e-mail: info@naec-epilepsy.org
www.naec-epilepsy.org

David.M Labiner, President
Nathan.B Fountain, VP
Susan T. Herman, Secretary/Treasurer
Jerry J. Shih, M.D, Board Member

NAEC educates public and private policy makers and regulators about appropriate patient care standards, reimbusement and medical services policies. NAEC is designed to complement, not compete with, the efforts of existing scientific and charitable epilepsy organizations.

8132 National Association of People with AIDS
8401 Colesville Rd
Suite 505
Silver Spring, MD 20910- 3349
240-247-0880
866-846-9366
FAX: 240-247-0574
e-mail: development@napwa.org
www.napwa.org

Frank Oldham, President/CEO
Stephen Bailous, Executive VP
Matt Lesieur, Vice President for Public Policy
Leslie Talley, Vice President for Development

The NAPWA believes in making a difference in the lives of our constituents. They also provide information and resources.

8133 National Association to Advance Fat Acceptance
PO Box 4662
Foster City, CA 94404-662
916-558-6880
FAX: 916-558-6881
www.naafa.org

Jason Docherty, Chair
Lisa Tealer, Director of Programs & Treasurer
Peggy Howell, Public Relations Director
Phyllis Warr, Membership and Member Services Director

Founded in 1969, the National Association to Advance Fat Acceptance (NAAFA) is a non-profit, all volunteer, civil rights organization dedicated to protecting the rights and improving the quality of life for fat people. NAAFA works to eliminate discrimination based on body size and provide fat people with the tools for self-empowerment through advocacy, public education, and support.

8134 National Ataxia Foundation
2600 Fernbrrok Ln
Suite 119
Minneapolis, MN 55447-4752
763-553-0020
FAX: 763-553-0167
e-mail: naf@ataxia.org
www.ataxia.org

Michael Parent, Executive Director
Susan Hagen, Patient Services Director
Susan Perlman, MD, Medical Director
Harry T. Orr, PhD, Research Director

The National Ataxia Foundation is a nonprofit, membership-supported organization established in 1957 to help ataxia families. The Foundation is dedicated to improving the lives of persons affected by ataxia through support, education, and research.

8135 National Autism Association
20 Alice Agnew Drive
Attleboro Falls,, MA 02763
877-622-2884
FAX: 774-643-6331
e-mail: naa@nationalautism.org
www.nationalautismassociation.org

Lori McIlwain, Co-Founder. Executive Director
Wendy Fournier, President
Katie Wright, VP
Rita Shreffler, Secretary, Founding Board Member

The mission of the National Autism Association is to educate and empower families affected by autism and other neurological disorders, while advocating on behalf of those who cannot fight for their own rights.

8136 National Brachial Plexus/Erb's Palsy Association
PO Box 23
Larsen, WI 54947-23
920-836-2151
FAX: 920-836-5813
e-mail: info@nbpepa.org
www.nbpepa.org

Brenda Copeland-Moore, President
Kris Kiesow, Treasurer
Cheryl Pratt, VP
Donna Schott, VP

To educate, inform, and assist those affected by Brachial Plexus Palsy by offering information, contacts, resources, parent matching, and assistance developing chapters or support groups throughout the United States. National Brachial Plexus/Erb's Palsy Association, Inc. Programs include parent matching services, assistance forming chapters, or support groups, provide support to families dealing with children with diagnosis of Brachial Plexus Injury & Erb's Palsy as well as other conditions.

8137 National Cancer Institute
9609 Medical Center Drive
Ste 300
Bethesda, MD 20892- 9760
301-496-0909
800-422-6237
TTY:800-332-8615
e-mail: cancergovstaff@mail.nih.gov
www.cancer.gov

Harold Varmos, Director

The National Cancer Institute coordinates the National Cancer Program, which conducts and supports research, training, health information dissemination, and other programs with respect to the cause, diagnosis, prevention, and treatment of cancer, rehabilitation from cancer, and the continuing care of cancer patients and the families of cancer patients.

8138 National Children's Leukemia Foundation
7316 Avenue U
Brooklyn, NY 11234-6250
718-251-1222
800-448-4673
FAX: 718-251-1444
e-mail: info@leukemiafoundation.org
www.leukemiafoundation.org

Yehuda Guttwein, President

Provides the cure for cancer and other life-threatening diseases throughout the world, and to insure that all persons, regardless of race, religion, ethnicity, gender, socioeconomic status or country of residence, have access to life-saving medical care. The NCLF supports medical research and direct patient care programs that ease the financial, social and psychological burdens of families with a diagnosis of cancer or other serious blood disorders.

8139 National Diabetes Information Clearinghouse
1 Information Way
Bethesda, MD 20892-3560
800-860-8747
FAX: 703-738-4929
TTY:866-569-1162
e-mail: ndic@info.niddk.nih.gov
www.diabetes.niddk.nih.gov

Michael T Sheppard CPA CAE, Executive Director

An information and referral service of the National Institute of Diabetes and Digestive and Kidney Diseases, one of the National Institutes of Health. The clearinghouse responds to written inquiries, develops and distributes publications about diabetes, and provides referrals to diabetes organizations, including support groups. The NDIC maintains a database of patient and professional education materials, from which literature searches are generated.

8140 National Digestive Diseases Information Clearinghouse
2 Information Way
Bethesda, MD 20892-3570
800-891-5389
FAX: 703-738-4929
TTY:866-559-1162
e-mail: nddic@info.niddk.nih.gov
www.digestive.niddk.nih.gov

Stephen P. James M.D., Executive Editor

Information and referral service of the National Institute of Diabetes and Digestive and Kidney Diseases. A central information resource on the prevention and management of digestive diseases, the clearinghouse responds to written inquiries, develops and distributes publications about digestive diseases, provides referrals to digestive disease organizations and support groups, and maintains a database of patient and professional education materials from which literature searches are generated.

8141 National Fibromyalgia Association
2121 S Towne Centre Pl
Suite 300
Anaheim, CA 92806-6124
714-921-0150
FAX: 714-921-6920
e-mail: shausen@fmaware.org
www.fmaware.org

Lynne Matallana, President
Mark Dobrilovic, Board of Director
John Fry, PhD, Board of Director
Michael Seffinger, DO, FAAFP, Board of Director

National Fibromyalgia Association's mission is to develop and execute programs dedicated to improving the quality of life for people with fibromyalgia.

8142 National Fragile X Foundation
1615 Bonanza St.
Suite 202, PO Box 3
Walnut Creek, CA 94596
925-938-9300
800-688-8765
FAX: 925-938-9315
e-mail: natlfx@fragilex.org
www.fragilex.org

Robert Miller, Executive Director
Linda Sorensen, MS, Associate Director
Jeffrey Cohen, Director of Government Affairs & Advocacy
David Salomon, Communications Coordinator

Unites the fragile X community to enrich lives through educational and emotional support, promote public and professional awareness and advance research toward improvement treatments and cure for fragile X syndrome.

8143 National Hemophilia Foundation
116 W 32nd St
Fl 11
New York, NY 10001-3212
212-328-3700
800-424-2634
FAX: 212-328-3777
e-mail: handi@hemophilia.org
www.hemophilia.org

Val Bias, CEO
Neil Frick, VP Research
John Indence, Vice President for Marketing & C
Joseph J. Kleiber, Senior Vice President for Chapte

The National Hemophilia Foundation is dedicated to finding better treatments and cures for bleeding and clotting disorders and to preventing the complications of these disorders through education,advocacy and research. Established in 1948, The National Hemophilia Foundation has chapters throughout the country. Its programs and initiatives are made possible through the generosity of individuals, corporations, and foundations as well as through the Centers for Disease Controll and Prevention (CDC)

8144 National Hydrocephalus Foundation
12413 Centralia St
Lakewood, CA 90715-1653
562-924-6666
888-857-3434
e-mail: debbifields@nhfonline.org
www.nhfonline.org

Debbi Fields, Executive Director
Michael Fields, President
Jaynie Dunn, Secretary
Sarah Dunn, Junior Director

Assembles and disseminates information pertaining to hydrocephalus, its treatments and outcomes. Establishes and facilitates a communication network among affected families and individuals.

8145 National Kidney and Urologic Diseases Information Clearinghouse
3 Information Way
Bethesda, MD 20892-3580
800-891-5390
FAX: 703-738-4929
TTY:866-569-1162
e-mail: nkudic@info.niddk.nih.org
www.kidney.niddk.nih.gov

Mel Eagle, Manager
Griffin P. Rogers M.D., Director

NKUDIC was established in 1987 to increase knowledge and understanding about diseases of the kidneys and urologic system among people with these conditions and their families, health care professionals, and the general public.

8146 National Organization for Albinism and Hypopigmentation
PO Box 959
E Hampstead, NH 03826-0959
603-887-2310
800-473-2310
FAX: 800-648-2310
e-mail: webmaster@albinism.org
www.albinism.org

Michael McGowan, Executive Director
Donna Appell, Vice-chair
Kelsey Thompson, Secretary
Doug DuBois, Board Member

Offers information and support to people with albinism, their families and the prodessionals who work with them.

8147 National Organization on Fetal Alcohol Syndrome
1200 Eton Ct NW
Washington, DC 20007-3239
202-785-4585
800-666-6327
FAX: 202-466-6456
e-mail: information@nofas.org
www.nofas.org

Tom Donaldson, President
Kathleen Tavenner Mitchell, VP
Brianna Montgomery, Program Manager
Andy Kachor, Media and Communications Coordin

Dedicated to eliminating birth defects caused by alcohol consumption during pregnancy and improving the qualtiy of life for those individuals and families affected.

8148 National Service Dog Center
Delta Society
875 124th Ave NE
Ste 101
Bellevue, WA 98005-2531
425-679-5530
FAX: 425-379-5539
e-mail: info@deltasociety.org
www.petpartners.org

Michelle Matheson, Director of Finance
R.Stephen Browning, President/CEO
Mary Margaret Callahan,, National Director of Program Development
Frances Pak,, Director of Operations

Pet Partners, formerly Delta Society, is a 501(c)(3)non-profit organization that helps people live healthier and happier lives by incorporating therapy, service and companion animals into their lives. We receive no government funding and rely on individuals, foundations and corporations for financial support.

8149 Okada Specialty Guide Dogs
543 Esteppe Rd
Front Royal, VA 22630
540-635-3937
FAX: 352-344-0210
e-mail: okada@okadadogs.com
www.okadadogs.com

Pat Putnam, Director

Trains dogs to aid deaf, hearing-impaired, Alzheimer's, seizure, amnesia and residential companion guide dogs.

8150 Ontario Cerebral Palsy Sports Association
7-46 Antares Dr
Nepean, ON, Canada K2E-7Z1
613-723-1806
866-286-2772
FAX: 613-723-6742
www.ocsa.on.ca

Amanda Fader, Executive Director
Don Sinclair, President
Steven Dukovich, VP
Don Borsk, Treasurer

Believes in the value of sport and that sport builds success in all aspects of life. It provides, promotes and coordinates competitive opportunities as well as encourages individual excellence through sport for athletes within the cerebral palsy family. To that end, OCPSA recruits, develops and supports athletes, coaches and volunteers.

8151 Ontario Federation for Cerebral Palsy
104-1630 Lawrence Avenue W
Toronto,, ON M6L-1C5
416-244-9686
877-244-9686
FAX: 416-244-6543
e-mail: info@ofcp.on.ca
www.ofcp.ca

Clarence Meyers, Executive Director
Gordana Skrba, Assistant Executive Director
Steve Chandler, Senior Manager
Syed Alam, Operations Manager

Assisting individuals and member groups in the development and provision of services and programs including accommodation in all parts of the province of Ontario.

8152 Overeaters Anonymous World Service Office
PO Box 44020
Rio Rancho, NM 87174-4020
505-891-2664
FAX: 505-891-4320
e-mail: info@oa.org
www.oa.org

Naomi Lippel, Manager

OA is not just about weight loss, obesity or diets; it addresses physical, emotional and spiritual well-being. It is not a religious organization and does not promote any particular diet. To address weight loss, OA encourages members to develop a food plan with a health care professional and a sponsor.

8153 People Against Cancer
604 East Street
PO Box 10
Otho, IA 50569
515-972-4444
800-662-2623
FAX: 515-972-4415
e-mail: info@PeopleAgainstCancer.net
www.peopleagainstcancer.com

Frank Wiewel, Executive Director

Publication of People Against Cancer, a nonprofit, grassroots, public benefit organization dedicated to 'New Directions in the War on Cancer.' We are a democratic organization of people with cancer, their loved ones and citizens working together to protect and enhance medical freedom of choice.

8 pages

8154 Prader-Willi Alliance of New York
PO Box 222
Baldwinsville, NY 13027
716-276-2211
800-442-1655
FAX: 315-320-0443
e-mail: alliance@prader-willi.org
www.prader-willi.org

Henry Singer, Director
Harry Persanis, Director
Daniel J. Maillet, Jr. Director
Catherine Maczko, Director

To provide information to the general public about Prader-Willi syndrome (PWS): Ýto promote awareness of PWS among the general public and medical professionals; to provide forms for discussion and professional interchange on the subject of PWS. To provide assistance, information, referral, and advocacy services to families and friends of persons suffering from PWS. To encourage and support research into the causes, cure and treatment of PWS.

8155 Prader-Willi Syndrome Association USA
8588 Potter Park Drive
Suite 500
Sarasota, FL 34238
941-312-0400
800-926-4797
FAX: 941-312-0142
e-mail: pwsausa@pwsausa.org
www.pwsausa.org

John Heybach, Co-Chair
Ken Smith, 0
David Agarwal, Board Member
Dottie Cooper, Interim Executive Director

National, nonprofit public charity that works for the benefit of individuals with Prader-Willi syndrome and their families. An organization of parents and others who are making a difference in the lives of those with Prader-Willi syndrome. Dedicated to serving individuals affected by Prader-Willi syndrome (PWS) their families, and interested professionals. To provide information, education, and support services to its members.

8156 Rasmussen's Syndrome and Hemispherectomy Support Network
8235 Lethbridge Rd
Millersville, MD 21108-1609
410-987-5221
FAX: 410-987-521
e-mail: rssnlynn@aol.com

Al & Lynn Miller, Founders

National not-for-profit organization dedicated to providing information and support to individuals affected by Rasmussen's Syndrome and Hemispherectomy. Publishes a periodic newsletter and disseminates reprints of medical journal articles concerning Rasmussen's Syndrome and its treatments. Maintains a support network that provides encouragement and information to individuals affected by Rasmussen's Syndrome and their families.

8157 Scientific Health Solutions
1621 N Circle Dr
Colorado Springs, CO 80909-2407
719-548-1600
800-331-2303
FAX: 719-572-8081
www.tomlevymd.com/serumtest.htm

Blanche Grube, Owner
Thomas Levy, President

SHS seeks to help those who are looking to avoid new dental toxicity by offering serum biocompatibility testing to help guide the choice of replacement dental materials. Every attempt is also made to help these people find dentists who are familiar with the testing, as well as with the general concepts of dental toxicity that are addressed on TomLevyMD.com

8158 Simon Foundation for Continence
PO Box 815
Wilmette, IL 60091-815
847-864-3913
800-237-4666
FAX: 847-864-9758
e-mail: cbgartley@simonfoundation.org
www.simonfoundation.org

Cheryle B Gartley, Founder/President
Anita Saltmarche, VP
Twila Yednock, Director of Special Events
Elizabeth LaGro, Director of Communications

The Simon Foundation is known throughout the world for its innovative educational projects and tireless efforts on behalf of people with loss of bladder and bowel control. Simon has led the way forward with many groundbreaking projects, for example: the first book written for laypersons, Managing Incontinence: A Guide to Living with the Loss of Bladder Control.

8159 Simonton Cancer Center
PO Box 6607
Malibu, CA 90264-6607
818-879-7904
800-459-3424
FAX: 310-457-0421
e-mail: simontoncancercenter@msn.com
www.simontoncenter.com

O Carl Simonton, Founder
Edward Gilbert, MD, Medical Director
Karen Smith Simonton, Executive / Program Director
Jessica Jedvaj, BA, Administrative Assistant

The Simonton Cancer Center is a non-profit organization dedicated to improving the health and lives of cancer patients and their families through psycho-social oncology.

8160 Spina Bifida Association
4590 Macarthur Blvd NW
Suite 250
Washington, DC 20007- 4226
202-618-4747
800-621-3141
FAX: 202-944-3295
e-mail: sbamar@sbamar.org
www.spinabifidaassociation.org

Cindy Brownstein, President and Chief Executive Of
Robin Austin, Communications Manager
Amanda Darnley, Director of Communications & Mar
Carmen J. Head, Director, Education & Support Se

Nonprofit organization. Mission is to promote the prevention of spina bifida and to enhance the lives of all affected. Addresses the specific needs of the spina bifida community and serves as the national representative of almost 60 chapters. Toll free 800 information and referral service. Legislative updates.

8161 Spina Bifida and Hydrocephalus Association of Canada
Suite 647-167 Av Lombard Avenue
Winnipeg,, MB R3B-0V3
204-925-3650
800-565-9488
FAX: 204-925-3654
e-mail: info@sbhac.ca
www.sbhac.ca

Colleen Tablot, President/Executive Director
Linda Randall, VP
Pauline Dooley, Treasurer
Lorelei Fletcher, Secretary

The Spina Bifida and Hydrocephalus Association of Canada has been working on behalf of people with spina bifida and/or hydrocephalus and their families.

8162 Taking Control of Your Diabetes (TCOYD)
1110 Camino Del Mar
Suite B
Del Mar, CA 92014-2649
858-755-5683
800-998-2693
FAX: 858-755-6854
e-mail: info@tcoyd.org
www.tcoyd.org

Sandra Bourdette, Co-Founder/Executive Director
Steven V Edelman, Founder/Director
Jill Yapo, Director of Operations
Roz Hodgins, Director, External Affairs

Taking Control of Your Diabetes works to educate and motivate people with diabetes to take a more active role in their condition and to provide innovative and integrative continuing diabetes education to medical professionals caring for people with diabetes.

8163 Tourette Syndrome Association
42-40 Bell Boulevard
Bayside, NY 11361-2874
718-224-2999
888-486-8738
FAX: 718-279-9596
e-mail: ts@tsa-usa.org
www.tsa-usa.org

Judit Ungar, President
Kevin St. P. McNaught, Vice President, Medical and Scie
Gary Frank, Executive Vice President
Dan Rostan, Vice President, Field Services

National, nonprofit membership organization. Mission is to identify the cause of, find the cure for, and control the effects of this disorder. A growing number of local chapters nationwide provide educational materials, seminars, conferences and support groups for over 35,000 members. Publishes brochures, flyers, educational materials and papers on treatment and research. Offers videos for purchase through a catalog of publications.

8164 United Cerebral Palsy
1825 K Street NW
Suite 600
Washington, DC 20006
202-776-0406
800-872-5827
FAX: 202-776-0414
e-mail: info@ucp.org
www.ucp.org

Tanneka Jones,, Director of Finance
Marc Irlandez, Director of Technology & Life La
Giselle Pole, Director of Development
Kaelan Richards, Director of Communications

UCP educates, advocates and provides support services to ensure a life without limits for people with a spectrum of disabilities. UCP works to advance the independence, productivity and full citizenship of people with disabilities through an affiliate network that has helped millions.

8165 United Cerebral Palsy of New York City
80 Maiden Lane
8th Floor
New York, NY 10038
212-683-6700
800-484-3827
e-mail: info@ucpnyc.org
www.ucpnyc.org

Linda B. Laul, Associate Executive Director, Pr
Mariette McBride, Assistant Executive Director for Adult and Clinical Services
Marianne Giordano, Assistant Executive Director for Education and Recreation Se
Vincent Siasoco, M.D., Medical Director

Has a more than 60 year history in the disability field and currently serves 14,000 individuals and family members through more than 75 programs. Its mission is to provide the highest quality services in health care, education, employment, housing and technology resources that support people with cerebral palsy and related disabilities in leading independent and productive lives.

8166 United Spinal Association
75-20 Astoria Boulevard
East Elmhurst, NY 11370
718-803-3782
FAX: 718-803-0414
unitedspinal.org

8167 Universal Institute: Rehab & Fitness Center
15-17 Microlab Rd
Ste 101
Livingston, NJ 07039
973-992-8181
800-468-5440
FAX: 973-992-9797
www.uirehab.com

Adam Steinberg, President
Lisa Lasso, VP CFO

Universal institute is a 15,000 square foot, state of the art rehabilitation facility that specializes in neurological disorders such as brain injuries, spinal cord injury, strokes, etc. We offer PT, OT, speech patholgy, cognitive remediation, aqua therapy and EMG biofeedback.

Camps

8168 ADA Camp Grenada
American Diabetes Association
1701 N. Beauregard St.
Alexandria, VA 22311
217-875-9011
800-DIA-ETES
800-342-2383
FAX: 217-726-2260
e-mail: volunteerupdates@diabetes.org.
diabetes.org

Dwight Holing, Chair
Larry Hausner, CEO
Debbie Johnson, CFO
Greg Elfers, Chief Field Development Officer

Camp Granada is an American Diabetes Association resident Camp located in Monticello, Illinois at the 4H Memorial Camp owned by the University of Illinois. For children with diabetes, ages 8-16. Activities include swimming, canoeing, wall climbing, tie-dying shirts, arts & crafts and fun filled evening programs.

8169 ADA Camp Kushtaka
American Diabetes Association
8216 Princeton-Glendale Rd.
PMB200
West Chester, OH 45069-1675
907-272-1424
800-342-2383
FAX: 907-272-1428
e-mail: pbell@diabetes.org
www.childrenwithdiabetes.com

Lori Cowie, Executive Director
Pam Bell, Organizer
Katherine Swartz, Program Director

ADA Camp Kushtaka is for children ages 7-17 with diabetes and their family (space permitting) and is located on the shores of Kenai Lake on the Kenai Peninsula in Cooper Landing. Camp is held in June and combines ongoing and informal diabetes management and education along with the fun of outdoor activities such as hiking, canoeing, crafts and swimming.

8170 ADA Camp Needlepoint
American Diabetes Association
1701 N. Beauregard St.
Alexandria, VA 22311
763-593-5333
800-DIA-ETES
800-342-2383
FAX: 952-582-9000
e-mail: cholten@diabetes.org
www.diabetes.org

Dwight Holing, Chair
Larry Hausner, CEO
Debbie Johnson, CFO
Greg Elfers, Chief Field Development Officer

Camping for children who have type 1 diabetes. Coed, ages 5-16.

8171 ADA Camp Sunshine
American Diabetes Association
PO Box 385
Huntsville, AL 35804
256-757-8114
FAX: 585-458-3810
www.diabetescamps.org

Terry Ackley, Exeuctive Director
Shelley Yeager, Director,Outreach & Development
Kathy Latimer, Administrative Assistant
Lisa Gier, Board Member

The American Diabetes Association New York Area's Camp is a residential camp for children with diabetes. The program is held on the Rotary Sunshine Campus in Rush, only 15 miles from Rochester. The camp is located on 133 acres of land in a rural setting including modern year round cabins, an Olympic-sized swimming pool, nature trails, athletic fields and a fishing pond. Ages 8-16; held during July.

8172 ADA Camp for Kids
American Diabetes Association
1701 N. Beauregard St.
Alexandria, VA 22311-3649
505-266-5716
888-342-2383
800-DIA-ETES
FAX: 505-268-4533
e-mail: lbrown@diabetes.org
www.diabetes.org/adacampnm

Dwight Holing, Chair
Larry Hausner, CEO
Debbie Johnson, CFO
Greg Elfers, Chief Field Development Officer

One-week camping session for children with diabetes. Coed, ages 8-13. Camp will be held at Manzano Mountain Retreat, one hour from Albuquerque, New Mexico. Please call for exact dates.

8173 ADA Teen Adventure Camp
American Diabetes Association
1701 N. Beauregard St.
Alexandria, VA 22311
312-346-1805
888-342-2383
800-DIA-ETES
FAX: 312-346-5342
e-mail: mejohnson@diabetes.org
www.diabetes.org/adacampteenadventure

Dwight Holing, Chair
Larry Hausner, CEO
Debbie Johnson, CFO
Greg Elfers, Chief Field Development Officer

Camping for teenagers with diabetes. Coed, ages 14 to 18. Camp dates are early in August. Located at the YMCA Camp Duncan in Ingleside, Illinois. Featured activities include archery and crafts, singing, outdoor movie night, and roller skating.

8174 ADA Triangle D Camp
American Diabetes Association
1701 N. Beauregard St.
Alexandria, VA 22311
312-346-1805
888-342-2383
800-DIA-ETES
FAX: 312-346-5342
e-mail: mejohnson@diabetes.org
www.diabetes.org/adacamptriangled

Dwight Holing, Chair
Larry Hausner, CEO
Debbie Johnson, CFO
Greg Elfers, Chief Field Development Officer

Triangle D Camp is a resident camp program located at the YMCA Camp Duncan in Ingleside, Illinois. Activities include swimming, row boating, canoeing, high ropes (11-13 yr. olds), climbing tower (9-10 yr. olds), Camp games, singing, archery, campfires, soccer, basketball, volleyball and diabetes education.

8175 ASCCA
Alabama Easter Seal Society
5278 Camp Ascca Drive
P.O. Box 21
Jacksons Gap, AL 36861
256-825-9226
800-THE-CAMP
FAX: 256-825-8332
e-mail: info@campascca.org
www.campascca.org

John Stephenson, Administrator
Matt Rickman, Camp Director
Joe Spavone, R.N., Director of Health Services
Allison Wetherbee, Director of Community Relations

Camp ASCCA is for children and adults with disabilities or health impairements. Camp ASCCA strives to help these individuals achieve equality, independence and dignity in a safe environment.

8176 Adventure Day Camp
3480 Commission Ct
Lake Ridge, VA 22192
703-491-1444
e-mail: office@princewilliamacademy.com
www.princewilliamacademy.com

Dr. Samia Harris, Founder & Executive Director
Rebecca Nykwest, Communications Director
Lindsay Chickering, Office Manager
Shiree Slade, Principal

Camping for children with asthma/respiratory ailments and cancer. Coed, ages 2-13.

8177 Agassiz Village
238 Bedford St
Suite B
Lexington, MA 02420-3477
781-860-0200
FAX: 781-860-0352
e-mail: csimmonds@agassizvillage.org
www.agassizvillage.org

Cliff Simmonds, Executive Director
Thomas Semeta, Camp Director
Warren Soar, Facility Director
Warren H Burroughs, Honorary Chairman

Agassiz Village offers a variety of activities for all campers, boys and girls, younger camper and teens, and programs for physically challenged children and teens. By participating in daily activities, campers build a cooperative and positive community of different races, ages, ethnic and cultural backgrounds while enhancing confidence and individuality. Camp is located in Poland, Maine. For ages 8-17.

8178 Arizona Camp Sunrise
American Cancer Society
PO Box 27872
Tempe, AZ 85285
602-952-7550
800-865-1582
FAX: 602-404-1118
e-mail: barb.nicholas@cancer.org
www.azcampsunrise.org

Barbara Nicholas, Director
Leigh Ansley, Manager
Melissa Lee, Camp Director
Jason Poulter, Technical Media Director

Provides one-week summer camping sessions to children aged 8-16 who have had, or currently have, cancer. The classes range from sports and outdoor games to dance and drama, arts, crafts, and cooking. Other activities planned for the campers include horseback riding, a trip to a lake, a dance, and learning to make friendship bracelets.

8179 Bearskin Meadow Camp
Diabetic Youth Foundation
5167 Clayton Road
Suite F
Concord, CA 94521
925-680-4994
FAX: 925-680-4863
e-mail: info@dyf.org
www.dyf.org

Mark McComb, President
Paula Gogin, Development Director
Janet Kramschuster, Interim Executive Director
Jennifer Goerzen, Resident Camp manager

Bearskin Meadow Campis is for children, teens and their families who are affected by diabetes. Bearskin teaches skills for blook glucose checking and techniques for adjusting insulin, food choices and how to have a fun, active life while living with diabetes.

8180 Becket Chimney Corners YMCA Camps and Outdoor Center
748 Hamilton Rd
Becket, MA 01223
413-623-8991
FAX: 413-623-5890
e-mail: cburke@bccymca.org
www.bccymca.org

Drew Lipsher, Chair
David Smith, Vice Chair
Christine Kalakay, Chief Financial Officer
Phil Connor, CEO

Half-week and one-week sessions for campers with asthma/respiratory ailments. Coed, ages 3 and up, families, seniors, single adults.

8181 Bright Horizons Summer Camp
Sickle Cell Disease Association of Illinois
8100 S. Western Avenue
Chicago, IL 60620
773-526-5016
866-798-1097
FAX: 773-526-5012
e-mail: sicklecelldisease-illinois@scdai.org
sicklecelldisease-illinois.org

Darryl H. Armstrong, Chair
TaLana Hughes, Executive Director
Anquineice Brown, Outreach Coordinator
Alana Burke, Case Manager

Camping for children with blood disorders, ages 7-13. The joys of learning include instruction in first aid, swimming and water safety, boating, horseback riding and bowling plus arts and crafts. In addition, there is a traditional menu of camp pleasures, like hayrides, cookouts, nature hikes and sing-a-longs.

8182 Camp Alpine
Alpine Alternatives
2518 E. Tudor Road
Suite 105
Anchorage, AK 99507
907-561-6655
800-361-4174
FAX: 907-563-9232
e-mail: info@alpinealternatives.org
ftp.akaccessiblemedia.org/

Margaret Webber, Executive Director

Our programs are designed to help people expand their horizons, master new skills, make new friends, and increase motor coordination. Most importantly, participants experience growth in self-confidence and independence that affects all aspects of an individual's life. Our services are open to all, regardless of type of disability or age. Activities include canoeing, hiking, swimming, outdoor games, sports, nature identification and much more.

8183 Camp Anuenue
250 Williams St. NW
Atlanta, GA 30303
808-595-7500
888-227-2345
FAX: 808-595-7502
e-mail: debra.glowik@cancer.org
www.cancer.org

Pamela K. Meyerhoffer, Chair
Robert E. Youle, Vice Chairman
Douglas K. Kelsey, Board Scientific Officer
Daniel P. Heist, Secretary/Treasurer

(1 week) June, children with or recovered from cancer.

8184 Camp Birchwood
Muscular Dystrophy Association
P.O.Box 670049
Chugiak, AK 99567
907-688-2734
FAX: 907-688-2734
e-mail: info@birchwoodcamp.org
www.birchwoodcamp.org

John Quinley, President
Doug Handlong, VP
Berneita Norris, Food Service Manager
Joyce Del Rosario, Office Manager

A summer camp at Birchwood Camp in Chugiak, Alaska for individuals ages 6-21 who are affected by any of the 40-plus neuromuscular diseases in MDA's program. Common activities include: swimming, hockey, baseball, soccer, football, boating, horseback riding, fishing, music, cooking, arts and crafts, movies, dancing, talent shows, Harley-Davidson motorcycle sidecar or three-wheeled cycle rides, a visit from fire fighters and time for socializing and laughing.

8185 Camp Boggy Creek
30500 Brantley Branch Rd
Eustis, FL 32736
352-483-4200
866-462-6449
FAX: 352-483-0589
e-mail: info@campboggycreek.org
www.boggycreek.org

J. Patterson Cooper, Chair
Wendy Durden, Vice Chair
June Clark, President/CEO
Paul Newman, Founder

Year-round sessions for children with a variety of chronic or life-threatening illnesses including cancer, hemophila, epilepsy, heart defects, HIV, spina bifida and asthma/respiratory ailments. Coed, ages 7-16.

8186 Camp Bon Coeur
Bon Coeur, Inc.
405 West Main St.
Lafayette, LA 70505-3765
337-233-8437
FAX: 337-233-4160
e-mail: info@heartcamp.com
www.heartcamp.com

Susannah Craig, Executive Director
Antonio Conner, MBA, President
Susan Randol, RN, MSN, Vice-President
Martha Wyatt, CPA, Treasurer

Two-week sessions June-July for children with heart defects. Coed, ages 8-16.

8187 Camp Breathe Easy
American Lung Association
404-231-9887
e-mail: annie@camptwinlakes.org
campbreatheeasy.com

Annie Garrett, Camp Director

Camp Breathe Easy is a seven-day, six-night overnight camp for children, ages 7-13, with asthma who need medication and are limited in summer camping opportunities. The children learn asthma self-management techniques and coping strategies to better handle their illness. Campers swim, repel off trees, fish, canoe, play soccer, basketball and miniature golf, and participate in ceramics and arts and crafts.

8188 Camp Carefree
American Diabetes Association
1846 West Seventh Street
Piscataway, NJ 08850-1918
732-752-1715
e-mail: director@campcarefreekids.org
www.campcarefreekids.org

Phyllis Woestemeyer, Director
Katie Nitchie, Camp Coordinator

Camp is located in Wolfeboro, New Hampshire. Sessions for campers with diabetes.

8189 Camp Carolina Trails for Children
American Diabetes Association
222 S Church St
Suite 336M
Charlotte, NC 28202-3247
704-373-9111
800-342-2383
888-342-2383
FAX: 704-373-9113
e-mail: enivens@diabetes.org
www.childrenwithdiabetes.com

Dianne Roth, Manager

The American Diabetes Association Camp Carolina Trails is an exciting week of summer fun for boys and girls entering grades 4 through 11. Camp includes many sports and activities such as swimming, hiking, canoeing and arts and crafts. It is held at

YMCA Camp Hanes on 400 acres next to hanging Rock State Park which is located at the base of Sauratown Mountain, just 30 minutes north of Winston-Salem, North Carolina. Camp for ages 10-17. Use address given in Virginia for more information.

8190 Camp Catch-a-Rainbow
American Cancer Society
250 Williams St. NW
Atlanta, GA 30303
808-595-7500
888-227-2345
FAX: 808-595-7502
e-mail: debra.glowik@cancer.org
www.cancer.org

Pamela K. Meyerhoffer, Chair
Robert E. Youle, Vice Chairman
Douglas K. Kelsey, Board Scientific Officer
Daniel P. Heist, Secretary/Treasurer

Camp Catch-a-Rainbow's programs are available completely free to any child in MI or IN who has or has had cancer, between the ages of 4 and 20, with their doctor's approval. Family Camp is reserved for those campers who have attended camp during that year's summer sessions and their families. Day, week, adult retreat, and family camp are available options.

8191 Camp Cheerful
Achievement Centers For Children
15000 Cheerful Ln
Strongsville, OH 44136-5420
440-238-6200
FAX: 440-238-1858
www.achievementcenters.org

Tim Fox, Executive Director
Bonnie Boenig, OTR/L, Director Therapy Services & Intensive Therapy Clinic
Donna Hefner McClure, M.S., Director of Education
Darla Motil, R.N., Director of Community Relations

Sessions for campers with developmental disabilities, mobility limitation and speech/communication impairment. Coed, ages 7-99.

8192 Camp Christmas Seal
American Lung Association of Oregon
102 W McDowell Rd
Phoenix, AZ 85003-1213
602-258-7505
FAX: 202-452-1805
e-mail: info@lungoregon.org
www.lungoregon.org

Kathryn A. Forbes, Chairman
John F. Emanuel, Vice Chair
Harold Wimmer, President/CEO
Penny J. Siewert, Secretary/Treasurer

Camp is located in Sisterhood, Oregon. Sessions for children with asthma/respiratory ailments. Coed, ages 8-15.

8193 Camp Classen YMCA
YMCA of Greater Oklahoma City
10840 Main Camp Rd
Davis, OK 73030
580-369-2272
FAX: 580-369-2284
www.itsmycamp.org

Ford C. Price, Chair
Tricia Everest, Vice Chairman
Mike Grady, President & CEO
Don Harris, Vice President & CFO

Camp is located in Davis, Oklahoma. Sessions for children and adults with diabetes. Coed, ages 8-17, families, seniors and single adults.

8194 Camp Conrad-Chinnock
Diabetic Youth Services
12045 E. Waterfront Drive
Playa Vista, CA 90094
310-751-3057
FAX: 888-800-4010
www.dys.org

Rocky Wilson, Executive and Camp Director
Dale Lissy, Camp Manager
Ryan Martz, Program Director
Tom Jenkins, Chief Operating Officer

Camp Conrad-Chinnock offers many recreational programs such as swimming, canoeing, arts & crafts to young adults and their families with diabetes. Dietary education programs and diabetes management are also available.

8195 Camp Courage North
Courage Center
3915 Golden Valley Rd
Golden Valley, MN 55422
763-588-0811
888-846-8253
FAX: 763-520-0577
e-mail: Information@CourageCenter.org
www.couragecenter.org

Jan Malcolm, CEO
Pamela J. Lindemoen, Executive Vice President of Oper
Stephen Bariteau, Chief Development Officer
Alice Johnson, Chief Financial Officer

Courage Center Camps - Camp Courage & Camp Courage North - are part of Courage Center, a non-profit rehabilitation and resource center for people of all ages and abilities who are experiencing barriers to health & independence. For more than 50 years, Courage Center camps have served children and adults with physical disabilities and those who are deaf and hard of hearing. In 2008, more than 800 people attended a Courage Center camp session. For more information, visit our web-site.

8196 Camp Del Corazon
11615 Hesby St
North Hollywood, CA 91601-3620
818-754-0312
888-621-4800
FAX: 818-754-0842
e-mail: information@campdelcorazon.org
www.campdelcorazon.org

Kevin Shannon, Co-Founder/President/Medical Director
Dan Levi, Board Member
Joel McHale, Board Member
Tom Arnold, Board Member

Active program for campers with heart disease, Camp del Corazon provides summer activities free of charge that include hiking and archery, arts and crafts, court and field games, waterfront activities and a beach barbecue.

8197 Camp Discovery
American Diabetes Association
PO Box 385
Huntsville, AL 35804
256-757-8114
FAX: 519-660-8992
e-mail: info@diabetescamps.org
www.diabetescamps.org

Mark Moyer, President
Terry Ackley, Executive Director
Philip De Rea, Treasurer
Janet Kramschauster, Secretary

Camp is located in Junction City, Kansas. Offers young people with diabetes a week of fun at rock springs 4-H Center. Special attention to diabetes makes Camp Discovery a safe environment for active youth while providing valuable diabetes managment education. Call the American Diabetes Association Kansas area office for more information. Coed, ages 8-17.

8198 Camp Eden Wood
Friendship Ventures
10509 108th St NW
Annandale, MN 55302
952-852-0101
800-450-8376
FAX: 952-852-0123
e-mail: info@friendshipventures.org
friendshipventures.org

Floyd Adelman, Chair
Jeff Bangsberg, Board Member
Robert Harnett, Board Member
Jerry Caruso, Board Member

Camp is located in Eden Prairie, Minnesota. Offers resident camp programs for children, teenagers and adults with developmental, physical or multiple disabilities, Down Syndrome, special medical conditions, Williams Syndrome, autism and/or other conditions. Fishing, creative arts, golf, sports and other activities are available. Respite care weekend camps year round for children, teenagers and adults. Guided vacations for teens and adults with developmental disabilities or other unique needs.

8199 Camp Floyd Rogers
Floyd Rogers Foundation
P.O.Box 31536
Omaha, NE 68131 402-341-0866
FAX: 402-341-0866
www.campfloydrogers.com

Buzz Wheeler, Camp Director

A camp for diabetic children. Coed, ages 8-18. 100 children come to Camp Floyd Rogers each summer. They come to enjoy activities, participate in special events, engage in innovative evening programs, and they meet other children their own age with diabetes. Camp Floyd Rogers offers young people an opportunity to share some of life's adventures with others who also happen to have diabetes.

8200 Camp Fun in the Sun
Inland NorthWest Health Services
P.O.Box 469
Spokane, WA 99210-0469 509-232-8138
www.campfuninthesun.org

Debbie Belknap, Registered Nurse
Colleen Carey, Endocrinologist
Joan Milton, Registered Dietitian
Laurie Payne, Registered Dietitian

Summer camp for children ages 8-18 whom have diabetes.

8201 Camp Glengarra
Girl Scouts - Foothills Council
33 Jewett Pl
Utica, NY 13501-4715 315-733-1909
FAX: 315-733-1909
e-mail: nbrown@girlscoutsfoothills.org
www.girlscoutsfoothills.org

Natalie Brown, Executive Director
Karen Lubecki, Director

Camp Glengarra is located on 500+ acres of fields and forests, about eight miles west of Camden. This Girl Scout Camp hosts a myriad of programs throughout the year as well as summer day and resident camp. Summer sessions for girls 5-17 with ADD or asthma/respiratory ailments.

8202 Camp Glyndon
American Diabetes Association
800 Wyman Park Dr
Suite 110
Baltimore, MD 21211-2837 410-265-0075
800-342-2383
FAX: 410-235-4048
e-mail: askada@diabetes.org
www.childrenwithdiabetes.com

Heather Magoon, Director

Camp is located in Nanjemoy, Maryland. One and two-week sessions July-August for children with diabetes and their families. Coed, ages 8-16.

8203 Camp Harkness
Arc of New London County
125 Sachem St
Norwich, CT 06360 860-889-4435
FAX: 860-889-4662
TTY:860-859-5493
e-mail: info@thearcnlc.org
www.thearcnlc.org/

Enrico DeMatto, President
Linda Rhodse, VP
Alan Messier, Treasurer
Wendy Mis, Secretary

In 1991 a group of parents and adults with spina bifida, were brought together with the mission to educate the public about spina bifida and issues affecting people who have this disability in addition To providing support and information and promoting programs that will help people with spina bifida. Since then SBAC has worked hard to support parents, adults with spina bifida and families

8204 Camp Hertko Hollow
101 Locust St
Des Moines, IA 50309 515-471-8523
888-437-8652
FAX: 515-288-2531
e-mail: a.wolf@camphertkohollow.com
www.camphertkohollow.com

Troy Norman, President
Brant Ausenhus, VP
Vicki Hertko, Treasurer
Steve Roy, Legal Counsel

Camp Hertko Hollow is a resident camp held at the Des Moines YMCA Camp site, located along the Des Moines River north of Boone, Iowa. Activities include horseback riding, swimming, canoeing, rappelling, crafts, ropes course, archery and riflery to name a few, plus special activities for different ages. Half-week and one-week sessions for children with diabetes. Coed, ages 6-16.

8205 Camp Hickory Hill
Central Missouri Diabetic Childrens Camp
P.O.Box 1942
Columbia, MO 65205 573-445-9146
e-mail: CampHickoryHill@gmail.com
www.camphickoryhill.com

David Bernhardt, President
Lisa Bernhardt, Camp Director
Nate Wisdom, Program Director
Frank La Mantia, Development Director

Educates diabetic children concerning diabetes and its care. In addition to daily educational sessions on some aspects of diabetes, campers participate in swimming, sailing, arts and crafts and overnight camping. Coed, ages 8-17.

8206 Camp Ho Mita Koda
Diabetes Association Of Greater Cleveland
3601 South Green Road
Suite 100
Cleveland, OH 44122 216-591-0800
FAX: 216-591-0320
e-mail: information@diabetespartnership.org
www.dagc.org

Roger Ruch, Chair
William Murman, Vice Chair
Christina R. Milano, President/CEO
Kyle Chones, Camp Director

Camp is located in Newbury, Ohio. Summer sessions for children with type 1 diabetes. Coed, ages 6-15. Type 2 diabetes, coed, ages 12-17. Bicycle adventure, coed, ages 13-19. Mini-day camp, ages 4-7, coed.

8207 Camp Hodia
1701 N 12th Street
Boise, ID 83702 208-891-1023
FAX: 208-891-1023
e-mail: alan@hodia.org
www.hodia.org

Natalie B. DelRio, Chair
Richard Christensen, Vice Chair
lLisa Gier, Executice Director
Vicki Cutshall, R.N., Director, Hodia Kids Camp

Camp is located in Alturas Lake, Idaho. One-week sessions for children with diabetes. Coed, ages 8-18. Ski Camp in Sun Valley in January, ages 12-18.

8208 Camp Honor
Hemophilia Association
826 N. 5th Ave.
Phoenix, AZ 85003 602-955-3947
888-754-7017
FAX: 602-955-1962
e-mail: info@hemophiliaz.org
www.hemophiliaz.org

Steven Helm, President
Jim Drurr, Vice President
Cindy Komar, CEO
Lindsey Bogard, Communications Director

Camp is located in Payson, Arizona at the Whispering Hope Ranch. One-week sessions for children with hemophilia or HIV and their siblings, as well as children of hemophiliacs. Coed, ages 7-17. Activities include swimming, canoeing, sports, archery and arts and crafts (to name a few fun things).

8209 Camp Independence

National Kidney Foundation
30 East 33rd Street
New York, NY 10016
770-452-1539
800-622-9010
FAX: 212-689-9261
e-mail: info@kidney.org
www.kidneyga.org

Gregory W. Scott, Chair
Beth Piraino, President
Bruce Skyer, CEO
Joseph Vassalotti, Chief Medical Officer

Camp Independence is Georgia's a overnight, week-long summer camp providing essential medical care, treatment & fun for kids with kidney disease and transplants. Camp Independence recognizes that campers are normal children but have special needs providing these children with opportunities for development & individual growth, peer support & normal life experiences. Activities include swimming, arts & crafts, fishing and horsebackriding, in addition to archery, games and sports, and ceramics.

8210 Camp Jened

United Cerebral Palsy Association New York
P.O.Box 483
Rock Hill, NY 12775-483
845-434-2220
FAX: 845-434-2253
www.campjened.org

Michael Branam, Executive Director

Camp is located in Rock Hill, New York. Sessions for adults with severe developmental and physical disabilities. Coed, ages 18-99.

8211 Camp John Warvel

American Diabetes Association
1701 N. Beauregard St.
Alexandria, VA 22311
312-346-1805
888-342-2383
800-DIA-ETES
FAX: 317-594-0748
www.diabetes.org

Dwight Holing, Chair
Larry Hausner, CEO
Debbie Johnson, CFO
Greg Elfers, Chief Field Development Officer

Camp is located in North Webster, Indiana. Provides an enjoyable, safe and educational out-of-doors experience for children with insulin-dependent diabetes. A unique learning atmosphere for children to acquire new skills in caring for their disease. The camp experience instills confidence for the child's self-management of diabetes. Offers one-week sessions and can accommodate 200 campers, boys and girls aged 7-16.

8212 Camp Joslin

Barton Center for Diabetes Education
30 Ennis Road
PO Box 356
North Oxford, MA 01537-0356
508-987-2056
FAX: 508-987-2002
e-mail: info@bartoncenter.org
www.bartoncenter.org

Thomas C. Lynch, Chair
John Peri-Okonny, 1st Vice chiar
Kristin Dyer, 2nd Vice Chair
Mark W. Fuller, Treasurer

Camp is located in Charlton, Massachusetts. For boys, ages 7-16, with diabetes. This program offers active summer sports and activities, supplemented by medical treatment and diabetes education. Coed Winter Camp and Coed Weekend Retreats are offered during the school year.

8213 Camp Joy

3325 Swamp Creek Rd
Schwenksville, PA 19473-1518
610-754-6878
FAX: 610-754-7880
e-mail: campjoy@fast.net
www.campjoy.com

Robert G Griffith, President

A special needs camp for kids and adults (ages 4-80+) with developmental disabilities such as: mental retardation, autism, brain injury, neurological disorder, visual and/or hearing impairments, Angelman and Down syndromes, and other developmental disabilities.

8214 Camp Ko-Man-She

American Diabetes Association
2555 S Dixie Drive
Suite 112
Dayton, OH 45409
937-220-6611
FAX: 937-224-0240
e-mail: dada@diabetesdayton.org
www.diabetesdayton.org

Terry Fague, President
Tyler Starline, VP
Susan McGovern, Executive Director
Robin Robertson, Administrative Assistant

Camp is located in Bellefontaine, Ohio. Summer sessions for children with diabetes. Coed, ages 8-17. Held in July.

8215 Camp Kweebec

157 Game Farm Rd.
Schwenksville, PA 19473
610-667-2123
FAX: 610-667-6376
e-mail: info@kweebec.com
www.kweebec.com

Les Weiser, Owner/Director
Maddy Weiser, Owner/Director
Rachel Weiser, Associate Director, Director of
Josh Weiser, Associate Director

Camp is located in Schwenksville, Pennsylvania. Sessions for children and adults with diabetes. Coed, ages 6-16, families, seniors and single adults.

8216 Camp L-Kee-Ta

940 Golden Valley Drive
Bettendorf, IA 52722
319-752-3639
800-798-0833
FAX: 319-753-1410
www.gseiwi.org

Teresa Colgan, Chair
Jill Dashner, 1st Vice chiar
Anna Gibney, Development Manager
Ann Hulett, Business Operations Coordinator

Camp is located in Danville, Iowa. Half-week and one-week sessions June-August for children with asthma/respiratory ailments. Girls, ages 7-18 and families.

8217 Camp Latgawa

Oregon-Idaho Conference Center
13250 S Fork Little Butte Creek Rd
Eagle Point, OR 97524- 5593
541-826-9699
e-mail: camplatgawa@hotmail.com
www.latgawa.gocamping.org

Eva LaBonty, Director

Camp Latgawa provides year round hospitality for groups up to 90 people. The bunk/dormitory style facilities are heated and have restrooms and showers either in the cabin or nearby.

8218 **Camp Libbey**
Maumee Valley Girl Scout Center
2244 Collingwood Blvd
Toledo, OH 43620-1147
419-243-8216
800-860-4516
FAX: 419-245-5357
e-mail: KelleeChancellor@girlscoutsofwesternohio.org
www.girlscoutsofwesternohio .org

Jody Wainscott, Chair
Ellen Iobst, 1st Vice Chair
Susan Gantz Matz, 2nd Vice Chair
Jerry Brose, Secretary
Camp for girls 7-18 with asthma/respiratory ailments, diabetes, epilepsy and muscular dystrophy is located in Defiance, Ohio.

8219 **Camp MITIOG**
Share, Inc
7615 N. Platte Purchase Drive
Kansas City, MO 64118
816-221-4450
877-221-4450
FAX: 816-221-1420
e-mail: midlands@midlandsmc.org
www.midlandsmc.org

Mike Hale, President/Financial Officer
Pam Mathena, Adm. Assistant to MMC Financial Officer
Donna Fletcher, Congregational Consultant
Don McLaughlin, Outreach Coordinator
Camp is located in Excelsior Springs, Missouri. One-week summer sessions for children with spina bifida. Coed, ages 6-16.

8220 **Camp Magruder**
Oregon-Idaho Conference Center
17450 Old Pacific Hwy
Rockaway Beach, OR 97136
503-355-2310
FAX: 503-355-8701
e-mail: director@campmagruder.org
www.campmagruder.org

Steve Rumage, Camp Director
Amy Wood, Program Services Director
Diana Gutzke, Reservations/ Guest Services
Mark Burley Manager, Maintenance Team
Camp is located in Rockaway Beach, Oregon. Sessions for children and adults with cancer and developmental disabilities. Coed, ages 9-18, families, seniors and single adults.

8221 **Camp Nejeda**
Camp Nejeda Foundation
910 Saddlebrook Road
P.O. Box 156
Stillwater, NJ 07875
973-383-2611
FAX: 973-383-9891
e-mail: information@campnejeda.org
www.campnejeda.org

Henry Anhalt, President
Scott Ross, VP
Denise Dadika, Board Member
William Curcio, Board Member
For children with diabetes, ages 7-15. Provides an active and safe camping experience which enables the children to learn about and understand diabetes. Activities include boating, swimming, fishing, archery, as well as camping skills.

8222 **Camp Not-A-Wheeze**
American Lung Association In Arizona
102 W McDowell Rd
Phoenix, AZ 85003-1213
602-258-7505
FAX: 202-452-1805
e-mail: info@lungoregon.org
www.lungarizona.org

Kathryn A. Forbes, Chairman
John F. Emanuel, Vice Chair
Harold Wimmer, President/CEO
Penny J. Siewert, Secretary/Treasurer
Camp Not-A-Wheeze is designed especially for kids ages 7-14 with moderate to severe asthma and was created to provide a traditional residential camp experience and teach children how to manage their asthma.

8223 **Camp Okizu**
Okizu Foundation
16 Digital Dr
Suite 130
Novato, CA 94949
415-382-9083
FAX: 415-382-8384
e-mail: info@okizu.org
www.okizu.org

John H. Bell, Chair
Michael D. Amylon, Vice Chair
Suzie Randall, Executive Director/Camp Director
Beth Dekker, Assistant Camp Director
Camp Okizu offers a place where children struggling with a life threatening illness and thier families can come to explore and enjoy a normal life experience. The camp also provides peer support, respite, mentoring, and a variety of other programs designed to help members of families affected by childhood cancer. The camp is open from April through October

8224 **Camp Pelican**
Louisiana Lions Camp
P.O.Box 290247
Kerrville, TX 78029
830-896-8500
FAX: 830-896-3666
e-mail: tlc@ktc.com
www.lionscamp.org

Tim Matakas, President
Kim Breaux, Vice President
Tessie Guillory, Treasurer
Autumn Gaspard, Secretary
Camp Pelican is an overnight residential camp for children with moderate to severe asthma or other pulmonary problems. Founded in 1977, Camp Pelican is jointly sponsored by the Louisiana Pulmonary Disease Camp Inc and the Louisiana Lions Camp. Over 100 children attend annually and participate in education, sports, arts and crafts, swimming and other camping activities. Medical staff including physicians, nurses, respiratory therapists and social workers participate in camp. Coed, ages 5-17.

8225 **Camp Rainbow**
Phoenix Childrens Hospital
1919 East Thomas Road
Phoenix, AZ 85016
602-933-1000
888-908-5437
888-908-KIDS
FAX: 602-546-0276
e-mail: rlyddon@phoenixchildrens.com
www.phoenixchildrens.org/

Jon Hulburd, Chair
Jacque Sokolov, MD, Vice Chair
Robert Meyer, President/CEO
David Lenhardt, Director
Camp is located in Prescott, Arizona. Offers one-week sessions for children who have had, or currently have, cancer. Boys and girls ages 7-17. Camp activities include swimming, horseback riding, arts and crafts, canoeing, performing arts, archery, rollerskating, fishing, an overnight camping trip and much more! It's a week filled with laughter, new experiences and new friends.

8226 **Camp Rap-A-Hope**
2701 Airport Blvd
Mobile, AL 36606
251-476-9880
FAX: 251-476-9495
e-mail: info@camprapahope.org
www.camprapahope.org

Laura Gibson, President
Melissa McNichol, Executive Director
Roz Dorsett, Assistant Director
West Sanders, Public Relations & Grant Development
Camp Rap-A-Hope is a one-week summer camp for children and teenagers who are battling cancer or have ever been diagnosed with cancer and are 7 to 17 years of age. It is free of charge. Camp Rap-A-Hope strives to make sure every camper gets the opportunity to develop new skills and self-confidence. Camp activities are appropriate for our campers' ages and abilities and include, but are not limited to: swimming, music, arts and crafts, archery, fishing, canoeing and horseback riding.

8227 **Camp Ronald McDonald for Good Times**
Ronald McDonald House For Charities-Southern Calif
1250 Lyman Place
Los Angeles, CA 90029
310-268-8488
800-625-7295
FAX: 310-473-3338
www.campronaldmcdonald.org

Edward Lodgen, President
Jodi Lesh, Vice President
Sarah Orth, Executive Director
Ken Teasdale, Treasurer

Free year-round residential camping for children with cancer and their families.

8228 **Camp Sawtooth**
Oregon-Idaho Conference Center
P.O.Box 68
Fairfield, ID 83327-68
800-593-7539
e-mail: sawtooth@gocamping.org
www.gocamping.org

David Hargreaves, Director

Camp located 35 miles north of fairfield, centrally located for all of southern Idaho.

8229 **Camp Seale Harris**
Southeastern Diabetes Education Services
500 Chase Park South
Suite 104
Birmingham, AL 35244
205-402-0415
FAX: 205-402-0416
e-mail: info@southeasterndiabetes.org
www.southeasterndiabetes.org

Tip McAlpin, Chair
Cindy Jamieson, Vice Chair
Rhonda McDavid, Executive Director
Nikki Carlisle, Coastal Programs Manager

A summer residential program that is located at Camp ASCCA (Alabama's Special Camp for Children and Adults), that encourages and motivates youth to reach their full potential despite diabetes, and teaches families how to serve as the primary educators and supporters for children and adolescents living with this illness. Fpur programs are offered: Senior Camp; Junior Camp; Family Camp; and Adventure Camps.

8230 **Camp Setebaid**
Setebaid Services
PO Box 196
Winfield, PA 17889-196
570-524-9090
866-738-3224
FAX: 570-523-0769
e-mail: info@setebaidservices.org
www.setebaidservices.org

Mark A. Moyer, President
David Langdon, VP
Peggy Coleman, Secretary
Jane Evans, Treasurer

Camping sessions for children with diabetes. Coed, ages 3-18 years. Family retreat for children with diabetes and their families.

8231 **Camp Sioux**
American Diabetes Association
106 Solid Rock Cir
Suite C
Park River, ND 58270
763-593-5333
FAX: 952-582-9000
e-mail: rbarnett@diabetes.org
www.diabetescamp.org

Sheila Chrspensen, Executive Director
Becky Barnett, Camp Director

The purpose of Camp Sioux is to provide a fun and safe camping experience for children living with diabetes. We want to give kids the opportunity to meet other kids just like them as well as help them gain confidence and independence in managing their diabetes.

8232 **Camp Smile-A-Mile**
P.O.Box 550155
Birmingham, AL 35255
205-323-8427
888-500-7920
FAX: 205-323-6220
e-mail: info@campsam.org
www.campsam.org

David L. Warren, President
Samuel H. Heide, VP
Ruan Weiss, VP
John C. Rives, Treasurer

Camp Smile-A-Mile is a non-profit organization for children who have or had cancer in Alabama. Camp Smile-A-Mile's mission is to provide challenging, unforgettable recreational and educational experiences for young cancer patients from across Alabama at no cost to their families. Our purpose is to provide these children with avenues for fellowship, to help them cope with their disease, and to prepare them for life.

8233 **Camp Sunrise**
Johns Hopkins Hospital
600 North Wolfe Street
CMSC 800
Baltimore, MD 21287-5904
410-955-5311
www.campsunrisemd.org

Sherryce Robinson, Mission Delivery Manager
Kira Elring, Regional Mission Director
Gloria Jetter, Regional Executive Director
Jack Shipkoski, CEO

Week long summer camp in White Hall, MD., for children ages 6-18 who have been diagnosed with or have survived cancer. Camp sunrise also has a 'day camp' program available for children ages 4-5. Camp activities include sports & games, swimming, arts & crafts, and nature hikes.

8234 **Camp Sweeney**
Southwestern Diabetic Fund
P.O.Box 918
Gainesville, TX 76241
940-665-2011
FAX: 940-665-9467
e-mail: info@campsweeney.org
www.campsweeney.org

Ernie Fernandez, Executive Director

Teaches self-care and self-reliance to children ages 7-18 with diabetes. Campers participate in such activities such as swimming, fishing, horseback riding and arts and crafts while learning about how to self manage their diabetes.

8235 **Camp Tall Turf**
816 Madison SE
Grand Rapids, MI 49507
616-452-7906
FAX: 616-452-7907
e-mail: info@tallturf.org
www.tallturf.org

Eric Brown, Chair
Ed Van Poolen, Vice Chair
Miriam DeJong, Director of Programs
Victoria P. Gibbs, Interim Executive Director

Camp is located in Walkerville, Michigan. Summer camping sessions for youth with asthma/respiratory ailments and ADD. Coed, ages 8-16.

8236 **Camp Taylor, Inc.**
5424 Pirrone Road
Salida, CA 95368
209-545-4715
FAX: 209-543-1861
e-mail: kimberlie@kidsheartcamp.org
www.kidsheartcamp.org

Kimberlie Gamino, Board Member
Rollin A. Podwys, Board Member
Steven Barbieri, Board Member
Charlie Liamos, Board Member

Camp Taylor is a place where children and young adults with heart disease and thier families can come for recreational activities and programs. The camp is open from May through September.

8237 Camp Vacamas
256 Macopin Rd
West Milford, NJ 07480
973-838-0942
877-428-8222
e-mail: info@vacamas.org
www.vacamas.org
Felix A. Urrutia, Executive Director
Kristin Short, Camp Director
Karen Wendolowski, Executive Secretary
Seth Friedman, MPA, Program Director
Disadvantaged children with asthma or sickle cell anemia, ages 8-16, are offered special programs in canoeing, backpacking, camping, music and leadership training. Sliding scale tuition. Year round programs for youth at risk groups. Conference center facility open for group rentals.

8238 Camp Waziyatah
530 Mill Hill Rd
Waterford, ME 04088-4011
207-583-2267
FAX: 509-357-2267
e-mail: info@wazi.com
wazi.com
Gregg Parker, Owner/Director
Mitch Parker, Owner/Director
Camp is located in Waterford, Massachusetts. Three, four and seven-week sessions June-August for campers with cancer and diabetes. Coed, ages 8-15 and families, single adults.

8239 Camp WheezeAway
American Lung Association Of Alabama
P.O.Box 3188
Bessemer, AL 35023-188
205-933-8821
800-586-4872
FAX: 251-491-1297
e-mail: kwaters@alabamalung.org
www.alabamalung.org
Kim Waters, Director
Camp WheezeAway is a 5 day overnight camp for children ages 8-12 with moderate to severe asthma, and is sponsored by the American Lung Association. Children are monitered while enjoying all the normal camp activities including ropes courses, canoeing, swimming, arts & crafts, horseback riding, fishing, tubing & more and above all learn to manage their asthma.

8240 Camps for Children & Teens with Diabetes
Diabetes Society
1165 Lincoln Ave
Suite 300
San Jose, CA 95125-3052
408-287-3785
800-989-1165
FAX: 408-287-2701
e-mail: info@diabetessociety.org
www.diabetessociety.org/camps
Sharon Ogbor, Executive Director
Thomas Smith, Director
Since 1974, sponsors up to 20 day camps, family camps and resident camps for children 4 through 17. These camps provide an opportunity for children with diabetes to go to camp, meet other children and gain a better understanding of their diabetes. The total experience can help campers develop more confidence in their abilities to control their diabetes effectively while enjoying the traditional camp experience. Camps are located throughout CA and parts of Nevada.

8241 Cedar Ridge Camp
4120 Old Routt Road
Louisville, KY 40299
502-267-5848
FAX: 502-267-0116
e-mail: info@cedarridgecamp.com
www.cedarridgecamp.com
Andrew Hartmans, Executive Director
Half-week, one and two-week sessions for children with diabetes, developmental disabilities and muscular dystrophy. Coed, ages 6-17.

8242 Champ Camp
American Lung Association In Alaska
7420 SW Bridgeport Road
Suite 200
Tigard, OR 97224
503-294-4094
800-586-4872
FAX: 503-294-4120
e-mail: info@lungmtpacific.org
www.aklung.org
Kathryn A. Forbes, Chairman
John F. Emanuel, Vice Chair
Harold Wimmer, President and CEO
Penny J. Siewert, Secretary/Treasurer
Champ Camp is a week long summer recreation and asthma education program at Camp Kushtaka on the beautiful shores of Kenai Lake. Campers are able to explore their skills in outdoor activities including canoeing, hiking, swimming, archery, and arts and crafts. More importantly, Champ Camp boosts self-confidence and instills a sense of responsibility. It teaches preventive measures to improve asthma management, and avoid asthmatic episodes as well as increases a camper's sense of independence.

8243 Clara Barton Diabetes Camp
Clara Barton for Girls with Diabetes
30 Ennis Road
PO Box 356
North Oxford, MA 01537-0356
508-987-2056
FAX: 508-987-2002
e-mail: info@bartoncenter.org
www.bartoncenter.org
Kevin Wilcoxen, Executive Director
Jesse Welch, Site & Facilities Director
Thomas Racine, Facilities Assistant
Brendan Duffy, Facilities Assistant
Girls, ages 3-17, with diabetes participate in a well-rounded camp program with special education in diabetes, health and safety. Activities include swimming, boating, sports, dance, music and arts and crafts. Two week adventure camp for high school girls offering camping, hiking, canoeing, etc. Also a minicamp (one week) for girls 6-12. Day camps are offered in Worcester, Boston, and New York City.

8244 Diabetes Camp
Tanager Place
1614 W Mount Vernon Road
Mount Vernon, IA 52314
319-363-0681
FAX: 319-365-6411
e-mail: dpirrie@tanagerplace.org
www.camptanager.org
Donald Pirrie, Camp Director
Provides children and adolescents with Diabetes a safe and healthy environment and healthy environment to enjoy a variety of recreational activities designed for fun and fitness. The camp held each July has an on-site 24-hour physician and nursing staff. Ages 6-13.

8245 EDI Camp
Wyman Center
600 Kiwanis Dr
St. Louis, MO 63025-2212
636-938-5245
FAX: 636-938-5289
e-mail: info@wymancenter.org
www.wymancenter.org
David Hilliard, President
Theresa Mayberry, Senior Vice President
Youngsters with diabetes learn how to care for themselves while participating in a wide variety of outdoor activities and trips. The camp, managed and financed by the American Diabetes Association Greater St. Louis Affiliate, offers camperships to children from the Greater St. Louis area, ages 7-16, but nonresidents may also apply.

8246 **Echoing Hills**
36272 County Road 79
Warsaw, OH 43844
740-327-2311
800-419-6513
FAX: 740-327-6371
e-mail: info@echoinghillsvillage.org
www.echoinghillsvillage.org

Buddy Busch, President/CEO
Summer camp for children and adults with cerebral palsy. Coed, ages 7-70.

8247 **Edward J Madden Open Hearts Camp**
250 Monument Valley Road
Great Barrington, MA 01230
413-528-2229
e-mail: hearts@openheartscamp.org
www.openheartscamp.org

Rick Farrell, President
David Zaleon, Executive Director
Jacqueline Reasor, Counselor
Jill Helme, Asst. Director
Eight week program for children who have had and are fully recovered from open heart surgery or a heart transplant. Four two week sessions by age group. Small camp - 25 campers per session.

8248 **FCYD Camp**
Foundation for Children and Youth with Diabetes
1995 W 9000 S
West Jordan, UT 84084
801-566-6913
www.fcydcamp.org

Nathan Gedge, Chair
David Okubo, President/Co-Founder
Elizabeth Elmer, Vice President
Sherrie Hardy, Director
Camping for children with diabetes. Coed, ages 1-18 and families.

8249 **Father Drumgoole Connelly Summer Camp**
MIV Mount Loretto
6581 Hylan Blvd
Staten Island, NY 10309-3830
718-317-2600
FAX: 718-317-2830
www.mountloretto.org

Stephen Rynn, Executive Director
Maryann Virga, Executive Assistant
Loretta Polanish, Executive Secretary
Ed Gani, Facilities Manager
Summer sessions for children with epilepsy, hearing impairment and developmental disabilities. Coed, ages 5-13.

8250 **Florida Diabetes Camp**
P.O.Box 14136
Gainesville, FL 32604
352-334-1321
FAX: 352-334-1326
e-mail: fccyd@floridadiabetescamp.org
www.floridadiabetescamp.org

Gary Cornwell, Executive Director
Chris Satkely, Assistant Director
Amy Soileau, Outreach Director
Robena Cornwell, Finance
Camp is located in Florida. One and two-week sessions June-August for children with diabetes. Coed, ages 6-18 and families. Camps throughout the year.

8251 **Friends Academy Summer Camps**
Duck Pond Rd
Locust Valley, NY 11560
516-393-4207
FAX: 516-465-1720
e-mail: camp@fa.org
www.fasummercamp.org

Rich Mack, Camp Director
Summer sessions for children with diabetes. Coed, ages 3-14, families.

8252 **God's Camp**
Episcopal Church of Hawaii
68-729 Farrington Hwy
Waialua, HI 96791-9314
808-637-6241
808-637-5505
FAX: 808-637-5505
e-mail: info@campmokuleia.com
www.campmokuleia.org

Debbie Alemeda, Manager
Episcopal Church tent camping, 5 nights, July. Church groups, family reunions, weddings, other organizations.

8253 **Growing Together Diabetes Camp**
ETMC
1000 S. Beckham
Tyler, TX 75701
903-597-0351
800-232-8318
e-mail: info@etmc.org
www.etmc.org

Marty Wiggins, Development Director
Vicki Jowell, Director
Elmer G. Ellis, President
Jerry Massey, Senior Vice President
A summer camp for youths ages 6 to 15 with Type 1 or Type 2 diabetes.

8254 **Happiness Is Camping**
2169 Grand Concourse
Bronx, NY 10453-2201
718-295-3100
FAX: 718-295-0406
e-mail: hicoffice@happinessiscamping.org
www.happinessiscamping.org

Kurt Struver, Executive Director
Richard G. Gorlick, M.D, Medical Director
Louis D'Agostino, President Of The Board
Antonio Dominiguez, Secretary
Happiness Is Camping, for children with cancer, was founded in 1980. About 400 children, girls and boys aged 6-15 years, attend the overnight camp, staying from one to all of the sessions, depending on their health.

8255 **Hemophilia Camp**
Tanager Place
1614 W Mount Vernon Road
Mount Vernon, IA 52314
319-363-0681
FAX: 319-365-6411
e-mail: dpirrie@tanagerplace.org
www.camptanager.org

Donald Pirrie, Camp Director
During the six-day camp children with Hemophilia and their siblings participate in individual and group activities designed for fun and fitness. The camp held each year in mid-June has a 24-hour physician and nursing staff. Ages 5-16.

8256 **Hole in the Wall Gang Camp**
565 Ashford Center Rd
Ashford, CT 06278
860-429-3444
FAX: 860-429-7295
e-mail: ashford@holeinthewallgang.org
www.holeinthewallgang.org

Raymond Lamontagne, Chairman
Ken Alberti, Chief Development Officer
James H. Canton, Chief Executive Officer
Kevin M. Magee, Chief Financial Officer
Low-cost eight-week sessions June-August for children with cancer and HIV. Coed, ages 7-15.

8257 **Kiwanis Camp Wyman**
Wyman Center
600 Kiwanis Dr
Eureka, MO 63025-2212
636-938-5245
FAX: 636-938-5289
e-mail: info@wymancenter.org
www.wymancenter.org

Keat Wilkins, Chairman
Dave Hilliard, President/CEO
Tom Etzkorn, VP,Executive Resource Officer
Mindy Sharp, MBA, SVP, Finance & Administration

Summer sessions for youth with diabetes. Coed, ages 8-16, run in conjunction with the American Diabetes Association. Call for program description.

8258 Makemie Woods Camp
Presbytery of Eastern Virginia
P.O.Box 39
Barhamsville, VA 23011
757-566-1496
800-566-1496
FAX: 757-566-8803
e-mail: makwoods@makwoods.org
www.makwoods.org

Mike Burcher, Director
Sherri Egerton, Program Director
Karen Broughman, Office Manager
Anthony Burcher, Storyteller in Residence
Residential Christian camp that tailors each group and individual goals. Counselors serve as teachers, friends and activity leaders. For children 8-18 with diabetes.

8259 Makemie Woods Camp/Conference Retreat
Presbytery of Eastern Virginia
P.O.Box 39
Barhamsville, VA 23011
757-566-1496
800-566-1496
FAX: 757-566-8803
e-mail: makwoods@makwoods.org
www.makwoods.org

Mike Burcher, Director
Sherri Egerton, Program Director
Karen Broughman, Office Manager
Anthony Burcher, Storyteller in Residence
Counselors serve as teachers, friends and activity leaders. The individual is important within the small group. No camper is lost in the crowd, but is an integral partner in the group process. Residential Christian Camp and conference center. Summer camp for children 8-18 and special camp for children with diabetes.

8260 Marist Brothers Mid-Hudson Valley Camp
PO Box 197
Esopus, NY 12429
212- 55- 123
e-mail: info@maristbrotherscenter.org
www.maristretreathouse.net

Don Nugent, Property Director
Qwen Ormsby, Executive Director
Matt Falon, Director of Operations
Mike Trainor, Facilities Director
Serves special people: children who have cancer or who are HIV positive, deaf or mentally retarded.

8261 Med-Camps of Louisiana
102 Thomas Road
Suite 615
West Monroe, LA 71291
318-329-8405
877-282-0802
FAX: 318-329-8407
e-mail: infos@medcamps.com
www.medcamps.com

Caleb Seney, Executive Director
Bethany Gerfers, Administrative Assistant
Kacie Hobson, Events & Volunteer Coordinator
Serves children with severe asthma and allergies and many more.

8262 Mountaineer Spina Bifida Camp
909 N. Sepulveda Blvd.
11th Floor
El Segundo, CA 90245
304-558-7098
877-242-9330
FAX: 310-280-5177
e-mail: info@kidscamps.com
www2.kidscamps.com

Milisa Galazzi, Director
Joey Waldman, Owner
Karen T. Safran, VP of Marketing
Is a non profit organization which pursues education and training and focuses on activities that promote independence and those that facilitate everyday life. The objectives are to build self esteem, promote independence and enhance the development of social skills.

8263 Muscular Dystrophy Association Free Camp
222 S. Riverside Plaza
Suite 1500
Chicago, IL 60606
907-276-2131
800-572-1717
FAX: 907-276-0946
www.mdausa.org

R. Rodney Howell, MD, Chairman
Steven M. Derks, President/CEO
Julie Faber, EVP/CFO
Pete Morgan, EVP/COO
MDA Camp provides a wide range of activities for those who have limited mobility or are in wheelchairs. The camp offers may outdoor sporting activities, art's & crafts and talent shows.

8264 NeSoDak
Lutherans Outdoors in South Dakota
3285 Camp Dakota Dr.
Waubay, SD 57273-1
605-947-4440
800-888-1464
FAX: 605-274-5024
e-mail: nesodak@losd.org
www.losd.org

Teri Gayer, Director
Layne Nelson, Executive Director
Nathan Skadsen, Program Director
Doug Nelson, Maintenance Director
NeSoDak provides a safe place for youth to build relationship, develop new skills, and live in a grace-filled community as they learn about Christ's love for them-all while enjoying time at the lake with a caring, well trained, energetic, and fun loving staff.

8265 Northwest Kiwanis Camp
P.O.Box 1227
Port Hadlock, WA 98339
360-732-7222
e-mail: nwkc@earthlink.net
weareugn.org/community-services/nw-kiwanis-ca

Kim Hammers, President
Carla Caldwell, Executive Director
Nikki Russell, Director, Development & Community Engagement
Debbie Reid, Administrative Assistant
Campers range from 6-60 in age, and includes those with developmental disabilities, cerebral palsy, autism, downs syndrome, and other physical and/or mental handicaps.

8266 Phantom Lake YMCA Camp
S110 W30240 YMCA Camp Road
Mukwonago, WI 53149
262-363-4386
FAX: 262-363-4351
e-mail: office@phantomlakeymca.org
www.phantomlakeymca.org

Ray Goodden, Chair
James Scharine, Vice Chair
Jodi Jacobsen, Secretary
Mike Hase, Treasurer
Summer camping for children with epilepsy, ages 7-15.

8267 Shady Oaks Camp
16300 Parker Road
Homer Glen, IL 60491
708-301-0816
FAX: 708-301-5091
e-mail: soc16300@sbcglobal.net
shadyoakscamp.org

Harry Burroughs, Chairman
Robert Szajkovics, President
Lori McAleavy, Vice President
Scott Steele, Executive Director
Shady Oaks Camp provides outdoor fun and recreation for children and adults with cerebral palsy and similar disabilities. Our camp is organized with the goal of providing stimulating life experiences that our campers may not have the opportunity to engage in elsewhere.

8268 **Sherman Lake YMCA Summer Camp**
Sherman Lake YMCA Outdoor Center
6225 N 39th St
Augusta, MI 49012 269-731-3000
FAX: 269-731-3020
e-mail: shermanlakeymca@ymcasl.org
www.shermanlakeymca.org

Luke Austenfeld, Executive Director
Jean Henderson, Business Manager
Lorrie Syverson, Director,Camping, Education & Retreat Services
Mark VanDaff, Facility Manager

Summer camping sessions for campers with ADD and spina bifida. Coed, ages 6-15 and families, seniors.

8269 **Strength for the Journey**
Oregon-Idaho Conference Center
1505 SW 18th Ave
Portland, OR 97201 503-802-9210
800-593-7539
FAX: 503-228-3196
e-mail: geneva@umoi.org
www.gocamping.org

Lisa Jean Hoefner, Executive Director
Geneva Cook, Camping Registrar
Eric Conklin, Office Assistant
Jennifer Aldrich, Assistant Treasurer

Camp is located near Sisters, Oregon. For adults living with HIV/AIDS.

8270 **Summer Camp for Children with Muscular Dystrophy**
Muscular Dystrophy Association - USA
222 S. Riverside Plaza
Suite 1500
Chicago, IL 60606 520-529-2000
800-572-1717
FAX: 520-529-5300
e-mail: mda@mdausa.org
www.mdausa.org

R. Rodney Howell, MD, Chairman
Steven M. Derks, President/CEO
Pete Morgan, EVP/COO
Julie Faber, EVP/CFO

Offers a wide range of activities such as adaptive sports, swimming, fishing, archery, scavenger hunts, dances & talent shows, art's & crafts, karaoke, and campfires.

8271 **Summer Camp for Physically & Mentally Challenged Children & Adults**
Kansas Jaycees' Cerebral Palsy Foundation
P.O.Box 267
Augusta, KS 67010 316-775-2421
FAX: 316-775-2421
e-mail: execdirector@cpranch.org
www.cpranch.org

Cheryl Schmeidler, Executive Director
Sarah Walker, Camp Director

Our mission is to provide a program which will allow individuals to enjoy their highest level of functioning and independence, consistant with their abilities, in a summer camp setting.

8272 **Suttle Lake Camp**
Oregon/Idaho Conference Center
The United Methodist Church
475 Riverside Drive
New York, NY 10115 541-595-6663
800-UMC-GBGM
800-862-4246
FAX: 541-595-2818
e-mail: info@umcmission.org
www.gbgm-umc.org

Deborah Mahaney, Executive Secretary
Denise Honeycutt, Deputy General Secretary
Roland Fernandes, Finance & Administration, General Treasurer
Rev. Shawn Bakker, Communications & Development

Camp is located in Sisters, Oregon. Camping sessions for children and adults with HIV. Coed, ages 6-18, families, seniors and single adults.

8273 **TSA CT Kid's Summer Event**
Tourette Syndrome Association of Connecticut (TSA)
c/o Massachusetts Chapter
39 Godfrey Street
Taunton, MA 02780 617-277-7589
e-mail: info@tsa-ma.org
www.tsact.org

Tom Meehan, Chairman
Peter Tavolacci, Vice-Chairman
Paul Nazario, Treasurer

TSA of Connecticut sponsors summer events for children with TS/Tourette Syndrome activities of which include minature golf in addition to an Annual Conference. The kids' program at this annual conference provides children who have TS a unique opportunity to meet other children like them who also struggle with TS. Entertainment includes puppeteers, magicians, learning karate from the experts, getting face paintings and more.
uniqu pages

8274 **Texas Lions Camp**
Lions Club Of Texas
P.O.Box 290247
Kerrville, TX 78029 830-896-8500
FAX: 830-896-3666
e-mail: tlc@ktc.com
www.lionscamp.com

Stephen Mabry, Executive Director

The primary purpose of the League shall be to provide, without charge, a camp for physically disabled, hearing/vision impaired and diabetic children from the State of Texas, regardless of race, religion, or national origin. Our goal is to create an atmosphere wherein campers will learn the can do philosophy and be allowed to achieve maximum personal growth and self-esteem. The camp welcomes boys and girls ages 7-16.

8275 **Twin Lakes Camp**
1451 E Twin Lakes Rd
Hillsboro, IN 47949-8004 765-798-4000
e-mail: outdoors@twinlakescamp.com
www.twinlakescamp.com

Jon Beight, Executive Director
Dan Daily, Program Director
Duane Bush, Guest Service
Donna Beight, Secretary

Provides a summer camp program for special needs children and young adults. Campers suffer from a wide range of maladies including crippling accidents, Spina Bifida, epilepsy, Cerebral Palsy, Muscular Dystrophy, Quadriplegia, Paraplegia, and other disabling diseases. Campers range in age from 8 to 27.

8276 **VACC Camp**
Miami Childrens Hospital
3200 W.W. 60 Ct
Suite 203
Miami, FL 33155-4076 305-662-8222
FAX: 786-268-1765
e-mail: bela.florentin@mch.com
www.vacccamp.com

Bela Florentin, Camp Coordinator
Ivette Hidalgo, MSN, ARNP, Camp Clinical Coordinator
Rose Ann Farrell, LCSW, Volunteer Assistant Coordinator
Javier Hern ndez, RRT, Volunteer Respiratory Therapist

VACC Camp gives families a fun opportunity to socialize with peers and enjoy activities not readily accessible to technology dependent children. The program includes swimming, field trips to local attractions, campsite entertainment, structured games, free play, and more - all to promote family growth and development while enhancing individual self-esteem and social skills. Parents have formal and informal opportunities to network among themselves.

8277 Wallowa Lake Camp
Oregon-Idaho Conference Center
84522 Church Ln
Joseph, OR 97846
541-432-1271
e-mail: wallowa@gocamping.org
www.wallowalakecamp.org

David Lovegren, Manager
Peggy Lovegren, Manager
Camp offers volleyball, badminton, horseshoes, baseball, crafts and wildlife viewing.

8278 Wisconsin Lions Camp
Wisconsin Lions Foundation
3834 County Road A
Rosholt, WI 54473
715-677-4969
FAX: 715-677-3297
e-mail: info@wisconsinlionscamp.com
wisconsinlionscamp.com

Evett J. hartvig, Executive Director
Elizabeth shelley, Administrative Assistant
Dale Schroeder, Facility Director
Meghan Postelnik, Office Asst.
Serves children who have either a visual, hearing or mild cognitive disability, as well as diabetes types I and II. Program activities include sailing, ropes course, hiking and canoe trips, environmental education, swimming, camping, canoeing, outdoor living skills and handicrafts. ACA accredited, located in central Wisconsin, near Stevens Point.

8279 Y Camp
YMCA of Greater Des Moines
1192 166th Drive
Boone, IA 50036
515-432-7558
FAX: 515-432-5414
e-mail: ycamp@dmymca.org
www.y-camp.org

David Sherry, Executive Director
Mike Havlik, Program Director- Environmental
Alex Kretzinger, Program Director- Summer Camp
Amy Joanning, Development Coordinator/Registrar
Camp is located in Boone, Iowa. Year-round one and two-week sessions for boys and girls with cancer, diabetes, asthma, cystic fibrosis, hearing impaired and other disabilities. Coed, ages 6-16 and families.

8280 YMCA Camp Fitch
The YMCA Of Youngstown - Metro Office
17 N Champion St
P.O. Box 1287
Youngstown, OH 44501
330-744-8411
FAX: 330-744-8415
e-mail: info@campfitchymca.com
www.youngstownymca.org

Thomas Fleming, Chair/ CVO
James B. Greene, 1st Vice chiar
Thomas Gacse, 2nd Vice chiar
Donald Harrison, 3rd Vice chiar
Camp is located in North Springfield, Pennsylvania. Camping sessions for children and adults with diabetes, hearing impairment, developmental disabilities, mobility limitation and speech/communication impairment. Ages 8-16, families and seniors.

8281 YMCA Camp Horseshoe
Ohio-West Virginia YMCA
PO Box 239
Point Pleasant, WV 25550-9408
304-675-5899
FAX: 304-478-4446
e-mail: horseshoe@hi-y.org
www.yla-youthleadership.org

David King, Executive Director
Summer camping for children with cancer, ages 7-18.

8282 YMCA Camp Ihduhapi
Minneapolis YMCA Camping Services
15200 Hanson Blvd.
Andover, MN 55304
763-230-9622
e-mail: info@campihduhapi.org
campihduhapi.org

Kerry Pioske, Camp Executive
Josh Cobb, Overnight Camp Director
Devin Hanson, Day Camp Director
Eric Wobschall, Building Superintendent
Camp is located in Loretto, Minnesota. Summer sessions for campers with asthma/respiratory ailments and epilepsy. Coed, ages 7-16.

8283 YMCA Camp Kitaki
Lincoln YMCA
570 Fallbrook Blvd.
Suite 210
Lincoln, NE 68521
402-434-9200
FAX: 402-434-9208
e-mail: info@ymcalincoln.org
www.ymcalincoln.org

Barb Bettin, President/CEO
J.P. Lauterbach, COO
Misty Muff, Chief Administrative Officer
Renee Yost, CFO
Camp is located in Louisville, Nebraska. Summer sessions for children with cystic fibrosis. Coed, ages 7-17 and families.

8284 YMCA Camp Orkila
YMCA of Greater Seattle
909 4th Ave
Seattle, WA 98104
206-382-5010
FAX: 206-382-4920
e-mail: dstankevich@seattleymca.org
www.seattleymca.org

John F. Vynne, Chair
David H. Wright, Vice Chair
Molly B. Stearns, Secretary
Nathaniel T. Brown, Treasurer
Camping for children with blood disorders and diabetes, ages 8-18.

8285 YMCA Camp Shady Brook
YMCA of the Pikes Peak Region (PPYMCA)
316 N. Tejon Street
Colorado Springs, CO 80903
719-329-7227
FAX: 719-272-7026
e-mail: campinfo@ppymca.org
www.campshadybrook.org

Sonny Adkins, Executive Director
Laura Petersen, Program Director
Patrick Casey, Facility Director
Michaela Eddleston, Conference & Retreat Director
Camp is located in Sedalia, Colorado. One-week sessions for campers with HIV. Boys and girls 7-16. Also families, seniors and single adults.

8286 YMCA Camp Weona
YMCA of Greater Buffalo
301 Cayuga Rd
Suite 100
Buffalo, NY 14225
716-565-6000
FAX: 716-565-6007
e-mail: contactus@ymcabuffaloniagra.org
www.ymcabuffaloniagara.org

John D. Murray, President/CEO
Camp is located in Gainesville, New York. Camping sessions for children and adults with epilepsy. Coed, ages 7-16, families and single adults. Nestled in 1,000 acres of hardwood and pine forests, Weona has miles of picturesque hiking trails, brooks, a heated outdoor pool and a world class adventure ropes course. Our indoor facilities include arts and crafts studios, environmental classrooms and a challenging rock climbing wall. It is the ideal setting for hands-on fun, adventure and learning.

8287 YMCA Camp jewell
YMCA of Greater Hartford
6 Prock Hill Road
P.O. Box 8
Colebrook, CT 06021
860-379-2782
888-412-2267
FAX: 860-379-8715
e-mail: camp.jewell@ghymca.org
www.ghymca.org

Eric Tucker, Executive Director
Camp is located in Colebrook, Connecticut. Two-week sessions for children with cancer. Coed, ages 8-16. Also families.

8288 YMCA Camp of Maine
305 Winthrop Center Rd
P.O. Box 446
Winthrop, ME 04364
207-395-4200
FAX: 207-395-7230
e-mail: info@maineycamp.org
www.maineycamp.org

Tom Christensen, CVO
Rebecca Henry, Vice CVO
Marty Allen, Treasurer
Heather Priest, Secretary
Activities include arts and crafts, nature study, hiking, and overnight camping, dancing, and singing. Summer session dates run from June through August; for ages 8-16.

8289 YMCA Outdoor Center Campbell Gard
4803 Augspurger Road
Hamilton, OH 45011
513-867-0600
877-224-9622
FAX: 513-867-0127
e-mail: camp@gmvymca.org
www.ccgymca.org

Pete Fasano, Executive Director
Darren Corns, Program Director
Tom Andrews, Facilities and Properties Manager
Wendi Moore, Office Manager
Camp is located in Hamilton, Ohio. Camping sessions for children with ADD, autism, developmental disabilities and blindness/visual impairment. Coed, ages 6-17 and families.

Print: Books

8290 A Woman's Guide to Living with HIV Infection
Johns Hopkins University Press
2715 N Charles St
Baltimore, MD 21218-4363
410-516-6900
800-548-1784
FAX: 410-516-6998
e-mail: jwehmueller@press.jhu.edu
www.press.jhu.edu

Rebecca A Clark M.D., PhD, Author
Robert T Maupin Jr. M.D. FACOG, Co-Author
Jill Hayes Hammer PhD, Co-Author
A resource for women with HIV that discusses coping with the diagnosis, finding a physician, recognizing symptoms, and preventing complications. Explains the latest treatment options and advice on coping with gynecologic infections. *$18.00*
328 pages Hardback

8291 ABC of Asthma, Allergies & Lupus
Global Health Solutions
2146 Kings Garden Way
PO Box 3189
Falls Church, VA 22043-2593
703-848-2333
800-759-3999
FAX: 703-848-0028
e-mail: information@watercure.com
www.watercure.com

Fereydoon Batmanghelidj MD, Author
Xiaopo Batmanghelidj, President
Kristin Swan, Administrator
This book introduces new approaches in preventing and treating asthma, allergies and lupus without toxic chemicals. It also offers new insight on how to prevent and treat children's asthma. *$ 17.00*
240 pages
ISBN 0-962994-26-x

8292 AIDS Sourcebook
Omnigraphics, Inc.
PO Box 31-1640
Detroit, MI 48231-8002
610-461-3548
800-234-1340
FAX: 610-532-9001
e-mail: info@omnigraphics.com
www.omnigraphics.com

Sandra J Judd, Editor
Basic consumer health information about the Human Immunodeficiency Virus (HIV) and Acquired Immunodeficiency Syndrome (AIDS), including facts about its origins, stages, types, transmission, risk factors, and prevention, and featuring details about diagnostic testing, antiretroviral treatments, and co-occurring infections. *$ 85.00*
600 pages 5th Edition 1911
ISBN 0-780811-47-8

8293 AIDS and Other Manifestations of HIV Infection
Elsevier Inc
30 Corporate Dr
Suite 400
Burlington, MA 01803-4252
781-313-4700
800-545-2522
FAX: 800-568-5136
e-mail: usbkinfo@elsevier.com
www.elsevier.com

Gary Wormser MD, Editor
A comprehensive overview of the biological properties of this etiologic viral agent, its clinicopathological manifestations, the epidemiology of its infection, and present and future therapeutic options. *$249.95*
1000 pages 2004
ISBN 0-127640-51-7

8294 AIDS in the Twenty-First Century: Disease and Globalization
Palgrav Macmillan
175 5th Ave
New York, NY 10010-7703
888-330-8477
FAX: 800-672-2054
e-mail: onlinesupportusa@palgrave.com
www.palgrave-usa.com

Gabriella Georgiades, Editor
Alan Whiteside, Author
Tony Barnett, Co-Author
The authors — exprets in the field for over 15 years — argue that it is vital to not only look at AIDS in terms of prevention and treatment, but to also consider consequences which affect households, communities, companies, governments, and countries. This is a major contribution toward understanding the global public health crisis, as well as the relationship between poverty, inequality, and infectious diseases. *$32.00*
464 pages
ISBN 1-403997-68-5

8295 Adult Leukemia: A Comprehensive Guide for Patients and Families
O'Reilly Media Inc
1005 Gravenstein Hwy N
Sebastopol, CA 95472-2811
707-827-7000
800-998-9938
FAX: 707-829-0104
e-mail: order@oreilly.com
www.oreilly.com

Linda Lamb, Editor
Barb Lackritz, Author
For the tens of thousands of Americans with adult leukemia, Adult Leukemia: A Comprehensive Guide for Patients and Families addresses diagnosis, medical tests, finding a good oncologist, treatments, side effects, getting emotional and other support, resources for further study, and much more. The book in-

cludes real-life stories from those who have battled leukemia themselves. *$29.95*
536 pages Paperback
ISBN 0-596500-01-7

8296 Advanced Breast Cancer: A Guide to Living with Metastic Disease
O'Reilly Media Inc
1005 Gravenstein Hwy N
Sebastopol, CA 95472-2811 707-827-7000
800-998-9938
FAX: 707-829-0104
e-mail: order@oreilly.com
www.oreilly.com
Linda Lamb, Editor
Musa Mayer, Author
This is the only book on breast cancer that deals honestly with the realities of living with metastic disease, yet offers hope and comfort. All aspects of facing the disease are covered, including: coping with the shock of recurrence, seeking information and making treatment decisions, communicating effectively with medical personnel finding support, and handling disease progression and end-of-life issues. A comprehensive guide, it also provides updated resources and treatment developments. *$24.95*
532 pages Paperback 1998
ISBN 1-565925-22-X

8297 Allergies Sourcebook
PO Box 31-1640
Detroit, MI 48231-8002 610-461-3548
800-234-1340
FAX: 610-532-9001
e-mail: info@omnigraphics.com
www.omnigraphics.com
Amy L Sutton, Editor
Basic comsumer health information about the immune system and allergic disorders, including rhinitis (hay fever), sinusitis, conjunctivitis, asthma, atopic dermatitis, and anaphylaxis, and allergy triggers such as pollen, mold, dust mites, animal dander, chemicals, foods and additives, and medications; along with facts about allergy diagnosis and treatment, tips on avoiding triggers and preventing symptoms, a glossary of related terms, and directories of resources for additional help and info. *$95.00*
608 pages 4th Edition 1911

8298 Alternative Approach to Allergies
Harper Collins Publishers
10 E 53rd St
New York, NY 10022-5244 212-207-7901
800-242-7737
FAX: 212-702-2586
e-mail: spsales@harpercollins.com
www.harpercollins.com
Theron G Randolph M.D., Author
Ralph W Moss PhD, Co-Author
Here is the book that revolutionized the way allergies and other common illnesses were diagnosed and treated.
ISBN 0-060916-93-1

8299 Alzheimer Disease Sourcebook
Omnigraphics
PO Box 8002
Aston, PA 19014-8002 800-234-1340
FAX: 800-875-1340
e-mail: info@omnigraphics.com
www.omnigraphics.com
Amy L. Sutton, Editor
Alzheimer Disease Sourcebook, Fifth Edition provides updated information about causes, symptoms, and stages of AD and other forms of dementia, including mild cognitive impairment, corticobasal degeneration, dementia with Lewy bodies, frontotemporal dementia, Huntington disease, Parkinson disease, and dementia caused by infections. *$95.00*
600 pages 1911
ISBN 0-780811-50-8

8300 Alzheimer Disease Sourcebook, 4th Edition
Omnigraphics
PO Box 8002
Aston, PA 19014-8002 610-461-3548
800-234-1340
FAX: 800-875-1340
e-mail: customerservice@omnigraphics.com
www.omnigraphics.com
Peter Ruffner, President, Co-Founder
Fred Ruffner, Founder
Basic consumer health information about alzheimer disease, other dementias, and related disorders, including multi-infarct dementia, dementia with lewy bodies, frontotemporal dementia (pick disease), Wernicke-Korsakoff syndrome (alcohol-related dementia), AIDS dementia complex, Huntington disease, Creutzfeldt-Jacob disease, and delirium. *$84.00*
603 pages
ISBN 0-780810-01-3

8301 American Academy of Pediatrics Guide to Your Child's Alleriges and Asthma
American Academy of Pediatrics
141 Northwest Point Blvd
Elk Grove Vlg, IL 60007-1098 847-228-0604
FAX: 847-434-8000
e-mail: newpubs@aap.org
www.aap.org
Judith Palfrey, President
Errol Alden, Executive Director
Consumer resource for parents who need answers and information about their children's allergies and asthma. Current advice on identifying allergies and asthma, preventing attacks, minimizing triggers, understanding medications, explaining allergies to young children, and helping children manage symptoms. *$15.00*
191 pages
ISBN 0-679769-82-X

8302 Amyotrophic Lateral Sclerosis: A Guide for Patients and Families
Demos Medical Publishing
11 West 42nd Street
15th Floor
New York, NY 10036 212-683-0072
800-532-8663
FAX: 212-683-0118
e-mail: support@demosmedical.com
www.demosmedpub.com
Richard Winters, Executive Editor
Beth Kaufman Barry, Publisher
Noreen Henson, Executive Director of Demos Heal
Reina Santana, Director of Special Sales & Righ
This comprehensive guide covers every aspect of the management of ALS. Beginning with discussions of its clinical features of the disease, diagnosis, and an overview of symptom management, major sections deal with medical and rehabilitative management, living with ALS, managing advanced disease and end-of-life issues, and reources that can provide support and assistance. *$29.95*
470 pages 2001
ISBN 1-888799-28-5

8303 Arthritis Sourcebook.
Omnigraphics
PO Box 31-1640
Detroit, MI 48231-8002 610-461-3548
800-234-1340
FAX: 610-532-9001
e-mail: info@omnigraphics.com
www.omnigraphics.com
Amy L Sutton, Editor
Basic consumer health information about osteoarthritis, rheumatoid arthritis, other rheumatic disorders, infectious forms of arthritis, and diseases with symptoms linked to arthritis, and facts about diagnosis, pain management, and surgical therapies. *$84.00*
567 pages 2nd Edition
ISBN 0-780806-67-2

8304 **Asthma Sourcebook.**
Omnigraphics
PO Box 31-1640
Detroit, MI 48231-8002
610-461-3548
800-234-1340
FAX: 610-532-9001
e-mail: info@omnigraphics.com
www.omnigraphics.com
Karen Bellenir, Editor
Provides information about asthma, including symptoms, remedies and research updates. *$84.00*
581 pages 2nd Edition
ISBN 0-780808-66-9

8305 **Asthma and Allergy Answers: A Patient Education Library**
Asthma and Allergy Foundation of America
8201 Corporate Dr
Suite 1000
Landover, MD 20785
202-466-7643
800-727-8462
FAX: 202-466-8940
e-mail: info@aafa.org
www.aafa.org
Amy Patterson, Senior Director of Administration & Governance
Jacqui Vok, Director of Programs and Services
William McLin, M.Ed., President/CEO
This resource contains 50 reproducible fact sheets for patients on a variety of popular asthma and allergy topics. Information is written in a patient-friendly question and answer format and packaged in a durable binder for easy storage and use. *$50.00*

8306 **Back & Neck Sourcebook.**
Omnigraphics
PO Box 31-1640
Detroit, MI 48231-8002
610-461-3548
800-234-1340
FAX: 610-532-9001
e-mail: info@omnigraphics.com
www.omnigraphics.com
Amy L Sutton, Editor
Basic consumer health information about back and neck pain, spinal cord injuries, and related disorders, such as degenerative disk disease, osteoarthritis, scoliosis, sciatica, spina bifida, and spinal stenosis, and featuring facts about maintaining spinal health, self-care, rehabilitative care, chiropractic care, spinal surgeries, and complementary therapies. *$84.00*
607 pages 2nd Edition
ISBN 0-780807-38-9

8307 **Being Close**
National Jewish Health
1400 Jackson St
Denver, CO 80206-2761
303-398-1002
877-225-5654
FAX: 303-398-1125
e-mail: allstetterw@njc.org
www.nationaljewish.org
Michael Salem M.D., President/CEO
William Allstetter, Director Media/External Relation
A booklet offering information to patients suffering from a respiratory disorder such as emphysema, asthma or tuberculosis, that discusses sexual problems and feelings.

8308 **Bittersweet Chances: A Personal Journey o f Living and Learning in the Face of Illness**
PublishAmerica
PO Box 151
Frederick, MD 21705-151
301-695-1707
FAX: 301-631-9073
e-mail: support@publishamerica.com
www.publishamerica.com
Dana Selenke Broehl, Author
Recounts Doug and Dana Broehl's journey of growth through the darkness of cystic fibrosis and the renewed hope of a double lung transplant. *$24.95*
189 pages Softcover
ISBN 1-413713-24-6

8309 **Blood and Circulatory Disorders Sourcebook**
Omnigraphics
PO Box 31-1640
Detroit, MI 48231-8002
610-461-3548
800-234-1340
FAX: 610-532-9001
e-mail: info@omnigraphics.com
www.omnigraphics.com
Amy L Sutton, Editor
Sandra J. Judd, Editor
Blood and Circulatory Disorders Sourcebook, Third Edition offers facts about blood function and composition, the maintenance of a healthy circulatory system, and the types of concerns that arise when processes go awry. It discusses the diagnosis and treatment of many common blood cell disorders, bleeding disorders, and circulatory disorders, including anemia, hemochromatosis, leukemia, lymphoma, hemophilia, hypercoagulation, thrombophilia, atherosclerosis, blood pressure irregularities, coronary *$84.00*
634 pages 2nd Edition
ISBN 0-780807-46-4

8310 **Blooming Where You're Planted: Stories From The Heart**
Meeting Life's Challenges
9042 Aspen Grove Lane
Madison, WI 53717-2700
608-824-0402
FAX: 608-824-0403
e-mail: help@MeetingLifesChallenges.com
www.makinglifeeasier.com
Shelley Peterman Schwatz, Editor
Author Shelley Peterman Schwarz takes you on her journey of self-discovery and change following her diagnosis of multiple sclerosis in 1979. Her personal stories are warm and humorous, and insightful. This 138-page book will motivate and inspire you to rise above life's challenges and live life to its fullest. *$12.95*
138 pages 1998
ISBN 0-891854-01-1

8311 **Brain Allergies: The Psychonutrient and Magnetic Connections**
McGraw-Hill
www.allergiesshop.com
William Philpott PhD, Author
Dwight Keating PhD, Author
Linus Pauling PhD, Author
A complete overview of the concept of brain allergies - the theory that exposure to certain foods and other substances triggers mental disorders in people so predisposed, and that such disturbances can be cured by eliminating these substances. *$16.95*
ISBN 0-658003-98-1

8312 **Brain Disorders Sourcebook**
Omnigraphics
PO Box 31-1640
Detroit, MI 48231-8002
610-461-3548
800-234-1340
FAX: 610-532-9001
e-mail: info@omnigraphics.com
www.omnigraphics.com
Sandra J Judd, Editor
Joyce Brennfleck Shannon, Editor
Brain Disorders Sourcebook, Third Edition provides readers with updated information about brain function, neurological emergencies such as a brain attack (stroke) or seizure, and symptoms of brain disorders. It describes the diagnosis, treatment, and rehabilitation therapies for genetic and congenital brain disorders, brain infections, brain tumors, seizures, traumatic brain injuries, and degenerative neurological disorders such as Alzheimer disease and other dementias, Parkinson disease, and am *$84.00*
600 pages 2nd Edition
ISBN 0-780807-44-0

8313 Breast Cancer Sourcebook
Omnigraphics
PO Box 31-1640
Detroit, MI 48231-8002
610-461-3548
800-234-1340
FAX: 610-532-9001
e-mail: info@omnigraphics.com
www.omnigraphics.com

Sandra J Judd, Editor
Amy L. Sutton, Editor
Breast Cancer Sourcebook, Fourth Edition, provides updated information about breast cancer and its causes, risk factors, diagnosis, and treatment. Readers will learn about the types of breast cancer, including ductal carcinoma in situ, lobular carcinoma in situ, invasive carcinoma, and inflammatory breast cancer, as well as common breast cancer treatment complications, such as pain, fatigue, lymphedema, hair loss, and sexuality and fertility issues. Information on preventive therapies, nutrition *$84.00*
600 pages 3rd Edition
ISBN 0-780810-30-3

8314 Breathe Free
Lotus Press
P.O.Box 325
Twin Lakes, WI 53181
262-889-8561
800-824-6396
FAX: 262-889-8591
e-mail: lotuspress@lotuspress.com
www.lotuspress.com

D Gagnon, Author
A Morningstar, Co-Author
A nutritional and herbal medicine self-help guide to treating a full range of respiratory conditions, including colds and flu. *$14.95*
179 pages
ISBN 0-914955-07-1

8315 Cancer Sourcebook
Omnigraphics
PO Box 31-1640
Detroit, MI 48231-8002
610-461-3548
800-234-1340
FAX: 610-532-9001
e-mail: info@omnigraphics.com
www.omnigraphics.com

Karen Bellenir, Editor
Cancer Sourcebook, Sixth Edition provides updated information about common types of cancer affecting the central nervous system, endocrine system, lungs, digestive and urinary tracts, blood cells, immune system, skin, bones, and other body systems. It explains how people can reduce their risk of cancer by addressing issues related to cancer risk and taking advantage of screening exams. *$84.00*
1105 pages 5th Edition
ISBN 0-780809-47-5

8316 Cancer Sourcebook for Women
Omnigraphics
PO Box 31-1640
Detroit, MI 48231-8002
610-461-3548
800-234-1340
FAX: 610-532-9001
e-mail: info@omnigraphics.com
www.omnigraphics.com

Amy L Sutton, Editor
Karen Bellenir, Editor
Cancer Sourcebook for Women, Fourth Edition offers updated information about gynecologic cancers and other cancers of special concern to women, including breast cancer, cancers of the female reproductive organs, and cancers responsible for the highest number of deaths in women. It explains cancer risks-including lifestyle factors, inherited genetic abnormalities, and hormonal medications-and methods used to diagnose and treat cancer. *$84.00*
687 pages 5th Edition
ISBN 0-780808-67-6

8317 Cardiovascular Diseases and Disorders Sourcebook, 3rd Edition
Omnigraphics
PO Box 8002
Aston, PA 19014-8002
610-461-3548
800-234-1340
FAX: 800-875-1340
e-mail: customerservice@omnigraphics.com
www.omnigraphics.com

Peter Ruffner, President, Co-Founder
Fred Ruffner, Founder
Cardiovascular Diseases and Disorders Sourcebook, Third Edition, provides information about the symptoms, diagnosis, and treatment heart diseases and vascular disorders. It includes demographic and statistical data, an overview of the cardiovascular system, a discussion of risk factors and prevention techniques, a look at cardiovascular concerns specific to women, and a report on current research initiatives. *$84.00*
687 pages Hard cover
ISBN 0-780807-39-6

8318 Childhood Cancer Survivors: A Practical Guide to Your Future
O'Reilly Media Inc
1005 Gravenstein Hwy N
Sebastopol, CA 95472-2811
707-827-7000
800-998-9938
FAX: 707-829-0104
e-mail: order@oreilly.com
www.oreilly.com

Linda Lamb, Editor
Nancy Keene, Author
Wendy Hobbie, Co-Author
Kathy Ruccione, Co-Author
More than 250,000 people have survived childhood cancer - a cause for celebration. Authors Keene, Hobbie, and Ruccione chart the territory of long-term survivorship: relationships; overcoming employment or insurance discrimination; maximizing health; follow-up schedules; medical late effects. The stories of over sixty survivors - their challenges and triumphs - are told. Includes medical history record-keeper. *$27.95*
464 pages Paperback 1906
ISBN 0-596528-51-5

8319 Childhood Cancer: A Parent's Guide to Solid Tumor Cancers
O'Reilly Media Inc
1005 Gravenstein Highway North
Sebastopol, CA 95472
707-827-7000
800-889-8969
FAX: 707-829-0104
e-mail: order@oreilly.com
www.oreilly.com

560 pages Paperback
ISBN 0-596500-14-9

8320 Childhood Diseases and Disorders Sourcebook, 2nd Edition
Omnigraphics
PO Box 8002
Aston, PA 19014-8002
610-461-3548
800-234-1340
FAX: 800-875-1340
e-mail: customerservice@omnigraphics.com
www.omnigraphics.com

Peter Ruffner, President, Co-Founder
Fred Ruffner, Founder
Sandra J Judd, Editor
Basic consumer health information about medical problems often encountered in pre-adolescent children, including respiratory tract ailments, ear infections, sore throats, disorders of the skin and scalp, digestive and genitourinary diseases, infectious diseases, inflammatory disorders, chronic physical and developmental disorders, allergies, and more. *$84.00*
600 pages Hard cover
ISBN 0-780810-31-0

8321 **Childhood Leukemia: A Guide for Families, Friends & Caregivers**
O'Reilly Media Inc
1005 Gravenstein Hwy N
Sebastopol, CA 95472-2811
707-827-7000
800-998-9938
FAX: 707-829-0104
e-mail: order@oreilly.com
www.oreilly.com
Linda Lamb, Editor
Nancy Keene, Author
The second edition of this comprehensive guide offers detailed and precise medical information for parents that includes day-to-day practical advice on how to cope with procedures, hospitalization, family and friends, school, and social, emotional, and financial issues. It features a wealth of tools for prents and contains significant updates on treatments and procedures. *$29.95*
528 pages 4th Edition 1910
ISBN 0-596500-15-7

8322 **Children with Cerebral Palsy: A Parents' Guide**
Woodbine House
6510 Bells Mill Road
Bethesda, MD 20817-1636
301-897-3570
800-843-7323
FAX: 301-897-5838
e-mail: info@woodbinehouse.com
www.woodbinehouse.com
Irvin Shapell, Owner
Beth Binns, Special Marketing Manager
Sarah Glenner, Office Receptionist;
Fran Marinaccio, Marketing Manager
A classic primer for parents that provides a complete spetrum of information and compassionate advice about cerebral palsy and its effect on their child's development and education. *$18.95*
481 pages
ISBN 0-933149-82-4

8323 **Chronic Fatigue Syndrome: Your Natural Gu ide to Healing with Diet, Herbs and Other Methods**
Random House Publishing
1745 Broadway
3rd Floor
New York, NY 10019-4305
212-782-9000
FAX: 212-572-6066
e-mail: ecustomerservice@randomhouse.com
www.randomhouse.com
Susanna Porter, Editor
Michael T Murray N.D.
Explains specific measures sufferers can take to improve stamina, mental energy, and physical abilities. *$15.00*
208 pages
ISBN 1-559584-90-6

8324 **Coffee in the Cereal: The First Year with Multiple Sclerosis**
Pathfinder Publishing
520-647-0158
800-977-2282
e-mail: bill@pathfinderpublishing.com
www.pathfinderpublishing.com
96 pages
ISBN 0-934793-07-7

8325 **Colon & Rectal Cancer: A Comprehensive Guide for Patients & Families**
O'Reilly Media Inc
1005 Gravenstein Hwy N
Sebastopol, CA 95472-2811
707-827-7000
800-998-9938
FAX: 707-829-0104
e-mail: order@oreilly.com
www.oreilly.com
Linda Lamb, Editor
Lorraine Johnston, Author
The fourth most common cancer, colon and rectal cancer is diagnosed in 130,000 new cases in the United States each year. Patients and families need uo-to-date and in-depth information to participate wisely in treatment decisions (e.g., knowing what sexual and fertility issues to discuss with the doctor before surgery). This book covers coping with tests and treatment side effects, caring for ostomies, finding supportt, and other practical issues. *$24.95*
544 pages Paperback 1999
ISBN 1-565926-33-1

8326 **Colon Health: Key to a Vibrant Life**
Norwalk Press
P.O.Box 190526
Boise, ID 83719-526
928-445-5567
FAX: 928-445-5567
e-mail: info@drnormanwalker.com
www.drnormanwalker.com
Norman Walker MD, Editor
Includes complete glossary of terms and index of referrals.

8327 **Complementary Alternative Medicine and Multiple Sclerosis**
Demos Medical Publishing
11 West 42nd Street
15th Floor
New York, NY 10036
212-683-0072
800-532-8663
FAX: 212-683-0118
e-mail: support@demosmedical.com
www.demosmedpub.com
Richard Winters, Executive Editor
Beth Kaufman Barry, Publisher
Noreen Henson, Executive Director of Demos Heal
Reina Santana, Director of Special Sales & Righ
Offers reliable information on the relevance, safety, and effectiveness of various alternative therapies that are not typically considered in discussions of MS management, yet are in widespread use. *$24.95*
304 pages
ISBN 1-932603-54-9

8328 **Conquering the Darkness: One Story of Recovering from a Brain Injury**
Paragon House
1925 Oakcrest Avenue
Suite 7
Saint Paul, MN 55113-2619
651-644-3087
800-447-3709
FAX: 651-644-0997
e-mail: info@paragonhouse.com
www.paragonhouse.com
Rosemary Yokoi, Publicity Director
Gordon Anderson, Executive Director
Deborah Quinn, Author
The course of recovery from a brain injury by a woman who lived through it. *$15.95*
276 pages 1998
ISBN 1-557787-63-8

8329 **Coping with Cerebral Palsy**
Rosen Publishing
29 East 21st Street
New York, NY 10010
800-237-9932
FAX: 888-436-4643
www.rosenpublishing.com
Laura Anne Gilman, Author
This second edition book provides parents of children and adults with cerebral palsy the answers to more than 300 questions that have been carefully researched. It represents 40 years of experience by the author and is presented in a highly readable, jargon-free manner. *$31.95*
ISBN 0-823931-50-1

8330 Curing MS: How Science is Solving the Mysteries of Multiple Sclerosis
Random House Publishing
1745 Broadway
3rd Floor
New York, NY 10019-4305
212-782-9000
FAX: 212-572-6066
e-mail: ecustomerservice@randonhouse.com
www.randomhouse.com
Howard L Weiner M.D., Author
Founder-director of the Multiple Sclerosis Center at Mass General Hospital discusses what ends up as a deconstruction of the last 30 years of his own and general MS research and of experience in treating patients with the puzzling disorder. Weiner summarizes what is currently known about treatments and the potential for a cure. *$14.95*
352 pages 1905
ISBN 0-307236-04-8

8331 Cystic Fibrosis: A Guide for Patient and Family
Lippincott Williams & Wilkins
16522 Hunters Green Parkway
PO Box 1620
Hagerstown, MD 21741-1620
301-223-2300
800-638-3030
FAX: 301-223-2400
e-mail: orders@lww.com
www.lww.com
David M Orenstein MD, Author
Text is designed specifically for patients with cystic fibrosis and their families. Explains the disease process, outlines the fundamentals of diagnosing and screening, and addresses the challenges of treatment for those living with CF. Includes new material on carrier testing, infection control, and more. *$51.50*
448 pages 3rd Edition
ISBN 0-781741-52-1

8332 Diabetes Sourcebook.
Omnigraphics
PO Box 31-1640
Detroit, MI 48231-8002
610-461-3548
800-234-1340
FAX: 610-532-9001
e-mail: info@omnigraphics.com
www.omnigraphics.com
Karen Bellenir, Editor
Diabetes Sourcebook, Fourth Edition contains updated information for people seeking to understand the risk factors, complications, and management of diabetes. It discusses medical interventions, including the use of insulin and oral diabetes medications, self-monitoring of blood glucose, and complementary and alternative therapies. *$84.00*
627 pages 4th Edition
ISBN 0-780810-05-1

8333 Digestive Diseases & Disorders Sourcebook
Omnigraphics
PO Box 8002
Aston, PA 19014-8002
610-461-3548
800-234-1340
FAX: 800-875-1340
e-mail: customerservice@omnigraphics.com
www.omnigraphics.com
Peter Ruffner, President, Co-Founder
Fred Ruffner, Founder
Digestive Diseases and Disorders Sourcebook provides basic information for the layperson about common disorders of the upper and lower digestive tract. It also includes information about medications and recommendations for maintaining a healthy digestive tract in addition to a glossary of important terms and a directory of digestive diseases organizations are also provided. *$84.00*
323 pages Hard cover
ISBN 0-780803-27-5

8334 Duchenne Muscular Dystrophy
Oxford University Press
198 Madison Ave
New York, NY 10016-4308
212-726-6000
800-445-9714
FAX: 919-677-1303
e-mail: custserv.us@oup.com
www.global.oup.com
William Lamsback, Editor
Alan Emery, Author
Francesco Muntoni, Co-Author
Identification of the genetic defect responsible for Duchenne Muscular Dystrophy and isolation of the protein dystrophin have led to the development of new theories for the disease's pathogenesis. This title incorporates these advances from the field of molecular biology, and describes the resultant opportunities for screening, prenatal diagnosis, genetic counselling and management. *$135.00*
282 pages 3rd Edition 2003
ISBN 0-198515-31-6

8335 Ear, Nose, and Throat Disorders Sourcebook
Omnigraphics
PO Box 31-1640
Detroit, MI 48231-8002
610-461-3548
800-234-1340
FAX: 610-532-9001
e-mail: info@omnigraphics.com
www.omnigraphics.com
Sandra J Judd, Editor
Ear, Nose and Throat Disorders Sourcebook, Second Edition, provides consumers with updated health information on the most common disorders of the ear, nose, and throat. The book also includes descriptions of current diagnostic tests, discussion of common surgical procedures, including cosmetic surgery on the nose and ears, a glossary of related medical terms, and a directory of sources for further help and information. *$84.00*
631 pages 2nd Edition
ISBN 0-780808-72-0

8336 Eating Disorders Sourcebook.
Omnigraphics
PO Box 31-1640
Detroit, MI 48231-8002
610-461-3548
800-234-1340
FAX: 610-532-9001
e-mail: info@omnigraphics.com
www.omnigraphics.com
Joyce Brennfleck Shannon, Editor
Provides general imformation, causes and treatments of eating disorders. *$84.00*
557 pages 2nd Edition
ISBN 0-780809-48-2

8337 Educational Issues Among Children with Spina Bifida
Spina Bifida Association of America
1600 Wilson Boulevard
Suite 800
Arlington, VA 22209
202-944-3285
800-621-3141
FAX: 202-944-3295
e-mail: sbaa@sbaa.org
www.sbaa.org
Ana Ximenes, Chair
Sara Struwe, President & CEO
Mark Bohay, National Web Initiatives & Development Manager
Elizabeth Merck, Development Manager
Children with spina bifida/ hydrocephalus often show unique learning strengths and weaknesses that affect their schoolwork. Parents and schools need to work together to help the young people meet their physical, social, emotional, and academic goals.

8338 Epilepsy, 199 Answers: A Doctor Responds to His Patients' Questions
Demos Medical Publishing
11 West 42nd Street
15th Floor
New York, NY 10036
212-683-0072
800-532-8663
FAX: 212-683-0118
e-mail: support@demosmedical.com
www.demosmedpub.com

Richard Winters, Executive Editor
Beth Kaufman Barry, Publisher
Noreen Henson, Executive Director of Demos Heal
Andrew N. Wilner MD, FACP, FAAN, Author

An epilepsy specialist answers questions about the causes, diagnosis, and treatments, and how to live and work with this brain disorder. Includes an epilepsy history timeline, patient health record form, resources, and a glossary. *$19.95*
180 pages
ISBN 1-932603-35-2

8339 Epilepsy: Patient and Family Guide
Demos Medical Publishing
11 West 42nd Street
15th Floor
New York, NY 10036
212-683-0072
800-532-8663
FAX: 212-683-0118
e-mail: support@demosmedical.com
www.demosmedpub.com

Richard Winters, Executive Editor
Beth Kaufman Barry, Publisher
Noreen Henson, Executive Director of Demos Heal
Orrin Devinsky, MD, Author

A guide for adults with epilepsy and for parents of children with the disorder explains the nature and diversity of seizures, the risks and benefits of the various antiepileptic drugs, and medical and surgical therapies. *$16.95*
408 pages
ISBN 1-932603-41-7

8340 Ethnic Diseases Sourcebook
Omnigraphics
PO Box 8002
Aston, PA 19014-8002
610-461-3548
800-234-1340
FAX: 800-875-1340
e-mail: customerservice@omnigraphics.com
www.omnigraphics.com

Peter Ruffner, President, Co-Founder
Fred Ruffner, Founder

Ethnic Diseases Sourcebook provides health information about genetic and chronic diseases that affect ethnic and racial minorities in the United States. Information about mental health services, women's health, and tips for improving health are also included, along with a glossary and a list of resources for additional help and informatio methods, treatment options, and current research initiatives. *$84.00*
648 pages Hard cover
ISBN 0-780803-36-7

8341 From Where I Sit: Making My Way with Cerebral Palsy
Scholastic
557 Broadway
New York, NY 10012-3962
124-484-2800
FAX: 212-343-6934
e-mail: contact@scholastic.co.in
www.scholastic.com

Dick Robinson, Chairman & CEO
Maureen O'Connell, Executive Vice President, Chief
Kyle Good, Senior Vice President, Corporate
Shelley Nixon, Author

An autobiographical account of a young woman explores how it feels to live with cerebral palsy while struggling to have a full life despite the challenges facing her every day. *$13.00*
136 pages
ISBN 0-590395-84-X

8342 Genetics and Spina Bifida
Spina Bifida Association of America
1600 Wilson Boulevard
Suite 800
Arlington, VA 22209
202-944-3285
800-621-3141
FAX: 202-944-3295
e-mail: sbaa@sbaa.org
www.sbaa.org

Ana Ximenes, Chair
Sara Struwe, President & CEO
Mark Bohay, National Web Initiatives & Development Manager
Elizabeth Merck, Development Manager

Spina bifida is a birth defect involving incomplete formation of the spine.

8343 Growing Up with Epilepsy: A Pratical Guide for Parents
Demos Medical Publishing
11 West 42nd Street
15th Floor
New York, NY 10036
212-683-0072
800-532-8663
FAX: 212-683-0118
e-mail: support@demosmedical.com
www.demosmedpub.com

Richard Winters, Executive Editor
Beth Kaufman Barry, Publisher
Noreen Henson, Executive Director of Demos Heal
Lynn Bennett Blackburn, PhD, Author

Developed to help parents with the uniques challenges that this disorder presents *$19.95*
168 pages
ISBN 1-888799-74-9

8344 Guide to Living with HIV Infection: Developed at the Johns Hopkins AIDS Clinic
Johns Hopkins Universty Press
2715 N Charles St
Baltimore, MD 21218-4363
410-516-6900
800-548-1784
FAX: 410-516-6998
e-mail: webmaster@jhupress.jhu.edu
www.press.jhu.edu

William Brody, President
John G Bartlett, M.D., Author
Ann K Finkbeiner, Co-Author

A handbook and reference for people living with HIV infection and their families, friends, and caregivers. *$19.95*
408 pages 6th Edition
ISBN 0-801884-85-6

8345 Handbook of Chronic Fatigue Syndrome
John Wiley & Sons
1 Wiley Drive
Somerset, NJ 08875-1272
732-469-4400
800-225-5945
FAX: 732-302-2300
e-mail: custserv@wiley.com
www.as.wiley.com

Leonard A Jason, Editor
Patricia A Fennell, Editor
Renee R Taylor, Editor

Discusses diagnosis and treatment as well as the history, phenomenology, symptomatology, assessment, and pediatric and community issues. Introduces phase-based therapy and nutritional approaches. *$ 110.00*
794 pages 2003
ISBN 0-471415-12-1

8346 Handbook of Epilepsy
Lippincott, Williams & Wilkins
Philadelphia, PA 19106-3713
215-521-8300
800-777-2295
FAX: 301-824-7390
www.lpub.com

J Lippincott, CEO

Pocket-sized reference provides concise, up-to-date, clinically oriented reviews of each of the major areas of diagnosis and management of epilepsy. *$42.95*

272 pages

ISBN 0-781743-52-4

8347 Healthy Breathing

National Jewish Health
1400 Jackson St
Denver, CO 80206-2761
303-270-2708
877-225-5654
FAX: 303-398-1125
e-mail: physicianline@njhealth.org
www.nationaljewish.org

Richard A. Schierburg, Chair
Robin Chotin, Vice Chair
Don Silversmith, Vice Chair
Michael Salem, CEO

Offers patients with lung or respiratory disorders information on exercise and healthy breathing.

8348 Heart of the Mind

New World Library
14 Pamaron Way
Novato, CA 94949
415-884-2100
800-972-6657
FAX: 415-884-2199
e-mail: ami@newworldlibrary.com
www.newworldlibrary.com

208 pages

ISBN 1-577311-56-6

8349 Hepatitis Sourcebook

Omnigraphics
PO Box 8002
Aston, PA 19014-8002
610-461-3548
800-234-1340
FAX: 800-875-1340
e-mail: customerservice@omnigraphics.com
www.omnigraphics.com

Peter Ruffner, President, Co-Founder
Fred Ruffner, Founder

Hepatitis Sourcebook provides basic consumer health information about hepatitis A, hepatitis B, hepatitis C, and other types of hepatitis, including autoimmune hepatitis, alcoholic hepatitis, nonalcoholic steatohepatitis, and toxin-induced hepatitis. It gives the facts about risk factors, prevention, transmission, screening and diagnostic methods, treatment options, and current research initiatives. *$84.00*

570 pages Hard cover

ISBN 0-780807-49-5

8350 Hip Function & Ambulation

Spina Bifida Association of America
1600 Wilson Boulevard
Suite 800
Arlington, VA 22209
202-944-3285
800-621-3141
FAX: 202-944-3295
e-mail: sbaa@sbaa.org
www.sbaa.org

Ana Ximenes, Chair
Sara Struwe, President & CEO
Mark Bohay, National Web Initiatives & Development Manager
Elizabeth Merck, Development Manager

The ability to walk is important in our society, despite recent advances in wheelchair design and wheelchair accessibility. It also is a desire of children with spina bifida.

8351 Hydrocephalus: A Guide for Patients, Families & Friends

O'Reilly Media Inc
1005 Gravenstein Hwy N
Sebastopol, CA 95472-2811
707-827-7000
800-998-9938
FAX: 707-829-0104
e-mail: order@oreilly.com
www.oreilly.com

Linda Lamb, Editor
Chuck Toporek, Author
Kellie Robinson, Author

Hydrocephalus is a life-threatening condition often referred to as, water on the brain, that is treated by surgical placement of a shunt system. Hydrocephalus: A Guide for Patients, Families and Friends educates families so they can select a skilled neurosurgeon, understand treatments, participate in care, know what symptoms need attention, discover where to turn for support, keep records needed for follow-up treatments, and make wise lifestyle choices. *$19.95*

379 pages Paperback 1999

ISBN 1-565924-10-X

8352 Hypertension Sourcebook

Omnigraphics
PO Box 8002
Aston, PA 19014-8002
610-461-3548
800-234-1340
FAX: 800-875-1340
e-mail: customerservice@omnigraphics.com
www.omnigraphics.com

Peter Ruffner, President, Co-Founder
Fred Ruffner, Founder

This Sourcebook describes the known causes and risk factors associated with essential (or primary) hypertension, secondary hypertension, prehypertension, and other hypertensive disorders. The book also provides information about blood pressure management strategies, including dietary changes, weight loss, exercise, and medications. *$ 84.00*

588 pages Hard cover

ISBN 0-780806-74-0

8353 Immune System Disorders Sourcebook.

Omnigraphics
PO Box 31-1640
Detroit, MI 48231-8002
610-461-3548
800-234-1340
FAX: 610-532-9001
e-mail: info@omnigraphics.com
www.omnigraphics.com

Joyce Brennfleck Shannon, Editor

Immune System Disorders Sourcebook provides information about inherited, acquired, and autoimmune diseases including primary immune deficiency, acquired immunodeficiency syndrome (AIDS), lupus, multiple sclerosis, type one diabetes, rheumatoid arthritis, and Graves' disease. Tips for coping with an immune disorder, caregiving, and treatments are presented along with a glossary and directory of additional resourcesories of additional resources. *$84.00*

643 pages 2nd Edition

ISBN 0-780807-48-8

8354 Informed Touch; A Clinician's Guide To TheEvaluation Of Myofascial Disorders

Inner Traditions/Bear And Company
One Park Street
PO Box 388
Rochester, VT 05767-0388
802-767-3174
800-246-8648
FAX: 802-767-3726
e-mail: customerservice@innertraditions.com
www.innertraditions.com

Rob Meadows, VP Sales/Marketing
Jessica Arsenault, Sales Associate
Donna Finando, LAc, LMT, Author
Steven Finando, PhD, LAc, Co-Author

A Clinician's guide to the evaluation and treatment of myofascial disorders. *$30.00*
224 pages
ISBN 0-892817-40-5

8355 Injured Mind, Shattered Dreams: Brian's Survival from a Severe Head Injury
Brookline Books
8 Trumbull Rd,
Northampton, MA 01060-4533
413-584-0184
800-666-2665
FAX: 413-584-6184
e-mail: brbooks@yahoo.com
www.brooklinebooks.com
Paperback
ISBN 0-91479 -95-6

8356 Interdisciplinary Clinical Assessment of Young Children with Developmental Disabilities
Brookes Publishing
P.O.Box 10624
Baltimore, MD 21285-0624
410-337-9580
800-638-3775
FAX: 410-337-8539
e-mail: custserv@brookespublishing.com
www.brookespublishing.com
Paul H. Brookes, Chairman
Jeffrey D. Brookes, President
Melissa A. Behm, Executive Vice President
George S. Stamathis, Vice President & Publisher
Offers insight from veteran team members on interdisciplinary team assessments. Professionals organizing a team as well as students preparing for practice will find advice on how practitioners gather information, approach assessment, make decisions, and face the challenges of their individual fields. Includes case studies and appendix of photocopiable questionnaires for clinicians and parents. *$44.95*
796 pages Hardcover
ISBN 1-557664-50-1

8357 Introduction to Spina Bifida
Spina Bifida Association of America
1600 Wilson Boulevard
Suite 800
Arlington, VA 22209
202-944-3285
800-621-3141
FAX: 202-944-3295
e-mail: sbaa@sbaa.org
www.sbaa.org
Ana Ximenes, Chair
Sara Struwe, President & CEO
Mark Bohay, National Web Initiatives & Development Manager
Elizabeth Merck, Development Manager
An aid for parents, family and nonmedical people who care for a child with spina bifida. *$7.00*

8358 It's All in Your Head: The Link Between Mercury Amalgams and Illness
Avery Publishing Group
299 W. Houston Street
New York, NY 10014
212-859-1100
FAX: 212-859-1150
e-mail: info@programexchange.com
programexchange.com
208 pages

8359 Joslin Guide to Diabetes: A Program for Managing Your Treatment
Joslin Diabetes Center
1 Joslin Pl
Boston, MA 02215-5306
617-732-2400
FAX: 617-732-2452
www.joslin.org
Richard S Beaser, M.D., Author
Amy Campbell,Ms, RD, CDE, Co-Author
Ralph M. James, Chairperson of the Board
John L. Brooks III, President/CEO
Discusses the causes of diabetes, the role of diet and exercise, meal planning and complications. Also provide information on drawing blood, mixing and injecting insulin, special challenges, living with diabetes. *$16.95*
352 pages Revised Edition

8360 Journey to Well: Learning to Live After Spinal Cord Injury
Altarfire Publishing
1835 Oak Terrace
Newcastle, CA 95658
www.altarfire.com
Margie Williams, Author
The author's close-up view of what life is like during and after such an incident, including her experience with institutional medicine and insurance companies (for better and for worse), and her determined - and ultimately successful - effort to rehabilitate herself and reconstruct her life. *$15.95*
251 pages
ISBN 0-965555-82-8

8361 Ketogenic Diet: A Treatment for Children and Others with Epilepsy
Demos Medical Publishing
11 West 42nd Street
15th Floor
New York, NY 10036
212-683-0072
800-532-8663
FAX: 212-683-0118
e-mail: support@demosmedical.com
www.demosmedpub.com
Richard Winters, Executive Editor
Beth Kaufman Barry, Publisher
Noreen Henson, Executive Director of Demos Heal
John M. Freeman, MD, Co Author
Patient education reference on the use of the ketogenic diet to conrol epilepsy in children. *$24.95*
328 pages Paperback
ISBN 1-932603-18-2

8362 Latex Allergy in Spina Bifida Patients
Spina Bifida Association of America
1600 Wilson Boulevard
Suite 800
Arlington, VA 22209
202-944-3285
800-621-3141
FAX: 202-944-3295
e-mail: sbaa@sbaa.org
www.sbaa.org
Ana Ximenes, Chair
Sara Struwe, President & CEO
Mark Bohay, National Web Initiatives & Development Manager
Elizabeth Merck, Development Manager
The Spina Bifida Association (SBA) serves adults and children who live with the challenges of Spina Bifida.

8363 Learning Among Children with Spina Bifida
Spina Bifida Association of America
1600 Wilson Boulevard
Suite 800
Arlington, VA 22209
202-944-3285
800-621-3141
FAX: 202-944-3295
e-mail: sbaa@sbaa.org
www.sbaa.org
Ana Ximenes, Chair
Sara Struwe, President & CEO
Mark Bohay, National Web Initiatives & Development Manager
Elizabeth Merck, Development Manager
The Spina Bifida Association (SBA) serves adults and children who live with the challenges of Spina Bifida.

8364 Let's Talk About Having Asthma
Rosen Publishing
29 E 21st St
New York, NY 10010-6209
212-420-1600
800-237-9932
FAX: 888-436-4643
www.rosenpublishing.com

Marianna Johnstone, Co-Author
Elizabeth Weitzman, Co-Author
Kelly Chambers, Marketing Assistant
Many kids suffer from asthma, which can overtake them suddenly, causing them terror as they struggle for breath. This book talks about the causes and treatments for asthma, as well as precautions sufferers should take. *$21.95*
ISBN 0-823950-32-8

8365 Leukemia Sourcebook
Omnigraphics
PO Box 8002
Aston, PA 19014-8002
610-461-3548
800-234-1340
FAX: 800-875-1340
e-mail: customerservice@omnigraphics.com
www.omnigraphics.com

Peter Ruffner, President, Co-Founder
Fred Ruffner, Founder
This Sourcebook provides health information about adult and childhood leukemias focusing on the diagnosis and treatments for leukemia, including chemotherapy, radiation, drug therapy, and transplantation of peripheral blood stem cells or marrow. Also included are tips for nutrition, pain and fatigue control, and recognizing possible long-term and late effects of leukemia treatment, along with a glossary and directories of additional resources. *$84.00*
564 pages Hard cover
ISBN 0-780806-27-6

8366 Life After Trauma: A Workbook for Healing
Guilford Press
72 Spring St
New York, NY 10012-4019
212-431-9800
800-365-7006
FAX: 212-966-6708
e-mail: info@guilford.com
www.guilford.com

Denaour Rosenbloom, Author
Mary Beth Williams, Co-Author
Barbar E Watkins, Co-Author
Laurie Anne Pearlman, Foreword
A self-help book on how to deal with trauma. *$19.95*
300 pages Paperback 1910
ISBN 1-606236-08-6

8367 Life Line
National Hydrocephalus Foundation
12413 Centralia St
Lakewood, CA 90715-1653
562-402-3523
888-857-3434
888-260-1789
FAX: 562-924-6666
e-mail: debbifields@nhfonline.org
www.nhfonline.org

Debbi Fields, Executive Director
Michael Fields, President/Treasurer
Jaynie Dunn, Secretary
Sarah Dunn, Junior Director
National Hydrocephalus Foundation quarterly newsletter. *$35.00*
12 pages Quarterly

8368 Lipomas & Lipomyelomeningocele
Spina Bifida Association of America
1600 Wilson Boulevard
Suite 800
Arlington, VA 22209
202-944-3285
800-621-3141
FAX: 202-944-3295
e-mail: sbaa@sbaa.org
www.sbaa.org

Ana Ximenes, Chair
Sara Struwe, President & CEO
Mark Bohay, National Web Initiatives & Development Manager
Elizabeth Merck, Development Manager
The Spina Bifida Association (SBA) serves adults and children who live with the challenges of Spina Bifida.

8369 Liver Disorders Sourcebook
Omnigraphics
PO Box 8002
Aston, PA 19014-8002
610-461-3548
800-234-1340
FAX: 800-875-1340
e-mail: customerservice@omnigraphics.com
www.omnigraphics.com

Peter Ruffner, President, Co-Founder
Fred Ruffner, Founder
Liver Disorders Sourcebook contains basic consumer health information about the liver, how it works, and how to keep it healthy through diet, vaccination, and other preventive care measures. Readers will learn about the symptoms and treatment options for such diseases as hepatitis, primary biliary cirrhosis, Wilson's disease, hemochromatosis, liver failure, cancer of the liver, and disorders related to drugs and other toxins. *$84.00*
580 pages Hard cover
ISBN 0-780803-83-1

8370 Living Beyond Multiple Sclerosis: A Woman's Guide
Hunter House
PO Box 2914
Alameda, CA 94501-914
510-865-5282
800-266-5592
FAX: 510-865-4295
e-mail: ordering@hunterhouse.com
www.hunterhouse.com

Judith Lynn Nichols, Author
Lily Jung, Foreword
This collection of e-mail conversations provides anecdotal and personal information contributed by women with multiple sclerosis. *$14.95*
256 pages
ISBN 0-897932-93-6

8371 Living Well with Asthma
Guilford Press
72 Spring St
New York, NY 10012-4019
212-431-9800
800-365-7006
FAX: 212-966-6708
e-mail: info@guilford.com
www.guilford.com

Cynthia L Divino, Author
Michael R Freedman, Co-Author
Samuel J Rosenberg, Co-Author
James D Crapo, Foreword
Meeting the needs of a growing clinical population, this reader-friendly, practical book offers a lifeline to asthma patients attempting to understand and cope with the psychological ramifications of their illness and its treatment. *$15.95*
213 pages Paperback
ISBN 1-572300-51-4

8372 Living Well with Chronic Fatigue Syndrome and Fibromyalgia

Harper Collins Publishers
10 E 53rd St
New York, NY 10022-5244
212-207-7901
800-242-7737
FAX: 212-702-2586
e-mail: spsales@harpercollins.com
www.harpercollins.com

Mary J Shomon, Author

From the author of Living Well With Hypothyroidism, a comprehensive guide to the diagnosis and treatment of chronic fatigue syndrome and fibromyalgia—vital help for the millions of people suffering from pain, fatigue, and sleep problems. *$14.95*

416 pages 2004
ISBN 0-060521-25-2

8373 Living Well with HIV and AIDS

Bull Publishing
PO Box 1377
Boulder, CO 80306-1377
303-545-6350
800-676-2855
FAX: 303-545-6354
www.bullpub.com

David Sobel, MPH, Author
Virginia Gonzalez MPH, Co-Author
Daina Laurent MPH, Co-Author
Kate Lorig RN, Co-Author

New drugs and drug combinations have turned HIV/AIDS into a long-term illness rather than a death sentence. Practical advice on mental adjustments and physical vigilance is outlined. *$18.95*

245 pages 3rd Edition
ISBN 0-923521-52-6

8374 Living With Spinal Cord Injury Series

Fanlight Productions C/O Icarus Films
32 Court St.
21st Floor
Brooklyn, NY 11201
718-488-8900
800-876-1710
FAX: 718-488-8642
e-mail: info@fanlight.com
www.fanlight.com

Barry Corbet, Producer
Jonathan Miller, President
Meredith Miller, Sales Manager
Anthony Sweeney, Acquisitions

The producer, himself injured in a helicopter crash, brings a unique perspective to this classic three-part series on coming to terms with spinal cord injury. These films offer enduring proof that a tough break doesn't have to mean a ruined life. *$210.00*

VHS 1973

8375 Living with Brain Injury: A Guide for Families

Delmar Cengage Learning
PO Box 6904
Florence, KY 41022-6904
800-354-9706
FAX: 800-487-8488
e-mail: esales@cengage.com
www.cengagesites.com

Richard C Senelick MD, Author
Karla Dougherty, Co-Author

A consumer text to aid people living with brain-injured survivors, includes facts on neuroplasticity, experimental rehabilitation research, and the process of rehabilitation itself. *$19.95*

225 pages Softcover 2001
ISBN 1-891525-09-3

8376 Living with Spina Bifida: A Guide for Families and Professionals

University of North Carolina at Chapel Hill
116 S Boundary St
Chapel Hill, NC 27514-3808
919-966-3561
800-848-6224
FAX: 919-962-2704
e-mail: uncpress@unc.edu
www.uncpress.unc.edu

Adrian Sandler MD, Author

A handbook that addresses patients' biopsychosocial and developmental needs from birth through adolescence and into adulthood. Sandler's holistic approach encourages families to focus more on the child and less on the disability while providing abundant information about this condition. *$20.95*

296 pages 2004
ISBN 0-807855-47-8

8377 Lung Cancer: Making Sense of Diagnosis, Treatment, and Options

O'Reilly Media Inc
1005 Gravenstein Hwy N
Sebastopol, CA 95472-2811
707-827-7000
800-998-9938
FAX: 707-829-0104
e-mail: order@oreilly.com
www.oreilly.com

Linda Lamb, Editor
Lorraine Johnston, Author

Straightforward language and the words of patients and their families are the hallmarks of this book on the number one cancer killer in the US. Written by a widely respected author and patient advocate, Lung Cancer: Making Sense of Diagnosis, Treatment, & Options has been meticulously reviewed by top medical experts and physicians. Readers will find medical facts simply explained, advice to ease their daily life, and tools to be strong advocates for themselves or a family member. *$ 27.95*

530 pages Paperback 2001
ISBN 0-596500-02-5

8378 Lung Disorders Sourcebook

Omnigraphics
PO Box 8002
Aston, PA 19014-8002
610-461-3548
800-234-1340
FAX: 800-875-1340
e-mail: customerservice@omnigraphics.com
www.omnigraphics.com

Peter Ruffner, President, Co-Founder
Fred Ruffner, Founder

Lung Disorders Sourcebook offers information about specific types of lung disorders, including diagnosis, treatment, and prevention issues. The book offers advice for preventing some types lung disorder that are acquired by asbestos, radon, and other environmental exposures. *$84.00*

657 pages Hard cover
ISBN 0-780803-39-8

8379 Lupus: Alternative Therapies That Work

Inner Traditions
PO Box 388
Rochester
VT, 05 0388-802-
800-246-8648
802-767-3726
TTY:customerserv
e-mail: info@innertraditions.com
www.innertraditions.com

Sharon Moore, Author

A comprehensive guise to noninvasive, nontoxic therapies for lupus - written by a lupus survivor. *$14.95*

256 pages 2000
ISBN 0-892818-89-1

8380 MAGIC Touch
MAGIC Foundation for Children's Growth
6645 North Ave
Oak Park, IL 60302-1057
708-383-0808
800-362-4423
FAX: 708-383-0899
e-mail: mary@magicfoundation.org
www.magicfoundation.org

Mary Andrews, CEO
Dianne Kremidas, Executive Director
Pam Pentaris, Office Manager
Jamie Harvey, Technical Education Teacher
Provides support and education regarding growth disorders in children and related adult disorders, including adult GHD. Dedicated to helping children whose physical growth is affected be a medical problem by assisting families of afflicted children through local support groups, public education/awareness, newsletters, specialty divisions and programs for the children.
36-40 pages Quarterly

8381 Management of Autistic Behavior
Sage Publications
2455 Teller Road
Thousand Oaks, CA 91320
805-499-0721
800-818-7243
FAX: 805-499-0871
e-mail: info@sagepub.com
www.sagepub.com

Sara Miller McCune, Founder, Publisher, Executive Chairman
Blaise R Simqu, President & CEO
Tracey A. Ozmina, Executive Vice President & Chief Operating Officer
Stephen Barr, Managing Director/SAGE London, President of SAGE Internation
Comprehensive and practical book that tells what works best with specific problems. *$51.00*
450 pages Paperback
ISBN 0-890791-96-1

8382 Management of Genetic Syndromes
John Wiley & Sons
111 River St
Hoboken, NJ 07030-5774
201-748-6000
201-748-6088
e-mail: info@wiley.com
www.as.wiley.com

Suzanne B Cassidy, Editor
Judith E Allanson, Editor
Edited by two of the field's most highly esteemed experts, this landmark volume provides: A precise reference of the physical manifestations of common genetic syndromes, clearly written for professionals and families, Extensive updates, particularly in sections on diagnostic criteria and diagnostic testing, pathogenesis, and management, A tried-and-tested, user-friendly format, with each chapter including information on incidence, etiology and pathogenesis, diagnostic criteria and testing, and d
$204.95
720 pages 3rd Edition
ISBN 0-470191-41-5

8383 Managing Post Polio: A Guide to Living Well with Post Polio
ABI Professional Publications
PO Box 149
St Petersburg, FL 33731-149
727-556-0950
800-551-7776
FAX: 727-556-2560
e-mail: webmaster@vandamere.com
www.abipropub.com

Lauro S Halstead MD, Editor
Edited by Lauro S. Halstead, M.D., Managing Post-Polio, 2nd Edition, provides a comprehensive overview dealing with the medical, psychological, vocational, and many other challenges of living with post-polio syndrome. With contributions from over 15 healthcare professionals, the majority of whom are polio survivors themselves, Managing Post-Polio distills and summarizes the wealth of information presented from over the past 20 plus years.
256 pages
ISBN 1-886236-17-8

8384 Meniere's Disease
Vestibular Disorders Association
5018 NE 15th Avenue
Portland, OR 97211
800-837-8428
FAX: 503-229-8064
e-mail: info@vestibular.org
www.vestibular.org

P. Ashley Wackym, Chair
Cynthia Ryan MBA, Executive Director
Tony Staser, Development Director
Kerrie Denner, Outreach Coordinator
VEDA's website contains a wealth of information on the symptoms, diagnosis and treatment of various types of vestibular disorders. *$5.00*

8385 Menopause without Medicine
Hunter House
PO Box 2914
Alameda, CA 94501-914
510-865-5282
800-266-5592
FAX: 510-865-4295
e-mail: ordering@hunterhouse.com
www.hunterhouse.com

Linda Ojeda PhD, Author
Menopause Without Medicine provides complete information on the symptoms of menopause - hot flashes, fatigue, sexual changes, depression and osteoporosis - and how to alleviate them.
$18.95
304 pages 5th Edition
ISBN 0-897934-05-3

8386 Movement Disorders Sourcebook
Omnigraphics
PO Box 8002
Aston, PA 19014-8002
610-461-3548
800-234-1340
FAX: 800-875-1340
e-mail: customerservice@omnigraphics.com
www.omnigraphics.com

Peter Ruffner, President, Co-Founder
Fred Ruffner, Founder
This Sourcebook provides health information about neurological movement disorders, their symptoms, causes, diagnostic tests, and treatments. Readers will learn about Essential Tremor, Parkinson's Disease, Dystonia, and many other early-onset and adult-onset movement disorders. Information about mobility and assistive technology aids is included, along with a glossary and a listing of additional resources. *$84.00*
600 pages Hard cover
ISBN 0-780810-34-1

8387 Multiple Sclerosis and Having a Baby
Inner Traditions
PO Box 388
Rochester, VT 05767-0388
802-767-3174
800-246-8648
FAX: 802-767-3726
e-mail: customerservice@innertraditions.com
www.innertraditions.com

Judy Graham, Author
Everything you need to know about conception, pregnancy and parenthood. *$12.95*
160 pages 2001
ISBN 0-892817-88-7

8388 Multiple Sclerosis: 300 Tips for Making Life Easier
Demos Medical Publishing
11 West 42nd Street
15th Floor
New York, NY 10036
212-683-0072
800-532-8663
FAX: 212-683-0118
e-mail: support@demosmedical.com
www.demosmedpub.com

Richard Winters, Executive Editor
Beth Kaufman Barry, Publisher
Noreen Henson, Executive Director of Demos Heal
Shelley Peterman Schwarz, Author

This latest book in the Making Life Easier series features tip, techniques and shortcuts for conserving time and energy so you can do more of the things you want to do. These tips should help increase the number of good days you have while encouraging you to develop your own techniques for making life easier. *$16.95*
128 pages
ISBN 1-932603-21-2

8389 Multiple Sclerosis: A Guide for Families
Demos Medical Publishing
11 West 42nd Street
15th Floor
New York, NY 10036
212-683-0072
800-532-8663
FAX: 212-683-0118
e-mail: support@demosmedical.com
www.demosmedpub.com

Richard Winters, Executive Editor
Beth Kaufman Barry, Publisher
Noreen Henson, Executive Director of Demos Heal
Rosalind C. Kalb, Ph.D., Author

Guide for living and coping with multiple sclerosis. *$24.95*
256 pages
ISBN 1-932603-10-7

8390 Multiple Sclerosis: A Guide for the Newly Diagnosed
Demos Medical Publishing
11 West 42nd Street
15th Floor
New York, NY 10036
212-683-0072
800-532-8663
FAX: 212-683-0118
e-mail: support@demosmedical.com
www.demosmedpub.com

Richard Winters, Executive Editor
Beth Kaufman Barry, Publisher
Noreen Henson, Executive Director of Demos Heal
Nancy J. Holland, RN, EdD,, Co Author

A must-have title for anyone who has recently been diagnosed with MS and a good idea for family members and friends. *$19.95*
256 pages
ISBN 1-932603-27-1

8391 Multiple Sclerosis: The Guide to Treatment and Management
Demos Medical Publishing
11 West 42nd Street
15th Floor
New York, NY 10036
212-683-0072
800-532-8663
FAX: 212-683-0118
e-mail: support@demosmedical.com
www.demosmedpub.com

Richard Winters, Executive Editor
Beth Kaufman Barry, Publisher
Noreen Henson, Executive Director of Demos Heal
Chris H. Polman, MD, FRCP, Co Author

A current guide to modern therapies. *$24.95*
216 pages
ISBN 1-932603-15-4

8392 Muscular Dystrophies
Oxford University Press
198 Madison Avenue
New York, NY 10016
212-726-6000
800-445-9714
FAX: 919-677-1303
e-mail: custserv.us@oup.com
www.oup.com

Alan E.H. Emery, Author

Describes the opportunities for management of more than 30 types of MD through respiratory care, physiotherapy and surgical correction of contractures, and examines the potential for effective treatment utilizing the new techniques of gene and cell therapy *$ 165.00*
330 pages
ISBN 0-192632-91-4

8393 Muscular Dystrophy in Children: A Guide for Families
Demos Medical Publishing
11 West 42nd Street
15th Floor
New York, NY 10036
212-683-0072
800-532-8663
FAX: 212-683-0118
e-mail: support@demosmedical.com
www.demosmedpub.com

Richard Winters, Executive Editor
Beth Kaufman Barry, Publisher
Noreen Henson, Executive Director of Demos Heal

Defines the available medical options at every stage of the disease and offers guidance even when it may seem that little or nothing can be done. Includes a glossary and suggestions for furhter reading. *$19.95*
144 pages Paperback
ISBN 1-888799-33-1

8394 Muscular Dystrophy: The Facts
Oxford University Press
198 Madison Avenue
New York, NY 10016
212-726-6000
800-445-9714
FAX: 919-677-1303
e-mail: custserv.us@oup.com
www.oup.com

Peter Harper, Author

A good first book for individuals and families faced with the likelihood or reality of a muscular dystrophy diagnosis. *$22.50*
178 pages
ISBN 0-192632-17-5

8395 My House is Killing Me! The Home Guide for Families with Allergies and Asthma
Johns Hopkins University Press
2175 N Charles St
Baltimore, MD 21218-4363
410-516-6900
800-548-1784
FAX: 410-516-6968
e-mail: webmaster@jhupress.jhu.edu
www.press.jhu.edu

Jeffrey C May, Author
Jonathan M Samet, M.D., Foreword
Kathleen Keane, Director

Chemical consultant May describes where and how the various parts of a residence can cause temporary or chronic illness for those with allergies or other sensitivities. *$20.95*
352 pages
ISBN 0-801867-30-9

8396 Neuropsychiatry of Epilepsy
Cambridge University Press
100 Brookhill Dr
West Nyack, NY 10994
845-353-7500
845-353-4141
www.cambridge.org

Michael R Trimble, Editor
Bettina Schmitz, Editor

Covers the practical implications of ongoing research, and offers a diagnostic and management perspective. Topics include cognitive aspects, nonepileptic attacks, and clinical aspects. For professionals treating epileptic patients. *$104.00*

232 pages 2nd Edition 1911
ISBN 0-521154-69-7

8397 Nick Joins In
Spina Bifida Association of America
1600 Wilson Boulevard
Suite 800
Arlington, VA 22209 202-944-3285
800-621-3141
FAX: 202-944-3295
e-mail: sbaa@sbaa.org
www.sbaa.org

Ana Ximenes, Chair
Sara Struwe, President & CEO
Mark Bohay, National Web Initiatives & Development Manager
Elizabeth Merck, Development Manager

When Nick, who is in a wheelchair, enters a regular classroom for the first time, he realizes that he has much to contribute. *$17.00*

8398 No More Allergies
Random House
1745 Broadway
3rd Floor
New York, NY 10019-4305 212-782-9000
FAX: 212-572-6066
e-mail: ecustomerservice@randonhouse.com
www.randomhouse.com

Markus Dohle, CEO
Gary Null PhD, Author

Null redefines a health problem that afflicts 40 million Americans: More than mere hay fever, contemporary allergic reactions include chronic fatigue syndrome, Alzheimer's disease, and even HIV infection. These conditions, he explains, occur when our immune systems break down. This ground-breaking book now prescribes effective solutions. *$23.00*

464 pages 1992
ISBN 0-679743-10-1

8399 No Time for Jello: One Family's Experience
Brookline Books
8 Trumbull Rd,
Northampton, MA 01060-4533 413-584-0184
800-666-2665
FAX: 413-584-6184
e-mail: brbooks@yahoo.com
www.brooklinebooks.com

Softcover
ISBN 0-91479 -56-5

8400 Nocturnal Asthma
National Jewish Health
1400 Jackson Street
Denver, CO 80206 303-270-2708
877-225-5654
FAX: 303-398-1125
e-mail: allstetterw@njc.org
nationaljewish.org

Rich Schierburg, Chair
Robin Chotin, Vice Chair
Michael Salem, M.D., President and CEO
Christine Forkner, CFO and Executive Vice President

Offers information to patients about how to understand and manage asthma at night.

8401 Obesity
Spina Bifida Association of America
1600 Wilson Boulevard
Suite 800
Arlington, VA 22209 202-944-3285
800-621-3141
FAX: 202-944-3295
e-mail: sbaa@sbaa.org
www.sbaa.org

Ana Ximenes, Chair
Sara Struwe, President & CEO
Mark Bohay, National Web Initiatives & Development Manager
Elizabeth Merck, Development Manager

The Spina Bifida Association (SBA) serves adults and children who live with the challenges of Spina Bifida. *$8.00*

8402 Obesity Sourcebook
Omnigraphics
PO Box 8002
Aston, PA 19014-8002 610-461-3548
800-234-1340
FAX: 800-875-1340
e-mail: customerservice@omnigraphics.com
www.omnigraphics.com

Peter Ruffner, President, Co-Founder
Fred Ruffner, Founder

Discusses diseases and other problems associated with obesity. *$78.00*

376 pages
ISBN 0-780803-33-6

8403 Occulta
Spina Bifida Association of America
1600 Wilson Boulevard
Suite 800
Arlington, VA 22209 202-944-3285
800-621-3141
FAX: 202-944-3295
e-mail: sbaa@sbaa.org
www.sbaa.org

Ana Ximenes, Chair
Sara Struwe, President & CEO
Mark Bohay, National Web Initiatives & Development Manager
Elizabeth Merck, Development Manager

The Spina Bifida Association (SBA) serves adults and children who live with the challenges of Spina Bifida. *$8.00*

8404 Official Patient's Sourcebook on Bell's Palsy
Icon Group International
9606 Tierra Grande Street
Suite 205
San Diego, CA 92126 FAX: 858-635-9414
e-mail: orders@icongroupbooks.com
www.icongroupbooks.com

ISBN 0-597835-20-9

8405 Official Patient's Sourcebook on Cystic Fibrosis
Icon Group International
9606 Tierra Grande Street
Suite 205
San Diego, CA 92126 FAX: 858-635-9414
e-mail: orders@icongroupbooks.com
icongroupbooks.com

356 pages
ISBN 0-597831-46-7

8406 Official Patient's Sourcebook on Muscular Dystrophy
Icon Group International
9606 Tierra Grande Street
Suite 205
San Diego, CA 92126 FAX: 858-635-9414
e-mail: orders@icongroupbooks.com
icongroupbooks.com

268 pages
ISBN 0-597832-10-2

8407 Official Patient's Sourcebook on Osteoporosis
Icon Group International
9606 Tierra Grande Street
Suite 205
San Diego, CA 92126
FAX: 858-635-9414
e-mail: orders@icongroupbooks.com
icongroupbooks.com

ISBN 0-597833-04-4

8408 Official Patient's Sourcebook on Post-Polio Syndrome: A Revised and Updated Directory
Icon Group International
9606 Tierra Grande Street
Suite 205
San Diego, CA 92126
FAX: 858-635-9414
e-mail: orders@icongroupbooks.com
icongroupbooks.com

124 pages
ISBN 0-597835-31-4

8409 Official Patient's Sourcebook on Primary Pulmonary Hypertension
Icon Group International
9606 Tierra Grande Street
Suite 205
San Diego, CA 92126
FAX: 858-635-9414
e-mail: orders@icongroupbooks.com
icongroupbooks.com

ISBN 0-597831-54-8

8410 Official Patient's Sourcebook on Pulmonary Fibrosis
Icon Group International
9606 Tierra Grande Street
Suite 205
San Diego, CA 92126
FAX: 858-635-9414
e-mail: orders@icongroupbooks.com
icongroupbooks.com

ISBN 0-597831-65-3

8411 Official Patient's Sourcebook on Scoliosis
Icon Group International
9606 Tierra Grande Street
Suite 205
San Diego, CA 92126
FAX: 858-635-9414
e-mail: orders@icongroupbooks.com
icongroupbooks.com

ISBN 0-597829-90-X

8412 Official Patient's Sourcebook on Sickle Cell Anemia
Icon Group International
9606 Tierra Grande Street
Suite 205
San Diego, CA 92126
FAX: 858-635-9414
e-mail: orders@icongroupbooks.com
icongroupbooks.com

ISBN 0-597831-57-2

8413 Official Patient's Sourcebook on Ulcerative Colitis
Icon Group International
9606 Tierra Grande Street
Suite 205
San Diego, CA 92126
FAX: 858-635-9414
e-mail: orders@icongroupbooks.com
icongroupbooks.com

ISBN 0-597834-09-1

8414 One Day at a Time: Children Living with Leukemia
Gareth Stevens Publishing
111 East 14th Street
Suite #349
New York, NY 10003
800-542-2595
FAX: 877-542-2596
e-mail: customerservice@gspub.com
www.garethstevens.com

56 pages Hardcover
ISBN 1-55532 -13-6

8415 Options: Revolutionary Ideas in the War on Cancer
People Against Cancer
P.O.Box 10
604 East Street
Otho, IA 50569
515-972-4444
800-662-2623
FAX: 515-972-4415
e-mail: info@PeopleAgainstCancer.org
www.peopleagainstcancer.com

Frank D. Wiewel, Executive Director/Founder

Publication of People Against Cancer, a nonprofit, grassroots public benefit organization dedicated to 'New Directions in the War on Cancer.' We help people to find the best cancer treatment. We are a democratic organization of people with cancer, their loved ones and citizens working together to protect and enhance medical freedom of choice.

8416 Osteoporosis Sourcebook
Omnigraphics
PO Box 8002
Aston, PA 19014-8002
313-961-1340
800-234-1340
FAX: 800-875-1340
e-mail: customerservice@omnigraphics.com
www.omnigraphics.com

Peter Ruffner, President, Co-Founder
Fred Ruffner, Founder

Discusses causes, risk factors, treatments and traditional and non-traditional pain management issues concerning osteoporosis. *$ 84.00*
568 pages Hard cover
ISBN 0-780802-39-1

8417 Parent's Guide to Allergies and Asthma
Allergy & Asthma Network Mothers of Asthmatics
Ste 150
PO Box 7474
Fairfax Station, VA 22039-7474
703-323-9170
800-756-5525
FAX: 703-323-9173
e-mail: custsvc@parent-institute.com
www.parent-institute.com

John H Wherry, Ed.D, President

A up-to-date, easy-to-read resource offering essential information on asthma and allergies.

8418 Partial Seizure Disorders: A Guide for Patients and Families
O'Reilly Media Inc
1005 Gravenstein Hwy N
Sebastopol, CA 95472-2811
707-827-7000
800-998-9938
FAX: 707-829-0104
e-mail: order@oreilly.com
www.oreilly.com

Linda Lamb, Editor
Mitzi Waltz, Author

Partial Seizure Disorders helps patients and families get an accurate diagnosis of this condition, understand medications and their side effects, and learn coping skills and other adjuncts to medication. It walks readers through developmental and school issues for young children; adult issues such as employment and driving; working with an existing health plan; and getting further help through advocacy and support organizations, articles, and online resources. *$19.95*
288 pages Paperback
ISBN 0-596500-03-3

8419 Penitent, with Roses: An HIV+ Mother Reflects
University Press of New England
1 Court St
Ste 250
Lebanon, NH 03766-1358
603-448-1533
800-421-1561
FAX: 603-448-7006
www.upne.com

Paula W Peterson, Author

Peterson, a married, middle-class, Jewish mother, was diagnosed with full-blown AIDS four years into her marriage and 11 months after her son was born. In seven poignant autobiographical essays and a collection of letters to her uninfected, four-year-old son, the author maintains an upbeat tone and describes her unsuccessful attempts to find the source of her infection (her husband tested negative), her relationships with her doctors, and her work as an HIV activist. *$ 26.95*

256 pages 2001
ISBN 1-584651-28-4

8420 Plan Ahead: Do What You Can
Spina Bifida Association of America
1600 Wilson Boulevard
Suite 800
Arlington, VA 22209
202-944-3285
800-621-3141
FAX: 202-944-3295
e-mail: sbaa@sbaa.org
www.sbaa.org

Ana Ximenes, Chair
Sara Struwe, President & CEO
Mark Bohay, National Web Initiatives & Development Manager
Elizabeth Merck, Development Manager
Folic aciid information for women at risk for recurrence. *$15.00*

8421 Post-Polio Syndrome: A Guide for Polio Survivors and Their Families
Yale University Press
PO Box 209040
New Haven, CT 6520-9040
203-432-0960
203-432-0948
e-mail: language.yalepress@yale.edu
www.yalepress.yale.edu

Julie K Silver M.D., Author
Laro S Halstead, M.D., Foreword
A guide for polio survivors, their families, and their health care providers offers expert advice on all aspects of post-polio syndrome. Based on the author's experience treating post-polio patients, Silver discusses issues of critical importance, including how to find the best medical care, deal with symptoms, sustain mobility, manage pain, approach insurance issues, and arrange a safe living environment. *$ 19.50*

304 pages 2002
ISBN 0-300088-08-3

8422 Prader-Willi Syndrome: Development and Manifestations
Cambridge University Press
32 Avenue of the Americas
New York, NY 10013-2473
212-924-3900
212-691-3239
www.cambridge.org

Joyce Whittington, Author
Tony Holland, Co-Author
Seeks to identify and provide the latest findings about how best to manage the complex medical, nutritional, psychological, educational, social and therapeutic needs of people with PWS. *$130.00*

230 pages 2004
ISBN 0-521840-29-3

8423 Preventing Secondary Conditions Associated with Spina Bifida or Cerebral Palsy
Spina Bifida Association of America
1600 Wilson Boulevard
Suite 800
Arlington, VA 22209
202-944-3285
800-621-3141
FAX: 202-944-3295
e-mail: sbaa@sbaa.org
www.sbaa.org

Ana Ximenes, Chair
Sara Struwe, President & CEO
Mark Bohay, National Web Initiatives & Development Manager
Elizabeth Merck, Development Manager
This report is for health professionals, parents and teachers. *$3.00*

8424 Prostate and Urological Disorders Sourcebook
Omnigraphics
PO Box 8002
Aston, PA 19014-8002
313-961-1340
800-234-1340
FAX: 800-875-1340
e-mail: customerservice@omnigraphics.com
www.omnigraphics.com

Peter Ruffner, President, Co-Founder
Fred Ruffner, Founder
Peter Ruffner, Co-Founder
Prostate and Urological Disorders Sourcebook provides information about prostate cancer and other prostate problems, such as prostatitis and benign prostatic hyperplasia. A glossary of andrological terms and a directory of resources for additional help and information are also included. *$84.00*

604 pages Hard cover
ISBN 0-780807-97-6

8425 Protecting Against Latex Allergy
Spina Bifida Association of America
1600 Wilson Boulevard
Suite 800
Arlington, VA 22209
202-944-3285
800-621-3141
FAX: 202-944-3295
e-mail: sbaa@sbaa.org
www.sbaa.org

Ana Ximenes, Chair
Sara Struwe, President & CEO
Mark Bohay, National Web Initiatives & Development Manager
Elizabeth Merck, Development Manager
Because awareness and proper action may help prevent an allergic reation, learning about latex allergy is especially important for parents, health care workers and anyone who is exposed to latex regulary. *$20.00*

8426 Questions and Answers: The ADA and Personswith HIV/AIDS
US Department of Justice
950 Pennsylvania Ave NW
Washington, DC 20530-9
202-307-0663
800-514-0301
FAX: 202-307-1197
TTY: 800-514-0383
www.ada.gov

Joanne Graham, Manager
Rebecca B. Bond, Chief
Zita Johnson Betts, Deputy Chief
James Bostrom, Deputy Chief
A 16-page publication explaining the requirements for employers, businesses and nonprofit agencies that serve the public, and state and local governments to avoid discriminating against persons with HIV/AIDS.

8427 Raynaud's Phenomenon
Arthritis Foundation
1330 W. Peachtree Street
Suite 100
Atlanta, GA 30309
404-872-7100
800-283-7800
FAX: 404-872-0457
arthritis.org

Daniel T. McGowan, Chair
Michael V. Ortman, Vice Chair
Ann M. Palmer, CEO/President
Peter W.C. Barnhart, Treasurer
The Arthritis Foundation is the largest national nonprofit organization that supports the more than 100 types of arthritis and related conditions. Founded in 1948, with headquarters in Atlanta, the Arthritis Foundation has multiple service points located throughout the country.

8428 Reaching the Autistic Child: A Parent Training Program
Brookline Books
8 Trumbull Rd,
Northampton, MA 01060-4533
413-584-0184
800-666-2665
FAX: 413-584-6184
e-mail: brbooks@yahoo.com
www.brooklinebooks.com

Softcover
ISBN 1-571290-56-7

8429 Respiratory Disorders Sourcebook
Omnigraphics
PO Box 8002
Aston, PA 19014-8002
313-961-1340
800-234-1340
FAX: 800-875-1340
e-mail: customerservice@omnigraphics.com
www.omnigraphics.com

Peter Ruffner, President, Co-Founder
Fred Ruffner, Founder
Sandra J Judd, Editor

Respiratory Disorders Sourcebook provides up-to-date information about infectious, inflammatory, occupational, and other types of respiratory disorders. Tips for managing chronic respiratory diseases and suggestions for ways to promote lung health are presented, and the book concludes with a glossary of related terms and a list of additional resources. *$84.00*
638 pages Hard cover
ISBN 0-780810-07-5

8430 SPINabilities: A Young Person's Guide to Spina Bifida
Spina Bifida Association of America
1600 Wilson Boulevard
Suite 800
Arlington, VA 22209
202-944-3285
800-621-3141
FAX: 202-944-3295
e-mail: sbaa@sbaa.org
www.sbaa.org

Ana Ximenes, Chair
Sara Struwe, President & CEO
Mark Bohay, National Web Initiatives & Development Manager
Elizabeth Merck, Development Manager

A cool and practical book for young adults becoming independent. *$22.30*

8431 Seizures and Epilepsy in Childhood: A Guide
John Hopkins University Press
2715 N Charles St
Baltimore, MD 21218-4363
410-516-6900
800-548-1784
FAX: 410-516-6998
e-mail: webmaster@jhupress.jhu.edu
www.press.jhu.edu

Kathleen Keane, Director
Eileen P G Vining MD, Co-Author
Diana J Pillas, Co-Author
John M Freeman, M.D., Co-Author

The award-winning Seizures and Epilepsy in Childhood is the standard resource for parents in need of comprehensive medical information about their child with epilepsy. *$54.00*
432 pages 3rd Edition
ISBN 0-801870-51-4

8432 Sexuality and the Person with Spina Bifida
Spina Bifida Association of America
1600 Wilson Boulevard
Suite 800
Arlington, VA 22209
202-944-3285
800-621-3141
FAX: 202-944-3295
e-mail: sbaa@sbaa.org
www.sbaa.org

Ana Ximenes, Chair
Sara Struwe, President & CEO
Mark Bohay, National Web Initiatives & Development Manager
Elizabeth Merck, Development Manager

Dr Sloan foucuses on sexual development, sexual activity and other important issues. *$11.00*

8433 Sinus Survival: A Self-help Guide
Penguin Group
375 Hudson St
New York, NY 10014-3658
212-366-2372
FAX: 212-366-2933
e-mail: insidesales@penguingroup.com
us.penguingroup.com

Robert S Ivker, Author

Self-help manual for sufferers of bronchitis, sinusitis, allergies, and colds. *$15.95*
336 pages Paperback 2000
ISBN 1-101798-02-6

8434 Social Development and the Person with Spina Bifida
Spina Bifida Association of America
1600 Wilson Boulevard
Suite 800
Arlington, VA 22209
202-944-3285
800-621-3141
FAX: 202-944-3295
e-mail: sbaa@sbaa.org
www.sbaa.org

Ana Ximenes, Chair
Sara Struwe, President & CEO
Mark Bohay, National Web Initiatives & Development Manager
Elizabeth Merck, Development Manager

Examines how spina bifida and hydrocephalus may influence development and learning social skills.

8435 Solving the Puzzle of Chronic Fatigue
Essential Science Publishing
1216 S 1580 W
Ste A
Orem, UT 84058-4906
801-224-6228
800-336-6308
FAX: 801-224-6229
e-mail: info@essentialscience.net
www.essentialsciencepublishing.com

Michael Rosenbaum, Author
Murray Susser, Co-Author

Although primarily a book about CFS, this comprehensive study also provides a detailed overview of candidiasis, including its causes and best approaches for treatment. *$14.95*
190 pages
ISBN 0-943685-11-7

8436 Son Rise: The Miracle Continues
New World Library
14 Pamaron Way
Novato, CA 94949
415-884-2100
800-972-6657
FAX: 415-884-2199
e-mail: ami@newworldlibrary.com
www.newworldlibrary.com

Barry Neil Kaufman, Author

Documents Raun Kaufman's astonishing development from a lifeless, autistic, retarded child into a highly verbal, lovable youngster with no traces of his former condition. Details Raun's extraordinary progress from the age of four into young adulthood, also shares moving accounts of five families that successfully used the Son-Rise Program to reach their own special children. *$14.96*
372 pages
ISBN 0-915811-53-7

8437 **Steps to Independence: Teaching Everyday Skills to Children with Special Needs**
Spina Bifida Association of America
1600 Wilson Boulevard
Suite 800
Arlington, VA 22209
202-944-3285
800-621-3141
FAX: 202-944-3295
e-mail: sbaa@sbaa.org
www.sbaa.org

Ana Ximenes, Chair
Sara Struwe, President & CEO
Mark Bohay, National Web Initiatives & Development Manager
Elizabeth Merck, Development Manager
A guide to help parents teach life skills to their disabled child. *$34.25*

8438 **Stroke Sourcebook**
PO Box 8002
Aston, PA 19014-8002
313-961-1340
800-234-1340
FAX: 800-875-1340
e-mail: customerservice@omnigraphics.com
www.omnigraphics.com

Peter Ruffner, President, Co-Founder
Fred Ruffner, Founder
Peter Ruffner, Co-Founder
Basic Consumer Health Information about Stroke, Including Ischemic, Hemorrhagic, and Mini Strokes, as Well as Risk Factors, Prevention Guidelines, Diagnostic Tests, Medications and Surgical Treatments, and Complications of Stroke.

8439 **Stroke Sourcebook, 2nd Edition**
Omnigraphics
PO Box 8002
Aston, PA 19014-8002
313-961-1340
800-234-1340
FAX: 800-875-1340
e-mail: customerservice@omnigraphics.com
www.omnigraphics.com

Peter Ruffner, President, Co-Founder
Fred Ruffner, Founder
Peter Ruffner, Co-Founder
Stroke Sourcebook, Second Edition provides updated information about stroke, its causes, risk factors, diagnosis, acute and long-term treatment, and recent innovations in poststroke care. Information on rehabilitation therapies, prevention strategies, and tips on caring for a stroke survivor is also included, along with a glossary of related terms and a directory of organizations that offer additional information to stroke survivors and their families. *$84.00*
626 pages Hard cover
ISBN 0-780810-35-8

8440 **Succeeding With Interventions For Asperger Syndrome Adolescents**
Autsim Society of North Carolina Bookstore
505 Oberlin Road
Suite 230
Raleigh, NC 27605-1345
919-743-0204
800-442-2762
FAX: 919-743-0208
e-mail: books@autismsociety-nc.org
www.autismbookstore.com

Tracey Sheriff, Chief Executive Officer
David Laxton, Director of Communications
Paul Wendler, Chief Financial Officer
Kristy White, Director of Development
This book includes a very useful outline of all the therapy sessions, which can be used as a template by a practitioner for creating their own interaction therapy intervention for adolescents.

8441 **Symptomatic Chiari Malformation**
Spina Bifida Association of America
1600 Wilson Boulevard
Suite 800
Arlington, VA 22209
202-944-3285
800-621-3141
FAX: 202-944-3295
e-mail: sbaa@sbaa.org
www.sbaa.org

Ana Ximenes, Chair
Sara Struwe, President & CEO
Mark Bohay, National Web Initiatives & Development Manager
Elizabeth Merck, Development Manager
The Spina Bifida Association (SBA) serves adults and children who live with the challenges of Spina Bifida.

8442 **Taking Charge**
Spina Bifida Association of America
1600 Wilson Boulevard
Suite 800
Arlington, VA 22209
202-944-3285
800-621-3141
FAX: 202-944-3295
e-mail: sbaa@sbaa.org
www.sbaa.org

Ana Ximenes, Chair
Sara Struwe, President & CEO
Mark Bohay, National Web Initiatives & Development Manager
Elizabeth Merck, Development Manager
Teenagers talk about life and physical disabilities. *$7.95*

8443 **Ten Things I Learned from Bill Porter**
New World Library
14 Pamaron Way
Novato, CA 94949
415-884-2100
800-972-6657
FAX: 415-884-2199
e-mail: ami@newworldlibrary.com
www.newworldlibrary.com

Shelly Ackerman, Author
Bill Porter worked for the Watkins Corp, selling household products door-to-door in one of Portland's worst neighborhoods. Afflicted with cerebral palsy and burdened with continual pain, Porter was determined not to live on government disability and went on to become Watkin's top-grossing salesman in Portland, the Northwest, and the US. This book was written by the woman who worked as Porter's typist and driver and later became his friend and cospeaker. *$20.00*
192 pages
ISBN 1-577312-03-1

8444 **Thyroid Disorders Sourcebook**
Omnigraphics
PO Box 8002
Aston, PA 19014-8002
313-961-1340
800-234-1340
FAX: 800-875-1340
e-mail: customerservice@omnigraphics.com
www.omnigraphics.com

Peter Ruffner, President, Co-Founder
Fred Ruffner, Founder
Thyroid Disorders Sourcebook provides essential information about thyroid and parathyroid function, diseases, and treatments. Also presented are symptoms, risk factors, diagnosis, treatments, thyroid effects on the body, and the impact of environmental conditions on the thyroid. *$84.00*
573 pages Hard cover
ISBN 0-780807-45-7

8445 Tourette Syndrome: The Facts
Oxford University Press
198 Madison Avenue
New York, NY 10016
212-726-6000
800-445-9714
FAX: 919-677-1303
e-mail: custserv.us@oup.com
www.oup.com

Mary Robertson, Co-Editor
Andrea Cavanna, Co-Editor
Johnathan Keats, Author
Jim Cullen, Author
The causes of the syndrome, how it is diagnosed, and the ways in which it can be treated. *$35.00*
122 pages
ISBN 0-198523-98-X

8446 Tourette's Syndrome: Finding Answers and Getting Help
O'Reilly Media Inc
1005 Gravenstein Hwy N
Sebastopol, CA 95472-2811
707-827-7019
800-889-8969
FAX: 707-824-8268
e-mail: order@oreilly.com
www.oreilly.com

416 pages Paperback
ISBN 0-596500-07-6

8447 Tourette's Syndrome: Tics, Obsessions, Compulsions: Developmental Psychopathology
John Wiley & Sons
111 River Street
Hoboken, NJ 07030-5774
201-748-6000
FAX: 201-748-6088
e-mail: info@wiley.com
www.wiley.com

Peter Booth Wiley, Chairman
Stephen M. Smith, President & CEO
John Kitzmacher, EVP, CFO
Ellis E. Cousens, Executive Vice President, COO
Contains 21 contributions compromising the work of researchers associated with the Yale Child Study Center, which has been at the forefront of research on Tourette's syndrome and associated disorders. *$85.00*
600 pages
ISBN 0-471113-75-1

8448 Treating Epilepsy Naturally: A Guide to Alternative and Adjunct Therapies
McGraw-Hill Company
P.O.Box 182605
Columbus, OH 43218
800-338-3987
FAX: 609-308-4480
e-mail: customer.service@mheducation.com
www.mcgraw-hill.com

David Levin, President and CEO
Patrick Milano, Chief Administrative Officer & CFO
Stephen Laster, Chief Digital Officer
David Stafford, SVP & General Counsel
Offers alternative treatments to replace and to complement traditional therapies and sound advice to find the right health practitioner. *$15.95*
288 pages
ISBN 0-658013-79-3

8449 Understanding Asthma
National Jewish Health
1400 Jackson Street
Denver, CO 80206
303-270-2708
877-225-5654
FAX: 303-398-1125
e-mail: allstetterw@njc.org
nationaljewish.org

Rich Schierburg, Chair
Robin Chotin, Vice Chair
Michael Salem, M.D., President and CEO
Christine Forkner, CFO and Executive Vice President
Offers a brief introduction to asthma and then goes into the physiology of asthma, the triggers of asthma, and diagnosis and monitoring of asthma.
27 pages

8450 Understanding Asthma: The Blueprint for Breathing
Allergy & Asthma Network Mothers of Asthmatics
8229 Boone Boulevard
Suite 260
Vienna, VA 22182
800-878-4403
FAX: 703-288-5271
www.aanma.org

Michael Amato, Chair
Tonya Winders, President & CEO
Brenda Silvia-Torma, Project Manager
Gary Fitzgerald, Managing Editor
A layman's guide to asthma facts based on a presentation from the first national asthma patient conference.

8451 Understanding Cystic Fibrosis
University Press of Mississippi
3825 Ridgewood Road
Jackson, MS 39211-6492
601-432-6205
800-737-7788
FAX: 601-432-6217
e-mail: press@ihl.state.ms.us
www.upress.state.ms.us

Leila W. Salisbury, Director
Craig Gill, Assistant Director/Editor-in-Chief
Anne Stascavage, Managing Editor
Vijay Shah, Acquiring Editor
A reference for CF patients and their families. *$14.00*
128 pages
ISBN 0-878059-67-9

8452 Understanding Multiple Sclerosis
University Press of Mississippi
3825 Ridgewood Road
Jackson, MS 39211-6492
601-432-6205
800-737-7788
FAX: 601-432-6217
e-mail: press@ihl.state.ms.us
www.upress.state.ms.us

Melissa Stauffer, Author
Craig Gill, Assistant Director/Editor-in-Chief
Anne Stascavage, Managing Editor
Vijay Shah, Acquiring Editor
Two psychologists discuss their roles with a member who has multiple sclerosis. Includes chapters on adolescents with multiple sclerosis, employment, and research. *$14.00*
136 pages
ISBN 1-578068-03-7

8453 Urologic Care of the Child with Spina Bifida
Spina Bifida Association of America
1600 Wilson Boulevard
Suite 800
Arlington, VA 22209
202-944-3285
800-621-3141
FAX: 202-944-3295
e-mail: sbaa@sbaa.org
www.sbaa.org

Ana Ximenes, Chair
Sara Struwe, President & CEO
Mark Bohay, National Web Initiatives & Development Manager
Elizabeth Merck, Development Manager
The Spina Bifida Association (SBA) serves adults and children who live with the challenges of Spina Bifida.

8454 Usher Syndrome
National Institute on Deafness & Other Communicati
31 Center Drive MSC 2320
Bethesda, MD 20892-2320
301-496-7243
800-241-1044
FAX: 301-770-8977
e-mail: nidcdinfo@nidcd.nih.gov
www.nidcd.nih.gov

James F Battey Jr MD PhD, Director
Judith A. Cooper, Deputy Director
Timothy J. Wheeles, Executive Officer
Tanya Brown, Executive Assistant

Explains what is Usher Syndrome, who is affected by Usher syndrome, what causes Usher syndrome, how is Usher syndrome treated, and what research is being conducted on Usher syndrome.

8455 What Everyone Needs to Know About Asthma
Allergy & Asthma Network Mothers of Asthmatics
8229 Boone Boulevard
Suite 260
Vienna, VA 22182
800-878-4403
FAX: 703-288-5271
www.aanma.org

Michael Amato, Chair
Tonya Winders, President & CEO
Brenda Silvia-Torma, Project Manager
Gary Fitzgerald, Managing Editor

Offers information and facts on gaining control of asthma, asthma triggers and monitoring asthma disorders.

8456 When the Road Turns: Inspirational Stories About People with MS
Health Communications
3201 SouthWest 15th Street
Deerfield Beach, FL 33442
954-360-0909
800-441-5569
FAX: 954-360-0034
www.hci-online.com

300 pages
ISBN 1-558749-07-1

8457 Young Person's Guide to Spina Bifida
Spina Bifida Association of America
1600 Wilson Boulevard
Suite 800
Arlington, VA 22209
202-944-3285
800-621-3141
FAX: 202-944-3295
e-mail: sbaa@sbaa.org
www.sbaa.org

Ana Ximenes, Chair
Sara Struwe, President & CEO
Mark Bohay, National Web Initiatives & Development Manager
Elizabeth Merck, Development Manager

Gives practical tips and suggestions for becoming independent and managing your health. *$19.00*

8458 Your Child and Asthma
National Jewish Health
1400 Jackson Street
Denver, CO 80206
303-270-2708
877-225-5654
FAX: 303-398-1125
e-mail: allstetterw@njc.org
nationaljewish.org

Rich Schierburg, Chair
Robin Chotin, Vice Chair
Michael Salem, M.D., President and CEO
Christine Forkner, CFO and Executive Vice President

A booklet offering information to parents and family about their child with asthma. Offers information on diagnosis, treatments, triggers and family concerns.

8459 Your Cleft Affected Child
Hunter House Inc. Publisher
PO Box 2914
Alameda, CA 94501-914
510-865-5282
800-266-5592
FAX: 510-865-4295
e-mail: ordering@hunterhouse.com
www.hunterhouse.com

Carrie T Gruman Trinker, Author

The book also provides in-depth information, guidance, and support on a wide variety of relevant topics, from feeding to surgery to helping a child cope until his/her cleft has been fully corrected.
$ 16.95
288 pages Paperback
ISBN 0-897931-85-4

8460 Your Guide to Bowel Cancer
Oxford University Press
2001 Evans Road
Cary, NC 27513
919-677-0977
800-445-9714
FAX: 919-677-1303
e-mail: custserv.us@oup.co
www.us.oup.com

ISBN 0-340927-46-1

Print: Journals

8461 AIDS: The Official Journal of the International AIDS Society
Lippincott Williams & Wilkins
2 Commerce Square
2001 Market St.
Philadelphia, PA 19103
215-521-8300
FAX: 215-521-8902
e-mail: customerservice@lww.com
lww.com

JA Levy, Co Editor
B. Autran, Co Editor
R. A Coutinho, Co Editor
J. P Phair, Co Editor

The latest groundbreaking research on HIV and AIDS. *$433.00*
18 per year

8462 American Journal of Orthopsychiatry
American Psychological Association
750 1st Street NorthEast
Washington, DC 20002-4242
202-336-5500
800-374-2721
FAX: 202-336-5502
TTY: 202-336-6123
www.apa.org

Nadine J. Kaslow, President
Norman B. Anderson, PhD, CEO & EVP
Bonnie Markham, Treasurer
Jennifer F. Kelly, Recording Secretary

Mental health issues from multidisciplinary and interprofessionals perspectives: clinical, research and expository approaches. *$45.00*
160 pages Quarterly

8463 Annals of Otology, Rhinology and Laryngology
Annals Publishing Company
4507 Laclede Ave
Saint Louis, MO 63108-2103
314-367-4987
FAX: 314-367-4988
e-mail: manager@annals.com
www.annals.com

Ken Cooper, President
Richard J. Smith, Editor
Monica L. Bergers, Editor's Assistant
Jim Cunningham, Advertising Representative

Original, peer-reviewed articles in the fields of otolaryngology - head and neck medicine and surgery, broncho-esophagology, audiology, speech, pathology, allery, and maxillofacial surgery. Official journal of the American Laryngological

Association/American Broncho-Esophagological Association. *$170.00*
112 pages Monthly

8464 Archives of Neurology
American Medical Association
P.O.Box 10946
Chicago, IL 60654 312-670-7827
800-262-2350
FAX: 312-464-4184
e-mail: subscriptions@jamanetwork.com
archpsyc.jamanetwork.com/public/contact.as px
Margaret Vanner, Manager
Mission is to publish scientific information primarily important to those physicians caring for people with neurologic disorders, but also for those interested in the structure and function of the normal and diseased nervous system. *$235.00*
198 pages Monthly

8465 Cleft Palate-Craniofacial Journal
Cleft Palate Foundation
810 E. 10th Street
Ste 102
Lawrence, NC 27514-2820 785-843-1234
800-242-5338
FAX: 785-843-1274
e-mail: membership@acpa-cpf.org
www.cpcjournal.org
Howard M. Saal, MD, President
Mark P. Mooney, PhD, President-Elect
Helen M. Sharp, PhD, CCC-SLP, Vice President
Ronal Reed Hathaway, DDS, MS, Vice President-Elect
A peer revived international multidisciplinary journal dedicated to current research on the care and treatment of children born with cleft lip and palate and other craniofacial anomalies. 6 issues/year

8466 Journal of Head Trauma Rehabilitation
Lippincott, Williams & Wilkins
P.O.Box 1620
Hagerstown, MD 21740 301-223-2300
800-638-3030
FAX: 301-223-2400
e-mail: orders@lww.com
www.lww.com
John D Corrigan PhD, ABPP, Editor
Scholarly journal designed to provide information on clinical management and rehabilitation of the head-injured for the practicing professional. Published bimonthly. *$113.96*

Print: Magazines

8467 Coping with Cancer Magazine
Media America
P.O.Box 682268
Franklin, TN 37068-2268 615-790-2400
FAX: 615-794-0179
copingmag.com
53 pages 6 x year

8468 CurePSP Magazine
Society for Progressive Supranuclear Palsy
Suite 201
30 E. Padonia Road
Timonium, MD 21093 410-785-7004
800-457-4777
FAX: 410-785-7009
e-mail: info@curepsp.org
www.psp.org
John T. Burhoe, Chair
Everett R. Cook, Vice Chair
Richard Gordon Zyne, President-CEO
Kathleen Matarazzo Speca, VP,Development & Donor Relations
Quarterly newsletter. The society's mission is to promote and fund research into finding the cause and cure for progressive supranuclear palsy (PSP). Provides information, support and advocacy to persons diagnosed with PSP, their families and caregivers. Educates physicians and allied health professionals on PSP and how to improve patient care.

8469 EpilepsyUSA
Epilepsy Foundation
8301 Professional Place
Landover, MD 20785-2353 301-459-3700
800-332-1000
FAX: 301-459-1569
e-mail: ContactUs@efa.org
epilepsyfoundation.org
Warren Lammert, Chair
Phil Gattone, President and CEO
May J. Liang, Secretary
Roger Heldman, Treasurer
Magazine reporting on issues of interest to people with epilepsy and their families. *$15.00*
22 pages Bi-Monthly

8470 MSFOCUS Magazine
Multiple Sclerosis Foundation
6520 North Andrews Avenue
Fort Lauderdale, FL 33309-2130 954-776-6805
888-MSF-CUS
888-225-6495
FAX: 954-938-8708
e-mail: support@msfocus.org, admin@msfocus.org
www.msfocus.org
Eric Schenck, President, Director
Charles Eader, Vice President, Treasurer
Jules Kuperberg, Executive Director
Alan Segaloff, Co- Executive Director
Contemporary national, nonprofit organization that provides free support services and public education for persons with Multiple Sclerosis, newsletters, toll-free phone support, information, referrals, home care, assitive technology and support groups.
48 pages Quarterly

8471 Orthotics and Prosthetics Almanac
American Orthotic & Prosthetics Association
330 John Carlyle Street
Suite 200
Alexandria, VA 22314 571-431-0876
FAX: 571-431-0899
e-mail: info@aopanet.org
www.aopanet.org
Anita L. Lampear, President
Charles H. Dankmeyer, Vice President
Thomas F. Fise, JD, Executive Director
Don DeBolt, Chief Operating Officer
Features articles covering current professional, patient care, government, business and National Office activities affecting the orthotics and prosthetics profession and industry. *$40.00*
80 pages Monthly
ISSN 1061-46 1

8472 PDF News
Parkinson's Disease Foundation
1359 Broadway
Suite 1509
New York, NY 10018 212-923-4700
800-457-6676
FAX: 212-923-4778
e-mail: info@pdf.org
www.pdf.org
Howard D. Morgan, Chair
Woodruff Atwell, Ph.D., Vice Chair
Stephen Ackerman, Treasurer
Isobel Robins Konecky, Secretary
8-12 pages Quarterly

8473 **POZ Magazine**
Smart + Strong
462 Seventh Ave
19th Floor
New York, NY 10018-7424
212-242-2163
800-973-2376
FAX: 212-675-8505
e-mail: webmaster@poz.com
www.poz.com

Megan Strub, Publisher
Oriol Gutierrez, Editor In-Chief
Jennifer Morton, Managing Editor
Kate Ferguson, Senior Editor
A health title written for individuals who are HIV+, their friends and families. POZ provides the latest treatment information, investigative journalism and survivor profiles.

8474 **SCI Life**
National Spinal Cord Injury Association
11300 Rockville Pike
Suite 803
Rockville, MD 20852
301-468-3902
FAX: 301-468-3904
e-mail: info@ilcreations.com
ilcreations.com

Quarterly/Free

8475 **Spine**
Lippincott, Williams & Wilkins
530 Walnut St
Philadelphia, PA 19106-3603
215-521-8300
FAX: 215-521-8411
e-mail: customerservice@lww.com
lww.com

James N Weinstein DO MSc, Editor
Publishes original papers on theoretical issues and research concerning the spine and spinal cord injuries. *$9.00*
26 Issues Year

8476 **Ventilator-Assisted Living**
International Ventilator Users Network
4207 Lindell Blvd
Suite 110
Saint Louis, MO 63108-2930
314-534-0475
FAX: 314-534-5070
e-mail: info@ventusers.org
www.ventusers.org

William G. Stothers, President/Chairperson
Saul J. Morse, Vice President
Joan L. Headley,MS, Editor
Marny E. Eulberg, Secretary
To enhance the lives and independence of ventilator-assisted living by promoting education, networking, and advocacy among these individuals and healthcare providers. Ventilator-Assisted Living supports Post-Polio Health International's educational, research, and advocacy efforts. Offers information about relevant events.
Quarterly

Print: Newsletters

8477 **ACPOC News**
Assoc of Children's Prosthetic-Orthotic Clinics
6300 N River Rd
Suite 727
Rosemont, IL 60018-4226
847-698-1637
FAX: 847-823-0536
e-mail: acpoc@aaos.org
www.acpoc.org

David B. Rotter,CPO, President
Jorge A. Fabregas, Vice President
Hank White,PT,PhD, Secretary-Treasurer
Anna Cuomo, Director
Quarterly publication from the Association of Children's Prosthetic/Orthotic Clinics. Included with membership.
40 pages Quarterly

8478 **AID Bulletin**
Project AID Resource Center
P.O. Box 5190
Kent, OH 44242-0001
330-672-3000
FAX: 330-672-4724
e-mail: info@kent.edu
www.kent.edu/

Beverly Warren, President
Todd A. Diacon, Provost & SVP
Gregg S. Floyd, Sr. Vice President
Greg Jarvie, Vice President
Has the latest news on upcoming conferences, literature, developments in programs and/or services for disabled persons who are substance abusers. Offers articles on their experiences, ideas and questions of others in this field which includes providers and consumers. *$7.50*

8479 **AIDS Alert**
AHC Media LLC
PO Box 550669
Atlanta, GA 30355
404-262-5436
800-688-2421
FAX: 404-262-5560
www.ahcpub.com/

Joy Daughtery Dickinson, Senior Managing Editor
Source of AIDS news and advice for health care professionals. Covers up-to-the-minute developments and guidance on the entire spectrum of AIDS challenges, including treatment, education, precautions, screening, diagnosis and policy. *$499.00*
Monthly

8480 **Adaptive Tracks**
Adaptive Sports Center
P.O.Box 1639
Crested Butte, CO 81224
970-349-2296
866-349-2296
FAX: 970-349-2077
e-mail: info@adaptivesports.org
www.adaptivesports.org

Christopher Hensley, Executive Director
Chris Read, CTRS, Program Director
Ella Fahrlander, Development Director
Mike Neustedter, Marketing Director
The Adaptive Sports Center (ASC) of Crested Butte, Colorado is a non-profit organization that provides year-round recreation activities for people with disabilities and their families. The ASC provides adaptive snowboarding downhill skiing, cross country skiing as well as backcountry trips. Summer activities include a variety of wilderness-based programs, multi-day trips into the back country, extensive cycling programs, canoeing, and white water rafting.
6 pages Quarterly

8481 **Arthritis Self-Management**
Rapaport Publishing, Inc.
150 W 22nd St
Ste 800
New York, NY 10011-2421
212-989-0200
FAX: 212-989-4786
e-mail: ASMcustserv@cdsfulfillment.com
www.arthritisselfmanagement.com

Richard A Rapaport, President
Maryanne Schott Turner, Director of Manufacturing
Richard Boland, Art Director
James Moorehead, Circulation Director
Arthritis Self-Management publishes practical 'how-to' information for the growing number of people with arthritis who want to know more about managing their condition. We focus on the day-to-day and long-term aspects of arthritis in a positive and upbeat style, giving our subscribers up-to-date news, facts, and advice to help them make informed decisions about their health. *$9.97*
BiMonthly

8482 Breaking Ground
Tennessee Council on Developmental Disabilities
404 James Robertson Pkwy
Suite 130
Nashville, TN 37243- 0228 615-532-6615
FAX: 615-532-6964
TTY:615-741-4562
e-mail: tnddc@tn.gov
www.tn.gov/cdd

Stephanie Brewer cook, Chair
Roger D. Gibbens,, Vice Chair
Wanda Willis, Executive Director
Errol Elshtain, Director of Development
Newsletter
20 pages 6 x Year

8483 Breaking New Ground News Note
Purdue University
225 West University Street
West Lafayette, IN 47907 765-494-4600
800-825-4264
FAX: 765-496-1356
engineering.purdue.edu/

Paul Jones, Project Manager
Bill Field, Project Director
Denise Heath, Project Asst.
Robert Stuthridge, Project Ergonomist
News, practical ideas and success stories of and for farmers and other agricultural workers with physical disabilities.
2 pages Quarterly

8484 Diabetes Self-Management
Rapaport Publishing, Inc.
150 W 22nd St
Ste 800
New York, NY 10011-2421 212-989-0200
FAX: 212-989-4786
e-mail: webeditor@diabetes-self-mgmt.com
www.diabetesselfmanagement.com
Richard A Rapaport, President
Maryanne Schott Turner, Director of Manufacturing
Richard Boland, Art Director
James Moorehead, Circulation Director
Publishes practical how-to information, focusing on the day-to-day and long-term aspects of diabetes in a positive and upbeat style. Gives subscribers up-to-date news, facts and advice to help them maintain their wellness and make informed decisions regarding their health. *$9.97*
BiMonthly

8485 Directions
Families of Spinal Muscular Dystrophy
925 Busse Road
Elk Grove Village, IL 60007 847-367-7620
800-886-1762
FAX: 847-367-7623
e-mail: info@fsma.org
www.fsma.org

Richard Rubenstein, Chair
Kenneth Hobby, President
Sue Kovach, Director of Finance
Megan Lenz, Communications Manager
$35.00
60-70 pages Quarterly

8486 IAL News
International Association of Laryngectomees
925B Peachtree Street NE
Suite 316
Atlanta, GA 30309 866-425-3678
www.larynxlink.com

Wade Hampton, President
Susan Reeves, Administrative Manager
Jodi Knott, Director, Voice Institute
Charles Rusky, Treasurer
Focuses on rehabilitation and well-being of persons who have had laryngectomy surgery.

8487 Informer
Simon Foundation
P.O.Box 815
Wilmette, IL 60091 847-864-3913
800-237-4666
FAX: 847-864-9758
e-mail: info@simonfoundation.org
simonfoundation.org
Cheryle Gartley, President and Founder
Elizabeth T. LaGro, VP, Communications & Education
Twila Yednock, Director of Special Events
Monica Liebert, Scientific Liason
Publishes items of interest to people with bladder or bowel incontinence, including medical articles, helpful devices, publications and a pen pal list. Quarterly newsletter.
Quarterly

8488 Moisture Seekers
Sjogren's Syndrome Foundation
6707 Democracy Boulevard
Suite 325
Bethesda, MD 20817 301-530-4420
800-475-6473
FAX: 301-530-4415
e-mail: tms@sjogrens.org
www.sjogrens.org

Kenneth Economou, Chair
Steven Taylor, CEO
Sheriese DeFruscio, VP of Development
Elizabeth Trocchio, Director of Marketing
Newsletter of the organization for lay people and professionals interested in Sjogren's Syndrome. Contains medical news, current research, and essential tips for daily living. *$25.00*
15-16 pages Monthly

8489 Momentum
National Multiple Sclerosis Society
Ste 6
421 New Karner Rd
Albany, NY 12205-3838 518-464-0850
800-344-4867
FAX: 518-464-1232
e-mail: nyr@nmss.org
www.nationalmssociety.org

Eli Rubenstein, Chair
Cynthia Zagieboylo, President & CEO
Sherri Giger, EVP, Marketing
Jennifer Douglas, EVP,Technology
News and information on research progress, medical treatments, patient services, therapeutic claims and activities.

8490 Options
People Against Cancer
P.O.Box 10
604 East Street
Otho, IA 50569 515-972-4444
800-662-2623
FAX: 515-972-4415
e-mail: info@PeopleAgainstCancer.org
www.peopleagainstcancer.com
Frank D. Wiewel, Executive Director/Founder
Publication of People Against Cancer, a nonprofit, grassroots public benefit organization dedicated to 'New Directions in the War on Cancer.' We help people to find the best cancer treatment. We are a democratic organization of people with cancer, their loved ones and citizens working together to protect and enhance medical freedom of choice.
8 pages Quarterly

8491 **PDF Newsletter**
Parkinson's Disease Foundation
1359 Broadway
Suite 1509
New York, NY 10018
212-923-4700
800-457-6676
FAX: 212-923-4778
e-mail: info@pdf.org
www.pdf.org

Howard D. Morgan, Chair
Woodruff Atwell, Ph.D., Vice Chair
Stephen Ackerman, Treasurer
Isobel Robins Konecky, Secretary

The Parkinson's Disease Foundation (PDF) is a leading national presence in Parkinson's disease research, education and public advocacy.
12-16 pages Quarterly

8492 **Parkinsons Report**
National Parkinson Foundation
200 SE 1st Street
Suite 800
Miami, FL 33131
305-243-6666
800-473-4636
800-4PD-INFO
FAX: 305-537-9901
e-mail: contact@parkinson.org
www.parkinson.org

John W. Kozyak, Chairman
Andrew B. Albert, Vice Chairman
Joyce Oberdorf, President and CEO
Leilani Pearl, VP,Marketing & Communications

Articles, reports and news on Parkinson's disease and the activities of the National Parkinson Foundation.
32 pages Qarterly

8493 **Post-Polio Health**
Post-Polio Health International
Ste 110
4207 Lindell Blvd
Saint Louis, MO 63108-2930
314-534-0475
FAX: 314-534-5070
e-mail: info@post-polio.org
www.post-polio.org

William G. Stothers, President
Saul J. Morse, Vice President
Joan L. Headley,MS, Executive Director
Marny E. Eulberg, Secretary

To enhance the lives and independence of polio survivors by promoting education, networking, and advocacy among these individuals and healthcare providers. Post-Polio Health supports Post-Polio Health International's educational, research, and advocacy efforts. Offers information about relevant events. *$30.00*
12 pages quarterly

8494 **Prader-Willi Alliance of New York Newsletter**
244 5th Avenue
Suite D-110
New York, NY 10001
716-276-2211
800-442-1655
FAX: 585-271-2782
e-mail: alliance@prader-willi.org
www.prader-willi.org

Amy McDougall, President
Rachel Johnson, Vice President
Nancy Finegold, Vice President
Nina Roberto, Executive Director

The Prader-Willi Foundation is a national, nonprofit public charity that works for the benefit of individuals with Prader-Willi syndrome and their families. *$20.00*
Quarterly

8495 **Quality Care Newsletter**
National Association for Continence
P.O.Box 1019
Charleston, SC 29402-1019
843-352-2559
800-BLA-DER
FAX: 843-352-2563
e-mail: memberservices@nafc.org
www.nafc.org

Donna Deng, Chairman
Nancy Hicks, Vice Chaiperson
Steven Gregg, Executive Director
Wendy Pokoski, Financial Administrator

Newsletter from NAFC. By donating $25 and becomming a Quality Care donor, you may receive our quarterly newsletter. *$25.00*
14-16 pages Quarterly

8496 **Rasmussen's Syndrome and Hemispherectomy Support Network Newsletter**
55 Kenosia Avenue
Danbury, CT 06810
203-744-0100
FAX: 203-798-2291
e-mail: rssnlynn@aol.com
http://www.rarediseases.org/rare-disease-info

Ronald J. Bartek, Chair
Sheldon M. Schuster, Vice Chair
Peter L. Saltonstall, President & CEO
Pamela Gavin, COO

National, not-for-profit organization dedicated to providing information and support to individuals affected by Rasmussen's Syndrome and hemispherectomy. Publishes a periodic newsletter and disseminates reprints of medical journal articles concerning Rasmussen's Syndrome and its treatments. Maintains a support network that provides encouragement and information to individuals affected by Rasmussen's Syndrome and their families.

8497 **SCI Psychosocial Process**
Amer Assn of Spinal Cord Injury Psych & Soc Wks
75-20 Astoria Blvd
East Elmhurst, NY 11370
718-803-3782
800-404-2898
FAX: 718-803-0414
e-mail: info@unitedspinal.org
http://www.unitedspinal.org/

David C. Cooper, Chairman
Patrick W. Maher, Vice Chairman
Joseph Gaskins, President and CEO
Denise A. McQuade, Secretary

Quarterly newsletter.

8498 **Special Care in Dentistry**
Blackwell Publishing
350 Main St
Malden, MA 02148
781-388-0200
FAX: 781-388-8210
www.blackwellpublishing.com

Peter Booth Wiley, Chairman
Stephen M. Smith, President & CEO
John Kitzmacher, EVP, CFO
Ellis E. Cousens, Executive Vice President, COO
$125.00
48 pages BiMonthly

8499 **TSA Newsletter**
Tourette Syndrome Association
42-40 Bell Boulevard
Bayside, NY 11361
718-224-2999
800-237-0717
FAX: 718-279-9596
e-mail: ts@tsa-usa.org
www.tsa-usa.org

Stephen M. McCall, President

National non-profit membership organization whose mission is to identify the cause of, find the cure for, and control the effects of this disorder. A growing number of local chapters nationwide provide educational materials, seminars, conferences and support groups for over 35,000 members.
Quarterly

8500 **Tethering Cord**
Spina Bifida Association of America
PO Box 5801
Bethesda, MD 20284
301-496-5751
800-352-9424
FAX: 202-944-3295
e-mail: sbaa@sbaa.org
www.ninds.nih.gov/

Caroline Lewis, Executive Officer
Story C. Landis, Director
Denise Dorsey, Chief Administrative Officer
Maryann Sofranko, Deputy Executive Officer

Tethered spinal cord syndrome is a neurological disorder caused by tissue attachments that limit the movement of the spinal cord within the spinal column. Attachments may occur congenitally at the base of the spinal cord (conus medullaris) or they may develop near the site of an injury to the spinal cord.

8501 **Tourette Syndrome Association Children's Newsletter**
42-40 Bell Boulevard
Bayside, NY 11361
718-224-2999
800-237-0717
FAX: 718-279-9596
e-mail: ts@tsa-usa.org
tsa-usa.org

Stephen M. McCall, President

National, nonprofit membership organization. Mission is to identify the cause of, find the cure for, and control the effects of this disorder. A growing number of local chapters nationwide provide educational materials, seminars, conferences and support groups for over 35,000 members.

8502 **Voice of the Diabetic**
NFB Diabetes Action Network
200 East Wells Street
Baltimore, MD 21230-4914
410-659-9314
888-581-4741
FAX: 410-685-5653
e-mail: editor@diabetes.nfb.org
www.nfb.org

Elizabeth Lunt, Editor
Marc Maurer, President
Fredric Schroeder, First Vice President
Ron Brown, Second Vice President

Newsletter containing personal stories and practical guidelines by blind diabetics and medical professionals, medical news, resource column and a recipe corner. We are a support and information network for all diabetics.
28 pages Quarterly

Non Print: Newsletters

8503 **Teens & Asthma**
American Lung Association
530 7th St SE
Washington, DC 20003
202-546-5864
FAX: 202-546-5607
e-mail: randrewn@aladc.org
www.epa.gov/

Rolando E Bates Jr, CEO

Tips from other teens with asthma to help those having it get on with the serious business of having fun with the rest of their lives.
Online/Free

Non Print: Video

8504 **Fragile X Family**
Fanlight Productions
c/o Icarus Films
32 Court Street, 21st Floor
Brooklyn, NY 11201
718-488-8900
800-876-1710
FAX: 718-488-8642
e-mail: info@fanlight.com, sales@icarusfilms.com
www.fanlight.com

Ben Achtenberg, Founder, Owner
Eric Kutner, Producer

Fragile X Family takes viewers inside the lives of a developmentally disabled family who are affected by Fragile X Syndrome, an inherited chromosomal disorder which is the second most common cause of mental retardation. *$149.00*
VHS/VIDEO
ISBN 1-572954-14-0

8505 **In the Middle**
Fanlight Productions
c/o Icarus Films
32 Court Street, 21st Floor
Brooklyn, NY 11201
718-488-8900
800-876-1710
FAX: 718-488-8642
e-mail: info@fanlight.com, sales@icarusfilms.com
www.fanlight.com

Ben Achtenberg, Founder, Owner

Documents the problems and joys shared by Ryanna, who has Spina Bifida, and her parents, teachers and classmates during her first year of being mainstreamed in a Head Start Program. *$99.00*

8506 **Narcolepsy**
Fanlight Productions
c/o Icarus Films
32 Court Street, 21st Floor
Brooklyn, NY 11201
718-488-8900
800-876-1710
FAX: 718-488-8642
e-mail: info@fanlight.com, sales@icarusfilms.com
www.fanlight.com

Ben Achtenberg, Founder, Owner
Jason Margolis, Producer

Presents the experiences of three individuals who lives and relationships have been disrupted by narcolepsy. Rental $50/day. *$199.00*
VHS/25 Minutes

8507 **Twitch and Shout**
Fanlight Productions
c/o Icarus Films
32 Court Street, 21st Floor
Brooklyn, NY 11201
718-488-8900
800-876-1710
FAX: 718-488-8642
e-mail: info@fanlight.com, sales@icarusfilms.com
www.fanlight.com

Ben Achtenberg, Founder, Owner
Laurel Chitden, Producer

This documentary provides an intimate journey into the startling world of Tourette Syndrome (TS), a genetic disorder that can cause a bizarre range of involuntary movements, vocalizations, and compulsions. Through the eyes of a photojournalist with TS, the film introduces viewers to others who have this puzzling disorder. This is an emotionally absorbing, sometimes, unsettling, and finally uplifting program about people who must contend with a society that often sees them as crazy or bad. *$225.00*

Sports

8508 National Sports Center for the Disabled
P.O.Box 1290
33 Parsenn Road
Winter Park, CO 80482
970-726-1518
FAX: 970-726-4112
e-mail: volunteer@nscd.org
www.nscd.org

Becky Zimmermann, President/CEO
Greg Voss, CFO
Diane Eustace, Marketing Director
Beth Fox, Operations Director

Innovative non-profit organization that provides year-round recreation for children and adults with disabilities. The world's largest adaptive ski program, teaching 25,000 lessons per winter at Winter Park Resort, Colorado. Also snowboarding, ski racing, showshoeing, cross-country skiing. Summer sports: rafting, sailing, camping, hiking, hand cycling, mountain biking, tandem biking, in-line skating, horseback riding, fishing, rock climbing. Sports symposium and clinics.

8509 Rehabilitation Institute of Chicago's Virginia Wadsworth Sports Program
345 East Suuperior St.
Chicago, IL 60611
312-238-1000
800-354-7342
800-354-REHA
FAX: 312-238-5017
e-mail: sports@ric.org
www.ric.org

Jude Reyes, Chair
mike P. Kransy, Vice Chair
Thomas Reynolds III, Vice Chair
Joanne C. Smith, President & CEO

RIC's Center for Health and Fitness is a full service fitness center for individuals with disablilties and the administrative offices for RIC's Wirtz Sports Program. Eighteen different sport and recreation programs are offered free of charge. The facility is adjacent to RIC's main building and also is the location of a branch of The National Center for Physical Activity and Disability (NCPAD), a joint project operated by the University of Illinois-Chigcago.

8510 US Paralympics
1 Olympic Plaza
Colorado Springs, CO 80901
719-866-2030
888-222-2313
FAX: 719-866-2029
e-mail: customerservice@donorsupportusoc.org
www.usparalympics.org

Jessica Galli, Track & Field
Derek Arneaud, Soccer
Willie Steward, Nordic Skiing
Muffy Davis, Alpine Skiing

A division of the US Olympic Committee focused on enhancing programs, funding and opportunities for persons with physical disabilities to participate in Paralymic sports.

Support Groups

8511 AAN's Toll-Free Hotline
Allergy and Asthma Network Mothers of Asthmatics
8229 Boone Boulevard
Suite 260
Vienna, VA 22182
800-878-4403
FAX: 703-288-5271
www.aanma.org

Michael Amato, Chair
Tonya Winders, President & CEO
Brenda Silvia-Torma, Project Manager
Gary Fitzgerald, Managing Editor

Offers answers to questions regarding allergies and asthma, provides referrals and support to assist the patient and his or her family.

8512 Breaking New Ground Resource Center
Purdue University
225 S University St
West Lafayette, IN 47907
765-494-5088
800-825-4264
FAX: 765-496-1356
e-mail: bng@ecn.purdue.edu
engineering.purdue.edu/

Bill Field, Project Director
Paul Jones, Project Manager
Steve Swain, Rural Rehab Specialist
Robert Stuthridge, Project Ergonomist

A resource center devoted to helping farmers and ranchers with physical disabilities. Resource materials and a free newsletter are available to anyone.

8513 Camp Candlelight
Epilepsy Foundation Arizona
Office Park 3
273 Azalea Rd #310
Mobile, AL 36609-1970
251-432-0970
800-626-1582
FAX: 251-432-0975
e-mail: tom.walsh002@chw.edu
http://www.epilepsyfoundationalabama.org

Jeff Matherne, President
Brian Finnigan, Vice President
Caroline Foster, Executive Director
David Toenes, Director,Client & Employment Services

Camp Candlelight provides children ages 8 to 15 a unique camp experience that mixes traditional summer camp with special sessions that teach campers about their seizures and gives them resources to manage the challenges that the seizures represent. Staff includes a neurologist, several nurses and a school psychologist, in addition to traditional camp staff who are given specialized training in responding appropriately to the needs of kids with epilepsy.

8514 Cancer Information Service
National Cancer Institute
BG 9609 MSC 9760
9609 Medical Center Drive
Bethesda, MD 20892-9760
301-496-8531
800-422-6237
800-4 C-NCER
FAX: 304-402-0181
e-mail: cancergovstaff@mail.nih.gov
www.cancer.gov

Barbara K. Rimer, Chairperson
Harold Varmus,MD, Director
Abby Sandler, Executive Secretary
Bruce A. Chabner, Chair

A nationwide network of 19 regional field offices supported by the National Cancer Institute which provides accurate, up-to-date information on cancer to patients and their families, health professionals and the general public. The CIS can provide specific information in understandable language about particular types of cancer, as well as information on second opinions and the availability of clinical trials.

8515 Clearinghouse on Disability Information: Office Special Education & Rehabilitative Service
U S Department of Education
400 Maryland Ave SW
Washington, DC 20202-1
202-245-7549
800-872-5327
FAX: 202-245-7614
www.ed.gov

Arne Duncan, Secretary Of Education
Tony Miller, Deputy Secretary
Martha Kanter, Under Secretary
Jo Anderson, Senior Advisor

Provides information to people with disabilities or anyone requesting information, by doing research and providing documents in response to inquiries. The information provided includes areas of federal funding for disability-related programs. Information provided may be useful to disabled individuals and their families, schools and universities, teacher's and/or school administrators, and organizations who have persons with disabilities as clients.

8516 Cornerstone Services
777 Joyce Rd
Joliet, IL 60436
815-741-7600
FAX: 815-723-1177
e-mail: jhogan@cornerstoneservices.org
cornerstoneservices.org

John R. Rogers, Chair
Vincent A. Benigni, Vice Chairperson
Ben Stortz, President/CEO
Don Hospell, Vice President/COO

Cornerstone Services provides progressive, comprehensive services for people with disabilities, promoting choice, dignity and the opportunity to live and work in the community. Established in 1969, the agency provides developmental, vocational, residential and behavior health services.

8517 Disability Network
Ste 54
3600 S Dort Hwy
Flint, MI 48507
810-742-1800
FAX: 810-742-2400
TTY:810-742-7647
e-mail: tdn@disnetwork.org
www.disnetwork.org

Bruce Chargo, Chairman
Diane Brown, Treasurer/ Vice Chairman
Mike Zelley, President & CEO
Linda F, Director, Finance, Operations

The Disability Network's mission is to realize consumer empowerment, self determination, full inclusion and participation of all people in the communities through independent living philosophy and the unequivocal implementation of the Americans with Disabilities Act

8518 Disability and Health: National Center for Birth Defects and Developmental Disabilities
Centers for Disease Control and Prevention
1600 Clifton Road
Atlanta, GA 30333
404-498-3012
800-232-4636
800-CDC-INFO
FAX: 404-498-3060
e-mail: cdcinfo@cdc.gov
www.cdc.gov/ncbddd/dh

Dr. Tom Frieden, Director
Sherri A. Berger, COO
Carmen Villar, Chief of Staff
Ileana Arias, Principal Deputy Director

Located within the new CDC, National Center for Birth Defects and Developmental Disabilities, the Disability and Health section, operates a ralatively small program that primarily supports: data collection on the prevalence of people with disabilities & their health status and risk factors for poor health and well-being; research on measures of disability, functioning and health; health promotion intervention studies; and dissemination of health information.

8519 Easter Seals
233 South Wacker Drive
Suite 2400
Chicago, IL 60606
312-726-6200
800-221-6827
FAX: 312-726-1494
www.easterseals.com

Richard W. Davidson, Chairman
Sandra L Bouwman, 1st Vice Chairman
Joseph G. Kern, 2nd Vice Chairman
Eileen H. Boone, Secretary

Easter Seals has been helping individuals with disabilities and special needs, and their families, live better lives for over 80 years. From child development centers to physical rehabilitation and job training for people with disabilities, Easter Seals offers a variety of services to help people with disabilities address life's challenges and achieve personal goals.

8520 Epilepsy Foundation
8301 Professional Place
Landover, MD 20785-2353
301-459-3700
800-332-1000
FAX: 301-459-1569
e-mail: ContactUs@efa.org
epilepsyfoundation.org

Warren Lammert, Chair
Phil Gattone, President and CEO
May J. Liang, Secretary
Roger Heldman, Treasurer

Offers information and referrals, support groups for dually diagnosed persons.

8521 Family Support Project for the Developmentally Disabled
3424 Kossuth Ave
Bronx, NY 10467-2410
718-519-5000
FAX: 718-519-4902
www.nyc.gov/html/hhc/ncbh/home.html

William Walsh, Vice President
Sheldon McLeod, COO

8522 Head Injury Hotline
Brain Injury Resource Center
P.O.Box 84151
Seattle, WA 98124-5451
206-621-8558
FAX: 206-329-0912
e-mail: brain@headinjury.com
www.headinjury.com

Hugh R. MacMahon, Neurology
Constance Miller, Founder
Paul M. Kuroiwa, Performance management consultant
B. Parker Lindner, Communications specialist

Disseminates head injury information and provides referrals to facilitate adjustment to life following head injury. Organizes seminars for professionals, head injury survivors, and their families.

8523 International Braille and Technology Center for the Blind
National Federation of the Blind
200 East Wells Street
Baltimore, MD 21230-4914
410-659-9314
FAX: 410-685-5653
e-mail: access@nfb.org
www.nfb.org

Marc Maurer, President
Fredric Schroeder, First Vice President
Ron Brown, Second Vice President
Marc Maurer, CEO

World's largest and most complete evaluation and demonstration center of all assistive technology used by the blind from around the world. Includes all braille, synthetic speech, print-to-speech scanning, internet and portable devices and programs. Available for tours by appointment to blind persons, employers, technology manufacturers, teachers, parents and those working in the assistive technology field.

8524 Lung Line Information Service
National Jewish Health
1400 Jackson Street
Denver, CO 80206
877-225-5654
877-225-5654
FAX: 303-398-1125
e-mail: allstetterw@njc.org
nationaljewish.org

Rich Schierburg, Chair
Robin Chotin, Vice Chair
Michael Salem, M.D., President & CEO
Christine Forkner, CFO and Executive Vice President

A free information service answering questions, sending literature and giving advice to patients with immunologic or respiratory illnesses. The Line is an educational service and not a substitute for medical care. Diagnosis or suggested treatment will not be provided for a caller's specific condition.

8525 National AIDS Hotline
Centers for Disease Control and Prevention
1600 Clifton Road
Atlanta, GA 30333
404-639-3311
800-232-4636
800-CDC-INFO
FAX: 404-498-3060
e-mail: cdcinfo@cdc.gov
www.cdc.gov

Dr. Tom Frieden, Director
Sherri A. Berger, COO
Carmen Villar, Chief of Staff
Ileana Arias, Principal Deputy Director

Offers free confidential information and publications on HIV infection and AIDS.

8526 PALS Support Groups
Parent Professional Advocacy League
10th Fl
45 Bromfield St
Boston, MA 02108
866-815-8122
FAX: 617-542-7832
e-mail: info@ppal.net
ppal.net

Earl N. Stuck, Chair
Lisa Lambert, Executive Director
Deborah A Fauntleroy, Associate Director
Meri Viano, Senior Regional Manager

Offers emotional support to parents and families of disabled children.

8527 PXE International
Ste 404
4301 Connecticut Ave NW
Washington, DC 20008- 2369
202-362-9599
FAX: 202-966-8553
e-mail: info@pxe.org
www.pxe.org

Patrick F. Terry, President
Sharon Terry, CEO
Terry M. Dermaid, Executive Director
Ian Terry, Webmaster

Provides support for individuals and families affected by psukdoxanthoma elasticum (PXE), and resources for healthcare professionals. PXE causes select elastic tissue to mineralize, and effects the skin, eyes, cardiovascular, and GI systems.

8528 Parent Assistance Network
Good Samaritan Hospital
10 E. 31st Street
Kearney, NE 68847
308-865-7100
800-235-9905
FAX: 308-865-2924
e-mail: sheilameyer@catholichealth.net
www.gshs.org

Randy DeFreece, President
Kent Barney, Chairman
Mary Henning, Vice Chairman
Julie Speirs, Secretary

Provides information and emotional support to all parents and especially to parents of children with disabilities in the central Nebraska area. Ongoing activities include parent support group meetings, parent-to-parent networking and referrals and Respite Care provider trainings.

8529 Post-Polio Support Group
Adventist Hinsdale Hospital
120 N Oak St
Hinsdale, IL 60521-3829
630-856-9000
FAX: 630-856-6000
www.keepingyouwell.com

David Crane, President

Information and support for polio patients and their families; meets the fourth Wednesday of each month.

8530 Prevent Child Abuse America
288 South Wabash Avenue
10th floor
Chicago, IL 60604
312-663-3520
800-244-5373
800-CHI-DREN
FAX: 312-939-8962
e-mail: mailbox@preventchildabuse.org
preventchildabuse.org

Fred M. Riley, Chair
David Rudd, Vice Chair
James Hmurovich, President & CEO
Robert Allen, Sr. Director, Administration

Through public education, community partnerships and support services, PCAMW helps everyone play a role in prevention. We share information on prevention stategies and effective parenting at community forums and events and advocate for polices and services that keep children safe. We operate PhoneFriend, a telephone support line for children at home without adult supervision and conduct personal safety workshops in schools, camps and libraries.

8531 Son-Rise Program
Option Institute
2080 South Undermountain Road
Sheffield, MA 01257
413-229-2100
877-766-7473
e-mail: happiness@option.org
www.autismtreatmentcenter.org

Samahria Lyt Kaufman, Co-Founder and Co-Director
Dane Griffith, Director of Administrative Services
Bears Kaufman, Co-Founder and Co-Director
Raun Kaufman, Director of Global Education

Internationally renowned and highly effective method for working with children challenged by autism, autism spectrum disorders, PDD and all other developmental difficulties. The program teaches parents, relatives, volunteers and professionals how to design and implement a child-centered, home-based educational program. Modality comprises an innovative and comprehensive system for learning and growth with specific impact in areas including eye contact, speech and communication and more.

8532 Special Children
1306 Wabash Ave
Belleville, IL 62220-3370
618-234-6876
FAX: 618-234-6150
e-mail: kathleencullan@sbcglobal.net
specialchildren.net

Kathleen Cullen, Administrator

A nonprofit agency serving children with developmental disabilities ages birth to 6 years

8533 Support Works
1607 Dilworth Rd W
Charlotte, NC 28203-5213
704-331-9500
e-mail: feedback@supportworks.org
www.supportworks.org

Joel Fisher, Manager

SupportWorks helps people find and form support groups. An 8 page publication Power Tools, clearly walks new group leaders through steps of putting together a healthy self-help group. SupportWorks also has a telephone conference program which allows people with similar diseases or other nonprofit issues to meet by phone conference for free or at very low cost.

8534 The Compassionate Friends
P.O.Box 3696
Oak Brook, IL 60522
630-990-0010
877-969-0010
FAX: 630-990-0246
e-mail: nationaloffice@compassionatefriends.org
compassionatefriends.org

Patrick O'Donnell, President
Georgia Cockerham, Vice President
Lisa Corrao, COO
Alan Pedersen, Executive Director

Peer support for bereaved parents, grandparents and siblings, offering over 600 chapters in the United States. The organization also offers a quarterly magazine, We Need Not Walk Alone, and TCF resources of brochures, DVDs, and memorial wristbands for the bereaved parent, grandparent and sibling.

8535 Toll-Free Information Line

Asthma and Allergy Foundation of America
8201 Corporate Drive
Suite 1000
Landover, MD 20785
202-466-7643
800-727-8462
800-7 A-THMA
FAX: 202-466-8940
e-mail: info@aafa.org
aafa.org

Lynn Hanessian, Chair
Yolanda Miller, SVP & COO
Lynda Mitchell, VP, Food Allergies
Nancy Kercher, Secretary

The Asthma and Allergy Foundation of America (AAFA) provides practical information, community based services and support through a national network of chapters and support groups. AAFA develops health education, organizes state and national advocacy efforts and funds research to find better treatments and cures.

8536 Visiting Nurse Association of America

2121 Crystal Drive
Suite 750
Arlington, VA 22202
571-527-1520
888-866-8773
FAX: 571-527-1527
e-mail: webadmin@vnaa.org
vnaa.org

Mary B. DeVeau, Chair
Linnea Windel, Vice Chair
Tracey Moorhead, President & CEO
Magaret Terry, VP of Quality & Innovation

The VNAA is the official national association for not-for-profit, community based home health organizations known as the Visiting Nurse Associations (VNA's). They created the profession of home health care more then 100 years ag. They have a united mission to bring compassionate, high-quality and cost-effective home care to individuals in their communities.

Speech & Language

Associations

8537 **American Speech-Language-Hearing Association**
2200 Research Blvd
Rockville, MD 20850-3289
301-296-5700
800-638-8255
FAX: 301-296-8580
TTY: 301-296-5650
e-mail: actioncenter@asha.org
www.asha.org

Patricia A. Prelock, PhD, CCC-SLP, President
Elizabeth S. McCrea, PhD, CCC-SLP, President-Elect
Donna Fisher Smiley, PhD, CC, Vice President for Audiology Practice
Howard Goldstein, PhD, CCC-SL, Vice President for Science and Research

The American Speech-Language Association is the professional, scientific, and credentialing association for 135,000 members and affiliates who are speech-language pathologists, audiologists, and speech, language, and hearing scientists in the United States and internationally. ASHA provides information for the public, professionals, students, and the research community related to hearing, balance, speech, language and swallowing disorders.

8538 **Aphasia Hope Foundation**
PO Box 26304
Shawnee, KS 66225-6304
913-839-8083
855-764-4673
e-mail: sandycaudell@aphasiahope.org
www.aphasiahope.org

Sandy Caudell, Program Director
Judi Stradinger, Executive Director

Aphasia Hope Foundation is a nonprofit foundation with a two-fold mission: 1.to promote research into the prevention and cure of aphasia and 2. to ensure that all survivors of aphasia and their caregivers are aware of and have access to the best prossible tratments.

8539 **Atlanta Aphasia Association**
1811 Windemere Drive
Atlanta, GA 30324
404-413-8299
e-mail: jlaures@gsut.edu
www.atlantaaphasia.org

Nancy Morris, President
Jacqueline Laures-Gore PhD, Co-President
Alan Morris, Secretary/Treasurer

The Altanta Aphasia Association has several purposes: to organize and provide resources to individuals with aphasia and those involved with aphasia at vaious levels; to educate the community about aphasia through resources, discussions and communication about research advances in stroke and aphasia; to promote socialization of those with aphasia through various functions; to provide support and training for the vocational needs of those with aphasia.

8540 **Autism Research Institute**
4182 Adams Ave
San Diego, CA 92116-2599
619-281-7165
866-366-3361
FAX: 619-563-6840
www.autism.com

Stephen Edelson, Executive Director
Jane Johnson, Managing Director
Valerie Paradiz, Director
Rebecca McKenney, Office Manager

Conducts research on the causes, diagnosis, and treatment of autism and publishes a quarterly newsletter that reviews worldwide research. Literature on causes and treatment available. Refers patients and families to health care professionals and clinics. Request publication list and sample newsletter, Autism Research Review.

8541 **Autism Services Center**
929 4th Ave
PO Box 507
Huntington, WV 25701-0507
304-525-8014
FAX: 304-525-8026
e-mail: candy@autismwv.org
www.autismservicescenter.org

Jimmie Moss, Director
Jodi Fields, Director
Barbara Bragg, Director
David Finley, Director

Provides developmental disabilities services with a specialty in autism. Services include case management, residential, personal care, assessments and evaluations, supported employment, independent living and family support.

8542 **Autism Treatment Center of America**
2080 S Undermountain Rd
Sheffield, MA 1257-9643
413-229-2100
877-766-7473
e-mail: correspondence@option.org
www.autismtreatmentcenter.org

Barry Neil Kaufman, Co-Founder/ Co-Originator/Senior Teacher/Trainer
Samahria Lyte Kaufman, Co-Founder/ Co-Originator/Senior Teacher/Trainer
Bryn Hogan, ATCA Senior Staff
William Hogan, ATCA Senior Staff

Since 1983, the Autism Treatment Center of America has provided innovative training programs for parents and professionals caring for children challenged by Autism, Autism Spectrum Disorders, Pervasive Developmental Disorders (PDD) and other development difficulties. The Son-Rise Program teaches a specific yet comprehensive system of treatment and education designed to help families and caregivers enable their children to dramatically improve in all areas of learning.

8543 **Communication Help, Education, Research, Apraxia Base (CHERAB)**
PO Box 8524
PSL, FL 34952-8524
772-335-5135
e-mail: help@cherab.org
www.cherab.org

Lisa Geng, Founder, President

The Cherab Foundation is a world-wide nonprofit organization working to improve the communication skills and education of all children with speech and language delays and disorders. Their area of emphasis is verbal and oral apraxia, severe neurologically-based speech and language disorders that hinder children's ability to speak.

8544 **Communication in Autism**
Federal Government
1 Communication Avenue
Bldg 1
Bethesda, MD 20892-3456
800-241-1044
FAX: 310-770-8977
TTY:800-241-1055
e-mail: nidcdinfo@nidcd.nih.gov
www.nidcd.nih.gov

James M. Anderson, M.D., Ph.D., Chairperson
James F. Battey, Jr. M.D., Ph., Director
Judith A. Cooper, Ph.D., Deputy Director
Timothy J. Wheeles, Executive Officer

The National Institute on Deafness and Other Communication Disorders (NIDCD) one of the National Institude of Health, supports and conducts research and research training on the normal and disordered processes of hearing, balance smell, taste, voice, speech and language.

8545 Deafness and Communicative Disorders Branch of Rehab Services Administration Office
Special Education And Rehab Services
400 Maryland Ave SW
Washington, DC 20202-1
202-245-7489
800-872-5327
FAX: 202-245-7614
TTY: 800-437-0833
e-mail: customerservice@inet.ed.gov
www.ed.gov

Arne Duncan, Secretary Of Education
Tony Miller, Deputy Secretary
Martha Kanter, Under Secretary
Jo Anderson, Senior Advisor
Promotes improved rehabilitation services for deaf and hard of hearing people and individuals with speech or language impairments. Provides technical assistance to public and private agencies and individuals.

8546 Hearing, Speech and Deafness Center (HSDC)
Hearing, Speech & Deafness Center (HSDC)
1625 19th Ave
Seattle, WA 98122-2848
206-323-5770
888-222-5036
FAX: 206-328-6871
TTY: 206-388-1275
e-mail: hsdc@hsdc.org
www.hsdc.org

Cherylyn McRae, Director of Development
David Webster, Director of Finance
Roger Mauldin, Interim CEO
Bryan Bullock, Billing Specialist & Facilities Manager
Our mission is to enrich lives of all adults and children who experience hearing loss, speech and language impairments or who are deaf, by providing professional services and by promoting community awareness and accessibility.

8547 International Fluency Association
Northern Illinois University
Dept. of Communicative Disorders
DeKalb, IL 60115-2899
e-mail: msugarman1@aol.com
www.theifa.org

David Shapiro, President
Manon Abbink-Spruit, Vice-President
Dorothy Ross, Treasurer
Norimune Kawai, Secretary
The International Fluency Association is a not-for-profit, international, interdisciplinary organization devoted to the understanding and management of fluency disorders, and to the improvement in the quality of life for persons with fluency disorders.

8548 Lindamood-Bell Home Learning Process
416 Higuera Street
San Luis Obispo, CA 93401
805-541-3836
800-233-1819
FAX: 805-541-8756
www.lindamoodbell.com

Nanci Bell, Founder/Director
Patricia C. Lindamood, Founder/Director
Founded in 1986 by Nanci Bell and Patricia Lindamood, Lindamood-Bell Learning Process is dedicated to enhancing human learning. Our critically acclaimed instructional programs teach children and adults to read, spell, comprehend, and express language.

8549 National Aphasia Association
350 Seventh Avenue
Suite 902
New York, NY 10001
800-922-4622
e-mail: naa@aphasia.org
www.aphasia.org

Donald Weinstein, Ph.D, Board President
Darlene S. Williamson, M.S., Vice President Programs
Daniel Martin, Vice President Strategic Planning
J. Tyler Entwistle, Treasurer/Vice President Budget & Finance
The National Aphasia Association (NAA) is a nonprofit organization that promotes public education, research, rehabilitation and support services to assist people with aphasia and their families.

8550 National Association of Special Education Teachers
1250 Connecticut Ave NW
Ste 200
Washington, DC 20036- 2643
202-296-7739
800-754-4421
FAX: 800-754-4421
e-mail: contactus@naset.org
www.naset.org

Dr Roger Pierangelo, Executive Director
Dr George Giuliani, Executive Director
The National Association of Special Education Teachers (NASET) is a national membership organization dedicated to rendering all possible support and assistance to those preparing for or teaching in the field of special education. NASET was founded to promote the profession of special education teachers and to provide a national forum for their ideas.

8551 National Black Association for Speech-Language and Hearing
700 McKnight Park Drive
Pittsburgh, PA 15237
412-366-1177
FAX: 412-366-8804
e-mail: nbaslh@nbaslh.org
www.nbaslh.org

Arnell Brady, Chair
Carolyn Mayo, Secretary
Linda McCabe Smith, Treasurer
The mission of the National Black Association of Speech-Language and Hearing is to maintain a viable mechanism through which the needs of black professionals, students and individuals with communication disorders can be met.

8552 National Center for Accessible Media
WGBH Educational Foundation
1 Guest St
Boston, MA 02135-2016
617-300-3400
FAX: 617-300-1035
TTY:617-300-2489
e-mail: access@wgbh.org
www.ncam.wgbh.org

Larry Goldberg, Director of Media Access and oversees
Geoff Freed, Director of technology projects and Web media standards
Madeleine Rothberg, Project Director
Bryan Gould, Project Manager of NCAM's Effective Practices for Describing
The Carl and Ruth Shapiro Family National Center for Accessible Media (NCAM) at Boston public broadcaster WGBH is a research and development facility dedicated to addressing barriers to media and emerging technologies for people with disabilities in their homes, schools, workplaces, and communities..

8553 National Cued Speech Association
Information Service
1300 Pennsylvania Avenue
Suite 190-713
Washington, DC 20004-1021
301-915-8009
800-459-3529
FAX: 301-915-8009
TTY: 800-459-3529
e-mail: sroffe@cuedspeech.org
www.cuedspeech.org

Shannon Howell, President
Penny Hakim, First Vice President
John Brubaker, VP Fundraising
Doug Dawson, Treasurer
The NCSA champions effective communication, language development and literacy through the use of cued speech. The NCSA envisions that individuals communicate effectively in the languageof their family and society. Families are informed about Cued Speech along with other communication options. Their rights are respected and instruction is provided to facilitate the

use of cued languages. Students achieve literacy through full access to language and education.

8554 **National Student Speech Language Hearing Association**
2200 Research Blvd
Rockville, MD 20850-3289
301-296-5700
800-498-2071
FAX: 301-296-8580
TTY: 301-296-5650
e-mail: nsslha@asha.org
www.asha.org/nsslha

Patricia A. Prelock, PhD, CCC-SLP, President
Elizabeth S. McCrea, PhD, CCC-SLP, President-Elect
Carlin F. Hageman, PhD, CCC-SLP, National Student Speech Language Hearing Association (NSSLHA
Lauren Zanfardino, Council Member

Founded in 1972, NSSLHA is the national organization for graduate and undergraduate students interested in the study of normal and disordered human communication. NSSLHA is the only official national student association recognized by the American Speech Language Hearing Association (ASHA).

8555 **National Stuttering Association**
119 W 40th St
Fl 14
New York, NY 10018-2514
212-944-4050
800-937-8888
FAX: 212-944-8244
e-mail: info@westutter.org
www.westutter.org

Sheryl Hunter, Esquire, Chairwoman
Kenny Koroll, Vice-Chairman
Bob Wellington, Treasurer and Chairman of the Finance Committee
Pattie Wood, Chair Family Programs

A nonprofit organization dedicated to bringing hope, dignity, support, education, and empowerment to children and adults who stutter and their families, and the professionals who serve them.

8556 **Providence Speech and Hearing Center**
1301 W Providence Ave
Orange, CA 92868-3892
714-923-1521
FAX: 714-639-2593
e-mail: pshc@pshc.org
www.pshc.org

Bruce May, President
Kevin Timone, Vice President - Fund Development
Randy Free, Vice President - Finance
Casey Immel, Treasurer

Mission is to provide the highest quality services available in the identification, diagnosis, treatment and prevention of speech, language and hearing disorders for persons of all ages.

8557 **Scottish Rite Center for Childhood Language Disorders**
Seattle Clinic
1207 North 152nd St
PO Box 4144
Olympia, WA 98501-144
360-357-5933
FAX: 206-324-3332
e-mail: hfray@ritecarewa.org
www.scottishrite.org

Jacqueline Brown, Clinical Director

Offers speech-language evaluations and treatment, hearing screening and consultations to children ages birth through adolescence. Bilingual services are also available.

8558 **Stern Center**
183 Talcott Road
Suite 101
Williston, VT 05495-9209
802-878-0230
FAX: 802-878-0230
www.sterncenter.org

Blanche Podhajski PhD, President
Edward R. Wilkens, Ed.D., Vice President for Development
Janna Osman, M.Ed., Vice President for Programs
Michael Shapiro, M.B.A., Chief Financial Officer

The Stern Center was founded as a nonprofit learning center dedicated to helping children and adults reach their full potential. Stern Center professionals evaluate and teach all kinds of learners, including those with learning disabilities such as dyslexia or attention deficit disorders. We evaluate and teach over 1,000 children and adults each year including those with learning disabilities, dyslexia, language disorders, autism, attention deficit disorders, and learning style differences.

8559 **Stuttering Foundation of America**
1805 Moriah Woods Blvd,
PO Box 11749, Suite 3
Memphis, TN 38111-0749
901-761-0343
800-992-9392
FAX: 901-761-0484
e-mail: info@stutteringhelp.org
www.stutteringhelp.org

Jane Fraser, President
Dennis Drayna, Director
Joseph R. G. Fulcher, Director
Frances Cook, Director

Provides resources, services, and support to those who stutter and their families, as well as support for research into the causes of stuttering.

8560 **Texas Speech-Language-Hearing Association**
2025 M Street NW,
Suite 800
Washington, DC 20036-2342
855-330-8742
888-729-8742
FAX: 512-494-1129
e-mail: tsha@assnmgmt.com
www.txsha.org

Judith Keller, President
Larry Higdon, Director
Melanie McDonald, President Elect
Tori Gustafson, Vice President

Mission is to encourage and promote the role of the speech-language pathologist and audiologist as a professional in the delivery of clinical services to persons with communications disorders. Encourages basic scientific study of processes of individual human communication with reference to speech, hearing and language.

8561 **The Childhood Apraxia of Speech Association**
416 Lincoln Ave
2nd Fl
Pittsburgh, PA 15209
412-343-7102
www.apraxia-kids.org

Mary Sturm, President
Sharon Gretz, Executive Director
Sue Freiburger, Secretary

The mission of the Childhood Apraxia of Speech Association is to strengthen the support systems in the lives of children with apraxia, so that each child has their best opportunity to develop speech.

8562 **The Davis Center**
19 State Route 10 E
Ste 25
Succasunna, NJ 07876
862-251-4637
FAX: 862-251-4642
e-mail: npdunn@thedaviscenter.com
www.thedaviscenter.com

Dorinne S Davis MA CCC-A FAAA, Director
Elizabeth Meade, Head Sound Therapist
Nancy Puckett-Dunn, Office Manger
Donna Warr, Office Assistant

The Davis Center's Sound Therapy Programs make positive changes for children and adults with autism, ADD/ADHD, auditory processing issues, Dyslexia, learning disabilities, and other learning and wellness challenges. Our programs address issues such as phonics, spelling, writing, reading comprehension, hearing only parts of words, following directions, discriminating between sounds, sound sensitivity, behavioral responses, focus, attention, and more.

8563 Wendell Johnson Speech And Hearing Clinic
University Of Iowa
116 Wendell Johnson Speech and Hear
Iowa City, IA 52242- 1025 319-335-8736
FAX: 319-335-8851
e-mail: linda-louka@uiowa.edu
www.uiow.edu

Ruth Bentler, Professor & Department Chair
Dorothy Albright, Secretary
Kathy Miller, Clerk
Elizabeth Walker, Audiologist

The clinic offers assessment and remediation for communication disorders in adults and children. The clinic also offers a Intensive Summer Residential Clinic for school age children needing intervention services because of speech, language, hearing and/or reading problems.

Camps

8564 CNS Camp New Connections
Mclean Hospital Child/Adolescent Program
Mailstop115
115 Mill Street
Belmont, MA 02478 617-855-2000
800-333-0338
FAX: 617-855-2833
e-mail: mcleaninfo@partners.org
mcleanhospital.org

Scott L. Rauch, MD, President & Chief Psychiatrist
Blaise Aguirre, Clinical Staff
Alan Barry, Clinical Staff
Susan L. Andersen, Research Staff

Four-week summer day camp for children ages 7-17 who have pervasive developmental disorders, Asperger's Syndrome, autism spectrum disorders and non-verbal learning disabilities. The camp is designed to help children develop social skills through fun activities including: communication games, swimming, field trips, drama, and arts and crafts. *$4500.00*

8565 Camp Royall
Autism Society of North Carolina
Ste 230
505 Oberlin Rd
Raleigh, NC 27605-1345 919-743-0204
800-442-2762
FAX: 919-743-0208
e-mail: jchampion@autismsociety-nc.com
www.autismsociety-nc.org

Sharon Jeffries-Jones, Chair
Elizabeth Phillippi, Vice Chair
Paul Wendler, Chief Financial Officer
David Laxton, Director of Communications

The best source in North Carolina for connecting people who live with autism (and those who care about them) with resources, support, advocacy and informantion tailored to thier unique needs.

8566 Camp Sisol
Jewish Community Center of Greater Rochester/JCC
1200 Edgewood Ave
Rochester, NY 14618 585-461-2000
e-mail: membership2@jccrochester.org
www.jccrochester.org

Marshall Lesser, Chair
Jeremy Wolk, President
Dan Goldstein, VP & Secretary
Leslie Berkoitz, Executive Director

Camp is located in Honeoye Falls, New York. Summer sessions for children with autism. Coed, ages 5-16.

8567 Childrens Beach House
100 West 10th Street
Suite 411
Wilmington, DE 19801-1674 302-655-4288
FAX: 302-655-4216
e-mail: inquiry@cbhinc.org
www.cbhinc.org

Martha P. Tschantz, President
Mary Helms, Vice President
Richard T Garrett, Executive Director
Nicholas Imhoff, Business Manager

Camp is located in Lewes, Delaware. Four-week sessions June-August for Delaware children with hearing impairment or speech/communication impairment. Coed, ages 6-12.

8568 Easter Seals Oklahoma
701 NorthEast 13th Street
Oklahoma City, OK 73104 405-239-2525
FAX: 405-239-2278
e-mail: sbusch@eastersealsoklahoma.org
www.eastersealsoklahoma.org

Rodney Burgamy, Chairman
David Adams, Board Member
Kristen Sorocco, Secretary
Jeb Reid, Treasurer

Adult day health center, and child development center.

8569 Meadowood Springs Speech and Hearing Camp
Institute for Rehab., Research, & Recreation Inc
P.O. Box 1025
Pendleton, OR 97801 541-276-2752
FAX: 541-276-7227
e-mail: info@meadowoodsprings.org
www.meadowoodsprings.com

Michael Ashton, Executive Director
Cliff Story, Property Manager
Missy Newcomb, Clinical Director
Audrey Black, Program Director

On 143 acres in the Blue Mountains of Eastern Oregon, this camp is designed to help young people who have diagnosed clinical disorders of speech, hearing or language. A full range of activities in recreational and clinical areas is available.

8570 New Horizons Summer Day Camp
YMCA
13821 Newport Avenue
Suite 200
Tustin, CA 92780 714-549-9622
FAX: 714-838-5976
www.ymcaoc.org

Robert Traut, Chair
Jeff Black, Vice Chair
Jeff McBride, President/CEO
Cara Owens, COO/VP,Operations

One-week sessions for children with ADD and speech/communication impairment. Coed, ages 5-14.

8571 Sequanota Lutheran Conference Center and Camp
P.O. Box 245
Jennerstown, PA 15547 814-629-6627
FAX: 814-629-0128
e-mail: contact@sequanota.com
www.sequanota.com

Carol Custead, President
David Shoemaker, Vice President
Nathan Pile, Executive Director
Loren Kurtz, Maintenance Director

Summer sessions for adults with developmental disabilities and speech/communication impairment.

8572 Talisman Summer Camp
64 Gap Creek Rd
Zirconia, NC 28790
828-697-6313
855-588-8254
855-LUV-TALI
e-mail: info@talismancamps.com
www.talismancamps.com

Doug Smathers, Camp Director/Owner
Linda Tatsapaugh, Operations Director/Owner
Robiyn Mims, Admissions Coordinator
Cory Greene, Program Manager
Camp is located in Black Mountain, North Carolina. Offers a program of hiking, rafting, climbing, and caving for learning disabled ADD/ADHD and autistic young people. Coed, ages 9-18.

8573 Wendell Johnson Speech & Hearing Clinic
University Of Iowa
250 Hawkins Dr
Iowa City, IA 52242-1025
319-335-8736
FAX: 319-335-8851
e-mail: kathy-miller@uiowa.edu
www.uiowa.edu

Chuck Wieland, President
Hans Hoerschelman, Vice President
Josh Smith, Budget Officer
Shannon Lizakowski, Secretary
The clinic offers assessment and remediation for communication disorders in adults and children. The clinic also offers a Intensive Summer Residential Clinic for school age children needing intervention services because of speech, language, hearing and/or reading problems.

8574 YMCA Camp Fitch
The YMCA Of Youngstown - Metro Office
17 N Champion St
P.O. Box 1287
Youngstown, OH 44501
330-744-8411
FAX: 330-744-8415
e-mail: info@campfitchymca.org
www.youngstownymca.org

Thomas Fleming, Chair/CVO
James B. Greene, 1st Vice Chair
Thomas Gacse, 2nd Vice Chairman
Timothy M. Hilk, President/CEO
Camp is located in North Springfield, Pennsylvania. Camping sessions for children and adults with diabetes, hearing impairment, developmental disabilities, mobility limitation and speech/communication impairment. Ages 8-16, families and seniors.

Print: Books

8575 Autism 24/7: A Family Guide to Learning at Home & in the Community
Autism Society of North Carolina Bookstore
Ste 230
505 Oberlin Rd
Raleigh, NC 27605-1345
919-743-0204
800-442-2762
FAX: 919-743-0208
e-mail: jchampion@autismsociety-nc.org
http://www.autismsociety-nc.org/

Sharon Jeffries-Jones, Chair
Elizabeth Phillippi, Vice Chair
Tracey Sheriff, Chief Executive Officer
Paul Wendler, Chief Financial Officer
Parents are encouraged to focus on skill sets and behaviors that most negatively affect family functioning, and replacing these behaviors with acceptable alternatives. *$19.95*

8576 Autism Handbook: Understanding & Treating Autism & Prevention Development
Oxford University Press
2001 Evans Road
Cary, NC 27513
919-677-0977
800-445-9714
FAX: 919-677-1303
e-mail: custserv.us@oup.co
http://www.oup.com/us/

320 pages
ISBN 0-195076-67-2

8577 Autism and Learning
Taylor & Francis
37-41 Mortimer St
London, UK W1T 3
http://www.informatandm.com

Stuart Powell, Author
Rita Jordan, Editor
This book is about how a cognitive perception on the way in which individuals with autism think and learn may be applied to particular curriculum areas.
160 pages Paperback
ISBN 1-853464-21-X

8578 Autism in Adolescents and Adults
Springer Publishing
233 Spring St
New York, NY 10013
877-283-3229

e-mail: ainy@aveda.com
http://aveda.edu/new-york

Eric Schopler, Editor
Gary B. Mesibov, Editor
This book is a great history lesson in the development of understanding about autism spectrum disorders, and is a testament to how far research and services in the field have come. This book contains lots of information about what general thinking and services used to be like, in an era when still little was understood about these disorders. *$ 63.00*
456 pages
ISBN 0-306410-57-5

8579 Autism...Nature, Diagnosis and Treatment
Autism Society of North Carolina Bookstore
Ste 230
505 Oberlin Rd
Raleigh, NC 27605-1345
919-743-0204
800-442-2762
FAX: 919-743-0208
e-mail: jchampion@autismsociety-nc.com
http://www.autismsociety-nc.org/

Sharon Jeffries-Jones, Chair
Elizabeth Phillippi, Vice Chair
Paul Wendler, Chief Financial Officer
David Laxton, Director of Communications
Covers perspectives, issues, neurobiological issues and new directions in diagnosis and treatment. *$49.00*

8580 Autism: Explaining the Enigma
Wiley Publishers
111 River Street
Hoboken, NJ 07030-5774
201-748-6000
FAX: 201-748-6088
e-mail: info@wiley.com
http://as.wiley.com

Peter Booth Wiley, Chairman
Stephen M. Smith, President & CEO
John Kitzmacher, EVP, CFO
Ellis E. Cousens, Executive Vice President, COO
Explains the nature of autism. *$27.95*

8581 Autism: From Tragedy to Triumph
Branden Publishing Company
17 Station St
Brookline, MA 2445-7995 617-730-5757
e-mail: branden@branden.com
http://www.yogainthevillage.com
Karen Wenc, Teaching Staff
Veronica Wolff, Teaching Staff
Annie Hoffman, Teaching Staff
Keith Beasley, Teaching Staff
A new book that deals with the Lovaas method and includes a foreward by Dr. Ivar Lovaas. The book is broken down into two parts — the long road to diagnosis and then treatment. *$12.95*

8582 Autism: Identification, Education and Treatment
Routledge
270 Madison Ave
New York, NY 10016-601 212-576-1411
http://books.google.co.in/books/about/Autism.
Dianne Zager, Editor
Chapters include medical treatments, early intervention and communication development in autism. *$36.00*
ISBN 0-805820-44-7

8583 Autism: The Facts
Oxford University Press
2001 Evans Road
Cary, NC 27513 919-677-0977
800-445-9714
FAX: 919-677-1303
e-mail: custserv.us@oup.co
http://www.oup.com/us/corporate/contact/?view
Simon Baron-Cohen, Co-Author
Patrick Bolton, Co-Author
$22.50
128 pages
ISBN 0-192623-27-3

8584 Autistic Adults at Bittersweet Farms
Routledge
12660 Archbold-Whitehouse Rd.
Whitehouse, OH 43571 419-875-6986
e-mail: mtilkins@bittersweetfarms.org.
http://www.bittersweetfarms.org/
Robert St. Clair, President
Matt Anderson, VP
Jan Toczynski, Secretary
Jon Ahlberg, Board Member
A touching view of an inspirational residential care program for autistic adolescents and adults. Also available in softcover. *$94.95*
Hardcover
ISBN 1-560240-42-3

8585 Beyond Baby Talk: From Sounds to Sentences, a Parent's Guide to Language Development
Prima Publishing
P.O.Box 1260
Rocklin, CA 95677-1260 916-787-7000
800-632-8676
FAX: 916-787-7001
www.primapublishing.com
Fernando Bueno, Editor in Chief
Julie Asbury, Managing Editor
Christopher Buffa, Sr. Editor
Andrea Hill, Community Manager
The authors discuss the best ways to help your child develop the all-important skill of communication and to recognize the signs of language development problems. *$15.95*
224 pages
ISBN 0-761526-47-1

8586 Breaking the Speech Barrier: Language Develpment Through Augmented Means
Brookes Publishing
P.O.Box 10624
Baltimore, MD 21285-0624 410-337-9580
800-638-3775
FAX: 410-337-8539
e-mail: custserv@brookespublishing.com
readplaylearn.com
Paul Brookes, Owner
This resource describes the creation of the System for Augmenting Language (SAL) for school-age youth with mental retardation and offers important insights into the language development of children who are not learning to communicate typically. *$39.95*
224 pages Paperback
ISBN 1-557663-90-0

8587 Breakthroughs: How to Reach Students with Autism
Aquarius Health Care Media
Ste 230
505 Oberlin Rd
Raleigh, NC 27605-1345 919-743-0204
800-442-2762
FAX: 919-743-0208
e-mail: jchampion@autismsociety-nc.org
http://www.autismtreatmentcenter.org/cont ents
Sharon Jeffries-Jones, Chair
Elizabeth Phillippi, Vice Chair
Tracey Sheriff, CEO
Paul Wendler, CFO
A hands-on, how-to program for reaching students with autism, featuring Karen Sewell, Autism Society of America's teacher of the year. Here Sewell demonstrates the successful techniques she's developed over a 20-year career. A separate 250 page manual ($59) is also available which covers math, reading, fine motor, self help, social adaptive, vocational and self help skills as well as providing numerous plan reproducibles and an exhaustive listing of equipment and materials resources. Video. *$99.00*

8588 Childhood Speech, Language & Listening Problems
Wiley Publishing
605 3rd Ave
New York, NY 10158-180 212-850-6000
FAX: 212-850-6088
http://books.google.co.in/books/about/Childho
Patricia McAleer Hamaguchi
Language pathologist Hamaguchi employs her 15 years of experience to show parents how to recognize the most common speech, language, and listening problems. *$16.95*
224 pages Paperback
ISBN 0-471387-53-3

8589 Cognitive Behavioral Therapy for Adult Asperger Syndrome
Autism Society of North Carolina Bookstore
Ste 230
505 Oberlin Rd
Raleigh, NC 27605-1345 919-743-0204
800-442-2762
FAX: 919-743-0208
e-mail: jchampion@autismsociety-nc.org
http://www.autismsociety-nc.org
Sharon Jeffries-Jones, Chair
Elizabeth Phillippi, Vice Chair
Tracey Sheriff, CEO
Paul Wendler, CFO
Text is prepared with case studies and examples from the author's own experiences working as a cognitive-behavioral therapist specializing in adults and adolescents with dual diagnosis, autism spectrum disorders, mood disorders, and anxiety disorders.

8590 Communication Development and Disorders in African American Children
Brookes Publishing
P.O.Box 10624
Baltimore, MD 21285-0624 410-337-9580
800-638-3775
FAX: 410-337-8539
e-mail: custserv@brookespublishing.com
readplaylearn.com
Paul Brooks, Owner
Research, Assessment, and Intervention. This text presents research on communication disorders and language development in African American children. Also addresses multicultural aspects of service delivery and intervention and discusses issues in assessing, diagnosing, and treating communication disorders. *$39.00*
400 pages Paperback
ISBN 1-55766-53-3

8591 Communication Development in Children with Down Syndrome
Brookes Publishing
P.O.Box 10624
Baltimore, MD 21285-0624 410-337-9580
800-638-3775
FAX: 410-337-8539
e-mail: custserv@brookespublishing.com
readplaylearn.com
Paul Brooks, Owner
This book offers an extensive, detailed explanation of communication development in children with Down syndrome relative to their advancing cognitive skills. It introduces a critical framework for assessing and treating hearing, speech, and language problems and provides explicit intervention methods and tested clinical protocols.
Paperback
ISBN 1-55766 -50-5

8592 Coping for Kids Who Stutter
Speech Bin
P.O.Box 1579
Appleton, WI 54912 419-589-1425
888-388-3224
FAX: 888-388-6344
e-mail: info@speechbin.com
www.speechbin.com
James R. Henderson, Chairman
Joseph M. Yorio, President & CEO
Rick Holden, EVP, Educators Publishing Service
Patrick T. Collins, EVP, Distribution
Informative book for children and adults about stuttering and how to manage it. *$15.95*
32 pages
ISBN 0-93785 -43-2

8593 Disorders of Motor Speech: Assessment, Treatment, and Clinical Characterization
Brookes Publishing
P.O.Box 10624
Baltimore, MD 21285-0624 410-337-9580
800-638-3775
FAX: 410-337-8539
e-mail: custserv@brookespublishing.com
readplaylearn.com
Paul Brooks, Owner
This book provides a probing examination of normal, dysarthric, and apraxic speech. Great for speech-language pathologists, neurologists, physical or occupational therapists, and physiatrists. *$47.00*
400 pages Hardcover
ISBN 1-55766 -23-1

8594 Employment for Individuals with Asperger Syndrome or Non-Verbal Learning Disability
Jessica Kingsley Publishers
440 Market Street
Suite 400
Philadelphia, PA 19106-2513 215-922-1161
866-416-1078
FAX: 215-922-1474
e-mail: orders@jkp.com
www.jkp.com
Laurie Schlesinger, Vp Of Sales & Marketing
Yvona Fast, Author
Most people with Non-Verbal Learning Disorder (NLD) or Asperger Syndrome (AS) are underemployed. This book sets out to change this. With practical and technical advice on everything from job hunting to interview techniques, from 'fitting in' in the workplace to whether or not to disclose a diagnosis, this book guides people with NLD or AS successfully through the employment mine field. There is also information for employers, agencies and careers counsellors on AS and NLD as 'invisible' disabili *$22.95*
272 pages
ISBN 1-843107-66-X

8595 Encounters with Autistic States
Jason Aronson
400 Keystone Industrial Park
Dunmore, PA 18512-1507 800-782-0015
448 pages Hardcover
ISBN 0-765700-62-

8596 Kitten Who Couldn't Purr
William Morrow & Company
1350 Avenue of the Americas
New York, NY 10019-4702 212-261-6500
FAX: 212-261-6925
http://www.goodreads.com/book/show/2319648.Th
Otis Chandler, CEO & Co-Founder
Eve Titus, Author
Jonathan the kitten doesn't know how to purr to say thank you, so he sets off to find someone to teach him. *$12.95*
32 pages

8597 Language Disabilities in Children and Adolescents
McGraw-Hill School Publishing
PO Box 182605
Columbus, OH 43218 800-338-3987
FAX: 609-308-4480
e-mail: customer.service@mheducation.com
mcgraw-hill.com
David Levin, President and CEO
Patrick Milano, Chief Administrative Officer & CFO
Stephen Laster, Chief Digital Officer
David Stafford, SVP & General Counsel
A comprehensive review of research in language disabilities.

8598 Language and the Developing Child
International Dyslexia Association
40 York Road
4th Floor
Baltimore, MD 21204 410-296-0232
800-ABC-D123
FAX: 410-321-5069
www.interdys.org
Hal Malchow, President
Ben Shifrin, Vice President
Elsa C. Hagen, Vice President
Suzanne Carreker, Secretary
This collection of papers introduces a new generation of teachers, clinicians and parents to the work of one of the key figures in the search for the causes and treatment of dyslexia. *$15.00*

8599 Late Talker: What to Do If Your Child Isn't Talking Yet
St Martin's Griffin
175 5th Ave
New York, NY 10010-7703
646-307-5151
888-330-8477
FAX: 212-674-6132
e-mail: customerservice@mpsvirginia.com
www.us.macmillan.com

Marilyn C Agin, Author

This handbook offers advice on ways to identify the warning signs of a speech disorder, information on how to get the right kind of evaluations and therapy, ways to obtain appropriate services through the school system and health insurance, at-home activities that parents can do with their child to stimulate speech, benefits of nutritional supplementation, and advice from experienced parents who've been there on what to expect and what you can do to be your child's best advocate. *$13.95*

256 pages Paperback
ISBN 0-312309-24-4

8600 Let Community Employment be the Goal for Individuals with Autism
Indiana Resource Center For Autism
1905 North Range Road
Bloomington, IN 47408-9801
812-855-6508
800-825-4733
FAX: 812-855-9630
e-mail: iidc@indiana.edu
www.iidc.indiana.edu/irca

Cathy Pratt, Director
Catherine Davies, Educational Consultant
Pamela Anderson, Outreach/Resource Specialist
Melissa Dubie, Research Associate

A guide designed for people who are responsible for preparing individuals with autism to enter the work force. *$7.00*

8601 Lollipop Lunch
Speech Bin-Abilitations
P.O.Box 1579
Appleton, WI 54912-1579
419-589-1425
888-388-3224
FAX: 888-388-6344
e-mail: info@speechbin.com
www.speechbin.com

James R. Henderson, Chairman
Joseph M. Yorio, President & CEO
Rick Holden, EVP, Educators Publishing Service
Patrick T. Collins, EVP, Distribution

Cleverly illustrated stories and activities for phonological and language development. *$19.95*

128 pages
ISBN 0-937857-54-8

8602 Management of Autistic Behavior
Sage Publications
2455 Teller Road
Thousand Oaks, CA 91320
805-499-0721
800-818-7243
FAX: 805-499-0871
e-mail: info@sagepub.com
www.sagepub.com

Sara Miller McCune, Founder, Publisher, Chairperson
Blaise R Simqu, President & CEO
Tracey A. Ozmina, Executive Vice President & Chief Operating Officer
Stephen Barr, Managing Director/SAGE London, President of SAGE Internation

This excellent reference is a comprehensive and practical book that tells what works best with specific problems. *$41.00*

450 pages

8603 Motor Speech Disorders
WB Saunders Company
14 Main Street
Southampton, NY 11968-2822
631-283-5050
800-523-1649
FAX: 631-283-2290
e-mail: info@saunders.com
www.wbsaunders.com

Joseph R Duffy PhD, Author

Professional text on rehabilitation techniques for motor speech disorders. *$74.00*

592 pages
ISBN 0-323024-52-5

8604 Neurobiology of Autism
Johns Hopkins University Press
National Library of Medicine
Building 38A
Bethesda, MD 20894
410-516-6900
888-346-3656
888-FIN- NLM
FAX: 410-516-6998
e-mail: info@ncbi.nlm.nih.gov
http://www.ncbi.nlm.nih.gov/pubmed/17919129

Pardo CA, Co-Author
Ebarhat CG, Co-Author

This book discusses recent advances in scientific research that point to a neurobiological basis for autism and examines the clinical implications of this research. *$28.00*

272 pages
ISBN 0-801880-47-5

8605 Nonverbal Learning Disabilities at Home: A Parent's Guide
Jessica Kingsley Publishers
400 Market Street
Suite 400
Philadelphia, PA 19106
215-922-1161
866-416-1078
FAX: 215-922-1474
e-mail: hello.usa@jkp.com
www.jkp.com

Jessica Kingsley, Chairman & Managing Director
Jemima Kingsley, Director
Octavia Kingsley, Production Director
Lisa Clark, Sr. Commissioning Editor

Explores the variety of daily life problems children with NLD may face, and provides practical strategies for parents to help them cope and grow, from preschool age through their challenging adolescent years. *$19.95*

272 pages Paperback
ISBN 1-853029-40-0

8606 Parent Survival Manual
Springer Publishing Company
11 West 42nd Street
8th Floor
New York, NY 10036
212-355-1501
FAX: 212-355-7370
e-mail: christieseducation@christies.edu
http://www.christieseducation.com

Craig Lickliter, Manager

A guide to crises resolution in autism and related developmental disorders. *$39.95*

8607 Perspectives: Whole Language Folio
Gallaudet University Bookstore
PO Box 35009
Charlotte, NC 28235-5009
202-651-5750
800-995-0550
FAX: 202-651-5744
http://www.cpcc.edu/disabilities/student-clas

Edwin A. Dalrymple, Chairman
Judith N. Allison, Vice Chair
Tony Zeiss, President
Ellen Zaremba, Administrative Assistant to the President

The 19 articles in this collection offer practical help to teachers seeking to emphasize whole language strategies in their classroom. *$9.95*
64 pages

8608 Please Don't Say Hello
Human Sciences Press
233 Spring St
New York, NY 10013 877-283-3229
e-mail: ainy@aveda.com
http://aveda.edu/new-york
Phyllis Terri Gold, Author
Paul and his family moved into a new neighborhood. Paul's brother was autistic. The children thought that Eddie was retarded until they learned that there were skills that he could do better than they could. *$10.95*
47 pages Paperback
ISBN 0-89885 -99-8

8609 Promoting Communication in Infants and Young Children: 500 Ways to Succeed
Speech Bin-Abilitations
P.O.Box 1579
Appleton, WI 54912-1579 419-589-1425
888-388-3224
FAX: 888-388-6344
e-mail: info@speechbin.com
www.speechbin.com
James R. Henderson, Chairman
Joseph M. Yorio, President & CEO
Rick Holden, EVP, Educators Publishing Service
Patrick T. Collins, EVP, Distribution
This practical reference for parents, caregivers and professional service providers how to promote communication development in infants and young children. Gives down-to-earth information and activities to help your youngest children succeed. It provides step-by-step suggestions for stimulationg children's speech and language skills. Paperback. *$14.95*
ISBN 0-937857-72-6

8610 Reading, Writing and Speech Problems in Children
International Dyslexia Association
40 York Road
4th Floor
Baltimore, MD 21204 410-296-0232
800-ABC-D123
FAX: 410-321-5069
www.interdys.org
Hal Malchow, President
Ben Shifrin, Vice President
Elsa C. Hagen, Vice President
Suzanne Carreker, Secretary
A tribute to the man who more than any other aroused the attention of the scientific community and who provided the sound educational principles on which much teaching of dyslexics today is based. *$27.00*
ISBN 0-89079 -79-1

8611 Relationship Development Intervention with Young Children
Taylor & Francis Group
73 Collier St.
London, N1 9BE 44- 0 -0 78
FAX: 44- 0 -0 78
e-mail: hello.usa@jkp.com
http://www.jkp.com/jkp/distributors.php
Jessica Kingsley, Chairman
Jemima Kingsley, Director
Octavia Kingsley, Production Director
Lisa Clark, Sr. Commissioning Editor
Social and emotional development activities for Asperger Syndrome, Autism, PDD and NLD. Comprehensive set of activities emphasizes foundation skills for younger children between the ages of two and eight. Covers skills such as social referencing, regulating behvior, conversational reciprocity, and synchronized actions. For use in therapeutic settings as well as schools and parents. *$22.95*
256 pages
ISBN 1-843107-14-7

8612 Riddle of Autism: A Psychological Analysis
Jason Aronson
Ste 200
4501 Forbes Blvd
Lanham, MD 20706 301-459-3366
800-462-6420
FAX: 301-429-5746
e-mail: customercare@nbnbooks.com
http://www.nbnbooks.com
Jason Brockwell, Sales Staff
Michael Sullivan, Sales
Mark Cozy, Sales Staff
Dennis Hayes, Director of Special Markets
Dr. Victor examines the myths that cloud an understanding of this disorder and describes the meanings of its specific behavioral symptoms. *$30.00*
356 pages Paperback
ISBN 1-568215-73-8

8613 Schools for Children with Autism Spectrum Disorders
Resources for Children with Special Needs
116 East 16th Street
5thFloor
New York, NY 10003 212-677-4650
FAX: 212-677-4070
e-mail: info@resourcesnyc.org
resourcesnyc.org
Ellen Miller-Wachtel, Chair
Shon E. Glusky, President
Rachel Howard, Executive Director
Stephen Stern, Director of Finance & Adminstration
Published every 24-36 months. *$20.00*
160 pages
ISBN 0-967836-53-0

8614 Self-Therapy for the Stutterer
Stuttering Foundation of America
1805 Moriah Woods Blvd.
Suite 3
Memphis, TN 38117 901-761-0343
800-992-9392
FAX: 901-761-0484
e-mail: info@stutteringhelp.org.
www.stutterhelp.org
Jane Fraser, President
Jean Gruss, Journalist
Robert M. Kurtz, Chairman & CEO
Malcolm Houg Fraser, Founder
A guide to help adults who stutter overcome the problem on their own. *$3.00*
191 pages Paperback
ISBN 0-933388-32-2

8615 Sex Education: Issues for the Person with Autism
Indiana Resource Center For Autism
1905 North Range Road
Bloomington, IN 47408-9801 812-855-6508
800-825-4733
FAX: 812-855-9630
e-mail: iidc@indiana.edu
www.iidc.indiana.edu/irca
Cathy Pratt, Director
Catherine Davies, Educational Consultant
Pamela Anderson, Outreach/Resource Specialist
Melissa Dubie, Research Associate
Discusses issues of sexuality and provides methods of instruction for people with autism. *$4.00*

8616 Son-Rise: The Miracle Continues
2080 South Undermountain Road
Sheffield, MA 01257
413-229-2100
800-714-2779
e-mail: sonrise@option.org
http://www.option.org

Samahria Lyt Kaufman, Co-Founder and Co-Director
Dane Griffith, Director of Administrative Services
Bears Kaufman, Co-Founder and Co-Director
Raun Kaufman, Director of Global Education

Part One is the astonishing record of Raun Kaufman's development from an autistic and retarded child into a loving, brilliant youngster who shows no traces of his former condition. Part Two follows Raun's development after the age of four, teaching the limitless possibilities of the Son-Rise Program. Part Three shares moving accounts of five other ordinary families who became extraordinary when they used the Son-Rise Program to reach their own unreachable children. *$12.95*
343 pages
ISBN 0-915811-53-7

8617 Sound Connections for the Adolescent
Speech Bin
P.O.Box 1579
Appleton, WI 54912-1579
419-589-1425
888-388-3224
FAX: 888-388-6344
e-mail: info@speechbin.com
www.speechbin.com

James R. Henderson, Chairman
Joseph M. Yorio, President & CEO
Rick Holden, EVP, Educators Publishing Service
Patrick T. Collins, EVP, Distribution

A resource to help older elementary and secondary students understand their sound systems an how it functions. It targets skills critical for academic achievement: phonological awareness, phonemic relationships, phonemic processing, listening and memory and teaches linguistic rules they need to succeed. *$19.95*
Paperback

8618 Talkable Tales
Speech Bin-Abilitations
P.O.Box 1579
Appleton, WI 54912-1579
419-589-1425
888-388-3224
FAX: 888-388-6344
e-mail: info@speechbin.com
www.speechbin.com

James R. Henderson, Chairman
Joseph M. Yorio, President & CEO
Rick Holden, EVP, Educators Publishing Service
Patrick T. Collins, EVP, Distribution

Read-a-rebus stories and pictures targeting most consonant phonemes for K-5 children. *$25.95*
128 pages
ISBN 0-93783 -44-0

8619 Teaching Children with Autism: Strategies for Initiating Positive Interactions
Brookes Publishing
P.O.Box 10624
Baltimore, MD 21285-0624
410-337-9585
888-337-8808
FAX: 410-337-8539
e-mail: custserv@healthpropress.com
http://www.healthpropress.com

Melissa A. Behm, President
Mary Magnus, Director

Stategies for initiating positive interactions and improving learning opportunities. This guide begins with an overview of characteristics and long-term strategies and proceeds through discussions that detail specific techniques for normalizing environments, reducing disruptive behavior, improving language and social skills, and enhancing generalization. *$32.95*
256 pages Paperback
ISBN 1-55766 -80-4

8620 Teaching and Mainstreaming Autistic Children
Love Publishing Company
9101 East Kenyon Avenue
Suite 2200
Denver, CO 80237
303-221-7333
FAX: 303-221-7444
e-mail: lpc@lovepublishing.com
http://www.lovepublishing.com/

Peter Knoblock, Author

Dr. Knoblock advocates a highly organized, structured environment for autistic children, with teachers and parents working together. His premise is that the learning and social needs of autistic children must be analyzed and a daily program designed with interventions that respond to this functional analysis of their behavior. *$24.95*
ISBN 0-89108 -11-9

8621 Techniques for Aphasia Rehab: (TARGET) Generating Effective Treatment
Speech Bin
P.O.Box 1579
Appleton, WI 54912-1579
419-589-1425
888-388-3224
FAX: 888-388-6344
e-mail: info@speechbin.com
www.speechbin.com

James R. Henderson, Chairman
Joseph M. Yorio, President & CEO
Rick Holden, EVP, Educators Publishing Service
Patrick T. Collins, EVP, Distribution

Practical treatment manual for use by aphasia clinicians. *$45.00*
384 pages
ISBN 0-93785 -50-5

8622 Understanding & Controlling Stuttering: A Comprehensive New Approach Based on the Valsa Hyp
National Stuttering Association
119 West 40th Street
14th Floor
New York, NY 10018
212-944-4050
800-937-8888
FAX: 212-944-8244
e-mail: info@westutter.org
www.nsastutter.org

Kenny Koroll, Chair
Tammy Flores, Executive Director
Stephanie Coopen, Family Programs Administrator
Mandy Finstad, Editor/Webmaster

Demonstrates how physical and psychological factors may interact to stimulate and perpetuate stuttering through a Valsalva-Stuttering cycle. *$25.00*
176 pages
ISBN 7-929773-01-3

8623 Verbal Behavior Approach: How to Teach Children with Autism & Related Disorders
Autism Society of North Carolina Bookstore
Ste 230
505 Oberlin Rd
Raleigh, NC 27605-1345
919-743-0204
800-442-2762
FAX: 919-743-0208
e-mail: jchampion@autismsociety-nc.com
http://www.autismsociety-nc.org

Sharon Jeffries-Jones, Chair
Elizabeth Phillippi, Vice Chair
Tracey Sheriff, CEO
Paul Wendler, CFO

Provides full descriptions of how to teach the verbal operants that make up expressive languate which include: manding, tacting, echoing and intraverbal skills. *$19.95*

8624 **Without Reason: A Family Copes with two Generations of Autism**
Books on Special Children
721 W Abram St
Arlington, TX 76013-6995
817-277-0727
800-489-0727
FAX: 817-277-2270
http://www.fhautism.com/

R. Wayne Gilpin, President
Jennifer Gilpin Yacio, Vice President and Editorial Director
David Reasor, CPA and Administrative Director
Teresa Corey, Conference Administrator

The author discovers his son has autism. He delves into problems of the autistic person and explains reasons for their actions.
$20.95
292 pages Hardcover

Print: Journals

8625 **American Journal of Speech-Language Pathology**
American Speech-Language-Hearing Association
2200 Research Boulevard
Rockville, MD 20850-3289
301-296-5700
800-638-8255
FAX: 301-296-8580
e-mail: nsslha@asha.org, productsales@asha.org
www.asha.org

Elizabeth S. McCrea, PhD, CCC-SLP, President
Barbara K. Cone, PhD, CCC-A, Vice President for Academic Affairs in Audiology
Carolyn W. Higdon, EdD, CCC-SLP, Vice President for Finance
Kaci Roger, Council Member

This is a quarterly journal of clinical practice for speech-language pathologists and language researchers. This journal will be online only beginning January 2010.

8626 **Journal of Speech, Language and Hearing Research**
American Speech-Language-Hearing Association
2200 Research Boulevard
Rockville, MD 20850-3289
301-296-5700
800-638-8255
FAX: 301-296-8580
e-mail: nsslha@asha.org, productsales@asha.org
www.asha.org

Elizabeth S. McCrea, PhD, CCC-SLP, President
Barbara K. Cone, PhD, CCC-A, Vice President for Academic Affairs in Audiology
Carolyn W. Higdon, EdD, CCC-SLP, Vice President for Finance
Kaci Roger, Council Member

This bimonthly journal contains basic, as well as applied research in normal and disordered communication processes. It will be available online only beginning January 2010.

8627 **Language, Speech, and Hearing Services in Schools**
International Fluency Association
Northern Illinois University
Dept. of Communicative Disorders
DeKalb, IL 60115-2899
www.theifa.org

David Shapiro, President
Norimune Kawat, Secretary
Rachel Everard, Treasurer
Shelley Brundage, Membership

This is a quarterly journal focusing on research appropriate to speech-language pathologists and audiologists in schools. The journal will only be available online beginning in January 2010.

Print: Magazines

8628 **Communication Outlook**
Artificial Language Laboratory
220 Trowbridge Road
East Lansing, MI 48824
517-353-8332
FAX: 517-353-4766
e-mail: artling@msu.edu
www.msu.edu

Lou Anna K. Simon, President
Satish Udpa, EVP for Administrative Services
Bill Beekman, VP & Secretary
Mark P. Haas, VP for Finance & Treasurer

Communication Outlook (CO) is an international quarterly magazine, which focuses on the techniques and technology of augmentative and alternative communication. CO provides information on technological developments for persons experiencing communication handicaps due to neurological, sensory or neuromuscular conditions. *$18.00*
32 pages Quarterly

Print: Newsletters

8629 **Access Audiology**
American Speech-Language-Hearing Association
2200 Research Boulevard
Rockville, MD 20850-3289
301-296-5700
800-638-8255
FAX: 301-296-8580
e-mail: nsslha@asha.org, productsales@asha.org
www.asha.org

Elizabeth S. McCrea, PhD, CCC-SLP, President
Barbara K. Cone, PhD, CCC-A, Vice President for Academic Affairs in Audiology
Carolyn W. Higdon, EdD, CCC-SLP, Vice President for Finance
Kaci Roger, Council Member

Dedicated to the specific needs of all professionals interested in hearing, balance, and the field of audiology. Each issue spotlights a specific topic of interest and relevance to audiologists.

8630 **Autism Research Review International**
Autism Research Institute
4182 Adams Avenue
San Diego, CA 92116-2599
619-281-7165
866-366-3361
FAX: 619-563-6840
e-mail: br@autismresearchinstitute.com
autism.com

Stephen Edelson, Executive Director
Jane Johnson, Managing Director
Valerie Paradiz, Director
Anthony Morgali, Producer

Provides clearly written summaries of articles selected from computer searches. *$18.00*
8 pages Quarterly

8631 **Communicologist**
Texas Speech-Language-Hearing Association
Ste 200
918 Congress Ave
Austin, TX 78701-2342
512-494-1128
888-729-8742
FAX: 512-494-1129
e-mail: tsha@assnmgmt.com
cisaustin.org

Judith Keller, President
Larry Higdon, Director
Melanie McDonald, President Elect
Tori Gustafson, Vice President

A forum for distributing current information relevant to the practices of speech-language pathology and audiology across the state. Provides TSHA membership with the latest news from the Executive Board and Task Forces, as well as information about regional associations, distinguished service providers, the TSHA

Annual Convention, and committee honors and nominations. Also contains advertisements of interest to the field.

8632 Connect
Hearing, Speech & Deafness Center (HSDC)
1625 19th Avenue
Seattle, WA 98122
206-323-5770
888-222-5036
FAX: 206-328-6871
e-mail: hsdc@hsdc.org
www.hsdc.org

Pamela Anderson, President
Ken Block, VP
David Webster, Director of Finance
Brayde Williamson, Director of Education
A newsletter that addresses concerns of those affected by speech and language disorders.
8 pages Quarterly

8633 NSSLHA Now
Ntn'l Student Speech Language Hearing Association
2200 Research Boulevard
Rockville, MD 20850-3289
301-296-5700
800-638-8255
FAX: 301-296-8580
e-mail: nsslha@asha.org, productsales@asha.org
www.asha.org

Elizabeth S. McCrea, PhD, CCC-SLP, President
Barbara K. Cone, PhD, CCC-A, Vice President for Academic Affairs in Audiology
Carolyn W. Higdon, EdD, CCC-SLP, Vice President for Finance
Kaci Roger, Council Member
Published three times per year.

8634 On Cue
National Cued Speech Association
1300 Pennsylvania Avenue, NW
Suite 190-713
Washington, DC 20004
301-915-8009
800-459-3529
www.cuedspeech.org

Shannon Howell, President
Penny Hakim, 1st Vice President
John Brubaker, VP Fundraising
Doug Dawson, Treasurer
Published several times a year and mailed to members of the Association.

8635 Stuttering & Your Child: Help For Parents
Stuttering Foundation of America
18005 Moriah Woods Blvd
PO Box 11749, Suite 3
Memphis, TN 38111-0749
901-761-0343
800-992-9392
FAX: 901-761-0484
e-mail: info@stutteringhelp.org
www.StutteringHelp.org

Jane Fraser, President
Dennis Drayna, Director
Joseph R. G. Fulcher, Director
Frances Cook, Director
The Stuttering Foundation provides resources, services and support to those who stutter and their families, as well as support research into the cause of stuttering. The Stuttering Foundation provides a referral list of speech-language pathologists and referrals to other information including research on stuttering, intensive workshops and camps. *$10.00*

8636 Stuttering Foundation Newsletter
Stuttering Foundation of America
P.O.Box 11749
Memphis, TN 38111-0749
901-761-0343
800-992-9392
FAX: 901-761-0484
e-mail: info@stutteringhelp.org
www.stutteringhelp.org

Jane Fraser, President
Jean Gruss, Journalist
Robert M. Kurtz, Chairman & CEO
Malcolm Houg Fraser, Founder

8637 Voice
Providence Speech and Hearing Association
1301 Providence Avenue
Orange, CA 92868
714-923-1521
855-901-7742
FAX: 714-744-3841
e-mail: pshc@pshc.org
www.pshc.org

Lewis Jaffe, President
Bret Rathwick, Vice President - Finance
Casey Immel, Treasurer
Marlene Woodworth, Secretary
People of all ages with speech and hearing problems by providing specialized products and services.

Non Print: Newsletters

8638 Access Academics & Research
American Speech-Language-Hearing Association
2200 Research Boulevard
Rockville, MD 20850-3289
301-296-5700
800-638-8255
FAX: 301-296-8580
e-mail: nsslha@asha.org, productsales@asha.org
www.asha.org

Elizabeth S. McCrea, PhD, CCC-SLP, President
Barbara K. Cone, PhD, CCC-A, Vice President for Academic Affairs in Audiology
Carolyn W. Higdon, EdD, CCC-SLP, Vice President for Finance
Kaci Roger, Council Member
Dedicated to the specific needs of academic and clinical faculty, PhD students and researchers. The e-newsletter was developed as part of the Focused Initiative on the PhD Shortage in Higher Education.

8639 Access SLP Health Care
American Speech-Language-Hearing Association
2200 Research Boulevard
Rockville, MD 20850-3289
301-296-5700
800-638-8255
FAX: 301-296-8580
e-mail: nsslha@asha.org, productsales@asha.org
www.asha.org

Elizabeth S. McCrea, PhD, CCC-SLP, President
Barbara K. Cone, PhD, CCC-A, Vice President for Academic Affairs in Audiology
Carolyn W. Higdon, EdD, CCC-SLP, Vice President for Finance
Kaci Roger, Council Member
An e-newsletter dedicated to the specific needs of speech-language pathologists in healthcare settings. Each issue of Access SLP Health Care features recent legislative activity impacting SLPs and provides information on clinical issues, continuing education opportunities, and ASHA web-based resources.

8640 **Access Schools**
American Speech-Language-Hearing Association
2200 Research Boulevard
Rockville, MD 20850-3289
301-296-5700
800-638-8255
FAX: 301-296-8580
e-mail: nsslha@asha.org, productsales@asha.org
www.asha.org

Elizabeth S. McCrea, PhD, CCC-SLP, President
Barbara K. Cone, PhD, CCC-A, Vice President for Academic Affairs in Audiology
Carolyn W. Higdon, EdD, CCC-SLP, Vice President for Finance
Kaci Roger, Council Member

Dedicated to the specific needs of school-based speech-language pathologists. Each Access Schools e-newsletter features recent legislative activity impacting school SLPs and provides information on clinical issues, continuing education opportunities, and ASHA web-based resources.

8641 **Stuttering**
Federal Government
31 Center Drive MSC 2320
Bethesda, MD 20892-2320
301-496-7243
800-241-1044
FAX: 301-402-0018
e-mail: nidcdinfo@nidcd.nih.gov
www.nidcd.nih.gov

James F. Battey, Director
Judith A. Cooper, Deputy Director
Timothy J. Wheeles, Executive Officer
Tanya Brown, Executive Assistant

Describes how speech is produced, treatments for stuttering and research supported by the federal government.

Non Print: Video

8642 **Autism: A World Apart**
Fanlight Productions
c/o Icarus Films
32 Court Street, 21st Floor
Brooklyn, NY 11201
718-488-8900
800-876-1710
FAX: 718-488-8642
e-mail: info@fanlight.com, sales@icarusfilms.com
www.fanlight.com

Ben Achtenberg, Owner, Founder
Nicole Johnson, Publicity Coordinator
Anthony Sweeney, Marketing Director

In this documentary, three families show us what the textbooks and studies cannot: what it's like to live with autism day after day; to raise and love children who may be withdrawn and violent and unable to make personal connections with their families. 29 minutes.
VHS/DVD
ISBN 1-572950-39-0

8643 **Autism: the Unfolding Mystery**
Aquarius Health Care Media
18 N Main St
Sherborn, MA 1770-1066
508-650-1616
e-mail: lkussmann@aquariusproductions.com

Lesile Kussmann, Owner

Explore what it means to be autistic, how you can recognize the signs of autism in your child, and hear about new treatments and programs to help children learn to deal with the disorder. *$145.00*
DVD

8644 **Getting Started with Facilitated Communication**
Facilitated Communication Institute, Syracuse Univ
370 Huntington Hall
Syracuse, NY 13244-1
315-443-9657
FAX: 315-443-9218
e-mail: fcstaff@syr.edu
www.thefci.syr.edu

Annegret Schubert, Producer

Describes in detail how to help individuals with autism and/or severe communication difficulties to get started with facilitated communication.
Video

8645 **I Just Want My Little Boy Back**
Autism Treatment Center Of America
2080 South Undermountain Road
Sheffield, MA 01257
413-229-2100
800-714-2779
e-mail: happiness@option.org
http://www.option.org

Samahria Lyt Kaufman, Co-Founder and Co-Director
Dane Griffith, Director of Administrative Services
Bears Kaufman, Co-Founder and Co-Director
Raun Kaufman, Director of Global Education

A great video for parents and professionals caring for children with special needs. Join one British family and their autistic son before, during and after their journey to America to attend The Son-Rise Program at The Autism Treatment Center of America. This informative, inspirational and deeply moving story not only captures the joy, tears, challenges and triumps of this amazing little boy and his family, but also serves as a powerful introduction to the attitude and principles of the program. *$25.00*

8646 **Understanding Autism**
Fanlight Productions
c/o Icarus Films
32 Court Street, 21st Floor
Brooklyn, NY 11201
718-488-8900
800-876-1710
FAX: 718-488-8642
e-mail: info@fanlight.com, sales@icarusfilms.com
www.fanlight.com

Ben Achtenberg, Owner, Founder
Nicole Johnson, Publicity Coordinator
Anthony Sweeney, Marketing Director

Parents of children with autism discuss the nature and symptoms of this lifelong disability and outline a treatment program based on behavior modification principles. 19 minutes
VHS/DVD
ISBN 1-572951-00-1

Support Groups

8647 **Autism Society of America**
4340 East West Highway
Suite 350
Bethesda, MD 20814-3067
301-657-0881
800-328-8476
FAX: 301-657-0869
e-mail: dallen@autism-society.org
www.autism-society.org

Mary Beth Collins, Director of Programs
Tonia Ferguson, Senior Director of Content
Scott Badesch, President/Chief Executive Officer
John Dabrowski, Chief Financial Officer

ASA is the largest and oldest grassroots organization within the autism community, with a nationwide network of chapters and over 20,000 members and supporters nationwide. ASA is the leading source of education, information and referral about autism and has been the leader in advocacy and legislative initiatives for more than four decades.

8648 **Cherab Foundation**
P.O.Box 8524
Port St Lucie, FL 34985-8524
772-335-5135
FAX: 772-337-4812
e-mail: help@cherab.org
www.cherab.org

Marilyn Agin, MD
Lisa Geng, Co Author

Helps to start, supports, and works together with other support groups and nonprofits (such as ECHO, VOICES, and Apraxia Network) that have mutual goals for helping children with apraxia and other speech disorders.

8649 Friends: National Association of Young People who Stutter
38 S Oyster Bay Rd
Syosset, NY 11791-5033
866-866-8335
e-mail: lcaggiano@aol.com
www.friendswhostutter.org

Lee Caggiano, President

A national organization created to provide a network of love and support for children and teenagers who stutter, their families, and the professionals who work with them.

8650 National Health Information Center
US Department of Health
P.O.Box 1133
Washington, DC 20013-1133
301-565-4167
800-336-4797
301-468-7394
FAX: 301-984-4256
e-mail: healthypeople@hhs.gov
http://www.healthypeople.gov

Jonathan Fielding, Chair
Shirika Kumanyika, Vice Chair

A health information referral service that puts health professionals and consumers who have health questions in touch with those organizations that are best able to provide answers.

8651 Speech Pathways
410 Meadow Creek Drive
Suite 206
Westminster, MD 21158
410-374-0555
800-961-2724
FAX: 410-374-8620
e-mail: kim.bell@speechpathways.net
speechpathways.net

Kimberly A. Bell, Owner
Karie Hadley, Therapist
Erica Hamilton, Therapist
Julie Kumpar, Therapist

We realize that parent and family support is critical to a child's success, in therapy as well as in life. We offer support at local and regional levels along with traditional speech and language services, and a wide variety of specialized pediatric programs. Our support groups/services are open to the larger community as well as to our clients.

Visual

Associations

8652 ACB Government Employees
American Council of the Blind
2200 Wilson Blvd
Ste 650
Arlington, VA 22201-3354
202-467-5081
800-424-8666
FAX: 703-465-5085
e-mail: info@acb.org
www.acb.org

Sarah Presley, President
Kim Charlson, Vice President
Marliana Lieberg, Secretary
Carla Ruschival, Treasurer
Members are present, former and retired employees of federal, state and local government agencies. Concerns of the organization include recruitment, placement and advancement of blind and visually impaired employees.

8653 ACB Radio Amateurs
American Council of the Blind
167 Green St
Reading, MA 01867
202-467-5081
800-424-8666
FAX: 202-467-5085
e-mail: acbra@acb.org
www.acbhams.org

Steve Dresser, President
Mike Duke, Vice President
Robert Rogers, Treasurer
Robert Spangler, Secretary
ACBRA is an organization of blind and sighted licensed radio amateurs who work together to make the hobby more accessible to people who are blind

8654 ACB Social Service Providers
American Council of the Blind
2200 Wilson Blvd
Ste 650
Arlington, VA 22201-3354
202-467-5081
800-424-8666
FAX: 703-465-5085
e-mail: info@acb.org
www.acb.org

Mitch Pomerantz, President
Kim Charlson, Vice President
Marliana Lieberg, Secretary
Carla Ruschival, Treasurer
Blind and visually impaired social workers, social service professionals, students pursuing careers in social work and other interested persons are members of this organization. ACBSSP works to promote full participation by visually impaired social services professionals in the field of social welfare.

8655 Achromatopsia Network
PO Box 214
Berkeley, CA 94701-214
510-540-4700
FAX: 510-540-4767
e-mail: achromatopsia@cox.net
www.achromat.org

Frances Futterman, President
The Achromatopsia Network is a nonprofit organization for individuals concerned with acrhomatopsia. It is committed to sharing information about achromatopsia and providing resources to meet the special needs of those affected by this eye condition; helping individuals and families concerned with achromatopsia to connect with one another; and promoting awareness and educating with a special emphasis on accomplishing this goal among those who provides services to the visually impaired.

8656 American Academy of Ophthalmology
655 Beach St.
PO Box 7424
San Francisco, CA 94120-7424
415-561-8500
866-561-8558
FAX: 415-561-8533
e-mail: customer_service@aao.org
www.aao.org

Randy Johnston, President
The American Academy of Ophthalmology is the largest national membership association of Eye M.D.s. Eye M.D.s are ophthalmologists, medical and osteopathic doctors who provide comprehensive eye care, including medical, surgical and optical care. More than 90 percent of practicing U.S. Eye M.D.s are Academy members, and the Academy has more than 7,000 international members.

8657 American Action Fund for Blind Children and Adults
1800 Johnston St
Ste 100
Baltimore, MD 21230-4914
410-659-9315
FAX: 410-685-5653
e-mail: actionfund@actionfund.org
www.actionfund.org

Barbara Loos, President
Ramona Walhof, Vice President
Sandra Halverson, Second Vice President/Medical Transcriptionist
James Omvig, Treasurer
A service agency which specializes in providing to blind people help which is not readily available to them from government programs or other existing service systems. The services are planned especially to meet the needs of blind children, the elderly blind, and the deaf-blind.

8658 American Council of Blind Lions
148 Vernon Avenue
Suite 650
Louisville, KY 40206-3354
502-897-1472
800-424-8666
FAX: 703-465-5085
e-mail: info@acb.org
www.acb.org/acbl

Mitch Pomerantz, President
Kim Charlson, First Vice President
Brenda Dillon, Second Vice President
Marlaina Lieberg, Secretary
A wonderful combination of Lionism and visual impairment nurtures the American Council of Blind Lions. ACBL's mission is awareness and highlights the great activities of the Knights of the Blind. The goals are to assist all clubs in their understanding of issues surrounding blind and visually impaired individuals.

8659 American Council of the Blind
2200 Wilson Blvd
Ste 650
Arlington, VA 22201-3354
202-467-5081
800-424-8666
FAX: 703-465-5085
e-mail: ebridges@acb.org
www.acb.org

Mitch Pomerantz, President
Kim Charlson, Vice President
Marliana Lieberg, Secretary
Carla Ruschival, Treasurer
A national membership organization whose members are visually impaired and fully sighted individuals who are concerned about the dignity and well-being of blind people throughout America. Formed in 1961, the Council has become the largest organization of blind people in the US with over 70 state affiliates and special interest chapters.

8660 American Foundation for the Blind
11 Penn Plz
Suite 300
New York, NY 10121-2018
212-502-7600
800-232-5463
FAX: 212-502-7777
e-mail: afbinfo@afb.net
www.afb.org

Carl Augusto, President/CEO
Paul Schroeder, Vice President
Rick Bozeman, Director
Scott Truax, Manager

The organizaton to which Helen Keller devoted her life, is a national nonprofit organization whose mission is to ensure that the ten million Americans who are blind or visually impaired enjoy the same rights and opportunities as other citizens.

8661 American Optometric Association
243 N Lindbergh Blvd
Saint Louis, MO 63141-7881
314-991-4100
800-365-2219
FAX: 314-991-4101
e-mail: MDJones@aoa.org
www.aoa.org

Ronald L Hopping, President
Mitchell Munson, President-Elect
David A. Cockrell, Vice President
Steven Loomis, Secretary-Treasurer

the AOA is the acknowledged leader and recognised authority for the eye and vision care in the world. The objectives of the AOA are centered on improving the quality and availiability of eye and vision care. The AOA fulfills its missions in accordance with health care and public policy related to eye care will uniformly recognise optometrists as primary health care providers and ensure the public has acess to the full scope of optometric care.

8662 American Printing House for the Blind
1839 Frankfort Avenue
PO Box 6085
Louisville, KY 40206- 0085
502-895-2405
800-223-1839
FAX: 502-899-2284
e-mail: info@aph.org
www.aph.org

Charles Barr, Chairman

The world's largest nonprofit organization creating educational, workplace and independent living products and services for people who are visually impaired. Also promotes independence of the blind and visually impaired persons by providing specialized materials, products, and services needed for educationand life.

8663 Associated Blind
212-683-4950
FAX: 212-683-4975
e-mail: memberservices@esightcareers.net
www.tabinc.org

Nancy O'Connell, Executive Director

Privately funded, non-profit agency, that was founded by a group of blind individuals as an organization promoting autonomy and self-determination. The mission is to assist individuals who are blind, visualy impaired or who have physical disabilities to become self-reliant and achieve financial independence through mainstream employment.

8664 Associated Services for the Blind
919 Walnut St
Philadelphia, PA 19107-5287
215-627-0600
FAX: 215-922-0692
e-mail: asbinfo@asb.org
www.asb.org

Patricia C. Johnson, President/Chief Executive Officer
Derby Ewing, Director, Human Services
Richard Forsythe, Director, Braille Division and Custom Audio
Linda Gaffney, Coordinator, Volunteer Services

ASB, a non-private, non-profit organization, promotes self esteem, independence, and self-determination in people who are blind or visually impaired. ASB accomplishes this by providing support through education, training and resources, as well as through community action and public education, serving as a voice and advocate for the rights of all people who are blind or visually impaired.

8665 Association for Education & Rehabilitationof the Blind & Visually Impaired
1703 N Beauregard St
Suite 440
Alexandria, VA 22311-1744
703-671-4500
877-492-2708
FAX: 703-671-6391
e-mail: jgandorf@aerbvi.org
www.aerbvi.org

Mr. Jim Adams, President
Ms. Christy Shepard, President-elect
Dr. Susan Jay Spungin, Secretary
Mr. Cliff Olstrom, Treasurer

The mission of AER is to support professionals who provide education and rehabilitation services to people with visual impairments, offering professional development opportunities, publications, and public advocacy.

8666 Association for Macular Diseases
210 E 64th St
8th Fl
New York, NY 10065-7471
212-605-3719
800-622-8524
FAX: 212-605-3795
e-mail: association@retinal-research.org
www.macula.org

Bernard Landou, President
Mary Fern Breheney, Board Member
Fern Breheney, Board Member
Joan R. Daly, Board Member

The Macula Foundation, Inc., a not-for-profit organization was established in 1978 to support basic and clinical research in vitreous retinal and macular diseases, a major cause of blindness of all age groups. Since it was formed, the Foundation has distributed grants and awards of approximately 15 million dollars earmarked for important clinical and scientific research and related teaching programs. Numerous research projects have been successful as a result of the Foundation.

8667 Blind Childrens Center
4120 Marathon St
Los Angeles, CA 90029-3584
323-664-2153
800-222-3566
FAX: 323-665-3828
e-mail: info@blindchildrenscenter.org
www.blindchildrenscenter.org

Lena French, Executive Director
Fernanda Armenta-Schmitt, PhD, Director of Education & Family Services/Assistant Executive
Muriel Scharf, Director of Development
Ross Vergara, Director of Finance

A family centered agency which serves children with visual impairments from birth to school-age. The center-based and home-based programs and services help the children aquire skills and build their independence. The center utilizes its expertise and experience to serve families and professionals worldwide through support services, education, and research.

8668 Blind Information Technology Specialists
American Council of the Blind
2200 Wilson Blvd
Ste 650
Arlington, VA 22201-3354
703-841-0048
800-424-8666
202-465-5085
FAX: 703-465-5085
e-mail: president@bits-acb.org
www.bits-acb.org

Richard Villa, President
Renee Zelickson, Vice President
Tom L. Jones, Secretary
Lynne Koral, Treasurer

BITS is a non profit organization which fosters the career development of blind computer professionals, promotes the use of computer technology by blind persons to improve the qualtiy of their personal and professional lives, and advocate for improved information access for all visually impaired people.

8669 Blinded Veterans Association
477 H St NW
Washington, DC 20001-2694 202-371-8880
800-669-7079
FAX: 202-371-8258
e-mail: bva@bva.org
www.bva.org

Samuel Huhn, President
Mark Cornell, Vice President
Robert Dale Stamper, Secretary
Roy Young, Treasurer
BVA locates blinded veterans who need assistance, guides them through the rehabilitation process, and acts as advocates for them before Congress and the Department of Veterans Affairs in the securing of all the benefits they have earned throught their service to the nation. Promotes access to technology and the practical use of the latest research. Its Field Service Program provides encouragement and emotional support through role models, who can demonstrate that the challenges can be overcome.

8670 Books for Blind and Physically Handicapped Individuals
Library of Congress
1291 Taylor St NW
Washington, DC 20011 202-707-5100
888-657-7323
FAX: 202-707-0712
TTY: 202-707-0744
e-mail: nls@loc.gov
www.loc.gov/nls

Frank Cylke, Director
Administers a national library service that provides braille and recorded books and magazines on free loan to anyone who cannot read standard print because of visual of physical disabilities who are eligible residents of the Unites States of America citizens living abroad.

8671 Braille Institute of America
741 N Vermont Ave
Los Angeles, CA 90029-3594 323-663-1111
800-272-4553
FAX: 323-663-0867
e-mail: tours@brailleinstitute.org
www.brailleinstitute.org

Lester M. Sussman, Chair
Percy Duran, Audit
Richard Larson, Development
Harvey Strode, Finance
Provides an environment of hope and encouragement for people who are blind and visually impaired through integrated educational, social and recreational programs and services. Provides assistance at 5 regional centers in Southern California and through 200 community outreach programs. In 2005-06, the Institute provided these services to more than 55,000 people. The Institute is operated and funded almost entirely through private individual and foundation sources.

8672 California State Library Braille and Talking Book Library
PO Box 942837
Sacramento, CA 94237-0001 916-634-0640
800-952-5666
FAX: 916-654-1119
e-mail: btbl@library.ca.gov
www.btbl.ca.gov

Mike Marlin, Director
The State Library stands as one of California's great public research institutions with a five-fold mission:serving the needs of elected officials and state agency employees;preserving the state's cultural heritage by collecting historic materials on California and the West;assisting public libraries through financial aid and consulting services;offering special services to disadvantaged and handicapped clients;ensuring that the general public has convenient and consistent access to resources.

8673 Canine Helpers for the Handicapped
5699 Ridge Rd
Lockport, NY 14094-9408 716-433-4035
FAX: 716-439-0822
e-mail: chhdogs@aol.com
www.caninehelpers.netfirms.com
Beverly Underwood, Executive Director
Laura Gates, Trainer
A nonprofit organization devoted to custom training Assistance Dogs to assist people with disabilities to lead more independent, secure lives.

8674 Caption Center
125 Western Ave
Boston, MA 02134 617-300-3600
FAX: 617-300-1020
TTY:617-300-3600
e-mail: access@wgbh.org
www.mattapanchc.org
Cristopher Brandon, Chair
Glenola Mitchell, Vice Chair
Dale L. Kurtz, Treasurer
Nelda M. Headley, Secretary
Has been pioneering and delivering accessible media to disabled adults, students and their families, teachers and friends for over 30 years. Each year, the Center captions more than 10,000 hours worth of broadcast and cable programs, feature films, large-format and IMAX films, home videos, music videos, DVDs, teleconferences and CD-Roms.

8675 Chicago Lighthouse for People who are Blind and Visually Impaired
1850 W Roosevelt Rd
Chicago, IL 60608-1298 312-666-1331
FAX: 312-243-8539
TTY:312-666-8874
e-mail: support@chicagolighthouse.org
www.chicagolighthouse.org
Bruce R. Hague, Chairman
Sandra C. Forsythe, Vice Chairman
Janet P. Szlyk, President
David Huber, Treasurer
A non profit agency committed to providing the highest quality educational, clinical, vocational, and rehabilitation services for children, youth and adults who are blind or visually impaired, including deaf blind and multi disabled. Also respects personal dignity and partners with individuals to enhance independent living and self sufficiency. This agency is a leader, innovator and advocate for people who are blind or visually impaired, enhancing the quality of life for all individuals.

8676 Clovernook Center for the Blind and Visually Impaired
7000 Hamilton Ave
Cincinnati, OH 45231-5240 513-522-3860
888-234-7156
FAX: 513-728-3946
TTY:513-522-3860
e-mail: contact@clovernook.org
www.clovernook.org
Alfred J. Tuchfarber, Chair
Wilbert F. Schwartz, Vice Chair
Mark Jackson, Treasurer
Thomas R. Flottman, Secretary
Mission is to promote independence and foster the highest quality of life for people with visual impairments, including those with additional disabilities. We provide comprehensive program services including training and support for independent living, orientation and mobility instruction, vocational training, job placement, counseling, recreation, and youth services. Meaningful employment opportunities are also provided to individuals who are blind or visually impaired.

8677 Clovernook Printing House, The Clovernook Center for the Blind and Visually Impaired

7000 Hamilton Ave
Cincinnati, OH 45231-5240 513-522-3860
888-234-7156
FAX: 513-728-3946
e-mail: contact@clovernook.org
www.clovernook.org

Alfred J. Tuchfarber, Chair
Wilbert F. Schwartz, Vice Chair
Mark Jackson, Treasurer
Thomas R. Flottman, Secretary

Clovernook also offers Braille Transcription Services including: Literary Books, Literary Magazines, Religious Materials, Instructional Manuals, ADA Conformance Materials, Literary Textbook Materials, Menus, Braille Alphabet Cards, and Forms. In addition, our Business Operations provide meaningful employment opportunities for individuals who are blind or visually impaired, while at the same time manufacturing high-quality products for customers across the country. *$145.00*

591 pages
ISBN 1-930956-48-7

8678 College of Optometrists in Vision Development

215 W Garfield Rd
Ste 200
Aurora, OH 44202-7884 330-995-0718
888-268-3770
FAX: 330-995-0719
e-mail: info@covd.org
www.covd.org

David A. Damari, President
Kara Heying, Vice President
Christine Allison, Secretary-Treasurer
Pamela R. Happ, Executive Director

The College of Optometrists in Vision Development (COVD) is an international membership association of eye care professionals including optometrists, optometry students, and vision therapists. Members of COVD provide developmental vision care, vision therapy and vision rehabilitation services for children and adults.

8679 College of Syntonic Optometry

2052 W. Morales Drive
Pueblo West, CO 81007-4202 719-547-8177
877-559-0541
FAX: 719-547-3750
e-mail: Syntonics@q.com
www.collegeofsyntonicoptometry.com

Larry Wallace, O.D., FCSO, Education Director
Mary Van Hoy, O.D., FCOVD,, President
Stefan Collier, F.O., FCSO, Vice President
John Pulaski, O.D., FCSO, Treasurer

An active and growing post-graduate educational organization. Established in 1933 its members include optometrists and other health professionals and supporters from around the world. Those who achieve a clinical level of experience and mastery are awarded the status of Fellow. Today, scientific as well as clinical verification of light's impact on health and healing and a growing public demand for functional and rehabilitative vision therapy continue to vitalise the college and its mission.

8680 Columbia Lighthouse for the Blind

1825 K St NW
Suite 1103
Washington, DC 20910-1261 301-589-0894
877-324-5252
FAX: 202-955-6401
e-mail: info@clb.org
www.clb.org

Tony Cancelosi, President
Anthony J. (Cancelosi, K.M., President/CEO

Offer programs that enable individuals who are blind or visually impaired to obtain and maintain independence at home, school, work and in the community. The programs and services include asistive technology training, career services, rehabilitation services, comprehensive low vision care and a wide range of children's programs.

8681 Council of Families with Visual Impairments

American Council of the Blind
1155 15th St NW
Ste 1004
Washington, DC 20005-2706 202-467-5081
800-424-8666
FAX: 202-467-5085
e-mail: cindy.vw@msn.com
www.acb.org

Jill Gaus, President
Lynn Jansen, Vice President
Debby Lieberman, Secretary
Mike Reese, Treasurer

A network of parents with blind or visually impaired children that offers support and outreach, shares experiences in parent/child relationships, exchanges educational, cultural and medical information about child development and more.

8682 Deaf-Blind Division of the National Federation of the Blind

200 East Wells Street
Baltimore, MD 21230-4914 410-659-9314
FAX: 410-685-5653
e-mail: nfb@nfb.org
www.nfb.org

Marc Maurer, CEO

The nation's largest and most influential membership organization of blind persons, with a two-fold purpose: to help blind persons achieve self-confidence and self respect and to act as a vehicle for collective self-expression by the blind. The NFB improves blind people's lives through advocacy, education, research, technology, and programs encouraging independence and self-confidence. It is the leading force in the blindness field today and is the voice of the nations blind.

8683 Eye Bank Association of America

1015 18th St NW
Suite 1010
Washington, DC 20036-5223 202-775-4999
FAX: 202-429-6036
e-mail: info@restoresight.org
www.restoresight.org

David Korroch, Chair
David Glasser, Chair-Elect
Donna Drury, Secretary
Woodford Van Meter, Treasurer

Established in 1961 by the American Academy of Ophthalmology's Committee on Eye Banks, the EBAA is a not-for-profit organization of eye banks dedicated to the restoration of sight through the promotion and advancement of eye banking. The EBAA has lead the transplantation field with the establishment of medical standards for the procurement and distribution of corneal tissue, accreditation of eye banks, and comprehensive education programs for doctors, technicians, and administrators.

8684 Fidelco Guide Dog Foundation

103 Vision Way
Bloomfield, CT 06002-1424 860-243-5200
FAX: 860-243-7215
e-mail: info@fidelco.org
www.fidelco.org

Stephen H. Matheson, Chairman
John H. Gotta, Vice Chairman
Glynis Cassis, Secretary
Mary P. CraigCraig, DVM, MBA,, Treasurer

The Fidelco Guide Dog Foundation, located in Bloomfield, Conn., is dedicated to providing increased freedom and independence to men and women who are blind by providing them with the highest quality guide dogs. We rely solely on the gifts and the generosity of individuals, foundations, corporations and organizations that partner with Fidelco to 'Share the Vision.'

8685 **Fight for Sight**
381 Park Ave S
Suite 809
New York, NY 10016-8806
212-679-6060
FAX: 212-679-4466
e-mail: info@fightforsight.com
www.fightforsight.com
Norman J. Kleiman, Ph.D., Board President
Gaby Kressly, BoardSecretary/Treasurer
Janice Benson, Asst Director
Amanda Angulo, Board Member
The mission is to support vision research, to find causes and cures for blindness, and to help save the sight of children through support of pediatric eye centers.

8686 **Foundation Fighting Blindness**
7168 Columbia Gateway Drive
Suite 100
Columbia, MD 21046
800-683-5555
TTY:8006835551
blindness.org

8687 **Guide Dog Users**
4851 N. Cedar Ave.
Apt 119
Fresno, CA 93726-2245
301-598-2131
866-799-8436
FAX: 301-871-7591
e-mail: treasurer@gdui.org
www.gdui.org
Laurie Mehta, President
Mary Beth Randall, First Vice President
Charles Crawford, Second Vice President
Sarah Calhoun, Secretary
Guide Dog Users Inc, (GDUI) an affiliate of the American Council of the Blind, is the largest guide dog consumer driven group in the world. Since 1972, members can excercise the privilege of shaping the initiatives and issues that most profoundly affect guide dog handlers. GDUI has 19 affiliate organizations throughout the US where members can personally interact and work together on local as well as global issues.

8688 **Guide Dogs for the Blind**
PO Box 151200
San Rafael, CA 94915-1200
415-499-4000
800-295-4050
FAX: 415-499-4035
e-mail: information@guidedogs.com
www.guidedogs.com
Bob Burke, Chair
Paul A. Lopez, President & CEO
George Kerscher, Vice Chair
Stuart Odell, Vice Chair, Finance
A nonprofit, charitable organization with a mission to provide Guide Dogs and training in their use to visually impaired people throughout the United States and Canada.

8689 **Guiding Eyes for the Blind**
611 Granite Springs Rd
Yorktown Heights, NY 10598-3499
914-245-4024
800-942-0149
FAX: 914-245-1609
e-mail: info@guidingeyes.org
guidingeyes.org
Wendy Aglietti, Chairman
Mary J. Conway, Vice Chair
Curt J. Landtroop, Vice Chair/Treasurer
Lorraine Miller, Secretary
An internationally recognized guide dog school that is dedicated to enriching the lives of blind and visually impaired men and women by providing them with the freedom to travel safely, thereby assuring greater independence, dignity and new horizons of opportunity

8690 **Guiding Eyes for the Blind: Breeding and Placement Center**
Guiding Eyes for the Blind
611 Granite Springs Rd
Yorktown Heights, NY 10598-3499
914-245-4024
800-942-0149
FAX: 914-245-1609
e-mail: infor@guidingeyes.org
www.guidingeyes.org
Bill Badger, President/CEO
Sue Dishart, Vice President
Carolyn Kihm, Director
Jerry Attard, Comptroller
Provides the means for blind and visually impaired individuals to achieve mobility, independence and companionship through the use of our professionally bred and trained guide dogs. Each month Guiding Eyes graduates approximately 12 guide dog/student teams from all over the US, Canada, and internationally. The guide dogs, 26 day residential training program, special needs program and lifetime follow-up services are offered at no cost to the students. Also provides at home training at no cost.

8691 **Horizons for the Blind**
125 Erick Street
A103
Crystal Lake, IL 60014-4404
815-444-8800
800-318-2000
FAX: 815-444-8830
TTY: 815-444-8800
e-mail: mail@horizons-blind.org
www.horizons-blind.org
Camille Caffarelli, Executive Director
Jeff T. Thorsen, First Vice President/Treasurer
Keith Myers, Second Vice President
Maryann Bartkowski, Secretary
Horizons for the Blind is a 501(c)(3) nonprofit organization dedicated to improving the quality of life for people who are blind or visually impaired, through our consumer products and services, the cultural arts, education and recreation.

8692 **Independent Visually Impaired Enterprisers**
American Council of the Blind
1155 15th St NW
Ste 1004
Washington, DC 20005-2706
202-467-5081
800-424-8666
FAX: 202-467-5085
e-mail: info@acb.org
www.ivie-acb.org
Jill Gaus, President
Lynn Jansen, Vice President
Debby Lieberman, Secretary
Mike Reese, Treasurer
Strives to broaden vocational opportunities in business for the visually impaired. Works to improve rehabilitation facilities for all types of business enterprises and publicizes the capabilities of blind and visually impaired business persons.

8693 **Institute for Families**
4650 Sunset Blvd
Mail Stop 111
Los Angeles, CA 90027- 6062
323-361-4649
FAX: 323-665-7869
e-mail: info@instituteforfamilies.org
www.instituteforfamilies.org
Margaret Yoshina, Executive Director
Jazmin Asbun, Administrative Assistant
Institute for Families offers counseling and support to families whose child has been diagnosed with cancer or other diseases that may impact vision. In addition to the counseling services, we provide books and videos to families and healthcare professionals as an additional resource to assist them during the difficult days after diagnosis.

8694 International Association of Audio Information Services (IAAIS)
1102 W Intl Airport Rd
Anchorage, AK 99518-1007 412-434-6023
800-280-5325
e-mail: lrk@ku.edu
www.iaais.org

Stuart Holland, President
Marjorie Williams, First Vice-President
Linda Hynson, Secretary
Andrea Pasquale, Treasurer
A volunteer driven membership organization of services that turn text into speech for people who cannot see, hold or comprehend the printed word and who may be unable to access information due to a disability or health condition. IAAIS shall encourage and support the establishment and maintenance of audio information services that provide access to printed information for individuals who cannot read conventional print because of blindess or any other visual, physical or learning disability.

8695 Jewish Braille Institute International
110 E 30th St
New York, NY 10016-7393 212-889-2525
800-433-1531
FAX: 212-689-3692
e-mail: library @jbilibrary.org
www.jbilibrary.org

Judy E. Tenney, Chairman of the Board
Dr. Ellen Isler, President and CEO
Israel A. Taub, Vice President and CFO
Frances Brandt, Treasurer
JBI International is a non-profit organization dedicated to meeting the Jewish and general cultural needs of the visually impaired, blind, physically handicapped and reading disabled - of all ages and backgrounds - worldwide. For nearly 80 years, JBI has provided people of all ages who are blind, visually impaired or reading disabled with books, magazines, and special publications in Braille, Large Print and in Audio format.

8696 Lighthouse International
111 E 59th St
New York, NY 10022-1202 212-821-9200
800-829-0500
FAX: 212-821-9707
TTY: 212-821-9713
e-mail: info@lighthouse.org
www.lighthouse.org

Ralph Caprio, Director, Facilities
Leslie Jones, Executive Director, Music School
William H. Seiple, PhD, Vice President of Research
Mark G. Ackermann, President and Chief Executive Officer
Since 1905, Lighthouse International has led the charge in the fight against vision loss through prevention, treatment and empowerment. Our founders, Winifred and Edith Holt, blazed a trail of firsts and opened up new doors of opportunity for people without sight. Today, we're proud to continue the Holt legacy on behalf of all those who look to the Lighthouse as a beacon of hope today - and will for many years to come.

8697 Lions Clubs International
300 W 22nd St
Oak Brook, IL 60523-8842 630-571-5466
FAX: 630-571-8890
TTY:630-571-6533
e-mail: lions@lionsclubs.org
www.lionsclubs.org

Benedict Ancar, Director
Jui-Tai Chang, Director
Jaime Garcia Cepeda, Director
Kalle Elster, Director
Our 46,000 clubs and 1.35 million members make us the world's largest service club organization. We're also one of the most effective. Our members do whatever is needed to help their local communities. Everywhere we work, we make friends. With children who need eyeglasses, with seniors who don't have enough to eat and with people we may never meet.

8698 Macular Degeneration Foundation
PO Box 531313
Henderson, NV 89053-1313 702-450-2908
888-633-3937
e-mail: liz@eyesight.org
www.eyesight.org

Liz Trauernicht, President/Director of Communications
Julie Zavala, VP/Asst Director of Operations
David Seftel, M.D., MBA, Executive Vice President/Director of Research Development
Ron Gallemore, Board Of Scientific Advisors
The Macular Degeneration Foundation is dedicated to those who have and will develop macular degeneration. We offer this growing community the latest information, news, hope and encouragement.

8699 National Alliance of Blind Students NABS Liaison
American Council of the Blind
1155 15th St NW
Ste 1004
Washington, DC 20005-2706 202-467-5081
800-424-8666
FAX: 202-467-5085
e-mail: info@acb.org
www.acb.org

Jill Gaus, President
Lynn Jansen, Vice President
Debby Lieberman, Secretary
Mike Reese, Treasurer
A student affiliate of the American Council of the Blind which is a national organization of blind and visually impaired high school and college students who believe that every blind and visually impaired student has the right to an equal and accessible education. Also encourages blind and visually impaired students to challenge their limits and reach their potential.

8700 National Association for Parents of Children with Visual Impairments (NAPVI)
PO Box 317
Watertown, MA 02471-317 617-972-7441
800-562-6265
FAX: 617-972-7444
e-mail: spedex.com@gmail.com
www.spedex.com/napvi

Susan LaVenture, Executive Director
Julie Urban, President
Venetia Hayden, Vice President
Kim Alfonso, Treasurer
A non profit organization of, by and for parents committed to providing support to the parents of children who have visual impairments . Also a national organization that enables parents to find information and resources for their children who are blind or visually impaired including those with additional disabilities. NAPVI also provides leadership, support, and training to assist parents in helping children reach their potential.

8701 National Association for Visually Handicapped (NAVH)
111 E 59th S
Fl 6
New York, NY 10022-1202 212-889-3141
800-829-0500
FAX: 212-821-9707
TTY: 212-821-9713
e-mail: info@lighthouse.org
www.lighthouse.org/navh

Mark G Ackerman, President & CEO
Barbara Gyde, Vice President
Ralph Caprio, Director
Karen Campbell, LCSW, Director of Social Services
NAVH is unique in the services it offers to the hard of seeing™ worldwide and is the only non-profit organization solely dedicated to providing assistance to this population. NAVH runs senior support groups, provides individual consultations, informational materials, training in the use of visual aids, and numerous other tools to ensure that the visually impaired can remain independent and lead fulfilling lives.

8702 National Association of Blind Educators
National Federation of the Blind
200 East Wells St
Baltimore, MD 21230-4914 410-659-9314
FAX: 410-685-5653
e-mail: nfb@nfb.org
www.nfb.org

Marc Maurer, CEO
Membership organization of blind teachers, professors and instructors in all levels of education. Provides support and information regarding professional responsibilities, classroom techniques, national testing methods and career obstacles. Publishes The Blind Educator, national magazine specifically for blind educators.

8703 National Association of Blind Lawyers
National Federation of the Blind
1660 South Albion Street
Denver, CO 80222-4046 303-504-5979
FAX: 303-757-3640
e-mail: slabarre@labarrelaw.com
www.nfb.org

Scott LaBarre, President
Membership organization of blind attorneys, law students, judges and others in the law field. Provides support and information regarding employment, techniques used by the blind, advocacy, laws affecting the blind, current information about the American Bar Association and other issues for blind lawyers.

8704 National Association of Blind Merchants
National Federation of the Blind
1837 S.Nevada Avenue
PMB #243
Colorado Springs, CO 80905-4286 719-423-2384
888-691-1819
866-543-6808
e-mail: kevanwirkey@blindmerchants.org
www.blindmerchants.org

Kevan Worley, President
Membership organization of blind persons employed in either self-employment work or the Randolph-Sheppard vending program. Provides information regarding rehabilitation, social security, tax and other issues which directly affect blind merchants. Serves as advocacy and support group.

8705 National Association of Blind Secretaries and Transcribers
National Federation of the Blind
200 East Wells St
Baltimore, MD 21230-4914 410-659-9314
FAX: 410-685-5653
e-mail: nfb@nfb.org
www.nfb.org

Marc Maurer, CEO
Membership organization of blind secretaries and transcribers at all levels, including medical and paralegal transcription, office workers, customer-service personnel and many other similar fields. Addresses issues such as technology, accomodation, career planning and job training.

8706 National Association of Blind Students
National Federation of the Blind
200 East Wells St
Baltimore, MD 21230-4914 410-659-9314
FAX: 410-685-5653
e-mail: nfb@nfb.org
www.nfb.org

Marc Maurer, CEO
For over 30 years this national organization of blind students has provided support, information, and encouragement to blind college and university students. NABS leads the way in offering resources in issues such as national testing, accessible textbooks and materials, overcoming negative attitudes about blindness from school personnel, developing new techniques of accomplishing laboratory or field assignments, and many other college experiences.

8707 National Association of Blind Teachers
American Council of the Blind
1155 15th St NW
Ste 1004
Washington, DC 20005-2706 202-467-5081
800-424-8666
FAX: 202-467-5085
e-mail: johnbuckley25@hotmail.com
www.blindteachers.net

Jill Gaus, President
Lynn Jansen, Vice President
Debby Lieberman, Secretary
Mike Reese, Treasurer
Works to advance the teaching profession for blind and visually impaired people, protects the interest of teachers, presents discussions and solutions for special problems encountered by blind teachers and publishes a directory of blind teachers in the US.

8708 National Association of Guide Dog Users
National Federation of the Blind
1003 Papaya Dr
Tampa, FL 33619-4629 813-626-2789
800-558-8261
888-624-3841
e-mail: president@nagdu.org
www.nagdu.org

Marion Gwizdala, President
Provides information and support for guide dog users and works to secure high standards in guide dog training. Addresses issues of discrimination of guide dog users and offers public education about guide dog use. Biennial newsletter available: Harness Up!

8709 National Association to Promote the Use of Braille
National Federation of the Blind
39481 Gallaudet Dr
Apt 127
Fremont, CA 94538 510-248-0100
877-558-6524
FAX: 818-344-7930
e-mail: mwillows@sbcglobal.net
www.nfbcal.org

Nadine Jacobson, President
Robert Jaquiss, Vice President
Linda Mentink, Second Vice President
Jennifer Dunnam, Secretary
Dedicated to securing improved Braille instruction, increasing the number of braille materials available to the blind and providing information of braille in securing independence, education and employment for the blind.

8710 National Braille Association
95 Allens Creek Rd
Bldg 1 Ste 202
Rochester, NY 14618- 3252 585-427-8260
FAX: 585-427-0263
e-mail: nbaoffice@nationalbraille.org
www.nationalbraille.org

David Shaffar, Executive Director
Jan Carroll, President
Whitney Gregory-Williams, Vice President
Heidi Lehmann, Secretary
The only national organization dedicated to the professional development of individuals who prepare and produce braille materials.

8711 National Braille Press
88 Saint Stephen St
Boston, MA 02115-4312 617-266-6160
888-965-8965
888-965-8965
FAX: 617-437-0456
e-mail: contact@nbp.org
www.nbp.org

Brian A. Mac Donald, President
Kimberley Ballard, Vice President
Tony Grima, Vice President of Braille Publications
Diane L. Croft, Publisher

The guiding purposes of National Braille Press are to promote the literacy of blind children through braille, and to provide access to information that empowers blind people to actively engage in work, family, and community affairs.

8712 National Center for Vision and Child Development
Lighthouse International
111 E 59th St
New York, NY 10022-1202
212-821-9200
800-829-0500
FAX: 212-821-9707
TTY: 212-821-9713
e-mail: info@lighthouse.org
www.lighthouse.org

Mark G Ackerman, President/CEO
Barbara Gyde, Vice President
Ralph Caprio, Director
The worldwide leader in helping people of all ages who are blind or partially sighted overcome the challenges of vision loss.

8713 National Diabetes Action Network for the Blind
National Federation of the Blind
1212 London Dr
Columbia, MO 65203-2012
573-875-8911
e-mail: ebryant@socket.net
www.nfb.org

Ed Bryant, Manager
Leading support and information organization of persons losing vision due to diabetes. Provides personal contact and resource information with other blind diabetics about non-visual techniques of independently managing diabetes, monitoring glucose levels, measuring insulin and other matters concerning diabetes. Publishes Voice of the Diabetic, the leading publication about diabetes and blindness.

8714 National Eye Institute
31 Center Drive MSC 2510
Bethesda, MD 20892-2510
301-496-5248
FAX: 301-402-1065
e-mail: 2020@nei.nih.gov
www.nei.nih.gov

Paul A Sieving MD PhD, Director
To conduct and support research for blinding eye diseases, visual disorders, mechanisms of visual function, and the preservation of sight.

8715 National Federation of the Blind
200 East Wells Street
at Jernigan Place
Baltimore, MD 21230-4998
410-659-9314
FAX: 410-685-5653
e-mail: nfb@nfb.org
nfb.org

John Berggren, Executive Director for Operation
John G. Paré Jr., Executive Director for Strategic Initiatives
Mark Riccobono, Executive Director, NFB Jernigan Institute
Joanne Wilson, Executive Director for Affiliate Action
The National Federation of the Blind (NFB) is the largest organization of the blind in the world. The Federation's purpose is to help blind people achieve self-confidence, self-respect, and self-determination. Their goal is the complete integration of the blind into society on a basis of equality.

8716 National Industries for the Blind
1310 Braddock Pl
Alexandria, VA 22314-1691
703-310-0500
FAX: 703-998-8268
e-mail: info@nib.org
www.nfb.org

Gary J. Krump, Chairperson
Ronald Tascarella, Vice Chairperson
Kristin Graham Koehler, Secretary
A nonprofit organization that represents over 100 associated industries serving people who are blind in thirty-six states. These agencies serve people who are blind or visually impaired and help them to reach their full potential. Services include job and family counseling, job skills training, instruction in Braille and other communication skills, children's programs and more.

8717 National Organization of Parents of Blind Children
National Federation of the Blind
200 East Wells St
Baltimore, MD 21230-4914
410-659-9314
FAX: 410-685-5653
e-mail: jim@riversedgehomes.com
www.nfb.org

Carlton Walker,, President
Barbara Cheadle,, President Emerita
Stephanie Kieszak-Holloway, First Vice-President
Andrea Beasley, Secretary
Support information and advocacy organization of parents of blind or visually impaired children. Addresses issues ranging from help to parents of a newborn blind infant, mobility and braille instruction, education, social and community participation, development of self confidence and other vital factors involved in growth of a blind child.

8718 New Eyes for the Needy
549 Millburn Avenue
PO Box 332
Short Hills, NJ 07078-332
973-376-4903
FAX: 973-376-3807
e-mail: neweyesfortheneedy@verizon.net
www.neweyesfortheneedy.org

Susan Dyckman, Executive Director
Marianne Muench Busby, Vice President
Barbara Daney, Treasurer
Suzanne Escousee, Secretary
New Eyes provides new prescription glasses for poor children and adults in the U.S. through a voucher system.

8719 Prevent Blindness America
211 W Wacker Drive
Suite 1700
Chicago, IL 60606
312-363-6001
800-331-2020
FAX: 312-363-6052
e-mail: info@preventblindness.org
www.preventblindness.org

James E. Anderson, Chair
Kira Baldanado, Director
Arzu Bilazer, Creative Director
Mary Bregantini, Senior Director
The nation's leading volunteer eye health and safety organization dedicated to fighting blindness and saving sight. Also touches the lives of millions of people each year through public and professional education, advocacy, certified vision screening training, community and patient service programs and research.

8720 Services for the Visually Impaired
8720 Georgia Ave
Suite 210
Silver Spring, MD 20910-3614
301-589-0894
FAX: 301-589-0884
e-mail: info@clb.org
www.clb.org

Ann Cook, Executive Director
Anthony J. (Cancelosi, CEO
Provides skills and resources to DC area residents who are blind or experiencing vision loss, and are also committed to helping people regain their indepence and maintaining it.

8721 Society For The Blind
1238 S Street
Sacramento, CA 95811
916-452-8271
FAX: 916-492-2483
e-mail: info@societyfortheblind.org
societyfortheblind.org

Shari Roeseler, Executive Director
Serving 26 counties in Northern California, Society for the Blind is a full service, nonprofit, agency providing services and programs for people who are blind or have low vision.

8722 **The Seeing Eye**
10 Washington Valley Rd
PO Box 375
Morristown, NJ 07963-0375
973-539-4425
FAX: 973-539-0922
e-mail: info@seeingeye.org
www.seeingeye.org

Peggy Gibbon,, Director of Canine Development
James A Kutsch Jr, President/CEO
Dolores Holle, VMD,, Director of Canine Medicine & Surgery
Randall Ivens, Director of Human Resources

An organization that concentrates on its mission to enhance the independence, dignity, and self confidence of blind people through the use of seeing eye dogs. The Seeing Eye will be an organization that concentrates on its mission to enhance the independence, dignity, and self confidence of blind people through the use of Seeing Eye dogs, and on improving its ability to fulfill this mission. We will maintain and nuture the spirit of our founders and adhere to the highest standards of respect

8723 **United States Association of Blind Athletes**
1 Olympic Plaza
Colorado Springs, CO 80909-3508
719-866-3224
FAX: 719-866-3400
e-mail: mlucas@usaba.org
www.usaba.org

Mark A. Lucas, Executive Director
Ryan Ortiz, Assistant Executive Director
John Potts, Goalball High Performance Director
Lacey Markle, Public Relations and Events Coordinator

USABA is a Colorado-based 501(c) (3) organization that provides life-enriching sports opportunities for every individual with a visual impairment. A member of the U.S. Olympic Committee, USABA provides athletic opportunities in various sports including, but not limited to track and field, nordic and alpine skiing, biathlon, judo, wrestling, swimming, tandem cycling, powerlifting and goalball (a team sport for the blind and visually impaired).

8724 **Vermont Association for the Blind and Visually Impaired**
60 Kimball Ave
South Burlington, VT 05403
802-863-1358
800-639-5861
FAX: 802-863-1481
e-mail: general@vabvi.org
www.vabvi.org

James Mooney, President
Thomas Chase, Vice President
Debbie Balserus, Secretary
Patricia Henderson, Treasurer

The Vermont Association for the Blind and Visually Impaired (VABVI), a non-profit organization founded in 1926, is the only private agency to offer free training, services and support to visually impaired Vermonters. Each year we serve hundreds of children from birth to age 22 and adults age 55 and over.

8725 **Vision World Wide**
Apt 302
5707 Brockton Dr
Indianapolis, IN 46220-5481
317-254-1332
800-431-1739
FAX: 317-251-6588
e-mail: info@visionww.org
www.visionww.org

Patricia L Prince, President

A non profit organization dedicated to improving the lives of the vision impaired through direct interaction and indirectly through the caregiving community. Also serve both the totally blind and those with various degrees and forms of vision loss.

8726 **Visions Center on Blindness (VCB)**
111 Summit Park Rd
Spring Valley, NY 10977-1221
212-625-1616
888-245-8333
FAX: 845-354-5130
e-mail: info@visionsvcb.org
www.visionsvcb.org

Nancy T. Jones, President
Richard P. Simon, Vice President
Burton M. Strauss, Treasurer
Carol Spawn Desmond, Secretary

VISIONS VCB is a 35-acre year round residential rehabilitation and training center in Rockland County, New York, 35 miles north of New York City in the Village of New Hempstead. Since it's founding over 85 years ago, VCB has become one of the largest and most comprehensive overnight training and vision rehabilitation facilities in the United States. Year round on weekends and during summer sessions, VCB serves 600 people of all ages.

8727 **Visually Impaired Veterans of America**
American Council of the Blind
1155 15th St NW
Ste 1004
Washington, DC 20005-2706
202-467-5081
800-424-8666
FAX: 202-467-5085
e-mail: bj2kiowa@worldnet.att.net
www.acb.org

Jill Gaus, President
Lynn Jansen, Vice President
Debby Lieberman, Secretary
Mike Reese, Treasurer

Maintain, promote and foster the well bring and rehabilitation of all visually Impaired Veterans of the Armed Forces of the United States of America who are eligible to receive from the Veterans Administration; develops and encourages the practice of high standards of personal professional conduct among Visually Impaired Veterans; maintain, promote, and foster public confidence and awareness In Visually Impaired Veterans.

8728 **Washington Ear**
12061 Tech Rd
Ste B
Silver Spring, MD 20904-7826
301-681-6636
FAX: 301-625-1986
e-mail: information@washear.org
www.washear.org

George Long, Chairman
Neely Oplinger, Executive Director
Freddie L. Peaco, President
Paul D'Addario, President-Elect

A non profit organization providing reading and information services for blind, visually impaired and physically disabled people who cannot effectively read print, see plays, watch television programs and films, or view museum exhibits. Ear free services strive to substitute hearing for seeing, improving the lives of people with limited or no vision by enabling them to be well-informed, fully productive members of their families, their communities and the working world.

Camps

8729 **Camp Barakel**
P.O.Box 159
Fairview, MI 48621-0159
989-848-2279
FAX: 989-848-2280
e-mail: info@campbarakel.org
www.campbarakel.org

Paul Gardner, Camp Director
Hannah Gardner, Music Coordinator
Jon Ford, Head Lifeguard
Stacy Ford, Adult Program Staff

Five-day Christian camp experience in mid-August for campers ages 18-55 who are physically disabled, visually impaired, upper trainable mentally impaired or educable mentally impaired, bus transportation provided from locations in Lansing, Flint and Bay City, Michigan.

8730 Camp Challenge
8914 US Highway 50 East
Bedford, IN 47421 812-834-5159
e-mail: info@gocampchallenge.com
www.gocampchallenge.com

Maria, Director of Engagement
One and two-week sessions for campers with developmental and or physical disabilities, hearing impairment and the blind/visually impaired. Ages 6-99 and families.

8731 Camp Lawroweld
Northern New England Conference
228 West Side Road
Weld, ME 04285 207-585-2984
FAX: 207-585-2985
e-mail: camplawroweld@gmail.com
www.lawroweld.org

Harry Sabnani, Executive Director
Camp is located in Weld, Maine. Week sessions July for campers who are blind or visually impaired, all ages. Other camps coed, ages 9-16 and families, single adults, June - September.

8732 Camp Lou Henry Hoover
Girl Scouts of Washington Rock Council
201 East Grove Street
Westfield, NJ 07090 908-518-4400
FAX: 908-232-4508
e-mail: girlscouts@gshnj.org
www.gshnj.org

Samantha Basek, Field Executive
Susan Brooks, CEO
Camp is located in Middleville, New Jersey. Sessions for girls who are blind/visually impaired, ages 7-18.

8733 Camp Merrick
PO Box 56
Nanjemoy, MD 20662 301-870-5858
FAX: 301-246-9108
e-mail: info@LionsCampMerrick.org
lionscampmerrick.org

Wayne Magoon, President
Ray Shumaker, Vice President
Julie Andrew, Board Member
Frank Culhane, Treasurer
Programs offered April-January for children who are blind/visually impaired, hearing impaired or diabetic. Coed, ages 6-15.

8734 Camp Winnekeag
257 Ashby Road
Ashburnham, MA 01430 978-827-4455
FAX: 978-827-4551
e-mail: sneconference@sneconline.org
www.campwinnekeag.com

Frank Tochterman, Religious Leader
Camp is located in Ashburnham, Massachusetts. Camping sessions for blind/visually impaired children. Coed, ages 8-16.

8735 Columbia Lighthouse for the Blind Summer Camp
Columbia Lighthouse for the Blind
1825 K Street NorthWest
Suite 1103
Washington, DC 20006 202-454-6400
FAX: 877-595-9228
e-mail: info@clb.org
clb.org

Tony Cancelosi, President
Anthony Cancelosi, CEO
Helps enable the blind or visually impaired to obtain and maintain independence at home, school, work and in the community. Programs and services include early intervention services, training and consultation in assistive technology, career placement services, comprehensive low vision care and a wide range of rehabilitation services. Highly acclaimed summer camp, picnics and holiday activities encourage blind and visualy impaired children to make new friends and experience the joys of childhood.

8736 Easter Seals Oklahoma
701 NorthEast 13th Street
Oklahoma City, OK 73104 405-239-2525
FAX: 405-239-2278
e-mail: sbusch@easterseals oklahoma.org
www.easterseals oklahoma.org

Rodney Burgamy, Chairman
David Adams, Board Member
Kristen Sorocco, Secretary
Jeb Reid, Treasurer
Adult day health center, and child development center.

8737 Enchanted Hills Camp for the Blind
Lighthouse for the Blind
214 Van Ness Avenue
San Francisco, CA 94102 415-431-1481
888-400-8933
FAX: 415-863-7568
e-mail: info@lighthouse-sf.org
lighthouse-sf.org

Joshua A. Miele, President
Chris Downey, 1st Vice President
Gena Harper, Secretary
Joseph Chan, Treasurer
Camp is located in Napa, California. Half-week, one and two-week sessions for blind, deaf/blind children and adults, ages 5 and up. This program offers a basic camping experience. Activities include music, art, dance, hiking and riding. Camperships are available to California residents.

8738 Highbrook Lodge
PO Box 1988
1909 East 101st Street
Cleveland, OH 44106- 8696 216-791-8118
FAX: 216-791-1101
www.clevelandsightcenter.org

William L. Spring, Chair
Thomas P. Furnas, 1st Vice Chair
Gary W. Poth, Treasurer
Sheryl King Benford, Secretary
Camp is located in Chardon, Ohio. Summer sessions for children, adults and familieswho are blind or have low vision. There are seven sessions held annually through June, July and August with an wide range of outdoor camp activities. Camp activities focus on gaining independent skills, mobility, orientation and self confidence in an accessable and traditional camp setting.
220-660/session

8739 Indian Creek Camp
Kentucky Tennessee Conference
150 Cabin Circle Drive
Liberty, TN 37095 615-548-4411
FAX: 615-548-4029
e-mail: info@indiancreekcamp.com
www.indiancreekcamp.com

Ken Wetmore, Director
Marty Sutton, Asst. Director
Toni Stephens, Program Director
Stephanie Rufo, Public Relations Director
Camp is located in Liberty, Tennessee. Summer sessions for children and adults who are blind/visually impaired. Coed, ages 7-17, families and seniors.

8740 Kamp A-Komp-Plish
9035 Ironsides Rd
Nanjemoy, MD 20662-3432 301-870-3226
301-934-3590
FAX: 301-870-2620
e-mail: recreation@melwood.org
www.kampakomplish.org

Jonathan Rondeau, Chief Program Officer
Bekah Carmichael, Director
Doria Fleisher, Associate Director
Marisa Cucuzella, Assistant Director

Camp is located in Nanjemoy, Maryland. Half-week, one-week and two-week sessions for blind/visually impaired children and those with developmental disabilities and mobility limitation. Coed, ages 8-16.

8741 Kamp Kaleo
46872 Willow Springs Road
Burwell, NE 68823 308-346-5083
e-mail: kampkaleo@gmail.com
www.kampkaleo.com

Gaylene O'Brien, Administrator
Sandy Denton, Minister Of Faith Development
Camp is located in Burwell, Nebraska. Summer sessions for campers who are blind/visually impaired or have developmental disabilities. Coed, ages 9-18 and families, seniors, single adults.

8742 National Camp for Blind Children
Christian Record Services
P.O. Box 6097
Lincoln, NE 68506-0097 402-488-0981
FAX: 402-488-7582
e-mail: infochristianrecord.org
www.christianrecord.org

Dan Jackson, Chair
Tom Lemon, Vice Chair
Larry Pitcher, President, Secretary
Al Burdick, Board Member
To enrich lives of those who are blind, visually impaired or physically challenged regardless of race, creed, economic status or gender. Also encourages each camper to achieve greater self-esteem and self confidence while seeking to excel in the use of his/her physical, mental, and spiritual capacities. Provides fee Christian publications and programs for people with visual impairments.
Monthly

8743 National Camps for Blind Children
Christian Record Services
P.O. Box 6097
Lincoln, NE 68506-0097 402-488-0981
FAX: 402-488-7582
e-mail: info@christianrecord.org
blindcamps.com

Dan Jackson, Chair
Tom Lemon, Vice Chair
Larry Pitcher, President, Secretary
Al Burdick, Board Member
Provides free Christian publications and programs, as well as new opportunities for people with visual impairments. Free services include subscription magazines available in braille, large print and audio cassette, full-vision books combining braille and print, lending library, gift bibles and study guides in braille, large print and audio cassette, national camps for blind children and scholarship assistance for blind young people trying to obtain a college education.

8744 Texas Lions Camp
Lions Club Of Texas
P.O.Box 290247
Kerrville, TX 78029 830-896-8500
FAX: 830-896-3666
e-mail: tlc@ktc.com
www.lionscamp.com

Stephen Mabry, Executive Director
The primary purpose of the League shall be to provide, without charge, a camp for physically disabled, hearing/vision impaired and diabetic children from the State of Texas, regardless of race, religion, or national origin. Our goal is to create an atmosphere wherein campers will learn the can do philosophy and be allowed to achieve maximum personal growth and self-esteem. The camp welcomes boys and girls ages 7-16.

8745 VISIONS Vacation Camp for the Blind
VISIONS Center on Blindness
111 Summit Park Road
Spring Valley, NY 10977 212-625-1616
888-245-8333
FAX: 845-354-5130
e-mail: cthorne@visionsvcb.org
www.visionsvcb.org

Nancy T. Jones, President
Richard P. Simon, Vice President
Burton M. Strauss, Treasurer
Carol Spawn Desmond, Secretary
Is a non profit agency that promotes the independence of people of all ages who are blind or visually imparied. Camp offers braille classes, computers with large print and voice output, support groups, discussions, mobility lessions, cooking classes, personal and home management training, large print and Braille books.

8746 Wendell Johnson Speech And Hearing Clinic
University Of Iowa
250 Hawkins Dr
Iowa City, IA 52242-1025 319-335-8736
FAX: 319-335-8851
e-mail: kathy-miller@uiowa.edu
www.uiowa.edu

Chuck Wieland, President
Hans Hoerschelman, Vice President
Josh Smith, Budget Officer
Shannon Lizakowski, Secretary
The clinic offers assessment and intervention for communication disorders in adults and children as well as an audiology clinic. The clinic also offers several summer programs for children with hearing, speech, language, autism and/or reading disorders, including a summer residential program for teens who stutter.

8747 YMCA Camp Chingachgook on Lake George
Capital District YMCA
1872 Pilot Knob Road
Kattskill Bay, NY 12844 518-656-9462
FAX: 518-656-9362
e-mail: chingachgook@cdymca.org
www.cdymca.org

George Painter, Executive Director
Billy Rankin, Senior Program Director
Dan Poole, Adventure Trip Director
Carol Lewis, Office Manager
Sailing programs for people with disabilities. Sessions for campers who are blind/visually impaired. Coed, ages 7-16, families, seniors and single adults.

Print: Books

8748 AFB Directory of Services for Blind and Visually Impaired Persons in the US and Canada
American Foundation for the Blind/AFB Press
2 Penn Plaza
Suite 1102
New York, NY 10121 212-502-7600
800-232-5463
FAX: 888-545-8331
e-mail: afbinfo@afb.net
www.afb.org

Carl Augusto, President & Chief Executive Officer
Rick Bozeman, Finance Director, Chief Financial Officer
Kelly Bleach, Chief Administrative Officer
Stacy Rollins, Executive Administrative Assistant to the President
Comprehensive print resource containing more that 2,500 local, state, regional, and national services throughout the US and Canada for persons who are blind or visually impaired. *$79.95*
624 pages Paperback/onlin
ISBN 0-891288-05-3

8749 About Children's Eyes
National Association for Visually Handicapped
111 East 59th Street
New York, NY 10022-1202
212-821-9384
800-829-0500
FAX: 212-821-9707
e-mail: info@lighthouse.org
lighthouse.org/navh

Mark G. Ackermann, President / CEO

How to identify the child with a visual problem. LightHouse acquired NAVH.

8750 About Children's Vision: A Guide for Parents
National Association for Visually Handicapped
111 East 59th Street
New York, NY 10022-1202
212-821-9384
800-829-0500
FAX: 212-821-9707
e-mail: info@lighthouse.org
lighthouse.org/navh

Mark G. Ackermann, President / CEO

Offers a better understanding of the normal and possible abnormal development of a child's eyesight. LightHouse acquired NAVH. *$.50*

8751 Access to Art: A Museum Directory for Blind and Visually Impaired People
American Foundation for the Blind/AFB Press
2 Penn Plaza
Suite 1102
New York, NY 10121
212-502-7600
800-232-5463
FAX: 888-545-8331
e-mail: afbinfo@afb.net
www.afb.org

Carl R. Augusto, President & Chief Executive Officer
Rick Bozeman, Finance Director, Chief Financial Officer
Kelly Bleach, Chief Administrative Officer
Stacy Rollins, Executive Administrative Assistant to the President

Details the access facilities of over 300 museums, galleries and exhibits in the United States. Also included are organizations offering art-related resources such as, art classes, competitions and traveling exhibits. *$19.95*
144 pages Large Print
ISBN 0-891281-56-8

8752 African Americans in the Profession of Blindness Services
Mississippi State University
P.O.Box 6189
Mississippi State, MS 39762
662-325-2001
FAX: 662-325-8989
TTY:662-325-2694
e-mail: nrtc@colled.msstate.edu
www.blind.msstate.edu

Jacqui Bybee, Research Associate II
Douglas Bedsaul, Research and Training Coordinator
Anne Carter, Research and Training Coordinator
Brenda Cavenaugh, Ph.D., Research Professor

This study investigated the level of participation by African Americans in vocational rehab. (VR) services to persons who are visually impaired. Using surveys and interviews with all state VR directors, national census data and national RSA data, it was found nationally that African Americans are substantially under-represented in the service provider ranks, yet over-represented as clients. *$20.00*
61 pages Paperback

8753 Age-Related Macular Degeneration
National Association for Visually Handicapped
111 East 59th Street
New York, NY 10022-1202
212-821-9384
800-829-0500
FAX: 212-821-9707
e-mail: info@lighthouse.org
lighthouse.org/navh

Mark G. Ackermann, President / CEO

A large booklet offering information and up-to-date research on Macular Degeneration. Also available in Russian. Revised in 2007. LightHouse acquired NAVH. *$5.00*

8754 American Anals of the Deaf Reference
800 Florida Ave NE
Washington, DC 20002-3600
202-651-5530
FAX: 202-651-5489
e-mail: gupress@gallaudet.edu
gupress.gallaudet.edu/annals

Stephanie Cawthon, Ph.D., Book Review Editor
Peter V. Paul, Ph.D., Editor, Literary Issues
Ye Wang, Ph.D., Senior Associate Editor
Feifei Ye, Ph.D., Associate Editor for Research Methodology

The controlled scope of GUPress operations allows the continuance of a highly focused commitment to individual titles that has contributed significantly to its 20 years of leadership in publishing on Deaf issues. Gallaudet University Press brings unmatched experience and knowledge to the marketplace for books on and for the Deaf community, its advocates, and scholars invested in the study of deaf society.

8755 Americans with Disabilities Act Guide for Places of Lodging: Serving Guests Who Are Blind
US Department of Justice
950 Pennsylvania Avenue NorthWest
Washington, DC 20530
202-307-0663
800-574-0301
FAX: 202-307-1197
TTY: 800-514-0383
www.ada.gov

Rebecca B. Bond, Chief
Zita Johnson Betts, Deputy Chief
Sally Conway, Deputy Chief
James Bostrom, Deputy Chief

A 12-page publication explaining what hotels, motels, and other places of transient lodging can do to accommodate guests who are blind or have low vision.

8756 Art and Science of Teaching Orientation and Mobility to Persons with Visual Impairments
American Foundation for the Blind/AFB Press
2 Penn Plaza
Suite 1102
New York, NY 10121
212-502-7600
800-232-5463
FAX: 888-545-8331
e-mail: afbinfo@afb.net
www.afb.org

Carl R. Augusto, President & Chief Executive Officer
Rick Bozeman, Finance Director, Chief Financial Officer
Kelly Bleach, Chief Administrative Officer
Stacy Rollins, Executive Administrative Assistant to the President

Comprehensive decription of the techniques of teaching orientation and mobility, presented along with considerations and strategies for sensitive and effective teaching. Hardcover. Paperback also available. *$48.00*
200 pages
ISBN 0-891282-45-9

8757 Awareness Training
Landmark Media
3450 Slade Run Drive
Falls Church, VA 22042
703-241-2030
800-342-4336
FAX: 703-536-9540
e-mail: info@landmarkmedia.com
landmarkmedia.com

Michael Hartogs, President
Peter Hartogs, VP New Business & Development
Richard Hartogs, VP Acquisitions
Beverly Weisenberg, Sales Representative

Covers disabilities of various types — vision, hearing, speech disorders, loss of limbs, loss of mobility, or mental/emotional limitations and how to integrate such individuals into various business and educational settings. It is a 4-part series designed to

identify and enable others to interact effectively with those suffering such disabilities. *$495.00*
Set of 4

8758 Babycare Assistive Technology
Through the Looking Glass
3075 Adeline Street
Suite 120
Berkeley, CA 94703
510-848-1112
800-644-2666
FAX: 510-848-4445
e-mail: tlg@lookingglass.org
www.lookingglass.org

Maureen Block, J.D., President
Thomas Spalding, Treasurer
Alice Nemon, Secretary
Mega Kirshbaum, Author
Available in braille, large print or cassette. Provides an overview of the baby care assistive technology work at Through The Looking Glass including a discussion of TLG's intervention model, the impact of babycare equipment and guidelines for equipment development. *$2.00*
8 pages

8759 Babycare Assistive Technology for Parents with Physical Disabilties
Through the Looking Glass
3075 Adeline Street
Suite 120
Berkeley, CA 94703
510-848-1112
800-644-2666
FAX: 510-848-4445
e-mail: tlg@lookingglass.org
www.lookingglass.org

Maureen Block, J.D., President
Thomas Spalding, Treasurer
Alice Nemon, Secretary
Mega Kirshbaum, Author
Examines the provision of babycare equipment through the lens of ithe infant/parent relationship, the lens of the family system, and through the lens of culture. Availiable in braille, large print or cassette. *$2.00*
7 pages

8760 Basic Course in American Sign Language
TJ Publishers
P.O. Box 702701
Dallas, TX 75370
972-416-0800
800-999-1168
FAX: 972-416-0944
TTY: 301-585-4440
e-mail: TJPubinc@aol.com
www.tjpublishers.com/

Tom Humphries, Author
Carol Padden, Co-Author
Terrance J O'Rourke, Co-Author
Accompanying videotapes and textbooks include voice translations. Hearing students can analyze sound for initial instruction, or opt to turn off the sound to sharpen visual acuity. Package includes the Basic Course in American Sign Language text, Student Study Guide, the original four 1-hour videotapes plus the ABCASI Vocabulary videotape. *$139.95*
280 pages

8761 Behavioral Vision Approaches for Persons with Physical Disabilities
Optometric Extension Program Foundation
7754 Braegger Road
Three Lakes, WI 54562
714-250-0176

e-mail: Info@depf.org
www.depf.org

Kristin R. Jungbluth, President
Eric J. Lindberg, VP
Barbara Kuntz, Secretary
Patricia S. Lindberg, Treasurer
A discussion of the behavioral vision/neuro-motor approach to providing directions for prescriptive and therapeutic services for the visually handicapped child or adult. *$49.50*
197 pages

8762 Belonging
Dial Books
375 Hudson St
New York, NY 10014-3657
212-366-2000
FAX: 212-414-3394
www.penguin.com/
Deborah Kent, Author
Meg attended special schools for the blind until she was ready for high school. She decided that she wanted to go to a regular high school. She and her mother practiced her walks to school and studied the layout of the building prior to school starting, but Meg was unprepared for the trip when there were 1,500 students. She adjusted quickly to the crowds and the pace of the new school.
200 pages Hardcover
ISBN 0-80370 -30-1

8763 Berthold Lowenfeld on Blindness and Blind People
American Foundation for the Blind/AFB Press
2 Penn Plaza
Suite 1102
New York, NY 10121
212-502-7600
800-232-5463
FAX: 888-545-8331
e-mail: afbinfo@afb.net
www.afb.org

Carl R. Augusto, President & Chief Executive Officer
Rick Bozeman, Finance Director, Chief Financial Officer
Kelly Bleach, Chief Administrative Officer
Stacy Rollins, Executive Administrative Assistant to the President
These writings of the pioneering educator, author and advocate range over a forty-year period include various ground-breaking papers for the blind educator, a rememberance of Helen Keller and other essays on education, sociology and history. *$21.95*
254 pages Paperback
ISBN 0-891281-01-0

8764 Blind and Vision-Impaired Individuals
Mainstream
Ste 830
3 Bethesda Metro Ctr
Bethesda, MD 20814-6301
301-961-9299
800-247-1380
FAX: 301-654-6714
e-mail: info@mainstreaminc.org
Charles Moster
Mainstreaming blind individuals into the workplace. *$ 2.50*
12 pages

8765 Blindness and Early Childhood Development Second Edition
American Foundation for the Blind/AFB Press
2 Penn Plaza
Suite 1102
New York, NY 10121
212-502-7600
800-232-5463
FAX: 888-545-8331
e-mail: afbinfo@afb.net
afb.org

Carl R. Augusto, President & Chief Executive Officer
Rick Bozeman, Finance Director, Chief Financial Officer
Kelly Bleach, Chief Administrative Officer
Stacy Rollins, Executive Administrative Assistant to the President
A review of current knowledge on motor and locomotor development, perceptual development, language and cognitive processes, and social, emotional and personality development. Paperback. *$34.95*
384 pages
ISBN 0-891281-23-8

8766 **Blindness: What it is, What it Does and How to Live with it**
American Foundation for the Blind/AFB Press
2 Penn Plaza
Suite 1102
New York, NY 10121
212-502-7600
800-232-5463
FAX: 888-545-8331
e-mail: afbinfo@afb.net
www.afb.org
Carl R. Augusto, President & Chief Executive Officer
Rick Bozeman, Finance Director, Chief Financial Officer
Kelly Bleach, Chief Administrative Officer
Stacy Rollins, Executive Administrative Assistant to the President
A classic work on how blindness affects self-perception and social interaction and what can be done to restore basic skills, mobility, daily living and an appreciation of life's pleasures. *$15.95*
396 pages Paperback
ISBN 0-891282-05-

8767 **Books are Fun for Everyone**
Nat'l Lib Svc/Blind And Physically Handicapped
1291 Taylor Street North West
Washington, DC 20011
202-707-5100
FAX: 202-707-0712
TTY:202-707-0744
e-mail: nls@loc.gov
www.loc.gov/nls
Karen Keninger, Director

8768 **Books for Blind & Physically Handicapped Individuals**
Nat'l Lib Svc/Blind And Physically Handicapped
1291 Taylor Street North West
Washington, DC 20011
202-707-5100
FAX: 202-707-0712
TTY:202-707-0744
e-mail: nls@loc.gov
www.loc.gov/nls
Karen Keninger, Director
A free national library program of braille and recorded materials for blind and physically handicapped persons.

8769 **Books for Blind and Physically Handicapped Individuals**
Nat'l Lib Svc/Blind And Physically Handicapped
1291 Taylor Street North West
Washington, DC 20011
202-707-5100
FAX: 202-707-0712
TTY:202-707-0744
e-mail: nls@loc.gov
www.loc.gov/nls
Karen Keninger, Director
A free national library program of braille and recorded materials for blind and physically handicapped persons is administered by the National Library Service for the Blind and Physically Handicapped Library of Congress.
Annual

8770 **Braille Book Bank, Music Catalog**
National Braille Association
95 Allens Creek Road
Building 1, Suite 202
Rochester, NY 14618
585-427-8260
FAX: 585-427-0263
e-mail: nbaoffice@nationalbraille.org
www.nationalbraille.org
Jan Carroll, President
Cindi Laurent, Vice President
David Shaffer, Executive Director
Heidi Lehmann, Secretary
Offers hundreds of musical titles in print form, braille and on cassette.
62 pages

8771 **Braille: An Extraordinary Volunteer Opportunity**
Nat'l Lib Svc/Blind And Physically Handicapped
1291 Taylor Street North West
Washington, DC 20011
202-707-5100
FAX: 202-707-0712
TTY:202-707-0744
e-mail: nls@loc.gov
www.loc.gov/nls
Karen Keninger, Director

8772 **Burns Braille Transcription Dictionary**
American Foundation for the Blind/AFB Press
2 Penn Plaza
Suite 1102
New York, NY 10121
212-502-7600
800-232-5463
FAX: 888-545-8331
e-mail: afbinfo@afb.net
afb.org
Carl R. Augusto, President & Chief Executive Officer
Rick Bozeman, Finance Director, Chief Financial Officer
Kelly Bleach, Chief Administrative Officer
Stacy Rollins, Executive Administrative Assistant to the President
A handy, portable guide that is a quick reference for anyone who needs to check print-to-braille and braille-to-print meanings and symbols. Paperback. *$21.95*
96 pages 96 pages
ISBN 0-891282-32-7

8773 **Can't Your Child See? A Guide for Parents of Visually Impaired Children**
Sage Publications
2455 Teller Road
Thousand Oaks, CA 91320
805-499-0721
800-818-7243
FAX: 805-499-0871
e-mail: info@sagepub.com
www.sagepub.com
Sara Miller McCune, Founder, Publisher, Executive Chairman
Blaise R Simqu, President & CEO
Tracey A. Ozmina, Executive Vice President & Chief Operating Officer
Stephen Barr, Managing Director/SAGE London, President of SAGE Internation
This second edition offers parents optimistic, practical guidelines for helping visually impaired children reach their full potential. *$26.00*
279 pages Paperback

8774 **Career Perspectives: Interviews with Blindand Visually Impaired Professionals**
American Foundation for the Blind/AFB Press
2 Penn Plaza
Suite 1102
New York, NY 10121
212-502-7600
800-232-5463
FAX: 888-545-8331
e-mail: afbinfo@afb.net
afb.org
Carl R. Augusto, President & Chief Executive Officer
Rick Bozeman, Finance Director, Chief Financial Officer
Kelly Bleach, Chief Administrative Officer
Stacy Rollins, Executive Administrative Assistant to the President
Profiles of 20 successful archivers who describe in their own words what it takes to pursue and attain professional success in a sighted world. Available in large print, cassette and braille. *$19.95*
96 pages
ISBN 0-891281-70-2

8775 Careers in Blindness Rehabilitation Services
Mississippi State University
P.O.Box 6189
Mississippi State, MS 39762 662-325-2001
FAX: 662-325-8989
TTY:662-325-2694
e-mail: nrtc@colled.msstate.edu
www.blind.msstate.edu

Jacqui Bybee, Research Associate II
Douglas Bedsaul, Research and Training Coordinator
Anne Carter, Research and Training Coordinator
Brenda Cavenaugh, Ph.D., Research Professor

In a follow-up study in a series examining the substantial under-representation of African Americans as professionals in blindness services, researchers questioned college students about their knowledge, opinions and interests in blindness services. *$15.00*
54 pages Paperback

8776 Cataracts
National Association for Visually Handicapped
111 East 59th Street
New York, NY 10022-1202 212-821-9384
800-829-0500
FAX: 212-821-9707
e-mail: info@lighthouse.org
lighthouse.org/navh

Mark G. Ackermann, President / CEO

A booklet offering information about Cataracts, diagnosis and treatment of this common condition. LightHouse acquired NAVH. *$ 4.00*

8777 Characteristics, Services, & Outcomes of Rehab. Consumers who are Blind/Visually Impaired
Mississippi State University
P.O.Box 6189
Mississippi State, MS 39762 662-325-2001
FAX: 662-325-8989
TTY:662-325-2694
e-mail: nrtc@colled.msstate.edu
www.blind.msstate.edu

Jacqui Bybee, Research Associate II
Douglas Bedsaul, Research and Training Coordinator
Anne Carter, Research and Training Coordinator
Brenda Cavenaugh, Ph.D., Research Professor

Issues regarding the efficacy of separate state agencies providing specialized vocational rehabilitation (VR) services to consumers who are blind have generated spirited discussions within the rehabilitation community throughout the history of the state-federal program. In this monograph, RRTC researches report results of their investigation of services provided to blind consumers in separate and general (combined) rehabilitation agencies. *$20.00*
45 pages Paperback

8778 Childhood Glaucoma: A Reference Guide for Families
NAPVI
1 North Lexington Avenue
White Plains, NY 10601 617-972-7441
800-562-6265
FAX: 617-972-7444
e-mail: napvi@guildhealth.org
www.napvi.org

Julie Urban, President
Venetia Hayden, Vice President
Susan LaVenture, Executive Director
Randi Sher, Secretary

A vaulable tutorial and resource covering all aspects from genetics through diagnosis, sibling relationships and more.
36 pages

8779 Children with Visual Impairments: A Guide For Parents
American Foundation for the Blind/AFB Press
105 East 22nd Street
New York, NY 10010 212-949-4800
childrensaidsociety.org

William D. Weisberg, Ph.D., President & CEO
Drema Brown, VP of Education
Katherine Eckstein, Chief of Staff
Beverly Colon, VP for Health & Wellness

Written by parents and professional, this book presents a comprehensive overview of the issues that are crucial to the healthy development of children with mild to severe visual impaiments. It also offers insight from parents about coping with the emotional aspects of raising a child with special needs. *$16.95*
416 pages
ISBN 0-933149-36-0

8780 Classification of Impaired Vision
National Association for Visually Handicapped
111 East 59th Street
New York, NY 10022-1202 212-821-9384
800-829-0500
FAX: 212-821-9707
e-mail: info@lighthouse.org
lighthouse.org/navh

Mark G. Ackermann, President / CEO

Designed to provide a foundation for a better understanding of teaching reading, writing, and listning skills to students with visual impairments from preschool age through adult levels. LightHouse acquired NAVH. *$57.95*
322 pages
ISBN 0-398066-93-2

8781 Communication Skills for Visually Impaired Learners
Charles C. Thomas
2600 South 1st Street
Springfield, IL 62704 217-789-8980
800-258-8980
FAX: 217-789-9130
e-mail: books@ccthomas.com
ccthomas.com

Michael P. Thomas, President
Randall Harley, Author
Mila Truan, Author
LaRhea Sanford, Author

This book has been designed to provide a foundation for a better understanding of teaching reading, writing, and listening skills to students with visual impairments from preschool age through adult levels. The plan of the book incorporates the latest research findings with the practical experiences learned in the classroom. *$57.95*
322 pages Paperback
ISBN 0-398066-93-2

8782 Comprehensive Examination of Barriers to Employment Among Persons who are Blind or Impaire
Mississippi State University
P.O.Box 6189
Mississippi State, MS 39762 662-325-2001
FAX: 662-325-8989
TTY:662-325-2694
e-mail: nrtc@colled.msstate.edu
www.blind.msstate.edu

Jacqui Bybee, Research Associate II
Douglas Bedsaul, Research and Training Coordinator
Anne Carter, Research and Training Coordinator
Brenda Cavenaugh, Ph.D., Research Professor

A multi-phase research project designed to: identify barriers to employment; identify and develop innovative successful strategies to overcome these barriers; develop methods for others to utilize these strategies; disseminate this information to rehabilitation providers; replicate the use of selected strategies in other settings. *$20.00*
90 pages Paperback

8783 Contrasting Characteristics of Blind and Visually Impaired Clients
Mississippi State University
P.O.Box 6189
Mississippi State, MS 39762 662-325-2001
FAX: 662-325-8989
TTY:662-325-2694
e-mail: nrtc@colled.msstate.edu
www.blind.msstate.edu

Jacqui Bybee, Research Associate II
Douglas Bedsaul, Research and Training Coordinator
Anne Carter, Research and Training Coordinator
Brenda Cavenaugh, Ph.D., Research Professor

This report examines cases in the National Blindness and Low Vision Employment Database to identify and profile environmental and personal characteristics of clients who are blind or visually impaired and who were achieving successful and unsuccessful retention of competitive jobs. A total of 787 cases were analyzed. *$15.00*
44 pages Paperback

8784 Dancing Cheek to Cheek
Blind Children's Center
4120 Marathon Street
Los Angeles, CA 90029-3584 323-664-2153
800-222-3567
FAX: 323-665-3828
e-mail: info@blindchildrenscenter.org
www.blindchildrenscenter.org

Scott E. Schaldenbrand, President
Mark Correa, Board Member
Midge Horton, Executive Director
Pamela Lansky, Co-Author

Beginning social, play and language interactions. *$ 10.00*
23 pages

8785 Development of Social Skills by Blind and Visually Impaired Students
American Foundation for the Blind/AFB Press
2 Penn Plaza
Suite 1102
New York, NY 10121 212-502-7600
800-232-5463
FAX: 888-545-8331
e-mail: afbinfo@afb.net
www.afb.org

Carl R. Augusto, President & Chief Executive Officer
Rick Bozeman, Finance Director, Chief Financial Officer
Kelly Bleach, Chief Administrative Officer
Stacy Rollins, Executive Administrative Assistant to the President

Offers an examination of the social interactions of blind and visually impaired children in mainstreamed settings and the community that highlights the need to teach social interaction skills to children and provide them with support. Paperback. *$45.95*
232 pages
ISBN 0-891282-17-4

8786 Diabetic Retinopathy
National Association for Visually Handicapped
111 East 59th Street
New York, NY 10022-1202 212-821-9384
800-829-0500
FAX: 212-821-9707
e-mail: info@lighthouse.org
lighthouse.org/navh

Mark G. Ackermann, President / CEO

A booklet offering information about Diabetic Retinopathy. LightHouse acquired NAVH.

8787 Diversity and Visual Impairment: The Influence of Race, Gender, Religion and Ethnicity
American Foundation for the Blind
2 Penn Plaza
Suite 1102
New York, NY 10121 212-502-7600
800-232-5463
FAX: 888-545-8331
e-mail: afbinfo@afb.net
www.afb.org

Carl R. Augusto, President & Chief Executive Officer
Rick Bozeman, Finance Director, Chief Financial Officer
Kelly Bleach, Chief Administrative Officer
Stacy Rollins, Executive Administrative Assistant to the President

Cultural, social, ethnic, gender, and religious issues can influence the way an individual perceives and copes with a visual impairment. *$45.95*
480 pages
ISBN 0-891283-83-8

8788 Do You Remember the Color Blue: The Questi Ons Children Ask About Blindness
Viking Books
375 Hudson Street
New York, NY 10014-3657 212-366-2000
FAX: 212-366-2933
e-mail: ecommerce@us.penguingroup.com
www.us.penguingroup.com

John Makinson, Chairman & CEO

The author answers thirteen thought-provoking questions that children have asked her over the years about being blind.
78 pages
ISBN 0-670880-43-4

8789 Don't Lose Sight of Glaucoma
National Eye Institute
2020 Vision Place
Building 31 Room 6a32
Bethesda, MD 20892-3655 301-496-5248
800-869-2020
FAX: 301-402-1065
e-mail: 2020@nei.nih.gov
www.nei.nih.gov

8790 Early Focus: Working with Young Children Who Are Blind or Visually Impaired & Their Families
American Foundation for the Blind/AFB Press
2 Penn Plaza
Suite 1102
New York, NY 10121 212-502-7600
800-232-5463
FAX: 888-545-8331
e-mail: afbinfo@afb.net
www.afb.org

Carl R. Augusto, President & Chief Executive Officer
Rick Bozeman, Finance Director, Chief Financial Officer
Kelly Bleach, Chief Administrative Officer
Stacy Rollins, Executive Administrative Assistant to the President

Describes early intervention techniques used with blind and visually impaired children and stresses the benefits of family involvement and transdisciplinary teamwork. Paperback. *$32.95*
176 pages
ISBN 0-891282-15-7

8791 Encyclopedia of Blindness and Vision Impairment Second Edition
Facts on File
132 West 31st Street
17th Floor
New York, NY 10001 800-322-8755
FAX: 800-678-3633
e-mail: CustServ@InfobaseLearning.com
www.factsonfile.com

Jill Sardenga, Author
Susan Shelly, Co-Author
Alan Shelly MD, Co-Author
Scott M Steidl MD, Co-Author

Designed to provide both laymen and professionals with concise, practical information on the second most common disability in the U.S. *$65.00*
340 pages Hardcover
ISBN 0-816042-80-2

8792 Equals in Partnership: Basic Rights for Families of Children with Blindness
NAPVI
1 North Lexington Avenue
White Plains, NY 10601
617-972-7441
800-562-6265
FAX: 617-972-7444
e-mail: napvi@guildhealth.org
www.napvi.org

Julie Urban, President
Venetia Hayden, Vice President
Susan LaVenture, Executive Director
Randi Sher, Secretary

A comprehensive compilation of educational advocacy materials to help parents better understand the special needs of their children with visual impairments and to assist them in accessing appropriate services for their children.

8793 Eye Research News
Research to Prevent Blindness
645 Madison Avenue
Floor 21
New York, NY 10022-1010
212-752-4333
800-621-0026
FAX: 212-688-6231
e-mail: inforequest@rpbusa.org
www.rpbusa.org

Diane S. Swift, Chair
Brian F. Hofland, PhD, President
David H. Brenner, VP & Secretary
Richard E. Baker, Treasurer & Asst. Secretary

Yearly publication from Research to Prevent Blindness. Free.
4 pages Yearly

8794 Eye and Your Vision
National Association for Visually Handicapped
111 East 59th Street
New York, NY 10022-1202
212-821-9384
800-829-0500
FAX: 212-821-9707
e-mail: info@lighthouse.org
lighthouse.org/navh

Mark G. Ackermann, President / CEO

A large booklet offering information, with illustrations, on the eye. Includes information on protection of eyesight, how the eye works and vision disorders. Available in Russian and Spanish also. LightHouse acquired NAVH. *$5.00*

8795 Eye-Q Test
National Association for Visually Handicapped
111 East 59th Street
New York, NY 10022-1202
212-821-9384
800-829-0500
FAX: 212-821-9707
e-mail: info@lighthouse.org
lighthouse.org/navh

Mark G. Ackermann, President / CEO

Five questions and answers to assist in knowing more about vision. Also available in Spanish and Russian. LightHouse acquired NAVH.

8796 Family Context and Disability Culture Reframing: Through the Looking Glass
Through the Looking Glass
3075 Adeline Street
Suite 120
Berkeley, CA 94703
510-848-1112
800-644-2666
FAX: 510-848-4445
e-mail: tlg@lookingglass.org
www.lookingglass.org

Maureen Block, J.D., President
Thomas Spalding, Treasurer
Alice Nemon, Secretary
Mega Kirshbaum, Author

This article provides an overview of the issues and guiding perspectives underlying 'Through the Lookingglass' eighteen years of work with families. Available in braille, large print or cassette. *$2.00*
5 pages

8797 Family Guide to Vision Care (FG1)
American Optometric Association
243 North Lindbergh Boulevard
Floor 1
Saint Louis, MO 63141-7881
800-365-2219
aoa.org

David A. Cockrell, OD, President
Andrea P. Thau, OD, Vice President
Barry Barresi, Executive Director
Christopher Quinn, OD, Secretary-Treasurer

Offers information on the early developmental years of your vision, finding a family optometrist and how to take care of your eyesight through the learning years, the working years and the mature years.

8798 Family Guide: Growth & Development of the Partially Seeing Child
National Association for Visually Handicapped
111 East 59th Street
New York, NY 10022-1202
212-821-9384
800-829-0500
FAX: 212-821-9707
e-mail: info@lighthouse.org
lighthouse.org/navh

Mark G. Ackermann, President / CEO

Offers information for parents and guidelines in raising a partially seeing child. LightHouse acquired NAVH. *$.60*

8799 Fathers: A Common Ground
Blind Children's Center
4120 Marathon Street
Los Angeles, CA 90029-3584
323-664-2153
800-222-3567
FAX: 323-665-3828
e-mail: info@blindchildrenscenter.org
www.blindchildrenscenter.org

Scott E. Schaldenbrand, President
Mark Correa, Board Member
Midge Horton, Executive Director
Fernanda Schmitt PhD, Co-Author

Exploring the concerns and roles of fathers of children with visual impairments. *$10.00*
50 pages

8800 Fighting Blindness News
Foundation Fighting Blindness
7168 Columbia Gateway Drive
Suite 100
Columbia, MD 21046
410-423-0600
800-683-5555
FAX: 410-363-2393
TTY: 800-683-5551
e-mail: info@FightBlindness.org
www.blindness.org

Gordon Gund, Chair
David Brent, Vice Chair of Research
Edward H. Gollob, President
Steve Alper, Director

Offers information on medical updates, donor programs, assistive devices, resources and clinical trial information for persons with visual impariments, blindness and retinal degenerative diseases.
2x Year

8801 First Steps
Blind Children's Center
4120 Marathon Street
Los Angeles, CA 90029-3584 323-664-2153
800-222-3567
FAX: 323-665-3828
e-mail: info@blindchildrenscenter.org
www.blindchildrenscenter.org

Scott E. Schaldenbrand, President
Mark Correa, Board Member
Midge Horton, Executive Director
Ferdinand Schmitt PhD, Co-Author
A handbook for teaching young children who are visually impaired. Designed to assist students, professionals and parents working with children who are visually impaired. Visit our website for many publications addressing training very young children who are blind or visually impaired. *$35.00*
203 pages

8802 Foundations of Orientation and Mobility
American Foundation for the Blind/AFB Press
2 Penn Plaza
Suite 1102
New York, NY 10121 212-502-7600
800-232-5463
FAX: 888-545-8331
e-mail: afbinfo@afb.net
www.afb.org

Carl R. Augusto, President & Chief Executive Officer
Rick Bozeman, Finance Director, Chief Financial Officer
Kelly Bleach, Chief Administrative Officer
Stacy Rollins, Executive Administrative Assistant to the President
This text has been updated and revised and includes current research from a variety of disciplines, an international perspective, and expanded contents on low vision, aging, multiple disabilities, accessibility, program design and adaptive technology from more that 30 eminent subject experts. *$79.95*
775 pages
ISBN 0-891289-46-3

8803 Foundations of Rehabilitation Counseling with Persons Who Are Blind r Visually Impaired
American Foundation for the Blind/AFB Press
2 Penn Plaza
Suite 1102
New York, NY 10121 212-502-7600
800-232-5463
FAX: 888-545-8331
e-mail: afbinfo@afb.net
www.afb.org
Carl R. Augusto, President & Chief Executive Officer
Rick Bozeman, Finance Director, Chief Financial Officer
Kelly Bleach, Chief Administrative Officer
Stacy Rollins, Executive Administrative Assistant to the President
Rehabilitation professionals have long recognized that the needs of people who are blind or visually impaired are unique and requie a special knowledge and expertise to provide and corrdinate rehabilitation services. *$59.95*
477 pages
ISBN 0-891289-45-3

8804 General Facts and Figures on Blindness
Prevent Blindness America
211 West Wacker Drive
Suite 1700
Chicago, IL 60606 800-331-2020
e-mail: info@preventblindness.org
www.preventblindness.org
Paul G. Howes, Chairman
Hugh R. Parry, President & CEO,Prevent Blindness America
Jerome Desserich, Vice President & Chief Financial Officer
Danielle Disch, Development Manager

8805 Get a Wiggle On
American Alliance for Health, Phys. Ed. & Dance
1900 Association Drive
Reston, VA 20191-1598 703-476-3400
800-213-7193
FAX: 703-476-9527
e-mail: aapar@aahperd.org
aahperd.org

Dolly D. Lambdin, President
E. Paul Roetert, CEO
Marybell Avery, Director
Frances E. Cleland, Director
Gives teachers and parents practical suggestions for helping blind and visually impaired infants grow and learn like other children. *$5.00*
80 pages
ISBN 0-88314 -77-2

8806 Gift of Sight
RP Foundation Fighting Blindness
1401 W Mount Royal Ave
Baltimore, MD 21217-4245 410-225-9409
800-683-5555
FAX: 410-225-3936

8807 Glaucoma
Glaucoma Research Foundation
251 Post Street
Suite 600
San Francisco, CA 94108 415-986-3162
800-826-6693
FAX: 415-986-3763
e-mail: question@glaucoma.org
glaucoma.org

Andrew L. Iwach, MD, Chair
Robert L. Stamper, MD, Vice Chair
Thomas M. Brunner, President and CEO
Bill Stewart, Secretary
Offers information on what glaucoma is, the causes, treatments, types of glaucoma, eye exams and prevention.

8808 Glaucoma: The Sneak Thief of Sight
National Association for Visually Handicapped
Fl 6
22 W 21st St
New York, NY 10010-6943 212-242-4438
800-3 C-NCOS
FAX: 631-736-0371
e-mail: customerservice@cancos.com
cancos.com
Denise Green, Owner
A pamphlet describing the disease, treatment and medications. Also available in Russian and Spanish. Revised in 1999. *$3.50*

8809 Guidelines and Games for Teaching Efficient Braille Reading
American Foundation for the Blind/AFB Press
2 Penn Plaza
Suite 1102
New York, NY 10121 212-502-7600
800-232-5463
FAX: 888-545-8331
e-mail: afbinfo@afb.net
www.afb.org

Carl R. Augusto, President & Chief Executive Officer
Rick Bozeman, Finance Director, Chief Financial Officer
Kelly Bleach, Chief Administrative Officer
Stacy Rollins, Executive Administrative Assistant to the President
Based on research in the areas of rapid reading and precision teaching, these guidelines represent a unique adaptation of a general reading program to the needs of braille readers. Paperback. *$ 24.95*
116 pages Paperback
ISBN 0-891281-05-4

8810 Guidelines for Comprehensive Low Vision Care
National Association for Visually Handicapped
111 East 59th Street
New York, NY 10022-1202
212-821-9384
800-829-0500
FAX: 212-821-9707
e-mail: info@lighthouse.org
lighthouse.org/navh

Mark G. Ackermann, President / CEO
A description of the proper method to conduct a low vision evaluation.LightHouse acquired NAVH. *$.50*

8811 Handbook for Itinerant and Resource Teachers of Blind Students
National Federation of the Blind
200 East Wells St
Baltimore, MD 21230-4914
410-659-9314
e-mail: nfb@iamdigex.net

Doris Willoughby, Author
Sharon L Monthei, Co-Author
The Handbook provides help to teachers, school administrators or other school personnel that have experience with blind or visually impaired students. The Handbook devotes 45 pages to Braille and how to teach Braille for parents and teachers. There are other chapters offering information on the law, physical education, fitting in socially, testing and evaluation, home economics, daily living skills and more. *$23.00*
533 pages Softcover
ISBN 0-962412-20-1

8812 Handbook of Information for Members of the Achromatopsia Network
P.O.Box 214
Berkeley, CA 94701-214
510-540-4700
FAX: 510-540-4767
e-mail: futterman@achromat.org
www.achromat.org

8813 Health Care Professionals Who Are Blind or Visually Impaired
American Foundation for the Blind
2 Penn Plaza
Suite 1102
New York, NY 10121
212-502-7600
800-232-5463
FAX: 888-545-8331
e-mail: afbinfo@afb.net
afb.org

Carl R. Augusto, President & Chief Executive Officer
Rick Bozeman, Finance Director, Chief Financial Officer
Kelly Bleach, Chief Administrative Officer
Stacy Rollins, Executive Administrative Assistant to the President
This resource is essential reading for older students and young adults who are blind or visually impaired, their families, and the professionals who work with them. *$21.95*
160 pages
ISBN 0-891283-88-9

8814 Heart to Heart
Blind Children's Center
4120 Marathon Street
Los Angeles, CA 90029-3584
323-664-2153
800-222-3567
FAX: 323-665-3828
e-mail: info@blindchildrenscenter.org
www.blindchildrenscenter.org

Scott E. Schaldenbrand, President
Mark Correa, Board Member
Midge Horton, Executive Director
Dori Hayashi MA, Co-Author
Parents of children who are blind and partially sighted talk about their feelings. *$10.00*
12 pages

8815 Heartbreak of Being A Little Bit Blind
National Association for Visually Handicapped
111 East 59th Street
New York, NY 10022-1202
212-821-9384
800-829-0500
FAX: 212-821-9707
e-mail: info@lighthouse.org
lighthouse.org/navh

Mark G. Ackermann, President / CEO
Summary of what it means to have impaired vision; includes illustrations. LightHouse acquired NAVH.

8816 Helen Keller National Center Newsletter
141 Middle Neck Road
Sands Point, NY 11050
516-944-8900
800-225-0411
FAX: 516-944-7302
e-mail: hkncinfo@hknc.org
www.hknc.org

Joseph McNulty, Executive Director
The center provides evaluation and training in vocational skills, adaptive technology and computer skills, orientation and mobility, independent living, communication, speech-language skills, creative arts, fitness and leisure activities.

8817 Helping the Visually Impaired Child with Developmental Problems
Teachers College Press
1234 Amsterdam Avenue
New York, NY 10027
212-678-3929
800-575-6566
FAX: 212-678-4149
e-mail: tcpress@tc.columbia.edu
www.teacherscollegepress.com

Mary Lynch, Manager
Brian Ellerbeck, Executive Acquisitions Editor
Marie Ellen Larcada, Senior Acquisitions Editor
Emily Spangler, Acquisitions Editor
This book aims to explore the human consequences of severe visual problems combined with other handicaps. The application of child development research to educational interventions, the need for educational and rehabilitative services that serve the human and the special needs of children and their families and the promise of technology in helping to expand communicative possibilities are also discussed. *$18.95*
216 pages Paperback
ISBN 0-807729-02-7

8818 History and Use of Braille
American Council of the Blind
2200 Wilson Boulevard
Suite 650
Arlington, VA 22201-3354
202-467-5081
800-424-8666
FAX: 703-465-5085
e-mail: info@acb.org
acb.org

Kim Charlson, President
Jeff Thom, 1st Vice President
Melanie Brunson, Executive Director
A system of touch reading and writing for blind persons in which raised dots represent the letters of the alphabet.

8819 How to Thrive, Not Just Survive
American Foundation for the Blind/AFB Press
2 Penn Plaza
Suite 1102
New York, NY 10121
212-502-7600
800-232-5463
FAX: 888-545-8331
e-mail: afbinfo@afb.net
www.afb.org

Carl R. Augusto, President & Chief Executive Officer
Rick Bozeman, Finance Director, Chief Financial Officer
Kelly Bleach, Chief Administrative Officer
Practical, hands-on guide for parents, teachers, and everyone involved in helping children develop the skills necessary for socialization, orientations and mobility, and leisure and recreational

activities. Some of the subjects covered are eating, dressing, personal hygiene, self-esteem and etiquette. *$24.95*
104 pages Paperback
ISBN 0-89128-48-7

8820 **Hub**
SPOKES Unlimited
1006 Main Street
Klamath Fals, OR 97601 541-883-7547
FAX: 541-885-2469
e-mail: spoks@internetcds.com
spokesunlimited.org

Wendy Howard, Executive Director
Celeste Wolf, Clerical Support Specialist II
Newsletter on rehabilitation, peer counseling, blindness, visual impairments, information and referral.

8821 **If Blindness Comes**
National Federation of the Blind
200 East Wells St
Baltimore, MD 21230-4914 410-659-9314
FAX: 410-685-5653
e-mail: nfb@iamdigex.net
www.nfb.org

Kenneth Jerrigan, Editor
An introduction to issues relating to vision loss and provides a positive, supportive philosophy about blindness. It is a general information book which includes answers to many common questions about blindness, information about services and programs for the blind and resource listings. Contact the Materials Center.

8822 **If Blindness Strikes Don't Strike Out**
2600 South 1st Street
Springfield, IL 62704 217-789-8980
800-258-8980
FAX: 217-789-9130
e-mail: books@ccthomas.com
www.ccthomas.com

Bob Stork, Owner

8823 **Imagining the Possibilities: Creative Approaches to Orientation and Mobility Instructio**
American Foundation for the Blind
2 Penn Plaza
Suite 1102
New York, NY 10121 212-502-7600
800-232-5463
FAX: 888-545-8331
e-mail: afbinfo@afb.net
afb.org

Carl R. Augusto, President & Chief Executive Officer
Rick Bozeman, Finance Director, Chief Financial Officer
Kelly Bleach, Chief Administrative Officer
Innovative and varied approaches to O&M techniques and teaching and dynamic suggestions on how to analyze learning styles are just some of the important topics included. *$49.95*
378 pages
ISBN 0-891283-82-X

8824 **Increasing Literacy Levels: Final Report**
Mississippi State University
P.O.Box 6189
Mississippi State, MS 39762 662-325-2001
FAX: 662-325-8989
TTY:662-325-2694
e-mail: nrtc@colled.msstate.edu
www.blind.msstate.edu

Jacqui Bybee, Research Associate II
Douglas Bedsaul, Research and Training Coordinator
Anne Carter, Research and Training Coordinator
Brenda Cavenaugh, Ph.D., Research Professor
This study is composed of three research projects to identify and analyze the appropriate use of and instruction in Braille, optical devices and other technologies as they relate to literacy and employment of individuals who are blind or visually impaired. *$20.00*
148 pages Paperback

8825 **Information Access Project**
National Federation of the Blind
200 East Wells St
Baltimore, MD 21230-4914 410-659-9314
FAX: 410-685-5653
e-mail: nfb@nfb.org
nfb.org

Marc Maurer, President
Assists entities covered by the ADA in finding methods for converting visually displayed information, such as flyers, brochures and pamphlets, to formats accessible to individuals who are visually impaired.

8826 **Information on Glaucoma**
Glaucoma Research Foundation
251 Post Street
Suite 600
San Francisco, CA 94108 415-986-3162
800-826-6693
FAX: 415-986-3763
e-mail: question@glaucoma.org
www.glaucoma.org

Andrew L. Iwach, MD, Chair
Robert L. Stamper, MD, Vice Chair
Thomas M. Brunner, President and CEO
Bill Stewart, Secretary

8827 **Intervention Practices in the Retention of Competitive Employment**
Mississippi State University
P.O.Box 6189
Mississippi State, MS 39762 662-325-2001
FAX: 662-325-8989
TTY:662-325-2694
e-mail: nrtc@colled.msstate.edu
www.blind.msstate.edu

Jacqui Bybee, Research Associate II
Douglas Bedsaul, Research and Training Coordinator
Anne Carter, Research and Training Coordinator
Brenda Cavenaugh, Ph.D., Research Professor
This study investigated the methods by which an individual can retain competitive employment after the onset of a significant vision loss. Interviews were conducted with 89 rehabilitation counselors across the US Strategies that contribute to successful job retention were identified as well as best rehabilitation practices in job retention. *$15.00*
60 pages Paperback

8828 **Know Your Eye**
American Council of the Blind
2200 Wilson Boulevard
Suite 650
Arlington, VA 22201-3354 202-467-5081
800-424-8666
FAX: 703-465-5085
e-mail: info@acb.org
acb.org

Kim Charlson, President
Jeff Thom, 1st Vice President
Melanie Brunson, Executive Director

8829 **Large Print Loan Library**
National Association for Visually Handicapped
111 East 59th Street
New York, NY 10022-1202 212-821-9384
800-829-0500
FAX: 212-821-9707
e-mail: info@lighthouse.org
lighthouse.org/navh

Mark G. Ackermann, President / CEO

A huge large print catalog of all the publications, fiction and non-fiction, cassette tapes, books-on-tape and videos available for the visually impaired from the loan library of the National Association for the Visually Handicapped. LightHouse acquired NAVH.

8830 Large Print Loan Library Catalog
National Association for Visually Handicapped
111 East 59th Street
New York, NY 10022-1202
212-821-9384
800-829-0500
FAX: 212-821-9707
e-mail: info@lighthouse.org
lighthouse.org/navh

Mark G. Ackermann, President / CEO
Listing of over 7,000 commercially published and NAVH large print books available through NAVH on a loan basis. Includes a limited selection of titles available for purchase. LightHouse acquired NAVH.

8831 Large Print Recipies for a Healthy Life
123601 Wilshire
Los Angeles, CA 90025
310-826-8280
800-481-EYES
FAX: 310-458-8179

Judith Caditz PhD, Author
$21.95
283 pages
ISBN 0-962236-82-9

8832 Learning to Play
Blind Children's Center
4120 Marathon Street
Los Angeles, CA 90029-3584
323-664-2153
800-222-3567
FAX: 323-665-3828
e-mail: info@blindchildrenscenter.org
www.blindchildrenscenter.org

Scott E. Schaldenbrand, President
Mark Correa, Board Member
Midge Horton, Executive Director
Presenting play activities to the pre-school child who is visually impaired. *$10.00*
12 pages

8833 Let's Eat
Blind Children's Center
4120 Marathon Street
Los Angeles, CA 90029-3584
323-664-2153
800-222-3567
FAX: 323-665-3828
e-mail: info@blindchildrenscenter.org
www.blindchildrenscenter.org

Scott E. Schaldenbrand, President
Mark Correa, Board Member
Midge Horton, Executive Director
Feeding a child with visual impairment. *$10.00*
28 pages

8834 Library Resources for the Blind and Physically Handicapped
Nat'l Lib Svc/Blind And Physically Handicapped
1291 Taylor St NW
Washington, DC 20011
202-707-5100
FAX: 202-707-0712
TTY:202-707-0744
e-mail: nls@loc.gov
www.loc.gov/nls

Karen Keninger, Director
NLS administers a national library service that provides braille and recorded books and magazines on free loan to anyone who cannot read standard print because of visual or physical disabilities and who are eligible residents of the United States or American citizens living abroad. The directory describes the cooperating libaries.
83 pages

8835 Library Services for the Blind
South Carolina State University
300 College Street NorthEast
P.O. Box 7491
Orangeburg, SC 29117
803-536-7045
FAX: 803-536-8902
e-mail: reference@scsu.edu
library.scsu.edu

Adrienne C. Webber, Dean, Library/Information Services
Ramona S. Evans, Administrative Specialist
Ruth A. Hodges, Reference & Information Specialist
Wanda L. Priester, Library Technical Asst.
News and information on developments in library services for readers who are blind and physically disabled.

8836 Lifestyles of Employed Legally Blind People
Mississippi State University
P.O.Box 6189
Mississippi State, MS 39762
662-325-2001
FAX: 662-325-8989
TTY:662-325-2694
e-mail: nrtc@colled.msstate.edu
www.blind.msstate.edu

Jacqui Bybee, Research Associate II
Douglas Bedsaul, Research and Training Coordinator
Anne Carter, Research and Training Coordinator
Brenda Cavenaugh, Ph.D., Research Professor
Results from a telephone survey show that visually impaired respondents are involved in a wide variety of activities with little restrictions on their range of activities. Sighted respondents tended to spend more time in child care, obtaining goods and services, attending to self-care activities and engaging in social activities, while visually impaired respondents spent more time in education and passive activities. This report is a study of expenditures and time use. *$ 10.00*
193 pages Paperback

8837 Lion
Lion's Clubs International
300 West 22nd Street
Oak Brook, IL 60523-8842
630-571-5466
FAX: 630-571-8890
TTY:630-571-6533
www.lionsclubs.org/

Joseph Preston, International President
Jitsuhiro Yamada, 1st Vice President
Robert E. Corlew, 2nd Vice President
Peter Lynch, Executive Director
Publication for the blind.

8838 Living with Achromatopsia
P.O.Box 214
Berkeley, CA 94701-214
510-540-4700
FAX: 510-540-4767
e-mail: futterman@achromat.org
www.achromat.org

Frances Futterman, Author
Consists entirely of comments from persons who know firsthand about living with achromatopsia.

8839 Low Vision Questions and Answers: Definitions, Devices, Services
American Foundation for the Blind/AFB Press
2 Penn Plaza
Suite 1102
New York, NY 10121
212-502-7600
800-232-5463
FAX: 888-545-8331
e-mail: afbinfo@afb.net
afb.org

Carl R. Augusto, President & Chief Executive Officer
Rick Bozeman, Chief Financial Officer
Kelly Bleach, Chief Administrative Officer
Stacy Rollins, Executive Administrative Assistant to the President
What does low vision mean? What do low vision services cost? What diseases cause low vision? Answers to these and other ques-

tions are presented in a comprehensive format with accompanying photographs. $50.00/pack of 25.
21 pages Pamphlet
ISBN 0-891281-96-7

8840 Low Vision: Reflections of the Past, Issues for the Future
American Foundation for the Blind/AFB Press
2 Penn Plaza
Suite 1102
New York, NY 10121
212-502-7600
800-232-5463
FAX: 888-545-8331
e-mail: afbinfo@afb.net
www.afb.org

Carl R. Augusto, President & Chief Executive Officer
Rick Bozeman, Chief Financial Officer
Kelly Bleach, Chief Administrative Officer
Stacy Rollins, Executive Administrative Assistant to the President
Background papers and a strategies section are used to identify the shifting needs of visually impaired persons and the resources that may be needed to address them. Paperback. *$34.95*
Paperback
ISBN 0-891282-18-1

8841 Mainstreaming and the American Dream
American Foundation for the Blind/AFB Press
2 Penn Plaza
Suite 1102
New York, NY 10121
212-502-7600
800-232-5463
FAX: 888-545-8331
e-mail: afbinfo@afb.net
www.afb.org
Carl R. Augusto, President & Chief Executive Officer
Rick Bozeman, Chief Financial Officer
Kelly Bleach, Chief Administrative Officer
Stacy Rollins, Executive Administrative Assistant to the President
Based on in-depth interviews with parents and professionals, this research monograph presents information on the needs and aspirations of parents of blind and visually impaired children. Paperback. *$34.95*
256 pages Paperback
ISBN 0-891281-91-7

8842 Mainstreaming the Visually Impaired Child
NAPVI
1 North Lexington Avenue
White Plains, NY 10601
617-972-7441
800-562-6265
FAX: 617-972-7444
e-mail: napvi@guildhealth.org
www.napvi.org

Julie Urban, President
Venetia Hayden, Vice President
Susan LaVenture, Executive Director
Randi Sher, Secretary
A unique, informative guide for teachers and educational professionals that work with the visually impaired. *$10.00*
121 pages Paper

8843 Making Life More Livable
American Foundation for the Blind
2 Penn Plaza
Suite 1102
New York, NY 10121
212-502-7600
800-232-5463
FAX: 888-545-8331
e-mail: afbinfo@afb.net
www.afb.org
Carl R. Augusto, President & Chief Executive Officer
Rick Bozeman, Chief Financial Officer
Kelly Bleach, Chief Administrative Officer
Stacy Rollins, Executive Administrative Assistant to the President
Shows how simple adaptations in the home and environment can make a big difference in the lives of blind and visually impaired older persons. The suggestions offered are numerous and specific, ranging from how to mark food cans for greater visibility to how to get out of the shower safley. Large print. *$24.95*
128 pages
ISBN 0-891283-87-0

8844 Meeting the Needs of People with Vision Loss: Multidisciplinary Perspective
Resources for Rehabilitation
22 Bonad Road
Winchester, MA 01890
781-368-9080
FAX: 781-368-9096
e-mail: orders@rfr.org
www.rfr.org

Susan L Greenblatt, Editor
Written by rehabilitation professionals, physicians, and a sociologist, this book discusses how to provide appropriate information and how to serve special populations. Chapters on the role of the family, diabetes and vision loss, special needs of children and adolescents, adults with hearing and vision loss. *$29.95*
ISBN 0-929718-07-0

8845 Model Program Operation Manual: Business Enterprise Program Supervisors
Mississippi State University
P.O.Box 6189
Mississippi State, MS 39762
662-325-2001
FAX: 662-325-8989
TTY:662-325-2694
e-mail: nrtc@colled.msstate.edu
www.blind.msstate.edu

Jacqui Bybee, Research Associate II
Douglas Bedsaul, Research and Training Coordinator
Anne Carter, Research and Training Coordinator
Brenda Cavenaugh, Ph.D., Research Professor
This monograph serves as a Model Program Operation Manual for Business Enterprise Program Supervisors who administer Randolph-Sheppard vending facilities under the Randolph-Sheppard Act. A wide variety of topics are covered including the role of the State Committee of Blind Venders, the role and responsibilities of the Vending Facility Operator, model qualification, for potential Facility Managers, guidelines for location of vending facilities and policies for closing vending facilities. *$20.00*
199 pages Paperback

8846 More Alike Than Different: Blind and Visually Impaired Children
American Foundation for the Blind/AFB Press
2 Penn Plaza
Suite 1102
New York, NY 10121
212-502-7600
800-232-5463
FAX: 888-545-8331
e-mail: afborders@abdintl.com
www.afb.org

Carl R. Augusto, President & Chief Executive Officer
Rick Bozeman, Chief Financial Officer
Kelly Bleach, Chief Administrative Officer
Stacy Rollins, Executive Administrative Assistant to the President
Offers photographs of blind and visually impaired children around the world learning to read and write, travel independently and performing basic living skills. Covers the most recent technological advances and demonstrates the universality of educational needs and goals. Paperback. $100.00/pack of 25.
ISBN 0-891281-69-0

8847 Mothers with Visual Impairments who are Raising Young Children
American Foundation for the Blind/AFB Press
2 Penn Plaza
Suite 1102
New York, NY 10121
212-502-7600
800-232-5463
FAX: 888-545-8331
e-mail: afbinfo@afb.net
www.afb.org

Carl R. Augusto, President & Chief Executive Officer
Rick Bozeman, Chief Financial Officer
Kelly Bleach, Chief Administrative Officer
Stacy Rollins, Executive Administrative Assistant to the President

Available in braille, large print or cassette. *$2.00*
16 pages

8848 Move With Me
Blind Children's Center
4120 Marathon Street
Los Angeles, CA 90029-3584
323-664-2153
800-222-3567
FAX: 323-665-3828
e-mail: info@blindchildrenscenter.org
www.blindchildrenscenter.org

Scott E. Schaldenbrand, President
Mark Correa, Board Member
Midge Horton, Executive Director
Nancy Chernus-Mansfield MA, Co-Author

A parent's guide to movement development for babies who are visually impaired. *$10.00*
12 pages

8849 National Eye Institute
National Institute of Health
31 Center Drive MSC 2510
Bethesda, MD 20892-2510
301-496-5248
FAX: 301-402-1065
e-mail: 2020@nei.nih.gov
www.nei.nih.gov

8850 National Library Services for the Blind& Physically Handicapped
Library of Congress
1291 Taylor Street North West
Washington, DC 20011
202-707-5100
FAX: 202-707-0712
TTY:202-707-0744
e-mail: nls@loc.gov
www.loc.gov/nls

Karen Keninger, Director

NLS is responsible for the selection, copyright clearance, and procurement of reading materials for blind and physically handicapped individuals. Distribution of the materials and relevant biblographic information either directly or through cooperating state and local network libraries. Design, development, and procurement of sound reproduction equipment and its distribution either directly or through cooperating agencies.

8851 Orientation and Mobility Primer for Families and Young Children
American Foundation for the Blind/AFB Press
2 Penn Plaza
Suite 1102
New York, NY 10121
212-502-7600
800-232-5463
FAX: 888-545-8331
e-mail: afbinfo@afb.net
www.afb.org

Carl R. Augusto, President & Chief Executive Officer
Rick Bozeman, Chief Financial Officer
Kelly Bleach, Chief Administrative Officer
Stacy Rollins, Executive Administrative Assistant to the President

Practical information for helping a child learn about his or her environment right from the start. Covers sensory training, concept development and orientation skills. Paperback. *$14.95*
48 pages
ISBN 0-891281-57-6

8852 Out of the Corner of My Eye: Living with Vision Loss in Later Life
American Foundation for the Blind/AFB Press
2 Penn Plaza
Suite 1102
New York, NY 10121
212-502-7600
800-232-5463
FAX: 888-545-8331
e-mail: afbinfo@fb.net
www.afb.org

Carl R. Augusto, President & Chief Executive Officer
Rick Bozeman, Chief Financial Officer
Kelly Bleach, Chief Administrative Officer
Stacy Rollins, Executive Administrative Assistant to the President

A personal account of students' vision loss and subsequent adjustment that is full of practical advice and cheerful encouragement, told by an 87 year old retired college teacher who has maintained her independence and zest for life. Available in paperback or on audio cassette. *$23.95*
120 pages
ISBN 0-891281-82-1

8853 Out of the Corner of My Eye: Living with Macular Degeneration
American Foundation for the Blind/AFB Press
2 Penn Plaza
Suite 1102
New York, NY 10121
212-502-7600
800-232-5463
FAX: 888-545-8331
e-mail: afbinfo@afb.net
www.afb.org

Carl R. Augusto, President & Chief Executive Officer
Rick Bozeman, Chief Financial Officer
Kelly Bleach, Chief Administrative Officer
Stacy Rollins, Executive Administrative Assistant to the President

A personal account of students' vision loss and subsequent adjustment that is full of practical advice and cheerful encouragement, told by an 87 year old retired college teacher who has maintained her independence and zest for life. *$29.95*
168 pages Paperback
ISBN 0-891238-31-2

8854 Pain Erasure: the Bonnie Prudden Way
Ballantine Books
1540 Broadway
New York, NY 10036-4039
212-751-2600
FAX: 212-572-4949

Bonnie Prudden, Author

Revolutionary breakthrough in pain relief involves trigger points-tender areas where muscles have been damaged from falls, childhood ailments, poor posture, and the stresses of daily life.

8855 Patient's Guide to Visual Aids and Illumination
National Association for Visually Handicapped
111 East 59th Street
New York, NY 10022-1202
212-821-9384
800-829-0500
FAX: 212-821-9707
e-mail: info@lighthouse.org
lighthouse.org/navh

Mark G. Ackermann, President / CEO

A reference booklet offering information on aids for the visually impaired. LightHouse acquired NAVH. *$.75*

8856 Pediatric Visual Diagnosis Fact Sheets
Blind Children's Center
4120 Marathon Street
Los Angeles, CA 90029-3584 323-664-2153
800-222-3567
FAX: 323-665-3828
e-mail: info@blindchildrenscenter.org
blindchildrenscenter.org

Scott E. Schaldenbrand, President
Mark Correa, Board Member
Midge Horton, Executive Director
Collection of fact sheets addressing commonly encountered eye conditions, diagnostic tests and materials. *$10.00*
10 pages

8857 Perkins Activity and Resource Guide: A Handbook for Teachers
Perkins School for the Blind
175 North Beacon Street
Watertown, MA 02472 617-924-3434
FAX: 617-972-7363
e-mail: info@perkins.org
www.perkins.org
Frederic M. Clifford, Chair of the Board
Philip L. Ladd, Vice Chair of the Board
Leslie Nordon, Secretary
Charles C.J. Platt, Treasurer
This is a comprehensive, two volume guide with over 1,000 pages of activities, resources and instructional strategies for teachers and parents of students with visual and multiple disabilities. *$80.00*

8858 Personal Reader Update
Personal Reader Department
9 Centennial Dr
Peabody, MA 01960-7906 978-977-2000
800-343-0311
FAX: 978-977-2409

8859 Preschool Learning Activities for the Visually Impaired Child
NAPVI
1 North Lexington Avenue
White Plains, NY 10601 617-972-7441
800-562-6265
FAX: 617-972-7444
e-mail: napvi@guildhealth.org
www.napvi.org

Julie Urban, President
Venetia Hayden, Vice President
Susan LaVenture, Executive Director
Randi Sher, Secretary
This guide for parents offers games and activities to keep visually impaired children active during the preschool years. *$8.00*
91 pages Paperback

8860 Reaching, Crawling, Walking....Let's Get Moving
Blind Children's Center
4120 Marathon Street
Los Angeles, CA 90029-3584 323-664-2153
800-222-3567
FAX: 323-665-3828
e-mail: info@blindchildrenscenter.org
www.blindchildrenscenter.org
Scott E. Schaldenbrand, President
Mark Correa, Board Member
Midge Horton, Executive Director
Orientation and mobility for preschool children who are visually imapired. *$10.00*
24 pages

8861 Reading Is for Everyone
Nat'l Lib Svc/Blind And Physically Handicapped
1291 Taylor Street North West
Washington, DC 20011 202-707-5100
FAX: 202-707-0712
TTY:202-707-0744
e-mail: nls@loc.gov
www.loc.gov/nls
Karen Keninger, Director

8862 Reading with Low Vision
Nat'l Lib Svc/Blind And Physically Handicapped
1291 Taylor Street North West
Washington, DC 20011 202-707-5100
FAX: 202-707-0712
TTY:202-707-0744
e-mail: nls@loc.gov
www.loc.gov/nls

Karen Keninger, Director

8863 Recording for the Blind & Dyslexic
20 Roszel Road
Princeton, NJ 08540 800-221-4792
FAX: 609-987-8116
e-mail: Custserv@LearningAlly.org
www.learningally.org/

Brad Grob, Chairman
Harold J. Logan, Vice Chairman
Andrew Friedman, President & CEO
Jim Halliday, Executive Vice President
Provides recorded and computerized textbooks, library services and other educational resources to people who cannot effectively read standard print because of visual impairment, dyslexia or other physical disability. RFB&D is now Learning Ally.

8864 Reference and Information Services From NLS
Nat'l Lib Svc/Blind And Physically Handicapped
1291 Taylor Street North West
Washington, DC 20011 202-707-5100
FAX: 202-707-0712
TTY:202-707-0744
e-mail: nls@loc.gov
www.loc.gov/nls
Karen Keninger, Director

8865 Resource List for Persons with Low Vision
American Council of the Blind
2200 Wilson Boulevard
Suite 650
Arlington, VA 22201-3354 202-467-5081
800-424-8666
FAX: 703-465-5085
e-mail: info@acb.org
acb.org
Kim Charlson, President
Jeff Thom, 1st Vice President
Melanie Brunson, Executive Director

8866 Rose-Colored Glasses
Human Sciences Press
233 Spring St
New York, NY 10013-1522 212-229-2859
800-221-9369
FAX: 212-463-0742

30 pages Hardcover
ISBN 0-87705 -08-8

8867 Say it with Sign
Harris Communications
15155 Technology Drive
Eden Prairie, MN 55344
952-388-2152
800-825-6758
FAX: 952-906-1099
e-mail: info@harriscomm.com
harriscomm.com

Robert Harris, Owner
Contains both the serious and fun side of signing and provides the basic signs that might be needed in an emergency situation.
$299.50
10-DVD set

8868 See A Bone
Facts on File
132 West 31st Street
14th Floor
New York, NY 10001
212-967-8800
800-683-5433
FAX: 212-760-0862
e-mail: info@northernleasing.com
northernleasing.com

Mark Donnell, President
$65.00
352 pages
ISBN 0-816042-80-2

8869 See What I Feel
Britannica Film Company
345 4th Street
San Francisco, CA 94107
415-928-8466
FAX: 415-928-5027
pacbikes.com

Dave Bekowich, Owner
A blind child tells her friends about her trip to the zoo. Each experience was explained as a blind child would experience it. A teacher's guide comes with this video.
Film

8870 Selecting a Program
Blind Children's Center
4120 Marathon Street
Los Angeles, CA 90029-3584
323-664-2153
800-222-3567
FAX: 323-665-3828
e-mail: info@blindchildrenscenter.org
www.blindchildrenscenter.org

Scott E. Schaldenbrand, President
Mark Correa, Board Member
Midge Horton, Executive Director
A guide for parents of infants and preschoolers with visual impairments. *$10.00*
28 pages

8871 Show Me How: A Manual for Parents of Preschool Blind Children
American Foundation for the Blind/AFB Press
2 Penn Plaza
Suite 1102
New York, NY 10121
212-502-7600
800-232-5463
FAX: 888-545-8331
e-mail: afbinfo@afb.net
www.afb.org

Carl R. Augusto, President & Chief Executive Officer
Rick Bozeman, Chief Financial Officer
Kelly Bleach, Chief Administrative Officer
Stacy Rollins, Executive Administrative Assistant to the President
A practical guide for parents, teachers and others who help preschool children attain age-related goals. Covers issues on playing precautions, appropriate toys and facilitating relationships with playmates. Paperback. *$12.95*
56 pages
ISBN 0-891281-13-4

8872 Sign of the Times
Fanlight Productions
c/o Icarus Films
32 Court Street, 21st Floor
Brooklyn, NY 11201
718-488-8900
800-876-1710
FAX: 718-488-8642
e-mail: info@fanlight.com, sales@icarusfilms.com
www.fanlight.com

Ben Achtenberg, Owner, Founder
Profiles a public school in the heart of Los Angeles - an American microcosm where over 300 languages are spoken, and where cultures and races collide. Fairfax High, publicized as the site of gang activity and murder, has long been a focus for bad press. But something very right is going on in this school. A Sign of the Times offers a positive example of how the American dream and American education are still alive

8873 Special Technologies Alternative Resources
210 McMorran Boulevard
Port Huron, MI 48060
810-987-7323
877-987-READ
e-mail: star@sccl.lib.mi.us
www.sccl.lib.mi.us/star.html

Arnold H. Larson, Chairman
Kathleen J. Wheelihan, Vice Chairman
Arlene M. Marcetti, Board Member
Stan Arnetti, Director
Addresses the needs of a very unique diverse group of people by offering a full range of library services for people who cannot read standard print. Provides reading material in specialized formats that permit individuals with disabilities to have access to the written word, delivering to customer's mailboxes free of charge. Talking Book Machines, recorded books and magazines, descriptive videos, large print editions and braille books and magazines.

8874 Standing on My Own Two Feet
Blind Children's Center
4120 Marathon Street
Los Angeles, CA 90029-3584
323-664-2153
800-222-3567
FAX: 323-665-3828
e-mail: info@blindchildrenscenter.org
www.blindchildrenscenter.org

Scott E. Schaldenbrand, President
Mark Correa, Board Member
Midge Horton, Executive Director
A guide to constructing mobility devices for children who are visually impaired. *$10.00*
38 pages

8875 Starting Points
Blind Children's Center
4120 Marathon Street
Los Angeles, CA 90029-3584
323-664-2153
800-222-3567
FAX: 323-665-3828
e-mail: info@blindchildrenscenter.org
www.blindchildrenscenter.org

Scott E. Schaldenbrand, President
Mark Correa, Board Member
Midge Horton, Executive Director
Basic information for the clasroom teacher of 3 to 8 year olds whose multiple disabilities include visual impairment. *$35.00*
157 pages
ISBN 0-891280-61-8

8876 Step-By-Step Guide to Personal Management for Blind Persons

American Foundation for the Blind/AFB Press
2 Penn Plaza
Suite 1102
New York, NY 10121
212-502-7600
800-232-5463
FAX: 888-545-8331
e-mail: afbinfo@afb.net
www.afb.org

Carl R. Augusto, President & Chief Executive Officer
Rick Bozeman, Chief Financial Officer
Kelly Bleach, Chief Administrative Officer
Stacy Rollins, Executive Administrative Assistant to the President

A manual of techniques in the areas of hygiene, grooming, clothing, shopping and child care. *$19.95*

136 pages Spiralbound
ISBN 0-891280-61-8

8877 Student Teaching Guide for Blind and Visually Impaired College Students

American Foundation for the Blind/AFB Press
2 Penn Plaza
Suite 1102
New York, NY 10121
212-502-7600
800-232-5463
FAX: 888-545-8331
e-mail: afbinfo@afb.net
www.afb.org

Carl R. Augusto, President & Chief Executive Officer
Rick Bozeman, Chief Financial Officer
Kelly Bleach, Chief Administrative Officer
Stacy Rollins, Executive Administrative Assistant to the President

A comprehensive resource designed to enable the student to enter the classroom of a university or college with confidence. Large print. *$14.95*

52 pages
ISBN 0-891281-42-8

8878 Survey of Direct Labor Workers Who Are Blind & Employed by NIB

Mississippi State University
P.O.Box 6189
Mississippi State, MS 39762
662-325-2001
FAX: 662-325-8989
TTY:662-325-2694
e-mail: nrtc@colled.msstate.edu
www.blind.msstate.edu

Jacqui Bybee, Research Associate II
Douglas Bedsaul, Research and Training Coordinator
Anne Carter, Research and Training Coordinator
Brenda Cavenaugh, Ph.D., Research Professor

This report is a follow-up to surveys by National Industries for the Blind in 1983 and 1987 and summarizes the results of a national survey of approximately 500 legally blind direct labor workers. *$10.00*

101 pages Paperback

8879 Talk to Me

Blind Children's Center
4120 Marathon Street
Los Angeles, CA 90029-3584
323-664-2153
800-222-3567
FAX: 323-665-3828
e-mail: info@blindchildrenscenter.org
www.blindchildrenscenter.org

Scott E. Schaldenbrand, President
Mark Correa, Board Member
Midge Horton, Executive Director

A language guide for parents of children who are visually impaired. *$10.00*

11 pages

8880 Talk to Me II

Blind Children's Center
4120 Marathon Street
Los Angeles, CA 90029-3584
323-664-2153
800-222-3567
FAX: 323-665-3828
e-mail: info@blindchildrenscenter.org
www.blindchildrenscenter.org

Scott E. Schaldenbrand, President
Mark Correa, Board Member
Midge Horton, Executive Director

a sequel to Talk to Me *$10.00*

15 pages

8881 Talking Books & Reading Disabilities

Nat'l Lib Svc/Blind And Physically Handicapped
1291 Taylor Street North West
Washington, DC 20011
202-707-5100
FAX: 202-707-0712
TTY:202-707-0744
e-mail: nls@loc.gov
www.loc.gov/nls

Karen Keninger, Director

8882 Talking Books for People with Physical Disabilities

Nat'l Lib Svc/Blind And Physically Handicapped
1291 Taylor Street North West
Washington, DC 20011
202-707-5100
FAX: 202-707-0712
TTY:202-707-0744
e-mail: nls@loc.gov
www.loc.gov/nls

Karen Keninger, Director

8883 Teaching Orientation and Mobility in the Schools: An Instructor's Companion

American Foundation for the Blind
2 Penn Plaza
Suite 1102
New York, NY 10121
212-502-7600
800-232-5463
FAX: 888-545-8331
e-mail: afbinfo@afb.net
www.afb.org

Carl R. Augusto, President & Chief Executive Officer
Rick Bozeman, Chief Financial Officer
Kelly Bleach, Chief Administrative Officer
Stacy Rollins, Executive Administrative Assistant to the President

This book, with its useful forms, checklists, and tips, will help O&M instructors and teachers of visually impaired students master the arts of planning schedules, organizing equipment and work routines, working with school personnel and educational team members, and effectively providing instruction to children with diverse needs. *$ 45.95*

176 pages
ISBN 0-891283-91-1

8884 Teaching Visually Impaired Children

Charles C. Thomas
2600 South 1st Street
Springfield, IL 62704
217-789-8980
800-258-8980
FAX: 217-789-9130
e-mail: books@ccthomas.com
www.ccthomas.com

Michael P. Thomas, President

A comprehensive resource for the classroom teacher who is working with a visually impaired child for the first time, as well as a systematic overview of education for the specialist in visual disabilities. It approaches instructional challenges with clear explanations and practical suggestions, and it addresses common concerns of teachers in a reassuring and positive manner. Also available in cloth. *$49.95*

352 pages Paper 2004
ISBN 0-398074-77-7

8885 Textbook Catalog
National Braille Association
95 Allens Creek Road
Building 1, Suite 202
Rochester, NY 14618
585-427-8260
FAX: 585-427-0263
e-mail: nbaoffice@nationalbraille.org
www.nationalbraille.org

Jan Carroll, President
Cindi Laurent, Vice President
David Shaffer, Executive Director
Heidi Lehmann, Secretary

Lists hundreds of scholarly, college and professional textbooks offered in large print, braille or on cassette for visually impaired readers.
80 pages

8886 Three Rivers News
Carnegie Library of Pitts. Library for the Blind
4724 Baum Boulevard
Pittsburgh, PA 15213
412-687-2440
800-242-0586
FAX: 412-687-2442
e-mail: clbph@clpgh.org
www.clpgh.org

Kathleen Kappel, Executive Director

Loans recorded books/magazines and playback equipment, large print books and described videos to western PA residents unable to use standard printed materials due to a visual, physical, or physically-based reading disability.
12 pages Quarterly

8887 To Love this Life: Quotations by Helen Keller
American Foundation for the Blind/AFB Press
2 Penn Plaza
Suite 1102
New York, NY 10121
212-502-7600
800-232-5463
FAX: 888-545-8331
e-mail: afbinfo@afb.org
www.afb.org

Carl R. Augusto, President & Chief Executive Officer
Rick Bozeman, Chief Financial Officer
Kelly Bleach, Chief Administrative Officer
Stacy Rollins, Executive Administrative Assistant to the President

Inspirational work that offers the penetrating observations of Helen Keller, the beloved deaf-blind champion of the rights of people with disabilities. Also available on cassette at $21.95 (ISBN# 0-89128-348-X) *$21.95*
144 pages Hardcover
ISBN 0-891283-47-1

8888 Touch the Baby: Blind & Visually Impaired Children As Patients
American Foundation for the Blind/AFB Press
2 Penn Plaza
Suite 1102
New York, NY 10121
212-502-7600
800-232-5463
FAX: 888-545-8331
e-mail: afbinfo@afb.net
www.afb.org

Carl R. Augusto, President & Chief Executive Officer
Rick Bozeman, Chief Financial Officer
Kelly Bleach, Chief Administrative Officer
Stacy Rollins, Executive Administrative Assistant to the President

A how-to manual for health care professionals working in hospitals, clinics and doctors' offices. Teaches the special communication and touch-related techniques needed to prevent blind and visually impaired patients from withdrawing from the healthcare workers and the outside world. $25.00/pack of 25.
13 pages
ISBN 0-891281-97-5

8889 Transition Activity Calendar for Students with Visual Impairments
Mississippi State University
P.O.Box 6189
Mississippi State, MS 39762
662-325-2001
FAX: 662-325-8989
TTY:662-325-2694
e-mail: nrtc@colled.msstate.edu
www.blind.msstate.edu

Jacqui Bybee, Research Associate II
Douglas Bedsaul, Research and Training Coordinator
Anne Carter, Research and Training Coordinator
Brenda Cavenaugh, Ph.D., Research Professor

The Transition Activity Calendar guides the student with a visual disability through the maze of college preparation. Beginning in junior high school, clearly written steps are listed for each grade level. Students planning to enter college after high school graduation can check-off their accomplishments each step of the way. The calendar helps students focus on their goals while providing reminders of tasks yet to be completed. It can be used in a self-directed manner or in a group format. *$4.25*
16 pages Paperback

8890 Transition to College for Students with Visual Impairments: Report
Mississippi State University
P.O.Box 6189
Mississippi State, MS 39762
662-325-2001
FAX: 662-325-8989
TTY:662-325-2694
e-mail: nrtc@colled.msstate.edu
www.blind.msstate.edu

Jacqui Bybee, Research Associate II
Douglas Bedsaul, Research and Training Coordinator
Anne Carter, Research and Training Coordinator
Brenda Cavenaugh, Ph.D., Research Professor

A report offering results from telephone interviews of college students with visual impairments and mail surveys of college officials which examines the transition experience of successful college students. General domains in the study include demographics, educational history, computers, specialized and adaptive equipment, resources, college preparation, problems adjusting to college and O&M skills. A literature review covers preparing for college, task timelines,and classroom, labs and tests. *$20.00*
151 pages Paperback

8891 Unseen Minority: A Social History of Blindness in the United States
American Foundation for the Blind/AFB Press
2 Penn Plaza
Suite 1102
New York, NY 10121
212-502-7600
800-232-5463
FAX: 888-545-8331
e-mail: abfinfo@abf.org
www.afb.org

Carl R. Augusto, President & Chief Executive Officer
Rick Bozeman, Chief Financial Officer
Kelly Bleach, Chief Administrative Officer
Stacy Rollins, Executive Administrative Assistant to the President

A lively narrative, with anecdotes, that recounts how the blind overcame discrimination to gain full participation in the social, educational, economic and legislative spheres. Hardcover. *$59.95*
573 pages Paperback
ISBN 0-891288-96-1

8892 Vision Enhancement
UN Printing
122
1790 E 54th St
Indianapolis, IN 46220-3454
317-254-1332
800-431-1739
FAX: 317-251-6588
e-mail: info@visionenhancement.org
www.visionww.org

Patricia L Price, Managing Editor

Designed to encourage and support individuals with vision loss, family members, and caregivers. *$25.00*
72-78 pages Quarterly

8893 Visual Impairment: An Overview
American Foundation for the Blind/AFB Press
2 Penn Plaza
Suite 1102
New York, NY 10121
212-502-7600
800-232-5463
FAX: 888-545-8331
e-mail: afbinfo@afb.net
www.afb.org
Carl R. Augusto, President & Chief Executive Officer
Rick Bozeman, Chief Financial Officer
Kelly Bleach, Chief Administrative Officer
Stacy Rollins, Executive Administrative Assistant to the President
An overall look at the most common forms of vision loss and their impact on the individual. Includes drawings as well as photographs that stimulate how people with vision loss see. Paperback. *$19.95*
56 pages
ISBN 0-891281-74-0

8894 Visual Impairments And Learning
Sage Publications
2455 Teller Road
Thousand Oaks, CA 91320
805-499-0721
800-818-7243
FAX: 805-499-0871
e-mail: info@sagepub.com
www.sagepub.com
Sara Miller McCune, Founder, Publisher, Executive Chairman
Blaise R Simqu, President & CEO
Tracey A. Ozmina, Executive Vice President & Chief Operating Officer
Stephen Barr, Managing Director/SAGE London, President of SAGE Internation
The major focus of this new, third edition is to present a new way of thinking about individuals with visual impairment so that they are viewed as participating members of a seeing world despite their reduced visual functioning. *$40.00*
213 pages
ISBN 0-890798-68-3

8895 Walking Alone and Marching Together
National Federation of the Blind
200 East Wells St
Baltimore, MD 21230-4914
410-659-9314
FAX: 410-685-5653
e-mail: nfb@iamdigex.net
www.nfb.org
Floyd Matson, Author
The history of the organized blind movement, this book spans more than 50 years of civil rights, social issues, attitudes and experiences of the blind. Published in 1990, it has been read by thousands of blind and sighted persons and is used in colleges, libraries and programs across the country as an important tool in understanding blindness and it's impact on both personal lives and the society at large. Braille $130, 2 track or 4 track cassette $40, Print $33.00. Contact Materials Center.

8896 What Do You Do When You See a Blind Person- and What Don't You Do?
American Foundation for the Blind/AFB Press
2 Penn Plaza
Suite 1102
New York, NY 10121
212-502-7600
800-232-5463
FAX: 888-545-8331
e-mail: afbinfo@afb.net
afb.org
Carl R. Augusto, President & Chief Executive Officer
Rick Bozeman, Chief Financial Officer
Kelly Bleach, Chief Administrative Officer
Stacy Rollins, Executive Administrative Assistant to the President
Examples of real-life situations that teach sighted persons how to interact effectively with blind persons. Topics covered include how to help someone across the street, how not to distract a guide dog and how to take leave of a blind person. *$25.00*
8 pages
ISBN 0-891281-95-5

8897 What Museum Guides Need to Know: Access for the Blind and Visually Impaired
American Foundation for the Blind/AFB Press
2 Penn Plaza
Suite 1102
New York, NY 10121
212-502-7600
800-232-5463
FAX: 888-545-8331
e-mail: afbinfo@afb.net
www.afb.org
Carl R. Augusto, President & Chief Executive Officer
Rick Bozeman, Chief Financial Officer
Kelly Bleach, Chief Administrative Officer
Stacy Rollins, Executive Administrative Assistant to the President
Explains how blind and visually impaired museum-goers experience art and offers pointers on greeting people, asking if help is needed and teaching about a specific work of art. Contains information on access laws, resources, training guides and guidelines for preparing large print, cassette and braille materials. *$14.95*
64 pages Paperback
ISBN 0-891281-58-4

8898 Work Sight
Lighthouse International
111 East 59th Street
New York, NY 10022-1202
212-821-9384
800-829-0500
FAX: 212-821-9707
e-mail: info@lighthouse.org
www.lighthouse.org
Mark G. Ackermann, President / CEO
Intended for employers and employees who have concerns about vision loss and job performance. *$25.00*

8899 World Through Their Eyes
Lighthouse International
111 East 59th Street
New York, NY 10022-1202
212-821-9384
800-829-0500
FAX: 212-821-9707
e-mail: info@lighthouse.org
www.lighthouse.org
Mark G. Ackermann, President / CEO
Intended to help nursing home staff understand how residents with impaired vision perceive the world. Concrete suggestions help staff provide better care to visually impaired residents. *$25.00*

8900 You Seem Like a Regular Kid to Me
American Foundation for the Blind/AFB Press
2 Penn Plaza
Suite 1102
New York, NY 10121
212-502-7600
800-232-5463
FAX: 888-545-8331
e-mail: afbinfo@afb.net
www.afb.org
Carl R. Augusto, President & Chief Executive Officer
Rick Bozeman, Chief Financial Officer
Kelly Bleach, Chief Administrative Officer
Stacy Rollins, Executive Administrative Assistant to the President
An interview with Jane, a blind child, tells other children what it's like to be blind. Jane explains how she gets around, takes care of herself, does her school work, spends her leisure time and even pays for things when she can't see money.
16 pages
ISBN 0-891289-21-6

Print: Journals

8901 **Journal of Visual Impairment and Blindness**
Sheridan Press,
450 Fame Ave
Hanover, PA 17331-1585
717-632-3535
800-352-2210
FAX: 717-633-8929
e-mail: pubsvc@tsp.sheridan.com
www.sheridanreprints.com
Sharon Shively, Editor
Published in braille, regular print and on ASC II disk and cassette, this journal contains a wide variety of subjects including rehabilitation, psychology, education, legislation, medicine, technology, employment, sensory aids and childhood development as they relate to visual impairments. $130 annual individual subscription, $180 annual institutional subscription.
64 pages Monthly
ISSN 0145-48 x

Print: Magazines

8902 **Blind Educator**
National Organization of Blind Educators
200 East Wells Street
Jernigan Place
Baltimore, MD 21230
410-659-9314
FAX: 410-685-5653
e-mail: nfb@nfb.org
www.nfb.org
Marc Mauer, President
Magazine specifically for blind educators.

8903 **Braille Forum**
American Council of the Blind
2200 Wilson Boulevard
Suite 650
Arlington, VA 22201-3354
202-467-5081
800-424-8666
FAX: 703-465-5085
e-mail: info@acb.org
www.acb.org
Kim Charlson, President
Jeff Thom, 1st Vice President
Melanie Brunson, Executive Director
Offered in print, braille, cassette, IBM computer disk and e-mail. $25 per format per year for companies and non-US residents.
48 pages Magazine

8904 **Braille Monitor**
Deaf-Blind Division of the Ntn'l Fed of the Blind
200 East Wells St
Baltimore, MD 21230-4914
410-659-9314
FAX: 410-685-5653
e-mail: nfbpublications@nfb.org
www.nfb.org
Marc Maurer, CEO
Barbara Pierce, Editor
The Braille Monitor is the leading publication of the National Federation of the Blind. It covers the events and activities of the NFB and addresses the many issues and concerns of the blind.

8905 **Dialogue Magazine**
Blindskills Inc
PO Box 5181
Salem, OR 97304-181
503-581-4224
800-860-4224
FAX: 503-581-0178
e-mail: info@blindskills.com
www.blindskills.com
B. T. Kimbrough, Executive Director
Publishes quarterly magazine in braille, large-type, cassette and email of news items, technology and articles of special interest to visually impaired youth and adults. Annual subscription cost $35 for braille, large print or cassette, $20 for email. *$28.00*
Quarterly

8906 **Future Reflections**
Deaf-Blind Division of the Ntn'l Fed of the Blind
200 East Wells Street
Baltimore, MD 21230-4914
410-659-9314
FAX: 410-685-5653
www.nfb.org
Marc Maurer, President
A magazine for parents and teachers of blind children.

8907 **Guide Magazine**
The Seeing Eye
P.O.Box 375
10 Washington Valley Road
Morristown, NJ 7963
973-539-4425
FAX: 973-539-0922
e-mail: info@seeingeye.org
seeingeye.org
James A. Kutsch, Jr., Ph.D., President & CEO
Robert Pudlak, CFO & Director of Administration & Finance
Glenn Cianci, Director of Facilities Management
Jean Thomas, Director of Donor & Public Relations
The Guide offers stories of inspiration from our graduates and news of the latest program developments.

8908 **JBI Voice**
Jewish Braille Institute of America
110 Est 30th Street
New York, NY 10016
212-889-2525
800-433-1531
FAX: 212-689-3692
e-mail: admin@jbilibrary.org
www.jbilibrary.org
Judy E. Tenney, Chairman
Thomas G. Kahn, Viec Chairman
Dr. Ellen Isler, President and CEO
Israel A Taub, Vice President and CFO
Monthly recorded magazine emphasizing Jewish current events and culture.

8909 **Jewish Braille Review**
Jewish Braille Institute of America
110 Est 30th Street
New York, NY 10016
212-889-2525
800-433-1531
FAX: 212-689-3692
e-mail: admin@jbilibrary.org
www.jbilibrary.org
Judy E. Tenney, Chairman
Thomas G. Kahn, Viec Chairman
Dr. Ellen Isler, President and CEO
Israel A Taub, Vice President and CFO
The JBI seeks the integration of Jews who are blind, visually impaired and reading disabled into the Jewish community and society in general. More than 20,000 men, women and children in 50 countries receive a broad variety of JBI services.

8910 **Merchant Messenger**
National Association of Blind Merchants
1837 South Nevada avenue
PMB #243
Colorado Springs, CO 80905
719-423-4384
888-691-1819
FAX: 719-527-0129
e-mail: markharris1222@sbcglobal.net
www.blindmerchants.org
Kevin Worley, President

8911 Musical Mainstream
Nat'l Lib Svc/Blind And Physically Handicapped
1291 Taylor Street North West
Washington, DC 20011
202-707-5100
FAX: 202-707-0712
TTY:202-707-0744
e-mail: nls@loc.gov
www.loc.gov/nls

Karen Keninger, Director
Articles selected from print music magazines.
Quarterly

8912 Opportunity
National Industries for the Blind
1310 Braddock Place
Alexandria, VA 22314-1691
703-310-0500
FAX: 703-998-8268
e-mail: services@nib.org
www.nib.org

The Honorabl Krump, Esq., Chairman
Louis J. Jablonski, Jr., Vice Chairman
Kevin A. Lynch, President and Chief Executive Officer
James M Kesteloot, Director
Offers information and articles on the newest technology, equipment, services and programs for blind and visually impaired persons.
Quarterly

8913 Providing Services for People with Vision Loss: Multidisciplinary Perspective
Resources for Rehabilitation
22 Bonad Road
Winchester, MA 01890-1302
781-368-9080
FAX: 781-368-9096
e-mail: orders@rfr.org
www.rfr.org

Susan L Greenblatt, Editor
A collection of articles by ophthalmologists and rehabilitation professionals, including chapters on operating a low vision service, starting self-help programs, mental health services, aids and techniques that help people with vision loss. *$19.95*
136 pages
ISBN 0-929718-02-0

Print: Newsletters

8914 AFB News
American Foundation for the Blind/AFB Press
2 Penn Plaza
Suite 1102
New York, NY 10121
212-502-7600
800-232-5463
FAX: 888-545-8331
e-mail: afbinfo@afb.net
www.afb.org

Carl R. Augusto, President & Chief Executive Officer
Rick Bozeman, Chief Financial Officer
Kelly Bleach, Chief Administrative Officer
Stacy Rollins, Executive Administrative Assistant to the President
National newsletter for general readership about blindness and visual impairments featuring people, programs, services and activities.
12 pages Quarterly

8915 ASB Visions Newsletter
Associated Services for the Blind
919 Walnut Street
Philadelphia, PA 19107
215-627-0600
FAX: 215-922-0692
e-mail: asbinfo@asb.org
www.asb.org

Patricia C. Johnson, President and CEO
Tim McGovern, Human Relations
Brian Rusk, Public Relations Officer
Derby Ewing, Director, Human Services
Newsletter associated services for the blind and visually impaired.

8916 Adaptive Services Division
District of Columbia Public Library
901G St NW,
Rm 215
Washington, DC 20001-4531
202-727-2142
FAX: 202-727-0322
TTY:202-559-5368
e-mail: lbph.dcpl@dc.gov
www.dclibrary.org

Venetia Demson, Chief, Adaptive Services
DC Regional Library for the blind, deaf and physically handicapped. Provides adaptive technology and training programs.
8 pages Quarterly

8917 Alumni News
Guide Dogs for the Blind
P.O.Box 151200
San Rafael, CA 94915-1200
415-499-4000
800-295-4050
FAX: 415-499-4035
guidedogs.com

Bob Burke, Chairman
Stuart Odell, Vice Chairman
Chris Benninger, President and CEO
Jay Harris, Secretary
Restricted to graduates only.

8918 Annual Report/Newsletter
National Accreditation Council for Agencies/Blind
Rm 1004
15 E 40th St
New York, NY 10016-401
212-683-5068
FAX: 212-683-4475

Ruth Westman, Executive Director
Provides standards and a program of accreditation for schools and organizations which serve children and adults who are blind or vision impaired.

8919 Association for Macular Diseases Newsletter
210 East 64th Street
New York, NY 10065
212-605-3719
FAX: 212-605-3795
e-mail: association@retinal-research.org
macula.org

Bernard Landou, President
Mary Fern Breheny, Board Member
Patricia Dahl, Board Member
Walter Ross, Editor-In-Chief
Not-for-profit organization promotes education and research in this scarcely explored field. Acts as a nationwide support group for individuals and their families endeavoring to adjust to the restrictions and changes brought about by macular disease. Offers hotline, educational materials, quarterly newsletter, support groups, referrals and seminars for persons and families affected by macular disease.

8920 Awareness
NAPVI
1 North Lexington Avenue
White Plains, NY 10601
617-972-7441
800-562-6265
FAX: 617-972-7444
e-mail: napvi@guildhealth.org
www.napvi.org

Julie Urban, President
Venetia Hayden, Vice President
Susan LaVenture, Executive Director
Randi Sher, Secretary
Newsletter offering regional news, sports and activities, conferences, camps, legislative updates, book reviews, audio reviews, professional question and answer column and more for the visually impaired and their families.
Quarterly

8921 **BTBL News**
Braille and Talking Book Library
P.O. Box 942837
Sacramento, CA 94237-0001
916-654-0261
800-952-5666
FAX: 916-654-1119
e-mail: btbl@library.ca.gov
www.btbl.ca.gov

Janet Coles, Editor
Christopher Berger, Senior Librarian
Olena Bilyk, Web Developer
Kim Brown, Communications Officer

BTBL News, the quarterly newsletter of the California Braille and Talking Book Library, features articles on topics of interest to library customers, including information about new services, existing services, events, staff and more.

8922 **Canes and Trails**
Guide Dogs for the Blind
P.O.Box 151200
San Rafael, CA 94915-1200
415-499-4000
800-295-4050
FAX: 415-499-4035
guidedogs.com

Bob Burke, Chairman
Stuart Odell, Vice Chairman
Chris Benninger, President and CEO
Jay Harris, Secretary

A quarterly newsletter for orientation and mobility specialists, rehabilitation professionals, teachers, and service providers in the field of blindness and visual impairment.

8923 **Community Connection**
Guide Dogs for the Blind
P.O.Box 151200
San Rafael, CA 94915-1200
415-499-4000
800-295-4050
FAX: 415-499-4035
guidedogs.com

Bob Burke, Chairman
Stuart Odell, Vice Chairman
Chris Benninger, President and CEO
Jay Harris, Secretary

A newsletter produced for our volunteers and other friends of Guide Dogs.

8924 **DVH Quarterly**
University of Arkansas at Little Rock
2801 S University Ave
Little Rock, AR 72204-1000
501-569-3000

Bob Brasher, Editor
Mary Boaz, Manager

Offers information on upcoming events, conferences and workshops on and for visual disabilities. Book reviews, information on the newest resources and technology, educational programs, want ads and more.
Quarterly

8925 **Deaf-Blind Perspective**
National Consortium on Deaf-Blindness
345 North Monmouth Avenue
Monmouth, OR 97361
503-838-8391
800-438-9376
FAX: 503-838-8150
TTY: 800-854-7013
e-mail: info@teachingresearchinstitute.org
www.tr.wou.edu

Ingrid Amerson, Child Development Center
Lyn Ayer, Center on Deaf & Blindness
Robert Ayres, Evaluation and Research
Cori Brownell, Center on Early Learning

A free publication with articles, essays, and announcements about topics related to people who are deaf-blind. Published two times a year (Spring and Fall) by the Teaching Research Institute of Western Oregon University, its purpose is to provide information and serve as a forum for discussion and sharing ideas.

8926 **Fidelco**
Fidelco Guide Dog Foundation
103 Vision Way
Bloomfield, CT 06002
860-243-5200
FAX: 860-769-0567
e-mail: info@fidelco.org
fidelco.org

Karen C. Tripp, Chairman
G. Kenneth Bernhard, Vice Chairman
Eliot D. Matheson, CEO
Diane R. Lindeland, VP, Finance

A newsletter published by Fidelco Guide Dog Foundation.

8927 **Focus**
Visually Impaired Center
1422 W Court St
Flint, MI 48503-5008
810-767-4014
FAX: 810-767-0020
www.vcflint.org

Charles Tommasulo, Executive Director

Newsletter offering information for the visually impaired person in the forms of legislative and law updates, ADA information, support groups, hotlines, and articles on the newest technology in the field.
Quarterly

8928 **Gleams Newsletter**
Glaucoma Research Foundation
2345 Yale Street
2nd Floor
Palo Alto, CA 94306
650-328-3388
800-826-6693
FAX: 415-986-3763
e-mail: info@glaucoma.org
auorthodontics.com

Tom Brunner, CEO

Offers updated medical & research information on glaucoma. Included are glaucoma treatmant and coping tips, legislative information, professional articles and book reviews.
6 pages Quarterly

8929 **Guide Dog News**
Guide Dogs for the Blind
P.O.Box 151200
San Rafael, CA 94915-1200
415-499-4000
800-295-4050
FAX: 415-499-4035
guidedogs.com

Bob Burke, Chairman
Stuart Odell, Vice Chairman
Chris Benninger, President and CEO
Jay Harris, Secretary

Read about changes to our teaching techniques, our new Adult Learning Program, vet tips, and find news about our graduates.

8930 **Guideway**
Guide Dog Foundation for the Blind
371 East Jericho Turnpike
Smithtown, NY 11787-2976
631-930-9000
800-548-4337
FAX: 631-930-9009
e-mail: info@guidedog.org
www.guidedog.org

James C. Bingham, Chairman
Alphonce J. Brown, Jr., Vice Chairman
Wells B. Jones, CEO
Jack Sage, Secretary

Offers updates and information on the foundation's activities and guide dog programs. In print form but is also available on cassette.
Monthly

8931 **Guild Briefs**
Catholic Guild for The Blind
65 East Wacker Place
Suite 1010
Chicago, IL 60601
312-236-8569
FAX: 312-236-8128
e-mail: info@guildfortheblind.org
www.guildfortheblind.org

Brett Christenson, President
Laura Rounce, Vice President
David Tabak, Executive Director
Toria Emas, Secretary
Monthly publication for individuals who are blind or visually impaired. It contains articles on topics such as service programs, scholarships, education, seniors, research, and government.
12 pages monthly

8932 **IAAIS Report**
Int'l Association of Audio Information Services
3920 Willshire Dr
Lawrence, KS 66049-3673
412-434-6023
800-280-5325
e-mail: aiblink@ak.net
www.iaais.org

Stuart Holland, President
Marjorie Williams, 1st Vice President
Linda Hynson, Secretary
Andrea Pasquale, Treasurer
Newsletter for persons interested in radio reading services. *$7.00*
Quarterly

8933 **Insight**
United States Association of Blind Athletes
1 Olympic Plaza
Colorado Springs, CO 80909
719-630-0422
FAX: 719-630-0616
e-mail: media@usaba.org
www.usaba.org

Mark A. Lucas, MS, Executive Director
Ryan Ortiz, Assistant Executive Director
John Potts, Goalball High Performance director
Matt Simpson, Membership & Outreach Coordinator
Covers news, announcements and activities of the association.
20 pages Quarterly

8934 **LampLighter**
Columbia Lighthouse for the Blind
1825 K Street NorthWest
Suite 1103
Washington, DC 20006
202-454-6400
FAX: 877-595-9228
e-mail: info@clb.org
clb.org

Tony Cancelosi, President
Anthony Cancelosi, CEO
Dedicated to helping the blind or visually impaired population.

8935 **Library Users of America Newsletter**
American Council of the Blind
2200 Wilson Boulevard
Suite 650
Arlington, VA 22201-3354
202-467-5081
800-424-8666
FAX: 703-465-5085
e-mail: info@acb.org
www.acb.org

Kim Charlson, President
Jeff Thom, 1st Vice President
Melanie Brunson, Executive Director
Published twice yearly, the newsletter contains much information about library services of particular interest to blind and visually impaired patrons, and is available in the following formats: Braille, audiocassette, large print and e-mail.

8936 **Light the Way**
Blind Children's Center
4120 Marathon Street
Los Angeles, CA 90029-3584
323-664-2153
800-222-3567
FAX: 323-665-3828
e-mail: info@blindchildrenscenter.org
blindchildrenscenter.org

Scott E. Schaldenbrand, President
Mark Correa, Board Member
Midge Horton, Executive Director
Newsletter of the Blind Childrens Center, a family-centered agency which serves young children with visual impairments. The center-based and home-based services help the children to acquire skills and build their independence. The center utilizes its expertise and experience to serve families and professionals worldwide through support services, education and research.

8937 **Lighthouse Publication**
Chicago Lighthouse
1850 West Roosevelt Road
Chicago, IL 60608-1298
312-666-1331
FAX: 312-243-8539
TTY:312-666-8874
e-mail: publications@chicagolighthouse.org
www.thechicagolighthouse.org

Janet P. Szlyk, Ph.D., President & Chief Executive Officer
Mary Lynne Januszewski, Executive Vice President/CFO
Melanie M. Hennessy, SVP
Terrence J. longo, Executive Vice President/COO

8938 **Lights On**
Fight for Sight
Ste 809
391 Park Ave S
New York, NY 10016-8806
212-679-6060
FAX: 212-679-4466
www.fightforsight.com

Mary Prudden, Executive Director
A newsletter published by Fight for Sight.

8939 **Long Cane News**
American Foundation for the Blind/AFB Press
2 Penn Plaza
Suite 1102
New York, NY 10121
212-502-7600
800-232-5463
FAX: 888-545-8331
e-mail: afbinfo@afb.net
www.afb.org

Carl R. Augusto, President & Chief Executive Officer
Rick Bozeman, Chief Financial Officer
Kelly Bleach, Chief Administrative Officer
Stacy Rollins, Executive Administrative Assistant to the President
SemiAnnual

8940 **Magnifier**
Macular Degeneration Foundation
P.O.Box 531313
Henderson, NV 89053
702-450-2908
888-633-3937
e-mail: liz@eyesight.org
www.eyesight.org

Liz Trauernicht, President & Director of Communications
Julie Zavala, VP & Asst. Director of Operations
David Seftel, EVP & Dircetor, R & D
Ron Gallamore, Board of Scientific Advisors
The Magnifier is the distributed without charge via email and by regular mail to those without access to the Internet. It features breaking news, clinical trails, clarifies recent reports in the media, announces new Internet resources and informs the public of important additions to the web site.

8941 NAVH Update
National Association of Visually Handicapped
111 East 59th Street
New York, NY 10022-1202
212-821-9384
800-829-0500
FAX: 212-821-9707
e-mail: info@lighthouse.org
lighthouse.org/navh

Mark G. Ackermann, President / CEO
A newsletter published by the National Association of Visually Impaired. LightHouse acquired NAVH.

8942 NBA Bulletin
National Braille Association
95 Allens Creek Road
Building 1, Suite 202
Rochester, NY 14618
585-427-8260
FAX: 585-427-0263
e-mail: nbaoffice@nationalbraille.org
www.nationalbraille.org

Jan Carroll, President
Cindi Laurent, Vice President
David Shaffer, Executive Director
Heidi Lehmann, Secretary
Published quarterly and included int he price of the regular and student NBA membership.

8943 NLS News
Nat'l Lib Svc/Blind And Physically Handicapped
1291 Taylor Street North West
Washington, DC 20011
202-707-5100
FAX: 202-707-0712
TTY:202-707-0744
e-mail: nls@loc.gov
www.loc.gov/nls

Karen Keninger, Director
Newsletter on current program developments.
Quarterly

8944 NLS Newsletter
Nat'l Lib Svc/Blind And Physically Handicapped
1291 Taylor Street North West
Washington, DC 20011
202-707-5100
FAX: 202-707-0712
TTY:202-707-0744
e-mail: nls@loc.gov
www.loc.gov/nls

Karen Keninger, Director
Newsletter on the service's volunteer activities.
Quarterly

8945 PBA News
Prevent Blindness America
211 West Wacker Drive
Suite 1700
Chicago, IL 60606
800-331-2020
e-mail: info@preventblindness.org
www.preventblindness.org

Paul G. Howes, Chairman
Hugh R. Parry, President & CEO,Prevent Blindness America
Jerome Desserich, Vice President & Chief Financial Officer
Danielle Disch, Development Manager
Newsletter is filled with the information you need to protect your eyes, preserve your sight, and educate yourself about your own eye condition or that of a family member. Publication offered three times yearly.
3 times yearly

8946 Planned Giving Department of Guide Dogs for the Blind
Guide Dogs for the Blind
P.O.Box 151200
San Rafael, CA 94915-1200
415-499-4000
800-295-4050
FAX: 415-499-4035
guidedogs.com

Bob Burke, Chairman
Stuart Odell, Vice Chairman
Chris Benninger, President and CEO
Jay Harris, Secretary
A newsletter published by Guide Dogs for the Blind.

8947 Playback
Recording for the Blind & Dyslexic
20 Roszel Road
Princeton, NJ 08540
800-221-4792
FAX: 609-987-8116
e-mail: Custserv@LearningAlly.org
www.learningally.org/

Brad Grob, Chairman
Harold J. Logan, Vice Chairman
Andrew Friedman, President & CEO
Jim Halliday, Executive Vice President
A publication dedicated to our unit's family of members, volunteers, supporters and staff. RFB&D is now Learning Ally.
3x Year

8948 Quarterly Update
National Association for Visually Handicapped
111 East 59th Street
New York, NY 10022-1202
212-821-9384
800-829-0500
FAX: 212-821-9707
e-mail: info@lighthouse.org
lighthouse.org/navh

Mark G. Ackermann, President / CEO
Quarterly newsletter offering information on new products for the visually impaired, advances in medical treatments, new books available in the NAVH large print loan library and any new/updated booklets. Free. LightHouse acquired NAVH.

8949 RP Messenger
Texas Association of Retinitis Pigmentosa
P.O.Box 8388
Corpus Christi, TX 78468-8388
361-852-8515
FAX: 361-852-8515
e-mail: tarp@homebiz101.com
www.geocities.com

Dorothy Steifel, Executive Director
A bi-annual newsletter offering information on Retinitis Pigmentosa. *$15.00*
BiAnnual

8950 SCENE
Braille Institute
527 North Dale Avenue
Anaheim, CA 92801
714-821-5000
800-272-4553
FAX: 714-527-7621
e-mail: oc@brailleinstitute.org
brailleinstitute.org

Lester M. Sussman, Chairman
Peter A. Mindnich, President
Jon K. Hayashida, OD, FAAO, Vice President, Programs & Services
Rezaur Rehman, Vice President, Finance
Offers information on the organization, question and answer column, articles on the newest technology and more for visually impaired persons.

8951 STAR
Special Technologies Alternative Resources
210 McMorran Boulevard
Port Huron, MI 48060
810-987-7323
877-987-READ
e-mail: star@sccl.lib.mi.us
www.sccl.lib.mi.us

Arnold H. Larson, Chairman
Kathleen J. Wheelihan, Vice Chairman
Arlene M. Marcetti, Board Member
Stan Arnetti, Director

A newsletter published by Special Technologies Alternative Resources.

8952 Seeing Eye Guide
The Seeing Eye
P.O.Box 375
10 Washington Valley Road
Morristown, NJ 07963
973-539-4425
FAX: 973-539-0922
e-mail: info@seeingeye.org
seeingeye.org

James A. Kutsch, Jr., Ph.D., President & CEO
Randall Ivens, Director of Human Resources
Robert Pudlak, CFO & Director of Administration & Finance
David Johnson, Director of Instruction & Training

A quarterly publication from Seeing Eye.
Quarterly

8953 Shared Visions
Vista Center for the Blind & Visually Impaired
413 Laurel St
Santa Cruz, CA 95060-4904
831-458-9766
800-705-2970
FAX: 831-426-6233
e-mail: information@vistacenter.org
doranblindcenter.org

Pam Brandin, Executive Director

A quarterly publication for Blind and Visually Impaired individuals from Vista Center for the Blind and Visually Impaired.

8954 Sharing Solutions: A Newsletter for Support Groups
Lighthouse International
111 East 59th Street
New York, NY 10022-1202
212-821-9384
800-829-0500
FAX: 212-821-9707
e-mail: info@lighthouse.org
www.lighthouse.org

Mark G. Ackermann, President / CEO

A newsletter for members and leaders of support groups for older adults with impaired vision. The letter provides a forum for support groups members to network and share information, printed in a very large type format.

8955 Sightings Newsletter
Schepens Eye Research Institute
20 Staniford Street
Boston, MA 02114
617-912-0100
FAX: 617-912-0110
www.schepens.harvard.edu

Michael Gilmore, Director
Mary E. Leach, Director of Public Affairs
Frances Ng, Director of Human Resources
Ojas P. Mehta, Director, Intellectual Property & Commercial Ventures

Publication of prominent center for research on eye, vision, and blinding diseases; dedicated to research that improves the understanding, management, and prevention of eye diseases and visual deficiencies; fosters collaboration among its faculty members; trains young scientists and clinicians from around the world; promotes communication with scientists in allied fields; leader in the worldwide dispersion of basic scientific knowledge of vision.

8956 Smith Kettlewell Rehabilitation Engineering Research Center
2318 Fillmore Street
San Francisco, CA 94115
415-345-2000
FAX: 415-345-8455
e-mail: rerc@ski.org
ski.org/rerc

John Brabyn, Ph.D., CEO/Executive Director
Ruth S. Poole, COO
Arthur Jampolsky, Director
Arthur Jampolsky,M.D., Founder

Reports on technology and devices for persons with visual impairments.

8957 Student Advocate
National Alliance of Blind Students NABS Liaison
Ste 1004
1155 15th St NW
Washington, DC 20005-2706
202-467-5081
800-424-8666
FAX: 202-467-5085
www.blindstudents.org

Melanie Brunson, Executive Director

A newsletter created by members of NABS and for any interested parties.

8958 TBC Focus
Chicago Public Library Talking Books Center
400 South State Street
Chicago, IL 60605
312-747-4300
800-757-4654
FAX: 312-747-1609
www.chipublib.org

Linda Johnson Rice, President
Christopher Valenti, VP
Christina Benitez, Secretary
Karim Adib, Director

Published quarterly by the Chicago Public Library Talking Book Center. Free of charge.
4 pages Quarterly

8959 Talking Books Topics
Nat'l Lib Svc/Blind And Physically Handicapped
1291 Taylor Street North West
Washington, DC 20011
202-707-5100
FAX: 202-707-0712
TTY:202-707-0744
e-mail: nls@loc.gov
www.loc.gov/nls

Karen Keninger, Director

New recorded books and program news
Bi-monthly

8960 Upstate Update
New York State Talking Book & Braille Library
222 Madison Avenue
Albany, NY 12230-1
518-474-5935
800-342-3688
FAX: 514-474-5786
TTY: 518-474-7121
e-mail: nyslweb@mail.nysed.gov
www.nysl.nysed.gov

Bernard A. Margolis, State Librarian & Asst. Commissioner for Libraries
Loretta Ebert, Research Library Director
Liza Duncan, Technical Services & Systmes

Books on audio cassette, cassette players, braille books, summer reading programs, braille writer, magnifiers, closed-circuit T.V., large-print photocopier, cassette books and magazines, children's books on cassette, reference materials on blindness and other handicaps.
4 pages Quarterly

8961 Visual Aids and Informational Material
National Association for Visually Handicapped
111 East 59th Street
New York, NY 10022-1202 212-821-9384
800-829-0500
FAX: 212-821-9707
e-mail: info@lighthouse.org
lighthouse.org/navh

Mark G. Ackermann, President / CEO
A complete listing of the visual aids NAVH carries such as magnifiers, talking clocks, large print playing cards, etc. LightHouse acquired NAVH. *$2.50*
65 pages

8962 Voice
Vermont Assn for the Blind & Visually Impaired
60 Kimball Avenue
South Burlington, VT 05403 802-863-1358
800-639-5861
FAX: 802-863-1481
e-mail: General@vabvi.org
vabvi.org

Thomas Chase, President
Stephen Pouliot, Executive Director
Kathleen Quinlan, Director of Operations
Lori Newsome, Office Manager
The Voice is a newsletter published by Vermont Association for the Blind and Visually Impaired.

8963 Voice of Vision
GW Micro
725 Airport North Office Park
Fort Wayne, IN 46825 260-489-3671
FAX: 260-489-2608
e-mail: sales@gwmicro.com
www.gwmicro.com

Dan Weirich, Owner
Offers product reviews, product announcements, tips for making systems or applications more accessible, or explanations of concepts of interest to any computer user or would-be computer user. This association newsletter is available in braille, in large print, on audio cassette and on 3.5 or 5.25 IBM format diskette.
Quarterly

Non Print: Newsletters

8964 Insight
Eye Bank Association of America
Ste 1010
1015 18th Street NorthWest
Washington, DC 20036 202-775-4999
FAX: 202-429-6036
e-mail: info@restoresight.org
www.restoresight.org

David Glasser, Chairman
Kevin Corcoran, President & Chief Executive Officer
Molly Georgakis, VP of Member Services
Patricia Hardy, Manager of Communications
An electronic newsletter.

8965 Listen Up
Recording for the Blind & Dyslexic
20 Roszel Rd
Princeton, NJ 8540-6206 609-452-0606
866-732-3585
FAX: 609-520-7990
www.learningally.org

John Kelly, CEO
RFB&D's bi-monthly electronic newsletter for members.

Non Print: Video

8966 Aging and Vision: Declarations of Independence
American Foundation for the Blind/AFB Press
2 Penn Plaza
Suite 1102
New York, NY 10121 212-502-7600
800-232-5463
FAX: 888-545-8331
e-mail: afbinfo@afb.net
www.afb.org

Carl R. Augusto, President & Chief Executive Officer
Rick Bozeman, Chief Financial Officer
Kelly Bleach, Chief Administrative Officer
Stacy Rollins, Executive Administrative Assistant to the President
A very personal look at five older people who have successfully coped with visual impairmant and continue to lead active, satisfying lives. Their stories are not only inspirational, but also provide practical, down-to-earth suggestions for adapting to vision loss later in life. 18 minute video tape. Also available in PAL, $52.95, 0-89128-276-9. *$42.95*
VHS
ISBN 0-891282-20-3

8967 Blindness, A Family Matter
American Foundation for the Blind/AFB Press
2 Penn Plaza
Suite 1102
New York, NY 10121 212-502-7600
800-232-5463
FAX: 888-545-8331
e-mail: afbinfo@afb.net
www.afb.org

Carl R. Augusto, President & Chief Executive Officer
Rick Bozeman, Chief Financial Officer
Kelly Bleach, Chief Administrative Officer
Stacy Rollins, Executive Administrative Assistant to the President
A frank exploration of the effects of an individual's visual impairment on other members of the family and how those family members can play a positive role in the rehabilitation process. Features interviews with three families whose 'success stories' provide advice and encouragement, as well as interviews with newly blinded adults currently involved in a rehabilitation program. 23 minute video tape. Also available in PAL, $49.95, 0-89128-271-8. *$43.95*
VHS
ISBN 0-891282-22-X

8968 Building Blocks: Foundations for Learning for Young Blind and Visually Impaired Children
American Foundation for the Blind/AFB Press
2 Penn Plaza
Suite 1102
New York, NY 10121 212-502-7600
800-232-5463
FAX: 888-545-8331
e-mail: afbinfo@afb.net
www.afb.org

Carl R. Augusto, President & Chief Executive Officer
Rick Bozeman, Chief Financial Officer
Kelly Bleach, Chief Administrative Officer
Stacy Rollins, Executive Administrative Assistant to the President
Presents the essential components of a successful early intervnetion program, including collaboration with family members, positive relationships between parents and professionals, public education, and attention to important programming components such as space exploration, braille readiness, orientation and mobility, play, cooking and music. Includes interviews with parents. Available in English or Spanish. 10 minute video tape. Also available in PAL, $33.95, 0-89128-268-8. *$26.95*
VHS
ISBN 0-891282-14-9

8969 Choice Magazine Listening
85 Channel Drive
Port Washington, NY 11050
516-883-8280
888-724-6423
888-724-6423
FAX: 516-944-5849
e-mail: choicemag@aol.com
www.choicemagazinelistening.org

Pamela Loeser, Editor in Chief
Ann Schlegel-Kyrkostas, Associate Editor
David Graham Pade, Associate Editor
Michael Tedeschi, Webmaster

A free audio anthology is available bi-monthly to visually impaired/physically disabled or dislexic persons nationwide. Playable on the special free 4-track cassette playback equipment which is provided by the Library of Congress through the National Library Service. Each issue features eight hours of unabridged magazine articles, short stories, poetry and media selections from over 100 sources. College level and older. Bimonthly distribution.
Bi-Monthly

8970 Juggler
Beacon Press
24 Farnsworth Street
Boston, MA 02210
617-742-2110
FAX: 617-723-3097
beacon.org

Helene Atwan, Executive Director

Andre was the young son of a wealthy, early Quebec fur trader. Because he was almost totally blind, he was overly protected by his family, and his movement outside his home was very limited.
Film

8971 Let's Eat Video
Blind Children's Center
4120 Marathon Street
Los Angeles, CA 90029-3584
323-664-2153
800-222-3567
FAX: 323-665-3828
e-mail: info@blindchildrenscenter.org
blindchildrenscenter.org

Scott E. Schaldenbrand, President
Mark Correa, Board Member
Midge Horton, Executive Director

Babies and toddlers with visual impairments lack one major avenue of exploration, and this significantly infulences their awareness, perceptions, and anticipation of the food which is presented to them. *$35.00*
VHS/DVD

8972 Look Out for Annie
Lighthouse International
111 East 59th Street
New York, NY 10022-1202
212-821-9384
800-829-0500
FAX: 212-821-9706
e-mail: info@lighthouse.org
www.lighthouse.org

Mark G. Ackermann, President / CEO

Depicts an older woman coping with her vision loss. It focuses on the emotional issues surrounding vision loss and conveys the idea that both the person with the vision disorder and their family and friends will need to make adjustments. *$25.00*
Video

8973 Not Without Sight
American Foundation for the Blind/AFB Press
PO Box 1020
Sewickley, PA 15143-920
412-741-1142
800-232-3044
FAX: 412-741-0609
e-mail: afborders@abdintl.com
www.afb.org

Carl R Augusto, President/CEO
Tracy Charlovich, Css

This video describes the major types of visual impairment and their causes and effects on vision, while camera simulations approximate what people with each impairmant actually see. Also demonstrates how people with low vision make the best use of the vision they have. 20 minute video tape, $49.95. *$42.95*
VHS 17 min
ISBN 0-891282-27-3

8974 Out of Left Field
American Foundation for the Blind/AFB Press
2 Penn Plaza
Suite 1102
New York, NY 10121
212-502-7600
800-232-5463
FAX: 888-545-8331
e-mail: afbinfo@afb.net
afb.org

Carl R. Augusto, President & Chief Executive Officer
Rick Bozeman, Chief Financial Officer
Kelly Bleach, Chief Administrative Officer
Stacy Rollins, Executive Administrative Assistant to the President

Illustrates how youngsters who are blind or visually impaired integrated with their sighted peers in a variety of recreational and athletic activities. 17 minute video tape. Also available in PAL, $33.95, 0-89128-270-X. *$29.95*
VHS 17 minutes
ISBN 0-891282-28-0

8975 See What I'm Saying
Fanlight Productions
c/o Icarus Films
32 Court Street, 21st Floor
Brooklyn, NY 11201
718-488-8900
800-876-1710
FAX: 718-488-8642
e-mail: info@fanlight.com, sales@icarusfilms.com
www.fanlight.com

Ben Achtenberg, Founder, Owner

The documentary follows Patricia, who is deaf and from a Spanish-speaking family, through her first year at the Kendall Demonstration Elementary School of Gallaudet University.
VHS/DVD

8976 See for Yourself
Lighthouse International
111 East 59th Street
New York, NY 10022-1202
212-821-9384
800-829-0500
FAX: 212-821-9706
e-mail: info@lighthouse.org
www.lighthouse.org

Mark G. Ackermann, President / CEO

This video features older adults with impaired vision who have been helped by vision rehabilitation. *$50.00*

8977 Shape Up 'n Sign
Harris Communications
15155 Technology Dr
Eden Prairie, MN 55344-2273
952-906-1180
800-825-6758
FAX: 952-906-1099
e-mail: info@harriscomm.com

Robert Harris, Owner

An aerobic exercise tape introducing the basic sign language for deaf and hearing children ages six to ten. *$29.95*
30 Minutes DVD

8978 Sight by Touch
Landmark Media
3450 Slade Run Drive
Falls Church, VA 22042
703-241-2030
800-342-4336
FAX: 703-536-9540
e-mail: info@landmarkmedia.com
landmarkmedia.com

Michael Hartogs, President
Peter Hartogs, VP New Business & Development
Beverly Weisenberg, Sales Rep
Richard Hartogs, VP Acquisitions

This video features the life and importance of Louis Braille. Vision-impaired performers and teachers demonstrate how Braille has benefitted their lives, and how improvements are constantly being made. *$195.00*
Video

8979 Taping for the Blind
3935 Essex Lane
Houston, TX 77027
713-622-2767
FAX: 713-622-2772
e-mail: info@tapingfortheblind.org
www.afb.org

Carl R. Augusto, President & Chief Executive Officer
Rick Bozeman, Chief Financial Officer
Robin Vogel, VP, Resource Development
Cynthia Fanzetti, Executive Director

An independent non profit educational organization funded by corporations, listeners and individuals, with a mission to turn sight into sound, enriching the lives of individuals with visual, physical and learning disabilities. Founded in 1967 to read materials not availiable through other sources onto standard audio cassettes in our custom recording division. In 1978, Houston Taping fFor The Blind signed on the air. Reading several dozen popular magazines and best selling books on the air.

8980 We Can Do it Together!
American Foundation for the Blind/AFB Press
2 Penn Plaza
Suite 1102
New York, NY 10121
212-502-7600
800-232-5463
FAX: 888-545-8331
e-mail: afbinfo@afb.net
afb.org

Carl R. Augusto, President & Chief Executive Officer
Rick Bozeman, Chief Financial Officer
Kelly Bleach, Chief Administrative Officer
Stacy Rollins, Executive Administrative Assistant to the President

This video illustrates a transdisciplinary team orientation and mobility program for students with severe visual and multiple impairments, covering both adapted communication systems used to teach mobility skills and basic indoor mobility in the school. For mobility instructors, administrators, teachers of the visually and severely handicapped, occupational, physical and speech therapists and parents. Discussion guide included. 10 minute video tape. Also available in PAL, $33.95, 0-89128-267-X. *$26.95*
VHS
ISBN 0-891282-13-0

Sports

8981 American Blind Bowling Association
1209 Somerset Road
Raleigh, NC 27610
919-755-0700
www.abba1951.org/contact.htm

Thomas Lester, President
A.J. Inglesby, 1st Vice President
James Benton, 2nd Vice President
Judy Mandelkow, Tournament Director

Promotes blind bowling throughout the US and Canada by sanctioning blind bowling leagues and conducting a National Tournament. Current membership exceeds 2,000 people in the United States and Canada.

8982 Basketball: Beeping Foam
Maxi Aids
42 Executive Boulevard
Farmingdale, NY 11735
631-752-0521
800-522-6294
FAX: 631-752-0689
TTY: 631-752-0738
e-mail: sales@maxiaids.com
www.maxiaids.com

Elliot Zaretsky, President

This sound making basketball enables the visually impaired to play basketball or other games. *$29.95*

8983 Blind Outdoor Leisure Development
P.O.Box 6639
Snowmass Village, CO 81615
970-923-0578
FAX: 970-923-7338
e-mail: possibilities@challengeaspen.com
challengeaspen.org

Jimmy Yeager, President
Jack Kennedy, VP
Grayson Stover, Secretary
Kevin Berg, Director

Outdoor recreation for the blind. Winter program of skiing with guides plus numerous summer programs for the visually impaired.

8984 Challenge Golf
otivation Media
1245 Milwaukee Ave
Glenview, IL 60025-2400
847-827-9057
FAX: 847-297-6829

Dorothy Bauer, Coordinator

A plain-language video, Challenge Golf is packed with information for beginners or veterans. Peter Longo covers 5 handicaps (one-arm, one-leg, in a seated position, blind, and arthritis) clearly and concisely, on how to play golf with a physical disability. In color, complete with special effects, graphs and real handicapped golfers at play. *$38.95*
Home Edition

8985 US Association of Blind Athletes
1 Olympic Plaza
Colorado Springs, CO 80909
719-630-0422
FAX: 719-630-0616
e-mail: media@usaba.org
www.usaba.org

Mark A. Lucas, MS, Executive Director
Ryan Ortiz, Assistant Executive Director
John Potts, Goalball High Performance director
Matt Simpson, Membership & Outreach Coordinator

Provides athletic opportunities and training in competitive sports for visually impaired and blind individuals throughout the US Competitions indlcude local, regional and national events, internation events, and the Winter and Summer Paralympic Games.

8986 United States Blind Golf Association
3094 Shamrock St N
Tallahassee, FL 32309-2735
864-987-9688
e-mail: info@usblindgolf.com
www.blindgolf.com

Jim Baker, President
Mike McKone, Vice President
Bill McMahon, Board Member
Jack Rupert, Board Member

Provides blind and vision impaired gold tournaments to members.

Support Groups

8987 Braille Institute Orange County Center
527 North Dale Avenue
Anaheim, CA 92801
714-821-5000
800-272-4553
FAX: 714-527-7621
e-mail: oc@brailleinstitute.org
brailleinstitute.org

Lester M. Sussman, Chairman
Peter A. Mindnich, President
Jon K. Hayashida, OD, FAAO, Vice President, Programs & Services
Rezaur Rehman, Vice President, Finance

Offers services, publications, information and programs free of charge to blind and visually impaired persons of all ages.

8988 Consumer and Patient Information Hotline
Prevent Blindness America
211 West Wacker Drive
Suite 1700
Chicago, IL 60606
800-331-2020
e-mail: info@preventblindness.org
www.preventblindness.org/

Paul G. Howes, Chairman
Hugh R. Parry, President & CEO,Prevent Blindness America
Jerome Desserich, Vice President & Chief Financial Officer
Danielle Disch, Development Manager

A toll-free line offering free information on a broad range of vision, eye health and safety topics including sports eye safety, diabetic retinopathy, glaucoma, cataracts, children's eye disorders and more.

8989 Department of Ophthalmology Information Line
Eye & Ear Infirmary
1855 W Taylor St
Chicago, IL 60612-7242
312-996-6590
FAX: 312-996-7770
e-mail: eyeweb@uic.edu
www.uic.edu

Jospeh White, President

Offers eye clinic and physician referrals to persons suffering from vision disorders as well as offers emergency information.

8990 Lighthouse International Information and Resource Service
111 East 59th Street
New York, NY 10022-1202
212-821-9384
800-829-0500
FAX: 212-821-9707
e-mail: info@lighthouse.org
lighthouse.org

Mark G. Ackermann, President / CEO

Provides information about eye diseases, low vision, age-related vision loss, adaptive technology, optical devices, large print and braille publishers, helps people find low vision services, vision rehabilitation services, and support groups across the U.S.; offers large selection of consumer products.

8991 National Association for Parents of Children with Visual Impairments (NAPVI)
1 North Lexington Avenue
White Plains, NY 10601
617-972-7441
800-562-6265
FAX: 617-972-7444
e-mail: napvi@guildhealth.org
www.napvi.org

Julie Urban, President
Venetia Hayden, Vice President
Susan LaVenture, Executive Director
Randi Sher, Secretary

In 1979, a group of parents responding to their own needs founded NAPVI, the National Association for Parents of the Visually Impaired, Inc. Never before was there a self-help organization specific to the needs of families of children with visual impairments. Since that time, NAPVI has grown and helped families across the US and in other countries.

8992 VUE: Vision Use in Employment
Carroll Center for the Blind
770 Centre Street
Newton, MA 02458-2597
617-969-6200
800-852-3131
FAX: 617-969-6204
e-mail: info@carrol.org
www.carroll.org

Joseph Abely, President
Brian Charlson, Director of Technology
Diane M. Newark, Chief Development Officer
Janet Perry, Human Resources Director

Provides engineering solutions plus training to help people keep jobs despite their vision loss.

8993 Washington Connection
American Council of the Blind
2200 Wilson Boulevard
Suite 650
Arlington, VA 22201-3354
202-467-5081
800-424-8666
FAX: 703-465-5085
e-mail: info@acb.org
acb.org

Kim Charlson, President
Jeff Thom, 1st Vice President
Melanie Brunson, Executive Director

Coverage of issues affecting blind people via legislative information, participates in law-making, legislative training seminars and networking of support resources across the US.

A

B

C

D

E

F

G

I

K

L

M

N

O

P

Q

R

S

T

U

V

W

X

Y

Z

Alabama

Alaska

Arizona

Arkansas

California

Colorado

Connecticut

Delaware

District of Columbia

Florida

Georgia

Hawaii

Idaho

Illinois

Indiana

Iowa

Kansas

Kentucky

Louisiana

Maine

Maryland

Massachusetts

Michigan

Minnesota

Mississippi

Missouri

Montana

Nebraska

Nevada

New Hampshire

New Jersey

New Mexico

New York

North Carolina

North Dakota

Ohio

Oklahoma

Oregon

Pennsylvania

Rhode Island

South Carolina

South Dakota

Tennessee

Texas

Utah

Vermont

Virginia

Washington

West Virginia

Wisconsin

Wyoming

AIDS

Accupressure

Aging

Alternative Therapies

Amputation

Amythrophic Lateral Sclerosis

Art & Music Therapies

Arthritis

Asthma

Attention Deficit Disorder

Autism

Behavioral Disorders

Birth Defects

Blind/Deaf

Brain Injuries

Cancer

Cerebral Palsy

Chiropractics

Chronic Disabilities

Cleft Palate

Cognitive Disorders

Cystic Fibrosis

Dementia

Dental Issues

Depression

Developmental Disabilities

Diabetes

Diet & Nutrition

Down Syndrome

Dyslexia

Education & Counseling

Emergency Alert

Environmental Disorders

Epilepsy

Head & Neck Injuries

Hearing Impairments

Hemophilia

Herbal Medicine

Human Interaction Disabilities

Immune Deficiencies

Incontinence

Language Disorders

Learning Disabilities

Lowe's Syndrome

Lung Disorders

Massage Therapy

Mental Disabilities

Mental Retardation

Multiple Disabilities

Multiple Sclerosis

Muscular Dystrophy

Neurological Impairments

Obesity

Orthopedical Disabilities

Pain Management

Parkinson Disease

Pediatric Issues

Phenylketonuria

Physical Disabilities

Polio

Prader-Willi Syndrome

Rare Disabilities

Respiratory Disorders

Severe Disabilites

Sexual Abuse & Related Conditions

Sjogren's Syndrome

Speech Disorders

Spina Bifida

Spinal Cord Injuries

Stroke

Theater & Dance Therapies

Tinnitus

Tourette Syndrome

Visual Impairments

Women

Grey House Publishing

2014 Title List

Visit **www.GreyHouse.com** for Product Information, Table of Contents and Sample Pages

General Reference

America's College Museums
American Environmental Leaders: From Colonial Times to the Present
An African Biographical Dictionary
An Encyclopedia of Human Rights in the United States
Constitutional Amendments
Encyclopedia of African-American Writing
Encyclopedia of the Continental Congress
Encyclopedia of Gun Control & Gun Rights
Encyclopedia of Invasions & Conquests
Encyclopedia of Prisoners of War & Internment
Encyclopedia of Religion & Law in America
Encyclopedia of Rural America
Encyclopedia of the United States Cabinet, 1789-2010
Encyclopedia of War Journalism
Encyclopedia of Warrior Peoples & Fighting Groups
From Suffrage to the Senate: America's Political Women
Nations of the World
Political Corruption in America
Speakers of the House of Representatives, 1789-2009
The Environmental Debate: A Documentary History
The Evolution Wars: A Guide to the Debates
The Religious Right: A Reference Handbook
The Value of a Dollar: 1860-2009
The Value of a Dollar: Colonial Era
This is Who We Were: A Companion to the 1940 Census
This is Who We Were: The 1920s
This is Who We Were: The 1950s
This is Who We Were: The 1960s
US Land & Natural Resource Policy
Working Americans 1770-1869 Vol. IX: Revolutionary War to the Civil War
Working Americans 1880-1999 Vol. I: The Working Class
Working Americans 1880-1999 Vol. II: The Middle Class
Working Americans 1880-1999 Vol. III: The Upper Class
Working Americans 1880-1999 Vol. IV: Their Children
Working Americans 1880-2003 Vol. V: At War
Working Americans 1880-2005 Vol. VI: Women at Work
Working Americans 1880-2006 Vol. VII: Social Movements
Working Americans 1880-2007 Vol. VIII: Immigrants
Working Americans 1880-2009 Vol. X: Sports & Recreation
Working Americans 1880-2010 Vol. XI: Inventors & Entrepreneurs
Working Americans 1880-2011 Vol. XII: Our History through Music
Working Americans 1880-2012 Vol. XIII: Education & Educators
World Cultural Leaders of the 20th & 21st Centuries

Business Information

Complete Television, Radio & Cable Industry Directory
Directory of Business Information Resources
Directory of Mail Order Catalogs
Directory of Venture Capital & Private Equity Firms
Environmental Resource Handbook
Food & Beverage Market Place
Grey House Homeland Security Directory
Grey House Performing Arts Directory
Hudson's Washington News Media Contacts Directory
New York State Directory
Sports Market Place Directory

Education Information

Charter School Movement
Comparative Guide to American Elementary & Secondary Schools
Complete Learning Disabilities Directory
Educators Resource Directory
Special Education

Health Information

Comparative Guide to American Hospitals
Complete Directory for Pediatric Disorders
Complete Directory for People with Chronic Illness
Complete Directory for People with Disabilities
Complete Mental Health Directory
Diabetes in America: A Geographic & Demographic Analysis
Directory of Health Care Group Purchasing Organizations
Directory of Hospital Personnel
HMO/PPO Directory
Medical Device Register
Older Americans Information Directory

Statistics & Demographics

America's Top-Rated Cities
America's Top-Rated Small Towns & Cities
America's Top-Rated Smaller Cities
American Tally
Ancestry & Ethnicity in America
Comparative Guide to American Hospitals
Comparative Guide to American Suburbs
Profiles of America
Profiles of... Series – State Handbooks
The Hispanic Databook
Weather America

Financial Ratings Series

TheStreet.com Ratings Guide to Bond & Money Market Mutual Funds
TheStreet.com Ratings Guide to Common Stocks
TheStreet.com Ratings Guide to Exchange-Traded Funds
TheStreet.com Ratings Guide to Stock Mutual Funds
TheStreet.com Ratings Ultimate Guided Tour of Stock Investing
Weiss Ratings Consumer Guides
Weiss Ratings Guide to Banks & Thrifts
Weiss Ratings Guide to Credit Unions
Weiss Ratings Guide to Health Insurers
Weiss Ratings Guide to Life & Annuity Insurers
Weiss Ratings Guide to Property & Casualty Insurers

Bowker's Books In Print® Titles

Books In Print®
Books In Print® Supplement
American Book Publishing Record® Annual
American Book Publishing Record® Monthly
Books Out Loud™
Bowker's Complete Video Directory™
Children's Books In Print®
El-Hi Textbooks & Serials In Print®
Forthcoming Books®
Law Books & Serials In Print™
Medical & Health Care Books In Print™
Publishers, Distributors & Wholesalers of the US™
Subject Guide to Books In Print®
Subject Guide to Children's Books In Print®

Canadian General Reference

Associations Canada
Canadian Almanac & Directory
Canadian Environmental Resource Guide
Canadian Parliamentary Guide
Financial Services Canada
Governments Canada
Health Services Canada
Libraries Canada
Major Canadian Cities
The History of Canada

Grey House Publishing | Salem Press | H.W. Wilson
4919 Route, 22 PO Box 56, Amenia NY 12501-0056

SALEM PRESS SALEM PRESS

2014 Title List

Visit **www.SalemPress.com** for Product Information, Table of Contents and Sample Pages

Literature

American Ethnic Writers
Critical Insights: Authors
Critical Insights: New Literary Collection Bundles
Critical Insights: Themes
Critical Insights: Works
Critical Survey of Drama
Critical Survey of Graphic Novels: Heroes & Super Heroes
Critical Survey of Graphic Novels: History, Theme & Technique
Critical Survey of Graphic Novels: Independents & Underground Classics
Critical Survey of Graphic Novels: Manga
Critical Survey of Long Fiction
Critical Survey of Mystery & Detective Fiction
Critical Survey of Mythology and Folklore: Heroes and Heroines
Critical Survey of Mythology and Folklore: Love, Sexuality & Desire
Critical Survey of Mythology and Folklore: World Mythology
Critical Survey of Poetry
Critical Survey of Poetry: American Poetry
Critical Survey of Poetry: British, Irish & Commonwealth Poets
Critical Survey of Poetry: European Poets
Critical Survey of Poetry: European Poets
Critical Survey of Poetry: Topical Essays
Critical Survey of Poetry: World Poets
Critical Survey of Science Fiction & Fantasy Literature
Critical Survey of Shakespeare's Sonnets
Critical Survey of Short Fiction
Critical Survey of Short Fiction: American Writers
Critical Survey of Short Fiction: British, Irish & Commonwealth Poets
Critical Survey of Short Fiction: European Writers
Critical Survey of Short Fiction: Topical Essays
Critical Survey of Short Fiction: World Writers
Cyclopedia of Literary Characters
Introduction to Literary Context: American Post-Modernist Novels
Introduction to Literary Context: American Short Fiction
Introduction to Literary Context: English Literature
Introduction to Literary Context: World Literature
Magill's Literary Annual 2014
Magill's Survey of American Literature
Magill's Survey of World Literature
Masterplots
Masterplots II: African American Literature
Masterplots II: Christian Literature
Masterplots II: Drama Series
Masterplots II: Short Story Series
Notable African American Writers
Notable American Novelists
Notable Playwrights
Short Story Writers

Science, Careers & Mathematics

Applied Science
Applied Science: Engineering & Mathematics
Applied Science: Science & Medicine
Applied Science: Technology
Biomes and Ecosystems
Careers in Chemistry
Careers in Communications & Media
Careers in Healthcare
Careers in Hospitality & Tourism
Careers in Law & Criminology
Careers in Physics
Computer Technology Inventors
Contemporary Biographies in Chemistry
Contemporary Biographies in Communications & Media
Contemporary Biographies in Healthcare
Contemporary Biographies in Hospitality & Tourism
Contemporary Biographies in Law & Criminology
Contemporary Biographies in Physics
Earth Science
Earth Science: Earth Materials & Resources
Earth Science: Earth's Surface and History
Earth Science: Physics & Chemistry of the Earth
Earth Science: Weather, Water & Atmosphere
Encyclopedia of Energy
Encyclopedia of Environmental Issues
Encyclopedia of Global Resources
Encyclopedia of Global Warming
Encyclopedia of Mathematics and Society
Encyclopedia of the Ancient World
Forensic Science
Internet Innovators
Introduction to Chemistry
Magill's Encyclopedia of Science: Animal Life
Magill's Encyclopedia of Science: Plant life
Magill's Medical Guide
Notable Natural Disasters
Solar System

Health

Addictions & Substance Abuse
Cancer
Complementary & Alternative Medicine
Genetics & Inherited Conditions
Infectious Diseases & Conditions
Magill's Medical Guide
Psychology & Mental Health
Psychology Basics

Grey House Publishing | Salem Press | H.W. Wilson
4919 Route, 22 PO Box 56, Amenia NY 12501-0056

2014 Title List

Visit **www.SalemPress.com** for Product Information, Table of Contents and Sample Pages

History and Social Science

A 2000s in America
50 States
African American History
Agriculture in History (check)
American First Ladies
American Heroes
American Indian Tribes
American Presidents
American Villains
Ancient Greece
Bill of Rights, The
Cold War, The
Defining Documents: American Revolution 1754-1805
Defining Documents: Civil War 1860-1865
Defining Documents: Emergence of Modern America, 1868-1918
Defining Documents: Exploration & Colonial America 1492-1755
Defining Documents: Manifest Destiny 1803-1860
Defining Documents: Reconstruction, 1865-1880
Defining Documents: The 1920s
Defining Documents: The 1930s
Defining Documents: World War I
Eighties in America
Encyclopedia of American Immigration
Fifties in America
Forties in America
Great Athletes
Great Events from History: 17th Century
Great Events from History: 18th Century
Great Events from History: 19th Century
Great Events from History: 20th Century, 1901-1940
Great Events from History: 20th Century, 1941-1970
Great Events from History: 20th Century, 1971-200
Great Events from History: Ancient World
Great Events from History: Middle Ages
Great Events from History: Modern Scandals
Great Events from History: Renaissance & Early Modern Era
Great Lives from History: 17th Century
Great Lives from History: 18th Century
Great Lives from History: 19th Century
Great Lives from History: 20th Century
Great Lives from History: African Americans
Great Lives from History: Ancient World
Great Lives from History: Asian & Pacific Islander Americans
Great Lives from History: Incredibly Wealthy
Great Lives from History: Inventors & Inventions
Great Lives from History: Jewish Americans
Great Lives from History: Latinos
Great Lives from History: Middle Ages
Great Lives from History: Notorious Lives
Great Lives from History: Renaissance & Early Modern Era
Great Lives from History: Scientists & Science
Historical Encyclopedia of American Business
Immigration in U.S. History
Magill's Guide to Military History
Milestone Documents in African American History
Milestone Documents in American History
Milestone Documents in World History
Milestone Documents of American Leaders
Milestone Documents of World Religions
Musicians & Composers 20th Century
Nineties in America
Seventies in America
Sixties in America
Survey of American Industry and Careers
Thirties in America
Twenties in America
U.S. Court Cases
U.S. Laws, Acts, and Treaties
U.S. Legal System
U.S. Supreme Court
United States at War
USA in Space
Weapons and Warfare
World Conflicts: Asia and the Middle East

WILSON

WILSON

2014 Title List

Visit **www.HwWilsonInPrint.com** for Product Information, Table of Contents and Sample Pages

Current Biography

Current Biography Cumulative Index 1946-2013
Current Biography Magazine
Current Biography Yearbook-2004
Current Biography Yearbook-2005
Current Biography Yearbook-2006
Current Biography Yearbook-2007
Current Biography Yearbook-2008
Current Biography Yearbook-2009
Current Biography Yearbook-2010
Current Biography Yearbook-2011
Current Biography Yearbook-2012
Current Biography Yearbook-2013
Current Biography Yearbook-2014

Core Collections

Senior High Core Collection
Middle & Junior High School Core
Children's Core Collection
Fiction Core Collection
Public Library Core Collection: Nonfiction

Sears List

Sears List of Subject Headings
Sears: Lista de Encabezamientos de Materia

The Reference Shelf

Aging in America
Revisiting Gender
The U.S. National Debate Topic, 2014/2015
Embracing New Paradigms in education
Marijuana Reform
Representative American Speeches 2013-2014
Reality Television
The Business of Food
The Future of U.S. Economic Relations: Mexico, Cuba, and Venezuela
Sports in America
Global Climate Change
Representative American Speeches, 2012-2013
Conspiracy Theories
The Arab Spring
U.S. National Debate Topic: Transportation Infrastructure
Families: Traditional and New Structures
Faith & Science
Representative American Speeches 2011-2012
Social Networking
Dinosaurs
Space Exploration & Development
U.S. Infrastructure
Politics of the Ocean
Representative American Speeches 2010-2011
Robotics
The News and its Future
American Military Presence Overseas
Russia
Graphic Novels and Comic Books
Representative American Speeches 2009-2010

Readers' Guide

Readers Guide to Periodicals Literature
Abridged Readers' Guide to Periodical Literature
Short Story Index

Indexes

Short Story Index
Index to Legal Periodicals & Books

Facts About Series

Facts About the Presidents, Eighth Edition
Facts About China
Facts About the 20th Century
Facts About American Immigration
Facts About World's Languages

Nobel Prize Winners

Nobel Prize Winners, 2002-2013

World Authors

World Authors 2000-2005
World Authors 2006-2013

Famous First Facts

Famous First Facts, Seventh Edition
Famous First Facts About American Politics
Famous First Facts About Sports
Famous First Facts About the Environment
Famous First Facts, International Edition

American Book of Days

The American Book of Days, Fifth Edition
The International Book of Days

Junior Authors & Illustrators

Tenth Book of Junior Authors & Illustrations

Monographs

The Barnhart Dictionary of Etymology
Celebrate the World
Indexing from A to Z
Radical Change: Books for Youth in a Digital Age
The Poetry Break
Guide to the Ancient World

Wilson Chronology

Wilson Chronology of Asia and the Pacific
Wilson Chronology of Human Rights
Wilson Chronology of Ideas
Wilson Chronology of the Arts
Wilson Chronology of the World's Religions
Wilson Chronology of Women's Achievements

Book Review Digest

Book Review Digest, 2014

Grey House Publishing | Salem Press | H.W. Wilson
4919 Route, 22 PO Box 56, Amenia NY 12501-0056